Guidelines for Client Teaching

Specific Nursing Care Plans

General Nursing Care Plans

MATERNITY AND GYNECOLOGIC CARE

The Nurse and the Family

MATERNITY AND GYNECOLOGIC CARE

The Nurse and the Family

IRENE M. BOBAK, R.N., M.S., Ph.D.

Professor,
San Francisco State University,
San Francisco, California

MARGARET DUNCAN JENSEN, R.N., M.S.

Professor Emeritus,
San Jose State University,
San Jose, California

MARIANNE K. ZALAR, R.N., Ed.D.

Associate Clinical Professor
Dept. of Family Health Nursing
University of California,
San Francisco, California
ZBS Research Associates
San Mateo, California

FOURTH EDITION

with 1011 illustrations

The C.V. Mosby Company

ST. LOUIS • BALTIMORE • TORONTO 1989

Mosby

Editor: Nancy L. Coon
Sr. Developmental editor: Susan R. Epstein
Developmental editor: Mary Espenschied
Project manager: Teri Merchant
Production editor: Deborah Vogel
Book design: John Rokusek

FOURTH EDITION

Printed in the United States of America

The C.V. Mosby Company
11830 Westline Industrial Drive, St. Louis, Missouri 63146

Library of Congress Cataloging-in-Publication Data

Bobak, Irene M.
Maternity and gynecologic care: the nurse and the family / Irene M. Bobak, Margaret Duncan Jensen, Marianne K. Zalar.—4th ed.

Includes bibliographies and index.
ISBN 0-8016-0469-9
1. Obstetrical nursing. 2. Gynecologic nursing. I. Jensen, Margaret Duncan. II. Zalar, Marianne K. III. Title.
[DNLM: 1. Family—nurses' instruction. 2. Gynecology—nurses' instruction. 3. Infant, Newborn—nurses' instruction. 4. Obstetrical Nursing. 5. Pregnancy—nurses' instruction. WY 157.3 B663m]
RG951.B667 1989
610.73'678—dc19

C/VH/VH 9 8 7 6 5 4 3 88-13555

Contributors

PRESENT EDITION

Iris E. Campbell, R.N., S.C.M., M.T.D., M.N.
Assistant Professor
Faculty of Nursing
University of Alberta
Edmonton, Canada

Diane S. Charsha, R.N.C., M.S.N.
MCH Clinical Specialist
Shore Memorial Hospital
Somers Point, New Jersey

Debra I. Craig, R.N., M.S.N.
Assistant Professor of Nursing
Point Loma Nazarene College
San Diego, California

Barbara A. Derwinski-robinson, R.N., M.S.N.
Associate Professor
Montana State University
Billings, Montana

Cheryl Harris, R.N., B.S.
Staff Nurse
Neonatal Intensive Care Unit
Children's Mercy Hospital
Kansas City, Missouri

Charlotte D. Kain, R.N.C., Ed.D.
Professor of Nursing
Montgomery County Community College
Blue Bell, Pennsylvania

Susan Weiner, R.N.C., M.S.N.
Perinatal Nurse Clinician
Thomas Jefferson University Hospital
Philadelphia, Pennsylvania

Beverly Gaglione, R.N., Ph.D.
Chairperson, Director of Nursing
Professor of Parent Child Nursing
East Stroudsburg University
East Stroudsburg, Pennsylvania

Carla D. Harris, R.N.C., M.S.N.
Nurse Practitioner, Associate Professor of Nursing
California State University
Instructional Design Associate
Huntington Beach, California

Beverly Horn, R.N., Ph.D.
Associate Professor, School of Nursing
University of Washington
Seattle, Washington

Linda Lee Miller, R.N., M.S.
Instructor, San Jose State University
San Jose, California

Barbara Petree, R.N., M.A.
Clinical Nursing Coordinator, Delivery Room
Stanford University Hospital
Stanford, California

Celeste Phillips, R.N., Ed.D.
Director of Nursing Education, Maternity Nursing Instructor
Cabrillo College
Aptos, California

M. Colleen Stainton, R.N., D.N.S.
Assistant Dean
Research and Development Professor, Faculty of Nursing
The University of Calgary
Alberta, Canada

Lucille Whaley, R.N., Ed.D.
Professor Emeritus, San Jose State University
San Jose, California
University of Southern California
Los Angeles, California

PREVIOUS EDITION

Joan Edelstein, R.N., P.N.P., Dr. P.H.
Associate Professor
San Jose State University
San Jose, California

Consultant Panel

Melanie Ashworth, R.N.
Stanford, California

Barbara L. Calder, R.N., B.S.N., M.C.Ed.
Assistant Professor
College of Nursing
University of Saskatchewan, Saskatoon
Saskatoon, Canada

Bruce Clayton, B.S., Pharm.D.
Department of Pharmacy Practice
University of Arkansas
Little Rock, Arkansas

Marilyn Daly, M.Ed.
Assistant Professor
Anatomy and Physiology
Biology Department
York College of Pennsylvania
York, Pennsylvania

Barbara Hayes, Nurse Midwife
Melbourne, Australia

Nyla Juhl, R.N., Ph.D.
Chair
Family and Community Nursing
College of Nursing
University of North Dakota
Grand Forks, North Dakota

Sheldon B. Korones, M.D.
Memphis, Tennessee

Jack Kundin, M.D.
San Mateo, California

Sylvia B. Lloyd, R.N., M.S.N.
Assistant Professor
Samuel Merritt College of Nursing
Oakland, California

Mary McMinn, R.N.
Instructor
Department of Nursing
Charles Stewart Mott Community College
Flint, Michigan

Linda Moore, R.N., M.S.N.
Instructor
California State University
Fresno, California

Mary Beth Moran, R.N., M.S.N.
Assistant Professor
College of Nursing
University of Oklahoma
Oklahoma City, Oklahoma

Cynthia E. Northrop, R.N., M.S., J.D.
Nurse Attorney; Private Law Practice
Adjunct Associate Professor
Teacher's College
Columbia University
New York, New York

Kathleen Patterson, R.N., M.S.
Lecturer
Department of Nursing
California State University
Fresno, California

Josy Petr, R.N., M.S.
Clinical Nurse Specialist
Adult Reproductive Health Associates in Reproductive Medicine
Flossmoor, Illinois

Celeste Phillips, R.N., Ed.D.
Director, Associate Degree Nursing Education
Cabrillo College
Santa Cruz, California

Nancy A. Prince, R.N.C., M.S.N.
Assistant Professor
Eastern Michigan University
Ypsilanti, Michigan

Fannie M. Rankin, R.N., B.S.
Certified Diabetes Educator
Mills-Peninsula Hospital
San Mateo, California

Barbara Rauh, R.N., C.N.A., B.S.N.
Director of Home Health Services
Southeast Missouri Hospital
Cape Girardeau, Missouri

M. Colleen Stainton, R.N., D.N.S.
Assistant Dean
Research and Development Professor
Faculty of Nursing
The University of Calgary
Alberta, Canada

Margretta M. Styles, R.N., Ed.D.
San Francisco, California

Paula Suter, R.N., M.A.
Cardiovascular Research Nurse
Stanford University Medical Center
Stanford, California

Susan Martin Tucker, R.N., B.S.N., P.H.N.
Director of Nursing
Kaiser Permanente Medical Center
East San Fernando Valley
Panorama City, California

Barbara Verner, R.N.
Clinical Supervisor
Kaiser Foundation Hospital
Los Angeles, California

Vivian Wahlberg, R.N., C.M., Dr. Med. Sc.,
Stockholm, Sweden

Francine Weatherby, R.N.C., Ph.D.
Assistant Professor
The University of Oklahoma Health Sciences Center
Oklahoma City, Oklahoma

Lucille Whaley, R.N., Ed.D.
Consultant, Parent-Child Nursing
Professor Emeritus
San Jose State University
San Jose, California

Sue Rodwell Williams, Ph.D., M.P.H., R.D.
President, SRW Productions, Inc., and
Director, The Berkeley Nutrition Group,
Berkeley, California;
Nutrition Consultant
Kaiser Permanente Medical Center
Oakland California;
Field Faculty
University of California
Berkeley, California

To the memory of my parents, Susan and Joseph Bobak, who provided a good beginning;

to my family and friends who encourage me and cheer me on;

to my colleagues who supply the professional inspiration;

to my students who motivate me.

I.M.B.

To my husband, Emil Nicholai Jensen, whose love, support, and encouragement have given meaning to my life.

M.D.J.

To my aunt, Mary Estok, who cared enough.

M.K.Z.

Preface

Maternity and Gynecologic Care: The Nurse and the Family is designed to be a comprehensive textbook as well as a resource for the practicing nurse concerning the care of the childbearing family and for the gynecologic care of women throughout the lifespan. The book addresses conditions commonly encountered by the nurse in day-to-day practice and problems that occur less frequently. Knowledge of normal conditions as well as common problems and unusual complications is essential to the delivery of safe, comprehensive, and holistic nursing care to women, fetuses, newborns, and families.

It is our philosophy that maternity and gynecologic nursing should combine scientific method and medical technology with the knowledge and sensitivity needed to provide holistic, individualized care to women and their families. This philosophy provided the impetus for writing the first edition of this text and continues to challenge us to develop each revision to incorporate the most current knowledge and techniques necessary to achieve the high standard of care we believe each client must receive.

We believe that the practice of nursing should be based on a scientific, problem-solving process designed to meet the needs of clients and their families. The five-step nursing process provides a logical, consistent framework for nursing practice that guides the nurse through the problem-solving process and focuses on setting and achieving client-centered goals. In maternity care, goals for the mother are a safe and satisfying pregnancy, a normal birth experience, and a healthy infant. The goal for the fetus is a healthy intrauterine existence; the goal for the neonate is a normal adjustment following birth. For the family and significant others, the goal of care is a childbirth experience that promotes parenting and the personal growth of all involved. In gynecologic care, the goals are promotion of wellness for the woman through knowledge of her body and its functioning throughout her lifespan, achievement of a partnership with the professional care provider in her own health care and maintenance, and obtainment of the ability to recognize conditions that require professional intervention. The goals for the family are health care experiences that promote personal support for involved individuals and active participation in future health maintenance and promotion activities.

Inherent in our philosophy is the wellness approach to nursing care. This approach views pregnancy and childbirth as a natural process rather than as an illness. The developmental changes a woman experiences throughout her life are also considered to be natural and normal. This focus provides a positive foundation for practice, as well as a logical organizing framework for teaching maternity and gynecologic nursing.

In keeping with this approach *Maternity and Gynecologic Care: The Nurse and the Family* emphasizes the normal childbirth experience and the normal changes that occur in the woman's reproductive system throughout her lifespan. We believe students need to thoroughly understand and recognize the *normal* processes and conditions before they can identify complications and comprehend their implications for care.

To truly meet the specific needs of each client the nurse must be knowledgeable about individual cultural influences and must include family members and significant others in the plan of care. We have therefore integrated both cultural and family considerations throughout the text to assist the nurse in recognizing and understanding the uniqueness of each client and administering individualized, family-centered care.

FEATURES

The fourth edition of *Maternity and Gynecologic Care: The Nurse and the Family* is designed to enhance learning and understanding and to facilitate easy retrieval of information. Special attention has been given to the reading level and presentation to provide information in a clear, logical, and readable manner. A two-color format has been incorporated in the design of the text to enhance understanding and highlight special content.

To ensure a logical and consistent presentation of material we have used the five-step nursing process as the organizing framework within the chapters. Each step of the process—assessment, nursing diagnoses, planning, implementation, and evaluation—is specially highlighted throughout the text for emphasis and clarity.

Detailed chapter outlines in the table of contents afford the reader the opportunity to quickly review each chapter's material. Each chapter begins with learning objectives that assist students by guiding their study. These objectives alert students to what they should accomplish by the end of the chapter. They also provide a basis for self-evaluation to determine the extent of understanding and competency. Key terms are also presented at the beginning of each chapter to alert students to new vocabulary that will be introduced in the chapter.

Each chapter ends with a brief summary to help students focus on the overall content presented. A list of key concepts follows to assist students in reviewing and evaluating their understanding of major points included in the chapter. Several study questions and suggested activities provide the learner with an opportunity to further consider the chapter's content and apply the knowledge gained. The references for each chapter document both classic and recent sources used and the bibliography provides an excellent resource for those seeking further information.

Nursing research has become an integral part of nursing education as well as practice, particularly in maternity and gynecologic nursing. The chapter on nursing research has been revised to focus on methods and applications appropriate to these areas. In addition, research highlights appear throughout the text, summarizing recent studies that illustrate the kinds of research currently being conducted.

Several special features are designed to meet the specific needs of the student and the beginning practitioner. These features facilitate understanding of the narrative and enhance the usefulness of the text as a practical resource. More than 50 nursing care plans assist the student in transferring the content presented to the planning of care. To administer individualized care the nurse must first be knowledgeable about the overall care for a particular condition or situation. *General nursing care plans* provide this information. *Specific nursing care plans* guide the student in tailoring care to meet the individual needs of a specific client. Both types of care plans follow the five-step nursing process and include client-centered goals for care as well as rationales for nursing actions.

Nearly 40 *guidelines for client teaching* illustrate strategies for organizing and relating health care content to individuals and families. Goals for teaching are gleaned for the nursing diagnoses and the client's health care needs. Content and teaching actions are designed to meet the desired goals. References and teaching aids served as further resources for developing teaching plans for clients. Sample teaching strategies encourage the nurse to develop individualized teaching plans.

Nearly 30 *procedures* provide the information necessary to competently perform technical skills. Equipment lists assist the nurse in preparing for the procedure. Step-by-step nursing actions ensure organized and systematic implementation; rationales for each step promote learning and understanding. Nursing actions for potentially life-threatening situations are provided in *emergency procedures.* These are highlighted and tabbed in the text and listed inside the front cover for easy retrieval. Also listed are the specially-boxed *danger signs* that alert the nurse to symptoms requiring immediate intervention.

Two additional features have been designed specifically with the learner's needs in mind. First, 16 tear-out *drug cards* provide essential drug information and nursing implications for commonly used maternal, newborn, and gynecologic drugs. Easily transported, the cards are designed for use in the clinical setting and serve as a quick reference. They supplement the use of a pharmacology text and hospital formulary.

Second, a *cervical dilation teaching guide* is printed on the inside back cover of the text. It assists the novice maternity nurse in visualizing different phases of cervical dilation in the childbearing client. It can also be used as a teaching aid when describing the birth process.

The *appendices* provide resource information for both students and practitioners. New to this edition is a resource guide that lists audiovisuals, community and national resources, nursing journals, and nursing organizations. The extensive *glossary* contains definitions of major obstetric, gynecologic, and nursing terms used in the text. The detailed *index* is an invaluable aid in assisting readers in finding information quickly.

ORGANIZATION

Maternity and Gynecologic Care: The Nurse and the Family is comprised of nine units organized to enhance learning and understanding. The first unit introduces concepts and issues basic to the practice of maternity and gynecologic nursing; the second unit provides information on sexuality and the reproductive system. Units III through VI present all of the normal, expected occurrences and nursing considerations throughout pregnancy, childbirth, and the postpartum period. Complications of childbearing, as well as problems occurring in the newborn, are thoroughly explained in Units VII and VIII. Unit IX focuses on women's health and gynecologic nursing.

Unit I, "Nursing Perspectives," describes the milieu within which contemporary nursing practice takes place. Chapter 1 identifies the major issues and challenges to nursing practice that emerge from a changing social and technologic context. Chapter 2 explains the deliberative combination of social, physical, and intellectual skills that make nursing a process involving the client, the nurse, and the environment. Chapter 3 describes the family as a unit of care. The skill, attitudes, and process of the nurse-client relationship are key components in developing a therapeutic setting for the care of clients and their families. Chapter 4 presents the legal implications inherent in the care of women and infants with specific reference to reproductive function. Chapter 5 presents an overview for incorporating nursing research as a component of a nursing process in maternity and gynecologic nursing.

Unit II, "Human Reproductive System," deals with the interplay of cultural, familial, and personal effects on inherited and biologic entities that affect the development of sexual potential. Chapter 6 is concerned with the biologic components of human sexuality over the lifespan. This chapter also includes a section on immunology to emphasize the importance of this body system in youth and age. Chapter 7 focuses on the psychosocial aspects of human sexuality, the origins of each person's sexual identity, and the developmental tasks of key periods in the life of the child, adolescent, and adult. Chapter 8 emphasizes the importance of the gynecologic examination in the care of clients before, during, and after their reproductive years.

Unit III, "Normal Pregnancy," details nursing care of the woman and her family throughout the course of a normal pregnancy. Chapter 9 focuses on the development of the fetus and reviews genetic factors. Chapter 10 presents the maternal anatomy and physiology relevant to pregnancy and maternal adaptations to the growing fetus. Chapter 11 focuses on the reactions of individual family members to pregnancy and the resulting dynamics within the family unit. Chapters 12, 13, and 14 deal with the knowledge and skills needed by the nurse to provide competent, comprehensive care of the pregnant woman and her family throughout each trimester of pregnancy. Chapter 15 highlights the nutritional needs of the mother and fetus during pregnancy, stressing the prevention of complications by early recognition of nutritional problems.

Unit IV, "Normal Childbirth," focuses on the collaborative care between the obstetric team and the pregnant woman and her family during the process of birth. Chapter 16 details the factors and processes of labor and the implications for nursing care. Chapter 17 reviews the nurse's role in the pharmacologic relief of pain and discomfort during labor and delivery. This chapter includes the physiologic basis for pharmacologic care and presents accepted drugs and modalities used. The second part of this chapter provides a basis for understanding techniques associated with intermittent monitoring of clients during the prenatal period and continuous monitoring of both mother and fetus during labor. Chapters 18, 19, and 20 present in detail the care of clients during the four stages of labor. The biologic and psychologic responses of the mother, fetus, and newborn to the stress of labor are emphasized, and general and specific nursing care measures are presented. Nursing considerations for other family members during the labor process are integrated throughout.

Unit V, "Normal Newborn," deals with the neonate's critical period of adjustment to extrauterine existence. The nurse must be knowledgeable about assessment and care of the newborn to ensure successful adaptation. Chapter 21 reviews basic knowledge of the biologic and behavioral characteristics of the newborn that nurses need for understanding, initiating, and teaching care of the newborn. Chapter 22 focuses on nursing care of the neonate. Information and techniques for accurate assessment and care are presented according to the five-step nursing process. Nursing interventions include promoting the newborn's growth and development through enriching social contacts as well as preparing parents to care for their infant. Chapter 23 centers on the nutritional needs of the newborn, which must be met to ensure optimum growth and development. Information is provided to prepare the nurse to assess nutritional status and teach parents about requirements and techniques to promote nutritional health in their newborn.

Unit VI, "Normal Postpartum Period," addresses a time of significant change for the childbearing family. The mother experiences physiologic changes as her body regains its nonpregnant status and psychologic changes as she adjusts to a new phase of motherhood with a separate but dependent infant. The family members have new roles to assume as the newborn becomes established as part of the family unit. Chapter 24 presents content basic to understanding the physiologic adjustments of the woman during the puerperium. Chapter 25 presents family responses to the birth of a child from the perspective of mother, father, sibling(s), and grandparents. It discusses adaptive and maladaptive adjustments of family members. The chapter also includes content related to the impact of the infant's responses and temperament on the parent-child relationship. Chapter 26 draws on content in the previous two chapters in the application of the nursing process to the care of the family during its adjustment in the puerperium.

Unit VII, "Complications of Childbearing," reviews in detail the maternal conditions that predispose or commit the maternity client to an abnormal rather than normal response to pregnancy. In Chapter 27 the high-risk client and the factors associated with diagnosis of high risk are identified. Techniques of biophysical monitoring of fetal health are emphasized. Chapter 28 focuses on loss and grief, states experienced by high-risk clients and families. The process associated with grief is discussed, as well as nursing care applicable in specific situations. Chapter 29 focuses on hypertensive states during pregnancy that may occur as a pregnancy-induced disease or may predate the pregnancy. Pregnancy-induced hypertension is recognized as the leading cause of maternal mortality. Chapter 30 contains content relevant to maternal infections during the antepartum, childbirth, and postdelivery periods. Maternal hemorrhagic conditions are identified in Chapter 31. Endocrine and metabolic disorders receive special attention in Chapter 32. Dystocia, and preterm and postterm labor are discussed in Chapter 33. Chapter 34 contains content about many medical, surgical, and psychosocial conditions that complicate pregnancy. Poverty, emotional complications, and abuse of psychoactive substances are included. Chapter 35 addresses the unique characteristics and needs of adolescent pregnancy and parenthood.

Unit VIII, "Complications of the Newborn," provides extensive information on the identification and care of the high-risk neonate. Chapter 36 presents guidelines for determining risk factors and details nursing interventions appropriate for a compromised neonate. Interventions include maintenance of respiration, oxygen therapy, and feeding measures. Chapter 37 describes complications associated with gestational age and birthweight. Chapter 38 focuses on birth trauma and the newborn of a diabetic pregnancy. Chapter 39 offers extensive content about infection and drug dependence. Chapter 40 presents complications of hyperbilirubinemia and congenital anomalies.

Unit X, "Women's Health and Gynecologic Care," encompasses preventive, curative, and rehabilitative nursing care throughout the lifespan. This care includes nursing skills that support women undergoing normal changes, such as menarche and menopause, as well as highly technical skills associated with care of the gynecologic-oncologic client. In Chapter 41 abnormal conditions associated with menstruation, such as dysmenorrhea, premenstrual syndrome, and endometriosis are discussed. Information about the climacterium enables nurses to help women make informed decisions regarding therapy and cope effectively with changes characteristic of this normal developmental event. The cause, effects on reproductive functioning, medical management, and nursing process are included for the conditions presented.

Chapter 42 contains content basic to understanding fertility management. It includes nursing care of clients relative to impaired fertility, control of fertility, surgical interruption of pregnancy, and termination of fertility.

Chapter 43 focuses on hazards to women's health in the environment and workplace. Two major social problems affecting many women—violence and poverty—are presented. Detection and diagnosis of the problems, care required, and community support available are also discussed.

Chapter 44 deals with neoplasia, which, particularly in malignant form, is part of the specialized oncologic care needed by gynecologic clients. The chapter reviews current concepts related to the medical management, the nursing process, the family, and community resources associated with care of the woman with neoplasia.

TEACHING AND LEARNING PACKAGE

To facilitate the teaching-learning process and help instructors and students in using the text to its fullest potential, we have developed the most comprehensive supplement package available.

1. The *Instructor's Manual with Test Bank* is keyed chapter by chapter to the text to help coordinate course objectives to chapter content. Unique to this manual are guidelines for maximizing the benefits of the text to students regardless of the duration of the maternity and gynecologic nursing course. The test bank includes over 500 questions directly related to the text. Answers include page references to enhance learning.
2. A *Computerized Test Bank* is available for use on the IBM PC or Apple IIe and IIc microcomputers. These questions, taken from the test bank in the *Instructor's Manual,* can be used as the basis for individual test construction. Directions for rearranging, adding, and deleting questions are included.
3. A set of two-color *Overhead Transparencies* includes more than 50 illustrations specially selected from the text for their instructional value during lectures and classroom discussions.
4. A *computer-assisted instruction (CAI)* program on maternal and fetal nutrition is available for IBM or Apple computers. This software reinforces material presented in the text regarding educating pregnant clients in proper nutrition and recommending food choices to ensure a healthy pregnancy and normal fetal development.
5. The new *Study Guide to Accompany Maternity and Gynecologic Care,* fourth edition, includes features that enable students to achieve maximum understanding of the content presented in the text. Keyed chapter-by-chapter to the text, the study guide includes learning objectives, key terms, comprehension exercises, clinical learning activities, and crossword puzzles.
6. The unique *Clinical Manual of Maternity and Gynecologic Nursing* provides practical, easily retrievable material in a handy, spiral-bound format. Following the organization of the fourth edition of *Maternity and Gynecologic Care: The Nurse and the Family,* each chapter includes an overview of current nursing research. Summaries of nursing actions provide comprehensive guidelines for care in a clear, tabular format. The manual provides a wealth of information vital to clinical practice, including nursing care plans, client teaching guidelines, procedures, danger signs, diagnostic lab test data, and drug and medication considerations.

We are fully aware of the increasingly important contribution men are making to the nursing profession, as well as the growing number of women entering the medical profession. We hope this trend will continue. The construction of the English language, however, sometimes makes it awkward to eliminate totally the feminine and masculine pronouns. Therefore to present material clearly and smoothly we have occasionally used the feminine pronoun to refer to the nurse and the masculine pronoun to refer to the physician.

Over the years we have received many comments and suggestions regarding our maternity nursing texts. We have incorporated many of these suggestions in the organization and development of this text. We welcome comments from instructors, students, and practitioners who use this text so that we may continue to be responsive to the needs of the profession.

ACKNOWLEDGEMENTS

We wish to thank everyone whose comments and suggestions prompted this collaborative effort and reviewers who provided valuable criticism of the manuscript.

We offer thanks for shared expertise and photographs to the staffs of Stanford University Medical Center, Stanford, California; Kaiser-Permanente Hospital and Santa Clara Valley Medical Center, Santa Clara, California; St. Luke's Hospital, Kansas City, Missouri; Jewish Hospital and Barnes Hospital, St. Louis, Missouri; Mills Memorial Hospital, San Mateo, California; Fountain Valley Community Hospital, Fountain Valley, California; and The Woman's Hospital of Texas, Houston, Texas.

We would like to thank the following photographers: Judith Bamber, San Jose, California; Joan Edelstein, San Jose, California; and M. Colleen Stainton, Calgary, Alberta, Canada. A special thank you goes to Marjorie Pyle, RNC, Lifecircle, Costa Mesa, California.

Several families in addition to our own have made unique contributions to the original photographs in this text, especially David and Carolyn Carlton and their son, Mathew.

We are indebted to these families, who embody the philosophical basis for our text—family centered nursing care.

This edition contains artwork by George Wassilchenko, Oral Roberts University, Tulsa, Oklahoma, whose precise, detailed anatomic drawings have made a substantial contribution to facilitating the study of complex theory. We look forward to a continuing association with this outstanding medical illustrator.

Special words of gratitude are extended to Nancy Coon and Suzi Epstein of the C.V. Mosby Company and Mary Espenschied for their encouragement, inspiration, and assistance in the preparation and production of this text. We acknowledge the assistance of our families, both concrete and supportive, and we thank each other for the stimulation, support, and mutual respect generated by this collaboration.

Irene M. Bobak
Margaret Duncan Jensen
Marianne K. Zalar

Contents in Brief

UNIT IX

Women's Health and Gynecologic Care

Contents

Unit I Nursing Perspectives

UNIT

I

Nursing Perspectives

Maternity and gynecologic nursing focuses on the woman, her infant, and her family as the clients of nursing. This unit describes the milieu within which contemporary nursing practice takes place. Chapter 1 identifies the major issues and challenges to nursing practice that emerge from a changing social and technologic context. Chapter 2 explains the deliberative combination of social, physical, and intellectual skills that make nursing a process involving the client, the nurse, and the environment. Chapter 3 describes the family as a unit of care. The skill, attitudes, and process of the nurse-client relationship are key components in developing a therapeutic setting for the care of clients and their families. Chapter 4 presents the legal implications inherent in the care of women and infants with specific reference to reproductive function. Chapter 5 presents an overview for incorporating nursing research as a component of the nursing process.

CHAPTER

1

Maternity and Gynecologic Nursing: Issues and Challenges

M. Colleen Stainton

Learning Objectives

Correctly define the key terms listed.

Examine maternity and gynecologic nursing in light of basic premises and principles of nursing practice.

Explain the context in which nursing care is carried out.

Identify the context variables to be assessed in each maternity-gynecologic client.

Evaluate the nurse as caregiver in terms of competence, social consciousness, commitment, health policy and planning, and political skills.

Discuss the identified issues for nursing in the future: integrating education, practice, and research; creating synchrony between knowledge and practice; developing a nursing science; credentialing specialty areas of practice; maintaining a care atmosphere in a high-technology cure milieu; and working in collaborative roles.

Key Terms

Alma-Ata declaration
basic premises
care atmosphere
collaborative roles
competence
context variables
credentialing
health care consumer
health policy and planning
integration: education, practice, research
nurse-specialists
nursing science
personal context
political skill
power of caring
principles of nursing practice
social consciousness
social context
synchrony between knowledge and practice

Recent studies of women's health show marked differences between men's and women's life expectancies and years of disability, as well as health differences between rich and poor women, and life-styles of women (Hancock, 1987). The health of women is a critical link to the health of children, families, and societies. Reproductive health is one aspect of women's health that has a ripplelike effect on other aspects of health and life-style. This book focuses on the reproductive processes that normally occur and on the prevention and care of pathophysiologic reproductive processes that occur in some women.

MATERNITY AND GYNECOLOGIC NURSING

Nursing, with its electric science and holistic philosophy, has a role in women's health from the time a woman is conceived until her death. Nursing practice requires knowledge and skill in helping women maintain psychologic and physiologic health as changes occur throughout the life span.

Maternity and gynecologic nursing is related to a dimension of nursing practice that occurs in settings where women are the primary entrants into the health care system. The nurse provides care to the clients in homes, clinics, hospitals, and rehabilitative areas. The clients in these care areas include the woman, her unborn and newborn infant, and those others the woman defines as significant in her interpersonal system (Fig. 1-1).

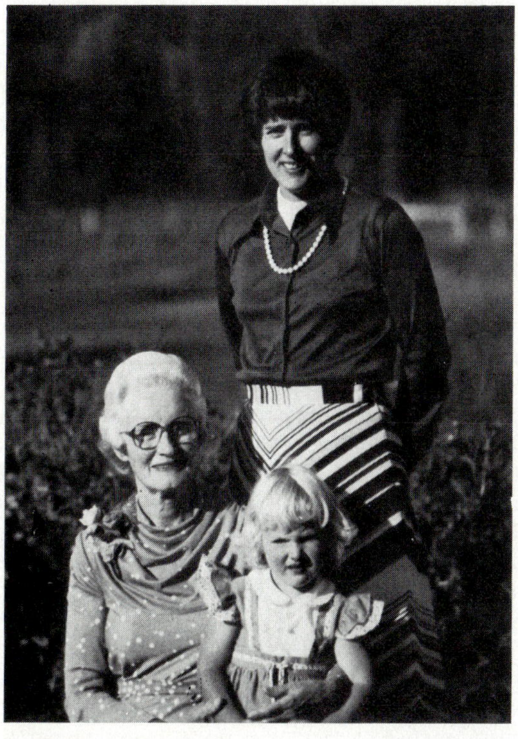

Fig. 1-1 Three generations. Each requires different aspects of maternity-gynecologic care throughout life span.
Courtesy Colleen Stainton.

The *purposes* of this book are to (1) provide a source of knowledge for basic nursing students seeking first licensure, (2) provide advanced knowledge for those specializing in maternity or gynecologic aspects of nursing practice, and (3) engender nursing attitudes that are sensitive to the contemporary social context of women and their reproductive function.

Basic Premises

The following four *major premises* provide the framework for nursing practice in maternity and gynecologic nursing:

1. Women are situated within a social context comprised of personal experience, future expectations, and a life-style. This context is based on a network of interpersonal relationships and social systems emanating from cultural practices and societal organizations, from which women derive knowledge about their bodies and health needs. Therefore episodes requiring maternity or gynecologic health care are interpersonally and intraculturally oriented events.
2. Nursing practice, including preventive, educational, curative, and rehabilitative functions, maintains and enhances significant relationships during episodes requiring maternity or gynecologic care.
3. All clients are entitled to readily accessible health care.
4. Highly specialized knowledge and intricate technology are most effective when applied with the client as collaborator in the decision-making process.

Principles of Nursing Practice

The following three *basic principles* guide nursing practice in the care of women:

1. Health promotion and disease prevention are more satisfying for the consumer and more cost-effective for society that remediation.
2. Nursing services are targeted toward helping women develop a sense of mastery of their bodies and their roles in the culture.
3. The health of one individual within a social system, such as a family, influences all the other members.

THE MATERNITY-GYNECOLOGIC CLIENT

Personal Context

A central relationship is that of the woman to her own body, both internally and externally. The reproductive organs and functions of human beings are essential to their role in society, their personal identities, and their overall physical and mental health. A woman's various body structures and functions are interrelated. In a state of good physical, social, and mental health, the complex biologic processes of the female body follow developmentally and cycle rhythmically through the specific processes associated with menarche, menstruation, sexual maturity, childbearing, lactation, and the climacteric without untoward change in other body functions, energy levels, or mental ability.

The *function* of the reproductive system is correlated with sexuality, body image, and self-esteem. Provision of nursing services related to reproductive function is both a significant and a sensitive dimension of practice. It relates to areas of health care that are personal and private and at the same time culturally relevant.

Social Context

A woman is deeply immersed in relationships to other persons, to a culture and some of its subcultures, and to society. *Person-to-person relationships are central to humanness.* A woman seeking health care brings her individual social context with her. The relationships within that context are known to be major factors in the level of health she is able to attain and maintain. The woman's sociocultural milieu and life-style determine and reflect her values, beliefs, commitments, attitudes, and patterns of functioning during episodes of loss, pain, joy, illness, and death (Hancock, 1987).

Recent work in gender differences points out deficits in developmental, psychologic, and sociologic theory with respect to women and is of particular interest to nurses working predominantly with women clients. Gilligan (1982, 1983) describes women as having a sense of interconnectedness to other people, a feeling of responsibility and caring that puts relationships in a primary and central place in a woman's sense of identity and world view. Chodorow (1978) attributes differences between men's and women's personalities and roles to the fact that both sexes are primarily reared by women caregivers in the early years. Boys are reared differently from girls, who are usually socialized to expect to do all of the child care; boys are valued for other abilities.

In developing a professional relationship, the nurse needs to work within the framework of the client and the relationships that pattern the woman's health practice. Life-style is a continuously changing phenomenon directly influenced by social, economic, political, and demographic features of a society (Belsky, 1981; Boss, 1980). For example, parenthood that occurs during the teen years or after age 30 creates special needs with implications for life-style changes (DeVore, 1983; Mercer, 1986). Similarly, the diagnosis of cancer in the reproductive tract does not automatically imply impending death but may require life-style modification to incorporate the regimen of chemotherapy. Eventual cure may require other life-style changes. Nurses play key roles in helping women, their families, and other members of their interpersonal systems in adapting during such events.

During the past 4 decades, economic growth, fertility control, educational and social opportunities, and the women's movement have increased the life-style options for women. Women's roles now involve more than reproduction. In many areas of the world, women are engaged in the work of the society; and Western women increasingly blend childbearing into other roles (Swanson-Kauffman, 1987).

Cultural traditions have been the major influence on how groups live together. Some cultures have been characterized by intergenerational families or households shared by several families made up of at least some blood relations. In the developing countries these patterns are changing because of the mobility of the young adults, who seek education or employment in urban areas, thus increasing the tendency toward nuclear families. In the Western world, the typical household consists of a nuclear family with husband, wife, and their children. Immigrant families throughout North America, the United Kingdom, and Europe tend to live in multiperson households consisting of various family groupings until they become economically established and culturally adapted.

Newcomers to the Western societies may experience stress in coping with unfamiliar expectations in the woman's role, such as household management and major responsibility for child care without the benefit of help from other family members or servants (Anderson, 1985; Meleis, 1987; Meleis and Rogers, 1987). This factor may be of particular importance when a woman or a family member enters the health care system for preventive or curative care or for childbearing. Cultural attitudes and values become crucial in coping with stressful life events, and in attaching to a new baby (Stainton, 1985).

Context variables provide a background for the assessment of a client, and they help the nurse understand the meaning of the woman's response to her body's functions and health problems. The assessment process is outlined in Chapter 2.

Context Variables

1. Health and illness behavior depend on cultural *values* and personal *preferences.* A nurse who unknowingly violates a belief can create stress in relationships within the woman's social system; not attending to preferences can reduce the effectiveness of the nurse-client relationship. Body and verbal language used in expressing feelings such as joy, love, pain, and grief are individually and culturally determined. Tolerance and a nonjudgmental attitude on the part of the nurse promote trust and honest expression of feelings. Also culture related are the social boundaries of touching. Attitudes toward touching another's or one's own body and public touching between males and females vary. Sensitivity to these issues is required in conducting examinations, teaching childbirth education classes, and providing tertiary care.

2. The *age* of the client generates specific needs for preventive and maintenance health care. For maternity and gynecologic nursing this age ranges from that of an unborn infant to an elderly woman. The increasing longevity of women expands their opportunities for having a variety of social roles during their lifetime and increases the potential for having to adapt to a chronic disease (Wilkins and Adams, 1983).

3. A woman's *attitude* toward her own health and the health of those close to her is affected by her interpersonal system and the level of social support it contains. This system may be characteristic of a nuclear, multigenerational, or cult family. It may be a household ranging from one person to many.

4. *Sexual patterns* will be individualized. The client may

be heterosexual, homosexual, bisexual, multipartnered, or celibate. These patterns may change over time.

5. The *major focus* of the woman's life and *sources of identity* will influence her life-style and health practices. The woman may be self-centered, family centered, career centered, or a blend of all three.

6. The degree of *legal autonomy* is an important consideration. Laws regarding informed consent and certain reproductive system procedures are state or province specific. For example, a teenager may or may not be able to seek contraceptives without parental permission. Legal autonomy also varies according to degree of mental competence determined by level of consciousness, retardation, or senility. Marital status may also affect legal autonomy. For example, a spouse's signature may be required for a married female to obtain sterilization. Such laws change as revisions are passed by governments.

The Woman as Health Care Consumer

The consumers in the health care system expect to participate in their own care as well-informed partners. "Knowledgeable consumers no longer comply with the power base of professionals and wish to be participants in the experience of their family members" (Stainton, 1981). Sophistication of the lay health consumer has resulted from the dissemination of scientific and other information to the public through extensive literature and other media resources. The nurse therefore needs not only to keep up to date with professional sources of information but also to be aware of the public sources. Assessment of a woman entering the health care system should include a discussion of her knowledge and attitudes acquired through her own investigation of the problem. The nurse can then amplify or clarify the woman's understanding of the concern. This approach forms the basis for the establishment of a plan of care.

THE NURSE AS CAREGIVER

Technical and Interpersonal Competence

Nurses are the minute-to-minute operators of many of the machines used in monitoring body functions, and the demands to attain and maintain a high level of technical skill cannot be denied. Technologic monitoring is done in both community- and hospital-based settings. The ability to use computer science and audiovisual aids is a necessary part of nursing practice. To work in collaboration with other team members, the nurse needs to be comfortable and creative in using these resources.

Home-based monitoring equipment has become increasingly available. The results from this equipment are entered into central computers and laboratories through sophisticated communication links. For example, fetal heart rate (FHR) and fetal movement of those at risk, as well as biochemical assays of pregnant women or women undergoing chemotherapy can be monitored from the client's setting (Fig. 1-2). Televised interactions between clients in rural areas and large health care centers are increasingly common as technologic capability advances. In addition,

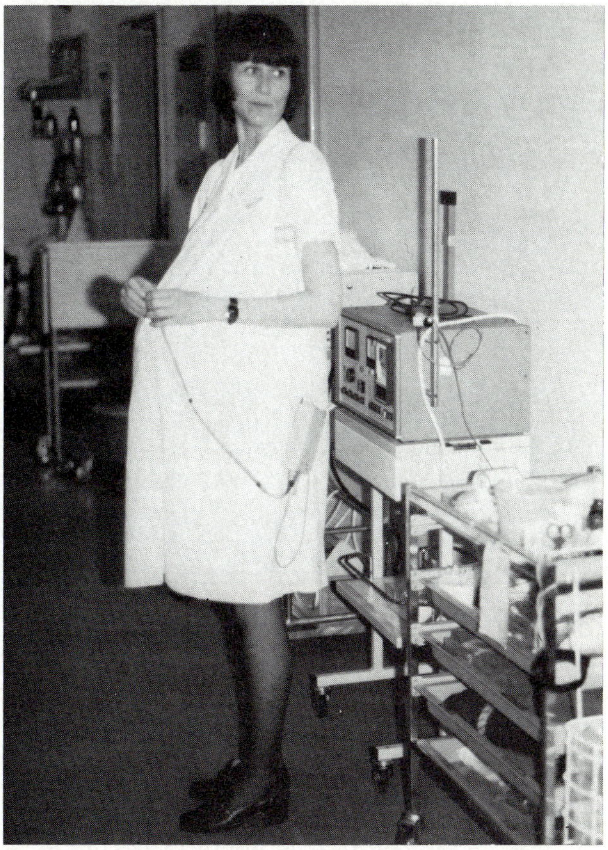

Fig. 1-2 Woman wearing portable fetal monitor while working. Courtesy Colleen Stainton.

the use of home-based computers in health care maintenance or monitoring has great potential. These capabilities facilitate a level of care previously unavailable or highly inconvenient.

Clients being monitored are often deeply concerned and frightened. They count on the nurse to understand these fears and to maintain interpersonal contact through touch, eye contact, listening, and responding to them as persons while precisely reading and recording machine outputs. They need anticipation of their fears and simple explanation designed to reassure them. Even the smallest premature infant attached to many monitoring devices needs human contact through voice and touch to survive and thrive.

Caring is the essence of nursing. It is expressed through the skillful combination of interpersonal and technical skills. In high-technology settings the warmth, hope, and shared concern of the nurse serve to balance the often dehumanizing aspects of the situation and help mobilize the client's energy for coping.

Much attention has been given to the importance of power in nursing. Benner (1984) suggests that the power of nursing is caring. Through nurses' own descriptions of their practice, Benner found that excellence requires commitment and involvement, as well as power. Six qualities of power associated with care were identified and are presented in the box on p. 6.

THE POWER OF CARING

Transforming Power

In the context of care a person may perceive new ways of seeing and coping so that her or his world is transformed into one of possibility and hope.

Reintegrative Power

Care can give the person's world back to her or him. Caring helps a client reestablish roles in the world by maximizing the ability to reestablish a meaningful life when the limitations seem insurmountable to the client.

Advocacy Power

The nurse interprets the situation for the client, the family, or other health team members and runs defense for the client by blocking obstacles to her or his ability to overcome a situational crisis.

Healing Power

The nurse establishes a healing relationship and a healing climate by reflecting an attitude of hope to self, clients, and other staff, finding a way to understand the situation that is clear and acceptable to the client and assisting the client to draw on her or his own social, emotional, and spiritual resources.

Participative Power

Engagement and involvement enable the nurse to experience whatever affirmation and strength is available in painful, difficult situations.

Problem-solving Power

A committed stance increases the nurse's sensitivity to cues and allows a search for solutions or the recognition of one when it is not being directly sought.

Modified from Benner, PE: From novice to expert: excellence and power in clinical nursing practice, Menlo Park, Calif, 1984, Addison-Wesley Publishing Co, Inc.

Social Consciousness

Social consciousness refers to an awareness of developing trends in the society that have a potential or actual effect on the welfare of its citizens. It implies an ability and willingness to take action to promote positive change. Awareness of developing trends that affect health care is each nurse's responsibility. Social action can be undertaken by nurses individually, but it is usually most effective when an organized group of nurses presents a unified stand that includes a plan for change.

The nature and scope of nursing are continuously evolving. The nurse working with the woman and her family can expect to be part of a field that involves complex biologic, psychologic, and social components. Rapidly advancing knowledge and technology have created concomitant legal, ethical, and moral issues with varied and changing perspectives. For example, the following new developments influence the issue of abortion*:

1. Increasing understanding of fetal life and early signs of individuality and personality (Stainton, 1985a).
2. Identification of the period between 28 and 32 weeks of gestation as the beginning of consciousness (Purpura, 1975).
3. Ability to diagnose and treat the fetus (Harrison et al., 1981).
4. Ethical considerations of rights when a well mother is carrying a fetus who is the client and whose treatment may pose threats to the mother's health or may inconvenience her (Fletcher, 1981).
5. Ability to visualize the young fetus and see the body organs functioning (Powledge, 1983).

Western society has become highly complex and achievement oriented. High-level technology and scientific discoveries, progressive education, and a high standard of living have resulted in many choices regarding reproduction and reproductive care. Self-actualization is the goal of many people who live in a society where independence, individuality, education, intelligence, attractiveness, and choice are highly valued. Some women and their partners prepare for and plan parenthood with rigid expectations for the outcome. They expect a satisfying pregnancy, a delivery that occurs as planned, and a child who is perfectly formed and of the desired sex (Stainton, 1985a).

Being successful in life's undertakings is a dominant theme in Western societies. To be successful includes the concepts of maintaining control, being self-reliant, and possessing power (Scott-Palmer and Skevington, 1981; Lederman, 1984; Stainton, 1985b). Maintaining control is applicable in all facets of an individual's life—whether they be emotional, physical, or environmental. Being self-reliant means being capable of making choices, assuming responsibility for one's actions, and showing initiative in solving problems. Possessing power means being able to manipulate the environment to ensure the safety, protection, and support of oneself and significant others. Stainton (1985b) found that parents' interpretation of a successful human being "was one who was self-reliant, social, independent and who could exercise power and control in achieving goals."

The role of mother, while still possessing the qualities of warmth, loving attention, and closeness, now reflects the cultural emphasis on success. Stainton (1985b) found that for mothers representative of upwardly mobile women in a Western society pregnancy was "a project of excellence, the product of which was a perfectly formed and healthy newborn." Control of conception, in vitro fertilization, embryonic implants, artificial insemination, and surrogate mothers add to the options available. Each choice adds to the potential and realized issues influencing both the nurse and the client and her family.

*Abortion is discussed in detail in Chapter 42.

DECLARATION OF BELIEF ABOUT THE NATURE AND PURPOSE OF NURSING

I BELIEVE in nursing as an *occupational force for social good,* a force that, in the *totality of its concern* for all human health states and for mankind's responses to health and environment provides a distinct, unique, and vital perspective, value orientation, and service.

I BELIEVE in nursing as a *professional discipline,* requiring a sound education and research base grounded in its own science and in the variety of academic and professional disciplines with which it relates.

I BELIEVE in nursing as a *clinical practice,* employing particular physiological, psychosocial, physical, and technological means for human amelioration, sustenance, and comfort.

I BELIEVE in nursing as a *humanistic field,* in which the fullness, self-respect, self-determination, and humanity of the nurse engage the fullness, self-respect, self-determination, and humanity of the client.

I BELIEVE that nursing's *maximum contribution* for social betterment is dependent on:

- The well-developed *expertise* of the nurse;
- The *understanding, appreciation,* and *acknowledgement* of that expertise by the public;
- The organizational, legal, economic, and political *arrangements* that enable the full and proper expression of nursing values and expertise;
- The ability of the profession to maintain *unity* within diversity.

I BELIEVE in *myself* and in my *nursing colleagues:*

- In our *responsibility* to develop and dedicate our minds, bodies, and souls to the profession that we esteem and the people whom we serve;
- In our *right* to be fulfilled, to be recognized, and to be rewarded as highly valued members of society.

From Styles, MM: On nursing: toward a new endowment, St Louis, 1982, The CV Mosby Co.

These advances and ensuing options must be mirrored against the spiraling costs of health care and the realization that low-income women may not receive even basic prenatal care, preventive care, or periodic health assessments. Many health problems need not be life threatening if they are diagnosed and treated at an early stage. Professionally skilled nurses who are socially conscious can lobby to be able to provide primary health care to offset gaps in health services. Advanced nursing practitioners provide less costly care that is more accessible and more relevant to the large majority of women (Calkin, 1984).

Social consciousness requires a belief system from which nurses direct their efforts on behalf of clients, agencies, communities, and the larger social system. One such system has been expressed by Styles (1982) (see box above). It provides a guiding framework for the development of programs and services for clients, as well as for the professional development of nurses themselves.

Commitment to Health Care For All

The International Conference on Primary Health Care at Alma-Ata in 1978 called for a worldwide commitment to health care for all by the year 2000. This call became the theme of the International Council of Nurses Congress in 1981. It emerged as the central issue in nursing at an International Conference on Clinical Decision Making in 1987. The mandate and the recommendations from Alma-Ata have set the framework for health and welfare program development in nations around the world (World Health Forum, 1981-1985) and will continue to do so throughout the next 2 decades (Mahler, 1981).

The overall recommendation from Alma-Ata was the development or extension of primary health care services. Primary health care takes place at the point of contact between the individual and the health system. It was described by the Alma-Ata conference group as follows:

> The services provided by primary health care will vary according to the country and the community, but will include at least: promotion of proper nutrition and an adequate supply of safe water; basic sanitation; maternal and child care, including family planning; immunization against the major infectious disease; prevention and control of locally endemic disease; education concerning prevailing health problems and the methods of preventing and controlling them; and appropriate treatment for common disease and injuries. The other levels of the health system provide more specialized services which become more complex as they become more central. (World Health Organization, 1978).

In order for the Alma-Ata mandate to be realized, *every* nurse must play a role in initiating and providing primary health care. This is a mandate that is not only applicable to the developing countries. Discrepancies exist between the health care available to rural and urban populations and to the rich and the poor in highly developed countries. Each nurse in each area can help reach the goal of health care for all by being cost conscious while providing care, identifying risk populations and finding ways to make services available to them, being willing to work for a time in rural or isolated areas, studying needs, and designing and testing innovative health care methods (e.g., Satz, 1982). Primary health care for all will ultimately result in a higher level of health with lowered health care costs.

Health Policy and Planning Ability

As a social force nurses have much to contribute in policy regarding health care. Individually and as organized professional groups, nurses are, and must continue to be, involved in decision making and policy development from the local to the international level. It is important for each nurse to know the persons who are planning and setting policy related to health care, to keep them informed on issues, and to support them politically. As nurses advance in skill and knowledge, it is critical for them to prepare not only at a specialized level of nursing practice but also for representation and policy development.

Political Skills

Political skills are an important feature of nursing's commitment to ensuring health care for all (Archer and Goehner, 1982; Wilson, 1981). Nursing as a professional practice is shaped by the society in which the practice occurs. The society is composed of many complex features that determine the prevailing modes of health care. Some of these features follow.

1. *Organization of health care delivery.* Health care delivery is influenced by legislation, ethical codes, policies, and short- and long-range plans.

2. *Socioeconomic and political climate.* This determines priorities for resource allocation at governmental, institutional, family/household, and personal levels.

3. *Organization of nursing as a professional group.* Nursing organizations set and control standards of practice required for licensure and specialist certification and standards of educational programs through approval and accreditation mechanisms. They also develop and disseminate a code of ethics. Policy statements and standards regarding social issues (e.g., the nurse's options in regard to assisting with abortion) and nursing functions (e.g., the nurse's role in the administration of intravenous drugs) are developed and distributed by nursing associations. Nursing is defined through these statements, which direct both educational and health care agencies in curriculum and protocol development.

Through its organizations nursing also lobbies government nationally and locally. Nurses should be informed of what their elected representatives are doing and the status of various issues. Professional nurses should keep memberships current, go to meetings, and read the publications of nursing organizations.

4. *Current scientific knowledge in the field.* Science provides increasing options in the area of pregnancy and childbirth and the possibility of prevention and cure from conditions that were previously chronic or fatal.

5. *Legal aspects of nursing.* Each state or province has a nurse practice act that governs the practice of nursing. Each act specifies the domain of nursing practice and licensure. Nurses participate in the formulation of these acts and are legally bound by them once they are passed through legislation. The statements defining nursing practice developed by the associations often form the basis for the laws governing nursing practice and education.

6. *Populations requiring health care.* Cross-cultural characteristics are a special feature of North American and European populations. Each country has high-risk populations that need targeting for primary health care. People of each culture have patterns of health and illness behavior characteristic of their group because of beliefs about health, life-style, and specific environmental hazards.

ISSUES FOR NURSING IN THE FUTURE

Several issues for nursing require resolution in the future. The processes and resolutions of each issue will influence caregivers and their clients in maternity and gynecologic services. Each issue is closely intertwined with the others—a reflection of their historical development and complexity.

Integrating Education, Practice, and Research

Until recently, nursing education was based on the apprenticeship model. Learning *to* nurse was done primarily in practice settings. The emphasis of nursing education has shifted, however, from many hours of practice to the study *of* nursing and theoretic applications. Contemporary nursing students will note, however, that an array of concepts and theories exist that are not entirely in harmony with the practice of nursing (Styles, 1983). For example, educators in nursing teach various nursing theories and concepts, such as loneliness, amelioration, family, crisis, attachment, and grief, and they describe human beings in terms of equilibrium, adaptation, and unity. Although it can be argued that these concepts and theories are all relevant to clients in all areas of nursing practice, beginning nurses have difficulty making the transfer, and experienced nurses do not use these concepts in describing their practice (Benner, 1983). A division exists between theoretic and practical knowledge. The development of research efforts to extract the theory embedded in expert nursing practice is an exciting part of this new paradigm (Benner and Wrubel, 1982).

Creating Synchrony Between Knowledge and Practice

Effort is being made to reunite theory development, education, research, and practice. Although some nurses in the past became skilled in conducting and using research and strengthening the educational programs, the nature and scope of nursing practice changed. Important questions relevant to the practice of nursing emerged. As a stronger knowledge base for both education and practice evolved from research, the interrelationships could be seen more readily (Fig. 1-3).

The advent of specialization in nursing, with graduate programs available and jobs for specialists in the complex marketplace, has led to the current transition in which the practice of nursing is once again becoming the focus. Education (basic, specialized, and continuing) and research (theory generating and theory testing) are more widely viewed *as basic* to excellent practice. Contemporary practitioners of nursing will feel the momentum of this transition as curriculums increasingly attend to the elements of nursing care that only can be learned in the practice arena, those elements identified by Benner (1983) as being embedded in practice and only available through learning by example from expert nurses. Part of this transition in maternity and gynecologic nursing is the perspective in which research is done to gain understanding of women's experiences during the reproductive continuum and to improve their care when they enter the health care system.

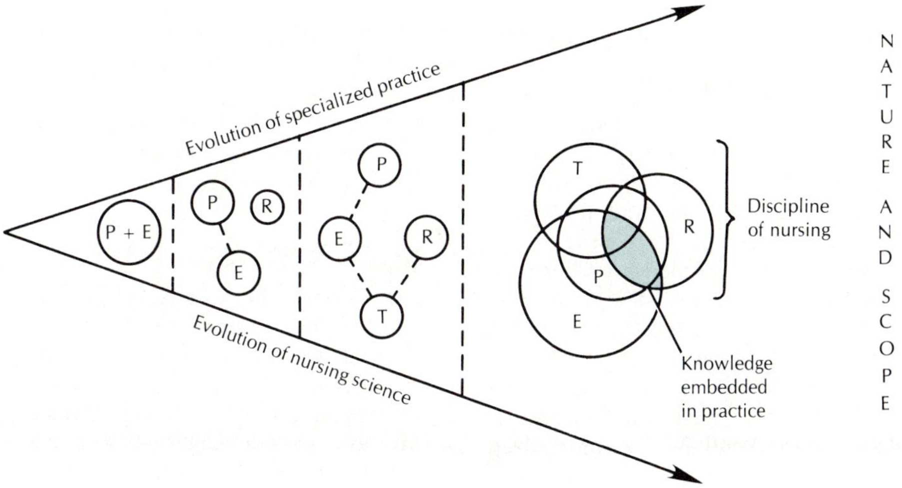

Fig. 1-3 Disintegration and reintegration of nursing knowledge and practice. *P*, practice; *E*, education; *T*, theory development; *R*, research.

Developing Nursing Science

Nursing practice in general is becoming a research-based profession recognized as a discipline with a perspective that makes a valuable contribution to science (Donaldson and Crowley, 1978; Stainton, 1982).*

Current nursing knowledge is a patchwork of related, but not integrated, knowledge and expertise. Because all nursing practice is specialized, it is important to develop and test theories that pertain to phenomena specific to areas of nursing practice such as maternity and gynecologic nursing (Meleis, 1987).

Although nursing has not had a research base for practice for long, research is now a part of every nurse's education and practice. Reva Rubin was one of the pioneers of clinical nursing research (1984). Her work forms the foundation for much of the research in maternal process during the maternity experience. Those currently entering the profession of nursing and those specializing are a part of this new thrust. This cadre of nurses will think and practice with a practice-research-theory triad at a level never before known in nursing. Increasingly, research questions already are being generated by clinicians, and research is becoming a part of nursing services in hospital and community settings. The work of nurse-researchers forms the foundation of the chapters of this book.

Credentialing Specialty Areas of Practice

One of the most pressing nursing issues to be resolved is the need to establish specialty areas of practice that form a meaningful fit with knowledge development and the relationship to practice. Specialization divides an area within a discipline into units that reflect distinctive characteristics. Specialists are, therefore those who have consciously and formally increased their knowledge and skill in a unit. Knowledge is achieved through study and research, and skill is developed through practice and experience. Specialization involves developing concepts, theories, and a typology of meanings peculiar to that area of practice.

Benner (1984) has identified areas of practical knowledge that nurses acquire as they become expert. These are described as the meanings that become common to nurses working with the same issues and that pervade all practice areas. One such example is that nurses typically try to develop a sense of possibility and hope for their clients, even when the situation is difficult. Although these areas of practical knowledge may describe and even define nursing care situations, they tend to be too broad for specialized practice with clients who are categorically grouped in the health care system according to biologic or psychologic need. Styles (1983) has challenged the National Federation for Specialty Nursing Organizations to come to terms with the poor fit between knowledge development, curriculums, credentials, and practice with respect to specialty nursing. The resolution of this issue is important, not only for nursing education and nursing practice but also for the ongoing development of nursing science. Women's health care is considered a specialty area by title, but in actuality it may be the same as the practice of the clinical nurse specialist in maternity or gynecology, the certified nurse-midwife (CNM), the family nurse practitioner (FNP), or other titles as set out in curriculums or practice settings. The evolution of nursing specialities and their credentialing is a continuing and important issue (American Nurses' Association, 1979; Field, 1982).

Maintaining a Care Atmosphere in a High-technology Cure Milieu

Nurses are inescapably involved in a health care system oriented toward those at risk and those who are ill. The onslaught of high-technology approaches in both the areas of prevention (e.g., ultrasound monitoring of a fetus) and cure (e.g., chemotherapy and radiation) has expanded the positive outcomes of reproductive care and raised the pos-

*For further review of the development of nursing as a science, see Stainton, MC: The birth of nursing science, Can Nurse 44(11):24, 1982.

sibility and hope for many people, ranging from those who previously were unable to conceive to those with metastatic cancer of the reproductive organs.

The nurse-client relationship can be enhanced by technologic resources. It is not farfetched to visualize a nurse available to a client by videophone or personalized pocket-size television. This is being done via satellite in some of the northern reaches of Canada through central areas in Ontario and Newfoundland. Imagine the security a new mother will feel if, when she has a problem with her newborn infant, she can dial a nurse, see her on a screen, have the nurse examine her infant or situation in the natural setting, and receive instant support and advice.

The nurse will often be communicating with whole families. Family members can provide vital information and are an important part of the health care of the woman involved. Wright and Leahey (1984) have developed and tested techniques for interviewing and assessing families. These techniques include the use of technologic devices such as videotape to increase the accuracy of data and feedback.

Working in Collaborative Roles

Nurses provide care in tandem with other members of the health care team in both community- and hospital-based settings. Education, practice, and research done cooperatively in the same settings and, when appropriate, collaboratively enrich the knowledge base of all professional groups. The woman seeking maternity or gynecologic care can be best served by those who are able to focus on the woman and work together. Nurses who have confidence that is derived from knowledge and skill and coupled with skepticism are autonomous. Such nurses can work effectively in collaboration with other members of the health care team.

Consultation and collaboration between nurse specialists can maximize the level of care received by the woman. Often a health care problem involves complex relationships between physiologic and psychosocial responses. For example, utilization of the expertise and experience of nursing colleagues on the psychiatric unit can assist in developing a plan of care designed to prevent or treat a depression that can occur if a woman is hospitalized for a long time.

SUMMARY

Theoretic and technical knowledge available to nursing is vast and increasing. Theories are constantly being tested and rejected, revised, or replaced by new ones, which are subsequently rejected or refined. A continuing evolution in the sciences guides reproductive function and nursing practice. Changes in knowledge and options cause new cultural meanings and possibilities to evolve concerning reproductive function and health care delivery. The nurse who provides maternity and gynecologic care is inescapably involved in these changes.

Gaining excellence and expertness in nursing practice amid the shifting social context requires the following:

1. A belief in the nature and purpose of nursing
2. A belief in the willingness and ability of each woman to participate in her health or illness management
3. The ability to apply the most current knowledge innovatively, individually, and inquisitively
4. A social consciousness that motivates interest, ability, and participation in issue resolution
5. Involved, powerful caring

KEY CONCEPTS

- Caring is the essence of nursing.
- Nursing practice requires knowledge and skill in helping women maintain psychologic and physiologic health as changes occur throughout the life span.
- Health and illness behavior depend on cultural values and personal preferences.
- The International Conference on Primary Health Care at Alma-Ata in 1978 called for a worldwide commitment to health care for all by the year 2000.
- Issues for nursing in the future include integrating education, practice, and research; creating synchrony between knowledge and practice; developing nursing science; credentialing specialty areas of practice; maintaining a care atmosphere in a high-technology cure milieu; and working in collaborative roles.
- In developing a professional relationship, the nurse works within the personal and social context of the woman and the relationships that pattern the woman's health practice.
- The nurse as caregiver requires technical and interpersonal competence, social consciousness, commitment to health care for all, health policy and planning ability, and political skills.
- Knowledgeable consumers no longer comply with the power base of professionals; they wish to be participants in the experience of their family members.

STUDY QUESTIONS AND ACTIVITIES

1. Discern, through interviews, the life-styles of three clients from differing economic or social groups.
2. Read and discuss the nurse practice act in your state or province.
3. Assess the local nursing community's readiness for contribution to at least three of the six political skills discussed in this chapter.
4. Discuss and compare the meaning of primary health care for nursing practice in rural and urban areas.

References

Anderson, JM: Perspectives on the health of immigrant women: a feminist analysis, Adv Nurs Sci 8:61, 1985

American Nurses' Association: The study of credentialing in nursing: a new approach, Kansas City, 1979, The Association

Archer, SE, and Goehner, PA: Nurses: a political force, Belmont, Calif, 1982, Wadsworth, Inc

Belsky, J: Early human experience: a family perspective, Dev Psychol 17:3, 1981

Benner, PE: Uncovering the knowledge embedded in clinical practice, Image 15(2):36, 1983

Benner, PE: From novice to expert: excellence and power in clinical nursing practice, Menlo Park, Calif, 1984, Addison-Wesley Publishing Co, Inc
Benner, PE, and Wrubel, J: Skilled clinical knowledge: the value of perceptual awareness, Nurse Educ 7(3):11, 1982
Boss, R: Normative family stress: family boundary changes across the lifespan, Fam Relations 29:445, 1980
Calkin, JD: A model for advanced nursing practice, J Nurs Adm 14:24, 1984
Chodorow, N: The reproduction of mothering: psychoanalysis and the sociology of gender, Berkeley, 1978, University of California Press
DeVore, NE: Parenthood postponed, Am J Nurs **83**:1160, 1983
Donaldson, S, and Crowley, DM: The discipline of nursing, Nurs Outlook 26:113, 1978
Field, PA: What this country needs now . . . nurses prepared to work with today's parents to revolutionize family-newborn care, Can Nurse 78(11):37, 1982
Fletcher, JC: The fetus as patient: ethical issues, JAMA 246:772, 1981
Gilligan, C: In a different voice, Cambridge, 1982, Harvard University Press
Gilligan, C: Do the social sciences have an adequate theory of moral development? In Haan, N, et al: Social science as moral inquiry, New York, 1983, Columbia University Press
Hancock, T: Health, women and the future, Health Care for Women International 8:249, 1987
Harrison, MR, et al: Management of the fetus with a correctable congenital defect, JAMA 246:774, 1981
Lederman, R: Psychosocial adaptation in pregnancy, Englewood Cliffs, NJ, 1984, Prentice Hall
Mahler, H: The meaning of "health for all by the year 2000," World Health Forum 2:5, 1981
Meleis, AI: Revisions is knowledge development: a passion for substance, Scholarly Inquiry for Nursing Practice 1:5, 1987
Meleis, AI, and Rogers, S: Women in transition: being versus becoming or being and becoming, Health Care for Women International 8:199, 1987
Mercer, RT: First-time motherhood: experiences from teens to forties, New York, 1986, Springer Publishing Co, Inc
Powledge, TM: Windows on the womb, Psychol Today 17:37, 1983
Purpura, D: Consciousness, Behav Today, p. 494, June 2, 1975
Rubin, R: Maternal identity and the maternal experience, New York, 1984, Springer Publishing Co, Inc
Satz, KJ: Integrating Navajo tradition into maternal-child nursing, Image 14(3):89, 1982
Scott-Palmer, J, and Skevington, SM: Pain during labor and menstruation: a study of locus of control, J Psychosom Res 25(3):1981
Stainton, MC: Parent-infant interaction: putting theory into nursing practice, Calgary, 1981, The University of Calgary
Stainton, MC: The birth of nursing science, Can Nurse 44(11):24, 1982
Stainton, MC: The fetus: a growing member of the family, Fam Relations **34**:321, 1985a
Stainton, MC: Origins of attachment: culture and cue sensitivity, unpublished doctoral dissertation, University of California, San Francisco, 1985b
Styles, MM: On nursing: toward a new endowment, St Louis, 1982, The CV Mosby Co
Styles, MM: The anatomy of a profession, Heart Lung 12:570, 1983
Swanson-Kauffman, KM: Overview of the balancing act: having it all, Health Care for Women International 8:1, 1987
Wilkins, R, and Adams, O: The healthfulness of life, Montreal, 1983, Institute for Research in Public Policy
Wilson, JB: Nurses and politics, Can Nurse 77:40, 1981
World Health Forum: An International Journal of Health Development, Health 2000, vols 2 to 6, 1981-1985
World Health Organization: Primary health care, Report of the International Conference of Primary Health Care, Alma-Ata, USSR, Sept. 6-12, 1978
Wright, LM, and Leahey, M: Nurses and families: a guide to family assessment and intervention, Philadelphia, 1984, FA Davis Co

Bibliography

Barnard, K: Knowledge for practice: directions for the future, Nurs Res 29:208, 1980
Barnard, KE: MCN keys to research: research utilization: the clinician's role, MCN 11(3):224, 1986
Bearinger, L, and Gephart, J: Priorities for adolescent health: recommendations of a national conference, MCN 12(3):161, 1987
Beck, CT: The conceptualization of power, Adv Nurs Sci 4(2):1, 1982
Bohny, BJ: Theory development for a nursing science, Nurs Forum 19(1):50, 1980
Carter, ER: Quality maternity care for the medically indigent, MCN 11(2):85, 1986
Daria, J, and Moran, S: Nursing in the 90s, Nurs '85, 15(12):26, 1985
Haller, KB: MCN keys to research: interrater reliability: essential for research and practice, MCN 12(1):78, 1987
Haller, KB: MCN keys to research: systematic documentation of practice, MCN 12(2):152, 1987
Haller, KB: MCN keys to research: readying research for practice, MCN 12(3):226, 1987
Lia-Hoagberg, B, et al: A computerized information system, MCN 12(1):11, 1987
Mercer, RT: Teenage motherhood: the first year, JOGN Nurs 9:16, 1980
Mercer, RT: Factors having an impact on maternal role attainment: the first year of motherhood, Springfield, Va, 1982, National Technical Information Service, US Department of Commerce
Neeson, JD, et al: Pregnancy outcome for adolescents receiving prenatal care by nurse practitioners in extended roles, J Adolesc Health Care 4:94, 1983
Vansintejan, GA, and Purdy, PJ: International family-planning training for nurse practitioners, JOGN Nurs 15(6):492, 1986

CHAPTER 2

The Client, the Nurse, and the Nursing Process

Learning Objectives

Correctly define the key terms listed.

Describe the maternity-gynecologic client, focusing on motivation, intercourse, pregnancy, birth, parenthood, gynecologic issues, and human responses.

Summarize the development of competence in nursing from novice to expert nurse.

Differentiate the roles of the nurse as teacher and counselor, technician, advocate, manager, and researcher, as well as the expanded roles.

Examine the nature and scope of maternity-gynecologic nursing.

Explain the stages of the nursing process.

Review the models of helping and coping.

Discuss the process of nurse-client relationships.

List the components of interpersonal communication.

Outline the teaching-learning process.

Key Terms

birthrate
body image
curative actions
decision-making process
functional health pattern
helping-coping models
home health care
locus of control
mortality
mutual goal setting
nurse competence
nursing process:
- assessment
- nursing diagnosis
- planning
- implementation
- evaluation

preventive actions
rehabilitative actions
self-awareness
self-esteem
social role
teaching-learning process
values clarification

Maternity and gynecologic nursing is a complex health service that is initiated in response to women and other members of their family seeking help for actual or potential health problems. Nursing activities range across the health-illness continuum from promotion of health to client rehabilitation. The greater scope and more sophisticated nature of the care offered today require a collaborative, team approach to maternity and gynecologic care involving the woman, her family, nurses, physicians, nutritionists, and other health professionals. No one group of health practitioners possesses either the competence or the time to act as the sole dispenser of health care—full utilization of all groups is needed.

This chapter discusses the woman, the nurse with a range of competence and roles, and the nursing process. Included is a description of the range and organization of nursing services offered and interpersonal communications, as well as a discussion of the process of the nurse-client relationship. The four models of helping and coping and the teaching-learning process enhance the nurse's skill in caring for women and their families through the nursing process.

MATERNITY-GYNECOLOGIC CLIENT

Motivation. Although reproduction is almost entirely a function of human sexuality, each person involved may perceive its components—intercourse, pregnancy, birth, and parenthood—separately, and endow each with a special meaning. The meaning attached to any one component can profoundly affect the outcome of the total process for woman, man, and child.

Gynecologic health issues can arise at any time during a woman's life span. Fertility management, menstrual cycle–related events, post-childbirth sequelae, neoplasia, and other situations affect women. Some occur concurrently with childbearing.

Intercourse. Both women and men may use intercourse or related sexual acts in a variety of ways. In a positive sense, it expresses tenderness and love, assuages loneliness, and provides physical relief of sexual tension; in a negative sense, it becomes a weapon to belittle or demean a partner through refusal, giving grudgingly of oneself, or taking another by force (rape). Some people have intercourse to demonstrate their sexual desirability to a peer group, hoping to enhance their social acceptance. It may form part of the experimenting process in moving toward adult sexuality. Increases in premarital intercourse and the less conventional practice of sharing partners appear to testify to the complex meaning that can be attached to the biologic act of intercourse.

Pregnancy can result from vaginal intercourse or deposit of sperm near the introitus. A pregnancy may or may not be wanted or accepted. Being accountable and responsible for the consequences of the sexual act demonstrate one facet of adulthood in the sexual sense.

Pregnancy. Pregnancy may represent a period of great creativity for a woman. She becomes aware of feelings and sensations she has never known before. She may feel a sense of fulfillment. She may see pregnancy as making her a complete woman. For most women the close relationship of mother and fetus is felt deeply.

Birth. The birth of a child often unifies a family. Many partners insist on sharing this important event by actively participating in the pregnancy and labor. For some people the sharing extends beyond the immediate participants; other family members, friends, and community members are included.

Parenthood. Parenthood, beginning as it does with the excitement of pregnancy and birth, can serve many human purposes. To some it is a life-fulfilling state, a chance to help their children become the adults of the future. Children born to such parents are wanted children, whose dependency is recognized and accepted. The children's achievements bring much pleasure to their parents. Their failures are also accepted, and love and support are forthcoming.

Some parents want children primarily for their own satisfaction. Such parents will expect their children to support the parents' self-concepts and need for love, acceptance, and success. But a young child is unable to live up to such expectations, so disappointment and frustration soon follow. Consequently the child may become a victim of neglect or even abuse.

Other pregnancies and resultant parenthoods are neither planned nor desired. Children born under these conditions may suffer parental and material deprivation. Edwards (1973) contends that one of the greatest needs such children have is parents who have learned the art of "gentle socialization of children," of creating a nurturing environment peopled with interested, concerned, and loving adults.

Unlike other manifestations of human sexuality, parenthood can be both a biologic and psychologic entity, or it can be entirely psychologic as in adoption. After a child is born, the parent by substitution or adoption can fulfill this socially and personally important role. These parents need the same preparation and support as biologic parents.

Gynecologic Issues. Fertility issues (premenstrual syndrome, infertility) or management (contraception, sterilization) may present a crisis situation for the woman and her family. Disorders such as sexually transmitted diseases or neoplasia affect clients' comfort, self-esteem, and relationships. A lack of knowledge of normal anatomy and physiology can be just as disruptive as a serious disorder.

Statistical Picture and Definitions

Potentially all sexually mature people in North America are candidates for reproductive health care. They come from all racial, ethnic, economic, and social groups. Approximately 70% are white, and 30% are nonwhite. They or their forebears were native-born Indians or Eskimos or came to this continent mainly from Europe, Africa, or Asia. Their age groups will vary from the adolescent, to the young adult, to individuals approaching middle age. Many, both women and men, will seek assistance concerning methods of contraception. Approximately 15% of all couples of childbearing age will seek help for infertility problems.

Approximately 3.9 million women, ranging in age from 12 to 52 years, give birth each year. Some of them will have the support of family, husbands, parents, children, and friends. Others will be alone. Some will be overjoyed by their pregnancies; others will be angry, defensive, or apathetic about their state. Most will be physically healthy; others, at least 500,000 a year, will be designated at *high risk* for either maternal, fetal, or familial reasons. Some of this latter group, through ignorance of current concepts of health care, will not seek medical attention until their or their infant's life is threatened.

The *fertility rate* is the number of births per 1000 women between the ages of 15 and 44 years (inclusive) calculated on a yearly basis. It is a more accurate means of comparing different population groups than the birthrate. The U.S. National Center for Health Statistics (1984) noted the fertility rate in 1984 was 65.4 (white women, 62.2; black women, 81.4) births per 1000 women of childbearing age.

The *birthrate,* the number of live births per 1000 population, was 15.5 in 1984. The decline in birthrate is expected to continue. The projected birthrate for the year 2000 is 13. In 1984, the birth rate by age of mother was:

Age	*Birthrate*
10-14	1.2
15-19	50.9
20-24	107.3
25-29	108.3
30-34	66.5
35-39	22.8
40-44	3.9
45-50	.2

The highest birthrates are in Utah (23.4) and Alaska (24.1). The lowest birthrate is in Connecticut (11.6).

A total of 770,400 live births, or 21% of those born in 1984, were born to single women (National Data Book, 1987). Among white women, 13.4% were single; among black and other women, 50.8 were single. The increase in the rate of childbearing among unmarried woman was attributed to the substantial rise in the rate for unmarried white women, which rose from 17.6 (in 1980) to 20.1 (in 1984), while the rate for unwed black women fell slightly.

Infant mortality is the yearly ratio of the number of deaths of infants before their first birthday per 1000 live births. Infant mortality nationwide in 1985 was 11.2, down by almost half from 1970. Among white infants, the mortality is 9.7; among black and other infants, 16.8; and among black infants, 19.2

Maternal mortality shows the number of maternal deaths per 100,000 live births. A *maternal death* is the death of a woman from *any* cause during pregnancy or within 42 days of the termination of pregnancy, regardless of the duration or site of the pregnancy. Maternal mortality has shown a remarkable decline. In 1930, 700 deaths occurred per 100,000 live births; in 1983 the rate was 8.0 per 100,000 live births. Among white women, the rate (1983) was 5.9; for black and all other women, 16.3; for black women, 18.3. The maternal mortality for women over 35 has also declined. In the years 1974 through 1978 there were 47.5 deaths per 100,000 live births to women over 35 years; in 1982 this was down to 24.2. The mortality included deaths from abortions.

A combination of factors stimulated this decline (WHO, 1976a; WHO, 1976b; WHO, 1977): availability of antimicrobial drugs for controlling infections, availability of blood and blood substitutes for treatment of hemorrhage, and formation of hospital and community committees to investigate causes and circumstances of each maternal death and to assign responsibility. In the over 35 category researchers suggested that the decline could be attributed to the higher socioeconomic status of such women having babies in recent years (San Francisco Chronicle, Jan. 2, 1986; National Data Book, 1987). The drop in maternal mortality also reflects the decrease in maternal deaths from abortion as states legalized the abortion procedure and safer techniques were employed.

Despite these efforts, mortality, both infant and maternal, for different segments of the population and different socioeconimic groups still shows inequities (National Data Book, 1987). Differences remain between white and nonwhite maternal mortality; the young and poor of any racial group also are vulnerable to maternity complications and maternal death. Many women still do not receive adequate prenatal care, and many women categorized as high risk are still without specialized treatment. Only 62.2% of black women and 79.6% of white women were receiving prenatal care during the first trimester (1984). Almost 20% of women under the age of 15 years received no prenatal care or delayed prenatal care. This delay in prenatal care and the large number of black low-birth-weight infants may have resulted in the finding that black infants were twice as likely to receive low Apgar scores at 1 minute and 5 minutes as white infants. The percentage of black low-birth-weight infants (12.4%) was twice as high as the percentage of white low-birth-weight infants (5.6%)(1984).

Neonatal mortality has been a traditional indicator of environmental influences. In the 1960s, professionals, local communities, and state and federal agencies identified factors that cause a higher mortality for the poor and designed programs to combat the problems (p. 19). The major contributing factor to a higher mortality for the poor was *inadequate nutrition.* A second factor was the *lack of prenatal care* because the poor did not realize the importance of early and continuous prenatal care, they could not afford care, private providers limited or excluded them from their practice, and impersonal treatment was delivered in overcrowded public clinics (Brook, 1980).

A third factor is related to the *availability of contraceptive techniques.* Contraceptive techniques are preventing many unwanted pregnancies; however, a large number of people are still not reached (Barnes, 1978). More than 3.5 million low- and marginal-income women and almost 2.5 million sexually active adolescents still lack family planning services (Chapter 35). Even among married couples some births continue to be unwanted and mistimed. More equal distribution and use of health resources among all citizens will be necessary to effect a beneficial change in maternal and child mortality and morbidity.

Statistics related to gynecologic conditions are presented in Unit IX.

Human Responses

Maternity-gynecologic clients and their families face biologic or psychosociocultural events that center on reproductive and gynecologic processes. These events elicit human responses that cluster around the tasks of decision making, adaptation, or participation in a critical life event. Underlying these tasks is the theme of perceived locus of control or power.

Decision Making and Informed Consent. The Patient's Bill of Rights* takes a firm position on the right of each person to be informed. Each client is entitled to information that covers every facet of her or his health needs, proposed care, anticipated outcome, and available alternatives. This right to know forms the legal basis of informed consent (Chapter 4). Holistic health concepts place emphasis on *education* and *self-care* rather than on dependence. Possession of information closes the competence gap between the client and the health care provider. Collaboration between care provider and recipient assumes "that individuals have the *capability to make decisions* about their health and that they ultimately have *control of their own health* by virtue of the choices they make" (Fogel and Woods, 1981).

Both client and nurse bring to the interaction a highly personal definition of health. In a collaborative relationship, "information is freely exchanged with clients and informed decision-making is ideally the client's domain." The nurse, in conjunction with the client, identifies the health care practices the client currently engages in. The nurse and client collaborate to identify the client's assets and deficits. A nursing diagnosis is formulated. Finally, the nurse *and* the client set the goals of care before the nursing care is implemented. In the absence of collaboration, knowledge deficits, noncompliance, ineffective individual or family coping, or other concerns may arise.

Adaptation. The response of a woman and her family to the biologic reality of pregnancy or a gynecologic condition is both physiologic and psychosociocultural and can be adaptive or maladaptive. The physiologic processes involved include the adaptation of the newborn to extrauterine existence and the adaptation of both the newborn and the mother to preexisting or presently existing physical and genetic insult. Psychosociocultural factors may overtax the coping mechanisms of the woman and her family. Anxiety about the ability to master new tasks, behaviors, attitudes, and sentiments inherent in the role may precipitate a crisis.

Without a nurturing environment there is potential for alterations in family processes or parenting or in health maintenance or for disturbance of self-concept. Anxiety and fear can result from lack of psychologic preparation. Properly timed teaching is a nursing care skill that can provide psychologic preparation and facilitate adaptation.

The occurrence of a reproductive tract disorder such as neoplasia, for instance, is traumatic at any time, especially during pregnancy. Fear and anxiety about potential or actual loss stress coping to the limit (Chapter 28). Family and individual strengths may be mobilized, however, resulting in a positive outcome (see Chapter 3).

Participation. Generally every person, regardless of level of income or social status, wishes to function in the best possible manner when confronted with a life event that has great personal implications. Many factors determine a person's ability to participate whole-heartedly in situations causing growth, joy, and pleasure to the self and others and, conversely, to face pain, separation, disability, or death adequately and well. Factors that influence a person's ability to cope with maturational and situational events include (1) the feelings a person has about her or his ability to maintain control, (2) the sharing of these critical life events with those who care, and (3) the nurturing provided by others in the environment.

Locus of Control. Powerlessness can be experienced by anyone, of any age, educational background, profession, or marital status. Powerlessness is defined as a state in which a person *perceives* a loss or a lack of personal control. The maternity client may feel powerless related to being pregnant. She may rejoice in the pregnancy but feel powerless relative to the events surrounding the child's birth. A sense of powerlessness can arise from many sources (Beck, 1982; Norton, 1985), such as lack of knowledge about available resources or choices (Carter, 1986), cultural or social limitations, or alterations in plans for meeting personal goals. Responses to perceived powerlessness vary and may include apathy, anxiety, anger, or depression.

While a person feels powerless, positive adaptation and readiness to learn is impaired. However, a person with internal locus of control feels she can affect outcome. She is freer to participate in decision making, learning, or in manipulating herself or her environment. Nurses can help people increase their control by providing information and by helping them learn how to solve problems. Sharing the pregnancy, labor, and delivery with people who care can contribute to a sense of control. Nurturing provided by others—nurses, physicians, family, friends—can help a woman gain internal locus of control.

MATERNITY-GYNECOLOGIC NURSE

Maternity-gynecologic nurses are in a unique position to effect change in the care women receive. Nurses have early, frequent, and continuing contact with the woman and her family. The nurse acts in a variety of roles to bring comprehensive health care to people during the childbearing years and beyond. As *clinicians,* nurses act as teachers, counselors, technicians, advocates, managers, and researchers. The degree to which nurses fulfill these roles depends on their level of competence.

Development of Competence. People solve problems in a number of ways, depending on the situation and their knowledge and experience. Benner's work (1983, 1984) describes how a body of practical knowledge is developed as the nurse acquires expertise. Implementation of the nursing process may be accomplished on several levels, depending on the practitioner's competence. Benner (1984) identifies the following five levels.

Novice. Novices are beginners who have no experi-

*The Patient's Bill of Rights must be posted in a prominent place in each hospital. Many hospitals include it in the packet of information given to each person admitted.

ence in the nursing care of the woman (family) for childbearing or gynecologic conditions. They may feel intimidated and be unable to see what nursing care they can provide. Benner (1984) states that novices "have little understanding of the contextual meaning of the recently learned textbook terms." The novice begins by learning rules for guiding practice. Yet even on the first day, unable to answer questions or determine the next course of action, the student has several years' experience in communicating with people, expressing concern, providing comfort, and seeking assistance. The presence of a caring human being is in itself valuable during a trying time.

Nursing students are not the only novices. The nurse who is new to a clinical area of practice or who is returning to nursing may also fall into this category. Highly competent practitioners in their first teaching experience are novice instructors.

Advanced Beginner. Once students have had some experience with clients under the guidance of instructors and preceptors, they can begin to synthesize clinical findings. This synthesis, rather than rules alone, provides the basis to guide nursing actions.

Competent Nurse. Nurses who have had experience working full time are able to more quickly establish priorities of need among their clients. Their organizational ability enables them to detect subtle cues in client behavior. These nurses have a feeling of mastery over situations likely to arise and can impart this feeling to clients and their families.

Proficient Nurse. Nurses with many years of experience can pick out the key components of a situation. They grasp the heart of the matter and can move forward and backward to focus on providing holistic care. Benner (1984) describes the proficient nurse as one who "learns from experience what typical events to expect in a given situation and how plans need to be modified in response to these events."

Expert Nurse. Benner (1984) describes the expert nurse as one who "with an enormous background of experience, now has an intuitive grasp of each situation and zeroes in on the accurate region of the problem without wasteful consideration of a large range of unfruitful, alternative diagnoses and solutions."

Teacher and Counselor. Maternity nursing emphasizes the preventive aspects of health care. Much of this is accomplished through teaching and counseling clients. As a teacher or counselor the nurse tries to help clients learn how to make the best possible health care decisions for themselves or their children. The nurse provides a nonjudgmental environment in which these decisions can take place and helps clients evaluate their efforts realistically. The nurse acts as a role model for the technical care of clients or their infants. With supportive teaching the nurse can help even the most anxious or uninformed client learn to provide safe care.

Technician. Technical skills are required for every stage of the nursing process. Such skills help nurses assess health status, create a safe, comfortable environment for clients and others, initiate therapeutic nursing actions, and efficiently use time, energy, and materials. The nursing profession has developed standards for nursing practice that provide criteria for evaluating the degree of competence a nurse has attained (Chapter 4). A competent nurse inspires confidence in clients. This confidence is an important part of the supportive care clients require.

Advocate. As health care becomes more complex, someone must act as liaison or advocate between the client and other personnel or health agencies. The maternity-gynecologic nurse encourages clients to become aware of their health care rights and responsibilities. The nurse is committed to a holistic view of health care and therefore often knows more about clients than do other health workers. The nurse is in a position to explain, interpret, defend, or protect clients' rights. As an advocate the nurse attempts to modify health services on a local or national level so they reflect a humanitarian approach to health care. Therefore participation in professional organizations and politics (such as health-related legislation) is an important feature of nursing's commitment to ensuring health care for all (Archer and Goehner, 1982; Wilson, 1981).

Manager. Nurse managers coordinate and facilitate the many services required in the health care of clients (Etheredge, 1985). Team leaders or charge nurses are examples of nurse managers since they direct the care of groups of clients and nursing personnel. They need to be knowledgeable about client care and able to communicate effectively with various types of health workers.

Researcher. Research has had an invaluable effect on shaping nursing practice and developing ideas for further inquiry that will keep our future practice alive. All nurses have the responsibility of adding knowledge through descriptive studies, the validation of knowledge using research design, and publication of results in professional literature. The idea of scientific research in nursing dates back to Florence Nightingale, who admonished nurses to develop the habit of systematically making and recording correct observations and then comtemplating their meaning. Observations should not be for curious facts but rather as the only means for discovering and verifying knowledge useful for saving lives. Nurses need to evaluate the effectiveness of establishing methods of clinical nursing by measuring the outcomes in the health status of clients. Current research findings need to be evaluated for relevance to practice. Modification of practice needs to be based on scientific data to ensure quality care.

Obstetric-gynecologic Nurse Practitioner. In 1979 the American College of Obstetrics and Gynecology (ACOG) and the Nurses' Association of the American College of Obstetrics and Gynecology (NAACOG) jointly defined the obstetric-gynecologic nurse practitioner as follows:

> A registered nurse who has satisfactorily completed a formal and accredited Obstetric-Gynecologic Nurse Practitioner educational program. The Obstetric-Gynecologic Nurse Practitioner will thus have been provided with special knowledge and skills in health maintenance, disease prevention, psychosocial and physical assessment, and management of health-illness needs in the primary care of women. This care is predominantly provided in an ambulatory setting. The Obstetric-Gynecologic Nurse Practitioner will provide such care interdependently with the physician and other members of the health care team.

Registered Nurse Certified (RNC). In 1981 the NAACOG Certification Cooperation (NCC) instituted a certification program for the in-hospital obstetric nurse and for the obstetric-gynecologic nurse practitioner (Nurses' Association of the American College of Obstetrics and Gynecology, 1982). This program requires a candidate to meet eligibility criteria based on educational or practice requirements and to successfully complete a 200-item multiple choice examination. Nurses who achieve certification are entitled to use RNC (registered nurse certified) after their name. Beginning with the 1983 examination, all nurses taking the examination for the obstetric-gynecologic nurse practitioner certification are required to be graduates from a nurse-practitioner program acceptable to the NCC. Also, since 1983 a neonatal nurse clinician/practitioner certification examination has been offered.

Since 1986, the two primary certifying agencies, the American Nurses' Association (ANA) and the National Association of Pediatric Nurse Associates and Practitioners have required a minimum of a baccalaureate degree to become a nurse practitioner; soon a master's degree probably will be required (Waters and Arbeiter, 1985).

Certified Nurse-midwife (CNM). Certified nurse-midwives are registered nurses who have additional knowledge and skill gained through an organized program of study and clinical experience recognized by the American College of Nurse Midwives (ACNM). Certification for entry into practice includes successful passage of a 6-hour essay examination and meeting other ACNM criteria. If certified as a nurse-midwife, participants may use the designation CNM after their names. They can perform tasks and care for the client in the same way as obstetric-gynecologic nurse practitioners. The primary focus of the CNM is in the area of management and care of mothers and babies throughout the maternity cycle (including delivery), so long as maternal progress meets criteria accepted as normal. The nurse-midwife is prepared to teach, interpret, and provide support as an integral part of services (Haire, 1981; Burst, 1980; Beebe, 1980; Rousch, 1979).

The issue of who should deliver the low-risk client does not arise out of clients' nonacceptance of the nurse-midwife or because of questionable competency but rather because legislative controls limit the practice. Some states have not yet changed their laws or codes to legitimize the nurse-midwife's practice and third-party payers such as Blue Cross do not cover the services.

In 1970 the ACOG, the NAACOG, and the ACNM issued a joint statement that in "medically directed teams, qualified nurse-midwives may assume responsibility for the complete care and management of uncomplicated maternity patients." This position has opened the door to the increased use of nurse-midwives in North America. In a number of states in the United States that have not permitted the full functioning of these nurses, legislative bills are pending that will provide the necessary license to practice.

The professional role of the midwife as defined by the World Health Organization (1976b) and amended by the Working Party on Midwifery Training in European Countries is as follows:

> A midwife is a person who is qualified to practice midwifery. She is trained to give the necessary care and advice to women during pregnancy, labor and the postnatal period, to conduct normal deliveries on her own responsibility and to care for the newly born infant. At all times she must be able to recognize the warning signs of abnormal or potentially abnormal conditions which necessitate referral to a doctor and to carry out emergency measures in the absence of a doctor. She may practice in hospitals, health units or domiciliary services. In any one of these situations she has an important task in health education with the family and the community.

NATURE AND SCOPE OF MATERNITY-GYNECOLOGIC NURSING

Maternity-gynecologic nursing involves actions that can be designated as preventive, curative, or rehabilitative in nature (Table 2-1) (ANA, 1982). It spans the lifetime of an individual from preconceptional planning for children through pregnancy and birth and the early adjustment of the family to a newborn child. These activities may be carried out in the home, clinic, or hospital.

The preventive aspects of maternity care include health promotion and prevention of disease states. Efforts are made to increase and strengthen the individual's ability to withstand the stress of everyday living. Nursing actions associated with these efforts represent many of the nurse's independent functions. They occur wherever nurse and client meet, whether the client is directly under the care of a physician or not. The nurse who teaches good nutrition, personal hygiene, and beneficial exercises to a pregnant woman is promoting the health of the woman and her developing fetus. The nurse who encourages a teenager to seek care for pregnancy or who discusses sexual adjustment with pregnant couples is acting to promote health and to prevent possible complications.

The early detection of physical and emotional disabilities in the mother or infant and initiation of corrective measures are essential components of maternity nursing. The checkpoints in prenatal evaluation correspond to the times during pregnancy when difficulties are known to occur. Women with diseases complicating pregnancy may be confined to a hospital for continuous evaluation and treatment. Cesarean birth may be chosen to safeguard mother or child.

Rehabilitative activities are directed toward returning an individual to her or his previous state with an equal or greater ability to function. The care given a pregnant teenager illustrates the rehabilitative aspects of maternity care. Nurses hope that through the physical and emotional support provided these young people they will be able to complete their development toward responsible adulthood. Nurses have provided the impetus to founding teenage clinics, high school programs for pregnant teenagers, and follow-up care to help teenagers give their children the mothering needed.

After a mastectomy or hysterectomy, women require sensitive and skillful care. Rehabilitative actions help her maintain or regain self-esteem, positive family processes and sexuality, and avoid social isolation.

• • •

Table 2-1 *Nature and Scope of Maternity Nursing*

Goal	Examples of Nursing Actions
Prevention	Health education of people: nutrition, general hygiene (rest, exercise, stress management, cleanliness), signs and symptoms of illness, community resources (clinics, etc.), environmental agents to avoid (drugs/chemicals, communicable disease, x rays)*
	Encouragement for women to keep scheduled appointments
	Development of a caring and trusting relationship with each client and her family
	Following assessment for level of knowledge and readiness to learn, health education regarding expected physical and psychologic changes and expected duration of those changes
Cure	Identification of family history or personal history of biophysical (e.g., genetic disorder), psychologic (e.g., recurrent depression), or social (e.g., poverty) risk factors
	Continuous assessment for detection of risk factors whenever nurse is in contact with childbearing family
	Education of client and family, supplemented by written information, regarding signs and symptoms of complications and emergency telephone numbers
	Maintenance of client records
Rehabilitation	Rapid notification of appropriate health team member (e.g., physician, nutritionist, social worker)
	Assisting physician to Explain (and reexplain) problem and its management to woman and family Carry out prescribed therapy Encourage client cooperation during therapy and follow-up Maintain records
	Maintenance of a trusting and caring relationship with woman and family
	Assisting woman and family to cope with grief associated with being termed ***high risk*** (a term that some people see as a stigma) or having her fetus considered to be at risk; careful assessment of perceptions, coping mechanisms, and support systems permits nurse to use crisis theory (see Chapter 3) as a format for care (see Chapter 28 for details)

*In the broader sense, each nurse participates in prevention through working for legislation and with community efforts to reduce hazards in the environment and to educate the public regarding health maintenance.

Nursing actions—preventive, curative, and rehabilitative—often overlap as nurses give care to any one client. The nurse responsible for the care of a premature infant in a neonatal intensive care unit makes continuous assessments of the infant's condition and modifies care to maintain an optimal state (curative). The nurse promotes the infants' future welfare by educating the parents regarding their child's care following discharge (preventive). Weaning the infant from oxygen therapy and respirators is essential before discharge (rehabilitative).

Home Health Care. One of the most drastic changes in health care delivery has been the establishment of a prospective payment system based on **diagnosis related groups (DRGs)**. The DRG categories allow pretreatment (prospective) billing for almost all United States hospitals reimbursed by Medicare. With hospitals now financially responsible when Medicare clients exceed the allotted admission stay, more clients are being discharged early. This has created an immense need for home care and other sources of community-based services. The exact impact DRGs will have on maternity-gynecologic care is uncertain, but with containment of health care cost a national priority, it is inevitable that some form of prospective payment will affect perinatal, maternity, and gynecologic clients. Nurses need to be aware of the changing economics and prepared to meet the challenges.

Prevention. Preventive nursing activities within the home have a long history. In her home the *gravida*, or new mother, is in her own environment. Cultural, ethnic, religious, socioeconomic, and interpersonal factors influencing the woman are evident. Knowledge of the woman's usual surroundings and life-style sheds light on factors that affect the plan and implementation of nursing care. The nurse must consider carefully those factors that influence the nurse-client relationship when establishing a therapeutic relationship in the home (Chapter 3). A model for data collection (Chapter 3) assists the nurse in understanding the family.

The nurse in the home can gain first-hand insight into such issues as nutrition, sanitation, child care and other responsibilities, discomforts of pregnancy, safety hazards, and the like. Anticipatory guidance and teaching of self-care measures are therefore more realistic. The home visit content is based on *what the woman wants and needs to know*. The nurse who has a preset plan will find the door closed firmly and the nurse-client relationship damaged.

Nurses who take their cues from the woman and attend to each need as it arises will find that by the end of the prenatal or postpartum period, for example, the necessary content will have been addressed, and the nurse will have discovered the excitement, challenge, and professional and personal satisfaction of home care.

A variety of prevention programs are also offered within the *community*. These programs provide a wide range of services, such as parent training classes, child care classes, telephone hot lines, career counseling, and many more.

Cure and Rehabilitation. Advances in technology and the availability of fewer family members for care within the home have traditionally caused activities related to cure and rehabilitation to occur primarily in the hospital setting.

Changing economic trends, however, have resulted in the early hospital discharge of clients who still require skilled nursing care (Arbeiter, 1984). One study demonstrated that early discharge can result in not only a savings in terms of money but also in terms of a beneficial effect on the client and family. This study proved that early discharge of very-low-birth-weight infants, with follow-up care in the home by a nurse specialist, is safe and cost effective (Brooten et al., 1986) (Chapter 37).

Government Resources. In 1935 Congress passed a broad Maternal and Child Health program under Title V of the Social Security Act. The program consisted of three proposals: (1) aid to dependent children, (2) maternal and child health services, including Crippled Children's Services (CCS) (now the Special Child Health Services), and (3) child welfare services. The first programs provided by Title V were prenatal and postnatal clinics, child health clinics, and training of professional personnel.

Since 1935 numerous other federal programs have been developed (U.S. House, 1984). Some of those that have had a major impact on maternal and child health include:

1. **Medicaid.** In 1965 Medicaid was created under Title XIX of the Social Security Act to reduce financial barriers to health care for the poor. It is the largest maternal-child health program. A major project under Medicaid is the Child Health Assessment Program (CHAP), which provides services for a large number of pregnant women and children.
2. **MCH Services Block Grant.** The Maternal and Child Health Services Block Grant provides health services to mothers and children, particularly those with low income or limited access to health services. Its primary purposes are to reduce infant mortality, reduce the incidence of preventable disease and handicapping conditions among children, and increase the availability of prenatal, delivery, and postpartum care to eligible mothers.
3. **Social Services Block Grant.** Established under Title XX of the Social Security Act, this block grant provides states with funds for child daycare, protective and emergency services, counseling, family planning, home-based services, information and referral, and adoption and foster care services.
4. **WIC.** In 1966 the Special Supplemental Food Program for Women, Infants, and Children (WIC) was passed. It provides nutritious food and nutrition education to low-income, pregnant, postpartum, and lactating women and to infants and children up to age 5. One nutrition program is the Food Stamp Program established in 1964. Food stamps are issued to people within a specified income for food purchase.
5. **Alcohol, Drug Abuse, and Mental Health Block Grant.** Established by the Omnibus Budget Reconciliation Act of 1981, the block grant provides funds to states for (1) projects to support prevention, treatment, and rehabilitation related to substance abuse and (2) grants to community mental health centers for the identification, assessment, and treatment of severely mentally disturbed children and adolescents.

THE NURSING PROCESS

The nursing process is usually described in five separate stages: assessment, diagnosis, planning, implementation, and evaluation (Fig. 2-1). Each stage has phases within it. The rate of progression through the phases depends on the nature of the health problem, the setting, the available resources, and the nurse's level of knowledge and skill.

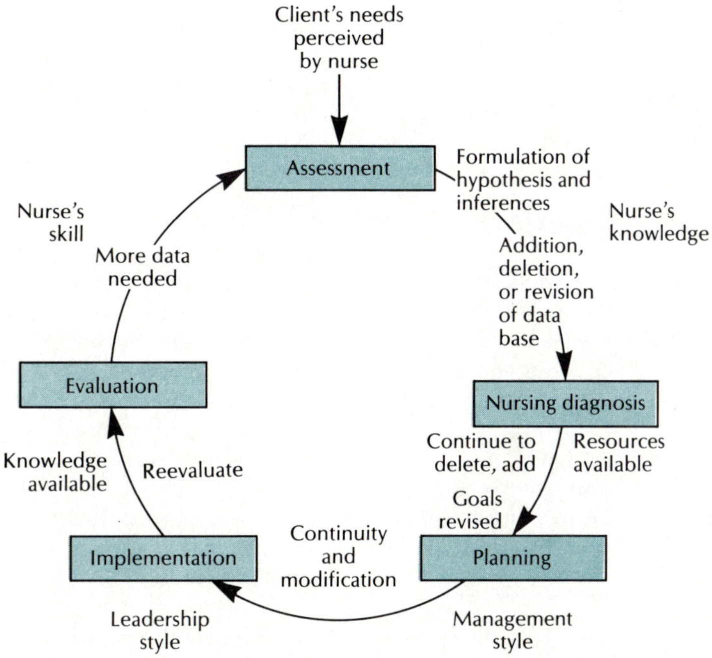

Fig. 2-1 Five stages of the nursing process.

Assessment

Assessment begins when the nurse is alerted to a client's need. The stimulus itself forms part of the data base. It may be the way the client walks into the clinic, the client's opening comment, a change in color, a raised temperature, or increased activity. The assessment stage involves at least two phases: data collection and formulation of inferences or hypotheses from the data.

Once alerted, the nurse attends to the client and begins the essential first phase in the assessment stage, the collection of sufficient accurate data to formulate a nursing diagnosis. Data is collected through interview, physical examination, and from laboratory tests. Sources of data collection include the client, her family and friends (if this is acceptable to the client or when the client is unable to provide essential information), and health care records.

An inference is a nurse's interpretation of the data collected. Inferences are subjective. The nurse's knowledge, skill, experience, values, and beliefs influence the formulation of inferences. See the discussion on models of helping and coping, values clarification, and cultural aspects of care for examples of factors that may influence the nurse's subjective judgments.

Nursing Diagnosis

A nursing diagnosis is a summary statement of the analyzed data (Kim et al., 1987; Gordon, 1982; Newman, 1984; Fadden, 1984; Tartaglia, 1985). The nursing diagnosis is a two-part statement (Carpenito, 1987). The first part consists of the diagnostic title, for example, parenting, alterations in, or coping, ineffective individual. The second part specifies the related etiologic or contributing factors. Following are two examples of nursing diagnoses: parenting, alterations in, related to breast-feeding difficulties; and, coping, ineffective individual, related to knowledge deficit about parenting.

Nursing diagnoses are sometimes organized within the Functional Health Framework developed by Gordon (1982).* The framework provides a means for organizing nursing assessment and standardizing data collection. The list of nursing diagnoses are grouped under functional health patterns in Table 2-2.

Controversy has arisen as a result of the difficulty in capturing all the possible human responses (Porter, 1986; Stainton, 1987) and expressing them in ways that have standardized meaning. There has also been a recognized need for nursing to diagnose wellness (Dvespohl, 1986; Houldin et al., 1987).

The nursing diagnosis statement indicates the nature and extent of the client's health problem. The second part of the statement gives direction to the nursing interventions and falls within the boundaries of nursing practice as stated in the nurse practice act. The diagnosis must also meet the standards of practice as set forth by the professional association.

The accuracy of the diagnosis depends on the *comprehensiveness of the data.* Three phases in processing the data are required to achieve accurate and meaningful nursing diagnoses: analysis, synthesis, and validation. *Analysis* is concerned with establishing categories of concerns or needs. *Synthesis* of the data is concerned with looking for relationships and patterns (Benner and Tanner, 1987). *Validation* can be done in three ways: (1) with the client, for relevance and completeness, (2) with others on the nursing team, so the diagnosis fits the data available, and (3) with a member or members of the client's interpersonal system.

Once the nursing diagnoses are established, the nurse takes time to explore the personal value judgments about the family that may affect and impede nursing interventions. The nursing diagnosis is crucial because it guides the selection and implementation of effective nursing interventions (Tartaglia, 1985).

Planning

Each diagnosis guides the nurse to select nursing actions. It is important to ask the client and family members how the client has coped with similar health problems or situations in the past. The client's self-care patterns should be incorporated into the nursing care plan as much as possible. Three essential phases in planning are (1) setting the goals in client-centered terms, (2) prioritizing the goals, and (3) selecting nursing actions that will help the client meet the goals.

Setting the Goals. Determination of the goal or goals is done with the client if possible. On some occasions this is not possible; for example, if the client is a newborn, unconscious, or too ill. In some cases the nurse assumes responsibility for clarifying the objectives of care with family members or through peer review in health care conferences. At times the nursing care plan is developed in conjunction with other health team members' plans so that the client's care is designed in a coordinated fashion. Attention is given to such factors as the client's time commitment, fatiguing factors, and child care considerations. Clients whose life-style and other responsibilities are considered in planning will be more likely to participate actively in their own health care plan.

Prioritizing the Goals. Prioritizing the goals is done on the basis of the immediacy of the problem (its life-threatening components) or the client's and nurse's preference. The nurse's preference is determined by the resources available, commitments to other clients, and the need for further data or plans of other health team members.

Once the goal is established, criteria used to measure (evaluate) progress toward the goal are selected. These outcome criteria are stated as objectively, specifically, and realistically as possible so they can be used both to direct nursing actions and as *outcome criteria.* For example, "Between 8 AM and 4 PM the client will drink between 800 and 1000 ml of fluids." This objective considers the client's wak-

*Further information is available from the North American Nursing Diagnosis Association (NANDA) Clearing House, School of Nursing, St Louis University, 3525 Caroline Ave, St Louis, MO, 63104.

Table 2-2 *Functional Health Patterns* and Related Nursing Diagnoses*

Functional Health Pattern	Nursing Diagnoses
Health perception–health management	Altered growth and development Altered health maintenance Noncompliance Potential for infection Potential for injury Health seeking behaviors
Nutritional-metabolic	Altered growth and development Fluid volume deficit Fluid volume excess Hyperthermia Hypothermia Altered nutrition: less than body requirements Altered nutrition: more than body requirements Altered oral mucous membrane Impaired skin integrity Impaired swallowing Impaired tissue integrity Ineffective thermoregulation Potential altered body temperature Potential for aspiration Ineffective breast-feeding
Elimination	Constipation Diarrhea Bowel incontinence Colonic constipation Perceived constipation Altered growth and development Functional incontinence Reflex incontinence Stress incontinence Total incontinence Urge incontinence Altered patterns of urinary elimination Urinary retention
Activity-exercise	Activity intolerance Ineffective airway clearance Ineffective breathing pattern Decreased cardiac output Diversional activity deficit Impaired gas exchange Altered growth and development Impaired home maintenance management Impaired physical mobility Feeding self care deficit Bathing/hygiene self care deficit Dressing/grooming self care deficit Toileting self care deficit Altered (specify type) tissue perfusion (cerebral, cardiopulmonary, renal, gastrointestinal, peripheral) Dysreflexia Fatigue Potential for disuse syndrome
Sleep-rest	Altered growth and development Sleep pattern disturbance
Cognitive-perceptual	Pain Chronic pain Altered growth and development Knowledge deficit (specify) Unilateral neglect Sensory/perceptual alterations (specify) (visual, auditory, kinesthetic, gustatory, tactile, olfactory) Altered thought processes Decisional conflict (specify)
Self-perception–self-concept	Anxiety Fear Altered growth and development Hopelessness Powerlessness Body image disturbance Personal identity disturbance Self-esteem disturbance Chronic low self-esteem Situational low self-esteem
Role-relationship	Impaired verbal communication Altered family processes Anticipatory grieving Dysfunctional grieving Altered growth and development Altered parenting Parental role conflict Impaired social interaction Social isolation Potential for violence: self-directed or directed at others
Sexuality-reproductive	Altered growth and development Rape trauma syndrome Sexual dysfunction Altered sexuality patterns
Coping–stress tolerance	Impaired adjustment Ineffective family coping: compromised Ineffective family coping: disabling Ineffective individual coping Altered growth and development Post-trauma response Defensive coping Ineffective denial
Value-belief	Altered growth and development Spiritual distress (distress of the human spirit)

*The functional health patterns were identified by M. Gordon in *Nursing Diagnosis: Process and Application* (New York, McGraw-Hill, 1982), with some minor changes by the authors. This nursing diagnosis list reflects the authors' adoption of the North American Nursing Diagnosis Association (NANDA) approved list from the Eighth National Conference (1988). The authors have deleted the listing of actual and potential next to a diagnostic category, since most diagnoses can be utilized as an actual or potential label.

ing time and provides for less intake of fluids after 4 PM to reduce possible interference with sleep from increased elimination.

Selecting Nursing Actions. Nursing actions that will help the client meet the goals may be developed by the nurse from a repertoire of known nursing interventions, from the literature, and by consulting with other nurses and the client. As the nurse's personal knowledge increases, an expanding repertoire of nursing skills enables her or him to make choices that finely tune the nursing actions to the client's needs and preferences.

Implementation

Nursing actions are selected on the basis of anticipated effectiveness; the goals and outcome criteria desired by client and nurse; the amount of risk involved for the client; the availability of resources, facilities, and personnel; and the client's ability to comply with the proposed care (Glass, 1983). The implementation phase includes referral to other team members. The coordination of care given by the various members is also an important consideration during this phase.

The overall management of the health care setting is an essential, indeed critical, aspect of the implementation phase. *Each nurse contributes to the setting by supporting colleagues through review of nursing care plans, willing consultation and assistance in client care, and appropriate praise.*

Evaluation

Evaluation is a joint process between nurse and family (Bloch, 1975). This phase involves assessing the client's progress toward or attainment of the goals using outcome criteria (Barba et al., 1978). The outcome of the evaluation phase determines the need for revision of goals, additional assessment data, or modification of nursing actions (Fig. 2-1).

INTERPERSONAL COMMUNICATION

The nurse's interpersonal skills and ability to communicate are basic to the application of the nursing process. With practice the nurse can develop a repertoire of communication techniques that facilitate the interchange. Contributing to the nurse's success as a communicator is the ability to establish a trusting relationship, empathize with the client, and develop mutually acceptable goals and therapy for care.

Trust

When individuals trust each other they feel secure. Travelbee (1971) has defined trust as "the assured belief that other individuals are capable of assisting in times of distress and will probably do so."

Certain descriptive terms occur again and again when people are asked to describe someone they would trust. These include *consistent, reliable, genuine, sincerely interested,* and *accepting.* Nurses can give care without trusting or being trusted; however, the level of care tends to be more mechanical because the focus is limited to physical aspects.

Empathy

Empathy, the ability "to sense the client's private world *as if* it were your own but without losing the *'as if'* quality" (Rodgers, 1961), is an important component of the intrapersonal process. An empathetic individual is sensitive to another's thoughts and feelings. Care is taken to communicate this awareness while retaining one's own identity. Sympathy differs from empathy. Sympathy includes a feeling *for* another person—"I feel sorry for her." Empathy implies getting *inside* another person, feeling what that person is feeling—"I sensed in her (the client) an awful loneliness." The ability "to walk in another's shoes" describes the important aspect of empathy.

The uniqueness of each individual precludes our complete understanding of another. Yet the potential for understanding grows with life experiences and with increased self-awareness. Self-awareness does not come easily; however, it is basic to becoming skilled in establishing meaningful relationships with clients.

Self-awareness. "Why did I say that?" and "Why did I do that?" are questions that all of us ask ourselves. Part of the answer to such questions lies in becoming aware of the effect values have on actions. Values as defined by Uustal (1978) are "general guides to behavior, standards of conduct that one endorses and tries to live up to or maintain."

Personal values arise as individuals concern themselves with establishing self-identity and attaining chosen life roles within their society and culture. Nurses hold values that are both personal and professional. The professional values are derived as the individual becomes part of a professional group and subscribes to and supports the standards of the group (e.g., American Nurses' Association nursing standards, Chapter 4). The more the values are in agreement, the fewer the possibilities of value conflict. However, to expect perfect harmony between sets of values is unrealistic. Each nurse needs to recognize value conflict when it occurs and know how to go about resolving it.

We are aware of some of the values that guide our behaviors. Nurses openly support efforts to include the family in nursing care because they believe the family acts as an important support system. On the other hand, some values that affect actions are not consciously held. Persons often behave in certain ways "because that is the way it should be." Many of the values that influence actions stem from concepts of *social roles* and of *the self.* A brief review of these two concepts precedes the discussion of the process of values and clarification.

Social Role. Social roles may be defined as socially prescribed patterns for behavior. Persons who share common attitudes and beliefs and assume responsibilities for certain tasks are performing a social role. These roles are learned in the process of social interaction, which begins at birth and continues throughout life. Individuals' concepts of a role (role expectations) govern how they expect others to act and how they expect to act. Every society sets up cultural norms for essential roles that serve as models for individuals to emulate in developing their personalized versions.

VALUE SYSTEMS

Every aspect of our lives conveys information about ourselves to others. The onlooker interprets and makes value judments about such things as the way people dress, where they were born, their accents, or their church affiliations. Each culture sets up behavior and speech patterns appropriate to different situations. These are known as normative patterns. Knowledge of these patterns is acquired by members of that culture as a result of mingling with various social groups and informally learning these patterns. The failure on the part of a stranger to that culture to recognize these communication patterns and operate within their context can lead to misunderstandings and the inability to carry on meaningful exchanges.

Once a person is committed to the idea of a role, it is incorporated into the self, and *values* are assigned to it. The value nurses place on certain aspects of their role can prove of great benefit to a client. The following situation as reported by a student is an example.

One of the infants in the nursery developed suspicious facial lesions. The mother had a history of herpes simplex II infection. The baby roomed-in with the mother. All infants in the nursery were considered as potentially infected and were isolated in the "B" room. The incoming babies were admitted to "A" room. I realized maintaining medical asepsis was vital to the babies' well-being and knew the problem would be enforcement. During report I noticed two doctors coming from "B" room and going in "A" room without changing gowns or scrubbing. I took it on myself to confront this "traffic" and afterward set up a routine for everyone to follow. I found it nerve-racking to stop doctors but realized the implications for the babies.

The student accepted the responsibility of acting as an advocate for her clients because she felt strongly (valued) that being an advocate was an important component of the nursing role. As a result her clients were protected from harm. As individuals come to value their concepts of social roles (role expectations) they may resist attempts to change the roles. Only minor modifications in attitudes, beliefs, and responsibilities are permitted. The role becomes traditional or stereotyped.

The traditional role of mother falls into the stereotyped category. In the traditional role the mother is expected to behave in a motherly fashion, that is, willingly give children love, attention, and physical care, even though she is simultaneously acting as career woman, lover, or wife. A nurse who expects a woman to function in the traditional role of mother can be upset if the client does not live up to the nurse's expectations. As a result the nurse may consciously or unconsciously withold supportive care, for example, be abrupt in contacts, avoid touching the client, or teach the client as little as possible. The following incident is illustrative of this.

Laura, a new mother, was a senior partner in a law firm. She announced she would be returning to work immediately and had hired a nurse to care for the baby. She did not appear for the informal discussion on baby care. When her nurse was questioned as to why Laura had not come, the nurse replied, "I did not tell her about it. I figured she's not interested. She's not going to be looking after the baby."

In this instance the nurse assumed the mother was not interested in her new baby because the mother did not conform to sterotyped mother-role behavior. The nurse's value judgment about the behavior prevented the nurse from functioning adequately in her role as a nurse.

The concept of a life role, with its various responsibilities and relationships, is not static. Change is inevitable as new life situations occur. If the initial adaptation to change results in a satisfactory outcome, subsequent alteration in role structure comes with less stress. Individuals can trust their ability to adjust, modify, or enlarge role commitments. The foundation for growth in the role is thereby established. The nurse is in a unique position to help women and men adapt to a new role through teaching. As people become proficient in the role, a favorable *self-concept* ensues.

Self-concept. The idea of the *self* develops slowly and has physical and social dimensions. Infants begin the process of awareness of their physical attributes and potential by defining the physical boundaries of themselves as they manipulate their bodies. The child and adult continue the process as they learn how to use their bodies effectively in health or after illness or surgery. The social concept of self develops through the assumption of social roles. Role taking continues through life. Two important components of self-concept are body image and self-esteem.

A subjective picture of one's physical appearance derived from one's own observations and by noting the response of others is known as *body image.* It represents the "sum of the conscious and unconscious attitudes the individual has toward his body. It includes present and past perceptions, as well as feelings about size, function, appearance, and potential" (Stuart and Sundeen, 1987). This picture is constantly changing as new perceptions and experiences occur. Adolescents become particularly conscious of their physical bodies as the body undergoes rapid change. Value judgments made about physical size, hair styles, and skin can be a source of pleasure or pain to the young person. The pregnant woman's body also reflects rapid change, and for some women this change can be disturbing.

The liking and disliking of the self is called *self-esteem.* Self-esteem develops as people attempt to master social roles (Satir, 1967). If individuals play out social roles well, they are applauded (rewarded) by people important to them (significant others) and as a result develop *high self-esteem.* If their efforts are not considered successful, the significant others may ignore them, criticize them, or blame them. As a result of these responses the person develops *low self-esteem.* Sullivan (1963) called this process "learning about the self from the mirror of other people." How individuals view themselves (self-esteem) conditions their responses to their world. Some people feel masterful; others are afraid. Some develop methods of coping with crisis, others "go to pieces" if their daily routines are interrupted. Some become part of a social group that acts as a support system, others remain alone. Clients often turn to nurses to help them develop the behaviors, attitudes, and responsibilities that are part of crucial life experiences such as parenthood or menopause.

Values Clarification

Values clarification is the process of identifying one's own values and beliefs. Once identified and recognized, the nurse can explore the ways values and beliefs can affect each phase of the nursing process. Hawley and Hawley (1975) noted that decisions were based largely on the values held by the decision maker. Decision making is a key component in the nursing process. Therefore nurses need to become aware of values, either their own or their clients, that can add to or detract from their efforts to make decisions congruent with therapeutic goals.

Uustal (1978) adapted the process of values clarification for nursing. Three major activities are involved in the process. They include choosing, prizing, and acting.

Choosing: Making choices about our values after consideration of alternatives.

EXAMPLE: I've thought and thought about going back to school just now, and I've come to the conclusion that I need to be with the kids at their ages. I have to put first things first. I talked it over with John, and he agrees. I can always go back to school later. After all, the kids will only be young once.

Prizing: Assigning a "value" to values, arranging our values in rank order, and acknowledging them publicly when appropriate.

EXAMPLE: Some principles I feel very strongly about, others I can adjust to circumstances. I try to let others know how I feel about certain things so they are forewarned about how I'll react if they try to make me change.

Acting: Behaving in a manner that is consistent with the individual's values. Through repetitious actions, a pattern of behavior can be discerned.

EXAMPLE: I could have said nothing about giving Mrs. Smith the Tylenol instead of aspirin. They are both stock drugs so they wouldn't be missed and physically they wouldn't hurt her. But I felt I had to be honest and report the error or I couldn't stand myself. In some things such as medications, even small differences could have adverse effects. I feel better that I acted according to my beliefs.

In the three examples cited above the individuals were making decisions and acting on the basis of professed values. Values clarification is part of everyday living. However, it can be used in a formal sense to assist in recognizing the effect values have on action. The following example illustrates how a student used the values clarification process after a conflict in nurse-client values prevented her from providing therapeutic care.

Before beginning Karen's care, I reviewed her record and found the following history. She was 20 years old and unmarried. She had had an abortion at 16 and again at 17. She had a baby at 19 and kept the baby. She was going to keep the baby from this pregnancy also. My reaction was one of shock. I felt resentment toward her and felt uncomfortable knowing I would have to interact with her. I remembered all I'd read and learned about single mothers and decided to accept this challenge. I did not want to let my feelings get in the way. My feelings stem from the fact that, as a result of a strict Catholic upbringing, I am fiercely against abortion. I consider it an act of murder. I was adopted. I am extremely sensitive to the fact that unwed girls are not giving their babies up for adoption, but rather bringing them home to an incomplete family.

After getting home I reflected on my behavior toward Karen. I failed in reaching my goal. I talked to Karen only when it was necessary. When I did talk to her, I kept it brief to be able to ignore her situation. I did not want to explore her home situation—if she had an adequate income or a significant other for emotional support, for fear of what I would learn. When I did ask her about future contraceptive plans, she said she had never used any and felt there was no need to. It tore me apart inside to think she may possibly bring more children into her insufficient family. In essence, I wanted as little to do with her as possible.

I now realize how much my personal views prevented me from performing therapeutic nursing care. I definitely want to work on this. I know it will be difficult to overcome my feelings.

In an effort to work through the value conflicts the student sorted the data as follows:

My Values	Client's Values as Assumed by the Nurse
Abortion is morally wrong	Abortion is an acceptable means of birth control
Family should consist of a wedded mother and father with children	Family without a father is all right
Methods of birth control (other than abortion) should be used if a person is sexually active to prevent children	Birth control other than abortion is not necessary

Table 2-3 *Example of Values Clarification Process Implemented by a Nursing Student*

Choosing Values	Prizing	Acting
Abortion morally wrong.	Part of my religious and moral beliefs.	Would request another client assignment and give reasons for my request. If client asked for information about abortions, would find client another resource person.
Sexually active adults need to assume responsible attitude toward possible pregnancy (through use of acceptable birth control, not abortion).	Part of my belief about being a responsible citizen.	Would include teaching and counseling about family planning in my care.
I feel every child should have a caring adult, social and economic support, and a place in society. A family should be formed through marriage and consist of a mother, father, and children.	I still feel the traditional family is the best. However, through reading and discussion, I can accept other family forms more readily.	I could work with single parents; I am going to act as volunteer this summer at "Center for Life," where counseling is given to pregnant women. The emphasis is on adoption, but community support systems for single parent families are explored if adoption alternative is not chosen.

As a result of the conflict in values, the nurse had the following responses:

1. Shock and disbelief but desire to give good care.
2. Inability to set up therapeutic nurse-client relationship:
   "I talked to Karen only when it was necessary. I wanted as little to do with her as possible."
3. Inadequate collection of data:
   "When I did talk to her, I kept it brief in order to be able to ignore her situation."
   "I did not want to explore her home situation if she had an adequate income or a significant other for emotional support—for fear of what I would learn."
   "When I did ask her about future contraceptive plans, she said she had never used any (abortion?) and felt there was no need to."
4. Feeling of guilt and anxiety over care given to client:
   "I now realize how much my personal views prevented me from performing therapeutic nursing care."
5. Desire to change approach to care:
   "I definitely want to work on this one. I know it will be difficult to overcome my feelings."

Once the data had been organized, the student used the values clarification process to help her with growth in the professional role. Table 2-3 illustrates how this student used values clarification to help her care for her clients more effectively in the future.

Language

The social or lay language of any culture contains elements that are known and recognized by all who speak it. Each subgroup in the culture, however, develops a language of its own. Subgroups may be determined by ethnic origin, age, or profession. The nurse learns a professional language as part of being initiated into the nursing group. For transactions between colleagues, a professional language facilitates precise, meaningful exchange of information.

Many clients are not familiar with medical terminology. Language that is not clear to both the sender and the receiver of communication will result in unmet goals. The nurse may have to translate or define terms unfamiliar to the client. Information must be given in familiar language with feedback for mutual understanding. Otherwise, much of what is said is either unclear or lost.

Language may also be used defensively. Nurses who maintain a joking relationship with clients regardless of the seriousness of the client's condition may be acting to defend themselves against the hurt and weight of involvement in the pain of others. Using language as a defense mechanism is often an unconscious act; the nurse is unaware of why she or he behaves in such a manner. According to Luft (1970), "The individual, like the group of which he is a part, has limited awareness of the sources of his own behavior and the effects of his behavior on others."

Communication Techniques

Certain communication techniques have proven successful as tools for strengthening therapeutic relationships. To become skilled in their use requires considerable practice. At first they may seem cumbersome or obvious. Gradually, however, they become part of the nurse's communication pattern and as such are useful in establishing the *meaning* of what one hears or says. Most of the techniques presented here are used together to elicit the information sought.

Listening. Listening is an active not a passive activity. It takes effort to hear what another says and to interpret and analyze its meaning. Nurses have to concentrate on the speaker, not on themselves, in an unbiased manner. A client may say something that triggers the listener's own values, reminding the nurse of personal concerns. Only practice will help the nurse cope with these interruptions to true listening. Listening is a sign of respect for another and acts as a powerful reinforcer.

Broad Opening Statements. Broad opening statements give the client an opportunity to select the topic for discussion. "What" questions can be helpful; for example, "What are you thinking about?" or "What were you able to do about . . . ?" "Why" questions tend to make a client defensive; for example, "Why did you miss last week's appointment?" This question might be more appropriately worded "I noticed you were not here for your appointment last week."

Closed questions that can be answered "yes" or "no" are to be avoided if the nurse is trying to find out what something means to a client. If the nurse is trying to discover how the client feels about not having a support person, a question such as "It must be hard to be on your own just now; how are you managing?" would be more effective. The nurse needs to be sensitive to a client's reluctance to discuss certain ideals or feelings and respect the need for privacy. The nurse can return to the topic when the bond between nurse and client is stronger.

Focusing. Focusing assists the client in identifying and expanding an area of importance. The nurse can encourage the client to describe how she perceives an event. The client might be asked to compare a present response with a similar past experience. The nurse can bring the primary problem into focus by developing a time frame for a sequence of events. The following example illustrates this technique:

Patricia, aged 14 years, came to the nurse in the clinic because she thought she was pregnant. During the interview with the nurse, Patricia gave a rambling report about how she loved her boyfriend, about her parents' angry divorce, and how they blamed everything on her. The nurse said, "Let me see if I can get the time frame worked out. Your parents got a divorce, and you feel they blame you. You have a loving boyfriend, you had intercourse, and now you feel you are pregnant. Let's talk about the possibility of your being pregnant first, and then we will go back to the others."

The nurse focused attention on the primary problem through identifying and analyzing the client's concerns.

Clarification. Clarification occurs when the nurse attempts to elicit the *meaning* of what the client is saying. Often the client will find it difficult to express emotional responses in other than a hesitant or fragmentary manner. The nurse needs to help the client clarify feelings as a first step in the client's recognition of the correlation between thought and action. Statements such as "Did you mean . . . ?" or "I can't quite follow you. Are you saying . . . ?" are helpful.

Restating. Restating is the repetition of a client's main thought or concern. Restating can bring attention to a thought that may otherwise be treated as trivial. It indicates also that the nurse is listening attentively. The following example illustrates this technique:

Marie talked to the nurse about her concerns over taking care of the baby. She said she had no experience with children as she had been an only child. Her mother found the care of one child enough and had not had any more. Marie said she was like her mother in so many ways, people often thought they were sisters. She wanted the home care nurse to come and check on how she was doing.

The nurse commented, "You said you were like your mother [restating]. Did you mean like your mother in finding the care of a baby difficult [clarification]?"

Validation. Validation of what is said and its meaning to the client conveys the nurse's understanding of not just content but also the feelings the client has about the content. If the nurse can reflect this accurately, the client senses the nurse's empathy, interest, and respect.

EXAMPLE

Client: I hate having to wear maternity clothes. It makes it so obvious you are pregnant. People treat you so differently, as though you weren't attractive anymore, just a dowdy old housewife.

Nurse: It is hard to see one's figure change—hard to get used to—it can make a person feel quite different about herself [validation].

The information the nurse gains from interviews or discussions with clients forms an important part of the data used to plan nursing care. The professional nurse assumes responsibility for obtaining data that is pertinent and verifiable. The techniques discussed above help the nurse attain this end.

Space. Hall's study (1966) of man's use of space showed that middle-class North Americans use space between communicators in definite ways. There are distances used to connote varying interpersonal relationships. Voice range and tone, the topic discussed, and body language employed are specific for each range. Hall described four distances as follows: *intimate,* 3 to 18 inches; *personal,* 1½ to 4 feet; *social,* 4 to 12 feet; and *public* beyond 12 feet. Voice tones progress from a murmur to a loud voice; topics discussed change from top secret to information considered in the public domain; and body language changes from caresses, stroking, and eye contact to exaggerated gestures and change in body stance (Table 2-4).

Personal involvement and concern are conveyed by interactions carried on within the intimate distance. The nurse can act as a model for personal involvement by showing an apprehensive new father how to enfold his infant in his arms and hold the baby close. At other times the nurse wishes to convey only professional concern even

Table 2-4 *Examples of Communication and Common Violations*

Topic	Space	Tone of Voice	Touch and Eye Contact	Common Violations
Secret or sensitive information exchanged with client; comforting parents whose infant has a defect; emotional responses of parents as they hold and admire child and express their love for child or each other	Intimate (3-18 in) Message: I accept you; I want to help you; I love you	Low, soft murmur	Nurse establishes eye contact with client; sits close to client in *en face* position; touches client (e.g., puts arm around shoulder); parents stroke, caress, kiss infant or each other	Condition of infant reported while nurse is standing at foot of mother's bed; sensitive information given out in loud voice during report at change of shift; healthy infants separated from parents before intimacy can take place
Report of health status; coaching during labor; assisting with feeding an infant; explanations of care; reports to other staff	Personal (1½-4 ft) Message: concern, warmth, friendliness	Soft, clear, concise	Eye contact maintained; nurse leans toward client; client discusses care with family; touch is with relaxed hand, gentle sure movements	Hurried, abrupt movements; voice loud, can be overheard by other clients, scolding tone; touch jerky, with flat of hand, poking with fingertips, grasps too firmly
Small group teaching of health care topics; discussion with parents in shared accommodation	Social (4-12 ft) Message: I like you; let us share this time	Louder, more definite, more formal	May stand or sit; eye contact maintained while talking; body gestures expansive, more formalized	Mumbling explanations; talking to one of a group only; gestures too unrestrained, "comes on too strong"; shouts
Lecture topics; sanitation, health insurance	Public (over 12 ft) Message: I have information for you	Loud, clear; may be used dramatically	Gestures exaggerated to be seen (e.g., arms flung out); eye contact moves over whole audience	Use of models, charts, etc. that can be seen only by those in the front row; ignoring questions

though the activities take place in the intimate distance. The nurse can use various techniques to indicate the professional versus the personal nature of an activity. When performing a vaginal examination, for example, the nurse begins by giving the purpose of the procedure. She then assumes a definite body set: face becomes impassive and preoccupied, the touch firm but gentle and precise, and the eyes directed away from the client's eyes. By acting in this manner, the nurse changes the connotation from personal to professional. She thereby minimizes client embarrassment. In addition to enhancing the nurse-client relationship, the body set accomplishes another objective—it permits the nurse to concentrate thought processes on what is being palpated by eliminating distracting stimuli.

At times the nurse consciously or unconsciously prevents true communication with clients by using space inappropriately. The nurse pauses at a client's doorway and calls, "How are you?" The reply is usually noncommittal. An individual is unable to discuss personal matters in a public distance range and may feel frustrated at being placed in this unsuitable position.

Another example of the use of space is the procedure adopted in a physician's or midwife's office. Once an examination is completed, the woman is given time to dress and is then seated in a chair by the practitioner's desk. A pattern of personal distance is established. Personal matters may be discussed in a soft voice while maintaining eye contact. A feeling that the practitioner has a warm and friendly interest in the client, as well as a professional one, is conveyed.

Another aspect of space is the concept of territoriality. This has been called *personal space* (Sommers, 1959). It moves with the individual, with the body as its center. Violations of personal space arouse defensive responses, either covert or overt. Some of the difficulty experienced by those anxious to replace traditional hospital maternity units with family-centered ones relates to the concept of personal space. Nurses and physicians had to share or give up space that was formerly theirs. Fathers, gandparents and siblings now occupy it. Until new patterns of space assignments are accepted, rules are used to soften the impact (e.g., visiting hours).

A final aspect of space is the way it is utilized. In North America we arrange furniture in a room in definite ways (normative pattern). The outer areas of a room are traditionally used for sitting, leaving the center clear for activity.

The pattern is often found in clinic waiting rooms. From a psychologic point of view, grouping of chairs or even single chairs would better answer the client's need to group together or to be alone. If clients change the chair arrangement of their own accord, the personnel often becomes uneasy and make comments regarding the liberties some will take—the message against nonconformity has been communicated.

Time. Another element in nonverbal communication is time, its meaning and use. Many aspects of North American culture are related to time. Appointments are made at definite times. Although a little leeway is allowed, the person is expected to be on time and, conversely, does not expect to be kept waiting. To be kept waiting is interpreted as a slight, an indication that one is of an inferior status. This can be particularly enraging if individuals suspect that there may be reasons to assume others are downgrading their status. One might see such reactions in government-sponsored health clinics. If clients are required to wait, they may suspect that the staff is looking down on them.

Clients who do not keep appointments are assumed to be shiftless and unconcerned. One of us (M.J.) visited an Indian village on the west coast of British Columbia to carry out a previously planned immunization program. Only a few older residents were found there; the others had left because the salmon were running. No offense was intended—one project could wait; the other could not. Being guided by the timing of natural events rather than by hours, days, weeks, months, or any other division of time seems incomprehensible to many North Americans. Communication can break down on such provocation.

Touch. Touch is another important nonverbal component of communication. On a social level people use touch to convey various messages about liking or disliking another person. Most people respect a firm handshake but are angered by a crushing one. People may hug friends but are offended if strangers press against them in an elevator. Mothers who are observed caring for their firstborn begin by using a tentative fingertip touch. As they become more secure in their role, they use the whole hand to support or manipulate the infant.

In person-to-person contacts with clients, nurses can use touch therapeutically. Massaging the back of a client confined to bed relieves muscle fatigue and contributes to client comfort. Even though the nurse may not speak a client's language she can express concern by holding the client's hand or stroking her brow.

Nurses must be aware of the importance of touch as means of nonverbal communication. Failure to touch or the way in which one touches can convey distaste for another. Nurses may avoid touching people they dislike or touch them as little as possible. When giving them nursing care, the nurse holds her hand stiffly or uses abrasive pressure rather than a caress. The recipients readily interpret the message, "I am distasteful to this person; she does not wish to be near me." These messages can interfere with the therapy being given.

Voice. Tone or rate, rhythm, and intensity of the voice are critical elements in communicating with others. Parents croon to their infants, mothers and fathers talk in high-pitched voices when alerting a newborn, and a nurse repeats instructions in a calm, gentle tone. These uses of voice tone convey love and acceptance. Conversely, talking loudly, mumbling, or speaking rapidly or hesitantly convey negative messages. Sometimes nurses will unconsciously raise the tone of their voice when speaking to clients who do not speak English. Unfortunately, not only do they not help the client comprehend, but they appear angry as well as incomprehensible to the client. The following nurse's report illustrates this concept.

> As I was in the neighborhood, I called at the Tam's house to let them know of changes in times the community clinic would be available. Mr. Tam, who acted as interpreter for the family, was not at home. I attempted to give the information to Mrs. Tam, whose English was limited. I suddenly realized that Mrs. Tam had moved away from me. She kept repeating, "Mr. Tam talk." I noticed I was talking very loudly as well as slowly. Once I realized what I was doing, I felt foolish. I wrote a note to Mr. Tam, thanked Mrs. Tam, and left.

Eye Contact. The manner in which people use eye contact is another important facet of every culture's nonverbal communication patterns. Ethnic groups vary considerably in the way eye contact is initiated and maintained. Some ethnic groups expect eye contact on first being introduced to another person and feel it is to be maintained during an ensuing conversation. If eye contact is avoided, uneasiness develops. The avoidance may be interpreted in a number of ways; for example, "She's not telling me the truth" or "I'm not worth being looked at." Other ethnic groups may avert their eyes when introduced as a token of respect. For some people, looking at a new baby is avoided unless they are also able to touch the child. They believe that if the child is not touched while being looked at, misfortune may befall that child. This belief is termed the *evil eye*.

A more detailed discussion on how North Americans use eye contact in establishing parent-child relationships is given in Chapter 25. As nurses we need to clarify our concepts of eye contact and validate the concepts with members of differing ethnic groups.

MODELS OF HELPING AND COPING

Nurses' helping effectiveness is influenced by their orientation to models of helping and coping. Nurses and the public they serve function in light of their assumptions about who is to blame for a problem and who is responsible for solving it. Four models are possible when assigning responsibility for both the problem and its solution, as shown below (Cronenwett and Brickman, 1983):

		Client responsible for problem: YES	Client responsible for problem: NO
Client responsible for solution	YES	Moral	Compensatory
	NO	Enlightenment	Medical

Moral Model

In the moral model of helping and coping, clients are seen as responsible for both the creation of and the solution to their own problems. One underlying assumption is that basically life is just; therefore people deserve what happens to them. The moral model is used by the couple who make the choice of having their baby at home among their family and friends (Cronenwett, 1980). If a complication occurs, the couple may perceive themselves as inferior, inadequate, or incompetent. Impairment to self-concept and potential for alterations in family processes or parenting, feeling of powerlessness, and spiritual distress may result. The nurse who also operates within the moral model may see the couple as responsible and may respond to them in a punitive nontherapeutic manner.

Compensatory Model

In the compensatory model of helping and coping the client is not held responsible for the problem but is expected to solve it with the help of others (Cronenwett, 1983). Clients see themselves and are seen as deprived through failure of the environment to provide them with goods and services to which they are entitled. Clients must be assertive and may need training to help them deal more effectively with their environment (Redman, 1988).

Helpers mobilize resources that compensate for the deficiencies in the environment. With deficiencies removed the client's competence is increased. The International Childbirth Education Association (ICEA) was formed to mobilize resources and create an environment that helps clients experience childbirth in a manner best suited to their priorities (Cronenwett and Brickman, 1983). The strength of this model is that it allows people to direct their energies outward without berating themselves (Redman, 1988). Operating within this model, clients in labor are not as apt to suffer the alteration in self-concept or spiritual distress that can accompany unexpected problems or outcomes.

The weak point of this model is that people can see themselves as continually solving problems they do not create. They find themselves constantly striving to overcome barriers (such as protocols established by the hospital staff) and may become bitter toward those they consider the source of their problem or discomfiture.

Medical Model

Health care providers are generally most familiar with this model. The medical model extends to all situations in which people are thought to be subject to forces such as disease that were and will continue to be beyond their control (Redman, 1988). Clients are seen as beings in need of treatment from the experts. The experts also prescribe the therapy and define what is a successful outcome. Input from clients is often not requested or heard (Cronenwett and Brickman, 1983). The helper's needs, rather than those of the client, are central to this model (Cronenwett and Brickman, 1983). The power lies with the helper.

According to Cronenwett and Brickman (1983) the majority of disagreements over policies affecting childbearing families in recent years originated between clients who favor a compensatory model and health care providers who function within the medical model. For most families, pregnancy remains a normal process. Therefore unless the client prefers it, the medical model may be dysfunctional.

The strength of the medical over the compensatory model lies in the freedom it provides to clients to accept help for unexpected problems during the childbearing or parenting experience. This model does allow people to claim help without blame for weakness; its deficiency is that it fosters dependency (Brickman et al., 1982; Redman, 1988).

Enlightenment Model

The central emphasis of the enlightenment model is on enlightening participants to the true nature of their problem; since their impulses are out of control, they must submit to discipline by agents of the community. The solution can be maintained only so long as this relationship is maintained. These assumptions can be a basis for coping whenever people are unable to control what they experience as undesirable behavior on their part. Its deficiency is that it can lead to fanatic concern with certain problems and can reconstruct people's lives around the behaviors and relationships in the model. It puts tremendous power in the hands of agents who control what participants believe is their ability to cope with their lives (Brickman et al., 1982; Redman, 1988).

Examples of external authorities are such agencies as Overeaters or Alcoholics Anonymous. Early natural childbirth movements often operated within the enlightenment model. That is, it was thought that women would be tempted by the medicated experience the physicians offered, and they needed an external force to help them resist this temptation. The early movement for breast-feeding at any cost is another example. Some teachers developed a fanatic attachment to the system for its own sake, rather than for the ultimate goal of a healthy mother and baby (Ewy and Ewy, 1970; Cronenwett and Brickman, 1983). Nurses must remain vigilant to prevent the "natural" (nonmedicated) childbirth or the breast-feeding itself from becoming *the goal;* these goals are inappropriate if they induce tremendous guilt or give rise to anxiety. Insistence on an inappropriate goal can lead to potential for alterations in parenting or family processes, potential for powerlessness, spiritual distress, or ineffective individual or family coping.

Use of Models in the Real World*

Real-world settings often contain a mixture of assumptions that characterize these models. Several points can be made about these models:

1. Problems between helpers and recipients can arise

*From Redman, KB: The process of patient education, ed 6, St Louis, 1988, The CV Mosby Co.

when each is operating on a different model. Indeed, we may have the wrong models in place in a number of areas.
2. There are some data to support the hypothesis that models in which people are held responsible for solutions are more likely to increase their competence.
3. Brickman et al. (1982) indicate a preference for the compensatory model, noting that it is the only one that justifies the act of helping (since the recipient is not responsible for problems) but still leaves clients with an active sense of control over their lives (since they have to use the help to find a solution).
4. Many questions remain. Are some helping models better than others or only for some clients? Has there been historic evolution of dominant models applied to different populations? There is now an emergence of the compensatory model in childbearing situations, over the previously predominant medical model.

The compensatory model is probably most congruent with the approach advocated here—one with mutual participation by client and nurse in the application of the nursing process.

NURSE-CLIENT RELATIONSHIPS: THE PROCESS

The nurse, aware that personal values and beliefs affect performance, is in a key position to help clients make logical decisions concerning health matters.

The nurse-client relationship is a dynamic *process* that evolves sequentially through four phases: preparation, initiation, consolidation and growth, and termination. Each phase accomplishes certain tasks and builds on a previous phase or phases.

The interactions between the client and nurse may be described as ones in which one person has "the intent of promoting the growth, development, maturity, improved functioning, and improved coping with the life of the other" (Rodgers, 1961). The process of developing a relationship is the same regardless of the time frame (short or long term) in which it takes place.

Preparation Phase

Before the first meeting with a client the nurse gathers as much data as possible and plans the first interaction. For example, reviewing the prenatal record before admission for labor alerts the nurse to prenatal client problems and allows the nurse to personalize the routines of admission.

Initiation Phase

The first meeting of client and nurse tends to set the stage for future contacts. The nurse attempts to establish a climate of trust, open communication, mutual understanding, and acceptance. The provision of *privacy* for the interview or examination encourages client to retain a sense of control and dignity. Clients vary in the amount of privacy they deem essential. For some the gynecologic examination is embarrassing as well as frightening. Some may prefer female medical or nursing personnel rather than male.

One nurse reported that in a clinic in Texas the women and their families did not appear to want privacy during interviews. They would initiate conversations concerning their ailments in the waiting room. However, the bathrooms, originally designed with doors opening into the lobby, had to be moved down a hallway because no client would enter them in view of others.

It is probably better to err on the side of providing too much privacy. Then, based on cues from clients, an appropriate level of privacy can be provided.

The dialogue begins with an exchange of names. The client determines which name preference she prefers: Mrs., Ms., Miss, or given name. With some clients, using a given name tends to set them at ease, while others may view this practice as presumptuous.

Contract for Care. The nurse establishes a contract for care based on client participation and mutual goal setting. The contract is not a formal one in the legal sense. Through discussion of expectations of nurse and client, conflict can be minimized and the client's sense of security increased.

Mutual Goal Setting. Determining appropriate nursing care for a particular client is largely the responsibility of the nurse. The extent to which the client accepts the therapy and complies with the recommended health regimen is an essential element in the success of the process. Formerly there was a tendency for medical and nursing personnel to dictate the form of therapy and the client's participation (medical model). Today many clients expect to share in planning their care and to make informed choices concerning therapy (compensatory model).

Nurse and client review the goals for care to arrive at mutual goals. Then they discuss the client behavior needed to achieve those goals.

EXAMPLE

Goal: Maintain the client's hemoglobin and hematocrit within normal limits.

Client actions:

1. Select an adequate diet that reflects client's likes, dislikes, and availability of nutrients.
2. Eat prescribed diet daily.
3. Take iron supplements as directed.

During discussion innovative solutions to client difficulties are often determined. Involving clients in the nursing care process increases their awareness of their responsibility for health. During the process of therapy, nurse and client mutually make periodic evaluations. At times, because of work related pressures, it is easy to resume old patterns of relationships (i.e., the all-knowing nurse and the dependent client). A conscious effort has to be made to maintain a partnership.

Compliance with Care. Once mutual goals have been established, the nurse may use various techniques to prompt compliance with the care. The atmosphere in which care is provided can be instrumental in the success of the therapy. Making clinics and hospitals more homelike can have a beneficial effect. A relaxed atmosphere encourages voicing of client needs and exchange of ideas.

Another effective technique to encourage compliance

with care is to ensure client understanding of therapy. Barriers to understanding can arise in various ways. Cultural differences can preclude understanding. Language differences may necessitate an interpreter. High anxiety levels can make it impossible for the client to "take in" the meaning of prescribed treatment. The nurse needs to repeat the teaching or counseling as often as it is needed.

Noncompliance with care may have serious consequences. Much of maternity care is preventive in nature. Preventive care depends on maintaining the health of mother and fetus, the prompt detection of disease, and the institution of remedial measures. Collaboration between nurse and client is essential for success. Client and nurse share accountability for successful health care. Each needs to participate in a responsible way in decisions about care.

Confidentiality. Confidentiality is a legal right of clients (Chapter 4). If a client volunteers information that the nurse feels must be shared with other medical personnel, the nurse must make this clear to the client. In some instances a client may not wish her obstetric history reviewed openly with her husband. She may have had an infant out of wedlock or an elective abortion of which her husband is not aware. The knowledge is relevant to her obstetric or gynecologic care, but otherwise such information is treated confidentially. The client needs assurance that personal data will be recorded and stored for future use in such a way that it is not available to the general public. Confidentiality engenders trust between client and nurse and is therefore a key element in communication.

During the initiation phase the nurse and client lay the groundwork for an individualized plan of care. Development of that plan occurs during the next phase.

Consolidation and Growth Phase

Throughout the consolidation and growth phase the nurse and client clarify goals, plan care, and put the plans into action. It is a phase based on mutual trust, growing insight into the reasons behind behaviors, and a working together for the client's benefit. Two important aspects of this phase are the closeness between the nurse and client and client dependency.

Closeness. Caplan (1961) noted that nurses can be adept at bridging distances between themselves and the client. The ability to become close to the client is an advantage in their roles as counselors. Closeness is demonstrated in many ways.

Nurses, through their involvement with clients and family members, are able to develop trusting relationships and act as emotional supports. Because clients see nurses as less remote than physicians, they feel freer to speak openly with them about their feelings and to ask questions.

Nurses touch clients; they stand close to them and seek eye contact. Nurses often comfort clients by putting an arm around them, stroking their hair, holding their hands. Closeness in space engenders feelings of safety in a client, much as parental closeness engenders feelings of safety in a child.

Nurses are present with clients in times of stress and crisis. They participate in the birth process with families and are there when clients face grief or despair. Nurses are also present to share the joy of birth and recovery from illness. Families' memories of important events often include their feelings about their nurses' support and concern.

Client Dependency. A certain amount of client dependency may be observed during the consolidation and growth phase. As long as dependency does not interfere with the client's ability to participate in care, it serves to cement the relationship. It is as though the client were saying, "If I need you, I know you will be there." As the nurse establishes a "safe" environment, the client becomes free to express anxieties or doubts openly, confident she will be heard by an understanding person. Dependency acts as a basis for future independent action as the client develops a feeling of self-esteem and respect for her own judgment.

Most of the care given to clients takes place during the consolidation and growth phase of the interpersonal relationship. During this phase the care given includes the following:

- Discussion of ongoing client problems and identification of stressors
- Evaluation of methods used by the client and her family to cope with present or potential crises and suggestions of alternatives as necessary
- Exploration of family and community support systems and plans for assistance in the care of other children, as well as the new baby

Gradually both client and nurse reveal more of their true feelings and perceptions and share their concepts of the purposes of therapy and the responsibilities of client and professional worker. Part of the nurse's functions will relate to the process of evaluation of client progress and consequent restructuring of plans.

Termination Phase

The termination phase serves as a summary for all that has gone before. Nurse and client review the goals they have accomplished and plan for future health care. This phase of the nurse-client relationship leaves a final impression of the health care system with the client. A positive impression can affect the client's future health maintenance. Satisfied clients are more likely to return for health care that is preventive rather than just curative.

DECISION MAKING

Many of the individuals who seek nurses' help will be concerned about making major *decisions* that will affect their lives and those of others. Sexually mature adults make many decisions concerning their sexuality. If a couple decides to have intercourse, they must decide whether the woman is to become pregnant or not. If the woman becomes pregnant, the woman or couple must decide to abort the fetus, become a parent, or give up the child for adoption. To maintain health, sexually mature adults make decisions about living health-sustaining life-styles, attaining the use of health facilities, or engaging the supervision of health professionals.

The values, beliefs, and attitudes of the individuals are factors in the decision-making process. Some persons make decisions based on carefully gathered information and consideration of consequences. Others make decisions without thought for the future, based on ignorance, prejudice, or myth. Nurses may assist clients with decision making in a number of ways.

Collection of Data. Sufficient valid data is needed as a basis for problem solving. The nurse can provide advanced and technical information at a level appropriate for client understanding, when the client is ready to hear it. The clinical significance of the information as it relates to her particular situation is shared with the client. Clients are referred to other resources for specialized information when the nurse is unable to provide it (e.g., genetic counseling, social services).

Consideration of Alternative Actions. The nurse can review with the client the risks and consequences of each action and the responsibilities each choice involves. A number of alternatives is discussed with the client. For instance, choices related to infant feeding are introduced early if possible. The parents therefore have ample time to discuss the advantages and disadvantages of breast- and bottle-feeding for their infant and themselves.

Formulation of Outcome Criteria. The nurse and client can consider reasonable standards for the behavior of the client, newborn child, or family members. Rigid adherence to impossible self-expectations can be destructive to self-concept as the following vignette demonstrates:

Janice and Peter had attended prenatal classes and were planning a "natural birth" without analgesia or anesthesia. Everything progressed as planned until just before delivery. The fetal heart rate slowed to 90 (normal rate: 120 to 160). The physician decided to use outlet forceps to hasten the infant's birth. Anesthesia was used to numb the vagina and perineum; forceps were applied; and the infant was delivered. The cord was wrapped three times around the infant's neck and was considered the probable cause of the slowing of the heart rate. In spite of the fact that Janice could not have foreseen or controlled the event, she and Peter were depressed by her inability to deliver their infant as planned.

Nurses teaching prenatal or other classes need to discuss what can happen. Such interactions with the childbearing family can help eliminate unrealistic expectations. Role playing "what if . . ." can be used as an effective learning technique.

Problem Solving and Decision Making. The nurse can encourage participation in decisions affecting an individual's welfare. Participation prompts a feeling of control over one's destiny, and self-esteem is increased. Therefore when possible, the *locus* or place of decision making is with the client. Once the client assumes responsibility for a decision, accountability for the outcome rests with the client. If a decision is considered to be detrimental to the well-being of the mother or child, every effort is made to have the client modify the decision.

At 5 PM Mrs. Peters phoned the delivery room at the hospital and reported that her membranes had ruptured, her contractions were coming every 5 minutes and were regular, and that she had considerable bloody mucus discharge. The nurse replied, "You sound as though you are in active labor. Because this is your third baby, you need to come to the hospital right away." Mrs. Peters said she would wait until her other children had had their dinner. The nurse replied that she should come at once.

The mother persisted with preparing the children's dinner. At 6 PM her contractions became very strong. She delivered her baby at home at 6:15 PM.

In this instance the mother made the decision not to go to the hospital when instructed (the *locus* of decision making was with the client), and the outcome (home birth) rested with her. In some instances, because of knowledge and expertise, the professional caregiver assumes responsibility for decisions. The nursing care of critically ill infants illustrates the decision-making responsibilities of the nurse-clinician. The nurse must decide when the infant needs assistance with respiration or other therapy. The nurse assumes responsibility for decisions because the *locus* of decision making is with the caregiver.

TEACHING-LEARNING: THE NURSE AND THE FAMILY

Early English leaders in nursing in the middle and late nineteenth century saw the importance of teaching families about sanitation, cleanliness, and care of the sick. Since much of the care of the sick at that time was done by the family, nurses' efforts to teach represented a way of extending their services (Redman, 1988).

Statements by the National League of Nursing Education reflect the concern during this century with preparing nurses for their teaching tasks. The following comment shows such a concern as early as 1918:

> Another limitation of the ordinary training is that it deals only or mainly with disease, neglecting almost entirely the preventive and educational factors which are such an essential element in the many new branches of public health work, such as school and visiting nursing, infant welfare, industrial welfare, and hospital social service (National League of Nursing Education, 1918).

The 1937 curriculum guide commented. "The nurse is essentially a teacher and an agent of health in whatever field [the nurse] may be working" (National League of Nursing Education, 1937).

The centrality of client teaching varies with formal philosophies of nursing (Redman, 1988). Kreuter (1957) identified teaching of self-care and counseling on health matters as nursing operations needed to provide care. Sister Olivia (1948) saw teaching as one of the tools of the nurse with the objective of promoting spiritual, mental, and physical health. Henderson (1964), Lambertsen (1964), and Peplau (1952) characterized nursing as an educative process and an educative instrument. Peplau (1977) sees a shift in emphasis from traditional mother-surrogate activities to more educative-nurturing ones. Hall (1964) saw some of the tenets of teaching as central to her philosophy of nurse-client interaction. Travelbee (1971) indicated that both the client and the nurse learn as a result of the interactive process and that if changes do not occur in either or both of the participants, a relationship has not been established.

King (1981) says one of the three fundamental health needs of human beings is usable health information at a time they need and can use it. Johnson (1980) (Behavioral System Model for nursing) sees teaching as one way to help people find new or better ways of behaving, contributing to an enlargement of choices. Kinlein's description of her practice, based on Orem's theory (self-care concept of nursing), provides a view of a truly nursing focus for client education (1977a). Kinlein proposes a health care system in which people are the primary givers of care to themselves—by virtue of choosing the health professional the person thinks would be most helpful at the time. Nursing's skills and strengths are teaching and counseling (Waters and Arbeiter, 1985).

Nursing is helping people in self-care practices with regard to their state of health (Redman, 1988). Instead of a practice focused on support of medical goals, the nursing focus in practice involves the use of nursing knowledge to help achieve the client's health goals (Kinlein, 1977b; Redman, 1988). Indeed, the client's knowledge, skills, and problem-solving ability form a self-care asset worth developing in and of itself.

Both teaching and nursing involve a helping relationship that has development of independence in the subject as the main objective. Teaching is one nursing action that can help the client toward self-care, with both the nurse and the client assuming responsibility toward that goal (Redman 1988).

High Priority of Health Education

A number of factors have converged to bring health teaching into prominence (Redman, 1988):

1. A change in emphasis from treatment of disease to the maintenance of health.
2. Emphasis on self-care and the individual's values, preferences, and personal definition of health (Redman, 1988).
3. A trend toward holistic health care (Gordon, 1981). The emphasis in holistic health is on education and self-care rather than on treatment or dependence. In addition, holistic health incorporates the view that the setting where health care takes place is a place for education. The holistic health care movement is part of a broad movement to create humane, democratic alternatives to large, impersonal, unresponsive services and institutions (Redman, 1988).
4. The consumerist movement to narrow the competence gap between helper and help recipient (Haug and Lavin, 1981).
5. Diagnosis related groups (DRGs) (p. 18) and shortened hospital stays including same-day surgery.
6. A Patient's Bill of Rights, American-Hospital Association (1975). Of the 12 rights listed, 7 are explicit about having information needs met.
7. Principles of medical ethics, American Medical Association, House of Delegates, 1980. This new version includes the statement, "A physician shall make relevant information available to patients and the public."

General Goals of Teaching

The goal of health education is teaching people to live life in the healthiest way possible. It is possible to prevent, promote, maintain, or modify a number of health-related behaviors through teaching (Redman, 1988). Following are some goals for the client to achieve as a result of the teaching-learning process:

1. Participation in management of the problem, decision making, self-care, treatment, and follow-through.
2. Integration of the illness into her or his life experience.
3. Self-strengthening through strengthening role performance in childbearing and parenting.
4. Acquisition of correct information as a basis for decision making and assurance.
5. Education of society to gain support for health-related legislation and environmental controls.

The goals of learning have been classified into three domains: cognitive (understanding), affective (attitudes), and psychomotor (motor skills) (Redman, 1988; Bloom, 1956). Each of these domains responds best to a particular method of learning. Facts and concepts are taught by written materials, audiovisual aids, lectures, and discussions. Attitudes can be examined and perhaps changed if necessary by discussion that provides insight into affective behavior. Motor skills are best learned through a demonstration of the skills, with subsequent practice until they are perfected (Redman, 1988).

The Teaching Process

The teaching process uses the same steps as those of the nursing process (Fig. 2-2).

Assessment. Need to learn. The first step is to identify the client's need for teaching. An individual may request information or express a desire to learn a task. The re-

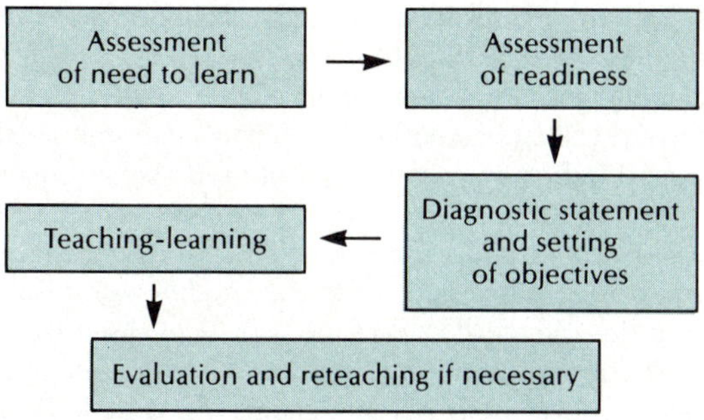

Fig. 2-2 The teaching process.
From Redman, BK: The process of patient education, ed 6, St Louis, 1988, The CV Mosby Co.

quested information may be about promoting health, preventing or treating a problem, or about a health facility and its services. Consumer groups, formed in response to needs perceived as unmet, define information to be shared with the public in general, as well as with involved clients. Health care providers recognize areas of learning commonly associated with various problems.

Readiness to learn. Learning requires *motivation*. People who are not convinced they need to learn will resist efforts to be taught. Several conditions affect motivation, one being the value systems that vary by cultural group and socioeconomic class (Redman, 1988). People vary in their *readiness* for health learning because of their intellectual capability, general educational background, and attitude toward responsibility (Redman, 1988; Loughrey, 1983; Taylor, 1984). According to Redman (1988), "There are two facets of readiness to learn: One is emotional readiness, or motivation, which determines the individual's willingness to put forth the effort necessary to learn. A second facet is experiential readiness, the individual's background of experiences, skills, and attitudes and his or her ability to learn that which is considered desirable" (Redman, 1988). A pattern of response receiving considerable attention is the theory of *learned helplessness* (Redman, 1988). Learned helplessness decreases motivation to learn. If the outcome is supposed to be independence, fear and inability to cope may be the unexpected result.

Some people feel that nothing they do can affect their environment or what happens to them. These people are described as having no *internal locus of control* or internal motivation.

Timing is another factor that affects a person's ability to learn. The person must feel an unmet need and yet be comfortable (physically and in that environment) and therefore able to learn (McHatton, 1985; Miller, 1985; Redman, 1988).

Diagnosis and Setting of Objectives. A nursing diagnosis can identify the existence of a knowledge deficit, for example, parenting, potential alterations in—related to knowledge deficit in physical care of the newborn. However, a well-stated learning objective is needed to specify exactly what a person is to learn. One such objective is "to give the baby a shampoo." The nurse validates the treatment with the parent. Subobjectives are present: (1) uses a safe method of holding the newborn, (2) protects the eyes from water and shampoo, (3) cleans the hair and scalp, (4) dries the hair, and (5) completes the shampoo without exposing the newborn to cold stress.

Planning and Implementation. Once the objective is known and validated, taking the woman's cultural or ethnic values and beliefs into consideration, the teaching method is chosen (Holden, 1985). The nurse plans teaching methods to cover all the domains. A discussion of giving a baby a shampoo identifies and helps the mother work through her attitudes (affective) about the activity. A discussion and demonstration presented at the woman's intellectual and educational level help her understand (cognitive). Giving the baby a shampoo with supervision helps the parent develop necessary motor skills (psychomotor). *The teaching is offered when the mother is comfortable and rested and has asked to learn the activity.* Most women tire easily in the early postpartum period, so the session should be limited by the woman's tolerance.

Evaluation. The nurse evaluates the effectiveness of teaching in several ways. For example, teaching is effective if:

1. The woman can shampoo the baby's hair, meeting each of the subobjectives.
2. The woman says she feels comfortable while giving the shampoo.
3. The woman says she understands related information.

If evaluation shows teaching was ineffective, the entire process is repeated beginning with assessment.

Teaching Tools

Teaching tools can be developed to help nurses present information. An example of a teaching tool to be used in this text is the guidelines for client teaching format found in the clinical chapters. The nurse changes the teaching tool as knowledge is built from interactions with clients.

SUMMARY

Nursing is a matrix of interwoven processes, competencies, and functions. Achieving excellence in becoming alert to meaningful cues and responding involves a comprehensive knowledge base and skillful use of the nursing process. Nurse-client responsibility is at the heart of providing nursing care. Although all human relationships have characteristics in common, the nurse-client relationship is initiated by the nurse for the benefit of the client. The nurse employs professional skills in communication and decision making to facilitate the process. The nurse's responsive dimensions, trust and empathetic understanding, are necessary ingredients of the nurse's role in therapeutic relationships. Awareness of client and nurse value systems contributes to acceptance of and progress toward mutually defined goals. Teaching is a central component of nursing care. Maternity and gynecologic nurses assume both traditional and new, expanded roles as they carry out the greater responsibilities such care engenders.

KEY CONCEPTS

- Although reproduction is almost entirely a function of human sexuality, each person involved may perceive its components—intercourse, pregnancy, birth, and parenthood—separately, and endow each with a special meaning.
- A lack of knowledge of normal anatomy and physiology and psychosocial effects can be just as disruptive as a serious disorder.
- Individuals have the capability to make decisions about their health and they ultimately have control of their own health by virtue of the choices they make.
- The degree to which maternity-gynecologic nurses fulfill nursing roles depends on their level of competence.
- Maternity-gynecologic nursing involves actions that

can be designated as preventive, curative, or rehabilitative.

- The nursing process involves both the client and the nurse in its five stages: assessment, diagnosis, planning, implementation, and evaluation.
- Nurses' helping effectiveness is influenced by their orientation to models of helping and coping.
- Self-awareness and values clarification are essential for nurses to provide holistic care to clients and their families.
- The nurse is essentially a teacher and an agent of health in whatever field the nurse may be working.

STUDY QUESTIONS AND ACTIVITIES

1. Assess your values and describe one incident in which you feel your value system prevented your delivery of therapeutic nursing care to a client. What can you do to increase your self-awareness?
2. After complete assessment of a client, develop a nursing care plan using the steps of the nursing process. In a group, compare and contrast individual care plans with emphasis on the rationale for interventions.
3. In a group, view a videotape of an interaction between a client and a nurse. Discuss observations of the essential factors of the nurse-client relationship. Identify the phase of the relationship.
4. Observe a teacher (prenatal instructor, group leader, nursing instructor) and identify the components of the teaching-learning process.
5. Go to a department store to buy an article of clothing. Note the many steps you take in making a choice. Compare with the decision-making process.

References

American College of Nurse-Midwives, American College of Obstetricians and Gynecologists, Nurses Association of the American College of Obstetricians and Gynecologists: Joint statement on maternity care, 1971. Statement superseded by joint statement on practice relationships between obstetrician/gynecologists and certified nurse-midwives, 1982

American College of Obstetricians and Gynecologists: Quality assurance in obstetrics and gynecology, Washington, DC, 1980, The College

American Hospital Association: A patient's bill of rights, Chicago, 1975, The Association

American Medical Association: Principles of medical ethics, Chicago, 1980, The Association

American Nurses Association: Nursing: a social policy statement, Kansas City, Mo, 1982, The Association

Arbeiter, JS: The big shift to home health nursing, RN 47:38, 1984

Archer, SE, and Goehner, PA: Nurses: a political force, Belmont, Calif, 1982, Wadsworth Publishing Co

Barba, M, et al: The evaluation of patient care through use of ANA's standards of nursing practice, Superv Nurse 9:42, 1978

Barnes, FEF: Ambulatory maternal health care and family planning services, Washington, DC, 1978, American Public Health Association

Beck, CT: The conceptualization of power, Adv Nurs Sci 4(2):1, 1982

Beebe, JE: NERCEN: a prototype of regional education efforts in nurse-midwifery (education exchange), JOGN Nurs 25(3):22, 1980

Benner, PE: Uncovering the knowledge embedded in clinical practice, Image 15(2):36, 1983

Benner, PE: From novice to expert: excellence and power in clinical nursing practice, Menlo Park, Calif, 1984, Addison-Wesley Publishing Co, Inc

Benner, PE, and Tanner, C: Clinical judgement: how expert nurses use intuition, Am J Nurs 87(1):23, 1987

Bloch, D: Evaluation of nursing care in terms of process and outcome: issues in research quality assurance, Nurs Res 24:256, 1975

Bloom, BS, editor: Taxonomy of educational objectives: the classification of educational goals. Handbook I: cognitive domain, New York, 1956, David McKay Co

Brickman, P, et al.: An attributional analysis of helping behavior. In Berkowitz, L, editor: Advances in experimental social psychology, vol 15, New York, 1982, Academic Press, Inc

Brook, C: Social, economic and biologic correlates of infant mortality in city neighborhoods, J Health Soc Behav 21(1): March 1980

Brooten, D, et al: A randomized clinical trial of early hospital discharge and home follow-up of very-low-birth-weight infants, N Engl J Med 315:934, 1986

Burst, H.: The American College of Nurse Midwives: a professional organization, J Nurse Midwife 25(1):Jan-Feb 1980

Caplan, G: An approach to community health, New York, 1961, Grune & Stratton, Inc

Carpenito, LJ: Nursing diagnosis: application to clinical practice, ed 2, Philadelphia, 1987, JB Lippincott Co

Carter, ER: Quality maternity care for the medically indigent, MCN 11(2):85, 1986

Cronenwett, LR: Elements and outcomes of a postpartum support group program, Res Nurs Health 3(3):33, 1980

Cronenwett, LR: Helping and nursing models, Nurs Res 32(6):342, 1983

Cronenwett, L, and Brickman, P: Models of helping and coping in childbirth, Nurs Res 32(2):84, 1983

Dvespohl, TA: Nursing diagnosis manual for the well and ill client, Philadelphia, 1986, WB Saunders Co

Edwards, M: Communications: dimensions in childbirth education, Pacific Grove, Calif, 1973, M Edwards

Etheredge, ML: Nurse-manager . . . try that title on for size, Nurs '85 15(8):26, 1985

Ewy, D, and Ewy, R: Preparation for childbirth: a Lamaze guide, New York, 1970, Signet

Fadden, TC, and Seiser, GK: Nursing diagnosis—a matter of form, Am J Nurs 84(4):470, 1984

Fogel, CI, and Woods, NF: Health care of women: a nursing perspective, St Louis, 1981, The CV Mosby Co

Glass, H: Interventions in nursing: goal- or task-oriented? Int Nurs Rev 30(2):53, 1983

Gordon, M: Historical perspective: The National Group for classification of nursing diagnoses. In Kim, MJ, and Moritz, DS, editors: Classification of nursing diagnoses, New York, 1981, McGraw Hill Book Co

Gordon, M: Nursing diagnosis: process and application, New York, 1982, McGraw-Hill Book Co

Haire, D: Improving the outcome of pregnancy through increased utilization of midwives, JOGN Nurs 26(11):5, 1981

Hall, LE: Nursing—what is it? Can Nurse 60:150, 1964

Hall, LE: Hidden dimensions, Garden City, NY, 1966, Doubleday Publishing Co

Haug, MR, and Lavin, B: Practitioner or patient—who's in charge? J Health Soc Behav 22:212, 1981
Hawley, RC, and Hawley, IL: Human values in the classroom: a handbook for teachers, New York, 1975, Hart Publishing Co
Henderson, V: The nature of nursing, Am J Nurs 64:62, 1964
Holden, JE: Don't just tell your patients—*teach* them, RN 48(7):29, 1985
Houldin, AD, Saltstein, SW, and Ganley, KM: Nursing diagnosis for wellness: supporting strengths, Philadelphia, 1987, JB Lippincott Co
Johnson, DE: The behavioral system model for nursing. In Riehl, J, and Roy, C, editors: Conceptual models for nursing practice, ed. 2, New York, 1980, Appleton-Century-Crofts
Kim, MJ, McFarland, GK, and McLane, AM: Pocket guide to nursing diagnosis, ed. 2 St Louis, 1987, The CV Mosby Co
King, IM: A theory for nursing: systems, concepts, process, New York, 1981, John Wiley & Sons Inc
Kinlein, ML: Independent nursing practice with clients, Philadelphia, 1977a, JB Lippincott Co
Kinlein ML: The self-care concept, Am J Nurs 77:598, 1977b
Kreuter, FR: What is good nursing care? Nurs Outlook 5:302, 1957
Lambertsen, EC: Nursing definition and philosophy precede nursing goal development, Mod Hosp 103:136, 1964
Loughrey, L: Dealing with an illiterate patient . . . you can't read him like a book, Nurs '83 13(1):65, 1983
Luft, J: Group processes: an introduction to group dynamics, ed 2, Palo Alto, Calif, 1970, National Press Books
McHatton, M: A theory of timely teaching, Am J Nurs 85(7):798, 1985
Miller, A: When is the time ripe for teaching? Am J Nurs 85(7):801, 1985
National Data Book and Guide to Sources: Statistical Abstract of U.S., 1987, ed 107, US Department of Commerce, Bureau of Census
National League of Nursing Education: Standard curriculum for schools of nursing, Baltimore, 1918, The Waverly Press, Inc
National League of Nursing Education: A curriculum guide for schools of nursing New York, 1937, The League
Newman, MA: Nursing diagnosis: looking at the whole, Am J Nurs 84(12):1496, 1984
North American Nursing Diagnosis Association (NANDA): Classification of nursing diagnoses: proceedings of the seventh conference, St Louis, 1987, The CV Mosby Co
Norton, SF, and Nichols, CW: Champions of choice, Am J Nurs 85(4):380, 1985
Nurses' Association of the American College of Obstetricians and Gynecologists: Certification's role in nursing (part 1), NAACOG Newsletter 9(3), May/June 1982
Nurses' Association of the American College of Obstetricians and Gynecologists: Standards for obstetric, gynecologic and neonatal nursing, The Nurses' Association of the American College of Obstetricians and Gynecologists, ed 2, 1981
Olivia, Sister M: Aims of nursing administration, Washington, D.C., 1947, The Catholic University of American Press. Cited by Brown, EL: Nursing for the future, New York, 1948, Russell Sage Foundation
Peplau, HE: Interpersonal relations in nursing, New York, 1952, GP Putnam's Sons
Peplau, HE: The changing view of nursing, Int Nurs Rev 24(2):43, 1977
Porter, EJ: Critical analysis of NANDA nursing diagnosis taxonomy. I. Image, J of Nurs Scholarship, 18:136, 1986
Redman, BK: The process of patient education, ed 6, St Louis, 1988, The CV Mosby Co
Rodgers, C: On becoming a person, Boston, 1961, Houghton & Mifflin Co
Rousch, R: The development of midwifery—male and female, yesterday and today, JOGN Nurs 24(3):27, 1979
San Francisco Chronicle, January 2, 1986.
Satir, V: Conjoint family therapy, Palo Alto, Calif, 1967, Science & Behavior Books
Sommers, R: Studies in personal space, Sociometry 20:247, 1959
Stainton, MC: Can we really get there from here? In Hannah, K, editor: Proceedings of clinical judgement and decision making: the future with nursing diagnosis, 1987
Stuart, GW, and Sundeen, SJ: Principles and practice of psychiatric nursing, ed 3, St Louis, 1987, The CV Mosby Co
Sullivan, HS: The interpersonal theory of psychiatry, New York, 1963, WW Norton & Co, Inc
Tartaglia, MJ: Nursing diagnosis: keystone of your care plan, Nurs '85 15(3):34, 1985
Taylor, JA: Are you missing what your patients can teach you? RN 47(6):63, 1984
Travelbee, J: Interpersonal aspects of nursing, ed 2, Philadelphia, 1971, FA Davis Co
US House of Representatives, Select Committee on Children, Youth, and Families: Federal programs affecting children, Washington, DC, 1984, US Government Printing Office
Uustal, DB: Values clarification in nursing application to practice, Am J Nurs 78:2058, Dec 1978
Waters, S, and Arbeiter, J: Nurse practitioners: how are they doing now? RN 48(10):38, 1985
Wilson, JB: Nurses and politics, Can Nurse 77:40, 1981
World Health Organization: Improvement in infant and perinatal mortality in the United States, 1965-1973, Washington, DC, 1976a, US Department of Health, Education and Welfare
World Health Organization: Technical report series no. 331, Geneva, 1976b, The Organization
World Health Organization: Population statistics, household and family characteristics, March 1977, Washington, DC, 1977, US Bureau of the Census, US Department of Commerce

Bibliography

Bentz, JM: Missed meanings in nurse/patient communication, MCN 5:55, 1980
Brody, DS: The patient's role in clinical decision-making, Ann Intern Med 93:718, 1980
Carpenito, LJ: Handbook of nursing diagnosis, New York, 1987, JB Lippincott Co
Field, L, and Winslow, EH: Moving to a nursing model, Am J Nurs 85:1098, 1985
Forsyth, DM: Looking good to communicate better with patients, Nurs '83 13:34, July, 1983
Foster, SD: Family and friends can enhance patient learning, MCN 13(2):91, 1988
Freebairn, J, and Gwinup, K: Ethics, values, and health, Irvine, Calif, 1980, Concept Media
Green, CP: Multiple role women: the real world of the mature RN learner, J Nurs Educ 26(7):266, 1987
Keleher, KC, and Mann, LI: Nurse-midwifery care in an academic health center, JOGN Nurs 15(5):369, 1986
Kim, MJ, et al: Pocket guide to nursing diagnoses, ed 2, St Louis, 1988, The CV Mosby Co
Lillesand, KM, et al: Nursing process evaluation: a quality assurance tool, Nurs Adm Q 7(3):9, 1983

Lutwak, RA, Ney, AM, and White, JE: Maternity nursing and Jewish law, MCN 13(1):44, 1988
McLane, AM: Classification of nursing diagnosis, St Louis, 1987, The CV Mosby Co
National Center for Health Statistics: Annual summary of births, deaths and marriages and divorces, Monthly Vital Statistics Report 31(13), 1985
Orr, I: Nursing audit, Senior Nurse 4:22, 1986
Putzier, DJ, and Padrick, KP: Nursing diagnosis: a component of nursing process and decision making, Top Clin Nurs 6:21, 1984
Rew, L: Nursing intuition: too powerful—and too valuable—to ignore, Nurs 87, 17(7):43, 1987
Rich, PL: With this flow sheet, less is more, Nurs '85 15(7):25, 1985.
Sandelowski, M: Women, health, and choice, Englewood Cliffs, NJ, 1981, Prentice-Hall
Smith, CE: Patient teaching: it's the law, Nurs 87, 17(7):67, 1987
Styles, MM: On nursing: toward a new endowment, St Louis, 1982, The CV Mosby Co
Tucker, SM, et al: Patient care standards: nursing process, diagnosis, and outcome, ed 4, St Louis, 1988, The CV Mosby Co
Wesley, HH, et al: A nursing minimum data set conference: executive summary, J Prof Nursing 4:217, 1986

CHAPTER

3

The Family, a Unit of Care

Learning Objectives

Correctly define the key terms listed.

Identify key factors in determining the quality of family health.

Explain the functions carried out by a family for the well-being of its members.

Distinguish the properties of family dynamics and the criteria for family decision making.

List three major family theories. Evaluate the components and implications for nursing of each theory.

Define and give examples of developmental and situational crises.

Identify factors that can alter one's perceptions of an event.

Differentiate between constructive and destructive coping mechanisms.

Relate the role of culture in the nursing care of individuals and families during the childbearing and child-rearing periods and for women with gynecologic problems.

Differentiate between a client care plan and a family care plan.

Key Terms

blended family
communal family
coping mechanisms
cultural context
developmental theories
extended family
family dynamics
family functions
family theories
homosexual family
interactional theories
maturational crisis
nuclear family
single-parent family
situational crisis
structural-functional theories
support systems

Every society sets up institutions to perform functions vital to its continuance. These institutions may be political, economic, social, or spiritual. Together they form the national social system.

One of the most important of these institutions is the family. The family represents a primary social group that influences and is influenced by other people and institutions. It is recognized as the fundamental social unit because most people have more continuous contact with this social group than with any other. The family assumes major responsibility for the introduction and socialization of persons. Despite the stresses and strains to which it now is subject, the family forms a social network that acts as a potent support system for its members.

FAMILY FRAMEWORKS

Families are defined in many ways. Definitions of the family involve delineation of family *structure, functions, composition,* and *affectional ties.* The United Nations (1969) describes the family as "those members of the household who are related, to a specific degree, through blood, adoption or marriage." Helvie (1981) defines the family as "a primary group of people living in a household in consistent proximity and intimate relationships." Because the concept of a family varies, the concept of *household* is sometimes substituted for that of the family. The term *household* is used to cover a number of family styles and refers to a group of people who share a common dwelling. Usually persons united by marriage, blood, or adoption form the core of the household; however, a household also may consist of a person or an unrelated group of people sharing the customary living arrangements of a family group. The concept of household encompasses not only traditional forms of family structure but also recently designated groups: (1) the never-married, (2) one parent and children living together as a one-parent family, (3) two homosexuals living together in a stable union, and (4) stable consensual unions, with or without children (WHO, 1978). Despite the difficulty of defining the family precisely, members of a family can readily describe its composition, who is kin and who is not, how the family has affected their lives, and what family style they believe in.

However the family is defined, the *family unit* is incomplete without an adult. From an adult's perspective the family can comprise persons of any age or sex bound by a blood or love relationship. From the child's perspective, the family is a set of relationships between the child's dependent self and one or more protective adults, as the following quotations indicate:

> "God and me, Mommie, Daddy, and J.R., Nana and Grandpa, Grandma and Grandpa, and Great Nana—people who love you and you have fun together." (Stacie, age 5)
>
> "A family is where everybody shares and cares for each other. A family is where there is love in the home. A family is where they go on vacations together. A family is where everybody shares with the work." (Robert, age 15)

Regardless of the form it assumes or the society in which it is found, the family possesses enduring characteristics that have far-reaching personal and societal effects. According to Blehar (1979):

> Despite disagreement about the state of the family and its definition, a consensus might be reached on three points: (1) the family is currently in a state of flux precipitated by economic and social pressures; (2) imperfect though it may be, it is difficult to imagine substituting an alternative that could perform all its functions as well; and (3) it is more desirable to bolster families than to attempt to supplant them with untried structures.

KEY FACTORS IN FAMILY HEALTH

Family-patterns, attitudes, and responses to change play a determining part in the health of individual members and their use of health services. Because the family acts as a primary force in generating support for clients, an understanding of this unit is essential to the formation of a nursing care plan.

Certain factors have proved important in determining the quality of family health. **Culture patterning** in areas such as childbearing, child rearing, or use of health services determines many health-related responses. **Family dynamics**, which encompass coordination of intrafamilial roles, distribution of power in the family, and the process of decision making, affects the use of health services. **Family responses to crisis**, including coping behaviors and the quality of personal responses and mutual concern, affect the level of support afforded family members. **Family socioeconomic characteristics** are important. Social class affects expectations, obligations, and rewards, all of which affect use of health services. In addition the family acts as the primary economic unit in which incomes may be pooled, expenditure decisions taken jointly, and services rendered internally.

FAMILY FUNCTIONS

As the family progresses through its life cycle, beginning with the commitment of two people to share a life and ending with the dissolution of the family through death or other separations, it carries out certain *functions* for the well-being of its members. The functions extend over five basic areas: biologic, economic, educational, psychologic, and sociocultural (WHO, 1978). The interdependent functions depend on the physical and mental health of family members. As a supportive structure for these functions, each family develops certain common *beliefs, values* and *sentiments* that are used as criteria in the choice of alternative actions.

Biologic Functions. Biologic functions include reproduction, care and rearing of children, nutrition, maintenance of health, and recreation. The ability to carry out such functions implies certain prerequisites: a healthy genetic inheritance, fertility management, care during the maternity cycle, good dietary behavior, intelligent use of health services, companionship, and nurturing of the elderly.

Economic Functions. Economic functions include earning enough money to carry out the other functions, determining the allocation of resources, and ensuring the financial security of family members. To accomplish these tasks the family must have the necessary skills, opportunities, and knowledge.

Educational Functions. Educational functions include the teaching of skills, attitudes, and knowledge relating to the other functions. To be able to do this, family members must have the necessary level of intelligence and the necessary knowledge, skills, and experience.

Psychologic Functions. The family is expected to provide an environment that promotes the natural development of personality, offers optimum psychologic protection, and promotes the ability to form relationships with people outside the family circle. These tasks require stable emotional health, common bonds of affection between individuals, and the ability to be mutually supportive, to tolerate stress, and to cope with crises.

Sociocultural Functions. Sociocultural functions are associated with the socialization of children. The socialization of children includes the transfer of values relating to behavior, tradition, language, and prevailing or previous social mores. It results in the conditioning of family members to a variety of behavior norms appropriate to all stages of adult life. To be able to do this, the family must possess accepted standards and be sensitive to the varying social needs of children according to their ages. It must also accept and exemplify behavioral norms and be willing to explain, defend, and promote them. Although certain functions are relegated to or emphasized more in one phase of the family's life cycle than another, (for example, the care and socialization of children are part of the childbearing and child rearing phase of the cycle), many of the functions are continuous for the survival and progress of the family.

FAMILY DYNAMICS

Families work cooperatively to accomplish family functions. To do this, family members assume appropriate social roles. Social roles are learned in the family, the first social group, and are learned in pairs, for example, mother-father, parent-child, and brother-sister. A social role does not exist by itself but is designed to mesh with that of a role partner. Pairing of roles enables social interactions to take place in an orderly, predictable manner—the roles are said to be complementary. Some families maintain a traditional pairing of roles, whereas other families have changed the behavior patterns to suit a change in family life-style. The process by which paired roles are brought into a new alignment is known as *negotiation.* Negotiation is essential if family equilibrium is to be maintained.

From the time it is formed, the family sets up *boundaries* between itself and the outside. People are extremely conscious of those considered members of their family and those who rank as outsiders—those who do not have kinship status. Some families isolate themselves from the community. Others have a wide community network to help in times of stress. Although boundaries exist for every family, family members set up *channels* through which they mediate external forces and attempt to protect the family from disturbances. The channels also ensure that the family receives its share of social resources.

Ideally the family provides a safe, intimate environment for the biopsychosocial development of children and its adult members. The family provides for the *nurturing* of the newborn and the gradual *socialization* of the growing child. It is the source of first relationships with others. The relationships children form with parents (or parenting persons) are the earliest and closest and persist throughout a lifetime. For better or worse, parent-child relationships influence a person's concepts of self-worth and ability to form later relationships. The family also interprets and mediates the child's perceptions of the complex outside world. The family provides the growing child with an identity that possesses both a past and a sense of the future. The family transmits cultural values and rituals from one generation to the next (Friedman, 1981).

Through everyday interactions the family develops and uses its own patterns of verbal and nonverbal *communication.* These patterns give insight into the feeling exchange within a family and act as reliable indicators of interpersonal functioning. Family members not only react to the communication or actions of other family members but also interpret and define them.

When assessing a family, nurses examine what is happening and who is doing what to whom. They also note how people perceive what is being done, what it means to them, and how this meaning is expressed. A baby cries to draw the attention of his or her mother, but the mother may interpret the crying as the baby's way of saying she is not a good mother.

Over time the family develops protocols for *problem solving,* particularly regarding decisions deemed important to the family, such as having a baby, buying a house, or sending children to college. The criteria used in making decisions are based on *family values* and *attitudes* concerning the appropriateness of the behavior of its various members and the moral, social, political, and economic events of the wider social system. The *power* to make critical decisions is conferred on a family member through tradition or negotiation. This power may be overt or covert and reflects the family's concepts of male or female dominance and cultural practices, social customs, and community norms. As a result family members are positioned into certain *statuses* or *hierarchies* and play out these statuses by assuming various *roles.* Most families have a member who "takes charge" or "is supportive" or "can't be expected to do anything."

FAMILY THEORIES

Many academic disciplines have studied the family and have developed theories that provide differing perspectives for assessing it. Knowledge of these theories provides the nurse with guides to understanding family functioning. They provide a basis for planning the day-to-day care of families and help predict certain future events that may necessitate a modification of care.

Structural-functional Theory

The structural-functional theory originated with the work of social anthropologists Malinowski (1945) and Radcliffe-Brown (1952), who documented the interrelatedness and interdependence of the national social system and all subsocial systems. According to this theory the family is a social system with components (family members) with specific roles and role behaviors, such as father role or mother role. Family dynamics are directed toward maintaining *equilibrium* between complementary roles to permit family functioning. Family structure is culturally determined. The United States represents a pluralistic culture in which varying family forms are recognized and accepted in differing degrees. Classification of families according to their structure provides insight into stresses that families may experience as they differ from the normative structures supported by the society.

Nuclear Family. The nuclear family is the form considered "normal" in contemporary Western society. Despite talk of new life-styles, it still represents 73% of all households (U.S. National Center for Health Statistics, 1982). This family group consists of parents and their still-dependent children. The family lives apart from either the husband's or wife's family of orientation and is usually economically independent.

The percentage of families with two wage earners rose dramatically during the last decade. In 1979 no fewer than 59.1% of married women with children ages 6 to 17 were in the labor force. According to Harris (1982) this change was caused by the fact that by the early 1960s families were "finding it increasingly difficult to achieve or hold onto middle-class standards of consumption for themselves and their children." Sidel (1986) reported that two-thirds of women aged 25 to 54 were employed in 1984.

Parents in the nuclear family are expected to play complementary roles of husband-wife and father-mother in giving emotional and physical support to each other and their children. Ideally the nuclear family provides for the care and socialization of children and social control for its members. It is held together by strong social bonds. It remains flexible enough to survive in an industrial world. During times of crisis the family can become an important area for social change.

The nuclear family has been described as isolated, but there is increasing evidence that kinship ties to previous family structures are not broken. Sons and daughters commonly remain in the same community as their families of orientation, although they establish their own nuclear families. Visiting relatives is part of their social life. The increased mobility of all segments of population means that grandparents, sisters, uncles, cousins, and other relatives can be more readily available to the isolated family. We often hear new mothers say, "My mother is going to fly in to help me for a week or so." In addition, friends and social groups from church or work provide support for the nuclear family and act in the role of absent families.

Extended Family. By definition the extended family includes three generations. It is family centered, its members live together as a group, and through its kinship network it provides supportive functions to all members. This family structure serves to prescribe the responsibilities and actions of family members. Some people believe the extended family impedes the mobility necessary in an industrialized society with its economic demands.

With an influx of new citizens from Southeast Asia, the Caribbean, and Mexico, the extended family is again playing an important role. The extended family provides the primary source of identity by maintaining language and cultural identification. It also provides economic support by "taking in" needy relatives and sharing food, shelter, and jobs, and it gives emotional support by maintaining kinship ties.

People who have experienced such a family may chafe at the bonds it creates, but when they leave, they may regret the absence of a wider sense of acceptance and recognition such a family provides. In changing to a more socially functional group, members of such "old-fashioned" families may need help in recognizing social institutions as an alternative family to which they can legitimately turn for help and sustenance in times of stress.

Communal Family. Communal family groupings vary from the highly formalized structure of the Amish community in Lancaster County, Pennsylvania, to the loosely knit groups found in the Santa Cruz Mountains near Boulder Creek, California. These latter communities are formed for specific ideologic or societal purposes. They are considered an alternative life-style for people who feel alienated from a predominantly economically oriented society. Some communes consist of nuclear groups living in an extended or expanded family community and are envisioned as persisting over time. Others may provide temporary shelter. In some communes all parents participate in caretaking activities for all children. In many of these groups the combination is fluid; individuals and families are free to come and go as their needs dictate.

The effect of such communities with regard to the children has yet to be determined. Groups that lack some permanence may perpetuate the difficulties associated with the highly mobile family seeking stability and continuity in social contacts. Communes composed solely of young adults and their children may be reproducing the ghettolike aspects of suburbia, with its limited contacts with diverse age, cultural, and economic groups.

Single-parent Family. The single-parent family is becoming an increasingly recognized structure in our society. The single-parent family may result from loss of a spouse by death, divorce, separation, or desertion; from the out-of-wedlock birth of a child; or from the adoption of a child. The 1984 U.S. Bureau of the Census reveals that 25.7% of all children 17 years old or younger live in a family with a single parent, another relative, or a nonrelative. This was the situation for 20% of white children and 59% of black children. As many as 85% of babies born to young unmarried mothers were kept by their mothers; 7% were given to other family members, leaving only 8% for adoption. Of the single parents, 95% are women, most commonly under 25 years of age and in a low-income bracket. Of the group with children under 6 years of age, almost 55% of the single parents are working; in the group with school-age children, about 65% are working mothers.

The single-parent family tends to be vulnerable economically and socially. Unless buttressed by a concerned society, it may create an unstable and deprived environment for the growth potential of children (Norton and Glick, 1986). Nutrition may be haphazard, communication and overt displays of affection curtailed, and discipline inconsistent (Hetherington, Cox, and Cox, 1977). For many of the adults involved this family structure represents a lonely existence in which decision making and other family tasks depend on a single adult (McLanahan, Wedemeyer, and Adelberg, 1981). Public policy is beginning to reflect recognition that a pluralistic society necessarily produces pluralistic forms of the family and that high levels of marital instability are probably to be expected in modern society. As with people who have broken away from the support of extended families, adults in single-parent families may need help in learning how to use community resources in developing or maintaining a satisfactory family life.

For other adults the single-parent family is a chosen lifestyle that provides a free and open system for development of parents and children. In these families, decision making and communication are seen as joint commitments between parent and child, and the parent-child relationship is considered a major source of life fulfillment.

Blended Family. The blended family includes stepparents and stepchildren. Separation, divorce, and remarriage are common phenomena in our society, in which approximately 40% of marriages end in divorce. Divorce and remarriage may occur at any time in the family life cycle and therefore will have different impacts on family function. Whatever the timing, effort is required to restabilize old family groups and constitute and stabilize new family groups. This emotional work must be accomplished before family and individual development can proceed.

Homosexual Family. Homosexual families are being recognized increasingly in Western society. Children in such families may be the offspring of previous heterosexual unions of the homosexual parent or be conceived by one member of a lesbian couple through artificial insemination. Lesbian couples have the same biologic and psychologic needs as do heterosexual couples. They seek quality care for themselves and their unborn and newborn child.

Implications for Nursing. Insights gained from the structural-functional approach can help the nurse become aware of family relationships. First the nurse can recognize the family's *relationship to the larger social system.* Some families establish rigid boundaries, outsiders are kept at a distance, and input from the community is curtailed. Other families are isolated, and when crisis strikes, they often find their inner resources inadequate as coping mechanisms. A third group of families maintains open boundaries through work, school, or community involvement. Energy can flow in both directions, and assistance often is given and accepted.

Second, noting the *internal relationships* of the family may reveal sources of strength or weakness. Commonly the socially conceptualized roles, such as husband and wife, may not fit reality. Hence people establishing or attempting to maintain the so-called normal family roles often face frustration. The interplay of traditionally designed complementary roles may be a source of role conflict. In many families today the husband's and wife's roles are interchangeable; that is, the wife assumes some instrumental functions (earning an income) and the husband assumes some expressive functions (caring for an infant). The ability to negotiate such exchanges is necessary to maintain equilibrium.

Third, the nurse needs to be aware of the development of *reciprocal relationships* within a family that can stunt a person's growth. Some families mold a family member to act as scapegoat; others designate a member to be forever dependent. As an example of the latter, some mothers of teenage parents use the situation to perpetuate the mother-daughter dominance.

The major drawback of the structural-functional theory is that its rigid adherence to roles and associated tasks requires a constant updating of the tasks assigned. In addition, this approach tends to "freeze the family in time."

Developmental Theory

The developmental theoretic approach to the study of the family incorporates ideas from a number of theoretic and conceptual approaches to the study of society and the individual (social systems approach, structural-functional approach, life cycle concepts of developmental needs and tasks, and concepts of interacting personalities). Familiar proponents of the life cycle concept are Duvall (1977) and Wright and Leahey (1984). The central theme in the developmental theory is noting "the changes in the process of internal development with the dimensions of time as central" (Bower and Jacobson, 1978). The family is described as a *small group, semiclosed* system that engages in interactive behavior within the larger cultural social system. The significant unit in this theory is the *person* rather than the role. The family process is one of *interaction* over the *life cycle* of the family.

Family members pass through phases of growth, from dependence through active independence to interdependence. The family also demonstrates variations in structure and function over time. Together these constitute the *family life cycle.* Stages and tasks of the family life cycle adapted from the developmental category of Duvall (1977), the Calgary Family Assessment Model (CFAM) (Wright and Leahey, 1984), and Streff (1981) are compared in Table 3-1.

Implications for Nursing. The developmental theory has provided many useful insights into family functioning. Knowledge of types of problems, identified during certain phases of the life cycle, can assist nurses in providing anticipatory guidance for families. For example, helping families prepare for changing family relationships as school-age children become adolescents may minimize the development of crisis situations.

Because the family as a group and the family as individuals are simultaneously engaged in developmental tasks (Duvall, 1977; Erikson, 1968), disharmony (dissonance) is possible if the developmental task of the family is not synchronous with the developmental task of the person. There are many examples of such dissonance. The adolescent father grappling with his need to break from his family ties is expected to establish monetary and other support for the new family he has created. The mother of the pregnant adolescent, a woman who is ready to move from family involvement in the care of her own children to community involvement, may resent having to assume responsibility for her daugher's child. As parents grow older, the original parent-child relationship may undergo role reversal. Some children find it difficult to accept their parents as depen-

Table 3-1 *Developmental Stages and Tasks of the Individual and Family Unit*

Duvall's Stage of the Family Life Cycle	Calgary Family Assessment Model	Streff's Developmental Task of the Family
Premarital-married couple	Marriage: the joining of families Establishment of couple identity Realignment of relationships with extended family Decisions about parenthood	Establishing relationship Defining mutual goals Developing intimacy Developing appropriate dependence, independence, interdependence pattern Establishing mutually satisfying relationship Negotiating boundaries of couple relationship and with individuals' families of origin Discussing issue of childbearing Making decision to conceive
Childbearing	Families with infants Integration of infants into family unit Accommodation of new parenting and grandparenting roles Maintenance of marital bond	Working out authority and responsibility issues Working out caretaker roles Having children Forming new unit Facilitating child's establishment of trust Acknowledging need for personal time and space while sharing with each other and child
Preschool	Families with preschoolers Socialization of children Adjustment to separation by parents and children	Continuing individual development as couple, parent, and family Experiencing changes in energy and time for individual and couple needs Promoting continued growth in each other and the relationship while encouraging child to develop autonomy and retain self-esteem Establishing own family tradition with each other and children without guilt related to breaks with traditions of families of origin
School age	Families with schoolchildren Development of peer relations by children Family adaptation to peers and school influences	One or both spouses establishing new roles in work settings or community or changes in child-rearing practices and gaining recognition for selves and children Children in school and after-school activities, relating with peers, self-esteem being enhanced or inhibited, and interfacing with activities in family
Teenage	Families with teenagers Development of increasing autonomy Refocus on midlife marital and career issues Beginning shift toward concern for older generation	Parents continue to develop roles in community and interests other than with children Children examine ways to experience freedom while expressing responsibilities for actions Struggles evolve with parents as emancipation process proceeds Family's value system may be challenged Couple relationship may be strong or weak, depending on how members respond to each other's needs

Adapted from Stuart, GW, and Sundeen, SJ: Principles and practices of psychiatric nursing, ed 3, St Louis, 1987, The CV Mosby Co.

Continued.

Table 3-1 *Developmental Stages and Tasks of the Individual and Family Unit—cont'd*

Duvall's Stage of the Family Life Cycle	Calgary Family Assessment Model	Streff's Developmental Task of the Family
Launching career	Families as launching centers Establishment of independent identities Renegotiation of marital relationship	Parents launching young adults with rituals marking rites of passage Change in relationship with children who are becoming adults or in new living situations; change in couple's relationship because of children's absence and increased time with one another
Middle-age parents	Middle-aged families Reinvestment in couple identity Realignment to include in-laws and grandchildren Dealing with disabilities of older generation	Energy channeled into guiding next generation via family or community activities, or couple may now be dealing with issues of aging of their own parents Children of middle-age parents may be adolescent
Aging family members	Aging families Shift to retirement Maintenance of couple and individual functioning	Persons have achieved satisfying relationships and feel sense of accomplishment and desire to continue to live fully until death instead of existing in state of despair Aging members are coping with bereavement and may now be living alone

dent, and, conversely, some parents resent the "interference" of children in their affairs. Awareness of the implications of situations such as these can be useful in helping the family develop appropriate coping mechanisms.

The developmental approach presents a concept of family that is fluid and changing and thus more in tune with reality. It is less difficult to plot the phases of the life cycle in the nuclear family than in an extended family. The extended family may involve many generations. Sometimes it is difficult to document the life cycle of a family; often we can only catch glimpses of it. It changes or disintegrates before we can grasp its significance.

Interactional Theory

Burgess (1926) first postulated the idea that the family could be perceived within an interactional framework. Mead (1934) presented the first concepts; Hills and Hansen (1960), Rose (1962), and Stryker (1959) made later additions.

The major theme of the interactional theory, also known as action theory or role theory, conceives of the family as a *unit of interacting personalities,* not bound necessarily by legal or contractural agreements, that exists as long as the interaction is taking place. The significant unit is *the individual.* The family process is one of *role taking.* This process is dynamic: family members are constantly testing the concept they have of the role of another and adjusting their own self-concept. The process is accomplished through *symbolic communication,* and all family behaviors stem from family members playing their many roles.

Implications for Nursing. The interactional theory is particularly useful as a basis for nurse-family interactions. It is broad enough and inclusive enough to encompass various insights into human nature. It transcends family configuration and cultural, ethnic, or social class boundaries of families, such as nuclear family or extended family, and emphasizes *communication* as a central process (Schvaneveldt, 1966). It helps the nurse understand the implications of family dynamics rather than always taking family actions at face value.

Family theories lend themselves to the systematic study of the family through research. Nurses also use the knowledge from family theories to assist in establishing working relationships with families. When nurses question "who is doing what work," they are using knowledge from the structural-functional theory. When they ask about the significance of events such as birth, children leaving home, or death, they are using family developmental approach. When they assess the effect the birth of a child may have on a husband-wife relationship, they are using interactional family theory.

FAMILY AND CRISIS

No family exists in a nonstress environment. For the family system, stress can arise internally or externally. Although many families cope with stress, the situation may become acute and take on the characteristics of a crisis. Crisis may be defined as a disturbance of habit: a disruption in a family's or an individual's usual means of maintaining control over a situation. If faced with a crisis, the family or person attempts to resolve the crisis using customary values and behaviors.

One of the goals of crisis intervention is to help the client learn new ways of dealing with conflicts or problems. Although the client may seek help for a specific problem, the strategies learned may be applied to future difficulties. The crises families or people experience can be centered around maturational or situational events.

Maturational Crisis

Maturational crises develop as a result of normal growth and development. They characteristically evolve over time and involve *role* and *status* changes. They include events such as birth, infancy, childhood, adolescence, adulthood, and old age. Each phase of the family life cycle produces characteristic crises or events capable of creating stress of such severity that it can affect the health of one or more family members.

The birth of a child represents one of the most important events in the life of a family. Births and the subsequent care of the children require parental, intellectual, and psychologic maturity, and this may account for periods of crisis in a family.

Nurses assist with the birth of children and can provide support as the adults undertake active parenting roles. Nurses can provide knowledge of human psychosocial development, which will help parents both to see their children realistically and to establish appropriate criteria for children's behavior. Nurses may use this unique relationship with a family to promote birth as a family-centered happening with great potential for growth for all participants.

Menopausal concerns often affect the entire family. Few opportunities are available to counsel women regarding normal changes, however, since nurses may not see these women except during an illness. The woman of 65 years of age and older is likely to be the concern of the nurse working in acute care, long-term care, and the community (Griffith-Kenny, 1986).

Situational Crisis

Situational crises include such events as preterm birth, mental or physical illness, loss of financial or social support, changed body image, experience of violence or serious illness, divorce, death, and grief. These crises involve a threat to a person's sense of integrity, or an actual or potential loss or deprivation of some kind. Anxiety or depression are characteristic responses. If the situational crisis causes severe strain, it can result in impairment of health.

Response to Crisis

In both maturational and situational crises the family plays a critical role in the alleviation of distress, successful adaptation, and healthy rehabilitation. The nurse's knowledge of a family's reactions to crisis prompts a more rational assessment of the family's ability to withstand the stress. The nurse can help the family mobilize its problem-solving abilities to deal with the problem (Chapter 2).

Aguilera and Messick (1986) have devised a stratagem for assessing a family's or an individual's potential or actual response to a crisis. They maintain that three key areas or components act as balancing factors affecting equilibrium: (1) the client's perception of the crisis event, (2) the client's coping mechanisms, and (3) the client's support system. The interplay between these three areas is critical for the outcome or resolution of a problem. A brief discussion of each of the three areas follows.

Perception of Event. What one person considers a crisis may or may not be perceived as a crisis by someone else. A factor such as *age* and *prior experience* can alter perception. For example, an event viewed as a crisis by an adolescent may not be seen as a crisis by a 30-year-old adult. *Emotional states, anxiety,* or *hostility* may color a person's perception. The highly anxious young mother of a firstborn child may become disorganized by her infant's crying, whereas a mother of four may accept the crying as normal.

Nursing intervention relative to a client's perception of a crisis-provoking event may be limited to helping the client state "what the problem is." However, if the event can have a negative effect on the client, the infant, or the family, more intervention is required as indicated in the following example.

In some cultures pregnancy is seen as such a natural event that no medical or nursing supervision is considered necessary. As complications of pregnancy can arise with detrimental effect for mother and child the nurse should encourage the family to participate in ongoing health care. Cultures define gynecologic conditions that are acceptable and those that are not. Menopause elevates a woman's status in some cultures (Chapter 41). In others, reproductive cancers are considered "dirty," and the women with these cancers are to be avoided. The nurse in such a situation could act as nurturer, information giver, or organizer.

Coping Mechanisms. Coping mechanisms can be defined as patterns of behavior that people or families have developed for dealing with threats to their sense of well-being (Stuart and Sundeen, 1987). Coping mechanisms may be constructive or destructive. *Constructive coping mechanisms* lead to a resolution of a problem. They vary with the level of anxiety being experienced. For mild anxiety the individual may resort to crying, sleeping, eating, exercise, or smoking and drinking. In interpersonal situations, avoiding eye contact or limiting close relationships to those who cause no anxiety may be successful.

If the threat and consequent level of anxiety become severe, people will resort to the use of task-oriented reactions, ego-oriented reactions or psychologic or physiologic conversions. Task-oriented behaviors are aimed at relieving the stress situations. They are consciously directed and have been objectively appraised by the person using them. Ego-oriented reactions are also known as ego-defense mechanisms. They include repression, projection, and displacement. These reactions protect the person from feelings of inadequacy and worthlessness. However, such responses can be used to the person's detriment. They can distort reality, interfere with interpersonal relationships, and limit working ability. If missed they become *destructive coping mechanisms.* Such habitual responses may be incorporated into the unconscious, and considerable effort may be required to bring such responses into conscious focus to enable the person to change or adapt them.

Psychologic or physiologic conversions are exaggerated or inappropriate coping mechanisms. Fear of crowds, of being alone, and of being in closed spaces are examples of psychologic conversions. An individual who reacts to stress with hypertension and eventual damage to the cardiovascular system is using physiologic conversion.

Nurses use knowledge of human coping mechanisms to assess the type of defense mechanism the person or family uses and the success of the mechanism in ameliorating problems. Attempts are made to substitute more beneficial behaviors if the defense is recognized as destructive. However, coping mechanisms, whether constructive or destructive, appear to be essential for all individuals and groups if they are to maintain emotional stability.

Support Systems. Support systems refer to the support that people may expect from others in their environment during a time of crisis. Caplan (1959), one of the developers of crisis intervention, maintains that the successful resolution of a crisis often depends on the client's support system. If a client's support system is strong, only minimal intervention may be necessary to resolve a crisis and help the client recover. If the client's support system is not strong, disorganization may occur and the client may not recover.

A client's support system may include family, friends, and significant others in the environment. Other people who function as part of support systems are health personnel, or "community caretakers" (Caplan, 1959). Community caretakers are people in the various agencies that represent the organized health resources of a community. These individuals are knowledgeable and experienced. They may be able to assist those who are unable to handle crises on their own or with the help of family and friends. The assistance may take the form of teaching or counseling, or it may involve helping the client learn the procedures for enlisting the aid of other community agencies.

Client education and support are now essential parts of all medical and nursing practice. Nurses have developed *parent education programs* to provide women and men with mechanisms for coping with the stress of labor. These programs also help parents learn about their infants' needs and about child-care activities, so that the parents are better able to cope with the changing needs of a growing child.

In addition to professionally led groups, *peer support groups* are now available to clients. Peer groups encourage interactions between people with similar problems. The groups promote interaction, encourage acceptance and support among members, and serve as a resource. Nurses and social workers have been leaders in originating such groups, in the hospital and in the community. They have worked with others in planning and establishing the groups.

CULTURAL CONTEXT OF THE FAMILY

The relationship of cultural patterns to family process is a central concern in nursing. The reproductive and gynecologic beliefs and practices of a culture are embedded in its economic, religious, kinship, and political structures. Concepts focus on four components of a cultural system: (1) the moral and value system, (2) the kinship system, (3) the knowledge and belief system, and (4) the ceremonial and ritual system. Nurses are becoming increasingly aware of the need to focus on cultural variations in perceptions of life events and use of health care systems because of cultural pluralism in North America and the rapid expansion of international nursing. Clients have a right to expect that their cultural needs relative to health care will be met, as well as their physiologic and psychologic needs. Newton (1972) suggested that health professionals distinguish between health practices based on necessity and those based on social custom. Those social customs need to be maintained and supported that help comfort or make more meaningful the reproductive and gynecologic events that occur to women and their families.

Culture has many definitions. Spradley (1981) defines culture as the "acquired knowledge people use to interpret experience and generate behavior." Each cultural group passes this knowledge to its members from generation to generation. Cultural knowledge includes beliefs and values about each facet of life from birth to death. A person's worldview results from his or her cultural knowledge and provides rules for interaction with others, with nature, and with the supernatural (Powers, 1982). These rules have been tested over time and relate to food, language, religion, art, health and healing practices, kinship relationships, and all other systems of behavior.

Subculture refers to a group existing within a larger cultural system that retains its own characteristics; individuals identify themselves as members of the group. A subculture may be an ethnic group or a group organized in other ways. For example, there is a subculture of nursing and a subculture of medicine.

Each subculture has rich and complex traditions regarding health practices that have proven effective over time. These traditions vary from group to group. Furthermore, nurses must always recognize that a wide range of diversity may exist within a group. Assessment of the beliefs and practices of a group and those within the group is essential for the health care provider striving to plan culturally sensitive health care.

Acculturation refers to changes that take place in one or both groups when people from different cultures come in contact with one another. People may retain some of their own culture and also reformulate cultural elements. Acculturation is contrasted with *assimilation,* in which a cultural group loses its identity and becomes a part of the dominant culture. An example of acculturation would be the adoption of food practices of ethnic groups in the United States. The original recipe for pizza, which is of Italian origin, has been accepted and adapted by many other groups.

Ethnocentrism is "being centered in one's own ethnic or cultural system, judging the world in general by the standards established in that particular system" (Downs, 1971). Socialization into the profession of nursing occurs within the framework of the Western health-care system. This system emphasizes the biomedical model, which in the United States is based primarily on the white, middle-class value system. The biomedical model presents pregnancy and childbirth as phenomena with inherent risks, most appropriately managed through specific knowledge and technology. The nurse encountering behavior in women incongruent with this model may become perplexed and label the women's behavior inappropriate and in conflict with good health practices. If the Western health-care system provides the only standards for judging, the behavior of the nurse is termed *ethnocentric*.

Cultural relativism, the opposite of ethnocentrism, involves learning about and applying the standards of another person's culture to activities within that culture. To be culturally relativistic means the nurse recognizes that people from different cultural backgrounds actually see the same objects and situations differently. There are reasons why people behave the way they do, and these reasons are for the most part culturally determined.

Cultural relativism does not require nurses to accept the beliefs and values of another culture; rather, nurses recognize that the behavior of others may be based on a system of logic different from their own. Cultural relativism is an affirmation of the uniqueness and value of every culture.

Childbearing in Various Cultures

Childbearing represents one facet of health that is related to all aspects of a woman's life. Although most cultures do not regard pregnancy or childbirth as illnesses, the conditions are considered times of heightened susceptibility to dangerous elements. Stern et al. (1980) noted that "pregnant women seek security measures and court benevolent gods with ritualized behavior, whether anointing their abdomens with herbal oils in an African village or practicing daily yoga in California." Perception of the time of greatest vulnerability varies among cultures, with some groups placing greatest emphasis on the prenatal stage and others on labor and delivery or the puerperium. Western health care culture places the greatest emphasis on the prenatal and labor and delivery stages and least on the postpartum stage.

Childbearing in all cultures is complete with norms and behavioral expectations for each stage of the perinatal cycle. All relate to each culture's view of how a person maintains health and prevents illness. Health practices reflect theories of balance and harmony among opposing forces. The intrinsic factors influencing balance and harmony include heat and cold. The extrinsic factors include air and water, food and drink, sleep and wakefulness, movement, exercise and rest, evacuation and retention, and passions of the spirits, or emotions. Thus for pregnant women of many cultures, maintenance of health during childbearing implies a balance and harmony in each women's relationship to her physical, social, and spiritual environment.

The North American Family. North American culture is focused around a nuclear family that includes married parents and children. Extended family relationships are recognized as existing, but their influence varies. Each nuclear family is considered a self-sufficient unit and ultimately responsible for its own functioning, especially child rearing.

Children in the North American family are desirable, but many parents do not define themselves in terms of being parents only. If a couple cannot or chooses not to have children, they are often accepted as being whole people and not incomplete in some way. Value is also placed on delaying the arrival of the first child until the married couple has adjusted to each other and until they are financially able to support a family. The desirable number of children in many North American families is small, usually two or three.

Infants are immediately accepted as members of the society into which they are born. Children are regarded as individuals with certain rights. They are not considered miniature adults, and they are allowed to engage in some behaviors that do not necessarily prepare them for adulthood. Play is valued for its own sake. On the other hand, early independence is encouraged.

Parents are the primary disciplinarians, and in the nuclear family they retain this function during the entire childhood. Parents may resent interference by others in the discipline of their child, even if the other person is a grandparent, aunt, or uncle. Discipline exists in the school system, but it is seen as a temporary extension of the parents' rights to discipline.

Parents are the major caregivers, with the mother assuming primary responsibility. Johnston (1980) points out that in the United States, parenting is not necessarily seen as intrinsically rewarding and enjoyable, but rather as a series of difficult, hygienic, and unrewarding activities. Children are enjoyed only when parental activities result in a child who gains weight, learns to walk and talk, or is toilet trained. Although recently father and mother are sharing more responsibility for care, in early infancy the father is often working and the mother remains at home to care for the infant. Other caregivers are used, but they are usually not kin. They may be baby-sitters or day-care workers, and they are paid for their services, usually by the hour.

Cultural Variations. Differences between the dominant culture of North America and other cultures in general are reflected in how the roles of parents are expressed and how children are viewed. In contrast to the dominant American value system, some cultures regard becoming a parent as the major way individuals define themselves as whole persons. Others believe the highest place in heaven can be reached only through marriage and childbearing. The greater the number of children, the higher the place in heaven. The Navajo woman's role is defined to a large extent in reproductive terms (Wright, 1982). For many blacks, pregnancy is necessary for a man and woman to be seen as whole persons (Carrington, 1978). Puerto Rican couples have their first child as soon as possible to indicate to themselves and the community that the husband is virile and the woman fertile (Murillo-Rohde, 1978). Among the Gadsup (Leininger, 1979) a woman becomes a woman and a man a man when each is married and has at least one child. For Mexican-Americans, childbearing is a privilege and an obligation of married women, and they are encouraged to have children as often as they can (Enriquez, 1982). Thus in many cultural groups parenthood is an ascribed status, and women have no social role without a family.

The importance of children within the family is part of the value system of many traditional cultures. Children are expected to contribute to the economic well-being of the family and to support the parents in their old age. They are regarded as "carriers of the culture." In some cultures, a family without children is abnormal, and a woman's failure to bear children is accepted as grounds for dissolution of a marriage.

FAMILY CARE PLAN

Assessment

To plan for the care of a family or particular family member, the nurse must remember that a family operates as a system. That is, no one family member has a problem—the whole family has a problem. Solutions to problems can evolve only through family participation.

Data Collection Process. The *process* of an assessment in planning family care is often more difficult and complicated than that involved in assessing the physical health of clients. It requires skill in communication and the ability to establish a trusting relationship. In every family group, areas of openness and privacy exist, and all groups resent interrogation by an outsider. The reasons for obtaining information must be explained to the client in a clear manner.

Information such as the address, marital status, and family members' ages can be obtained readily because it is generally given freely. Other information is attained by (1) *observing* and noting relationships, attitudes, and stress responses (who is doing what), (2) *listening* to conversation about community and family involvements or hopes and aspirations, and (3) *being aware* of matters such as why persons have missed appointments or refused to use existing health care facilities.

Cultural Considerations. Cross-cultural variations in reproductive practices occur with respect to interpersonal relationships, family and kinship relationships, and folk practices. Clients have a right to expect that their cultural needs relative to reproduction will be met, as well as their physiologic and psychologic needs. A culture's reproductive beliefs and practices are embedded in that culture's social system and can truly be understood only as they relate to that group's economic, religious, kinship, and political structures. To expect the nurse to have this kind of knowledge for each cultural group is unrealistic. How, then, can information presented in this chapter be used effectively by the nurse?

Stern (1980) developed a model for improving communication between individuals and families from a variety of ethnic and cultural backgrounds and Western health care providers. Identified in this model are barriers in communication that exist on three levels: approach, custom, and language. Such a model, if generalized to other cultures, is useful for nurses.

Approach includes numerous factors one considers in interpersonal relationships. The American approach to most issues in health care is to address the problem directly. With many cultures (Stern, 1980) engaging in small talk is vital before a serious discussion. Commenting on flowers or pictures and having tea or a cold drink are equated with showing respect. To begin talking to an expectant mother about the need for prenatal care before commenting on the other children, the pretty chair, or the weather might set up an atmosphere of distrust. In some cultures, women prefer a caregiver of the same sex. Therefore it is critical that the initial encounter be with a woman. Showing respect and patience are essential in building trust and effecting cultural change.

Custom includes practices and behaviors characteristic of a culture. Understanding that a cultural reason exists for all behaviors and making a sincere effort to ascertain the person's rationale for behavior are important steps in establishing trust. The clients themselves may be the most helpful in assisting the nurse to understand their cultural logic and individual differences. Assessment of health beliefs and practices is essential for the health care professional who is striving to achieve a holistic approach to care. For the client, adherence to a particular cultural custom provides a sense of constancy with one's cultural heritage.

Language is an important factor. Stern (1980) emphasizes the use of clear, jargon-free English. An interpreter, either a family member or a member of the same cultural group, may be used. When an interpreter is being used, it is important to address questions and responses to the client and not to the interpreter.

The following questions illustrate ways to elicit cultural explanations regarding childbearing or gynecologic conditions:

1. What do you and your family think you should do to keep healthy during pregnancy?
2. What are the things you can do or not do to affect your health and the health of your baby?
3. Who are the persons you want with you during your labor?
4. What are considered abnormal signs during menopause?
5. What things or actions are important to you and your family to do after the baby is born?
6. What do you and your family expect from the nurse or nurses caring for you?
7. How do you and your family feel about your hysterectomy?
8. How will family members participate in your pregnancy, childbirth, and parenting?

A nurse cannot be expected to know all there is to know about every culture and subculture, as well as their many life-styles. Understanding one's own culture is necessary to come to a better realization of why we believe as we do. Understanding clients' cultures, through interview, study, contact, and a demonstrated sincere interest, is invaluable. This understanding enables nurses to render culturally sensitive and relevant nursing care.

Model for Data Collection. The following outline is an assessment model based on a guide developed by faculty members of San Jose State University Department of Nursing in 1982.

I. Family identification
   A. *Composition.* Who are the family members currently living in the household? Are they kin or nonkin? What are their ages?
   B. *Social history.* What is the social background of

each member regarding education, income, occupation, marital status, ethnicity, and culture?

C. *Community and neighborhood.* What is the general tone of the neighborhood? Are resources such as water, electricity, and sewers available? Is the area one of affluence or poverty? What are the residents of the neighborhood like (e.g., friendly, noncommittal)?

II. Individual and family data

A. *Health history.* What is the family's health history? What actions has the family used in the past when one of its members was ill? What are the family's present reasons for seeking care?

B. *Family dynamics.* How well does the family work together to accomplish family functions? What social roles does each family member assume? How are roles within the family negotiated? What are the family's boundaries? What channels do family members use to interface with the community? What communication patterns are employed? What are the family's protocols for problem solving? What are the family's values and attitudes as reflected in problem solving and decision making; for example, who has the power? What aspects of family theories are represented by this family: structural-functional, developmental, or interactional?

1. *Techniques* used in assessing individual and family dynamics include interviewing and observation. Robbins and Schacht (1982) have devised four basic steps nurses can use in observing communication behavior and inferring hierarchies within families.

a. Observe the interactions of the entire family and remember that an observer has a part in the iteractions.

b. Outline the interactions just as a camera would record them, without inferred meaning. This outline may be written on paper.

c. Review the interactions: who spoke first, who spoke with whom, and when, who summed up, who spoke or acted for whom, and who followed whose advice.

d. Proceed with the appropriate intervention, exchanging information within the family's communication system.

2. *Recording* the assessment data under the following headings can reveal patterns that provide guidelines to planning nursing care:

a. Communication patterns: direct or indirect, open or closed?

b. Leadership: patriarchial, matriarchial, egalatarian, democratic?

c. Hierarchies: who possesses the power and over what areas?

d. Roles and relationships: who is the breadwinner, decision maker, leader, nurturer?

e. Values: are values based on materialism, importance of family, religion, ethnic or cultural patterns?

f. Beliefs regarding health and illness: do the beliefs reflect myths, old wives' tales, cultural influences?

g. Priorities: are the priorities housing, jobs, food, other?

III. Family strengths: following is a checklist to assist the nurse in identifying present and potential family strengths and weaknesses based on health history and family dynamics:

A. Ability to maintain a healthy life-style and general health status.

B. Ability to provide for the family's physical, emotional, spiritual, and cultural needs:

1. Physical: providing adequate space, equipment, material goods, food, etc.
2. Emotional: helping family members recognize and develop their capacity for sensitivity to each other's needs.
3. Spirtual: sharing of basic beliefs and spiritual or religious values.
4. Cultural: sharing of basic beliefs and cultural values.

C. Child-rearing practices and discipline (if appropriate).

1. Capability of both parents to respect each other's views and decisions on child-rearing practices.
2. If a single parent, capacity of the parent to be consistent and effective in raising the child or children.

D. Communication: ability to communicate and express a wide range of emotions and feelings both verbally and nonverbally.

E. Support, security, and encouragement:

1. Capacity of the family to provide its members with feelings of security and encouragement.
2. Ability to achieve balance in the pattern of family activities.

F. Growth-producing relationships: family's ability to maintain and build friendships and relationships in the neighborhood.

G. Responsible community relationships: capacity of the family members to assume responsibility through participation in social, cultural, or community activities.

H. Growing with and through children: capacity of parents to recognize that children may be a force for growth in the parents' lives.

I. Self-help and accepting help: family members' ability to seek and accept help when *they* think they need it.

J. Flexibility of family functions and roles: family members' ability to "fill in" for one another during times of illness or when needed.

K. Crisis as a means of growth: family members' ability to unite and become supportive during a crisis or traumatic experience.

L. Family unity, loyalty, and intrafamily cooperation: family members' ability to recognize and use family traditions and rituals that promote unity and pride.

Analysis, Synthesis, Validation. Following the data-gathering phase the nurse analyzes and synthesizes the findings. Inferences about the data are formulated. Because inferences are subjective and based not only on the nurse's competence level but also on individual values and beliefs, the nurse needs to validate the interpretation of the data with the client. Validation of inferences is followed by the development of nursing diagnoses.

Nursing Diagnoses

Nursing diagnoses are formulated to reflect the family's perception of its needs, as well as the nurse's perception. *It is important to determine the family's perception of its nursing care needs rather than that of any one family member.*

Once the nursing diagnoses are established, the nurse takes time to explore personal value judgments about the family that may affect and impede nursing interventions. It is also essential for the nurse to validate the diagnoses. In addition to direct validation with the family, a review of the literature, an analysis of norms, and discussion with other persons involved in the family are means of validation.

Planning

Setting Goals. The next step is to set goals and outcome criteria related to each diagnosis. These are established as a joint enterprise between nurse and family. They are evaluated for realism and acceptance by family members. Goals for care are both short and long range. Once agreed on, the goals are assessed to determine priority. Certain health needs require immediate attention, for example, unexplained vaginal bleeding. Other health needs require more time to resolve, for example, anger over birth of a child of undesired sex.

Selecting Nursing Actions. Working with the available data, the nursing diagnoses, and the health goals, the nurse proceeds to organize a plan for implementing the most appropriate interventions. The nurse identifies the nursing role, that is, whether the role is teacher, direct care provider, or referrer. The nurse plans for the best use of resources available to the family, both internal and community support systems. The nurse must determine whether the resources are appropriate and whether the family is able or willing to use them.

Implementation

The selected nursing actions are implemented; they are preventive, curative, or rehabilitative, and are tailored to the individual needs of the family and its members.

Evaluation

Evaluation is a joint process between nurse and family. Mutually determined goals and outcome criteria need to be stated precisely so that the degree to which goals are met can be determined. The criteria need to be realistic and flexible enough to permit modification as circumstances change.

SUMMARY

The family is the fundamental social unit of every society. It has many functions. One function is to serve as a crucial support system for the individual. Family dynamics are complex. Family theories provide guides to understanding family functioning and its developmental stages and tasks. The family faces and must cope with maturational and situational crises. Families function within a cultural context. All of the components of the nurse and individual client relationship and of the nursing process are utilized when the client-family unit is the focus of care.

KEY CONCEPTS

- The family forms a social network that acts as a potent support system for its members.
- In both maturational and situational crises the family plays a critical role in the alleviation of distress, successful adaptation, and healthy rehabilitation.
- Balancing factors affecting equilibrium in a family include the client's perception of the crisis event, the client's coping mechanisms, and the client's support system.
- Ideally, the family provides a safe, intimate environment for the biopsychosocial development of children and its adult members.
- Sometimes it is difficult to document the life cycle of a family; often we can only catch glimpses of it.
- The reproductive and gynecologic beliefs and practices of a culture are embedded in its economic, religious, kinship, and political structures.
- Differences between the dominant culture of North America and other cultures in general are reflected in how the roles of parents are expressed and how children are viewed.
- North American culture is a pluralistic one in which varying family forms are recognized and accepted in differing degrees.

STUDY QUESTIONS AND ACTIVITIES

1. Develop a family care plan for a childbearing family or a family in which a woman has a gynecologic problem.
2. Select a family whose cultural origins are different from your own. Interview an adult member of the family regarding cultural variations related to childbearing and childrearing. Pay particular attention to taboos.
3. Select one of the family theories and analyze a childbearing, childrearing family or family in which a woman has a gynecologic problem using the major concepts identified in the theory.
4. Compare strengths, stressors, coping patterns, and implications for nursing between two structural functional family classifications.

References

Aguilera, DC, and Messick, JM: Crisis intervention: theory and methodology, ed 4, St Louis, 1986, The CV Mosby Co

Blehar, MC: Families and public policy. In Corfman, E, editor: Families today, vol 2, National Institute of Mental Health, Division of Scientific and Public Information, Science Monograph No 1, Washington, DC, 1979, US Government Printing Office

Bower, F, and Jacobson, M: Family theories: frameworks for nursing practice. In Archer, S, and Fleshman, R, editors: Community health nursing: patterns and practice, N Scituate, Mass, 1978, Duxbury Press

Burgess, EW: The family as a unit of interacting personalities, Family 7:3, March, 1926

Caplan, G: Concepts of mental health and consultation, Children's Bureau, US Department of Health, Education and Welfare, Washington, DC, 1959, US Government Printing Office

Carrington, BW: The Afro-American. In Clark, AL, editor: Culture/childbearing/health professionals, Philadelphia, 1978, FA Davis Co

Downs, JF: Cultures in crisis, Beverly Hills, Calif, 1971, Glencoe Press

Duvall, ER: Marriage and family development, ed 5, Philadelphia, 1977, JB Lippincott Co

Enriquez, MG: Studying maternal-infant attachment: a Mexican-American example. In Kay, MA, editor: Anthropology of human birth, Philadelphia, 1982, FA Davis Co

Erikson, EH: Identity: youth and crisis, New York, 1968, WW Norton & Co, Inc

Friedman, MM: Family nursing theory and assessment, New York, 1981, Appleton-Century-Crofts

Griffith-Kenney, J: Contemporary women's health: a nursing advocacy approach, Menlo Park, Calif, 1986, Addison-Wesley Publishing Co

Harris, M: America now: the anthropology of a changing culture, New York, 1982, Simon & Schuster, Inc

Helvie, C: Community health nursing: theory and process, New York, 1981, Harper & Row, Publishers, Inc

Hetherington, EM, Cox, M, and Cox, R: Beyond father absence: conceptualizations of the effects of divorce. In Hetherington, EM, and Parke, R, editors: Contemporary readings in child psychology, New York, 1977, McGraw-Hill Inc

Hills, R, and Hansen, D: The identification of conceptual frameworks used in family study, Marriage Fam Living 22:311, 1960

Johnston, M: Cultural variations in professional and parenting patterns, JOGN Nurs 9:9, 1980

Leininger, M: The Gadsup of New Guinea and early childcaring behaviors with nursing implications. In Leininger, M, editor: Transcultural nursing '79, New York, 1979, Masson Publishing USA, Inc

Malinowski, B: The dynamics of cultural change, New Haven, Conn 1945, Yale University Press

McLanahan, SS, Wedemeyer, NV, and Adelberg, T: Network structure, social support, and psychological wellbeing in the single-parent family, J Marriage Fam 43:601, Aug, 1981

Mead, GH: Mind, self and society, Chicago, 1934, The University of Chicago Press

Murillo-Rohde, I: The Puerto Rican: Part II. In Clark, A, editor: Culture/childbearing/health professionals, Philadelphia, 1978, FA Davis Co

Newton, N: Childbearing in broad perspective: pregnancy, birth and the newborn baby, Boston, 1972, Delacorte Press

Norton, A, and Glick, P: One parent families: a social and economic profile, Fam Relations 35(1):9, 1986

Powers, BA: The use of orthodox and Black-American folk medicine, Adv Nurs Sci 4:35, 1982

Radcliffe-Brown, A: Structure and function in a primitive society, New York, 1952, Free Press

Robbins, M, and Schacht, T: Family hierarchies, Am J Nurs 82:284, 1982

Rose, A: Human behaviors and social processes: an interactional approach, Boston, 1962, Houghton Mifflin Co

Schvaneveldt, J: The international framework in the study of the family. In Nye, FA, and Bernardo, FM, editors: Emerging conceptual frameworks in family analysis, New York, 1966, Macmillan Publishing Co

Sidel, R: Women and children last, New York, 1986, Viking Penguin Inc

Spradley, BW: Community health nursing, Boston, 1981, Little, Brown & Co, Inc

Stark, S: Mormon childbearing. In Kay, MA, editor: Anthropology of human birth, Philadelphia, 1982, FA Davis Co

Stern, PN, et al: Culturally-induced stress during childbearing: the Filipino-American experience, Issues Health Care Women 2(3-4):67, 1980

Streff, M: Examining family growth and development: a theoretical model, Adv Nurs Sci 3(4):61, 1981

Stryker, S: Symbolic interaction as an approach to family research, Marriage Fam Living 21:111, May, 1959

Stuart, GW, and Sundeen, SJ: Principles and practice of psychiatric nursing, ed. 3, St Louis, 1987, The CV Mosby Co

United Nations: Principles and recommendations for the 1970 population census, New York, 1969

US National Cancer for Health Statistics, US Bureau of the Census, US Department of Commerce, Washington, DC, 1982, The Center

Wright, A: Attitudes toward childbearing and menstruation among the Navajo. In Kay, MA, editor: Anthropology of human birth, Philadelphia, 1982, FA Davis Co

Wright, LM, and Leahey, M: Nurses and families: a guide to family assessment and intervention, Philadelphia, 1984, FA Davis Co

World Health Organization: Health and the family: studies in the demography of family life cycles and their health implication, Geneva, 1978, The Organization

Bibliography

Afeck, LB, and Hickey, J: Health classes for migrant workers' families, Am J Nurs, July, 1972

Affonso, DD: The Filipino American. In Clark, AL, editor: Culture/childbearing/health professionals, Philadelphia, 1978, FA Davis Co

Alvarez, R: Delivery services for latino community mental health, Los Angeles, 1975, University of California, Los Angeles

Bampton B, et al: Initial mothering patterns of low income black primiparas, JOGN Nurs, May, 1981

Branch, M, and Paxton, P: Providing safe nursing care for ethnic people of color, New York, 1976, Appleton-Century-Crofts

Carrington, BW: The Afro-American. In Clark, AL, editor: Culture/childbearing/health professionals, Philadelphia, 1978, FA Davis Co

Chung, JJ: Understanding the Oriental maternity patient, Nurs Clin North Am 12:67, 1977

Clark, AL, and Howland, IH: The American Samoan. In Clark, AL, editor: Culture/childbearing/health professionals, Philadelphia, 1978, FA Davis Co

D'Angelo, P: Son of Italy, New York, 1975, Arno Press

Demmi, L, and Eoxsey, K: Encountering the recent influx of Cuban refugees in the emergency department, JEN 7:11, 1981

Doherty, W: Family interventions in health care, Fam Relations 34(1):129, 1985

Flynn, M: Coordination of social and health care for the elderly: the British and Irish examples, Gerontologist, 20:300, 1980

Griffith, S: Childbearing and the concept of culture, JOGN Nurs 11:181, 1982

Grosso, C, et al: The Vietnamese American Family . . . and grandma makes three, MCN 6:177, 1981

Henderson, G, and Primeaux, M: Transcultural health care, Menlo Park, Calif, 1981, Addison-Wesley Publishing Co, Inc

Hollingsworth, AO, et al: The refugees and childbearing: what to expect, RN 43:45, 1980

Kendall, K: Maternal and child care in an Iranian village. In Leininger, M, editor: Transcultural nursing '79, New York, 1979, Masson Publishing USA, Inc

Kiple, K, and King, V: Another dimension to the black diaspora: diet, disease, and racism, Cambridge, 1981, Cambridge University Press

Kniep-Hardy, M, and Burkhardt, MA: Nursing the Navajo, Am J Nurs, 77:95, 1977

Lee, PA: Health beliefs of pregnant and postpartum Hmong women, Nurs Res 8(1):83, 1986

Leininger, M: Cultural diversities of health and nursing care, Nurs Clin North Am 12:5, 1977

Lifton, RJ, Kato, S, and Reich, MR: Six lives/six deaths, New Haven, 1979, Yale University Press

McGoldrick, M: Normal families: an ethnic perspective. In Walsh, F, editor: Normal family processes, New York, 1982, The Guilford Press

Meleis, AI, and Sorrell, L: Bridging cultures: Arab American women and their birth experiences, MCN 6:171, 1981

Monroe, P, Garand, J, and Price, S: Family health plan choices: the health maintenance organization option, Fam Relations 34(1):71, 1985

Muecke, M: Caring for the southeast Asian refugee patients in the USA, Am J Public Health 73:431, 1983

Orque, MS, et al: Ethnic nursing care: a multicultural approach, St Louis, 1983, The CV Mosby Co

Perry, DS: The umbilical cord: transcultural care and customs, J Nurse Midwife 27(4):25, 1982

Primeaux, M: American Indian health care practices, Nurs Clin North Am 12(1):55, 1977

Sklare, M: Understanding American Jewry, New Brunswick, Conn, 1982, Center for Modern Jewish Studies, Brandeis University

Sue, S, and Wagner, NW editors: Asian-Americans: psychological perspectives, Ben Lomond, Calif, 1973, Science & Behavior Books

The Single Parent Family, Special issue of Family Relations, Fam Relations 35:1, Jan, 1982

Tien, JL: Do Asians need less medication? Issues in clinical assessment and psychopharmacology—a nursing perspective, J Psychosoc Nurs Ment Health Serv 22:19, 1984

Tien, JL, and Johnson, H: Black mental health client's preference for therapists: a new look at an old issue, Int J Soc Psychiatry 31(4):258, 1985

US Department of Health, Education and Welfare: The Indian health program, Washington DC, 1972, US Government Printing Office

Vogel, VJ: American Indian Medicine, Oklahoma, 1970, University of Oklahoma Press

Wake, S, and Sporakowski, M: An intergenerational comparison of attitudes towards supporting aged parents, J Marriage Family 34:42–48

Welch, S, Comer, J, and Steinman, M: Some social and attitudinal correlates of health care among Mexican-Americans, J Health Soc Behav 14:205, 1973

White, E: Giving health care to minority patients, Nurs Clin North Am 27: March, 1977

Zepeda, M: Selected maternal infant care practices of Spanish-speaking women, JOGN Nurs 11:371, 1982

CHAPTER

4

Legal and Ethical Issues

Cheryl Harris

Learning Objectives

Correctly define the key terms listed.

Identify examples of duty: the standard of care.

List three ways in which a nurse may commit professional malpractice.

Describe examples of liability and causation.

Summarize the independent practice of nursing.

Assess risk management through practices of prevention and appropriate reporting, and discovery procedures.

Discuss two purposes for maintaining accurate client records.

List 10 steps in a bioethical decision-making model.

Explore ethical dilemmas in relation to in vitro fertilization and embryo transplantation, elective abortion, neonatal intensive care, and AIDS.

Assess mother surrogates and genetic counseling in relation to legal-ethical issues.

Key Terms

Legal Terms

abandonment
breach
civil law
discovery and privileged communication
duty: standard of care
expert witness
incident report
informed consent
liability and causation
malpractice
nurse practice act
professional competency and currency
professional liability insurance
professional negligence
quality assurance
reasonable prudent person
risk management
tort

Ethical Terms

beneficence
cost-containment
ethical dilemmas
ethical perspective
ethics committee
nonmalfeasance
value systems

The field of maternity and newborn care (perinatal nursing)—in which birth and death, life and the capacity to make life are encountered on a daily basis—perhaps offers more legal and ethical challenges to the professional nurse than does any other area of nursing.

This chapter introduces the nurse to basic legal and ethical issues that influence women's health care and suggests nursing-practices that promote quality professional care. The chapter contains three major divisions: (1) *legal issues,* a broad overview of the legal responsibilities and potential liabilities incurred by perinatal nurses, (2) *risk management,* a system of nursing behavior designed to improve the quality of nursing care, as well as to minimize the risk of legal liability, and (3) *ethical issues,* a discussion of some ethical dilemmas that may be encountered by the perinatal nurse. Reading material suggested for further investigation is listed in the bibliography.

LEGAL ISSUES

Laws affect nursing in many ways. Activities required of the nurse by law include eye prophylaxis for the newborn and the reporting of venereal disease and child abuse. Criminal law affects nursing when the professional nurse exceeds the scope of nursing and practices medicine without a license or aids and abets an unlicensed individual to practice medicine. This discussion, however, is concerned with civil law that seeks to compensate parties who have been injured or damaged by the negligence of a professional nurse. This civil law has been termed the *law of torts.* A tort is a civil offense.

The visual sequence of events preceding a legal claim for damages caused by negligence is as follows:

1. The state licenses a professional nurse to practice nursing according to the guidelines established by the state's nurse practice act.
2. A member of the general public enters into a relationship with a professional nurse in which the nurse offers and delivers health care services.
3. By virtue of the license to practice, the nurse has certain duties and obligations. These duties and obligations are called the standards of care.
4. The nurse fails to fulfill these duties and obligations and breaches a standard of care. The nurse need not *intend* to do harm. Harm may be inflicted unintentionally through negligence.
5. As a direct or indirect but foreseeable result of that breach, an actual injury is sustained. The injury must be actual rather than potential or "at risk for" injury. Actual injury includes both physical harm and emotional distress.
6. The client or client's family may be compensated for the injury by monetary damages assessed against the nurse. "General damages" include the cost of health care and rehabilitation, income lost from absence from work, and income lost from the impaired ability to work. "Special damages" include pain and suffering experienced by the injured party.

Duty: the Standard of Care. The standard of care, or external code of behavior or expected performance, for a professional nurse is that average degree of skill, care, and diligence exercised under similar circumstances by the reasonably prudent nurse with similar background, training, and experience (Black, 1979). Major points of the American Nurses' Association, Standards of Maternal-Child Health Nursing are presented in the box below.

The Organization for Obstetric, Gynecologic, and Neonatal Nurses (NAACOG) has published standards that are presented as recommendations and general guidelines (NAACOG, 1986). Examples of standards for obstetric nursing, neonatal nursing, and gynecologic nursing are on p. 56, whereas standards for electronic fetal monitoring appear in Chapter 17.

Standard of care is measured and applied by the courts in the form of verdicts in lawsuits or settlements. To be successful in a lawsuit against a nurse, the plaintiff must first define the nurse's duty or standard of care and then prove that the nurse failed to conform to that standard of care. Standards of care reflect minimum requirements for performance.

To determine the standard of care for professional nursing, the appropriate starting point is the state's **nurse prac-**

ANA STANDARDS OF MATERNAL-CHILD HEALTH NURSING

Standard I: The nurse helps children and parents attain and maintain optimum health.

Standard II: The nurse assists families to achieve and maintain a balance between the personal growth needs of individual family members and optimum family functioning.

Standard III: The nurse intervenes with vulnerable clients and families at risk to prevent potential development and health problems.

Standard IV: The nurse promotes an environment free of hazards to reproduction, growth and development, wellness, and recovery from illness.

Standard V: The nurse detects changes in health status and deviations from optimum development.

Standard VI: The nurse carries out appropriate interventions and treatment to facilitate survival and recovery from illness.

Standard VII: The nurse assists clients and families to understand and cope with developmental and traumatic situations during illness, childbearing, childrearing, and childhood.

Standard VIII: The nurse actively pursues strategies to enhance access to and utilization of adequate health care services.

Standard IX: The nurse improves maternal and child health nursing practice through evaluation of practice, education, and research.

American Nurses' Association: Standards of maternal and child health nursing practice, Kansas City, Mo, 1983, American Nurses' Association.

NOTE: This chapter's content relates only to the United States.

tice act and the state regulations pertaining to nursing practice. These laws and regulations define the scope of nursing practice, standards for nursing education, and the point of articulation between the profession of nursing and the profession of medicine. To exceed the legal base of nursing practice is, by definition, to violate the standard of care and to be negligent. For instance, if a particular state declares it illegal for the nurse to dispense medication without a physician's order and the professional nurse hands a woman a month's supply of birth control pills, that action is a violation of the standard of care. If there are no written policies or procedures to permit such nursing interventions, the nurse's actions are negligent.

Standards of care are determined by the nursing profession in its definition of nursing practice, policies and protocols for nursing practice, standards of nursing education, and proscription of activities considered outside of nursing. Standards of care are further delineated by nursing specialist organizations and joint boards of medicine and nursing who define appropriate behavior in special and specific circumstances.

Other standards of care established by the profession are the policies and protocols governing nursing practice in a particular agency or unit of an institution. These **policies** and **protocols** define behavior expected of all professionals within their domain. They may act to expand behavior expected in a particular situation beyond the customary practice of nursing and into the practice of medicine. For instance, special or standardized procedures may permit a nurse in an intensive care unit to initiate drug therapy if a client displays a particular symptom. They may also permit a nurse to dispense birth control pills under special circumstances where otherwise that behavior would be illegal (Calif. Bus. and Prof. Code).

Professional nurses have a legal obligation to know and understand the standard of care or duty imposed on them. Ignorance of a policy or protocol will not be accepted as an excuse for failure to follow it. This is one reason why it is critical for nurses to keep current in their specialties.

Some recent cases have established the duty of the nurse to oversee the behavior of other professionals and to report situations in which other professionals' behavior fails to conform with the established standard of care (Cushing, 1985). For instance, when a physician writes an erroneous drug order, the nurse has a duty to report the error and obtain a corrected order (Annas, Glantz, and Katz, 1981). When the client is exposed to danger as a result of action by other professionals, the nurse has a duty to protect that client. That duty extends beyond mere reporting of the incident and requires the nurse to follow up on reporting until the client is returned to safety (Darling, 1965). Labor and delivery room nurses occasionally deal with this situation when they call for physician assistance and fail to get it. They must continue to ask for physician assistance until they do get it. The nurse's responsibility extends beyond the care of clients directly assigned to her or him and encompasses the behavior of other professionals functioning in the same area.

Breach: Failure to Conform to the Standard of Care. In a court of law the standard of care is established by the testimony of expert witnesses who generally are leaders in their field. Their credentials include administrative responsibility, teaching, and research in addition to clinical competence. These expert witnesses are presented with the actual situation or with a hypothetical situation that is an exact duplicate of the case under consideration. They are then asked to state what behavior is required of the nurse and what behavior would fail to conform to the standard of care. The judge or jury makes the final determination regarding whether the defendant-nurse in the actual situation had breached the standard of care.

When the standard of care is breached and that breach is a cause of injury to the client, the nurse may be guilty of professional malpractice. The legal definition of *malpractice* is "professional misconduct, improper discharge of professional duties, or failure to meet the standard of care of a professional which resulted in harm to another" (Black, 1979). Professional malpractice is a form of negligence. The legal definition of *negligence* is "carelessness, failure to act as an ordinary, prudent person, or action contrary to what a reasonable person would have done" (Black, 1979). These definitions state the three ways in which a nurse might commit professional malpractice:

1. By performing a duty carelessly or improperly
2. By failing to perform a duty when it is indicated
3. By performing an unauthorized act

Liability and Causation. Professional nurses are liable for the consequences of their actions. The best synonym for *liable* is *responsible.* Nurses are responsible for both the direct and indirect results caused by their actions. If a client falls out of bed as a consequence of the nurse's failure to put up the side rails, the nurse is responsible for the harm to the client directly caused by that failure to act. If the nurse fails to report the improper behavior of another health care professional and a client is injured by that other person, the nurse is responsible for that injury indirectly caused by the failure to act.

Until the last 10 years, courts rarely found nurses to be independently liable for their actions (Fiesta, 1983). Most courts found that nurses acted on the basis of orders given and were not autonomous or independent providers of services. The nurse functioned either as an agent of the physician, in which case the physician assumed all liability, or as an employee of the hospital, in which case the hospital assumed all liability. The legal doctrine that assigns liability for the entity controlling the nurse is *respondeat superior* (Black, 1979). It literally means "let the master answer" and assigns liability for nursing action to the employer of the nurse. This sort of liability of the hospital and physician is called vicarious liability.

Within the last 10 years, however, a change in the legal perspective of nursing practice has occurred. Increasingly, nurses are viewed as autonomous health care providers who practice independently in certain clearly defined situations. Recent cases have found nurses to be independently liable and did not assign the liability to physicians and hospitals where nurses were acting outside of the direction of physicians and hospitals (Black, 1979).

It is important for the professional nurse to understand the distinction between the dependent practice of nursing, which is the implementation of the physician-directed management of care, and the independent practice of nursing. Based on the California Nurse Practice Act, the California Nurses' Association's definition of the **independent practice of nursing** is:

1. Direct and indirect client care services that ensure the safety, comfort, personal hygiene, and protection of clients and the performance of disease prevention and restorative measures.
2. The performance of skin tests and immunization techniques and the withdrawal of human blood from veins and arteries.
3. The observation of signs and symptoms, reactions to treatment, and general behavior or physical condition and the determination of whether such observations exhibit abnormal findings and the appropriate reporting and referral of such abnormalities (Calif. Bus. and Prof. Code).

The independent practice of nursing encompasses those decisions and actions taken by the nurse based on nursing judgment and a nursing management plan rather than on a management plan directed by the physician. The indepe-

Table 4-1 *Standards for Obstetric, Gynecologic, and Neonatal Nursing*

	Nursing Practice	Health Education
Clinical Area	Comprehensive obstetric, gynecologic, and neonatal (OGN) nursing care is provided to the individual, family, and community within nursing care is provided to the individual, family, and community within the framework of the nursing process.	Health education for the individual, family, and community is an integral part of obstetric, gynecologic, and neonatal nursing practice.
Obstetric Nursing	*Examples:*	*Examples:*
Antepartum	Assessments for risk, need for referrals, maternal and fetal well-being, administers medications, provides emotional support.	Teaching of maternal adaptations, both physical and psychologic, nutrition, hygiene, family dynamics.
Intrapartum	Assessments and interventions for maternal and fetal well-being, progress of labor (physical and psychologic), care and comfort, newborn immediately following birth.	Teaching of labor process, health care during the intrapartum period, control of discomfort, participation of family.
Postpartum	Assessments and interventions for postdelivery recovery, family interaction, and integration of newborn into family unit.	Teaching of involutional process, parenting skills, family dynamics, infant care, fertility management.
Neonatal Nursing		
Normal/low risk newborn	Assessment and interventions for respirations, temperature, maturity level, infection, family contact, nutrition.	Teaching of newborn care, protection and safety, nutrition, family dynamics, parenting skills, newborn characteristics and responses.
High-risk newborn	Assessment and interventions for respirations, temperature, maturity level, infection, family-newborn interaction.	Teaching of neonatal pathophysiologic processes and care needs, family dynamics, parenting skills.
Gynecologic Nursing		
Ambulatory	Assessment and intervention for gynecologic conditions, nutritional status, sexual concerns, self-care.	Teaching of reproductive anatomy and physiology, health promotion and maintenance.
Inhospital	Assessment for intervention for gynecologic conditions, nutritional status, sexual concerns, self-care, altered health patterns.	Teaching of content specific to condition, health maintenance and promotion related to specific condition.

Adapted from Standards for obstetric, gynecologic, and neonatal nursing, ed 3, Washington, DC, 1986, The Organization for Obstetric, Gynecologic, and Neonatal Nurses (NAACOG).

dent practice of nursing may theoretically become the basis for future independent liability of the nurse.

Risk Management

Risk management is an evolving concept stemming directly from the large losses sustained by hospitals, physicians, nurses, and professional liability insurance carriers. These losses result from lawsuits for malpractice. The risk management process seeks to minimize losses by identifying risks, establishing preventive practices, developing reporting mechanisms, and delineating procedures for managing a lawsuit once it has been filed. The nurse should be familiar with the concepts of risk management and their implications for nursing practice. Effective risk management minimizes the risk of a lawsuit against the nurse.

Practices involved in risk management also lead to improved nursing care. The nurse should view these concepts as a system of checks and balances that ensure a high quality of client care.

Preventive Practices

Quality Assurance. Quality assurance is an umbrella term used to encompass those activities that review and

Policies and Procedures	Professional Responsibility	Personnel
The delivery of obstetric, gynecologic, and neonatal care is based on written policies and procedures.	The obstetric, gynecologic, and neonatal nurse is responsible and accountable for maintaining knowledge and competency in individual nursing practice and for being aware of professional issues.	Obstetric, gynecologic, and neonatal staff are provided to meet client-care needs.
Examples: Policies and procedures for scope of practice, nursing orders and standards of care, health education, monitoring.	*Examples:* Current concepts, trends, and scientific advances for the care of the antepartum client and her family.	*Examples:* Orientation program addresses skills and knowledge needs and quality assurance. Staffing is appropriate.
Policies and procedures for above actions, and for nurse's role regarding informed consents and implementation of independent nursing actions in emergency situations.	Current concepts, trends, and scientific advances for the care of the intrapartum client and her family.	Orientation program addresses skills and knowledge needs for unit and quality assurance. Staffing is appropriate.
Policies and procedures for above actions, and for postdelivery recovery and nursing research.	Current concepts, trends, and scientific advances for the care of the postpartum client and her family.	Orientation program addresses skills and knowledge needs for the unit and quality assurance. Staffing is appropriate.
Policies and procedures for scope of practice and standard of care, health education, research, emergency care.	Current concepts, trends, and scientific advances for the care of the normal/low-risk neonate and her/his family.	Orientation program addresses skills and knowledge needs for the unit and quality assurance. Staffing is appropriate.
Policies and procedures for special assessment and interventions of the high-risk newborn and her/his family.	Current concepts, trends, and scientific advances for the care of the high-risk newborn and her/his family.	Orientation program addresses skills and knowledge needs for the unit and quality assurance. Staffing is appropriate.
Policies and procedures ror assessment and intervention for the ambulatory client.	Current concepts, trends, and scientific advances for the care of the ambulatory gynecologic client.	Orientation program addresses skills and knowledge needs for the unit and quality assurance. Staffing is appropriate.
Policies and procedures for assessment and intervention for the inhospital client.	Current concepts, trends, and scientific advances for the care of the hospitalized gynecologic client.	Orientation program addresses skills and knowledge needs for the unit and quality assurance. Staffing is appropriate.

evaluate actual client care and institute remedial actions to bring client care into conformity with the standard of care (ACOG, 1980). Quality assurance includes chart review, chart audit, peer review, and performance evaluations.

The first step in quality assurance is to establish the acceptable standard of care. For example, one standard might be the taking and recording of vital signs once during every 8-hour shift. Another example might be the requirement of a minimum of graduate level nursing education for a clinical nurse specialist. A third example might be a rate statement, such as no more than 10 minutes' delay in administering a timed medication. These standards often take the form of policies and protocols.

The second step in quality assurance is to construct a test of the standard. Examples of testing procedures include the following:

1. Review of case management of all clients who develop decubiti
2. Chart review of all women admitted to labor and delivery room for adequacy of nursing history
3. Chart audit of random sample of charts of postpartum women to determine frequency of entry of vital signs
4. Quarterly performance evaluation of all labor and delivery nursing personnel using the job description as a standard of performance

After the test has been constructed and administered, its results are reviewed and compared with the standard of care. If the test results show a failure to conform to the standard of care, remedial action is defined, and a repeat test or evaluation is scheduled. The goal of quality assurance is to establish that all professional conduct meets the applicable standard of care.

Informed Consent. The concept of informed consent is also a form of risk management. The concept of informed consent originates with the right of persons to consent to all forms of touching. Violation of that right is called battery. Informed consent is established by law and includes the right to consent to diagnostic and therapeutic measures and to refuse them (Calif. Adm. Code). Informed consent includes the provision of information about the procedure, its risks, its anticipated results, and any alternatives to it. It is usually the responsibility of the person performing the procedure to obtain informed consent.

Many problems have arisen from the process of informed consent (Cushing, 1984). The major problem for providers is that the only test for informed consent is the client's assertion that she or he understands and agrees. If at a later date the client denies that she or he understood, the provider may have to prove that the consent process was adequate. Unfortunately the only documentation of the procedure may be a short "informed consent obtained" statement on the chart.

The professional nurse should be aware of these issues regarding informed consent:

1. Responsibility for obtaining informed consent rests with the person performing the procedure and is usually not delegated to the nurse. The nurse may, however, contribute to the education process by providing background information about the procedure or by witnessing the signature process.
2. Consent must be obtained from a competent individual. The client must not be a minor and must be in a state of mind unaffected by drugs or injury. There are special considerations if the client is a minor or mentally incompetent, or if obtaining consent during an emergency.
3. The information process must be geared to the client's level of understanding. It must be done in the language and with the words that the client is capable of understanding.
4. Blanket consents (I consent to everything) and blanket releases (I release everyone from liability) are traditionally disregarded by the courts. They may be seen as an effort to misinform or deceive the client.
5. The consent is only as good as its documentation. The best documentation is by the client in her or his own handwriting included in the chart. Oral consents are also legal and binding. They are, however, difficult to prove several years later in the process of a lawsuit.
6. Client's refusal should be carefully documented and thereafter respected.

As with any surgical procedure, an informed consent is required for voluntary sterilization. Since a couple's ability to produce children is such an emotionally charged situation, many institutions require the consent of the spouse before performing a sterilization procedure (Rhodes and Miller, 1984).

Professional Liability Insurance. Professional liability insurance is a risk management concept because it may prevent nurses from incurring large losses that result from a legal settlement or judgment against them. Insurance is provided by contract based on the periodic payment of a premium. Coverage is limited by a ceiling amount per lawsuit or settlement and by an aggregate total per year. The insurance policy should be investigated carefully for the type of coverage, limits of coverage, and exceptions to coverage. Some policies do not cover nurses in expanded roles. Others do not cover independent nurses or self-employed nurses.

Employed nurses are confronted with the issue of whether to carry insurance in addition to the protection offered by their employers. The main argument against such coverage is that it adds to the cost of litigation because it involves an additional insurance company who will hire more lawyers and perhaps delay the proceedings. The main argument for carrying added coverage is to supplement coverage offered by the employer. It allows the nurse as an individual to find legal representation. Personal insurance will cover the nurse for activities outside the scope of employment. It will ensure that the nurse's interests, as well as the interests of the hospital and the physician, are represented.

Professional Competency and Currency. Maintaining professional competency and currency is a critical issue in risk management and in prevention of liability risk. The standard care for a professional is conduct required of the average member of the profession with a similar background under similar circumstances. The average member of the profession maintains a level of competency that does not incorporate ignorance of the standard of care. When *expert witnesses* establish the standard of care, it is inferred that the average professional is informed and competent in that standard. Ignorance may not be claimed as a defense.

Occasionally nurses are placed in situations in which their professional competency is impeded by an outside factor. Two common situations are "short staffing" and "floating." Professional nurses have a duty to report situations in which the standard of care is breached by circumstances inherent in the situation (Horsley, 1981). The duty extends to the point that communication is clearly given to a person who has the power to remedy the situation. The duty may require the nurse to ask for assistance, supervision, and orientation. Ultimately the nurse may have to try to reject the assignment. Unfortunately the professional nurse may be caught in a conflict with another professional duty, that of not abandoning the client. In trying to resolve this situation the nurse should make these points clear:

1. The breach of the standard of care was reported to a supervisor who was potentially able to remedy the situation.
2. Rejection of the assignment would have placed the client in greater danger from **abandonment**.

One further issue that relates to the nurse's competency is that of mental impairment from excessive fatigue, drugs, or alcohol. A nurse must never endanger a client's condition through the nurse's use of such substances or extreme lack of sleep.

Quality of Nurse-client Relationship. A final concept of prevention is the **quality of the relationship** between the nurse and the client. It has been clearly documented that clients who feel angry, frustrated, and depersonalized by their health care are more likely to sue when an injury occurs (Wecht, 1982). It is also clear that anger and frustration are common accompaniments to illness and adjustment to the post-illness state. No nurse can make every client happy all of the time, but every nurse possesses the judgment and skill necessary to support a client through illness to recovery. It is helpful to identify early those situations in which the client seems unusually upset and in which that upset is directed toward the staff. Involvement of the client in the management plan, special attention to comfort measures, and perhaps changes in nursing assignments may help the client feel less victimized and more in control of the situation.

Reporting Practices. A major aspect of risk management is appropriate **documentation of client care** and effective communication of those incidents that may give rise to a malpractice suit. Documentation of client care is accomplished by charting occurrences and observations on the client record. Communication of problem situations is accomplished by incident reports. It is critical to be aware of the differences between the client record and incident reports.

The two main purposes for keeping client records are (1) to produce a clear and accurate history of the client in relation to the illness or problem and the management plan and (2) to enhance communication between the many health care providers who may provide services in any given situation. Therefore charting must be accurate, objective, and comprehensive.

Errors. A major issue in accuracy is how to deal with **errors.** Here are some guidelines to follow:

1. Never change someone else's charting. If it is clearly inaccurate, place a note in the chart signed by you with the correct information. Do not state that "Ms. X charted in error." Merely make the correct observation. Bring the inaccuracy to the attention of the professional who made it so that the needed correction may be made.
2. To change an error in your own charting, draw one line clearly through the error and write ERROR over it. Do not obliterate the error. Make the necessary correction and sign and date it in a separate notice that is *legibly* written.
3. Never make accusations of error directly in the chart. The appropriate place for those notations may be in an incident report.
4. Always sign your full professional name and title.

Objectivity. Objectivity in charting may be problematic when conclusions rather than observations are charted. The most troublesome conclusions are those that cast aspersions on the character or reputation of the client such as alcoholism, substance abuse, violent nature, or irresponsibility. Those conclusions may be appropriate in charting when they represent a confirmed diagnosis or when they are items in a differential diagnosis. Otherwise it is far more accurate and objective to chart the actual behavior observed. Those observations are then available to support a subsequent diagnosis should it be appropriate. For instance, instead of charting that the client was drunk, chart that the client was unsteady, unable to walk, and had an odor of alcohol on his breath.

Comprehensiveness. No nurse completes client assignments with charts tucked under one arm for immediate recording. There is delay in virtually all charting. Delay may contribute to gaps and omissions in charting with the result that the charting is not comprehensive. Here are some guidelines to follow:

1. Never chart out of time sequence or try to squeeze a note in between two other notes. Place the accurate time and date next to the note currently being made and chart the circumstances accounting for delay in the charting.
2. Chart significant observations or changes immediately. Make sure the time and date are accurate.
3. Never chart that something is done before it is done, especially with medications.
4. When the nurse is too involved with client care to chart, such as in emergency situations, have a recorder note events and changes. This should include accurate times and names of persons giving care. The recorder should not be a member of the family or a casual observer but rather a person with professional responsibility for charting.
5. Omissions in charting may be interpreted to mean that the care did not occur. When vital signs are not charted and the client claims the vital signs were not taken, there is no evidence that they actually were taken (Cushing, 1982). Therefore it is critical to chart all observations to avoid omitting essential information.

In the event of a lawsuit the client record is the only

piece of evidence created at the time of the event that documents the actual circumstances and chain of happenings. Because the chart is compiled by health care providers, inaccuracies such as lack of comprehensiveness or objectivity in the chart would imply defects in the quality of care given. Health care providers can only fall back on their recollections of the event, which may be hazy or absent with the passage of time. Providers' allegations of quality care tend to sound self-serving on the witness stand when their recollections are contested by the word of the injured client. There is simply no substitute for a careful, accurate, objective client record.

Incident Reports. Incident reports document situations in which the health care professional and the institution may incur liability. These reports are submitted only to hospital or agency administrators, specifically to risk managers and insurance claims agents. They may document errors or omissions in care that breach the standard of care, irresponsible or negligent professional behavior, and unfortunate outcomes in client care such as injury, disability, or death.

Incident reports are considered to be confidential communication between the institution's staff and administration. They are *not* included in the client's chart.* If an incident report is found in the client's chart, that report may be used by the plaintiff-client against the hospital and nurse. Incident reports may be found to be privileged. If written as confidential documents between the institution's attorney and the client-institution, they are protected from disclosure by attorney-client privilege. The confidential and privileged nature of the incident report makes it the preferred vehicle for documentation of breach of the standard of care. It is the means by which effective change can take place within the institution to remedy situations exposing it to liability.

Here are some guidelines for the use of incident reports (Cushing, 1985):

1. Never write "An incident report has been filed" in the client's record or place a copy of the report in the client's record.
2. The report should be written accurately and clearly, giving all the essential facts. Accusations and admissions should be avoided.
3. The report should be submitted to the appropriate member of the hospital administration. The more copies distributed, the weaker the assertion that the report is confidential and privileged. In some states, incident reports are available for *discovery* in a lawsuit.

Discovery and Privileged Communication. Discovery occurs after a lawsuit has been filed. It is the process by which both the plaintiff and the defendent attempt to "discover" everything they can about the event in dispute. Both sides in the lawsuit attempt to bring every fact in the dispute into play. Both sides are wary of surprises. There is a legally required exchange of information between the plaintiff and the defendant so that each side has a reasonable opportunity to develop a fair case.

All records, conversations, and events are discoverable unless they are privileged. Attorney-client privilege may protect the incident report from disclosure. The physician-client relationship (and some nurse-client communications) is ordinarily privileged except when the client makes it an object under dispute. Then all relevant aspects of the relationship are discoverable by the other side.

Here are some guidelines to follow in relation to the process of discovery:

1. All unprivileged documents are discoverable, including private journals. If the nurse has made a private record of the event and of her participation in the event, the other side may require its disclosure. Records of the nurse's participation in the event should be in the form of an incident report submitted to the appropriate member of the administration. In some states, this incident report protected from disclosure by the attorney-client privilege.
2. Conversations are discoverable. No outside discussion of the event should occur without representation of the institution's attorney. This prohibition includes discussions with the client, the client's family, the client's attorney and colleagues, and friends of the nurse. If, however, the incident is discussed in a recognized peer review/quality assurance activity, that discussion may be privileged under a special legal exception. If asked to participate in such a discussion, the nurse should inquire whether the discussion is privileged before participating.
3. If the nurse has received an official request (a subpoena) for information from the plaintiff-client, full cooperation should be given to comply with the request in good faith. Compliance with the request for information should be reviewed by the institution's attorney before material is submitted.
4. All communication with the client and the client's attorneys and investigators should be made in the presence of the institution's attorney or the nurse's representative with her or his knowledge and consent.
5. Nurses should be aware of their rights to hire an attorney on their own to represent their interests. However, the hospital has the obligation to defend its employees and should provide an attorney to be present during all contacts with the client and the client's attorneys after a lawsuit has been filed.

Mother Surrogates

The incidence of infertility has increased over the past decades. In response to these problems, some couples have taken advantage of controversial solutions to address their desire for children. Legal complications are possible with some choices made by these couples. In the highly publicized Stern-Whitehead Baby M case in New Jersey, both the natural father and the surrogate mother claimed custody of the baby. A lengthy and traumatic court case resolved the initial issue, when custody of Baby M was granted to her natural father and his wife.

As a result of the controversy inherent in payments for a surrogate mother's services and the delicate and complex ethical issues, commercial surrogacy has been banned in Great Britain (Brahams, 1987). George Annas of The Hastings Center (1986) believes commercial surrogacy is de-

*Opinion on this important matter may be changing.

humanizing to infants and exploits women. He also states that the courts in Kentucky view surrogate mother arrangements as equivalent to baby selling and therefore illegal under current statutes of that state.

Genetic Counseling

Genetic counseling is often provided for a couple following the birth of an infant with an inherited problem. The purpose of counseling is to give parents accurate information about recurrence risks in subsequent children. Since complete accuracy in genetic counseling is important, a nurse who has not received graduate training in this field risks legal liability if she engages in providing genetic counseling to parents.

ETHICAL ISSUES

Ethical dilemmas occur in every field of nursing practice; perinatal nursing is not immune. Technical advances in the medical field have proceeded at a breakneck pace, often outstripping society's ability to consider the ethical implications of these new techniques. Fetal experimentation, neonatal intensive care, amniocentesis resulting in a recommendation for abortion, genetic engineering, and the humane treatment of persons with AIDS are just a few areas in which nurses must determine an ethical stance. For this reason, it is important for nurses to develop a rational, systematic, well-considered *ethical perspective* with which to analyze these ethical questions. This section will not address all of the ethical decisions a nurse must make, but it should help nursing students develop this aspect of their practice.

During their early years, nurses begin to form their ethical and moral values within their own family structure and through religious affiliations. Nurses have responsibilities and commitments to use ethical conduct in relationships with clients, other nurses, physicians, and their employing institution (Curtin 1982). Inherent in the values of most nurses are **beneficence** (the practice of doing good) and **nonmalfeasance** (to do no harm). In some circumstances, it is difficult to prevent these two principles from conflicting. For example, in newborn intensive care, some treatment is painful. Decisions must be made about whether future quality of life justifies the pain inflicted on the infant and her or his parents during treatment.

Several different professional associations, including The American Nurses Association, have developed codes of ethics for nurses to follow (see box, above right). These frameworks for ethical conduct are helpful when applied to a given client circumstance in which ethical questions have arisen.

According to a study by Berseth et al. (1984), newborn intensive care nurses are often reluctant to assist in making ethical decisions about various critical issues in neonatal intensive care. These nurses believe that the physician and parents of the child should make such decisions. However, nurses who serve as primary care givers have unique insights about the entire family unit and therefore could be helpful if they joined in the dialogue of decision making.

Thompson and Thompson (1985) have presented a

CODE FOR NURSES

1. The nurse provides services with respect for human dignity and the uniqueness of the client unrestricted by considerations of social or economic status, personal attributes, or the nature of health problems.
2. The nurse safeguards the client's right to privacy by judiciously protecting information of a confidential nature.
3. The nurse acts to safeguard the client and the public when health care and safety are affected by the incompetent, unethical, or illegal practice of any person.
4. The nurse assumes responsibility and accountability for individual nursing judgments and actions.
5. The nurse maintains competence in nursing.
6. The nurse exercises informed judgment and uses individual competence and qualifications as criteria in seeking consultation, accepting responsibilities, and delegating nursing activities to others.
7. The nurse participates in activities that contribute to the ongoing development of the profession's body of knowledge.
8. The nurse participates in the profession's efforts to implement and improve standards of nursing.
9. The nurse participates in the profession's efforts to establish and maintain conditions of employment conducive to high quality nursing care.
10. The nurse participates in the profession's effort to protect the public from misinformation and misrepresentation and to maintain the integrity of nursing.
11. The nurse collaborates with members of the health professions.

*Reprinted with permission of the International Council of Nurses.

A BIOETHICAL DECISION MODEL*

Step One	Review the situation to determine health problems, decision needed, ethical components, and key individuals
Step Two	Gather additional information to clarify situation
Step Three	Identify the ethical issues in the situation
Step Four	Define personal and professional moral positions
Step Five	Identify moral positions of key individuals involved
Step Six	Identify value conflicts, if any
Step Seven	Determine who should make the decision
Step Eight	Identify range of actions with anticipated outcomes
Step Nine	Decide on a course of action and carry it out
Step Ten	Evaluate/review results of decision/action

*Thompson, JE, and Thompson, HO: Ethics in Nursing, New York, 1981, Macmillan Publishing Co, Inc, with permission.

bioethical model for a logical reasoning process that nurses may use to make ethical decisions (see box, bottom, p. 61). Through use of the 10 steps described in this bioethical model, the nurse will be able to analyze critically ethical situations as they arise. Thompson and Thompson suggest that nurses and other professionals form small discussion groups to address ongoing ethical problems within their area of practice.

Within the scope of maternity and newborn intensive care are numerous subjects with ethical questions.

In Vitro Fertilization and Embryo Transplantation

A recent ethical dilemma brought to focus by modern obstetrics is the technique of in vitro fertilization with subsequent embryo transplantation, the results of which are known as test-tube babies. Since the first live birth with this technique in 1978, numerous infants have been born as a result of this procedure.

In March 1979, the Ethics Advisory Board of the Department of Health, Education, and Welfare recommended that in vitro fertilization be considered not only ethically acceptable but also an inevitable treatment for infertility. Several questions were raised concerning the possible disrespect for human life, for example, discarding of fertilized eggs. Steinfels (1979) suggests that the developed eggs can be discarded at 14 days or less after fertilization because normal uterine implantation will have occurred by that time.

Another ethical question raised by Smith (1982) concerns the relative cost of in vitro fertilization. In countries with limited medical resources, decisions need to be made regarding how funds should be spent. Should they be allocated for renal dialysis for an adult who requires this accepted and proven method of treatment or for relief of the infertility problem faced by a couple who has been attempting to have a child for years?

The issue of in vitro fertilization is legally, ethically, and morally significant. As the use of this technique proliferates, questions will probably increase.

Elective Abortion

"Pro-life" and "pro-choice" public groups have dramatically focused ethical and legal attention on the issue of abortion. Fromer (1982) reminds us that, like it or not, nurses are very much involved in abortion issues. Nurses may assist as an abortion is performed or may refuse to do so. Nurses are asked to give advice about abortions and to provide information about where a client may obtain one. To provide service to a client seeking an abortion, nurses must understand their personal ethical position on abortion (Thompson and Thompson, 1981).

From an ethical perspective, abortion is essentially the removal of the woman's support from the fetus. This leads to fetal death, since the fetus cannot sustain its life without the mother. Bok (1978) suggests that if an abortion is performed after the diagnosis of a fetal defect, the parents have consented to remove support from that particular fetus. This raises the issue of abortion for the fetus's sake.

Camenisch (1976) notes that initially it might seem reasonable to abort a seriously malformed fetus for its own sake to prevent the suffering anticipated from its malformation. But he argues that we must use this argument with care. The concern for the fetus it expresses may obscure the role of the interests of parents, society, and other affected parties. But most problematic is that in following this argument we do not offer the fetus the better life we seek for those whose ills we can treat. Here we "treat" the problem by eliminating the patient. And it is not clear what sort of benefit that is, nor whether it can be a benefit in the absence of a beneficiary. It is not even clear that we know what that tradeoff means. Therefore he concludes that while concern for the future of a malformed fetus should influence our deliberations, it is not clear that that concern provides conclusive grounds for abortion.

Summarizing the abortion controversy is difficult, but basically the pro-choice proponents believe that the mother's rights take precedence and that she should have freedom of choice and privacy. Many pro-choice advocates believe that abortions should be used only as a last resort, with contraception and adoption being other alternatives. Most pro-life proponents believe that the fetus is human from the moment of conception and as such should be protected from abortion, which ends life.

Neonatal Intensive Care

Hundreds of neonatal intensive care units (NICUs) are available throughout the United States. They are confronted with difficult ethical questions and legal problems of all types.

Some of the ethical dilemmas in decision making are ironically caused by the dramatic advances in neonatal-perinatal care. The medical and nursing knowledge base has increased rapidly in a relatively short time. Infants who would have automatically died 10 years ago now have a good chance to survive with few undesirable consequences. In essence, the joint disciplines of perinatology and neonatology have pushed back the point of viability to unimagined degrees. A premature infant of less than 1500 g (3 lb, 5 oz) had a slim chance of survival in 1965. Whereas an infant of 1000 g (2 lb, 3 oz) has a good chance today. The advances in neonatal surgery have significantly improved the outcome for many infants born with heart defects or other congenital anomalies. This section will explore some of the issues faced by nurses who work in an NICU.

Costs of Treatment. One ethical problem that arises not only in the NICU but in all areas of perinatal care involves societal pressures about money. Newborn intensive care and fetal surgery are costly. Considering the dwindling public funds available for health care, many persons question the appropriateness of diverting monies from preventive programs (such as immunization programs for the poor) to the care of one critically ill infant. The hospitalization cost for one NICU baby can easily exceed $100,000. Federal, state, and local funds used for this type of care will not be available for other health care programs.

Veatch (1986) describes the ethical dilemmas of *cost-containment* caused by diagnosis related groups (DRGs).

For example, if a hospital discovers that DRG 386 (extreme prematurity, neonates) is "losing money" for the hospital, they might decide to close their NICU, transfer out severely affected neonates, or change their guidelines for resuscitation based on a higher birth weight. Veatch believes the ethics of cost-containment decisions deserve examination.

Unpredictable Prognoses. Many infants who receive care in the NICU have an unpredictable prognosis, which presents ethical dilemmas for all personnel. For example, neonatal asphyxia has a variable outcome depending on the severity of the original episode. If the infant suffers a subsequent cardiac arrest, the appropriate care might be in question. Is resuscitation of the infant ethically correct? How long should resuscitation efforts be continued? Is there an ethical imperative to save all infants?

The NICU is designed to facilitate diagnosis and treatment of infants with immediate and acute but essentially life-threatening problems, such as aspiration pneumonia or respiratory distress syndrome. Proper care can result in a dramatic reduction in morbidity and mortality in these infants. However, an ethical question arises as to whether it is appropriate to use equipment and intensive care skills to keep an infant with a poor prognosis alive while "neglecting" an infant with a better prognosis.

Cohen (1977) discusses violation of the ethical principle of aiding one client while harming another. He suggests that if one assumes the obligation to provide intensive care to a client, terminating this care later because another client has a higher potential for survival violates the original obligation. However, he recognizes the difficult dilemma that intensive care personnel face when they do not want to sustain infants who are beyond salvage (e.g., an infant who has suffered a massive intracranial hemorrhage). Persons who care for these infants have difficulty deciding which infant would be better served if allowed to die.

Steinfels (1978) poses the question of whether the emphasis on neonatal intensive care for smaller and smaller premature infants has resulted in decreased efforts in the prevention of prematurity. Although a birth weight of 1000 g was formerly the lower limit of saving premature infants, many NICUs now use heroic efforts to save infants weighing as little as 600 to 700 g. Steinfels also suggests that more attention be paid to the impact on the family of the premature infant who is saved but severely impaired.

Silverman (1981) suggests that many parents may believe that producing an infant with severe handicapping conditions is worse than having an infant who dies. Furthermore, he deplores the "rescuer" role of many health professionals. In this role providers make unrestrained heroic efforts to prolong even the most fragile life with no concern for the parents' wishes. Silverman asserts that because parents will have the day-to-day responsibilities for consequences of neonatal intensive care, they should be among the primary decision makers regarding the care of their infant.

Since outcome for neonates is often difficult to predict, Rhoden (1986) suggests the adoption of guidelines to help make decisions in life and death situations. She describes guidelines adopted by other countries as they make decisions about neonatal care. Every case must be decided on an individual basis, but Rhoden suggests that such guidelines can help in the decision-making process for many of the infants who receive care in NICUs.

Many authorities have suggested that an ethics committee composed of clergy, ethicists, lawyers, physicians, nurses, and lay persons could review each case. Watchko (1983) recommends a model in which the physician and parent would make the original decision and then review their decision with an ethics committee. If disputes resulted about what was correct, the courts would be asked to intervene. In this solution, the parents represent a non-institutional perspective and are subject to review by other family members, social agencies, such as churches, and close friends. The physician, who represents an institutional viewpoint, is subject to peer review. The hospital-based committee serves as a consultant. If the courts are involved, they assume the primary authority.

AIDS

Acquired immune deficiency syndrome (AIDS) was first identified and brought to public attention in 1981. The epidemic of this lethal syndrome poses physical, emotional, legal, and ethical challenges to nurses regardless of their area of practice. Maternity nurses who manage health issues for pregnant women and their newborns with AIDS must examine their own values.

Brown (1987) states that the AIDS epidemic has an impact on nurses at all levels of practice from staff nurses, to administrators, to educators. Nurses are confronted with many different ethical issues involved in AIDS, such as the client's right to human dignity, privacy, and confidentiality. Often the nurse may have conflicts within herself about the client who lives an alternative life-style, or who is a drug abuser. Nurse administrators must confront issues of resource allocation and personnel management for those under their supervision. Nurses must be educated about the physical nature of this disease process to assist their clients, as well as to protect themselves from contracting this incurable disease.

Steele (1986) notes that AIDS is a "catastrophic health problem". She recommends that nurses must examine their own reactions and engage in values clarification to help society cope with this crisis. Finally, Steele reminds all nurses that they may be in a position to help AIDS victims develop a high quality of life for whatever time they have remaining, since they know that their disease is always fatal.

SUMMARY

A wide variety of ethical and legal issues arise in maternity and newborn nursing. This chapter presents a review of current ethical and legal positions involved in the care of clients. Many of the ethical dilemmas are a result of the rapid advances taking place in all specialties. The new medical technology and expanded roles for nurses have increased the chances of survival for normal infants and improved the care for all newborns. Because family-centered maternity health care raises ethical and legal questions of monumental proportions, it is essential for all nurses who care for women, new mothers, and their infants to understand these issues.

KEY CONCEPTS

- The conduct of all legally competent individuals is held to a standard of care—that degree of care exercised by a reasonably prudent person under similar circumstances.
- Professional nurses are liable for the consequences of their actions.
- The independent practice of nursing encompasses those decisions and actions taken by nurses based on *nursing judgment* and *nursing management* plan.
- The concept of risk management seeks to minimize losses by establishing preventive practices, appropriate reporting practices, and discovery procedures.
- In the event of a lawsuit, the client record is the only piece of evidence created at the time of the event.
- Ethical dilemmas occur in every field of nursing practice.
- Nurses have responsibilities and commitments to use ethical conduct in relationships with clients, other nurses, physicians, and their employers.
- Inherent in the values of most nurses are beneficence and nonmalfeasance.

STUDY QUESTIONS AND ACTIVITIES

1. Determine from the nursing service at your hospital if a "conscience clause" for nurses is written into the policies. If so, read and discuss it with your student group.
2. Determine what policy is written or unwritten concerning "no-code" and withholding of treatment in the neonatal intensive care unit at your hospital.
3. Research recent medical malpractice suits to determine the type and frequency of obstetric-related suits. Report on such questions as: How often was the nurse named as defendant? and Are there any areas of obstetric practice that seem particularly hazardous in relation to lawsuits?
4. Interview several registered nurses on the subject of "floating." Obtain answers to these questions for discussion with the group:
   a. Does their facility make a practice of floating nurses?
   b. How do they personally feel about floating?
   c. What do they do if they feel unqualified to float to a certain area?
   d. What pressures have they felt relative to floating?
   e. Have any of them floated to an area and had a serious problem develop while there?

References

American College of Obstetricians and Gynecologists: Quality assurance in obstetrics and gynecology, Washington, DC, 1980, The College

American Nurses Association: Standards of maternal-child health nursing practice, Kansas City, Mo, 1983, American Nurses Association

Annas, GJ: The Baby Broker Boom, Hastings Center Rep 16(3):30, 1986

Annas, G, Glantz, L, and Katz, B: The rights of doctors, nurses and allied health professionals, Cambridge, Mass, 1981, Ballinger Publishing Co

Berseth, CL, Kenny, JD, and Durand, R: Newborn ethical dilemmas: Intensive care and intermediate care nursing attitudes, Crit Care Med 12(6): June, 1984

Black, HC: Black's law dictionary, St. Paul, 1979, West Publishing Co

Bok, S: Ethical problems of abortion, Hastings Center Rep 19(4):19, 1978

Brahams, D: The Hasty British Ban on Commercial Surrogacy, Hastings Center Rep 17(1):16, 1987

Brown, ML: AIDS and Ethics: concerns and considerations, Oncol Nurs Forum 14(1):69, 1987

California Administrative Code, Section 70707

California Business and Professions Code, section 2725. California Administrative Code, section 1470 et seq

Camenisch, PF: Abortion of the fetus' own sake, Hastings Center Rep 6(2):38, 1976

Cohen, CV: Ethical problems of intensive care, Anesthesiology 47:217, 1977

Curtin, L, and Flaherty, MJ: Nursing ethics: theories and pragmatics, Bowie, Md, 1982, Robert Brady Co

Cushing, M: Gaps in documentation, Am J Nurs 82:1899, Dec, 1982

Cushing, M: Incidents reports: for your eyes only, Am J Nurs 85:873, Aug, 1985

Cushing, M: Informed consent—an MD responsibility? Am J Nurs 84:437, April, 1984

Cushing, M: Lesions from history: the picket-guard nurse, Am J Nurs 85:1073, Oct, 1985

Darling v. Charleston Community Memorial Hospital, 211 NE 2nd 253 (IL 1965)

Fiesta, J: The law and liability: a guide for nurses, New York, 1983, John Wiley & Sons, Inc

Fromer, MJ: Abortion ethics, Nurs Outlook 30(4):234, 1982

Horsley, JE: Short-staffing means increased liability for you, RN 44(2):73, 1981

NAACOG: Standards for Obstetric, Gynecologic and Neonatal Nursing, ed 3, Washington, DC, 1986

Rhoden, NK: Treating baby Doe: the ethics of uncertainty, Hastings Center Rep 16(4): Aug, 1986

Rhodes, A, and Miller, R: Nursing and the law, ed 4, Rockville, Md, 1984, Aspen Publishers, Inc

Silverman, WA: Mismatched attitudes about neonatal death, Hastings Center Rep 11(6):12, 1981

Smith, PK: Ethics and in-vitro fertilization, Br Med J 284:1287, 1982

Steele, SM: AIDS: clarifying values to close in on ethical questions, Nursing and Health Care 7:5, May, 1986

Steinfels, M: New childbirth technology: a clash of values, Hastings Center Rep 8:9, Feb, 1978

Steinfels, M: In vitro fertilization: "ethically acceptable" research, Hastings Center Rep 9:5, June, 1979

Thompson, JE, and Thompson, HO: Ethics in nursing, New York, 1981, Macmillan Publishing Co, Inc

Thompson, JE, and Thompson, HO: Ethical decision making for nurses, Norwalk, CT, 1985, Appleton-Century-Crofts

Veatch, RM: DRGs and the ethical reallocation of resources, Hastings Center Rep 16(3): June, 1986

Watchko, JF: Decision making on critically ill infants by parents, Am J Dis Child 137:795, 1983

Wecht, C, editor: Legal medicine 1982, Philadelphia, 1982, WB Saunders Co

Bibliography

American Nurses Association: Nursing: a social policy statement, Kansas City, Mo, 1982, American Nurses Association

Annas, GJ: Baby M: babies (and justice) for sale, Hastings Center Rep 17(3):13, 1987

Barnard K: Maternal-child health nursing: a perspective on service, research and training. Zero to Three: Bulletin of the National Center for Clinical Infant Programs 2(4):1, 1982

Buley, DD: When the burden of proof falls on you, Nurs '86 16:41, Feb, 1986

Creighton, H: Law every nurse should know, Philadelphia, 1981, WB Saunders Co

Creighton, H: Liability of nurse floated to another unit, Nurs Management 13(3):54, 1982

Cuddihy N: On nurse-midwifery legislation, J Nurse Midwife 29(2):55, 1984

Cushing, M: Legal side: first, anticipate the harm . . ., Am J Nurs 85:137, Feb, 1985

Cushing, M: Legal side: how a suit starts, Am J Nurs 85:655, June, 1985

Cushing, M: Legal side: how courts look at nursing practice acts, Am J Nurs 86:131, Feb, 1986

Driscoll, ME: AIDS: legal aspects of occupational exposure, Calif Nurs Review 10(3):10, 1988

Erlen, JA, and Holzman, IR: Anencephalic infants: should they be organ donors? Pediatr Nurs 14(1):60, 1988

Ethics Grand Rounds: When refusing treatment jeopardizes another life, Nurs '88 18(5):145, 1988

Fromer, MJ: Ethical issues in sexuality and reproduction, St Louis, 1983, The CV Mosby Co

Greenlaw J: Documentation of patient care: an often underestimated responsibility, Law Med Health Care 29:172, Sept, 1982.

Huttman, BR: Dilemmas: not murder—just nothing, Am J Nurs 85:959, Sept, 1985

Isil, OA: Legal risks and perinatal health care, NAACOG update series, lesson 13, vol 1, 1984

Kim M, McFarland G, and McLane A: Pocket Guidé to Nursing Diagnoses, ed 2, St Louis, 1987, The CV Mosby Co

LaBar, C: Filling in the blanks on prescription writing, Am J Nurs 86:30, Jan, 1986

Lagerloff, J: Ethics: maternal-fetal conflict, Calif Nurs Rev 10(1):34, 1988

LaRocco, SA: Dilemmas in practice: a case of patient abuse, Am J Nurs 85:1233, Nov, 1985

Larson, DR: Ethics: Should anencephalic neonates be organ donors? AORN J 47(3):778, 1988

Northrop, CE, and Kelly, ME: Legal issues in nursing, St Louis, 1987, The CV Mosby Co

Penticuff, JH: Ethics in obstetric and gynecologic nursing, NAACOG update series, lesson 26, vol 1, 1984

Roland, R: Technology and motherhood: reproductive choice reconsidered, SIGNS 12(3):512, 1987

Shaffer, MK, and Pfeiffer, IL: Dilemmas in practice: nursing research and patients' rights, Am J Nurs 86:23, Jan, 1986

Smith, SJ, and Davis, AJ: Ethical dilemmas: conflict among rights, duties, and obligations, Am J Nurs 80:1463, Aug, 1980

Styles, M: On nursing, St Louis, 1982, The CV Mosby Co

Trandel-Korenchuk, D: Informed consent: client participation in childbirth decisions, JOGN Nurs 11:379, Nov-Dec, 1982

Swider, SM, Mcelmurry, BJ, and Yarling, RR: Ethical decision making in a bureaucratic context by senior nursing students, Nurs Res 34(2):109, 1985

Van Lier, DJ, and Roberts, JE: Promoting informed consent of women in labor, JOGN Nurs 15(5):419, 1986

CHAPTER

5

Nursing Research

Marianne K. Zalar

Learning Objectives

Correctly define the key terms listed.

Summarize why it is essential for the practicing nurse to be involved in clinical research.

Discuss four criteria for selecting research topics.

Explore the role of the nurse as a consumer of nursing research.

Formulate the kinds of questions a nurse needs to answer when evaluating a research study.

Identify at least one resource available to practicing nurses for assistance in evaluating published research studies.

Evaluate a published research study using Tanner's guidelines for evaluating nursing clinical research.

Examine the value of nursing research in nursing practice.

Assess the role of the nurse as a clinical researcher.

Key Terms

clinical nursing research
clinical relevance
collaborative research
conceptual utilization
consumer of research
evaluating research findings
external validity
generalizability of findings
implementation of findings
instrumental utilization
instrumentation
internal consistency
internal validity
replication of research
research utilization
sample
variable

Maternity and gynecologic nursing care traditionally has been based on empirical wisdom rather than on scientifically based research. The more nursing practice is based on nursing research, however, the higher the quality of the practice, thus making it imperative that practicing nurses be involved in clinical nursing research.

In past decades, nursing leaders have increasingly recognized that clinical nursing research is essential for advancing the profession and for resolving important client care questions (Lindeman, 1973). The nurse at the bedside (the clinician) is in the best position to identify researchable clinical problems, to collect research data as a part of practice, and to implement clinically significant findings (Zalar et al., 1985). In fact, *the clinician is the only one who can implement nursing research findings.*

Brown et al. (1984) analyzed 137 substantive studies published from 1952 to 1980 in 4 nursing research journals. They found that research studies related to clinical practice increased from 29% in 1952-53 to 63% in 1980. Of the 40 studies analyzed from 1980 research publications, 18% were in the speciality area of obstetrics and gynecology.

With the assistance of an experienced researcher, practicing maternity-gynecologic nurses can learn to translate clinical problems to researchable problems, design research proposals, analyze findings, critique research reports, and implement research projects and findings. Practicing nurses may never wish to become full-time nurse-researchers, but with the help of experienced researchers, they can do a great deal toward resolving the innumerable unanswered questions in clinical nursing.

MATERNITY-GYNECOLOGIC NURSES AS CLINICAL RESEARCHERS

Clinical research emerges from the needs of maternity-gynecologic clients. The wide variety of roles performed by maternity-gynecologic nurses facilitates the selection of research topics. Therefore the orientation toward nursing care provides the focus for clinical research, which is directed by the nurse's orientation as clinician, personal counselor, and health educator.

Nurses' primary orientation toward care rather than cure provides the framework for differentiating nursing research from medical research. Disease entities that provide the basis for medical clinical research are insufficient as study topics of nursing care research, because their study does not take into consideration the roles performed by nurses in practice. Ideally, nursing and medicine participate in collaborative research in which the nurse studies the care and cost components for a particular population of clients and the physician studies the cure components. Such interdisciplinary collaborative research has the potential for making impressive contributions to health care.

Purpose of Maternity and Gynecologic Nursing Research

Maternity and gynecologic nursing research is conducted to (1) gain a better understanding of biopsychosocial responses of pregnant women and new families, their newborn infants, and reproductive issues for women, (2) improve quality and decrease cost of nursing care, (3) improve nursing interventions, and (4) test nursing theories. The following examples of nursing research will demonstrate how maternity-gynecologic nurses have dealt with these issues.

Understanding Psychophysiologic Dynamics. In 1986 Blank explored early psychophysiologic mother-infant interaction. She measured the maternal anxiety and perception of infant satiety, anxiety, and feeding behavior of 65 healthy, postpartum, bottle-feeding mothers. She found a significant direct relationship between infant prefeed cortisol and postfeed glucose, but not between infant formula consumption and postfeed glucose. The mothers completed the Blank Infant Tenderness Scale and the State-Trait Anxiety Inventory. As a result, it was found that a relatively mild maternal anxiety at feeding time is associated with both increased formula intake and decreased postfeed cortisol. The decreased postfeed cortisol is indicative of a feeling of security.

A prefeed heel stick was performed for baseline serum glucose and cortisol. Another heel stick for serum glucose and cortisol was done at 1 hour postfeeding. Pearson correlations indicated a significant direct relationship between infant formula consumption and postfeed glucose.

The contribution of this type of research is important because nurses are responsible for assessing mother-infant relationships and identifying infant growth and development problems. They are in a position to scientifically assess the need for intervention in selected disruptive situations.

Quality and Cost of Care Issues. Measel and Anderson (1979) conducted a series of investigations in which restless premature infants developing intestinal distension would become relaxed and could be tube-fed successfully if allowed to suck on a pacifier during and after each feeding. A sample of 59 premature infants was randomly assigned to treatment and control groups. Treated infants showed readiness for bottle feeding 3.4 days earlier than the control group and were discharged 4 days sooner. Findings were identical with regard to weight gain and readiness for bottle feeding when the study was replicated. The 30 infants in this replicated study were discharged 8 days sooner than the control group.

The actual cost savings were reported to be $104,000. The implications nationally for cost saving from this seemingly simple nursing intervention are staggering.

The purpose of nursing research is to document the benefits of alternative models of treatment and care, providing the alternative is truly substitutive and not additive (Fagin, 1982). This study is a dramatic example of nursing research impacting quality of care with resulting cost savings.

Improving Nursing Interventions. A study to investigate prevention and control of postpartum breast engorgement was done by comparing four treatments: compression binder, standardized support bra, fluid limitation, and a pharmacologic preparation (Brooten et al., 1983). The researchers found that women using the pharmacologic preparation experienced less breast engorgement, pain, and leaking of colostrum and milk than did women in any of the nonpharmacologic treatment groups. In addition, it was found that the highest incidence of breast pain occurred between the third and fifth days postpartum regardless of the treatment used.

These kinds of studies demonstrate the importance for the nurse of constantly reviewing and evaluating nursing policies and procedures. As stated in the introduction, nursing practice must be based on scientific research rather than on empirical wisdom. At the same time, however, it is important to remember that the experience alone of expert maternity-gynecologic nurses can generate important research questions.

Testing Theories. The research on maternal handling patterns originated with Rubin (1963), who observed postpartum mothers handling their newborn infants. Rubin reported that the mothers initially used their fingertips when handling their newborns; only after several days did they use their palms; and later they used their arms and upper torsos. Tulman (1985) tested this theory by studying the pattern of newborn handling by 36 newly delivered women during their infants' first postpartum bedside visit and the pattern of newborn handling by 36 female nursing students at the beginning of their first clinical day in a hospital normal newborn nursery. The sequence of use of fingers, palms, arms, and trunk was different for mothers and students. Although the mothers did not follow the sequence of handling reported in the literature, the students did, thus casting doubt on the specificity of a pattern of maternal handling of the newborn infant as a means of assessing maternal attachment.

The findings from this study demonstrate the importance of testing nursing theories. Certainly the findings from one study neither support nor negate a theory; however, they do provide the direction for future study. Collaboration between nursing clinicians and theorists plays an important role in the enhancement of the nursing profession.

Clinical Problems

The standard definition of a problem is a question raised for inquiry, consideration, or solution; a source of perplexity, distress, or vexation. Diers (1971) has defined a problem as a "difference between two states of affairs, a discrepancy between the way things are and the way they ought to be, or between two sets of facts, or what one knows and what one needs to know to eliminate the problem." Problems may be expressed as concerns, gripes, or hunches. A problem becomes important in maternity-gynecologic nursing when the discrepancy between the way things are and the way they should be makes a difference in client care.

To analyze a problem for its researchability, first identify the problem (gripe, concern, or hunch), then identify the scope of the discrepancy between what is and what ought to be, and finally, identify the potential consequence for client care of resolving the problem. If the discrepancy between the way things are and the way they ought to be is great enough, a research topic has emerged.

Research Topics

Following are four criteria for selecting research topics (Diers, 1971):

1. *Is the problem researchable?* The issue must be a question of facts. An opinion question, that is, one that can be answered by yes or no, is not answerable by scientific research.
2. *Does the nurse have access and control over the phenomenon in question?* The nurse evaluates the question for availability of research subjects and control over implementation of findings from the study. It would be inappropriate for a nurse to design a research protocol to study a treatment regimen that is controlled by the physician or that requires an unavailable sample of clients. For example, the nurse who wants to study the effect of prenatal education on length of labor may not have access to pregnant clients of certain physicians.
3. *Is the question of sufficient importance and magnitude?* Research takes time. The nurse must consider whether the personal, economic, and time commitments are warranted. In addition, the nurse analyzes the question for scope and importance. For example, is the question too broad to study in a reasonable period? Will the findings make a difference in client care?
4. *Are methods available for studying the problem?* The nurse must be able to translate the problem into measurable terms. In addition, to learn if differences exist between groups or treatments being studied, the measurable variables must be narrow enough to be manipulated.

Nursing Diagnoses. A study topic can appropriately emerge from a nursing diagnosis, which is a clinical nursing judgment about an individual, family, or community that is derived through a deliberate, systematic process of data collection and analysis. It emphasizes clients and their potential or actual health problems. The nursing diagnosis focuses on the nurse's and client's goals for the client or family in relation to the delivery of care. It provides the basis for prescriptions for definitive therapy that nurses, by virtue of their education and experience, are capable and licensed to provide and for which the nurse is accountable. It is expressed concisely, and it includes the cause of the condition when known. Because diagnoses, therapy, and outcomes are interrelated, the nursing diagnosis provides an ideal focus for process, outcome, process-outcome, or related studies.

Examples of nursing diagnoses that may become research topics for maternity-gynecologic nurses are listed below:

1. Pain related to perineal repair (e.g., episiotomy). Potential research question related to comparing hot and cold sitz baths for comfort.
2. Potential for injury related to initiation of breast-feeding. Potential research question related to length of time the infant is at the breast during each feeding in the first 24 hours and the incidence of fissures on the nipples and degree of sore nipples.
3. Potential for stress incontinence related to poor perineal muscle tone. Potential research question related to stress incontinence and the use of Kegel's exercises.

4. Anxiety related to lack of knowledge about surgical procedures (hysterectomy). Potential research question related to group versus individual teaching at a hospital or clinic and degree of expressed anxiety.
5. Potential for impaired skin integrity of healthy term newborns related to type (e.g. pH) of soap used. Potential research question related to the presence of skin rash and the use of two more types of soap.
6. Potential for ineffective thermoregulation related to method of temperature assessment used. Potential research question comparing axillary and rectal temperatures.

Other Sources. Several other sources may be used for study topics:

1. *Nursing functions.* The introduction of diagnosis related groups (DRGs) has made nurses' documentation of clients' daily nursing resource requirements imperative for maintaining the nursing department's standards of care. Areas for nursing research include documentation of the average time for nursing functions such as teaching breast feeding, performing nonstress tests, and initial ambulation after delivery.
2. *Input from clients.* Clients and their families may also provide valuable input when a clinical research proposal is being designed. Areas for nursing research could include accommodations for labor and recovery, methods of assisting with loss and grief, and involvement with self-medication postpartum.
3. *Outcome measures in home care.* Clients are being discharged earlier and sicker than in the past. As a result, home care has become an important issue for maternity-gynecologic nurses. Areas for nursing research include the impact of home care services, the relationship of the nursing process to nursing outcomes, evaluation of quality of nursing care, and quality of life as an outcome measure.

MATERNITY-GYNECOLOGIC NURSES AS RESEARCH CONSUMERS

As consumers of research, clinicians read research reports to determine the scientific merit and clinical utility of the studies and apply research findings where appropriate. Mallick (1983) believes that the role of the research consumer depends on the nurse's appreciation of the importance of the role, understanding of the research process, and ability to critically analyze research with clinical application as the goal. Nurses who critique nursing research learn that few research studies are without flaws. In addition, they learn that gaining an adequate understanding of a clinical phenomenon may require investigation of a number and variety of additional research studies.

Tanner (1987) developed an effective set of pragmatic guidelines for clinicians to use for evaluating research for use in practice. These guidelines, which are divided into five steps, emphasize the potential utility in clinical practice, the critical components of scientific merit, and practical considerations. The evaluator is directed to answer a series of questions for each of the five steps relevant to the study, followed by a decision based on the response to the questions. These decision points are of particular value to the busy clinician because if the study does not meet certain criteria, the reader may elect not to continue with the evaluation.

Potential Utility in Clinical Practice

Research might be used for *instrumental utilization* or for *conceptual utilization* (Caplan and Rich, 1975) (see box below). Instrumental utilization refers to cases in which the user can describe the specific way in which the research knowledge is being used for decision making. Conceptual utilization refers to the influence of one or more studies on a decision maker's thinking about an issue, without putting the information to any specific, documented use.

For example, a maternity nurse who works on a postpartum unit and is concerned about finding an improved intervention for reducing breast pain and engorgement in

CRITERIA FOR EVALUATING A STUDY FOR CLINICAL RELEVANCE*

1. What was the problem that was studied? Does this study have the potential to help solve a problem that you currently face in your practice?
2. Does the study have the potential to help you with any of the following types of decisions?
   a. Deciding on appropriate observations to make in order to rule in or rule out particular diagnoses
   b. Identifying the extent to which patients may be at risk for certain problems or complications
   c. Deciding on the intervention most likely to produce desired outcomes, reduce the probability of complications, or both
3. Is a theory or proposition that might serve to guide practice tested by the study? What kinds of decisions might be guided by this theory?
4. Did the investigator test an intervention in this study? If yes, describe the intervention. Do you see the potential for using the intervention in your practice? Consider the following: (a) under nursing control and (b) feasible in your setting, given staffing patterns and cost constraints.
5. How did the investigator measure the dependent variables or outcomes? Do you see the potential for using any of these measures in your practice? Consider the following: (a) under nursing control, (b) would be of assistance to nurses in their assessment of patients or evaluation of outcomes, and (c) feasible in your setting, given staffing patterns and cost constraints.

Decision Point

If the answer to any *one* of questions 1 to 5 is yes, then the study deserves further consideration. It has potential for use in practice. If you answered no to *all* of the questions, then the study is probably not relevant to your practice and there is no need to evaluate it further (unless you are reviewing the study for other reasons).

*From Tanner, CA: Heart Lung, 16(4):424, 1987.

non-breast-feeding mothers would be reviewing research findings for instrumental utilization.

On the other hand, a nursing student during the maternity rotation who wants to learn more about parenting roles would check the course reading list and read the listed report of a study that attempted to determine how closely a group of new parents' anticipated roles matched their actual involvement in parenting, as measured by the amount of time spent in various activities with their infants (Humenick and Bugen, 1987). Conceptual utilization is the intent of this type of evaluation because the student wants to learn more about childbearing families and does not necessarily want to change nursing practice.

Critical Components of Scientific Merit

After particular studies have been judged clinically relevant, they are evaluated for scientific merit. The areas to be evaluated include conceptualization and internal consistency (see box below), methodologic rigor, and generalizability.

Conceptualization and Internal Consistency. According to Tanner (1987):

> The conceptualization ought to make sense to clinicians who wish to use the study in their practice and it ought to provide the basis for the study design and reporting of findings. The results ought to be reported in a way that clearly addresses the research question. In short, the report should make sense and hang together.

For example, in the study of breast pain and engorgement of nonnursing mothers carried out in a sample of 68 newly delivered women, the investigators compared the four treatments by measuring changes that directly pertained to the conceptualization of the problem and were easy for clinicians to observe. They measured chest circumference, increased breast-tissue tension, extension of engorgement into the axilla, pain experienced, amount of pain relief sought, and leakage of colostrum or milk.

Methodologic Rigor. If the study has demonstrated conceptual and internal consistency, the review of the study for methodologic rigor is the next step in the process (see box, p. 71, at left). There are two major areas for evaluation: *internal validity* and *methodologic soundness.*

Internal validity answers the question of whether the experimental treatment made a difference in the specific experimental instance. Campbell and Stanley (1963) identified eight different classes of extraneous variables that might produce effects that confound the effect of the experimental stimulus. These classes of extraneous variables are discussed in every basic research textbook and are worth reviewing by maternity-gynecologic nurses who evaluate nursing research studies.

The methodology section of a research report includes the sample, instrumentation, and analysis.

1. *Sample* is a subset of the population selected in the data source. When the sample is too small or is not selected randomly, the validity of the findings are negatively affected.
2. *Instrumentation* is the mechanism used to measure the independent or dependent variable(s) in a research study. Instruments are investigator-developed—questionnaire, an open-ended interview guide, or a standardized test (e.g., laboratory test results, IQ test). Documentation of the validity and reliability of the instruments in the methods section of the report enhances credibility of the findings. Unless evaluators are familiar with the particular instrument used in the study, they cannot know whether the instrument is accurate and stable or whether it measures what it claims to measure.
3. *Analysis* is used to report the findings. Descriptive and inferential statistical techniques are most commonly used in research report analysis. A statistician or nurse researcher may be needed to help interpret findings when complex statistics are used in a study.

Generalizability of Results. As stated earlier, internal validity asks the question whether the experimental treatments made a difference. External validity asks the question of *generalizability:* To what populations, settings, treatment variables, and measurement variables can this effect be generalized (Campbell and Stanley, 1963)? This is an important question for the maternity-gynecologic nurse who considers changing nursing practice as a result of research

CRITERIA FOR EVALUATION OF SCIENTIFIC MERIT: CONCEPTUALIZATION AND INTERNAL CONSISTENCY*

1. Overall, does the report hang together and make sense to you?
2. Does the underlying conceptualization make sense? Specifically:
   a. Is there justification for the study?
   b. Do the study questions relate to the justification?
3. Overall, do the methods fit with the conceptualization or justification for the study and with the study questions in the following areas: (a) subjects and setting, (b) sampling procedures, (c) instruments, (d) procedures, and (e) analysis?
4. Do the investigators answer the questions that they posed?

Decision Point

If there are major conceptual problems (e.g., the underlying justification doesn't make sense) or if there is no internal consistency in the report (i.e., the methods do not fit with the conceptualization or the research questions are not adequately or properly addressed), then you have several possible options: (1) to continue with more detailed evaluation of the study, hoping that additional reading will clarify the confusing aspects of the report; (2) to seek consultation from a person with some expertise in research methods who may be able to clarify some of your questions; or (3) to evaluate the report no further, because it is sufficiently confusing that its usefulness in practice is jeopardized.

*From Tanner, CA: Heart Lung, 16(4):424, 1987.

CRITERIA FOR EVALUATION OF SCIENTIFIC MERIT: BELIEVABILITY OF RESULTS*

The questions that follow are screening questions and serve to alert the reader to major methodologic issues:

1. Are the methods used likely to lead to believable, internally valid results? Specifically:
   a. What subjects were studied and how were they selected? If a convenience sample was used, did the investigator control for sample characteristics that might influence the results of the study?
   b. If an intervention was tested with different treatment groups, were the subjects randomly assigned to these groups? If not, did the investigator control for possible initial differences between the groups?
   c. Does the author discuss reliability of the measures? Is reliability satisfactory?
   d. Does the author discuss validity of the measures? Are you confident of the instrument validity?
2. Are the conclusions drawn by the author based on the data presented and believable in light of the methods used? Specifically:
   a. Does the author stay within the boundaries indicated by the subjects, the types of interventions attempted, and the measures used?
   b. If there were statistically significant findings (e.g., a positive correlation between two variables, a difference between two treatment groups), does the author have a reasonable explanation? Based on your knowledge and experience, what other explanation might there be for these results?
   c. If the findings were not as expected or were not statistically significant, does the author provide a reasonable explanation? Could any of the following be possible explanations for these results: small sample size, invalid or insensitive measures, an unusually heterogeneous sample, or an insufficiently strong intervention?

Decision Point

The set of questions in item 1, above, identify critical issues in methodology. If any one of these aspects is not adequately addressed in the research report, it *may* be grounds for the reader to decide on nonutilization—depending on the risk involved in using the results and depending on the availability of other studies that corroborate the results of this study.

If the methodologic issues in item 1 are adequately addressed, the reader then evaluates whether the conclusions drawn are appropriate. There frequently will be explanations or conclusions other than those which the author provides; negative review on this aspect is not sufficient by itself to decide on nonutilization. However, if results can be clearly attributed to factors other than those raised in the original research question, additional caution in using the study is warranted.

*From Tanner, CA: Heart Lung, 16(4):424, 1987.

SCIENTIFIC MERIT: GENERALIZABILITY OF THE RESULTS*

1. Is the sample and setting similar or dissimilar to the sample and setting to which you wish to generalize (target population)?
2. Have other studies been conducted that address the same problem, test the same intervention, evaluate the same measure, or test the same theory (replications)? Were the results similar to the results obtained in the present study?

Decision Point

In the ideal situation, there will be considerable similarity between the study sample and the target population, *and* the study will have been replicated. The nurse can have confidence in the study findings and have more confidence in using the study in his or her practice. More frequently, one or both of the criteria are not met. If, however, the study has met other criteria, and if it is possible to systematically evaluate the use of the study in practice, then utilization is recommended. Failure to meet the criteria of generalizability, alone, is not sufficient justification for a nonutilization decision.

*From Tanner, CA: Heart Lung, 16(4):424, 1987.

findings (see box above). There must be some degree of certainty that clients will respond to the treatment in the same way as the subjects in the reported study.

Sample size, randomization, and representativeness are key issues in making this determination. The degree of certainty is greatly increased if the clients for whom the change is intended have the same characteristics as the study sample (representativeness), if the study sample was randomly selected (everyone in the population had an equal chance of being selected), and if the sample size was large enough to predict a relationship between the experimental treatment and client outcome.

Regretfully, few clinical nursing studies have a sufficient sample size or have a randomly selected sample. For example, it is difficult to obtain a random sample of laboring women because of the inability to control when a woman's labor will begin. Therefore, since most clinical studies use convenient samples, it becomes necessary to increase sample size to obtain credibility.

Another mechanism for increasing credibility and generalizability of research findings is through *replication.* Replication is accomplished by repeating the exact same study with a representative sample. The more often the study is replicated with the same findings the greater the probability that the findings are credible.

Practical Considerations

After the clinician has determined that a study has instrumental or conceptual potential for utilization and has met the criteria for scientific merit, there are some practical

OTHER FACTORS TO CONSIDER IN UTILIZATION*

Instructions

The following questions can be addressed either from the standpoint of the individual nurse's making a judgment as to whether to use research in the care of a particular patient or from the standpoint of instituting a major change in practice throughout the institution. If the intended scope is the latter, then the reader will need to anticipate a major effort in planning, with involvement of multiple group. In either case, the following questions must be addressed before the research base is implemented in practice:

1. What is the feasibility of doing systematic evaluation of the research-based practice?
2. What is the risk of changing practice based on the research?
3. As important as the preceding considerations, what is the risk of maintaining current practice (i.e., not trying the practice suggested by the research)?
4. What is the cost of changing practice on the basis of this research?
5. What are the benefits of changing practice?

Decision Point

If the benefits outweigh the costs, the risks are minimal, and it is feasible to systematically evaluate the outcomes, even with a single patient, then it is appropriate to proceed to use the research in clinical practice. This is true even if not all the criteria for scientific merit have been met. If costs or risks are high, and if some aspect of scientific merit is questionable, then additional research should be conducted before practice is changed on the basis of the research.

*From Tanner, CA: Heart Lung, 16(4):424, 1987.

issues that must be considered before implementation of the intervention. The first issue is the risk and cost/benefit ratio. Preparation and number of staff, based on type and number of antepartum and postpartum mothers is an important issue. The second issue is systematic evaluation, the importance of which in nursing clinical practice cannot be overemphasized.

In summary, the guidelines for evaluating research findings provide a valuable tool for busy clinicians to review nursing research as a basis for maternity and gynecologic nursing practice. A review of the literature, however, may not yield adequate studies to provide the necessary basis for changing practice. Therefore to answer the clinical question, the nurse may need to replicate a study or conduct a new study.

RESEARCH-RELATED ACTIVITIES

The combined efforts of clinicians, administrators, managers, and researchers are necessary to conduct clinical research and to utilize findings in the clinical setting. The nursing administrator plays an important role in facilitating clinical research by legitimizing clinicians' research activities. The nurse manager plays the key role in both the conduct of research and utilization of research findings. A manager who is committed to research as an integral component of practice encourages staff nurses on the unit, arranges scheduling so staff nurses can attend research courses, is actively involved in the identification of practice-relevant research problems, and facilitates policy and procedure changes when indicated by the research findings.

SUMMARY

Nurse-clinicians have the greatest responsibility to the profession of nursing because of their impact on quality health care provided to clients and their families. Clinical research as an integral component of nursing care provides a mechanism for making changes in care. Nurse faculty, nurse administrators, and nurse-researchers must provide the assistance necessary for nurses to base practice on sound scientific theories.

KEY CONCEPTS

- The more nursing practice is based on nursing research, the higher the quality of the practice.
- The nurse at the bedside is in the best position to identify researchable clinical problems, to collect research data as a part of practice, and to implement clinically significant findings.
- The clinician is the only one who can implement nursing research findings.
- The wide variety of roles performed by maternity-gynecologic nurses in relation to the client facilitate the selection of research topics.
- Nurses' primary orientation toward care rather than cure provides the framework for differentiating nursing research from medical research.
- A problem becomes important when the discrepancy between the way things are and the way they should be make a difference in client care.
- As consumers of research, clinicians read research reports to determine the scientific merit and clinical utility of the studies and apply research findings where appropriate.
- Evaluating research findings provides a valuable tool for busy clinicians to review nursing research as a basis for maternity and gynecologic nursing practice.
- The combined efforts of clinicians, administrators, managers, and researchers are necessary to conduct clinical research to utilize findings in the clinical setting.

STUDY QUESTIONS AND ACTIVITIES

1. Select a nursing diagnosis and—
   a. Identify an area for a potential research study
   b. Review the literature to learn if the identified area has been researched
   c. If studies have been done, select one of the studies and evaluate it using Tanner's guidelines.

2. Review at least two studies using Tanner's guidelines for evaluating clinical research studies.
3. Attend at least one hospital inservice education program that focuses on intended changes in either policy or procedures where nursing research findings have played a role in decision making.

References

Blank, DM: Relating mothers' anxiety and perception to infant satiety, anxiety, and feeding behavior, Nurs Res 35(6):327, 1986

Brooten, DA, Brown, LP, Hollingsworth, AO, et al: A comparison of four treatments to prevent and control breast pain and engorgement in nonnursing mothers, Nurs Res 32(4):225, 1983

Brown, JS, Tanner, CA, and Padrick, KP: Nursing's search for scientific knowledge, Nurs Res 33(1):26, 1984

Campbell, DT, and Stanley, JC: Experimental and quasi-experimental designs for research, Chicago, 1963, Rand McNally College Publishing Co

Caplan, N, and Rich, RF: The use of social science knowledge in policy decisions at the national level, Ann Arbor, 1975, Institute for Social Research, University of Michigan

Diers, D: Finding clinical problems for study, J Nurs Adm 1(15):15, 1971

Fagin, CM: The economic value of nursing research, Am J Nurs 12(12):1844, 1982

Humenick, SS, and Bugen, LA: Parenting roles: expectation versus reality, MCN 12(1):36, 1987

Lindeman, CA: Nursing research: a visible, viable component of nursing practice, J Nurs Adm 3(92):18, 1973

Mallick, MJ: A constant comparative method for teaching research critique to baccalaureate nursing students, Image 15(4):120, 1983

Measel, CP, and Anderson, GC: Nonnutritive sucking during tube feeding: effect on clinical course in premature infants, JOGN Nurs 8(5):265, 1979

Rubin, R: Maternal touch, Nurs Outlook 11:828, 1963

Tanner, CA: Evaluating research for use in practice: guideline for the clinician, Heart Lung, 16(4):424, 1987

Tulman, LJ: Mothers' and unrelated persons' initial handling of newborn infants, Nurs Res 34(4):205, 1985

Zalar, MK, Welches, LJ, and Walker, DD: Nursing consortium approach to increase research in service settings, J Nurs Adm 15(7):36, 1985

Bibliography

Brink, PJ, and Wood, MJ: Basic steps in planning nursing research, North Scituate, Mass, 1978, Duxbury Press

Fox, DJ: Fundamentals of research in nursing, New York, 1966, Appleton-Century Crofts

Gordon, M: Determining study topics, Nurs Res 29(2):83, 1980

Kaempfer, SH: A care orientation to clinical nursing research, Oncol Nurs Forum 9(4):36, 1982

Nurses Association of the American College of Obstetrics and Gynecology: Model for utilization of NAACOG standards, 1977, NAACOG Committee on Practice

Nurses Association of the American College of Obstetrics and Gynecology: 1986: standards for obstetrics and gynecology, ed 3, 1986, NAACOG Ad Hoc Committee to Revise Standards

Treece, EW, and Treece, JW, Jr: Elements of research in nursing, ed 4, St Louis, 1986, The CV Mosby Co

Polit, D, and Hungler, B: Nursing research: principles and methods, ed 3, Philadelphia, 1987, JB Lippincott Co

Waltz, C, and Bausell, RB: Nursing research: design, statistics, and computer analysis, Philadelphia, 1981, FA Davis Co

Wilson, HS: Research in nursing, Menlo Park, Calif, 1985, Addison-Wesley Publishing Co, Inc

Wilson, HS: Introducing research in nursing, Menlo Park, Calif, 1987, Addison-Wesley Publishing Co, Inc

Woods, NF, and Catanzaro, M: Nursing research: theory and practice, St Louis, 1988, The CV Mosby Co

UNIT

II

Human Reproductive System

Human sexuality pervades all our perceptions and affects our responses throughout life. Each person's sexual potential develops through an interplay of cultural, familial, and personal effects on inherited and biologic entities. Chapter 6 is concerned with the biologic components of human sexuality over the life span. This chapter also includes a section on immunity to emphasize the importance of this body system in youth and age. Chapter 7 focuses on the psychosocial aspects of human sexuality, the origins of each person's sexual identity, and the developmental tasks of key periods in the life of the child, adolescent, and adult. Chapter 8 emphasizes the importance of the gynecologic examination in the care of clients before, during, and after their reproductive years.

CHAPTER 6

Anatomy and Physiology

Learning Objectives

Correctly define the key terms listed.

Identify the internal, external, and accessory structures of both the female and male reproductive tracts.

Explain the functions of the structures of both the female and male reproductive tracts.

Summarize the menstrual cycle in relation to hormonal response, ovarian response, and endometrial response.

Discuss the clinical significance of human sexual response.

Compare the sexual response cycle of the female and male as related to comparable reproductive structures of each.

Review expected changes in the reproductive structures over the life span of a woman.

List six physiologic defense mechanisms that comprise the body's first line of defense.

Differentiate between naturally acquired and artificially acquired immunity.

Compare and contrast T lymphocyte response and B lymphocyte response.

Relate factors affecting the functioning of the immune defense system.

Key Terms

acquired immunity
allergic response
B lymphocyte response
climacteric
complement cascade
endometrial cycle
hypothalamic-pituitary cycle
interferon
living ligature
menarche
menopause
menstruation
mittelschmerz
myotonia
orgasm
ovarian cycle
ovulation
particularistic immunity
prostaglandins
pubarche
spinnbarkheit
squamocolumnar junction
T lymphocyte response
universalistic immunity
vasocongestion
withdrawal bleeding

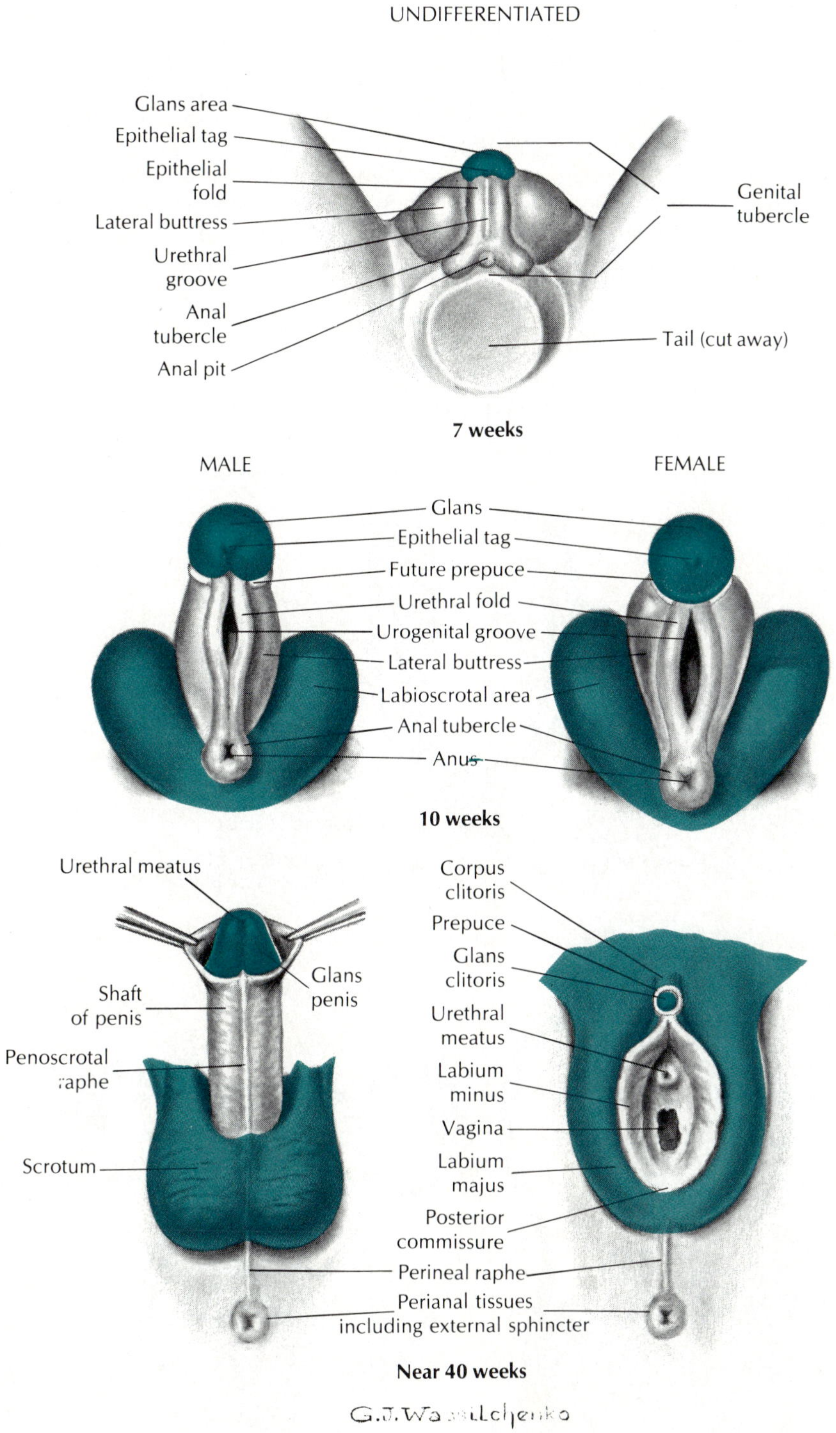
UNDIFFERENTIATED
Glans area
Epithelial tag
Epithelial fold
Lateral buttress
Urethral groove
Anal tubercle
Anal pit
Genital tubercle
Tail (cut away)
7 weeks
MALE
FEMALE
Glans
Epithelial tag
Future prepuce
Urethral fold
Urogenital groove
Lateral buttress
Labioscrotal area
Anal tubercle
Anus
10 weeks
Urethral meatus
Glans penis
Shaft of penis
Penoscrotal raphe
Scrotum
Corpus clitoris
Prepuce
Glans clitoris
Urethral meatus
Labium minus
Vagina
Labium majus
Posterior commissure
Perineal raphe
Perianal tissues including external sphincter
Near 40 weeks

Fig. 6-1 Homologues of external genitals.

Nurses providing maternity-gynecologic health care to women require a greater depth and breadth of knowledge of female anatomy and physiology than is usually taught in general courses. Often, the reproductive tract, including the breasts, is the last system taught, if there is time. Knowledge of the anatomy and physiology of the structures, both female and male, involved in reproduction is basic to planning for, implementing, and evaluating nursing care of the maternity-gynecologic client and her family.

Although the female and male reproductive systems differ markedly in appearance, their structures are homologous (having the same embryonic origin) (Figs. 6-1 and 6-2). Each structure performs a vital role in the continuation of the human species and the generation and maintenance of secondary sexual characteristics. Through hormonal influences the genitals, pelvis, and breasts acquire the unique adaptations necessary to childbearing. Both female and male reproductive systems consist of the following four principal components:

1. External genitals
2. A pair of primary sex glands (gonads)
3. Ducts leading from the gonads to the body's exterior
4. Secondary (accessory) sex glands

In the usual course of events, life begins and is sustained for 9 months within the protective environment of the female. Therefore the female reproductive system will be considered first, beginning with the external genital structures.

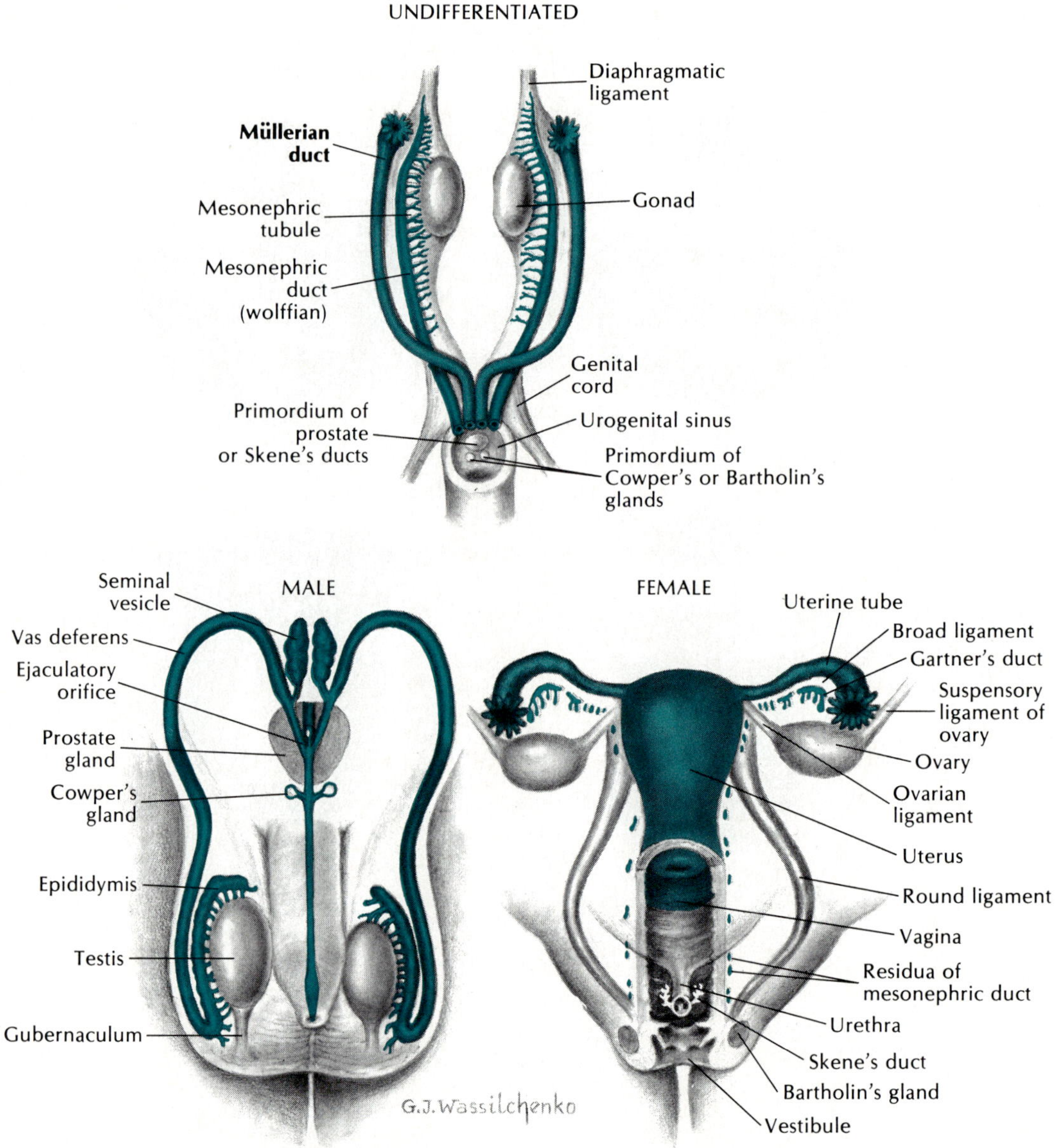

Fig. 6-2 Homologues of internal genitals.

FEMALE REPRODUCTIVE SYSTEM

The female reproductive system consists of internal organs, located in the pelvic cavity and supported by the pelvic floor, and external genitals, located in the perineum. The female's internal and external reproductive structures develop and mature in response to estrogens and progesterones, starting in fetal life and continuing through puberty and throughout the childbearing years. The reproductive structures atrophy (decrease in size) with age or a drop in ovarian hormone production. An extensive and complex innervation and a generous blood supply support the functions of these structures. The appearance of the external genitals varies greatly from woman to woman, since the size, shape, and color are determined by heredity, age, and race and the number of children a woman has borne.

External Structures

The external female genitals (vulva, pudenda) are located in the perineum. The external structures are presented in the following order:

1. Mons pubis (mons veneris)
2. Labia majora (sing., labium majus) and minora (sing., labium minus)
3. Clitoris
4. Prepuce of clitoris
5. Vestibule
   a. Urethral or urinary orifice (meatus)
   b. Lesser vestibular, paraurethral, or Skene's glands
   c. Hymen and vaginal introitus, or orifice
   d. Greater vestibular, vulvovaginal, or Bartholin's glands
6. Fourchette
7. Perineum

The external genitals are illustrated in Fig. 6-3.

Mons Pubis. The mons pubis, or mons veneris, is the rounded, soft fullness of subcutaneous fatty tissue and loose connective tissue over the symphysis pubis. It contains many sebaceous (oil) glands and develops coarse, dark, curly hair at pubarche, about 1 to 2 years before the onset of the menses. Menarche occurs on the average at 13 years of age. In 75% of women the pattern of hair growth (the escutcheon) is a triangular shape with the base along the top of the symphysis pubis. The escutcheon in males is more diamond shaped. In 25% of women, pubic hair extends upward toward the umbilicus along the linea alba. Characteristics of pubic hair vary from sparse and fine among Oriental women to thick, coarse, and curly among black women. The functions of the mons are to play a role in sensuality and to protect the symphysis pubis during coitus.

Labia Majora. The labia majora are two rounded

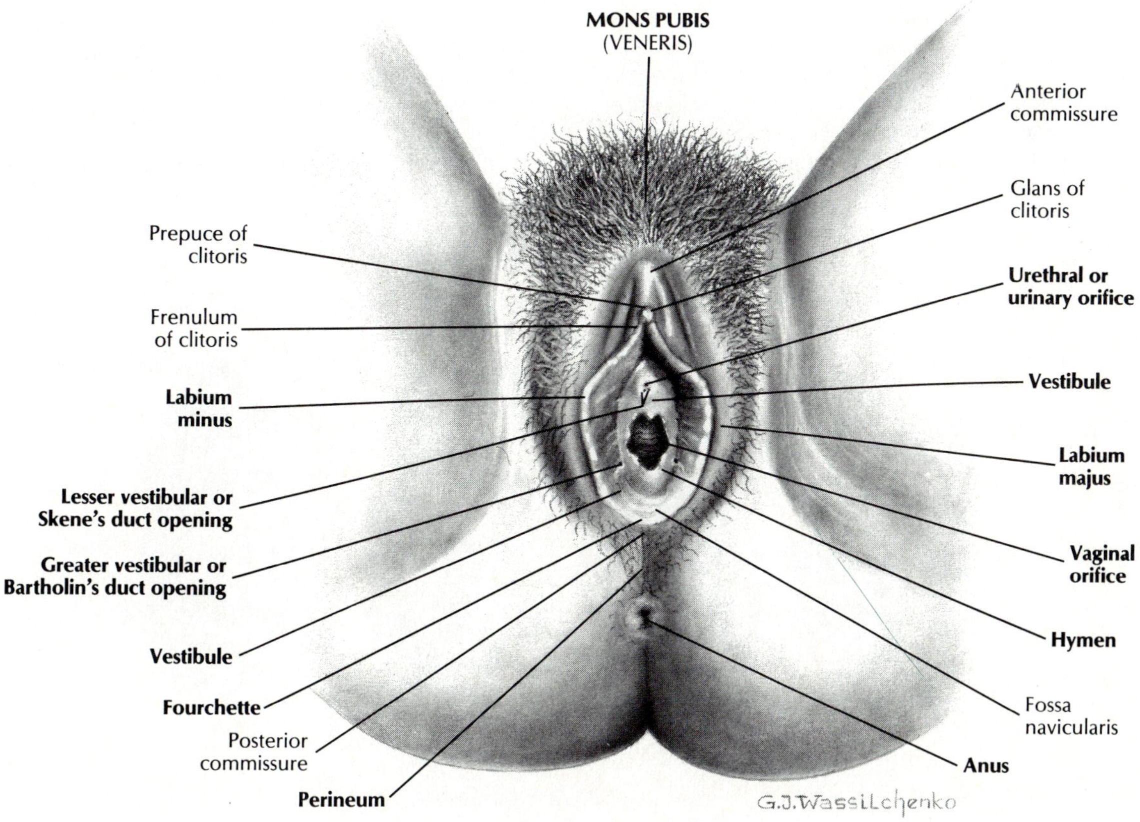

Fig. 6-3 External female genitals.

lengthwise folds of skin-covered fat and connective tissue that merge with the mons. They extend from the mons downward around the labia minora, ending in the perineum in the midline. The labia majora function as protection for the labia minora, urinary meatus, and vaginal introitus. In the woman who has never experienced vaginal childbirth the labia majora come together in the midline, obscuring the vaginal introitus. Some labial separation and even gaping of the vaginal introitus follow childbirth and perineal or vaginal injury.

On their lateral surfaces the labial skin is thick, usually pigmented darker than the surrounding tissues, and covered with coarse hair (similar to that of the mons) that thins out toward the perineum. The medial (inner) surfaces of the labia majora are smooth, thick, and without hair. They contain an abundant supply of sebaceous glands and sweat glands and are highly vascular. The extreme sensitivity of the labia majora to touch, pain, and temperature is caused by the extensive network of nerves; thus they function during sensual arousal.

Labia Minora. The labia minora, located between the labia majora, are narrow, lengthwise folds of hairless skin extending downward from beneath the clitoris and merging with the fourchette. Whereas the lateral and anterior aspects of the labia are usually pigmented, their medial surfaces are similar to vaginal mucosa: pink and moist. Their rich vascularity gives them a reddish color and permits marked turgescence (swelling) of the labia minora with emotional or physical stimulation. The glands in the labia minora also lubricate the vulva. A rich nerve supply makes them sensitive, enhancing their erotic function. The space between the labia minora is called the vestibule.

Clitoris. The clitoris is a short, cylindric, erectile organ fixed just beneath the arch of the pubis; the visible portion is about 6 × 6 mm or less in the unaroused state. The tip of the clitoral body is called the glans and is more sensitive than its shaft. In healthy women the length of the clitoral body varies from 2 mm to 1 cm, and the width is usually estimated at 4 to 5 mm. When sexually aroused, the glans and shaft increase in size.

Sebaceous glands of the clitoris secrete smegma, a fatty substance with a distinctive odor, which serves as a pheromone (an organic compound that provides communication with other members of the same species to elicit a certain response, which in this case is erotic stimulation of the human male). The term *clitoris* comes from a Greek word meaning "key" because the clitoris was seen as the key to female sexuality.

Its rich vascularity and innervation make the clitoris highly sensitive to temperature, touch, and pressure sensation. The clitoris contains more nerve endings than does its male homologue, the glans penis. Its main function is to stimulate and elevate levels of sexual tension.

Prepuce of Clitoris. Near the anterior junction the right and left labia minora separate into medial and lateral portions. The lateral portions unite above the clitoris to form its prepuce, a hoodlike covering; the medial portions unite below the clitoris to form its frenulum. Sometimes the prepuce covers the clitoris. As a result this area has the appearance of an opening that can be mistaken for the urethral meatus if the nurse does not identify vulvar structures carefully. Attempts to insert a catheter into this sensitive area can cause considerable discomfort.

Vestibule. The vestibule is an ovoid or boat-shaped area formed between the labia minora, clitoris, and fourchette. The vestibule contains the openings to the urethra, paraurethral (lesser vestibular, Skene's) glands, the vagina, and the paravaginal (greater vestibular, vulvovaginal, or Bartholin's) glands. The thin, almost mucosal, surface of the vestibule is easily irritated by chemicals (feminine deodorant sprays, bubble bath salts), heat, discharges, and friction (tight jeans).

Although not a true part of the reproductive system, the *urinary* (urethral) *meatus* is considered here because of

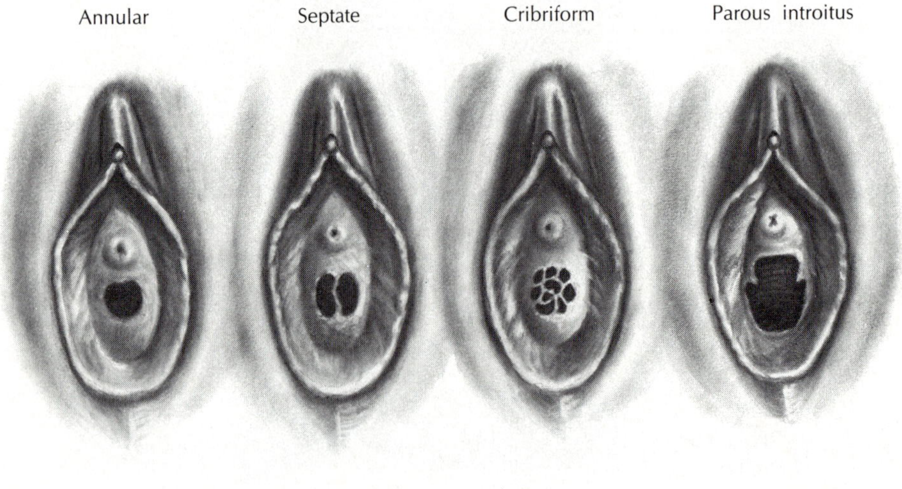

Fig. 6-4 Hymen and parous introitus.

its closeness and relationship to the vulva. The meatus is a pink or reddened opening of varying shapes, often with slightly puckered margins. The meatus marks the terminal, or distal, part of the urethra. It is usually located about 2.5 cm (1 in) below the clitoris.

The *lesser vestibular* (paraurethral, Skene's) *glands* are short tubular structures situated posterolaterally just inside the urethral meatus, at about the 5 and 7 o'clock positions around the meatus. They produce a small amount of mucus, which functions as lubrication.

The *hymen* (Fig. 6-4) is a partial, rarely complete, elastic but tough mucosa-covered fold around the *vaginal introitus.* In virginal females the hymen may be an impediment to vaginal examination, insertion of menstrual tampons, or coitus. The hymen may be elastic and allow distension, or it may be torn easily. Occasionally the hymen covers the orifice completely, resulting in an imperforate hymen that prevents passage of menstrual flow, instrumentation (e.g., with a speculum), or coitus. A hymenotomy may be necessary in some cases. After instrumentation, use of tampons, coitus, or vaginal delivery, residual tags of the hymen (hymenal caruncles or carunculae myrtiformes) may be seen.

One common myth is that one can tell by the condition of the hymen whether a female is a virgin. Sexually active and even parous females may have intact hymens. For other women the hymen may be torn during strenuous physical work or exercise, masturbation, or use of tampons. Some cultural groups cleanse the infant girl so vigorously that the hymen is torn, leaving only vaginal tags in its place. Therefore the "test for virginity"—evidence of bleeding following sexual intercourse—is an unreliable criterion.

The *greater vestibular* (vulvovaginal, Bartholin's) *glands* are two compound glands at the base of the labia majora, one on either side of the vaginal orifice. Each gland is drained by several ducts, about 1.5 cm long. Each opens into the groove between the hymen and the labia minora. Usually the gland openings are not visible or palpable. The glands secrete a small amount of clear, viscid mucus, especially during coitus. The alkaline pH of the mucus is supportive of sperm.

Fourchette. The fourchette is a thin, flat, transverse fold of tissue formed where the tapering labia majora and minora merge in the midline below the vaginal orifice. A small depression, the fossa navicularis, lies between the fourchette and the hymen.

Perineum. The perineum is the skin-covered muscular area between the vaginal introitus and the anus. The perineum forms the base of the perineal body (see Fig. 6-17). The terms *vulva* and *perineum* occasionally but inaccurately are used interchangeably.

Internal Structures

The internal reproductive organs are discussed in the order that reflects the path of the ovum. Supportive tissues are discussed along with the internal reproductive organs they support. Internal organs include the ovaries, uterine tubes, uterus, and vagina. A brief description of the bony pelvis follows.

Ovaries: Female Gonads

Location and Support. One ovary is located on each side of the uterus, below and behind the uterine tubes. The ovaries are held in place by two ligaments, the *mesovarian* portions of the uterine broad ligament, which suspend them from the lateral pelvic side walls at about the level of the anterosuperior iliac crest, and the *ovarian* ligaments (Figs. 6-6 and 6-10), which anchor them to the uterus. The ovaries are movable with palpation.

Structure. The ovaries are similar in origin (homologous) to the testes in the male. Each ovary is composed of two layers around a central zone (Fig. 6-5). Each ovary re-

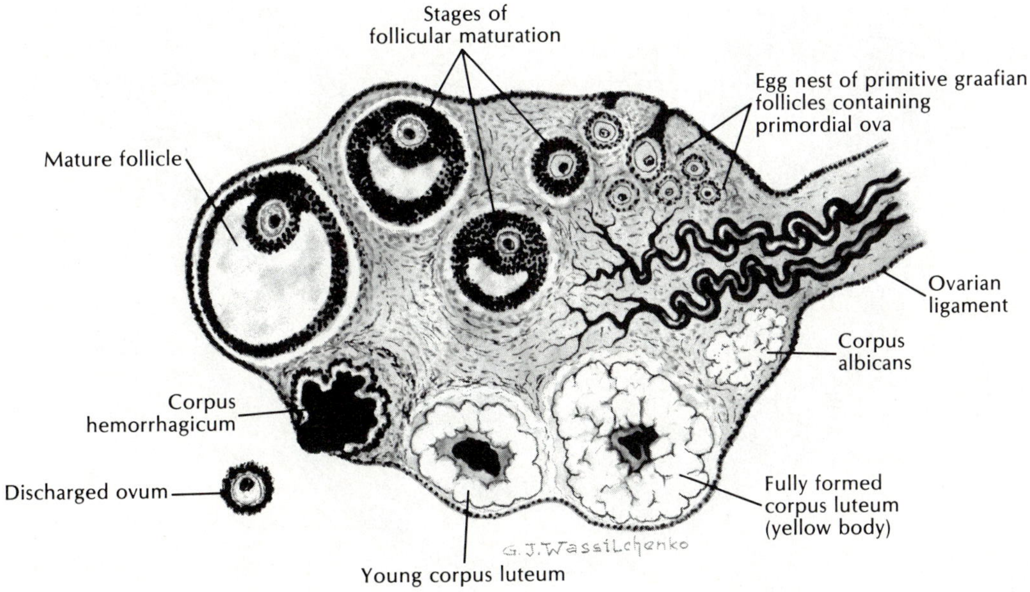

Fig. 6-5 Cross section of ovary.

sembles a large almond in size and shape. Each is whitish and rounded but flattened, weighs about 3 g, and measures approximately 3 × 2 × 1 cm. At the time of ovulation, ovarian size may double temporarily. The oval-shaped ovaries are firm in consistency and slightly tender. The surface of the ovary is smooth before menarche. After sexual maturity, scarring from repeated ruptures of follicles and ovulation roughens the nodular surface.

Blood Vessels and Lymphatics. Ovarian arteries carry a rich blood supply from the aorta to the ovaries. The left ovarian vein empties into the left renal vein, but the right ovarian vein drains into the inferior vena cava. The ovarian lymphatics drain into the iliac and periaortic nodes.

Innervation. The nerve supply to the ovaries is through T-10 to L-1, together with fibers of the pelvic sympathetic nervous system.

Functions. The two functions of the ovaries are ovulation and hormone production. At birth the normal female's ovaries contain countless thousands of primordial (primitive) ova. At intervals during the reproductive life (generally monthly), one or more ova mature and undergo ovulation. The ovary is also the major site of production of steroid sex hormones (estrogens, progesterone, and androgens) in amounts required for normal female growth, development, and function.

Uterine Tubes (Oviducts)

Location and Support. The paired uterine (fallopian) tubes are attached to the uterine fundus (Figs. 6-6, 6-7, and 6-10). The tubes extend laterally, enter the free ends of the broad ligament, and curl around each ovary.

Structure. The tubes are approximately 10 cm (4 in) long and 0.6 cm (¼ in) in diameter. Each tube has an outer coat of peritoneum, a middle, thin muscular coat, and an inner mucosa. The smooth muscle fibers are arranged in an inner circular and an outer longitudinal layer. The mucosal lining consists of columnar cells, some of which are ciliated and others of which are secretory. The mucosa is at its thinnest during the time of menstruation. Each tube, along with its mucosa, is continuous with the mucosa of the uterus and of the vagina.

The structure of the uterine tube changes along its length. Four distinctive segments can be identified (Figs. 6-6 and 6-7): (1) the infundibulum, (2) the ampulla, (3) the isthmus, and (4) the interstitial part. The *infundibulum* is the most distal portion. Its funnel, or trumpet-shaped opening is encircled with fimbriae. The infundibulum has been described as a ruffled petunia or a sea anemone. The fimbriae become swollen, almost erectile, at ovulation. The *ampulla* makes up the distal and middle segment of the tube. It is in the ampulla that the sperm and the ovum meet and fertilization occurs.

The *isthmus* is proximal to the ampulla. It is small and firm, much like the round ligament. The *interstitial* (or intramural) portion passes through the myometrium between the fundus and the body of the uterus and has the smallest lumen. Before the fertilized ovum can pass through this lumen or tunnel, measuring less than 1 mm in diameter, it has to discard its crown of granulosa cells.

Blood Vessels and Lymphatics. Ovarian and uterine vessels service the tubes. Lymphatics terminate in two glands alongside the aorta and the inferior vena cava.

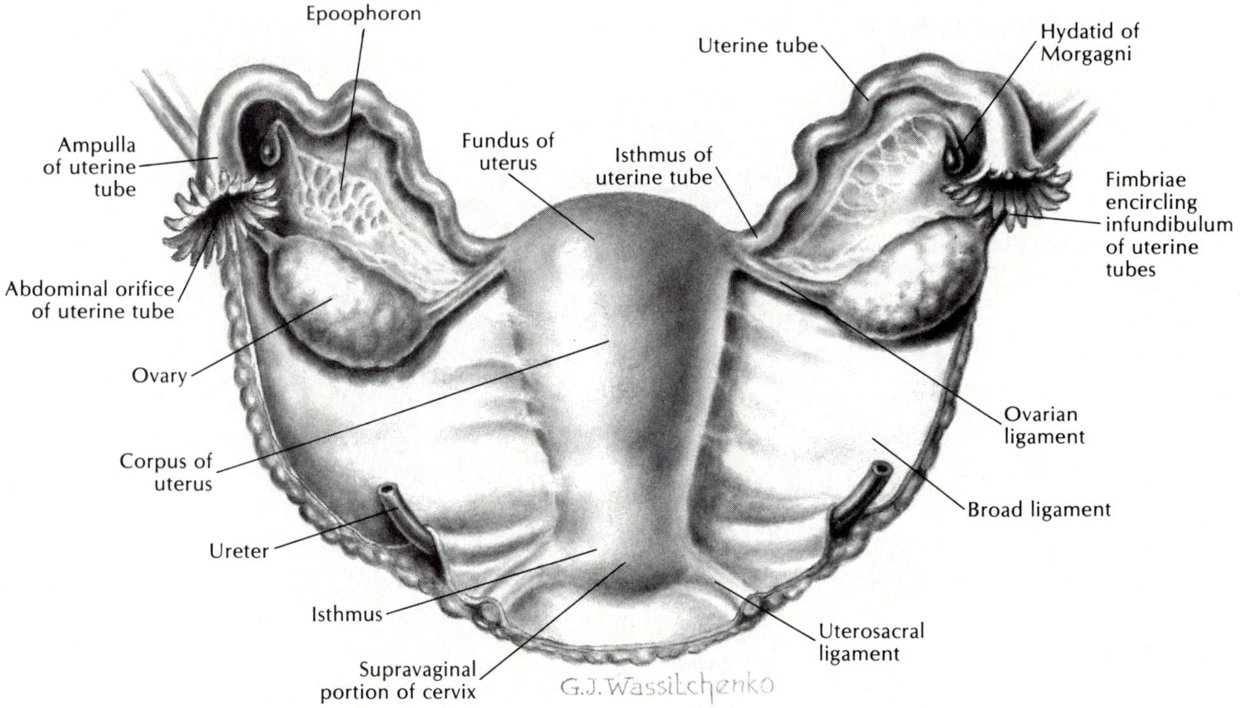

Fig. 6-6 Uterus and adnexa, posterior view.

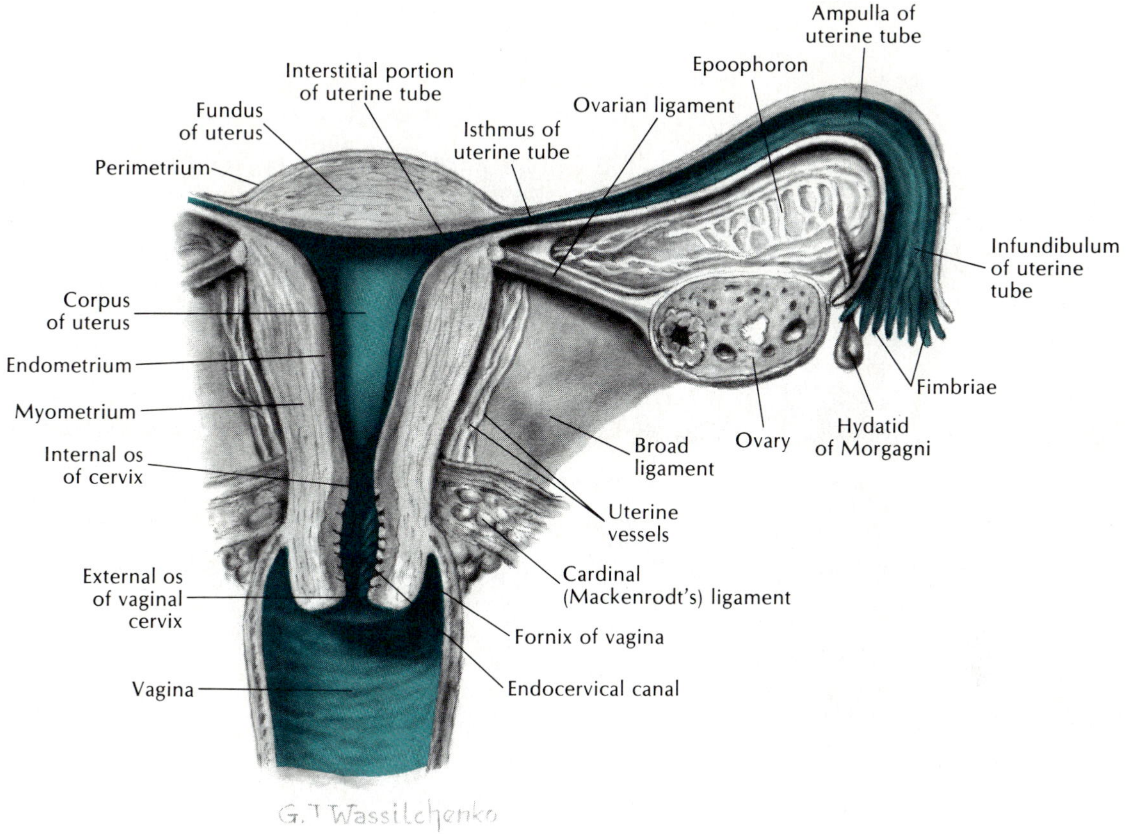

Fig. 6-7 Cross section of uterus, adnexa, and upper vagina.

Innervation. The nerve supply has several sources. Most nerve fibers originate and terminate in segments T-10 to L-1. The exact role of this diversified innervation is not understood.

Functions. The uterine tubes provide a passageway for the ovum. The fingerlike projections (fimbriae) of the infundibulum pull the ovum into the tube with wavelike beckoning motions. The ovum is propelled along the tube, partially by the cilia but primarily by the peristaltic movements of the muscular coat, toward the uterine cavity. Peristaltic motion is influenced by estrogen and prostaglandins. Peristaltic activity of the uterine tubes and the secretory function of their mucosal lining are greatest at the time of ovulation. The columnar cells secrete a nutrient to sustain the ovum while it is in the tube.

Ureters. Although the ureters are not part of the reproductive tract, they are discussed here because of their anatomic proximity to the reproductive organs (see Figs. 6-6, 6-9, and 6-14). As the ureters leave the kidney, they pass just behind the ovarian blood vessels close to the uterine tubes and in front of the uterine blood vessels.

Uterus

Location. Between birth and puberty the uterus descends gradually into the true pelvis from the lower abdomen. After puberty the uterus is usually located in the midline in the true pelvis behind the symphysis pubis and urinary bladder and in front of the rectum.

Position. For most women, with the urinary bladder empty, the uterus is anteverted (tipped forward) and slightly anteflexed (bent forward), with the corpus lying over the top of the posterior wall of the bladder. The cervix is directed downward and backward toward the tip of the sacrum so that it is usually at approximately a right angle to the plane of the vagina. For other women the uterus may be in the midposition or tipped backward (retroverted) (Fig. 6-8). The uterus that is bent more than usual so that the fundus is closer to the cervix is said to be anteflexed, or retroflexed (Fig. 6-8).

A full bladder pushes the uterus back toward the rectum. A full rectum moves the uterus forward against the bladder. Uterine position also changes, depending on the woman's position (e.g., lying supine, prone, on her side, or standing), her age, and pregnancy.

The free mobility permits the uterus to rise slightly during the sexual response cycle so that the cervix is placed in a position to increase the likelihood of fertilization.

Support. The uterus is supported by ligaments and by muscles of the pelvic floor, including the perineal body. A total of 10 ligaments stabilize the uterus within the pelvic cavity: four paired ligaments (broad, round, uterosacral, and cardinal) and two single ligaments (anterior and posterior) (Figs. 6-6, 6-7, 6-9, and 6-10).

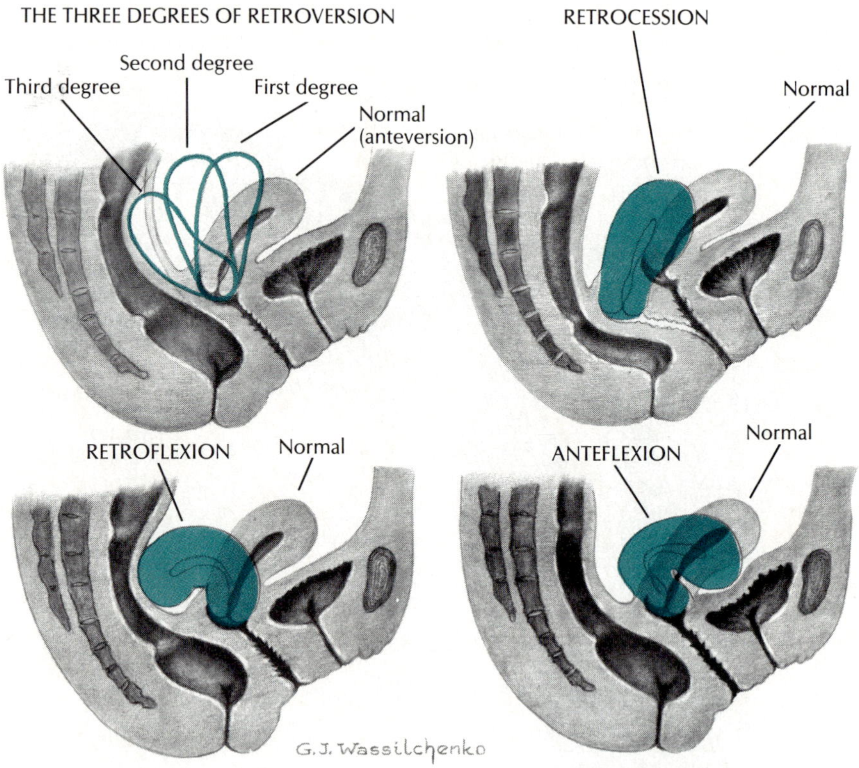

Fig. 6-8 Uterine positions.

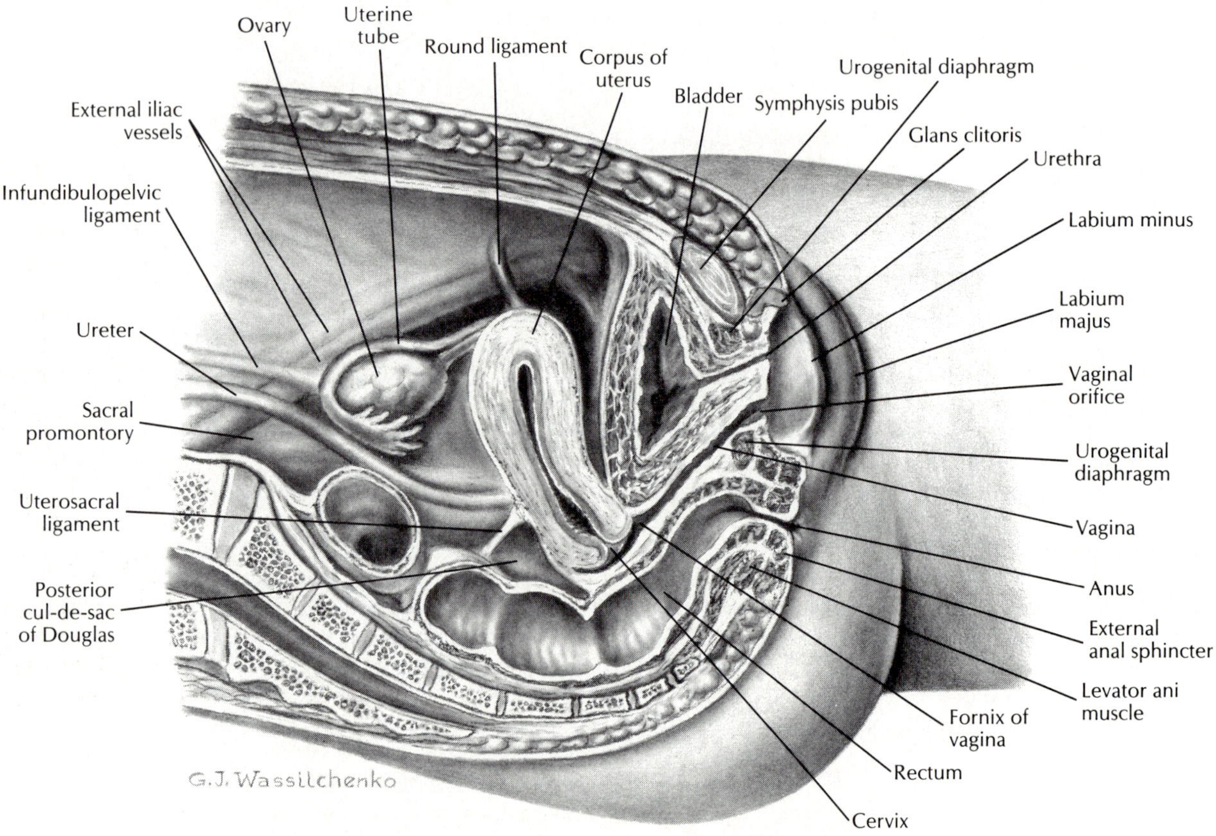

Fig. 6-9 Midsagittal view of female pelvic organs, with woman lying supine.

The paired *broad ligaments* are double folds of parietal peritoneum that extend winglike from the sides of the uterus to the pelvic walls. These ligaments divide the pelvic cavity into anterior and posterior components. In the upper portion of the broad ligaments are suspended the uterine tubes, ovaries, round ligaments, and ovarian ligaments. This upper portion consists of loose connective tissue that does *not* influence uterine position.

The two *round ligaments* are composed of smooth muscle and connective tissue. The round ligaments extend from the upper outer angles formed where the uterine tubes join the uterine corpus (at the cornua), through the inguinal canals, and end in the labia majora. In the nonpregnant state it is a lax cord; in pregnancy it is stretched and increases in diameter (see discussion of round ligament pain, Table 13-2).

The single *anterior* (uterovesical or pubocervical) *ligament* is a continuation of parietal peritoneum that forms the anterior fold of the broad ligament, extending from the anterior surface of the supravaginal cervix of the uterus to the posterior surface of the bladder. The pouch formed by the fold of peritoneum is shallower than the posterior pouch.

The denser connective tissue of the lower portion of the broad ligaments is sometimes known as the *cardinal, transverse,* or *Mackenrodt's ligaments* (Figs. 6-7 and 6-10). The uterine blood vessels and the ureters are enclosed within the cardinal ligaments, where they are connected to the lateral margin of the uterus. The cardinal ligaments form the upper portion of the posterior ligament.

The single *posterior* (or rectovaginal) *ligament* is a continuation of parietal peritoneum (posterior fold of broad ligament) extending from the posterior surface of the uterus to the rectum. The posterior ligament forms the deep rectouterine pouch also known as the *cul-de-sac of Douglas* (Figs. 6-9 and 6-17). An incision into this area is referred to as a *culdotomy.*

The two *uterosacral ligaments* are cordlike folds of peritoneum extending from the supravaginal cervical portion of the uterus to the fascia over the second and third sacral vertebrae and passing on each side of the rectum (Figs. 6-6, 6-9, and 6-10). These ligaments hold the uterus in position by maintaining traction on the cervix.

In summary the main uterine supports are the ligaments surrounding the supravaginal cervix:

1. Anterior (pubocervical)
2. Cardinal (transverse, Mackenrodt's)
3. Posterior (rectovaginal)
4. Uterosacral

Structure, Shape, Size, and Divisions. The uterus is a flattened, hollow, muscular, thick-walled organ that looks somewhat like an upside-down pear (Fig. 6-6). Its length, width, and thickness vary, averaging about 7.5 × 3.5 × 2 cm (3 × 1½ × ¾ in.). In the adult woman who has never been pregnant the uterus weighs 60 g (2 oz). The uterus normally is symmetric in shape and nontender, smooth, and firm to the touch. The degree of firmness varies with several factors; for example, it is spongier during the secretory phase of the menstrual cycle, softer during pregnancy, and firmer after menopause.

The uterus has three parts: the *fundus,* the upper, rounded prominence above the insertion of the uterine tubes; the *corpus,* or main portion, encircling the intrauterine cavity; and the *isthmus,* the slightly constricted portion that joins the corpus to the cervix and is known as the lower uterine segment during pregnancy.

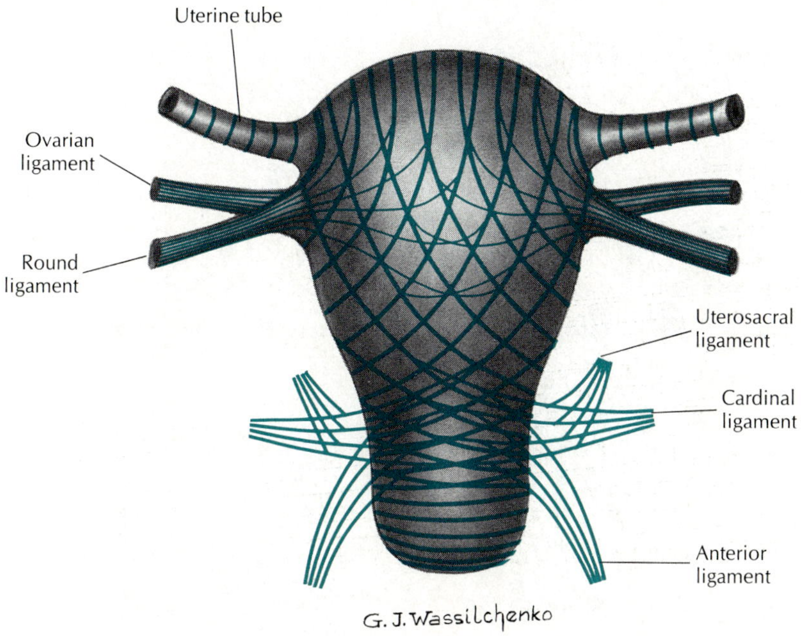

Fig. 6-10 Schematic arrangement of directions of muscle fibers. Note that uterine muscle fibers are continuous with supportive ligaments of uterus.

Uterine Wall. The wall of the uterus is made up of three layers: the endometrium, the myometrium, and a partial outer layer of parietal peritoneum (Fig. 6-7).

The highly vascular *endometrium* is a lining of mucous membrane composed of three layers: a compact surface layer, a spongy middle layer of loose connective tissue, and a dense inner layer that attaches the endometrium to the myometrium. (The upper two layers are also referred to as the functional layer; and the inner layer, as the basal layer.) During menstruation and following delivery the compact surface and middle spongy layers slough off. Just after menstrual flow ends, the endometrium is 0.5 mm thick; near the end of the endometrial cycle, just before menstruation begins again, it is about 5.0 mm (less than ¼ in) thick.

Layers of smooth muscle fibers that extend in three directions (longitudinal, transverse, and oblique) make up the thick *myometrium* (Fig. 6-10). The smooth muscle fibers interlace with elastic and connective tissues and blood vessels throughout the uterine wall and blend with the dense inner layer of the endometrium. The myometrium is particularly thick in the fundus, thins out as it nears the isthmus, and is thinnest in the cervix.

The *outer* myometrial layer, found mostly in the fundus, is made up of longitudinal fibers and is therefore well suited for expelling the fetus during the birth process. In the thick *middle* myometrial layer the interlaced muscle fibers form a figure-eight pattern encircling large blood vessels. Contraction of the middle layer produces a hemostatic action (Fig. 6-11). Only a few circular fibers of the *inner* myometrial layer are found in the fundus. Most of the circular fibers are concentrated in the cornua, the place where the uterine tubes join the uterine body, and around the internal os. The sphincter action of this layer prevents the regurgitation of menstrual blood out of the uterine tubes during menstruation. Their sphincter action around the internal cervical os helps retain the uterine contents during pregnancy. Injury to this sphincter can weaken the internal os and result in an incompetent internal cervical os (see Chapter 31).

For clarity and interest, each muscle layer and its function were described individually. It must be remembered that the myometrium works as a whole. The structure of the myometrium, which gives strength and elasticity, presents an example of adaptation to function:

1. To thin out, pull up, and open the cervix and to push the fetus out of the uterus, the fundus must contract with the most force.
2. Contraction of interlacing smooth muscle fibers that surround the blood vessels controls blood loss after abortion and childbirth. Because of their ability to close off (ligate) blood vessels between them, the smooth muscle fibers of the uterus are referred to as the **living ligature** (Fig. 6-11).

Muscle fibers of the uterine myometrium are continuous with the muscle layers in the uterine tubes and vagina and with muscle fibers in the ovarian, round, and cardinal ligaments; they are minimally continuous with those in the uterosacral ligaments.

The *parietal peritoneum,* a serous membrane, coats all the uterine corpus except for the lower one fourth of the anterior surface, where the bladder is attached, and the cervix. Because parietal peritoneum does not completely cover this organ, it is possible for diagnostic tests and surgery involving the uterus to be performed without entering the abdominal cavity.

Cervix. The lowermost portion of the uterus is the cer-

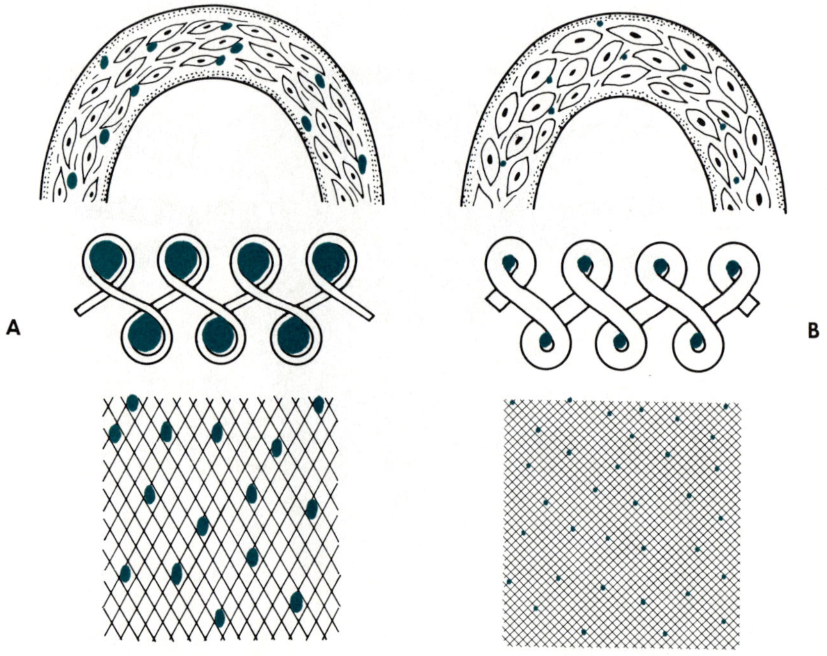

Fig. 6-11 The living ligature: interlacing smooth muscle fibers of the thick middle myometrium. Color denotes blood vessels. **A,** Relaxed muscle fibers. **B,** Contracted muscle fibers ligating the blood vessels.

vix, or neck. The attachment site of the uterine cervix to the vaginal vault divides the cervix into the longer supravaginal (above the vagina) portion (Fig. 6-6) and the shorter vaginal portion (Fig. 6-7). The length of the cervix is about 2.5 to 3 cm, of which about 1 cm protrudes into the vagina in the nongravid woman.

The cervix is composed primarily of fibrous connective tissue with some muscle fibers and elastic tissue. The cervix of the nulliparous woman is a rounded, almost conical, rather firm, spindle-shaped body approximately 2 to 2.5 cm in external diameter. The narrowed opening between the uterine cavity and the endocervical (canal inside the cervix that connects the uterine cavity with the vagina) canal is the internal os. The narrowed opening between the endocervix and the vagina is the external os. The external os is a small circular opening in women who have not borne children. Childbirth changes the circular os to a small transverse opening dividing the cervix into an anterior and a posterior lip (Fig. 6-12).

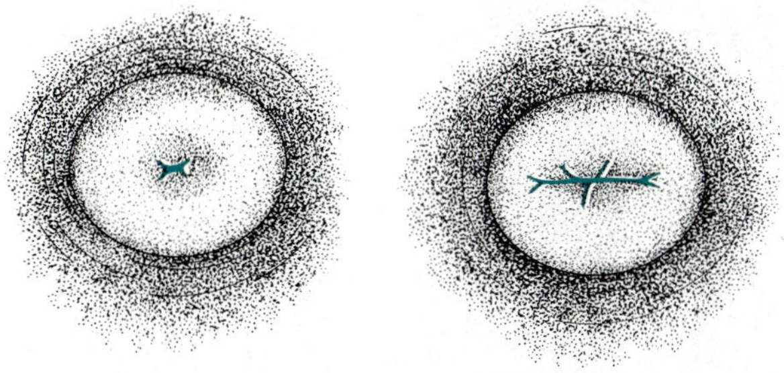

Fig. 6-12 External cervical os as seen through speculum. **A**, Nonparous cervix. **B**, Parous cervix.

When the woman is not ovulating or pregnant, the tip of the cervix feels firm, much like the end of one's nose, with a dimple in the center. The dimple marks the site of the external os.

The most significant characteristic of the cervix is its ability to stretch during vaginal childbirth. Several factors contribute to cervical elasticity: high connective tissue and elastic fiber content, numerous infoldings in the endocervical lining, and a muscle fiber content of about 10%.

Canals. There are two cavities within the uterus, which are known as the uterine and cervical canals (Fig. 6-13). The uterine canal in the nonpregnant state is compressed by thick muscular walls so that it is only a potential space, flat and triangular in shape. The base of the triangle is formed by the fundus. The uterine tubes open into either end of the base. The apex of the triangle points downward and forms the internal os (opening) of the cervical canal.

The endocervical canal with its many infoldings has a surface layer of tall, columnar, mucus-producing cells. *Columnar epithelium* is beefy red, deeper, and rougher looking than the epithelial outer covering of the cervix (Fig. 6-13). After menarche (the start of menstruation) *squamous epithelium* covers the outside of the cervix (ectocervix). This external covering of flat cells gives a glistening pink color to the cervix. A deeper bluish red color is seen when

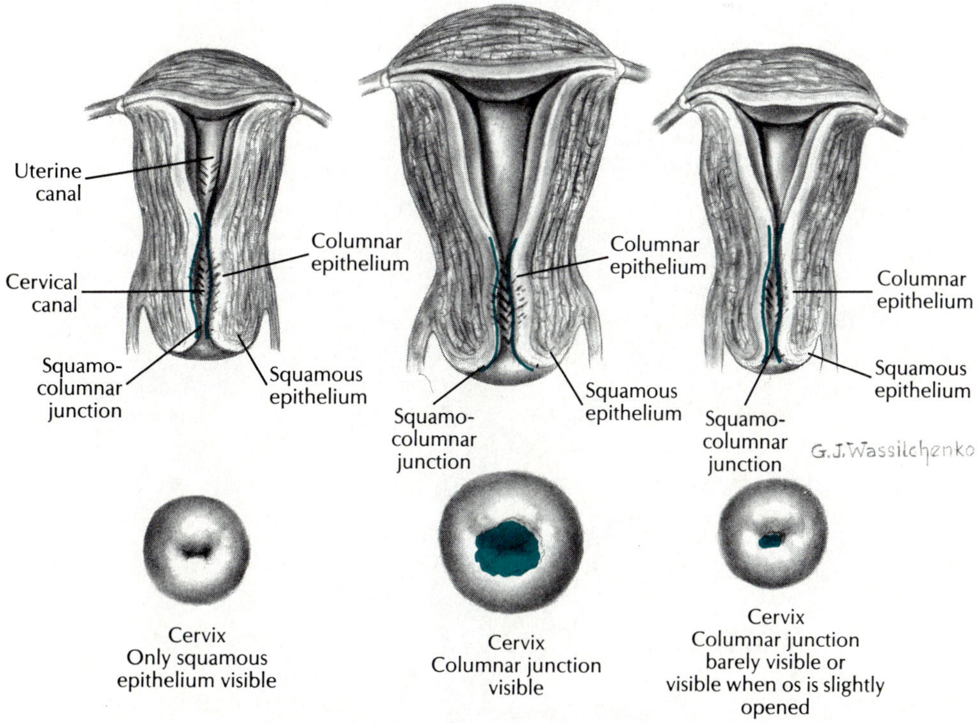

Fig. 6-13 Uterine and cervical canals and the squamocolumnar junction. Color denotes columnar epithelium.

Fig. 6-14 A, Pelvic blood supply. B, Blood supply of perineum and uterus.

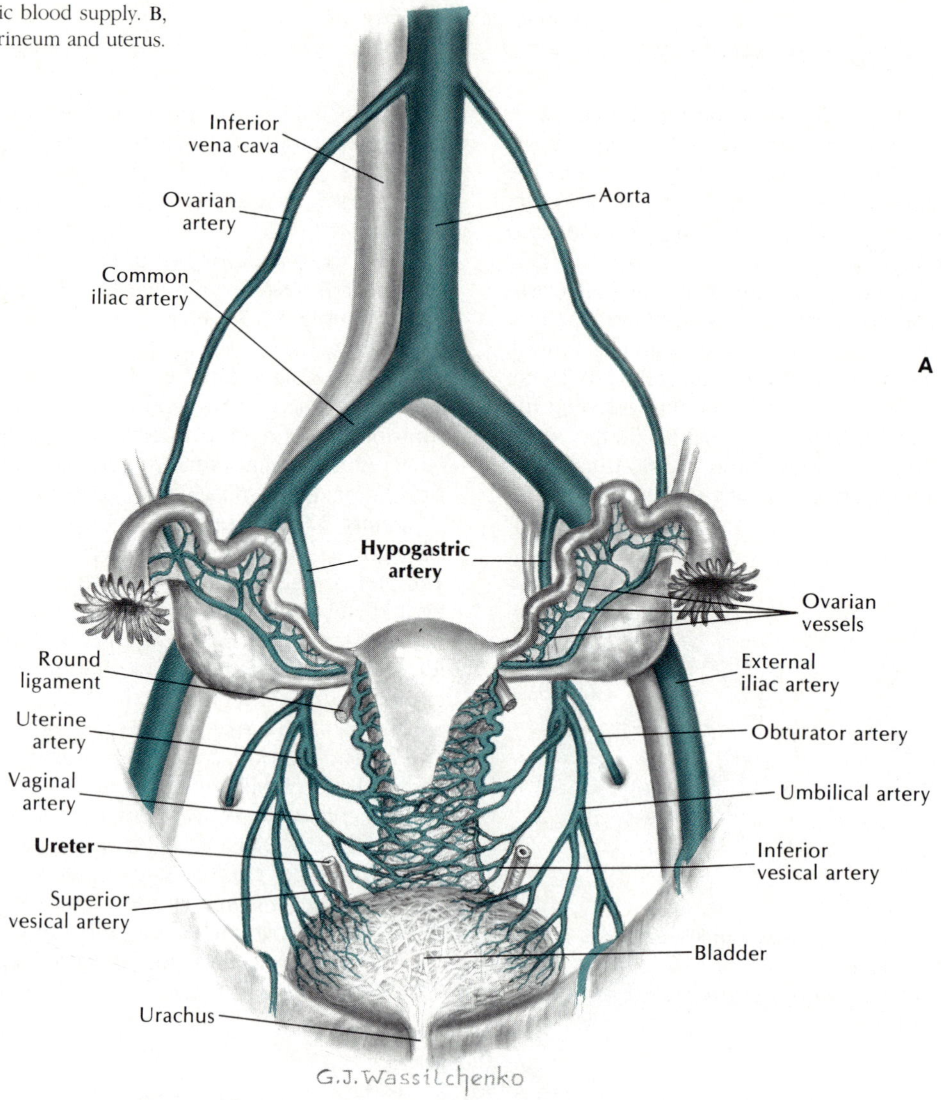

Inferior vena cava
Ovarian artery
Common iliac artery
Aorta
A
Hypogastric artery
Ovarian vessels
Round ligament
External iliac artery
Uterine artery
Obturator artery
Vaginal artery
Umbilical artery
Ureter
Inferior vesical artery
Superior vesical artery
Bladder
Urachus
G.J. Wassilchenko

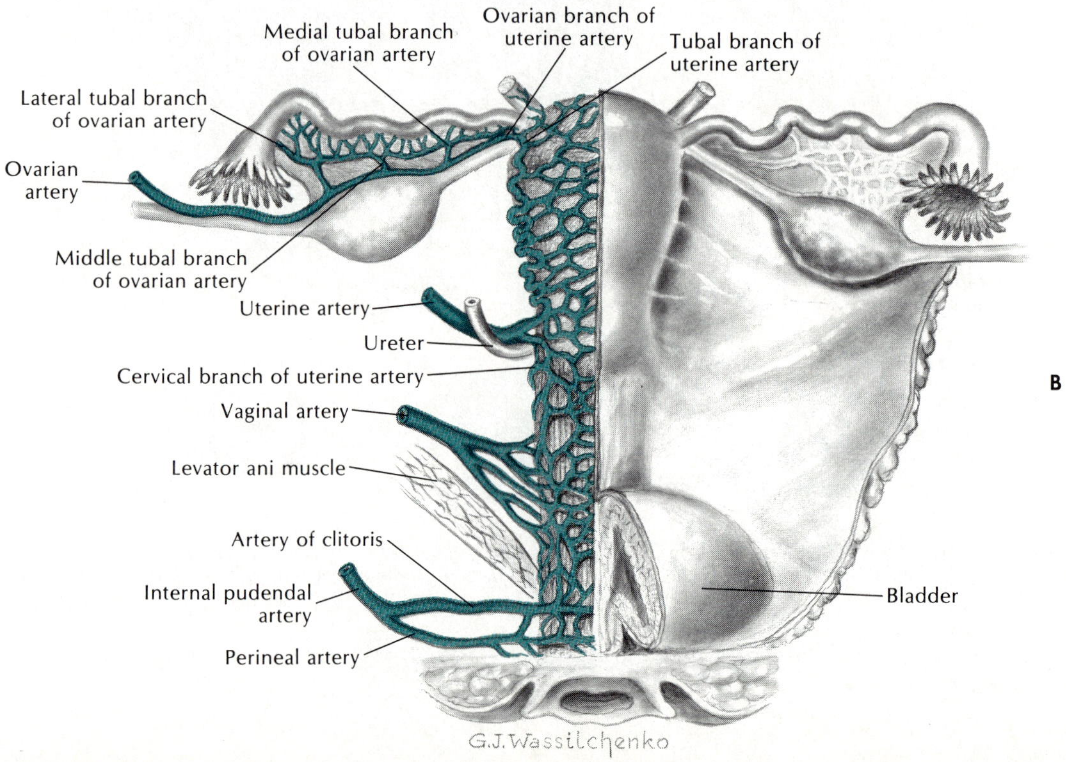

Medial tubal branch of ovarian artery
Ovarian branch of uterine artery
Tubal branch of uterine artery
Lateral tubal branch of ovarian artery
Ovarian artery
Middle tubal branch of ovarian artery
Uterine artery
Ureter
Cervical branch of uterine artery
B
Vaginal artery
Levator ani muscle
Artery of clitoris
Internal pudendal artery
Bladder
Perineal artery
G.J. Wassilchenko

the woman is ovulating or pregnant. A reddened (hyperemic) cervix may indicate inflammation.

The two types of epithelium meet at the *squamocolumnar junction* (Fig. 6-13). This junction line is usually just inside the external cervical os but may be found on the ectocervix in some women. The squamocolumnar junction is the most common site of neoplastic cellular changes. Therefore cells for cytologic study, the Papanicolaou smear, are scraped from this junction.

The columnar epithelial cells produce odorless and nonirritating mucus in response to ovarian endocrine hormones—estrogen and progesterone.

Blood Vessels. The abdominal aorta divides at about the level of the umbilicus and forms the two iliac arteries. Each iliac artery divides to form two arteries, the major one of which is the hypogastric artery. The uterine arteries branch off from the *hypogastric arteries.* The closeness of the uterus to the aorta ensures an ample blood supply to meet the needs of the growing uterus and conceptus.

In addition the ovarian artery, a direct subdivision of the aorta, first supplies the ovary with the blood and then proceeds to join the uterine artery, thus further adding to the blood supply (Fig. 6-14).

In the nonpregnant state the uterine blood vessels are coiled and tortuous. With advancing pregnancy and an enlarging uterus, these blood vessels straighten out. The uterine veins follow along the arteries and empty into the internal iliac veins.

Lymphatics. The lymphatics of the uterus are extensive. They are contained in three networks: at the base of the endometrium, within the myometrium, and just under the peritoneal coat of the uterus. There are *no* lymphatics in the more superficial layers of the endometrium. Lymphatic drainage occurs mainly at the isthmus along the uterine vessels. Near the uterine fundus, drainage joins that of the ovarian and tubal lymphatics to nodes around the aorta. Some lymphatics may drain into femoral, iliac, and hypogastric nodes.

Innervation. The internal genitals have a rich supply of afferent and efferent autonomic nerves, both motor and sensory.

Motor Nerves. Parasympathetic fibers from the sacral nerves are probably responsible for producing vasodilation and inhibiting muscular contraction. Efferent sympathetic motor nerves arise from the ganglia of T-5 (thoracic 5) to T-10, come together over the sacrum, and reach the uterus through ganglia that lie near the base of the uterosacral ligaments. These efferent sympathetic motor nerves are believed to cause vasoconstriction and muscular contraction. The autonomic nerves just described (parasympathetic and efferent sympathetic motor) regulate the action of the uterus, but the uterus has an intrinsic motility (i.e., it can contract and relax even if the nerves to it are cut). This means that even if a woman suffers an accident that injures the spinal cord at or above T-5, she may still be able to have uterine contractions sufficient to deliver an infant vaginally.

Sensory Nerves. Sensory fibers, carrying pain sensation from the uterus, come together in the paracervical areas and proceed upward to pass just below the division (bifurcation) of the aorta, and then travel to the spinal cord at the level of T-11 and T-12. Because of this arrangement, pain that originates in the ovary or in the ureters may mimic pain that originates in the uterus, any of which may be felt in the flank and down to the inguinal and vulvar areas.

Functions. The three functions of the uterus are essential for the survival of the species but not for the individual. These functions include cyclic menstruation with rejuvenation of the endometrium, pregnancy, and labor.

Vagina

Location and Support. The vagina is a tubular structure located in front of the rectum and behind the bladder and urethra (Fig. 6-9). The vagina extends from the introitus, the external opening in the vestibule between the labia minora of the vulva, to the cervix. When the woman is standing, the vagina slants backward and upward. It is supported mainly by its attachments to the pelvic floor musculature and fascia.

Structure. The vagina is a thin-walled, collapsible tube capable of great distension. Because of the way the cervix protrudes into the uppermost portion of the vagina, the length of the anterior wall of the vagina is only about 7.5 cm, while that of the posterior wall is about 9 cm. The recesses formed all around the protruding cervix are called fornices: right, left, anterior, and posterior. The posterior fornix is deeper than the other three (Figs. 6-7 and 6-17).

The smooth muscle walls are lined with glandular mucous membrane. During the reproductive years this mucosa is arranged in transverse folds called *rugae.*

The vaginal mucosa responds promptly to estrogen and progesterone stimulation. Cells are lost from the mucosa, especially during the menstrual cycle and pregnancy. Cells scraped from the vaginal mucosa can be used to estimate steroid sex hormone levels.

Vaginal Fluid. Vaginal fluid is derived from the lower or upper genital tract. The continuous flow of fluid from the vagina maintains relative cleanliness of the vagina. Therefore vaginal douching in normal circumstances is not necessary. A spread of vaginal mucus from the posterior vaginal fornix and a scraping from the squamocolumnar junction of the cervix (Figs. 6-13 and 8-15), fixed in ethyl ether and alcohol and then treated with trichrome nucleocytoplasmic stain, constitute the *Papanicolaou (Pap) smear* used throughout the world for cytologic cancer detection.

Blood Vessels and Lymphatics. The copious blood supply to the vagina is derived from the descending branches of the uterine artery, the vaginal artery, and the internal pudendal arteries (Fig. 6-14). The venous return of vaginal blood is through the pudendal, vaginal, and uterine veins. The lymphatics of the upper vagina drain to the rectovaginal, septal, presacral, external iliac, and hypogastric nodes. The lower vaginal lymphatics are directed to the superficial inguinal nodes.

Innervation. The vagina is relatively insensitive. There is some innervation from the pudendal and hemorrhoidal nerves to the lowest one third. Because of this minimal innervation and lack of special nerve endings the vagina is the source of little sensation during sexual excitement and

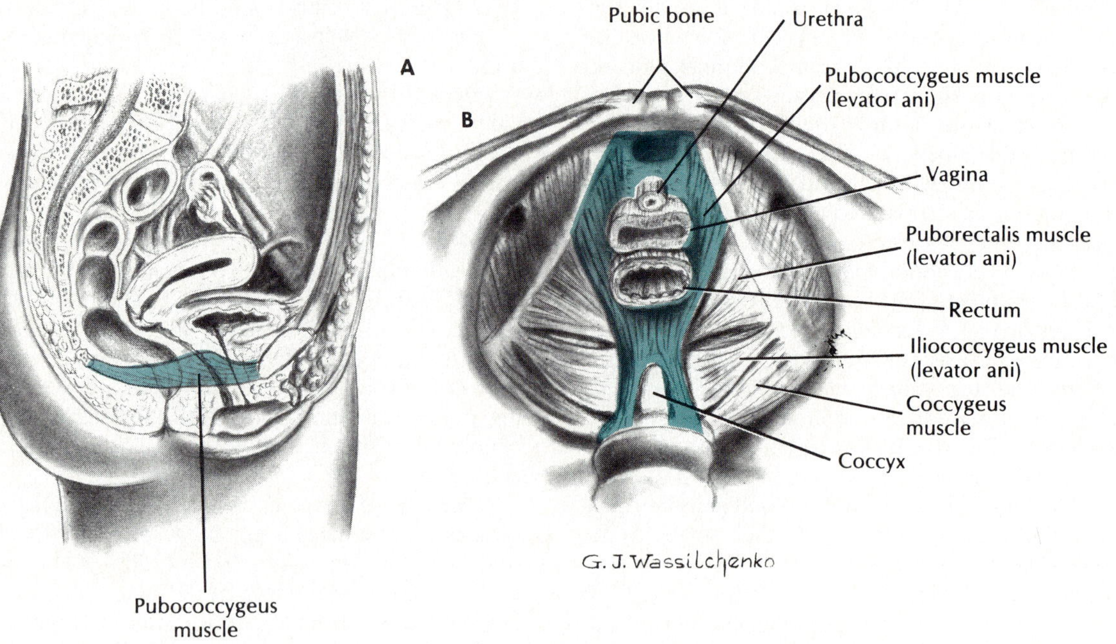

Fig. 6-15 Upper pelvic diaphragm. **A**, Pubococcygeus portion of the levator ani muscles, midsaggital view. **B**, View from above.

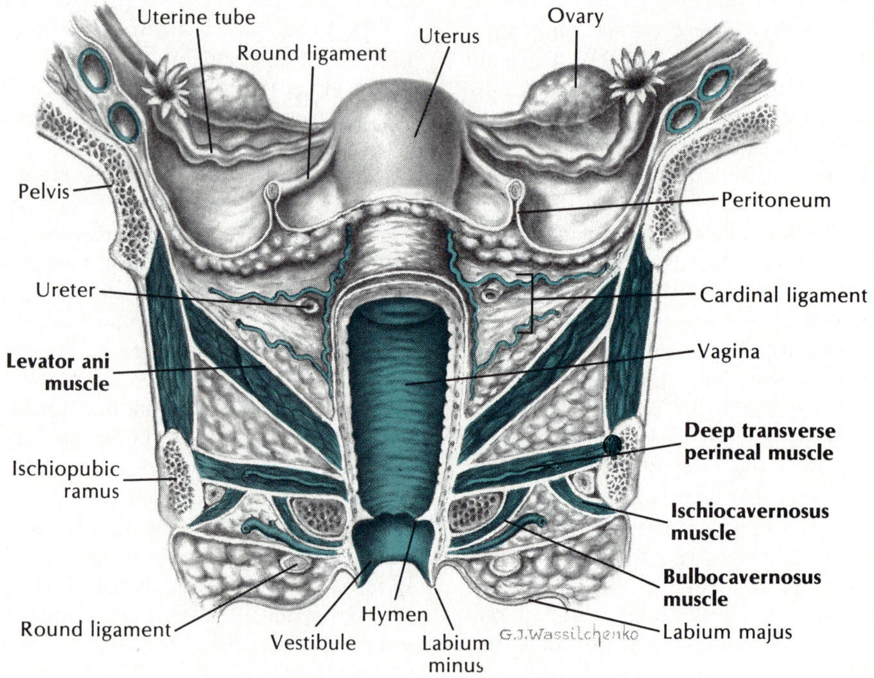

Fig. 6-16 Levator ani muscles of upper pelvic diaphragm and urogenital (lower pelvic) diaphragm, anterior view.

coitus and less pain during the second stage of labor than if this tissue were well supplied with nerve endings. The nerve supply is mainly autonomic. Sensations arising in the vagina terminate at the level of S-2, S-3, and S-4.

G-Spot. The G-spot is an area on the anterior vaginal wall beneath the urethra defined by Grafenberg as analogous to the male prostate gland. During sexual arousal it may be stimulated to the point of orgasm with ejaculation into the urethra of fluid similar in nature to prostatic fluid (Droegemueller et al., 1987; Ladas, Whipple, and Perry, 1982).

Functions. The vagina functions as the organ for copulation (coitus) and as the birth canal.

Pelvic Floor and Perineum. The pelvic floor and perineum are composed of the pelvic diaphragm, the urogenital diaphragm or triangle, and the muscles of the external genitals and anus. The perineum is sometimes defined as including all the muscles, fascia, and ligaments of the upper (pelvic) and lower (urogenital) diaphragms. The perineal body adds strength to these structures.

Upper Pelvic Diaphragm. The upper pelvic diaphragm, composed of muscles and their fascia and ligaments, extends across the lowest part of the pelvic cavity like a hammock (Fig. 6-15). The largest and most significant portion of the diaphragm is formed by the pair of broad, thin *levator ani muscles* that extend sheetlike between the ischial spines and coccyx, and the sacrum. The levator ani group of muscles is made up of three muscle pairs: puborectalis, iliococcygeus, and pubococcygeus muscles. The pubococcygeus muscle is particularly significant for women. It plays a role in sexual sensory function, in bladder control, in controlling perineal relaxation during labor, and in expulsion of the fetus during birth.

The second paired muscles of the upper pelvic diaphragm are the closely joined *coccygeus muscles.* These muscles extend from the ischial spines to the coccyx and lower sacrum. The several parts of the pelvic diaphragm provide a slinglike support to abdominal and pelvic viscera.

The strength and resilience of this sling are derived from the way in which the layered parts of this sling are interwoven and interlaced. The layers are not fixed; that is, they slide over each other. This unique arrangement strengthens the supportive capacity of the pelvic diaphragm, allows for dilation of the vagina during the birth process and for its closure after delivery, and assists with constriction of the urethra, vagina, and anal canal, which pass through the diaphragm.

Lower Pelvic (Urogenital) Diaphragm. The lower pelvic diaphragm is located in the hollow of the pubic arch and consists of the transverse perineal muscles, which originate at the ischial tuberosities and insert into the perineal body. The strong muscle fibers provide support to the anal canal during defecation and to the lower vagina during delivery. The deep transverse perineal muscles join to form a central seam, or raphe. Some of their fibers encircle the urinary meatus and vaginal sphincters.

The *perineum* is located below the upper and lower pelvic diaphragm. Its muscles and fascia reinforce the strength of the pelvic diaphragm and aid in constricting the urinary, vaginal, and anal openings. The *bulbocavernosus muscle* (Fig. 6-16) fibers originate in the perineal body and surround the vaginal opening as the muscle fibers pass forward to insert into the pubis.

The *ischiocavernosus muscles* originate in the tuberosities of the ischium and continue at an angle to insert next to the bulbocavernosus muscles (Fig. 6-16). These muscle fibers contract to cause erection of the clitoris.

Anal sphincter muscle fibers originate at the coccyx, separate to pass on either side of the anus, fuse, and then insert into the transverse perineal muscles.

The bulbocavernosus, transverse perineal, and anal sphincter muscle fibers can be strengthened through Kegel's exercises (see Chapter 8).

Perineal Body. The *perineal body,* the wedge-shaped mass between the vaginal and anal openings, serves as an anchor point for the muscles, fascia, and ligaments of the upper and lower pelvic diaphragms (Fig. 6-17). The skin-covered base of the body is known as the perineum. The perineal body, about 4 cm wide by 4 cm deep, is continuous with the septum between the rectum and vagina. This tissue is flattened and stretched as the fetus moves through the birth canal.

The Bony Pelvis. The nurse needs to be thoroughly familiar with the bony pelvis to understand the female reproductive tract and perineum. The pelvis serves three primary purposes: (1) Its bony cavity produces a protective cradle for pelvic structures. (2) Its architecture is of special importance in accommodating a growing fetus throughout pregnancy and during the birth process. (3) Its strength provides stable anchorage for the attachment of supportive muscles, fascia, and ligaments.

Bony Structures. In a study of the bony pelvis the following structures and *landmarks* are especially important (Fig. 6-18):

1. Iliac crest and superior, anterior iliac spine
2. Sacral promontory
3. Sacrum
4. Coccyx
5. Symphysis pubis
6. Subpubic arch
8. Ischial spines
9. Ischial tuberosities

The pelvis (Fig. 6-18, *A*) is made up of four bones: (1) and (2) the right and left innominate bones, each of which is made up of the right or left pubic bone, ilium, and ischium, which fuse after puberty; (3) the sacrum; and (4) the coccyx. The two *innominate bones* (hip bones) form the sides and front of the bony passage, and the *sacrum* and *coccyx* form the back.

Below the *ilium* is the *ischium,* a heavy bone terminating posteriorly in the rounded protuberances known as the *ischial tuberosities* (Fig. 6-18, *B*). The tuberosities bear the body's weight in the sitting position. The *ischial spines,* the sharp projections from the posterior border of the ischium into the pelvic cavity, may be blunt or prominent.

The *pubis,* forming the front portion of the pelvic cavity, is located beneath the mons. In the midline the two pubic bones are joined by strong ligaments and a thick cartilage to form the joint called the symphysis pubis. In the female the angle formed by the subpubic arch optimally measures slightly more than 90 degrees.

The *sacrum* is formed by five fused vertebrae. The up-

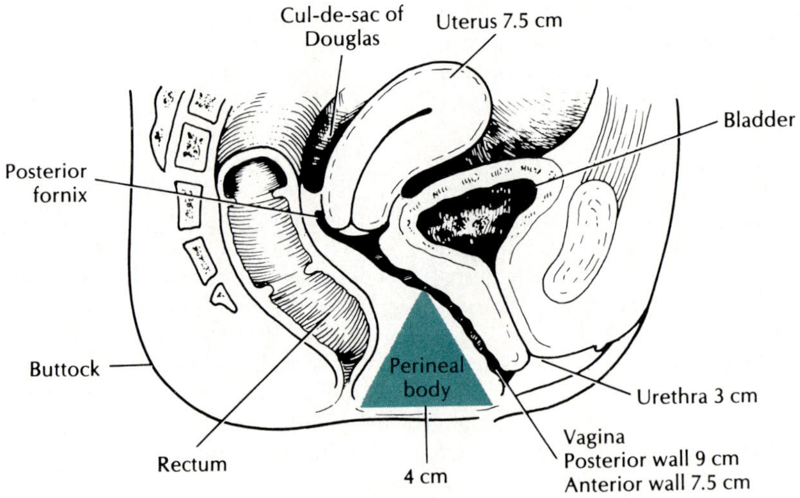

Fig. 6-17 Perineal body. Location and size relative to surrounding tissues, with woman sitting.

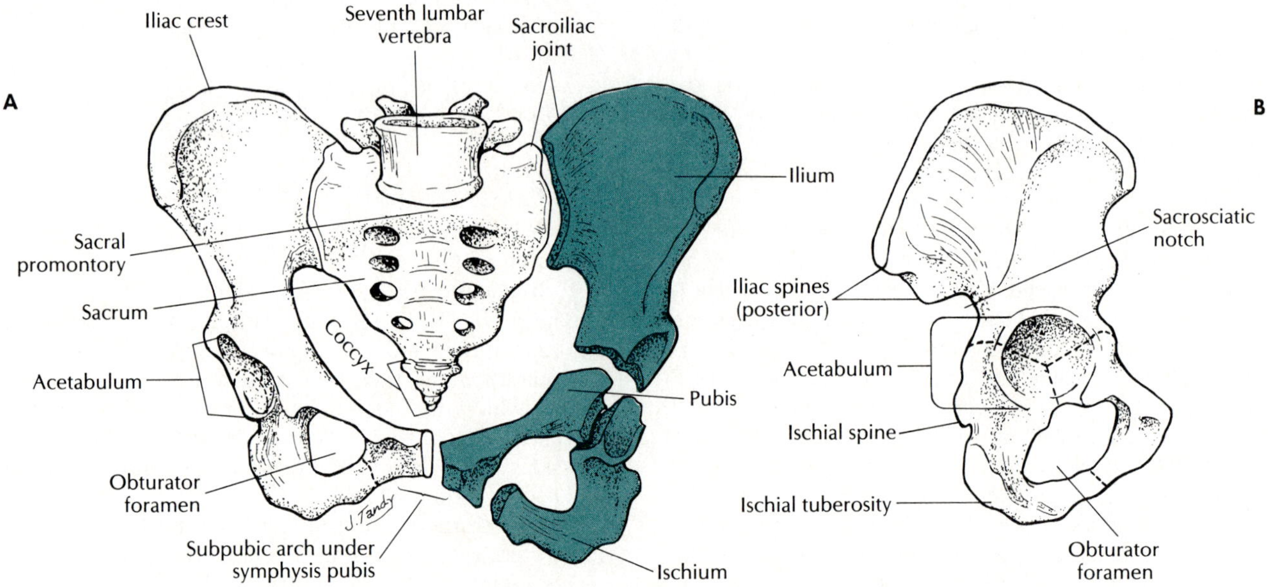

Fig. 6-18 Adult female pelvis. **A**, Anterior view. The three embryonic parts of the left innominate bone are lightly shaded. **B**, External view of right innominate bone (fused).

per anterior portion of the body of the first sacral vertebra, the promontory, forms the posterior margin of the pelvic brim.

The *coccyx* (tailbone), composed of three to five fused vertebrae, articulates with the sacrum. The coccyx projects downward and forward from the lower border of the sacrum.

False and True Pelves. The pelvis is divided into two sections, the shallow upper basin, or false pelvis, and the deeper lower, or true, pelvis (Fig. 6-19). The *false pelvis* lies above the linea terminalis (brim, inlet) and varies considerably in size in different women. The *true pelvis* consists of the brim, or inlet, and the area below.

Pelvic Planes. Pelvic planes include those of the *inlet,* the *midpelvis,* and the *outlet.* The cavity of the mid true pelvis resembles an irregularly curved canal (Fig. 6-20) with unequal anterior and posterior surfaces. The anterior surface is formed by the length of the symphysis (4.5 cm). The posterior surface is formed by the length of the sacrum (12 cm).

Pelvic Variations. Age, sex, and race are responsible for the greatest variations in pelvic shape and size. There is considerable change in the pelvis during growth and development. Pelvic ossification is complete at about 20 years of age or slightly later. Smaller people have smaller, lighter bones than larger people.

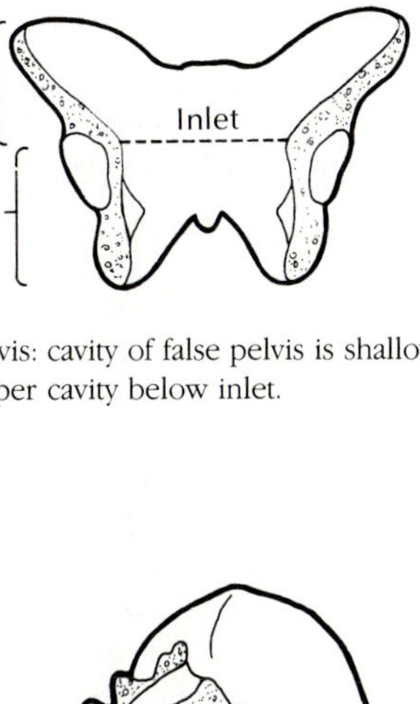

Fig. 6-19 Female pelvis: cavity of false pelvis is shallow basin above inlet; true pelvis is deeper cavity below inlet.

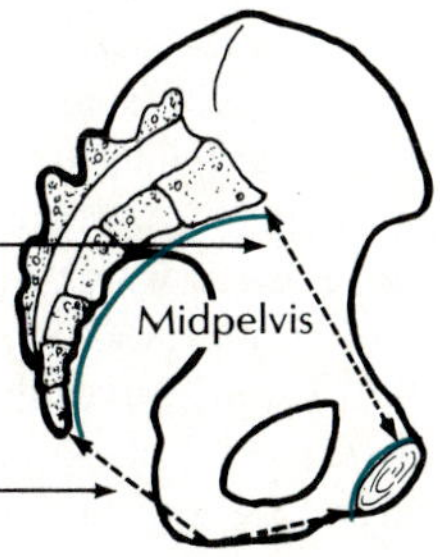

Fig. 6-20 Female pelvis: cavity of true pelvis is an irregularly curved canal.

Breasts

Location and Support. The breasts are paired mammary glands located between the second and sixth ribs (Fig. 6-21). About two thirds of the breast overlies the pectoralis major muscle, between the sternum and mid axillary line, with an extension to the axilla referred to as the tail of Spence. The lower one third of the breast overlies the serratus anterior muscle. The breasts are attached to the muscles by connective tissue or fascia.

The breasts of healthy mature women are approximately equal in size and shape but are often not absolutely symmetric. The size and shape vary depending on the woman's age, heredity, and nutrition. However, the contour should be smooth with no retractions, dimpling, or masses. The breasts of women who have never given birth to a child are usually shaped like half cones or hemispheres. If a woman has breast-fed at some time, her breasts may be pendulous.

Structure. True glandular tissue is called *parenchyma;* supporting tissues, the fat and fibrous connective tissue are called *stroma.* It is the relative amount of stroma that determines the size and consistency of the breast.

Estrogen stimulates growth of the breast by inducing fat deposition in the breasts, development of stromal tissue (i.e., increase in its amount and elasticity), and growth of the extensive ductile system. Estrogen also increases the vascularity of breast tissue.

Once ovulation begins in puberty, progesterone levels increase. The increase in progesterone causes maturation of mammary gland tissue, specifically the lobules and acinar structures. During adolescence fat deposition and growth of fibrous tissue contribute to the increase in the size of the gland. Full development of the breast is not achieved until after the end of the first pregnancy or in the early period of lactation.

Each mammary gland is made up of 15 to 20 lobes, which are divided into lobules. Lobules are clusters of acini. An acinus is a saclike terminal part of a compound gland emptying through a narrow lumen or duct. In discussions of mammary glands the correct anatomic term (*acinus*) is often used interchangeably with *alveolus.* The acini are lined with epithelial cells that secrete colostrum and milk. Just below the epithelium is the myoepithelium (myo, muscle), which contracts to expel milk from the acini (Fig. 6-22).

The ducts from the clusters of acini that form the lobules merge to form larger ducts draining the lobes. Ducts from the lobes converge in a single nipple (papilla) surrounded by an areola. Just as the ducts converge, they dilate to form common lactiferous sinuses, which are also called ampullae. The lactiferous sinuses serve as milk reservoirs. Many tiny lactiferous ducts drain the ampullae and exit in the nipple.

The glandular structures and ducts are surrounded by protective fatty tissue and are separated and supported by fibrous suspensory *Cooper's ligaments.* Cooper's ligaments

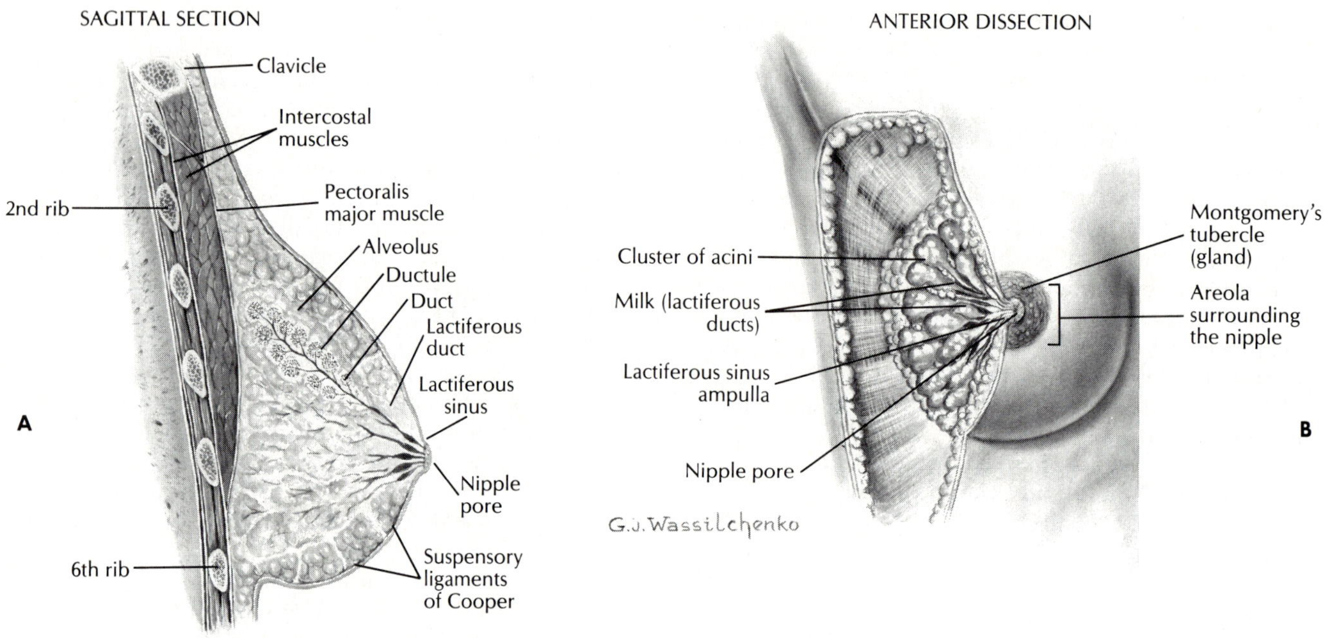

Fig. 6-21 Position and structure of mammary gland. **A**, Sagittal section. **B**, Anterior dissection.
A, Sagittal section from Seidel et al: Mosby's guide to physical assessment, St Louis, 1987, The CV Mosby Co.

provide support to the mammary glands while permitting their mobility on the chest wall.

The round nipple is usually slightly elevated above the breast. On each breast the nipple projects slightly upward and laterally. It contains 15 to 20 openings from lactiferous ducts. The nipple (mammary papilla) is surrounded by fibromuscular tissue and covered by wrinkled skin. Except during pregnancy and lactation, there is no discharge from the nipple.

The nipple and surrounding areola are usually more deeply pigmented than the skin of the breast. The rough appearance of the areola is caused by sebaceous glands, the glands of Montgomery (Fig. 6-21) directly beneath the skin. These glands secrete a fatty substance that is thought to lubricate the nipple. Smooth muscle fibers in the areola contract to stiffen the nipple to make it easier for the breast-feeding child to grasp.

Blood Vessels and Lymphatics. The vascular supply to the mammary gland is abundant. In the nonpregnant state the skin does not have an obvious vascular pattern. The normal skin is smooth without tightness or shininess.

The skin covering the breasts contains an extensive superficial lymphatic network that serves the entire chest wall and is continuous with the superficial lymphatics of the neck and abdomen (Fig. 6-23). In the deeper portions of the breasts the lymphatics form a rich network as well. The primary deep lymphatic pathway drains laterally toward the axillae.

Functions. Besides their function of lactation, breasts function as organs for sexual arousal in the mature adult.

Changes in Response to the Menstrual Cycle. The breasts change in size and nodularity in response to cyclic ovarian changes throughout reproductive life. Increasing levels of both estrogen and progesterone in the 3 to 4 days

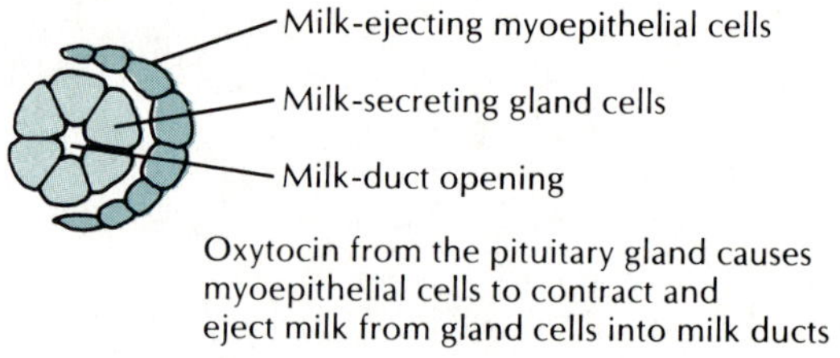

Fig. 6-22 Acinus in cross section.

before menstruation increase vascularity of the breasts, induce growth of the ducts and acini, and promote water retention. The epithelial cells lining the ducts proliferate in number, the ducts dilate, and the lobules distend. The acini become enlarged and secretory, and lipid (fat) is deposited within their epithelial cell lining. As a result, breast swelling, tenderness, and discomfort are common symptoms just before the onset of menstruation. After menstruation, cellular proliferation begins to regress, acini begin to decrease in size, and retained water is lost.

After breasts have undergone changes numerous times in response to the ovarian cycle, the proliferation and involution (regression) are not uniform throughout the breast. In time, after repeated hormonal stimulation, small persistent areas of nodulations may develop. This normal physiologic change must be remembered when breast tissue is examined. Nodules may develop just before and during menstruation, when the breast is most active. The physiologic alterations in breast size and activity reach their minimal level about 5 to 7 days after menstruation stops. Therefore is is easiest to detect pathologic changes at this time (Fig. 6-24).

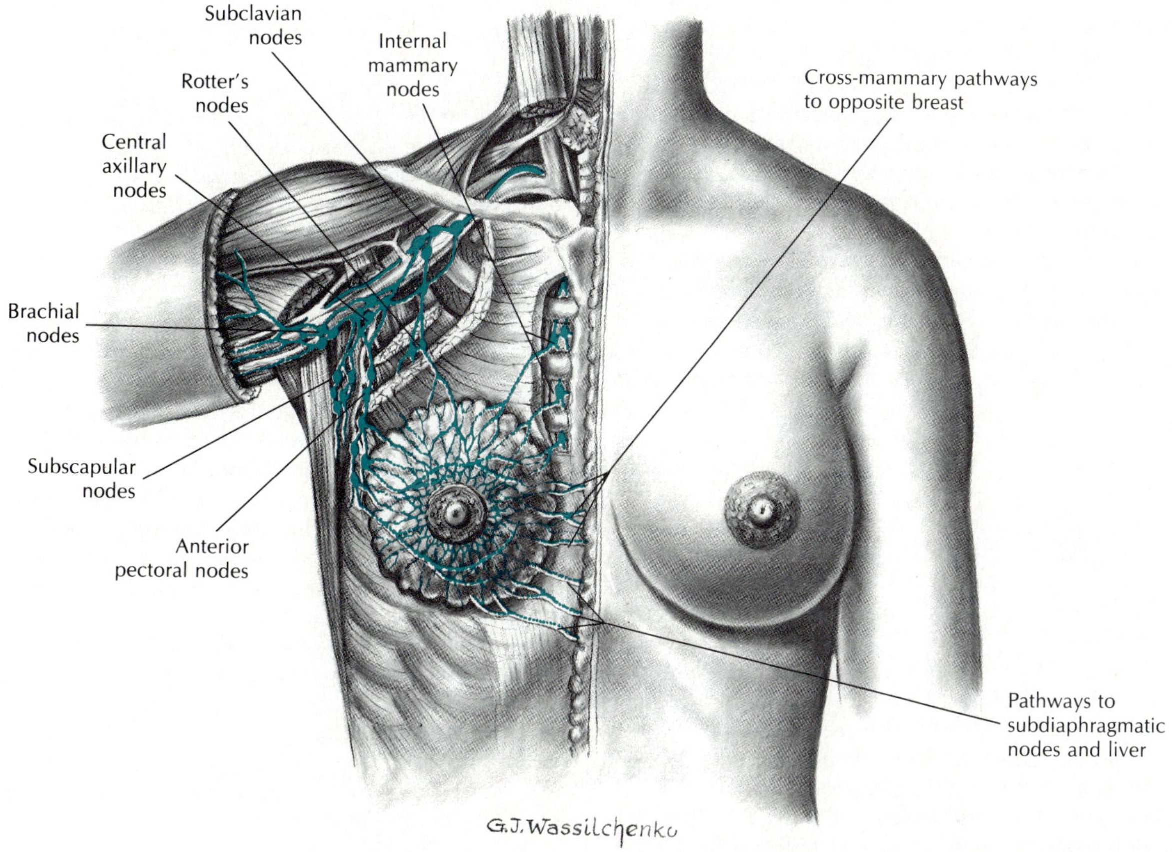

Fig. 6-23 Mammary gland: lymphatic drainage.

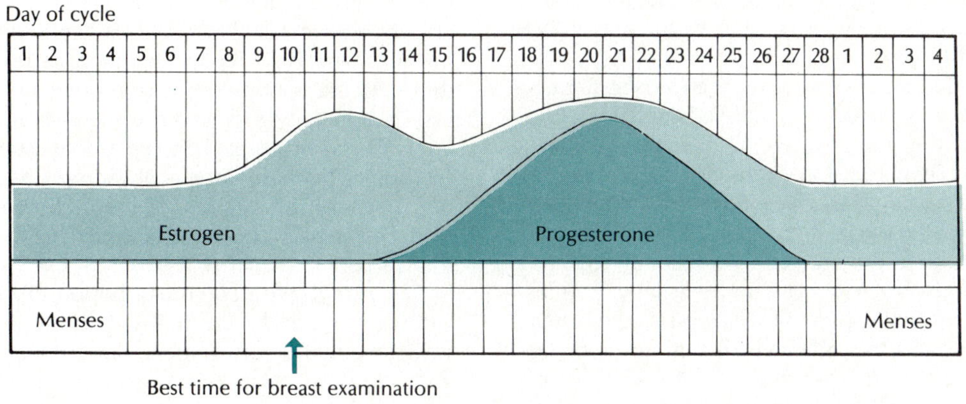

Fig. 6-24 Changes in breast tissue in response to menstrual cycle.

Menstrual Cycle

Menstrual Myths. Many myths have their origin in the mystery that surrounded the woman, her hidden reproductive organs, and her uniqueness in adding new members to society. As a consequence a vast store of folklore, fancies, and superstitions have evolved. Because of their recurring nature, menstrual cycles were thought to be under the control of the moon. Before the discovery of ovulation in humans, it was thought that an egg was produced during menstruation only when fruitful intercourse had occurred. Not until the nineteenth century was knowledge available about the existence of the human egg, ovulation, and ovarian functioning.

An awareness of some myths about menstruation is necessary to use the nursing process effectively with both female and male clients. The most common myths in existence today include the following:

1. During menstruation the woman is vulnerable and therefore needs to be protected.
2. The menstruating woman can pose a danger.
3. Menstrual blood has healing powers, is an aphrodisiac, or is capable of bestowing fertility.

The menstruating woman is seen as being vulnerable to physical and psychologic stress. Recall some of the myths you may have heard: "Don't wash your hair," "Don't take a bath," "Watch out, you'll catch cold," "That's too heavy for you to carry now."

As late as the second half of this century the many behavioral changes falsely attributed to women during their menstrual cycles have been used to argue, for example, why it would be unwise to have a woman for president of the United States. Historical literature contains many references to dangers attributed to menstrual women. Should a menstruating woman walk through a farmer's fields, the crops would not grow and the flowers would wilt; if she tried to bake bread, the dough would not rise. The danger also exists for her husband so that physical contact, especially sexual intercourse, was and in some places still is prohibited. In many cultures the menstruating woman is kept in a separate menstrual hut or in separate quarters. Following a ritualized "cleansing" the woman returns to her place in her family.

Menarche. Although young girls secrete small, rather constant amounts of estrogen, a marked increase occurs between 8 and 11 years of age. Moreover, increasing amounts and variations in gonadotropin and estrogen secretion develop into a cyclic pattern at least a year before menarche or the first menstrual period. This occurs in most girls in North America at about 13 years of age.

Initially periods are irregular, unpredictable, painless, and anovulatory in the majority of young girls. After one or more years a hypothalamic-pituitary rhythm develops, and adequate cyclic estrogen is produced by the ovary to mature a number of graafian follicles. Approximately 14 days *before* the beginning of the next menstrual period, pituitary follicle-stimulating hormone (FSH) rises, a surge of luteinizing hormone (LH) is released by the anterior hypophysis, and ovulation (extrusion of the ovum) occurs.

Ovulatory periods tend to be regular, monitored by progesterone. In some women ovulatory periods are associated with slight uterine cramping (dysmenorrhea), which may be an effect of progesterone or prostaglandins or both. This discomfort is rarely serious and is readily relieved by a hot water bottle, exercise, or simple analgesics. When viewed in its proper perspective slight cramping may be reassuring to the girl and her parents as an indication of normal ovulatory function.

Although pregnancy may occur in exceptional cases of true (constitutional) precocious puberty, most pregnancies in young girls occur well after the normally timed menarche. *However, all girls would benefit from knowing that pregnancy can occur at any time after the onset of menses.*

Endometrial Cycle

Menstruation. Menstruation is periodic uterine bleeding that begins with the shedding of secretory endometrium approximately 14 days after ovulation. **The first day of the menstrual discharge has been designated as *day 1* of the cycle.** The average duration of menstrual flow is 5 days (range of 3 to 6 days), and the average blood loss is approximately 50 ml (range of 20 to 80 ml), but there is great variation. During menstruation the average daily loss of iron is 0.5 to 1 mg. If the woman's usual blood loss is over 80 ml, she will most likely need iron supplementation to prevent secondary anemia.

For about 50% of women, menstrual blood does not appear to clot. The menstrual blood clots within the uterus, but the clot is liquefied before it is discharged from the uterus. If the discharge leaves the uterus too rapidly, liquefaction may not be complete so that clots will appear in the vagina. Uterine discharge includes mucus and epithelial cells in addition to blood.

It is generally assumed that the purpose of the menstrual cycle is to prepare the uterus for pregnancy. When pregnancy does not occur, menstruation follows. The individual's age, physical and emotional status, and environment influence the regularity of her periods.

Phases. The four phases of the menstrual cycle are (1) the menstrual phase, (2) the proliferative phase, (3) the secretory phase, and (4) the ischemic phase (Fig. 6-25). During the *menstrual phase,* shedding of the functional two thirds of the endometrium (the compact and spongy layers) is initiated by periodic vasoconstriction of the spiral arterioles most marked in the upper layers of the endometrium. The basal layer is always retained, and regeneration begins near the end of the cycle from cells derived from the remaining glandular remnants or stromal cells in the basalis.

The *proliferative phase* is a period of rapid growth that extends from about the fifth day to the time of ovulation, which would be, for example, day 10 of a 24-day cycle, day 14 of a 28-day cycle, or day 18 of a 32-day cycle. The endometrial surface is completely restored in approximately 4 days or slightly before bleeding ceases. From this point on an eightfold to tenfold thickening occurs, with a leveling off of growth at ovulation. Early in the proliferative phase the functional layer is moderately dense and only slightly vascular. Three or four days before ovulation the glands develop and vascularity is increased. The proliferative

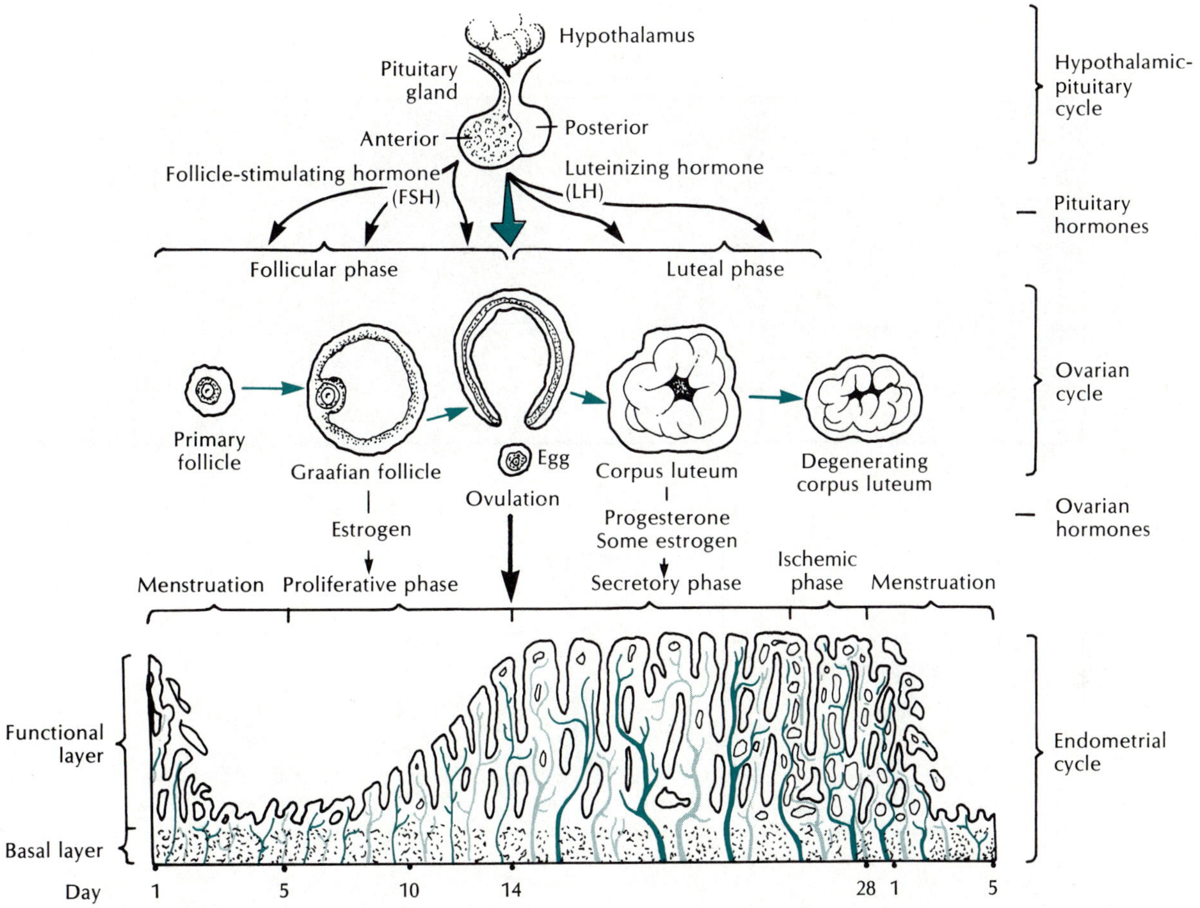

Fig. 6-25 Menstrual cycle.

phase depends on estrogen stimulation derived from ovarian (graafian) follicles.

The *secretory phase* extends from the day of ovulation to about 3 days before the next menstrual period. After ovulation, larger amounts of progesterone are produced. This hormone causes the glands to become tortuous, serrated, and widened. An edematous, vascular, functional endometrium is now apparent. The cells lining the glands secrete a thin, glycogen-containing fluid.

At the end of the secretory phase the fully matured secretory endometirum reaches the thickness of heavy, soft velvet. It becomes luxuriant with blood and glandular secretions, a suitable protective and nutritive bed for a fertilized ovum, should one be available.

Implantation (nidation) of the fertilized ovum generally occurs about 7 to 10 days after ovulation. If fertilization and implantation do not occur, the corpus luteum (yellow body) regresses. With the rapid fall in progesterone and estrogen levels the spiral arteries go into a spasm. During the *ischemic phase* the blood supply to the functional endometrium is blocked and necrosis develops. The functional layer separates from the basal layer, and menstrual bleeding begins, marking day 1 of the next cycle.

Hypothalamic-pituitary Cycle. Toward the end of the normal menstrual cycle, blood levels of estrogen and progesterone fall. Low blood levels of these ovarian hormones stimulate the hypothalamus to secrete gonadotropin-releasing hormone (Gn-RH). Gn-RH in turn stimulates anterior pituitary secretion of FSH. FSH stimulates development of ovarian graafian follicles and their production of estrogen. Estrogen levels begin to fall, and hypothalamic Gn-RH triggers the anterior pituitary release of LH. A marked surge of LH and a smaller peak of estrogen precede the expulsion of the ovum from the graafian follicle by about 24 to 36 hours. LH peaks about the twenty-third or twenty-fourth day of a 28-day cycle. If fertilization and implantation (nidation) of the ovum have not occurred by this time, regression of the corpus luteum follows. Therefore the levels of progesterone and estrogen decline, menstruation occurs, and the hypothalamus is once again stimulated to secrete Gn-RH.

Ovarian Cycle. The primitive graafian follicles contain immature oocytes (primordial ova; Fig. 6-5). Before ovulation, from 1 to 30 follicles begin to mature in each ovary under the influence of FSH and estrogen. The preovulatory surge of LH affects a selected follicle. Within the chosen follicle the oocyte matures, ovulation occurs, and the empty follicle begins its transformation into the corpus luteum. This *follicular phase* (preovulatory phase; Fig. 6-25) of the ovarian menstrual cycle varies in length from woman to

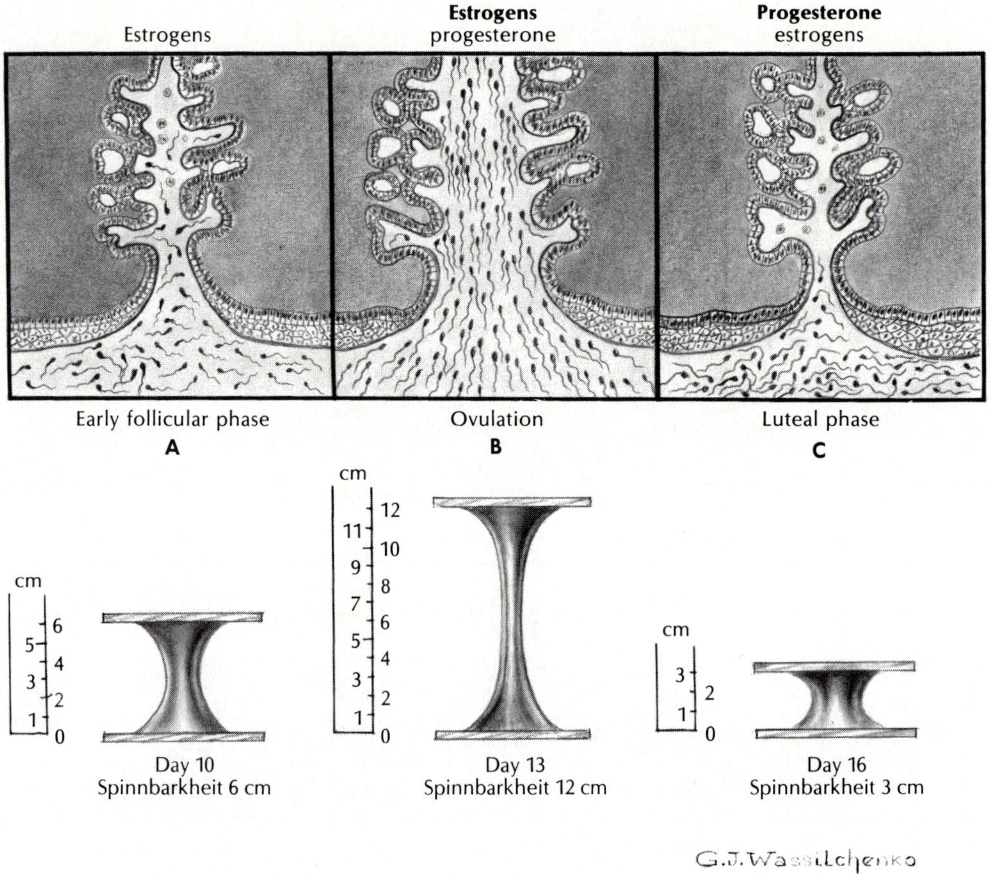

Fig. 6-26 Changes in cervix and in cervical mucus during menstrual cycle. **A**, Changes in opening of the cervix that facilitate sperm migration. **B**, Characteristic stretchable quality of cervical mucus demonstrated between two glass slides.

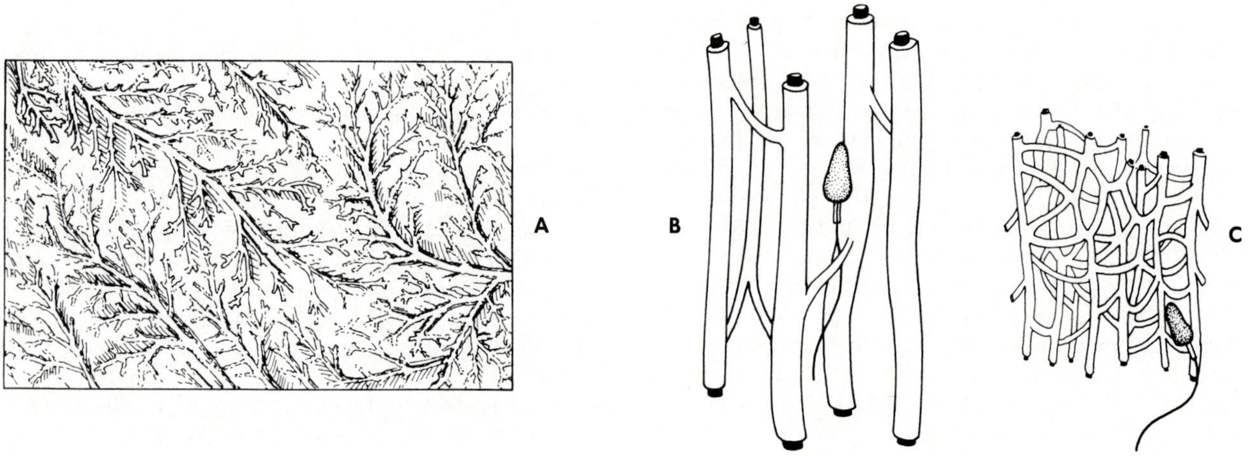

Fig. 6-27 Cervical mucus changes during menstrual cycle. **A**, Fern pattern under estrogen influence. **B**, Mucus receptive to sperm passage under estrogen influence. **C**, Mucus nonreceptive to sperm passage under progesterone influence.

From Fogel, CI, and Woods, NF: Health care of women: a nursing perspective, St Louis, 1981, The CV Mosby Co.

woman. Almost all variations in cycle length are the result of variations in the length of the follicular phase. On rare occasions (1 in 100 menstrual cycles), more than one follicle is chosen and more than one oocyte matures and undergoes ovulation (see discussion of twins, Chapter 33).

After ovulation, estrogen levels drop. For 90% of women, only a small amount of *withdrawal bleeding* occurs so that it goes unnoticed. In 10% of women there is sufficient bleeding for it to be visible, resulting in what is known as *midcycle bleeding*.

The *luteal phase* begins immediately after ovulation and ends with the start of menstruation. This postovulatory phase of the ovarian cycle usually *requires 14 days* (range of 13 to 15 days). The corpus luteum reaches its peak of functional activity 8 days after ovulation, secreting both of the steroids, estrogen and progesterone. Coincident with this time of peak luteal functioning the fertilized egg is implanted in the endometrium. If no implantation occurs, the corpus luteum regresses, and steroid levels drop. Two weeks after ovulation, if fertilization and implantation do not occur, the functional layer of the uterine endometrium is shed through menstruation.

Other Cyclic Changes. When the hypothalamic-pituitary-ovarian axis is functioning properly, other tissues undergo predictable responses. Before ovulation the woman's basal body temperature (BBT) is lower, often below 37° C (98.6° F); after ovulation, with rising progesterone levels, her BBT rises. Changes in the cervix and cervical mucus follow a generally predictable pattern (Figs. 6-26 and 6-27). At the time of ovulation, cervical mucus is thin and clear. It looks, feels, and stretches like egg white. This stretchable quality is termed *spinnbarkheit* (Fig. 6-26). Some women experience localized lower abdominal pain called *mittelschmerz* that coincides with ovulation.

These and other cyclic changes enhance fertility awareness and form the basis for the symptothermal method used for conception and contraception. The subjective and objective signs are biologic markers of the phases of the menstrual cycle (Table 6-1). Examination of women with infertility problems includes a thorough documentation of the presence or absence of these biologic markers (see Chapter 42).

Climacteric. The climacteric (perimenopause) is a transitional phase during which ovarian function and hormone production are declining. This phase spans the years from the onset of premenopausal ovarian decline to the postmenopausal time when symptoms stop. Menopause (from the French *meno,* menstruation, and *pause,* stop) refers only to the last menstrual period. However, unlike menarche, menopause can be dated with certainty only at one year after menstruation ceases. The average age at natural menopause is 51.4 years, with a range of 35 to 60 years. Menopause is an unmistakable biologic marker for the end of reproductive function (see Chapter 41).

Changes in reproductive organs and hormones occurring during the climacteric may be viewed as reversals of endocrine events that began at puberty (Fig. 6-28). One of the initiating events of the climacteric may be the diminishing number of primordial follicles in the ovary. During the reproductive period, 400 follicles mature and several thousand more atrophy. Eventually fewer and fewer follicles exist, producing less and less estrogen, and fewer and fewer corpus lutea are present, producing less and less progesterone. The level of gonadal hormone production decreases gradually, until there is no longer enough to stimulate endometrial growth and initiate endometrial sloughing. Circulating pituitary gonadotropin levels rise as ovarian hormone concentrations decrease. Levels of FSH and LH remain high after menopause has occurred.

Diminishing levels of ovarian estrogen gradually affect target organs. The cells of reproductive organs and surrounding tissues shrink in size or atrophy slowly. The *uterus* becomes smaller in size or involutional. The endometrium becomes thinner. *Menstrual cycles* become irregular or cease abruptly. Several patterns of irregular menstrual cycles may occur. Some women state that their menses come regularly but are lighter and last fewer days. Other women note that they may skip one cycle every few months. A few women describe irregular cycles that are also heavier in flow.

As estrogen stimulation is withdrawn from the muscles that support the uterus, the *levator ani* (Figs. 6-9, 6-15, and 6-16), which already may have been stretched or torn during childbirth, undergoes further relaxation and loss of tone. The *vaginal walls* grow thinner, smoother, and shorter. The *vestibular glands* (Fig. 6-3) produce less mucus. Lubrication during coitus takes longer, since the vagina produces less fluid. The *labia* lose subcutaneous fat. Microscopic examination of the cells of the *cervix* and *vagina* shows changes in the numbers of the three kinds of cells that make up reproductive tissue. Superficial cells, which predominate during the reproductive phase, decrease in number; intermediate cells increase in number; and eventually parabasal cells predominate, as in childhood.

Urethral atrophy is related to withdrawal of ovarian hormones. The terminal portion of the *urethra* has the same embryonic origin as the vagina. Consequently the cells of the distal urethra shrink in size, shortening the urethra after menopause. *Bladder walls* become thin, and bladder support weakens.

Estrogen and calcitonin are needed to maintain equilibrium between the breaking down or resorption of bone and continuous bone formation. Estrogen inhibits bone resorption by raising calcitonin levels, which control the rate of bone formation. Decreasing estrogen levels lower calcitonin concentration. Concurrently levels of parathyroid hormone rise, enhancing bone breakdown. Estrogen also increases the metabolism of vitamin D, which is essential for absorption of calcium from the intestine; as estrogen levels decline, calcium uptake declines. As a result, *bone density* decreases.

Vasomotor instability, evidenced by hot flushes ("hot flashes"), can be annoying. The dilation of blood vessels may be caused by surges of anterior pituitary hormones (FSH or LH), which would connect hot flushes with hormonal disturbances in the hypothalamus, the heat regulatory center of the brain. An accompanying release of prostaglandins may contribute to dilation of the blood vessels.

Later in the postmenopausal period the outer portion of the ovary ceases production of hormones. The core retains its ability to produce androstenedione, a weak male hor-

Table 6-1 *Markers (Signs and Symptoms) of the Phases of the Menstrual Cycle*

Marker	Preovulation	Ovulation	At Least 2 Days After Ovulation up to Menses
Subjective Signs			
Physical discomfort			
Breasts	Unreported	Unreported	Heaviness, fullness; enlarged, tender*
Abdomen	Dysmenorrhea: uterine cramping; nausea, vomiting, and diarrhea; dizziness	Intermenstrual pain (mittelschmerz) occurs 1.7 days after peak of cervical mucus and 2.5 days before increase in BBT	Premenstrual syndrome: backaches; feeling of increasing pelvic fullness
General	Increased weight; feeling of heaviness	Unreported	Headache†; acne
Affective changes‡			
Moods	Some depression may persist from premenses	Sense of well-being	Premenstrual syndrome (PMS): increased irritability, passivity, depression
Libido	Unreported	Increases sexual desire	Unreported
Energy levels	Unreported	Unreported	Spurt of energy, followed by fatigue
Objective Signs			
BBT	36.2-36.3° C (97.2-97.4° F)	34-36 hr before BBT drops 0.2-0.3° F; 24-48 h after, BBT rises 0.7-0.8° F	≥36.7° C (98° F)
Respiration	Unreported	Unreported	Hyperventilation with decrease in alveolar P_{CO_2}
Heart rate	Unreported	Unreported	Increased slightly
Breasts	Time of least hormonal effect and smallest breast size	Increased nipple erectility; increased areolar pigmentation	Increased nodularity; enlarged
Cervix (Figs. 6-26 and 6-27) Mucus characteristics	"Dry" (no mucus) progressing to clear, opaque, watery, slippery mucus and increasing spinnbarkheit; increasing numbers of vaginal and cervical cells and lymphocytes	Abundant, thin, clear (egg white) mucus with spinnbarkheit (4 cm often up to 10 cm) that dries in a fern pattern (arborization); facilitates sperm transport	Cloudy, sticky, impenetrable to sperm; dries in granular pattern
Mucus pH	About 7.0	7.5	Unreported
Os	Gradual, progressive widening	Open, with mucus seen spilling out	Gradual closing of os
Color of exocervix	Pink	Hyperemic (red)	Gradual return to pink
Body	Firm to touch (like tip of nose)	Soft (like earlobe)	Gradual return to firm

*Sociocultural influences may affect symptoms reported by women. Breast tenderness is rarely reported by Japanese women.

†Headaches reported with greater frequency by Nigerian women.

‡NOTE: Literature usually attributes negative premenstrual symptoms to biology, while good moods and rational behavior are not. When men and women are compared in activity patterns, mood changes, and symptoms, similar variability has been found in *both* men and women even though the changes in women are given more attention by society.

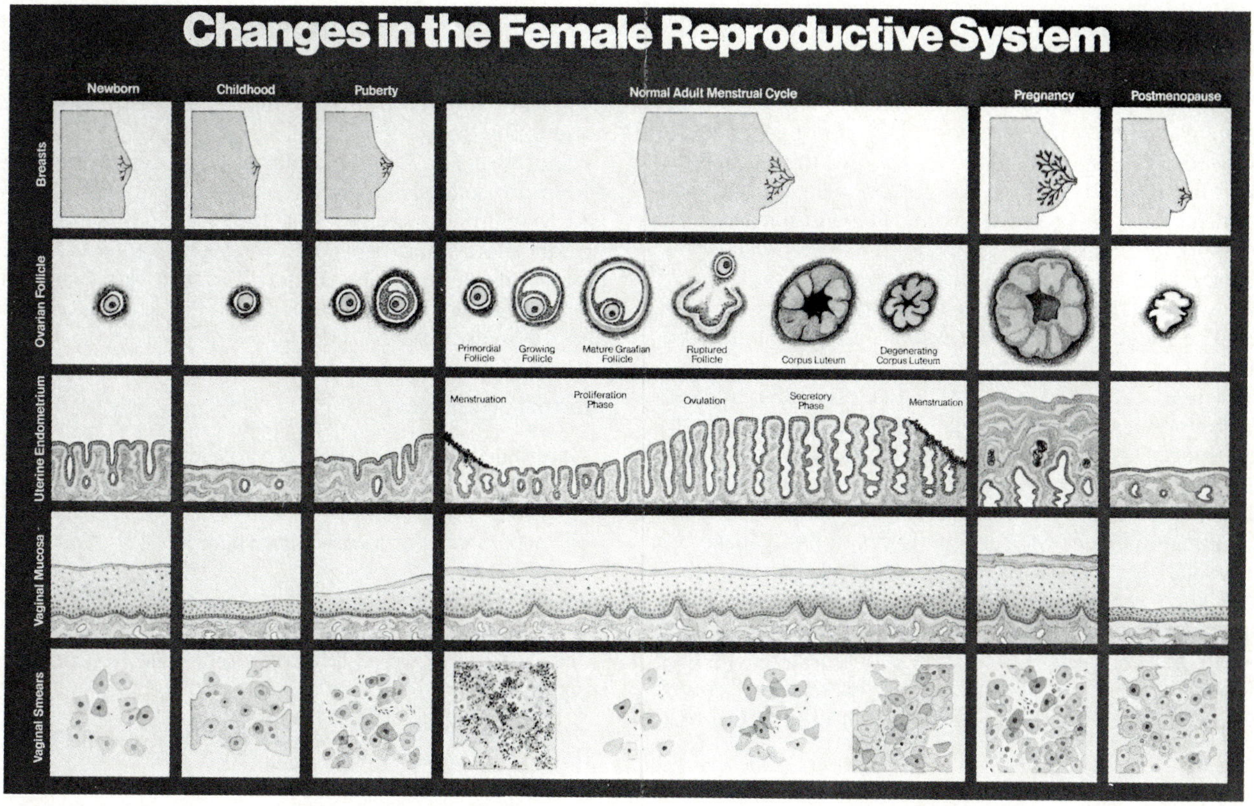

Fig. 6-28 Summary of changes in female reproductive system over life span.
Courtesy Merrill-National Laboratories, Division of Richardson-Merrill, Inc, Cincinnati

mone that can be converted into estrone. Estrone is the chief estrogen present during the postmenopausal period. While the ovary's core continues to function, it produces 20% of the circulating androstenedione; the adrenal gland produces the remaining 80%. The ovarian core also produces another male hormone, testosterone. Following menopause the female hormone influence declines, while the male hormone influence remains static or increases in response to high levels of FSH and LH. At this time some women may note a growth of dark, coarse facial hairs on the chin, as well as increased amounts of fuzzy facial hair. After the ovarian core ceases to function, the adrenal gland is the sole producer of steroid hormones.

The conversion of androstenedione into estrone occurs in body fat. Therefore obese women tend to have higher postmenopausal concentrations of estrone than do women with less subcutaneous fat.

MALE REPRODUCTIVE SYSTEM

The male reproductive tract consists of external genitals and internal organs, located in the pelvic cavity. The male's reproductive system begins to develop in response to testosterone during early fetal life. Essentially no testosterone is produced during childhood. Resumption of testosterone production at the onset of puberty stimulates growth and maturation of reproductive structures and secondary sex characteristics.

External Structures

The structures that make up the external genitals are presented in the following order:

1. Mons pubis
2. Penis
3. Scrotum

Mons Pubis. At maturity, pubic hair is long, dense, coarse, and curly, forming a diamond-shaped pattern from the umbilicus to the anus.

Penis. The penis, an organ of copulation and urination, consists of the shaft or body and the glans (Fig. 6-29). The shaft of this external male reproductive organ, which enters the vagina during coitus, is composed of three cylindric layers and erectile tissue, two lateral *corpora cavernosa* and a *corpus spongiosum,* which contains the urethra. These corpora terminate distally in the smooth, sensitive *glans penis,* which is the counterpart of the female glans clitoris.

Skin and fascia loosely envelop the penis to permit enlargement during erection. The glans is the enlarged end of the penis that contains many sensitive nerve endings and a urethral meatus at the tip (usually). The *prepuce* (foreskin), an extended fold of skin, covers the glans in uncircumcised males (Fig. 6-30). In the newborn the foreskin is not retractable and may not be retractable for 4 to 6 months or even as long as 13 years. It is easily retractable in the adolescent and the adult. With sexual arousal, neurocirculatory factors cause considerable increase in blood flow to the erectile tissue of the corpora, and enlargement and erection of the penis occur.

The *urethra* is an exiting passageway for both urine and semen (Figs. 6-29 and 6-30). The urethra consists of four anatomic segments: the *prostatic,* or posterior, segment is encircled by the prostate gland and houses the ejaculatory ducts that connect the seminal vesicles with the urethra. The next segment is known as the *membranous* urethra and is located within the perineum. Cowper's glands are located on either side of the membranous urethra. The *bulbous* urethra is found in the region of the bulb of the urethra. The longest portion, the *penile* urethra, extends the entire length of the male organ.

Scrotum. The *scrotum,* a wrinkled, pouchlike fullness of skin, muscles, and fascia (Fig. 6-30), is divided internally by a septum, and each compartment normally contains one *testis,* one *epididymis,* and one *vas deferens* (seminal duct). The left side of the scrotum hangs somewhat lower (about 1 cm) than the right. Six separate layers of tissue make up the scrotal sac. The skin is abundantly supplied with sebaceous and sweat glands and is sparsely covered with hair. Under the skin is found the *cremaster* fascia and thin smooth muscle layer. Contraction and relaxation of this smooth muscle result in retraction of the testes to protect them from external trauma and cold. During hot external (environmental) or internal (fever) temperature the cremaster muscle relaxes, dropping the testes away from the body. Conversely, cold external temperature stimulates contraction of the cremaster muscle to bring the testes close to the body.

The purpose of this mobility is to maintain the testes within an optimal temperature range for the production and viability of sperm. Hot tubbing, tight underwear (jockey shorts) and pants, and long-term sitting (long-distance truck drivers) present too hot an external environment or prevent testicular mobility so that spermatogenesis and sperm are jeopardized.

Internal Structures

Internal structures include the following:

1. Testes: male gonads
2. Ducts of the testes
3. Accessory reproductive tract glands
   a. Seminal vesicles
   b. Prostate glands
   c. Bulbourethral glands

Figs. 6-29 and 6-30 illustrate the male reproductive structures.

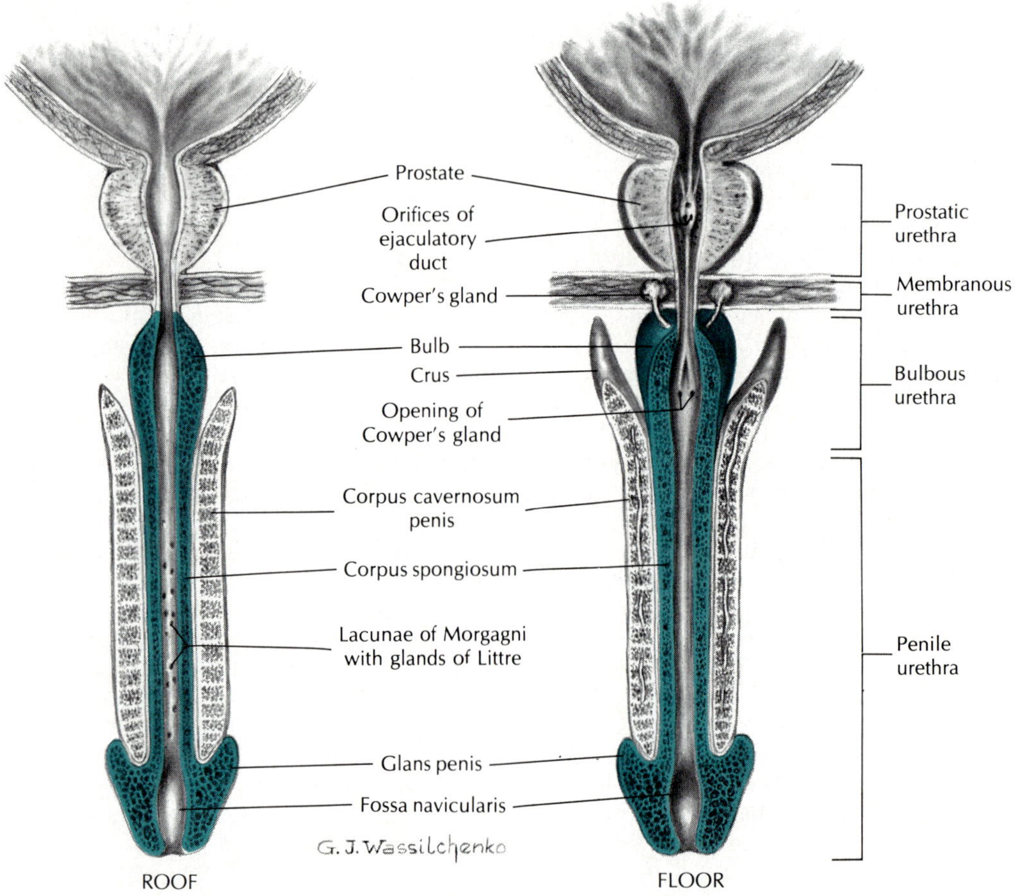

Fig. 6-29 Anatomy of urethra and penis.

Testes: Male Gonads

Location and Support. The testes are two small ovoid glands located within the scrotal sac. Both are suspended by attachment to scrotal tissue and the spermatic cord. Originally located in the abdomen, the testes descend through the inguinal canal by the end of the seventh lunar month of fetal life. At term birth one or both of the testes may still be within the inguinal canals with final descent into the scrotal sac occurring in the early postnatal period. The testes must be within the scrotum for spermatogenesis to occur.

Structure. The testes are similar in origin (homologous) to the ovaries in the female. Each testis is whitish, somewhat flattened from side to side, measures about 4 or 5 cm in length, and weighs 10 to 15 g. White fibrous tissue encases each testis and divides it into several lobules. Within each lobule are one to three long (about 75 cm), narrow, coiled *seminiferous tubules* and clusters of *interstitial cells* (Leydig's cells). Spermatids attach to the germinal epithelium (Sertoli cells) within the seminiferous tubules and develop into sperm. The interstitial cells are large connective and supportive tissue (stromal) cells responsible for the production of the androgen hormone testosterone.

Functions. The two principal functions of the testes are spermatogenesis and hormone production. Primitive sex cells (spermatogonia) are present in the seminiferous tubules of the male newborn. Spermatogenesis, the maturation process that results in sperm, begins during puberty and normally continues throughout a man's lifetime. The testes secrete the steroid sex hormone testosterone in the amounts that are required for normal male growth, development, and function.

Ducts (Canals) of the Testes. For sperm to exit the body they must travel the full length of the duct system in succession: seminiferous tubules, epididymides (pl.), vasa deferentia (pl.), ejaculatory ducts, and the urethra. The seminiferous tubules are mentioned above. Each testis has one tightly coiled tube, about 6 m (20 ft) in length. The tube, the *epididymis* (Fig. 6-30) lies along the top and side of each testis. The epididymides are storage sites for maturing sperm and produce a small part of the seminal fluid (semen). Seminiferous tubules are continuous with the epididymides, which in turn connect to the vasa deferentia.

Accessory Reproductive Tract Glands. Accessory reproductive glands secrete fluids that support the life and function of sperm. These glands include the paired *seminal ves-*

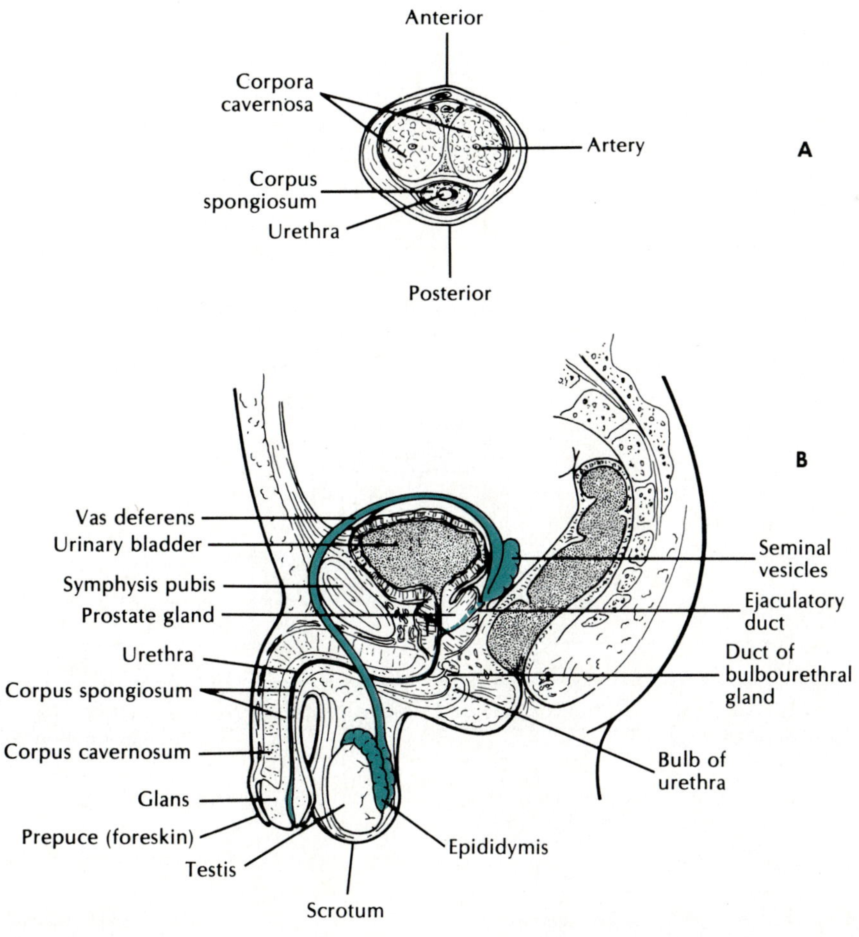

Fig 6-30 Fascial planes of male lower genitourinary tract. **A,** Transverse section of penis. **B,** Relationship of bladder, prostate, seminal vesicles, penis, urethra, and scrotal contents.

icles, located along the lower posterior surface of the bladder; the *prostate gland,* which surrounds the prostatic urethra; and the *bulbourethral* (or Cowper's) *glands,* located below the prostate, one at either side of the membranous urethra (Figs. 6-29 and 6-30).

Semen

The components of semen derive from several sources. Each component of semen and its origin, function, and percent of total volume are presented in Table 6-2. At the time of ejaculation, 3 to 5 ml of semen is released.

FEMALE AND MALE DEVELOPMENT AND RESPONSE PATTERNS: A COMPARISON

Hypothalamic-pituitary-gonadal Axis

The hypothalamus and anterior pituitary gland in females and males regulate the production of FSH and LH. The target tissue for these hormones is the gonad. In the female the ovary produces ova and secretes estrogen and progesterone; in the male the testis produces sperm and secretes testosterone. A feedback mechanism between hormone secretion from the gonads, hypothalamus, and anterior pituitary aids in the control of the production of sex cells and steroid sex hormone secretion (Figs. 6-25 and 6-31).

Table 6-2 *Composition of Semen*

Origin	Component	Functions	Percent of Ejaculate
Testes and epididymides	Some fluid	Vehicle for sperm transport	Under 5%*
	Sperm (hundreds of millions)	Fertilization of ova to perpetuate species	
Seminal vesicles	Seminal fluid containing:		30%
	Fructose	Energy source	
	Prostaglandins	Increase motility of uterus	
	Thick mucus	Vehicle for sperm transport	
	Coagulation protein	Entrap sperm	
Prostate gland	Prostatic secretion containing:		60%
	Alkaline fluid	Supports and enhances sperm motility	
	Thin mucus	Vehicle for sperm transport	
	Fibrinolysin	Liquefies semen for 10 minutes after ejaculation, to release sperm	
	Citrate, acid phosphatase, spermine, spermidine, zinc, magnesium		
	Immunoglobulins (IgG and IgA)		
Bulbourethral glands	Alkaline fluid	Support and enhance sperm motility	Under 5%
	Fibrinolysin	Assist in liquefying semen to release entrapped sperm	

*Vasectomy affects only the production of this portion of the ejaculate so that there is no noticeable change in volume, even after sperm are no longer available for transport through the remaining canal system.

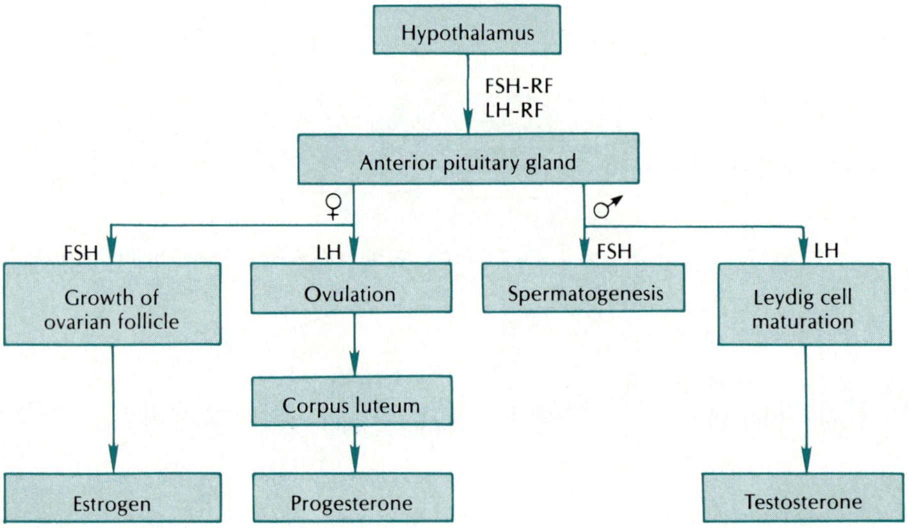

Fig. 6-31 Hypothalamic-pituitary-gonadal axis; comparison of female and male (RF = releasing factor).

Table 6-3 *Stages of Sexual Development: Female*

Age	Stages
0-12	I. Preadolescent. Female pelvic contour evident; breasts flat; labia majora smooth; labia minora poorly developed; hymenal opening small or absent; mucous membranes dry and red; vaginal cells lack glycogen.
8-13	II. *Breasts:* Elevation of nipple; small mound beneath areola, which is enlarging and begins pigmentation. *Labia majora:* Thickened, more prominent, and wrinkled; *labia minora* easily identified because of increased size along with clitoris; urethral opening more prominent; mucous membranes moist and pink; some glycogen present in vaginal cells. *Hair:* First appears on mons and then on labia majora about time of menarche; still scanty, soft, and straight. *Skin:* Increased activity of sebaceous and merocrine sweat glands, and initial function of apocrine glands in axilla and vulva begin.
9-14	III. Rapid growth peak is passed; menarche most often at this stage and invariably follows peak of growth acceleration. *Breasts:* Areola and nipple further enlarge, and pigmentation more evident; continued increase in glandular size. *Labia minora:* Well developed, and vaginal cells have increased glycogen content; mucous membranes increasingly pale. *Hair:* In pubic area thicker, coarser, often curly (considerable normal variation including a few girls with early stage II at menarche). *Skin:* Further increased activity of sabaceous and sweat glands with beginning of acne in some girls; adult body odor.
12-15	IV. *Breasts:* Projection of areola above breast plane, and areolar (Montgomery) glands apparent (this development is absent in about 20% of normal girls); glands easily palpable. *Labia:* Both majora and minora assume adult structure; glycogen content to vaginal cells begins cyclic characteristics. *Hair:* In pubic area more abundant; axillary hair present (rarely present at stage II, often present at stage III).
12-17	V. *Breasts:* Mature histologic morphology, nipple enlarged and erect, areolar (Montgomery's) glands well developed, globular shape. *Hair:* In pubic area more abundant and may spread to thighs (in about 10% of women it assumes "male" distribution with extension toward umbilicus). Facial hair increased often in form of slight mustache. *Skin:* Increased sebaceous gland activity and increased severity of acne if present before.

Reproduced with permission from Lowrey, GH: Growth and development of children, ed 8, Chicago, 1986, Year Book Medical Publishers.

Table 6-4 *Stages of Sexual Development: Male*

Age	Stages
0-14	I. Preadolescent
10-14	II. Increasing size of *testes* and *penis* is evident (testis length reaches 2 cm or more). Scrotum integument is thinner and assumes an increased pendulous appearance. *Hair:* First appearance of pubic hair in area at base of penis. *Skin:* Increased activity of sebaceous and apocrine sweat glands, and apocrine glands on axilla and scrotal area begin.
11-15	III. *Testes* and *penis:* Further increase in size and pigmentation apparent. Leydig's cells (interstitial) first appear at stage II and are now prominent in testes. *Hair:* In pubic area more abundant and present on scrotum; still scanty and fine textured; axillary hair begins. *Breasts:* Button-type hypertrophy in 70% of boys at stages I and III. *Larynx:* Changes in voice as a result of laryngeal growth begin. *Skin:* Increasing activity of sebaceous and sweat glands with beginning of *acne,* adult body odor.
12-16	IV. Rapid growth peak is passed; nocturnal emissions begin. *Testes:* Further increase in size; length 4 cm or greater; increase in size of *penis* greatest at stages III and IV. *Hair:* Pubic hair thicker and coarser and in most ascends toward umbilicus in typical male pattern; axillary hair increases; facial hair increased over lip and upper cheeks. *Larynx:* Voice deepens. *Skin:* Increasing pigmentation of scrotum and penis; *acne* often more severe. *Breasts:* Previous hypertrophy decreased or absent.
13-17	V. *Testes:* Length greater than 4.5 cm. *Hair:* Pubic hair thick, curly, heavily pigmented, extends to thighs and toward umbilicus. Adult distribution and increase in body hair (chest, shoulders, thighs, etc.) continue for more than another 10 years. Baldness, if present may begin. *Skin:* Acne may persist and increase. *Larynx:* Adult character of voice.

Reproduced with permission from Lowrey, GH: Growth and development of children, ed 8, Chicago, 1986, Year Book Medical Publishers.

Stages of Sexual Development

Stages of the development of secondary sexual characteristics of the female and the male are described in Tables 6-3 and 6-4. Although the first outward appearance of maturing sexual development occurs at an earlier age in females, both females and males achieve physical maturity at about the age of 17. However, great variation is possible between individuals' rates of development.

Physiologic Response to Sexual Stimulation

Anatomic and reproductive differences notwithstanding, women and men are more alike than different in their physiologic response to sexual excitement and orgasm.* For example, the glans clitoris and the glans penis are homologues with the same number of nerve endings (see Fig. 6-1). This explains why the clitoris is so sensitive to sexual stimulation. Not only is there little difference between female and male sexual response, but it is now accepted that the physical response is essentially the same where the source of stimulation is coitus, fantasy, or mechanical or manual masturbation.

Currently there are two theories to explain the physiologic response to sexual stimulation. The first and most widely used theory is the four-phase response cycle described by Masters and Johnson. The second is Helen Kaplan's biphasic sexual response cycle.

Four-phase Response Cycle. Physiologically, sexual response, according to Masters and Johnson (1966), can be analyzed in terms of two processes: vasocongestion and myotonia.

1. *Vasocongestion.* Sexual stimulation results in reflex dilation of penile blood vessels (erection) and circumvaginal blood vessels (lubrication), causing engorgement and distension of the genitals. Venous congestion is localized primarily in the genitals, but it also occurs to a lesser degree in the breasts and other parts of the body.
2. *Myotonia.* Arousal is characterized by increased muscular tension, resulting in voluntary and involuntary rhythmic contractions. Example of sexually stimulated myotonia are pelvic thrusting, facial grimacing, and spasms of the hands and feet (carpopedal spasms).

The response cycle is arbitrarily divided into four phases: excitement phase, plateau phase, orgasmic phase, and resolution phase. One moves through the four phases progressively, and there is no sharp dividing line between any two phases. However, there are specific body changes that take place in sequence. The time, intensity, and duration for cyclic completion also vary for individuals and situations.

The following descriptions and drawings of the female and male genitals show the major body changes during the four phases of the response cycle.

Excitement Phase: Women. The first observable reaction to sexual stimulation is vaginal lubrication, which has the biologic function of preparing the vagina for penile penetration. The inner two thirds of the vaginal barrel lengthen and distend. The cervix and fundus are pulled upward.

The external genitals become congested and darker in color. The clitoris increases in diameter and in tumescence (vascular congestion and swelling) (Fig. 6-32, *A*).

Excitement Phase: Men. The first observable reaction to sexual stimulation is erection of the penis (increase in length and diameter). The scrotal skin becomes congested and thick. The testes elevate because of contraction of the cremasteric musculature (Fig. 6-32, *B*).

Plateau Phase: Women. The wall of the outer one third of the vagina becomes greatly engorged, along with the labia minora, forming the "orgasmic platform." The clitoris retracts under the clitoral hood to protect the clitoris from intense, direct stimulation (Fig. 6-33, *A*).

Plateau Phase: Men. Preorgasmic emission of two or three drops of mucoid substance is released from Cowper's glands. The testes continue to elevate until they are situated close to the body to facilitate ejaculatory pressure (Fig. 6-33, *B*).

Orgasmic Phase: Women. Strong, rhythmic (every 0.8 second), muscular contractions occur in the orgasmic platform (Fig. 6-34, *A*). The number of contractions ranges from 3 to 15. The uterus also contracts rhythmically.

This phase may be subjectively described as follows:

Stage 1: sensation of "suspension," followed by "intense sensual awareness, clitorally oriented and radiating upward into the pelvis"

Stage 2: "suffusion of warmth" especially in the pelvic area

Stage 3: "pelvic throbbing" located in the vagina and lower pelvis

Orgasmic Phase: Men. Testes are held at maximum elevation (Fig. 6-34, *B*). Rhythmic contractions of the penis and rectal sphincter occur at 0.8-second intervals for the first three to four major responses.

This phase may be subjectively described as follows:

Stage 1: point of "inevitability," which occurs just before ejaculation and lasts 2 or 3 seconds; awareness of presence of fluid in the urethra

Stage 2: ejaculation with rhythmic contractions capable of expelling semen up to 60 cm (24 in)

Resolution Phase: Women. Blood returns from the engorged walls of vagina, and the labia majora and minora rapidly return to their unexcited state. The clitoris rapidly returns from under the hood; however, return to normal size may take longer. Uterus descends, and cervix dips into seminal pool (Fig. 6-35, *A*).

Resolution Phase: Men. In the first stage of the resolution phase 50% of erection is lost rather rapidly. The second stage can last much longer, depending on the maintenance of physical condition (Fig. 6-35, *B*).

Refractory Period. The *refractory* period is the time necessary to complete the cycle again. The time varies from a few minutes to a few days, depending on the age and state of physical and emotional health.

Biphasic Response. Kaplan (1974) has presented an alternative to the four-phase sexual response cycle of Masters and Johnson. She believes clinical and physiologic evidence suggests that sexual response is biphasic, with the

*See Chapter 7 for a discussion of the psychologic components of human sexuality.

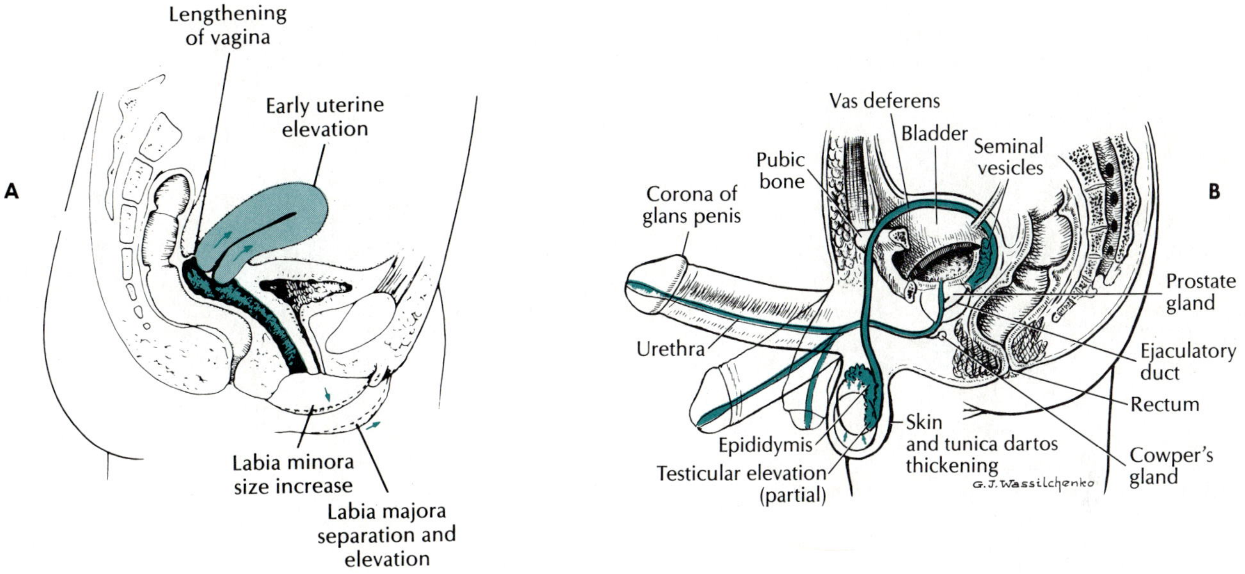

Fig. 6-32 Pelvic organs during excitement phase. **A**, Female. **B**, Male.
A, From Fogel, CI, and Woods, NF: Health care of women: a nursing perspective, St Louis, 1981, The CV Mosby Co.

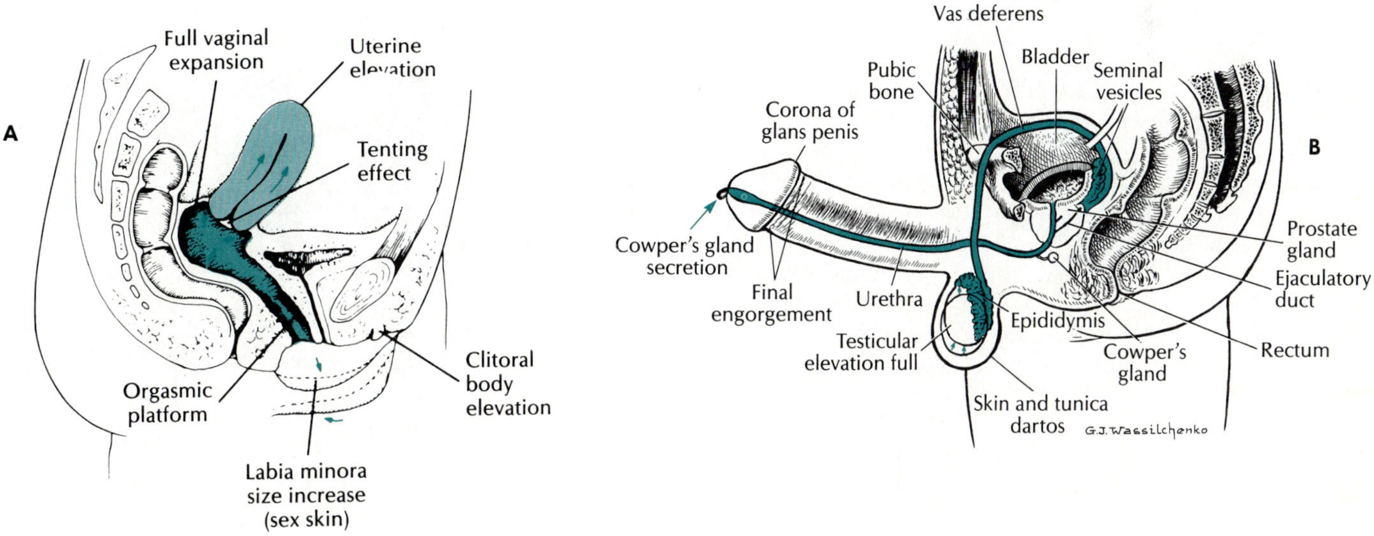

Fig. 6-33 Pelvic organs during plateau phase. **A**, Female. **B**, Male.
A, From Fogel, CI, and Woods, NF: Health care of women: a nursing perspective, St Louis, 1981, The CV Mosby Co.

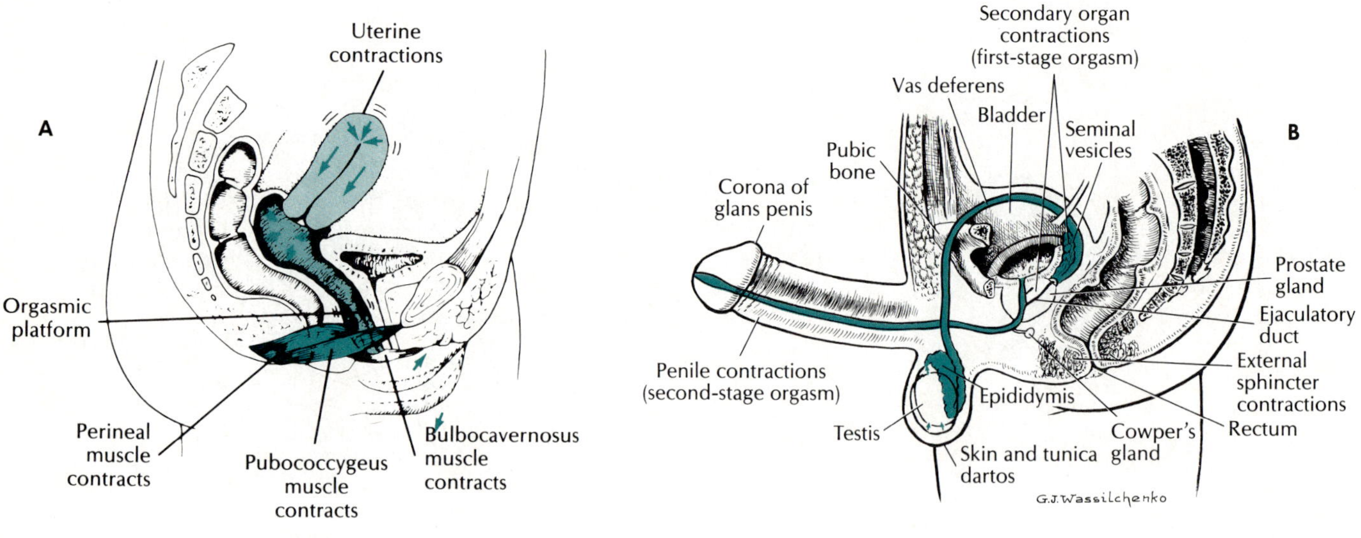

Fig. 6-34 Pelvic organs during orgasmic phase. **A**, Female. **B**, Male.
A, From Fogel, CI, and Woods, NF: Health care of women: a nursing perspective, St Louis, 1981, The CV Mosby Co.

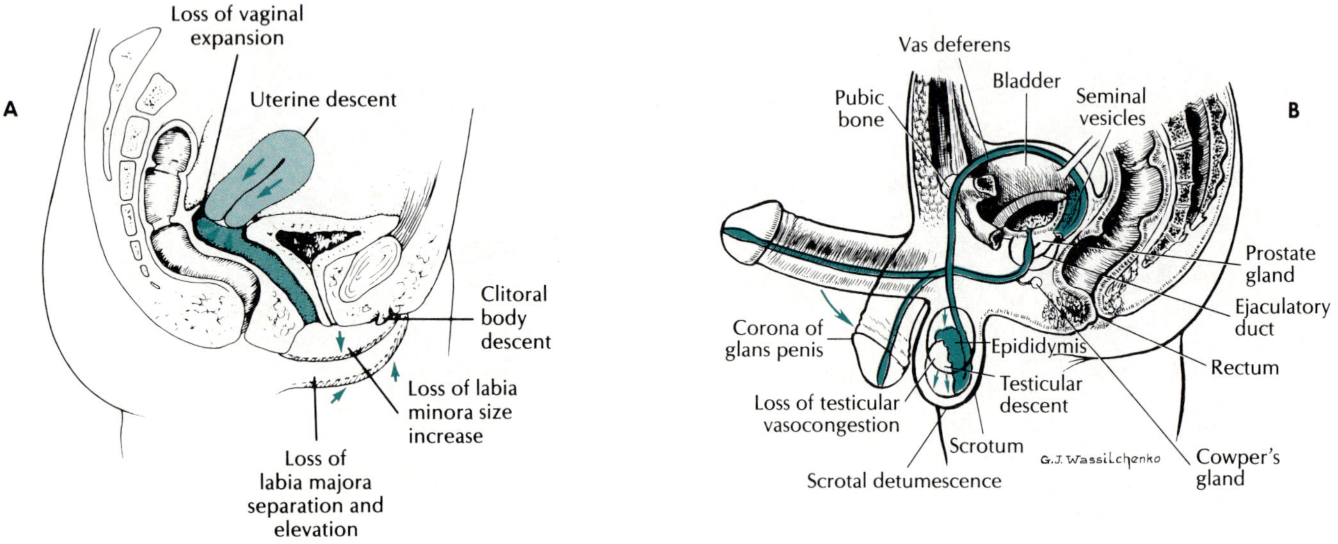

Fig. 6-35 Pelvic organs during resolution phase. **A**, Female. **B**, Male.
A, From Fogel, CI, and Woods, NF: Health care of women: a nursing perspective, St Louis, 1981, The CV Mosby Co.

following two distinct and relatively independent components:

1. Genital vasocongestive reaction—produces vaginal lubrication and swelling in the female and penile erection in the male
2. Reflex clonic muscular contractions—constitute orgasm in both sexes

Phase 1: Vasocongestive Reaction. Erection in the male is local vasocongestive response. During erection the corpora cavernosa become engorged with blood. Special valves in the penile veins are closed by reflex action, preventing loss of blood. This mechanism is regulated by the parasympathetic division of the autonomic nervous system. This system controls the diameter and valves of the penile blood vessels, thus causing erection or loss of erection. Once erection has occurred, excitement can be maintained for some time. Men are physically capable of losing and regaining several erections during love play.

Kaplan calls the vasocongestive reaction in females the "lubrication-swelling" phase. During this phase, dilation of the circumvaginal venous plexus causes a transudate on the walls of the vagina, which results in lubrication. The tissues become the "orgasmic platform" (analogous to erection in the male). In addition the uterus becomes engorged and begins to rise slightly out of the pelvic cavity so that the cervix is placed in a position to increase the likelihood of fertilization.

Phase 2: Reflex Clonic Muscular Contractions. The visceral aspects of the ejaculatory reflex are under control of the sympathetic division of the autonomic nervous system, as opposed to the parasympathetic division that is involved with erection. Male orgasm has two phases: *emission* and *ejaculation*. Emission comprises contractions of the vasa deferentia, the prostate, the seminal vesicles, and the internal part of the urethra. Masters and Johnson (1966) have called the subjective response to emission "ejaculatory inevitability." Ejaculation is the external mechanism that causes spurts of semen to be forced outward from the penis.

The biphasic nature of the response cycle is dramatically explained by the impact of aging on the refractory period. For example, a man's frequency of ejaculation may be reduced, but his ability to have erections may remain relatively the same.

The woman, like the man, has orgasms consisting of a series of reflex, involuntary rhythmic contractions of the orgasmic platform.

Clinical Significance. There are four important findings from the research of Masters and Johnson that have significance for nurses working with pregnant women and their families. These findings concern (1) multiple orgasm, (2) simultaneous orgasm, (3) clitoral versus vaginal orgasm, and (4) variations in orgasmic patterns.

Multiple Orgasm. Since women never physically have a refractory period, they are capable of having one orgasm after another until exhausted. Multiple orgasms are most commonly reported by women in their late thirties and early forties. Some women have reported being multiply orgasmic for the first time during the second trimester of pregnancy. The reason is that because of the increased vasocongestion of pregnancy, total completion of the resolution phase never occurs.

Simultaneous Orgasm. Many couples have considered simultaneous orgasm the ultimate goal of sexual bliss. The findings of Masters and Johnson and of others show the illogic of such goals, because many couples progress through the response cycle at different rates. The myth of the desirability of simultaneous orgasm has harmed many relationships because of the difficulty of achieving this goal. Although possible, simultaneous orgasm is the exception rather than the rule and is achieved when the woman reaches orgasm easily.

Clitoral versus Vaginal Orgasm. Freud taught that women transfer sexual sensation from the clitoris to the vagina when they reach psychosexual maturity. A clitoral orgasm was considered therefore to be an immature orgasm. This belief existed until Masters and Johnson demonstrated that an orgasm is a total body response to sexual stimulation, with the most intense response located in the pelvic area. The response is essentially the same regardless of whether it is experienced through coitus, masturbation, or mechanical stimulation. The clitoris is defined as the "transmitter and conductor" of erotic sensation. Hite (1976) reported that 30% of the women in her sample of 300 were orgasmic during intercourse without additional clitoral stimulation.

Variations in Orgasmic Patterns. There are many response patterns for both women and men. These patterns vary in both intensity and duration.

Prostaglandins

Prostaglandins (PGs) are oxygenated fatty acids now classified as hormones. The different kinds of PGs are distinguished by letters (PGE, PGF), numbers (PGE_2), and letters of the Greek alphabet ($PGF_{2\alpha}$).

PGs are produced in most organs of the body but most notably by the prostate and the endometrium. Therefore semen and menstrual blood are potent prostaglandin sources. PGs are metabolized quickly by most tissues. They are biologically active in minute amounts in the cardiovascular, gastrointestinal, respiratory, urogenital, and nervous systems. They also exert a marked effect on metabolism, particularly on glycolysis. Prostaglandins play an important role in many physiologic, pathologic, and pharmacologic reactions. $PGF_{2\alpha}$, PGE_1, and PGE_2, are most commonly used in reproductive medicine.

Role in Reproductive Functions. Prostaglandins affect smooth muscle contractility and modulation of hormonal activity. Indirect evidence supports PGs' effects on the following events:

1. Ovulation
2. Fertility
3. Changes in the cervix and cervical mucus that affect receptivity to sperm
4. Tubal and uterine motility
5. Sloughing of endometrium (menstruation)
6. Onset of abortion, spontaneous and induced
7. Onset of labor, term and preterm

After exerting their biologic actions, newly synthesized

PGs are rapidly metabolized by tissues in such organs as the lungs, kidneys, and liver.

PGs may play a key role in ovulation. If PG levels do not rise along with the surge of LH, the ovum remains trapped within the graafian follicle. Following ovulation, PGs may influence production of estrogen and progesterone by the corpus luteum.

The introduction of PGs into the vagina or into the uterine cavity (from ejaculated semen) increases the motility of uterine musculature, which may assist the transport of sperm through the uterus and into the oviduct. High concentration of PGs in the semen (about 55 μg/ml) may be necessary for normal fertility in males.

PGs produced by the woman cause regression (return to an earlier state) of the corpus luteum, regression of the endometrium, and sloughing of the endometrium, which results in menstruation. PGs increase myometrial response to oxytocic stimulation, enhance uterine contractions, and cause cervical dilation. They may be one factor in the initiation or maintenance of labor or both. In addition, prostaglandins may be involved in the following pathologic states: male infertility, dysmenorrhea, hypertensive states, preeclampsia-eclampsia, and anaphylactic shock. Further discussion of PGs relevant to abortion may be found in Chapter 31; for a discussion of PGs' role in pregnancy and childbirth, see Chapter 10.

IMMUNOLOGY

Beverly Gaglione

Viewing life as an opportunity to grow and develop through interactions with other systems in the environment enables the nurse to appreciate those factors that monitor and mediate the self-other relationships. A systems theory approach to the concept of immunity is useful in understanding the numerous and complex physiologic factors that serve to maintain the integrity of the body's organization when nonself cells or substances affect the various patterns of the body.

Two different types of immunity are addressed in Table 6-5: universalistic (or nonspecific) and particularistic (or specific). *Universalistic immunity* consists of those physiologic defense mechanisms that are common to nearly all humans. It provides general protection against the deleterious effects of nonself cells and substances. *Particularistic immunity* refers to those defense mechanisms that are unique to an individual because of personal experiences in the environment. This type of immunity is not only peculiar to an individual but also unique in that it involves resistance to certain specific foreign cells and substances.

Universalistic (Nonspecific) Immunity

The following immune defense mechanisms are shared by all healthy human beings. Those physiologic defense mechanisms that comprise the body's first line of defense (i.e., those that prevent invasion of the body by foreign cells and substances) include the following:

1. Intact skin, which has a slightly acidic pH and secretes sodium chloride (perspiration) through its sweat glands—both of which discourage many microorganisms but at the same time encourage other bacteria (*resident flora*) that function to keep pathogenic bacteria and other nonself matter in check.
2. A ciliated respiratory tract, the operation of which protects the lungs and bronchi from microorganisms, debris, and dirt.
3. A viscous mucous membrane, which lines all the portals (entrances and exits) of the body, including the eye. The character of the mucous membrane inhibits the growth and activity of invading microorganisms. The outward flow of tears, urine, and vaginal secretions hinders the inward movements of microorganisms.
4. The enzyme lysozyme, which is found in tears, saliva, milk, mucus, and other body fluids and is capable of lysing, or breaking down, the cell walls of many different types of bacteria.
5. The very acidic pH of the stomach, which creates a hostile environment for nonself cells and substances, and the resident bacteria of the colon, which discourage the colonization and growth of pathogenic bacteria in the intestines.
6. Eyelids, which can close to protect the eye.

Table 6-6 provides examples of immunologic problems associated with pregnant and parturient women, newborns, and postpartum and perimenopausal women when there is a dysfunction of the first line of defense.

If foreign cells and substances do manage to penetrate the body's first line of defense, a *second line of defense* is present in all healthy human beings. The various mechanisms of this line of defense include the following:

1. The body has the capability of producing an inflammatory response and "fighting" cells. This response begins with the release of histamine from mast cells, which causes local vasodilation—distending the capillary beds—resulting in the characteristic warm, reddened inflammatory response. Serous fluid and white blood cells then pass through the distended capillaries and present themselves at the site of invasion, drawn by chemotactic substances released by the invaded cells. Other white blood cells position themselves in strategic places in the body to detect and fight invasive substances. Table 6-7 details the various types of leukocytes (white blood cells) and their roles in the body's defense system.

2. A complementary mechanism of defense acts in a series of steps. The initial step catalyzes subsequent phases, and the overall effect is like a pile of dominoes that have begun to fall against one another. The name of this general mechanism, *complement cascade,* is derived from its function: to complement. The mechanism is comprised of 11 different proteins; the whole effect of their interaction results in chemotaxis (in this instance chemically attracting white blood cells to the site of invasion), triggers the release of histamine from mast cells, neutralizes viruses, and lyses cell membranes of invading cells. Although the complement cascade is said to be a nonspecific defense, it is set into motion by a specific antigen-antibody response. The specific antibody does not have the ability to lyse the invading cell, but the complement cascade results in a multifaceted, combined specific and nonspecific attack on the antigenic substance.

Table 6-5 *Application of Systems Theory to Concept of Immunology*

Principles of Systems Theory	Examples from Human Physiology	Immunologic Effect
A system is characterized by degrees of openness—extent to which that system is able to be influenced by another system.	*Skin:* Its integrity being intact.	U* Provides physical and mechanical barrier to microorganisms and some substances.
	Skin: Its selective permeability.	P† Permits absorption of substances to which one can be sensitive; involves IgE antibody.
	Skin: Its NaCl perspiration.	U Inhibits certain bacterial flora from colonizing and overwhelming system.
	Placenta: Its selective permeability.	P IgG humoral antibodies cross placental barrier and provide particularistic (passive natural) immunity, whereas IgM and IgA antibodies do not.
A system exhibits patterns or regularities that permit predictions to be made about behavior and operation of system.	*Vagina:* In a state of good health, fecund woman maintains acidic pH.	U Inhibits growth of certain bacteria and fungi.
	Vagina: Under influence of systemic antibiotic therapy or steroid therapy, resident Döderlein bacilli are reduced in number.	P *Candida albicans* (fungus) establishes itself on mucosa.
	Complement cascade: Series of events initiated by antigen-antibody reaction.	U Results in chemical attraction of leukocytes and phagocytes to site of invasion; degranulation of mast cells (releasing histamine); neutralization of viruses; and lysis of invading cells.
Behavior of whole system is affected by that of its parts and by its interactions with other systems.	*Bone marrow:* Treatment with certain antineoplastic drugs suppresses function of marrow.	U Depression of number and function of phagocytes, monocytes, and B and T lymphocytes, resulting in compromised site of immunocompetency.
	Exposure to German measles (rubella), polioviruses, etc.	P Development of IgM humoral antibodies upon first exposure to antigen, to provide protection against invading viruses.
A system is affected by space and time dimensions.	*T-cell receptor sites:* Only certain places in body have these receptor sites.	U T-cell receptor sites are essential for cell-mediated type of immune response. Fact that a woman can be host to embryo formed from mate's sperm cell and surrogate mother's ovum, and can continue pregnancy to term‡ is evidence of the female reproductive tract's immune unresponsiveness to foreign protein substances.
	Repeated exposure to an antigen (as through booster injection or second allograft from same donor) is example of effect of time on immune response.	P Because of existence of memory B and T lymphocyte cells, there is accelerated and stronger antibody or cytotoxic response to substances that body has previously experienced.
Changes occur within system and between systems via communication.	*Histocompatibility complex molecules* permit recognition of self from nonself cells and substances.	U Stimulates initiation of or inhibition of foreign tissue rejection response
	Antigens (antibody generators) are introduced into body via air currents (respiratory tract), pulsating circulating blood, flagellated movements of some cells, etc.	P Antigens in blood stimulate development of B lymphocyte, humoral antibody, whereas antigens in tissue stimulate T lymphocyte, cell-mediated cytotoxic antibody response.
Nature of systemic change is such that it is progressively more complex and innovative.	Once triggered into effect, *complement cascade,* a complex of 11 proteins, appears to be unidirectional, sustained by enzymes that catalyze subsequent steps.	U Sum effect of cascade is multifaceted attack on antigenic substance. End result of cascade is lysis of invading cell's wall.
	When *blood levels* of appropriate antibiotic drug therapy (according to culture and sensitivity tests) are inadequately maintained, offending microorganism is not effectively brought under control.	P Antigenic bacteria develop resistant strains to antibiotic and may then actually thrive in environment of once effective antibiotic, resulting in overwhelming attack on body system.

*U, Universalistic or nonspecific effect, a protective immunologic mechanism that is common to all healthy human beings.

†P, Particularistic or specific effect, a protective mechanism that is unique to an individual's system and experience.

‡Bustillo et al., 1984.

Table 6-6 ***Examples of Potential Obstetric, Neonatal, or Gynecologic Immunologic Problems Associated With Dysfunction of Universalistic First Line of Defense Mechanisms***

Client Type	First Line of Defense Dysfunction	Immunologic Problem
Obstetric		
Antepartum phase	pH of stomach and mouth altered toward more basic reaction secondary to self-medication with $NaHCO_3$ for heartburn (pyrosis).	Prone to invasion of pathologic bacteria in gastrointestinal tract.
Intrapartum phase	Episiotomy, especially a third- or fourth-degree extension of perineal laceration.	Possibility of contamination of suture line (by direct extension) and infection of perineum, vagina, uterus, fallopian tubes, and peritoneum with coliform bacteria.
Postpartum phase	If soap or other drying agent is mistakenly applied to "clean" or "disinfect" nipples and areola area of breasts, lubricating glands of Montgomery may cease to function adequately. Also, if breast pads with plastic liners are used, moisture will remain against nipple, predisposing it to maceration and cracking.	In case of drying, this may lead to change in secretion of fatty acids and thus to increased susceptibility to tissue breakdown, colonization and invasion of bacteria. With cracking of nipple and subsequent break in integrity of skin comes likelihood of invasion of pathogenic bacteria, leading to mastitis.
Neonatal	If child is born with facial paralysis (Bell's palsy) secondary to birth injury from forceps, eye on affected side may remain open (until closed and protected by nurse).	Surface of eye could dry out and be prone to injury and microbial invasion.
Gynecologic	A postmenopausal woman can be expected to have a decrease in vaginal secretions secondary to altered hormonal (estrogenic and progesteronic) influence over mucosal and endometrial secretions.	Prone to vaginitis.

Table 6-7 ***Role of White Blood Cells in Body's Defense System***

Type of White Blood Cell (WBC)	Percentage (%) of Total WBC*	Role Played in Immunity
Granulocytes	51-78	These cells have granules or lysosomes that function to degrade material ingested by WBCs.
Neutrophils ("segs" or polymorphonuclear neutrophils)	50-70	These granulocytes travel in blood to site of invasion; then they adhere to endothelium of blood vessel and proceed to pass through blood vessel to area of invasion and inflammation. Here they act by phagocytosis and lysis.
Eosinophils	1-4	Found mostly in tissues of skin, lungs, and gastrointestinal tract, these cells act as phagocytes.
Basophils	0-1	These noncirculating cells are found in connective tissue, where they release heparin and possibly other chemotactic substances that augment and complement inflammatory and allergic response.
Mononuclear (nongranular) leukocytes	22-48	No granules are found in cytoplasm of these cells. They are also known as *agranulocytes.*
Monocytes	2-8	Monocytes travel to site of invasion (like neutrophils) and act as macrophages (very large phagocytes). Some reside in spleen, lymph nodes, connective tissue, and lungs, where they screen out and destroy foreign or damaged self tissues in that environment.
Lymphocytes	20-40	
B type	95%-98% of *circulating* lymphocytes	B lymphocytes travel through body in blood and lymph systems. They proliferate during viral or bacterial infection and form plasma cells (from which *specific* antibodies are made) and memory cells (also *specific* antibodies from which clones are made during subsequent exposure to same antigenic substance). B lymphocytes provide humoral immunity. (See Table 6-9 for more detailed information about role and action of various humoral antibodies.)
T type T "killer" or cytotoxic cells T-helper cells T-suppressor cells	Approximately 2% of *circulating* antibodies	These lymphocytes act primarily against nucleated cells including body's own cells that may be altered by a foreign substance. When stimulated by an antigen, these lymphocytes also form *specific* monocloned T "killer" (cytotoxic) cells and memory cells. T lymphocytes provide cell-mediated immunity. (See Table 6-9 for more detailed information on role of various subpopulations of T lymphocyte.)

*These percentages are based on the total number of *circulating* white blood cells found in serum; hence it is clear that basophils, eosinophils, and T lymphocytes will be underrepresented in the serum, since they are located in other sites in the body.

3. *Interferon,* a nonspecific (undifferentiated by viral type) protein, made by any of the body's own cells in response to a viral infection. Interferon is released by cells that have already been invaded by a virus and is used by the noninfected body cells to avert the destructive effects of the viral attack. In the chain of simultaneously occurring body defenses, interferon release takes place after tissue has been invaded but before the development (in sufficient quantity) of the specific antibodies that will neutralize or otherwise destroy the invading substances. The time dimension of systems theory is relevant in this context: Once a specific antibody is needed, it takes a certain period of *time* before an effective circulating level, or quantity, of the appropriate antibody is reached. Until that time the white blood cells and the interferon attempt to hold the invading substance in check.

Interferon continues to be released for the first 24 hours after a cell is invaded by a virus. It is important to realize that the interferon does not arrest a de facto viral infection or invasion that is already established within a cell; it is only of benefit to those cells that have not yet succumbed to the attacking virus. Apparently, the half-life of interferon is of such short duration (most sources indicate that it provides protection only for one 24-hour period) that its use artificially (by injection) is not only impractical but expensive. At present, its production in laboratories and by genetic engineers entails considerable work and expense.

4. Finally, the secondary line of defense mechanisms in the human immune system consists of the lymph vessels, lymph nodes, spleen, tonsils, and thymus. The lymph vessels transport interstitial fluid to the lymph nodes and back to the circulatory system. Lymph fluid contains the agents of trauma, phagocytes, and body tissue that has been damaged from the invasive substances. These by-products of the invasion reach the lymph nodes and are trapped there. This fact makes it clear why lymph nodes adjacent to a cancer site, for example, in breast cancer, are usually excised during surgery, since the nodes are expected to harbor stray cancer cells. Lymphocytes, primarily produced by the bone marrow and the thymus gland, are in abundance in the lymph nodes, along with macrophages (Table 6-7). These two types of cells attack the invading agents lodged in the lymph nodes. Lymphocytes and macrophages are also found in large quantities in the spleen and the tonsils. Because of their location, the tonsils function to trap airborne invasive agents, whereas the spleen functions to tap invasive agents borne by the blood. The thymus gland, located behind the sternum, is an organ that plays a vital role in the development of T lymphocytes. (T lymphocytes take their name from the thymus gland.) The thymus is normally active in fetal life and in early childhood but usually atrophies after puberty. The roles played by the T and B lymphocytes and their specific antibodies are detailed below.

Particularistic (Specific) Immunity

As defined earlier, particularistic or specific immunity refers to those defense mechanisms developed by an individual in response to environmental stresses or opportunities, the effect of which confers a degree of resistance or nonsusceptibility to specific foreign microorganisms or substances. Table 6-8 depicts four different categories of particularistic immunity, based on distinctions between resistance that is naturally versus artificially acquired and resistance that is obtained actively or acquired passively.

Actively Acquired Immunity. An actively acquired immunity is obtained by engaging the body in the process of *producing antibodies* specific to the dimensions or characteristics of an antigenic substance. The type of resistance conferred by actively acquired immunity is usually of long duration, sometimes lasting for a lifetime.* The length and strength of the immune response are increased through repeated exposure to small amounts of the antigenic substance. This is the rationale that underlies the sequence of "booster" injections in an immunization series. Repeated or "booster" exposure to small amounts of the antigen or to attenuated (weakened, not so virile) antigen encourages the antibody population to increase. (See Table 6-10 for information regarding the correct interpretation of a titration test.)

Passively Acquired Immunity. An immunity that is passively acquired provides protection to the body in the event of exposure to specific antigens. The body does not produce its own antibodies in this case; it receives them passively. In general, immunity that is passively acquired is of short duration, since the immune globulin received is of the "fighter" type, not the "memory" type (see Table 6-7 and the discussion that follows); hence its life span is limited.

Naturally Acquired Immunity. A naturally acquired immunity is developed in response to one's individual experiences throughout life. The body of a person exposed to the viruses that produce diseases such as mumps, German measles, and hepatitis has first-hand experience with the invading agents. Therefore that person's specific immune defenses are stimulated to develop the particular antibodies to fight the invading agents. The passively acquired natural immunity entails a degree of uniqueness because the antibodies received from one's mother (via placenta or colostrum) depend on the antigens to which the mother was exposed and the subsequently developed antibodies; the length of pregnancy†; and whether or not the child was breast-fed.

Artificially Acquired Immunity. An artificially acquired immunity can be said to be iatrogenic, since the antigens (in the case of active artificial immunity) and the antibodies (in the case of passive artificial immunity) introduced into the body are considered to be "legend" drugs, which require a physician's prescriptive order before they can be administered. As pharmcologic categories of drugs, these antigens (e.g., attenuated poliovirus and attenuated rubella virus) and these antibodies (e.g., immune Rh_O (Du) im-

*For detailed information about susceptibility and resistance factors (length of immunity following exposure to the antigen) to communicable diseases, refer to the 1981 edition of *Control of Communicable Diseases in Man,* an official report of the American Public Health Association, Washington, D.C.

†Prematurely born infants receive less antibody protection than do term-birth neonates because the placental transfer of IgG antibodies is greater during the last several weeks of pregnancy (Korones, 1986).

mune globulin and hepatitis B immune globulin) are known as *biologicals* since they are produced from living cells. Before administering these products, it is extremely important to check carefully the expiration dates and lot numbers of the items, since the material can deteriorate or become contaminated.

T Lymphocyte Response. Two different types of lymphocytes are responsible for the development of the antibody-specific immune responses in the body. They are known as T lymphocytes and B lymphocytes. The T lymphocytes, derived from thymus tissue, are activated against eukaryotic (nucleated) cells, and they exert their action at the level of tissues that are invaded by some nonself substance or cells. The type of specific immunity effected by T lymphocytes is known as *cell-mediated immunity.* Facilitating the body in their job of identifying nonself cells and then attracting cytotoxic (killer) T lymphocytes specific to the offending invading substance are special molecules—known as major histocompatibility complex (MHC) molecules—and T-helper (T_H) cells. The MHC molecule is a coded section of a cell that identifies that cells as "self" or "nonself." The MHC code for all your healthy cells is the same. Your best friend's MHC code is different from yours. (In the future with improved technology, nurses may not be identifying newborns by footprinting them but by obtaining a specimen for MHC code discernment.) Hence it is understandable why one person's body tends to reject grafted or transplanted tissue from another person (as an allograft)—unless that person is an identical twin. It is this cell-mediated T lymphocyte specific immune reaction that is involved when a body rejects transplanted organs or tissue.

T-Helper Cells. When a virus or another nonself substance invades a person's cells, the MHC complex becomes somewhat altered. This alteration triggers a "nonself" identity and release of some chemotactic substance(s) that at-

Table 6-8 *Types of Particularistic (Specific) Acquired Immunity*

	Active	Passive
Naturally acquired	Body produces an antibody specific to stimulating antigen that has entered body via dysfunction of primary line of defense. EXAMPLE: Exposure to measles (rubeola) or German measles (rubella) virus stimulates production of IGM antibodies (see Table 6-9) and memory antibodies that provide protection and resistance to virus on subsequent exposure. Experience with these diseases and their specific antibodies usually confers a permanent type of immunity (long lasting).	Body receives specific antibodies made by another person and transmitted via a "natural" process (placental transmission or through colostrum). EXAMPLE: IgA antibodies are received by infants from their mother's colostrum and IgG antibodies are received in utero, especially during last several weeks of pregnancy, from mother's circulating humoral antibodies. (Table 6-9 provides more detail regarding different types of immunoglobulins and humoral antibodies.) This type of immunity is transient, lasting only for several months.
Artificially acquired	Body produces antibody specific to stimulating antigen injected into body. Usually antigen is attenuated (weakened, so as not to produce a full-blown virulent disease). EXAMPLES: Sabin trivalent oral polio virus consists of three types of live but weakened polio virus. When administered, it stimulates production of IgM antibodies and memory cells specific to three types of antigens. When nonpregnant woman is given rubella vaccine, she is injected with live but attenuated German measles virus. It takes about 3 months for her to develop full immunity to rubella virus subsequent to injection. She must not become pregnant in this 3-month period, since her body is still considered to be "fighting" rubella virus as it develops IgM antibodies against it.	Body is injected with IgG antibodies produced by another person or animal, to provide protection against antigens to which body has been exposed. EXAMPLE: When a woman who is Rh negative delivers a baby who is Rh_o (Du) immune positive, or if such a woman has an abortion (miscarriage), she is at risk of being exposed to fetal Rh-positive erythrocytes (secondary to microfracture of placental tissue, with escape of fetal blood cells and their uptake by maternal circulation). If permitted to respond "naturally" to these fetal Rh-positive antigen cells, mother would develop long-lasting "fighter" antibody cells against Rh-positive cells. This would pose a problem to subsequent Rh-positive children she would conceive, since her "fighter" antibodies would cross placenta and attack cells of her fetus. Thus woman is given anti–Rh-positive antibodies, so that she will not produce her own antibodies. *Timing* of injection of Rh_o (Du) immune globulin is of utmost importance. If it is given too late after delivery (after 72 hours), mother will have begun process of forming her own long-lasting antibodies against Rh-positive cells. Once a woman has developed long-lasting immunity against Rh-positive cells, she is no longer a candidate for immune globulin, and her Rh-positive offspring are prone to erythroblastosis fetalis.

tracts the T-helper cells. The T-helper cells function to activate cytolytic or cytotoxic (killer) T cells that are specifically made to the dimensions or characteristics of the invading antigenic substance. In addition the T-helper cell activates the B lymphocytes in their development of specific circulating antibodies, and so it also indirectly triggers the complement cascade.

Killer T Cells: Memory Cell and Fighter Cell. Killer T cells are of at least two types: a memory cell and a fighter cell. The killer T cells are capable of producing monoclones to specific antigens. The memory cell retains the instructions for producing clones of the specific killer T cell. Because of this conservative strategy, the body reacts more quickly (see Table 6-5) to a repeated exposure to an antigen. This principle is operational when a person receives a second tissue or organ transplant from the same donor: the graft or tissue rejection response is accelerated and stronger with subsequent exposure to the same antigen. The mechanism for making the specific antibody (killer cell) is already in place, and therefore the antigen-antibody reaction is almost immediate.

The immune response memory cells (of both the T and B lymphocytes) are stored in lymph nodes and the spleen. The lymph nodes and the spleen often enlarge during the active acute phase or invasive acute phase of invasive attack. These tissues are the focal sites for the replicating monoclones of the requisite T and B specialized lymphocyte cells.

The "fighting" killer T cells act in several different ways: by neutralizing the antigen, by invading it, or by triggering the auxiliary macrophages and interferon responses.

T-Suppressor or T-Regulator Cell. Another type of T cell is the T-suppressor or T-regulator cell. This cell apparently functions via negative feedback to prevent the killer T cells and even the B lymphocytes from becoming activated or to limit their action.

B Lymphocyte Response. The B lymphocytes are derived from bone marrow. They produce antigen-specific antibodies that circulate in the blood. Therefore the B lymphocytic defense mechanism is known as the *effector* of the humoral immunity system. When stimulated by an antigen, the immature (undeveloped or unspecified) B lymphocyte differentiates into plasma cells and memory cells. The antigen-specific antibodies are released by the plasma cells during the first exposure to the antigen. These antibodies function by binding with their antigen and neutralizing, agglutinating, or opsonizing it. The antigen-antibody complex also triggers the complement cascade. The cascade ultimately results in lysis of the cell membrane of the offending invading agent. The memory B lymphocytes continue to circulate (they stay unbound); they travel to the lymph nodes, the spleen, or to both to replicate monocloned antibodies in the event of repeated exposure to the specific antigenic substance.

Primary Humoral Response. Primary humoral response occurs after the initial contact with a specific anti-

Table 6-9 *Role and Action of Specific Antibodies Produced by B and T Lymphocytes*

Antibody Type	Immunity Type	Role and Action
T-killer (cytotoxic) lymphocyte	Cell-mediated	Activated against foreign protein (as allografts); intracellular infections (viral, mycobacterial, protozoal, and fungal infections that have not only gained entrance to body but also have lodged within cells in tissue); and self (own) cells that have undergone subtle but significant enough change so as to alter the histocompatibility complex code of cells; converting it to nonself status.
B lymphocyte	Humoral (circulating)	
IgA		These antibodies scout, screen, and protect mucosal surfaces of respiratory tract, gastrointestinal tract, and genitourinary tract. They are developed principally in response to viral antigens. They are also found circulating in saliva, colostrum, tears, synovial fluid, and bile, so they are also known as "secretory" immunoglobulins (found in secretions of the body).
IgD		Although these antibodies have been identified by researchers, their role and function have not been discerned to date.
IgE		These antibodies function during hypersensitivity (allergic) responses. They regulate release of histamine from mast cells when allergens bind with their corresponding IgE antibodies. They are also said to have an antihelminthic role (eradicating worms from gastrointestinal tract).
IgG		The B lymphocyte antibodies make up greatest number of all five classes of immunoglobulins. Primarily found circulating in serum, they are concerned with secondary humoral response, chiefly to invading viruses and bacteria. This is only type of B lymphocyte antibody that crosses placental barrier and provides natural passively acquired immunity to fetus and neonate. Activates complement cascade when specific antibody binds with antigen.
IgM		These large-size antibodies found in serum are manifested during primary humoral response to invading viral and bacterial organisms. They activate complement cascade phenomenon after binding with antigen.

Table 6-10 *Using Laboratory Test Data Regarding Activated Immune Defense System to Determine Approach to Health Care*

Test Performed	Purpose of Test	Nursing Care Implications
Agglutination and titer levels (blood test)	These two tests permit quantitative and qualitative determination of presence of antibodies to antigen. In quantitative phase, fact of clumping (agglutination) or no clumping is indicative of antibody-antigen reaction (depending on structure of test, absence or presence of clumping may be read as positive test for antigen-antibody reaction). *It is a test of this type that is performed as immunologic test for pregnancy (searching for antibody reaction to antigen known as human chorionic gonadotropin),* which is formed by fetal tissue. Qualitative or titration test indicates degree of response aroused in body by antigen. Commonly physician will order two tests of titration separated by a time interval *(as before delivery and after delivery, in case of indirect Coombs' test)* to determine if there has been a change—most notably a rise—in titer levels, which would indicate recent experience with antigen in question. *In case of testing for immunity (resistance) to rubella,* titration test is essential to determine if client has adequate number of antibodies to provide protection in event of repeated exposure to rubella virus. Most labs consider a titration at level of 1:10 as adequate to ensure a state of immunity against rubella. NOTE: The titration levels conferring immune status differ from disease to disease.	A positive test indicates that exposure has occurred to antigenic substance. *In case of direct Coombs' test* (for detection of specific maternal antibodies—IgG—on fetal erythrocytes, antigenic substances): positive test result should alert nurse to fact that neonate is at risk for hyperbilirubinemia, oxygen deficit (secondary to hemolysis of red blood cells), and all sequelae of erythroblastosis fetalis (see Chapter 40). *In case of indirect Coombs' test* (for detection of anti-Rh antibodies appearing in mother's serum): if test result is positive and if serial dilutions of serum indicate there is considerable anti-Rh antibody activity in mother's system, mother would not be a candidate for Rh_o (Du) immune globulin, since she had already developed the IgM and IgG antibodies against Rh. *If pregnant woman has positive titration test for rubella at 1:4 dilution* (1 part serum to 4 parts diluent) but not positive test at 1:8 dilution, she does not have adequate antibody protection against rubella virus. Woman is then susceptible to acquiring disease if exposed to virus. Compounding risk is fact that rubella that can be demonstrated to have occurred during first trimester of pregnancy (on basis of interval-titration tests) poses a hazardous risk to fetus (see Chapters 30 and 39). Postpartum woman who has demonstrated negative rubella titration test is good candidate to receive rubella vaccine, provided she practices some form of contraception for 3 months following injection of live, attenuated vaccine—until she has developed state of immunity to the disease. Client should also sign informed consent before receiving rubella vaccine, to indicate that she is aware of her responsibilities and risks associated with artificially induced active immunity therapy.
Complement (C3, C4) activity (blood test)	Instead of testing for activation of entire complement cascade, usually test is performed for two aspects of cascade sequence, to determine if they have been triggered. In event of immune response, levels of C3 and C4 (2 of 11 proteins involved in cascade) decrease, indicating their having been used.	This is a nonspecific test. It is possible that there may be "normal" test result yet immune response occurring in body. In combination with other tests (e.g., LE [lupus erythematosus] prep, ANA [anti-nuclear antibody] and RF [rheumatoid factor] tests), this test may be used to determine progression of the autoimmune disease processes.
C reactive protein (blood test)	This is a nonspecific test indicative of inflammatory process. It is sometimes used to rule out viral infection because protein is not present in cases of virally-caused inflammation.	Because this test is nonspecific, caution must be used in interpreting results. *It is possible for pregnancy or drug therapy with estrogenic birth control pills to produce false positive test.* Also, test may be positive in other types of inflammatory situations, as during acute myocardial infarction, acute phase of rheumatic disease, or rheumatoid arthritis.

Table 6-10 *Using Laboratory Test Data Regarding Activated Immune Defense System to Determine Approach to Health Care—cont'd*

Test Performed	Purpose of Test	Nursing Care Implications
Culture and sensitivity (C & S)	This test permits identification of type of antigen probably responsible for infectious process. Details about Gram's stain, type of environment (aerobic or anaerobic) that supports growth of antigen, and other characteristics of agent can be determined. Once a bacteria, virus, or fungus has been identified, test continues, to evaluate effectiveness (or sensitivity) of variety of antibiotic drugs in inhibiting growth of agent. Occasionally a C & S test is performed during a phase of antibiotic therapy, when client has not shown improvement with prescribed medication.	Nurse is responsible for collecting correct amount of specimen for culture, in appropriate type container. It is preferable that specimen is collected before antibiotic therapy is initiated, because this therapy could affect and invalidate test results. Once results of test are available, it is imperative that client receive medication to which antigenic organisms are sensitive (and not resistant). If client has been receiving a drug to which organism is resistant, nurse must contact physician and report test result immediately.
Immunoelectrophoresis of serum proteins: IgA, IgD, IgE, IgG, IgM (blood test)	Normally this test is used to detect changes in any of immunoglobulins. *In case of a newborn,* this test may be performed to learn if IgM antibodies are present in the cord blood. (*Note:* These large IgM antibodies do not cross placental barrier.)	*If infant is born with suspicion of intrauterine acquired infection,* nurse should save placenta and cord for laboratory analysis (for IgM antibodies and other tests). A positive IgM cord blood test necessitates contacting physician immediately and initiating protective and supportive care to infected infant (see Chapters 36 and 39).
Immunofluorescent antibody (IFA) tests (blood test)	In *direct* test (searching for *antigen*), a fluorescent-labeled antibody is mixed with sample of blood. If antigen is present, it binds with antibody and can be detected with ultraviolet light microscope. In *indirect* test (searching for *antibody*), known antigen is mixed with blood sample and then fluorescein anti-immunoglobulin antibodies are mixed in. If a fluorescein-bound antibody-antigen complex is seen, no antibodies were present and so there was no exposure to that antigen (supposedly, unless immune system is compromised or defective).	*Two tests of this type have significance for maternity clients:* fluorescent treponemal antibody (FTA-ABS) test for syphilis exposure and IFA test for toxoplasmosis. (See Chapter 30 regarding care of pregnant women with these infections.) If congenital syphilis of infant is suspected or confirmed, isolation techniques should be instituted for care of infant until such time that she or he is adjudged noncontagious on basis of drug therapy specific to the spirochete.
Sedimentation (erythrocyte) rate (blood test)	During acute systemic inflammatory process, erythrocytes gain in density and therefore fall or settle more rapidly when placed in test tube with anticoagulant. The more quickly cells settle, the more acute and active inflammatory process is said to be.	Change in rate of sedimentation should signal need to reevaluate those limitations placed on client. (This is not a reliable test during pregnancy when sedimentation rate is normally elevated.)
White blood cell count (WBC) and differential	Total count of white blood cells indicates number of leukocytes circulating in serum. An increase is expected during infectious and inflammatory processes. Decreases are associated with certain diseases or certain therapies (antineoplastic drugs or radiation). Differences in the percentages of the various types of leukocytes is associated with activation of or disturbances in the immune responsiveness specific to the role of the type of WBC that is altered (see Table 6-7).	Client with increased levels, indicating active immune response, needs supportive care (adequate rest, fluids, and nutrition) to fight invading organisms successfully. Client with decreased levels or with a number of immature WBCs (on differential assessment) would need protective care, since resistance level (immune responsivity) would be low, and thus client would be prone to overwhelming infection(s). At times, protective or reverse isolation must be practiced, along with blood transfusions and passive artificial immunity therapy. If a client with leukopenia is on drug therapy for any condition, nurse must check to be sure that drug therapy does not coincidentally further deplete number of WBCs (by depressing bone marrow function) as side effect; if it does, conference with physician is indicated for alternate drug therapy or supportive therapy to restore client's immune responsiveness.

Continued.

Table 6-10 *Using Laboratory Test Data Regarding Activated Immune Defense System to Determine Approach to Health Care—cont'd*

Test Performed	Purpose of Test	Nursing Care Implications
White blood cell count WBC and differential—cont'd		NOTE: Some elevation of WBC in pregnancy (up to 16,000/cu mm) and during labor and early postpartum period (up to 25,000/cu mm) is normal. Neonates are expected to have high levels of WBCs (18,000-40,000) during first few weeks of extrauterine life. As in children (up to about age 8), lymphocytes in infants become more prevalent than neutrophils. This is probably because of activity of thymus gland in infancy and early childhood. An increase in number of neutrophils is considered a healthy response to invasion, indicating intact and well-functioning immune system. If eosinophil content is increased, nurse should assist in assessment of sources of allergy or possible parasitic infestation. If lymphocyte count is decreased or if the subpopulations of T-helper and T-suppressor cells are reversed, client has compromised or deficient immune responsiveness and is in need of protective, supportive care.

gen. It generally takes between 48 to 72 hours before the corresponding B lymphocyte antibody specific to fight that antigen is ready in a quantity sufficient to be effective.

Secondary Humoral Response. A secondary humoral response entails a short response time to the antigen because of the presence of the memory cells, which reduces the production time. Therefore the response time is generally within 24 to 48 hours, and the strength of the response is greater.

There are five known classes of B lymphocyte antibodies. They are called immunoglobulins (Ig). The gamma globulins of the type IgG are the most widely studied; they are used prophylactically to confer passively acquired immunity status for a short-term period for select clients. (See Table 6-8.) Table 6-9 specifies the role and action of the specific antibodies produced by the B and the T lymphocytes.

Assessment of Immune Responsiveness

If the area of invasion is not quickly resolved by nonspecific and specific defense mechanisms, or if it is not confined to an area (as by abscess formation) it may spread in either a contiguous fashion or systemically, through the blood or lymph circulation. In turn this may be manifested as lymphadenitis (inflammation of the lymph nodes), lymphadenopathy, or septicemia. Symptoms of these processes include swollen and tender lymph nodes (secondary to the accumulation of the agents of trauma, the phagocytes, and the body's own cellular or lymphoid debris resulting from the attack), fever, anorexia, fatigue and lethargy, and leukocytosis (with increased demand there is an increased supply of the necessary white blood cells). In addition to ordering culture and sensitivity tests to determine the causative invading agent (if possible) and the appropriate effective drug therapy to assist the body in combating the infection, a physician commonly orders other types of laboratory tests to determine the body's responsiveness to the invasion. Nurses need to understand the reason(s) why these various tests are performed and the significance of the outcomes of the tests. The laboratory data provide additional assessment information that guides the nurse and the physician in their approach to the care of the client. Table 6-10 provides information about various laboratory tests of immunologic responsiveness that should be monitored, and the special nursing care implications that are associated with the tests or their outcomes. Those tests that have specific relevance to maternity, gynecologic, or neonatal clients are italicized in the table.

Factors Affecting the Functioning of the Immune Defense System

Age: Variations Across the Life Span. Although the healthy term neonate is expected to have the first-line defense mechanisms functional, the newborn does not sweat, has no tears, and is not born with resident skin or intestinal flora. For example, the lack of intestinal flora is responsible for the newborn's inability to synthesize vitamin K and thus places the neonate at risk for hemorrhagic disease. Resistance to infection is lowered following hemorrhage for anyone, regardless of age. When the integrity of the skin is broken by an internal fetal scalp electrode, the newborn is predisposed to a blood or tissue invasion by foreign cells or substances. The preterm, small-for-gestational-age, and postterm infants have different qualities of skin that increase their susceptibility to invasive agents. Infants whose birth is traumatic or who are born with depleted nutritional stores, have even greater susceptibility to infection.

The term infant is expected to have passively acquired natural immunity of IgG antibodies via placental transfer that confer resistance to those specific antigens against which the maternal antibodies were developed (Table 6-8). The preterm infants may be deficient in this type of immunity, especially if born before week 36 of gestation. The breast-fed infant who receives colostrum will have additional naturally acquired passive protection of IgA antibodies from the mother.

The newborn is capable of leukocyte activity and will develop IgM antibodies as the initial humoral response to exposure to an antigenic bacteria or virus. The fetus is capable of forming IgM antibodies in response to an intrauterine infection (See Table 6-10, immunoelectrophoresis tests). IgA antibodies produced by the infant (in the process of active natural immune responsiveness) are apparent in mucous membranes, secretions, and tears within a few months after birth.

Theorists have offered immunologic explanations about diseases (e.g., rheumatoid arthritis and adult-onset diabetes mellitus) that generally propose that the body's defense system has been overwhelmed or exhausted after operating efficiently for so many years. This model offers a "compensation, then decompensation," entropic view of physiology rather than the continually compensating, negentropic view* that is characteristic of a systems theory orientation. Some researchers argue that there is a kind of "programming" for dysfunction of the immune system, established and detectable early in life, but more manifest among the elderly. The fact that the thymus gland begins to atrophy after puberty can be used to support this hypothesis.

Environment. The environment of each person is significant in determining the challenges posed to one's immune system. The various component factors of one's environment—the quality of air, water, and food, the ventilation, refrigeration, crowding, and cleanliness in the setting—contribute to the risks that a person encounters from nonself microorganisms and substances. With the infectious diseases of tuberculosis and toxoplasmosis, one can readily appreciate the influence of environment in acquisition and transmission. Not every person is exposed to the tubercle bacillus or to the parasite that causes toxoplasmosis. However, if one lives in a setting in which tubercle bacillus is endemic (e.g., an urban, overcrowded area with poor ventilation), then the risks of exposure are much greater. The cat owner whose pet harbors the toxoplasmosis parasite is at increased risk of acquiring the disease, especially if the person has contact with the cat's feces (i.e., through emptying the litter pan). Although the exact mode of transmission of the parasite from animal to man is not known, it is recognized that the infection can be transmitted from mother to fetus via placental transfer.

The environment of the newborn in a hospital setting is a factor over which a nurse can exert some control, in order to effect fewer challenges to the neonate's immune defense system. Persons who harbor infectious diseases should be barred from the nursery, and the medical aseptic technique employed in the nursery environment should be meticulous (Chapter 22). This is not to suggest that the normal newborn should be provided with a sterile environment but that there is no reason to overtax a relatively meager set of immune defense mechanisms. An overwhelming systemic infection, such as that caused by herpes virus in the neonate, can not only interfere with healthy growth and development of the parent-child relationship because of prolonged separation but also threaten the newborn's life. For this reason the environment into which a fetus will be born must be assessed for its risk potential in posing harm to the newborn.

Nutritional Status. The notion of environment as a factor in immune responsiveness can also be applied to the internal environment of a person. The adequacy of the diet consumed contributes to the supportive mechanisms of the body that enhance resistance factors to invading organisms and substances. A diet sufficient in protein maintains the correct osmotic fluid pressure in the blood, sustaining the adequate hydration of the body's tissues. Nutritional intake that is adequate with regard to vitamins, minerals, fluid, and the basic four food groups is supportive of an intact, functionally competent immune defense system. The body retains the ability to make immunoglobulins even if the dietary patterns are low in daily consumption of protein and calories. However, the synthesis of the proteins that comprise the complement (and are responsible for the complement cascade) are more sensitive to malnourishment and especially protein deficits. Nutritional deficiency states also negatively affect the production of interferon and T lymphocytes. The health of lymphoid tissue has been associated with the adequacy of zinc intake.

Breast milk is supportive of the body's immune defense system because it favors the growth of the *Lactobacillus bifidus* in the infant's intestinal tract. This microorganism converts lactose (milk sugar) into lactic acid. Lactic acid diminishes the growth of pathogenic organisms in the intestine. Also, breast milk provides the necessary amounts of protein, calories, and essential minerals (such as zinc) for healthy functioning of the immune system (Chapter 23).

Life-Style. Certain infectious diseases are associated with the patterns of living that people establish for themselves. For instance, the sexually transmitted diseases of syphilis and gonorrhea are more likely to be acquired by people with multiple sex partners. Many other aspects comprise the concept of *life-style* besides sexual preference patterns and sexual behavior. These factors include the numerous health behaviors that people practice—such as their patterns of rest, exercise, food and drug intake, relaxation, work performance, self-care, and use of health care professionals. It is important for the nurse to assess carefully the numerous details about clients' life-styles because these factors affect the clients' susceptibility to invasion by

**Negentrophy* is a systems theory term for negative entropy, which indicates that instead of deteriorating a system increases in complexity over time.

nonself substances. For instance, a pattern of heavy alcohol consumption is associated with certain nutritional deficiencies (notably the B vitamin complex) that decrease the individual's immune responsiveness to vaccines and depress the cell-mediated and humoral lymphocytic activity (Whitney and Cataldo, 1983). Individuals who assume responsibility for their health and who practice health maintenance and preventive strategies (as acquiring artificial active immunity) are more likely to enjoy a competent immune defense system.

Health Problems Associated with Compromised or Deficient Immune System Responsiveness

Four different types of health problems are associated with compromised or deficient immune systems (Table 6-11): (1) acquired immune deficiency syndrome (AIDS); (2) severe combined immunodeficiency disease (SCID); (3) intentionally induced immunosuppression secondary to transplant surgery or treatment; and (4) unintentionally induced immunosuppression secondary to the sequelae accompanying antineoplstic drug or radiation therapy. Table 6-11 distinguishes between those problems that have been contracted directly (actively) or indirectly (passively). All four types create problems of lowered resistance to invasive agents and therefore of increased susceptibility to infections. The types of infection and other problems to which the afflicted clients are prone differ somewhat. These differences are identified in the table.

Principles of Nursing Care for the Client With Compromised Immune Responsiveness

When clients have any degree of compromised immune responsiveness, the nurse must take steps to ensure their protection from sources of infection in the hospital and the home environment. Scrupulous attention must be given to practicing medical asepsis by all caregivers who come in contact with the client to prevent superimposed iatrogenic nosocomial infections. In some cases reverse or protective isolation should be instituted to further protect the client.

To devise an individualized plan the nurse assesses for factors that place a person at risk, such as the client's age, overall health status, environment, and life-style. The client requires supportive therapy to maintain good fluid and nutritional status and to maintain the integrity of this first-line defense mechanism. In some situations the client is further protected with passive immunity support via IgG antibody injections. Those clients who have a poor prognosis (as those with AIDS and SCID) and their families also need to have supportive psychosocial care and opportunities to discuss and design their own future. Specific care needs that are induced for clients with problems of immune responsiveness are discussed in Chapters 30, 39, and Unit IX.

Relationship Between Allergic and Immunologic Phenomena

An allergen is a foreign substance that induces or generates an allergic reaction in the body. That reaction can be mild (manifested as erythema, local swelling, and pruritis), moderate, or, severe (manifested as anaphylaxis, with shock and constricted bronchioles leading to oxygen deficit and even death). The allergic reaction is caused by the histamine released from mast cells by the action of IgE humoral antibodies.

The IgE antibodies, developed from B lymphocytes, are formed as a sensitivity response to certain allergens in the environment. Upon repeated exposure to those allergens, the IgE antibody specific to that foreign substance binds with it and causes the rupture and consequent degranulation of the mast cell. The histamine so released produces peripheral vasodilation, causing local flushing, decrease in blood pressure, and capillary distension (which encourages the movement of intravascular fluid into the interstitial spaces, resulting in edema). It also constricts the smooth muscle of the bronchi, compromising the exchange of oxygen and carbon dioxide in the body.

Although antihistamines have a role to play in the treatment of mild allergic phenomena, they cannot be effective in situations of severe manifestations of allergy (as anaphylaxis). In these cases epinephrine (Adrenalin) is the drug of choice (by injection), to reverse the pathophysiologic condition by dilating the bronchi; by constricting the blood vessels, causing an increase in blood pressure; and by increasing the rate and strength of the heartbeat (and therefore the circulation of oxygen through the body).

The desensitization process—by which minute amounts of the allergen are gradually introduced into the client's system (increasing the exposure, but in amounts that are too small to produce allergic symptoms)—is technically an immunologic treatment aimed at assisting the body to become immune to the allergen by developing IgM antibodies specific to the substance.

Some clients have developed a sensitivity to certain foods, soaps, or drugs as allergens. Although it should be standard procedure for the nurse to assess all clients for sensitivity to foreign foods and substances (including adhesive tape), occasionally the nurse is involved in producing an inadvertant allergic reaction in a client. Such an incident may even occur while the nurse is administering a protective immunization to a client (as the rubella vaccine), since the vaccine is currently derived from duck egg or human (foreign protein) culture.

It is essential that nurses appreciate the complex operation of the immune system and that they fully understand how to (1) support the healthy defense mechanisms of clients; (2) protect those clients whose immune responsiveness is impaired; and (3) avoid the unintentional stimulation of potentially dangerous (allergic) defense mechanisms.

SUMMARY

Basic knowledge about the female and male reproductive systems is a prerequisite to understanding the process of conception. A systematic investigation of the human reproductive system provides the maternity-gynecologic nurse with a firm foundation for gaining insight into the client's needs and health concerns. The nurse has been provided with information on the similarities and differ-

Table 6-11 *Examples of Four Different Types of Immunodeficiency Problems*

	Active (Direct Transmission)	Passive (Indirect Transmission)
Naturally acquired	EXAMPLE: Acquired immune deficiency syndrome (AIDS) via exposure to antigen through direct sexual contact.* *Immunologic symptoms:* There is normal humoral type of immunity (because this disease characteristically afflicts people after they have had a functionally effective immune system) but reversal of subpopulation of T cells: ratio of T-helper to T-suppressor cells is reversed. This causes failure of cell-mediated immune system to be triggered; consequently this also fails to stimulate B lymphocytes and complement cascade from functioning. *Prone* to unusual or rare problems such as Kaposi's sarcoma and opportunistic infections as *Pneumocystis carinii* pneumonia (PCP). It must be remembered that immunity to common microorganisms is developed, and that circulating humoral antibodies continue to provide protection from those common invaders. *Treatment:* No therapy has been effective in curing or reversing pathophysiology to date.	EXAMPLE: Severe combined immunodeficiency disease (SCID), acquired via heredity from birth, either by autosomal-recessive transmission or by sex-linked transmission (X-linked lymphopenic agammaglobulinemia).† *Symptoms:* There are impaired or absent humoral and cell-mediated immune defense mechanisms. *Prone* to continual bouts of infection with "ordinary" type of microorganisms. It becomes manifested shortly after birth, when influence of the mother's passively transmitted IgG (via placenta) and IgA (via colostrum) antibodies wear off. *Treated* with IgG injections, reverse isolation (one child literally existed within a series of sterile "bubble" compartments until 2 weeks before he died at age 12), and bone marrow transplants (frequently not successful; usual problem is graft vs. host rejection).
Artificially acquired (iatrogenic)	EXAMPLE: Intentionally induced immunosuppression that occurs secondary to treatment with certain drugs (e.g., corticosteroids, azathioprine [Imuran], and/or cyclosporin) to decrease T-cell activation and consequent rejection of transplanted foreign protein tissue (allografts). Recently, a number of different types of organs have been transplanted—kidneys, hearts, and livers (e.g., cases in which infant is born with biliary atresia; see Chapter 40). Success of this kind of surgery has been possible only with adjunct therapy of immunosuppression, which enables donor cells to be accepted rather than rejected by the recipient cells. *Problems:* Client needs protective, supportive nursing care and gradual withdrawal from immunosuppressive agent. Compounding problems experienced by these clients, in addition to pain and fear associated with surgery, are untoward side effects associated with immunosuppressive drug therapy. These include hypersensitivity, anemia, thrombocytopenia, alopecia, steatorrhea, and lesions of mouth (with azathioprine); and hirsutism, edema, hyperglycemia (with corticosteroids).	EXAMPLE 1: Unintentionally induced immunosuppression that occurs secondary to antineoplastic therapy with radiation and/or certain chemotherapeutic drugs that depress bone marrow function. Antineoplastic therapy commonly affects rapidly proliferating bone marrow cells, as well as cancer cells for which therapy is given. White blood cells are thereby depressed and unable to engage in phagocytosis, T cell–mediated immunity and, missing cell-mediated type, humoral type is not triggered, nor is complement cascade. CONDITION EXAMPLE: Maternity client with treated choriocarcinoma (Chapter 44) *Treatment:* Includes supportive and replacement therapy (with blood products), as well as citrovorum (Leucovorin) calcium therapy, a form of folic acid which, if given within 1 hour of methotrexate, protects bone marrow against destructive effects of chemotherapy. *Problems:* Compounding problems experienced by these clients, in addition to dread of cancer therapy (in some cases) and fear of prognosis of cancer diagnosis, are multiple side effects associated with antineoplastic therapy. These may include allergic reactions, depressed clotting factors, abnormal liver function, anemia, nausea and vomiting, alopecia, heart muscle toxicity, and stomatitis. Added to this list are those problems associated with common, rare, and opportunistic infections. EXAMPLE 2: AIDS acquired through acceptance of blood or blood products from an AIDS-afflicted client. Hemophiliacs are especially prone to acquisition of AIDS via this mechanism.

*Since AIDS is transmitted by direct sexual contact as well as indirectly through blood products, the disease is presented here in two different places in the typologic schema.

†See Whaley, LF, and Wong, DL: Nursing care of infants and children, ed 3, St Louis, 1987, The CV Mosby Co.

ences of the female and male reproductive organs, growth and development patterns, and human sexual response. Immunology was presented in considerable depth because of its important role in life processes.

KEY CONCEPTS

- Female and male reproductive structures are homologus, and each system has four principal components.
- The myometrium of the uterus is uniquely designed to expel the fetus and promote hemostasis following birth.
- The uterus has an intrinsic motility allowing uterine contractions even after spinal cord injury.
- Normal feedback regulation of the menstrual cycle depends on an intact hypothalamic-pituitary-gonadal mechanism.
- The female's reproductive tract structures and breasts respond predictably to changing levels of sex steroids across the life span.
- Prostaglandins play an important role in reproductive functions by their affect on smooth muscle contractility and modulation of hormones.
- The structure of the endometrium permits regeneration without scarring following menstruation and childbirth.
- Ovulation occurs 14 days before the first day of menstruation.
- The body has the capability of producing an inflammatory response and "fighting" cells.
- Factors such as age, life-style, environment, and nutrition affect the functioning of the immune defense system.

STUDY QUESTIONS AND ACTIVITIES

1. Using a teaching model, identify the external structures of both female and male reproductive tracts.
2. Assess the factors of the immune response in an assigned client, using the information in this chapter.
3. In group discussion, describe myths and misunderstandings encountered regarding menstruation and menopause.
4. Assess some of the popularized books on sexual response and bring findings to class for a discussion of how this material relates to anatomic and physiologic facts, accepted theories of sexual response, and the challenges of client education for the maternity-gynecologic nurse.

References

American Public Health Association: Control of communicable diseases in man: an official report, Washington, DC, 1981, The Association

Bustillo, M, et al: Nonsurgical ovum transfer as a treatment of infertile women, JAMA 251:1171, 1984

Droegemueller, W, et al.: Comprehensive gynecology, St Louis, 1987, The CV Mosby Co

Hite, S: The Hite report: nationwide study of female sexuality, New York, 1976, Dell Publishing Co, Inc

Kaplan, HS: The new sex therapy, New York, 1974, Brunner/Mazel, Inc

Korones, SF: High-risk newborn infants: the basis for intensive nursing care, ed 4, St Louis, 1986, The CV Mosby Co

Ladas, AK, Whipple, B, and Perry, JD: The G-spot and other recent discoveries about human sexuality, New York, 1982, Rinehart & Winston

Lowrey, GH: Growth and development of children, ed 8, Chicago, 1986, Year Book Medical Publishers

Masters, WH, and Johnson, VE: Human sexual response, 1966, Little, Brown & Co

Whaley, LF, and Wong, DL: Nursing care of infants and children, ed 3, St Louis, 1987, The CV Mosby Co

Whitney, EN, and Cataldo, CB: Understanding normal and clinical nutrition, New York, 1983, West Publishing Co

Bibliography

Anthony, CP, and Thibodeau, GA: Textbook of anatomy and physiology, ed 11, St. Louis, 1983, The CV Mosby Co

Bates, B: A guide to physical examination and history taking, ed 4, Philadelphia, 1987, JB Lippincott Co

Danforth, D, and Scott, JR, editors: Obstetrics and gynecology, ed. 5, Philadelphia, 1986, JB Lippincott Co

Delaney, J, et al: The curse: a cultural history on menstruation, New York, 1976, New American Library

Fogel, CI, and Woods, NF: Health care of women: a nursing perspective, St Louis, 1981, The CV Mosby Co

Guyton, AC: Textbook of medical physiology, ed 7, Philadelphia, 1986, WB Saunders Co

Kaiser, HB: Allergy and immunology: new discoveries, new treatments, better results, Contemp OB/GYN 21:90 (special issue), May 1983.

Lein, A: The cycling female: her menstrual rhythm, San Francisco, 1979, WH Freeman and Co

Malasanos, L, Barkauskas, V, Moss, M, and Stoltenberg-Ollen, K: Health assessment, ed 3, St Louis, 1985, The CV Mosby Co

Moore, KL: The developing human, ed 2, Philadelphia, 1977, WB Saunders Co

Moore, KL: Before we are born: basic embryology and birth defects (revised reprint), Philadelphia, 1977, WB Saunders Co

Pritchard, JA, et al: Williams obstetrics, ed 17, Norwalk, Conn., 1985, Appleton-Century-Crofts

Ryan, KJ: Interpreting the controls of the menstrual cycle, Contemp OB/GYN 26(3):107, 1985

Whitley, N: A manual of clinical obstetrics, Philadelphia, 1985, JB Lippincott Co

Willson, JR, Carrington, ER, and Ledger, WJ: Obstetrics and gynecology, ed 8, St Louis, 1988, The CV Mosby Co

Woods, NF: Relationship of socialization and stress to perimenstrual symptoms, disability, and menstrual attitudes, Nurs Res 34(3):145, 1985

CHAPTER 7

Psychosocial Nature of Human Sexuality

Learning Objectives

Correctly define the key terms listed.

Explain two theories of human development.

Relate the four developmental tasks of sexual identification in childhood.

Review the nurse's role in parental counseling regarding sex education.

Delineate the six developmental tasks of adolescence.

Differentiate expected behaviors in the three phases of adolescence.

List the developmental tasks of the three phases of adulthood.

Critique some commonly held myths regarding human sexuality.

Assess personal belief system regarding sexuality and the impact such beliefs have on one's ability to counsel and teach sexually related material.

Explore the role of the nurse as counselor in adult sexuality.

Key Terms

androgenous personality
autonomy
cognitive development
concrete operations stage
core gender identity
developmental task
ego integrity
gender preference
generativity
heterosexuality
homosexuality
identity
industry
initiative
intimacy
masturbation
personality development
preoperational stage
promiscuous
sensorimotor stage
sex role standard
sexuality
taboo
trust

A holistic approach to sexual development takes into account the psychosocial nature of human sexuality, as well as the biologic nature. These spheres are interdependent and involve processes that progress in an orderly manner to the ultimate physical and psychologic maturity of an individual. The purpose of this chapter is to trace the psychosocial development of sexuality from birth through adulthood. A brief description of cognitive development as proposed by Piaget is included in the presentation. Intellectual response is a critical factor in developing a socially responsible use of sexual potential. As a person's sense of sexual identity is influenced by mastery of psychologic developmental tasks, Erikson's stages of personality development are presented. Social forces that strengthen the concepts of femaleness or maleness are reviewed. The review begins with gender identity in the young child and progresses through the life cycle. Family members are the first significant others in the child's sexual, cognitive, and personality development. As the child matures and ventures into the wider world, peer, educational, and other social groups provide environments that may promote or retard development.

COGNITIVE DEVELOPMENT

Cognition is the process by which people recognize, accumulate, and organize the knowledge of their world and use this knowledge to solve problems and change behavior. A young woman is used for an example. The process begins when she *perceives* or recognizes an event as a problem. She then searches her *memory* to see if the problem is similar to any past experience. Next she *generates ideas* as to a possible solution. Finally she *evaluates* the accuracy of the choice. Obviously the richer the source of ideas, concepts, and past experiences used in successful resolution of problems, the greater the odds for success in resolving current difficulties. Both innate intellectual ability and the quality of the environment are decisive factors in cognitive development.

Piaget (1950), a Swiss scientist, developed theories about how adult thought develops. He contends that two mental activities, *organization* and *adaptation,* continue throughout life. Adaptation derives from two complementary processes: *assimilation,* the absorption of new information interpreted in terms of existing structures, and *accommodation,* the changing of existing structure to fit new information. According to Piaget, cognitive development progresses in an orderly and sequential manner through four stages. The process is one of gradual evolution, with each stage building on the specific attainments of the previous one. Table 7-1 summarizes cognitive and personality development across the life span.

Sensorimotor Stage (Birth to 2 Years). Reflex activity dominates the beginning of the sensorimotor stage. It gives way to repetitive and finally to imitative behavior. Any problem solving is the result of trial and error, but a sense of "what causes what" begins to emerge. Discovery can be exciting as a child becomes aware of her or his own body, as well as other familiar objects. Language begins in a limited fashion, mostly single or double words such as "mine" or "me too." By the end of this period an object can exist without being present (object permanence). As a result, hide-and-seek is no longer frightening but has become a pleasurable game.

Preoperational Stage (2 to 7 Years). During the preoperational stage children are extremely self-centered or egocentric. As Whaley and Wong (1987) express it, "they are unable to see things from any perspective other than their own; they cannot see another's point of view, nor can they see any reason to do so." They live in a well-defined world made up of what they see, hear, or otherwise experience. Characteristically, children are "centered" in that they see one aspect of a situation but are unable to take any other factors into account. They are unaware of the transition process between one static state (the beginning) and another static state (the end). Gradually their language becomes more complex, and single words progress to phrases and then to sentences. Children grow dramatically through direct experience and an increasing ability to use symbolic communication. Behavior appears to assume *cyclic trends* of equilibrium and disequilibrium.

Concrete Operations Stage (7 to 12 Years). The concrete operations stage is characterized by a gradual increase in problem-solving ability. The method of reasoning used is inductive. Solutions to problems are not based on abstractions but are derived from what has been perceived and categorized. The "social self" appears. Children are no longer exclusively egocentric but can relate to the feelings and thoughts of others.

Formal Operations Stage (12 to 18 Years). Progress through the formal operations stage may be erratic and difficult for the adolescent. By the end of this stage, successful people can consider hypotheses and analyze scientifically. They can deduce conclusions from a set of observations, consider alternatives, and assess risks. In short, they are capable of reasoning logically by using abstractions and of assuming responsibility for the actions taken as solutions to their problems. Piaget notes that formal thinking involves two major dimensions: the use of propositional logic (the ability to think about a problem and thus rearrange aspects of it until it becomes clear) and the ability to separate fantasy from fact.

PERSONALITY DEVELOPMENT

Personality is a complex of characteristics that distinguishes a particular individual in her or his relationships with others. It includes emergent tendencies to act and to interact and thereby influence the individual's environment.

Erikson (1959) proposed a theory of personality development that defines the process in stages. Each stage focuses on a central conflict and depends on the one before it. These problems are envisioned as conflicts between opposites; for example, trust versus mistrust. As each conflict is resolved or mastered to a greater or lesser degree, the individual is ready to move on to the next level. Unresolved conflicts can hamper a person's further development and may persist in residual form throughout life. (See Table 7-1.)

Table 7-1 *Summary of Cognitive and Personality Development*

Stage	Significant Others	Cognitive Development (Piaget)	Personality Development (Erikson)
Infancy (birth to toddlerhood)	Maternal person	Sensorimotor: reflex→repetition→imitation	Trust vs. mistrust
Early childhood (2-7 yr)	+ Parental persons and other family members	Preoperational, direct experience (seeing, hearing, feeling) within a well-defined world	Initiative vs. guilt
Middle childhood (7-12 yr)	+ Neighborhood and school	Concrete thinking (not abstract), humanized (limited inductive reasoning)	Industry vs. inferiority
Adolescence (12-18 yr)	+ Peer groups and models of leadership	Formal thinking (deductive and abstract reasoning) may be limited up to 15 yr	Identity vs. identity confusion
Early adulthood	+ Partners in friendship, sex, competition, and cooperation	Formal thinking includes problem solving and separation of fantasy and fact	Intimacy and solidarity vs. isolation
Young and middle adulthood	+ Divided labor and shared household	Formal thinking includes problem solving and separation of fantasy and fact	Generativity vs. self-absorption
Later adulthood	+ Humankind, family, and friends	Formal thinking includes problem solving and separation of fantasy and fact	Ego integrity vs. despair

Trust Versus Mistrust (Birth to 1 Year). Basic trust develops as a response to being loved and cared for by a giving and concerned adult. The period from birth to 1 year is a time of "taking in" for the infant, who needs nurturing, security, and a feeling of continuity to develop trust. If such care makes up the bulk of the infant's experiences, trust takes precedence over mistrust. Successful completion of this stage results in a sense of trust in the child's responses to others throughout life.

Autonomy versus Shame and Doubt (1 to 3 Years). A sense of autonomy develops with the gradual unfolding of the child's control of body, self, and people in the immediate environment. If those who provide care applaud the child's efforts toward self-control and increasing motor skills, autonomy will result. Conversely, feelings of self-doubt and shame can occur if the child experiences frequent failures and frustrations.

Initiative versus Guilt (3 to 6 Years). The stage of initiative versus guilt ushers in an active exploratory phase in children's development. They learn much from their world by playing games and asking endless questions. They show more evidence of being guided by an inner conscience: the "parent" has been increasingly internalized. This is a time for fears and phobias. Children's developmental tasks revolve around directing their efforts toward purposeful activity and achieving a balance between daring and caution.

Industry versus Inferiority (6 to 12 Years). During the period of industry versus inferiority, children develop a sense of being a productive worker. They need opportunities to complete activities and be rewarded for their efforts. Introduction to formal schooling takes place now, and success or failure in this respect can set the stage for later career choice.

Identity versus Identity Confusion (12 to 18 Years). The period of adolescence comes after a period of relative calm. During this time of transition between childhood and adulthood, adolescents have certain tasks to perform: they must establish sexual roles, select an occupation, become independent of the family, and develop a social rather than egocentric response to people and the wider society. The adolescent must accept a new body image that includes the ability to reproduce. Successful mastery of these tasks helps adolescents develop a sense of self and identity that both they and society can accept. With this sense comes the ability for devotion and fidelity. Without it people know not "who they are" or "where they are going," and identity confusion persists.

Intimacy Versus Isolation (Early Adulthood). Once people have sense of identity, they can move toward intimate relationships with others. This can be expressed on a personal level as friendship, sexual intimacy, or the intimacy of parent-child relationships. On a social level love of fellow humans is expressed in concern for the welfare of others. Without this sense of freedom to love and be loved, people are isolated and may develop a sense of alienation from family, friends, and society.

Generativity versus Self-absorption (Young and Middle Adulthood). During the period of generativity versus self-absorption, people are concerned with creating the next generation and providing the necessary nurturing and caretaking. The tasks in this stage include preparation for assuming the role of parent, participating in the birth of children, and adapting to the reality of parenthood. Some people may become substitute parents in myriad ways: adopting children, being friends to adolescents, teaching, or nursing. Self-absorption is minimized when involvement of the self with others takes place. Growth of the personality as a person seeks balance between commitment to self and commitment to others leads to a sense of productiveness and fulfillment.

Ego Integrity versus Despair (Late Adulthood). Staying productive and involved in the welfare of others increases the satisfaction of elderly people. (In the United States old age arbitrarily begins at 65 years.) In most cases an elderly person's physical and mental abilities gradually decline, imposing limitations and curtailing her or his sphere of activity. As people confront the limitations, they must balance acceptance against despair. Wisdom and a sense of satisfaction in their accomplishments come to those who succeed in the search for personal meaning.

DEVELOPMENT OF SEXUALITY

Sexual identity begins at conception. At that time, through the chance combination of an ovum and a sperm, a person's biologic sex is determined. Thereafter, intrauterine and extrauterine environmental influences both play their part in the realization of each person's sexual potential. Biophysical, psychologic, sociocultural, and ethical factors all contribute to the molding of an individual's sexuality.

Sexuality pervades the whole of a person's life; it is more than a sum of isolated physical acts. It is a purposeful force in human nature, observable in everyday life in endless variations. It may find expression in the love of parent for child and child for parent, of friend for friend, or a woman for man and man for woman. It can be the source of pleasure or pain, fulfillment or deprivation, and sharing or exploitation. Recognition of the power of such drives has prompted each culture throughout history to develop social codes, religious dogmas, or legal restraints. These help delineate the sex role models and patterns to be followed in the process of achieving adult sexuality.

We are born into a sexually oriented world, and from birth onward we assume socially defined sexual roles that reflect the basic pattern prescribed by the society. These roles are learned informally through being part of a social group. Development of a concept of sexual roles and sexual identity begins at an early age and continues as a series of developmental tasks throughout a person's life span.

Infancy and Childhood

Developmental Tasks. One of the first questions parents ask when their child is born is "Is it a boy or a girl?" The answer sets in motion a series of social influences that will be reflected in the child's concept of "who I am" and "what I can do." The tasks relative to forming a sexual identity include developing core gender identity, acquiring prescribed sex role standards, identifying with the parent of the same sex, and establishing gender preference.

Core Gender Identity. Core gender identity is the earliest and most stable form of gender identity. By 2 years of age children can differentiate between girls and boys through awareness of dissimilarities in hair and clothing and some awareness of anatomic differences. Core gender identity is developed in normal children by the time they have reached 3 or 4 years of age.

Efforts to determine the importance of biologic versus environmental contributions to a person's gender identity have generated much controversy and research. Some studies indicate certain different biologic responses in female and male newborns and suggest differences in the infants' responses to the environment and readiness for various learning experiences. Other studies reveal the importance of gender labeling on the eventual acceptance of gender identity. Infants whose sex was uncertain at birth accepted the sex role assigned by their parents and identified with that role (Maccoby, 1974).

From the child's perspective, knowing oneself as either a girl or a boy begins before full realization of the implications of sexual identity. The infant establishes her or his gender identity from interactions with the parents. It is largely accomplished by acceptance of parental labeling; for example, "Be a good boy," "That's my girl," and "That is my big boy."

Communication, verbal or nonverbal, provides the child with cues about the sex-appropriateness of her or his behavior. A sense of trust in sexual identity develops through the early reaffirmations of femaleness or maleness.

Sex Role Standards. The term *sex role standards* refers to the various behaviors, attitudes, and attributes that differentiate the roles. Even 2-year-olds are exposed to this conditioning, because parents choose for them the kinds of clothing, toys, and activities that reflect the parents' expectations of sex role standards.

The child learns by observing the behavior of mothers, fathers, brothers, and sisters. The child formulates a concept of who should perform what tasks, who provides the comforting, who provides the active play, and who is nurturing when there is sickness. The feelings children develop about themselves as people in general and as sexual people in particular are directly related to their experiences with their bodies and the attitudes and values they derive from many sources. One of the most important ways children learn about their bodies is through exploratory sexual behavior (sex play). *Sex play* is defined by Kinsey et al. (1948, 1953) as "actual genital play." Four categories of sex play are listed as follows:

1. *Self-exploration and self-manipulation*: most common forms of sex play. Fondling of penis and manual stimulation of the clitoris are most common. Infants begin the process of exploring their bodies even by 2 to 3 months of age. As they grow they discover they are able to experience sexual pleasure through self-stimulation. Parents who feel masturbation is harmful will rebuke even young children and forbid them "to play with themselves."
2. *Same-sex comparisons*: comparison of size and shape. Prepubescent homosexual behaviors do not necessarily lead to adult homosexuality. Children need reassurance that their genitals are similar to those of others.
3. *Coital play*: when a boy lies on top of a girl. The activities are largely experimental, imitative, and exploratory.

Children become aware of parental sleeping arrangements, bathing, and privacy. They begin differentiating sex role behaviors and will play at being Mommy and Daddy.

4. *Exhibitionism*: showing and handling genitals in public, especially in the presence of companions. Most children engage in sex play activities only sporadically, especially when these activities are ignored by adults. For example, one out of four boys who had engaged in sex play had done so only during one year, and some had participated in such play only once before puberty (Kinsey et al., 1948). Kinsey et al. (1948, 1953) found that 9 years of age was the peak age for girls, when 14% engaged in some form of sex play. For boys the peak was 12 years of age, when 38% were similarly involved.

During early childhood (2 to 7 years) children are vulnerable to shaming experiences. Parents often use the sense of shame or guilt to encourage children to limit acting out sexually to appropriate places. Children need to be encouraged to develop self-control without loss of self-esteem or the feeling that sexual activity is sinful. During middle childhood the child interacts more freely outside the family. Biologic drives are less pronounced as the child strives for body competence and mastery. Sex role mastery centers on competitiveness, such as "being the fastest runner," or "throwing the ball farther than anyone else."

In Western society the adjectives used to describe a female predominantly express a mothering capacity, that is, "gentle, loving, submissive, patient, warm, and concerned." These qualities suit a person whose central reason for being is assumed to be the care and nurturing of the young and, by extension, anyone who needs such care. Those adjectives used to describe the male, namely, "dominant, aggressive, impatient, objective, and ambitious," portray a person capable of independent, decisive action. These are seen as the qualities needed in the marketplace and the basis for career orientation.

In reality, people of both sexes possess these qualities in common. Some personalities lean more toward the socially defined concept of either female or male; others have no clear demarcation of roles. These latter people, termed *androgynous personalities,* use those qualities most needed at the moment without feeling guilty about usurping another's role. A male nursing student made the following comment during a discussion of mothering:

> It is not a case of one or the other, it is what the time calls forth. The most nurturing behavior of "mothering," if you want to call it that, that I've ever seen was in Vietnam when a man was trying to get a wounded friend out of range of fire. He protected him, covering him with his own body, gave him his food and water. No mother could have shown more devotion.

A common way children prepare for a future parenting role is through sibling caretaking. Older children from either the nuclear or extended family care for younger children. Older children are used to provide role flexibility for mothers and for the development of caretaking skills by children. Stereotyped sex roles, so important in many cultures, are maintained when children assume child care responsibilities for younger family members (Weisner and Gallimore, 1977).

Identification With Parent of Same Sex. As a child comes to identify with the parent of the same sex the child internalizes the values, attitudes, and ideals of that parent. The exact method by which the process of identification is accomplished is not yet known. The child does perceive physical and psychologic similarities and is told about similarities by others. Adoption of the same-sex parent's behavior may be motivated by fear of loss of the love of this important person or by awareness of that person's power to control rewards. For a girl to forgo identification with her father, she must love her mother sufficiently to form a positive identification with her. A boy needs to relinquish his early identification with his mother and form a strong commitment to his father.

Gender Preference. Gender preference implies not only a knowledge of one's gender and the appropriate sex role but also a liking for it. Development of gender preference involves three main elements: (1) success in the role, (2) liking the same-sex parent, and (3) reinforcement from family, ethnic group, and social institutions as to the value of the role (Newman and Newman, 1975). As with other attitudes, fluctuations in preference can and do occur as people face situations in which one sex role either enhances or hinders personal goals. Deep-seated sex preferences on the part of parents can affect initial parent-child relationships if the child is not of the preferred sex. The parenting lag that results can last a day or a lifetime, depending on whether the parent succeeds or fails in resolving conflicting emotions. Certain ethnic groups have welcoming rituals for one sex and not for the other. These seemingly innocuous societal and personal preferences eventually lead a person to make value judgments about the worthiness of her or his sex. As a result the individual's self-esteem is either increased or diminished.

By the time puberty occurs the person has completed most of the developmental tasks of early childhood. Acceptance of childhood sexual identity will have consequences for self-esteem, peer relations, and selection of skills and interest. The concomitant development of moral standards such as honesty and fidelity results in a linkage between sexual identity (role) and moral commitments. Feelings of self-acceptance or guilt can be generated by either upholding or violating standards in these spheres.

Table 7-2 describes the sex-related behaviors of infancy, early childhood, and late childhood. In addition, the function for each behavior is given. As the reader will see from this table and the following two tables, human sexuality is a developmental process throughout the life cycle.

Implications for Nursing A knowledgeable maternity nurse has many opportunities to help young parents provide a supportive environment for their children's sexual development. *Nurses and parents must be careful not to ascribe adult motives to the sexual behaviors of children.* Katchadourian and Lunde (1972) stated: "It is particularly important not to label the sex play of children as deviant or perverse, no matter what it entails. To do so would be like calling a child who believes in ghosts and fairies delusional or mentally ill." Kolodny et al. (1979) caution nurses that contradictory messages about the body (parental encouragement to be aware of the body but to exclude the genitals from awareness) are among the earliest recognizable common determinants of adult sexual problems. For example, parents tell their children to "wash behind their ears" and then remind them to "wash down there." Parents and many health professionals respond to their own insecurities about sex when confronted by the overt but innocent sexuality of children.

Adolescence

Adolescence, the transitional period between childhood and adulthood, begins with puberty. The onset of puberty varies for each person. Biologically the first visible signs of puberty are the development of the secondary sexual characteristics. Menstruation can be a first indication of puberty. Shortly thereafter most teenagers experience a rapid increase in linear growth. Concomitantly, emotional changes such as moodiness, tearfulness, or withdrawal are suddenly noticeable in a previously serene youngster. For example, one mother related, "My daughter (aged 12) asked me where I had put her baby teeth. When I replied that I had thrown them away, she burst into tears and cried that I didn't think much of her to throw away something so precious."

It is not until adolescence that the socially and parentally defined sex role is openly questioned. In recent years changes in the concepts of what constitutes female and male roles have had great impact on teenagers. Conflict can result when the teenager chooses standards consistent with the peer group's attitude rather than with parental expectations.

Developmental Tasks. Erikson (1959) has described the adolescent stage of development as the one in which the

Table 7-2 *Infancy and Childhood Sexual Development*

Age	Behavior	Function
Infancy (birth to 18 mo)	Oral exploration, sucking, mouthing; explores own body	Erotic attachments and pleasures achieved from self-stimulation are forerunners of future development
	Quality and quantity of touch by caretaker; color of clothes, blankets, room; style of clothes	Beginning of formation of core gender identity
	Mothers look at and talk to girls more than boys and respond to girl's irritability more quickly; boys are touched, held, rocked, and kissed more as infants	Parental acceptance of general societal roles for females and males
	Boys: erection in first few days of life; girls: vaginal lubrication	Reflex response, not yet eroticized
Early childhood (18 mo to 3 yr)	Act of releasing contents of bowel and bladder is source of enjoyment	Learns to associate genitals with privacy, and cleanliness or dirt
	Phallic exhibitionistic period (discovers genitals and finds they can bring pleasure)	Beginning of lifelong association between sexual feelings and genitals
	Sporadic investigation of playmate's genitals; sex play probably more homosexual than heterosexual	Knowledge seeking; experimental, imitative, exploratory play, precursor to future sociosexual encounters
Middle childhood (3 to 5 yr)	Observes relationship between parents (kiss, hug, talk to each other)	Works through beginning relationships with parent of opposite sex; much of warmth the child experiences from close relationships with parents is later transferred to relationships with persons of opposite sex
	Self-exploration and self-manipulation	Learns erotic potential
Late childhood (5 to 11 yr)	Transition from home environment to school	Develops meaningful relationships with peers of same sex; solidifies sexual identity with homosocial relationships
	Begins to read, watch movies and television	Latent erotic inquiry develops; moral categories are learned
	Learns "dirty" words	Cognitive and affective meanings of words and symbols are not understood and possibly may be distorted by child
	May be labeled as "tomboy" or "sissy"	Early gender distinction; learns early that male role is more important than female role

Adapted by Marianne Zalar from Sadock, BJ, Kaplan, HD, and Freedman, AM: The sexual experience, Baltimore, 1976, The Williams & Wilkins Co.

major task is achieving identity versus identity confusion. A person's identity has many dimensions, including intellectual, interpersonal, and sexual. It is now recognized that the adolescent developmental process proceeds in sequence through three phases. These phases—early, middle, and late adolescence—put a characteristic stamp on the manner of accomplishing the developmental tasks. The developmental tasks of adolescence may be defined as follows (adapted from Havighurst, 1972):

1. *Achieving awareness and acceptance of body image.* The body image is well established by about 15 years of age. Adolescents must cope with normal but rapid changes in physical appearance and alterations in functional capacity. They must accept their physique and learn to use their bodies effectively. Deviations from the "norm" are a source of stress and may or may not be incorporated into the adolescent's body image.
2. *Achieving emotional independence of parents and other adults.* The movement away from dependence on parents that was begun with the school years is completed in this period of development. Successful accomplishment results in affection and respect for one's parents without a childish dependence on them.
3. *Achieving new and more mature relations with age mates of both sexes.* Adolescents accomplish a satisfactory social adjustment through social activities and experimentation with the peer group. Here they learn to behave as adults as they create, on a small scale, the society of their elders. The influence of the peer group increasingly takes precedence over that of the family.
4. *Achieving a feminine or masculine social role.* Although sex is biologically determined, the feminine and masculine roles are culturally established behavior sets that must be learned.
5. *Establishing a life-style that is personally and socially satisfying.* This includes the choice of a career, as well as contemplation of sexual relationships, marriage, family interdependence, and parenthood.
6. *Acquiring a set of values and an ethical system as a guide to socially responsible behavior.* This includes assuming responsibility for her or his own behavior and recognizing the effect that behavior may have on another's welfare.

Table 7-3 outlines the sexual behaviors and sexual functions of early, middle, and late adolescence.

Early Adolescence. Early adolescence begins approximately between 11 and 13 years and merges with midadolescence at 14 or 15 years (Johnson, 1983). It is characterized by an increase in height and the appearance of the secondary sexual characteristics.

In terms of cognitive powers early adolescent thought represents a mixture of two stages, the concrete operational stage and the beginning of the formal operational stage (Piaget, 1950). Although there is a greater capacity for logical reasoning, adolescent thought is still based largely on concrete evidence rather than on abstractions. Some adolescents never reach the final level of cognition (the ability to deal with abstractions), whereas others move smoothly through the intervening period.

Young adolescents tend to see the world around them only in relation to the effect it has on *them.* As their capacity for abstract thought increases, they become intensely interested in themselves, their thoughts, ideas, and fantasies, and what effect they have on others. As a result they are introspective, self-conscious, and easily hurt by real or imagined slights. They feel that everyone is looking at them critically so they demand privacy. The slamming of the bedroom door, the NO ADMITTANCE signs put on retreats, and the long periods of self-enforced isolation from the family are typical of this phase.

The major task of early adolescence is acceptance of a new body image. The rapid changes in appearance cause adolescents to spend much time thinking about their bodies and comparing their physiques with those of others. Girls are interested in their developing breasts and often want to wear brassieres before they are needed. They tend to idealize body structure and feel depressed when their skin, hair, and legs do not compare favorably with the "ideal."

Parents are still in control, and the young adolescent is aware of vulnerability and need for dependence. However, parents and brothers and sisters notice a beginning of the critical appraisal to which they will be increasingly subjected. The adolescent becomes aware of the status of the family in the community and is anxious that her or his family measure up to certain standards.

This is the time of intense relationships with members of the same sex, and these relationships are used primarily for support and mutual understanding. Young adolescents have endless face-to-face and telephone conversations about hypothetical activities; for example, "If Peter speaks to me, I will say . . . ." Through these conversations they weigh alternatives, assess risks, evaluate results and in fact practice the problem-solving approach.

Vocational choice is not a source of conflict. The young adolescent's choice is often unrealistic or idealistic. Young adolescents fantasize about what they are able to do, and although their increasing cognitive powers make them accept this as daydreaming, they are defensive about their abilities. They do like to work for money and often take newspaper routes or baby-sit.

Midadolescence. Midadolescence begins around 14 or 15 years and merges with late adolescence at about age 17. Almost all adolescents have reached their growth peak by midadolescence. Many aspects of the body have attained their adult form. For example, in boys the development of the lower jaw alters the contour of the face from the round, childish one to that of the adult. Both boys and girls generally accept their bodies, although this acceptance is tempered by a desire to look otherwise. As a result the interest in their bodies is expressed through efforts to improve themselves. Grooming, makeup, and the right clothes become all important. Stabilizing the body image is important in developing a sense of identity. Adolescents of this age can remember that they looked much the same a year ago; body structure has begun to assume permanence.

The midadolescent phase is characterized by increasing competence in abstract thought (Johnson, 1983). The adolescent is capable of perceiving future implications of current acts and decisions. The ability to think in this manner fluctuates. In times of stress the adolescent reverts to concrete operations.

The major task during this phase is emancipation from the family. Adolescents vacillate between acting like responsible adults and acting like dependent children. Their ability to step into the adult role, even if briefly, increases their resentment of being considered children. Role experimentation becomes a central process in the search for identity. Adolescents "try out" many roles in fantasy. They may select movie stars or sports heroes as role models. Vocational choice is related to the midadolescents' concern about obtaining the life-style they desire. The settled occupations of their parents and their parents' friends may seem too confining and limiting to their activities. They want to

Table 7-3 *Adolescent Sexual Development*

Age	Behavior	Function
Early adolescence (12 to 15 yr)	Talking; being given greater autonomy and less direct adult supervision	Enlargement of the testing of superego formation
	Greater involvement in and importance of peer groups, especially same sex (homosocial peer involvement); social recognition of sexual interest even if premature in terms of biologic development	Reflects commitment to anticipated roles
	Masturbation, necking, petting, and especially heterosexual intercourse	Commonly generates feelings of anxiety and guilt
	Boys	Directly linked to sexual pleasure
	Capacity to ejaculate; first orgasm within 2 years of puberty for all but a few boys	
	Pattern of masturbation initiated	Leads to independent commitment to sexuality (i.e., capacity to engage in sexual activity without social or emotional attachments); exploring of biologic capacities
	Active fantasy life	Helps reinforce commitments to heterosexual behavior
	Girls	
	Menstruation	Serves as direct reminder that intercourse can result in pregnancy
	Masturbation to orgasm rare at this age	
	Homosocial peer involvement	Reflects a commitment to anticipated roles as girlfriend, wife, and mother
Middle adolescence (15 to 18 yr)	Rating and dating system becomes central aspect of adolescent society	Heterosociality becomes fairly normative in terms of both adult and youth culture expectations
	Masturbation, especially for boys, is an important sexual outlet	Represents way station in transition from infantile to adult sexuality and from narcissism to object relatedness
	Sociosexual activity colored by homosocial attachments (activity involves sharing stories about scoring, going steady, etc.)	Role confirmation
	Petting, genital involvement without coitus; when there is coital involvement, relationships are usually not serious and do not generate numerous repetitions	Associated with involvement in peer social life (i.e., general popularity, frequency of dating, number of partners dated)
Late adolescence (18 to 20 yr)	Premarital intercourse virtually normative	Period of maximal interpersonal and intrapsychic sexual self-consciousness
	Beginning of superficial problems of sexual competence (i.e., secondary impotence, premature ejaculation, penis size, failure to achieve orgasm)	One's sexual status is a matter of public concern
	Unresolved problems of relating erotic to sentimental (residual of good girl vs. bad girl syndrome, masturbation)	
	Girl's anxieties about unintended pregnancy and concern for effect on her reputation if relationship does not culminate in marriage	

Adapted by Marianne Zalar from Sadock, BJ, Kaplan, HD, and Freedman, AM: The sexual experience, Baltimore, 1976, The Williams & Wilkins Co.

do something new, different, and monetarily rewarding.

There is a definite movement away from the family. Mid-adolescents are critical of their parents, and the parents' appearance, behavior, dress, and social manners are all subjected to intense scrutiny and disparagement. Brothers and sisters are considered a nuisance, and the adolescent sees herself as being treated unfairly in terms of other members of the family. An adult outside the family group—a nurse, a physician, a coach, or a school counselor, for example—may be taken as a role model. There is increased participation in the adult world. Adolescents become advocates of various ideologies and enjoy debating the merits of current ideas. Many show evidence of leadership potential as they engage in developing their cognitive skills. Rebellion is usually couched in verbal terms rather than physical ones and is more destructive than constructive. Running away is a common phenomenon for adolescents between the ages of 15 and 17 years as an attempt to solve problems and to prove they are not children.

Peer relationships now dominate over family ones. The adolescent looks to the peer group for definitions of the behavioral code. There is a strong need to affirm the newly developed self-image through the affirmation of peers. Most conflicts with parents reflect this change, and communication patterns that were once open may become closed.

There is a change from relationships with members of the same sex to heterosexual relationships. Adolescents test their ability to attract the opposite sex. They continue to define the parameters of femininity and masculinity. They tend to develop plural or rapidly changing serial relationships. As one mother remarked, "I couldn't keep up with the girls' names. I use to just say 'Hello there.' I was afraid I'd call Brenda, Linda or make some other terrible mistake."

Late Adolescence. The late adolescent phase extends from age 17 through 21. The upper limit of the phase depends on cultural, economic, and educational factors (Johnson, 1983). The late adolescent is physically mature. Most late adolescents have achieved a stable body image, and the agonizing over this or that real or fancied disability is largely over.

Cognitive development in late adolescence reflects the decentering of thought and production of a life plan, as described by Elkind (1968) and Piaget (1972). They have established abstract thought processes. They are future oriented and capable of perceiving and acting on long-range options.

One of the major tasks confronting the late adolescent is to become a fully *independent* productive citizen. This occurs as the adolescent moves from being an idealistic reformer to an achiever. Adolescents finally realize that criticism alone will not bring about changes and that ideals must be linked to a commitment and work. They become self-supporting or begin their professional education. They have become socially functioning adults (Handwerker and Hodgman, 1983). The choice of career pattern is reasonably set. Whatever it may be, it will establish the adult lifestyle. Although young women are now assuming the right to choose careers rather than early marriage, many still suspend the final shaping of a career until after commitments to parenthood are fulfilled.

Late adolescents are more tolerant of their families, in part perhaps because they sense the ending of the intense dependent relationship. If, on the whole, parents have permitted growth through role experimentation and have supported the need for increasing independence, the conflicts of parent and child seem to fade. On the other hand, the now self-supporting person may feel totally alienated and break all family ties.

Late adolescents' relationships are still peer-centered, but they realize that with the changes in locale necessitated by job or education these early friendships may end and be replaced by others. The need for approval by the peer group is still strong.

The late adolescent is capable of forming stable relationships. She or he is ready for mutuality and reciprocity in caring for another, in contrast to the former self-centered orientation. Marriage and family become part of present or future plans.

Adolescent Sexuality. The adolescent's heightened sexual awareness brings to the surface sexual concerns. These include myths about masturbation and concerns about possible homosexuality, sexual activity and the presence, frequency, and content of sexual fantasies and dreams. Although sexually mature, they are trying to cope with emerging sensations and social situations while they are still psychologically immature.

Masturbation. Young adolescents may fear that any deviation from normal, particularly of the genitals, has resulted from masturbation. The adolescent needs to learn that masturbation is a normal, universal behavior that causes neither physical nor mental harm. It is a natural part of learning about human sexuality and can be a useful means of relieving sexual tension (Brookman, 1983).

Masturbation is also a common mode of discharge of tension for adolescents, particularly when alone, unhappy, or frustrated. It serves to fuse psychological and physical sexuality. It is not always associated with sexual fantasies. The value of masturbation may be lessened by the shame and guilt that accompany it. Male adolescents often fear discovery of evidence of ejaculation and females often fear changes in their genitals as a result of masturbation. Fears are not limited to discovery by others but also are caused by the expansive experience of orgasm, with the resulting feelings of loss of ego boundaries. If masturbation is used as a continual source of comfort or with inappropriate exposure (exhibitionism), it is indicative of disturbance (Stuart and Sundeen, 1987).

Mutual masturbation can also serve the purposes of tension release and fusing of identity. If mutual masturbation is the primary focus of the relationship, without the enrichment of other aspects of a relationship, then it may be maladaptive. Mutual masturbation is often acceptable to adolescents as long as it does not lead to intercourse. It can help dispel anxieties about sexuality by assuring adolescents that they are sexually adequate (Josselyn, 1971).

Homosexuality. Homosexual experience to some degree is part of the psychosexual development of many individuals. The adolescent who is overly affectionate with

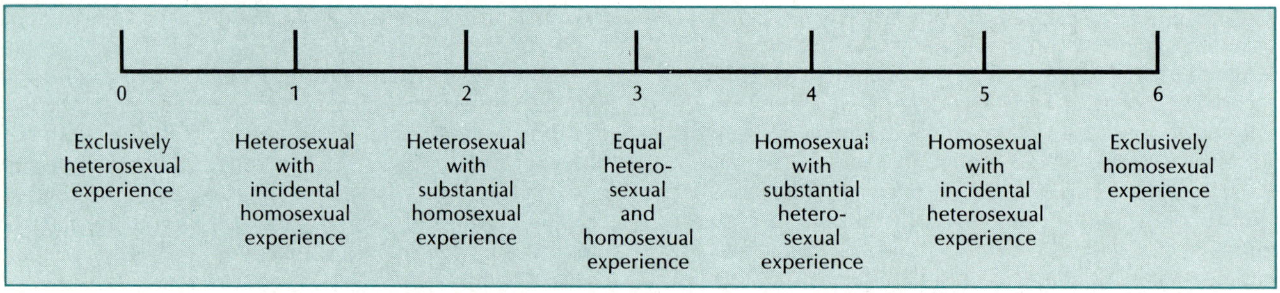

Fig. 7-1. Sexual preference scale by Kinsey (1948).

same-sex peers or adults may cause considerable parental concern. This is a result of society's unresolved position on the meaning or acceptance of homosexuality. Fantasies about sexual encounters with members of the same sex can be very disturbing to the adolescent. Memories of early same-sex explorations compound the adolescent's fear of becoming homosexual. The fear is probably a reaction to society's negative valuation of homosexuality.

For many years the medical profession, including psychiatry, has searched for causes of homosexuality. The message in looking for the cause of a condition is that it is a maladaptive state that can be treated or cured. Many theories of the cause of homosexuality have been formulated; however, no cause has ever been established. Today emphasis is placed on learning more about homosexuality and viewing it as a sexual preference or mode of sexual expression (Kinsey, 1948) (Fig. 7-1).

Marmor (1980) defined the homosexual person as "one who is motivated in adult life by a definite preferential erotic attraction to members of the same sex and who usually (but not necessarily) engages in overt sexual relations with them." Marmor's definition excludes transitory incidental homosexual activity in adolescence and in primarily heterosexual persons.

The incidence of homosexuality in the United States today has been conservatively estimated at 10% to 15% of the population (APA, 1987). If these estimates are accurate, nurses come into contact with homosexuals on a daily basis. Despite this high incidence of homosexuality, nurses generally know little about homosexuality and almost always assume that all clients are heterosexual (Stuart and Sundeen, 1987).

Sexual Activity. Adolescents are surrounded by mixed messages. Parents, religious groups, teachers, health professionals, and others tell them to refrain about sexual contact, to control sexual impulses, and to keep away from temptation. Many of these same adults are asking adolescents to refrain from activities they themselves openly practice. At the same time books, movies, music, and advertisements are laden with sexually stimulating messages.

Questions about whether and when to be sexually active and whether one needs to have sex to be popular become a major part of the lives of adolescents. They express confusion about love and how one expresses love, and concern about sexual adequacy. Pajama parties and locker room discussions are often the only outlet the adolescent has to discuss some of these concerns and to obtain information—and a great deal of misinformation—about sex.

Interest in dating stems from the adolescent's need for companionship and emotional and physical closeness. Intimacy includes hand-holding, kissing, embracing, petting, and sexual intercourse. Approximately two thirds of all teenage males and one half of all teenage females have had intercourse at least once (Brookman, 1983). Many younger adolescents may use intercourse as a means of conforming to peer group expectations, as a challenge to parents, as experimentation, or as a means of relieving loneliness or stress. Some adolescents develop sincere commitments to one another that may persist and lead to marriage. Many have "a series of close committed single-partner relationships, each lasting weeks, months, or longer" (Brookman, 1983). Few adolescents are promiscuous; that is, they do not have multiple partners with little or no commitment.

Adolescents are hesitant to talk to adults, especially parents, because the adult often discounts or invalidates their feelings. Some parents are threatened by their adolescent's budding sexuality. They (and some nurses) deal with their own uncertainty about sex by ignoring the reality of adolescent sexuality or by becoming hostile and punitive. At times little attention is given to the teenager who is reluctant to engage in dating at all. The young person who fails to show any interest may need careful evaluation.

Implications For Nursing. Health professionals need to be knowledgeable and comfortable with their own sexuality to work effectively with adolescents. Glossing over important issues and making broad generalizations about sexual concerns can be more confusing than helpful. Nurses who counsel young people about specific sexual issues need (1) knowledge of sexual anatomy, physiology, and behavior; (2) recognition of the importance of local peer influences; and (3) understanding of the adolescent's family and ethnocultural background. The approach to adolescents is based on their intellectual and psychosocial maturation. Provision of privacy and reassurance of confidentiality are essential to building trust and confidence between adolescent and nurse. The adolescent usually is willing to express concerns if the discussions are held in a comfortable and nonjudgmental setting.

An increased incidence of adolescent pregnancy and the increased number of adolescents with sexually transmitted diseases make sex education and sex counseling a major task for nurses working with adolescents (see Chapter 35). Information about their bodies' sexual responses, contraception, pregnancy, and sexually transmitted disease can be made available to them to help them become sexually responsible adults.

It is important for nurses working with adolescents to be aware of adolescents' concern about masturbation and homosexuality. Factual information about masturbation can be given to adolescents, but it is not appropriate for the counselor to advocate masturbation. The decision should be made by each person and rightly includes personal values, such as religious belief.

Brookman (1983) states that reassurance concerning homosexuality may be offered by sharing these points:

1. Strong attraction to same-sex adults is a normal event for most adolescents, representing displacement of such feelings for parents onto others in the separation-individuation process.
2. Strong attraction to same-sex peers is the first step in the shifting of a person's love-object relationship from the parents to age mates. It is also an intermediate early-adolescent stage in the development of the capacity to form intimate interpersonal relationships.
3. Exhibitionism, voyeurism, and mutual masturabtion are common experimental experiences, especially among boys age 8 to 13. Group masturbation and ejaculation, often as a contest, are common methods of declaring maturity and superiority in the peer group.
4. In many cultures, the expression of affection between same-sex friends and relatives through embracing and kissing is a normal and accepted practice for males, as well as females.
5. People who have had a homosexual episode in adolescence do not necessarily retain a homosexual preference as adults. There is nothing predictive in such an act alone.
6. Adult sexual identity is not solidified until late adolescence, but as this is most influenced by early childhood factors, ultimate sexual gender preference is well established, albeit nascent, by the advent of adolescence.

It is important to note that some adult homosexuals report awareness of their homosexuality as early as adolescence. The nurse counseling such adolescents needs to be accepting and comfortable in communicating with people who exhibit a sexual preference that may differ from their own. The incidence of sexually transmitted diseases and other infections encountered in sexual relationships makes it essential to secure appropriate medical and counseling sources for all individuals. Nurses who are not comfortable with these clients need to refer them to other professionals or agencies who can help them. "Counseling support from within the gay community can be a valuable adjunct to whatever the health professional can provide" (Brookman, 1983).

Adulthood

Adulthood encompasses the period from adolescence to a person's death. Three phases are discernable: early, middle, and late adulthood. Table 7-4 outlines the sexual behaviors and sexual functions of these three phases.

Early Adulthood. Early adulthood encompasses that portion of the life cycle devoted to parenting, consolidation of relationships, whether marital or nonmarital, and commitment to a life work. The young adult has attained physical and intellectual maturity. Stature and reproductive growth are virtually complete. The process of aging, beginning in the twenties and continuing in the thirties and forties, causes minimal overt change.

Cognitive powers include the ability to think abstractly, to be future oriented and to act on long-range options (Piaget, 1950). Personality development is related to the task of developing intimacy and solidarity as opposed to existing in isolation (Erikson, 1959). Intimacy involves learning to give and receive love, choosing whether to marry and choosing a sexual partner or partners (Duvall, 1977).

Body image remains a concern for the young adult, particularly in terms of body contour and size (Woods, 1984). Nonacceptance of one's body may inhibit the establishment of sexual relationships.

Family ties are important, but the relationship of parent and child takes on an adult quality. The young adult is expected to be moving toward financial and social independence from the family. She or he is also expected to choose a vocation and obtain the necessary education for it. Establishing a career and advancing in it are major concerns throughout this part of the life cycle.

Social groupings include varying age levels and are often based on similar interests. The need for strong friendships with peers diminishes as individual friendships assume permanence.

Sexuality. Early adulthood has been described as a period of maximum sexual self-consciousness (Offer and Simon, 1976). There is social acceptance and legitimization of sexual experiences. The tasks of sexual development for the young adult include maintaining a long-term commitment to a sexual relationship, practicing responsible reproductive health care, and making rational decisions about childbearing.

1. *Commitment to a relationship* is strengthened by the need to give and receive pleasure. Commitments vary in length and type. For example, some couples remain monogamous throughout their marriage. Others have open marriages, in which the couple agrees that one or both may participate in other sexual encounters. Some couples remain in relationships without formal marriage. Relationships can be terminated by divorce or death. Finally, serial monogamy is practiced by many people in the United States. Serial monogamy is characterized by repeated marriages and divorces. The person is married to only one person at a time but is married a number of times throughout her or his life.
2. *Responsible reproductive health care* includes such actions as women having a Papanicolaou smear at prescribed intervals or both women and men avoiding sexually transmitted diseases.
3. *Rational decisions about childbearing* are important to ensure that every child is a wanted child. The couple is responsible for using a reliable contraceptive technique when pregnancy is not desired. Unwanted children often become targets of abuse and neglect.

Myths. In a culture characterized by a rapid increase in knowledge and technology, many people still are misinformed about human sexuality. Listed below are common myths about reproduction and birth control (McCary, 1982; Stuart and Sundeen, 1987):

1. A couple must have simultaneous climaxes if conception is to take place
2. A woman can become pregnant only through penile penetration or artificial insemination
3. Urination by the woman after coitus or having sexual intercourse in a standing position will prevent pregnancy
4. The woman determines the sex of the child
5. Excessive masturbation is harmful
6. Sex during menstruation is unclean and harmful
7. Advancing age means the end of sex

Middle and Late Adulthood. These phases of the life cycle represent the greatest maximizing of early potential and then a gradual lessening of biopsychosocial attainment through the normal process of aging (Chapter 41). Changes in family structure from events such as children leaving home, death of a spouse or role reversal in dealing with aging parents necessitate major changes in life-style. The critical task for these years is maintaining feelings of self-esteem versus despair. The need to love and be loved, to be successful and to feel meaningful prompts involvement in community service and in leisure pursuits.

Cognitive powers continue unabated until physical insults such as Alzheimer's disease or cerebral vascular accident cause a decline. Body image remains an important concern. Western society's accent on health and youth make grooming, weight, nutrition, and exercise a continuous part of adult's daily life.

Sexuality. The sexual developmental tasks of middle and late adulthood focus primarily on adapting to the physical and emotional changes in sexual performance caused by the aging process. The childbearing years are coming to an end. This is a relief for many couples because the threat of pregnancy can be removed from their lovemaking. Others may mourn the loss of the chance for another child.

The fear of growing older in a youth-oriented society can be a source of depression and anxiety. Bodily changes,

Table 7-4 *Adult Sexual Development*

Age	Behavior	Function
Early adulthood (23 to 30 yr)	Formal engagement and marriage	Sexual access legitimized and regularized; as sexual access ceases to be a problem, more attention focused on activity
	Sexual dysfunction problems become more meaningfully symptomatic	Problems with gender competence, regularization of sexual access plus sheer density of interaction may result in declining eroticism especially for men
	Pregnancy and child rearing	Many pressures (fatigue, economic, time, occupational) contribute to decreased eroticism
	Beginning of extramarital affairs	More common among men of low socioeconomic class because of weaker commitment to occupational success and resulting loss of homosocial masculinity
Middle adulthood (30 to 46 yr)	Rates of marital intercourse decline	Maximal involvement in careers, family, and child rearing
	Men's interest in marital competence decreases	Much of decline caused by (1) de-eroticization of wife-mother role and (2) husband's alternative attachments
	Women's interest in marital competence increases	Commitment to the sensual and away from continuing confirmation of emotional attachment
	Period of rising extramarital activity	For men, homosocial validation of masculinity; for women, justification
Late adulthood (46 to 65 yr)	Imperative to continue sexual activity	Harder for either sex to continue to function because of long sexual abstinence
	Loss of sexual partner through death or illness	Frequently have guilt feelings about sexual fantasies
	Performance problems (particularly erectile difficulties)	Source of anxiety
	Menopause	Can be freedom from pregnancy worries and also source of concern in youth-oriented society
Old age (65 + yr)	Sexual feelings still experienced although desire and ability have decreased somewhat	Result in guilt feelings because of cultural taboo against sexuality among aged persons

Adapted by Marianne Zalar from Sadock, BJ, Kaplan, HD, and Freedman, AM: The sexual experience, Baltimore, 1976, The Williams & Wilkins Co.

lower hormone production, and menopause may contribute to anxiety and depression.

The research of Masters and Johnson (1966) has shown that aging does not decrease libido or the capacity to be orgasmic. Men and women are capable of sexual activity well into their old age. Disinterest and abstinence are probably caused by loss of a partner, boredom, ill health, or cultural attitudes about the appropriateness.

Many older people do not understand the impact of aging on their physical response to sexual stimulation. They see these changes as an indication they should terminate sexual activity rather than merely as a need to make minor adaptations. For example, lubrication in women is slower and decreased in amount; in men, erection is slower and erectile firmness decreased. Love play will probably need to be extended, with more direct genital stimulation to produce lubrication and erection. Woman have a shortened orgasmic phase and men's need to ejaculate decreases, resulting in decreased force and volume of ejaculation. These physiologic changes require adaptations in sexual behavior and not cessation of sexual activity.

Mims and Swenson (1980) have stated:

> Sexual fulfillment throughout adulthood and into old age is not only possible but likely. The feeling that older people are not interested in sex (except if they are abnormal—the "dirty old man" syndrome) is largely caused by our inability to imagine our parents or our grandparents as sexually active people. The greatest danger of such attitudes is that they tend to comprise a "self-fulfilling prophecy": if people believe that sexual interest ceases with advancing age, they will find that it does cease. Or, if sexual interest persists, people may believe themselves to be abnormal, sinful, or psychologically sick.

Implications for Nursing. The nurse is in a unique position to help adults with health maintenance and detection of problems concerning sexuality. Contacts with adults occur at clinics or hospitals when people seek counseling or care for contraception. Giving nursing care during the pregnancy cycle is an important part of the maternity-gynecologic nurse's role.

The role of sex educator is an important one for nurses working with families during the childbearing and child rearing years. Parents often need help with teaching their children about sex because adults commonly are misinformed about many aspects of reproduction and how their bodies function. Parents therefore need accurate sex information to teach their children to be healthy, responsible sexual beings.

Besides helping with childhood and adult sexuality, the nurse can help prepare clients for the sexual problems and changes occurring with age. Many nurses have not been aware of the importance of sex education for older people because of the myth that the elderly are no longer interested in sex.

Sexual dysfunction problems often begin after children are born. The mother especially may become so involved with child rearing that her relationship with her husband suffers. At the same time the husband may be actively involved in career establishment, thereby leaving little energy for home life. The nurse needs to be aware of how the demands of parenting can adversely affect the marital relationship. Simple counseling provided during these early years may prevent serious marital problems in later years.

The older woman, in particular, who has been able to move gracefully into old age and who continues to recognize herself as a sexual being is probably better able to accept the sexuality of the young. The pregnancy of a daughter then may be accepted as a continuation of her own sexuality rather than as a threat or reminder of her lost youth.

A knowledgeable, nonjudgmental nurse who recognizes personal sexual biases can contribute a great deal to the sexual health of young families. The nurse can recognize potential problems within the marriage and either intervene or refer the couple for further counseling.

SUMMARY

By the time puberty occurs a person has completed most of the developmental tasks of early childhood. Acceptance of childhood sexual identity will have consequences for self-esteem, peer relations, and selection of skills and interest. The concomitant development of moral standards such as honesty and fidelity results in a linkage between sexual identity (role) and moral commitments. Feelings of self-acceptance or guilt can be generated by either upholding or violating standards in these spheres.

By the end of late adolescence the individual is ready to move into the adult world. At this point late adolescents have developed intellectually and socially. Their independence is reflected in their ability to become productive citizens, to establish long-term intimate relationships with others and to emancipate themselves from their families. Their self-image is realistic and they have the capacity to give as well as receive love.

Adulthood represents the longest period in the life cycle. During this time childhood potential is realized and key social roles are assumed. The importance ascribed to the roles of man/woman, husband/wife, and parent/child reflect society's concern with the biopsychosocial nature of adult sexuality.

KEY CONCEPTS

- Nurses need to know themselves and to be aware of their own feelings and values regarding sexuality before they can adequately and competently help clients meet their needs.
- Nurses need to understand that everyone's feelings and values regarding sexuality are not going to match their own feelings and values.
- The atmosphere in which the child is raised will affect future attitudes and behaviors.
- Sexual identity begins early, reflects societal tasks, and involves four developmental tasks: gender identity, gender preference, identification with same sex parent, and sex role standards.
- Exploratory sexual behaviors are the foundation for adult sexuality.

- The maternity-gynecologic nurse can help parents provide age-appropriate sex education.
- Adolescence can best be understood in three phases, involving six developmental tasks: achieving more mature relations with age mates of both sexes, achieving a feminine or masculine social role, accepting one's physique, achieving emotional independence of parents and other adults, establishing a satisfying life-style, and acquiring a new set of values.
- Mixed messages about sexuality, peer pressures, and confusion about the relationship of love and sex may cause conflicts.
- Needs for information about masturbation, contraception, pregnancy, and venereal disease may be complicated by a lack of communication with parents.
- Responsible sexuality includes commitment to a relationship, responsible reproductive health care, and rational decisions about childbearing.

STUDY QUESTIONS AND ACTIVITIES

1. List four or five behaviors appropriate for each of the following stages of psychosocial development.
   A. Late childhood (ages 5 to 11 years)
   B. Early adolescence (ages 12 to 15 years)
   C. Middle adolescence (ages 15 to 18 years)
   D. Late adolescence (ages 18 to 20 years)
   E. Adulthood (ages 20 to 30 years and over 50 years)
2. Assess at least three assigned clients to determine the stage of sexual development and list observed behaviors that support assessment findings.
3. List attitudes that may inhibit or facilitate support of a client's sexual expression.
4. Identify attitudes that may make it difficult for nurses to support the sexuality of the following:
   A. Children
      (1) Preschool age group (ages 3 to 5 years)
      (2) School age group (ages 5 to 11 years)
      (3) Adolescents (ages 12 to 15 years)
   B. Older parent group (40 years old or over)
   C. Mentally or physically impaired persons
   D. Drug-dependent persons (alcoholics, heroin addicts)
5. Write down personal belief systems and discuss how these may affect one's ability to counsel and teach sexuality-related material.

References

American Psychiatric Association: Diagnostic and statistical manual of mental disorders, ed. 3, revised, (DSM-III-R), Washington, DC, 1987, The American Psychiatric Association.

Brookman, R: Adolescent sexuality and related health problems. In Hoffman, A, editor: Adolescent medicine, Menlo Park, Calif, 1983, Addison-Wesley Publishing Co, Inc

Duvall, ER: Family development, ed 5, Philadelphia, 1977, JB Lippincott Co

Elkind, D: Cognitive development in adolescence. In Adams, JF, editor: Understanding adolescence, Boston, 1968, Allyn & Bacon, Inc

Erikson, E: Identity and the life cycle; selected papers. In Psychological issues, New York, 1959, International Universities Press

Handwerker, L, and Hodgman, C: Approach to adolescence by Perinatal Staff. In McAnarney, E, editor: Premature adolescent pregnancy and parenthood, New York, 1983, Grune & Stratton, Inc

Havighurst, RJ: Developmental tasks and education, ed 3, New York, 1972, David McKay Co, Inc

Johnson, R: Adolescent growth and development. In Hoffman, A, editor: Adolescent medicine, Menlo Park, Calif, 1983, Addison-Wesley Publishing Co, Inc

Josselyn, I: Adolescence, New York, 1971, Harper & Row, Publishers, Inc

Katchadourian, HA, and Lunde, DT: Fundamentals of human sexuality, New York, 1972, Holt, Rinehart and Winston

Kinsey, AC, et al: Sexual behavior in human male, Philadelphia, 1948, WB Saunders Co

Kinsey, AC, and others: Sexual behavior in human female, Philadelphia, 1953, WB Saunders Co

Kolodny, RC, et al: Textbook of human sexuality for nurses, Boston, 1979, Little, Brown & Co, Inc

Maccoby, EE, and Jacklin, C: The psychology of sex differences, Stanford, Calif, 1974, Stanford University Press

Marmor, J, editor: Homosexual behavior: a modern reappraisal, New York, 1980, Basic Books Inc, Publishers

Masters, WH, and Johnson, VE: Human sexual response, Boston, 1966, Little, Brown & Co, Inc

McCary, JL: Human sexuality, ed 4, New York, 1982, Van Nostrand Reinhold Co, Inc

Mims, FH, and Swenson, M: Sexuality, a nursing perspective, New York, 1980, McGraw-Hill Book Co

Newman, B, and Newman, R: Development through life: a psychosocial approach, Homewood, Ill, 1975, The Dorsey Press

Offer, D, and Simon, W: Sexual development. In Sadock, B, Kaplan, H, and Freedman, A, editors: The sexual experience, Baltimore, 1976, The Williams & Wilkins Co

Piaget, J: The psychology of intelligence, Boston, 1950, Routledge & Kegan Paul

Piaget, J: Intellectual evolution from adolescence to adulthood, Hum Dev 15:1012, 1972

Stuart, GW, and Sundeen, SJ: Principles and practice of psychiatric nursing. ed 3, St Louis; 1987, The CV Mosby Co

Weisner, TS, and Gallimore, R: My brother's keeper: child and sibling caretaking, Curr Anthropol 18:169, 1977

Whaley, LF, and Wong, DL: Nursing care of infants and children, ed 3, St Louis, 1987, The CV Mosby Co

Woods, NF: Human sexuality in health and illness, ed 3, St Louis, 1984, The CV Mosby Co

Bibliography

Alan Guttmacher Institute: Teenage pregnancy: the problem that hasn't gone away, New York, 1981, The Institute

Anderson, ML: Talking about sex with less anxiety, J Psychosoc Nurs Ment Health Serv 18(6):10, 1980

Forrest, JD: American women—a sexual profile, Contemp OB/GYN 29 (special issue): 75, April, 1987

Gordon, S, Scales, P, and Everly, K: The sexual adolescent: communicating with teenagers about sex, ed 2, N Scituate, Mass, 1979, Duxbury Press

Hacker, SS: Students'questions about sexuality: implications for nurse educators, Nurse Educator 10(4):28, 1984

Havens, B, and Swenson, I: Menstrual perceptions and preparation among female adolescents, JOGN Nurs 15(5):406, 1986

Krozy, R: Becoming comfortable with sexual assessment, Am J Nurs 78(4):1036, 1980

Lion, E, editor: Human sexuality in nursing processes, New York, 1982, A Wiley Medical Publication

Marsman, JC, and Herold, ES: Attitudes toward sex education and values in sex education, Fam Relations 35(3):357, 1986

Masters, WH, et al: Human sexuality, Boston, 1982, Little, Brown & Co

Nass, GD, Libby, RW, and Fisher, MP: Sexual choices: an introduction to human sexuality, ed 2, Monterey, Calif, 1984, Wadsworth Health Science Division

Sarrel, LJ, and Sarrel, PM: Sexual unfolding: sexual development and sex therapies in late adolescence, Boston, 1979, Little, Brown & Co

Sherwen, LN: Psychosocial dimensions of the pregnant family, New York; 1987, Springer Publishing Co Inc

Storch, ML (1987).Taking a sexual history, Contemp OB/GYN, 29 (special issue): 111, April 1987

CHAPTER

8

Gynecologic Examination

Learning Objectives

Correctly define the key terms listed.

List four factors influencing the client's contact with the health care system.

Formulate reasons for entering a gynecologic health care system.

Identify and discuss each of the eight components of the gynecologic interview.

Determine some adaptations that are necessary when assessing the older woman and the woman with a handicap.

Relate how a woman is prepared for the gynecologic examination.

Summarize the assessment of the thyroid gland, breasts, abdomen, and external genitals.

Explain supine hypotension and vasovagal syncope.

Review the assessment of the internal pelvic structure.

Summarize the procedure for the clean catch urine specimen and Papanicolaou smear.

Delineate guidelines for client teaching for prevention of urinary tract infections, breast self-examination, Kegel's exercises, and vaginal douching.

Key Terms

cancer warning signals
chief concern
historian
Kegel's exercises
lithotomy position
nonjudgmental
Papanicolaou smear
proscription
review of systems
sexism
supine hypotension
support
vaginal douching
vasovagal syncope

THE GYNECOLOGIC CLIENT

Women's health care needs change with age, developmental level, and role expectations. About 40% of women seeking maternity-gynecologic care are adolescents. The number of women in their seventh and eighth decades seeking gynecologic care, however, is increasing as the life span lengthens. The nurse can help each woman learn about her body and become an active participant in her health care. Teaching a *woman,* in most cases, however, translates into teaching a *family.*

The changing status and roles for women affect their life needs and ability to cope with problems. Some stressors commonly affecting women include working outside the home, physical disabilities, changing residences, becoming separated or divorced, raising children (sometimes alone), and outliving their mates.

Culture, religion, socioeconomic status, personal circumstances, the uniqueness of the individual and stage of development are among the factors that influence a person's recognition of need for care and responses to the health care system and therapy. For many, modesty and fear of the unknown make the health assessment—the interview, the physical examination, but particularly the pelvic examination—an ordeal. The woman, whether a young adolescent or a mature woman, may be ignorant of generative and sexual function. Indeed, knowledge and visual exploration of genital anatomy may be forbidden in certain groups.

Every society has developed extensive expectations with prescriptions and proscriptions for attitudes and behaviors concerning such vital events as pregnancy, childbirth, and management of fertility. For instance, in some cultures, virginity at marriage may be an absolute requirement, with the size of the hymenal opening being used by some groups as a criterion for determining virginity. Therefore, to avoid disrupting the hymen, examination of the vaginal vault is limited to a one-finger internal examination and to the use of the smallest available speculum (see Fig. 8-13). The use of tampons and douches must be avoided in the medical management of these women. In another example, the mother of one nursing student came to my office with a copy of the text on maternity. She said that her daughter is forbidden to use the book because "she is not married yet" (the student was 22 years of age).

On the other hand, nonmarital sexual activity, often with multiple partners of the same or opposite sex, is increasingly acceptable in the United States; this affects the incidence of infection, cervical neoplasia and dysplasia, and unplanned pregnancy. In this day of assumed enlightenment, many persons are uninformed, governed by myths, and afraid to appear stupid by asking questions or to be put in the position of being judged.

Signs and symptoms of disease also have different meanings to different people (see discussions of menstruation [Chapter 6] and sexual myths [Chapter 7]). Attitudes toward health promotion and disease prevention vary, for example, women seek preventive care more than men; frequency of preventive services increases with socioeconomic status (Fogel and Woods, 1981). For others, health care is sought only after illness has occurred.

Reasons for Entering a Gynecologic Health Care System

Many women postpone examinations until there is a specific need such as pregnancy, contraception, pelvic pain, abnormal uterine bleeding, incapacitating vaginal discharge (especially pruritic), or lumps and masses.

Other minor or embarrassing signs and symptoms (urinary incontinence, dyspareunia [painful intercourse], annoying vaginal discharge) are only elicited by sensitive and careful interviewing and examination. Many women are unaware of the role of psychologic and physical stressors in the initiation, aggravation, or continuation of some gynecologic disorders.

Other women use a minor symptom as a ticket for admission to the health care system. Underlying their spoken reason for coming in (chief or primary complaint) may be such motives as wanting to become sexually active or such concerns as fear of cancer or sexually-transmitted disease, pregnancy, or need for counseling for generative or sexual functioning or for perimenopausal events.

ATTITUDES OF HEALTH CARE PROVIDERS

Learning occurs best in a safe environment in which the atmosphere is *nonjudgmental* and *sensitive* and the interaction is *strictly confidential.* The *woman's vulnerability* must be recognized and accepted; confidentiality is assured for the woman regardless of her age. The right of minors who wish to keep parents from learning of their medical problems must be respected (see Chapter 7). Some states have passed legislation requiring that in cases where a minor is diagnosed as having venereal disease or as being pregnant, this information may not be given to parents even if they request it.

The role of the physician and nurse has changed from that of authoritarian and controller to that of facilitator and consultant in problem solving. The woman's desire to become actively involved and to make informed, competent decisions relevant to her health care requires that the physician and nurse provide the woman with support, counsel, and information sufficient to understand the problem, if one arises, as well as the nature of therapy and available alternatives.

The recipient of health care needs to perceive the nurse's actions as supportive (Chapter 2). Support and reassurance must begin with the woman's first contact with the health care system. Women must be viewed as competent and treated with courtesy, attention, and friendliness by the entire staff. The data base is obtained in an unhurried manner, and the questions phrased in a sensitive and nonjudgmental manner. The examiner's body language fits the verbal communication.

Nursing is an interactive process that involves establishing a relationship with another individual within the broad goal of maintaining and enhancing health. The nursing student or new graduate may not be comfortable in this new role. However, clients can sense and benefit from the nurse's genuine concern and caring even when interview and physical examination skills are not yet well developed.

Sexism in Health Care. Sexism in the delivery of health

services has been brought to the public's attention. Traditional orientation reflects biases about women rooted in attitudes, values, and practices 150 years old (Griffith-Kenney, 1986; Ehrenreich and English, 1978). Investigators have exposed evidence of sexist bias in diagnosis (Broverman et al., 1970; Ehrenreich and English, 1978; McCranie et al., 1978), in treatment such as unnecessary surgery (Corea, 1977; Larned, 1977), in prescription of medications (Cooperstock, 1971; Waldron, 1977), and in hospital admissions for psychiatric problems (Tudor et al., 1977). Advertisements in medical journals perpetuate the gender stereotypes of males as physician-healers and women as those in need of help. When women are asked how they feel, they address different issues than those that the male caregiver might imagine women to be concerned about (McBride and McBride, 1981).

In light of heightened awareness of traditional biases, the American Board of Internal Medicine (1985) has suggested a series of questions that may be used by the interviewer. These questions are designed to give full concern to the client's feelings and needs; for example, "Would you prefer to talk to an older or younger, female or male physician?"

Contemporary orientation, reflecting a more holistic approach to women's health, is gaining acceptance. "Nursing has been in the forefront in providing services that acknowledge women's capacity for health, self-growth, integrity, and participation in the process of health care" (Griffith-Kenny, 1986). Nursing research, advocacy, teaching, role modeling, and political and social activism provide avenues for nurses to ensure a holistic approach to health care delivery.

Both the health care provider and the consumer are served best by constant vigilant watch for the adverse influence of sexism in education for the provision of health care, the dispensing of health care services, and the use of health care services (Howell, 1974; Marieskind, 1975; Ruzek, 1978).

Goals for Client. When identified before assessment, goals for the woman direct the interaction with her. Some examples of goals are:

1. Woman is psychologically and emotionally ready for the examination.
2. Woman's anxiety, embarrassment, and feelings of vulnerability are avoided or minimized.
3. Woman's self-esteem and dignity are enhanced.
4. Woman is physiologically prepared for the examination.
5. Woman's personal motivation and goals in relation to health maintenance and promotion are heightened.
6. Any adverse sequelae are avoided, such as vasovagal syncope.

Examiner Goals. The examiner's goals are two: to meet the goals for the client and to compile a complete data base without too much stress in the situation.

Assessment and Mutuality. Clients appreciate knowing why certain questions are asked and examinations are performed. Sharing this information with the client is the first step in intervention and accomplishes the following:

1. Increases woman's self-esteem (e.g., "I am worthy of examiner's time and trust in my ability to understand").
2. Increases client's knowledge base of reportable signs and symptoms for herself and others.
3. Demystifies health care so that client can perceive extent of her control as a participant in her health maintenance and care.
4. Assists her in developing her problem-solving and decision-making skills.
5. Adds to her repertoire of coping mechanisms by adding to her knowledge base.

Other techniques use communication skills such as reflection, silences, and verbalization of fears that the client may find hard to verbalize herself (out of embarrassment or other reasons) (Chapter 2).

Sequence of Health Assessment. In the process of health assessment, the data base is gathered to provide insight into the client's biophysical, socioeconomic, interpersonal, and environmental situation. This information is needed to explore how these overall experiences interrelate in her present situation and influence her future goals. The examiner and woman must share their perceptions and interpretations of the data to arrive at mutual goals before a plan of care can be developed. Implementation of this process is modified by many factors, such as the woman's age (adolescence to mature womanhood), possession of a handicap or disability, level of understanding or education (capability to understand or presence of a language barrier), cultural background, and the initiation of a trust relationship with the client (Chapter 2).

Several excellent guides are available to provide assistance in obtaining, organizing, and recording data (Malasanos et al., 1985; Bates, 1987; Seidel et al., 1987). The information gathered varies somewhat; however, there is general agreement that at least the data sought by the following guide is included (same guide is used for the assessment of the maternity client in Chapter 12):

1. Interview: the history
   a. Identifying information
   b. Source and reliability of information
   c. Chief concern
   d. Present problem or illness
   e. Past medical history
   f. Family history
   g. Social and experiential history
   h. Review of systems
2. Physical examination
3. Laboratory tests
   a. Blood: VDRL or other test for syphilis, complete blood count (CBC) with hematocrit, hemoglobin, and differential values; blood type and Rh; antibody screen (Kell, Duffy, rubella, toxoplasmosis, anti-Rh); sickle cell; level of folacin when indicated
   b. Urine: Clean-catch urine specimen tested for glucose, protein, and acetone; microscopic assessment for pus, red blood cells, and casts; culture and sensitivity as necessary
   c. Skin test: Tine or PPD (purified protein derivative [of tuberculin]) for exposure to tuberculosis
   d. Cervical and vaginal smears for cytologic evaluation and for diagnosis of infections

INTERVIEW: THE HISTORY

Individual variations in knowledge, maturation, life experience, cognitive abilities, and personality affect the interview process. Ethnicity, chronologic age, or presence of a disability or socially unacceptable disease are potential stereotyping traps for the unaware interviewer. Some older adults experiencing confusion or memory loss may need extra time to understand and answer questions. Short sentences, simple language, and conferences with other family members may be appropriate. Older women bring to the interview a lifetime of experience that may be a source of richness, wisdom, meaning, and perspective (Seidel et al., 1987). Women may have serious and handicapping physical or emotional disorders—deafness, blindness, depression, or mental retardation. Every woman is entitled to be respected and involved to the fullness of her capacity.

The following general outline is presented only as a guide for history taking. This guide should be adapted by the interviewer to accommodate the nurse's and client's individuality.

Biographic Information (Admission Form). At a woman's first visit she fills out a form with biographic and historical data before meeting with the examiner. The examiner scans the admission form and welcomes her to the office. When the woman and examiner are comfortable, the examiner begins with the interview, clarifying, expanding, or completing the admission form. The nurse ensures that the client's name, identification number, age, mental status, racial origin, ethnic background, address, phone numbers, occupation, and date of visit are recorded. Names of next of kin are noted for dependent adults. Identifying data should appear on all pages of the document.

Source and Reliability of Information. Old records are considered reliable sources. The nurse records a subjective judgment about the reliability of the person giving the history—the client, the parent, or other historian.

Chief Concern. The chief concern is the verbatim response to the question, "What problem or symptom(s) brought you here today?" The onset and duration of the problem is also noted.

Present Problem or Illness. No single outline is applicable to all cases. The interviewer may feel most comfortable asking questions related to the chief concern. Other interviewers prefer to complete the history before returning to the present. It may be useful to ask the client to sketch out the problem first. Using this method, the interviewer can see the relative importance of the features surrounding the problem from the client's perception.

The client's state of health before the onset of the present problem is determined. In addition, the earliest symptomatology noted before the initial episode may reveal its cause. If the problem is of long standing, the reason for seeking attention at this time is elicited. Identification of associated symptoms and factors that precipitate, exacerbate, or relieve the condition provide important data. The client is requested to describe how the problem has affected her usual life-style. The course of the problem is plotted from the onset to the present. The findings are summarized and reviewed with the client/historian to confirm or correct the information obtained. When more than one significant problem is present, each one is treated in the same manner.

*Past Medical History**

1. **General health and strength**
2. **Childhood illnesses**: measles, mumps, whooping cough, chickenpox, scarlet fever, acute rheumatic fever, diphtheria, poliomyelitis
3. **Major adult illnesses**: tuberculosis, hepatitis, hypertension, diabetes, myocardial infarction, tropical or parasitic diseases, sexually transmitted diseases, other infections; any nonsurgical hospital admissions (dates and reasons)
4. **Immunizations**: polio; diphtheria; pertussis; and tetanus toxoid; influenza; cholera; typhus; typhoid; last PPD or other skin tests; unusual reactions to immunizations: tetanus or other antitoxin made with horse serum
5. **Surgery**: dates, hospital, diagnosis, complications
6. **Serious injuries**: resulting in disability; if the present problem has potential medicolegal relation to an injury, give full documentation
7. **Medications**: current and recent medications, including dosage; both prescription, over-the-counter, and home remedy; old, left-over prescriptions
8. **Allergies**: especially to medications, but also to environmental allergens and foods
9. **Transfusions**: reactions; date and number of units transfused

*Family History**

1. Do any members of the client's family have illnesses with features similar to the client's illness?
2. What is the health status or cause of death of parents and siblings, with ages at death?
3. Is there a history of: heart disease, high blood pressure, cancer, tuberculosis, stroke, diabetes, gout, kidney disease, thyroid disease, asthma and other allergic states, blood diseases, sexually transmitted diseases, any familial disease?
4. What are the ages and health status of spouse and children?
5. If there is a hereditary disease in the family, such as hemophilia, Tay-Sachs disease, or sickle cell anemia, what is the condition of the grandparents, aunts, uncles, and cousins? A pedigree diagram is often helpful in recording this information.

*Social and Experiential History**

1. **Personal status**: birthplace, where raised, home environment as youth (e.g., parental divorce or separation, socioeconomic class, cultural background), education, position in family, marital status, general life satisfaction, hobbies, interests, perception of "being healthy"
2. **Nutrition**: diet; regularity of eating; quantity of cof-

*Adapted from Seidel, HM, et al.: Mosby's guide to physical examination, St Louis, 1987, The CV Mosby Co.

fee, tea, and alcohol consumed; use of vitamin and mineral supplementation
3. **Activity-exercise**: quantity and type
4. **Sleep-rest**: regularity of sleeping, hours, usual times for sleep-rest
5. **Coping-stress tolerance**: typical stressors, estimate of level of stress on a typical day at home or work, usual ways of coping, relaxing, use of illicit drugs (frequency, type, and amount)
6. **Sexuality**:
   a. Times and frequency of coitus
   b. Contraceptive history: type, when used, any problems, time and reasons for discontinuation
   c. Attitudes concerning range of acceptable sexual behavior as defined by such factors as culture, religion, family, and peer group
      (1) Is it all right for married people to masturbate?
      (2) How do your ideas and feelings about sex differ from those of your partner?
   d. Sexual self-concept (how one sees oneself sexually influences how one relates to others)
   e. Level of knowledge, including understanding of how the body functions, sexual anatomy and physiology, and myths and misinformation about sex
   f. Sexual behavior: marital or alternative relationship
   g. Marital relationships
7. **Home conditions**: housing, economic condition, type of health insurance if any, pets and their health
8. **Occupation**: description of usual work and present work if different; conditions and hours, physical or mental strain; duration of employment, present and past exposure to heat and cold, industrial toxins (especially lead, arsenic, chromium, asbestos, beryllium, poisonous gases, benzene, and polyvinyl chloride or other carcinogens); any protective devices required; exposure to cigarette smoke
9. **Environment**: travel and other exposure to contagious diseases, residence in tropics, water and milk supply, other sources of infection if applicable
10. **Military record**: dates and geographic area of assignments
11. **Religious preference**: determine any religious proscriptions concerning health care
12. **Culture and ethnic**: determine any proscriptions or prescriptions affecting health care

*Review of Systems.** It is probable that all of the questions in each system will not be included every time you take a history. Nevertheless, some questions regarding each system should be included in every history. These essential questions are listed in bold type in the outline that follows. More comprehensive and detailed questions relating to each system are listed afterward and need to be included whenever the client gives positive responses to the first group of questions for that system. Keep in mind that these lists do not represent an exhaustive list of questions that might be appropriate within an organ system. Even more detailed questions may be required depending on the client's problem.

1. **General constitutional symptoms**: energy level, feelings of well-being, fever, chills, malaise, fatigability, night sweats; weight (average, preferred, present, change, appetite)
2. **Skin**: rash or eruption, itching, pigmentation or texture change; excessive sweating; abnormal nail or hair growth
3. **Musculoskeletal**: joint stiffness, pain, restriction of motion, swelling, redness, heat, bony deformity, muscle tone and cramping, vascularity, bone fragility, flat feet, curvature of spine
4. **Head**
   a. General: frequent or unusual headaches, dizziness, syncope, severe head injuries
   b. Eyes: visual acuity or problems, pain, discharge; use of eye drops or other eye medications; history of trauma or familial eye disease; prescription glasses or contact lenses; last visit to ophthalmologist
   c. Ears: hearing loss, pain, discharge, tinnitus, vertigo
   d. Nose: sense of smell, frequency of colds, obstruction, epistaxis, postnasal discharge, sinus pain
   e. Throat and mouth: hoarseness or change in voice; frequent sore throats, bleeding or swelling of gums; recent tooth abscesses or extractions; soreness of tongue or buccal mucosa, ulcers; disturbance of taste, dentures, last visit to a dentist, frequency of dental care, problems with chewing or swallowing
   f. Neck: pain, restriction of movement, swelling
5. **Endocrine**: thyroid enlargement or tenderness, heat or cold intolerance, unexplained weight change, diabetes, polydipsia, polyuria, changes in facial or body hair, increased hat and glove size, skin striae
   a. Menses: regularity, duration and amount of flow, dysmenorrhea, last menstrual period (LMP), previous menstrual period (PMP), last normal menstrual period (LNMP), intermenstrual discharge or bleeding, itching, date of last Papanicolaou smear, age at menopause, libido, frequency of intercourse, sexual difficulties
   b. Pregnancies: number, miscarriages, abortions, duration of pregnancy in each and any complication during any pregnancy or postpartum period; use of oral or other contraceptives
   c. Breasts: pain, tenderness, discharge, lumps, mammograms
6. **Respiratory**: pain relating to respiration, dyspnea, cyanosis, wheezing, cough, sputum (character and quantity), hemoptysis, night sweats, exposure to TB; date and result of last chest x-ray study; frequency and types of infection; number of cigarettes smoked per day and for how many years
7. **Cardiovascular**: history of congenital heart disease, rheumatic fever, hypertension, hypotension, pain; dyspnea; palpitations; number of pillows (to elevate head) needed to sleep comfortably; estimate of exercise tolerance, past ECG or other cardiac tests

*Adapted from Seidel, HM, et al.: Mosby's guide to physical examination, St Louis, 1987, The C.V. Mosby Co.

8. **Hematologic**: blood type, Rh factor, anemia, tendency to bruise or bleed easily, thromboses, thrombophlebitis, any known abnormality of blood cells, transfusions
9. **Immune**: lymph nodes—enlargement, tenderness, suppuration, infections (type, response to therapy, complications), autoimmune disorders
10. **Gastrointestinal**: appetite, digestion, intolerance for any class of foods, dysphagia, heartburn, nausea, vomiting, regularity of bowels, constipation, diarrhea, change in stool color or contents (clay-colored, tarry, fresh blood, mucus, undigested food), flatulence, hemorrhoids, hepatitis, jaundice, dark urine; history of ulcer, gallstones, polyps, tumor; previous x-ray studies (where, when, findings)
11. **Genitourinary**: dysuria, flank or suprapubic pain, urgency, frequency, nocturia, hematuria, polyuria, hesitancy, dribbling, loss of force of stream, passage of stone; edema of face, stress incontinence, hernias, sexually transmitted disease (inquire what kind and symptoms)
12. **Neurologic**: syncope, seizures, weakness or paralysis, abnormalities of sensation or coordination, tremors, loss of memory; unusual frequency, distribution, or severity of headaches, serious head injury in past
13. **Psychiatric**: depression, mood changes, difficulty concentrating, nervousness, tension, suicidal thoughts, irritability, sleep disturbances, drug or alcohol abuse

The Older Woman.* Older adults can present a special challenge in organizing the information obtained from the history. They may have multiple health problems that are often chronic, progressive, debilitating, and overlapping with the process of aging. Disease symptoms may be less dramatic in older people, producing vague or nonspecific signs and symptoms. Confusion, for example, may be the only symptom of an infection or a cerebrovascular accident. Pain is often an unreliable symptom, because some older people seem to lose pain perception and experience pain in a different manner from the classic expectations. The excruciating pain usually associated with pancreatitis, for example, may be perceived by the older person as a dull ache, and myocardial infarction can occur without the cardinal symptom of pain. Conversely, older adults have a higher risk of developing painful conditions or injuries. Since many conditions may be present simultaneously, the cause of pain may be difficult to isolate.

Some clients fail to report symptoms, because they are afraid that the complaint will be attributed to old age or feel that nothing can be done. They may have lived with a chronic condition for so long that they have incorporated the symptoms as part of their expectation of daily living.

The tendency for multiple problems to be treated with multiple drugs places the older person at risk for iatrogenic disorders. A complete medication history is essential, with special attention to interactions of drugs, diseases, and the aging process.

Functional assessment should be included as part of the older adult's history. In the review of systems, questions that address functional capacity in the following areas are included:

Self-care Activities	*Instrumental Activities*
Walking	Driving a car
Getting out of bed	Using public transportation
Bathing	Dialing a telephone
Combing hair	Hanging up clothes
Shaving	Obtaining groceries
Dressing	Preparing meals
Eating (chewing)	Taking medications as prescribed
Getting to bathroom by self	

Other dimensions of functional capacity that should also be explored include social resources, economic resources, recreational activity, sleep patterns, sexuality, environmental control, and use of the health care system. The interrelationship of physical health, mental health, social situation, and the environment is particularly evident in the older population.

The Woman With a Disability. Clients with serious and handicapping physical or emotional disorders—the deaf, the blind, the depressed, the physically disabled, the mentally retarded, the brain injured—must all be respected and the assessment approach adapted to their needs. Clients who are emotionally restricted may not be able to give an effective history, but they must be respected, and the history should be obtained from *them* to the extent possible. Their points of view and their attitudes matter. Still, when necessary, the family, other health professionals involved in care, and the client's record must be queried to get the complete story. Each client must be fully respected and fully involved to the limit of emotion, cognitive capacity, or physical handicap.

Some of the most common communication barriers can be overcome if the following are kept in mind:

1. When families are available, they often can advise on communication techniques that have been used successfully at home.
2. Translators may be found for language barriers most of the time.
3. The deaf often read, write, and read lips. The interviewer must speak slowly and enunciate each word clearly and in full view. A translator who signs may be available.
4. The blind usually can hear. Talking louder to them to make a point does not help. The blind cannot see gestures.
5. Communicate directly with the client with a disability. Maintain eye contact. Learn about the disability from *her*.

Concluding Questions. At the conclusion of obtaining the history, the client is asked, "Is there anything else that you think would be important for me to know?" If several complaints are mentioned and discussed in the history, it is often useful to ask, "What problem concerns you most?" In certain situations, such as vague, complicated, or contradictory histories, it may be helpful to ask, "What do you think is the matter with you?"

*Adapted from Seidel, HM, et al: Mosby's guide to physical examination, St Louis, 1987, The CV Mosby Co.

THE PHYSICAL EXAMINATION

Once the history has been taken, it is necessary to move on to the physical examination—the laying on of hands. The manner in which the interview has been conducted sets the stage for this portion of the examination. Usually the woman is guided to discuss any fears she may have regarding the examination: fear of pain, fear of discovery of disease, fear from negative memories of previous examinations or perhaps unfortunate experiences with coitus, and fear of the unknown. The examiner needs to determine the client's needs for basic information regarding the structure of the genital organs and provide this information, along with a demonstration of the equipment that may be used and an explanation of the procedure itself. The interaction requires an unhurried, sensitive, and gentle approach with a matter-of-fact attitude.

It is important that the examiner assures the cleanliness of the facilities, equipment, supplies, and hands. All equipment necessary for the procedure should be in place to avoid interrupting the examination (Fig. 8-1).

The Basic Examination

The woman is assured of privacy for the examination without unexpected intrusions. She is given a cover gown and drape for modesty. The environment is comfortably warm and pleasant.

The physical examination begins with assessment of vital signs, height and weight, and blood pressure. Because the bladder must be empty before pelvic examination, the urine specimen is obtained. Obtaining a clean catch urine specimen is described in Procedure 8-1.

Each examiner has developed a routine for proceeding with the physical examination; most choose the head-to-toe progression. Heart and breath sounds are evaluated and extremities are examined. Distribution, amount, and quality of body hair is of particular importance because the findings reflect nutritional status, endocrine function, and general emphasis on hygiene. The thyroid gland is assessed carefully. The typical basic examination is usually completed without much difficulty for the healthy woman.

Care During the Examination. The examiner needs to remain alert to the woman's clues that (1) give direction to the remainder of the assessment and that (2) indicate imminent untoward response such as supine hypotension, vasovagal syncope, and possible cardiac arrest.

Vasovagal Syncope. Vasovagal syndrome (see box, p. 145) is a poorly defined but real emergency. It occurs without warning, is of brief duration but without predictable effects, and **can be fatal.** Those who have an attack should be managed by basic principles of cardiopulmonary resuscitation (CPR) (Queenan, 1982).

The syndrome occurs when two conditions are operative: (1) There is an actual or a potential threat of physical harm. Often the experience the woman is facing is either a new one or one that was hard for her to face on a previous occasion. (2) The injury or potential harm is one that the woman is expected to face with ease,* for example, venipuncture or gynecologic examination.

The vasovagal response is biphasic: the *sympathetic nervous system* (fight or flight) discharges and pulse rate, blood pressure (especially systolic), cardiac output, and vascular resistance increases. The woman appears apprehensive and pale but says she is "fine." Then, if the woman

*Men are more susceptible than women in our society. Men are not supposed to be afraid.

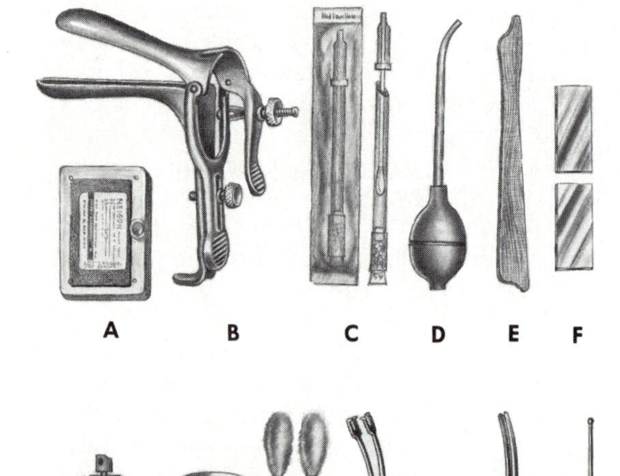

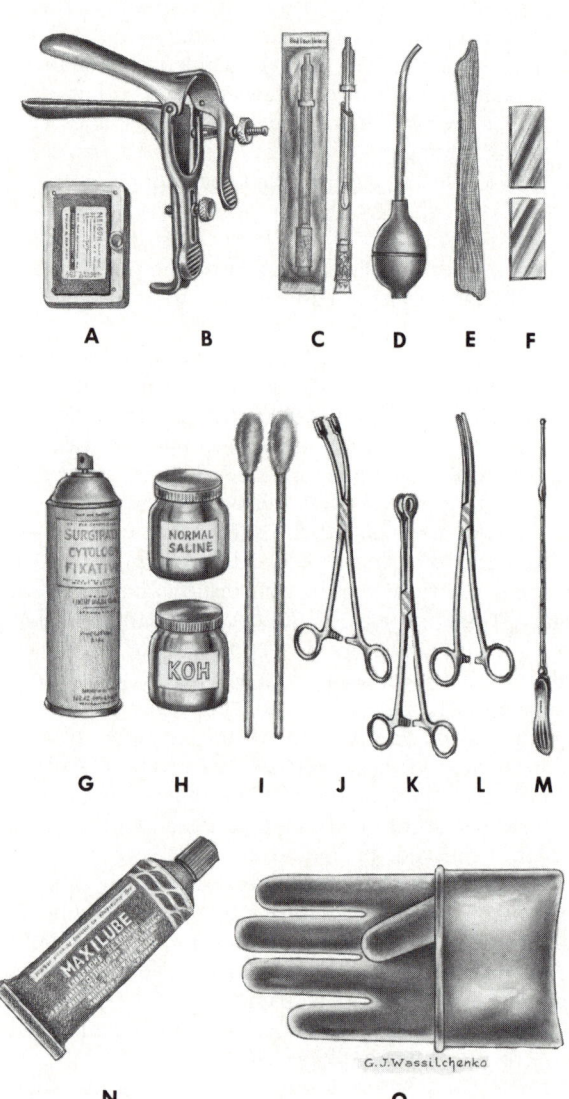

Fig. 8-1 Equipment used for pelvic examination. **A,** Thayer-Martin medium for isolation of *Neisseria gonorrhoeae.* Cylindrical container *(arrow)* is for pellet that releases carbon dioxide; medium and specimen are refrigerated until transport to laboratory. **B,** Vaginal speculum. **C,** Culturette, modified Stuart's bacterial transport medium with self-contained sterile swab. **D,** Vaginal pipette with rubber bulb. **E,** Plastic spatula for Papanicolaou smear and cytology. **F,** Slides for cytology specimens (Pap smear) or for wet mounts for diagnosing cause of vaginitis. **G,** Spray can of fixative for slide specimens. When dry, slides are packaged in cardboard for transport to laboratory. **H,** Normal saline and 10% potassium hydroxide (KOH) for wet mounts of vaginal fluids. **I,** Cotton pledget stick. **J,** Tenaculum. **K,** Ring (sponge or stick) forceps. **L,** Tissue forceps. **M,** Uterine sound (slightly curved for insertion). **N,** Sterile lubricant; may be antiseptic. **O,** Glove for vaginal and rectal examinations (sterile for vaginal, clean for rectal).

Procedure 8-1

Clean-Catch Urine Specimen

DEFINITION

Collection of urine during midstream micturition.

PURPOSE

To obtain an uncontaminated specimen of urine for routine urinalysis during the first visit, and evaluation for glucose and protein at subsequent visits.

EQUIPMENT

Packaged clean-catch urine set, or specimen cup with lid; toilet paper, moistened.

NURSING ACTIONS	RATIONALE
Instruct woman to wash her hands before touching her genitals or collecting specimen.	To teach hygienic self-care.
Instruct woman to wash her labia with moistened toilet paper or prepackaged wipes, then spread her labia and wipe from front to back using each wipe only once, then	To minimize contamination of the specimen.
begin voiding, and obtain in a clean container 30 to 60 ml (1 to 2 oz) of urine after urine has been flowing a few seconds.	To obtain an adequate specimen volume.
Remind woman to wash her hands after collection and final wiping with toilet paper.	To reinforce hygienic practice. To clean hands from any possible urine spillage.
Label container and fill in name and data for laboratory; that is, to be tested for glucose, protein, and acetone; microscopic assessment for pus, red blood cells, and casts; culture and sensitivity as necessary.	To ensure proper identification of client, specimen, purpose, and date/time obtained. To assess for potential complications such as infection and preeclampsia.
Instruct the woman to bring a specimen each time she comes for prenatal follow-up care. Ideally, the specimen is obtained immediately after rising in the morning. A clean container must be used. It does not have to be refrigerated.	To support health teaching and involve woman in her care. To ascertain current date base. Urinalysis profiles important information regarding health status, for example, excess protein may indicate preeclampsia.
Record findings on the appropriate forms.	To allow continuity of care by formation of a current data base.

perceives the threat as overwhelming and just cannot face it, the *parasympathetic nervous system* (conservation and withdrawal) discharges, and all physical changes reverse suddenly—decreasing pulse, blood pressure, cardiac output, and vascular resistance. The woman is diaphoretic and feels weak, muscle tone relaxes, and she complains of lightheadedness and vertigo and loses consciousness. Vomiting, bowel movement, and seizures may occur. The symptoms are summarized in the Danger Signs box. Nursing actions are presented in the Emergency Procedure.

The Thyroid Gland. The thyroid gland is the largest endocrine gland in the body and the only one accessible to direct physical examination. The thyroid gland is fixed to the trachea and thus ascends during swallowing. This distinguishes thyroid structures from other neck masses. The techniques used to examine the thyroid gland include observation, palpation, and auscultation (Malasanos et al., 1986; Seidel et al., 1987; Bates, 1987). Although there are several techniques used for palpation of the thyroid, the underlying principles for each technique include movement of the gland while the client swallows, adequate exposure of the gland by relaxation and manual displacement of surrounding structures, and comparison of one side of the gland with the other.

DANGER SIGNS

Vasovagal Syncope

1. **Shock**
   a. Apprehension
   b. Pallor
   c. Diaphoresis
   d. Generalized weakness
   e. Lightheadedness
   f. Vertigo
2. **State of Consciousness**
   a. Vomiting
   b. Seizures
   c. Incontinence, bowel or bladder
   d. Loss of consciousness
3. **Cardiopulmonary Arrest**
   a. Absence of breathing
   b. Absence of heart beat

EMERGENCY PROCEDURE

VASOVAGAL SYNCOPE

DEFINITION

Transient loss of consciousness resulting from a sudden fall in blood pressure caused by decreased peripheral resistance, decreased cardiac output, reduced venous return, and slowing of the heart. Occurs suddenly.

PURPOSE

To prevent death.

EQUIPMENT

Crash cart (emergency cart).

NURSING ACTIONS	RATIONALE
Alert physician.	To provide essential immediate care.
Assess for signs of shock; decreased blood pressure and increased pulse; apprehension; pallor; diaphoresis; generalized weakness; lightheadedness; vertigo.	To determine the extent of shock response.
Assess level of consciousness: partial to total loss of consciousness, seizures and vomiting, and incontinence of bowel or bladder.	To determine client's state of consciousness and related responses that may place client at additional risk (e.g., vomiting).
Ensure adequate airway:	To permit oxygenation.
Extend head or use jaw-thrust maneuver.	
Suction as required.	To keep airway unobstructed.
Provide oxygen when airway is clear.	To increase tissue perfusion and prevent cellular death.
Begin seizure precautions.	To protect client from injury.
Assist with cardiopulmonary resuscitation (CPR):	To prevent death.
Airway.	To identify and remove obstruction.
Breathing: mouth to mouth or artificial intermittent pressure breathing with oxygen (1:5 compressions with help; 2:15 compressions when alone):	To verify need for and provide external respiratory assistance to maintain oxygenation.
Circulation: external cardiac compression 60 to 80 per minute.	To verify need for and assist with external support to perfuse tissues.
Assist with drugs:	
Atropine sulphate, 0.4 to 1.0 mg, intravenously.	To reduce cardiac vagal tone, increase rate of sinus and atrial pacemakers, and improve atrioventricular conduction.
Epinephrine HCl, 0.5 to 1.0 mg. (5 to 10 ml of a 1:10,000 solution) intravenously (USP-DI, 1986); or 1 mg (10 ml of a 1:10,000 solution) endotracheally.	To stimulate alpha and beta receptors; for example, to increase heart rate, force of myocardial contractions, and peripheral vascular resistance.
Assist with direct current defibrillation, 200 to 400 J (Phipps, Long, and Woods, 1987).	To restore normal cardiac rhythm.

Assessment of thyroid function or possible dysfunction includes more than observation of the area where the thyroid gland is located. Metabolic rates and rhythms, including menstrual regularity in the woman of childbearing age, are governed by the thyroid gland. The effects of thyroid activity are widespread. Therefore observations of behavior, appearance, skin, eyes, hair, and cardiovascular status are important.

Several findings require further attention. Examples of suspicious findings include the following:

1. Observation: unusual bulging.
2. Palpation:
   a. Enlargement may indicate thyroiditis. Symmetrical enlargement is normal in the presence of a deficiency of dietary iodine (Malasanos et al., 1986).
   b. Consistency that is coarse and gritty may indicate inflammation.
   c. Nodules are counted. They are described as smooth or irregular, soft or hard. Solitary nodules are suggestive of carcinoma (Malasanos et al., 1986).
3. Auscultation: If enlargement is present, the gland is assessed with the bell of a stethoscope. Vascular sounds are increased in a hypermetabolic state. The accelerated blood flow causes a vibration heard as a vascular bruit or soft, rushing sound (Seidel et al., 1987).

The Gynecologic Examination

Many women are intimidated by the gynecologic portion of the physical examination. The nurse in this instance can take an advocacy approach that supports a partnership relationship between the client and the care provider.

The Breasts. The gynecologic examination includes an evaluation of the breasts primarily to establish a data base of normal findings. However, the practitioner needs to be alert to the possibility of carcinoma at all times. See Chapter 44 for incidence across the life span. Early detection of potential malignancies has been and continues to be the single most important factor in the successful treatment of this disease. Since professional assessment is done only periodically, each woman is advised to do a breast self-examination (BSE) on a monthly basis at the time when the breast is least affected by menstrual changes, 4 to 10 days after the last menstrual period (Fig. 6-23) (women who no longer menstruate can use the first of every month for BSE).

Anatomy and physiology of the breast are presented in several sections of this text.* As the examiner proceeds through the examination, the woman is taught about BSE, or if she already follows a routine for BSE, her knowledge and technique are refreshed.

At the start of the examination, the breasts are observed for symmetry, contour, color, size, and surface characteristics such as vascularity, moles, and nevi (Fig. 8-2). The nipples are checked for areolar pigmentation and discharge and for response to stimulation (i.e., erection, flattening, or inversion). The woman then presses her hands against her waist to cause pectoral contraction and repeats the assessment above (Fig. 8-3).

When the woman raises her arms above her head, the position of the nipple and any dimpling (localized skin retraction) of the surface are noted. Breast may appear symmetrical at rest, but elevating the breast reveals lesion (Fig. 8-4).

If the woman's breasts are pendulous, and problems exist, leaning forward to allow the breast to hang loose may reveal dimpling or other irregularities.

For the next part of the examination, the woman lies flat with her arm abducted and her hand under her head to help flatten breast tissue evenly over the chest wall, facilitating inspection and palpation (Fig. 8-5). A pillow placed under the shoulder of the breast to be examined helps further position breast tissue. Each breast is examined separately. The examiner can use both hands; however, in self-examination, the woman uses the hand opposite to the side being examined. The fingers are held flat against the breast, and the tissue is palpated gently against the chest wall (Fig. 8-6). The examination may be done either by using a circular method, quadrant by quadrant, or a spoke-wheel pattern (Fig. 8-7). The presence of regions of tenderness are distinguished, as are thickened or firm zones. Any masses are noted for location, size, consistency, and mobility or fixation to the skin or chest wall. Palpation of the breast includes glandular tissue, areolar areas, and the nipples. Normally breast tissue is slightly lobular; hard fixed masses are abnormal. In Fig. 8-8 the client demonstrates the proper technique for self-examination of the nipple. No examination is complete without assessing those parts of the breast known as the tail of Spence (Fig. 8-9) and the axillary lymph nodes. The lymph nodes are palpated while the client is in a sitting position. Easy access is gained to the axillary nodes with the client's arms at her sides and muscles relaxed Fig. 8-10. To gain the necessary muscle relaxation, the examiner supports the client's arm. The lymph nodes are assessed by using a rotary motion with two or three finger tips.

Although malignancy may occur anywhere in the breast, the most common site is the upper outer quadrant. One method for recording findings is illustrated in Fig. 8-11.

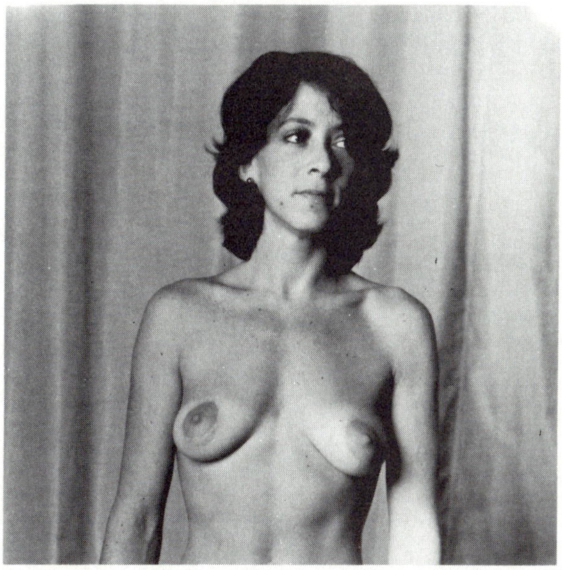

Fig. 8-2 Observe breasts with client's arms at her side.
From Potter, PA, and Perry, AG: Fundamentals of nursing, ed 2, St Louis, 1989, The CV Mosby Co.

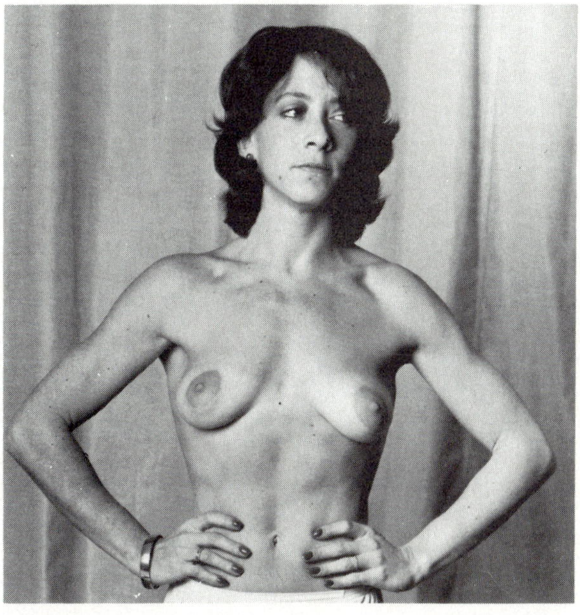

Fig. 8-3 Pressing hands against hips contracts pectoral muscles, accentuating any existing tissue retraction.
From Potter, PA, and Perry, AG: Fundamentals of nursing, ed 2, St Louis, 1989, The CV Mosby Co.

*Anatomy, physiology, growth, development across the life span, Chapter 6; maternal adaptation to pregnancy, Chapter 10; during the post-delivery period, Chapter 24; during lactation, Chapter 23.

The Abdomen. The examination of the abdomen is done carefully and systematically. In Table 8-1, assessment factors and probable clinical significance of findings are discussed for inspection, auscultation, percussion, and palpation. The nurse's skill in assessment and recording add invaluable information that, when combined with the findings from the physician, laboratory, and other technicians, form a comprehensive data base. The content presented here also is intended to assist the nurse in providing anticipatory guidance for preventive and rehabilitative care.

Pelvic Examination. The woman is assisted into the lithotomy position for the pelvic examination. When she is in the lithotomy position, the woman's hips and knees are flexed with the buttocks at the edge of the table and her feet supported by heel or knee stirrups. Some women prefer to keep their shoes or socks on, especially if the stirrups are not padded.

Many women express feelings of vulnerability and strangeness when in the lithotomy position. During the procedure the nurse assists the woman with relaxation techniques—the physician's and nurse's behavior toward her to this point adds to her ability to relax. One method of assisting the woman to relax is to have her place her hands on her chest at about the level of the diaphragm, breathe deeply and slowly (in through her mouth and out through her O-shaped mouth), concentrate on the rhythm

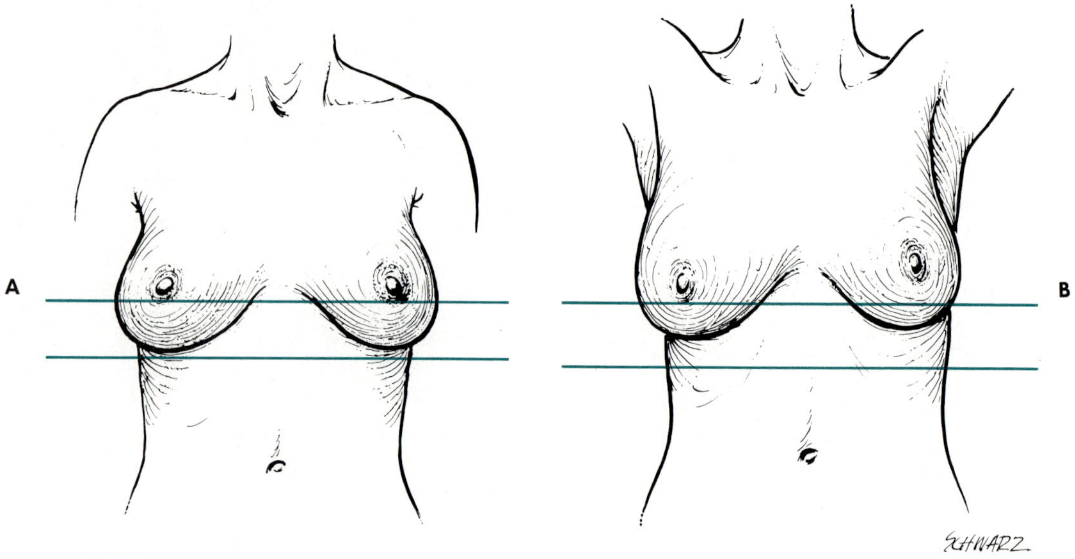

Fig. 8-4 **A**, Breasts appear symmetrical at rest. **B**, Breasts do not elevate symmetrically with arm raising.
From Malasanos, L, et al: Health assessment, ed 3, St Louis, 1986, The CV Mosby Co.

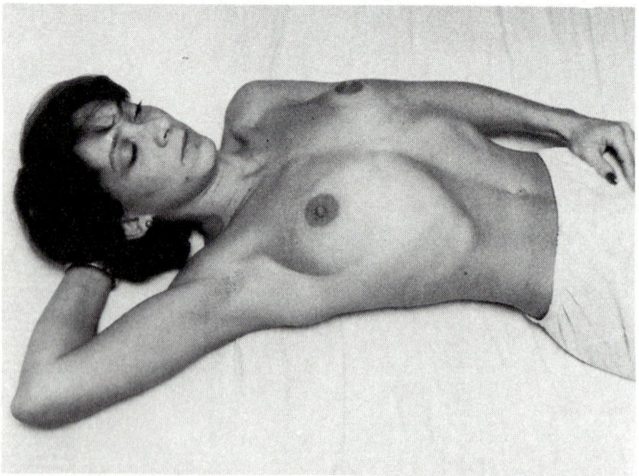

Fig. 8-5 Proper position for inspection and palpation of right breast. Reverse arm positions for left breast.
From Potter, PA, and Perry, AG: Fundamentals of nursing, ed 2, St Louis, 1989, The CV Mosby Co.

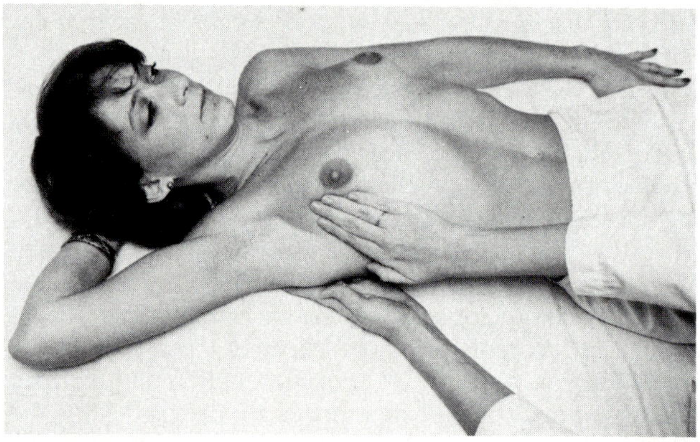

Fig. 8-6 Each breast is examined using a rotary motion of the fingertips.
From Potter, PA, and Perry, AG: Fundamentals of nursing, ed 2, St Louis, 1989, The CV Mosby Co.

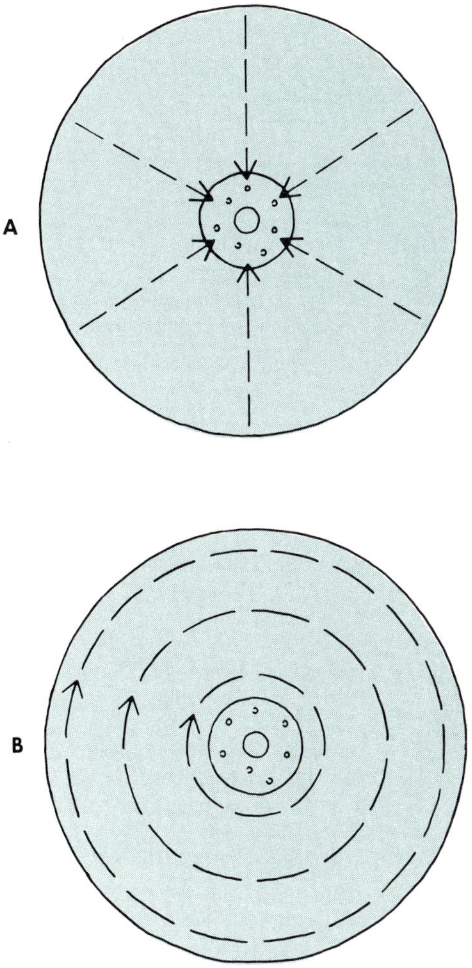

Fig. 8-7 Two methods of systematic breast palpation. **A**, Palpation in wedge sections (spoke-wheel fashion) from breast periphery to center. **B**, Palpation along concentric circles from periphery to center. It usually takes three circles to cover all breast tissue.
From Malasanos, L, et al: Health assessment, ed 3, St Louis, 1986, The CV Mosby Co.

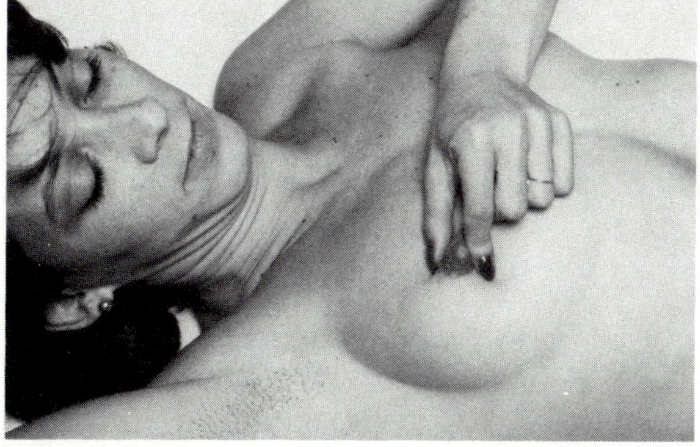

Fig. 8-8 The client palpates the nipple for presence of discharge.
From Potter, PA, and Perry, AG: Fundamentals of nursing, ed 2, St Louis, 1989, The CV Mosby Co.

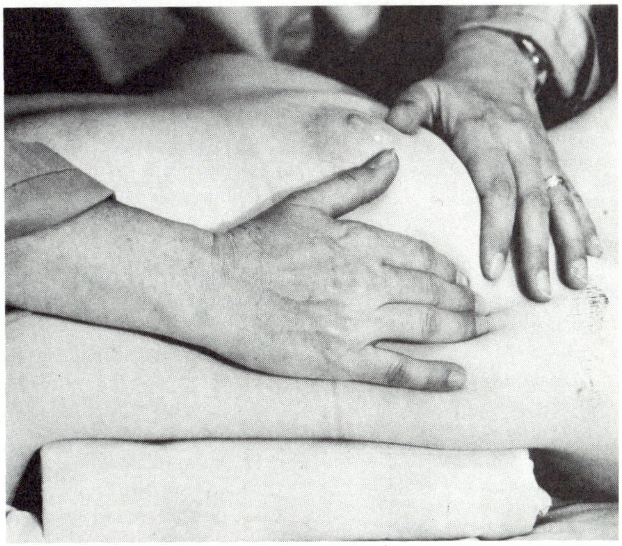

Fig. 8-9 Palpation of the axillary tail of Spence.
From Malasanos, L, et al: Health assessment, ed 3, St Louis, 1986, The CV Mosby Co.

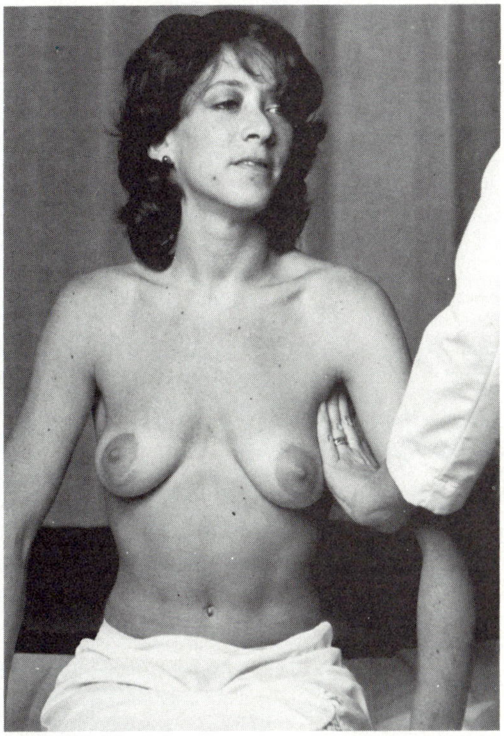

Fig. 8-10 The examiner supports the client's arm and palpates axillary lymph nodes.
From Potter, PA, and Perry, AG: Fundamentals of nursing, ed 2, St Louis, 1989, The CV Mosby Co.

Table 8-1 *Abdominal Assessment*

Assessment Factor	Possible Clinical Significance	Nursing Actions
Inspection		
Skin	Skin:	Describe
Color	Color:	Color
General	General physical condition: pale	Pattern, if color varies
Hyperpigmentation	Linea nigra	Presence, height
Rashes	Infection, allergy, poor hygiene, drug use, nutritional status	Color, size in centimeters, raised or flat, location, and distribution; use palpation as necessary
Lesions	Spider nevi, infections, infestations, moles	
Scars	May result in adhesion or obstruction	
Striae	Old (silver): obesity, pregnancy; reddish: pregnancy, Cushing's syndrome	Color
Dilated veins	Possible vena cava obstruction	Distribution, amount
Turgor	Nutritional status	Degree of turgor, rule out edema
Texture	Nutritional status	Dry, moist
Hair distribution	Hirsutism (endocrine imbalance)	Pattern, amount if unusual
Umbilicus	Displaced upward: pregnancy	Describe
Color	Discoloration: suspect intraperitoneal bleeding	Refer immediately
Contour	Hernia, pregnancy	Reducible? Tender?
Location	Previous surgery may have caused adhesion or obstruction	Position, length, healing of scar
Signs of inflammation	Current infection, cellulitis	Discharge, odor, color, duration, pain
Contour and symmetry: abdominal, inguinal, femoral regions	Protuberant: adipose, gas distension, tumor, ascites, pregnancy	Record: flat, scaphoid (concave), rounded, protuberant isolated bulges; whether bulges are reducible
	Hernias: umbilical, incisional, diastasis recti hernia over linea alba, ovoid bulge in groin	Possible inguinal hernia; check if reducible
	Bulges: full bladder, pregnancy, masses, enlarged lymph nodes	
Peristalsis	Normally seen in a thin person, may indicate intestinal obstruction	Observe across abdomen—from one side, then from other side; use good lighting
Pulsations	Normally seen in epigastrium	Record location and intensity
Auscultation		
Normal	Normal: clicks, gurgles, "growling" (borborygmi with hyperperistalsis); frequency of sounds: 5 to 34/min	Auscultate all four quadrants and epigastrium Perform before percussion and palpation
Increased	Increased: diarrhea, early obstructive process	Listen for 2 minutes or more over suspicious area
Decreased	Decreased or absent: paralytic ileus	
High pitched	High-pitched tinkling with abdominal cramps: possible intestinal obstruction	
Percussion		
Fat	Fat: scattered dullness or tympany; umbilicus sunken	Unless pregnancy is far advanced, percuss all four quadrants first, then liver, spleen, stomach, and bowel; or percuss all areas, then percuss and palpate each organ before proceeding to the next; note distribution or absence of sounds
Tympany	Tympany: normally predominates over abdomen; stomach: left lower anterior rib cage; gaseous distension: generalized tympany	
Dullness	Dullness:	
	Supra pubic: full bladder	Have woman void to facilitate examination
	Liver:	
	Obscured upper border: right pleural effusion	Note level of lower border in midclavicular line; note upper border; measure boundaries if enlarged
	Obscured lower border: gas in colon	Describe boundaries; refer

Table 8-1 *Abdominal Assessment—cont'd*

Assessment Factor	Possible Clinical Significance	Nursing Actions
Dullness—cont'd	Solid tumor (ovarian): dullness over symphysis pubis, tympany around dullness: umbilicus not displaced upward Ascites Supine: dullness down both flanks, meeting over symphysis pubis surrounding tympanic area over umbilicus Left lateral: dullness on dependent half, tympany over superior half	
Palpation		
Irregular uterine contours	Uterine anomaly, myomata	Describe size, location, and consistency; refer
Adnexa	Adnexa Fullness, unilateral pelvic pain over mass, possible left shoulder pain: probable ectopic pregnancy Mass: possible ovarian cyst, tumor	Adnexa Describe size in centimeters; characteristics—smooth, irregular, nodular, hard, soft, fluctuant, motility, tenderness, pulsating or not. Rebound tenderness? Ballotable? Refer
Guarding of abdomen caused by pain over McBurney's point	Possible appendicitis (Fig. 34-2 and Chapter 34)	Assess vital signs, describe responses, submit ordered laboratory tests

of breathing, and relax all body muscles with each exhalation (Malasanos et al., 1986; Chapter 14). This breathing technique is particularly helpful for the adolescent or the virginal woman whose introitus may be especially tight, or for whom the experience may be new and may provoke tension.

Some women relax when they are encouraged to become involved with the examination with a mirror placed so that the area being examined can be seen by the client. This type of participation helps with health teaching as well. Distraction is another technique that can be used effectively. For example, placement of interesting pictures or mobiles on the ceiling over the head of the table.

The nurse is reminded that the woman *must not squeeze her eyes closed or clench her fists;* tightening these muscles permits the tightening of the perineal muscles.

Many women find it distressing to attempt to converse in the lithotomy position. Most clients appreciate an explanation of the procedure as it unfolds as well as coaching for the type of sensations they may expect. But in general women prefer not to have to respond to questions until they are again upright and at eye level with the examiner. Questioning during the procedure, especially if they cannot see their questioner's eyes, may make women tense.

Supine Hypotension. When a woman is lying in the lithotomy position, the weight of abdominal contents may compress the vena cava and aorta, resulting in a drop in blood pressure. Pallor, breathlessness and clammy skin are other objective signs. Symptoms are summarized in the danger signs box. Nursing actions are presented in the emergency procedure. If the woman is unable to tolerate the lithotomy position, the left lateral or semi-Fowler's position may be used for genital examination (Fig. 8-12).

External: Inspection. The examiner sits at the foot of the table for the inspection of the external genitals and for the speculum examination. To facilitate open communication and to help the woman relax, the woman's head is raised on a pillow and the drape is arranged so that eye to eye contact can be maintained. In good lighting, external genitals are inspected for sexual maturity (developing hair pattern and labial maturity in the young woman and the thinning hair pattern and labia in the perimenopausal woman), the clitoris, labia, and perineum. After childbirth

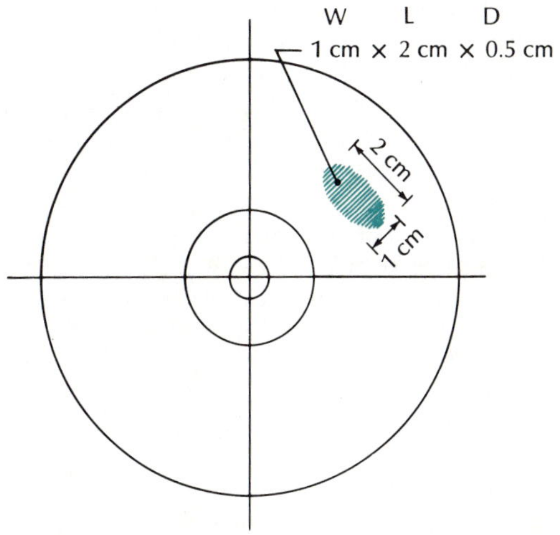

Fig. 8-11 Diagram of mass within upper outer quadrant of left breast.

From Malasanos, L, et al: Health assessment, ed 3, St Louis, 1986, The CV Mosby Co.

EMERGENCY PROCEDURE

SUPINE HYPOTENSION

DEFINITION

While lying in lithotomy position, weight of abdominal contents may compress the vena cava and aorta. Compression of these major vessels results in a drop in blood pressure, pallor, breathlessness, clammy skin, and other signs of shock.

PURPOSE

Reduce compression of the large vessels to allow the woman's symptoms to abate and to bring all body functions back into homeostasis.

EQUIPMENT

None.

NURSING ACTIONS	RATIONALE
Remove woman from lithotomy position, and position her on her side until signs and symptoms abate (Fig. 18-9).	To take the weight of the abdominal contents off of the vena cava and aorta.
Provide the woman with a frank explanation.	To provide knowledge that reduces fear of the unknown and forms basis for self-care.

DANGER SIGNS

Supine Hypotension

1. **Blood pressure drops**
2. **Pallor**
3. **Breathlessness**
4. **Clammy skin**

or other trauma there may be healed scars. Normal findings are discussed in Chapter 6, other observations that would *not* be within normal limits include:

1. Hair in excessive amount, especially if associated with excessive amounts on her trunk, face, or extremities; no hair growth in the woman who is older than 16 years; furunculosis, pediculosis.
2. Clitoral size that is more than 0.5 to 1 cm or that is atrophied.
3. Abnormal masses in the frenulum.
4. Enlargement or asymmetry of the labia. These findings may be associated with such conditions as varicosities, neoplasms, inflammation, edema, trauma (hematoma after delivery or rape), or cysts (of canal of Nuck).
5. Asymmetric pigmentation change, increased or decreased, on the labia. Leukoplakia appears as white, adherent patches on the skin that look like spots of white paint. Some causes of changes in pigmentation may be neoplasms, moles, inflammation, or skin disorder. Erythema may be caused by inflammation or a reaction to some chemical (deodorant panty liners, deodorant spray, contraceptive foam). Excoriations may result from nervous scratching or a condition that causes pruritus. Ulcerations may reflect neoplasia, infection, or trauma. Growths or warts may be seen and need to be assessed for cause, for example, malignant neoplasm.
6. Lumps along the inguinal canal may be enlarged lymph nodes that may accompany new or repeated sexually transmitted disease or other disorder. (When the examination is over, ask the woman to stand up without a drape over the lower abdomen for assessment for inguinal hernia that may only be seen when she is upright. If the woman's abdomen protrudes, because of pregnancy or obesity, she may be unable to see her inguinal area and therefore not notice if a bulge appears in the inguinal area when she is standing. The bulge may be a hernia. If one appears, the examiner assesses for reducibility.)

External: Palpation. The examiner proceeds with the examination using palpation,* as well as inspection. The examiner wears two gloves for this portion of the assessment. The labia are spread apart to expose the structures in the vestibule: urinary meatus, Skene's glands, vaginal orifice, and Bartholin's glands. To assess the Skene's glands, the examiner inserts one finger into the vagina and "milks" the area of the urethra (Fig. 8-13). Any exudate from the *urethra,* or the *Skene's glands* is cultured. Masses and erythema of either structure are assessed further. Ordinarily, the openings to the Skene's glands are not visible; prominent openings may be seen if the glands are infected (e.g.,

*As a sign of caring and to assist the woman to feel more at ease, the woman should receive a verbal cue and a cue through touch on a nonemotionally charged body part (e.g., knee) before experiencing touch on her genitals. The back of the hand, lightly touching the inner aspect of the thigh, often works well.

A

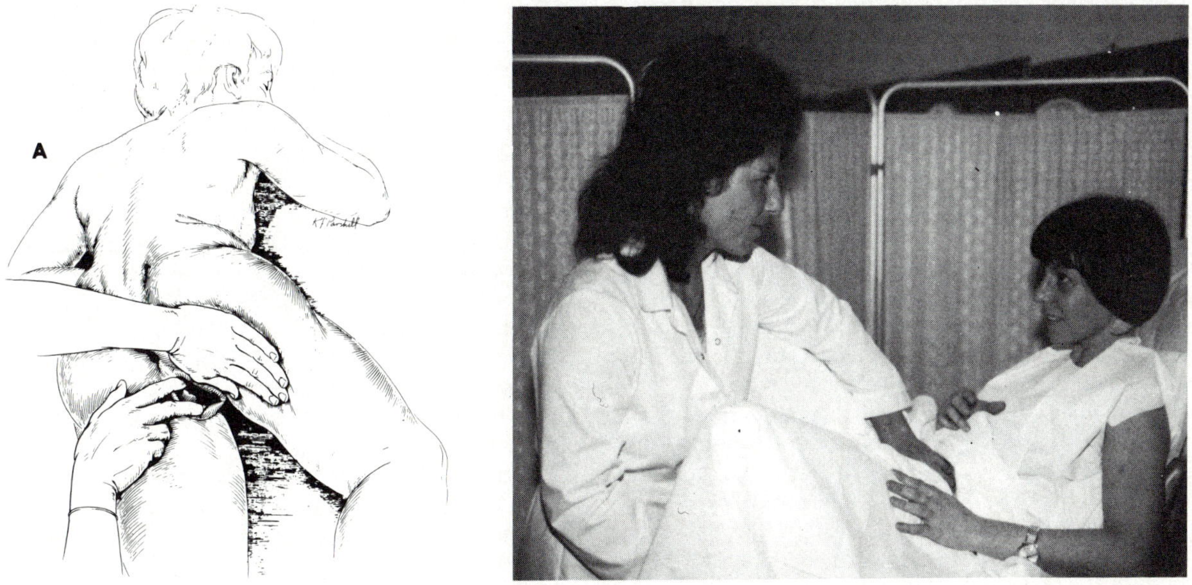

B

Fig. 8-12 Alternate positions for examination of genitals. **A**, Left lateral position. **B**, Semi-Fowler's position.

(**A**, from Malasanos, L, Barkauskas, V, Moss, M, and Stoltenberg-Allen, K: Health assessment, ed 3, St Louis, 1986, The CV Mosby Co. **B**, photograph by Irene M. Bobak)

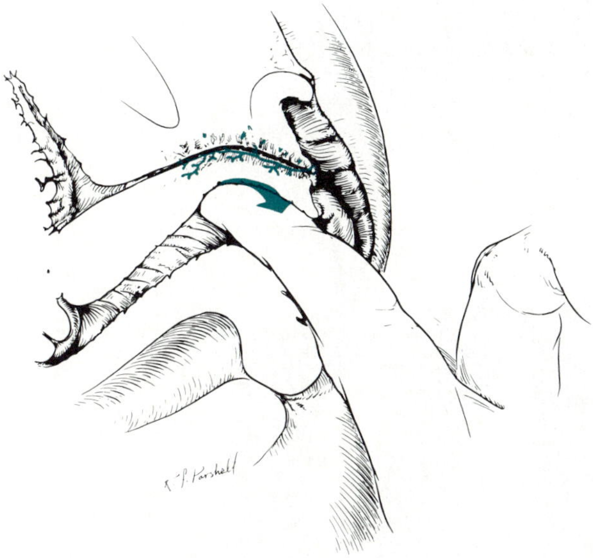

Fig. 8-13 Palpation of Skene's glands.

From Malasanos, L, et al: Health assessment, ed 3, St Louis, 1986, The CV Mosby Co.

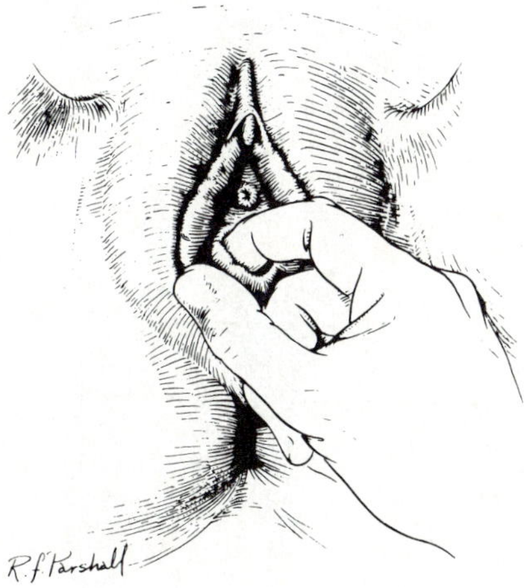

Fig. 8-14 Palpation of Bartholin's glands.

From Malasanos, L, et al: Health assessment, ed 3, St Louis, 1986, The CV Mosby Co.

with gonorrhea). During the examination, the examiner keeps in mind the findings from the review of systems, such as, history of burning on urination.

The *vaginal orifice* is examined. Carunculae myrtiformes (hymenal tags) are normal findings. With one finger still in the vagina, the examiner repositions the index finger near the posterior part of the orifice. With the thumb outside the posterior part of the labia majora, the examiner compresses the area of *Bartholin's glands* located at the 8 o'clock and 4 o'clock positions and looks for swelling, discharge, and pain (Fig. 8-14).

The *support* of the anterior and posterior *vaginal wall* is assessed. The examiner spreads the labia with the index and middle finger and asks the woman to strain down. Any bulge from the anterior wall (urethrocele or cystocele) or posterior wall (rectocele) is noted and compared to the history, such as, difficulty to start the stream of urine or constipation (Chapter 41).

The *perineum* (area between the vagina and anus) is assessed for scars from old lacerations or episiotomies, for thinning, fistulas, masses, lesions, and inflammation. The *anus* is assessed for hemorrhoids, hemorrhoidal tags, and integrity of the anal sphincter. Occasionally, following traumatic delivery with lacerations that extended into the anal sphincter, the muscle may not have been correctly repaired; for example, the examiner will see a "dimple" over two ends of separated muscle and the "wink" reflex is incomplete. If the anal sphincter was not repaired correctly, the woman may have given a history of incontinence, for instance. The anal area is also assessed for lesions, masses, abscesses, tumors. If there is a history of sexually transmitted disease, the examiner may want to culture the anal canal at this time.

Throughout the genital examination, the examiner notes the odor. Odor may indicate infection and poor hygienic practices.

Internal: Vaginal Speculum. When the woman made the appointment for her examination, she was asked to refrain from douching or using vaginal medications for the previous 24 hours. These actions cloud diagnosis based on secretions, cells, and odor. In addition, douching removes vaginal secretions, making insertion of the vaginal speculum more difficult. Some women have a hard time complying with this request; they cannot go to the doctor feeling unclean in the genital region.

Vaginal specula consist of two blades and a handle. Specula come in a variety of types and styles (Fig. 8-15). Vaginal specula are used to view the vaginal vault and cervix. The pelvic examination is detailed in Procedure 8-2. Fig. 8-16 describes the insertion of a vaginal speculum.

A

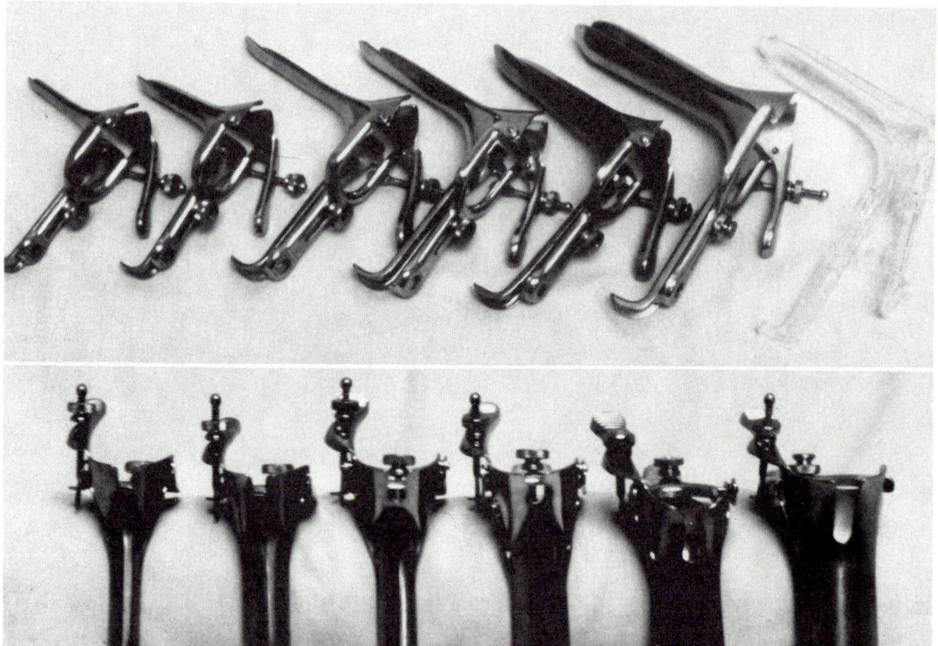

B

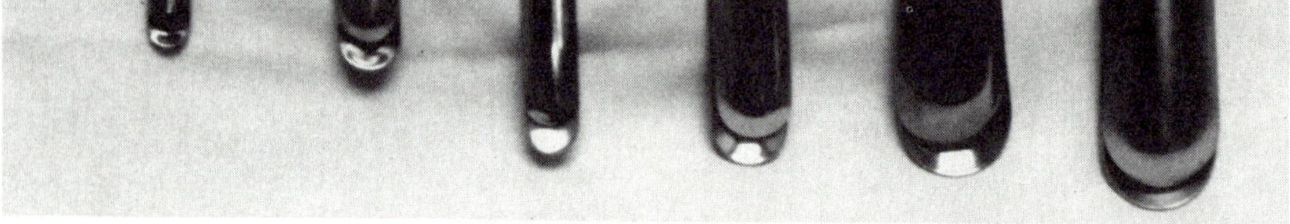

Fig. 8-15 Vaginal specula. From left to right: **A**, Short-billed pediatric, pediatric, small Pederson, Pederson, small Graves, large Graves, plastic Graves. **B**, Short-billed pediatric, pediatric, small Pederson, Pederson, small Graves, large Graves.

From Seidel, H, et al: Mosby's guide to physical examination, St Louis, 1987, The CV Mosby Co.

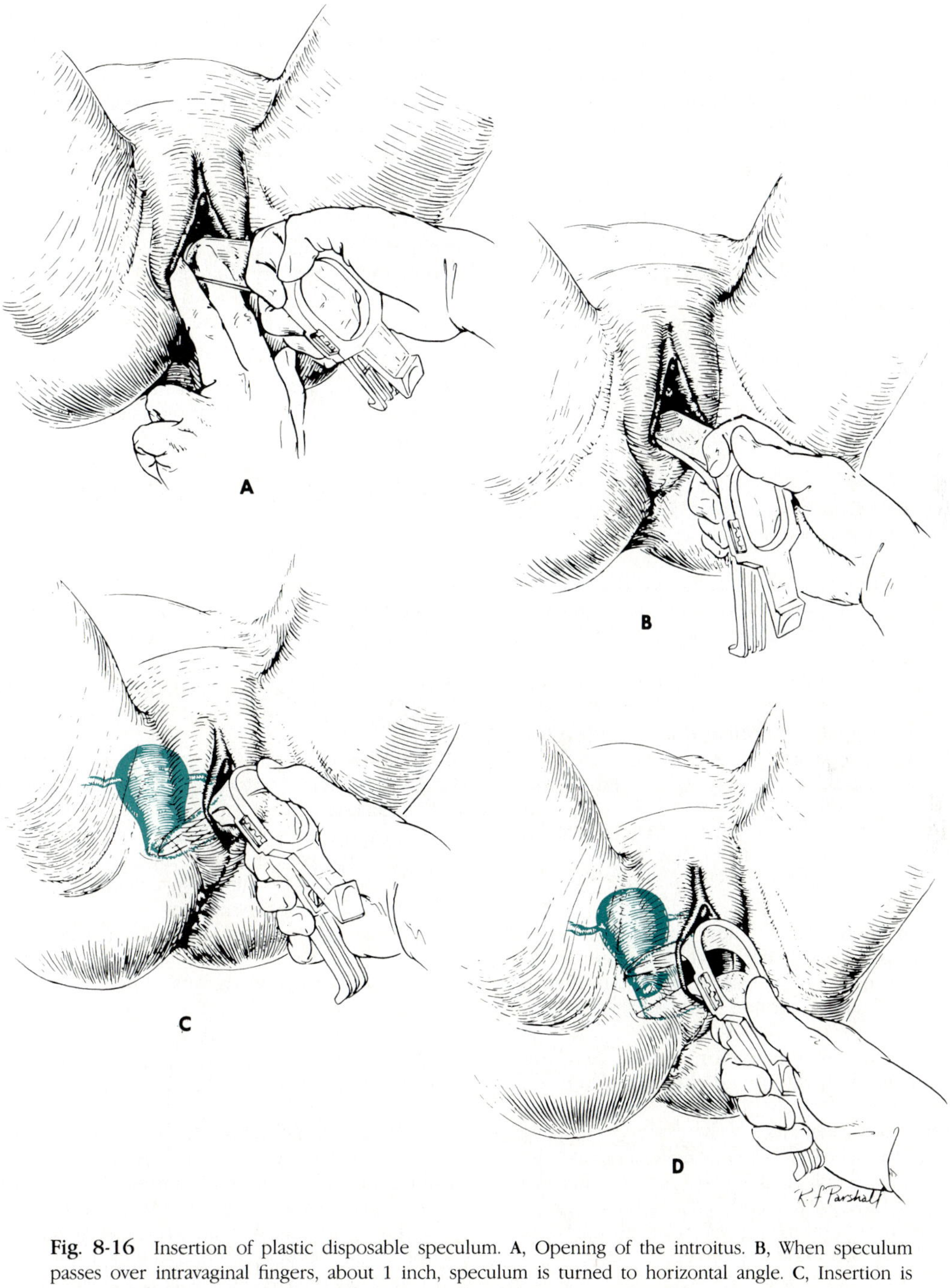

Fig. 8-16 Insertion of plastic disposable speculum. **A**, Opening of the introitus. **B**, When speculum passes over intravaginal fingers, about 1 inch, speculum is turned to horizontal angle. **C**, Insertion is continued to back of vagina at a 45-degree angle to the examination table. **D**, Speculum blades are opened to reveal cervix. Blades are secured by compressing them, moving top one forward until click is heard.

From Malasanos, L, et al: Health assessment, ed 3, St Louis, 1986, The CV Mosby Co.

Procedure 8-2

PELVIC EXAMINATION

DEFINITION

Inspection and palpation of the internal and external structures comprising the female reproductive system. Examination may be done manually or with aid of instrumentation.

PURPOSE

To provide a data base for medical diagnoses, medical therapy, nursing diagnoses, and nursing care. To involve the woman as an active participant in her own health supervision, maintenance, and care.

EQUIPMENT

To obtain specimens for screening potential problems. Gynecologic table and drapes.
Supplies as neccessary (see Fig. 8-1).

NURSING ACTIONS	RATIONALE
Wash hands.	To minimize chance for nosocomial infection.
Ask client to empty her bladder before the examination (obtain clean-catch urine specimen as needed; see Procedure 8-1).	To increase woman's comfort and facilitate accurate assessment.
Instruct woman to remove her clothing (from the waist down if only the pelvic exam is to be done) and put on a cover gown; provide privacy for this.	To provide adequate exposure for thorough gynecologic examination. To show respect.
Explain purpose of the procedure and how it is done. Describe sensations to expect. Inform the client who will do the procedure, and about how long it will take. Ask her if she wishes a mirror to watch.	To reduce anxiety related to knowledge deficit. To provide woman with chance to have more control over situation and to learn more about her body.
Assist the woman into the lithotomy postion (the woman's hips and knees are flexed with the buttocks at the edge of the table with her feet supported by heel or knee stirrups), and drape appropriately.	To increase her comfort and facilitate examination; however, other positions can be used (Fig. 8-12). To meet her need for modesty and provide warmth.
Adjust pillow under client's head.	To increase her comfort and help relax her abdominal musculature.
Lubricate examiner's fingers with water or water-soluble lubricant before bimanual examination (Fig. 8-18).	To reduce friction and discomfort and to avoid other types of lubricant that can distort findings.
Warm speculum in warm water.	To increase client's comfort since warm metal is less shocking to the mucous membrane.
During the examination, support client. Explain the procedure during inspection of external genitals, insertion of speculum for examination of vagina and cervix (Fig. 8-16), and bimanual examination of internal organs (Fig. 8-18).	To reduce her anxiety by keeping her informed. To increase her knowledge about her body.
Refrain from questioning the woman extensively. Hold question until she is sitting up and at eye level with the examiner.	To prevent tension that can develop if she is questioned, especially if she cannot see the questioner's eyes.
Assist with relaxation techniques. Have the woman place her hands on her chest at about the level of the diaphragm, breathe deeply and slowly (in through her mouth and out through her O-shaped mouth), concentrate on the rhythm of breathing, and relax all body muscles with each exhalation (Malasanos et al., 1986).	To decrease common feeling of vulnerability and strangeness when in lithotomy position. To help her relax perineum during the examination. NOTE: This breathing technique is particularly helpful for the adolescent or the woman whose introitus may be especially tight. Others for whom the experience may be new or tension provoking can also benefit from using this technique.
Encourage woman to become involved with the examination if she shows interest. For example, a mirror can be placed so that the area being examined can be seen by the woman.	To assist the interested woman and to motive other women to be participants in their own care. To provide health teaching.
Distract the attention of the tense woman by placing interesting mobiles or pictures on the ceiling or wall near her head.	To provide distraction that is an effective method of reducing tension.

Procedure 8-2—cont'd

Remind the woman not to squeeze her eyes closed, clench her fists, or squeeze the nurse's hand.	To help her relax her perineum, since tightening these muscles encourages tightening of the perineal muscles.
Assess woman for and treat imminent untoward responses (see emergency procedure: vasovagal syncope, p. 146; emergency procedure: supine hypotension, p. 152).	To ensure the safety and health of the woman.
Instruct woman to bear down when speculum is being inserted (Fig. 8-16).	To open the vaginal introitus and relax perineal muscles for easier insertion of the speculum.
Apply gloves and assist examiner with collection of specimens for cytology such as Papanicolaou smear (see Procedure 8-3). After handling specimens, remove gloves and wash hands.	To implement universal precautions when handling body fluids (see Chapter 30). To reduce possibility of contamination of specimens. To minimize nosocomial infections.
Assist woman at completion of examination to a sitting position and then a standing position.	To attain a sitting position comfortably without strain. To reduce possibility of transient or orthostatic hypotension that may occur if position is changed rapidly.
Provide tissues to wipe lubricant from perineum.	To provide comfort and promote cleanliness.
Provide privacy for woman while she is dressing.	To show respect and to promote feelings of security and worth.
Inform woman as to the next step in the assessment protocol.	To supply information to reduce tension that arises from facing the unknown.
Record findings on the appropriate forms.	To provide permanent record of data base to foster continuity of care.

Cervix. The speculum blades are opened to reveal the cervix and are locked into the open position. The cervix is inspected: position and appearance of os, position, color, lesions, bleeding, and discharge. Cervical findings not within normal limits (for example, ulcerations, masses, inflammation, excessive protrusion into the vaginal vault), anomalies (for example, cock's comb, hooded, or collared cervix), and polyps are noted.

Collection of Specimens. Collection of specimens for cytologic examination is an important part of the gynecologic examination. **Infection** can be diagnosed through examination of specimens collected during the pelvic examination. These infections include gonorrhea, *Chlamydia trachomatis,* and herpes simplex types 1 and 2. Once the diagnoses have been made, treatment can be instituted.

Papanicolaou Smear. Carcinogenic conditions, potential or actual, can be determined by examination of cells from the cervix collected during the pelvic examination (Procedure 8-3).

Gonorrheal Culture. A culture for gonorrhea is done to screen women for gonorrheal infection that could compromise the woman, her fetus if she is pregnant, and her partner. The woman is told the reason for the test (e.g., test for vaginal infection). If she is pregnant, the test is done routinely at the first prenatal visit and repeated toward the end of pregnancy (week 36).

The specimen is obtained at the same time as the Papanicolaou smear, and the same precautions regarding use of digital examinations and lubricant are followed. A specimen is obtained from the endocervical canal using a sterile cotton-tipped applicator (Fig. 8-17). The applicator is rolled on a culture plate with a special medium (Thayer-Martin). The plate is then incubated.

Chlamydia Trachomatis Smear. Smears of urethral or cervical secretions are collected during the pelvic examination, following the same precautions used for the Papanicolaou smear. A fluorescein-conjugated monoclonal antibody test system for the detection of chlamydia antigen is available. Slides containing the smears are incubated for 30 minutes with fluorescein-labeled antibodies. The physician then examines the slides using a fluorescent microscope.

Tissue cultures are still sometimes used, although they are more expensive and it takes longer to obtain results with them than with the monoclonal tests.

*Herpes Simplex, Types 1 and 2 Culture.** If an open lesion is present at the time of the initial pelvic examination, a viral culture is obtained from the lesion and is repeated at intervals. A positive Papanicolaou smear may be caused by the presence of herpes simplex, type 2.

Vagina. For assessing vaginal discharges other than blood, Chapters 10 and 30. After the specimens are obtained, the vagina around the cervix is viewed by rotating the speculum. The speculum blades are unlocked and partially closed. As the speculum is withdrawn, it is rotated and the vaginal walls inspected for color, lesions, rugae, fistulas, and bulging.

Incontinence. Incontinence of urine during straining is not a normal finding and is noted. A variety of factors can cause incontinence, including pubococcygeal muscles that are weak from lack of exercise (Kegel's) or trauma from childbirth (see guidelines for client teaching: Kegel's exercises, p. 162).

Internal: Bimanual Palpation. The examiner stands

*See also Chapter 30

Procedure 8-3

PAPANICOLAOU SMEAR (PAP SMEAR, PAP TEST)

DEFINITION

A laboratory technique of cytologic examination.

PURPOSE

To detect abnormalities of cell growth. During gynecologic examination cells from the squamocolumnar junction, the cervix, and the vagina are examined. Identification of endometrial or ovarian cancer *cannot* be obtained with this test.

EQUIPMENT

See Fig. 8-1.

NURSING ACTIONS	RATIONALE
Instruct the woman that optimum time for test is near the time of ovulation in her menstrual cycle.	To facilitate specimen collection since cervical os is somewhat open and mucus is plentiful (see Table 6-1, Fig. 6-26) and menstrual flow does not distort findings.
Instruct woman not to douche, use vaginal medications, or engage in intercourse at least 24 hours before the procedure.	To avoid altering findings that can lead to misdiagnosis. To prevent discomfort since douching removes vaginal secretions that provide lubrication.
Explain to client the purpose of the test and what sensations she will feel as the specimen is obtained (i.e., pressure, not pain). Inform her of who will perform the test.	To reduce tension that develops when people face the unknown.
Wash hands and apply gloves.	To prevent contamination of slides from other sources, and after slides are prepared to implement universal precautions when handling body fluids (see Chapter 30).
Assist examiner with test. The cytologic specimen is obtained before any digital examination of the vagina is made, or endocervical bacteriological specimens are taken with cotton swabbing of the cervix.	To prevent cell distortion by lubricant.
Instruct woman to fold her hands over her midriff and breathe as described in Procedure 8-2.	To promote comfort and reduce tension through relaxation and distraction.
Explain to woman that the specimen is taken by placing the S-shaped end of cervical spatula just within the cervical canal at the external os (see Fig. 6-13). The blade is rotated 360 degrees so that the surface at the squamocolumnar junction is firmly scraped. If the junction is inside the cervical canal, a swab may be used to obtain cells (see Fig. 6-13). If gross exudate is present, the excess is gently pushed away from the os with the end of the spatula.	To obtain cells from the squamocolumnar junction, the most common site of dysplasia and neoplasia (see Chapter 44).
Explain to woman that the specimen is spread on a slide without rubbing or drying, sprayed lightly with fixative, and allowed to dry.	To prepare the first slide, which contains mainly cells from the endocervix and ectocervix.
Explain to woman that some mucus is obtained from the posterior fornix (vaginal pool) with the rounded end of the spatula, spread on another slide, sprayed, and dried.	To prepare the second slide with mucus that may contain cells from the endometrium, endocervix, and vagina.
Label the slides with the woman's name and site. Include on the form to accompany the slides the woman's name, age, parity, and chief complaint or reason for taking the cytologic specimens.	To minimize chance of loss or mismatching specimens.
Place slides in carrying container, remove gloves, and wash hands.	To prevent cross-contamination.
Send the specimens to the pathology laboratory promptly for staining, evaluation, and a written report, with special reference to abnormal elements, including cancer cells.	To prevent delay that may cause change in specimen and a false report
Advise the woman that repeat smears may be necessary if specimen is not adequate.	To reduce anxiety if asked to return.
Instruct the woman concerning routine checkups for cervical or vaginal cancer (see Chapter 12, First trimester, and Chapter 44, Neoplasia).	To provide health maintenance information as part of procedure to reach as many people as possible.
Record the examination, date, and any untoward reactions on the woman's record.	To maintain concise, complete recording for providing care for clients.

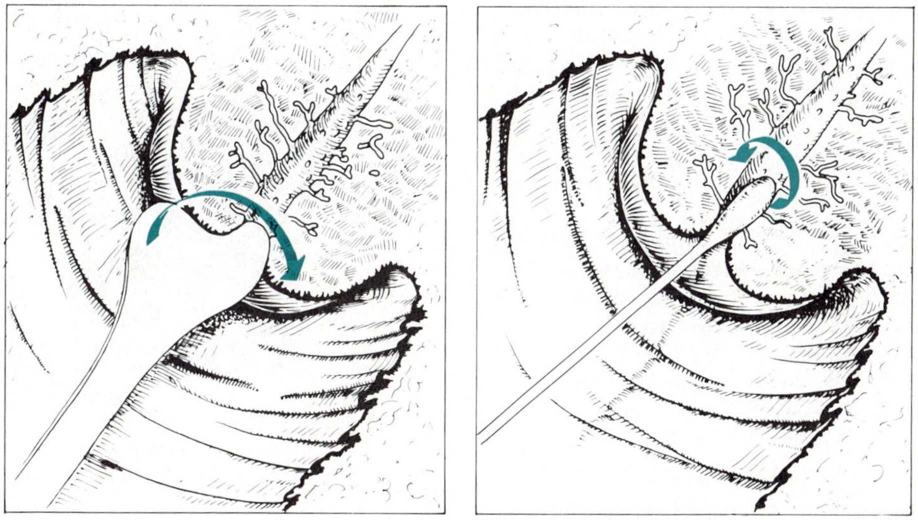

Fig. 8-17 A, Cervical smear. B, Endocervical smear.
From Malasanos, L, et al: Health assessment, ed 3, St Louis, 1986, The CV Mosby Co.

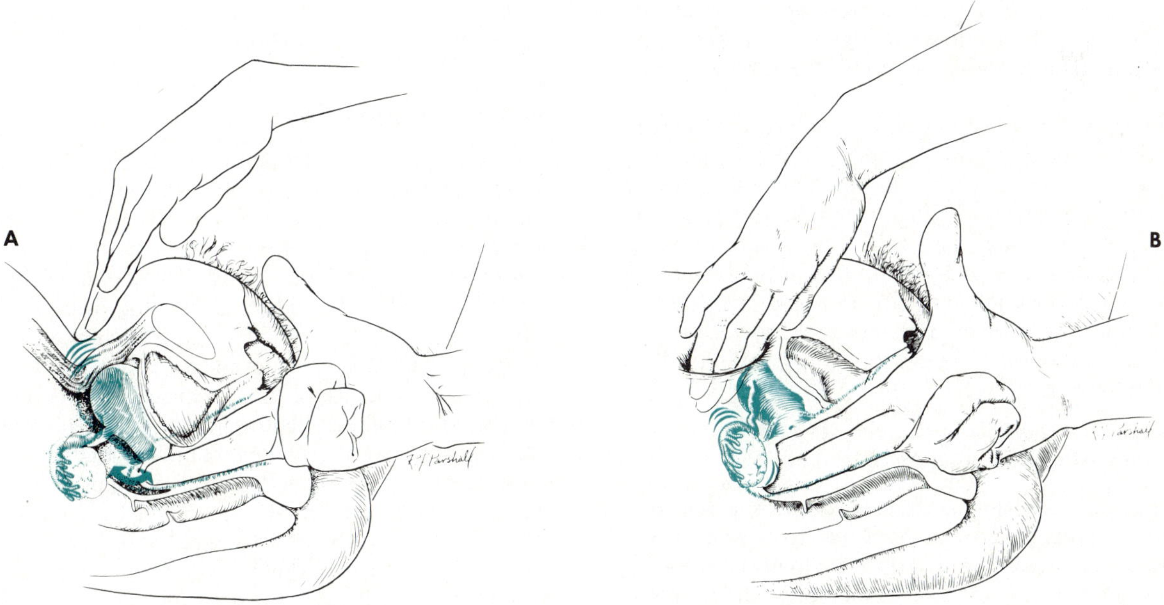

Fig. 8-18 Bimanual (abdominovaginal) palpation of uterus, A, and adnexa, B.
From Malasanos, L, et al: Health assessment, ed 3, St Louis, 1986, The CV Mosby Co.

for this part of the examination. A small amount of lubricant is dropped* onto the fingers of the gloved hand for the internal examination. Thumb and forefinger of (usually) ungloved hand separate the labia. Then for most women, 2 lubricated fingers (index and middle) of the gloved hand are slipped into the vagina while continuing gentle downward pressure. To avoid tissue trauma and contamination, the thumb of the gloved hand is abducted and the ring and little fingers are flexed into the palm.

The vagina is palpated for distensibility, lesions, and tenderness. The cervix is examined for position, shape, consistency, motility, and lesions. The fornix around the cervix is palpated.

The other hand is placed on the abdomen halfway between the umbilicus and symphysis pubis and exerts pressure downward toward the pelvic hand. Upward pressure from the pelvic hand traps reproductive structures for assessment by palpation (Fig. 8-18, *A*). The uterus is assessed for position (Fig. 6-8), size, shape, consistency, regularity, motility, masses, and tenderness.

Moving the abdominal hand to the right lower quadrant and the fingers of the pelvic hand in the right lateral fornix, the adnexa is assessed for position, size, tenderness, and masses (Fig. 8-18, *B*). If the ovary is felt when the female is young, it is usually smooth; when the woman is mature, it is somewhat nodular because of healed ruptured follicles; when the woman is 3 to 4 years past menopause, it is atrophied and usually no longer palpable. The examination is repeated on her left side.

Just before the intravaginal fingers are withdrawn, the woman is asked to tighten her vagina around the fingers as much as she can. If the muscle response is weak, the woman is assessed for her knowledge about Kegel's exercises (see guidelines for client teaching: Kegel's exercises, p. 162).

Internal: Rectovaginal Palpation. To prevent contamination of the rectum from organisms in the vagina (e.g., gonorrhea) it is best to change gloves, add fresh lubricant, and then reinsert the index finger into the vagina and the middle finger into the rectum. (Fig. 8-19). Insertion is facilitated if the woman strains down. The maneuvers of the abdominovaginal examination are repeated. The rectovaginal examination permits assessment of the rectovaginal septum, the posterior surface of the uterus, and the region behind the cervix.

Conference After Examination

After the pelvic examination, the woman is assisted into a sitting position, given tissues or wipes to cleanse herself, and privacy to dress. The woman often returns to the examiner's office for a discussion of findings, prescriptions for therapy, and counseling.

LIFE-CYCLE VARIATIONS

Developmental Stages. Newborn genitals are discussed in Chapters 21 and 22 and developmental stages are discussed in Chapters 6 and 9. Young or virginal females may need a one-finger examination. A small Pederson vaginal or a nasal speculum may facilitate vaginal inspection (Fig 8-15). Pediatric clients especially are assessed for ambiguous genitals, foreign bodies in the vagina, labial adhesions, and precocious or delayed puberty.

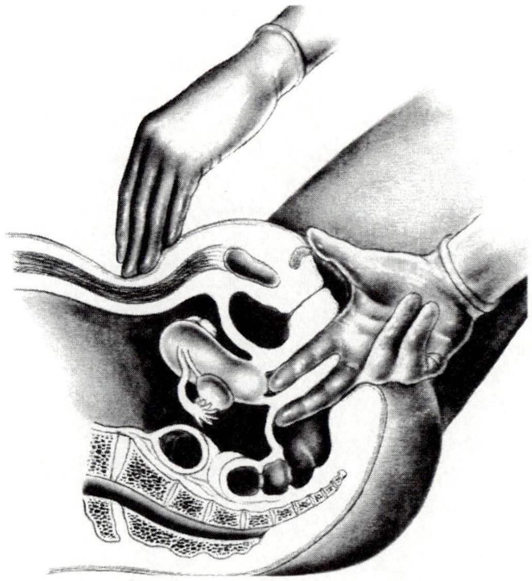

Fig. 8-19 Rectovaginal palpation.
From Seidel, H, et al: Mosby's guide to physical examination, St Louis, 1987, The CV Mosby Co.

Pregnancy. Maternal anatomic and physiologic adaptations to pregnancy are discussed in Chapter 10; recovery from childbirth is discussed in Chapters 20 and 24.

Older Adults. Changes in the genitals attributed to aging are discussed in Chapters 6 and 41.

NURSING DIAGNOSES

Knowledge of the nursing process is essential to making an informed gynecologic health assessment. Clinical reasoning involves systematic assessment of the client. Analysis of data includes identification of the defining characteristics (signs and symptoms), clustering of the defining characteristics, and naming the cluster in nursing diagnosis terminology (Appendix C). The next step is identification of the causes or related factors from the assessment data.

Once a nursing diagnosis is confirmed and a cause identified when possible, client-centered goals are formulated collaboratively with the client, nursing interventions are implemented, and expected outcomes are projected. Nursing interventions are aimed at modifying (i.e., ameliorating, reducing, increasing, or changing) the related factors, which will eventually modify the defining characteristics of nursing diagnoses. Expected outcomes are client centered and focus on the achievement of the woman's goals as demonstrated in clients by the modification of defining characteristics and by the eventual change in or elimination of the nursing diagnosis (Kim et al., 1987).

Guidelines for client teaching are developed from nursing diagnoses of potential concerns for many women. Guidelines for client teaching for prevention of urinary tract infection, Kegel's exercises (exercises for the pelvic floor), breast self-examination (BSE).

*If the contaminated glove touches the tube, the tube is discarded.

Guidelines For Client Teaching

PREVENTION OF URINARY TRACT INFECTION

ASSESSMENT

Woman is unaware of self-care measures to prevent urinary tract infection (UTI).

Woman may be pregnant, which predisposes her to UTI, and UTI may be a factor in preterm labor.

Woman may be experiencing postmenopausal urinary tract changes that predispose her to UTI.

NURSING DIAGNOSES

Potential for injury related to UTI urinary elimination, potential for altered patterns related to UTI.

Potential for pain related to UTI.

Knowledge deficit related to preventive actions.

GOALS

Short-term

Woman will be able to verbalize preventive methods.

Woman will learn preventive method.

Intermediate

Woman will routinely incorporate preventive methods in ADL.

Long-term

Woman will prevent UTI and the complications that may arise from it.

References and teaching aids

Texts.

Hospital- or clinic-prepared instructions.

Illustrations.

CONTENT/RATIONALE	TEACHING ACTION
Teach the woman general hygiene measures:	
Always wipe front to back after urinating or moving bowels. Use a clean piece of toilet paper for each front to back wipe. Wiping in the opposite way, from back to front, may carry bacteria from the rectal area (anus) to the urethral opening and increase risk of infection. Use soft, absorbent toilet tissue, preferably white and unscented. Harsh, scented, or printed toilet paper may cause irritation.	Using an illustration, show woman locations of urinary meatus, vagina, and anus. Provide explanation and rationale for action.
Change tampons, panty shields, or sanitary napkins often. Bacteria can multiply in menstrual blood or on soiled panty shields.	Encourage discussion about perineal hygiene, for example, feelings regarding odors, vaginal discharges, stress incontinence, touching oneself.
Wear underpants and panty hose with a cotton crotch. Avoid wearing tight-fitting slacks or panty shields for long periods. A build up of heat and moisture in the genital area may contribute to the growth of bacteria.	Explain how nylon and synthetic fibers retain heat and moisture.
Explain to the woman proper fluid and food intake:	
Drink 2 to 3 quarts (8 to 12 glasses) of liquid a day; 8 to 10 ounces of cranberry juice a day may be included, since cranberry juice is more acidic than other fluids and can lower the pH of the urinary tract. A more acidic urinary tract is a less hospitable medium to developing bacteria.	Elicit feelings or ideas concerning cultural, ethnic, religious, or other factors affecting food and fluid intake. Discuss rationale. Discuss fluid intake if woman is edematous, has PIH, or has difficulty sleeping at night as a result of nocturia.
Include lactobacilli in diet. Yogurt that contains the live culture and acidophilus milk may help prevent UTI, as well as vaginal infections. Lactobacilli, which are normally found in the vagina and the urinary tract, maintain the normal pH balance.	Provide rationale for including these foods in the woman's diet. Discuss food preferences.
Teach woman proper urination practices:	
Urinate frequently. Maintain fluid intake to ensure urination; do not limit fluids to reduce frequency of urination. Do not ignore signals that indicate the need to use the bathroom. Holding urine increases the time bacteria are in the bladder and allows them to multiply. Plan ahead when in situations where you will be unable to urinate for a long period of time, for example, before a long car ride, try to urinate in advance. Always urinate before going to bed at night.	Elicit information about daily schedule, for example, if working, can she get to the bathroom often. Provide rationale.
Urinate before and after intercourse, then drink a large glass of water to urinate again. This helps eliminate a medium for bacteria that are introduced during intercourse.	Provide an explanation concerning the introduction of bacteria during intercourse. Discuss rationale.
Post climacteric counseling (See Chapter 41).	See Chapter 41.

EVALUATION The nurse can be reasonably assured that care was effective if the woman does not develop an UTI.

Guidelines For Client Teaching

KEGEL'S EXERCISES (EXERCISES FOR THE PELVIC FLOOR)

ASSESSMENT

1. Woman is pregnant, postpartum, or postmenopausal.
2. Woman has problems with urinary dribbling.
3. Vaginal laxity noted on pelvic examination.
4. Woman indicates interest in learning.

NURSING DIAGNOSES

Knowledge deficit.
Stress incontinence.
Potential for altered sexuality patterns.

GOALS

Short-term

To meet knowledge deficit.
To begin exercises to prevent loss of tone or regain tone.

Intermediate

To exercise routinely.

Long-term

To gain and maintain muscle tone.

REFERENCES AND TEACHING AIDS

Texts.

Hospital or clinic-prepared instructions, illustrations.

CONTENT/RATIONALE	TEACHING ACTIONS
Rationale: To strengthen the muscles around the reproductive organs and improve muscle tone. Many women are not aware of the muscles of the pelvic floor until it is pointed out that these are the muscles used when urinating and during sexual intercourse and are therefore consciously controlled. Since pelvic floor muscles encircle the outlet through which the baby must pass, it is important that they be exercised, because an exercised muscle can stretch and contract readily at the time of birth. To help the pelvic floor muscles return to normal functioning, Kegel's exercises should be started immediately after delivery. After menopause occurs, muscle tone around the reproductive organs may decrease (Chapter 41). Kegel's exercises can strengthen these muscles and improve muscle tone. If practiced on a regular basis, the exercises help prevent prolapsed uterus and stress incontinence.	Initiate teaching of exercises. Show illustrations with location of muscles (Figs. 6-15 and 6-16). Encourage discussion and questions.
The exercise:	
A. The muscles that stop the flow are the pubococcygeal muscles. Doing Kegel's exercises during urination helps the woman know whether she is doing them correctly. If she can stop the stream of urine, her tone is good.	A. Teach woman to locate pubococcygeal muscles by practicing stopping the flow and starting it again while urinating.
B. After a woman has located the correct muscles, Kegel's exercises can be done in the following ways: 1. *Slow:* Tighten the muscle, hold it for the count of three, and relax it. 2. *Quick:* Tighten the muscle, and relax it as rapidly as possible. 3. *Push out-pull in:* Pull up the entire pelvic floor as though trying to suck up water into the vagina. Then bear down as if trying to push the imaginary water out. This uses abdominal muscles also.	B. Validate with the woman that she has located the muscles. Teach the three ways of performing the exercise.
Practice: This exercise needs to be practiced several times a day to be effective. It must be done every day for the rest of the woman's life. This exercise can be done 10 times in a row at least 3 times or more a day. Although some people recommend doing this exercise as many as 100 times in a row, this only fatigues the pelvic floor muscles.	Emphasize the benefits of the exercise.
A good time to practice is during trips to the bathroom, but additional practice at other times is even more beneficial.	Emphasize that, since it is not obvious when a woman is practicing, she might practice any time and anywhere.

EVALUATION The nurse can be reasonably assured that teaching was effective if the woman reports increased muscle tone to control urine flow and during sexual intercourse.

Guidelines For Client Teaching

BREAST SELF-EXAMINATION

ASSESSMENT

Woman states she does not know how to examine her breasts.
Woman has potential risk for developing breast lumps and cancer because of history (see Chapter 44).

NURSING DIAGNOSIS

Knowledge deficit related to self-care: breast self-examination (BSE).

GOALS

Short-term

Woman will verbalize reasons why BSE is important.
Woman will verbalize steps of BSE and rationale for each step.
Woman will demonstrate BSE procedure correctly.

Intermediate (By first postpartum check-up or by next gynecologic examination)

Woman verbalizes steps of BSE and rationale.
Woman states she has examined her breasts once.
After weaning: woman will be familiar with the normal feel and appearance of her breasts.

Long-term

Woman performs BSE every month.

References and teaching aids.

American Cancer Society's pamphlet, *How to examine your breasts.*
Mirror.
Model for practicing palpation and recognition of masses.

CONTENT/RATIONALE	TEACHING ACTION
To provide content and rationale for BSE during the menstrual cycle; see p. 94, and Fig. 6-24. Breast anatomy is discussed in Chapter 6; benign and malignant disorders are discussed in Chapter 44.	Encourage questions to uncover anxieties, concerns, and knowledge gaps about BSE. Review content and rationale, as needed. Encourage questions.
To perform observation:	Demonstrate for woman.
Woman sits in front of mirror and observes her breasts while assuming four positions. 1. Arms relaxed at her sides. 2. Hands pressed against her waist (Fig. 8-3). 3. Arms over head (Fig. 8-4). 4. Leaning forward.	Assist woman to assume postures correctly.
Review normal and suspicious characteristics (p. 146).	Review, compare with woman's breasts and with pamphlet. Assist woman with verbalization of her observations of herself.
To perform palpation: Palpation is performed with the woman in the supine position and a pillow under the shoulder on the side of the breast to be examined (Fig. 8-5).	Using a teaching model or illustration, demonstrate methods of systematic breast palpation.
Examination is performed in a systematic manner (Figs. 8-6, and 8-7) and includes the nipple (Fig. 8-8). Palpation of axillary lymph nodes is most easily done by the practitioner (Fig. 8-10). However, the woman can learn too.	Demonstrate palpation on model and on woman's breast; observe return demonstration. Assist woman to supine position with pillow under shoulder on side to be examined. Assist woman through self-examination and verbal description of her findings. Encourage and answer questions.
To know how to report findings: Findings are described by their characteristics (e.g., color, discharge) and by their location (Fig. 8-11).	Review characteristics while referring to pamphlet or other printed matter.
When woman notes reportable signs or symptoms, she needs to note the phase of her menstrual cycle (if she is still cycling).	Using an illustration such as Fig. 8-11, show woman how to locate lesion.

EVALUATION Teaching of the cognitive and motor aspects of BSE is considered effective when the woman verbalizes and demonstrates the steps of the procedure. Teaching related to the affective/psychologic aspect of BSE may be considered effective if the woman performs BSE routinely *and* reports any findings immediately.

SUMMARY

The gynecologic client's perception of gynecology-related anatomy and function, reasons for entering the health care system, and social and other factors influence the client's contact with the health care system. The gynecologic health assessment includes the interview, physical assessment, and diagnostic testing. The physical assessment focuses on the thyroid gland, the breasts, the abdomen, and the reproductive structures, both internal and external.

The older woman and the woman with a handicap require some adaptations in the health assessment process but merit the same respect and consideration as all individuals.

Some data collected may prove irrelevant for the individual client's current or future health management. However, the data may be invaluable to some future researcher's epidemiologic investigation of a disorder: its incidence, cause, clinical manifestations, therapy, and prognosis.

KEY CONCEPTS

- Culture, religion, socioeconomic status, personal circumstances, the uniqueness of the individual and stage of development are among the factors that influence a person's recognition of need for care and responses to the health care system and therapy.
- The changing status and roles for women affect their health, needs, and ability to cope with problems.
- Assessment is more comprehensive, and client learning is best in a safe environment in which the atmosphere is nonjudgmental and sensitive, and the interaction is strictly confidential.
- Every client is entitled to be respected and fully involved in the assessment process to the fullness of her capacity.
- A health assessment includes a comprehensive interview and physical examination and diagnostic testing.
- Every nurse must be competent to identify and respond appropriately to supine hypotension and vasovagal syncope.
- Nursing diagnoses are derived from the data from the health assessment and form the basis for planning, implementing, and evaluating nursing care, e.g. (client teaching).

STUDY QUESTIONS AND ACTIVITIES

1. Visit a clinic and participate in a complete gynecologic examination with a client. Observe the intake procedure, the client's emotional condition, and the health teaching that occurs.
2. Discuss in a group personal experiences and reactions to gynecologic examinations.
3. Direct a client in collecting a clean catch urine specimen.
4. Role play with a classmate counseling a woman about having a pelvic examination and a Papanicolaou smear.
5. Utilize each of the client teaching tools at least once, either with a client or in a simulated situation with classmates.

References

American Board of Internal Medicine: A guide to awareness and humanistic qualities in the internist, 1985, American Board of Internal Medicine

Bates, B: A guide to physical examination, ed 4, Philadelphia, 1987, JB Lippincott Co

Berger, KJ, and Fields, WL: Pocket guide to health assessment, Reston, V, 1980, Reston Publishing Co, Inc

Broverman, JK, et al: Sex-role stereotypes and clinical judgments of mental health, J Consult Clin Psychol **34(1)**:1, 1970

Cooperstock, R: Sex differences in the use of mood-modifying drugs: an explanatory model, J Health Soc Behav **12**:238, 1971

Corea, G: The hidden malpractice: how American medicine treats women as patients and professionals, New York, 1977, William Morrow & Co, Inc

Ehrenreich, B, and English, D: For her own good: 150 years of the experts advice to woman, New York, 1978, Anchor Press

Fogel, CI, and Woods, NF: Health care of women: a nursing perspective, St Louis, 1981, The CV Mosby Co

Griffith-Kenney, J: Contemporary women's health, Menlo Park, Calif, 1986, Addison-Wesley Publishing Co, Inc

Howell, MC: What medical schools teach about women, N Engl J Med **291**:304, 1974

Kim, MJ, et al: Pocket guide to nursing diagnoses, ed 2, St Louis, 1987, The CV Mosby Co

Larned, D: The epidemic in unnecessary surgery. In Dreifus, C, editor: Seizing our bodies: the politics of women's health, New York, 1977, Random House

Malasanos, L, et al.: Health assessment, ed 3, St Louis, 1986, The CV Mosby Co

Marieskind, HI: Gynecological services and the women's movement: restructuring obstetrics and gynecology, Paper presented at American Public Health Association 103rd Annual Meeting, Nov 16-20, 1975

McBride AB, and McBride WL: Theoretical underpinnings for women's health, *Women Health,* 6(1/2):37, 1981

McCranie, EW, et al: Alleged sex-role stereotyping in the assessment of women's physical complaints: a study of general practitioners, Soc Sci Med **12**:111, 1978

Phipps, WJ, Long, BC, and Woods, NF: Medical-surgical nursing: concepts and clinical practice, ed 3, St Louis, 1987, The CV Mosby Co

Queenan, JT, editor: Managing ob/gyn emergencies: a contemporary ob/gyn book, Oradell, NJ, 1982, Medical Economics Books

Ruzek, SB: The women's health movement: feminist alternatives to medical control, New York, 1978, Praeger Publishers

Seidel, HM, et al: Mosby's guide to physical examination, St Louis, 1987, The CV Mosby Co

Tudor, W, et al: The effect of sex role differences on the social control of mental illness, J Health Soc Behav **18**: 98, 1977

United States Pharmacopeia Dispensing Information, St Louis, 1986, The CV Mosby Co

Waldron, I: Increased prescribing valium, librium, and other drugs: an example of the influence of economic and social factors on the practice of medicine, Int J Health Serv 7(1):91, 1977

Bibliography

Callan, CM: What to tell patients about douching, Contemp OB/GYN 27:178, 1986 (Special issue)

Capraro, VJ, et al: The gyn exam for newborns, young children, and adolescents, Contemp Obstet Gynecol **20**(4):43, 1982

Chesler, P: Women and madness, New York, 1972, Doubleday & Co, Inc

Collier, P: Health behaviors of women, Nurs Clin North Am **17**(1):121, 1982

Coslow, F, and Steinberg, MC: Relaxation techniques in ambulatory care practice, Nurse Pract **8**(9):26, 1983

Dan AJ, Graham EA, and Beecher CP editors: *The menstrual cycle,* vol 1, *A synthesis of interdisciplinary research,* New York: 1980, Springer Publishing Co, Inc

Harris, BA: Significant changes in obstetrics, 1976-1986. The Female Patient, 11(9):104, 1986

Henderson, G, and Primeaux, M, editors: Transcultural health care, Menlo Park, Calif, 1981, Addison-Wesley Publishing Co, Inc

Herschberger, R: Adam's rib, New York, 1970, Harper & Row, Publishers, Inc

Knor, ER: Decision making in obstetrical nursing, Philadelphia, 1987, BC Decker Inc

Lovell, MC: Silent but perfect "partners": medicine's use and abuse of women, Adv Nurs Sci **3**:25, 1981

Meneilly, GS and Minaker, KL: Obtaining the geriatric history. Contemp OB/GYN 28(3):177, 1986

Mercer, RT: Nursing research: The bridge to excellence in practice, *Image* 15:47, 1984

Muff, J, editor: *Socialization, sexism, and stereotyping. Women's Issues in Nursing,* St Louis, 1982, The CV Mosby Co

Muhlenkamp, AF, Waller, MM, and Bourne, AE: Attitudes toward women in menopause: a vignette approach, *Nurs. Res.* **32**:20, Jan/Feb 1983

NAACOG Technical Bulletin: Adolescent gynecology—initial pelvic exam. No 5, Nov 1979

Norris, C: Self care, Am J Nurs **79**:486, 1979

Orque, MD, Bloch, B, and Monrroy, LS: Ethnic nursing care: a multicultural approach, St Louis, 1983, The CV Mosby Co

Roland, CG: The insidious bias of medical language, Nurs Dig **5**(1):53, 1977

Rutledge, DN: Factors related to women's practice of breast self-examination, Nurs Res, 36(2):117, 1987

Sandelowski, M: Women, health, and choice, Englewood Cliffs, NJ, 1981, Prentice-Hall, Inc

Scherger, JE: Changing gloves between vaginal and rectal examination: an additional reason. JAMA 257(2):191, 1987

Scully, D, and Bart, P: A funny thing happened on the way to the orifice: women in gynecology textbooks, Am J Soc **78**:1045, 1973

Swartz, WH: The semi-sitting position for pelvic examination (letter), JAMA **251**(9):1163, 1984

Symposium: The periodic exam, Contemp OB/GYN 28(5):172, 1986

Tucker, SM, et al: Patient care standards: nursing process, diagnosis and outcome, ed 4, St Louis, 1988, The CV Mosby Co

Tunnadine, P: The role of genital examination in psychosexual medicine, Clin Obstet Gynecol 7:283, 1980

Wawrzyniak, MN: The painless pelvic, MCN 11(3):178, 1986

Willard, MD, Heaberg, GL, and Pack, JB: The educational pelvic examination: women's responses to a new approach, JOGN Nurs 15(2):135, 1986

Woods, NF: Women's health: perspectives for nursing research, Nurs Clin North Am **17**(1):113, 1982

UNIT III

Normal Pregnancy

Conception initiates a phenomenal process with far-reaching effects. The maturation of a new person follows a blueprint determined generations ago. Reproduction bridges the gap between past and future and introduces significant alterations in present family structures. Chapter 9 focuses on the infant before birth, reviews the genetic factors that affect the developmental process, and the fetus's readiness for extrauterine life. Chapter 10 presents the maternal anatomy and physiology relevant to pregnancy and maternal adaptations to the growing fetus. Chapter 11 is concerned with family responses to the birth of a child. All family members respond to pregnancy in light of their own needs. Chapters 12, 13, and 14 deal with the knowledge, skills, and procedures basic to the care of clients during the prebirth period. The care is discussed under the five components of the nursing process: assessment, formation of nursing diagnoses, planning, implementation, and evaluation. Chapter 15 discusses the nutrition needs of mother, fetus, and child. Recognition of nutrition problems and prevention of complications are stressed.

Research highlights begin with this unit. The following abstracts represent examples of available *nursing* research within the last few years:

Chapter 9: The fetus: a growing member of the family.
Chapter 10: Comparisons of cardiac output in supine and lateral positions.
Chapter 11: Network structure, social support, and psychological outcomes of pregnancy.
Chapter 13: Automobile seat belt practices of pregnant women.
Chapter 14: Identifying priorities for prepared childbirth research.
Chapter 15: Unique aspects of Korean-American mothers.

CHAPTER 9

Genetics, Conception, and Fetal Development

Learning Objectives

Correctly define the key terms listed.

Summarize the process of fertilization.

Explain the fundamental principles of genetics.

Evaluate fetal changes in each of the three stages of development.

Review the functions of the placenta.

Discuss at least four functions of amniotic fluid.

Identify at least three organs and tissues arising from each of the three primary germ layers.

List at least three developmental changes of each organ system and its correlating timetable.

Explain the importance of pulmonary surfactant and the L/S ratio.

Explore the potential effects of teratogens on the embryo and fetus week by week during gestation.

Key Terms

amniotic fluid
capacitation
chorionic villi
chromosome
conception (fertilization)
decidua
diploid
ductus arteriosus
embryo
fetal circulation
fetal heart rate (FHR)
fetal membranes
fetus
foramen ovale
gametogenesis
genes
gestational age
haploid
hematopoiesis
human chorionic gonadotropin (hCG)
implantation
karyotype
lanugo
last menstrual period (LMP)
lecithin/sphingomyelin (L/S) ratio
meconium
Mendel's laws
neural tube
placenta
placental barrier
quickening
surfactant
trophoblast
viability
zygote

The maternity nurse is in the unique position of providing nursing care to the unborn. Gravidas and their families have many questions about fetal development, such as "When is our baby due?" "How big is my baby now?" "My friend had a baby with blue eyes, but both of them have brown eyes. Is that possible?" "My baby jerks every couple of minutes for a short time sometimes. My mother said the baby is hiccuping. Is that so?" "How does the baby breathe in there?" "Everyone smokes in the office where I work. Will it hurt the baby?" "Will having sex (late in pregnancy) put holes in the baby's head or in his heart?" These questions commonly crop up in prenatal classes and private conversations with the woman or her partner. The wide media coverage of substances that affect the unborn can be disturbing to parents. The knowledgeable nurse can advise parents based on understanding of conception and normal fetal development. This chapter is designed to help nurses answer these questions. It gives a brief overview of the genetic basis of inheritance and normal embryonic and fetal development from conception to full-term gestation.

GENETICS

Genes and Chromosomes

The biologic and behavioral characteristics of each human being are determined by the action of thousands of minute particles of hereditary material contained within the nuclei of all living cells. Each of these particles or *genes,* has a specific function in the control or regulation of cellular activity. Alone or in combination with other genes, they are responsible for all human traits or characteristics, for the orderly pattern and timing of development from conception to death, and for continuity of the species through consistent transmission of these traits from generation to generation.

The genes are composed of tiny segments of *deoxyribonucleic acid* (DNA), which enables them to duplicate themselves exactly during cell division. Each body cell contains two sets of genes arranged in a line to form larger structures, the *chromosomes,* within the cell nucleus. Each cell nucleus contains two sets of chromosomes consisting of two matching sets of genes, one set obtained from each parent during the process of fertilization. When members of a pair of genes are alike and produce the same effect they are called *homozygous;* when they are not alike and produce different effects, they are said to be *heterozygous* (Fig. 9-1).

Chromosomes cannot be seen except under a microscope. For analysis they are stained, magnified, and photographed. Then each individual chromosome is cut out and arranged in a **karyotype** according to size and shape. They appear as structures with either an X or a Y shape. Fig. 9-2 illustrates the chromosomes in a body cell.

Cell Division

Somatic cells divide by the process of *mitosis,* in which the cell components, including the genetic material, divide and are distributed equally to the two newly formed cells (Fig. 9-3). Each new cell contains the same composition and genetic potential as the original cell.

The process of cell division in the reproductive cells is called *gametogenesis.* Gametogenesis takes place by *meiosis,* or *reduction division,* to form **gametes.** It consists of two successive divisions. In the *first* division the pairs of homologous chromosomes randomly separate from each other to form two nonidentical cells containing 23 nonhomologous chromosomes. In the *second* meiotic division the individual chromosomes split to form two identical cells, each with the same genetic complement of 23 chromosomes (Fig. 9-4).

Gametogenesis

Spermatogenesis. Meiosis in the male gonad is a continuous process that begins about the time of puberty and lasts until senescence. A primitive diploid germ cell (spermatogonium) matures to form a *primary spermatocyte,* which divides to form two *secondary spermatocytes,* each with a haploid complement (23) of chromosomes. These subsequently divide equally to form the spermatids, which gradually differentiate into small, highly motile *spermatozoa,* or sperm (Figs. 9-5 and 9-7).

Each normal sperm carries a haploid number of chromosomes, either 22 autosomes and an X chromosome or 22 autosomes and a Y chromosome. The male supplies the genetic material (an X or a Y sex chromosome) that determines the sex of the child.

Oogenesis. Unlike spermatogenesis, the process of meiosis in the ovaries is not a continuous process. Oogenesis begins during intrauterine life, and the female gametes have already enlarged and developed into *primary oocytes* at the time of birth (Fig. 9-6). These primary oocytes (approximately 500,000 in number) have begun the first meiotic division but remain suspended at this stage until, one at a time, they are stimulated to complete the division.

When oogenesis continues, the primary oocyte with a diploid complement of chromosomes completes the first meiotic division. However, there is an unequal distribution of the cellular contents. Although the chromosome complement is reduced to the haploid number and equally divided between the two cells, there is unequal distribution of the cytoplasm. The result is one large *secondary oocyte* containing the bulk of the cellular contents and a small, nonfunctioning *first polar body.* The second meiotic division begins at ovulation when the secondary oocyte divides to form a large, nonmotile *ovum* and a *second polar body.* The polar bodies, unable to support reproduction, soon disintegrate. The ovum (Fig. 9-7) does not complete the second meiotic division until triggered by the entrance of the sperm at fertilization. Each normal ovum contains 22 autosomes and an X chromosome. An ovum fertilized by a sperm bearing a Y chromosome results in a male zygote, whereas an ovum fertilized by an X-bearing sperm results in a female zygote.

When the sperm and the ovum meet and form a zygote (fertilized ovum), the diploid number of chromosomes (44 autosomes and 2 sex chromosomes) is restored (Fig. 9-8). At that moment the sex of the new human is determined, and the blueprints for the growth, development, and maturation of a new individual are laid down.

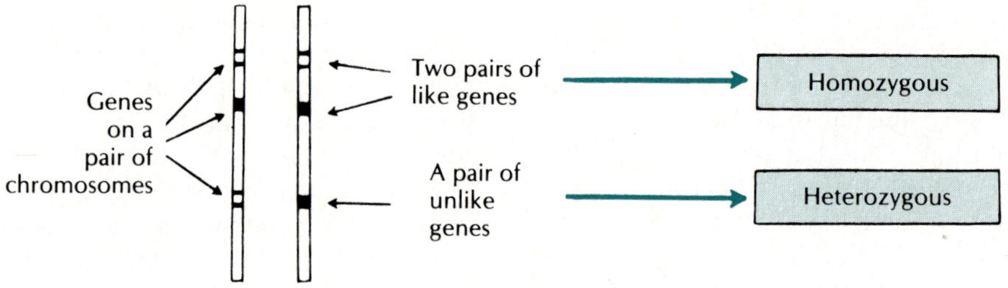

Fig. 9-1 Genes on a pair of chromosomes illustrating like and unlike gene pairs.
From Whaley, LF: Understanding inherited disorders, St Louis, 1974, The CV Mosby Co.

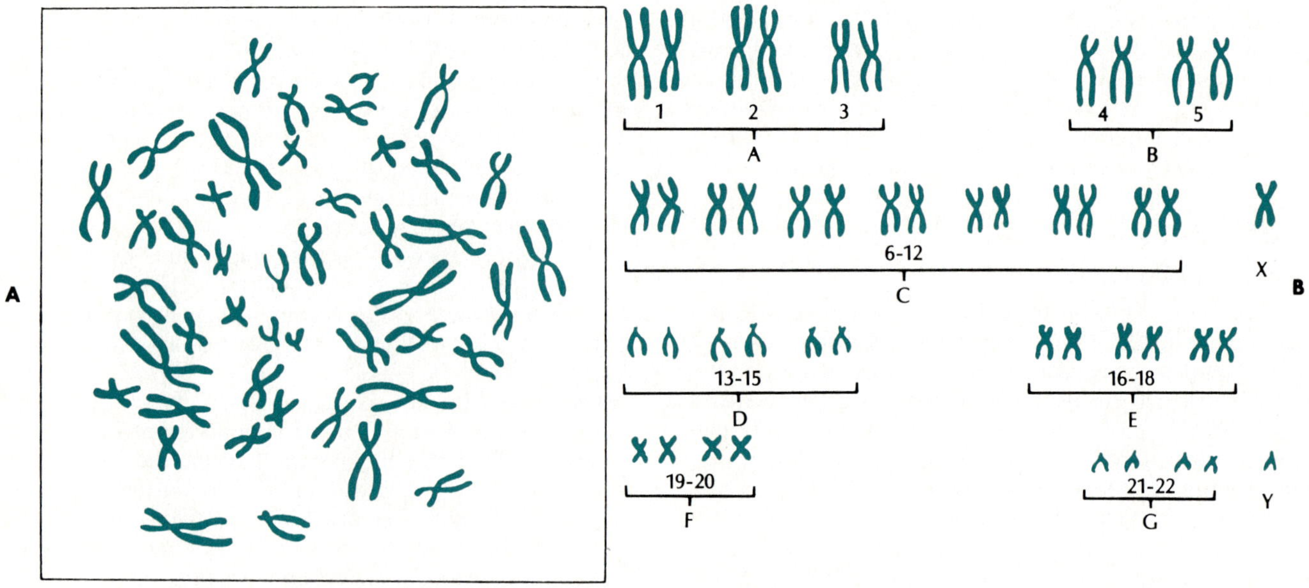

Fig. 9-2 Male chromosomes during cell division. **A**, Example of photomicrograph. **B**, Chromosomes arranged in karyotype.
From Whaley, LF, and Wong, DL: Nursing care of infants and children, ed 3, St Louis, 1987, The CV Mosby Co.

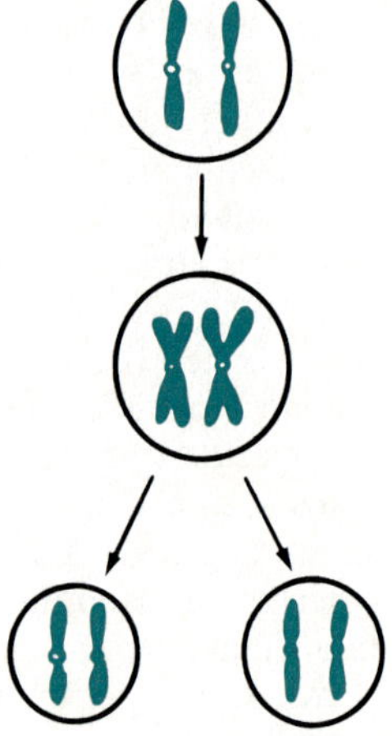

Fig. 9-3 Mitosis in somatic cell.
From Whaley, LF, and Wong, DL: Nursing care of infants and children, ed 3, St Louis, 1987, The CV Mosby Co.

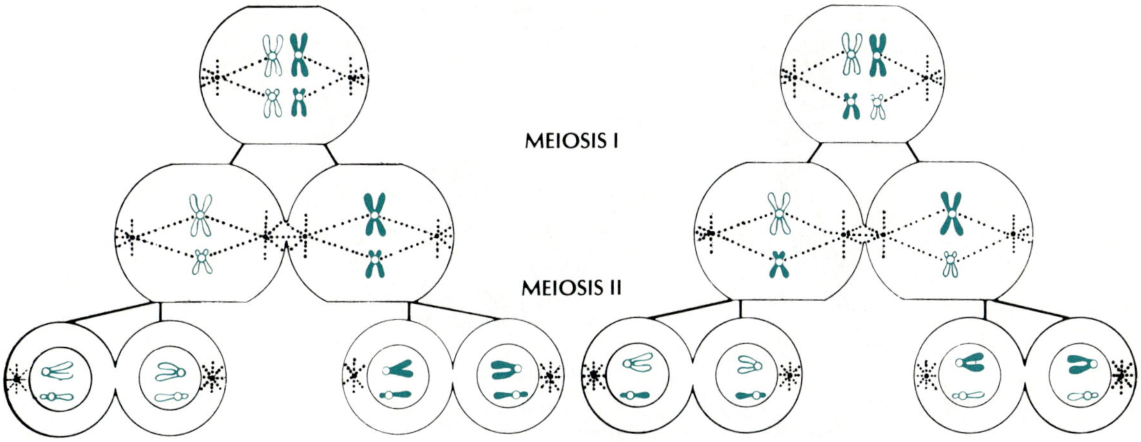

Fig. 9-4 Process of meiosis: a premeiotic germ cell with two sets of chromosomes forms four germ cells, each with a single set of chromosomes. Two alternative arrangements of chromosome pairs on first meiotic spindle are diagrammed.
From Sandberg EC: Synopsis of obstetrics, ed 10, St Louis, 1987, The CV Mosby Co.

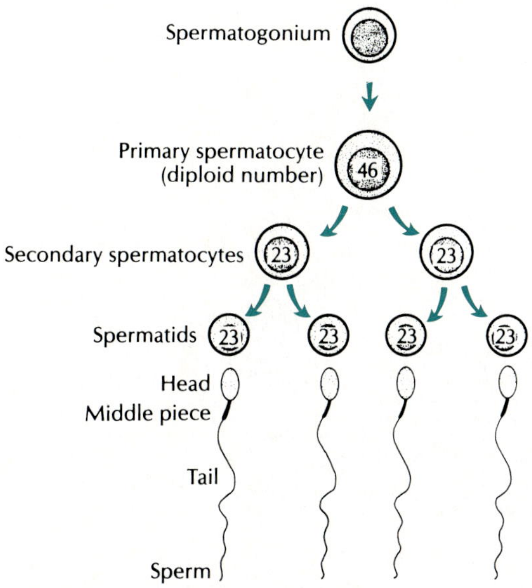

Fig. 9-5 Spermatogenesis. Gametogenesis of the male produces four mature gametes, the sperm.

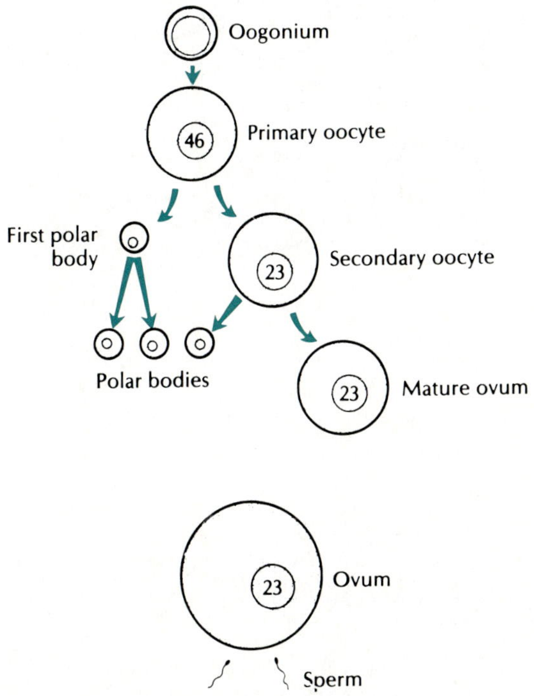

Fig. 9-6 Oogenesis. Gametogenesis in the female produces one mature ovum and three polar bodies. Note the relative difference in overall size between the ovum and sperm.

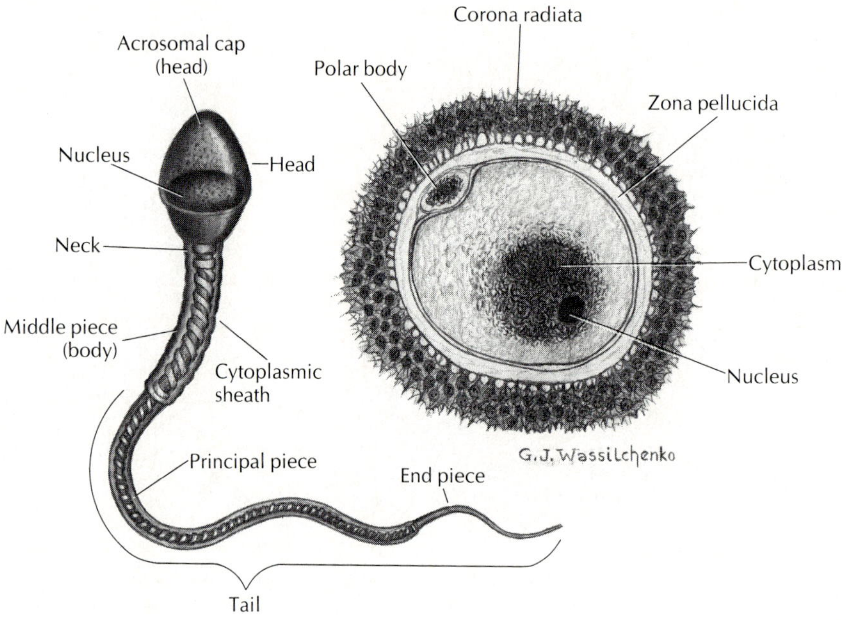

Fig. 9-7 Sperm and ovum.

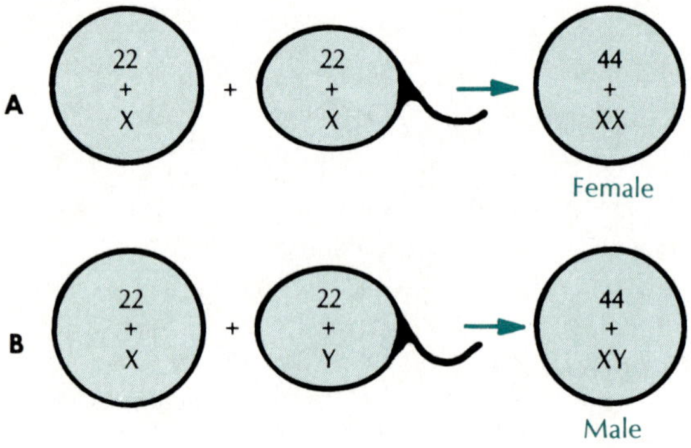

Fig. 9-8 Fertilization. **A**, Ovum fertilized by X-bearing sperm to form female zygote. **B**, Ovum fertilized by Y-bearing sperm to form male zygote.

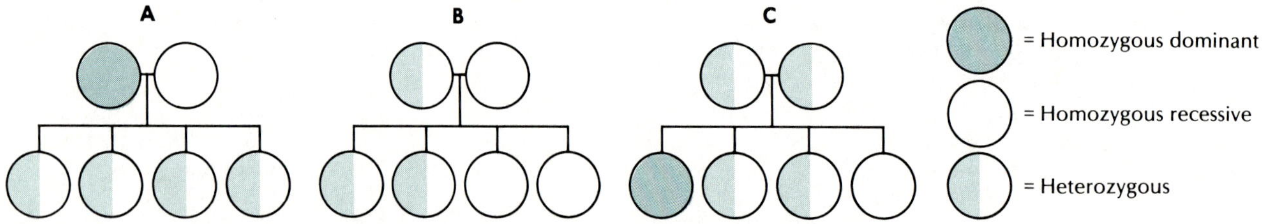

Fig. 9-9 Possible offspring in three types of matings. **A**, Homozygous-dominant parent and homozygous-recessive parent. Children all heterozygous, displaying dominant trait. **B**, Heterozygous parent and homozygous-recessive parent. Children 50% heterozygous display dominant trait; 50% homozygous display recessive trait. **C**, Both parents heterozygous. Children 25% homozygous dominant trait; 25% homozygous display recessive trait; 50% heterozygous display dominant trait.

Gene Transmission in Families

The genes act in predictable fashion during gamete formation and fertilization, and it is on this orderly performance that the science of genetics rests. A knowledge of the way in which genes combine, segregate, and recombine is essential to an understanding of their distribution in families. The fundamental principles of genetics, or Mendel's laws, are briefly summarized as follows:

principle of dominance Not all genes that determine a given trait operate with equal vigor. When two genes at a given locus produce a different effect (e.g., the gene for eye color), they may compete for expression in the individual. As a result, one may mask or conceal the effect of the other. The characteristic that is manifest in the individual (and the gene that produces the effect) is referred to as *dominant;* that which is hidden and not manifest is *recessive* (Fig. 9-9).

principle of segregation The paired chromosomes, bearing genes derived from each parent, are separated when gametes are formed during meiosis. Each gene segregates in pure form, and chance alone determines which gene (paternally derived or maternally derived) will travel to a specific gamete.

principle of independent assortment The members of one pair of genes are distributed in the gametes in random fashion, independent of other pairs.

CONCEPTION (FERTILIZATION)

During sexual intercourse 2 to 5 ml of semen, usually containing more than 300 million sperm, is ejaculated into the female vagina. By flagellar movement the sperm make their way through the fluids of the cervical mucus (if the mucus is receptive), across the endometrium, and into the uterine tube to meet the descending ovum in the ampulla of the tube (see Chapter 6 for further discussion).

Before fertilization the sperm undergo a physiologic change called *capacitation* and a structural change called *acrosome reaction.* Capacitation refers to the removal of a protective coating from the sperm. Enzymes produced by the lining of the uterine tubes assist in capacitation of the sperm. The acrosome reaction refers to the small perforations that form in the anterior head of the sperm. Enzymes (e.g., hyaluronidase) escape through these perforations and digest a path for the sperm through the corona radiata and zona pellucida of the ovum. Only one sperm is required for actual fertilization, but the presence of many increases the chances for one to penetrate.

Fertilization (conception), the fusion of a *sperm* and an *ovum* (oocyte), is a process that requires about 24 hours. To fertilize an egg the sperm must pass through the *corona radiata* and *zona pellucida* and enter the egg; then female and male pronuclei undergo changes that result in a **zygote.**

In general, the process of fertilization takes place as follows: The cells of the corona radiata are dispersed by enzyme action of tubal mucosa and sperm. With the aid of its tail movements, the sperm can pass through this outermost covering of the egg. The acrosomes of several sperm release enzymes that digest a pathway through the zona pellucida. One sperm (usually) attaches to and fuses with the egg's plasma membrane, which then breaks down at the point of contact. At the moment that a sperm makes contact with the egg's plasma membrane, the oocyte reacts in two ways: a "zona reaction" (as yet not understood) occurs, preventing the entry of more sperm, and the oocyte matures (its nucleus is now known as the female pronucleus). The head and tail of the sperm enter the egg, leaving the sperm's plasma membrane (cytoplasmic sheath) attached to that of the oocyte. The tail of the sperm degenerates rapidly; its head enlarges to form the male pronucleus. The female and male pronuclei come together in the center of the oocyte and lose their cell membranes.

The fertilized ovum begins to divide, differentiate, and grow into a person, a replica of humanity's continuing generations and yet a unique individual. The growth that takes place from conception to birth is more rapid than at any other time in a person's life. The zygote weighs 15 ten-millionths of a gram; a 7-pound term baby weighs about 3175 g. In those 9 months the zygote increases in size by more than 200 billion times.

Multiple Pregnancy

Twins. Twins produced from a single ovum are termed *monozygotic,* or identical, and are always of the same sex. Those produced from separate ova are *dizygotic,* or fraternal, and may be of the same or opposite sex. Monozygotic twinning is a random occurrence. Dizygotic twinning (multiple ovulation), on the other hand, is an autosomal-recessive trait carried by the daughters of mothers of twins. Dizygotic twinning occurs more commonly as maternal age at conception increases.

Dizygotic, but not monozygotic, twins tend to repeat in families. If twins occur in the first pregnancy, a repetition of twinning or some other form of multiple birth is about five times more likely to occur at the next pregnancy than it is in the general population (Moore, 1977a, b).

Monozygotic Twins. In monozygotic twinning, one ovum is fertilized. Therefore these twins share identical genetic material. These twins are of the same sex, genetically identical, and similar in physical appearance. Environmental factors, for example, anastomosis of placental vessels, may cause physical differences. Monozygotic twinning usually begins around the end of the first week after fertilization and results from division of the inner cell mass into two embryonic primordia. If the blastomeres (cells resulting from the cleavage of a fertilized ovum [zygote]) separate, two implantations result (Fig. 9-10, *A*). If they do not separate, two identical embryos, each in its own amniotic sac, develop within one chorionic sac (Fig. 9-10, *B*). The twins have a common placenta and often some placental vessels join.

Rarely, later division of embryonic cells results in monozygotic twins that are in one amniotic and one chorionic sac (Fig. 9-10, *C*). Such twins are rarely delivered alive because the umbilical cords are commonly entangled so that circulation ceases and one or both fetuses die.

Dizygotic Twins. In dizygotic twinning, two ova are fertilized at the same time or within hours of each other. The resulting twins may be of the same sex or of different sexes. They are no more alike genetically than brothers or sisters born at different times. Dizygotic twins always have two amnions and two chorions, but the chorions and placentas may be fused (Fig. 9-11).

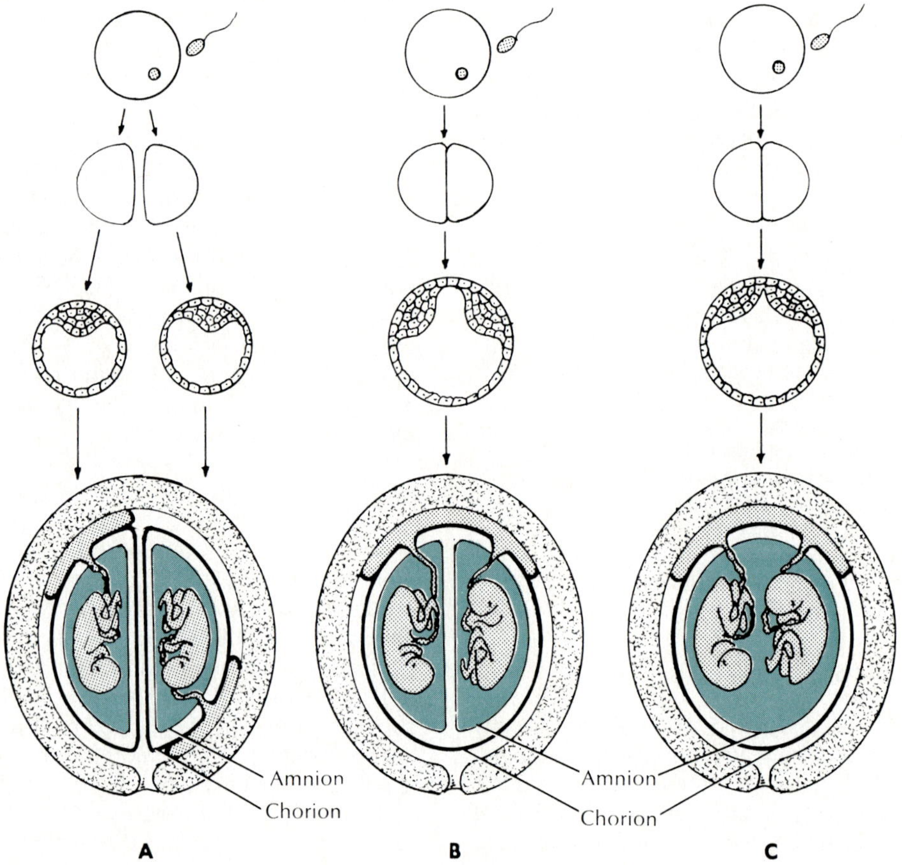

Fig. 9-10 Formation of monozygotic twins. **A,** One fertilization: blastomeres separate, resulting in two implantations, two placentas, and two sets of membranes. **B,** One blastomere with two inner cell masses, one fused placenta, one chorion, and separate amnions. **C,** Later separation of inner cell masses, with fused placenta and single amnion and chorion.

From Whaley, LF: Understanding inherited disorders, St Louis, 1974, The CV Mosby Co.

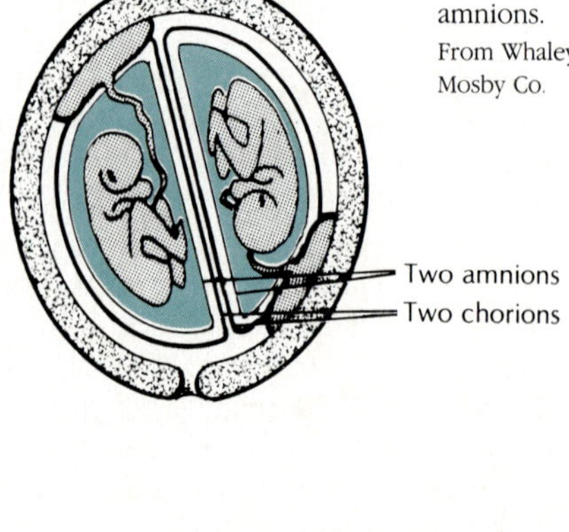

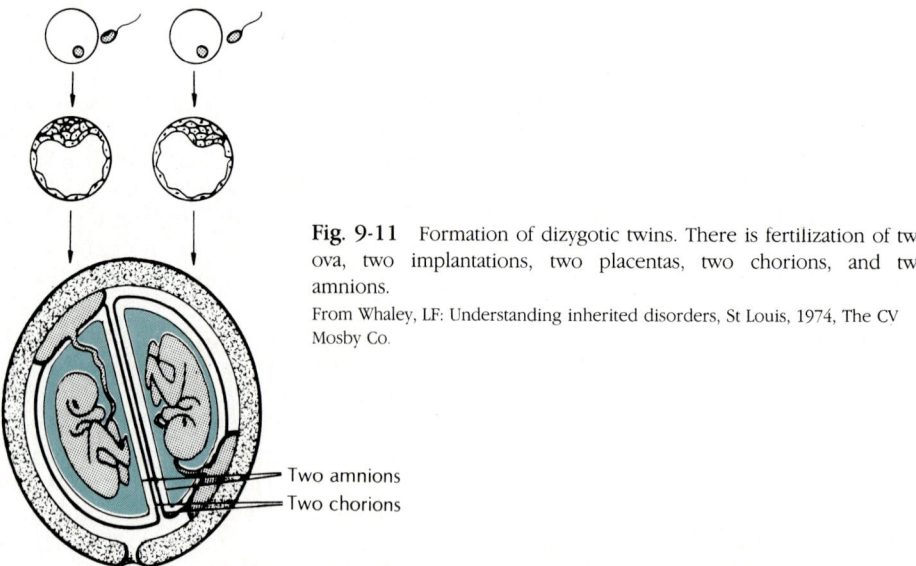

Fig. 9-11 Formation of dizygotic twins. There is fertilization of two ova, two implantations, two placentas, two chorions, and two amnions.

From Whaley, LF: Understanding inherited disorders, St Louis, 1974, The CV Mosby Co.

Other Multiple Pregnancies. *Triplets* occur once in about 7600 pregnancies and may be derived from (1) one zygote and be identical, (2) two zygotes and consist of identical twins and a single infant, or (3) three zygotes and be of the same sex or of different sexes (Fig. 9-12, *A*). In the last case, the infants are no more similar than those from three separate pregnancies. Similar possible combinations occur in *quadruplets* (Fig. 9-12, *B*), *quintuplets, sextuplets, septuplets,* and so forth. Types of multiple births higher than triplets are rare. They have occurred more often in recent years following the administration of gonadotropins to women with ovulatory failure or to women who undergo in vitro fertilization (Chapter 42).

Table 9-1 *Comparison of Gestational Time Units*

	Reference Point	
	Fertilization	Last Menstrual Period (LMP)
Days	266	280
Weeks	38	40
Calendar months	8¾	9
Lunar months	9½	10

From Moore, KL: Before we are born: basic embryology and birth defects, Philadelphia, 1974, WB Saunders Co.

GESTATION

Time Units

The chronology of pregnancy may be referred to in several ways, for example, 10 lunar months (of 4 weeks each), 40 weeks of gestation, or 9 calendar months (3 trimesters of 3 months each). **In this chapter, conceptional age in weeks refers to the time since fertilization.** In clinical practice however, the term *gestational age* or **menstrual age** refers to the time since the first day of the last menstrual period (LMP).

There is a difference of 2 weeks in calculating the duration of pregnancy, depending on the reference point used (Table 9-1). Calculation from the LMP (for a 28-day cycle) is 2 weeks longer than that from the time of fertilization. A graphic representation of the differences is seen in Fig. 9-13. The first square is "day 1 of menses" or day 1 of LMP. Note that 2 weeks pass before fertilization. These 2 weeks are added when discussing menstrual age of the pregnancy. The third row of squares identifies the onset of development after fertilization on the first day of the third week of the menstrual cycle.

The date of birth is calculated as about 266 days after fertilization, or 280 days after the onset of the last normal menstrual period (LNMP). From fertilization to the end of the embryonic period, age is best expressed in days. Thereafter age is commonly given in weeks. Because ovulation and fertilization are usually separated by not more than 12 hours, these events are more or less interchangeable in expressing prenatal age.

Developmental Stages

The fusion of the nuclei of the two gametes is called conception, fertilization, fecundation, or impregnation. Fusion initiates the first of the three stages of human prenatal development: ovum, embryo, and fetus.

Ovum. The conceptus is called an ovum during the period from conception until primary villi appear. Villi appear approximately 12 to 14 days after fertilization or about 4 weeks since LMP (see "primary villi" in Fig. 9-13, week 2, day 13). By the end of this period, implantation (nidation) is complete. The conceptus is totally within the endometrium and is covered by surface epithelium.

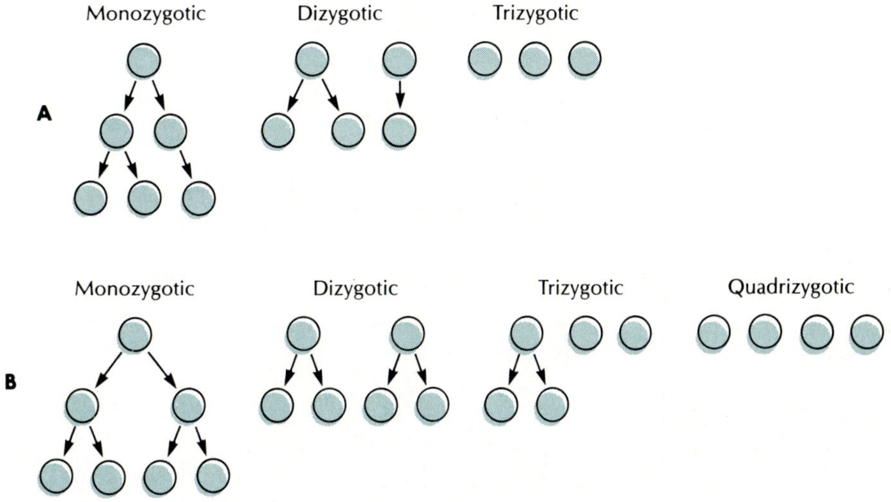

Fig. 9-12 **A**, Formation of triplets, and **B**, quadruplets indicating variety of mechanisms that can produce multiple births. Quadruplets can be formed from one to four ova.
From Whaley, LF: Understanding inherited disorders, St Louis, 1974, The CV Mosby Co.

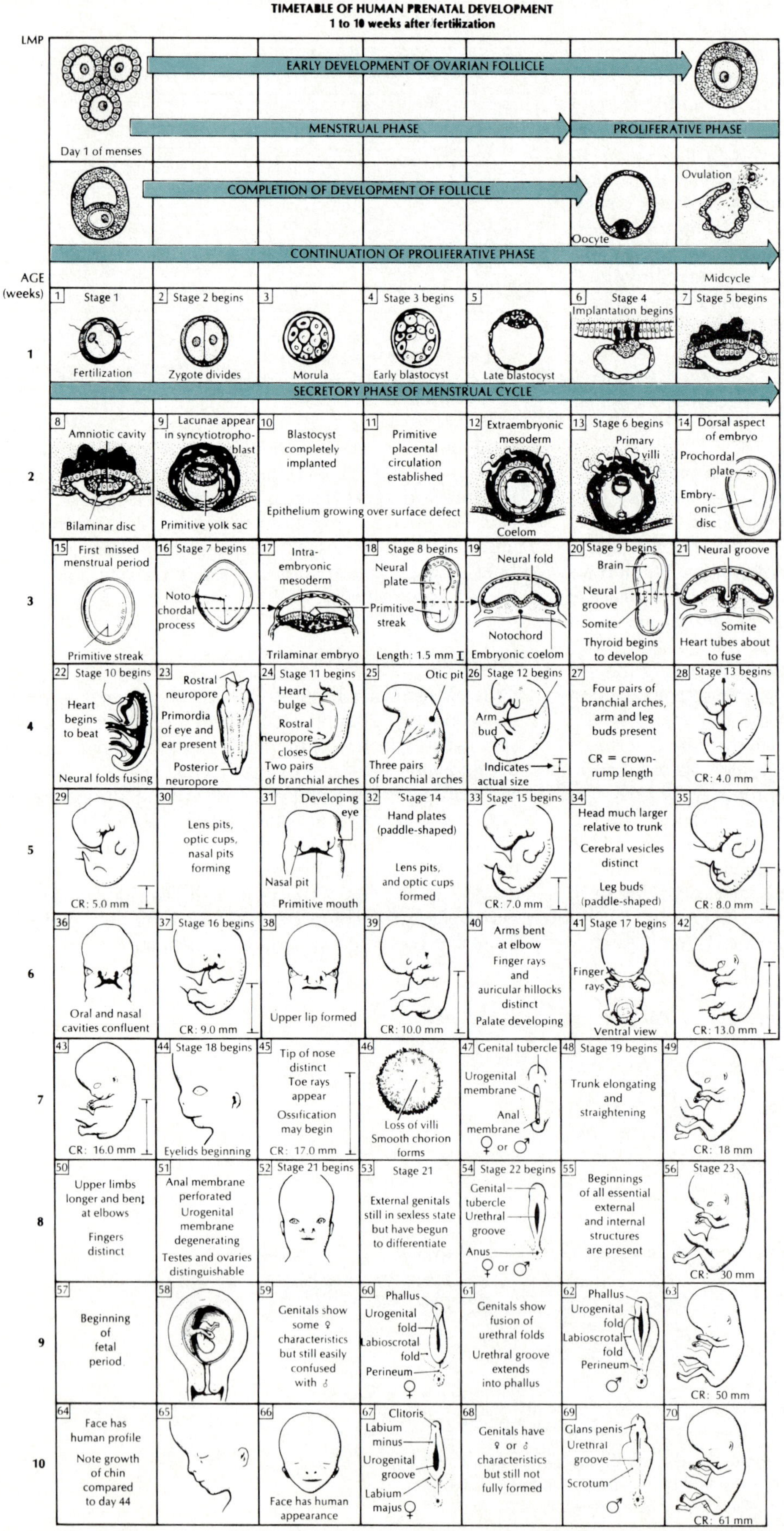

Fig. 9-13 Timetable of human prenatal development from LMP and weeks 1 to 10 following fertilization. Within large boxes are small boxes with numbers in upper left corner. These numbers refer to days since fertilization.
From Moore, KL: The developing human: clinically oriented embryology, ed 2, Philadelphia, 1977, WB Saunders Co.

Embryo. The organism is called an *embryo* during the period from the end of the ovum stage until it measures approximately 3 cm (2.5 in) from crown to rump, normally 54 to 56 days (10 weeks since LMP). This period is characterized by rapid cell division and is the most critical time in the development of an individual (Fig. 9-14). All the principal organ systems are being established and are highly vulnerable to environmental agents (e.g., **teratogens** such as viruses, drugs, radiation, or infection). There are at least two means by which malformations of embryos and fetuses can result from exposure to teratogenic agents. Such teratogens may cause cellular necrosis, or they may destroy cell function by biochemical paralysis. Developmental interference during this time can result in major congenital (existing before birth) abnormalities (Chapters 30, 40, and Appendix G). By the end of this period the beginnings of all the main systems have been established. The embryo attains characteristics that establish it as unquestionably human and is then referred to as a *fetus,* a Latin word meaning *offspring.*

Fetus. The embryo becomes a fetus at the end of the embryo stage and remains a fetus until the pregnancy is terminated (see Fig. 9-13, week 9, day 57). Changes occurring during the fetal period, although important, are not as dramatic as those in the preceding period, because the fetus is less vulnerable to the teratogenic effects of drugs, viruses, or radiation—*malformations.* However, these noxious agents may interrupt normal *functional development* of organs, especially the central nervous system (Fig. 9-14).

Viability

The capability of a fetus to survive outside the uterus at the earliest gestational age is called viability. Until recently it was believed that viability was reached when the fetus weighed more than 1000 g and had reached at least 28 weeks' gestational age. Improvement in maternal and neonatal care now suggests that a new standard of viability must be established (see Chapter 4). On the basis of the limits of available clinical technology, current published literature about fetal lung development, and the age at which the respiratory system is capable of supporting satisfactory gas exchange, fetal viability can be first expected at approximately 22 to 23 weeks' gestation. Since there is a problem with accuracy in estimating gestational age, it is difficult to establish definite criteria.

Survival outside the uterus depends on two factors: (1) the maturity of the fetal central nervous system (CNS) for directing rhythmic respirations and controlling body temperature and (2) the maturity of the lungs.

The Decidua

As part of the morphologic changes in the endometrium during the secretory phase (phase of the corpus luteum) of the menstrual cycle (see Fig. 9-13, week 1), the blood vessels enlarge and the entire lining becomes more succulent and richer in glycogen. After conception the vascularity of the uterine wall increases greatly under the influence of the ovarian hormones, principally progesterone.

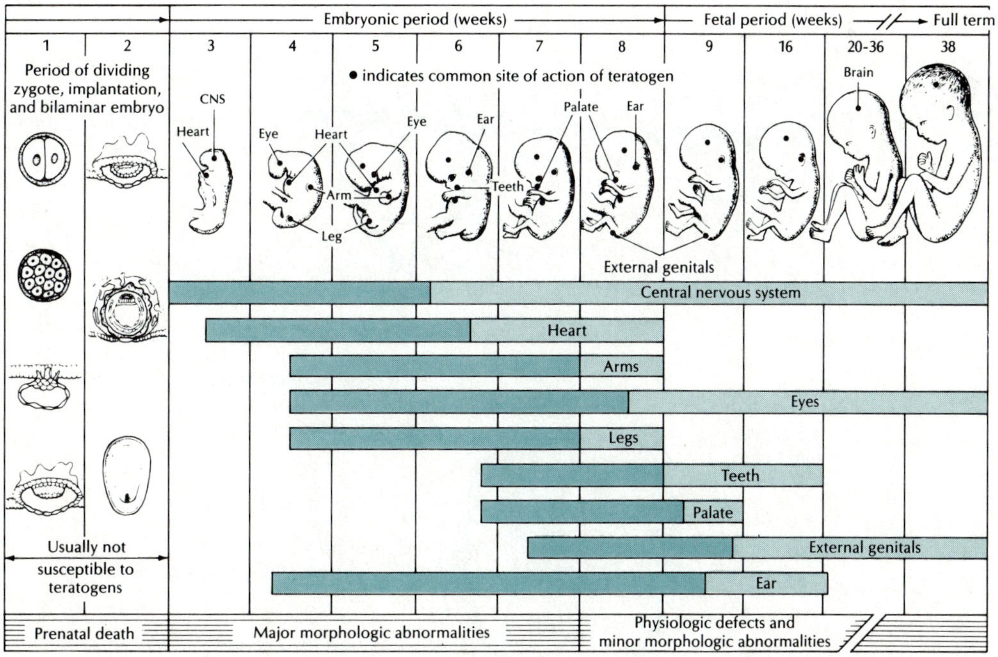

Fig. 9-14 Sensitive, or critical, periods in human development. Dark color denotes highly sensitive periods; light color indicates stages that are less sensitive to teratogens.

From Moore, KL: The developing human: clinically oriented embryology, ed 2, Philadelphia, 1977, WB Saunders Co.

After implantation the endometrium is called the *decidua,* which means "to cast off," or "to discard," since this is actually what happens after the infant is born: the prepared lining of the endometrium *is* cast off in a vaginal discharge called lochia (see Chapter 20).

This decidua is divided into three areas (Fig. 9-15):

1. *Decidua vera (parietalis)* is that part of the endometrium not directly associated with the development of the embryo.
2. *Decidua basalis* is the portion of the decidua vera where nidation takes place; that is, the area where chorionic villi (frondosum) invade the maternal blood vessels and develop into the placenta.
3. *Decidua capsularis* is the portion of the decidua vera that covers the blastocyst after nidation occurs, isolating it from the other portions of the uterus. It appears to fuse with the chorion, a fetal membrane, as pregnancy advances.

Implantation (Nidation)

The ovum is released from the ovary at ovulation and passes into the uterine tube where it is met and fertilized by a sperm. After conception the zygote, propelled by ciliary action and irregular peristaltic contractions, starts to move through the uterine tube into the uterine cavity (Fig. 9-16). During the 3- to 4-day period it takes to travel down the uterine tube, the zygote begins a process of rapid cell division called *mitosis,* or *cleavage.* The initial division of the zygote results in two *blastomeres* which subsequently divide into progressively smaller blastomeres. At the end of 3 to 4 days, the developing individual comprises about 16 blastomeres arranged in a ball-like structure called a *morula.* After the morula enters the uterus, a cavity forms within the dividing cells, changing the morula into a *blastocyst.* The blastocyst remains free in the uterus for 1 or 2 days, and then the exposed cells of the *trophoblast* (cellular wall of the blastocyst) implant, generally in the endometrium of the anterior or posterior fundal region.

Cells of the attaching portion of the trophoblast secrete proteolytic (causing breakdown of proteins) and cytolytic (causing breakdown of cells) enzymes to help them burrow their way into the compact layer of the endometrium. This burrowing into the endometrium is called *nidation,* or *implantation.* Slight bleeding, called **implantation bleeding,** occurs in some women. In almost all cases, trophoblastic burrowing stops before it reaches the myometrium. About 7 to 10 days elapse between fertilization and the completion of implantation (Fig. 9-13).

During the first few weeks after nidation, trophoblasts (primary villi) appear over the entire blastodermic vesicle. Trophoblasts are vascular processes that have the power of cytolysis and are able to tap maternal blood vessels as sources of nourishment and oxygen for the embryo. These villi are the first stage of the developing **chorionic villi** (fingerlike projections) that secrete the **human chorionic gonadotropic hormone** (hCG) and synthesize proteins and glucose for approximately 12 weeks. By 12 weeks, the fetal liver can supply its own glucose and insulin. The hCG stimulates continued secretion of progesterone and estrogen by

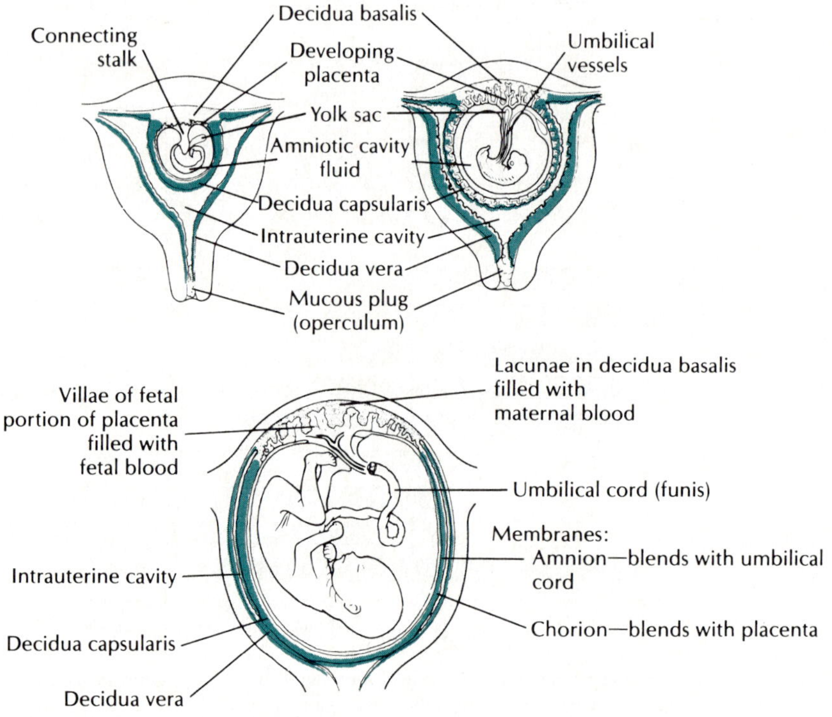

Fig. 9-15 Development of fetal membranes. Note gradual obliteration of intrauterine cavity as decidua capsularis and decidua vera meet. Also note thinning of uterine wall. Chorionic and amniotic membranes are in apposition to each other but may be peeled apart.

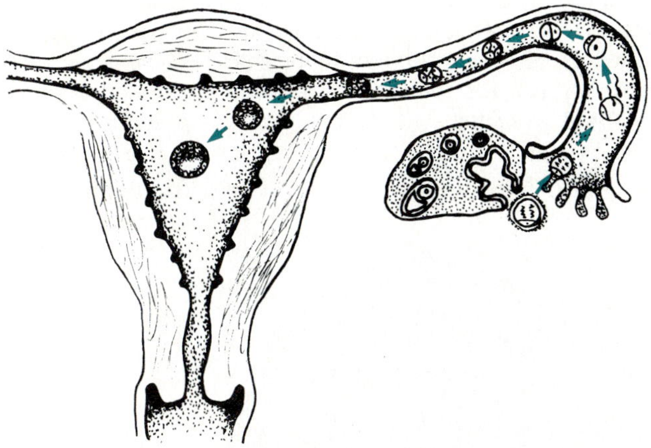

Fig. 9-16 Diagrammatic summary of the ovarian cycle, fertilization and development during the first week. See Fig. 9-13, day 14 since LMP and week 1.

the corpus luteum, thus preventing ovulation and menstruation during pregnancy.

Chorionic villi invasion of the endometrium by enzyme action occasionally opens a maternal vein and artery causing lacunae (small blood lakes) in the decidua basalis. This rich blood supply causes the adjacent villi to multiply rapidly. These villi become the *chorion frondosum,* or fetal portion, of the future placenta.

Placenta

Structure. The maturing placenta (Greek for "flat cake") develops into 15 or 20 subdivisions called *cotyledons.* Each of these is partially separated from other cotyledons by fenestrated septa (windowed partitions); thus in essence each cotyledon is a functioning unit.

Growth of the thickness of the placenta continues until 16 to 20 weeks' gestation. The placental circumference continues growing until later pregnancy. The fully developed placenta *(afterbirth)* is a reddish, discoid organ 15 to 20 cm (6 to 10 in) in diameter and 2.5 to 3 cm (about 1 in) thick (Fig. 9-17). The weight of a term placenta is 400 to 600 g (1 lb to 1 lb, 5 oz) or approximately one sixth the weight of the newborn. About four fifths of the placenta by weight is of fetal origin; the remainder is maternal.

The maternal surface of the placenta, the area originally adherent to the decidua basalis of the uterus, is rough and beefy red. The cotyledons stand out as segments with shallow clefts between. The fetal surface of the placenta is shiny and slightly grayish. The umbilical vessels that enter the cord can be seen as a branching system just beneath the membranes (Fig. 9-17). The fetal membranes cover the fetal surface of the placenta and extend from the placental margins to envelop the fetus and its amniotic fluid.

In multiple pregnancy, one or more placentas will be present. The number depends on the number of fertilized ova and the manner of ovum segmentation (see discussion of multiple pregnancy).

Functions. The placenta has many unique properties. Most of these properties—endocrine, metabolic, and immunologic—are derived from the trophoblasts. Understanding placental functions gives insight into prenatal life and is helpful in providing nursing care to the unborn and the newborn.

Placental function depends almost entirely on maternal circulation. Maternal circulation depends on the woman's blood pressure, condition of her blood vessels, maternal position, and uterine contractions. **Optimal circulation to the placenta and fetus is possible when the woman is lying on her left side** (see Fig. 18-9).

Endocrine Function. During pregnancy a new group of *protein* hormones of placental origin is seen. One of these, hCG, is the basis for pregnancy tests. At one time it was thought that the placenta was one of the four steroid-producing glands. It may be that the placenta relies for much of the synthesis of steroid hormones on precursors from the mother and fetus (Danforth and Scott, 1986). *Steroid* hormones include estrogens and progesterone. Among the actions of placental hormones are the maintenance of pregnancy and the initiation of labor.

Metabolic, Respiratory, and Renal Function. The intervillous space serves as the depot from which materials are transferred actively or passively through the chorionic epithelium to the fetal vessels. In this space substances from the fetus enter the maternal circulation. Because this process of transfer supplies the fetus with oxygen, as well as nutrients, and provides for elimination of metabolic waste products, the chorionic villi and the intervillous space function as a lung, gastrointestinal tract, and kidney for the fetus.

Immunologic Function. "The placenta and fetus appear to defy the laws of transplantation immunology" (Pritchard et al., 1985). "The placenta corresponds to a natural homograft in that it is a transplant of living tissue within the same species, yet it does not normally evoke the usual immune response reaction to homografts, resulting in destruction and rejection of the graft" (Willson et al., 1983). This quality of the placenta is of major interest. If the "secret" of the placenta can be unlocked, the problem of rejection in organ transplants and other immune phenomena may be eliminated.

Protective Function. Only two layers of cells separate maternal and fetal circulation for the first 12 weeks of gestation. During the second and third trimesters, only one cell layer separates the two blood streams. This so-called *placental barrier* is a partial (semipermeable) barrier; it provides only limited protection to the fetus. Throughout pregnancy it either actively or passively permits, facilitates, and adjusts the amount and rate of transfer of a wide range of substances to the fetus.

Transfer

General Concepts. The placenta is a complex organ of transfer. Its major function is to transfer oxygen and a great variety of nutrients from the mother to the fetus. Conversely, it conveys carbon dioxide and other metabolic wastes from the fetus to the mother. The placenta, and to a limited extent the attached membranes, supply all material for fetal growth and energy production while removing all products of fetal catabolism.

There is no continuous direct communication between the fetal blood in the vessels of the chorionic villi and the maternal blood in the intervillous space. Although maternal and fetal circulations are independent, development of occasional breaks in the chorionic villi permits the escape of varying numbers of fetal erythrocytes into the maternal circulation. This *leakage* is the clinically significant mechanism by which some Rh-negative women become sensitized by the erythrocytes of their Rh-positive fetus (see Chapter 40). The transfer of substances from mother to fetus and from fetus to mother depends primarily on the

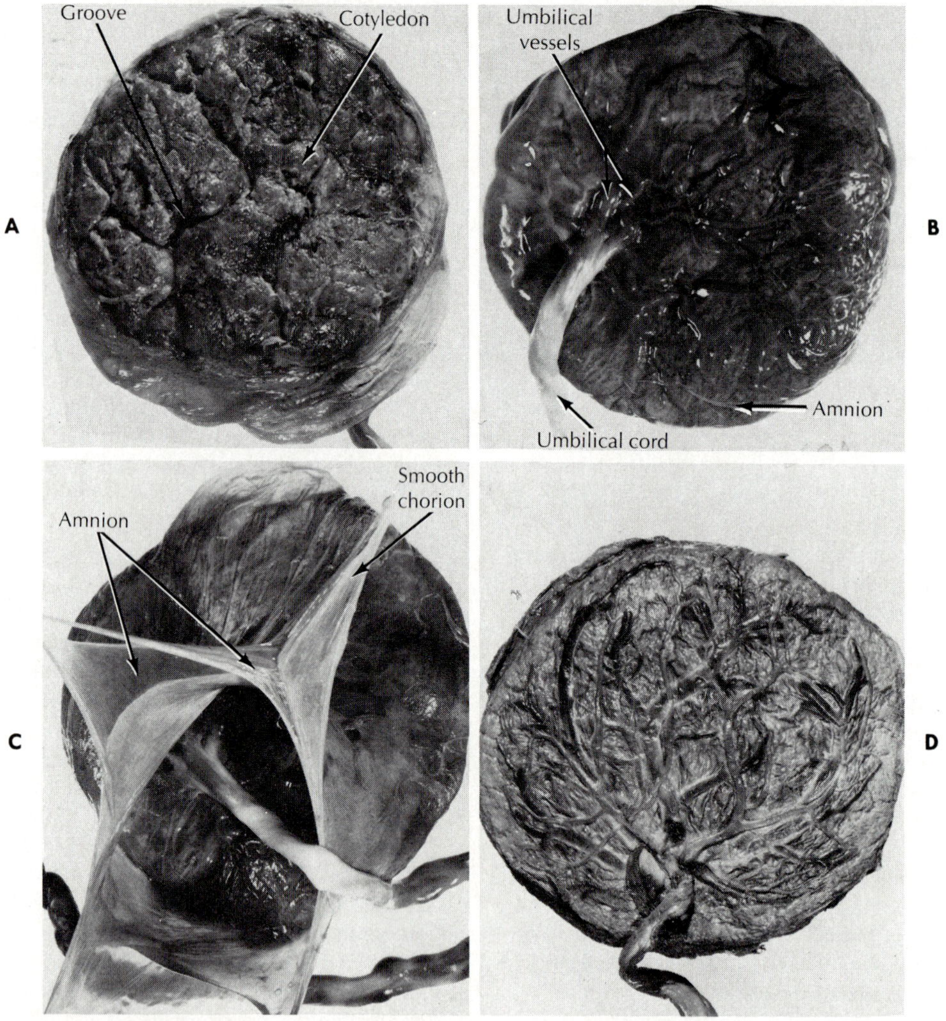

Fig. 9-17 Photographs of full-term placentas. **A,** Maternal (or uterine) surface, showing cotyledons and grooves. **B,** Fetal (or amniotic) surface, showing blood vessels running under amnion and converging to form umbilical vessels at attachment of umbilical cord. **C,** Amnion and smooth chorion are arranged to show that they are (1) fused and (2) continuous with margins of placenta. **D,** Placenta with a marginal attachment of the cord, often called a battledore placenta because of its resemblance to bat used in medieval game of battledore and shuttlecock.

From Moore, KL: The developing human: clinically oriented embryology, ed 2, Philadelphia, 1977, WB Saunders Co.

mechanisms that permit the transport of such substances through the intact chorionic villus.

At least nine variables determine the effectiveness of the human placenta as an organ of transfer (Pritchard et al., 1985):

1. The concentration in the maternal plasma of the substance under consideration and in some instances the extent to which it is bound to another compound
2. The rate of maternal blood flow through the intervillous space
3. The area available for exchange across the villous epithelium
4. In case the substance is transferred by **diffusion** the physical properties of the tissue barrier, interposed between blood in the intervillous space and blood in the fetal capillaries
5. For any substance actively transported, the capacity of the biochemical machinery of the placenta for effecting **active transfer**
6. The amount of the substance metabolized by the placenta during transfer
7. The area for exchange across the fetal capillaries in the placenta
8. The concentration in the fetal blood of the substance, exclusive of any that is bound
9. The rate of fetal blood flow through the villous capillaries

Unfortunately, in human pregnancy many of these processes cannot be measured accurately in either the mother or the fetus.

Transfer by Diffusion. Most substances with a molecular weight less than 500 can diffuse readily through the placental tissue. Molecular weight clearly has a bearing on the rate of transfer by diffusion; generally the smaller the molecule, the more rapid is the rate. Diffusion, however, is not the only mechanism of transfer of compounds with a low molecular weight. The placenta actually facilitates the transfer of a variety of such compounds, especially those that are in low concentration in maternal plasma but that are essential for the rapid growth of the fetus.

Simple diffusion appears to be the mechanism involved in the transfer of oxygen, carbon dioxide, water and most but not all electrolytes. Anesthetic gases are highly lipid soluble and pass through the placenta within minutes of administration by simple diffusion, according to the concentration gradient.

Insulin, steroid hormones from the adrenal glands, and hormones from the thyroid may cross the placenta but do so at slow rates. Substances of high molecular weight do not usually traverse the placenta, but there are pronounced exceptions, such as immune γ-globulin G (IgG) with a molecular weight of about 160,000. IgG crosses the placenta with considerable efficiency. All four major subclasses of IgG appear to cross the placenta from mother to fetus but whether by the same or different transport systems is not clear. Near term, the immunoglobulin IgG is present in approximately the same concentrations in cord and maternal sera. IgA and IgM of maternal origin are effectively excluded from the fetus.

Selective Transfer. Although diffusion is an important method of placental transfer, the chorionic villus exhibits enormous selectivity in transfer, maintaining different concentrations of a variety of metabolites on the two sides of the villus.

Selectivity may occur by *active transport* and *pinocytosis.* Active transport is carrier-mediated or "facilitated," often by enzyme action. It results in the transfer of glucose, amino acids, calcium, iron, and other substances of higher molecular weight. Pinocytosis is a mechanism by which minute particles, including free fatty acids, may be engulfed and carried across the cell. For pinocytosis, a virtually continuous system of vesicles and vacuoles may be found that extend from the placenta's syncytial surface to the capillary endothelium.

The concentrations of a number of substances that are not synthesized by the fetus are several times higher in fetal than in maternal blood. *Ascorbic acid* is one example of this phenomenon. This crystalline substance of relatively low molecular weight chemically resembles the pentose and hexose sugars and might be expected to traverse the placenta by simple diffusion. The concentration of ascorbic acid, however, is two to four times higher in fetal plasma than in maternal plasma.

The unidirectional transfer of *iron* across the placenta provides another example of the unique capabilities of the human placenta for transport. Iron is transported actively from maternal to fetal plasma, and in the human fetus the amount transferred appears to be independent of maternal iron status (Pritchard et al., 1985). The human placenta actively concentrates *iodide* on the fetal side.

The placenta is known to concentrate a large number of *amino acids* intracellularly from maternal plasma. The actual uptake of amino acids by the placenta occurs by diffusion and active transport. Fetal uptake of amino acids most likely depends on this concentrating capacity of the placenta.

Infections. Because of their small size, some viruses traverse the placenta with ease; the larger bacteria rarely involve the fetus except when inflammation of the placenta develops.

Many viruses, including those responsible for rubella, chickenpox, measles, mumps, poliomyelitis, cytomegalic inclusion disease, coxsackie virus disease, and western equine encephalitis, may cross the placenta and infect the fetus. *Treponema pallidum, Toxoplasma* and *Plasmodium* species, and *Mycobacterium tuberculosis* may similarly produce intrauterine infection. With protozoal and bacterial, but not necessarily viral, infections, there is almost always histologic evidence of involvement of the placenta (Pritchard et al., 1985).

Placentitis is generally the result of an intranatal infection from an ascending invasion of bacteria from vagina and cervix associated with ruptured membranes and prolonged labor but may occur even if membranes are intact. Maternal, fetal, and neonatal infections are discussed in Chapters 30 and 39.

Malignancies. Rarely, malignancies in the pregnant woman can be transferred to the placenta and to the fetus.

Approximately 50 percent of these are malignant melanomas or hematopoietic in origin (Chapter 44).

Drugs. Many drugs cross the placenta readily (e.g., caffeine, alcohol, nicotine, carbon monoxide, pesticides, the over 1000 other toxic substances and gases* inhaled from cigarette smoke, antibiotics, antihistamines, sedatives, analgesics, narcotics, and anesthetics). Most drugs promptly cross the placenta, and many are deleterious to the human fetus.

Examples of these drugs are given in Appendix G. Because medications, as well as vaccines and excessive amounts of certain vitamins, may contain elements harmful to the fetus, all but essential medications should be avoided, particularly during the first trimester.

Oxygen. For a discussion of oxygen transfer, see the discussion of fetal hemoglobin, p. 186.

Fetal Membranes

Two closely applied by separate membranes line the uterine cavity and surround the developing embryo-fetus (Fig. 9-15). Both membranes, the *amnion* (inner membrane) and the *chorion* (outer membrane), arise from the zygote. As the chorion develops, it blends with the fetal portion of the placenta, the amnion blends with the fetal umbilical cord, or *funis.* These deceptively strong, translucent membranes contain not only the fetus but also the amniotic fluid, and they are continuous with the margins of the placenta.

Chorion. The outer membrane, the **chorion**, forms a large portion of the connective tissue thickness of the placenta on its fetal side. It is the structure in and through which the major branching umbilical vessels travel on the surface of the placenta. On its surface near the insertion of the umbilical cord are the remnants of the yolk sac (see discussion below). Ordinarily the chorion does not have a fetal blood supply except in the case of velamentous insertion of the cord. Its vascular support is primarily provided by blood vessels arising from the decidua. On its fetal surface it is juxtaposed to the outer layer of amnion.

Amnion. The inner avascular membrane, the **amnion**, is bathed by amniotic fluid on one side and on the other side is contiguous with the chorion laeve. The chorion laeve, also a thin membrane of fetal origin, is contiguous with the maternal decidua vera (parietalis). Direct communication between the fetus and avascular amnion is established by way of the amniotic fluid. There is some evidence to support the formation of large quantities of prostaglandins by amnion cells. Fetal urine appears to stimulate PGE_2 production by amnion cells. Thus the fetal kidney and fetal urine appear to be important components of a fetal signal in the initiation and maintenance of labor in women (Pritchard et al., 1985).

Amniochorion. In the human, the chorion laeve and amnion form an avascular **amniochorion** that serves important functions that include solute and fluid transport, as well as prostaglandin formation at the time of parturition. Other functions of the amniochorion seem to be to retain and assist in the formation of amniotic fluid.

*Hydrogen cyanide is present in cigarette smoke. This is the same gas used to execute prisoners in gas chambers.

Amniotic Fluid

Origin, Composition, and Volume. During pregnancy the amniotic fluid volume increases at an average rate of 25 ml per week during the first trimester, and 50 ml per week during the second trimester. The full-term fetus is immersed in about 1000 ml (range of 800 to 1200 ml) of clear, slightly yellowish liquid that has a faint characteristic (not foul) odor. The specific gravity of amniotic fluid is 1.007 to 1.025, and the pH is neutral to slightly alkaline (7.0 to 7.25). It contains albumin, urea, uric acid, creatinine, lecithin, sphingomyelin, bilirubin, fat, fructose, inorganic salts, epithelial cells, a few leukocytes, various enzymes, and lanugo hairs. Amniotic fluid, replaced every 3 hours, is thought to have multiple origins and a composition that changes during pregnancy. Early in pregnancy it probably originates from maternal serum, but as pregnancy proceeds, a greater proportion of it is derived from fetal urine.

Functions. Amniotic fluid accomplishes numerous functions for the fetus, including the following:

1. Protects the fetus from direct trauma by distributing and equalizing any impact the mother may receive
2. Separates the fetus from the fetal membranes
3. Allows freedom of fetal movement and permits musculoskeletal development
4. Facilitates symmetric growth and development of the fetus
5. Protects the fetus from the loss of heat and maintains a relatively constant fetal body temperature
6. Serves as a source of oral fluid for the fetus
7. Acts as an excretion-collection repository for substances from the fetal urinary, respiratory, and alimentary tracts

Diagnostic Value. There is still much to be learned about amniotic fluid. However, study of its components has provided a great deal of knowledge about the sex, state of health, and maturity of the fetus. Amniocentesis (Chapter 27) has made it possible to detect diseases and abnormalities that may suggest the options of therapeutic abortion or intrauterine treatment.

There is great variation within the normal volume; however, more than 2 L (hydramnios) or less than 300 ml (oligohydramnios) is usually associated with fetal disease or abnormality (see Chapter 40).

Umbilical Cord

The umbilical cord (funis) is the lifeline that links the embryo and the placenta. It extends from the umbilicus to the fetal portion of the placenta and is attached either centrally or eccentrically. At term this light gray, smooth, vascular attachment is 50 to 55 cm long, slightly longer than the fetus, and is approximately 2 cm in diameter.

The surface of the cord is composed of thin squamous epithelium and is an extension of the skin of the fetus; however, *it contains no pain receptors.* The cord normally contains two umbilical arteries and one umbilical vein. The vein carries oxygenated blood to the fetus, and the arteries return deoxygenated blood to the placenta. Commonly these vessels are longer than the cord and consequently become coiled on themselves, giving the cord a lumpy appearance. They are supported by a loose connective tissue containing a cushioning mucoid material called **Wharton's jelly.** This jelly prevents kinking of the cord in utero and interference with circulation to the fetus.

Approximately 400 ml of blood flows through the cord every minute. The pressure exerted by this rapid flow makes the cord relatively stiff and not flexible as it is after birth. If fetal movements cause the cord to loop, its stiffness prevents the loops from kinking and from knotting tightly. The higher water content of Wharton's jelly causes the cord to shrink quickly after birth. In addition, several naturally occurring prostaglandins in Wharton's jelly have a vasoconstrictive effect that inhibits bleeding from the umbilical cord stump when it is cut after birth.

The Yolk Sac

By 9 weeks, the yolk sac has shrunk to a pear-shaped remnant, about 5 mm in diameter, which is connected to the midgut by the narrow yolk stalk (Fig. 9-15). The human yolk sac is nonfunctional as far as yolk storage is concerned. However, its development is essential for several reasons (Moore, 1977a): (1) It appears to have a role in the transfer of nutrients to the embryo during the second and third weeks while the uteroplacental circulation is being established. (2) Blood develops on the walls of the yolk sac beginning in the third week and continues to form here until hematopoietic activity begins in the liver during the sixth week. (3) During the fourth week the dorsal part of the yolk sac is incorporated into the embryo as the primitive gut; this gives rise to the epithelium of the trachea, bronchi and lungs, and of the digestive tract. (4) Primordial germ cells appear in the wall of the yolk sac early in the third week and subsequently migrate to the developing sex glands or gonads, where they become the primitive germ cells (spermatogonia or oogonia). Although the yolk sac and allantois (not discussed here) are vestigial structures, their formation is essential for normal embryonic development. Both are important early sites of blood formation, and part of the yolk sac is incorporated into the embryo as the primitive gut.

The yolk sac shrinks as pregnancy advances and eventually becomes very small. The yolk stalk usually detaches from the gut by the end of the fifth week. In about 2% of adults, the intraabdominal part of the yolk stalk persists as a diverticulum of the ileum known as *Meckel's diverticulum* (Moore, 1977a).

EMBRYONIC DEVELOPMENT AND FETAL MATURATION

Fetal maturation takes place in an orderly and predictable pattern (Fig. 9-13 and Table 9-2). There is steady increase in overall growth, and organ systems develop from the three primary germ layers: the ectoderm (ecto = outside), the entoderm (ento = inner), and the mesoderm (meso = middle). The *ectodermal* germ layer gives rise to such tissues as the skin and nails, the nervous system, and tooth enamel. The *entodermal* germ layer develops into such tissues as epithelial inner linings of the gastrointestinal and respiratory tracts, endocrine glands, and auditory canal. The *mesodermal* germ layer forms tissues such as the connective tissue, teeth (except for the enamel), muscles and blood and vascular systems.

Cardiovascular System

The first system to function in the developing human is the cardiovascular system. Blood vessel formation begins early in the third week; it follows the first missed menstrual period of the mother. The cardiovascular system must form early to bring nourishment and oxygen from the mother to the embryo. The cardiovascular system is functional (heart is beating) before the mother's menstrual period is 1 week late. At this time (3 weeks since conception), circulation of blood begins the fetomaternal exchange of oxygen, nutrients, and waste products. This exchange is necessary because the fetal lungs and digestive system are not functional until after birth.

Fetal Circulation. The single umbilical vein carries oxygen-enriched blood from the placenta (Fig. 21-2). Upon entering the liver, the vein gives off a number of branches and then enters the ductus venosus. About half the oxygenated blood bypasses the liver through the ductus venosus into the inferior vena cava. There it mixes with deoxygenated blood from the fetal lower extremities, abdomen, and pelvis. Most of this blood then enters the right atrium and is pumped through the foramen ovale into the left atrium, where it mixes with a small amount of deoxygenated blood returning from the lungs through the pulmonary veins. The blood then flows into the left ventricle and exits through the ascending aorta. *As a result, the vessels leading to the heart, head, neck, and upper limbs receive well-oxygenated blood.* This circulatory pattern is the reason for the embryo's cephalocaudal (head-to-tail) development, which persists in subsequent motor development, making it possible for the infant to manipulate his hands long before being able to walk.

A small quantity of oxygenated blood from the inferior vena cava remains in the right atrium and mixes with deoxygenated blood from the superior vena cava and coronary sinus. It then flows into the right ventricle and pulmonary artery, passing through the ductus arteriosus into the aorta; a small amount is diverted to the nonfunctional lungs.

The paired umbilical arteries return most of the mixed blood from the descending aorta to the placenta. There the fetal blood simultaneously gives up carbon dioxide and waste materials and takes up oxygen and nutrients from the maternal blood. The remaining blood circulates through the lower part of the fetal body and ultimately enters the inferior vena cava.

The pattern of blood flow* is as follows (Fig. 21-2):

*The four structures that differentiate fetal circulation from extrauterine circulation are shown in bold type. The foramen ovale and ductus arteriosus allow fetal blood to bypass the fetal lungs.

Table 9-2 *Milestones in Human Development Before Birth Since LMP*

4 Weeks	8 Weeks	12 Weeks	16 Weeks
External Appearance			
Body flexed, C-shaped; arm and leg buds present; head at right angles to body	Body fairly well formed; nose flat, eyes far apart; digits well formed; head elevating; tail almost disappeared; eyes, ears, nose, and mouth recognizable	Nails appearing; resembles a human; head erect but disproportionately large; skin pink, delicate	Head still dominant; face looks human; eyes, ears, and nose approach typical appearance on gross examination; arm-leg ratio proportionate; scalp hair appears
Crown-To-Rump Measurement (cm), Weight (g)			
0.4-0.5, 0.4	2.5-3, 2	6-9, 19	11.5-13.5, 100
Musculoskeletal System			
All somites present	First indication of ossification—occiput, mandible, and humerus; fetus capable of some movement, definitive muscles of trunk, limbs, and head well represented	Some bones well outlined, ossification spreading; upper cervical to lower sacral arches and bodies ossify; smooth muscle layers indicated in hollow viscera	Most bones distinctly indicated throughout body; joint cavities appear; muscular movements can be detected
Circulatory System			
Heart develops, double chambers visible, begins to beat; aortic arches and major veins completed	Main blood vessels assume final plan; enucleated red cells predominate in blood	Blood forming in marrow	Heart muscle well developed; blood formation active in spleen
Gastrointestinal System			
Stomach at midline and fusiform; conspicuous liver; esophagus short; intestine a short tube	Intestinal villi developing; small intestines coil within umbilical cord; palatal folds present; liver very large	Bile secreted; palatal fusion complete; intestines have withdrawn from cord and assume characteristic positions	Meconium in bowel; some enzyme secretion; anus open
Respiratory System			
Primary lung buds appear	Pleural and pericardial cavities forming; branching bronchioles; nostrils closed by epithelial plugs	Lungs acquire definite shape; vocal cords appear	Elastic fibers appear in lungs; terminal and respiratory bronchioles appear
Renal System			
Rudimentary ureteral buds appear	Earliest secretory tubules differentiating; bladder-urethra separates from rectum	Kidney able to secrete urine; bladder expands as a sac	Kidney in position; attains typical shape and plan
Nervous System			
Well-marked midbrain flexure; no hindbrain or cervical flexures; neural groove closed	Cerebral cortex begins to acquire typical cells; differentiation of cerebral cortex, meninges, ventricular foramens, cerebrospinal fluid circulation; spinal cord extends entire length of spine	Brain structural configuration roughly complete; cord shows cervical and lumbar enlargements; fourth ventricle foramens developed; sucking present	Cerebral lobes delineated; cerebellum assumes some prominence
Sensory Organs			
Eye and ear appearing as optic vessel and otocyst	Primordial choroid plexuses develop; ventricles large relative to cortex; development progressing; eyes converging rapidly; internal ear developing	Earliest taste buds indicated; characteristic organization of eye attained	General sense organs differentiated
Genital System			
Genital ridge appears (fifth week)	Testes and ovaries distinguishable; external genitals sexless but begin to differentiate	Sex recognizable; internal and external sex organs specific	Testes in position for descent into scrotum; vagina open

Modified from Whaley, LF, and Wong, DL: Nursing care of infants and children, ed 3, St Louis, 1987, The CV Mosby Co.

20 Weeks	24 Weeks	28 Weeks	32 Weeks	36 Weeks	40 Weeks
Vernix caseosa appears; lanugo appears; legs lengthen considerably; sebaceous glands appear	Body lean but fairly well proportioned; skin red and wrinkled; vernix caseosa present; sweat glands forming	Lean body, less wrinkled and red; nails appear	Subcutaneous fat beginning to collect; more rounded appearance; skin pink and smooth; has assumed delivery position	Skin pink, body rounded; general lanugo disappearing; body usually plump	Skin smooth and pink, copious vernix caseosa; moderate to profuse hair; lanugo on shoulders and upper body only; nasal and alar cartilage apparent
16-18.5, 300	23, 600	27, 1100	31, 1800-2100	35, 2200-2900	40, 3200+
Sternum ossifies; fetal movements strong enough for mother to feel		Astragalus (talus, ankle bone) ossifies; weak, fleeting movements minimum tone	Middle fourth phalanxes ossify; permanent teeth primordia seen; can turn head to side	Distal femoral ossification centers present; sustained, definite movements, fair tone; can turn and elevate head	Active, sustained movement; good tone; may lift head
	Blood formation increases in bone marrow and decreases in liver				
Enamel and dentine depositing; ascending colon recognizable					
Nostrils reopen; primitive respiratory-like movements begin	Alveolar ducts and sacs present; lecithin begins to appear in amniotic fluid (weeks 26-27)	Lecithin forming on alveolar surfaces	L/S ratio = 1.2:1	L/S ratio ≥ 2:1	Pulmonary branching only two thirds complete
				Formation of new nephrons ceases	
Brain grossly formed; cord myelination begins; spinal cord ends at level S-1	Cerebral cortex layered typically; neuronal proliferation in cerebral cortex ends	Appearance of cerebral fissures, convolutions fast appearing; indefinite sleep-wake cycle; cry weak or absent; weak suck reflex		End of spinal cord at level (L-3); definite sleep-wake cycle	Myelination of brain begins; patterned sleep-wake cycle with alert periods; cries when hungry or uncomfortable; strong suck reflex
Nose and ears ossify	Can hear	Eyelids reopen; retinal layers completed, light receptive; pupils capable of reacting to light	Sense of taste present; aware of sounds outside mother's body		
	Testes at inguinal ring in descent to scrotum		Testes descending to scrotum		Testes in scrotum; labia majora well developed

1. Placenta
   ↓
   Umbilical vein ↗ Liver, sinusoids, hepatic veins ↘ / ↘ Ductus venosus → Inferior vena cava
2. Inferior vena cava→Right atrium→**Foramen ovale**→Left atrium→Left ventricle→Aorta
3. Inferior vena cava→Right atrium→Right ventricle→Pulmonary artery→Small amount to nonfunctional lungs but most of it through **Ductus arteriosus**→Aorta→Hypogastric arteries→**Umbilical arteries**→Placenta

FHR and Fetal Hemoglobin. Following are a number of compensatory circulatory factors that benefit the fetus (these values are those of the fetus near term):

1. The fetal heart rate (FHR) is 120 to 160 beats/min, and the fetal cardiac output is approximately 350 to 500 ml/kg/min, or about that of the adult at rest.
2. The hemoglobin of the fetus is primarily fetal hemoglobin (HgF), a type synthesized before birth. HgF is capable of maintaining a high oxygen saturation at a lower pressure (P_{O_2}). It has been estimated that HgF can carry as much as 20% to 30% more oxygen than can maternal hemoglobin.
3. The hemoglobin concentration of the fetus is about 50% higher than that of the mother.

As a result of these compensatory circulatory factors, greater amounts of oxygen can be transported to the fetal tissues.

Hematopoietic System

Hematopoiesis (formation and development of blood cells) occurs in the yolk sac between weeks 3 and 6. Hematopoietic activity begins in the liver about the sixth week of gestation, when vascular channels have been formed. Later, blood formation occurs in the spleen, bone marrow, and lymph nodes.

Platelets are present in the circulation by the eleventh week of gestation. The isoagglutinogens (e.g., the Rh factor) that determine blood grouping are present in the red blood cells soon after the sixth week. Because of the early appearance of red blood cells, the Rh-negative woman needs to be protected against isoimmunization after each pregnancy that lasts longer than 6 weeks after fertilization, as well as after the birth of each child who is Rh positive (for extensive discussion, see Chapters 6 and 40 and Table 6-8).

Respiratory System

As previously mentioned the fetal lungs do not function until after delivery. Simple diffusion (passing from higher to lower concentration across a semipermeable membrane) across the placenta explains the exchange of oxygen and carbon dioxide in the fetus (see p. 181).

Developmental Phases. Development of human lungs occurs in four overlapping phases (from conception):

1. *Pseudoglandular period* (5 to 17 weeks' gestation): formation of bronchi and terminal bronchi
2. *Canalicular period* (13 to 25 weeks' gestation): enlargement of lumens of bronchi and terminal bronchioles, development of respiratory bronchioles and alveolar ducts, increased vascularity of lung tissue
3. *Terminal sac period* (24 weeks gestation to birth): growth of primitive alveoli (terminal air sacs) from alveolar ducts; fetuses younger than 24 weeks are not likely to survive if born before the terminal sac period begins
4. *Alveolar period* (late fetal period to approximately 8 years of age): formation of characteristic pulmonary alveoli as the lining of the terminal air sacs thins, with the number of alveoli increasing 6 to 8 times between birth and age 8 years.

Pulmonary Surfactants. During the terminal sac period *pulmonary surfactants* are produced in increasing amounts by the alveolar cells. Surfactants (surface factors or wetting agents), substances that minimize surface tension, designate a group of surface-active phospholipids. Of this group, *lecithin* (phosphatidylcholine) may be the crucial antiatelectasis factor responsible for alveolar stability. This biochemical compound is present on the surface of the alveolar cells, creating the minimum surface tension necessary to keep these spaces open on expiration following birth. In extrauterine life, lungs must remain partially expanded at all times.

The effect of decreased surface tension, caused by the presence of lecithin in the lining layer of alveoli, can be compared to powdering rubber gloves so that they do not stick together and to the Teflon coating on cooking utensils. The active ingredient in sprays used to keep foods from sticking to frying pans is lecithin. If insufficient surfactants are present, the lungs cannot be properly inflated, and respiratory distress syndrome (RDS) may develop.*

Pulmonary surfactants migrate from the lung fluid and mix with amniotic fluid in the upper respiratory tract and then flow into the amniotic fluid. The presence of surfactants in the amniotic fluid is used as a biochemical marker for determining the degree of fetal lung maturity. Lung maturity is the capacity of lungs to accommodate to normal ventilation after birth. Lecithin builds up in the amniotic fluid from about the twenty-fourth week, while sphingomyelin, another pulmonary phospholipid, remains unchanged. Hence, by determining the amount of lecithin present in relation to sphingomyelin, or the **lecithin-sphingomyelin (L/S) ratio**, an appraisal of fetal lung maturity is possible (Table 9-3).

No consistent relationship exists between fetal weight, age, and pulmonary maturity. Up to 10% of mature fetuses have been reported as having low L/S ratios, whereas normal ratios have been reported in premature infants (Korones, 1986).

Following is a list of maternal diseases that have been shown to alter the normal developmental schedule of pulmonary maturity; that is, the attainment of an L/S ratio of 2 or more was either accelerated (pulmonary maturity before 35 weeks) or delayed (pulmonary maturity after 35 weeks). Maternal conditions associated with accelerated development of pulmonary maturity are generally those that cause diminished maternal blood flow to the placenta and therefore an insufficiency or impairment, to varying extent, of

*Some diseases in adults result in decreased lecithin production and the development of adult respiratory distress syndrome (ARDS).

Table 9-3 *Secretion of Pulmonary Surfactant since LMP*

Gestation Age (weeks)	L/S Ratio*	Lung Maturity
26-27	Secretion into alveolar space begins	Viability attained
30-32	1.2 to 1	
35	2 to 1	Maturity attained

*Lecithin-sphingomyelin ratio.

oxygen transport to the fetus (Korones, 1986). The resultant fetal distress apparently increases the blood level of corticosteroid, which triggers elaboration of surfactant in alveolar cells.

The following disorders are associated with alteration from normal time of appearance of mature L/S ratio*:

Accelerated maturity can be expected in the presence of the following:

1. Maternal conditions
   a. Hypertension, regardless of origin (preeclampsia, other hypertensive states)
   b. Sickle cell disease
   c. Narcotic addiction
   d. Diabetes mellitus with vascular involvement
   e. Chronic retroplacental hemorrhage (e.g., partial premature separation of placenta [abruptio placentae])
   f. Hyperthyroidism
   g. Corticosteroids,† aminophylline
   h. Maternal infections (see Chapter 30)
2. Fetal conditions such as prolonged rupture of fetal membranes (48 to 72 or more hours before delivery), intrauterine infection, or both

Decelerated maturity can be anticipated in the presence of the following:

1. Maternal conditions
   a. Diabetes mellitus (e.g., gestational diabetes) (Chapter 32)
   b. Chronic glomerulonephritis
2. Fetal conditions
   a. Rh disease, particularly with hydrops fetalis (Chapter 40)
   b. Smaller of identical twins (nonparasitic) (Chapter 37)

Numerous other variables may affect the outcome of predictions of pulmonary maturity based on the L/S ratio. Some have already been demonstrated. Extensive investigation will no doubt uncover others. For example, the presence of maternal blood in amniotic fluid tends to lower the L/S ratio. Thus a mature ratio in bloody fluid is a valid result; an immature ratio may be incorrect. The presence of meconium in amniotic fluid affects results in an unpredictable way; it may either raise or lower the L/S ratio from its true value by a mechanism that is not understood. In some instances a ratio of 2 or more may be associated with postnatal RDS caused by events that transpire after collection of the sample (Chapter 40). As data accumulate, new insights will evolve regarding accuracy and error in the predictive value of the L/S ratio (Korones, 1986).

Maternal Oxygenation. A reduction in the rate and depth of maternal respiration may be reflected in fetal oxygenation. Excessive amounts of barbiturate, narcotic analgesia, or maternal hypoxia during anesthesia may reduce the fetal Po_2. Moreover, heavy maternal sedation by those drugs that readily cross the placenta may depress the fetal CNS respiratory center to further jeopardize the baby at birth. Breathing of pure oxygen (10 to 12 L/min) by the mother before delivery and again before cessation of pulsation in the cord after delivery may aid the infant.

Respiratory Movement. *Periodic fetal hiccup* can be seen and palpated, and rhythmic fetal respiratory movements can be demonstrated by ultrasonography in advanced pregnancy. Fetal cellular wastes (squamae) and lanugo fragments are commonly found in the fetal respiratory passages. Hence respirations at birth appear to be an extension of intrauterine respiratory movement.

Renal System

The placenta is the major fetal excretory organ and effectively eliminates waste products from fetal blood. The placenta, in collaboration with maternal lungs and kidneys, maintains fetal water, electrolyte, and acid-base balance. Kidneys are *not* necessary for fetal growth and development but are important in the control of the composition and volume of amniotic fluid. An infant may be born without kidneys. However, renal excretory and regulatory functions must begin immediately after delivery to maintain life and health.

In preparation for extrauterine existence the fetal kidneys develop rapidly. They appear in the fifth week and begin to function during the eighth week. Urine is excreted into and mixes with the amniotic fluid that the fetus swallows.

Neurologic System

Development of the Brain. The *neural plate* (a thickened area of embryonic ectoderm), from which the infant's nervous system develops, appears during the third week of gestation. The *neural tube** and *neural crest* evolve from this structure, the first differentiating into the CNS (the brain and cord) and the second into the peripheral nervous system.

The brain, which is formed at the cranial end of the neural tube, consists of the forebrain, midbrain, and hindbrain. The longest part of the neural tube ultimately becomes the spinal cord.

*Adapted from Korones, SB: High-risk newborn infants: the basis for intensive nursing care, ed 4, St Louis, 1986, The CV Mosby Co.

†This finding was the basis for corticosteroidal (β-methasone) therapy to stimulate fetal lung maturity when premature delivery is anticipated (Chapters 33, 37).

*The nurse may need to explain to parents about neural tube defects, one of several malformations that can be identified in utero through amniocentesis (see test for α-fetoprotein).

The human brain is only partially developed and functional at birth. It grows in three stages: first, prenatally by hyperplasia (an increase in cell number); second, during the first 6 months of life by a combination of hyperplasia and hypertrophy (an increase in size of existing cells); and third, thereafter until puberty by hypertrophy. An adequate supply of protein and calories is required for this process, particularly during the first and second stages. Prenatal maternal anemia and malnutrition compromise fetal brain development: if the fetus does not receive adequate nutrition early in development, there is a smaller number of cells developed; if the fetus continues to receive inadequate nutrition, the existing cells are smaller in size.

The late fetal and early neonatal phases of maturation are especially critical to later achievement. Disease, trauma, or unfavorable environmental factors may irreparably alter the development of the CNS (Fig. 9-14).

Hypoxia attributable to maternal causes (e.g., premature separation of the placenta), fetal causes (e.g., cord entanglement), or iatrogenic causes (e.g., maternal hypotension after being given spinal anesthesia) may be critical to the infant. Many of the survivors of severe asphyxia develop cerebral palsy, mental retardation, or other neurologic deficits. Newborns of 36 weeks' gestational age or younger are less sensitive to hypoxia but are more sensitive to birth trauma than mature newborns. Fortunately, however, the infant has remarkable powers of recuperation, and many depressed babies appear to recover satisfactorily. See Chapter 21 for more information on newborn neurologic function.

Neuromuscular Behavior. Fundamental to the successive development of behavior patterns is the development of neuromuscular structure and functioning. Behavior advances through five stages: (1) myogenic (originating in the muscle) response, (2) neuromotor (muscle movement stimulated by nerves) response, (3) reflex response, (4) integration of simple reflexes, and (5) integration and control from higher centers. Fetal development of the nervous system parallels fetal behavior.

Response to Stimulation. Studies revealed that before the middle of the seventh week since LMP, "the human embryo appears incapable of any type of reflex activity" in response to stimulation (Hooker, 1952). During the next 6½ weeks increasing sensitivity was evidenced. By 13½ weeks all areas of the body except the top and back of the head appeared to be sensitive. Stimulation of parts of the body were found to cause a response. For example, lips were pressed together when stroked, the tongue moved when the inside of the mouth was touched, and stimulation of the palm resulted in finger closing and wrist flexion.

Movement. At 9 weeks since LMP the whole fetus moves in a jerky, rather convulsive manner, but between 10 and 12 weeks, periods of quiet or resting can be noted (Van Dongen and Goudie, 1980); and "instead of the mechanical, stereotyped movement seen earlier, the various activities are graceful and flowing—the fetus is very active" (Hooker, 1952). In one study using ultrasonography the fetus was seen to propel himself around in the amniotic fluid by using paddling movements with the feet, to roll over, turn somersaults, place his hands behind his head and over his ears, suck his thumb, and grasp the umbilical cord (Freud, 1983). Respiratory efforts have been visualized at 18½ weeks, swallowing with tongue movements by 12½ weeks, and sucking by 29 weeks. By 16 weeks fetal muscle movement is strong enough to activate receptors on the maternal abdominal wall; the mother usually interprets this as "the baby moving" and professionals refer to it as "quickening."

Behavioral States. Active and inactive periods noted first between 10 and 12 weeks since LMP develop a sequential pattern by 28 weeks. Stainton (1983a) identifies three behavioral states—active, quiet, and sleeping—from data acquired from 23 expectant parents during interviews about their knowledge of their unborn child in the last trimester of pregnancy (see research highlight, p. 189). Both mothers and fathers described times when the fetus was responsive to their voices or to rubbing of the mother's abdomen by kicking and moving. Parents noted times when the fetus was quiet but awake and aware. At other times parents said that calling in a loud voice or shaking the abdomen did not result in more than a brief movement. In those pregnancies in which the father's style was expressive (May, 1980), the father's descriptions validated the mother's. Brazelton (1982) notes that most mothers can delineate three behavioral states in the fetus: active "alert," deep sleep with little or no movement, and intermediate sleep with irregular startlelike movement.

Sensory Awareness

Touch. Most pregnant women can verify that the fetus touches the uterine wall during pregnancy. In doing so the fetus experiences touch. Fetal response to touch through the uterine wall has not been studied through ultrasonic observation, but parental reports of its effect are consistent. Pregnant women are often seen to be rubbing their abdomens and describe success in assisting their unborn infant to "calm down" or "settle down" when upset (Stainton, 1983b). Prospective fathers also have reported being able to "calm" a restless fetus by patting or rubbing the mother's abdomen (Stainton, 1983a).

Fetal response to painful stimuli can be demonstrated. A fetoscope placed on the mother's abdomen with pressure will usually result in fetal movement away from the site, thus requiring someone to hold the fetus in position to ensure accurate assessment. The insertion of an amniocentesis needle near or touching the fetus will also provoke a moving away movement (Liley, 1972).

If procedures recognized as painful to a newborn or adult are being considered for the fetus (e.g., intrauterine correction of a defect), fetal anesthesia is warranted. Anesthesia is administered to the mother, and by placental transfer the fetus is anesthetized. Anesthesia is provided during intrauterine transfusions requiring puncture of the fetal abdominal wall and during insertion of catheters to drain urine from the fetus with urinary tract anomalies (Harrison et al., 1981).

Hearing. The fetus is able to hear both internal and external sounds by the fifth month of pregnancy (Liley, 1972). The fetus lives in an environment bombarded with

RESEARCH HIGHLIGHT

The Fetus: A Growing Member of the Family

Purpose

An exploratory study using a constant, comparative analysis was done by Stainton (1985) to identify parents' perceptions about and interpretations of fetal behavior.

Sample/Methodology

Focused, semistructured interviews of 25 couples (none expecting their first child and 16 expecting their second child) were conducted in the expectant parents' home during the eighth or ninth month of pregnancy.

Findings

Five categories of information developed out of the experiential data given by the parents. All couples differentiated between the real appearance of their fetus and their "dream baby." Both parents communicated verbally or nonverbally with the unborn infant and it was reciprocated. All but two couples attributed a gender to the fetus. All unborn infants had a predictable sleep/wake cycle and expectant parents had knowledge of their unborn infant's emotions, preferences, sensitivities, and response patterns defined by the researcher as temperament.

Implications

These findings suggest that birth may be best approached as a turning point on a continuum of an interrelated history between parents and their newborn. The language surrounding childbirth, which has traditionally included terms such as *beginning relationship, the brand new baby, the new mother* may need revision to acknowledge the prebirth relationship and parental caring about and for their infant during pregnancy. Findings from this and future research will be of particular value to childbirth educators and others who work with expectant parents.

Stainton, MC: The fetus: a growing member of the family, Fam Relations 34(7):321, 1985.

sound. Pulsations of maternal blood flow through the large abdominal vessels supplying the lower body areas, placenta, and uterus and the noise emanating from the mother's digestive tract has been measured to be as high as 85 decibels (Walker et al., 1971; Henshall, 1972). Clements (1977) found that 4- to 5-month-old fetuses discriminated between musical sounds by kicking and moving violently when the music of Beethoven, Brahms, or rock groups was played and quieting with Vivaldi or Mozart.

The sensitive hearing of the fetus has prompted researchers to investigate to what extent the fetus, while in utero, can hear, learn to recognize, and record sounds that contribute to its later social responses, particularly with its mother. Numerous studies (Condon, 1977; Eisenberg, 1979; Simner, 1971) point to a selective listening to the mother's voice sounds and rhythms during intrauterine life that prepares the newborn for recognition and interaction with her or his primary caregiver. Parents have reported feeling gentle movements in response to talking or singing to their fetus (Stainton, 1983a). One mother reported that her baby began "irritable jerky movements" when she changed from vacuuming a carpet to moving the vacuum over a hardwood floor (Stainton, 1983a).

Taste. Taste buds are well developed in the fetus. The fetus has a larger number of taste buds than either a child or an adult and they are more widely distributed (Liley, 1972). Apparently the fetus can distinguish between sweet and sour tastes. In addition, cold solutions can induce hiccups in the fetus.

Sight. Until recently, newborns were thought to be only slightly light sensitive and unable to see. It is now known that light enters the uterus, especially in late pregnancy when the tissues are thin, and that both rods and cones are present at birth (Dobson, 1976). Fetal movement has been elicited through the use of bright light directed on the uterus (Grimwade et al., 1971). Als et al. (1979) found that during the last trimester the fetus would startle when a bright light was directed on the mother's abdomen near the head and turned actively but smoothly toward a soft light. These findings were based on reports by mothers and confirmed with ultrasound.

Summary. In summary, the fetus is well equipped with sensory devices to assist in the accumulation of information to promote continued development. The human newborn is not inexperienced at birth—she or he possesses a repertoire of behaviors that meet needs and provide protection. The behavioral state at birth is derived from a gradual development during the fetal period of life. Awareness of fetal response is stimulating research into the concept of prebirth parenting and the effects that mother-father-fetus interactions may have on subsequent parent-child relationships.

Gastrointestinal System

The digestive system forms during the fourth week. The middle portion of the intestine projects out into the umbilical cord during the fifth week of development because there is not enough room in the abdomen (the liver and kidneys are taking up considerable space at this time). The intestines return to the abdomen during the tenth week. Failure of the intestines to return to the abdomen results in a condition known as *omphalocele.*

Intrauterine nutrition and elimination occur through the placenta, making it unnecessary for the slowly developing gastrointestinal system to function before birth. During the second trimester the fetus begins to swallow amniotic fluid.

Metabolism. While in utero the fetus exists in a nondemanding physical environment. Constant ambient temperature, minimal physical activity, depressed muscle tone, and effective insulation against heat loss all contribute to a relatively low metabolic rate. The fetus maintains a temperature about 0.4° C (0.7° F) above maternal temperature. Oxygen consumption is about one third that of the neonate. Most of the caloric intake is used to accomplish growth and development.

The fetus receives its glucose, its main source of energy, from the mother. **Maternal insulin does not pass to the fetus; the fetus secretes insulin.** The fetus synthesizes glycogen and anabolizes (forms) his own fat rather than receiving these nutrients in these forms from the mother.

Meconium. As term approaches, increasing amounts of meconium (the end product of fetal metabolism) are found in the fetal intestinal tract. Normal meconium is a sterile, dark, greenish brown, semisolid residue of bile and embryonic secretions, plus cellular waste (squamous epithelial cells) and hair swallowed in utero. The presence of meconium in amniotic fluid before delivery usually, but not always, indicates fetal hypoxia (see Chapter 18).

Hepatic System

Liver function begins at about the fourth week after conception. Hematopoiesis starts at about the sixth week of intrauterine life; this activity is primarily responsible for the rapid growth and relatively large size of the liver during the second month of gestation.

The fetal liver at term is proportionately much larger than the liver of the 1-year-old infant. It is a metabolic and glycogen storage organ that also secretes bile and acts as a depot for iron. Full liver function is not achieved until well after delivery, however. For example, coagulation factors contributed to or produced by the liver and fibrinogen are low at the time of delivery but adjust in early infancy. The production of fetal liver enzymes is limited, especially in the fetus of less than 36 weeks' since conception.

Endocrine System

The fetal *adrenal cortex,* or outer part of the gland, produces cortisol. Increasing amounts of cortisol may be important in the initiation of labor.

The *thyroid* gland is the first endocrine gland to develop in the fetus. By the fourth week the thyroid can synthesize thyroxine.

By the twelfth week insulin may be extracted from the beta cells of the fetal *pancreas.* The fetus must supply whatever is needed for its metabolism of glucose. Insulin is the primary hormone regulating the rate of fetal growth. If the mother is diabetic, the response of the beta cells of the fetal pancreas to repeated stimuli of hyperglycemia (caused by high levels of maternal glucose) will be hyperplasia (increased amount of tissue) of all body structures except the brain. This is thought to account for the large size of the infants of diabetic mothers and the hyperinsulinism found in these newborns immediately after birth.

Reproductive System

Until the end of the ninth week, female and male external genitals appear somewhat similar (see Fig. 6-1). It is not until the twelfth week that external genitals are well enough developed to be easily distinguishable.

Female Genital Development and Function. The fetal ovary (see Fig. 6-5) has many primordial (primitive) follicles and produces small but increasing amounts of estrogen. It is the high level of maternal estrogen that stimulates the fetal endometrium; the rapid drop in maternal estrogens in fetal circulation following birth is followed by withdrawal bleeding. *Withdrawal bleeding* accounts for the brief mucoid vaginal discharge and even slight bloody spotting that may be noted in female neonates.

During childhood a small but continuing secretion of estrogen occurs. Before puberty a much greater production of estrogen accounts for the development of female secondary sex characteristics (see Table 6-3).

Male Genital Development and Function. Early in embryonic development, the gonads of the genetically male fetus (fetus with a Y chromosome) play a critical role in the formation of the genital tract. As the gonads evolve in the testicular pattern, presumably under the influence of maternal hCG, LH, and fetal adrenal hormones, the testes produce androgenic hormones that result in growth and differentiation of male genitals.

After delivery a slow increase in the production of androgen and traces of estrogen continue until just before puberty, when much larger amounts of testosterone, in particular, are secreted. This increase causes development of the male secondary sex characteristics (see Table 6-4).

Immune System

Near term, the fetus passively acquires natural immunity of IgG antibodies via placental transfer (p. 181). The fetus will develop IgM antibodies in response to maternal bacterial or viral infection. An in-depth discussion of the immune defense system across the life span is presented in Chapter 6. See Chapter 21 for discussion of the immune system in the newborn.

SUMMARY

Nurses need to understand basic genetic concepts and the ways hereditary factors interact with the constantly changing environment. This includes knowledge about the genetic basis of inheritance and normal development from conception through full-term gestation. Fig. 9-18 summarizes fetal development, maternal events, common discomforts, examples of remedies, and drug substances to avoid. It was taken from a brochure prepared for coaching parents through pregnancy.

Text continued on p. 196.

Fig. 9-18 Summary of fetal development, maternal events, common discomforts, examples of remedies and drug substances to avoid.

Week 1	Week 2	Week 3	Week 4	Week 5	Week 6	Week 7	Week 8
Baby's Development The ovum becomes fertilized, divides, and burrows into the uterus.	The embryonic disk (ectoderm, entoderm, mesoderm) is formed. These three primitive germ layers will generate every organ and tissue in your baby's body.	The first body segments appear, which will eventually form the primitive spine, brain, and spinal cord.	Heart, blood circulation and digestive tract take shape. The embryo is now one fifth of an inch long, the head one third of its total length.	The heart starts to pump blood; limb buds appear. Major divisions of the brain can now be discerned.	Eyes begin to take shape, external ears develop from skin folds.	Development is proceeding rapidly. The face is now complete with eyes, nose, lips, and tongue—even primitive milk teeth. Tiny bones and muscles appear beneath the thin skin.	The embryo is now a little more than an inch long, its tiny heart beating at about 40 to 80 times a minute.
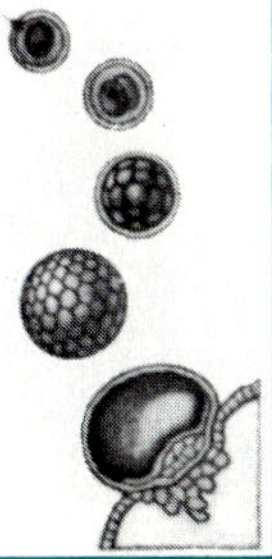	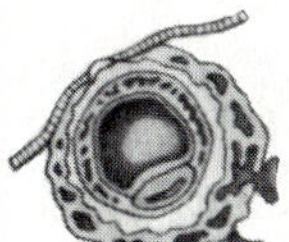	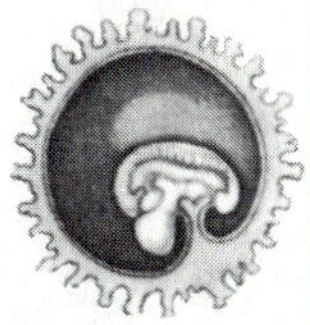	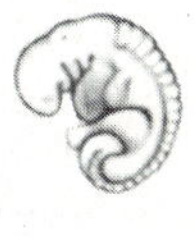	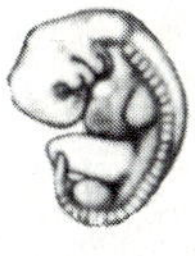	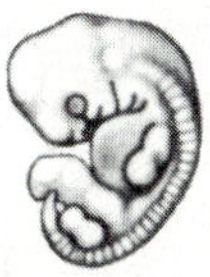	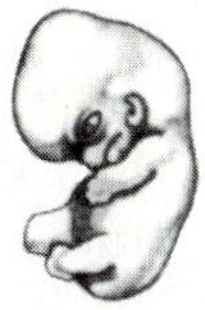	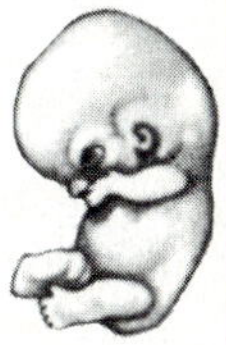
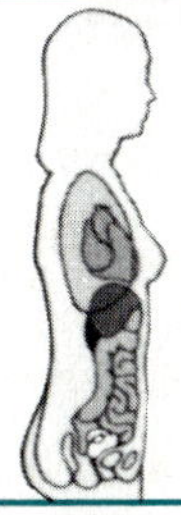	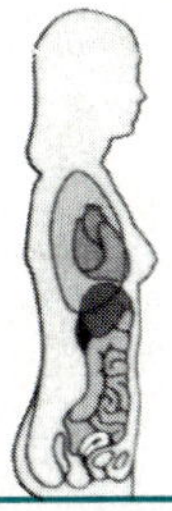	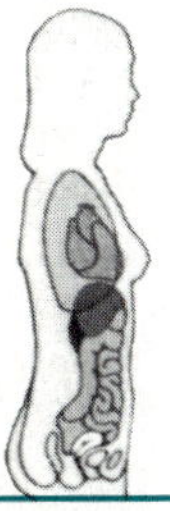	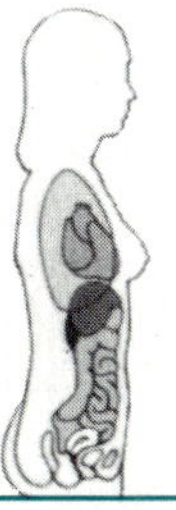	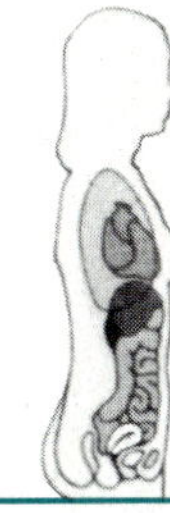	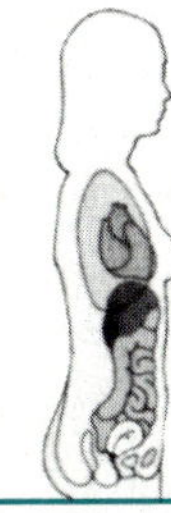	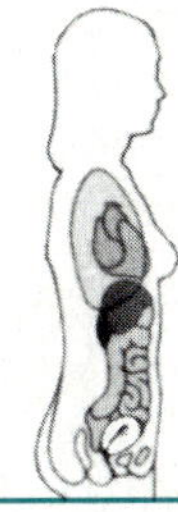	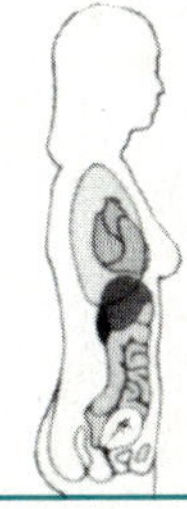
Maternal Events Ovaries increase production of "pregnancy-maintaining" hormone, progesterone.	First missed period	Placenta grows to cover one fifteenth of the uterine interior. Breast may begin to feel tender. No weight gain.			Exchange of fetal and maternal metabolites across the placenta begins, yet the two circulations are completely separate.	No noticeable weight gain.	The placenta now covers about one third of the uterine lining.
Common Discomforts		**Morning sickness** occurs because increased hormonal activity slows down your digestive system, apparently to enhance the absorption of nutrients for your baby.	**Fatigue** is thought to be caused by a change in ovarian hormone production (progesterone and relaxin), the purpose of which is to relax pelvic ligaments, stimulate breast growth, and soften the cervix.		**Urinary frequency** is caused by the uterus compressing the bladder against the pelvic bones, thus reducing its capacity, and also by hormonal changes that affect the water balance in your body.		
Remedies		Eat a few dry crackers before arising. Frequent, small, low-fat meals during the day should also help. Drink liquids between meals.	Exercise regularly, get plenty of sleep with frequent naps during the day.		You can decrease pressure on the bladder at night by sleeping on your side. Also, drink no fluids after 6 p.m.		
Drug Substance to Avoid		**Antiemetics** • cyclizine (Migral®, Marezine®) • meclizine (Antivert®, Bonine®) • trimethobenzamide (Tigan®) (Avoid throughout pregnancy.)	**Stimulants** • amphetamines • excessive caffeine (Avoid throughout pregnancy.)				
Acceptable Alternatives None: Avoid all drugs not prescribed by a physician for a specific condition. Avoid X-rays.							

Continued.

Fig. 9-18, cont'd. Summary of fetal development, maternal events, common discomforts, examples of remedies and drug substances to avoid.

	Week 9	Week 10	Week 11	Week 12	Week 13	Week 14	Week 15	Week 16
Baby's Development	Genitalia is now well defined; the baby's sex is determined. Eyelids finish forming and seal shut. The embryo has become a fetus.	The fetus assumes a more human shape as the lower body rapidly develops. Blood and bone cells form. The first movements begin.	Organs begin to function. The pancreas is producing insulin; the kidneys, urine.	The lungs have taken shape; primitive breathing motions begin. The swallowing reflex has been mastered as the fetus sucks its thumb while floating weightlessly in the amniotic fluid.		The musculoskeletal system has matured. The nervous system begins to exercise some control over the body; blood vessels rapidly develop.	With hands ready to grasp, the fetus—now weighing about 7 ounces—kicks restlessly against the amniotic sac.	All organs and structures have been formed and a period of simple growth begins.
	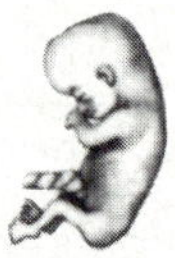	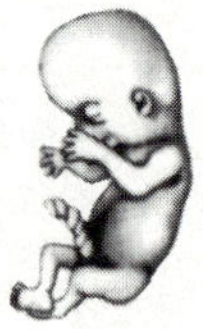	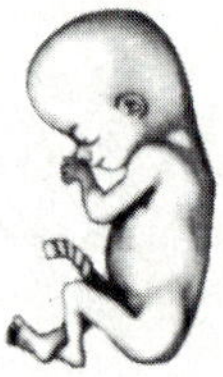	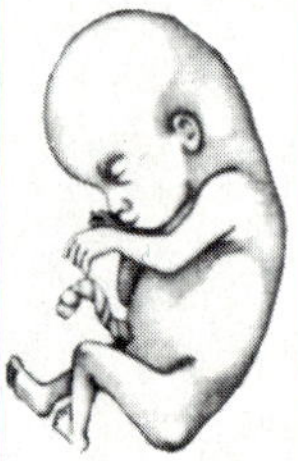	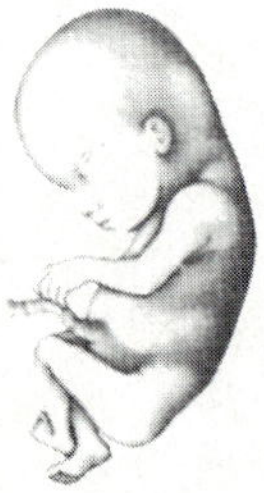	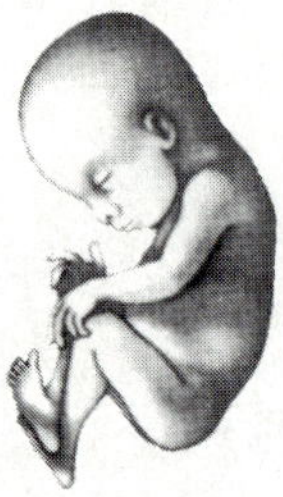	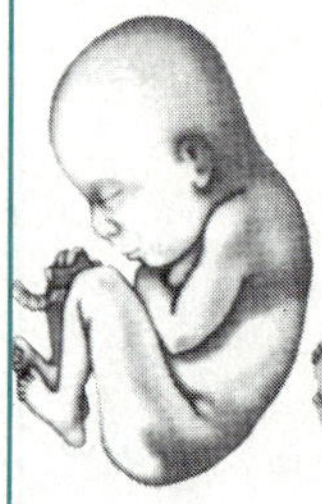	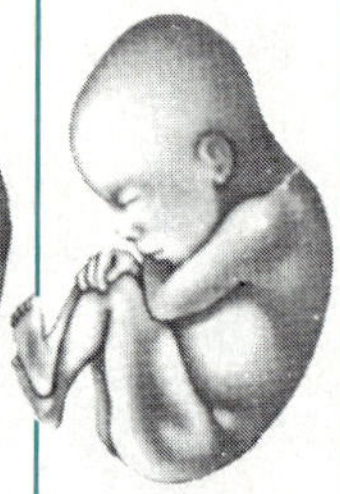
	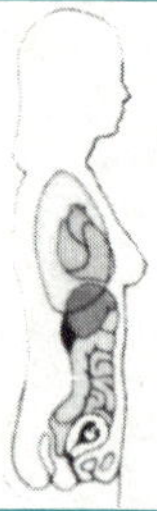	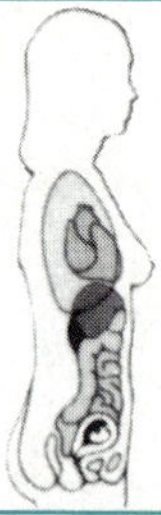	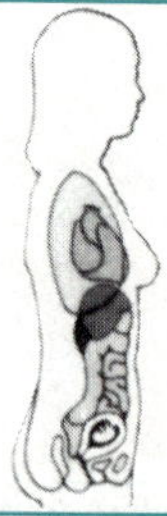	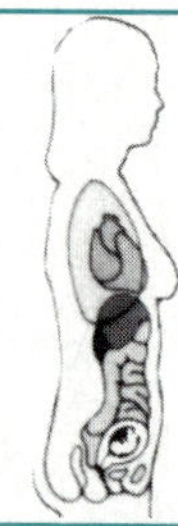	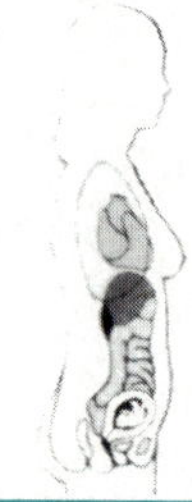	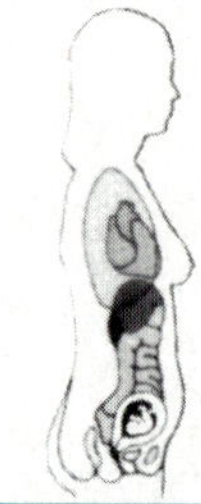	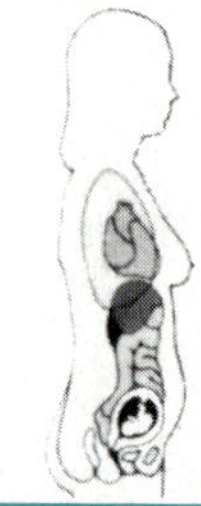	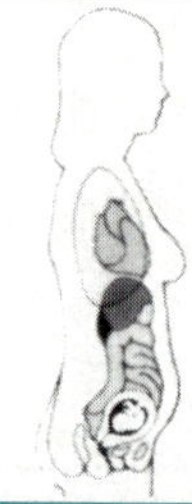
Maternal Events	Maternal blood volume has increased 30-40%.	The sensation of these first movements has been described by some women as if something were blowing bubbles through a straw in their stomachs.	2 to 3 pound weight gain. Possible increase in perspiration.	The placenta has reached complete functional maturity, acting as the baby's lungs, kidneys, liver, and digestive and immune systems.		3 to 4 pound weight gain. Belly beginning to show.		The fetal heartbeat can now be heard with an amplified stethoscope. Placenta begins producing the estrogen hormone.
Common Discomforts		**Sleeplessness** may result from the discomfort or anxieties of pregnancy.				Vaginal secretions are the result of an increased supply of blood and glucose to the vaginal mucosa. Severe itching, irritation, and malodor suggest an infection is present.		**Headaches** may occur while your body becomes adjusted to changes in blood volume and vascular tone. Emotional tension may also be a factor.
Remedies		A glass of warm milk before bedtime can work wonders. It's also good for your baby!				If infection is suspected, consult a health professional. Otherwise, cleanse daily with warm water, keeping the area dry to prevent chafing. Apply yogurt for vulvar itch.		Change body positions slowly. Resting with a damp cloth on the forehead helps some women. Drinking milk and/or eating a small snack also produces relief in some.
Drug Substances to Avoid		• tranquilizers • narcotics • antihistamines • alcohol • barbituates (Avoid throughout pregnancy.)				Vaginal Anti-infectives • metronidazole (Flagyl®) (Avoid throughout pregnancy.)		**Analgesics** • salicylates (aspirin) • phenacetin/caffeine • propoxyphene (Darvon®) • Indomethacin (Indocin®) **Tranquilizers** (Avoid throughout pregnancy.)
Acceptable Alternatives	None: Avoid all drugs not prescribed by a physician for a specific condition. Avoid X-rays.					• AVC™ Cream • Nystatin vaginal tablets (Mycostatin®) • Miconazole vaginal cream (Monistat®)		**TYLENOL**® brand acetaminophen

	Week 17	Week 18	Week 19	Week 20	Week 21	Week 22	Week 23	Week 24
Baby's Development		An oily coating protects the fetus. Fine hair covers the body and keeps the oil on the skin.	Eyebrows, eyelashes, and head hair develop.	The fetus is now following a regular schedule of sleeping, turning, sucking, and kicking—and has settled upon a favorite position within the uterus.		The skeleton is developing rapidly as the bone-forming cells increase their activity.	Eyelids begin to open and close.	The fetus now weighs about 27 ounces.
	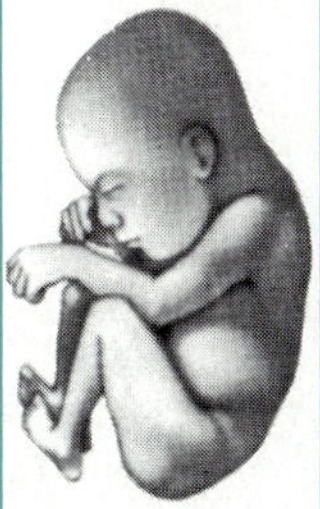	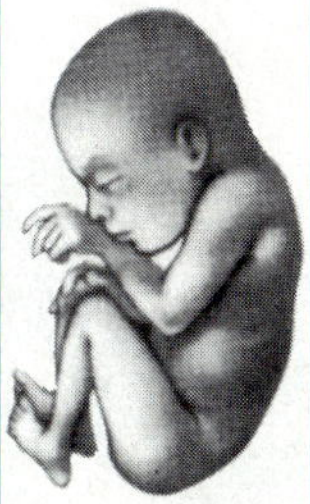	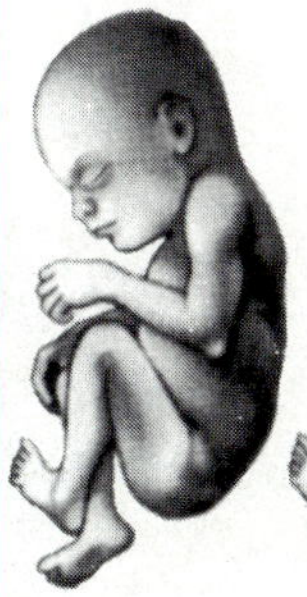	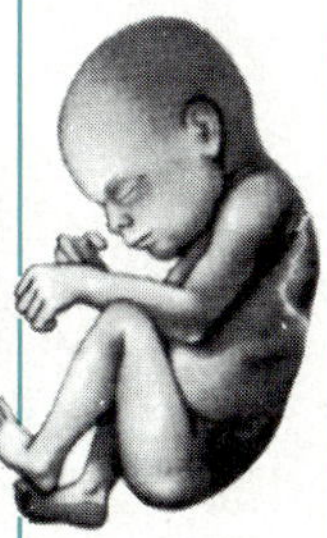	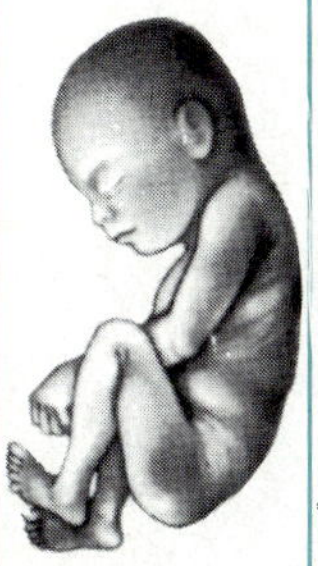	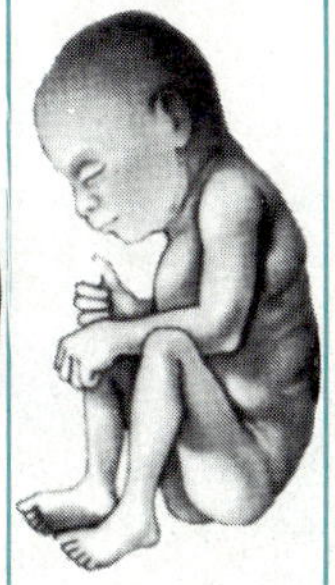	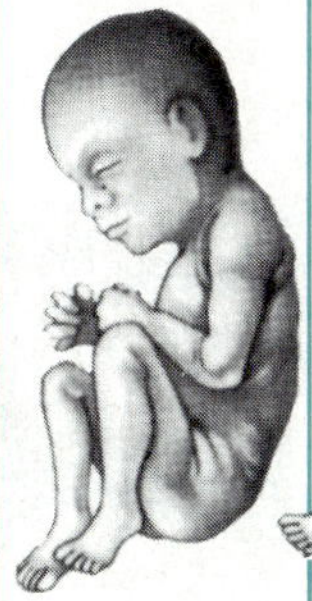	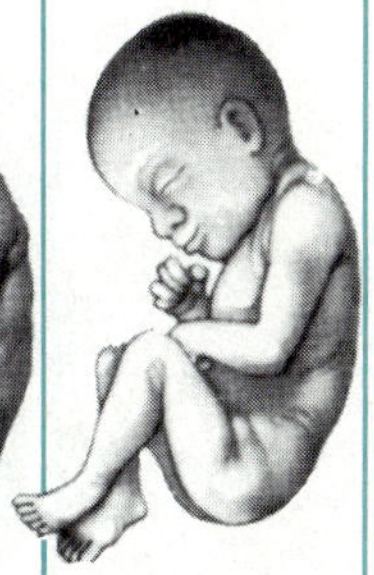
	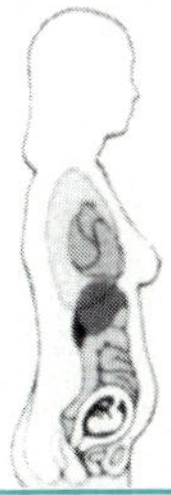	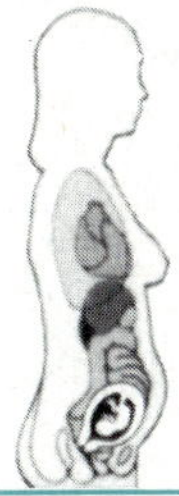	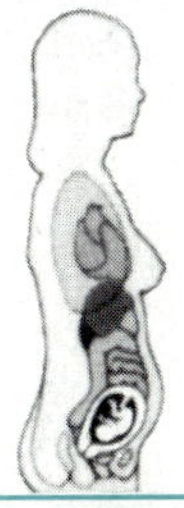	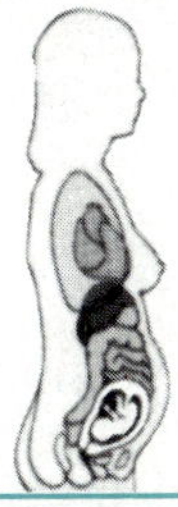	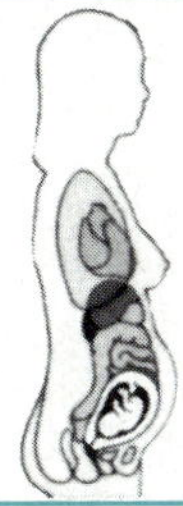	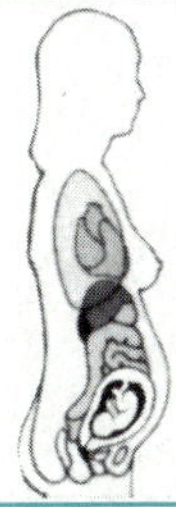	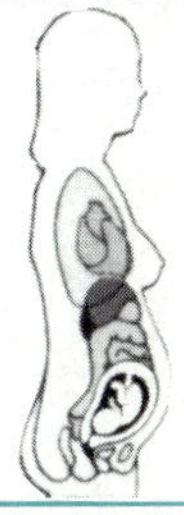	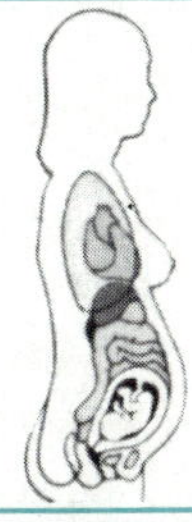
Maternal Events		3 to 4 pound weight gain.	Breasts begin secreting colostrum in preparation for nursing.	The placenta reaches its largest size relative to the fetus, covering one-half of the uterine lining. There is 400 ml of fluid now present in the amniotic sac.		3 to 4 pound weight gain.		The placenta becomes thicker rather than wider. Mother can now sense when baby's awake.
Common Discomforts		**Faintness or dizziness** when standing suddenly. This is caused by reduced blood flow to the brain as your body adjusts to new circulatory patterns. Possible shortness of breath.	**Varicose veins** are often the result in rising blood pressure in the lower extremities. This is caused by the enlarged uterus cutting off blood flow back from the legs to the heart.	**Allergies,** such as hay fever, are a common problem for some people.		**Skin changes** such as darkened nipples, stretch marks, splotches on cheeks and forehead, acne, redness on palms of hands and soles of feet are mainly due to increased hormone levels in the blood.		**Nosebleeds** sometimes occur because of increased blood volume and nasal congestion.
Remedies		Try to sit with your feet up, whenever possible; rise slowly and support yourself.	Whenever sitting, rest legs on footstool with feet elevated; avoid pressure on lower thighs. Many women find support stockings helpful.	Air conditioning (with a clean filter) often helps, and a pollen mask can be worn to screen out allergens.		Be patient. Virtually all of these effects will subside soon after childbirth.		Apply a little petroleum jelly in each nostril; that should stop the bleeding. A humidifier may also help. Do not irritate nasal mucosa.
Drug Substances to Avoid		• tranquilizers • alcohol (Avoid throughout pregnancy.)		**Most antihistamines** • hydroxyzine (Atarax®) • trimeprazine (Temaril®) (Avoid throughout pregnancy.)		Tetracycline (for acne) (Avoid throughout pregnancy.)		
Acceptable Alternatives (occasional use)		• smelling salts • aromatic spirits of ammonia		Chlorpheniramine for congestion; nasal spray for stuffy nose, occasionally. Calamine Lotion for rashes.		If nipples or abdomen itch, a lanolin-based cream or baby oil can provide relief. A mild soap can remove the excessive facial oil produced by acne.		Pseudoephedrine or nasal spray may be used occasionally for stuffy nose, if necessary.

Continued.

Fig. 9-18, cont'd. Summary of fetal development, maternal events, common discomforts, examples of remedies and drug substances to avoid.

Week 25	Week 26	Week 27	Week 28	Week 29	Week 30	Week 31	Week 32
Baby's Development	To a certain extent, the baby can now breathe, swallow, and regulate its body temperature, but still depends greatly upon maternal support. 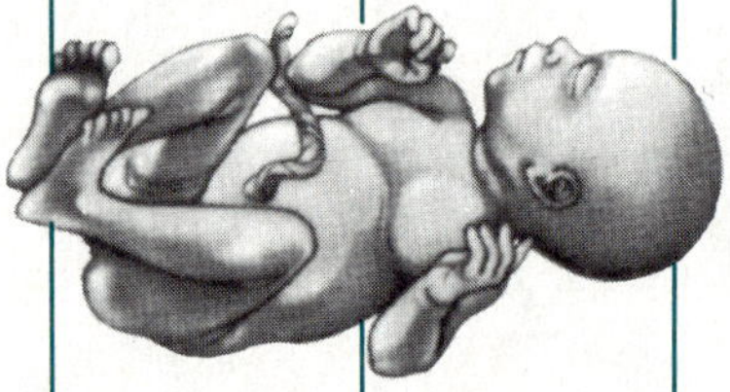	A substance called *surfactant* forms in the lungs, preparing them to function independently at birth.	Baby is two-thirds grown.	Fat deposits are building up beneath the skin to insulate the baby against the abrupt change in temperature at birth.	The digestive tract and the lungs are now nearly fully matured, and the skin becomes less red and wrinkled. 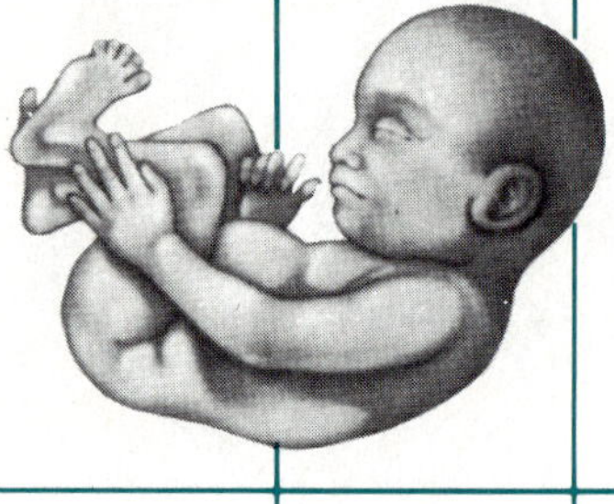	The baby has grown to about 14 inches.	
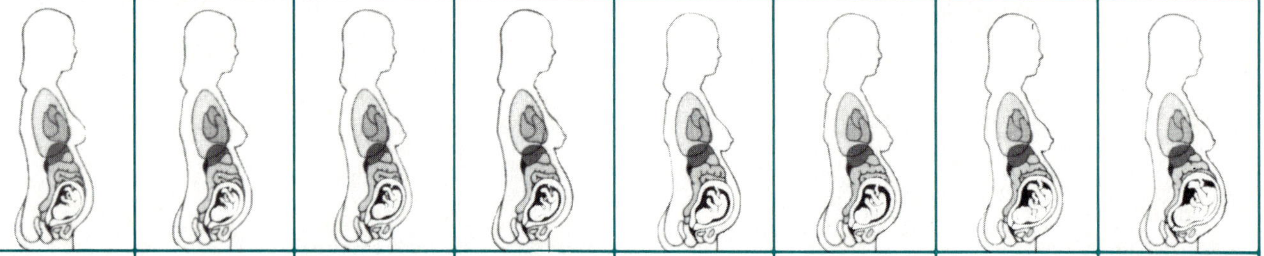							
Maternal Events	3 to 4 pound weight gain.	Respiratory movements can be detected by ultrasound. Mother sometimes feels baby's breathing as "hiccups."	The volume of amniotic fluid decreases to make room for growing fetus.		3 to 5 pound weight gain.		Mother may have trouble sleeping because of baby's activity.
Common Discomforts		**Leg and muscle cramps** may be caused by fatigue, by pressure exerted on the nerves by the uterus, or by too little calcium or too much phosphorus in the diet.	**Heartburn** often occurs as the stomach emptying time is delayed, causing a burning sensation in the throat.		**Swollen ankles.** The pressure of the uterus on the large veins returning blood to the heart may induce water retention.	**Constipation** is another result of the decelerated digestive process. As food moves slowly through your intestines, more water is extracted, leaving the stool drier and harder.	**Hemorrhoids** may also develop.
Remedies		Exercise regularly, walking especially. Elevate legs and flex toes when resting. Increase milk consumption.	Drink milk between small, frequent meals. This problem will disappear soon after your baby's birth.		Elevate legs—once or twice a day for an hour or so—with your hips. Sleep on your left side.	Eat foods containing roughage, such as raw fruits, vegetables, cereals with bran. Drink liquids and exercise frequently.	Soaking in a warm bath or sitting on soft pillows should soothe the symptoms of hemorrhoids.
Drug Substances to Avoid		• salicylates (aspirin) • tranquilizers (Avoid throughout pregnancy.)	**Antacids** • calcium carbonate • magnesium trisilicate (Gaviscon®) • sodium bicarbonate (baking soda) • cimetidine (Tagamet®) (Avoid throughout pregnancy.)		**Most diuretics** ("water pills") (Avoid throughout pregnancy.)	**Laxatives** • mineral oil • castor oil (Avoid throughout pregnancy.)	
Acceptable Alternatives (occasional use)		Calcium supplements with little or no phosphorus.	• Maalox® • Mylanta® (also for "gas")			For Constipation: • Metamucil® • Senokot® • teaspoon of milk of magnesia at bedtime	For Hemorrhoids: • Nupercainal® suppositories or cream • Anusol® • Medicone®

Week 33			To Term
Baby's Development	Virtually the entire uterus is now occupied by the baby, and its activity is restricted. 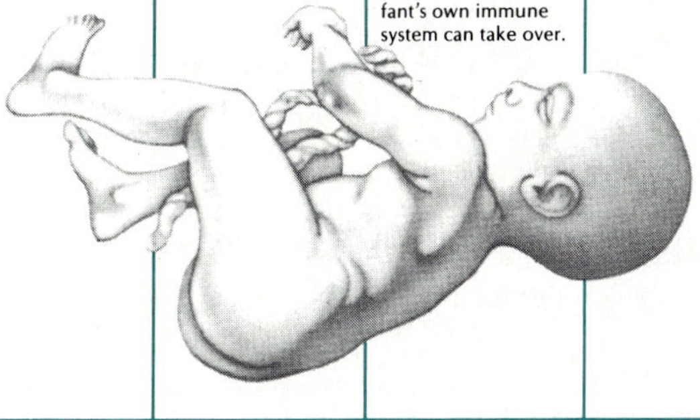	Maternal antibodies against measles, mumps, rubella, whooping cough and scarlet fever are transferred to the baby, providing protection for about 6 months until the infant's own immune system can take over.	
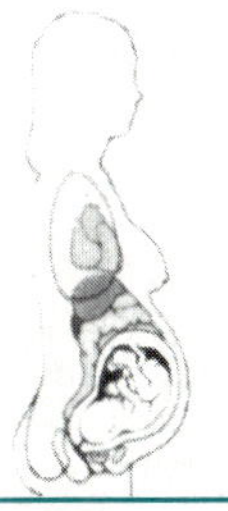	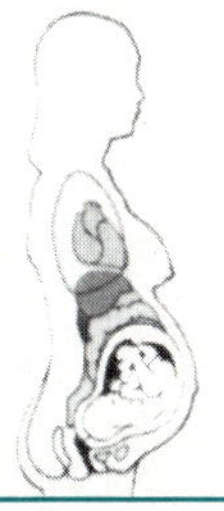	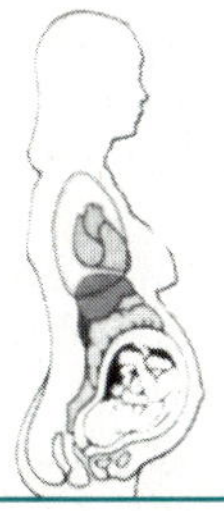	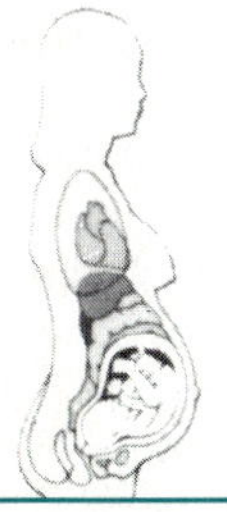
Maternal Events	The placenta is nearly 4 times as thick as it was 20 weeks ago and weighs about 20 ounces.	Preparing for birth, the baby descends deeper into the mother's pelvis. 3 to 5 pound weight gain.	In 9 short months, the miracle is complete: you have transformed a single, microscopic fertilized cell into a 6000 billion celled human being.
Common Discomforts	**Backaches** are often caused by muscles and ligaments relaxing in preparation for the stretching required in delivery. Also by the added off-center weight of the enlarged uterus.	**Urinary frequency** is caused—for the second time in your pregnancy—by the uterus compressing the bladder against the pelvic bones, thus reducing its capacity.	**Uterine contractions** become perceptible as the cervix and lower uterine segment prepare for labor.
Remedies	Back exercises, such as the "pelvic tilt," can help strengthen back and abdominal muscles. Wear low-heeled shoes or flats; avoid heavy lifting.	You can decrease pressure on the bladder at night by sleeping on your side. Urinate frequently.	
Drug Substances to Avoid	**Analgesics** • salicylates (aspirin) • propoxyphene (Darvon®) • phenacetin/caffeine • indomethacin (Indocin®) • codeine (Avoid throughout pregnancy.)		
Acceptable Alternatives (occasional use)	**TYLENOL®** brand acetaminophen		

KEY CONCEPTS

- Genes are responsible for all human traits, for the orderly pattern and timing of development from conception to death, and for continuity of the species through consistent transmission of these traits from generation to generation.
- At fertilization, a zygote is formed, the sex of the new human is determined, and the blueprints for the growth, development, and maturation of a new individual are laid down.
- Genes act in predictable fashion during gamete formation and fertilization (Mendel's laws).
- Human gestation is approximately 280 days since last menstrual period; 266 days after fertilization.
- The placenta is the most accurate record of the infant's prenatal experience.
- In the human, the chorion laeve and amnion form an avascular amniochorion that serves important functions that include solute and fluid transport, as well as prostaglandin formation at the time of parturition
- Fetal maturation takes place in an orderly and predictable pattern.
- There are sensitive, or critical, periods in human development during which tissues are highly vulnerable to environmental agents, for example, teratogens.
- The L/S ratio provides one method of assessing for fetal lung maturity in most instances.
- The fetus is well equipped with sensory devices to assist in the accumulation of information to promote continued development. The human newborn possesses a repertoire of behaviors that meet needs and provide protection.

STUDY QUESTIONS AND ACTIVITIES

1. Visit a biology lab to examine specimens of human embryos. Compare the differing stages of development.
2. Obtain a placenta with membranes from the delivery area, examine carefully; explain the structures and their development.
3. Visit local pharmacies and other stores to find what over-the-counter drugs are available to pregnant women (including alcohol and tobacco). List at least three different preparations that might affect the embryo or fetus and describe both their effects and the method of transport of the drug to the fetus.
4. Visit a prenatal clinic and conduct a class on the effects of over-the-counter drugs on the fetus. Prepare handouts for the clients. Include stages of fetal development in your discussion.

References

Als, H, et al: Dynamics of the behavioral organization of the premature infant: a theoretical perspective. In Field, TM, et al, editors: Infants born at risk, New York, 1979, Spectrum Press

Benirschke, K: The placenta: how to examine it and what you can learn, Contemp OB/GYN, 17:117, 1981

Brazelton, TB: Joint regulation of neonate-parent behavior. In Tronick, EZ: Social interchange in infancy: affect, cognition, and communication, Baltimore, 1982, University Park Press

Clements, M: Observations on certain aspects of neonatal behavior in response to auditory stimuli. Paper presented at the Fifth International Congress of Psychosomatic Obstetrics and Gynecology, Rome, 1977

Condon, WS: A primary phase in the organization of infant responding behavior. In Schaffer, HR, editor: Studies in mother-infant interaction, New York, 1977, Academic Press, Inc

Danforth, DN, and Scott, JR, editors: Obstetrics and gynecology, ed 5, Philadelphia, 1986, JB Lippincott Co

Dobson, V: Spectral sensitivity of the 2-month infant as measured by visually evoked cortical potential, Vision Res 16:367, 1976

Eisenberg, RB: Stimulus significance as a determinant of infant responses to sound. In Thoman, EB, editor: Origins of the infant's social responsiveness, The Johnson & Johnson Baby Products Co, Pediatric Round Table, 2, Skillman, New Jersey, 1979

Freud, E: Prenatal attachment and bonding, Paper presented to the First International Congress on Pre- and Peri-natal Psychology, Toronto, July 8, 1983

Grimwade, JC, et al: Human fetal heart rate change and movement in response to sound and vibration, Am J Obstet Gynecol 109:86, 1971

Harrison, MR, Management of the fetus with a correctable congenital defect, JAMA 246:774, 1981

Henshall, WR: Intrauterine sound levels, Am J Obstet Gynecol 112:576, 1972

Hooker, D: The prenatal origin of behavior, Lawrence, 1952, University of Kansas Press

Korones, SB: High-risk newborn infants: the basis for intensive nursing care, ed 4, St Louis, 1986, The CV Mosby Co

Liley, AW: The foetus as a personality, Aust NZJ Psychiatry 6:99, 1972

May, KA: A typology of detachment/involvement styles adopted during pregnancy by first-time expectant fathers, West J Nurs Res 2:445, 1980

Moore, KL: Before we are born: basic embryology and birth defects, rev ed, Philadelphia, 1977a, WB Saunders Co

Moore, KL: The developing human, ed 2, Philadelphia, 1977b, WB Saunders Co

Pritchard, JA, MacDonald, PC, and Gant, NF: Williams obstetrics, ed 17, Norwalk, Conn, 1985, Appleton-Century-Crofts

Simner, ML: Newborn's response to the cry of another infant, Dev Psychol 5:136, 1971

Stainton, MC: A comparison of pre-natal and post-natal perceptions of their babies by parents, Paper presented to the First International Congress on Pre-and Peri-natal Psychology, Toronto, July 8, 1983a

Stainton, MC: Interview data, 1983b

Van Dongen, LG, and Goudie, EG: Fetal movement patterns in the first trimester of pregnancy, Br J Obstet Gynaecol 87:191, 1980

Walker, D, et al: Intrauterine noise: a component of the fetal environment, Am J Obstet Gynecol 109:91, 1971

Willson, JR, Carrington, ER and Ledger, WJ: Obstetrics and gynecology, ed 8, St Louis, 1988, The CV Mosby Co

Bibliography

Athey, PA, and Hadlock, FP: Ultrasound in obstetrics and gynecology, St Louis, 1981, The CV Mosby Co

Berger, T, et al: Factors affecting human sperm penetration of zona-free hamster ova, Am J Obstet Gynecol 145:397, 1983

Bernhardt, J: Sensory capabilities of the fetus, MCN 12(1):44, 1987

Chatterjee, MS: Paternal age and Down's syndrome, Contemp OB/GYN 21:171, May 1983

England MA: Color atlas of life before birth: normal fetal development 1983. Distributed in North America and Canada by Year Book Medical Publishers, Inc, by arrangement with Wolfe Medical Publications, Ltd

Ericson, AJ: What is a teratogen? Childbirth Education: 44, Winter 1986/1987

Fanaroff, AA, and Martin, RJ, editors: Neonatal-perinatal medicine: diseases of the fetus and infant, ed 4, St Louis, 1987, The CV Mosby Co

Health status of Vietnam veterans, III: reproductive outcomes and child health, JAMA 259(18):2715, 1988

Lowrey, GH: Growth and development of children, ed 8, Chicago, 1986, Year Book Medical Publishers, Inc

Lowrey, GH: Growth and development of children, ed 8, Chicago, 1986, Year Book Medical Publishers, Inc

McCoshen, JA: The role of cervical mucus in reproduction, Contemp OB/GYN 29(5):94, 1987

Page, EW, et al: Human reproduction: essentials of reproductive and perinatal medicine, ed 3, Philadelphia, 1981, WB Saunders Co

Plauche, WC: Phosphatidylglycerol and lung maturity, Am J Obstet Gynecol 144:167, 1982

Schreiber, JR: New insights into follicular development, Contemp OB/GYN 22(6):125, 1983

Sopelak, VM: Studying the microenvironment of the ovarian follical, Contemp OB/GYN 27(5):179, 1986

Whaley, LF: Understanding inherited disorders, St Louis, 1974 The CV Mosby Co

Williams, SR: Basic nutrition and diet therapy, ed 8, St Louis, 1988, The CV Mosby Co

Wohlgemuth, DJ, and Balke, EM: Changes in egg and sperm before and during fertilization, Contemp Obstet Gynecol 20(5):196, 1982

CHAPTER

10

Anatomy and Physiology of Pregnancy

Learning Objectives

Correctly define the key terms listed.

Describe various pregnancy tests.

Explain the expected maternal anatomic and physiologic adaptations to pregnancy.

Identify the maternal hormones produced during pregnancy, as well as their target organs. Relate their major effects on pregnancy.

List signs and symptoms of pregnancy.

Describe gravidity and parity using the 5-digit and 2-digit systems.

Compare and contrast the abdomen, vulva, and cervix of the nullipara and multipara.

Key Terms

amenorrhea	hypertrophy
ballottement	leukorrhea
Braxton Hicks' sign	lightening
Chadwick's sign	linea nigra
diastasis recti abdominis	monoclonal antibodies
chloasma	Montgomery's tubercles
epulis	operculum
ferning	palmar erythema
friability	pyrosis
funic souffle	quickening
Goodell's sign	radioimmunoassay
Hegar's sign	striae gravidarum
hirsutism	telangiectasis
hyperplasia	uterine souffle

Pregnant Woman

gravidity	parity
multigravida	multipara
nulligravida	nullipara
primigravida	primigravida
	parturient

A healthy pregnancy with a physically safe and emotionally satisfying outcome for both mother and infant is the goal of maternity care. Consistent health supervision and surveillance are of utmost importance. Many maternal adaptations are unfamiliar to pregnant women and their families. The knowledgeable maternity nurse can help the pregnant woman recognize the relationship between her physical status and the plan for her care. Sharing information encourages the pregnant woman to participate in her own care, depending on her interest, need to know, and readiness to learn.

Essential to the study of maternity care is an understanding of the following terms used to describe the pregnant woman:

gravida A woman who is pregnant.
parturient A woman in labor.
gravidity Pregnancy without regard to the outcome.
parity The number of *pregnancies* in which the fetus or fetuses have reached viability, not the number of fetuses delivered. Whether the fetus is born alive or is stillborn after viability is reached does not affect parity.
nulligravida A woman who has never been pregnant.
primigravida A woman who is pregnant for the first time.
multigravida A woman who has had two or more pregnancies.
nullipara A woman who has *not* completed a pregnancy with a fetus or fetuses who have reached the stage of fetal viability (legal definition: 22 to 23 weeks of gestational age).
primipara A woman who has completed one pregnancy with a fetus or fetuses who have reached the stage of fetal viability.
multipara A woman who has completed two or more pregnancies to the stage of fetal viability.

This information is abbreviated as gravidity/parity. For example, "I/O" means that a woman is pregnant for the first time (primigravida) and has not carried a pregnancy to viability (nullipara).

Another abbreviation commonly employed in maternity centers is even more detailed. It consists of five digits with hyphens for separation. The first digit represents the total number of pregnancies, including the present one; the second digit represents the total number of deliveries; the third indicates the number of premature babies; the fourth identifies the number of abortions, and the fifth is the number of children currently living. If a woman pregnant only once with twins delivers at the thirty-fifth week and the babies survive, the abbreviation that represents this information is "1-1-2-0-2." During her next pregnancy the abbreviation is "2-1-2-0-2." Additional examples are given in Table 10-1.

Table 10-1 *Gravidity and Parity Using Five-Digit and Two-Digit Systems*

Condition	Five-digit System A* B C D E	Two-digit System F
Judith is pregnant for the first time.	1 - 0 - 0 - 0 - 0	I/0
She carries the pregnancy to term and the neonate survives.	1 - 1 - 0 - 0 - 1	I/I
She is pregnant again.	2 - 1 - 0 - 0 - 1	II/I
Her second pregnancy ends in abortion.	2 - 1 - 0 - 1 - 1	II/I
During her third pregnancy, she delivers viable twins.	3 - 2 - 0 - 1 - 3	III/II

**A,* Times uterus has been pregnant; *B,* number of deliveries, *C,* number of premature deliveries; *D,* number of abortions (spontaneous or elective); *E,* number of living children; *F,* gravidity/parity; corresponds to A and B of the 5-digit system.

PREGNANCY TESTS

Early detection of pregnancy allows early initiation of care. Some tests will diagnose pregnancy as early as 8 days after ovulation or about 22 days since the last menstrual period (LMP). Other tests are accurate from 4 to 18 days after the missed menstrual period. All tests that are in current use detect the presence of human chorionic gonadotropin (hCG). A first-voided morning urine specimen contains levels of hCG approximately the same as those in serum, whose levels increase exponentially between days 21 and 70 (counting from the first day of the LMP). Random urine samples usually have lower levels. The ability to recognize the beta subunit of hCG is the newest innovation in the evolution of endocrine tests for pregnancy. The wide variety of tests precludes discussion of each, however, several categories of tests are described here. The nurse should read the manufacturer's directions for the test to be used.

Latex agglutination inhibition (LAI) tests are easy to do and give results in 2 minutes. They are accurate from 4 to 10 days following missed menses. Examples of this type of test include the Gravindex slide, Pregnosticon slide, and UCG Beta slide.

Hemagglutination inhibition (HAI) tests are more sensitive than LAI tests but require 1 to 2 hours to obtain results. Except for one test, Neocept, which gives accurate results at or before missed menses, all HAI tests are accurate about 4 days following missed menses. Also on the market is e.p.t., (early pregnancy test) an HAI in-home test available for consumer purchase (Doshi, 1986).

The *radioreceptor assay* is one of the newest categories of pregnancy tests. This 1-hour serum test requires fairly sophisticated equipment. Radioreceptor assays are usually accurate at time of missed menses (14 days after conception) (Brucker and MacMullen, 1985). Biocept G is an example of this type of test.

Radioimmunoassay pregnancy tests for the beta subunit of hCG use radioactively labeled markers, which require the testing to be done in a laboratory. Depending on the degree of sensitivity required, the test time ranges from 1 to 48 hours. Radioimmunoassays are the most sensitive pregnancy tests available today (Brucker and MacMullen, 1985). Pregnancy can be diagnosed 8 days after ovulation or 6 days before missed menses.

Direct agglutination tests use monoclonal antibodies against the hCG molecule (see ELISA testing, Chapter 12).

This simple one-step procedure gives accurate results at or before missed menses depending on the test used.

Enzyme immunoassays use complex monoclonal anti-hCG with enzymes.* A visible color change makes the results easy to read. This new test holds promise for the future. Confidot is an immunoenzymatic assay home pregnancy test. The manufacturers of Confidot claim that this self-administered test confirms pregnancy approximately 10 days after fertilization, about 4 days before missed menses.

Interpretation of the results of pregnancy tests requires some judgment. The type of pregnancy test and its degree of *sensitivity* (ability to detect low levels of a substance) and *specificity* (ability to discern the absence of a substance) are interpreted in conjunction with the woman's history, which includes the date of the last normal menstrual period (LNMP), usual cycle length, and results of previous pregnancy tests. It is important to know if the woman is a substance abuser. Interactions with other drugs can give false results. Improper collection of the specimen, hormone-producing tumors, and laboratory errors may be responsible for false reports (Doshi, 1986). Where there is any question, serial testing may be the answer (Batzer, 1985). Speed and convenience need to be weighed against sensitivity and specificity.

Developing *monoclonal antibodies* for these pregnancy tests entails fusing a single antibody-producing cell with a myeloma cell to create a hybridoma. By these means, unlimited quantities of an antibody with high affinity for luteinizing hormone (LH) or hCG can be generated in cell culture. Only the most specific antibodies with superior binding ability are selected for cloning and mass production (Batzer, 1986).

ADAPTATIONS TO PREGNANCY

This chapter provides the basis for preventive, curative, and rehabilitative maternity care. Maternal adaptations are attributed to the **hormones** of pregnancy and to **mechanical pressures** arising from the enlarging uterus and other tissues. These adaptations serve to protect the woman's normal physiologic functioning, to meet the metabolic demands pregnancy imposes on her body, and to provide for fetal developmental and growth needs. Although pregnancy is a normal phenomenon, problems can occur. The nurse needs an adequate foundation in normal maternal physiology to accomplish the following:

1. Identify potential or actual deviation from normal adaptation to initiate remedial care
2. Help the mother understand the anatomic and physiologic changes during pregnancy.
3. Allay the mother's (and family's) anxiety, which may result from lack of knowledge
4. Teach the mother (and family) signs and symptoms that must be reported to the physician

Among the expected adjustments to pregnancy are changes that are found in some disease states; for example, low hemoglobin levels, a high erythrocyte sedimentation rate, dyspnea at rest, and alterations in cardiac function and endocrine balance. These changes reflect the body's effort to protect the mother and the fetus. An understanding of these changes is necessary for anyone who participates in the care of the mother and the fetus.

Some of the adaptations are recognized as signs and symptoms of pregnancy. These signs and symptoms appear in **bold print** throughout the chapter. A summary of the signs and symptoms of pregnancy and their order of appearance are presented in Table 12-2.

REPRODUCTIVE SYSTEM AND BREASTS

Hypothalamus-pituitary-ovarian Axis

During pregnancy, elevated levels of estrogen and progesterone suppress secretion of follicle-stimulating hormone (FSH) and LH. The maturation of a follicle and ovulation of an ovum do not occur. Menstrual cycles cease. Although the majority of women experience **amenorrhea**, at least 20% have some slight, painless spotting during early gestation for unexplained reasons. A great majority of these women continue to term and have normal infants.

After implantation, the fertilized ovum and the chorionic villi produce hCG, which maintains the corpus luteum's production of estrogen and progesterone for the first 8 to 10 weeks of pregnancy until the placenta takes over their production. (Danforth and Scott, 1986).

Uterus

Enlargement. The phenomenal uterine growth in the first trimester occurs in response to the hormonal stimulus of high levels of estrogen and progesterone. Enlargement results from (1) increased vascularity and dilation of blood vessels, (2) hyperplasia (production of new muscle fibers and fibroelastic tissue) and hypertrophy (enlargement of preexisting muscle fibers and fibroelastic tissue), and (3) development of the decidua (see Fig. 10-1). By 7 weeks the uterus is the size of a large hen's egg; by 10 weeks, the size of an orange (twice its nonpregnant size); by 12 weeks, the size of a grapefruit. Table 10-2 compares uterine measurements for the nonpregnant and pregnant uterus at 40 weeks' gestation. After the third month uterine enlargement is primarily the result of mechanical pressure of the growing fetus (Seidel et al., 1987).

Table 10-2 *Comparison of Measurements for Nonpregnant and Pregnant Uterus at 40 Weeks**

Measurement	Nonpregnant	Pregnant (40 Weeks)
Length	6.5 cm (2½ in)	32 cm (12½ in)
Width	4 cm (1½ in)	24 cm (9½ in)
Depth	2.5 cm (1 in)	22 cm (8½ in)
Weight	60-70 g (2½ oz)	1100-1200 g (2½ lb)
Volume	≤10 ml	5000 ml

*Note that references vary as to the exact values but all references agree on the magnitude of the growth the uterus undergoes during pregnancy.

*Read package inserts for a description of "monoclonal anti-hCG with enzymes."

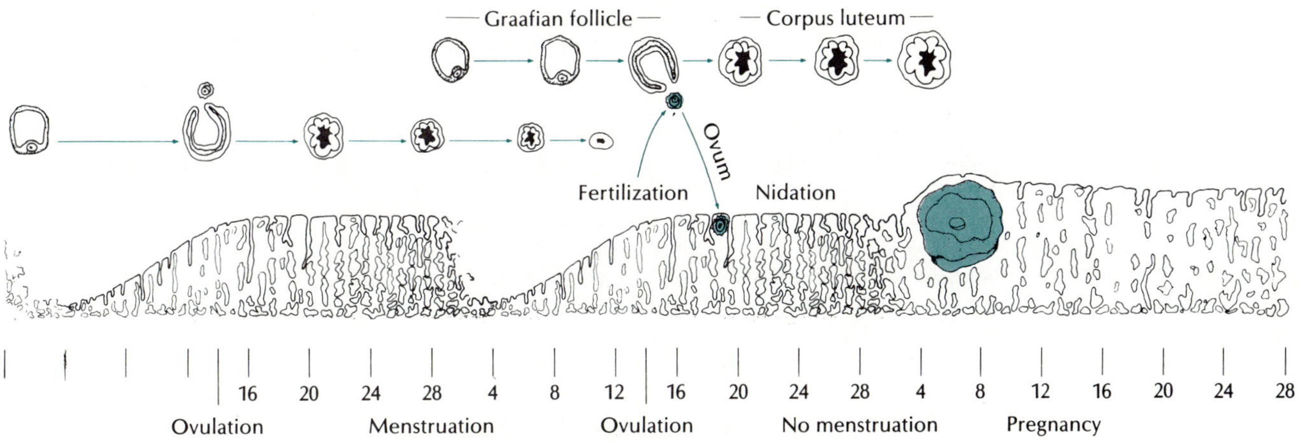

Fig. 10-1 Changes in endometrium and corpus luteum if pregnancy occurs (in days).

As the uterus increases in size, it also changes in weight, shape, and position. The muscular walls strengthen and become more elastic. At conception the uterus is shaped like an upside-down pear. During the second trimester it is spheric or globular. Later, as the fetus lengthens, the uterus becomes larger and more ovoid, and it rises out of the pelvis into the abdominal cavity. In the nonpregnant woman, the uterine cavity holds about 10 ml of fluid; during pregnancy, its capacity increases to 5 to 10 L or more (Pritchard, MacDonald, and Gant, 1985).

A reasonably accurate correlation of **uterine enlargement** and the duration of amenorrhea in weeks counting from the sixth week to term is possible in most normal pregnant women. Variation in the positions of the fundus or the fetus, variations in the amount of amniotic fluid present, or the presence of more than one fetus reduces the accuracy of this estimation of the duration of pregnancy.

The pregnancy may "show" after the fourteenth week, although this depends to some degree on the woman's height and weight. **Abdominal enlargement** may be less apparent in the primigravida with good abdominal muscle tone (see Figure 10-2). Posture also influences the type and degree of abdominal enlargement seen.

Consistency. During the early weeks of pregnancy an increase in uterine blood flow and lymph causes pelvic congestion and edema. As a result, the uterus, cervix, and isthmus soften perceptibly and progressively, and the cervix takes on a bluish color **(Chadwick's sign).**

At about the seventh to eighth week the following patterns of **uterine softening** are noted: isthmic softening and compressibility (**Hegar's sign**; Fig. 10-3), cervical softening **(Goodell's sign)**, easy flexion of the fundus on the cervix **(McDonald's sign)**, softening and slight fullness of the fundus near the area of implantation **(Braun von Fernwald's sign)**, or a soft lateral bulge with cornual implantation **(Piskacek's sign).** After the eighth week, general enlargement and softening of the uterine corpus and cervix are likely.

The nonsteroid ovarian hormone relaxin may act synergistically with progesterone (Danforth and Scott, 1986; Pritchard, MacDonald, and Gant, 1985). Relaxation occurs not

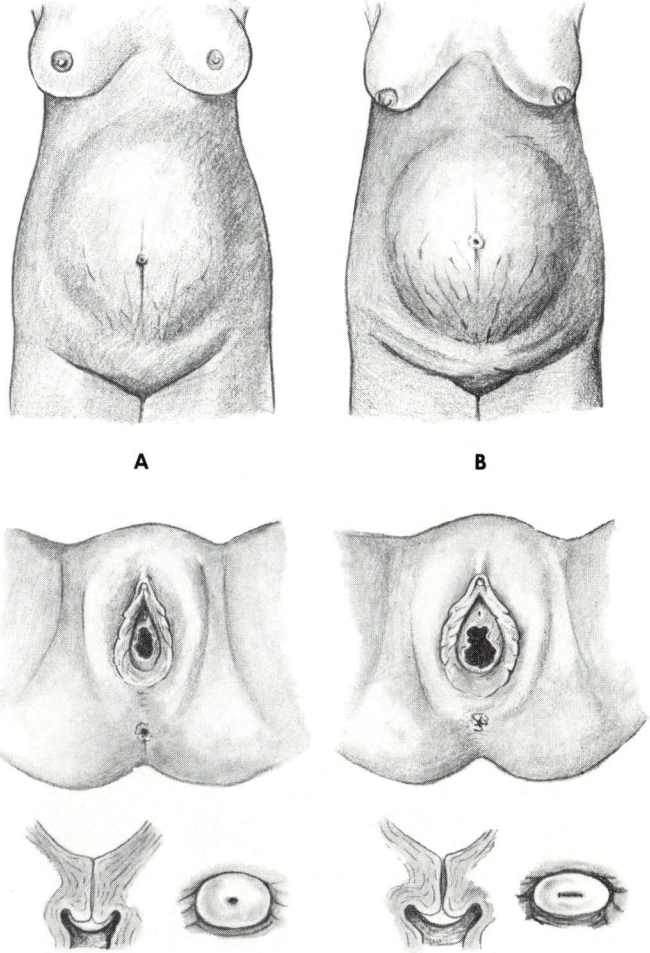

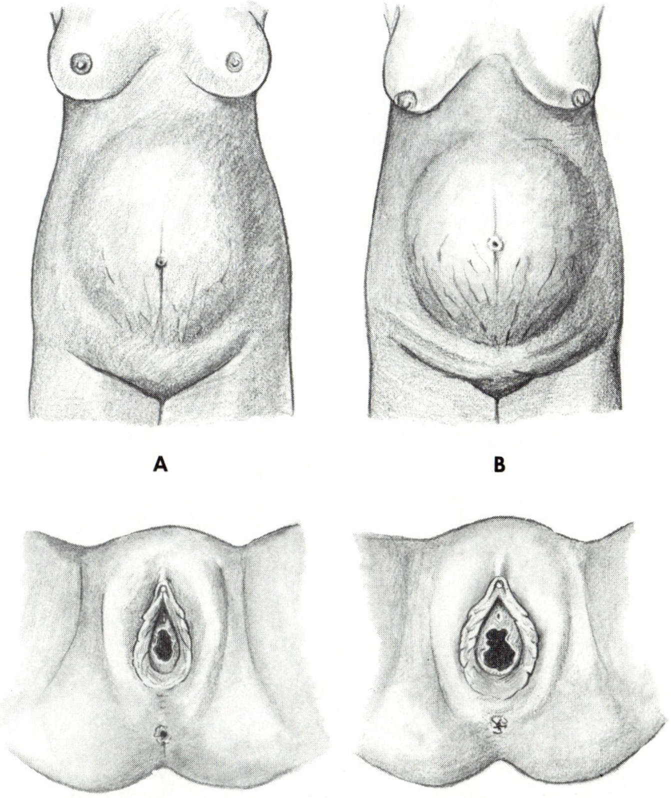

Fig. 10-2 Comparison of abdomen, vulva, and cervix in nullipara, **A**, and multipara, **B**, at the same stage of pregnancy and parturition.

only in the uterus but throughout various parts of the body, such as on the joints and walls of blood vessels.

Position. As the uterus grows it is elevated out of the pelvic area and may be palpated above the symphysis pubis sometime between the twelfth and fourteenth weeks of pregnancy (Fig. 10-4). The softness of the isthmus results is exaggerated uterine anteflexion during the first 3 months of pregnancy. The fundus presses on the urinary bladder, which along with edema of the bladder wall, causes the woman to experience urinary frequency. The uterus rises gradually to the level of the umbilicus at about 22 to 24 weeks and nearly reaches the xiphoid process at term. Between weeks 38 and 40, fundal height drops as the fetus begins to engage in the pelvis (lightening).

Generally the uterus is rotated to the right as it elevates, probably because of the presence of the rectosigmoid colon on the left side. However, the extensive hypertrophy (enlargement) of the round ligaments keeps the uterus in line. Eventually the growing uterus touches the anterior abdominal wall and displaces the intestines to either side of the abdomen. When a pregnant woman stands, the major part of her uterus rests against the anterior abdominal wall and contributes to altering her center of gravity.

Contractility. Soon after the fourth month of pregnancy, uterine contractions can be felt through the abdominal wall. These contractions are referred to as the **Braxton Hicks' sign**, a probable sign of pregnancy. Braxton Hicks contractions are a continuation of the irregular, painless contractions that occur intermittently throughout each menstrual cycle. The contractions are felt as uterine firmness through the abdominal wall or are evident because they raise and push the uterus forward. Contractions facilitate uterine blood flow and thereby oxygenation of the products of conception. Although Braxton Hicks' contractions are not ordinarily painful, some women do complain they are annoying. After the twenty-eighth week, contractions become much more definite, especially in slender women. Generally these contractions cease with walking or exercise. Rarely they may be perceived as painful. They may become strong enough during the last few weeks to be confused with the contractions of beginning labor.

Blood Flow. In a normal term pregnancy, one sixth of the total maternal blood volume is within the uterine vascular system. The rate of blood flow through the uterus averages 500 ml/min, and oxygen consumption of the gravid uterus averages 25 ml/min. Maternal arterial pressure, contractions of the uterus, and maternal position are three factors known to influence blood flow to this organ throughout pregnancy. Estrogens appear to have a regulatory rather than a direct influence on uterine blood flow, and protein synthesis is also probably a necessary step to increasing flow. The fetus may have some control over its blood supply (Resnik, 1982).

Intrauterine Sounds. Using an ultrasound device or a fetal stethoscope, the physician or nurse may hear (1) the **uterine souffle** or bruit, a rushing sound of maternal blood going to the placenta that is synchronous with the maternal pulse, (2) the **funic souffle**, which is synchronous with the fetal heart rate and caused by fetal blood coursing through the umbilical cord, and (3) the **fetal heart**

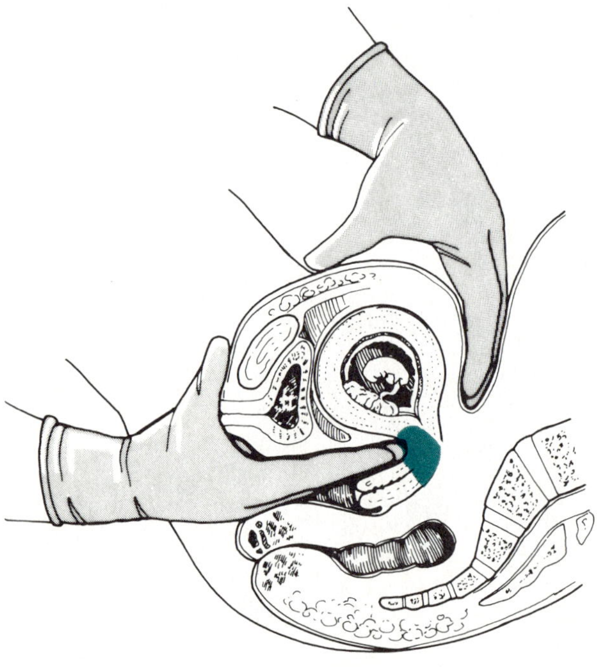

Fig. 10-3 Hegar's sign. Bimanual examination for assessing softening of isthmus while the cervix is still firm.

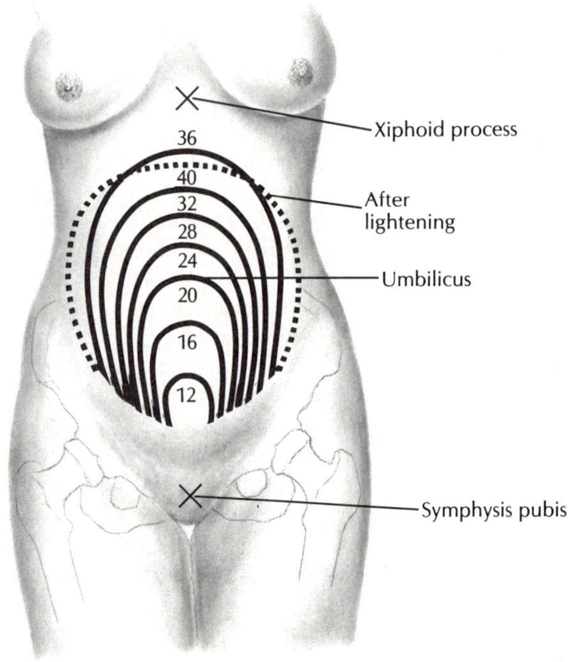

Fig. 10-4 Height of fundus by weeks of normal gestation with a single fetus. Dotted line indicates height after lightening.
Adapted from Malasanos, L, et al: Health assessment, ed 3, St Louis, 1985, The CV Mosby Co.

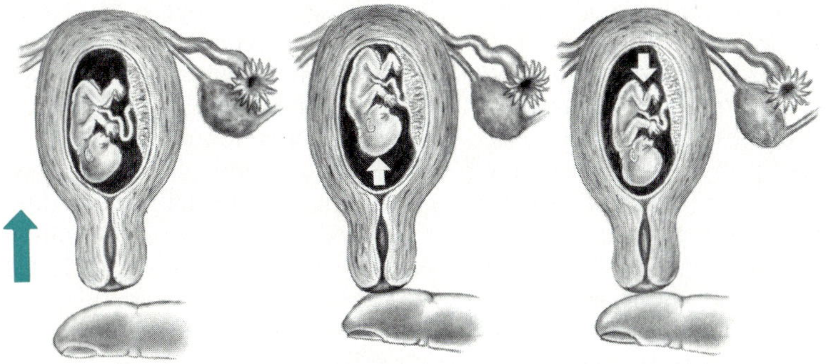

Fig. 10-5 Internal ballottement (18 weeks).

rate (FHR). For further discussion, see Chapter 17.

Ballottement. Passive movement of the unengaged fetus is called **ballottement.** Ballottement can be identified generally between the sixteenth and eighteenth week. Ballottement is a technique of palpating a floating structure by bouncing it gently and feeling it rebound. The examiner's finger within the vagina taps gently upward; the fetus rises. Then the fetus sinks, and a gentle tap is felt on the finger (Fig. 10-5). Internal ballottement of a fetus within a uterus is a probable objective sign of pregnancy.

Quickening. The first recognition of fetal movements, or "feeling life," by the multiparous woman may occur as early as the fourteenth to sixteenth week. The primigravidas may not notice these sensations until the eighteenth week or later. **Quickening** is commonly described as a flutter and is difficult to distinguish from peristalsis. Noting the week in which quickening occurs provides a tentative clue in dating the duration of gestation.

Cervix. A softening of the cervical tip may be observed about the beginning of the sixth week in a normal, unscarred cervix. The softening of the cervix during pregnancy (Goodell's sign) is brought about by increased vascularity, slight hypertrophy, and hyperplasia of the muscle and its collagen-rich connective tissue, which becomes loose, edematous, highly elastic, and increased in volume. The glands near the external os proliferate beneath the stratified squamous epithelium, giving the cervix the velvety consistency characteristic of pregnancy. The changes in the cervix, as well as those of the vagina, help prepare the birth canal for the fetus's passage through it (Fig. 10-6). **Friability** is increased; that is, the cervix bleeds easily when scraped or touched. Increased friability is the cause of the few drops of blood seen after coitus with deep penetration or vaginal examination. These few drops are usually within normal limits.

The cervix of the nullipara is rounded. Lacerations of the cervix almost always occur during the birth process. With or without lacerations, following childbirth the cervix becomes more oval in the horizontal plane, and the external os appears as a transverse slit (see Fig. 10-2).

Vagina and Vulva

Internal Structures. Pregnancy hormones prepare the vagina for distension during labor by producing a thickened vaginal mucosa, loosened connective tissue, hypertrophied smooth muscle, and an increase in the length of the vaginal vault. Increased vascularity results in a violet-bluish color to the vaginal mucosa and cervix. The deepened color, termed **Chadwick's sign** or **Jacquemier's sign**, may be evident as early as the sixth week, but is easily noted at the eighth week of pregnancy. Desquamation (or exfoliation) of the vaginal, glycogen-rich cells occurs under estrogen stimulation. The cells that are shed contribute to the thick, whitish vaginal discharge, leukorrhea.

During pregnancy the pH of vaginal secretions becomes less acidic. The pH changes from 4 to 5 to about 5.5 to 6.5. *The rise in pH makes the pregnant woman more vulnerable to vaginal infections,* especially yeast infections. A diet of large quantities of sugars can make the vaginal environment even more suitable for a yeast infection.

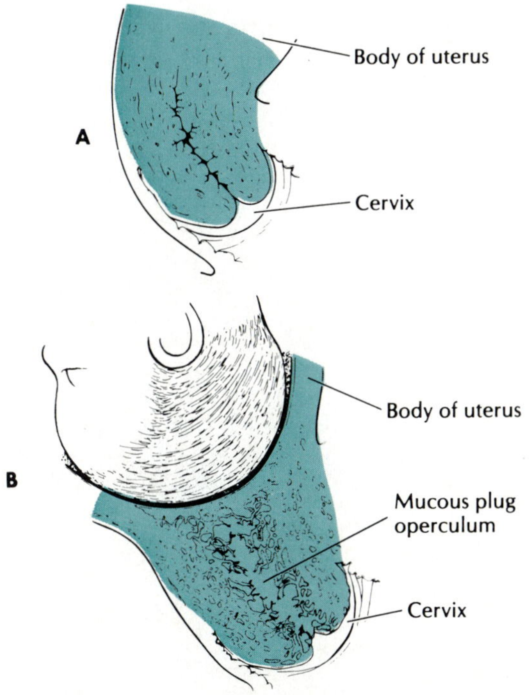

Fig. 10-6 A, Cervix in nonpregnant woman. B, Changes in cervix during pregnancy.

The increased vascularity of the vagina and other pelvic viscera results in a marked increase in sensitivity. The *increased sensitivity may lead to a high degree of sexual interest and arousal,* especially during the second trimester of pregnancy. The increased congestion plus the relaxed walls of the blood vessels and the heavy uterus may result in edema and varicosities of the vulva. The edema and varicosities usually resolve during the postpartum period.

External Structures. External structures of the *perineum* are enlarged during pregnancy because of an increase in vasculature, hypertrophy of the perineal body, and deposition of fat (Fig 10-7). The labia majora of the nullipara approximate and obscure the vaginal introitus; those of the parous woman separate and gape after childbirth and perineal or vaginal injury. Torn residual tags of the hymen remain after the use of tampons, coitus, and vaginal delivery. Fig. 10-2 compares the nullipara and the multipara in relation to several characteristics: pregnant abdomen, vulva, and cervix.

Leukorrhea is a white or slightly gray mucoid discharge with a faint musty odor. Increased estrogen and progesterone stimulation of the cervix produces copious mucoid fluid. The fluid is whitish because of the presence of many exfoliated vaginal epithelial cells caused by normal pregnancy hyperplasia. This vaginal discharge is never pruritic or blood stained. Because of the progesterone effect, *ferning* (see Fig. 6-27) does *not* occur in the dried cervical mucous smear. The mucus fills the endocervical canal, resulting in the formation of the mucous plug (operculum) (Fig. 10-6). The operculum acts as a barrier against bacterial invasion during pregnancy.

Breasts

Fullness, heightened sensitivity, tingling, and **heaviness** of the breasts begin as early as the sixth week of gestation. Breast sensitivity varies from mild tingling to frank pain (mastodynia). **Nipples** and **areolae** become more **pigmented,** a **secondary pinkish areola** develops, and nipples become more erectile. Hypertrophy of the sebaceous (oil) glands embedded in the primary areola, called **Montgomery's tubercles,** may be seen around the nipples. These sebaceous glands may have a protective role in that they keep the nipples lubricated. Suppleness of the nipples is jeopardized if the protective oils are washed off with soap.

The richer blood supply dilates the vessels beneath the skin. Once barely noticeable, the blood vessels now become visible, often appearing in an intertwining blue network beneath the surface of the skin. Venous congestion in the breasts is more obvious in primigravidas. Striae may appear at the outer aspects of the breasts.

During the second and third trimesters, growth of the mammary glands accounts for the progressive increase in breast size. The high levels of luteal and placental hormones in pregnancy promote proliferation of the lactiferous ducts and lobule-alveolar tissue, so that the palpation of the breasts reveals a generalized, coarse nodularity. The increase in glandular tissue displaces connective tissue, and as a result the tissue becomes softer and looser. Overstretching of the fibrous suspensory Cooper's ligaments supporting the breasts may be prevented with a well-fitted maternity brassiere.

Although development of the mammary glands is functionally complete by midpregnancy, lactation is inhibited until a drop in estrogen level occurs after delivery of the fetus and placenta. A thin, clear, viscous precolostrum secretion, however, may be expressed from the nipples by the end of the sixth week (Seidel et al., 1987).* This secretion thickens as term approaches and is then known as **co-**

*References differ as to the gestational week during which precolostrum can be expressed. Some references cite week 16 as the earliest time at which fluid may be expressed from the breasts.

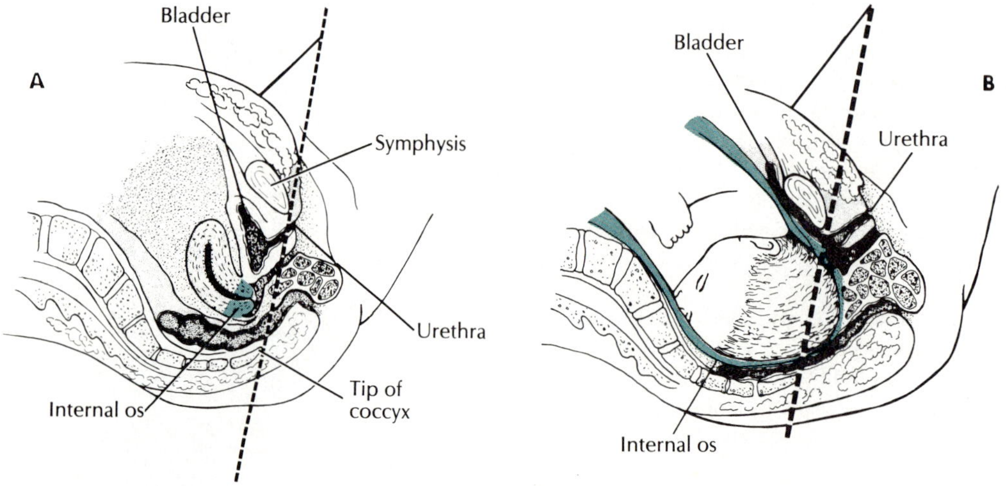

Fig. 10-7 A, Pelvic floor in nonpregnant woman. B, Pelvic floor at end of pregnancy. Note marked projection (growth of tissue) below line joining tip of coccyx and inferior margin of symphysis. Note elongation of bladder and urethra as a result of compression. Fat deposits are increased.

lostrum. Colostrum, the creamy, white to yellowish premilk fluid, may be expressed from the nipples during the third trimester. See discussion of prolactin in this chapter.

GENERAL BODY SYSTEMS

Cardiovascular System

Maternal adjustments to pregnancy involve extensive changes in the cardiovascular system, both anatomic and physiologic. Cardiovascular adaptations serve to protect the woman's normal physiologic functioning, to meet the metabolic demands pregnancy imposes on her body, and to provide for fetal developmental and growth needs.

Anatomic Changes: Cardiac Size and Position. Slight cardiac hypertrophy (enlargement) or dilation is probably secondary to increased blood volume and cardiac output. As the diaphragm is displaced upward, the heart is elevated upward and rotated forward to the left (Fig. 10-8). The apical impulse (PMI) is shifted upward and laterally about 1 to 1.5 cm (½ in). The degree of shift depends on the duration of pregnancy and the size and position of the uterus.

Auscultatory Changes. Auscultatory changes accompany the changes in heart size and position. Increases in blood volume and cardiac output also contribute to auscultatory changes common in pregnancy. There is more audible splitting of S_1 and S_2, and S_3 may be readily heard after 20 weeks of gestation. Additionally, grade II systolic ejection murmurs may be heard over the pulmonic area.

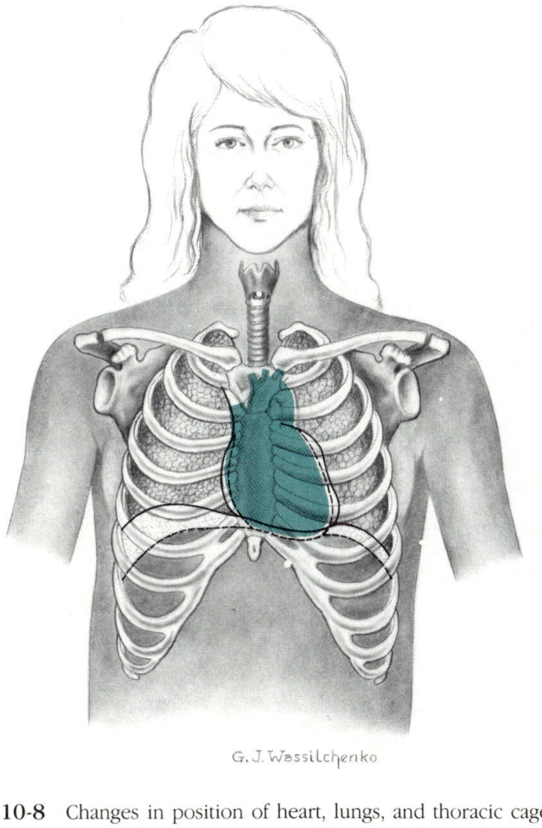

Fig. 10-8 Changes in position of heart, lungs, and thoracic cage in pregnancy. *Broken line,* Nonpregnant. *Solid line,* Change that occurs in pregnancy.

Pulse and Blood Pressure. Between 14 and 20 weeks, *pulse* increases slowly up to 10 to 15 beats per minute, which then persists to term. Palpitations may occur. *Arterial blood pressure* (brachial artery) varies with age. Blood pressure findings vary with the position of the woman. It is highest when she is sitting, lowest when she is lying in the left lateral recumbent position, and intermediate when she is supine. During the first half of pregnancy, there is a decrease in both systolic and diastolic pressure of 5 to 10 mm Hg. The decrease in blood pressure is probably the result of peripheral vasodilation from hormonal changes during pregnancy. During the third trimester, maternal blood pressure should return to the values obtained during the first trimester. Edema of the lower extremities and varicosities results from obstruction of the iliac veins and inferior vena cava by the uterus and causes increased *venous pressure.*

Blood Volume and Composition. The degree of blood volume expansion varies considerably (Pritchard, MacDonald, and Gant, 1985). Blood volume increases by approximately 1500 ml* (normal value: 8.5% to 9% of body weight). The increase is made up of 1000 ml *plasma* plus 450 ml red blood cells (RBCs). The increase in volume starts about the tenth to twelfth week, peaks at about 25% to 40% at the thirty-second to thirty-fourth week, then decreases slightly to the fortieth week. The increased volume is a protective mechanism. It is essential for (1) the hypertrophied vascular system of the enlarged uterus, (2) adequate hydration of fetal and maternal tissues when the woman assumes an erect or supine position, and (3) fluid reserve for blood loss during the delivery and puerperium. Peripheral vasodilation maintains a normal blood pressure despite the increased blood volume in pregnancy.

During pregnancy there is an accelerated production of RBCs (normal 4 to 5.5 million/mm^3). The percentage of increase depends on the amount of iron available. The RBC mass increases by 30% to 33% by term if an iron supplement is taken. It increases by only 17% in some women if no supplement is taken. For the discussion of iron therapy see Nutrition, Chapter 15.

Normal *hemoglobin* values (12 to 16 g/dl blood) and *hematocrit* values (37% to 47%) decrease. The decrease is more noticeable during the second trimester, when rapid expansion of blood volume takes place. If the hemoglobin value drops to 10 g/dl or less, or if the hematocrit drops to 35% or less, the woman is considered anemic.

The total *white cell count* increases during the second trimester and peaks during the third trimester. This increase is primarily in the leukocytes; the lymphocyte count stays about the same throughout pregnancy. See Appendix E for laboratory values during pregnancy.

Cardiac Output. Cardiac output increases from 30% to 50% by the thirty-second week of pregnancy; it declines to about a 20% increase at 40 weeks. The elevated cardiac output is largely a result of increased stroke volume and in response to increased tissue demands for oxygen (normal value is 5 to 5.5 L/min) (Fig. 10-9). The cardiac output de-

*Expansion of blood volume: primigravidas, 1250 ml; multigravidas, 1500 ml; twin pregnancies, 2000 ml.

creases with the woman in the supine position (see Chapter 8). Cardiac output increases with any exertion such as labor and delivery.

Circulation and Coagulation Times. The circulation time decreases slightly by week 32. It returns to near normal near term.

There is a greater *tendency to coagulation* during pregnancy because of increases in various clotting factors. Fibrinolytic activity (the splitting up or the dissolving of a clot) is depressed during pregnancy. During the postpartum period, fibrinolytic activity is depressed, and the woman is again more vulnerable to thrombosis.

Respiratory System

Structural and ventilatory adaptations occur during pregnancy to provide for both maternal and fetal needs. Maternal oxygen requirements increase in response to the acceleration in metabolic rate and the need to add to the tissue mass in the uterus and breasts. The conceptus requires oxygen and a way to eliminate carbon dioxide.

Anatomic Changes. Elevated levels of estrogen cause the ligaments of the rib cage to relax, permitting increased chest expansion (Fig. 10-8). In preparation for the enlarging uterus, the length of the lungs decreases. The transverse diameter of the thoracic cage increases by about 2

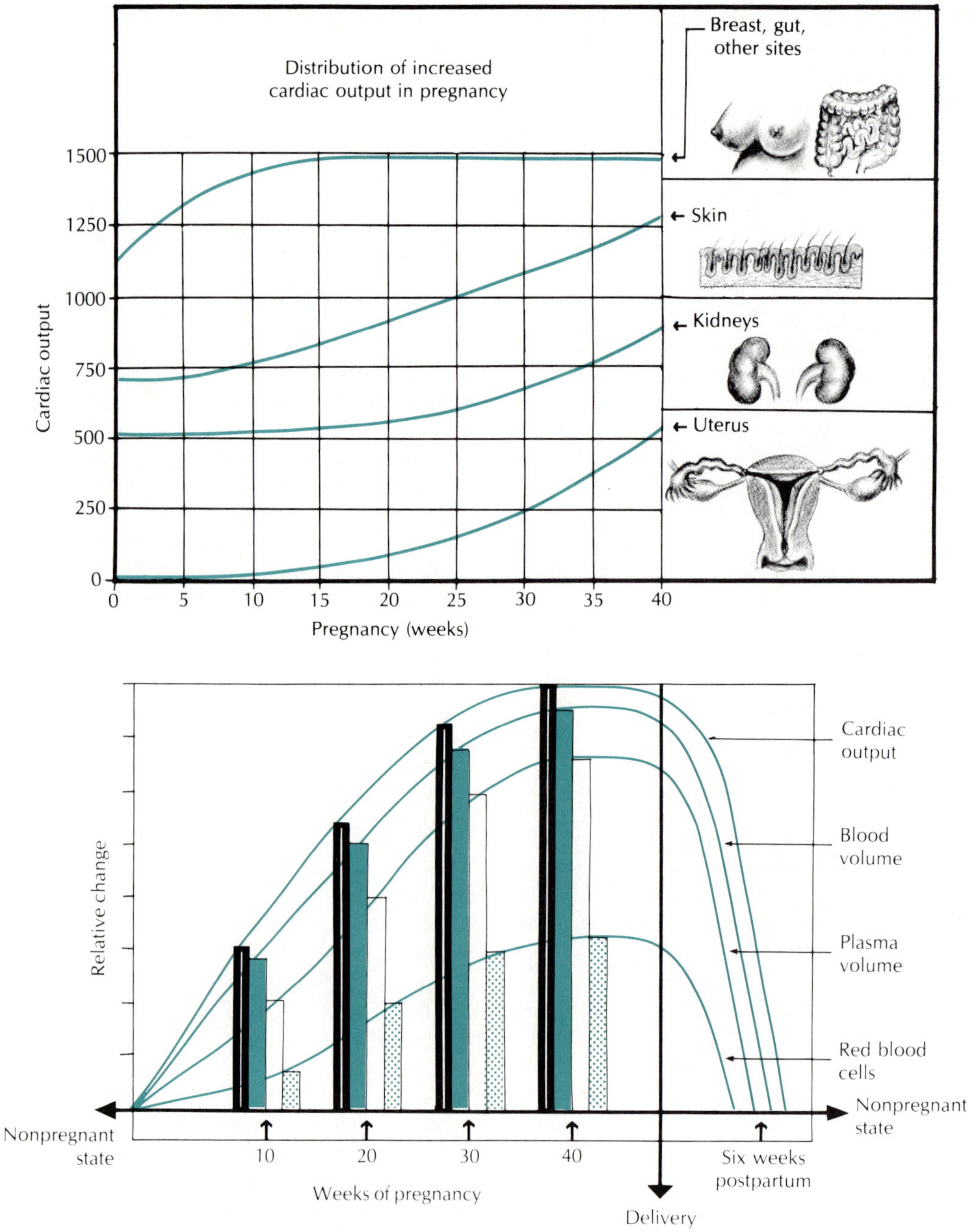

Fig. 10-9 Distribution of increased cardiac output in pregnancy.

cm (¾ in), and the circumference increases by 5 to 7 cm (2 to 2¾ in) (Pritchard, MacDonald, and Gant, 1985). The costal angle of approximately 68 degrees before pregnancy increases to about 103 degrees in the third trimester. The lower rib cage appears to flare out. After delivery, the chest may not return to its prepregnant state (Seidel et al, 1987).

The level of the diaphragm is displaced by as much as 4 cm (1½ in) during pregnancy. With advancing pregnancy, thoracic breathing replaces abdominal breathing, and descent of the diaphragm with inspiration becomes less possible.

Increased vascularization in response to elevated levels of estrogen also occurs in the upper respiratory tract. As the capillaries become engorged, edema and hyperemia develop within the nose, pharynx, larynx, trachea, and bronchi. This congestion within the tissues of the respiratory tract gives rise to several conditions commonly seen during pregnancy. These conditions include nasal and sinus stuffiness, epistaxis (nosebleed), changes in the voice, and marked inflammatory response to even a mild upper respiratory infection.

Increased vascularity also swells tympanic membranes and eustachian tubes, giving rise to symptoms of impaired hearing, earaches, or a sense of fullness in the ears.

Pulmonary Function. The pregnant woman breathes deeper (increases *tidal volume,* the amount of gases exchanged with each breath) but increases her respiratory rate only slightly (about two breaths per minute). The increase in respiratory tidal volume associated with the normal respiratory rate results in an increase in respiratory minute volume by approximately 26%. The increase in the respiratory minute volume is the *hyperventilation of pregnancy,* which is responsible for a decreased concentration of carbon dioxide in alveoli. The hyperventilation of pregnancy is apparently caused by the increased levels of progesterone, since it has been mimicked in males given progestrone (Danforth, 1986). There is a more efficient exchange of lung gases in the alveoli. The oxygen-carrying capacity of the blood is increased accordingly.

During pregnancy, changes in the respiratory center result in a lowered threshold for carbon dioxide. Progesterone and estrogen are presumed to be responsible for the increased sensitivity of the respiratory center. In addition, pregnant women experience increased awareness of the need to breathe; some may complain of dyspnea at rest.

Although pulmonary function is not impaired by pregnancy, diseases of the respiratory tract may be more serious during gestation (Pritchard, MacDonald, and Gant, 1985). One important factor may be the increased oxygen requirements.

Basal Metabolism Rate. The basal metabolism rate (BMR) usually rises by the fourth month of gestation. It is increased by 15% to 20% by term. The BMR returns to nonpregnant levels by 5 to 6 days postpartum. The elevation in BMR reflects increased oxygen demands of the uterine-placental-fetal unit, as well as oxygen consumption from increased maternal cardiac work. Peripheral vasodilation and acceleration of sweat gland activity assist in dissipating the excess heat resulting from the increased metabolism during pregnancy. Gravidas may experience heat intolerance, which is annoying to some women. **Lassitude** and **fatigability** after only slight exertion are described by many women in early pregnancy. These feelings may persist, along with a greater need for sleep. Lassitude and fatigability may be caused in part by the increased metabolic activity (see discussion of thyroid gland later in this chapter).

Acid-base Balance. By about the tenth week of pregnancy, there is a decrease of about 5 mm Hg in Pco_2. Progesterone may be responsible for increasing the sensitivity of the respiratory center receptors so that tidal volume is increased and Pco_2 falls, the base excess (HCO_3, or bicarbonate) falls, and pH rises (becomes more basic). These alterations in acid-base balance indicate that *pregnancy is a state of respiratory alkalosis* compensated by mild metabolic acidosis.

Renal System

The kidneys are vital excretory organs. Their purpose is to maintain the body's internal environment in the relatively constant homeostatic state necessary for the efficient functioning of the body at the cellular level. The kidneys are responsible for maintenance of electrolyte and acid-base balance, regulation of extracellular fluid volume, excretion of waste products, and the conservation of essential nutrients.

Anatomic Changes

Renal Pelves and Ureters. Changes in renal structure result from hormonal activity (estrogen and progesterone), pressure from an enlarging uterus, and an increase in blood volume. As early as the tenth week of pregnancy, the renal pelvis and the ureters dilate. Dilation of the ureters is more pronounced above the pelvic brim, occurring most commonly on the right side as a result of the position of the uterus. In most women the ureters below the pelvic brim are of normal size. The smooth muscle walls of the ureters undergo hyperplasia and hypertrophy and relaxed muscle tone. The ureters elongate, become tortuous, and kink. In the latter part of pregnancy, the right renal pelvis and ureter dilate more than on the left as a result of the displacement of the heavy uterus to the right by the sigmoid colon.

Because of these changes, a larger volume of urine is held in the pelves and ureters and urine flow rate is slowed. Urinary stasis or stagnation has several consequences:

1. There is a lag between the time urine is formed and when it reaches the bladder. Therefore clearance test results may reflect substances contained in glomerular filtrate several hours before.
2. Stagnated urine is an excellent medium for the growth of microorganisms. In addition, the urine of pregnant women contains greater amounts of nutrients, including glucose. Therefore, during pregnancy, women are more susceptible to urinary tract infection.

Bladder and Urethra. Bladder irritability, nocturia, and **urinary frequency** and **urgency** (without dysuria) commonly are reported in early pregnancy. Near term, bladder symptoms may return.

Urinary frequency results from increased bladder sensitivity and later from compression of the bladder (Fig. 10-7). In the second trimester the bladder is pulled up out of the true pelvis into the abdomen. The urethra lengthens to 7.5 cm (3 in) as the bladder is displaced upward. The pelvic congestion of pregnancy is reflected in hyperemia of the bladder and urethra. This increased vascularity causes the bladder mucosa to be traumatized and bleed easily. There is a decrease in bladder tone, which permits distension of the bladder to approximately 1500 ml. At the same time the bladder is compressed by the enlarging uterus, resulting in the urge to void even if the bladder contains only a small amount of urine.

The causes of dilation of the urine collection and transport system are not fully understood. It has been thought that dilation occurred mainly in response to the high levels of progesterone during pregnancy. There is some evidence that dilation is in response to mechanical pressure as well. Early in pregnancy pressure results from dilated blood vessels, and later, from the enlarging uterus compressing ureters as they pass over the pelvic brim.

Renal Function Changes. In normal pregnancy, renal function is altered considerably. Glomerular filtration rate (GFR) and renal plasma flow (RPF) increase early in pregnancy (Pritchard, MacDonald, and Gant, 1985). The woman's kidneys must manage the increased metabolic and circulatory demands of the maternal body and also excretion of fetal waste products. Changes in renal function are caused by pregnancy hormones, an increase in blood volume, the woman's posture, physical activity, and nutritional intake.

Renal function is most efficient when the woman lies in the left lateral recumbent position and least efficient when the woman assumes a supine position. When the pregnant woman is lying supine, the heavy uterus compresses the vena cava and the aorta, and cardiac output decreases. The result is a drop in maternal blood pressure and fetal heart rate (vena cava or hypotensive syndrome) and a drop in the volume of blood to the kidneys (see Fig. 10-9). When cardiac output drops, blood flow to the brain and heart is continued at the expense of other organs, including the kidneys and uterus.

Fluid and Electrolyte Balance

Sodium Balance. Selective renal tubular reabsorption maintains sodium and water balance regardless of changes in dietary intake and losses through sweat, vomitus, or diarrhea. From 500 to 900 mEq of sodium is normally retained during pregnancy to meet fetal needs. The need for increased maternal intravascular and extracellular fluid volume requires additional sodium to expand fluid volume and to maintain an isotonic state. To prevent excessive sodium depletion, the maternal kidneys undergo a significant adaptation by increasing tubular reabsorption. As efficient as the renal system is, it can be overstressed by excessive dietary sodium intake or restriction or by use of diuretics. *Severe hypovolemia and reduced placental perfusion are two consequences.*

Water Balance. The capacity of the kidneys to excrete water during the early weeks of pregnancy is more efficient than later in pregnancy. Occasionally in early pregnancy the extent of water loss may cause some women to feel thirsty. The pooling of fluid in the legs in the latter part of pregnancy decreases renal blood flow and GFR. The diuretic response to the water load is triggered when the woman lies down, preferrably on her left side, and the pooled fluid reenters general circulation. This pooling of blood in the lower legs is sometimes referred to as **physiologic edema,** which requires no treatment.

Nutrient Excretion Including Glucose. Under normal circumstances the kidney reabsorbs almost all of the glucose and other nutrients from the plasma filtrate. In pregnant women tubular reabsorption of glucose is impaired so that glucosuria does occur at varying times and to varying degrees. Normal values are 0 to 20 mg/dl. That is, during any one day the urine is sometimes positive and sometimes negative. When it is positive, the amount of glucose varies from 1+ to 4+.

In nonpregnant women, blood glucose levels must be at 160 to 180 mg/dl before glucose is "spilled" into the urine (not reabsorbed). During pregnancy, glucosuria occurs when maternal glucose levels are lower than 160 mg/dl. Why glucose, as well as other nutrients such as amino acids, is wasted during pregnancy is not understood, nor has the exact mechanism been discovered. Although glucosuria may be found in normal pregnancies (indeed 1+ levels may be seen with increased anxiety states), the possibility of diabetes mellitus must be kept in mind (see Chapter 32).

Proteinuria. Albumin and globulin are proteins that are not normal constituents of urine at any time. Small (trace) amounts of protein may occasionally be found in concentrated urine or in first-voided urine following sleep. However, a measurable amount (over 150 mg in 24 hours) of protein in the urine is a significant sign of renal disease at any time.

Integumentary System

Alterations in hormonal balance and mechanical stretching are responsible for several changes in the integumentary system during pregnancy. General changes include increases in skin thickness and subdermal fat, hyperpigmentation, hair and nail growth, accelerated sweat and sebaceous gland activity, and increased circulation and vasomotor activity. There is greater fragility of cutaneous elastic tissues, resulting in striae gravidarum, or stretch marks. Cutaneous allergic responses are enhanced.

Pigmentation is caused by the anterior pituitary hormone melanotropin, which is increased during pregnancy. Facial melasma, also called **chloasma** or **mask of pregnancy,** is a blotchy, brownish hyperpigmentation of the skin over the malar prominences and the forehead, especially in dark-complexioned expectant women. Chloasma appears in 50% to 70% of pregnant women, beginning after the sixteenth week and increasing gradually to delivery. The sun intensifies this pigmentation in susceptible women. Chloasma caused by normal pregnancy usually fades after delivery. Darkening of the nipples, areolae, axillae, and vulva occurs at about the same time.

The **linea nigra** is a pigmented line extending from the symphysis pubis to the top of the fundus in the midline; this line is known as the linea alba before hormone-induced pigmentation. In primigravidas the extension of the linea nigra, beginning in the third month, keeps pace with the rising height of the fundus; in multigravidas the entire line often appears earlier than the third month.

Striae gravidarum, or stretch marks, which appear in 50% to 90% of gravidas during the second half of pregnancy, may be caused by action of adrenocorticosteroids. Striae reflect separation within the underlying connective (collagen) tissue of the skin. These slightly depressed streaks tend to occur over areas of maximal stretch (i.e., abdomen, thighs, and breasts). The stretching sometimes causes a sensation that resembles itching. Tendency to the development of striae may be familial. After delivery they usually fade, although they never disappear completely. In the multipara, in addition to the reddish striae of the present pregnancy, glistening silvery lines representing the cicatrices (scars) of previous striae are commonly seen.

Angiomas or telangiectasias are commonly referred to as **vascular spiders**. They are tiny, stellate or branched, slightly raised and pulsating end-arterioles. The spiders, a result of elevated levels of circulating estrogen, are usually found on the neck, thorax, face, and arms. They are also described as focal networks of dilated arterioles radiating about a central core. The spiders are bluish in color and do not blanch with pressure. Striae may be evident on the breasts as a result of stretching as they increase in size. Vascular spiders appear during the second to the fifth month of pregnancy in 65% of white women and 10% of black women. The spiders usually disappear after delivery.

Pinkish red, diffuse mottling or well-defined blotches are seen over the palmar surfaces of the hands in about 60% of white women and 35% of black women during pregnancy (Pritchard, MacDonald, and Gant, 1985). These pigmentation changes and **palmar erythema** may also be seen in women taking oral hormonal contraceptives.

Epulis (gingival granuloma gravidarum) is a red, raised nodule on the gums that bleeds easily. This lesion may develop around the third month and usually continues to enlarge as pregnancy progresses. Treatment by excision is initiated only if it becomes excessive in size, causes pain, or bleeds excessively.

By the sixth week some women notice **thinning and softening of the fingernails and toenails.** Nail polish and nail polish remover may need to be discontinued and the nails kept short to prevent breakage. **Oily skin** and **acne vulgaris** may occur during pregnancy. For other women the skin clears and looks radiant. **Hirsutism** is commonly reported. An increase in fine hair growth may occur. The fine hair tends to disappear after pregnancy. Growth of coarse or bristly hair does not usually disappear after pregnancy. Some women comment that their hair is thickest and most abundant during pregnancy.

Musculoskeletal System

The gradually changing body and increasing weight of the pregnant woman cause marked alterations in posture (Fig. 10-10) and walking. The great abdominal distension that gives the pelvis a forward tilt, decreased abdominal muscle tone, and increased weight bearing in late pregnancy require a realignment of the spinal curvatures. The woman's center of gravity shifts forward. An increase in the normal lumbosacral curve develops, and a compensatory curvature in the cervicodorsal region (exaggerated anterior flexion of the head) is required to maintain balance. Large breasts and a stoop-shouldered stance will further accentuate the lumbar and dorsal curves. Locomotion is more

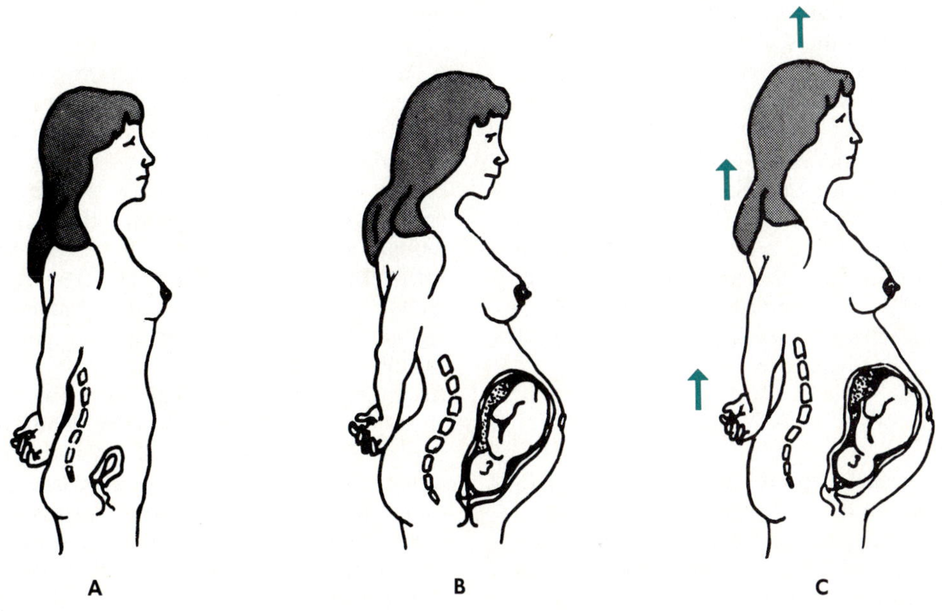

Fig. 10-10 Postural changes during pregnancy. **A**, Nonpregnant. **B**, Incorrect posture. **C**, Correct posture.

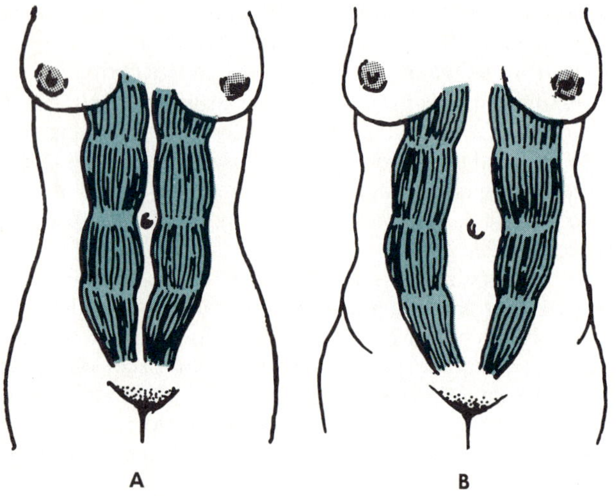

Fig. 10-11 Possible change in rectus abdominis muscles during pregnancy. **A**, Normal position in nonpregnant woman. **B**, Diastasis recti in pregnant woman.

difficult, and the waddling gait of the gravid woman, called "the proud walk of pregnancy" by Shakespeare, is well known. The ligamentous and muscular structures of the mid and lower spine may be severely stressed. These and related changes often cause musculoskeletal discomfort.

The young, well-muscled woman may tolerate these changes without complaint. However, older women or those with a back disorder or a faulty sense of balance may have a considerable amount of back pain during and just after pregnancy.

Slight relaxation and increased mobility of the pelvic joints are normal during pregnancy. This is secondary to exaggerated elasticity and softening of connective and collagen tissue, and the result of increased circulating steroid sex hormones. These adaptations permit enlargement of pelvic dimensions. The degree of relaxation varies, but considerable separation of the symphysis pubis and the instability of the sacroiliac joints may cause pain and difficulty in walking. Obesity and multiple pregnancy tend to increase the pelvic disability.

The muscles of the abdominal wall stretch and ultimately lose some tone. During the third trimester the rectus abdominis muscles may separate (Fig. 10-11), allowing abdominal contents to protrude at the midline. The umbilicus flattens or protrudes. After delivery, the muscles gradually regain tone. However, **diastasis** (separation) **of the rectus abdominis muscles** may persist. The maternal pelvis is discussed in detail in Chapter 16.

Neurologic System

Little is known regarding specific alterations in function of the neurologic system during pregnancy, aside from hypothalamic-pituitary neurohormonal changes. Specific physiologic alterations resulting from pregnancy may cause the following neurologic or neuromuscular symptomatology:

1. Compression of pelvic nerves or vascular stasis caused by enlargement of the uterus may result in sensory changes in the legs.
2. Dorsolumbar lordosis may cause pain because of traction on nerves or compression of nerve roots.
3. Edema involving the peripheral nerves may result in *carpal tunnel syndrome* during the last trimester. The edema compresses the median nerve beneath the carpal ligament of the wrist. The syndrome is characterized by paresthesia (abnormal sensation such as burning or tingling because of a disorder of the sensory nervous system) and pain in the hand, radiating to the elbow. The dominant hand is usually affected most.
4. Acroesthesia (numbness and tingling of the hands) is caused by the stoop-shouldered stance assumed by some women during pregnancy. The condition is associated with traction on segments of the brachial plexus.
5. Tension headache is common when anxiety or uncertainty complicates gestation. However, vision problems such as refractive errors, sinusitis, or migraine may also be responsible for headaches.
6. "Lightheadedness," faintness, and even syncope (fainting) are common during early pregnancy. Vasomotor instability, postural hypotension, or hypoglycemia may be responsible.
7. Hypocalcemia may cause neuromuscular problems such as muscle cramps or tetany.

Gastrointestinal System

The functioning of the gastrointestinal tract during pregnancy presents a curiously interesting picture. The appetite increases. Intestinal secretion is reduced. Liver function is altered, and absorption of nutrients is enhanced. The colon is displaced laterally upward and posteriorly. Peristaltic activity (motility) decreases. As a result bowel sounds are diminished, and constipation, nausea, and vomiting are common. Blood flow to the pelvis increases as does venous pressure, contributing to hemorrhoid formation in later pregnancy.

Mouth. The gums are hyperemic, spongy, and swollen. They tend to bleed easily because the rising level of estrogen cause selective increased vascularity and connective tissue proliferation (a nonspecific gingivitis). There is no increase in secretion of saliva. Women do complain of **(ptylism)** (excessive salivation). This perceived increase is thought to be caused by the decrease in unconscious swallowing by the woman when nauseated. Epulis and bleeding gums are discussed under Integumentary System.

Teeth. The pregnant woman requires about 1.2 g of calcium and approximately the same amount of phosphorus every day during pregnancy. This is an increase of about 0.4 g of each of these elements over nonpregnant needs. With a well-balanced diet (see Chapter 15), these requirements are satisfied. Serious dietary deficiency, however, may deplete the mother's osseous stores of these elements but does not draw on calcium in her teeth. Demineralization of teeth does not occur during pregnancy. Hence the old adage "for every child a tooth" is untrue. Poor dental hygiene during pregnancy or anytime and gingivitis may contribute to dental caries, which could result in the loss of a tooth.

Esophagus, Stomach, and Intestine. Herniation of the upper portion of the stomach *(hiatal hernia)* occurs after the seventh or eighth month of pregnancy in about 15% to 20% of gravidas. This condition results from upward displacement of the stomach, which causes a widening of the hiatus of the diaphragm. It occurs more often in multiparas and older or obese women.

Increased estrogen production causes decreased secretion of hydrochloric acid. Therefore peptic ulcer formation or flare-up of existing peptic ulcers is uncommon during pregnancy.

Increased progesterone production causes decreased tone and motility of smooth muscles, so that there is esophageal regurgitation, decreased emptying time of the stomach, and reverse peristalsis. As a result the woman may experience "acid indigestion" or *heartburn* (pyrosis).

In response to increased needs during pregnancy, iron is absorbed more readily in the small intestine. In general, if the individual is deficient in iron, iron absorption is increased.

Increased progesterone (causing loss of muscle tone and decreased peristalsis) results in an increase in water absorption from the colon. **Constipation** may result. In addition, constipation is secondary to hypoperistalsis (sluggishness of the bowel), unusual food choice, lack of fluids, abdominal distension by the pregnant uterus, and displacement of intestines with some compression. *Hemorrhoids* (varicose veins of the rectum and anus) may be everted or may bleed during straining at stool. Bowel habits and a characteristic type of stool are established early in life. Variations will be noted with concern and may be perceived as a disease process. A mild ileus (sluggishness, lack of movement) that follows delivery, as well as postdelivery fluid loss and perineal discomfort, contributes to continuing constipation.

Gallbladder and Liver. The gallbladder is quite often distended by hypotonic during pregnancy. Decreased emptying time and thickening of bile are typical. These features, together with slight hypercholesterolemia from increased progesterone levels, may account for the common development of *gallstones* during pregnancy.

Hepatic function is difficult to appraise during gestation. However, only minor changes in liver function develop during pregnancy. Occasionally, intrahepatic cholestasis (retention and accumulation of bile in the liver, caused by factors within the liver) in response to placental steroids, occurs late in pregnancy and may result in *pruritus gravidarum* (severe itching) with or without jaundice. Oatmeal baths and lotions help ease the itching. These distressing symptoms subside promptly after delivery.

Abdominal Discomfort. Intraabdominal alterations that can cause discomfort include pelvic heaviness or pressure, round ligament tension, flatulence, distension and bowel cramping, and uterine contractions. In addition to displacement of intestines, pressure from the expanding uterus increases venous pressure in the pelvic organs. Although most abdominal discomfort is a consequence of normal maternal alterations, the physician is constantly alert to the possibility of disorders such as bowel obstruction or an inflammatory process.

Appendicitis (see Fig. 34-2) may be difficult to diagnose. The *appendix* is displaced upward and laterally, high and to the right, away from McBurney's point.

Endocrine System

Profound endocrine changes occur that are essential for pregnancy maintenance, normal fetal growth, and postpartum recovery. Metabolic changes and weight gain are discussed in detail in Chapter 15. Each hormone, its source and principal effects, and clinical significance are described in Table 10-3.

Thyroid Gland. During pregnancy there is slight enlargement of the thyroid gland caused by hyperplasia of the glandular tissue and increased vascularity (Pritchard, MacDonald, and Gant, 1985; Danforth and Scott, 1986). Oxygen consumption and BMR increase secondary to the metabolic activity of the products of conception. For a discussion of changes in thyroid hormone production see Pritchard, MacDonald, and Gant (1985); and Danforth and Scott (1986).

Parathyroid Gland. Pregnancy induces a slight secondary hyperparathyroidism, a reflection of increased requirements for calcium and vitamin D. When the needs for growth of the fetal skeleton are greatest (during the last half of pregnancy), plasma parathormone levels are elevated; that is, the peak level occurs between 15 and 35 weeks' gestation.

Pancreas. The fetus requires significant amounts of glucose for its growth and development. To meet its need for fuel, the fetus not only depletes the store of maternal glucose but also decreases the mother's ability to synthesize glucose by siphoning off her amino acids. Maternal blood glucose levels fall. Maternal insulin does *not* cross the placenta to the fetus. As a result, in early pregnancy, the pancreas decreases its production of insulin.

However, as pregnancy continues, the placenta grows and produces progressively larger amounts of hormones (i.e., [hPL] hCS, estrogen, and progesterone) (Table 10-3). Cortisol production by the adrenals also increases. Estrogen, progesterone, hPL, and cortisol collectively decrease the mother's ability to utilize insulin. Cortisol stimulates increased production of insulin but also increases the mother's peripheral resistance to insulin (i.e., the tissues cannot use the insulin). Insulinase is an enzyme produced by the placenta to deactivate maternal insulin. Decreasing the mother's ability to utilize her own insulin is a protective mechanism that ensures an ample supply of glucose for the needs of the fetoplacental unit.

The result is an added demand for insulin by the gravida. The normal beta cells of the islets of Langerhans in the pancreas can meet the demand for insulin that continues to increase at a steady rate until term (for a discussion of gestational diabetes mellitus, see Chapter 32).

Pituitary Prolactin. In pregnancy, serum prolactin begins to rise in the first trimester and increases progressively

Table 10-3 *Hormonal Factors in Pregnancy*

Hormone and Source	Principal Effects	Clinical Significance
Fetoplacental Unit		
Estrogen: produced by ovary and adrenal cortex as in prepregnant state; however, principal source is placenta; synthesized from precursors from fetal liver and adrenals; increase in level of E_3 (estriol) by end of fourth week, by end of pregnancy, 300 × normal; however, low potency of E_3 means estrogenic activity only 30 × normal	Level of circulating estriol rises in pregnancy and so increases in urine and amniotic fluid	Urinary excretion of 30-40 mg/24 hr of estriol by end of pregnancy—an indication of fetal well-being (must be repeated, i.e., serial): Significant decrease indicates fetus in jeopardy (or fetal death) Excessive increase may indicate multiple pregnancy, erythroblastosis fetalis
	Enlargement of uterus: Hypertrophy of musculature Proliferation of endometrium Increase in blood supply	Probable sign of pregnancy Continued growth indicates pregnancy advancing
	Enlargement of breast Growth of glandular tissue ducts, alveoli, nipples	Breast tenderness
	Deposition of fat	
	Enlargement of genitals	Growth of vagina permits passage of infant
	Nutrient metabolism altered: Increases elastic properties of connective tissue (relaxation of pubic joints and pelvic ligaments; cervix enlarges, softens, is stretchable [theory])	Softening of connective tissue: Backache, tenderness over pubic area, flank pain Cervical dilation
	Decreased secretion of HCl, pepsin	Digestive upsets, nausea, decreased absorption of fat
	Affects thyroid function: thyroxine production increases, but so does production of thyroxine-binding globulin	No major increase in free thyroxine (BMR rises primarily as result of increased oxygen consumption with growth of uterus, fetus, placenta)
	Interferes with folic acid metabolism	
	Increase in total body proteins	Positive nitrogen balance: protein available for fetal growth
	Sodium and water retention by kidney tubules	Increased plasma volume and interstitial fluid volume→edema, fluid reserve
	Hematologic changes: Hypercoagulability of blood Decrease in fibrinolytic activity Increase in sedimentation rate (SR)	Safety mechanism vs. hemorrhage Tendency for thrombosis to occur (legs) Affects use in clinical diagnosis using SR tests (no diagnostic value)
	Vascular changes: Telangiectasias (spider nevi) Palmar erythema	No clinical significance; changes usually disappear after pregnancy
	Stimulation of production of melanin-stimulating hormone	Hyperpigmentation (chloasma, linea nigra, areolar tissue, genitals)
Progesterone: produced by corpus luteum (Fig. 10-1) for 2 months and by placental trophoblastic cells from about 8-10 days after conception; rises steadily through pregnancy	Promotes development of decidual (secretory) cells in endometrium	Glycogen deposits support nutrition of embryo
	Decreases contractility of gravid uterus	Prevents uterine contractions from causing spontaneous abortion
	Promotes development of secretory portions of lobular-alveolar system	Prepares breasts for lactation
	Nutrient effects: Favors maternal fat deposition	Nutritional significance: Energy available for maternal and fetal needs
	Reduced gastric motility, sphincters relaxed	Regurgitation (heartburn); small, frequent feedings tolerated
	Increases sodium excretion	Hyponatremia may develop
	Increases sensitivity of respiratory center to CO_2	Respiratory rate increases; decreased alveolar and arterial P_{CO_2} (feeling of breathlessness)

Table 10-3 *Hormonal Factors in Pregnancy—cont'd*

Hormone and Source	Principal Effects	Clinical Significance
Progesterone—cont'd		
	Reduces tone of smooth muscle	Colonic activity diminishes (constipation) Reduced tone of bladder and ureters (distension, urinary stasis, urinary tract infections) Vascular tone decreases (venous dilation; stasis in lower limbs with edema, varicosities) Decreased tone in gallbladder: reduced motility; incidence of gallbladder disease increases
	Raises body temperature 0.5° C	Feelings of warmth, perspiration increases
Human chorionic gonadotropin (hCG): produced by syncytiotrophoblast; peak level by day 60-70 of gestation, levels fall after fourth month, disappear 2 weeks after pregnancy ends	Maintenance of corpus luteum in early pregnancy	Corpus luteum not necessary after first few weeks—placenta produces sufficient hormones
	Exerts interstitial-cell-stimulating effect on testes of male fetus	Testosterone levels in male fetus rise
	May have immunologic properties	May inhibit lymphocyte response to foreign protein, the fetal portion of placenta
	May cause allergic response	May be cause of hyperemesis gravidarum Diagnostic value: Persistence of hCG after spontaneous abortion symptomatic of hydatidiform mole or choriocarcinoma Basis for hormone test for pregnancy Decreased level in threatened abortion Increased level with multiple pregnancies
Human placental lactogen (hPL) or chorionic growth hormone (CGH) (also called human chorionic somatomammotropic hormone [hCS]) produced by syncytiotrophoblast; detectable by week 5 or 6; rises steadily, disappears 2 weeks after delivery	Similar action to pituitary growth hormone: Glucose metabolism: Decreases use of glucose for energy by maternal organism by increasing lipolysis to make fatty acids available for energy (carbohydrate sparer)	Glucose metabolism changes result in: Glucose available for fetal energy needs (only energy source for fetus)
	Glycogen deposition increased, cells saturated (inhibits glyconeogenesis), causing blood glucose levels to rise	Diabetogenic effect in mother (increased blood glucose levels stimulate beta cells of islets of Langerhans to produce more insulin)—may "burn out," producing diabetes mellitus
	Carbohydrates and insulin required for hormone activity	Fetal pancreas produces insulin by week 12; maternal insulin does not cross placenta; fetal pancreas may overproduce if continuous hyperglycemic stimulus is present; at birth infant becomes hypoglycemic and brain growth is endangered
	Protein metabolism: Increases protein synthesis Decreases breakdown and utilization of protein for energy (mobilizes free fatty acids; if excessive, may cause ketosis)	Protein metabolism: Protein available for fetal and maternal growth needs
	Acts synergistically with hydrocortisone and insulin in development of alveoli of breast (lactogenic effect)	Preparation of breasts for lactation
	Amount secreted depends on size of placenta	Research to determine whether level of circulating hPL (hCS, CGH) an indicator of normal pregnancy

Continued.

Table 10-3 *Hormonal Factors in Pregnancy—cont'd*

Hormone and Source	Principal Effects	Clinical Significance
Origin: Multiple Organs		
Prostaglandins: widely distributed in human body, including seminal fluid, brain, nerves, most endocrine organs, endometrium, decidua, and amniotic fluid	Reproductive system: play a role in erection, ejaculation, ovulation, formation of corpus luteum, uterine motility, parturition, and milk ejection Cardiovascular system: play a role in platelet aggregation, blood pressure increase	Prostaglandins are used to induce labor in second-trimester abortions; may be used (research in progress) for induction of labor at term
Ovary, Corpus Luteum		
Relaxin	Present in many mammalian species and may serve to: Promote cervical softening Remodel collagen	Same as principal effects
Pituitary		
Pituitary growth hormone: produced by anterior pituitary	Decreases markedly during pregnancy and rises slowly to prepregnancy level 6-8 weeks after delivery	May be reason why insulin requirements decrease after delivery (hPL ↓ with delivery of placenta)
Follicle-stimulating hormone (FSH): produced by anterior pituitary	Decreases markedly during pregnancy; remains low for 10-12 days after delivery Increases then to follicular-phase concentrations during third week after delivery	Ovulation ceases during pregnancy See Hypothalamic-pituitary-ovarian function, Chapter 42
Prolactin (PRL): produced by anterior pituitary	Lactation: stimulates production of fat, lactose, and casein by mammary glandular cells after placenta is delivered May play role in regulation of fluid exchange across fetal membranes, lung maturation, and pregnancy maintenance	Milk not produced prenatally despite high levels because high levels of estrogen have a local inhibitory effect on mammary gland
Melanocyte-stimulating hormone: produced by anterior pituitary	Causes darkening of integument and nevi: chloasma; linea nigra; darkening of nipples, areolae, and vulva	Pigmentation changes are objective, presumptive signs of pregnancy; usually fade after delivery
Beta-endorphins and encephalins: produced by middle lobe of pituitary	Display analgesic properties	Discomfort is lessened or made more tolerable
Oxytocin: produced by *posterior* pituitary	Causes uterus to contract Action suppressed by action of progesterone until production of oxytocin exceeds that of progesterone Stimulates myoepithelial cells in mammary glands to eject milk	May be used to induce or augment labor Spurt of oxytocin during expulsive phase of labor to ensure efficient muscle contraction during and immediately after birth Sensory receptors in nipple stimulate release of oxytocin via reflex arc. During lactation oxytocin stimulates myoepithelial cells in the mammary gland to eject milk
Thyroid Gland		
Thyroxine: produced by thyroid gland with stimulation from anterior pituitary	Gland enlargement with 20% increase in function: BMR increased to 25% near term; BMR returns to nonpregnant level within 1 week after delivery; return to normal size, within 6 weeks	Woman may experience palpitations, tachycardia, emotional lability, heat intolerance, fatigability, and increased perspiration

to term. It is generally believed that although all the hormonal elements (estrogen, progresterone, thyroid, insulin, and free cortisol) necessary for breast growth and milk production are present in elevated concentrations during pregnancy, the high levels of estrogen inhibit active alveolar secretion by blocking the binding of prolactin to breast tissue, thus inhibiting the milk-producing effect of prolactin on the target epithelium (Danforth and Scott, 1986).

Endocrine System and Maternal Nutrition

Progesterone causes the deposit of fat in subcutaneous tissues over the abdomen, back, and upper thighs. The fat serves as an energy reserve for both pregnancy and lactation. Several other hormones affect nutrition. *Aldosterone* conserves sodium. *Thyroxin* regulates metabolism. *Parathyroid hormone* controls calcium and magnesium metabolism. *Human placental lactogen (hPL)* acts as a growth hormone. *Human chorionic gonadotropin (hCG)* induces nausea and vomiting in some women in early pregnancy.

SUMMARY

The intimate union of mother and fetus is referred to as the fetoplacental maternal unit. Because the maternal organism responds as a total unit to the developing fetus, the intrauterine environment of the fetus is maintained at an optimal level only to the extent that the mother's systems can adjust to the developing organism.

Adaptation to pregnancy involves all of a woman's body systems. The mother's physical response is assessed in relation to normal expected alterations. Subjective symptoms and objective signs arising from these changes serve as a basis for diagnosis of pregnancy.

KEY CONCEPTS

- The biochemical, physiologic, and anatomic adaptations that occur during the short span of human pregnancy are profound and return almost completely to the pre-pregnancy state following delivery and lactation.
- Maternal adaptations are attributed to the hormones of pregnancy and to mechanical pressures arising from the enlarging uterus and other tissues.
- The understanding of these adaptations to pregnancy remains a major goal, for without such knowledge it is difficult, if not impossible, to understand the disease processes—pregnancy-induced or coincidental—that can threaten women during pregnancy and the puerperium.
- The ability to recognize the beta subunit of hCG through monoclonal antibody technology has revolutionized endocrine tests for pregnancy.
- Adaptations to pregnancy protect the woman's normal physiologic functioning, meet the metabolic demands pregnancy imposes on her body, and provide for fetal developmental and growth needs.
- The rise in pH of the pregnant woman's vaginal secretions makes her more vulnerable to vaginal infections.
- Increased vascularity and sensitivity of the vagina and other pelvic viscera may lead to a high degree of sexual interest and arousal.
- Some adaptations to pregnancy result in discomforts such as fatigue, urinary frequency, nausea, and breast sensitivity.
- Balance and coordination are affected by changes in joints and the woman's center of gravity as pregnancy progresses.

STUDY QUESTIONS AND ACTIVITIES

1. Spend several hours observing and participating at a prenatal clinic.
   a. What anatomical adaptations to pregnancy did you observe or assess?
   b. Were any physiologic adaptations to pregnancy apparent? If so, what?
   c. What complaints or questions were asked by clients (gravidas and spouse, or other) related to anatomic or physiologic changes?
2. Interview three pregnant women (and spouse, or other, if present) at different stages of their pregnancy:
   a. How does each feel about changes in her body related to anatomic and physiologic adaptations?
   b. Which changes do they find pleasant?
   c. Which changes do they find uncomfortable or troublesome?
   d. What is their level of understanding of these adaptations?
   e. Does the nurse in the clinic function as a teacher?
3. Prepare a class for expectant mothers (parents) in which they discuss adaptations.
4. Explore own emotions and attitudes regarding the changes a woman's body undergoes during pregnancy.
5. Observe demonstrations of the various pregnancy tests described in the text; then choose one test and prepare an explanation suitable for client education of how that test works.

References

Batzer, FR: Guidelines for choosing a pregnancy test, Contemp OB/GYN 26:37, October 1985 (special issue)

Batzer, FR: Test kits for ovulation and pregnancy, Contemp OB/GYN 28:7, October 1986 (special issue)

Brucker, MC, and MacMullen, NJ: What's new in pregnancy tests? JOGN Nurs 14:353, Sept-Oct 1985

Danforth, DN, and Scott, JR editors: Obstetrics and gynecology, ed 5, Philadelphia, 1986, JB Lippincott Co, Inc

Doshi, ML: Accuracy of consumer performed in-home tests for early pregnancy detection, Am J Public Health, 76:512, 1986

Pritchard, JA, MacDonald, PC, and Gant, NF: Williams obstetrics, ed 17, Norwalk, Conn, 1985, Appleton-Century-Crofts

Resnik, R: What controls uterine blood flow? Contemp OB/GYN 19(6):111, 1982

Seidel, HM, et al: Mosby's guide to physical examination, St Louis, 1987, The CV Mosby Co

Bibliography

Barron, WM, and Lindheimer, MD: Basics: renal function during pregnancy, Contemp OB/GYN 21(5):179, 1983

Calguneri, M, et al: Changes in joint laxity occurring during pregnancy, Ann Rheum Dis 41:126, 1982

Diamond, S: Headaches, Clinical Symposia, CIBA 33:2, 1981

Gibbs, CE: Sudden sensorium derangement during pregnancy, Contemp OB/GYN 20:39, 1982

Goodlin, RC, et al: Clinical signs of normal plasma volume expansion during pregnancy, Am J Obstet Gynecol 145:1001, 1983

Malasanos, L, et al: Health assessment, ed 3, St Louis, 1985, The CV Mosby Co

Miller, BK: How to spot . . . and treat . . . carpal tunnel syndrome . . . early, Nursing '80 10:50, 1980

National Foundation—March of Dimes: Maternal assessment: urine evaluation, series 2, Prenatal care, module 2, part A, White Plains, New York, 1979

News: Monoclonals: new frontiers in reproductive medicine in Technology 1986, Contemp OB/GYN 26:75, October 1985

Ozanne, P, et al: Erythrocyte aggregation during normal pregnancy, Am J Obstet Gynecol 146:576, 1983

Patterson, JA: Lab tests to establish prenatal profile, Contemp Obstet Gynecol 18:29, 1981 (special issue)

Rosen, T, and Mills, J: Tattletale lesions: could this be a "stretchmark"? RN 46(2):49, 1983.

Samples, JT, et al: The dynamic characteristics of the circumvaginal muscles, JOGN Nurs 17(3):194, 1988

Stauffer, RA, et al: Gallbladder disease in pregnancy, Am J Obstet Gynecol 144:661, 1982

Urban, DJ, et al: Nurse specialization in reproductive endocrinology, JOGN Nurs 11(3):167, 1982

van Geelen, JM: The urethral pressure profile in pregnancy and after delivery in healthy nulliparous women, Am J Obstet Gynecol 144:636, 1982

Walls, JL: Diagnosis and treatment of meralgia paresthetica, Nurs Pract 9:43, 1984

Walters, CA, et al: Human myometrium: a new potential source of prolactin, Am J Obstet Gynecol 147:639, 1983

Willson, JR, Carrington, ER, and Ledger, WJ: Obstetrics and gynecology, ed 8, St Louis, 1988, The CV Mosby Co

CHAPTER 11

Family Dynamics of Pregnancy

Learning Objectives

Correctly define the key terms listed.

Examine maternal adaptation to pregnancy in regard to acceptance, identification with motherhood role, family relationships, and anticipation of labor.

Examine paternal adaptation to pregnancy in regard to acceptance, identification with fatherhood role, family relationships, and anticipation of labor.

Discuss sibling adaptation to pregnancy.

Discuss grandparent adaptation to pregnancy.

Evaluate pregnancy after age 35.

Determine appropriate content for classes designed for the first, second, third, and "fourth" trimesters of pregnancy.

Review "Education for choice."

Explain parent preparation for cesarean birth.

Explain sibling preparation for the birth of a child.

Explain grandparent preparation for the birth of a child.

Key Terms

ambivalence
announcement phase
body boundaries
claiming
couvade
developmental tasks
educational diagnosis
expressive style
fantasy child
focusing phase
grandparental adaptation
informed choice
instrumental style
maternal adaptation
mitleiden
mood changes
moratorium phase
observer style
paternal adaptation
readiness for pregnancy
sibling adaptation
support

Pregnancy involves all family members. "Conception is the beginning, not only of a growing fetus but also of the family in a new form with an additional member and with changed relationships" (Grossman et al., 1980). Family members react to pregnancy and interpret its meaning in light of their own needs, as well as the needs of the others affected. The process of family adaptation to pregnancy takes place within a cultural environment. "Culture provides the medium through which life experiences are interpreted" (Glass, 1983; Stainton, 1985b). (Chapter 2 discusses cultural influences in greater depth.)

The role of women has changed in Western societies, since women have moved out of the home and participated actively in the economic, social, and political life of their communities.

The changing role of mother has resulted in a corresponding role change for many men. The role of father now includes more direct participation in preparation for birth, in the birth process, and in caring for the child.

Pregnancy confronts both mother and father with new tasks. They need to prepare a nurturing and safe environment for the unborn, as well as newly born child. During pregnancy, parents' identities change and the possibilities and responsibilities of their new roles are explored. In addition, the process of negotiating and preparing for new roles (sibling roles, grandparent roles) for family members is undertaken by the mother and father.

MATERNAL ADAPTATION

Pregnant women, a varied population, ranging from teenagers to women in their forties, use the 9 months of pregnancy to adapt to the maternal role. The maternal role is a complex, social and cognitive process that is not intuitive but is learned (Rubin, 1967a). In becoming a mother the teenager shifts from being mothered to mothering. The adult moves from "well-established routines to the unpredictable context created by an infant" (Mercer, 1981). Pregnancy for the primigravida is the "period of transition between two lifestyles—two states of being: the woman without child and the woman with child" (Lederman, 1984). For the multigravida the transition is from woman with child to woman with children.

Pregnancy can be described as a developmental change as modifications take place in the woman's self and body in preparation for a new level of caring and responsibility. The dynamic interaction between intrapsychic and biologic processes functions to change the woman's self-concept in readiness for parenthood. The woman is involved in a reassessment of her "self-image, beliefs, values, priorities, behavior patterns, relationships with others and problem-solving skills" (Lederman, 1984). As a result of adapting to the maternal role the mother moves from being self-contained and independent to being committed to a life-long concern for another human being. There appears to be a gradual unfolding characterized by a "progressive emphasis in the mother's way of thinking away from the single self and toward the mother-baby unit" (Lederman, 1984). Most women are successful in adapting during the period of pregnancy. They experience stress but not necessarily intense conflict (Grossman et al., 1980; Leifer, 1980; Wolkind and Zajicek, 1981).

To accomplish the changes in herself the mother undertakes certain developmental tasks. These have been described as identifying with the role of mother, accepting the pregnancy, reordering the relationships between mother and daughter and between husband and wife, establishing a relationship with the unborn child, and preparing for the birth experience (Deutch, 1945; Caplan, 1959; Rubin, 1967a, b; Lederman, 1984; Stainton, 1985b). The mental processes accompanying the developmental tasks continue throughout pregnancy. In normal circumstances the mental processes are progressive toward a period of readiness, just before term, in which birth seems to be an essential prerequisite to further development of feelings toward the child. Studies of the interpersonal context of pregnancy have shown a relationship between the accomplishment of these developmental tasks and the extent to which the pregnant woman perceives her social relationships to be supportive of the pregnancy and of her (Ballou, 1978; Entwistle and Doering, 1981; Leifer, 1980; Mercer, 1982).

Identification with Motherhood Role

The process of identifying with the motherhood role begins early in each woman's life, with the memories she has of being mothered as a child (Sherwen, 1987). She may have used stepping-stone roles to begin understanding what being a mother entails: playing with dolls, babysitting, or taking care of siblings.

For many women pregnancy and caring for children is regarded as one of the most important goals of their lives. These women have always wanted a baby, liked children, and looked forward to motherhood. They are highly motivated to become parents. Such motivation affects the acceptance of pregnancy and eventual prenatal and parental adaptation (Grossman et al., 1980; Lederman, 1984). Other women seem not to have considered in any detail what motherhood means to them. During the 9 months of pregnancy, conflicts need to be resolved so that these women can envision themselves as being concerned, loving parents. These conflicts might include not wanting the pregnancy or child or whether to maintain or relinquish a career. How a woman's social group views the feminine role can make the woman lean more toward motherhood or a career, toward being married or single, or toward being independent rather than interdependent.

Acceptance of Pregnancy

An initial step in adapting to the maternal role is acceptance of the idea of pregnancy and assimilation of the pregnant state into the woman's way of life (Lederman, 1984). The degree of acceptance is reflected in the woman's readiness for pregnancy and her emotional responses.

Readiness for Pregnancy. For many women the availability of birth control measures permits a pregnancy to be viewed as a joint commitment between responsible partners. Planning for conception is done with consideration for other children, if present, financial stability, and for some, the effect on the woman's career. Planning reflects the cultural emphasis on control as a factor in achieving a pregnancy with the best possible outcome. However, even with a planned pregnancy concerns about changes in lifestyle can occur. Researchers have found that planning a pregnancy does not necessarily relate to the woman's acceptance of pregnancy (Entwistle and Doering, 1981). For other women pregnancy occurs as a natural outcome of the marital relationship and may or may not be desired, depending on circumstances. For the adolescent, pregnancy can result from sexual experimentation combined with nonuse of contraception.

Realization that pregnancy signals the end of girlhood and the beginning of womanhood and that it is accompanied by new tasks and responsibilities comes as a surprise to some women and can be a source of stress to many. More than any other happening, pregnancy functions as a rite of passage indicative of reaching maturity in a society that has no other obvious rituals. In many states the pregnant woman is legally an adult regardless of age. She may give personal consent for any type of care for herself or for her newborn. She is entitled to financial and other aid from a government source if needed and, if unwed, is considered the sole legal guardian of her child. As such she retains the right to care for the child herself, place the child in a foster home, or give the child up for adoption.

The early symptoms of pregnancy can be used to confirm the idea of pregnancy or dismiss it if denial seems necessary, even before the medical diagnosis of pregnancy has been made. Examples of conversational cues that indicate acceptance or denial are given in Table 11-1. Women prepared to accept a pregnancy are prompted by early symptoms to seek medical validation of the pregnancy. Women who have strong feelings of "not me," "not now," and "not sure" may postpone seeking supervision and care (Rubin, 1970). Once pregnancy is confirmed, the first overt reactions to its biologic reality may be manifested. A woman's emotional response to the confirmation of her suspicions may range from great delight to shock, disbelief, and despair. The reaction of many women to confirmation of their pregnancy is the "someday but not now" response:

> There is a real pleasure in finding oneself functionally capable of becoming pregnant. There is pleasure in learning that others are pleased with the promise of having, and being given, a child. But these feelings exist independently of the question of time. Personally and privately she is not ready, not now. (Rubin, 1970)

Caplan (1959) also reports that the majority of his clients were dismayed initially at finding themselves pregnant. However, dismay gave way to an eventual acceptance of pregnancy that paralleled the growing acceptance of the reality of a child. He cautions against equating nonacceptance of the pregnancy with rejection of the child. Women can separate the state of physical pregnancy from the idea of being a parent. Thus a woman may dislike being pregnant but feel love for the child to be born.

Emotional Responses

Predominant Mood. Women who are happy and pleased about their pregnancies often view pregnancy as biologic fulfillment and part of their life plan. They exhibit high self-esteem. They tend to be confident about outcomes for themselves, their babies, and other family members.

Even though a general state of well-being predominates, an emotional lability expressed as rapid mood changes is commonly encountered in pregnant women.

Mood Changes. Disconcerting to the mother-to-be and those around her are the rapid mood changes occasioned by an increased sensitivity to actions and words of persons who are significant to her. Increased irritability, explosions of tears and anger, and feelings of great joy and cheerfulness alternate, apparently with little or no provocation. According to one father-to-be:

> "I sometimes think she is crazy—we're going somewhere she wants to go, out to dinner or a concert. She goes upstairs happy as a lark and in 2 minutes is down again in a regular temper, won't go, and shouts at me. I really feel bewildered by it all."

Table 11-1 *Conversational Cues Regarding Possible Pregnancy*

Symptom	Acceptance	Denial
Amenorrhea	"I'll wait one more time; the doctor will think I'm crazy if I go in right away."	"This has happened before. My periods are always irregular. When I went away to college I didn't menstruate for nearly a year."
Tingling and tenderness of breasts	"This is always the second symptom I have. Then I'm pretty sure I'm pregnant."	"My breasts always hurt just before I menstruate." "I am gaining weight. I need a new bra." "My breasts are finally developing. I thought they never would."
Nausea and vomiting	"I didn't think I'd be one who gets sick, but you never know."	"I must have the flu—that's what I'll say if old Smith (teacher) says anything. I've had to go out of the room three mornings in a row."
Urinary frequency	"I have to go at the worst times, but now I don't care. I just say, 'Jane take over the class' and go."	"I'm so nervous all the time it makes me want to go to the bathroom constantly. It is so hard to explain to your teacher."
Feeling of fatigue	"When I'm first pregnant I could just sleep all the time."	"Mother asks how come I'm so tired. She doesn't know how hard I work at tennis."

Many reasons, such as sexual concerns or fear of pain during delivery, have been postulated to explain this seemingly erratic behavior. It may be that the profound hormonal changes that are part of the maternal response to pregnancy are also responsible for mood changes, much as they are before menstruation or during menopause.

Openness in Dealing with Others. Openness about her feelings toward herself and others becomes a noticeable trait in the woman as pregnancy progresses (Caplan, 1959). The layer of reserve that society has hitherto imposed is lifted. The woman exhibits a willingness to talk about matters previously not discussed or discussed only within the family confines. She seems to believe that expression of her thoughts and ideas or description of her symptoms will be of interest to and welcomed by the listener. She appears to enter into a trusting relationship with the outsider she deems protective. This openness, coupled with a readiness for learning, makes working with pregnant women a delight and increases the likelihood of supportive care being therapeutically effective.

Responses to Discomfort of Pregnancy. Not all women suffer from discomforts associated with pregnancy. When the child is wanted, the discomforts experienced tend to be considered as irritations, and the measures taken to relieve them are usually successful. The women derive pleasure from thinking about the unborn child, and this feeling of closeness to the child helps them adjust to the discomfort.

In some instances the woman who commonly complains about physical discomforts may be asking for help with conflicts regarding the mothering role and its responsibilities. Further assessment of coping measures and tolerance is indicated (Lederman, 1984).

Responses to Changes in Body Image. The woman develops a feeling of an overall increase in the size of her body and of occupying more space. This feeling intensifies as pregnancy advances (Jessner, 1970). There is a gradual loss of definite **body boundaries** that serve to separate the self from the nonself. These boundaries provide a feeling of safety: "I looked in the mirror and wondered if it were really me. I had a sudden feeling that I was ballooning outward, there was no end, and I did not know how to bring it together and be myself again." Fawcett (1978) describes this feeling as an awareness of the "perceived zone of separation between self and nonself." The way a woman thinks about her body and her attitude toward pregnancy are related (Rubin, 1968; Lederman, 1984; Strang, 1985). The woman's expanding abdomen may become an object of ridicule and shame or a source of pride.

Men respond in a variety of ways to their wife's changing shape. Some say their wife is most beautiful when pregnant, whereas others make derisive comments about the pregnant contours and are repulsed by them.

A woman who resents losing her shape may make derogatory comments about her abdomen. Commonly women such as this begin wearing maternity clothes before they actually need to. These negative feelings may be countered, however, by a "Mother Earth" feeling, one of being a protective shield for the fetus (Deutch, 1945; Colman, 1969; Rubin, 1970).

For most women the feeling of liking or not liking their bodies in the pregnant state is temporary and does not cause significant changes in their perception of themselves.

Ambivalence During Pregnancy. Ambivalence is defined as simultaneous conflicting feelings, such as love and hate toward a person, thing, or state of being. Ambivalence is a normal response experienced by persons preparing for a new role. Most women have some ambivalent feelings during pregnancy.

Even for women who are pleased to be pregnant, feelings of hostility toward and a wishing away of the pregnancy or unborn child come and go. Such things as a husband's chance remark about the attractiveness of a slim, nonpregnant woman or hearing about a colleague's promotion when the decision to have a child means relinquishing a job can give rise to ambivalent feelings. Daily events such as body sensations, feelings of dependence, or realization of the responsibilities associated with child care can trigger such feelings.

Intense feelings of ambivalence that persist through the third trimester may indicate unresolved conflict with the motherhood role (Lederman, 1984). If the birth of a healthy child ensues, memories of these ambivalent feelings are dismissed. If a child with a defect is born, some women look back at the times of not wanting the child and feel intensely guilty. Even the most enlightened persons tend to give credence in times of stress to the "magical powers of thought." The woman sees her feelings of ambivalence as being instrumental in causing a defect in her child.

Dependence versus Independence. For some women recognition of increasing dependency needs when independence has been attained may give rise to conflict. Independence implies individuation, an ability to stand on one's own. The woman's feelings of being a self-reliant person, someone in control of her own destiny, have become part of her expectations of herself. Pregnancy alters this state: the mother can never be alone. Her baby is always with her as part of her body consciousness. She needs nurturing and support from her husband through birth and child rearing. Adaptation to dependency requires many women to change their self-image as they move from independence to mutual dependency.

Mother-daughter Relationship

The woman's relationship to her mother has proved significant in adapting to pregnancy and motherhood (Deutch, 1945; Caplan, 1959; Rubin, 1967a, b; Ballou, 1978; Leifer, 1980; Mercer, Hackleg, and Bostrom, 1982). Lederman (1984) noted the importance of four components in the gravida's relationship with her mother: the mother's availability, the mother's reactions to the daughter's pregnancy, the mother's respect for her daughter's autonomy, and the willingness to reminisce.

In Lederman's study, the availability of the gravida's mother referred to both past and present. During childhood the availability of the mother was perceived as her being there, loving and supportive. Women with such mothers used them as role models for themselves. For other women in the study the mother was perceived as not being available. However, some of these mothers became available during the pregnancy; that is, they showed interest in the daughters and were emotionally supportive as one adult to another. "With the common bond of motherhood and mutual availability, subjects often described a closeness that appeared to facilitate the development and adaptation of both individuals" (Lederman, 1984).

The mother's reaction to the daughter's pregnancy signified her acceptance of the grandchild and of her daughter. If the mother is supportive, the daughter has an opportunity to discuss pregnancy and labor and her feelings of joy or ambivalence with a knowledgeable and accepting woman. Rubin (1975) noted that if the gravida's mother is not pleased with the pregnancy, the daughter begins to have doubts about her self-worth and the eventual acceptance of her child by others.

Mothers who were able to respect their daughters' autonomy prompted feelings of self-confidence in their daughters. These mothers were capable of accepting the daughters as adults, ones who would be self-reliant and in control. The coming child helped the grandmother-to-be move toward a grandmother role. Some grandmothers use the birth of their grandchildren as a second chance at mothering. Grandparents who had helped their children become independent were seen as being willing to help rather than interfere or dominate.

Reminiscing about the gravida's early childhood and sharing the grandmother-to-be's account of her childbirth experience helped the daughter anticipate labor and delivery and prepare for the event (Levy and McGee, 1975). Hearing about themselves as young children gave the gravidas feelings that their parents had loved and wanted them. As a result they drew closer to their parents. They began to feel that in spite of the errors they might make in their own mothering experiences they would continue to be loved by their children.

Wife-husband Relationship

The father of her child is usually the most important of the pregnant woman's significant others (Richardson, 1983). There is increasing evidence that the woman who is nurtured by her male partner during pregnancy has fewer emotional and physical symptoms, fewer labor and childbirth complications, and an easier postpartum adjustment (Lederman, 1979; Grossman et al., 1980; May, 1982b). Women have expressed two major needs within the wife-husband relationship during pregnancy (Richardson, 1983). The first need relates to the wife's securing indications that she is loved and valued. "The woman repeatedly stressed the importance of feeling that her husband accepted and valued her in her changing roles as wife and mother-to-be. She carefully monitored his attitudes and feelings for indications of acceptance throughout pregnancy" (Richardson, 1983). The second expressed need was related to securing her husband's acceptance of the child. The ever-present reality of being pregnant and the increasing reality of the child impel the woman to prepare for the time when the child will be born. The need to feel secure concerning the father's interest in the child results from the woman's role in assimilating the child into the family. Rubin (1975) states that "as the childbearer, it devolves on the pregnant woman to ensure the necessary social and physical accommodation within the family and within the household for a new member."

The marital relationship is not a static one but evolves over time. The addition of a child changes forever the nature of the bond between wife and husband. Lederman (1984) reported that wives and husbands grew closer during pregnancy. Pregnancy had a maturing effect on the wife-husband relationship as the partners merged into new roles and discovered new aspects of one another. The partners who trusted and supported each other were able to share mutual dependency needs. Women expressed a need for the fathers' active involvement in preparation for birth. To most women the husband was seen as a stabilizing influence, a good listener to expressions of doubts and fears, and a source of physical and emotional reassurance (Grossman et al., 1980). Most women were aware of the developmental needs of their husbands during pregnancy. They were sympathetic toward the husband's need for reassurance as to his importance to the wife. Wives recognized that the husbands could feel jealous of the closeness of the mother and unborn baby.

Communication between the couple is important during pregnancy. Since pregnancy is a developmental crisis, it is a time of emotional upheaval for both the man and the woman. Partners who do not understand the seemingly rapid physiologic and emotional changes of pregnancy can become confused by the other's behavior. Talking to each other about the changes they are experiencing is of primary importance. Increased communication can lead to the recognition of issues. With increased understanding of the other's point of view, couples are more able to define problems and offer the needed support. The marital bond is strengthened as a result.

Parental Concerns. Parental concern for the health of the child seems to vary during the course of pregnancy (Leifer, 1980). The first concern appears in the first trimester and relates to abortion. One woman expressed her feelings as follows: "I spotted [blood] off and on. The doctor said, 'If you are going to hold it, you will; if you abort it, it is probably just as well.' How could he say 'it'? He was talking about my baby." As the child becomes more of a reality; with movement and an audible heartbeat, parental anxiety is focused on possible defects in the mental or physical abilities of the child. Parents talk openly about these anxieties and press for confirmation that the child will be all right. Less identifiable in the later stages of pregnancy is fear about the death of the child; this possibility is evidently remote for parents. Death of the infant comes as a great shock; little or no anticipatory grieving has been done.

Concerns couples have about sexual expression during pregnancy are addressed in Chapter 12.

Mother-child Relationship

Incorporating an infant into an existing family system requires emotional attachment to the child. Researchers have found that attachment to the child begins during the prenatal period (Rubin, 1975; Leifer, 1977; Cranley, 1981a,b; Stainton, 1983, 1985b). Women use fantasizing and daydreaming to prepare themselves for motherhood. They think of themselves as mothers and what mothering qualities they would like to possess. Expression of desires to be warm, loving, and close to their child are common. Maternal commitment to the unborn child is based on a collegial mother-daughter relationship and a mutually supportive husband-wife relationship.

Development of the Relationship. The mother-child relationship progresses through pregnancy as a developmental process (Shereshefsky and Yarrow, 1973; Rubin, 1975; Leifer, 1980). Three **developmental tasks** are identified in the evolution of the relationship:

1. To accept the biologic fact of pregnancy. The woman needs to be able to state, "I am pregnant." The mother has to incorporate the idea of a child into her body and self-image.
2. To accept the growing fetus as distinct from the self and as a person to nurture. The woman can now state, "I am going to have a baby."
3. To prepare realistically for the birth and parenting of the child. The woman expresses the thought, "I am going to be a mother" and defines the nature and characteristics of the child.

Early in pregnancy the mother's thoughts center around herself and the immediate reality of the pregnancy itself. Ballou (1978) found that at this time the child is viewed as "part of one's self." Lumley (1980a,b, 1982a) discovered that the majority of women think of their fetus as "unreal" during the early period of pregnancy. Evidently the pregnancy is experienced as "something happening to *me*."

During the second trimester the egocentric state of the first trimester is balanced by a growing awareness of the child as a separate being. The differentiation of the child from the woman's self permits the beginning of the mother-child relationship. Gilligan (1982) notes that "we experience relationship only insofar as we differentiate other from self."

By the fifth month most women have accomplished the task of identifying the unborn child as a separate person. The mother's sensing of her child as separate from herself encourages not only *caring* but also *responsibility*. With acceptance of the reality of the child (hearing the heartbeat and feeling the child move) and with a subsidence of early symptoms, the woman enters a quiet period. At this time she becomes more introspective, and the fantasy or dream child takes shape. Researchers have noted that women whose pregnancies were planned and who were pleased with their pregnant state felt attachment to the child earlier than other women (Leifer, 1980; Cranley, 1981a,b; Lumley, 1982b). Sometimes a pregnant woman holds her abdomen and gently rocks it as though rocking the child. Conversation reveals the intensity of this intimate mother-baby relationship as women talk freely about their children and their hopes and aspirations for the children's futures. Pet names may be given: "I called all my babies 'Herman' before they were born." Sexual preferences surface: "I just knew I was going to have a boy this time." Some women even begin to plan the child's career: "I saw her as a ballet dancer."

The child becomes precious to the woman, and the feeling that "I am going to have a baby" supersedes all else. The mother seems to withdraw from other relationships

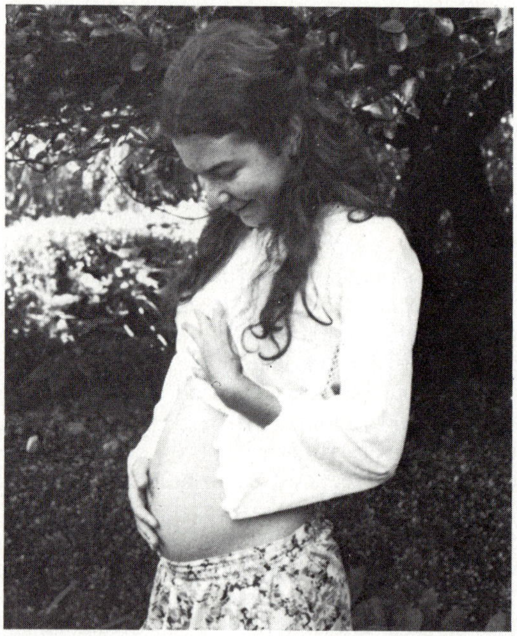

Fig. 11-1 Mother talks to her baby: "How are you doing in there?"

and to concentrate her interest on the unborn child. Husbands and other children seem to sense the withdrawal; sometimes husbands comment on feeling "left out," and children become more demanding in their efforts to redirect the mother's attention to themselves.

In the last months of pregnancy the quiet period is superseded by an active period. The active period is more oriented to reality on the part of the mother toward her parental role and toward her child. As discussed in Chapter 9 the unborn child is capable of response to sound, light, and tactile stimulation. Some parents interact a great deal with their child during pregnancy and perceive the child to respond to tactile, verbal, and other environmental stimuli in an individualized, personalized manner (Fig. 11-1) Stainton (1985a, b) reports the following instances:

> Particularly, "when I am driving, there is some movement the baby does in the lower left side, so I assume it is with the hands. It won't stop until I reposition myself, so I assume he or she needs more room," reported one. Another described "wiggling its feet or pushing against my rib cage when I slouch until I straighten up."

Mothers also deal with discomfort caused by the unborn baby's stretching or positioning. According to one woman, a verbal command such as "Hey, that's too high" resulted in the fetus's shifting position. Another unborn baby consistently moved enough to waken the mother at 4 AM but settled as soon as the mother emptied her bladder (Stainton, 1985b).

Anticipation of Labor

Many women prepare actively for the birth process. They read books, view films, and attend parenting classes. Talking to other women (mothers, sisters, friends, strangers) is a traditional source of information for the gravida. At times the other women tend to recount problems they experienced with deliveries. Such descriptions can frighten nulliparas. The woman who has given birth has her own history of labor and delivery that can either comfort her or make her fearful.

Anxieties. Anxiety can arise from concern about "a safe passage" for herself and her child during the birth process (Rubin, 1975). This may not be expressed overtly, but cues are given as the nurse listens to the plans women make for care of the new baby and other children in case "anything should happen." These feelings persist despite statistical evidence about the safe outcome of pregnancy for the mother. Many women express fear about the pain of delivery. They may fear mutilation because of their ignorance of their body structure and the birth process. Women express concern over what behaviors will be appropriate during the birth process and how the persons who will be caring for them will accept them and their actions. Lederman (1984) found women's fear of loss of control and concomitant loss of self-esteem in labor had physical and emotional dimensions. The women feared a physical loss of control over her body, that is, not being able to work with contractions, failing to relax or breathe properly. Loss of control was also related to medical decisions regarding physical care made without the women's knowledge (Highley and Mercer, 1978). Associated with loss of control over the body was loss of emotional control. Women worried about crying or becoming hysterical or hostile to their husbands or the staff.

The women's reactions to possible loss of control in labor affected their plans for use of analgesics and anesthesia during labor. These responses varied from complete rejection to total acceptance. The use of drugs during labor was also related to concern about the safety of the child.

Anxiety about reaching the hospital in time for the birth, practical concerns for the care of children at home, and the uncertainty of being able to plan specific dates for outside help or the partner's vacation combined to make the last few weeks a time of tension. The tension was compounded by a lack of adequate rest. Generally speaking everyone wishes to function in the best possible manner when confronted with a life event that has great personal implications. The ability to participate wholeheartedly in situations that result in growth, joy, and pleasure to the self and others and, conversely, to face pain, separation, disability, or death adequately come in part from the feelings one has about the ability to maintain control, in part from sharing these critical periods with those who care, and in part from the nurturing provided by others in the environment. The best preparation for labor was found to be "a healthy sense of the realistic—an awareness of work, pain, and risk balanced by a sense of excitement and expectation of the final reward" (Lederman, 1984).

Readiness for Childbirth. Toward the end of the third trimester a recurrence of symptoms brings the physical nature of pregnancy back to the woman's focus of attention. Breathing is difficult, and movements of the fetus become vigorous enough to disturb the mother's sleep. Backaches, frequency and urgency of urination, constipation, and varicose veins can become troublesome. The bulkiness and consequent awkwardness of her body impede the woman's ability to care for other children, perform routine housekeeping duties, and assume a comfortable position for sleep and rest.

By the ninth lunar month the majority of women become impatient for labor to begin whether the birth is anticipated with joy, dread, or a mixture of both. They have a strong desire to come to the end of the state of pregnancy, "to be over and done with it." Women at this stage are ready to move on to the next stage of pregnancy: childbirth and assuming different aspects of the maternal role.

PATERNAL ADAPTATION

Expectant fathers, like the expectant mothers, have been preparing for parenthood throughout their lives (Sherwen, 1987). Subconsciously or consciously men give thought to having a wife and children. During courtship and early marriage a couple's discussion of future plans may even include the number, spacing, and names of their children-to-be (Bobak, 1968).

The father's thoughts and feelings during pregnancy are similar to the mother's. His beliefs about the ideal mother and father and his cultural expectations of appropriate behavior during pregnancy will affect his response to his partner's need for him. Fathers try to anticipate the changes in their lives the child will bring. They wonder how they will react to less freedom, noise, disorder, and caretaking activities. They question their ability to share the love for prior offspring with their unborn child.

The response of the father to pregnancy varies as does the mother's. To one man the pregnant state of his partner may mean freedom to engage in nurturing behavior. To another, it represents a time of loneliness and alienation as the woman becomes physically and emotionally engrossed in the unborn child. He may seek comfort and understanding outside the home or become interested in a new hobby or involved with his work. Some men view pregnancy as a proof of their masculinity. To others, pregnancy as a result of intercourse with a woman has no meaning in terms of responsibility to either mother or child. However, for most women and men pregnancy functions as a time of preparation for the parental role, of fantasy, of great pleasure, and of intense learning.

How fathers adjust to the parental role is the subject of increasing contemporary research. In older societies the man is expected to subject himself to various behaviors and taboos associated with pregnancy and giving birth (Bobak, 1968; May 1982b). These practices are known as **couvade** (French, "to hatch"). By enacting the couvade through definite patterns of socially prescribed behaviors, the man's new status is recognized and endorsed. In addition, his responses are channeled into acceptable modes of expression. His behavior acknowledges his psychosocial as well as biologic relationship to the mother and child. In Western societies, particularly those of the United States and Canada, participation of fathers in childbirth has risen dramatically over the last 15 years (May, 1982b). The father in the role of labor coach is now well established in North American cultures.

The man's responses to becoming a father change during the course of pregnancy, as do those of the mother. Phases of the developmental pattern become apparent. Emotional responses, concerns, and informational needs span the entire experience but seem to be more obvious in one phase than another. May (1982c) describes three phases: the announcement phase, the moratorium phase, and the focusing phase. These phases characterize the three **developmental tasks** experienced by the expectant father.

The early period, the *announcement phase,* may last from a few hours to a few weeks. The developmental task is to accept the biologic fact of pregnancy. The man needs to be able to state, "She is pregnant and I am the father." Men react to the confirmation of pregnancy with joy if the pregnancy is desired or dismay if the pregnancy is unplanned or unwanted. Realization of the reality of the pregnant state seems to come more slowly for the male partner. The woman experiences the early symptoms of pregnancy, but the man sees little physical change in his wife in the first trimester of pregnancy. On seeing a sonograph of his son at 12 weeks, one man remarked, "Until I saw his picture, it was all unreal. I knew intellectually my wife was pregnant, but it didn't mean anything to me. It was amazing—in a few minutes I became a father."

The second phase, the *moratorium phase,* is the period of adjusting to the reality of pregnancy. The developmental task is to come to terms with the reality of pregnancy and be able to state, "We are going to have a baby, and we are changing." Men appear to put conscious thought of the pregnancy aside for a time. Fathers seem to become more introspective. They engage in many discussions about their relationships with different family members and friends and about their own philosophy of life, religion, childbearing, and child-rearing practices. Depending on the man's readiness for the pregnancy, this phase may be relatively short or persist until the last few months (May, 1982c).

The third phase, the *focusing phase,* begins in the last trimester and is characterized by the father's active involvement in both the pregnancy and his relationship with his child. The developmental task is to negotiate with his partner the role he is to play in labor and to prepare for the next stage of parenthood. The man needs to be able to state, "I know my role during the birth process, and I am going to be a parent." In this phase the man concentrates on "his own experience of pregnancy, and in doing so he feels more in tune with his wife. He begins to redefine himself as a father and the world around him in terms of his future fatherhood" (May, 1982c).

Identification With Fatherhood Role

Every father brings to pregnancy concepts developed over his lifetime that affect his response to his wife's pregnancy, just as her concepts do. Certain experiences have been found to be particularly important in modifying the manner in which the father adjusts to pregnancy and the parental role (Cronenwett and Kunst-Wilson, 1981; Kunst-Wilson and Cronenwett, 1981; Lederman, 1984).

The father's perceptions of the male and father role within his social group will guide his selection of the tasks and responsibilities he will assume. His memories of fathering by his own father and the experiences he has had with child care will affect his response (Bobak, 1968). Some men are highly motivated to nurture and love a child. They may be highly excited and pleased about the anticipated role of father. If men have reasonable self-esteem and control of financial resources and working conditions, they seem more able to incorporate the fatherhood role into their life plans. Lederman (1984) notes that fatherhood identification is a crucial developmental step. "It can temporarily reactivate conflicts with his own parents, intensify feelings of separation, heighten dependency needs, and rekindle feelings of sibling rivalry. The husband who can look at these temporary regressions honestly is more likely to effect attachment and bonding with his newborn."

House (1981) delineated four types of support necessary for the man in the process of preparing for fatherhood:

1. *Emotional support.* During adult life the man's primary source of support is his spouse (Lein, 1979). This support has to be modified to permit nurturing of a third family member and to permit the additional nurturing his wife needs. Therefore the father needs to seek support from family and friends (see research highlight).
2. *Instrumental support.* The father needs to know on whom he can depend for help if necessary, for example, sisters, brothers, parents, or particular friends.
3. *Informational support.* The father needs to know who is available (e.g., professionals or relatives) to provide "tips" on how to solve immediate problems.
4. *Appraisal support.* The father needs to find others to provide comparison information, that is, criteria against which he can measure his performance.

The experience of pregnancy acts as a maturing factor in a man's life. Both husband and wife have to negotiate new role commitments with each other.

Acceptance of Pregnancy

Readiness for Pregnancy. May (1982c) found in her study that fathers' readiness for pregnancy was reflected in three areas: "(1) a sense of relative financial security, (2) stability in the couple relationship, and (3) a sense of closure to the childless period in their relationship."

Many men express concern for the family's *economic security.* Today the majority of young married women, as well as men, are employed outside the home. Although pregnant women and mothers with young children may be employed in a work setting, many childbearing and child-rearing women have a phase of unemployment. Length of leave from employment is determined by a combination of factors, such as the couple's economic status, the policies of the employer, and the couple's value system. Some men attempt to compensate for anticipated needs by keeping their current jobs even though they had planned a change. They may put more effort into earning rapid promotions by working overtime or by taking on extra work. The concern for providing financially may extend beyond the immediate future. Some men acquire new or additional insurance at this time (Bobak, 1968).

RESEARCH HIGHLIGHT

Network Structure, Social Support, and Psychological Outcomes of Pregnancy

Purpose

This study measured social network characteristics and perceived social support during the third trimester of pregnancy and at 6 weeks postpartum.

Sample

A convenient sample of 50 primigravid couples participated in this study.

Methodology

The Social Network Inventory was developed by the investigator to measure emotional, material, information, and comparison support. In addition, the Postpartum Self-Evaluation Questionnaire (Lederman et al., 1981) was administered 4 weeks postpartum.

Findings

A greater percentage of relatives in the network and more overlap with the spouse's network were important factors associated with positive postpartum outcomes for men, but not for women. Emotional and instrumental support were important variables in explaining 6-week postpartum outcomes. Informational and appraisal supports were not significant variables during this period.

Implications

The findings from this study can influence the delivery of nursing care in the following ways. First, father participation in child care positively influenced the mother's perception of the quality of her relationship with her spouse. If both can be helped to plan and enact roles that are mutually satisfactory, the quality of the marital relationship will not suffer because of the birth of the child. Second, in this study few primigravid couples were a part of networks whose members were in the same stage of family development. Nurses may compensate for this deficit by suggesting opportunities for postpartum appraisal support. Finally, fathers in this study expressed significantly less confidence than did mothers in their ability to cope with the tasks of parenting. Nurses need to recognize fathers' real need for emotional support regarding their parental role.

Cronenwett, LR: Network structure, social support, and psychological outcomes of pregnancy, Nurs Res 34(2):93, 1985

Those couples who have a *stable relationship* before pregnancy tend to draw closer as a result of their coming parental roles. Pregnancy and parenthood are not remedies for marital problems and conflicts. Those couples who were reasonably conflict free when pregnancy occurred appeared to have agreement on "value systems, areas of responsibility, sex roles, and child care" (Lederman, 1984).

For men their wives' pregnancies bring *to closure the childless period* in their lives. For many men pregnancy is a hoped for and welcome idea. They view having children and being a father as an integral part of their life plan. For some of them the desire to control the time when pregnancy occurs is as culturally relevant as it is to their wives. Couples who plan mutually for pregnancy are more accepting of pregnancy (Lederman, 1984). For some couples pregnancy is unplanned. If the husband had expected to remain childless, a pregnancy can mean alterations in life plans and life-styles. Some men find the change in expectations difficult to accept. They do not necessarily become reconciled to the pregnancy (May, 1982c).

Emotional Responses. *Styles of involvement* in pregnancy vary among men. Style refers to the "general patterns of feelings and behaviors that reflect the way men see themselves in relation to pregnancy" (May, 1980). Men's reactions to pregnancy and their involvement in it depend to some extent on their basic personality structure. Their personality structure is reflected in the style in which they project themselves. Three styles characteristic of men studied during their wives' first-time pregnancy have been described by May (1980, 1982a): the observer style, the expressive style, and the instrumental style.

Observer style was defined as a detached approach to involvement in the pregnancy. Both fathers who wanted the pregnancy and those who did not fall into this category. Those who were happy about the pregnancy were interested in being supportive of their wives and desirous of being good fathers. However, because of cultural values or feelings such as shyness they needed to distance themselves from such activities as prenatal classes, decisions about breast-feeding, or choosing professional care. They appeared to need an "emotional buffer zone." They recognized that by nature they were unemotional and matter-of-fact and that pregnancy had not changed them (May, 1982c).

The other group who were not happy about the pregnancy, reported feelings of ambivalence about pregnancy and the inevitable role of father (May, 1982c). These men believed they needed time to adjust to the idea of pregnancy and fatherhood. They responded to the feelings of ambivalence by becoming involved in careers and resisting their wives' attempts to involve them in preparations for the coming child. "Men established an emotional distance from the pregnancy in relation to the amount of ambivalence they experienced. Women often sensed this distance and attempted to involve their partners more closely. Often the man responded by withdrawing more" (May, 1982c).

Expressive style was defined as a strong emotional response to pregnancy and a desire to be a full partner in the project (Fig. 11-2). These husbands and wives were mutually responsive in their relationships. The husbands showed awareness of their wives' needs for support and were conscious of the times when they were not able to give the wives the support needed. They experienced the same emotional lability that characterizes pregnant women. They were excited and pleased about the baby but also worried about their ability to be a good father. These fathers may experience the discomforts usually associated with women in pregnancy, such as nausea, lassitude, and various aches and pains. **Mitleiden** (suffering along), or psychosomatic symptoms of expectant fathers, has long been recognized as a phenomenon of expectant fatherhood. In 1627 Bacon observed, "That loving and kinde Husbands, have a Sense of their Wives Breeding Childe, by

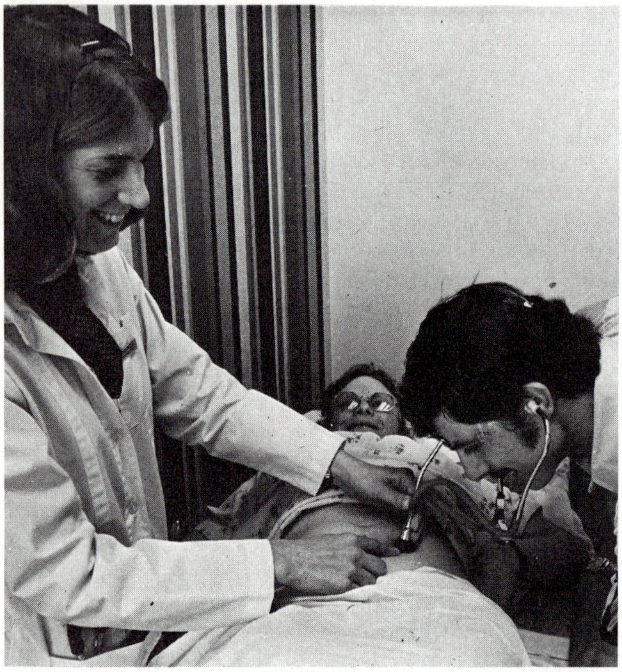

Fig. 11-2 Nurse helps husband listen to the fetal heartbeat during a prenatal examination.
Courtesy Stanford University Hospital.

some Accident in their owne Body." And another author in the 1600s commented, "It often falls out, that when the woman is in good health, the husband is sick, yea sometimes being many miles off" (Hunter and Macalpine, 1963). The husband alone may suffer these discomforts. The symptoms can be a positive force that brings the couple closer together and assists the father in becoming more responsive to his wife's and child's needs for love and care.

Instrumental styles were adopted by men who emphasized tasks to be accomplished and who saw themselves as "caretakers or managers of the pregnancy" (May, 1980). They asked questions, became interested in the role of labor coach, and planned for photographs during pregnancy, birth, and the neonatal period. They felt responsible for the outcome of pregnancy and were protective and supportive of their wives.

Description of the three styles of involvement emphasize the differences in the ways men can experience pregnancy. Each needs to feel free to define his role in pregnancy just as the woman does. Freedom to choose a role is particularly applicable in the man's preparation for labor. Not all men are able or willing to attend childbirth classes or act as labor coaches. This can arise from cultural conditioning or personal expression of supportive roles.

Husband-wife Relationship

The marital relationship is a reciprocal one. Both partners are required to respect each other's need for support and limitations. Much of what is known about the effect of pregnancy on the husband-wife relationship has resulted from the wife's appraisal of her husband's response. Husbands' responses vary from close involvement with the wife to almost no contact (May, 1980). The responses reflect personal style and cultural concepts.

Ballou (1978) found the husband's role in pregnancy to be one of nurturance and responding to his wife's feelings of vulnerability in both her biologic state and in her relationship with her own mother. The husband's support during pregnancy is thought by his spouse to be an indicator of his involvement in the pregnancy and his preparation for attachment to their child (Caplan, 1959; Grossman et al., 1980; Leifer, 1980; Lederman, 1984).

In psychoanalytic literature some aspects of the father's behavior are identified as indicators of rivalry. Rivalry between the expectant father and his pregnant wife is not new. In Greek legend, Zeus, angered by his wife's superior wisdom after she conceived, swallowed her and later gave birth to Athena, who emerged full grown from his forehead. In the same instant he both punished and replaced his wife. Direct rivalry with the fetus may be evident, especially during sexual activity. Husbands may protest that fetal movements prevent sexual gratification, making comments such as, "We can't have sex with 'that' kicking around in there" (Bobak, 1968).

The wife's increased introspection may be a source of anxiety to her husband. He may experience a sense of uneasiness as she becomes preoccupied with thoughts of the child and of her mother, with her growing dependence on her male physician, and with her reevaluation of their relationship. He may sense that his wife's support—his key support—is being withdrawn (Bobak, 1968).

Deciding on the infant's feeding method is of concern when the partners' preferences differ or when one partner has intense reactions. Recognized benefits and disadvantages of one method over another appear to be irrelevant. Some expectant mothers are startled by the husband's strong insistance on one method or the other. Some men insist that the wife breast-feed; others are adamantly set against breast-feeding. When the husband refuses to voice an opinion, the wife experiences uneasiness. Inwardly she accuses him of disinterest or feels uncertain about choosing the right way. The wife seems to ask for his support for whatever choice is made (Bobak, 1968).

All these activities speak to the father's involvement and concerns in becoming a father to his own child. Throughout the pregnancy his memories of being fathered as a child emerge. These memories, coupled with his expectations of *himself,* help define his role as father.

Father-child Relationship

Research indicates that the father-child attachment can be as strong as the mother-child relationship (Greenberg and Morris, 1974; Jones, 1981; Cronenwett, 1982); fathers can be as competent as mothers in nurturing their infants (Parke and Sawin, 1976). Paternal behavior toward children does not differ significantly from maternal behavior (Field, 1978), with the exception of sociophysical play with their infants.

Men prepare for fatherhood in many of the same ways as women do for motherhood—reading, fantasizing, and daydreaming about the baby. They may adjust working commitments to include new responsibilities. Many fathers plan vacations to coincide with the births of the children, enabling them to spend time with their new families.

Daydreaming is a form of role playing. This form of anticipatory psychologic preparation for the infant is most common in the last weeks before delivery. Rarely do men confide their daydreams unless they are reassured that daydreams are normal and fairly common. Questions such as the following assist the nurse and the parent in identifying concerns and informational needs and allow for reality testing:

1. What do you expect the child to look and act like?
2. What do you think being a father will be like?
3. Have you thought about the baby's crying? Changing diapers? Burping the baby? Being awakened at night? Sharing your wife with the baby?

Occasionally just asking the questions suffices. The father may not wish to share his answers with the nurse at the moment but may need time to think them through or discuss them with his spouse.

If an expectant father can imagine only an older child and has difficulty visualizing or talking about the infant, this area needs to be explored. Information about his unborn child's ability to respond to light, sound, and touch and encouragement to feel and talk to the fetus can be given. Plans for seeing, holding, and examining his newly born child can be made.

As the birth day approaches, questions regarding fetal and newborn behaviors increase: "What do they do in there (in utero)?" "Is he hiccuping?" "Does he suck his thumb?" "How is he breathing?" "What does a newborn baby look like?" Some fathers express shock or amazement about the small size of clothes and furniture for the baby. Other fathers protest, "He'll only be real to me when I can hold him in my arms."

Some fathers become involved with the coming newborn by means of activities such as picking the child's name and anticipating the child's sex. As early as the first month the name of the child may be selected. Family tradition, religious mandate, and continuation of one's own name or names of relatives and friends are important in the selection process. The names chosen are tried on for fit; for example, the father might emphatically state, "I just can't picture myself as being a father to a boy named John." Some strive for originality in the name because "a common name just won't do." Armed with several names, one husband said he would decide on his final choice only after he saw the baby, pointing out that "to be named Eric, he *must* be blue eyed and blond" (Bobak, 1968).

At the time of birth most parents are able to accept the sex of the child born to them. Occasionally disappointment is evident and voiced. The parents may experience a grief reaction and a sense of loss at birth as they release the fantasized child and begin to accept the real child.

Anticipation of Labor

The days and weeks immediately preceding the expected day of delivery are characterized by anticipation and anxiety. Many husbands (and couples) describe the dimension of time as heavy, slowed down, and distorted. Boredom and restlessness are common. Expectant fathers and their wives focus on the birth process.

During the last 2 months of pregnancy many expectant fathers experience a surge of energy to create and achieve in the home and on the job. These behaviors could be interpreted as tangible evidence of sharing the wife's childbearing experience while channeling the anxiety of other feelings of the final weeks before birth. Furthermore, these behaviors earn recognition and compliments from friends, relatives, and the wife, and some may even coincide with the wife's nesting activities. Dissatisfaction with present living space increases. The need to alter the environment is acted on wherever possible (Bobak, 1968).

The father's anxieties may be expressed by refusal to think about the coming event, by planning other activities during his wife's labor, or by sleeping and resting to the exclusion of all else. The expectant mother's reactions to the observed behaviors in her mate vary. A prevailing reaction is concern about the possibility of being deserted physically or emotionally when she is feeling most vulnerable.

A major concern of the father is his ability to get the mother to a medical facility in time for the birth. It is a convenient and acceptable focus for his fear and anxiety. Initially some fathers fantasize several ridiculously humorous situations and then move on to plan what they will do. Many rehearse the routes to the hospital, timing each route at different times of the day. Suitcase, car, and essential telephone numbers are readied (Bobak, 1968).

In addition, many fathers want to be able to recognize labor and determine when it is appropriate to leave for the hospital or call the physician or midwife. The concern here is twofold: getting to the hospital in time and not appearing ignorant.

Many fathers have questions about the labor suite's physical environment and staffing—furniture, nursing staff, location, and availability of physician and anesthesiologist. Other fathers' interests lie in knowing what is expected of them when their wives are in labor.

The father has fears of mutilation and death for his wife and child. While he harbors these fears within, he cannot listen or help his mate with her unspoken or overt apprehensions. Words such as "dropped," "rupture of bag of waters," "bloody show," "tears and stitches," and "labor pains" have violent overtones (Bobak, 1968).

With the exception of parent education classes a father has few opportunities to learn to be involved, active, and a needed partner in this rite of passage into parenthood. The unprepared, unsupported father may add to the mother's fears. Tensions and apprehensions are readily transmitted and may increase the mother's difficulties. His own self-doubts and fear of inadequacy may be realized if he is not supported. Self-confidence comes from achieving realistic goals and earning the approval of others.

SIBLING ADAPTATION

The mother with other children faces additional demands when she becomes pregnant. She spends much time and energy reorganizing her relationships with existing children. There is a recognized need to prepare siblings for the birth of the anticipated child and to begin the process of role transition in the family. Parents attempt to include the children in the pregnancy. They are sympathetic to older children's protests against losing their places in the family hierarchy. No child willingly gives up a familiar position (Richardson, 1983).

The response of siblings to pregnancy varies with age and dependency needs. The 1-year-old infant seems largely unaware of the process. However, the 2-year-old child notices the change in mother's appearance and may comment, "Mommy's fat." The 2-year-old child's need for sameness in the environment makes the child aware of any change. Younger children exhibit more "clinging" behavior. Some revert to dependent behaviors in toilet training or eating.

By the third or fourth year of age children like to be told the story of their own beginning and accept its being compared with the present pregnancy. They like to listen to heartbeats and sometimes worry about how the baby is being fed and what she or he wears. Parents often take older children with them to antepartum visits, particularly in the last few weeks (Fig 11-3). Children's responses to feeling the unborn baby moving in utero are often ones of delight. Other mothers report the child's affectional reactions to the baby in utero. One mother reported, "Near the end [of the pregnancy] he began to kiss my belly. I was surprised by that" (Walz and Rich, 1983). Interference with established routines can cause anger. One 4-year-old boy resented not being able to fit on his mother's lap anymore and was not above shoving at his mother's abdomen. His father resolved the issue by making the child a small ski he could slide down his mother's bosom and over her abdomen ("over the hump"). He could still sit close by, touch her, and accept her abdomen as part of his life. Sharing possessions with the unborn child is often short lived. Mothers have noted that cribs or toys donated to the coming child are mostly reclaimed.

A

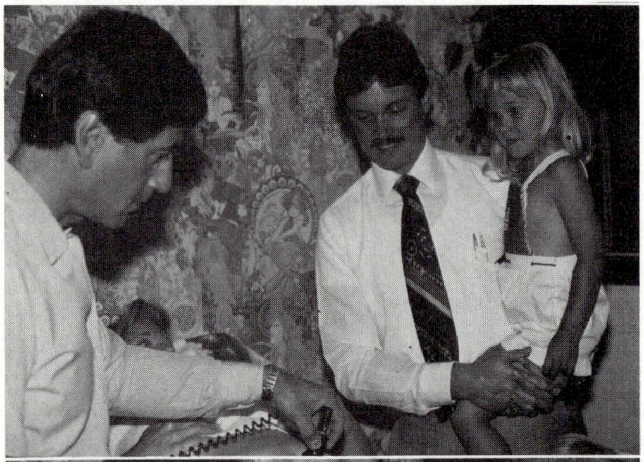

B

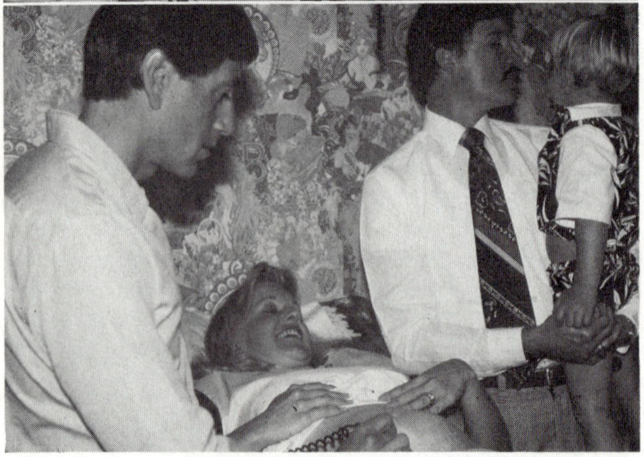

Fig. 11-3 Father and siblings accompany mother on prenatal visit. **A**, Daughter's attention is focused on nurse listening to baby's heart. **B**, Son is reluctant to watch as fetal heart rate is assessed.

School-age children take a more clinical interest in their mother's pregnancy. They may want to know in more detail, "How did the baby get in there?" and "How will it get out?" Children in this age group notice pregnant women in stores, churches, and schools and sometimes seem shy if they need to approach a pregnant woman directly. On the whole they look forward to the new baby, see themselves as "mothers" or "fathers," and enjoy being included in the preparations of buying baby supplies and readying a place for the baby. Because they still think in concrete terms and base judgments on the here and now, they respond positively to their mother's current good health and do not seem to be anxious about a future injury to her or to the unborn child. They need help to cope with any adverse change in the physical or mental status of the parent or newborn, since they do not anticipate such a change.

For early and middle adolescents preoccupied with the establishment of their own sexual identity, the overwhelming evidence of the sexual activity of their parents may prove difficult to accept. They reason that if they are "too young" for such activity, certainly their parents are "too old." All the uncertainties about the status of their parents and the appearance of their mothers are compounded by the pregnancy. They seem to take on a critical parental role and may ask, "What will people think?" or "How can you let yourself get so fat?" Many pregnant women with teenage children will confess that their teenagers are the most difficult factor in their current pregnancy.

On the positive side, just as the parents will someday catch a glimpse of the fine person their adolescent will become, so are parents-to-be suddenly confronted by a warm, sensitive person who is able to restore the mother's self-esteem, as illustrated by the following example:

> "I came home one day feeling very pregnant, tired, and heavy and dreading the idea of making dinner and being helpful—you know—the mother bit! Mary [age 15 years] was cooking some hamburger, had the table set for dinner, and even had a flower centerpiece. For some reason I just started to cry. She came to me and hugged me and said, 'I think you're doing the loveliest thing in the world, having a baby.' I'll always remember that—she was really *my* mother for the moment."

Late adolescents do not appear to be unduly disturbed. They think that they soon will be gone from home. Parents usually report that offspring in this group are comforting and act more as other adults than as children. One mother delivering her tenth baby remarked, "The only complaint my oldest daughter made was, 'Mother, I'm getting married in August, so don't you dare be too pregnant to come to the wedding.' "

GRANDPARENT ADAPTATION

The definition of "grand" is extensive and includes descriptions such as impressive or imposing; stately, majestic, dignified; highest, or very high, in rank or official dignity; of great importance or distinction; first-rate, very good, splendid; princely, regal, royal, and exalted. A grandparent is an ancestor, one generation more remote—a founder or originator of a family. Grandparents are a vital link between generations (Horn and Manion, 1985).

Every pregnancy affects all family relationships. In particular, a first pregnancy is undeniable evidence that one is now old enough to have a child who is soon to bear a grandchild. Many think of a "grandparent" as old, white-haired, and becoming feeble of mind and body. Being "old" carries a stigma for some in predominantly youth-oriented societies. Some people face grandparenthood when still in their 30s and 40s. A mother-to-be announcing her pregnancy to her mother may be greeted by, "How *dare* you do that to me! *I* am not ready to be a grandmother!" Both daughter and mother may be startled and hurt by the outburst.

However, most grandparents are delighted with the prospect of a new baby in the family. It reawakens their feelings of their own youth, the excitement of giving birth, and their delight in the behavior of the parents-to-be when they were infants. They set up a memory store of first smiles, first words, and first steps, which can be used later for "claiming" the newborn as a member of the family. Satisfaction comes with the realization that continuity between past and present is guaranteed.

Recent research indicates the importance of the grandparent-grandchild relationship. Grandparents act as a potential resource for families. Their support can strengthen family systems by widening the circle of support and nurturance (Barranti, 1985). The parent acts as negotiator in establishing the grandparent-grandchild relationship (Greene and Polivka, 1985). Many women report that their pregnancies bridged the final gap between them and their own mothers. The estrangement that began in adolescence disappeared as the now-pregnant daughter experienced joys, concerns, and anxieties similar to those her mother had felt before her.

PARENTHOOD AFTER 35

The following discussion relates to the older woman (over 35 years). Adolescent clients, both mother and father, are discussed in Chapter 35.

Two groups of older parents are now discernible in the population of women having a child late in their childbearing years. One group is made up of multiparous women who have many children or who have a child during the menopausal period. The other group of older parents includes relative newcomers to maternity care. These are women who have deliberately delayed childbearing until their 30s or early 40s.

Multiparas

Multiparas may be women who have never used contraceptives because of personal choice or lack of knowledge concerning contraceptives, or they may be women who have used contraception successfully during the childbearing years. As menopause approaches these latter women may cease to menstruate regularly, stop using contraception, and consequently become pregnant. The older multipara often experiences displacement, feeling that pregnancy alienates her from her peer group and that her age interferes with close associations with young mothers (Hogan, 1979). Other parents welcome the unexpected infant as evidence of continuing maternal and paternal roles.

Including the family in preparation for the birth is important. The other children in the family may be teenagers. Women often welcome the professional person's support and suggestions concerning how to best involve them. Because older siblings often assume aspects of the parental role, the child develops in a "multiparent" household.

Nulliparas

The number of primigravidas aged 35 to 40 has increased by 40%. Births in this age group have increased by 37% over the last 10 years. It is no longer uncommon to see primigravidas in their late 30s or even in their early 40s. Reasons include advanced education, career priorities, and better contraceptive measures.

These women choose parenthood as opposed to the alternative, a child-free life-style. They often are successfully established in a career and a life-style with a partner that includes time for self-attention, establishment of a home with accumulated possessions, and freedom for travel. When questioned as to why they chose pregnancy late in life, many reply, "because time is running out." Sheehy (1977) points out that age 35 brings a biologic boundary into view. Deutch (1945) refers to the late desire for a child as a biologic "closing of the gates."

The dilemma of choice includes recognition that being a parent will have both positive and negative consequences. Couples need to discuss the consequences of childbearing and child rearing before committing themselves to a lifelong venture. Partners in this group seem to share the preparation for parenthood, the planning for a family-centered birth, and the desire to be loving and competent parents. The reality of child care may prove difficult for these parents. The mother who is accustomed to the stimulation of and contact with other adults may find the isolation with her infant difficult to accept. Anger and resentment toward the father (or infant) can result, even if they "prepare" themselves for these aspects of parenting. (Unit VII deals with the physical risks of the older gravida.)

Only one study of the psychologic dimension of older primigravidas has been reported in the nursing literature. Using grounded theory, Winslow (1987) reported findings from a group of 12 married primigravidas, aged 35 to 40. All of these women were white, well-educated, and articulate. Despite its limitations, the study identified important dimensions for consideration in planning care for the primigravida after 35. The four phases these women worked through can provide a basis for understanding the older primigravida. The box below summarizes these phases.

The women in this group approached pregnancy as a project. The early periods were characterized by *planning* and control. The "right time" for pregnancy seemed to be influenced by five factors: commitment and love relationship with the father, increasing possibility of infertility or genetic defects with advancing age, presence of a sense of accomplishment and satisfaction with life to date, desire for a baby, and rejection of remaining childless.

Seeking *safe passage* marked the second phase. The women sought information from books and friends about pregnancy. One learning approach that did not provide them with the greater control they were seeking, however, was childbirth education courses for parents-to-be (Winslow, 1987). They actively sought to rule out fetal disorders, and they were careful in searching for the best possible maternity care.

The *reality of now* refers to the transition period between 24 to 34 weeks. The women in this group were aware of movement from one role and life-style to another. Overall, they felt a sense of physical well-being. Simultaneously, they noted that they had begun to perceive themselves differently. During this phase they identified sources of stress in their lives at that time and anticipation of childbirth was the only problem identified that related to pregnancy.

Anticipating the future occupied considerable time and energy during the latter part of pregnancy. Their concerns centered on issues such as having enough energy and stamina to meet the demands of parenting, fitting a new role into the established role as a working woman, meeting the need to alter their relationships with their husbands, and restructuring their lives to include care of the baby.

See prebirth classes below, and Chapter 25 for further discussion of pregnancy after age 35.

PREBIRTH EDUCATION

In its publication *Guidelines for Childbirth Education* (1981) the Nurses' Association of the American College of Obstetricians and Gynecologists (NAACOG) defines *childbirth education* as follows:

> The process designed to assist parents in making the transition from the role of expectant parents to the role and responsibilities of parents of a new baby which includes the period from the time of conception to approximately three months after birth.

This statement implies that childbirth education is more than preparation for a labor and birth experience. It is also *preparation for parenting* to enhance parental *competence.*

The goal of teaching in preparation for birth and parenting is to enable the nurse and clients to enter each other's worlds, recognize mutual values, and learn more about each other and themselves. Concerns are shared, and mutual learning goals are accepted. We indoctrinate when we teach a "set of beliefs" and teach them in such a way that their validity seems beyond question. To avoid indoctrination, it is important to consider all sides of the issues. *Learning is a lifelong search for truth.*

Comprehensive parent education programs are needed to meet the numerous and varied learning needs of expectant and new parents. Classes in preparation for the birth itself are only one part of preparation-for-parenthood programs. Such programs recognize that pregnancy is not a disease state but a state of wellness. During pregnancy people move from the role of expectant parents to the role and responsibilities of parents of a new baby. Pregnancy can be a meaningful growth experience.

Traditionally, teaching has occurred within a formalized

PREGNANCY AS A PROJECT—A CONCEPTUAL FRAMEWORK

TIME		NAME	DOMINANT CONCEPT	GOAL
Preconception	1	Planning for pregnancy	Planned change	To become pregnant at the "right time"
Up to 20 weeks	2	Seeking safe passage	Control	To attain an optimal outcome for self and baby
Last half of pregnancy	3	The reality of now	Transition	To savor the moment
	4	Anticipating the future	Uncertainty	To integrate motherhood with important parts of one's previous life

Winslow, W: First pregnancy after 35: what is the experience? MCN 12(2):93, 1987.

structure in North America. However, it also has been recognized that all of life educates and that teaching occurs in many ways. Too often, education for birth and parenting has been limited to a classroom. Formal classes may be effective for people socialized into structured education, but structured education can be ineffective for people who have not found the classroom atmosphere stimulating.

Nurses have limitless opportunities to teach parents in formal classes, in small group sessions, in office and clinic waiting rooms, and at home. Education for childbirth and for parenting is an integral part of the nursing process.

Teaching can be defined as a deliberate intentional action taken to help another person learn to do what that person cannot presently do. **Learning** involves measurable behavior change resulting from practice and experience.

Like the nursing process, teaching is a process involving assessment, formulation of diagnoses (educational), planning, implementation, and evaluation (Fig. 11-4).

Assessment

Assessment involves data collection for the purpose of identifying client needs. Pertinent data include the ages of the learners, their culture or ethnicity, and their readiness to learn. This data gathering is a continuous collection of information from a variety of valid and reliable sources. Examples of sources include group discussion, observation, and formal pen-and-pencil assessment of learning needs; personal interviews (Winslow, 1987); client health records; other health-care team members; family members; and review of pertinent literature.

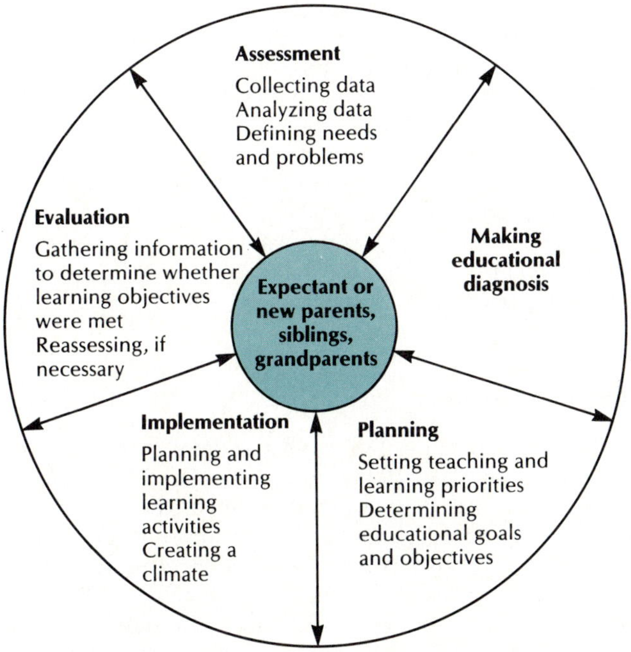

Fig. 11-4 The teaching process parallels the nursing process. Arrows indicate direction of communication.

Educational Diagnosis

An educational diagnosis can be formulated after the collected data have been analyzed and learning needs and problems defined. An educational diagnosis identifies the client's learning needs and suggests a plan of action. It must be kept in mind that the special needs of all pregnant women must be met (Mercer, 1979). For example, those experiencing first pregnancy after age 35 and who have had successful careers require a greater amount of sophistication in childbirth courses than younger primigravidas. Winslow (1987) found that a population of primigravidas, aged 35 to 44, felt out of place and did not receive the caliber or quality of information they had hoped for in the classes they attended.

Planning

Planning involves specifics. The nurse establishes teaching and learning priorities for the identified needs using her or his personal philosophy of childbirth and parent education as a guide. Educational goals are then identified as the nurse works with the family. Next, educational objectives are established. These are statements related to the goal. They are specific, measurable, attainable, and agreed on by the family and the nurse.

Implementation

Implementation involves carrying out the learning activities designed to meet the learning objectives. The emphasis is on principles, content, level, and scope of learning. Implementation encompasses selecting instructional methods. These methods include (1) discussion, (2) role playing, (3) repetition, (4) testing, (5) rewards, and (6) the use of audiovisual materials. The physical and emotional needs of the learner are given priority. An atmosphere conducive to learning is created in a climate of friendliness and acceptance.

Evaluation

Evaluation determines teaching effectiveness in relation to the stated objectives. Methods commonly used by nurses to evaluate client learning are (1) direct observation, (2) client records, (3) reports, (4) tests, (5) interviews and questionnaires with clients and their families, (6) interviews and questionnaires with staff, and (7) research using statistical comparisons. Effective evaluation occurs as a result of careful planning.

Parent Education Programs

A typical preparation-for-parenthood program recognizes that expectant parents and their families have different interests and information needs as the pregnancy progresses. Consequently, the program is designed to meet the information needs of parents at the three major stages of pregnancy and after birth.

First Trimester Classes. Early pregnancy ("early bird") classes provide fundamental information. Classes are developed around the following areas: (1) early fetal development, (2) physiologic and emotional changes of pregnancy, (3) human sexuality, and (4) the nutritional needs of the mother and fetus. Environmental and workplace hazards have become important concerns in recent years. Even though pregnancy is considered a normal process, exercises, danger signs, drugs, and self-medication are topics of interest and concern.

Second Trimester Classes. Midpregnancy classes emphasize the woman's participation in self-care. Classes provide information on (1) preparation for breast-and formula-feeding, (2) basic hygiene, (3) common complaints and simple, safe remedies, (4) infant health, and (5) parenting.

Third Trimester Classes. Late pregnancy classes are designed to meet the needs of the entire family: (1) couple discussion groups, (2) expectant father discussion groups, (3) sibling classes, (4) grandparents' classes, and (5) newborn care classes. Special classes are developed for teenage parents, for parents expecting a cesarean delivery (Hart, 1980), and for parents of twins. Refresher courses for those who feel they are prepared through previous childbirth experience but would like to review a few things are also available (Mercer, 1979).

Throughout the series of classes there is discussion of support systems that people can use during pregnancy and after birth; such support systems help parents function independently and effectively. During all the classes the open expression of feelings and concerns about any aspect of pregnancy, birth, and parenting is welcomed.

Postpartum ("Fourth" Trimester) Classes. After-birth classes help parents meet the tasks and responsibilities of their new roles. Topics for discussion can include (1) coping mechanisms for the reality of parenting, (2) use of support systems, and (3) infant care and growth of development. Birth control methods and adapting to new roles (wife-lover ⇌ mother and husband-lover ⇌ father) are explored.

Parent Preparation for Cesarean Birth

Concerned professional and lay groups in the community have established councils for cesarean birth in an attempt to meet the needs of women and their families. Such groups advocate including preparation for cesarean birth in all parenthood preparation classes (Fawcett and Henklein, 1987). This is encouraged even if parents-to-be "tune out" such discussions and feel later that they have been betrayed by not having been made aware of this eventuality. No woman can be guaranteed a vaginal delivery, even if she is in good health and there is no indication of danger to the fetus before the onset of labor. Every woman needs to be aware of and prepared for this possibility. The unknown and unexpected is ego weakening. Each woman or couple needs accurate data to build new coping abilities or to strengthen old ones. "Walking through," role playing, or worry work before a crisis situation increases one's sense of control in that situation and serves to minimize the sense of loss experienced.

Childbirth educators stress the importance of emphasizing the similarities as well as differences between cesarean and vaginal births. Also, in support of the philosophy of family-centered birth, many hospitals have changed policies to permit fathers to share in cesarean births as they have vaginal ones (see Chapter 33). Women undergoing cesarean birth stress that the continued presence and support of their partners have helped them experience a positive response to the whole process:

> Knowing that he would be there and that he would be among the first to hold and nurture our baby made a tremendous difference to me. Even though "I" as the woman couldn't participate as directly as I had anticipated, "we" as the family could. I felt a sense of control, not a sense of being a passive . . . well . . . organ.

In many hospitals today care of parents experiencing a cesarean birth is family centered rather than surgery centered. As education on cesarean birth is being incorporated into prenatal classes, couples are becoming aware of options available to them if a cesarean delivery is necessary. Some of the alternatives available to women and their families who experience cesarean birth include the following:

1. Cesarean delivery that is performed in the labor and delivery area, rather than in the general surgery area
2. The choice of regional instead of general anesthesia, whenever possible
3. The option of having a support person (preferably father) present during the birth
4. The opportunity for skin-to-skin contact with baby and parents immediately after birth
5. Initiation of early rooming-in with help from staff until mother is able to assume responsibility for baby care
6. Encouragement of breast feeding
7. Extended and unlimited visiting privileges for the immediate family members

Cesarean delivery is a birth experience and must be incorporated as such. The goal is a positive birth experience brought about by cooperation among parents, physicians, and hospital personnel.

Sibling Preparation

Sibling preparation has a definite place in family-centered maternity care (Johnsen and Gaspard, 1985). Many expectant parents are concerned about an older child's response to the birth of a new sister or brother. Parents want to provide as much support as possible for the older child or children (see also Chapters 17, 19, 20, and 25). For the preschool child, becoming a big sister or brother is a complex and growth-oriented adaptation. The older child's responses are influenced by many variables that include techniques of preparation, the father's role, the parents'

Guidelines For Client Teaching

SIBLING PREPARATION

ASSESSMENT

1. Couple expecting second child in 3 months. Four-year-old son asking many questions about the baby in "mommy's tummy". Child resistant to living at aunt's house during mother's hospitalization.
2. Parents express desire for preparation of older sibling.

NURSING DIAGNOSES

Knowledge deficit related to older sibling's capabilities and needs.
Impaired verbal communication related to older child's development level.
Altered family process related to addition of new family member.

GOALS

Short-term

Child and parents feel less anxious about the mother's impending hospitalization.
Child begins to develop realistic expectations of newborn.
Parents begin to develop strategies to prepare the older child for the mother's hospitalization and newborn sibling.

Intermediate

Child begins to prepare for role transition to be brother.
Parents begin to develop strategies for caring for older sibling and new child.
Parents begin to prepare for role transition necessitated by addition of new member to family.

Long-term

Child develops realistic expectations of newborn.
Child and parents learn new coping skills.
Parents successfully make role transition necessitated by addition of new member to the family.

REFERENCES AND TEACHING AIDS

Audiovisual materials: films, slides, doll, cassette recordings, materials with which to draw pictures.
See bibliography for list of references available to parents and small children.
Enroll and attend a sibling class.
Sibling visitation while mother is hospitalized.

CONTENT/RATIONALE	TEACHING ACTION
To allay anxiety related to an unknown environment (Johnsen and Gaspard, 1985): Have older sibling: Visit hospital classroom. Dress up in hospital clothing. Learn hospital "rules," such as walk slowly, and talk quietly. Tour maternity area, see and touch telephone that he can use to talk to his mother. See naked newborn.	Prepare a room to convey warmth and friendliness. Explain hospital clothing, then change to scrub outfit worn by fathers and nurses. Help child try on hospital gowns, masks, and caps. During tour, answer questions and expect child to abide by hospital "rules."
To help child form realistic expectations of the newborn: Have older sibling practice in new role: By listening to stories about what newborns can do and how older children react to new born babies. By holding a doll with care to support the head. By exploring what he can do when the baby cries. Hear sound of newborn cries and cooing as they vary with hunger, contentment, desire for company, and complaining about a dirty or wet diaper.	Read stories and employ role-playing. Ask open-ended or leading questions. Help child with holding the doll. Demonstrate ways to console a crying baby, such as singing and talking. Caution against picking up baby. Caution against touching the baby's head. Play cassette of baby sounds and encourage questions and discussion.
To help child substitute acceptable behavior for unacceptable behavior with the newborn: Have older sibling practice through role-playing: When newborn gets a present and older child does not. When parent spends time with the newborn. When the child gets angry with the newborn.	Role-play situation demonstrating positive responses to newborn in selected situations. Involve older child with problem-solving in selected situations.
To help child recognize his feelings: Have older sibling: Watch a film depicting jealousy, anger, and being left out (Johnsen and Gaspard, 1985).	Show film and encourage discussion.
Participate in discussion of film and how to ask for help when needed.	Lead discussion; encourage comments.
Participate in drawing a picture to show how he feels and what he understands of his mother's pregnancy and the coming baby.	Provide equipment, space and directions for drawing, such as "draw a picture of your family." Ask child to tell a story about his picture.

EVALUATION The nurse can be reasonably assured that the teaching plan has been effective when all goals have been met. Older sibling demonstrates realistic expectations of the newborn and remains reassured about parental love. Child and parents learn new coping skills. Parents and sibling successfully make the role transition necessitated by addition of a new family member.

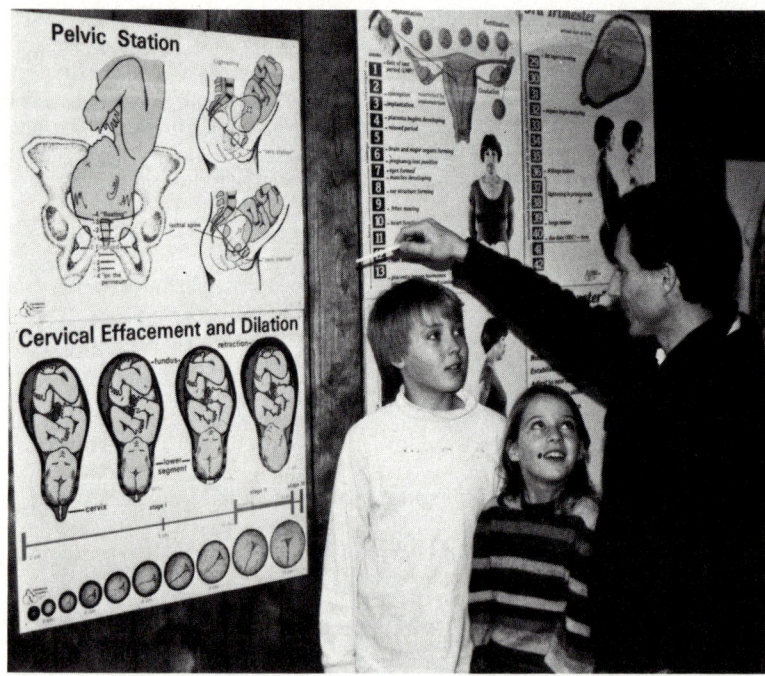

Fig. 11-5 Sibling preparation class.
Community Birth Center, Community Hospital, Santa Cruz, Calif.

GRANDPARENTS' TOUR AND CLASS

Objectives

Participants will be able to:

1. State policies and procedures of labor and delivery, nursery, and family-centered unit.
2. Explain purpose and reason for Bililites and infant warmers.
3. Describe circumcision and cord care.
4. Summarize total care of family unit at hospital.

Outline

I. Meet in administrative office and move to classroom
  A. Slides on family-centered care
  B. Discussion of options available to couple of today
    1. LeBoyer
    2. Birthing room
    3. Lamaze
  C. Changing role of father in family unit
    1. Education
    2. Participation
  D. Changing role of grandparent
    1. Mobility
    2. Transient society
    3. Retirement

II. Tour through labor and delivery area
  A. Science and technology and birth process
    1. Why fetal monitoring
    2. Why IVs
  B. Complications in labor
  C. Anesthesia of today
  D. Gown and mask for delivery room
    1. Position of father
    2. Explanation of warmer

III. Nursery
  A. Transitional care nursery (use check sheet to explain care)
  B. General nursery: Bililites
  C. Intensive care nursery and family-centered care

IV. Skylight room: visiting anytime at mother's choice

V. Family-centered care
  A. Visit to empty room on family unit
  B. Explanation of channel 5 (in-hospital)

VI. Return to classroom for demonstrations and explanations (coffee and doughnuts)
  A. Cord care (demonstrate with doll)
  B. Circumcision care
  C. Temperature regulation of newborn
  D. Bonding
  E. Breast-feeding
  F. Normal newborn skin conditions (use pictures)

VII. Questions and answers

Courtesy Jane Rohan, Education Department, The Woman's Hospital of Texas, 7600 Fannin St, Houston, Texas, 77054.

attitudes, the effect of the child's separation from the mother who is hospitalized, and the hospital's visitation policy (Honig, 1986).

Professional groups of clinics and hospitals are developing classes to prepare children for the birth of a new brother or sister (Fig. 11-5). A general teaching plan used for young children is found in the guidelines for client teaching: sibling preparation for childbirth. The general plan can be modified to fit needs of children of different ages and the needs of children who will be present during the birth.

Grandparent Preparation

The proliferation of literature, visual aids, and classes for expectant and new parents projects these as *the* sources for information. Rapid advances in technology, increased mobility of families, and establishment of nuclear families sometimes thousands of miles distant have added to the reliance of these sources for information and guidance (Newell, 1984).

Fortunately, childbirth educators are becoming more aware of the unique role of the grandparent and are forming classes for grandparents (Hassid, 1984; McKay and Phillips, 1984; Horn and Manion, 1985). An outline for such classes, developed by childbirth educators at The Woman's Hospital of Texas (Houston), is presented on p. 234. The various grandparental roles are acknowledged (Kornhaber and Woodward, 1981): (1) historian who transmits the history of the family and provides continuity with the present, (2) resource person and shares knowledge gleaned from experience, (3) role model, and (4) support person.

Grandparents' anxieties and concerns and their relationships with expectant parents and with grandchildren should be opened to discussion during courses for expectant parents as well (see guidelines for client teaching: grandparent preparation, p. 236). The expectant parents may use this opportunity to begin to resolve conflicts and perceived differences with their parents, a task that can enhance their ability to relate to their own children. In addition, another potential problem can be averted. Consider the difficulty a child faces when a beloved grandparent is belittled by a beloved parent; the child is caught in the middle (Satir, 1972) thus negatively influencing the relationship with the parent and that with the grandparent. To be truly *family-oriented,* maternity care must consider the grandparent when implementing the nursing process with childbearing families. (See also Chapter 25). The grandparents' classes represent one method of facilitating the adjustment to the grandparenting role, of incorporating the grandparents into the family system, and of encouraging communication between the generations (Maloni, McIndoe, and Rubenstein, 1987).

EDUCATION FOR CHOICE

Birth is a life event that has significant impact on human behavior. Childbirth requires sensitive management and attention to the psychosocial health of the family.

In June 1978 the American College of Obstetricians and Gynecologists (ACOG) published a joint statement, "The Development of Family-Centered Maternity/Newborn Care in Hospitals." The statement was prepared by the Interprofessional Task Force on Health Care of Women and Children, which included representatives from the American Academy of Pediatrics (AAP), the American College of Nurse-Midwives (ACNM), the American Nurses' Association (ANA), ACOG, and the Nurses' Association of the American College of Obstetricians and Gynecologists (NAACOG). These five organizations endorsed the concept of family-centered childbirth and supported efforts to develop alternative childbirth centers along the lines described in the statement. The American Hospital Association added its support. The definition of family-centered care in the joint statement follows:

> Family-centered maternity/newborn care can be defined as the delivery of safe, quality health care while recognizing, focusing on, and adapting to both the physical and psychological needs of the client-patient, the family, and the newly born. The emphasis is on the provision of maternity/newborn health care which fosters family unity while maintaining physical safety.

The statement recommends significant changes in hospital maternity care, including the following:

1. The option of a homelike birthing room where woman remains (with her family if desired)
2. Flexible rooming-in with maximum mother-child contact during the first 24 hours
3. Breast feeding and handling of the baby immediately after delivery
4. Allowing the father or other support persons to be present throughout the labor, delivery, and recovery periods
5. Allowing siblings to visit in a special family room
6. Optional early discharge from the hospital with careful follow-up after discharge
7. Childbirth preparation classes offered by the hospital

The alternative birth movement is the practical application of the family-centered concept of maternity-newborn care. However, family-centered care requires more than just a proper physical environment. The attitude of the health care providers is the most important aspect of family-centered care. Family-centered care recognizes birth as a vital life event and not a surgical procedure. The philosophic approach to family-centered care and alternative childbirth programs is that which gives people the right to make informed choices regarding their childbirth experiences.

Organizations such as ICEA and ASPO and the National Association of Parents and Professionals for Safe Alternatives in Childbirth (NAPSAC) have increased the public's knowledge of prepared childbirth techniques and their impact on birth outcomes. The prepared childbirth movement has fostered greater acceptance of birth as a normal, rather than a pathologic, event and has encouraged expectant parents to become more knowledgeable about and accountable for their participation. As women began to experience childbirth awake and aware, they began to feel greater self-esteem and control over their lives. Also, the

Guidelines For Client Teaching

GRANDPARENT PREPARATION

ASSESSMENT

1. Expectant parents voice concerns about role of grandparents and request assistance (depends on grandparent's readiness to learn).
2. Expectant grandparents request information about hospital policies and procedures, modern childbirth methods, new parents' needs, and their own roles.
3. Expectant grandparents would like to provide support to expectant parents before and after the birth of the baby.

NURSING DIAGNOSES

Knowledge deficit related to hospital policies, childbirth methods, and how to provide support to expectant parents.

Altered family processes related to addition of a new family member.

Potential for ineffective individual coping related to need for role change.

GOALS

Short-term

Grandparents are oriented to hospital routines and policies.

Grandparents are oriented to childbirth method and experience expected by their children.

Grandparents learn current techniques of infant care.

Intermediate

Grandparents prepare for role change from parents to grandparents.

Grandparents begin to define mutually acceptable role-relationship with their children.

Grandparents relive and come to terms with own childbirth experience.

Long-term

Grandparents develop and maintain mutually satisfying role-relationship with children and new grandchild.

Grandparents become effective and supportive grandparents and parents.

REFERENCES AND TEACHING AIDS

Audiovisual materials: films, slides, charts.

List of references available to the general public.

Tour of maternity unit; introduction to gowns, shoe covers, and caps.

Values clarification or attitude awareness exercise (Horn and Manion, 1985).

CONTENT/RATIONALE	TEACHING ACTION
To explore values and attitudes: Values-clarification, attitude awareness exercise: When I think about myself as a grandparent, I feel ______. Children bring a couple ______. Breast feeding is ______. Pacifiers are ______. Labor is ______. During their child's labor and delivery, grandparents should ______. The happiest (most satisfying) memory of my (my wife's) labor and childbirth was ______. The unhappiest (least satisfying) memory of my (my wife's) labor and childbirth was ______.	Develop and administer values and attitudes exercise. Use exercise as a basis for starting small-group discussion. Encourage members of group to compare and contrast own experiences, values, and attitudes.
To explore knowledge base of science and technology concerning the birth process: Conduct grandparents class. Use prioritized list of topics they wish to discuss as focus.	Elicit topics the grandparents wish to discuss, write on a chalkboard, and ask group to prioritize list; encourage questions. Use appropriate audiovisual materials: charts, films, slides.
To expand learning and orient to environment of maternity area, provide: Tour of unit. Hands-on experience with equipment and supplies. Introduction of personnel. Description of personnel's services and responsibilities.	Offer or conduct a tour of the maternity area including restrooms, waiting room, telephones, cafeteria, and selected supplies (gowns, shoe-covers) and equipment (fetoscope). Introduce the grandparents to available personnel and review their roles. Return group to classroom.
To bring closure to class: Review the grandparent's questions. Discuss their comparisons. Summarize the experience.	Encourage questions. Encourage the grandparent's to compare and contrast their own experiences with the class content. Provide printed material. Thank the group for their interest.

EVALUATION Teaching has been effective when grandparents develop and maintain a mutually satisfying role-relationship with their children and grandchildren. Goals have been met when grandparents become effective and supportive to their children and grandchildren.

social significance of the birth experience became very clear to many women and their mates.

Consumer response has been varied, demonstrating the intensely personal quality of every birth experience and the need for safe, sensible choices in care during this important life event (Periscope, 1987). Some couples wish to exercise maximum control over the birth of their child, with minimal technology and intervention by the health care team. Other couples choose a more traditional approach. The key element in optimal care of the childbearing family is **informed choice** about the place of birth, the plan of care, and the people present. In fact, the ICEA has always subscribed to the motto, "Freedom of choice based on knowledge of alternatives."

Choice and the Nurse

Understanding why families choose alternatives to traditional hospital birth (see Chapter 14) is imperative. Cohen (1982) compared women who chose two different childbirth alternatives: a hospital or a freestanding alternative birth center (ABC). He found that women choosing the birth center planned to emphasize autonomy and independence rather than intimacy in their child rearing. Also, their closest relationships were much more supportive and involved in the birth than those women choosing hospital births. Women delivering at the Childbearing Childrearing Center (CCC) at the University of Minnesota, Minneapolis (Rising and Lindell, 1982) reported the three major reasons they chose the center were (1) to have control over their experience, (2) to have family-centered care, and (3) to have no routine procedures administered. Kieffer (1980) compared the attitudes of 109 women before and after experiencing birth using the birthing room concept. The four highest ranking reasons for choice of the birth room were (1) philosophy, (2) no separation of mother and baby, (3) personal involvement in the birth, and (4) freedom to make choices regarding labor and birth. These studies seem to indicate that attitudes toward issues of choice in the childbirth experience are related to the degree of control that families expect to exert over the birth event (Fullerton, 1982).

Most people who choose home birth are very sincere and concerned about their own safety and the health and safety of their unborn child (Searles, 1981). In fact, there are probably as many sincere and well-considered reasons for choosing home birth as there are home births. For many individuals experiencing home birth, birth is a very special, intensely personal event to be shared only with family and friends, and not with assorted hospital personnel who are strangers. For many others, birth is an intensely spiritual experience for which a hospital setting is totally inappropriate. Still others do not relish giving up responsibility for their births to hospital personnel; instead, these people want to control their own experience. Most people choosing home birth understand fully the risk involved but also understand that there are risks in hospital birth.

The nurse's concern is to encourage expectant couples to explore the birth alternatives available to them so they can make a responsible, informed decision. It is the nurse's responsibility to become actively involved in ensuring that a variety of options for safe childbirth are available in communities.

SUMMARY

Pregnancy represents a developmental crisis in a person's and a family's lives. The concept of crisis implies events that necessitate change in outlook, role responsibilities, and everyday living. The ability to respond to changes with new behaviors and new self-concepts is fostered not only by intrinsic strengths but also by extrinsic strengths, such as the love and support of outsiders. Nurses can act as one source of extrinsic strength. The knowledge they possess of the responses of all family members to a pregnancy enables them to use their responses as the cornerstones of nursing-care plans.

The nurse encourages the childbearing family to participate in prenatal classes. Attendance at such classes permits sharing of experiences with other couples and families. The couple is reassured by knowing that their thoughts, feelings, and concerns are common to others. Classes can increase confidence and self-assurance and help parents develop new coping skills.

The long-term contact nurses have with clients and their families provides unique opportunities for informed supportive nursing that may have a long-term effect on family life.

KEY CONCEPTS

- Pregnancy involves all family members, who react to pregnancy and interpret its meaning in light of their own needs, as well as the needs of the others affected.
- The process of family adaptation to pregnancy takes place within a cultural environment.
- Pregnancy presents several developmental tasks to the mother- and father-to-be as they prepare for new levels of caring and responsibility.
- Since pregnancy is a developmental crisis, it is a time of emotional upheaval for both the man and the woman, necessitating adequate communication between them.
- The parent-child, sibling-child, and grandparent-child relationships start during the pregnancy.
- Childbirth education is a process designed to assist parents in making the transition from the role of expectant parents to the role and responsibilities of parents of a new baby, which includes the period from the time of conception to approximately 3 months after birth.
- The nursing process and the teaching process are parallel.
- Maternity care should be family-centered regardless of the method of birth and the place of birth.
- The goal of preparation for childbirth and parenting is "education for choice."

STUDY QUESTIONS AND ACTIVITIES

1. Through discussions with assigned appropriate clients, discuss characteristics of adaptation to pregnancy: maternal, paternal, sibling, and grandparental.
2. Through discussion with an expectant couple, identify ambivalent feelings experienced throughout the pregnancy.
3. Focus discussion of students and peers who have experienced childbirth on emotional responses, body image, and realization of role changes.
4. Check libraries and bookstores for popularized accounts of pregnancy and childbirth processes (the "how-to" approach). Choose one book to critique for the class in terms of its accuracy compared with the discussion of the possible effect such books might have on the pregnant woman and her husband.

References

American College of Obstetricians and Gynecologists: The development of family-centered maternity/newborn care in hospitals, Washington, DC, 1978, The College

Ballou JW: The psychology of pregnancy, Lexington, Mass, 1978, DC Heath & Co

Barranti, C: The grandparent/grandchild relationship: family resource in an era of voluntary bonds, Fam Relations 34:3, July 1985

Bobak, I: Fathers, Unpublished research, 1968

Caplan, G: Concepts of mental health and consultation, Washington, DC, 1959, US Department of Health, Education, and Welfare

Cohen, RL: A comparative study of women choosing two different birth alternatives, Birth 9:1, Spring 1982

Colman, AD: Psychological state during the first pregnancy, Am J Orthopsychiatry 39:778, 1969

Cranley, MS: Development of a tool for the measurement of maternal attachment during pregnancy, Nurs Res 30:281, 1981a

Cranley, MS: Roots of attachment: the relationship of parents with their unborn, Birth Defects 17(6):59, 1981b

Cronenwett, LR: Father participation in child care: a critical review, Res Nurs Health 5:63, 1982

Cronenwett, LR: Network structure, social support, and psychological outcomes of pregnancy, Nurs Res 34(2):93, 1985

Cronenwett, LR, and Kunst-Wilson, W: Stress, social support, and the transition of fatherhood, Nurs Res 30:196, 1981

Deutch, H: The psychology of women, vol 2, New York, 1945, Bantam Books, Inc

Entwistle, DR, and Doering, SG: The first birth: a family turning point, Baltimore, 1981, Johns Hopkins University Press

Fawcett, J, and Henklein, JC: Antenatal education for cesarean birth: extension of a field test, JOGN Nurs 16(1):61, 1987

Fawcett, J: Body image and the pregnant couple, MCN 3:227, 1978

Field, T: The three Rs of infant-adult interactions: rhythms, repertoires, and responsitivity, J Pediatr Psychol 3:131, 1978

Fullerton, JDT: The choice of in-hospital or alternative birth environment as related to the concept of control, J Nurse Midwife, 27:2, March/April 1982

Gilligan, C: In a different voice: psychological theory and women's development, Cambridge, Mass, 1982, Harvard University Press

Glass J: Prebirth attitudes and adjustment to parenthood: when preparing for the worst helps family relations, Fam Relations 32:377, 1983

Greenberg, M, and Morris, N: Engrossment: the newborn's impact upon the father, Am J Orthopsychiatry 44:520, 1974

Greene, R, and Polivka, J: The meaning of grandparent day cards: an analysis of the intergenerational network, Fam Relations 34:2, April 1985

Grossman, FK, et al: Pregnancy, birth, parenthood, San Francisco, 1980, Jossey-Bass, Inc, Publishers

Hart, G: Maternal attitudes in prepared and unprepared cesarean deliveries, JOGN Nurs 9:243, 1980

Hassid, P: Textbook for childbirth educators, ed 3, New York, 1984, JB Lippincott Co

Highley, BL, and Mercer, RT: Safeguarding the laboring woman's sense of control, Matern Child Nurs J 3(1):39, 1978

Hogan, LR: Pregnant again—at 41, Matern Child Nurs J 4:174, 1979

Honig, JC: Preparing preschool-aged children to be siblings, MCN 11(1):37, 1986

Horn, M, and Manion, J: Creative grandparenting: bonding the generations, JOGN Nurs 14:233, May/June 1985

House, JS: Work, stress and social support, Reading, Mass, 1981, Addison-Wesley Publishing Co, Inc

Hunter, R, and Macalpine, I, editors: Three hundred years of psychiatry: 1535-1860, London, 1963, Oxford University Press

Jessner, L, et al: The development of parental attitudes during pregnancy. In Anthony, EJ, and Benedek, T, editors: Parenthood, Edinburgh, 1970, Churchill Livingstone, Inc

Johnsen, NM, and Gaspard, ME: Theoretical foundations of a prepared sibling class, JOGN Nurs 14:237, May/June 1985

Jones, C: Father to infant attachment, effects of early contact and characteristics of the infant, Res Nurs Health 4:193, 1981

Kieffer, MJ: The birthing room concept at Phoenix Memorial Hospital. II. Consumer satisfaction during one year, JOGN Nurs 9:158, May/June 1980

Kornhaber, A, and Woodward, KL: Grandparents/grandchildren: the vital connection, Garden City, NY, 1981, Anchor Press/Doubleday

Kunst-Wilson, W, and Cronenwett, L: Nursing care for the emerging family: promoting paternal behavior, Res Nurs Health 4:201, 1981

Lederman, R: Psychosocial adaptation in pregnancy, Englewood Cliffs, NJ, 1984, Prentice-Hall, Inc

Lederman, R, et al: Relationship of psychological factors in pregnancy to progress in labor, Nurs Res 28:2, 1979

Lederman, RP, Weingarten, CT, and Lederman, E: Postpartum self-evaluation questionnaire: measures of maternal adaptation. In Lederman, R, Raff, B, and Carroll, P, editors: Perinatal parental behavior: nursing research and implications for newborn health, New York, 1981, Alan R Liss, Inc

Leifer, M: Psychological changes accompanying pregnancy and motherhood, Genet Psychol Monogr 95:57, 1977

Leifer, M: Psychological effects of motherhood: a study of first pregnancy, New York, 1980, Praeger Publishers

Lein L: Male participation in home life: impact of social supports and breadwinner responsibility on the allocation of tasks, Fam Coord 28:489, 1979

Levy, JM, and McGee, RK: Childbirth as a crisis, J Pers Soc Psychol 31:171, 1975

Lumley, J: The development of maternal-fetal bonding in first pregnancy. In Zichella, L, editor: Emotions and reproduction, New York, 1980a, Academic Press, Inc

Lumley J: The image of the fetus in the first trimester, Birth Fam J 7:5, 1980b
Lumley, J: Attitudes to the fetus among primigravidas, Aust Pediatr J 18:106, 1982a
Lumley, J: Maternal-fetal bonding. II. Implications for the next three months, unpublished manuscript, Melbourne, 1982b, Monash University
Maloni, JA, McIndoe, JE, and Rubenstein, G: Expectant grandparents class, JOGN Nurs 16(1):26, 1987
May, KA: A typology of detachment and involvement styles adopted during pregnancy by first-time expectant fathers, Western J Nurs Res 2:445, 1980
May, KA: The father as observer, Matern Child Nurs J 7:319, 1982a
May, KA: Father participation in birth: fact and fiction, J Calif Perinat Assoc 2:41, Fall 1982b
May, KA: Three phases of father involvement in pregnancy, Nurs Res 31:337, 1982c
McKay, S, and Phillips, CR: Family-centered maternity care: implementation strategies, Rockville, Md, 1984, Aspen Systems Corp
Mercer, RT: "She's a multip . . . she knows the ropes," MCN 4:301, Sept/Oct 1979
Mercer, RT: A theoretical framework for studying factors that impact on the maternal role, Nurs Res 30:2, March/April 1981
Mercer, RT, Hackley, K, and Bostrom A: Factors having an impact on maternal role attainment in the first year of motherhood, San Francisco, 1982, University of California, San Francisco, Dept of Family Health Care Nursing
Newell, NJ: Grandparents: the overlooked support system for new parents during the fourth trimester, NAACOG Update Series, 1:lesson 21, 1984
Nurses' Association of the American College of Obstetricians and Gynecologists: Guidelines for childbirth education, Washington, DC, 1981, The Association
Parke, RD, and Sawin, DB: The father's role in infancy: a reevaluation, Fam Coord 25:365, 1976
Periscope: Alternative birthing study publishes findings, Calif Perinatal Assn, p 4, Winter 1987
Richardson, P: Women's perceptions of change in relationships shared with children during pregnancy, Matern Child Nurs J 12:2, Summer 1983
Rising, SS, and Lindell, SG: The Childbearing Childrearing Center: a nursing model, Nurs Clin North Am 17:1, March 1982
Rubin, R: Attainment of the maternal role. I. Processes, Nurs Res 240:237, 1967a
Rubin, R. Attainment of the maternal role. II. Models and referents, Nurs Res 16:342, 1967b
Rubin, R: Body and image and self-esteem, Nurs Outlook 16:20, June 1968
Rubin, R: Cognitive style in pregnancy, Am J Nurs 70:502, 1970
Rubin, R: Maternal tasks in pregnancy, Matern Child Nurs J 4: Spring 1975
Satir, V: Peoplemaking, Palo Alto, Calif, 1972, Science & Behavior Books
Searles, C: The impetus toward home birth, J Nurse Midwife 26:3, May/June 1981
Sheehy, G: Passages: predictable crises of adult life, New York, 1977, Bantam Books, Inc
Shereshefsky, PM, and Yarrow, LJ, editors: Psychological aspects of a first pregnancy and early postnatal adaptation, New York, 1973, Raven Press
Sherwen, LN: Psychosocial dimensions of the pregnant family, New York, 1987, Springer Publishing Co, Inc
Stainton, MC: A comparison of prenatal and postnatal perceptions of their babies by parents, paper presented to the First International Congress on Pre- and Peri-natal Psychology, Toronto, July 8, 1983
Stainton, MC: The fetus: a growing member of the family, Fam Relations 34:321, 1985a
Stainton, MC: Origins of attachment: culture and cue sensitivity, unpublished doctoral dissertation, University of California, San Francisco, 1985b
Strang, V: Body image, attitudes during pregnancy and the postpartum period, JOGN Nurs 14:4, July-Aug 1985
Walz, B, and Rich, O: Maternal tasks of taking on a second child in the postpartum period, Matern Child Nurs J 12:3, fall, 1983
Winslow, W: First pregnancy after 35: what is the experience? MCN 12(2):92, 1987
Wolkind, S, and Zajicek, E: Pregnancy: a psychological and social study, New York, 1981, Grune & Stratton, Inc

Bibliography

Austin, SE: Childbirth classes for couples desiring VBAC (vaginal birth after cesarean), MCN 11(4):250, 1986
Avant, KC: Stressors on the childbearing family, JOGN Nurs 17(3):179, 1988
Brown, MA: Social support and symptomatology: a study of first-time expectant parents, doctoral dissertation, Seattle, 1983, University of Washington, Dissertation Abstracts International, 44, 111B, 1983
Brown, MA: Marital support during pregnancy, J Obstet Gynecol Neonatal Nurs 15 (6): 475, 1986
Brown, MA: Social support during pregnancy: a unidimensional or multidimensional construct? Nurs Res 35(1):4, 1986
Brown, MA: Social support, stress and health: a comparison of expectant mothers and fathers, Nurs Res 35:72, 1986
Clinton, J: Couvade patterns, predictors, and nursing management, W J Nurs Res 7:221, 1985
Clinton, JF: Expectant fathers at risk for couvade, Nurs Res 35(5):290, 1986
Clinton, JF: Physical and emotional responses of expectant fathers throughout pregnancy and the early postpartum period, Int J Nurs Stud 24(1):59, 1987
Cox, M: Many professional women apply career lessons to job of childbirth, Wall Street Journal 25, 39, Aug 17, 1984b
Dubin, B: Images of the body, Lecture at University of California, Feb 15, 1985
Fawcett, J, and York, R: Spouses' physical and psychological symptoms during pregnancy and the postpartum, Nurs Res 35(4):144, 1986
Fawcett, J, et al: Spouses' body image changes during and after pregnancy: a replication and extension, Nurs Res 35(4):220, 1986
Griffin, S: Childbearing and the concept of culture, JOGN Nurs 11:181, 1982
Howley, C: The older primipara: implications for nurses, JOGN Nurs 10:182, 1981
Humenick, SS: Pregnant adult learners, NAACOG Update Series 1: lesson 24, 1984
Imprints, Birth and Life Bookstore, P.O. Box, 70625, Seattle, WA 98107, Sept, 1983 (a source of books on birth and life)
Jordan B: Birth in four cultures, Montreal, 1983, Eden Press

Josselyn, IM: Psychology of fatherliness, Smith College Studies Social Work 26:1, Feb 1956
Keuscher, MB, and Oliver, M: A overview of childbirth education, J Calif Perinatal Assoc 2(1):79, 1982
Krugen, S, and Maetzold, LD: Practices of tradition for pregnancy, Matern Child Nurs J 12:135, 1983
Libresco, M: Creative teaching: beyond lecture and demonstration, In Humenick, SS, editor: Expanding horizons in childbirth education, Washington, DC, 1983, ASPO/Lamaze (PO Box 33429 Farragut Station, Washington DC 20033)
Mercer, RT: Patterns of maternal role attainment over the past year, Nurs Res 34:119, 1985
Mercer, RT, et al: Theoretical models for studying the effect of antepartum stress on the family, Nurs Res 35(6):339, 1986
Miller, SJ: Prenatal nursing assessment of the expectant family, Nurse Pract 11(5):40, 1986
Moore, D: Prepared childbirth and marital satisfaction during the antepartum and postpartum periods, Nurs Res 32:73, March/April 1983
Moore, L, et al: Self-assessment: a personalized approach to nursing during pregnancy, JOGN Nurs 15(4):311, 1986
Mueller, LS: Pregnancy and sexuality, JOGN Nurs 14(4):289, 1985
Nicholas and the baby (16 mm film or ¾ inch videocassette), Centre Productions, Inc, Suite A, 1312 Pine St, Boulder, Colo 80302 (Film available for preparing older preschool and school-age children for participation in the birth experience)
Norton, SF, and Nichols, CW: Champions of choice, Am J Nurs 85(4):380, 1985
Rankin, SH, and Duffy, KL: Patient education issues, principles, and guidelines, Philadelphia, 1983, JB Lippincott Co
Redman, BK: The process of patient education, ed 6, St Louis, 1988, The CV Mosby Co
Stainton, MC: Parent infant interactions: putting theory into nursing practice, Calgary, 1981, The University of Calgary
Strang, VR, and Sullivan, PL: Body image attitudes during pregnancy and the postpartum period, JOGN Nurs, 14(4):332, 1985
Strickland, OL: The occurrence of symptoms in expectant fathers, Nurs Res 36:(3):184, 1987
Swanson, J: The marital sexual relationship during pregnancy, JOGN Nurs vol 9: Sept/Oct 1980
Thomas, BS: Identifying priorities for prepared childbirth research, Obstet Gynecol Neonatal Nurs 13(6):400, 1984
Waller, MM: Siblings in the childbearing experience, NAACOG Update Series 1: lesson 17, 1984
Weiss, SJ: The language of touch, Nurs Res 28:76, 1979
Wiles, LS: The effect of prenatal breastfeeding education on breastfeeding success and maternal perception of the infant. J Obstet Gynecol Neonatal Nurs 13 (4):253, 1984

CHAPTER 12

First Trimester

Learning Objectives

Correctly define the key terms listed.

Summarize health assessment of the gravida in the first trimester.

Assess the presumptive, probable, and positive manifestations of pregnancy.

Outline the schedule of visits for a woman with a normal pregnancy.

Evaluate cultural influences of the woman's (family's) response to pregnancy and the use of the health care system.

List the 11 physical danger signs of the prenatal period.

Describe signs of potential parenting disorders.

Formulate possible nursing diagnoses and type of data base expected to support these diagnoses.

Review planning of care and establishing goals with gravidas and their families.

Discuss implementation and evaluation of care during the first trimester.

Key Terms

amenorrhea
ballottement
breast fullness
cultural variations
estimated date of delivery (EDD)
evil eye
first trimester
gestational age
imitative magic
last menstrual period (LMP)
"morning sickness"
Nägele's rule
physical danger signs
positive signs
presumptive signs and symptoms
probable signs and symptoms
taboos
urinary frequency

The prenatal period is a preparatory one both physically, in terms of fetal growth and maternal adaptations, and psychologically, in terms of anticipation of parenthood. Becoming a parent represents one of the maturational crises of our lives and as such can represent a time of growth in responsibility and concern for others. It is a time of intense learning for the parents and for those close to them, as well as a time for development of family unity.

During a woman's life, pregnancy is unique because only then does the healthy woman seek ongoing health care. Regular prenatal visits, ideally beginning soon after the first missed menstrual period, offer opportunities to ensure the health of the expectant mother and her infant. This is done by supervising the course of normal pregnancy. Prenatal health supervision permits diagnosis and treatment of maternal disorders that may have preexisted or may develop during the pregnancy. It is designed to follow the growth and development of the fetus and to identify abnormalities that may interfere with the course of normal labor. The woman and her family can seek support for stress and learn parenting skills.

The professionals who have contact with the gravida and her family will include a cross section of health workers such as nurse, physician, nutritionist, and social worker. It is essential that these persons collaborate to provide holistic care for their clients. The initial visit of the woman to either the physician's office or an obstetric clinic is important in setting the tone for her care. The woman needs to feel welcomed and important. The initial visit may include diagnosing the pregnancy and establishing the data base, depending on the duration of gestation. If pregnancy is too early and cannot be verified, her next appointment is scheduled in 2 weeks. Misdiagnosis can lead to serious emotional and legal consequences.

The woman's desire for pregnancy is evaluated. If she is pregnant and does not wish to continue the pregnancy, she is referred for abortion counseling (see Chapter 42). If she is not pregnant and does not wish to be, she is referred for fertility management, if appropriate (see Chapter 42).

If the woman is pregnant and plans to carry the pregnancy to term, prenatal care is instituted. The nursing care presented follows the process of nursing: assessment, formulation of nursing diagnoses, planning, implementation, and evaluation.

DIAGNOSIS OF PREGNANCY

The clinical diagnosis of pregnancy before the second missed period may be difficult in at least 25% to 30% of women. Physical variability, lack of relaxation, obesity, or tumors, for example, may confound even the experienced obstetrician or midwife. Accuracy is most important, however, because social, medical, or legal consequences of an inaccurate diagnosis, either positive or negative, can be extremely serious. A correct date for the last menstrual period (LMP), the date of intercourse, or the basal body temperature (BBT) record may be of great value in the accurate diagnosis of pregnancy. Reexamination in 2 to 4 weeks may be required for verifying the diagnosis.

Great variability is possible in the subjective and objective symptoms of pregnancy. The diagnosis of pregnancy is classified as follows: presumptive, probable, and positive (Table 12-1).

The *positive signs* of pregnancy are (1) demonstration of a **fetal heart** distinct from that of the mother, (2) appreciation of **fetal movement** by someone other than the mother, and (3) **visualization of the fetus** with a technique such as ultrasound (Danforth and Scott, 1986).

The nurse is referred to Chapter 10 for an in-depth discussion of the symptomatology reflecting maternal adaptations to pregnancy. Many of the signs and symptoms of pregnancy are clinically useful in the diagnosis of pregnancy. The *presumptive signs* and symptoms of pregnancy can be caused by conditions other than gestation. Therefore no one manifestation can be relied on for a final impression, nor are combinations of several manifestations diagnostic. Table 12-2 outlines the differential assessment of signs and symptoms of pregnancy.

The positive signs used to confirm the diagnosis of pregnancy include certain pregnancy tests (see Chapter 10). Enzyme-linked immunosorbent assay (ELISA) testing is the most popular testing procedure for pregnancy (Batzer, 1985; Danforth and Scott, 1986). It uses a specific monoclonal antibody produced by hybrid cell-line technology (News, 1985). An enzyme rather than a radioactive compound identifies the antigen of the substance to be measured. The enzyme induces a simple color-change reaction. The endpoint of the test can be read with either the eye or a spectrometer.

ELISA testing has many advantages. The antigen enzyme conjugate and test reagents are stable, the equipment needs are simple, and there are no nuclear waste products. As an office or home procedure it requires minimal time and offers results in 5 minutes coupled with sensitivities from 25 to 50 mIU/ml of human chorionic gonadotropin (hCG) in the specimen. ELISA technology is the basis for the new over-the-counter tests. The manufacturer provides directions for collection of specimen (serum, plasma, or urine), care of specimen, testing procedure, and reading of results.

ESTIMATED DATE OF DELIVERY

Following the diagnosis of pregnancy the woman's first question usually concerns when she will deliver. This date has traditionally been termed the *estimated date of confinement* (EDC). To promote a more positive perception of both pregnancy and delivery, however, the term *estimated date of delivery* (EDD) is usually used. Because the precise date of conception generally must remain conjectural, many formulas or rules of thumb have been suggested for calculating the EDD. None of these rules of thumb are infallable, but Nägele's rule is reasonably accurate and is the method usually used.

Nägele's Rule

Nägele's rule is as follows: add 7 days to the first day of the LMP, subtract 3 months, and add 1 year. The formula becomes EDD + ([LMP + 7 days] − 3 months) + 1 year. For example, if the first day of the LMP was July 10, 1989, the EDD is April 17, 1990. In simple terms, add 7 days to the LMP and count forward 9 months.

Table 12-1 *Signs and Symptoms of Pregnancy in Order of Appearance**

Presumptive	Probable	Positive
Subjective Symptoms		
Amenorrhea (4 weeks)† Nausea, vomiting (4 weeks) Breast sensitivity (6 weeks) Urinary symptoms (6 weeks) Lassitude/fatigue Constipation Weight gain Fingernail changes Quickening (16-20 weeks) Mood swings	Same as presumptive symptoms; when combined with probable signs, strong suspicion of pregnancy	No symptoms positively diagnostic of pregnancy
Objective Signs		
Elevation of BBT Integumentary changes Pigmentation Striae gravidarum Telangiectases (spider nevi) Acne, hirsutism Epulis Breast changes (8 weeks) Enlargement Secondary areolae Montgomery's tubercles Precolostrum (16 weeks) Abdominal enlargement Pelvic changes Vagina (Chadwick's sign; leukorrhea) (8 weeks) Cervix (softening; Goodell's sign; dried mucus in granular pattern) (6-8 weeks) Uterine softening (Hegar's sign) (6 weeks) Relaxation of bony pelvic joints and ligaments Vulval varicosities (10 weeks)	Uterine enlargement: Size of large hen's egg (7 weeks) Size of an orange (10 weeks) Size of a grapefruit; uterus becomes an abdominal organ (12 weeks) Uterine contractions (Braxton Hicks' sign) (20 weeks) External ballottement (24 weeks) Internal ballottement (14 weeks) Uterine souffle Laboratory tests (except radioimmunoassay of beta subunit of hCG‡; this endocrine test provides definitive results)	FHT‡ Echocardiography (5 weeks) Real-time ultrasound imaging (heart motion can be visualized at 7 weeks) Electronic device (8-12 weeks) Electrocardiogram (12 weeks) Auscultation of fetal heart (17-18 weeks) Palpation of fetal movement (about 20 weeks) Ultrasonographic (echographic) evidence of gestational sac confirms presence of intrauterine gestation (6 weeks); fetal breathing movements can be visualized by 11 weeks; detection of FHT (8-12 weeks); by week 14 the fetal head and thorax can be visualized, and subsequently the placenta can be localized Laboratory tests Immunologic (6 weeks) Radioimmunoassay (can diagnose pregnancy as early as 23 days after first day of last menstrual period, about 5 days before next menstrual period would have been due) Home pregnancy test (9 days after end of missed period) Clinical test Progesterone withdrawal

*Clinical diagnosis of pregnancy depends on the ability to interpret presumptive, probable, and positive physical signs and symptoms.
†Time of appearance of symptoms is provided when predictable.
‡FHT, Fetal heart tones; hCG, human chorionic gonadotropin.

Nägele's rule assumes that the woman has a 28-day cycle and that the pregnancy occurred on the fourteenth day. An adjustment is in order if the cycle is longer or shorter than 28 days. With the use of Nägele's rule, only about 4% to 10% of gravidas will deliver spontaneously on the EDD. Most women will deliver during the period extending from 7 days before to 7 days after the EDD (Appendix D).

Assessment

The process of assessment continues throughout the prenatal period. It begins when a woman makes contact with health professionals because she suspects she is pregnant. Assessment techniques include the interview, the physical examination, and laboratory tests.

A checklist of care needs spanning pregnancy is a valuable tool. It provides the team of care providers with a communication tool to prevent gaps and identify areas of repeated concern for clients. When shared with clients, the checklist items validate their universality among gravidas and their families. Knowledge that items are common to many offers some reassurance. Reading the checklist also reminds clients of otherwise forgotten data. A checklist for the first trimester is on p. 244. Chapters 13 and 14 include checklists for the second and third trimesters.

Table 12-2 *Differential Assessment of Signs and Symptoms of Pregnancy*

Symptoms	Possible Causes of Diagnostic Error
Abdominal enlargement	Obesity, abdominal muscle relaxation, tumors, ascites, ventral abdominal hernia
Amenorrhea	Emotional factors: severe emotional shock, tension, fear of or strong desire for pregnancy
	Endocrine factors: adrenal or ovarian neoplasms, thyroid or pituitary disorders, lactation, menopause
	Metabolic factors: anemia, malnutrition, diabetes mellitus, degenerative disorders
	Systemic disease: acute or chronic infection (tuberculosis, brucellosis) or malignancy
	Local causes (cervical obstruction; jogging)
Braxton Hicks' contractions	Contractions of muscles of abdominal wall
Breast sensitivity (mastalgia; mastodynia)	Infectious processes: mastitis, cystic mastitis, premenstrual tension
	Pseudocyesis (false pregnancy)
	Estrogen excess associated with anovulatory periods or ovarian tumors
Cervical and uterine changes in shape, size, consistency	Tumors, adenomyosis, cervical stenosis with hematometra or pyometra, tubo-ovarian cysts
	Normal-size uterus displaced by a pelvic tumor (fibroid or myoma)
Clinical and laboratory findings	Poor thermometer, faulty use of thermometer, inaccurate recording
Elevation of BBT	Corpus luteum cyst
Pregnancy tests	Drug ingestion: progesterone
	False results, incorrect interpretation of results
	Elevation of hCG levels for a few days after spontaneous abortion
	Elevation of hCG: hydatidiform mole, choriocarcinoma
Lassitude and fatigue	Psychologic: emotional disorders
	Pathologic: anemia, infection, malignant disease
Epulis	Infection, dental calculus, vitamin C deficiency
Hyperpigmentation of skin	Local causes (excessive sunlight, tanning)
	System diseases (Addison's disease)
	Use of oral contraceptives
Leukorrhea	Infections: vaginal, cervical
	Tumors
Nausea or vomiting	Emotional factors: anxiety, pseudocyesis, anorexia nervosa
	Gastrointestinal disorders: hiatal hernia, ulcers, enteritis, appendicitis
	Systemic disease: acute infection—influenza, encephalitis
	Allergies
Nipple discharge (milklike)	Drug ingestion: oral contraceptives, psychotropic drugs
	Tumors
	Syndromes (also associated with amenorrhea): hypothalamic or anterior pituitary disorders
Pseudocyesis	Emotional factors
	Pituitary tumor
Quickening	Peristalsis; "gas"
Souffle	Heard over vascular tumors or aneurysms or in thin women; may be abdominal aortic pulsation

FIRST TRIMESTER CHECKLIST

- Diagnosis and expected date of delivery
- Schedule and events of visits
- Counseling for self-care:
  - Adaptations/discomforts
    - Breast changes
    - Urinary frequency
    - Nausea and vomiting
    - Fatigue
    - Psychosocial responses and family dynamics
  - Exercise and rest
  - Relaxation
  - Nutrition
  - Sexuality
  - Danger signs
  - Resources
    - Education
    - Dental evaluation
    - Medical service
    - Social service
    - Emergency room
- Diagnostic tests
  - Specify
- Other

Interview

The initial assessment interview establishes the therapeutic relationship between nurse and client (see Chapters 2 and 8). It is planned, purposeful communication that focuses on specific content. Two sources are usually used in collecting data: the client's subjective interpretation of health status and the nurse's objective observations. During the interview the nurse observes the client's affect, posture, body language, skin color, and other physical and emotional signs. These observations become important data in the assessment.

Often the client will be accompanied by a family member or members. The nurse builds a relationship with these persons as part of the social context of the client. They also are helpful in recalling and validating information related to the client's health problem. With the client's permission, those accompanying her can be included in the initial prenatal interview. Wright and Leahey (1984) offer excellent guidance to the nurse in developing skills for interviewing families and assessing the interaction between family members. Observations and information about the client's family are part of the interview. For example, if the client is accompanied by small children, the nurse can inquire about her plans for child care during the forthcoming labor and delivery.

The interview provides information about the client's biopsychosocial status. Although the format for interviewing or recording the client's health history may differ, the information obtained is universal.

Reason for Client's Request for Care. The client's description of the purpose for the request for care is quoted verbatim in the record. For example, "I think I am pregnant," or "My legs get so swollen I can hardly walk." This statement does not constitute a diagnosis, since the client's condition needs to be confirmed by the nurse or physician before any care is instituted. Recording the chief purpose of a visit in the client's own words alerts other personnel to the "priority of need" as seen by the client.

Past Medical History. The interviewer will record such information as the woman's menstrual history, sexual activity, and previous pregnancies and their outcomes. The conduct of the *present pregnancy* is predicated on the reports of previous pregnancies.

The past medical history describes medical or surgical conditions that may affect the course of pregnancy or that may be affected by the pregnancy. For example, the pregnant woman who has diabetes or epilepsy will require special care. Because most clients are anxious during the initial interview, reference to cues such as a Medic Alert bracelet will help the client explain allergies, chronic diseases, or medications being used (e.g., cortisone, insulin, or anticonvulsants). If the woman is using any *pharmaceuticals,* she is asked to list them and describe their use.

Previous surgeries are described. Abortion may predispose the woman to incompetent cervix; uterine surgery or extensive repair of the pelvic floor may necessitate cesarean birth; appendectomy rules out appendicitis as cause of right lower quadrant pain; spinal surgery contraindicates spinal or epidural anesthesia. Any *injury* involving the pelvis is noted particularly.

Often clients who have adapted well to chronic or handicapping conditions forget to mention them because they are so integrated into their life-style. Special shoes or a limp may indicate a pelvic structural defect, which is an important consideration in pregnancy. The nurse who observes these special characteristics and can inquire about them sensitively obtains individualized data that will provide the basis for a comprehensive nursing care plan. Observations are vital components of the interview process because they prompt the nurse and the client to focus on the specific needs of the client and her family.

Family History. The family history provides information about the client's immediate family, including parents, siblings, and children. This helps identify familial or genetic disorders or conditions that could affect the present health status of the woman. A description of a detailed family history is presented in Chapter 8.

Social and Experiential History. *Situational factors* such as the family's ethnic and cultural background and socioeconomic status are determined in the social and experiential history. *Perception of this pregnancy* is explored. Is this pregnancy wanted or not, planned or not? Is the woman (couple) pleased, displeased, accepting, or nonaccepting. Is the pregnancy "hers" or "theirs?" What problems arise because of the pregnancy: financial, career, and living accommodations? The *family support* system is determined (see Chapter 3). What primary support is available to the mother? Are there changes needed to promote adequate support for the mother? What are the existing relationships between mother, father, siblings, and in-laws? What preparations are being made for the care of the woman and dependent family members during labor and for the care of the infant after birth? Is community support needed, for example, financial, educational? What are the woman's (couple's) ideas about childbearing, expectations of infant's behavior, and outlook on life and the female role? Questions that need to be asked include, What will it be like to have a baby in the home? How is your life going to change by having a baby? What plans do having a baby interrupt? During interviews throughout the pregnancy the nurse remains alert for potential parenting disorders (see box below).What is the woman's (couple's) attitude toward health care, particularly during childbearing? What is expected of the physician and how is the relationship between the woman (couple) and nurse viewed?

SIGNS OF POTENTIAL PARENTING DISORDERS

Parents

Depression—mother extremely depressed over pregnancy
Fear and loneliness—mother alone, anticipates delivery with fear: careful explanations do not seem to dissipate fear
Nonsupport of mother by husband or family
Decision change—mother or father originally wanted an abortion or seriously considered relinquishment
Abusive or neglectful background of either parent
Living conditions of parents—overcrowded, isolated, unstable, or intolerable
Lack of modern facilities—telephone, electricity, fresh running water
Lack of support systems for parents—no close relatives or friends

Child or Pregnancy

Undue concern—mother appears overly concerned with sex of baby
Denial of pregnancy—mother not willing to gain weight, make plans for baby, refuses to talk about situation
"One-too-many-children"—child may be one too many for mother to handle
Unresolved ambivalence—intensity of ambivalence concerning child or pregnancy heightened at term
Stressful behavior—mother appears uncomfortable around crying infants
Unrealistic expectations—mother, or parents, rigid with infant's behavior

Coping mechanisms and patterns of interacting are identified (see Chapters 3 and 11). Early in the pregnancy the nurse determines the woman's (couple's) knowledge of pregnancy, maternal changes, fetal growth, care of self, and care of the newborn, including feeding. It is important to ask about attitudes toward unmedicated or medicated childbirth, as well as to inquire about parental knowledge of availability of parenting skills classes. Before planning for nursing care, the nurse needs information about the woman's (couple's) decision-making abilities and living habits (e.g., exercise, sleep, diet, diversional interests, personal hygiene, clothing).

Attitudes concerning the range of *acceptable sexual behavior* during pregnancy are explored. Questions such as the following could be asked: What has your family (partner, friends) told you about sex during pregnancy? or What are your feelings about sex during pregnancy? *Sexual self-concept* is given more emphasis by employing questions such as, How do you feel about the changes in your appearance? How does your partner feel about your body now? Do maternity clothes make pregnant women attractive?

Review of Systems. During this portion of the interview, symptomatology indicative of pregnancy is elicited. In addition, preexisting or concurrent problems are identified and described (Chapter 8). The woman is questioned about physical symptoms she has experienced such as shortness of breath or pain. Pregnancy affects and is affected by all body systems (see Chapter 10); therefore knowledge of the present status of body systems is important in planning care. For each sign or symptom expressed, the following additional data should be obtained: body location, quality, quantity, chronology, setting, aggravating or alleviating factors, and associated manifestations (onset, character, course).

Physical Examination

The initial physical examination provides the baseline for assessing subsequent changes. For example, the pregnant woman's weight and blood pressure are assessed against normative data; but, in addition, the rate of her weight gain and rise or fall in her blood pressure are important notations. A rapid weight gain in excess of the norm for the gestation period may signal the possibility of a multiple pregnancy, developing edema, or both.

The examiner uses a formalized sequence in conducting a physical examination. A cephalocaudal or system-by-system approach and a checklist will prevent omitting any key information. As the examination proceeds, the client can be questioned about pertinent health concerns or symptoms. The techniques used are observation, palpation, percussion, and auscultation (Seidel et al., 1987; Malasanos et al., 1985). Refer to Chapter 8 for general guidelines and for the examination of the thyroid, breasts, abdomen (Table 8-1), and pelvis.

The woman's knowledge and skill in breast self-examination (BSE) are assessed. If the woman is considering breast-feeding, the nipples are examined for erectility. The woman's knowledge of measures to prevent urinary tract infection is reviewed.

The pelvic examination (Procedure 8-2) may be deferred to the next prenatal visit if the woman is anxious, tense, or refuses to have one at this visit. The vagina enlarges, and supporting structures are more relaxed as pregnancy advances. The tone of the pelvic musculature and need for and knowledge of Kegel's exercises (p. 162) are assessed. During the pelvic examination the nurse remains alert for symptomatology of supine hypotension and vasovagal syncope, pp. 152 and 146.

Early in pregnancy, before the uterus is an abdominal organ, the fetal heart tones (FHTs) can be heard with an ultrasound fetoscope or an ultrasound stethoscope (Fig. 18-13, *C, D*). The instrument is placed in the midline just anterior to the symphysis pubis. Firm pressure is needed as the scope is used. The woman and her family can be offered the opportunity to listen to the FHTs.

Laboratory Tests

The data obtained from laboratory examination of specimens add important information concerning the symptomatology of pregnancy and health status. Both nursing and medical diagnoses stem from such information.

Specimens are collected at the initial visit so that results of their examination will be ready for the next scheduled prenatal visit (Table 12-3). A clean-catch urine specimen (Procedure 8-1) is tested. Tine or purified protein derivative of tuberculin (PPD) tests are administered for exposure to tuberculosis. During the pelvic examination cervical and vaginal smears for cytology (Papanicolaou smear [Procedure 8-3] and herpes simplex type 2) and for infection (Chlamydia organisms, gonorrhea [Fig. 8-15]) are obtained. Blood is drawn to test for a variety of conditions: venereal disease research laboratory (VDRL) test for syphilis; complete blood count (CBC) with hematocrit, hemoglobin, and differential values; blood type and Rh factor; antibody screen (Kell, Duffy, rubella, toxoplasmosis, and anti-Rh); sickle cell anemia; level of folacin when indicated; urine is tested for glucose, protein, and acetone; culture and sensitivity tests are ordered as necessary.

Fetal Development

A summary of the development of the fetus is presented in the box on p. 247.

Nursing Diagnoses

Each client and family will have a unique set of responses to pregnancy. To attend to these responses the nurse begins by formulating appropriate nursing diagnoses (Chapter 2). Following are examples of nursing diagnoses arising from analysis of assessment findings during the first trimester:

- Anxiety, potential, related to
  - Concern about herself
  - Physical changes with pregnancy
  - Her (or other's) feelings about the pregnancy
- Pain, related to
  - Early discomforts of pregnancy

Table 12-3 *Laboratory Tests in Prenatal Period*

Laboratory Test	Purpose
Hemoglobin/hematocrit, WBC, differential	To detect anemia
Hemoglobin electrophoresis	To identify women with hemoglobinopathies (e.g., sickle cell anemia)
Blood type, Rh, and irregular antibody	To identify those fetuses at risk for developing erythroblastosis fetaiis or hyperbilirubinemia in neonatal period
Rubella titer	To determine immunity to rubella
VDRL/FTA-ABS*	To identify women with untreated syphilis
AIDS antibody, hepatitis	To screen high-risk population
Urinalysis, including microscopic examination of urinary sediment; pH, specific gravity, color, glucose, albumin/protein, RBC, WBC, casts, acetone; hCG	To identify women with unsuspected diabetes mellitus, renal disease, hypertensive disease of pregnancy; infection; pregnancy
Urine culture	To identify women with asymptomatic bacteriuria
Renal function tests: BUN,† creatinine, electrolytes, creatinine clearance, total protein excretion	To evaluate level of possible renal compromise in women with a history of diabetes, hypertension, or renal disease
Papanicolaou smear	To screen for cervical intraepithelial neoplasia and herpes simplex type 2
Vaginal or rectal smear for *Neisseria gonorrhoeae, Chlamydia*	To screen high-risk population for asymptomatic infection
Tuberculin skin testing	To screen high-risk population
Cardiac evaluation; ECG, chest x-ray film, and echocardiogram	To evaluate cardiac function in women with a history of hypertension or cardiac disease

*FTA-ABS, fluorescent treponemal antibody absorption test.
†BUN, blood urea nitrogen.

FETAL DEVELOPMENT AT 13 WEEKS

1. Differentiation of tissues complete as period of organogenesis ends
2. Human appearance
3. Sex distinguishable
4. Skeleton ossifying
5. Tooth buds forming
6. Respiratory activity evident
7. Insulin secreted (since eighth week)
8. Kidneys secreting
9. Intestine returns to abdomen
10. Head is one-third of total length
11. Length: 9 cm (3½ in)
12. Weight: 15 g (½ oz)
13. Fetus less susceptible to malformation from teratogenic agents

- Altered family processes related to
  - Family's response to diagnosis of pregnancy
- Knowledge deficit, related to
  - Maternal and familial adaptations to pregnancy
  - Maternal and familial adaptations to EDD
- Altered nutrition: less than body requirements, related to
  - "Morning sickness"
- Altered sexuality patterns, related to
  - Discomforts of early pregnancy

See nursing care plans in this chapter, pp. 260-262.

Planning

Planning care for clients during the first trimester of the prenatal period is based on the biopsychosocial assessment of the client and her family. For each client a plan is developed that relates specifically to her clinical and nursing problems. The information in this chapter is general in nature; that is, not all women will experience all problems discussed nor require all facets of the care described. The nurse selects those aspects of care relevant to the client and the client's family based on the following goals:

Goals directed to the maternity population as a whole:

1. To develop health services that are available to all pregnant women, their fetuses, and their families.
2. To develop standards of maternity care applicable to all women and their families (Tucker et al., 1988; NAACOG, 1986; Appendix B).
3. To develop nursing strategies with sound scientific bases.

Goals related to physiologic care:

1. To diagnose pregnancy and determine the EDD.
2. To provide clients with pertinent knowledge of the adaptation of the maternal body to a developing fetus as a basis for understanding the rationale and necessity for modalities of care.
3. To provide clients with information and counseling, including those relating to nutritional needs, sexual needs, activities of daily living, and discomforts of pregnancy.

4. To detect deviations, by risk factor analysis, from the normal progress of pregnancy and to initiate prompt remedial therapy.
5. To alert clients to symptoms that indicate deviations from normal progress and protocols for reporting them.

Goals related to psychosocial care:

1. To identify information needs/readiness for learning.
2. To encourage participation by clients and their families in their care during the first trimester of pregnancy.
3. To provide support for clients and their families as they experience the first trimester of pregnancy.
4. To establish an environment that promotes an emotionally satisfying pregnancy.

The general nursing care plan on p. 260 provides general guidelines for students participating in or observing a nurse during a client's first prenatal visit. The specific nursing care plan on p. 262 for a gravida with morning sickness and fatigue demonstrates how the general care plan is adapted for the individual client.

Implementation

Nurses assume many caregiving roles during the prenatal period. The clinician's role can be categorized as both supportive and teacher/counselor/advocate.

Supportive Activities

The nurse-client relationship is critical in setting the tone for further interactions (see Chapter 2). The techniques of listening with an attentive expression, touching, and using eye contact have their place, as does recognition of the client's feelings and her right to express them. The intervention may occur in various formal or informal settings. For certain persons, involvement in goal-directed health groups is neither feasible nor acceptable. Encounters in hallways or clinic examining rooms, home visits, or telephone conversations may provide the only opportunities for contact and can be used effectively. Sometimes women seek information about a particular problem repeatedly, not so much for the advice given, but to direct the nurse's attention toward themselves. The nurse can help these women by asking for a client-generated solution and a report of its effectiveness.

In supporting a client it must be remembered that both the nurse and the client are contributing to the relationship. The nurse has to accept the client's responses as a factor in trying to be of help. An example of one nurse-client relationship follows:

Mrs. __________________ had been very forthright in saying that this pregnancy was unplanned but had countered this statement with comments such as "All things happen for the best," "We always wanted the boys to have a family to turn to," and "Children bring their own love." Over a period of time, as our relationship developed to one of *mutual* trust, she complained increasingly of her fear of pain, her hating to wear maternity clothes, and her having to give up helping the family. Finally I ventured to say, "Sometimes when a pregnancy is unplanned, women resent it very much and are angry about it." Her relief was evident. She said, "Oh, you don't know how angry I've been." As a result the whole tenor of support being offered changed, and the plan was adjusted to meet her real needs.

The nurse also needs to accept the fact that the woman must be a willing partner in a purely voluntary relationship. As such, the relationship can be refused or terminated at any time by the pregnant woman or her family.

Supportive care involves developing, augmenting, or changing the mechanisms used by women and families in coping with stress. An effort is made to promote active participation by the individuals in the process of solving their own problems. Clients are helped to gather pertinent information, explore alternative actions, make decisions as to choice of action, and assume responsibility for the outcomes. These outcomes may be any or all of the following:

1. Living with a problem as it is
2. Mitigating effects of a problem so that it can be accepted more readily
3. Eliminating the problem through effecting change

Expectations of success in the area of emotional supportive care must of necessity be flexible. It is not within the province of any outsider to assure another person a rewarding, satisfying experience. The mother and persons significant to her are crucial elements in this process. Many of their problems are beyond the scope or capabilities of any professional worker. In describing her work with young and poor persons, Edwards (1973) notes: "They did not usually change their living situation and I was not instrumental in modifying home or drug problems." However, this did not deter her from encouraging clients to use the decision-making process as a means of coping with problems rather than merely complaining about injustice.

At other times a successful outcome can be readily documented. A woman who early in her pregnancy had predicted a severe depressive state in the postdelivery period was elated when such a state did not materialize. She remarked to the nurse who had provided support during the pregnancy and birth, "You're the best nerve medicine I've ever had!"

Teacher/Counselor/Advocate

Health maintenance is an important aspect of prenatal care. Client participation in the care ensures prompt reporting of untoward responses to pregnancy. Client assumption of responsibility for health maintenance is prompted by understanding of maternal adaptations to the growth of the unborn child and a readiness to learn. Nurses in their roles of teacher/counselor/advocate provide clients with the information necessary for compliance with health care measures.

The expectant mother needs information about many subjects, including diet, exercise, sleep, bowel habits, smoking, alcohol ingestion, medication usage, and sexual relations. It is impossible to impart at one visit all of the information the woman and her family may need at the time her pregnancy is diagnosed. She can be given printed information at this time, either in the form of notes that are prepared by the obstetrician or as a listing of the books pertaining to pregnancy that have been written for lay persons. If the latter, the obstetrician, nurse, or nurse-midwife should have read the books carefully to be certain they supply the kind of information desired.

Nutritional intake is an important factor in the maintenance of maternal health during pregnancy and in the provision of adequate nutrients for embryonic/fetal development. Assessing nutritional status and providing nutritional information are part of the nurse's responsibilities in prenatal care. For detailed information concerning maternal and fetal nutritional needs, see Chapter 15.

Formal classes in childbirth and parenthood education have proved successful for some women and families. "Early bird" classes provide fundamental information to meet the needs of most expectant parents during the first trimester (Chapter 11). Allowing the expectant mother or family the opportunity to ask questions and express any anxieties or fears she or they may have is also important.

Schedule for Care. During the initial visit, women appreciate knowing the schedule for return prenatal visits. Most women can expect to return every 4 weeks until the twenty-eighth week of pregnancy, every 2 weeks until the thirty-sixth week of pregnancy, and then every week from week 37 until delivery. More frequent visits may be needed to accommodate the woman's individual needs.

The initial prenatal visit is usually lengthy. Women can be reassured by knowing what to expect on subsequent visits (see Chapters 13 and 14).

Danger Signs. One of the first responsibilities of persons involved in the care of the pregnant woman is to alert her to signs and symptoms that indicate a potential complication of pregnancy. The client needs to know how to report such danger signs (see box, above right). When one is stressed by a disturbing symptom, it is difficult to remember specifics. Therefore the gravida and her family are reassured if they receive a printed form listing the signs and symptoms that warrant an investigation and the phone numbers to call in an emergency.

Discomforts of Pregnancy. Women pregnant for the first time are confronted with symptoms that would be considered abnormal in the nonpregnant state. Much of prenatal care requested by such women relates to explanations of the causes of the discomforts and what measures can be taken to relieve them. The discomforts are fairly specific to each trimester of pregnancy. Information about the physiology, prevention, and treatment of discomforts experienced during the first trimester are given in Table 12-4.

Nurses can anticipate these symptoms and provide anticipatory guidance for women. Women who have a knowledge of the physical basis for the discomforts of pregnancy are less apt to become overly anxious concerning their health. An understanding of the rationale for treatment promotes their participation in their own care. Nurses need to use terminology the woman (or couple) can understand.

The effectiveness of measures to relieve discomforts of pregnancy is a valid subject for nursing research. The study by Dilorio (1985) involving first trimester nausea in pregnant teenagers is a good example of how the nurse can incorporate research into practice (see research highlight).

DANGER SIGNS

Potential Complication of Pregnancy

1. Visual disturbances—blurring, double vision, or spots
2. Swelling of face, fingers or over sacrum
3. Headaches—severe, frequent, or continuous
4. Muscular irritability or convulsions
5. Epigastric pain (perceived as severe stomach ache)
6. Persistent vomiting—beyond first trimester, severe vomiting at any time
7. Fluid discharge from vagina—bleeding or amniotic fluid (anything other than leukorrhea)
8. Signs of infections—chills, fever, burning on urination, diarrhea
9. Pain in abdomen—severe or unusual
10. Change in fetal movements—absence of fetal movements after quickening, any unusual change in pattern or amount

RESEARCH HIGHLIGHT

First Trimester Nausea in Pregnant Teenagers

Purpose

To study the incidence and characteristics of nausea and vomiting among pregnant teenagers, as well as to gather information on the types and effectiveness of measures used by teenagers to control nausea and vomiting.

Sample

78 teenagers who attended three county health department maternity clinics.

Methodology

Dilorio* developed a 15-item questionnaire to collect data from the teenagers.

Findings

The measure the teenagers most commonly used to control nausea and vomiting was to lie down (63%). Other measures used were eating crackers and drinking soda; and a minority of the teenagers (9.1%) took a drug to help control symptoms.

Implications

These findings suggest that lying down may be a commonsense approach to counteract orthostatic hypotension and may be the reason lying down was effective in controlling the symptoms. Therefore Dilorio suggests controlled studies to determine if a relationship exists between orthostatic hypotension, and nausea and vomiting during pregnancy.

*Dilorio, C: First trimester nausea in pregnant teenagers: incidence, characteristics, intervention, Nurs Res 34(6):372, 1985.

Table 12-4 *Discomforts During the First Trimester*

Discomfort	Physiology	Treatment
Breast changes, new sensations: pain, tingling	Hypertrophy of mammary glandular tissue and increased vascularization, pigmentation, and size and prominence of nipples and areolae caused by hormone stimulation	Supportive maternity brassiere with pads to absorb discharge may be worn at night; wash with warm water and keep dry; see Maternal physiology and sexual counseling
Urgency and frequency of urination	Vascular engorgement and altered bladder function caused by hormones; bladder capacity reduced by enlarging uterus and fetal presenting part	Kegel's exercises; limit fluid intake before bedtime; reassurance; wear perineal pad; refer to physician for pain or burning sensation
Languor and malaise; fatigue (early pregnancy, usually)	Unexplained, may be due to increasing levels of estrogen, progesterone, and hCG or to elevated BBT; psychologic response to pregnancy and its required physical/psychologic adaptations	Reassurance; rest as needed; well–balanced diet to prevent anemia
Nausea and vomiting, "morning sickness"—occurs in 50% to 75% of pregnant women; starts between first and second missed periods and lasts until about fourth missed period; may occur any time during day; if mother does not have symptoms, expectant father may; may be accompanied by "bad taste" in mouth	Cause unknown (may result from hormonal changes, possibly hCG; may be partly emotional, reflecting pride in, ambivalence about, or rejection of pregnant state)	Avoid empty or overloaded stomach; maintain good posture—give stomach ample room; stop or decrease smoking; eat dry carbohydrate on awakening; remain in bed until feeling subsides, or alternate dry carbohydrate 1 hour with fluids such as hot tea, milk, or clear coffee the next hour until feeling subsides; eat 5 to 6 small meals per day; avoid fried, odorous, spicy, greasy, or gas-forming foods; consult physician if intractable vomiting occurs; reassurance
Ptyalism (excessive saliva)—may occur starting 2 to 3 weeks after first missed period	Elevated estrogen levels (?); may be related to reluctance to swallow because of nausea	Astringent mouth wash; chewing gum; support
Psychosocial dynamics (Chapter 11): mood swings, mixed feelings	Hormonal and metabolic adaptations; plus feelings about female role, sexuality, timing of pregnancy, and resultant changes in one's life and life-style	Treatment same as prevention; both partners need reassurance and support; support significant other who can reassure woman about her attractiveness, etc.; improved communication with her partner, family, and others; refer to social worker, if needed, or supportive services (financial assistance, food stamps)

Employment. Many women continue to work during pregnancy. A recent American study found an employment rate of 60% among pregnant women (Marbury and others, 1984). Pregnant women, particularly those with young children, who have regular jobs in addition to home responsibilities are carrying one of the heaviest loads of all workers (Bryant, 1985).

Whether the expectant mother can or should work and for how long depends on the physical activity involved, industrial hazards, and medical or obstetric complications. A prime consideration is the avoidance of a fetotoxic environment (e.g., chemical dust particles or gases such as inhalation anesthesia). Operating room personnel who are pregnant need to be aware of the dangers of their working environment to the fetus.* The latest Occupational Safety and Health Administration New Hazard Communication Standard (labeled the federal right-to-know law), November, 1985, requires chemical manufacturers to assess exposure health hazards and inform employees of those hazards (NAACOG, 1985). Nurses who are pregnant are not to be assigned to the care of infants or others with infectious diseases that can be dangerous to the fetus (e.g., measles or cytomegalovirus [CMV]).

The Pregnancy Discrimination Act of 1978 designates the conditions under which a woman can obtain maternity leave.

> Women affected by pregnancy, childbirth, or related medical conditions shall be treated the same for all employment related purposes, including receipt of benefits under fringe benefit programs, as other persons not so affected but similar in their ability or inability to work.*

Part of the anticipatory guidance given during pregnancy should include discussion of maternity leave and discussion of plans to return to work (Leap and others, 1980). The following questions need to be reviewed with the client (Brucker and Reedy, 1983):

1. Does the client's employer cover her health care?

*Since most operating rooms have rectified the problem of escaping gases, this problem has greatly diminished.

*Public Law 95-555; 92 Stat. 2076; Oct. 31, 1978, and the 1979 amendment to Title VII, the Pregnancy Discrimination Act.

2. What policies for leave are granted by the employer?
3. What provisions are made for coverage of the infant's health care (coverage for infants is not addressed in the Pregnancy Discrimination Act)?
4. What should be done if the company policy is at variance with the Pregnancy Discrimination Act? (One answer is that the U.S. Department of Labor investigates and handles complaints regarding Pregnancy Discrimination Act violations or suspected violations.)

Employment during the later pregnancy and postpartum periods is discussed in subsequent chapters.

Physical Activity. A number of researchers have recommended moderate exercise during pregnancy (Bullard, 1981; Dean, 1981; Hutchinson et al., 1981; Jopke, 1983) (see box below). However, activities continued to the point of exhaustion or fatigue compromise uterine perfusion and fetoplacental oxygenation (Dale et al., 1982). If the woman is accustomed to jogging, she may continue; however, she should not reach the point of fatigue. Heat stress may also endanger the fetus. Furthermore, as gestation advances the woman's center of gravity changes, her bony pelvic support loosens, her coordination usually decreases, and she no-

EXERCISE TIPS FOR PREGNANT WOMEN

Consult your health-care provider when you know or suspect you are pregnant. Discuss your medical and obstetric history, your current regimen, and the exercises you would like to continue throughout pregnancy.

Seek help in determining an exercise routine that is well within your limit of tolerance, especially if you have not been exercising regularly. Don't push too hard.

Consider decreasing weight-bearing exercises (jogging, running) and concentrate on non-weight-bearing activities such as swimming, cycling, or stretching. The latter cut down on bouncing motions, decrease the workload, and may be better tolerated by the fetus. If you are a runner, you may wish to walk instead, starting in your seventh month.

Because strenuous exercise during the last few weeks of pregnancy increases the risk of low birthweight, stillbirth, and infant death, reduce exercise sharply 4 weeks before your due date.

Avoid risky activities such as surfing, mountain-climbing, sky-diving, and racquetball. As your pregnancy progresses, your increasing weight, a shift of your center of gravity, and the softening and mobility of your joints and ligaments may alter coordination. Activities requiring precise balance and coordination may be dangerous.

Exercise regularly at least 3 times a week, as long as you are healthy, to improve muscle tone and increase or maintain your stamina. Sporadic exercises may put undue strain on your muscles.

Limit activity to shorter intervals. Exercise for 10 to 15 minutes, rest for 2 to 3 minutes, then exercise for another 10 to 15 minutes. During exercise, blood flow is redistributed from the internal organs to the skeletal muscle system. The decreased blood flow to the uterus may be risky for the fetus if it continues too long. This decrease reverses rapidly when exercise stops.

Decrease your exercise level as your pregnancy progresses. The normal alterations of advancing pregnancy, such as decreased cardiac reserve and increased respiratory effort, may produce physiologic stress if you exercise strenuously for a long time. Your greater body weight calls for a larger energy output, so you will feel more fatigue. If you are a runner, switch to walking during the last 4 weeks before delivery.

Take your pulse every 10 to 15 minutes while you are exercising. If it's more than 140 beats per minute, slow down until it returns to a maximum of 90.

Avoid becoming overheated for extended periods. It's best not to exercise for more than 35 minutes, especially in hot, humid weather. As your body temperature rises, the heat is transmitted to your fetus. Prolonged or repeated fetal temperature elevation may result in birth defects, especially if done during the first 3 months.

Limit the time you spend in hot tubs, saunas, or hot baths. Here are some guidelines:

- Hot tub: water temperature 39.0° C (102.2° F) for less than 15 minutes or 41.0° C (105.8° F) for less than 10 minutes
- Sauna: room temperature 81.4° C (178.5° F) for less than 5 minutes.
- Hot bath: water temperature 39.0° C (102.2° F) for less than 15 minutes.

Ask your health club about the temperature of its hot tubs and saunas, and measure your water temperature at home.

Warmup and stretching exercises prepare your joints for more strenuous exercise and lessen the likelihood of strain or injury to your joints.

A cool-down period of mild activity after exercising will help bring your respiration, heart, and metabolic rates back to normal and avoid pooling of blood in the exercise muscles.

Rest for 10 minutes after exercising, lying on your left side. As the uterus grows, it puts pressure on your inferior vena cava, a major vein carrying blood to your heart, on the right side of your abdomen. Lying on your left side takes the pressure off the vena cava and promotes return circulation from your extremities and muscles to your heart, increasing blood flow to your placenta and fetus.

Drink two or three 8-ounce glasses of water after you exercise, to replace the body fluids you lost through perspiration. While exercising, drink water whenever you feel the need.

Increase your caloric intake to replace the calories burned during exercise. Eat enough to satisfy your hunger and support a weight gain of 1 pound a week, beginning in your fourth month. Choose such high-protein foods as fish, cheese, eggs, or meat.

Take your time. This is not the time to be competitive or train for activities requiring long endurance.

Wear a supportive bra. Your increased breast weight may cause changes in posture and put pressure on the ulnar nerve.

Wear supportive shoes. As your uterus grows, your center of gravity shifts and you compensate by arching your back. In addition, your pelvic muscles and ligaments soften and become more mobile. These natural changes may make you feel off balance and more likely to fall.

Stop exercising immediately if you experience shortness of breath, dizziness, numbness, tingling, abdominal pain, or vaginal bleeding, and consult your health-care provider.

From Paglone, A and Worthington, S: Cautions and advice on exercise during pregnancy, Contemp OB/GYN **25**:160, May 1985 (special issue).

tices a sensation of awkwardness. Awkwardness may cause her to lose balance and fall injuring herself (see guidelines for client teaching: exercise).

Exercises such as those depicted in Fig. 12-1 are taught either at prenatal classes or by the nurse in the clinic or the physician's office. The exercises promote comfort and assist in preparing the woman for labor. Posture and how to lift and move objects safely also are discussed and demonstrated to counteract the awkwardness and prevent the discomfort experienced starting in the second trimester of pregnancy (Chapter 13, guidelines for client teaching: body mechanics).

***Flying Exercise* (Fig. 12-2).** The posture and breathing techniques involved in this exercise assist the woman with discomforts such as heartburn and dyspnea. Relaxation often results as well.

1. Sit tailor or Indian fashion. *Keep back straight throughout exercise.*
2. Raise arms over head. Elbows are straight and palms are held toward each other.

Guidelines For Client Teaching

EXERCISE

ASSESSMENT

1. Gravida requests information about relaxation, rest, relief of discomforts (e.g., backache, heartburn, insomnia), and exercises.

NURSING DIAGNOSES

Potential pain related to emotional or physical tension.
Knowledge deficit related to exercise in pregnancy.

GOALS

Short-term

Woman increases self-care skills by learning at least two exercises.
Woman relieves a current discomfort.
Woman learns limits of safe exercise for self.

Intermediate

Woman reports positive results from exercises used (e.g., increase in comfort, sense of well-being).
Woman appreciates the role of appropriate exercise in health maintenance.

Long-term

Woman continues to exercise appropriately across the life span as one self-care activity in health maintenance.

REFERENCES AND TEACHING AIDS

Illustrations
Cassettes of "New Age" music (e.g., sounds of waterfalls, birds, ocean waves) or other appropriate music.
Full-length mirror, floor mat or comfortable seats, pillows.
Lay references available at bookstores everywhere.

CONTENT/RATIONALE	TEACHING ACTION
To identify maternal anatomic and physiologic adaptations since these affect and are affected by exercise: Factors to consider: Energy level may be low because of poor sleeping and increased energy cost of increase in metabolic rate and weight and emotional adjustment. Change in center of gravity, stretching of abdominal muscles, strain on muscles in general, and relaxation of joints. Altered coordination, balance, and concentration and occasional faintness. Fetal needs for oxygen. Prepregnancy established exercise routine and body condition and current state of health.	Encourage discussion of woman's exercise habits, reasons for and results of exercises she now uses, current discomforts and methods being employed to alleviate them, and exercises she wishes to learn.
To promote sense of well-being:	Encourage woman to listen to her body.
Follow the exercise tips for pregnant women in box on p. 251.	Discuss content of box on p. 251 in light of gravida's individual needs.
Learn and practice pelvic tilt (rock) (Fig. 12-1).	Assess gravida's ability to assess her pulse. Demonstrate.
Use "Flying exercise" for relief of heartburn and dyspnea (Fig. 12-2).	Guide gravida through exercise. Use illustrations such as Figs. 12-1 and 12-2.

EVALUATION The nurse can be reasonably assured that care was effective when goals for care have been met. The woman demonstrates exercises appropriately. Woman states she uses exercises as needed and that doing so relieves her discomfort.

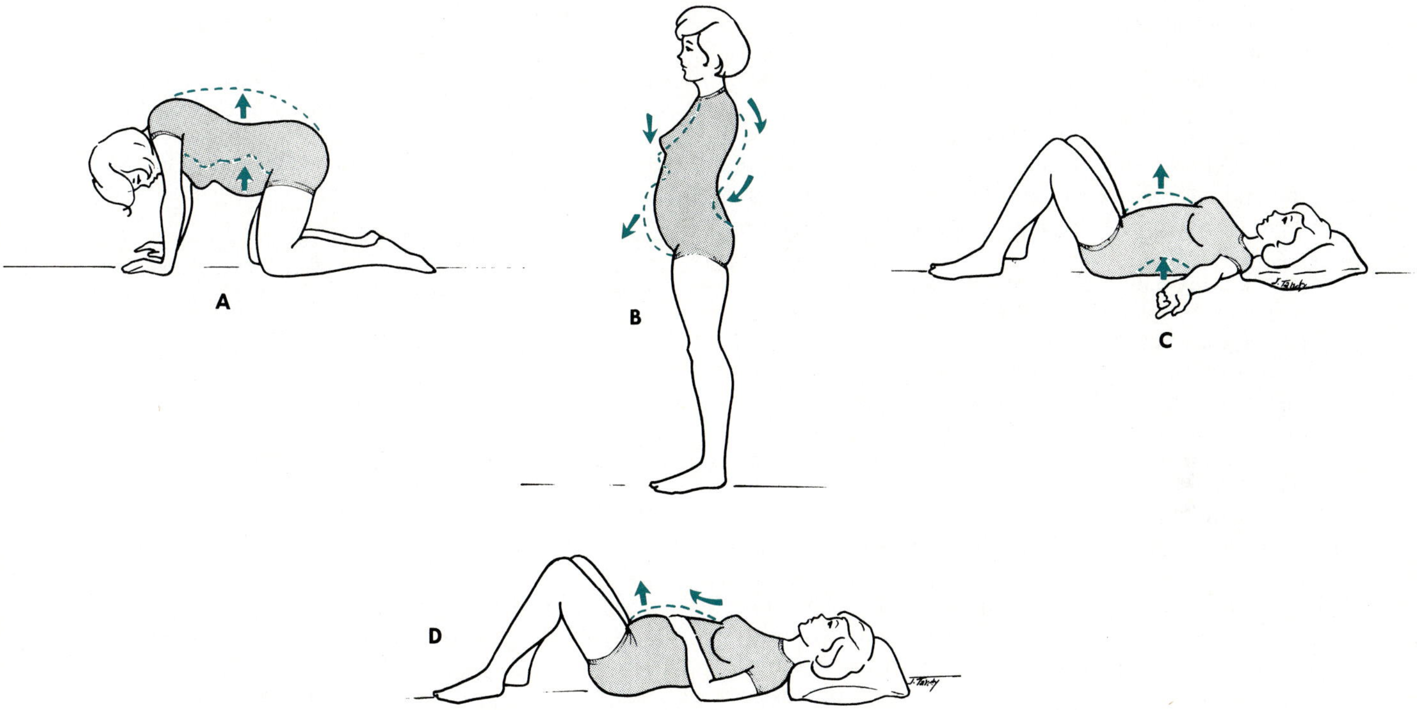

Fig. 12-1 Exercises. **A-C**, Pelvic rocking relieves low backache (excellent for relief of menstrual cramps as well). **D**, Abdominal breathing aids relaxation and lifts abdominal wall off uterus.

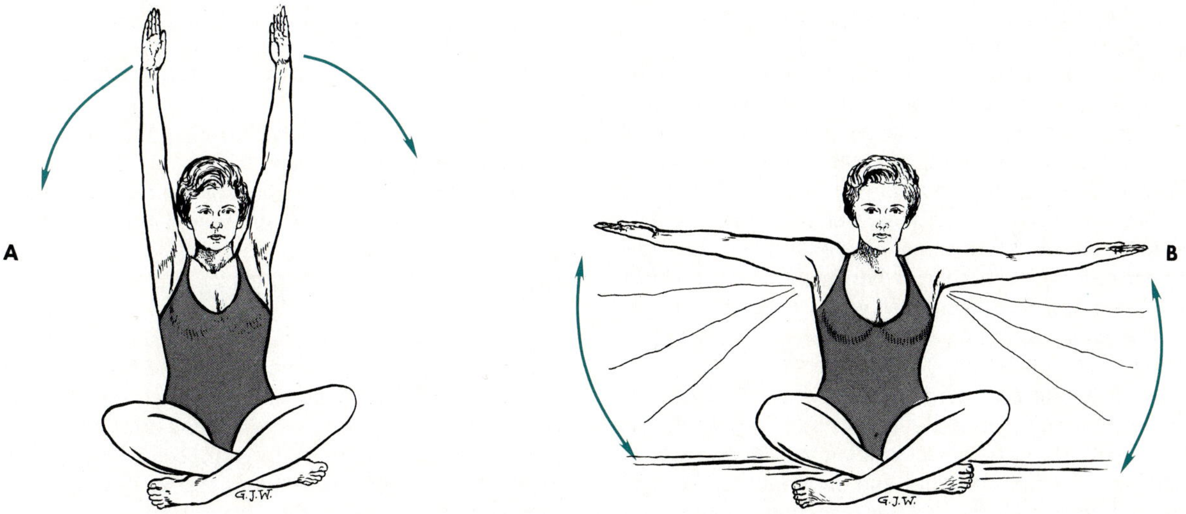

Fig. 12-2 Flying exercise promotes relaxation and reduces discomforts such as heartburn and dyspnea.

3. With palms facing upward, lower arms out to sides.
4. Reach behind back and try to bring backs of hands together briskly; repeat five times.
5. With hands in lap, shrug shoulders (upward toward ears) while breathing in through the nose.
6. Passively and slowly let out breath while letting go of shoulders.

Dental Health. Dental care during pregnancy is especially important. Nausea during pregnancy may lead to poor oral hygiene, and dental caries may develop. No physiologic alteration during gestation can cause dental caries. Calcium and phosphorus in the teeth are fixed in enamel. Therefore the old adage "for every child a tooth" need not be true.

There is no scientific evidence that filling teeth or even dental extraction with the use of local or nitrous oxide-oxygen anesthesia causes abortion or premature labor. Antibacterial therapy should be considered for sepsis, however, especially in gravidas who have had rheumatic heart disease or nephritis. Extensive dental surgery is postponed until after delivery for the woman's comfort, if possible (Martin and Reeb, 1982, 1983).

Medications: Prescribed or Over-the-counter (OTC) Drugs. Although much has been learned in recent years about fetal drug toxicity (Appendix G), the possible teratogenicity of many drugs is still unknown. This is especially true for new medications and combinations of drugs. Moreover, certain subclinical errors or deficiencies in intermediate metabolism in the fetus may convert an otherwise harmless drug into a hazardous one. The greatest danger of causing developmental defects in the fetus from drugs exists from fertilization through the first trimester (i.e., the period of organogenesis) (Chapter 9). Self-treatment must be discouraged. All drugs, including aspirin, should be limited, and a careful record of therapeutic agents used should be kept (Howard and Hill, 1979; McKay, 1980; Luke, 1982). Hazards of one artificial sweetner are discussed in Chapter 15. See guidelines for client teaching, p. 256.

Immunization. There has been some concern over the safety of various immunization techniques during pregnancy. The recommendations of the American College of Obstetricians and Gynecologists (1982) with appropriate updating for specific immunizations during pregnancy are summarized in Table 12-5 (Pritchard et al., 1985):

Table 12-5 *Immunizations During Pregnancy*

Immunization	Comments
Cholera	Only to meet international travel requirements
Hepatitis A	After exposure; newborns of mothers who are incubating or ill should receive 1 dose after birth
Hepatitis B	Hepatitis B hyperimmune globulin to infant soon after delivery, followed by vaccination
Influenza	Evaluate pregnant woman for immunization according to criteria applied to others
Measles	Live virus vaccine contraindicated on theoretic grounds during pregnancy; pooled immune globulins for postexposure prophylaxis
Mumps	Contraindicated on theoretic grounds during pregnancy
Plague	Should be used only if substantial risk of infection
Poliomyelitis	Not recommended routinely for adults but mandatory in epidemics or when traveling to endemic area
Rabies	Same as nonpregnant
Rubella	Contraindicated although teratogenicity of vaccine appears to be negligible
Tetanus-diphtheria	Give toxoid if no primary series or no booster in 10 years; for postexposure prophylaxis with unvaccinated tetanus immune globulin and toxoid
Typhoid	Recommended if traveling in endemic region
Varicella	Varicella-zoster immune globulin may be given; indicated for newborns whose mothers developed varicella within 4 days before or 2 days after delivery
	Immunize before travel to high-risk area but postpone travel if possible

Substance Abuse. Occasional alcoholic beverages *may* not be harmful to the mother or her infant. Excesses must be avoided; regular drinkers or those who drink heavily during pregnancy have infants who demonstrate fetal alcohol syndrome (see Chapter 39; Appendix G).

Cigarette smoking or continued exposure to a smoke-filled environment (even if the mother does not smoke) is associated with fetal growth retardation and an increase in perinatal and infant morbidity and mortality. Laboratory studies indicate a lowered Po_2 level in both mother and fetus during exposure to cigarette smoke. Smoking may result in a lessened supply of milk during lactation, and harmful substances may be transferred to the infant in the milk.

Any mind-altering substance has a deleterious effect on the fetus and should not be used (see Chapter 39, and Appendix G). Marijuana, heroin, and cocaine are well-known examples of such substances.

Radiation. For a discussion of the dangers of radiation during pregnancy, see Chapter 9, and Appendix G.

Sexual Counseling During Pregnancy

Sexual counseling includes countering misinformation, providing reassurance of normalcy, and suggesting alternative behaviors. The uniqueness of each couple is considered within a biopsychosocial framework.

Counseling couples concerning sexual adjustment during pregnancy demands self-assessment by the nurse as well as a knowledge of the physical, social, and emotional responses to sex during pregnancy (Zalar, 1976). Not all maternity nurses are comfortable dealing with the sexual concerns of their clients. Nurses who are aware of their personal strengths and limitations in dealing with sexual content are in a better position to make referrals when necessary.

A significant number of clients merely need *permission* to be sexual during pregnancy. Many other clients need *information* about the physiologic changes that occur during pregnancy and to have myths associated with sex during pregnancy debunked. Giving permission and providing information are within the purview of the maternity nurse and should be an integral component of providing health care. See guidelines for client teaching, p. 257.

A few couples must be referred for either *sex therapy* or *family therapy*. Couples with sexual dysfunction problems of long standing that are intensified by pregnancy are referred for sex therapy. When a sexual problem is a symptom of a more serious interactional problem, the couple would benefit from family therapy.

Obtaining a History. The history provides a baseline for sexual counseling. History taking is an ongoing process. Receptivity to changes in attitudes, body image, marital relationships, and physical status is relevant throughout pregnancy. When changes occur, unexpected problems may develop that require intervention. The history reveals the client's knowledge of female anatomy and physiology, attitudes about sex during pregnancy, as well as perceptions of the pregnancy, the health status of the couple, and the quality of their marital relationship. Identification of the couple's subjective experience provides the direction and focus of sexual counseling.

Countering Misinformation. Many myths and much of the misinformation related to sex and pregnancy are masked behind seemingly unrelated issues. For example, a question about the baby's ability to hear and see in utero may be related to the baby's role as an observer in lovemaking. The counselor must be extremely sensitive to questions behind the question when counseling in this highly charged emotional area.

Fetal heart rate (FHR) decreases during orgasm; however, fetal distress has not been noted. Although it has been suggested that premature delivery may be induced by the effect of oxytocin released during maternal response, by orgasmic contractions, or by prostaglandins in the male ejaculate, researchers have not validated these hypotheses. When possible the couple is counseled together. Expectant parent education classes can also be an effective way to explore these kinds of concerns because of the support and sharing offered by the group.

Providing Reassurance of Normalcy. Couples are relieved to learn that their fears and concerns do not make them "weird" or "crazy." A breast-feeding mother may welcome the knowledge that her erotic response to suckling is normal. At the same time the father may be relieved to know that many fathers are jealous of their suckling infants.

It is important for the counselor to view sexuality in its broadest sense. Kissing, hugging, massaging, petting, and increased gentleness and sensitivity are valid forms of sexual expression and signs of affection. Each of these behaviors is pleasurable in itself and is not always a preliminary behavior leading to intercourse. When a couple cannot have, or chooses not to have, penile-vaginal intercourse, the need for closeness and intimacy can be expressed in many other ways.

Suggesting Alternative Behaviors. To date research has not proved conclusively that coitus and orgasm are contraindicated at any time during pregnancy for the obstetrically and medically healthy woman (Mill and others, 1981; Naeye, 1981; Flood and Naeye, 1984). However, a history of more than one spontaneous abortion or a threatened abortion in the first trimester, impending miscarriage in the second trimester, or premature rupture of membranes, bleeding, or abdominal pain during the third trimester warrant precaution against coitus and orgasm. Naeye (1979) suggests that improved genital hygiene and perhaps other actions may reduce the risk of intrauterine infection. Until we have more data, "a reasonable policy might be to recommend the avoidance of intercourse and orgasm in the third trimester in women with a poor reproductive history or in those who, on pelvic examination, have premature ripening of the cervix." In an interview Naeye commented further that he "was not prepared to recommend prolonged abstinence during pregnancy, since this can cause serious marital discord."

Solitary and mutual masturbation and oral-genital intercourse may be used by couples as *alternatives to penile-vaginal intercourse*. Men who enjoy cunnilingus may feel "turned off" by the normal increase in amount and odor of vaginal discharges during pregnancy. Couples who practice cunnilingus should be cautioned concerning the blowing of air into the vagina, particularly during the last few weeks of pregnancy. There have been cases reported of maternal death from air emboli caused by forceful blowing of air into the vagina. If the cervix is slightly open (as it may be near term), there is the possibility that air will be forced between the membranes and the uterine wall. Some air may enter the maternal placental lakes, thus gaining entrance into the maternal vascular bed.

The woman or couple should also be cautioned against masturbatory activities when orgasmic contractions are contraindicated. Studies have shown that orgasm is often more intense when induced by masturbation. After being cautioned against orgasm, some women require reassurance if they experience erotic dreams.

Pictures of possible variations of *coital position* are often helpful. The female-superior, side-by-side, and rear-entry positions are possible alternative positions to the traditional male-superior position. The woman astride (superior position) allows her to control the angle and depth of penile penetration as well as to protect her breasts and abdomen. The side-by-side position is the one of choice, especially during the third trimester, since it requires reduced energy and pressure on the pregnant abdomen. For other positions, the reader is referred to Bing and Colman (1977) and McCary (1982).

Multiparous women have reported severe *breast tenderness* in the first trimester. A coital position that avoids direct pressure on the woman's breasts and decreased breast fondling during love play can be recommended. The woman should also be reassured that this condition is normal and temporary. *Lactating mothers* lose milk in uncontrolled spurts in response to sexual stimulation. The couple that is forewarned can be prepared for this eventuality.

Some women complain of lower abdominal cramping and backache after orgasm during the first and third trimes-

Guidelines For Client Teaching

PRECAUTIONS FOR DRUG USE DURING PREGNANCY

ASSESSMENT

1. Woman expresses/demonstrates knowledge deficit regarding hazards of substance abuse, including smoking and ingestion of alcohol during pregnancy.
2. Woman states she sees no harm in over-the-counter (OTC) drugs or vitamins.

NURSING DIAGNOSES

Knowledge deficit related to drug use or abuse during pregnancy, including OTC medications, alcohol, and cigarette smoking.

Potential for fetal injury related to exposure to hazardous chemicals.

Potential for altered fetal growth and development related to exposure to hazardous chemicals.

Potential for altered nutrition related to drug-abuse.

GOALS

Short-term

Gravida will discuss the use of *any* drug with her physician beforehand.

Woman states she is aware that even OTC medications can be harmful to her pregnancy and fetus.

Woman indicates she knows the hazards of alcohol and cigarettes during her pregnancy.

Intermediate

Woman states she understands the reasons for not using any drug that was not prescribed by her physician at this time (even OTC medications).

Woman is educated about teratogenesis.

Woman reduces or stops smoking and alcohol consumption during pregnancy.

Woman adjusts dietary intake to supply appropriate amounts of nutrients.

Long-term

Woman understands consequences of drug, alcohol, and cigarette use.

Woman does not self-medicate.

REFERENCES AND TEACHING AIDS

Printed instructions prepared by nurses, physicians, or others.

Charts and pamphlets showing the development of the fetus at various times.

Pamphlets from the March of Dimes discussing drug, alcohol, and cigarette use and abuse during pregnancy.

CONTENT/RATIONALE	TEACHING ACTION
To provide information about fetal development: Pregnancy is divided into trimesters of 3 months each. During these first months (the period of organogenesis) human development goes from ovum to embryo to fetus. This period of life is characterized by rapid cell division. All principle organ systems are being established at this time and are extremely vulnerable to the effects of chemical teratogens.	Using charts and visual aids show client how the baby is formed at this time. Discuss the rapid cell division and growth that is going on inside of her.
Interference at this time can result in major congenital malformations or abnormalities.	Discuss how environmental agents such as drugs, alcohol and smoking can interrupt normal development of the organs. Allow woman time to ask questions. Use simple, easy-to-understand language. Provide basic information.
To provide information about the use of prescription drugs: Information concerns the subject of self-medication with OTC drugs that are usually seen as harmless. Combinations of drugs may cause problems too.	Inform the woman that her physician is aware of the consequences of drug use at this time, therefore, physician would not prescribe any medication that would harm her baby or her pregnancy. Discuss how OTC drugs either alone or in combination could be troublesome. Caution the woman strongly about taking any drug without first checking with her doctor.
To alert woman to hazards of alcohol and smoking: No safe level of alcohol consumption has yet been established. The period of greatest susceptibility and dose-response relationship are not known (Beckman and Brent, 1986).	Discuss the prudence of alcohol consumption at this time. Explain this is still an area of questionable unknowns.
Cigarette smoking or second-hand smoking (exposure to smoke-filled rooms) is associated with fetal growth retardation, decreased placental perfusion, and possible decrease in milk production. Harmful substances from cigarette smoking are transferred in breast milk to baby and inhaled by baby.	Discuss how smoking can effect the woman's fetus and pregnancy. If the woman is a smoker, discuss the options she has on ways to stop. If she is resistant to stop, then try to offer ways in which she can cut down.

EVALUATION The nurse may be reassured that teaching was effective if the woman does not use OTC drugs, alcohol, other drugs of abuse, or smoke during pregnancy. She is able to verbalize understanding that these chemicals are harmful to her and her fetus.

Guidelines For Client Teaching

SEXUAL COUNSELING DURING PREGNANCY

ASSESSMENT

1. Woman experiencing adaptations to pregnancy (fatigue, nausea).
2. Woman indicates breasts hurt when touched.
3. Woman and husband request information.
4. This is woman's first pregnancy, with no history of vaginal bleeding or uterine cramping.

NURSING DIAGNOSES

Knowledge deficit, alternative positions.
Altered sexuality patterns.
Potential for anxiety if reactions are perceived as abnormal.
Potential for ineffective individual coping.

GOALS

Short-term

To validate and assure the universality of their responses.
To meet information needs.
To problem-solve regarding solutions and needed changes.

Intermediate

To continue to make adjustments regarding sexuality throughout pregnancy.
To verbalize mutual satisfaction with their choices.

Long-term

To continue to make mutually acceptable adjustments regarding sexuality across the life span.

REFERENCES AND TEACHING AIDS

Bing, E, and Colman, L: Making love during pregnancy, New York, 1982, FA Davis Co.
Rakowitz, E, and Rubin, GS: Lovemaking in pregnancy. Lamaze Parents' Magazine, 1985 edition, ASPO Lamaze, 55 Northern Blvd, Greenvale, LI, NY, 11548-1390.
Plastic learning models, illustrations.

CONTENT/RATIONALE	TEACHING ACTION
*To broaden knowledge base regarding sexuality and sexual expression during pregnancy**:	
Discuss maternal physiologic adaptations to pregnancy: breasts, nausea, fatigue, abdominal changes, perineal enlargement, leukorrhea, pelvic vasocongestion, and orgasmic responses (Chaper 10).	Provide a safe, open, nonjudgmental atmosphere (Chapter 2).
Discuss maternal and paternal responses to pregnancy (Chapter 11).	Remain alert to personal beliefs and values to avoid decreasing one's effectiveness in providing sexual counseling.
Identify clients' cultural prescriptions and proscriptions.	Validate feelings, give permission.
Discuss responses to interview questions.	Ask about things they have heard, read; what they want to discuss.
Inform couple that, although her libido may be depressed during first trimester, it increases during the second and third trimesters.	Time the discussions to clients' phase in childbearing cycle and readiness to learn.
In subsequent visits and postpartum, discuss: 1. Breast-feeding and: father's responses, mother's fantasies and sexual feelings during breast-feeding, milk spurt during orgasm. 2. Resumption of sexual relationship after delivery.	
To encourage problem-solving and experimentation in mutual sexual gratification: Discuss: 1. Alternative behaviors (e.g., mutual masturbation, foot massage, cuddling). 2. Alternative positions (e.g., female-superior, side-lying).	Provide comfortable environment, offer alternatives, show illustrations.
To prevent potential intrauterine infection and reduce anxiety of injury to fetus: 1. Inform that intercourse is safe as long as it is not uncomfortable for the woman and the membranes have not ruptured. 2. Review signs of ruptured membranes (Chapter 18). 3. Caution against use of hot tubbing. Extreme temperatures that increase maternal temperature can compromise fetal well-being. 4. Discuss cultural prescriptions and proscriptions unique to their situation.	Show illustrations of fetus in utero with closed cervix and intact membranes.

EVALUATION The nurse can be assured that teaching was effective when the woman (couple) verbalizes increased knowledge and uses it to make mutually accepted adjustments regarding sexuality throughout pregnancy.

*For alterations in sexual practice if she or her sexual partner have tested positive for AIDS virus (HIV) see Chapter 30.

ters. A back rub can often relieve some of the discomfort, as well as provide a pleasant experience. A tonic contraction, often lasting up to a minute, replaces the rhythmic contractions of orgasm during the third trimester. Changes in FHRs without fetal distress have been reported.

Well-informed nurses who are comfortable with their own sexuality and the sexual counseling needs of pregnant couples can offer counseling in a valuable but often neglected area. They can establish an open environment in which couples can feel free to introduce their concerns about sexual adjustment and seek support and guidance (Mueller, 1985).

Cultural Variation in Prenatal Care

Prenatal care as we know it is a phenomenon of Western medicine. The Western biomedical model of care encourages women to seek prenatal care as early as possible in their pregnancy by visiting a physician or clinic. Visits are usually routine and follow a systematic sequence, with the initial visit followed by a monthly and then weekly visits. Monitoring weight and blood pressure; testing blood and urine; teaching specific information about diet, rest, and activity; and preparing for childbirth are common components of prenatal care.

This model not only is unfamiliar but commonly seems strange to many groups (Artschwager, 1982). Even when the prenatal care described is familiar, some practices may conflict with a subcultural group's beliefs and practices. Because of these and other factors, such as lack of money, lack of transportation, and poor communication on the part of health care providers, many groups do not participate in the prenatal care system. Their behavior may be misinterpreted by nurses as uncaring, lazy, or ignorant. For example, Muecke (1976) points out that the Northern Thai do not focus on the prenatal period at all. They only focus on the childbirth and postpartum periods. According to their beliefs, they personally perceive themselves as having little influence on pregnancy until the time of birth. For them spiritual influences, apart from human beings, control what occurs before birth. Western prenatal care, which does not deal with the spiritual influences, appears irrelevant.

Horn's research (1982) with a group of Northwest Coast Indians elicited the strongly held belief that visible preparation for the coming infant was commonly associated with the infant's death. Women could identify many instances when preparation such as buying infant clothes or preparing a crib was followed by the death of the infant. A high infant mortality supported this belief. Another group not favoring preparation by the mother before birth is the Arab-American population. Meleis and Sorrell (1981) stress that Egyptian and Arab mothers do not have a layette or room set aside for newborns at the time of birth. They believe that planning ahead has the potential of defying God's will. Also planning ahead only to have those plans not materialize can be disappointing. Women on the Caribbean island of St. Kitt prefer not discussing the coming infant, mentioning its name, or referring to it directly until it is christened (Gussler, 1982). Until the time of christening, spirits of the dead would come and make the infant ill or kill it. This same concern for the dead spirit's influence was expressed by the Muckleshoot, who kept a candle burning to keep the spirits from coming to get the baby. Kendall (1979) tells of a pregnant Iranian woman's grandmother who prepared a complete set of clothing for her expected grandchild during the sixth or seventh month of pregnancy. She placed among the clothing a triangular scarf with beads, amulets, and shells to ward off the *evil eye* and thus protect the newborn infant.

A concern for *modesty* is also a deterrent for prenatal care for many persons. Exposing one's body parts, especially to a man, is a major violation of modesty. Puerto Ricans (Parken, 1978), Mexicans (Kay, 1982), and Japanese (Bernstein and Kidd, 1982) express great concern over body exposure. Arab women also value modesty (Meleis and Sorrell, 1981). Besides being fully clothed, the Arab woman is expected to manifest modesty through diffidence, shyness, and bashfulness when interacting with men and strangers. For many women invasive procedures such as vaginal examination may be so threatening that they cannot be discussed, even with one's own husband. Thus many Arab women prefer a midwife over a male physician. Recent immigrants such as Southeast Asians also prefer a midwife (Gallo and others, 1980; Hollingsworth and others, 1980).

For numerous cultural groups a physician is deemed appropriate only in times of illness. A physician is considered inappropriate when pregnancy is considered a normal process and the woman is in a state of health. Even when problems with pregnancy develop according to beliefs of Western medicine, they may not be perceived as problems but may be considered normal. Muecke (1976) notes that Thai women do not perceive weakness, fainting spells, palpitations, tremors, and diarrhea as abnormal. Many Muckleshoot women view puffiness of hands, eyes, and feet and frequent headaches as normal (Horn, 1982).

Although pregnancy is considered normal by many, certain practices are expected of women of all cultures to ensure a good outcome. *Prescriptions* tell women what to do, and *proscriptions* establish *taboos.* The purposes of these practices are to (1) prevent maternal illness from a pregnancy-induced imbalanced state, (2) protect the vulnerable fetus, and (3) protect other persons from illness caused by a woman in state of imbalance. Prescriptions and proscriptions discussed in the chapter are related to emotional response, clothing, activity and rest, sexual activity, and dietary practices.

Emotional Response. Virtually all cultures emphasize the importance of a socially harmonious and agreeable environment. Absence of stressful relationships is important for a successful outcome for mother and baby. Harmony with other persons must be fostered. Visits from extended family members may be required to demonstrate continued pleasant and noncontroversial relationships. If dissonance exists in any relationship with others, it is usually dealt with in culturally prescribed ways. For example, a pregnant woman on the Muckleshoot reservation described how she became ill after eating chili, a food to avoid during pregnancy because of its spiciness. The pregnant woman's mother had specifically warned her about eating chili. Thus the woman had created disharmony in two areas, physiologic and social, by eating a proscribed food and by not following the mother's abmonitions. To remedy the situation and to reestablish harmony, the pregnant woman attended a Shaker prayer service. She prayed for herself and was "brushed off"; that is, a church member symbolically brushed the problem away by touching her shoulder lightly. She believed she had now regained a state of physiologic and social harmony.

Imitative magic functions in other proscriptions in addition to food. Mexicans advise against pregnant women witnessing an eclipse of the moon because they believe it may cause a cleft palate in the infant. Exposures to an earthquake may result in premature delivery or miscarriage. A breech may occur if the earthquake was exceptionally strong (Clark, 1970). Snow (1974) notes that among blacks a pregnant woman must not ridicule someone with an affliction for fear her child might be born with the same handicap. A mother should not hate a person lest her child resemble that person, and dental work should not be done during pregnancy because it may cause a baby to have a harelip. Carrington (1978) describes a widely held folk belief in many cultures that includes refraining from raising one's arm above one's head and refraining from tying knots, so that the umbilical cord does not wrap around the baby's neck and become knotted.

Clothing. Although most cultural groups do not prescribe specific clothing for pregnancy, modesty is an expectation for many (Clark, 1970; Meleis and Sorrell, 1981). Spanish-speaking people of the Southwest wear a cord beneath the breast and knotted over the umbilicus. This cord, called a *muneco,* is thought to prevent morning sickness and ensure a safe delivery (Brown, 1976). Amulets, medals, and beads may be worn to ward off evil spirits.

Physical Activity and Rest. Norms that regulate physical activity of mothers during pregnancy vary tremendously. Many groups (Carrington, 1978; Horn, 1982; Stringfellow, 1978) encourage women to be active, to walk, and to engage in normal although not strenuous activities to ensure that the baby is healthy and not too large. On the other hand, the Filipino woman is cautioned that any activity is dangerous, and others willingly take over work (Affonso, 1978; Stern, 1981). The belief among Filipinos is that inactivity constitutes a protection for mother and child. The mother is encouraged to simply produce the succeeding generation. Health care providers could misinterpret this behavior as laziness or noncompliance with the health regimen desired in prenatal care. Again it is important for the nurse to find out the meaning of activity and rest for each culture.

Sexual Activity. In most cultures sexual activity is not prohibited until the end of pregnancy. Among blacks sexual relations are viewed as natural because pregnancy is a state of health (Carrington, 1978). Mexican-Americans view sexual activity as necessary to keep the birth canal lubricated (Kay, 1982). On the other hand, Vietnamese have definite proscriptions about sexual intercourse, requiring abstinence as early as the sixth month (Hollingsworth and others, 1980; Stringfellow, 1978). Sexual taboos are more common after delivery.

Diet. Nutritional information given by Western health care providers may be a source of conflict for many cultural groups. The conflict is commonly not known by the health care providers unless they have an understanding of dietary beliefs and practices of the persons for whom they are caring (see Chapter 15).

Evaluation

Maternal and fetal goals are continuously evaluated according to measurable, established criteria. The clinical findings that represent normal response are presented as outcome criteria in the general and specific nursing care plans that follow. These criteria are used as a basis for selecting appropriate nursing actions and evaluating their effectiveness.

Text continued on p. 263.

General Nursing Care Plan

INITIAL PRENATAL VISIT

ASSESSMENT	NURSING DIAGNOSIS (ND)/ PLAN (P)/GOAL (G)	RATIONALE/ IMPLEMENTATION	EVALUATION
Woman suspects pregnancy; needs confirmation of diagnosis. Sexual intercourse without contraception. Missed menstrual period(s).	ND: Knowledge deficit related to diagnosis of pregnancy. P: Meet woman's knowledge needs. G: The woman will become knowledgeable about diagnosis of pregnancy and her status (pregnant or not).	*To confirm the diagnosis the nurse will:* Establish a client data base. Take a nursing history. Do a preliminary health history. Obtain laboratory data as deemed necessary by physician. Provide time to discuss physician's diagnosis and explanations.	Woman verbalizes understanding of diagnostic measures. Woman learns whether she is pregnant.
Woman asks when she will have the baby.	ND: Knowledge deficit related to estimated date of delivery (EDD). P: Meet woman's knowledge needs. G: The woman will become knowledgeable about her EDD.	*To determine the EDD the physician and nurse will:* Calculate EDD based on: Information from the client data base. Information from nursing history. Naegle's rule. Ultrasound. Fundal height measurements. *To inform the woman the nurse will:* Explain how the EDD is determined. Reinforce physician's explanation that it is not 100% accurate.	Woman verbalizes understanding of the EDD and asks relevant questions. Woman understands that she may give birth just before or after the EDD.
Woman needs a schedule for subsequent prenatal visits.	ND: Knowledge deficit related to schedule of prenatal visits throughout pregnancy. P: Meet woman's knowledge needs. G: The woman will schedule appointments throughout pregnancy G: The woman will keep scheduled appointments. G: The woman understands the importance of regular visits	*To educate the woman the nurse will:* Inform the woman of the schedule for prenatal visits. Discuss the importance of adhering to the schedule unless otherwise informed.	Woman schedules appointments as per plan. Woman keeps scheduled appointments. Woman understands and verbalizes rationale of appointment schedule.

General Nursing Care Plan—cont'd

ASSESSMENT	NURSING DIAGNOSIS (ND)/ PLAN (P)/GOAL (G)	RATIONALE/ IMPLEMENTATION	EVALUATION
Woman asks what she should do differently and how her body will change now that she's pregnant.	ND: Knowledge deficit related to the psychologic and physiologic adaptations to pregnancy. ND: Knowledge deficit related to self-care behavior. P: Meet woman's knowledge needs. G: The woman will be able to identify her body's physiologic and psychologic adaptations to pregnancy. G: The woman will use self-care behaviors to maintain an optimum level of wellness for herself and the fetus.	*To determine the woman's present level of health the nurse will:* Interview woman and gain the information for the prenatal health assessment. *To teach the woman about changes resulting from pregnancy the nurse will:* Explain normal psychologic and physiologic adaptations to pregnancy. *To teach the woman how to care for herself properly the nurse will:* Inform the woman of self-care techniques. Explain the purpose and importance of each technique.	Woman verbalizes understanding of physiologic and psychologic adaptations to pregnancy. Woman asks appropriate questions regarding physiologic and psychologic adaptations to pregnancy. Woman verbalizes that she feels well. Physical assessment confirms that woman and fetus are healthy.
Woman says that making love has become uncomfortable.	ND: Altered sexuality patterns related to discomforts of early pregnancy. P: Meet woman's knowledge needs. G: Woman will understand how physiology of pregnancy affects intercourse.	*To teach about physiological affects of pregnancy on intercourse the nurse will:* Discuss sexuality and sexual behaviors during pregnancy. Discuss those symptoms the woman is experiencing that affect intercourse and foreplay.	The woman will ask appropriate questions and verbalize understanding of information discussed.
Woman indicates she is unaware of signs and symptoms that could signal danger to her and her fetus during pregnancy.	ND: Knowledge deficit of signs and symptoms, potential for danger to mother and fetus. P: Meet woman's knowledge needs. G: The woman will gain knowledge about danger signs during pregnancy.	*To determine possible medical implications the nurse will:* Obtain information about preexisting or concurrent medical conditions. *To teach the woman about possible danger signs the nurse will:* Discuss danger signs with the woman. Inform the woman of signs and symptoms she should consider abnormal. Provide the woman with a printed paper with danger signs of pregnancy and phone number of physician, hospital, and clinic.	The woman verbalizes understanding of problems or danger signs that should be reported.

Specific Nursing Care Plan

NAUSEA (MORNING SICKNESS) AND FATIGUE

Ruth Piper has just been diagnosed as being 8 weeks pregnant. During her initial prenatal visit she tells the nurse that she is experiencing nausea and dry heaves in the morning on awakening (sometimes being awakened by the nausea). She states that this is interfering with her morning routine and sometimes making her late to work. Ruth also reports that at 4 PM, when she gets home from work, she is so tired that she can't fix dinner for herself and her husband; all she wants to do is go to bed for the night. This break in her routine is upsetting her and she asks for help.

ASSESSMENT	NURSING DIAGNOSIS (ND)/ PLAN (P)/ GOAL (G)	RATIONALE/ IMPLEMENTATION	EVALUATION
Ruth says she is experiencing nausea and dry heaves on awakening.	ND: Pain related to change in hormone levels and the body's adaptation to pregnancy. ND: Sleep pattern disturbance related to nausea (morning sickness) of pregnancy. P: Meet Ruth's knowledge needs and provide for discussing feelings and concerns. G: Ruth will be free of nausea and dry heaves. G: Ruth will resume normal sleep-rest pattern.	*To teach Ruth how to reduce nausea the nurse will:* Take a 24-hour diet history. Inform Ruth to keep crackers or other dry carbohydrates at the bedside. Eat one or two crackers dry on awakening, before getting out of bed. Discuss eating Ruth's meals dry and drinking between meals. Caution Ruth to avoid eating fried or greasy foods, especially before bed. Discuss eating small, frequent meals instead of 3 large ones.	Ruth verbalizes understanding of instructions. Nausea lessens or stops; dry heaves stop. Ruth resumes normal sleep-rest pattern.
Ruth states she is extremely fatigued.	ND: Fatigue related to early pregnancy. ND: Activity tolerance, decreased, related to fatigue of early pregnancy. ND: Knowledge deficit related to common discomforts of pregnancy. P: Meet Ruth's knowledge needs and provide time for discussing feelings and concerns. G: Ruth will learn how to deal with the fatigue of early pregnancy. G: Ruth will be able to increase her activity level. G: Ruth will be able to resume activities of daily living (ADL) without undue fatigue.	*To teach Ruth how to deal with fatigue the nurse will:* Discuss ways to deal with the fatigue of pregnancy. Suggest ways to help Ruth assume ADL.	Ruth verbalizes understanding of instructions. Ruth will be able to resume ADL. Ruth will resume self-care. Ruth will increase activity level.

SUMMARY

The prenatal period is one of growth and change in the woman's personal and social context. Achieving a goal of a safe and satisfying pregnancy for a woman and her family require a mutual effort on the part of the woman and the professionals involved. Practitioner and client need a clear understanding of their objectives, roles, and capabilities. Nursing care provided during this period can act as a stimulus for the continued use of the health care system by the woman and her family. Nursing actions reflect the changes experienced by the woman as she progresses through the first trimester of pregnancy. For further clarification see the general and specific nursing care plans in this chapter.

KEY CONCEPTS

- The prenatal period is a preparatory one both physically, in terms of fetal growth and maternal adaptations, and psychologically, in terms of anticipation of parenthood.
- Important components of the initial prenatal visit include detailed and carefully recorded findings from the interview, a comprehensive physical examination, and selected laboratory tests.
- Through assessment, formulation of nursing diagnoses, and planning, mutually derived with the client and her family when appropriate, individualized care may be implemented; evaluation of care is an ongoing process.
- Maternal physical and familial adaptations to pregnancy generate needs that the nurse-clinician can anticipate and meet by providing support, and teaching/counseling/advocacy, and by performing manual skills.
- Cultural prescriptions and proscriptions influence responses to pregnancy and to the health care delivery system.
- Even in normal pregnancy the nurse must remain alert to hazards such as supine hypotension and vasovagal syncope, 11 danger signs, and signs of potential parenting disorders.

STUDY QUESTIONS AND ACTIVITIES

1. In an actual or simulated clinical setting, complete an initial prenatal interview (history) and comprehensive physical examination.
2. Participate in the first prenatal visit of a client and use the nursing process to develop a specific nursing care plan for her needs.
3. Discuss how the nurse's role as support person would differ for a woman with a supportive family who was pleased with her pregnancy as opposed to a woman facing pregnancy without such support.
4. In small groups discuss cultural influences based on data from interviews with clients or from personal experiences.
5. Practice taking a sexual history with a classmate. Discuss results in small groups.

References

Affonso, DD: The Filipino American. In Clark A, editor: Culture/childbearing/health professionals, Philadelphia, 1978, FA Davis Co

Artschwager, M: Anthropology of human birth, Philadelphia, 1982, FA Davis Co

Batzer, FR: Guidelines for choosing a pregnancy test, Contemp OB/GYN 26:37 Oct 1985 (special issue)

Bernstein, JL, and Kidd, YA: Childbearing in Japan. In Kay, MA, editor: Anthropology of human birth, Philadelphia, 1982, FA Davis Co

Bing, E, and Colman, L: Making love during pregnancy, New York, 1977, Bantam Books, Inc

Brown, MS: A cross-cultural look at pregnancy, labor, and delivery, Obstet Gynecol Nurs 5:35, 1976

Brucker, MC, and Reedy, NJ: Maternity leaves and the Pregnancy Discrimination Act, JOGN Nurs 12:341, 1983

Bryant, H: Antenatal counseling for women working outside the homes, Birth 12:4, Winter 1985

Bullard, JA: Exercise and pregnancy, Can Fam Physician 27:977, 1981

Carrington, BW: THe Afro-American. In Clark, AL, editor: Culture/childbearing/health professionals, Philadelphia, 1978, FA Davis Co

Clark, M: Health in the Mexican-American culture: a community study, Berkeley, 1970, University of California Press

Dale, E, et al: Exercise during pregnancy: effects on the fetus, Can J Appl Sport Sci 7:98, June 1982

Danforth, DN, and Scott, JR, editors: Obstetrics and gynecology, ed 5, Philadelphia, 1986, JB Lippincott Co

Dean, J: Pregnancy and exercise: how much and what kind? On this the experts agree: more research is needed, Sportwest 1:30, Dec 1981

Edwards, M: Communications: dimensions in childbirth education, Pacific Grove, Calif, 1973, M Edwards

Flood, B, and Naeye, R: Factors that predispose to premature rupture of fetal membranes, JOGN Nurs 13:4, March/April 1984

Gallo, AM, et al: Little refugees with big needs, RN 43:45, 1980

Gussler, J: Poor mothers and modern medicine in St. Kitts. In Kay, MA, editor: Anthropology of human birth, Philadelphia, 1982, FA Davis Co

Hollingsworth, AO, et al: The refugees and childbearing; what to expect, RN 43:45, 1980

Horn, BM: Northwest coast Indians: the Muckleshoot. In Kay, MA, editor: Anthropology of human birth, Philadelphia, 1982, FA Davis Co

Howard, FM, and Hill, JM: Drugs in pregnancy, Obstet Gynecol Surv 34:643, 1979

Hutchinson, PL, et al: Metabolic and circulatory responses to running during pregnancy, Phys Sportsmed 9:55, Aug 1981

Jopke, T: Pregnancy: a time to exercise judgement, Phys Sportsmed 11:139, July 1983

Kay, MA, editor: Anthropology of human birth, Philadelphia, 1982, FA Davis Co

Kendall, K: Maternal and child care in an Iranian village. In Leininger, M, editor: Transcultural nursing, '79, New York, 1979, Masson Publishing USA

Leap, TL, et al: Equal employment opportunity and its implications for personnel practices in the 1980s, Labor Law J 31:669, 1980

Luke, B: Does caffeine influence reproduction? MCN 7:240, July/Aug 1982

Malasanos, L, et al: Health assessment, ed 3, St Louis, 1986, The CV Mosby Co
Marbury, MC, et al: Work and pregnancy, Occup Med vol. 26, 1984
Martin, BJ, and Reeb, RM: Oral health during pregnancy: a neglected nursing area, MCN 7:350, 1982
Martin, BJ, and Reeb, RM: The nurse as the first line of defense against periodontal disease, JOGN Nurs 12:333, 1983
McCary, JL: Human sexuality: physiological factors, ed 4, New York, 1982, Van Nostrand Reinhold Co, Inc
McKay, S: Smoking during the childbearing years, MCN 5:46, Jan/Feb 1980
Meleis, AI, and Sorrell, L: Bridging cultures: Arab American women and their birth experiences, MCN 6:171, 1981
Mill, J, et al: Should coitus late in pregnancy be discouraged, Lancet 1:136, 1981
Muecke, MA: Health care systems as socializing agents: childbearing the North Thai and Western ways, Soc Sci Med 10:377, 1976
Mueller, L: Pregnancy and sexuality, JOGN Nurs 14:4, July/Aug 1985
NAACOG: Reproductive health hazards: women in the workplace, vol 11, Feb 1985, NAACOG, 600 Maryland Ave, SW Suite 2000, Washington, DC 20024
NAACOG: Standards for obstetrics, gynecologic, and neonatal nursing, ed 3, 1986, NAACOG, 600 Maryland Ave, SW Suite 2000, Washington, DC 20024
Naeye, RL: Coitus and associated amniotic-fluid infections, N Engl J Med 301:1198, 1979
Naeye, RL: Coitus and antepartum hemorrhage, Br J Obstet Gynecol 88:765, 1981
News: Monoclonals: new frontiers in reproductive medicine in Technology 1986 Contemp OB/GYN 26:75, Oct 1985
Paglone, A, and Worthington, S: Cautions and advice on exercise during pregnancy, Contemp OB/GYN 25:160, May 1985 (special issue)
Parken, M: Culture and preventive health care, JOGN Nurs 7:40, 1978
Pritchard, J, et al: Williams obstetrics, ed 17, Norwalk, Conn, 1985, Appleton-Century-Crofts
Seidel, HM, et al: Mosby's guide to physical examination, St Louis, 1987, The CV Mosby Co
Snow, L: Folk medical beliefs and their implications for care of patients, Ann Intern Med 81:82, 1974
Stern, PM: Solving problems of cross-cultural health teaching: the Filipino childbearing family, Image 13:47, 1981
Stringfellow, L: The Vietnamese. In Clark, A, editor: Culture/childbearing/health professionals, Philadelphia, 1978, FA Davis Co
Tucker, SM, et al: Patient care standards, ed 4, St. Louis, 1988, The CV Mosby Co
Wright, LM, and Leahey, M: Nurses and families: a guide to family assessment and interaction, Philadelphia, 1984, FA Davis Co
Zalar, MK: Sexual counseling for pregnant couples, MCN 1:176, May/June 1976

Bibliography

Afaf Ibraheim Meltas, L: Arab American women and their birth experiences, MCN 6:171, May/June 1981
Alexander, LL: The pregnant smoker: nursing implications, JOGN Nurs 16(3):167, 1987
Bash, D: Jewish religious practices related to childbearing, J Nurse Midwife 25(5):39, 1980
Bentz, JM: Missed meanings in nurse/patient communication, MCN 5:55, Jan/Feb 1980
Bond, MB: Reproductive hazards in the workplace, Contemp OB/GYN 28(3):57, 1986
Brown, MA: Marital support during pregnancy, JOGN Nurs 15(6):475, 1986
Chenger, P, and Kovacik, A: Dental hygiene during pregnancy: a review, MCN 12(5):342, 1987
Dameron, GW: Helping couples cope with sexual changes pregnancy brings, Contemp Obstet Gynecol 21:23, Feb 1983
Engstrom, JL: Measurement of fundal height, JOGN Nurs 17(3):172, 1988
Foster, SD: MCN patient teaching, MCN 12(2):131, 1987
Gray, JD, et al: Prediction and prevention of child abuse, Semin Perinatol 3:86, Jan 1979
Gross, C, et al: The Vietnamese American family—and grandma makes three, MCN 6:177, May/June 1981
Lee, PA: Health beliefs of pregnant and postpartum Hmong women, West J Nurs Res 8(1):83, 1986
Miller, SJ: Prenatal nursing assessment of the expectant family, Nurse Pract 11(5):40, 1986
Moore, L, et al: Self-assessment: a personalized approach to nursing during pregnancy, JOGN Nurs 15(4):311, 1986
Petitti, DB: Nausea and pregnancy outcome, Birth 13(4):223, 1986
Poole, CJ: Fatigue during the first trimester of pregnancy, JOGN Nurs 15(5):375, 1986
Queenan, JT, moderator: Managing pregnancy in patients over 35, Contemp OB/GYN 29(5):180, 1987
Wheeler, LA: Sexuality during pregnancy and the puerperium, Perinatal Press 3:131, Oct 1979
Winslow, W: First pregnancy after 35: what is the experience? MCN 12(2):92, 1987
Ziskin, DE, and Neese, GJ: Pregnancy gingivitis: history, classification, etiology, Am J Orthod 32:390, 1980

CHAPTER 13

Second Trimester

Learning Objectives

Correctly define the key terms listed.

Discuss maternal and fetal assessment.

Outline the schedule and events of prenatal visits.

Formulate possible nursing diagnoses and the type of data base expected to support these diagnoses.

Review planning of care and establishing goals with gravidas and their families.

Summarize the care implemented during the second trimester of pregnancy.

Explain the evaluation of the nursing care.

Explore and give the rationale for standards for maternity care and employment.

Key Terms

body mechanics
carpal tunnel syndrome
chloasma
conscious relaxation
constipation
effleurage
fetal gestational age
fetal health status
fetal heart rate (FHR)
fundal height
hemorrhoids
leg edema
leukorrhea
linea nigra
mean arterial pressure (MAP)
nipple cup
nipple preparation
pelvic tilt (rock)
pinch test
round ligament pain
striae gravidarum
tailor sitting position
varicosities

By the second trimester the pregnancy usually has been positively diagnosed. The woman and her family have had time to adjust to the pregnancy, and the initial visit or two have been completed. For many women, discomforts common to the first trimester are resolving, but it is still too early to focus intently on the labor and birth.

For most women no apparent major problems are identified. For them, a common pattern for return visits is scheduled. Throughout the second trimester, monthly visits are sufficient, although additional visits may be warranted should the need arise.

Assessment

Maternal

Interview. Follow-up visits are less extensive than the initial prenatal visit (see general nursing care plan, p. 283). At each visit, the woman is asked for a summary of events since the previous visit. She is asked about her general well-being, complaints or problems, or questions she may have. The interviewer can reinforce teaching about danger signs by inquiring about them at each visit. Personal and family needs are identified and explored (Chapters 11 and 14). Success or failure of self-care measures are discussed; and learning needs and readiness for learning are assessed.

Careful, precise, and concise recording of client responses and laboratory results contribute to the continuous supervision vital to the mother and fetus. A checklist of care needs during the second trimester of pregnancy is a valuable tool. It provides the team of care providers with a communication tool to prevent gaps and identify areas of repeated concern for clients. A sample checklist for the second trimester is shown in the box, above right .

SECOND TRIMESTER CHECKLIST

- Schedule and events of visits
- Counseling for self-care:
  - Adaptations/discomforts
    - Skin changes
    - Palpitations
    - Faintness
    - GI distress
    - Varicosities
    - Neuromuscular and skeletal distress
  - Safety (seat belts)
  - Exercise and rest
  - Relaxation
  - Nutrition
  - Sexuality
  - Personal hygiene
  - Danger signs
  - Preparation for
    - childbirth } classes
    - parenthood } classes
- Fetal growth and development
- Diagnostic tests
  - Specify
- Other

Physical Examination. Reevaluation is constant. Each woman reacts differently to pregnancy. Careful monitoring of pregnancy and reactions to care is vital. A data base updated at each contact with a client reveals patterns in movement and content.

At each visit temperature, pulse, and respirations are measured; blood pressure (right arm, woman sitting) is taken; weight and the determination of whether weight gain (or loss) is compatible with overall plan for weight gain are evaluated (see Chapter 15); and presence and degree of edema are noted. These findings reflect the status of maternal adaptations.

When the interview or physical examination findings are suspicious, an in-depth examination is performed.

Assessment of Blood Pressure. Careful interpretation of blood pressure is important in risk-factor analysis for all gravidas. Blood pressure is evaluated on the basis of absolute values and length of gestation and is interpreted in the light of modifying factors.

Absolute values of a systolic blood pressure ≥ 140 mm Hg and a diastolic blood pressure ≥90 mm Hg are suggestive of hypertension. A rise in systolic blood pressure ≥30 mm Hg over baseline and in diastolic blood pressure ≥15 mm Hg over baseline are also significant regardless of whether absolute values are less than 140/90. For example, if a woman's blood pressure normally is 105/60, a change to 120/75 must be viewed as potential for hypertension.

The **mean arterial pressure** (MAP) reaches its lowest point in the second trimester at about 22 weeks, then rises slowly to term (Page, Villee, and Villee, 1981). An MAP of ≥90 in the second trimester is associated with an increase in the incidence of pregnancy-induced hypertension (PIH) in the third trimester. The MAP is estimated by adding one third of the *pulse pressure* to the diastolic pressure. Pulse pressure is the difference between the systolic and diastolic values.

Example

Blood pressure: 106/70 at 22 weeks
Pulse pressure (106 − 70): 36 ÷ 3 = 12
MAP: (diastolic) 70 + 12 = 82

MAP readings of 82 at 22 weeks are within the normal range for the length of gestation.

Additional factors must be considered. These factors include maternal position, maternal anxiety, and size of cuff. **Maternal position** affects readings. Brachial blood pressure is highest when the woman is sitting and lower when she is in the lateral recumbant position. Therefore the same maternal position and the same arm are used at each visit. The position and arm used are noted along with the reading.

Some degree of compression of the vena cava occurs in all women who lie on their back during the second half of pregnancy. Some women experience a fall of ≥30 mm Hg systolic. After 4 to 5 minutes a reflex bradycardia is seen, cardiac output is reduced by half, and the woman feels faint (see box, vasovagal syncope, p. 145).

Maternal anxiety can elevate readings. If an elevated reading is found, the gravida is given time to rest, and the reading is repeated.

The **proper size cuff** is absolutely necessary for accurate readings. The cuff should be 20% wider than the diameter of the extremity around which it is wrapped: about 12 to 14 cm (about 6 in) for average-sized individuals and 18 to 20 cm (about 8 in) for obese individuals. Too small a cuff yields a false high reading; too large a cuff yields a false low reading.

Laboratory Tests. Routine laboratory tests during the second trimester are limited. A clean-catch urine specimen is used to detect glucose, acetone, and albumin/protein. Urine for culture and sensitivity and blood samples are obtained only if signs and symptoms warrant. Hematocrit (HCT) or packed cell volume (PCV) may be done at each visit in some offices.

Fetal

Fundal Height. During the second trimester the uterus becomes an abdominal organ. Measurement of the height of the uterus above the symphysis pubis is used as one indicator of the progress of fetal growth. It also provides a gross estimate of the duration of pregnancy.

A pliable (not stretchable) tape measure or a pelvimeter may be used to measure fundal height. The height of the fundus is measured from the notch of the pubic symphysis over the top of the fundus without tipping the corpus back.

To increase measurement reliability and facilitate management, the same person examines the gravida at each of her prenatal visits, and one protocol is established for use by all examiners providing care to a group of gravidas. The protocol must include the gravida's position on the table and the measuring device and method used. The gravida's position is supine with the knees slightly bent and the head and shoulders slightly elevated. Early in pregnancy, her bladder should be empty. If a pliable measuring tape is used, it should be specified whether the measurement is taken with the tape following the exact contour of the uterus to the fundus or whether the measurement is read with the palm of the hand at the fundus and the tape elevated between the forefinger and middle finger (Fig. 13-1). *McDonald's rule* adds precision to the measurement of fundal height during the second and third trimesters. It is calculated as follows:

Height of fundus (cm) × $2/7$ (or + 3.5) =
Duration of pregnancy in lunar months
Height of fundus (cm) × $8/7$ =
Duration of pregnancy in weeks

Measurement of fundal height may aid in identification of high-risk factors. A stable or decreased fundal height may indicate intrauterine growth retardation; an excessive increase could mean multiple gestation or hydramnios (see Unit VIII). Among the factors that affect the accuracy of measurement are obesity (subtract 1 cm from the measurement if the gravida weighs 90 kg [200 pounds] or more),

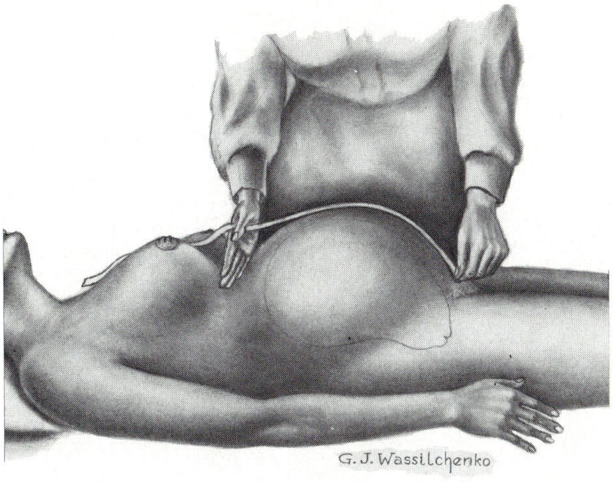

Fig. 13-1 Measurement of fundal height from symphysis.

the amount of amniotic fluid, multiple gestation, the fetal size and attitude, the tilt of the uterus, and the width of the examiner's finger if fingerbreadths are used.

Fetal Gestational Age. In a normal pregnancy, fetal gestational age is estimated by determining the duration of pregnancy and the date of delivery. In some centers ultrasonography is used with all pregnancies, and a more exact estimation of gestational age can be made (see box, p. 268). Ultrasonography may be used to establish the duration of pregnancy if the woman is unable to give a precise date for her last menstrual period (LMP) or if the size of the uterus does not conform to the stated date of the LMP. For a discussion of the use of ultrasound for estimation of gestational age of the fetus or detection of fetal anomalies, see Chapter 27. Ultrasonography is not, however, a universally recommended procedure (see Chapter 27).

Fetal Health Status. Assessment of fetal health status includes consideration of fetal movement, fetal heart rate (FHR), and abnormal maternal or fetal symptoms.

The mother is instructed to note the extent and timing of fetal movements and to report immediately if the pattern changes or if movement ceases. Regular movement has been found to be a reliable determinant of fetal health (Cohen, 1985).

The FHR is checked on routine visits once it has been heard (see Fig. 13-2).

Early in this trimester, the FHR may be heard with the ultrasound stethoscope (Fig. 13-2, *C*) or the ultrasound fetoscope (Fig. 17-13, *C*). Before the fetus can be palpated by Leopold's maneuvers (Chapter 14), the scope is moved around the abdomen until the FHR is heard. Each nurse develops a set pattern for searching the abdomen, for example, starting first in the midline about 2 to 3 cm (1 in) above the umbilicus followed by the left lower quadrant, and so on. The FHR is counted and the quality and rhythm noted (Chapter 17). Later in the second trimester, the FHR can be determined with the fetoscope or stethoscope (Fig. 13-2, *A*, *B*).

Normal rate and rhythm is another good indicator of fetal health. Absence of FHR, once heard, requires immediate investigation.

CORRELATION OF DATA IN DETERMINING FETAL GESTATIONAL AGE*

Menstrual History

LNMP: Date ________ Duration ________ Amount ________
LMP: Date ________ Duration ________ Amount ________
PMP: Date ________ Duration ________ Amount ________
Menarche ________ Interval ________ Duration ________
History of menstrual irregularity ________

Contraceptive History

Type of contraceptive ________
When stopped ________

Pregnancy Test

Date ________ Type ________ Result ________

Clinical Evaluation

First uterine size estimate: Date ________ Size ________
FHT first heard: Date ________ Dopptone ________ Fetoscope ________
Date of quickening ________
Current fundal height ________ EFW ________
Current week of gestation ________
Ultrasound: Date ________ Week of gestation ________ BPD ________
Reliability of dates ________

Impression

EDD ________ Estimated gestational age ________
Estimation based on ________
Comments ________
Signature ________ Date ________

**LNMP,* Last normal menstrual period; *PMP,* previous menstrual period (before LMP); *EFW,* estimated fetal weight; *BPD,* biparietal diameter.

A B C

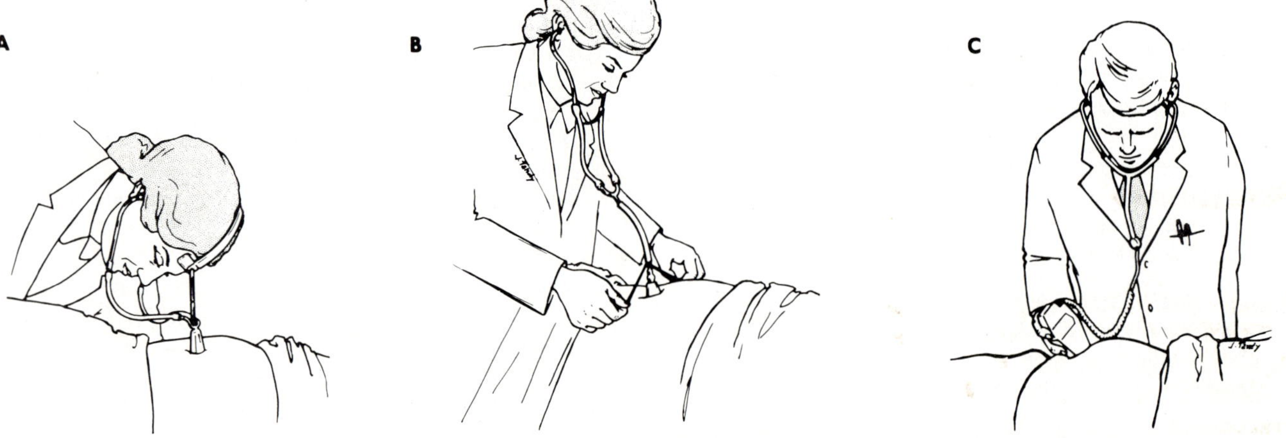

Fig. 13-2 Detecting fetal heartbeat. **A,** Fetoscope. **B,** Stethoscope with rubber band. **C,** Ultrasound stethoscope.

FETAL DEVELOPMENT AT 26 WEEKS

1. Viable at week 24
2. Fetal movements obvious
3. FHR readily heard
4. Scalp hair, eyebrows, eyelashes, fine downy lanugo and vernix cover the skin
5. Eyelids still fused
6. Skin is red, shiny, and thin
7. Face is wrinkled, giving an "old man appearance"
8. Length is 30 cm (12 in)
9. Weight is 600 g (1¼ lb)
10. Uterus at or just above level of umbilicus

The second trimester is a period of rapid growth. The box above summarizes fetal development.

Intensive investigation of fetal health status is initiated if any maternal or fetal complications arise (e.g., maternal hypertension, premature rupture of membranes, or irregular or absent FHR). (For a discussion of electronic fetal monitoring, see Chapter 17; for other monitoring techniques of the fetus at risk, see Chapter 27).

Nursing Diagnoses

Each individual is affected differently by pregnancy. Careful monitoring of the pregnancy and responses to care is of utmost importance. It is particularly difficult to distinguish discomforts of the second and third trimesters. Multiparous women tend to demonstrate some discomforts in pregnancy earlier than nulliparous women do. Continuous assessment, analysis, and formulation of diagnosis is imperative. The following are only a few examples of nursing diagnoses that can emerge from the data base.

- Anxiety, potential for, related to
  - Discomforts of pregnancy
  - Changing family dynamics
  - Fetal well-being
- Pain, potential for, related to
  - Discomforts of pregnancy
- Knowledge deficit, related to
  - Self-care measures for rest and relaxation
  - Personal hygiene (increased sweating, oily skin, leukorrhea)
  - Preparation for parenthood
- Altered family processes related to
  - Lack of understanding of second trimester changes
  - Changing sexual relationship or marital support
- Potential for injury related to
  - Nonuse of safety harness in automobiles

Planning

Planning care for clients during the second trimester of pregnancy is given direction from the nursing diagnosis. A plan is developed mutually with each client to the extent possible. The plan is individualized, relating specifically to her needs. The information in this chapter is general in nature; not all women will experience all problems discussed nor require all facets of care described.

The specific nursing care plan (see p. 284) serves as a guide for students developing a plan of care that reflects individual needs of the client.

The nurse continues to foster the growing relationship between care provider and client. Goals are the same as those for the mother, fetus, and family given in Chapter 12 for the first trimester (see p. 247).

Implementation

Nurses assume many caregiving roles during the second trimester of the prenatal period. The clinician's roles can be categorized as both supportive and as teacher/counselor/advocate. Midpregnancy classes focus on parental needs during this time (Chapter 11).

Supportive Role

The same guidelines as those discussed in Chapter 12 (see p. 248) are pertinent in the second trimester as well. The manner in which the nurse implements the roles of teacher/counselor/advocate and the consideration shown the mother while technical tasks are performed also support and reassure the gravida and her family.

Teacher/Counselor/Advocate

Changes Normal for Pregnancy. Several new discomforts or changes are experienced by women as maternal adaptations continue in the second trimester. Clear separation of discomforts and changes by trimester is impossible. Check Chapters 12 and 14 if a discomfort or change is not found in Table 13-1.

Clothing. Comfortable, loose clothing is best. Washable fabrics (e.g., absorbent cottons) are often preferred. Since maternity clothes are expensive and rarely wear out, hand-me-downs or used clothes from garage sales can suffice. Tight brassieres and belts, stretch pants, garters, tight-top knee socks, panty girdles, and other constrictive clothing should be avoided. Tight clothing over the perineum encourages vaginitis and miliaria (heat rash). Impaired circulation in the lower extremities favors varices.

A well-fitted maternity girdle, frequently readjusted, may be used for backache by obese women or those with a multiple pregnancy. The woman should be cautioned to begin fastening the girdle from the pubic symphysis upward to support the uterus from below. An old, even very large, girdle meant for the nonpregnant woman is unsuitable during pregnancy because it pushes the abdomen (uterus) inward. A nonmaternity girdle may also aggravate backache and leg ache.

Maternity brassieres are constructed to accommodate the increased breast weight, chest circumference, and size of breast tail tissue (under the arm). These brassieres have drop flaps over the nipples to facilitate breast-feeding. A good brassiere can help prevent neckache and backache (see guidelines for client teaching: body mechanics, p. 272).

Text continued on p. 273.

Table 13-1 *Problems Related to Maternal Adaptations to Pregnancy*

Discomfort	Physiology	Prevention/Treatment
Pigmentation deepens (striae gravidarum, chloasma, linea nigra, fingernails, hair, nipples and areolae); acne, oily skin	Melanocyte-stimulating hormone (from anterior pituitary) (Table 10-3)	Not preventable; usually resolved during puerperium; reassurance given to women and their families about these manifestations of pregnant state
Spider nevi (telangiectasias)—appear during trimesters 2 or 3 over neck, thorax, face, and arms (in that order) in two thirds of women	Focal networks of dilated arterioles (end-arteries) from increased concentration of estrogens	Not preventable; reassurance that they fade slowly during late puerperium; rarely disappear completely
Palmar erythema occurs in 50% of pregnant women; may accompany spider nevi	Diffuse reddish mottling over palms and suffused skin over thenar eminences and fingertips may be caused by genetic predisposition or hyperestrogenism	Not preventable; reassurance that condition will fade within 1 wk after giving birth
Pruritus (noninflammatory)	Unknown cause; various types as follows:	Keep fingernails short and clean; refer to physician for diagnosis of cause
	Nonpapular	Not preventable; symptomatic: Keri baths; mild sedation
	Closely aggregated pruritic papules	Not preventable; as for nonpapular type
	Increased excretory function of skin and stretching of skin possible factors	Distraction; tepid (not hot) baths with sodium bicarbonate or oatmeal added to water; lotions and oils; change of soaps or reduction in use of soap; loose clothing
Palpitations	Unknown; should not be accompanied by persistent cardiac irregularity	Not preventable; reassurance; refer to physician if accompanied by symptoms of cardiac decompensation
Supine hypotension (vena cava syndrome) and bradycardia	Posture induced by pressure of gravid uterus on ascending vena cava when woman is supine; reduces uterine-placental and renal perfusion	Side-lying position or semi-sitting posture, with knees slightly flexed (see box, supine hypotension, p. 152)
Faintness and, rarely, syncope (orthostatic hypotension): may persist throughout pregnancy	Vasomotor lability or postural hypotension from hormones; in late pregnancy may be caused by venous stasis in lower extremities	Moderate exercise, deep breathing, vigorous leg movement; avoid sudden changes in position* and warm crowded areas; move slowly and deliberately; keep environment cool; avoid hypoglycemia by eating 5 to 6 small meals per day; elastic hose; sit down as necessary; if symptoms are serious, refer to physician
Food cravings (see Chapter 15)	Cause unknown; cravings determined by culture or geographic area	Not preventable; satisfy craving unless it interferes with well-balanced diet; report unusual cravings (eg., pica: laundry starch, clay, dirt) to physician
Heartburn (pyrosis, or acid indigestion): burning sensation in lower chest or upper abdomen, occasionally with burping and raising of a little sour-tasting fluid; may also occur in first trimester	Progesterone slows GI tract motility and digestion, reverses peristalsis, relaxes cardiac sphincter, and delays emptying time of stomach; stomach displaced upward and compressed by enlarging uterus	Limit or avoid gas-producing or fatty foods and large meals; maintain good posture; keep torso upright; bend down at knees to reach below the waist; sips of milk for temporary relief; hot tea, chewing gum; physician may prescribe antacid between meals (NOTE: *Do not* use baking soda or Alka-Seltzer or patent medicines); flying exercise; refer to physician for persistent symptoms

*Caution woman to rise slowly and sit on edge of bed or to assume hands-and-knees posture before rising, and to get up slowly after sitting or squatting.

Table 13-1 *Problems Related to Maternal Adaptations to Pregnancy—cont'd*

Discomfort	Physiology	Prevention/Treatment
Constipation	GI tract motility slowed because of progesterone, resulting in increased resorption of water and drying of stool; intestines compressed by enlarging uterus; predisposition to constipation because of oral iron supplementation	Six glasses of water per day; roughage in diet; moderate exercise; maintain regular schedule for bowel movements; use relaxation techniques and deep breathing; *do not* take stool softener, laxatives, other drugs, or enemas without first consulting physician; *never* ingest mineral oil, since this inhibits absorption of fat-soluble vitamins
Flatulence with bloating and belching	Reduced GI motility because of hormones, allowing time for bacterial action that produces gas; swallowing air	Chew solid foods slowly and thoroughly; avoid gas-producing foods, fatty foods, large meals; exercise; regular bowel habits
Varicose veins (large distended, tortuous, superficial veins); may be associated with aching legs and tenderness; may be present in legs and vulva; hemorrhoids (piles) are varicosities in the perianal area	Hereditary predisposition; relaxation of smooth muscle walls of veins because of hormones, causing pelvic vasocongestion; condition aggravated by enlarging uterus, gravity, and bearing down for bowel movements; thrombi from leg varices rare but may be produced by hemorrhoids	Avoidance of obesity, lengthy standing or sitting, constrictive clothing, and constipation and bearing down with bowel movements; moderate exercises; rest with legs and hips elevated (Fig. 13-3); support stockings applied before rising; thrombosed hemorrhoid may be evacuated; relieve swelling and pain with hot sitz baths, local application of astringent compresses
Leukorrhea: often noted throughout pregnancy	Hormonally stimulated cervix becomes hypertrophic and hyperactive, producing abundant amount of mucus	Not preventable; *do not douche;* hygiene; perineal pads; reassurance; refer to physician if accompanied by pruritis, foul odor, or change in character or color
Headaches (through week 26)	Emotional tension (more common than vascular migraine headache); eye strain (refractory errors); vascular engorgement and congestion of sinuses from hormone stimulation	Emotional support; prenatal teaching; conscious relaxation; refer to physician for constant "splitting" headache, after assessing for pregnancy induced hypertension (PIH)
Carpal tunnel syndrome (involves thumb, second and third fingers, lateral side of little finger)	Compression of median nerve from changes in surrounding tissues: pain, numbness, tingling, burning; loss of skilled movements (typing); dropping of objects	Not preventable; elevation of affected arms, splinting of affected hand may help; surgery is curative
Periodic numbness, tingling of fingers (acrodysesthesia): occurs in 5% of pregnant women	Brachial plexus traction syndrome from drooping of shoulders during pregnancy (occurs especially at night and early morning)	Maintain good posture; wear good supportive maternity brassiere; reassurance that condition will disappear if lifting and carrying baby does not aggravate it
Round ligament pain (tenderness)	Stretching of ligament caused by enlarging uterus	Not preventable; reassurance, rest, good body mechanics to avoid overstretching ligament; relieve cramping by squatting or bringing knees to chest
Joint pain, backache, and pelvic pressure; hypermobility of joints	Relaxation of symphyseal and sacroiliac joints because of hormones, resulting in unstable pelvis; exaggerated lumbar and cervico-thoracic curves caused by change in center of gravity from enlarging abdomen	Maternity girdle; good posture and body mechanics; avoid fatigue; wear low-heeled shoes; conscious relaxation; firm mattress; local heat and back rubs; pelvic rock exercise; rest; reassure that condition will disappear 6-8 wk after delivery

Guidelines For Client Teaching

BODY MECHANICS DURING PREGNANCY

ASSESSMENT

1. Pregnant woman's center of gravity changes.
2. Woman has poor posture resulting in frequent backaches.
3. Woman needs instruction on proper body mechanics to perform activities of daily living (ADL) comfortably and safely.

NURSING DIAGNOSES

Pain: backache, related to poor posture and body mechanics.
Knowledge deficit related to self-care.
Potential for injury related to poor body mechanics.

GOALS

Short-term

Woman will identify potential sources of backaches.
Woman will learn and use good posture.

Intermediate

Woman will learn and use proper body mechanics.

Long-term

Woman will continue to use good posture and proper body mechanics throughout pregnancy.

REFERENCES AND TEACHING AIDS

Printed instructions and diagrams.
Full-length mirror, floor mat, straight-backed chair.
Many references available for lay people such as Marshall, C: From here to maternity, Citrus Heights, Calif, 1986, Conmar Publishing Co (P.O. Box 641, 95610).

CONTENT/RATIONALE	TEACHING ACTION
To understand maternal adaptations that could predispose to backache:	
Softening and relaxation of pelvic joints occur in response to circulating steroid hormones.	Use illustrations such as Fig. 10-10 to describe maternal adaptations, and correct/incorrect body alignment and center of gravity.
Abdominal muscles are stretched and weakened and the anterior portion of pelvis gradually tilts downward as the uterus increases in size and weight.	Use illustrations such as Figs. 10-10 and 10-4 to describe change in abdominal musculature.
Curvature of lumbarsacral vertebras increases as woman leans backward to maintain her balance.	
Shortening of and strain on back muscles and ligaments results in backache if the woman does not learn to correct this curvature.	
An improperly fitted maternity bra that provides inadequate support to the enlarging breasts and poor posture adds to the strain on muscles and ligaments high in the back, thus aggravating backache.	Use illustration of breast changes (Fig. 10-10) to emphasize increase in size and weight.
To develop a kinesthetic sense for good body alignment during pregnancy, practice the following:	
Pelvic tilt (rock) in standing position against a wall, or lying on floor. Using a solid surface makes it easier to feel lumbar curve.	In front of mirror, demonstrate pelvic tilt exercise and good posture.
Pelvic tilt (rock) on hands and knees, and while sitting in straight-back chair.	In front of mirror, guide woman through exercise and aligning body into good posture. Emphasize *feel* of movements and posture (see Figs. 12-1 and 13-4,*A*) by voice and touch.
Abdominal muscle contractions during pelvic tilt while standing, lying, or sitting helps strengthen rectus abdominis.	
Good posture to restore proper body alignment—head, shoulders, lumbarsacral curve, knees, and feet placement.	Use illustrations as needed (Figs. 10-10 and 13-4, *A*).
To learn good body mechanics, practice the following:	
Leg muscles are used to reach objects on or near floor. Bend at the knees, not the back. The back is kept straight. Knees are bent to lower body to squatting position. Feet are kept 12 to 18 inches apart for a solid base to maintain balance (Fig. 13-4, *B*).	Use illustrations, demonstrate and evaluate return demonstration (Fig. 13-4, *B*).

Guidelines For Client Teaching—cont'd

CONTENT/RATIONALE	TEACHING ACTION
Lift with the legs. To lift heavy object (young child), one foot is placed slightly in front of the other and kept flat as woman lowers herself on one knee. She lifts the weight holding it close to her body, and never higher than chest high. To stand up or sit down, one leg is placed slightly behind the other as she raises or lowers herself.	See Fig. 13-4, *C*
To prevent round ligament pain and strain on abdominal muscles, see Table 13-1	Use Table 13-1 for providing anticipatory guidance on several discomforts of pregnancy.
To learn self-care techniques to prevent and/or relieve backache:	Discuss with woman and her family.
Several comfort measures provide comfort directly and by reducing tension: warm showers, heating pad, rest as needed,* and massage, vibrator.	Review comfort measures and discuss which would work for her.
NOTE: Avoid hot-tubbing (see exercise tips, p. 251).	
Reduce lumbar curve with any of the following:	Encourage and answer questions.
Correct posture.	Practice sitting, pelvic rock and abdominal contraction.
Maternity girdle to support weak abdominal muscles.	
For prolonged standing (e.g., ironing, out-of-home employment), place one foot on low footstool or box; change positions often.	
Move car seat forward so that knees are bent and higher than hips. If needed, use a small pillow to support low back area.	
Sit in chairs low enough to allow both feet on floor and preferably, with knees higher than hips.	
Practice pelvic tilt and abdominal contraction.	
Wear sturdy, supportive, low heeled (no more than 1 inch) shoes.	
Ensure a good night's sleep. Use a firm mattress, or if preferred, a water bed. Sleep in side lying positon, supported by pillows, as needed (e.g., under abdomen, between knees).	Discuss which method woman can implement.

EVALUATION Teaching has been effective when all goals have been attained. Woman uses good posture and body mechanics on subsequent visits. Woman wears appropriate clothing and shoes. Woman verbalizes the self-care measures she continues to use. Woman states she no longer has backache or other muscle strain.

*It is recommended that employers have a place where women can lie down during their breaks (see box. p. 277).

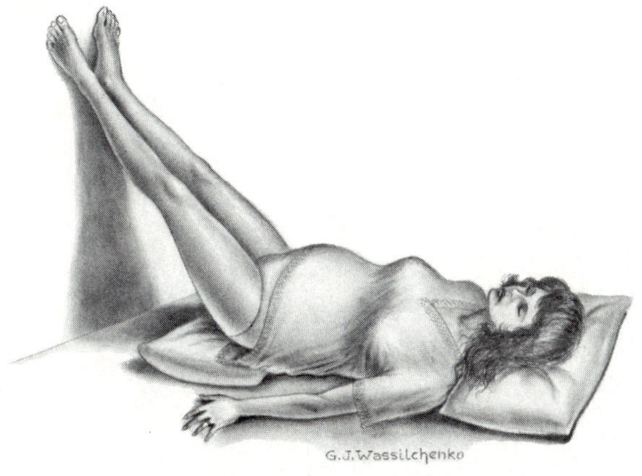

Fig. 13-3 Position for resting legs and reducing swelling, edema, and varicosities. Encourage woman with vulvar varicosities to include pillow under her hips.

Elastic hose or leotards may give considerable comfort to women with large varicose veins or swelling of the legs. Comfortable shoes that provide firm support and promote good posture and balance are advisable. Very high heels and platform shoes are not recommended because of the woman's changed center of gravity. She has a tendency to lose her balance. In the third trimester her pelvis tilts forward and her back arches. Leg aches and leg cramps are aggravated by nonsupportive shoes.

Bathing and Swimming. Tub bathing is permitted even in late pregnancy, because water does not enter the vagina unless under pressure. However, tub bathing is contraindicated after rupture of the membranes. Baths can be therapeutic because they relax tense tired muscles, help counter insomnia, and make the pregnant woman feel fresh. Physical maneuverability presents a problem (increased chance of falling) late in pregnancy. Swimming is also permitted during normal pregnancy, although diving is discouraged because of possible traumatic injury.

Physical Activity. Physical activity promotes a feeling of well-being in the pregnant woman. It improves circulation, assists relaxation and rest, and counteracts boredom as it does in the nonpregnant woman. Exercise tips for pregnancy are presented in detail in Chapter 12. Guidelines for client teaching of Kegel's exercises to strengthen the muscles around the reproductive organs and improve muscle tone are found in Chapter 8.

Rest and Relaxation. The pregnant woman is encouraged to plan regular rest periods particularly as pregnancy advances (Fig. 13-5). The side-lying position is recommended to promote uterine perfusion and fetoplacental oxygenation by eliminating pressure on the ascending vena cava (supine hypotension). During shorter rest periods, the woman can assume the position in Fig. 13-3 to promote venous drainage from the legs and relieve edema and varicose veins. The mother is shown how to rise slowly to minimize the hypotension secondary to changes in position common in the latter part of pregnancy. The nurse can alert the woman to several methods for relaxation (see guidelines for client teaching: relaxation, p. 275; and box, learning to relax, p. 276).

Conscious Relaxation Guide. Relaxation is the release of the mind and body from tension through conscious effort and practice. The ability to relax consciously and intentionally can be beneficial for the following reasons:

1. Relief of normal discomforts related to pregnancy
2. Reduction of stress and therefore diminished pain perception during the childbearing cycle
3. Heightened self-awareness and trust in own ability to control one's responses and functions
4. Coping with stress in everyday life situations, pregnant or not

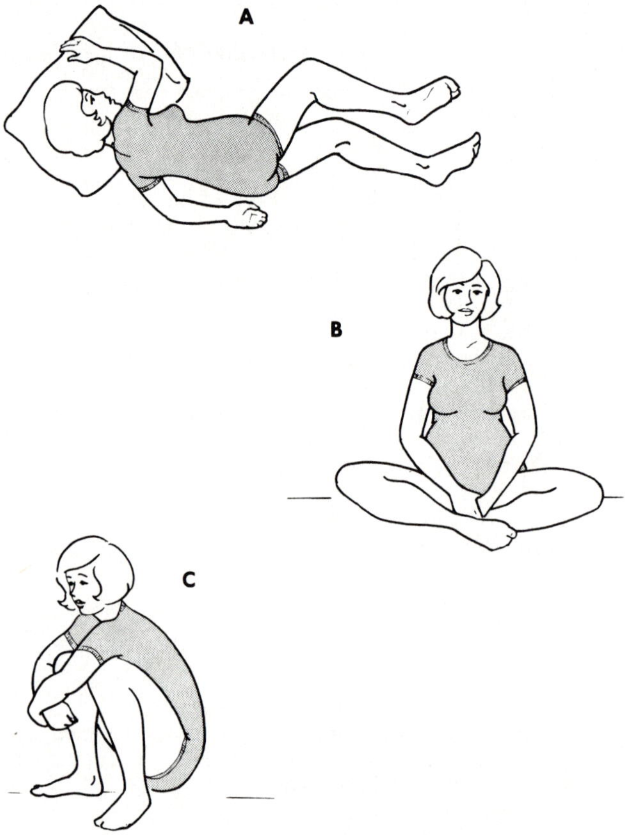

Fig. 13-5 Positions for rest and relaxation. **A,** Side-lying position. Some women prefer to support upper leg with pillows. **B,** Tailor sitting position aids in relaxing muscles of pelvic floor. **C,** Squatting helps relax the pelvic floor. All these positions can be assumed during labor.

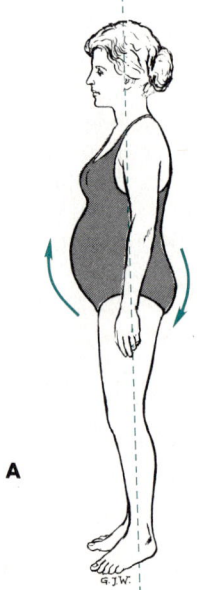

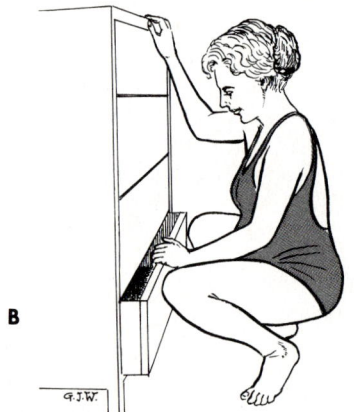

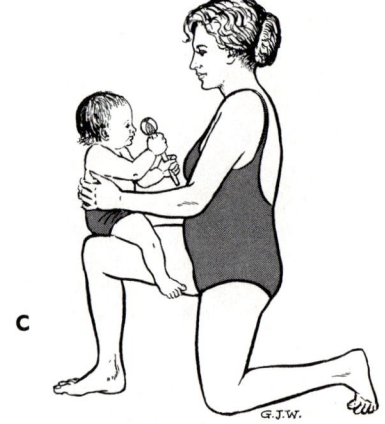

Fig. 13-4 Correct body mechanics. **A,** Standing. **B,** Stooping. **C,** Lifting.

Guidelines For Client Teaching

RELAXATION

ASSESSMENT

1. Gravida states she "just can't relax."
2. Gravida asks for information.
3. Gravida appears tired or tense.

NURSING DIAGNOSES

Pain related to emotional or physical tension.
Knowledge deficit related to self-care through relaxation techniques.

GOALS

Short-term

Woman learns sources of tension.
Woman increases self-care skills by learning at least two methods of relaxation.

Intermediate

Woman reports success with methods learned.
Woman expands self-care skills by learning additional relaxation measures to prevent or reduce stress.

Long-term

Woman utilizes and reports success with relaxation measures in labor and postpartum.
Woman continues to use and expand skills with relaxation within her family, across the life span.

REFERENCES AND TEACHING AIDS

Illustrations.
Cassettes of "New Age" music (e.g., sounds of waterfalls, birds, ocean waves).
Full-length mirror, floor mat or comfortable seats, pillows.
Many lay references available at bookstores everywhere.
Preparation for parenthood classes.

CONTENT/RATIONALE	TEACHING ACTION
To identify sources of tension:	
Maternal adaptation to pregnancy underlies many discomforts.	Validate the universality of tension and need for active relaxation.
The change in center of gravity, increase in weight and metabolic rate, and awkwardness increase tension on muscles and ligaments. Fetal activity interrupts rest.	Utilize gravida's readiness to learn to teach self-care skills that could last a lifetime for her and if she teaches it, for her family.
Psychosocial adaptations require energy.	
The combined sources often interrupt sleep and rest. Decreased resilience throughout pregnancy is characteristic.	
To present a variety of methods from which gavida can choose the most appropriate for her:	
Conscious relaxation with active imagery, see p. 276.	Keep abreast of a variety of methods.
Learning to relax, see p. 276.	Present each without imposing own preferences.
Exercises are relaxing for many people, see guidelines for client teaching: exercises, p. 252, and exercise tips, p. 251.	Use illustrations. Play cassettes. Demonstrate.
Use of good body mechanics aids relaxation, see guidelines for client teaching: body mechanics, p. 272.	Assist woman through practice. Refer clients to classes for therapeutic touch, acupressure and massage, yoga, and hypnosis per client requests.
Knowledge of common discomforts and self-care measures (Table 13-1) and answers to common questions (p. 269) can contribute to relaxation.	
Exercises to stretch and rest back muscles at home or at work:	Alert clients that if unable to relax because of persistent physical or emotional discomfort, that physician must be notified.
Stand behind a chair. Support and balance self using the back of the chair (Fig. 13-6). Squat for 30 seconds; stand for 15 seconds. Repeat 6 times, several times per day, as needed.	
While sitting in chair, lower head to knees for 30 seconds. Raise up. Repeat 6 times, several times per day, as needed.	

EVALUATION The nurse can be reasonably reassured that teaching was effective when the goals for care are met. The woman demonstrates relaxation techniques appropriately. Woman states she uses the techniques and feels that they bring her relief.

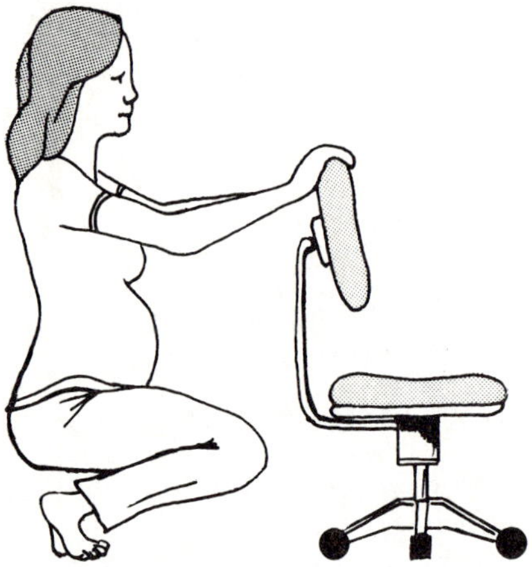

Fig. 13-6 Squatting for muscle relaxation and strengthening, and for keeping leg and hip joints flexible.

The techniques for conscious relaxation are numerous and varied. See box below for one technique. The following guidelines can be used by anyone:

1. Preparation: Loosen clothing, assume a comfortable sitting (Fig. 13-7) or side-lying position with all parts of body well-supported with pillows.
2. Beginning: Allow self to feel warm and comfortable. Inhale and exhale slowly, and imagine peaceful relaxation coming over each part of the body starting with the neck and working down to the toes. Often persons who learn conscious relaxation speak of feeling relaxed even if some discomfort is present.
3. Maintenance: Imagine (fantasize or daydream) to maintain the state of relaxation. With *active imagery* the person imagines herself as moving or doing some activity and experiencing its sensations. With *passive imagery,* one imagines watching a scene, such as a lovely sunset.
4. Awakening: The return to the wakeful state is gradual. The person begins slowly to take in the stimuli from the surrounding environment.
5. Further retention and development of the skill: Regular practice for regular periods of time each day, for exam-

LEARNING TO RELAX

First Level

1. Take three slow, deep breaths. At the height of the inhalation breath, pause for about 2 seconds before releasing the air. Breathe naturally and rhythmically in through your nose and out your mouth with lips slightly pursed. Imagine a balloon inflating and deflating in your belly.
2. Close your eyes tightly and frown. Relax the tensed muscles.
3. Grit your teeth and then relax, letting your tongue drop from the roof of your mouth.
4. Bend your neck forward, then drop your chin on your chest.
5. Raise your shoulders at attention, then let them drop forward into a comfortable slump.
6. Clench your right hand as if squeezing a ball, then relax. Repeat with left hand.
7. Take a very deep breath. Fill your lungs and hold your breath for 2 to 3 seconds, then exhale fully.
8. Pull in your stomach muscles as tightly as possible and let go.
9. Squeeze the muscles in your buttocks and perineum (Kegel's exercise), then relax.
10. Tense the muscles in your right leg, then relax. Repeat with your left leg.
11. Flex your right foot. Point your toes toward your body and then relax. Repeat with left foot.
12. Feel the feeling of having your whole body relaxed.

Second Level

1. Do slow, rhythmic breathing.
2. Tense face muscles and then relax.
3. Tense neck and shoulders; relax.
4. Clench hands and tense arms, then relax.
5. Tense abdomen and buttocks, then relax.
6. Tense legs and feet, then relax.

Third Level

1. Use rhythmic breathing.
2. Relax your face.
3. Relax upper body.
4. Relax lower body.

Use visualization to aid in relaxing. See relaxation as a white light of energy flowing in through the top of your head. As the white light advances downward, see the tension being pushed out of your body through your finger tips and toes until it disappears.

The only difference in the three levels of relaxation is practice. As you become more aware of your body and learn to relax, you can hasten the process to reach the relaxed state. It becomes second nature.

Marshall, CC: From here to maternity, Citrus Hgts, Calif, 1986, Comar Publishing Co. Courtesy Comar Publishing Co.

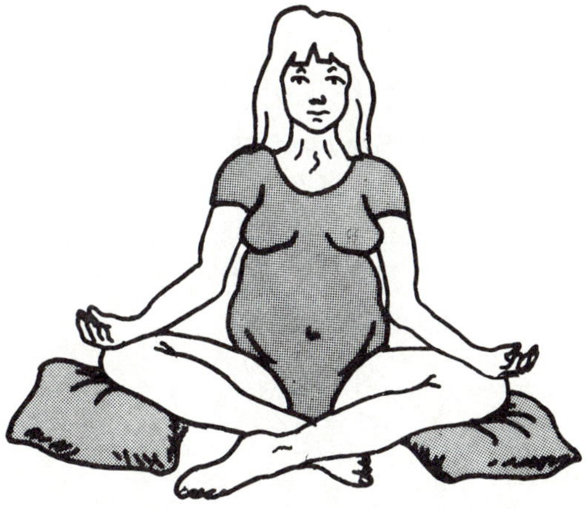

Fig. 13-7 One position suitable for conscious relaxation.

ple, at the same hour for 10 to 15 minutes each day, is refreshing, revitalizing, and invigorating.

Employment. Continued assessment during the prenatal period is necessary to determine if working is causing undue fatigue or stress. It may be possible for the woman to change the type of work being done with a recommendation from her physician (Bryant, 1985). Some women may lose interest in work as they become more introverted during the second trimester of pregnancy. This response may be difficult to accept for the woman who has always been competent and independent before pregnancy.

Activities that depend on a good sense of balance should be discouraged, especially during the last half of pregnancy. Commonly, excessive fatigue is the deciding factor in the termination of employment. Women in sedentary jobs need to walk around at intervals and should neither

STANDARDS FOR MATERNITY CARE AND EMPLOYMENT (U.S. CHILDREN'S BUREAU)

1. Facilities for adequate prenatal medical care should be readily available for all employed pregnant women, and arrangements should be made by those responsible for providing prenatal care, so that every woman has access to such care. Local health departments should make the services of prenatal clinics available to industrial plants, and the personnel management or physicians and nurses within the plant should make available to employees information about the importance of such services and where they can be obtained.
2. Pregnant women should not be employed on a shift including the hours between 12 midnight and 6 AM. Pregnant women should not be employed more than 8 hours a day or more than 48 hours per week, and it is desirable that their hours of work be limited to not more than 40 hours per week.
3. Every woman, especially a pregnant woman, should have at least two 10-minute rest periods during her work shift, for which adequate facilities for resting and an opportunity for securing nourishing food should be provided.
4. It is not considered desirable for pregnant women to be employed in the following types of occupations, and they should, if possible, be transferred to lighter and more sedentary work:
   a. Occupations that involve heavy lifting or other heavy work.
   b. Occupations that involve continuous standing and moving about.
5. Pregnant women should not be employed in the following types of work during any period of pregnancy:
   a. Occupations that require a good sense of bodily balance, such as work performed on scaffolds or stepladders and occupations in which the accident risk is characterized by accidents causing severe injury, such as operation of punch presses, power-driven woodworking machines, or other machines having a point-of-operation hazard.
   b. Occupations involving exposure to toxic substances considered to be extra hazardous during pregnancy, including the following:
      Aniline
      Benzene and toluene
      Carbon disulfide
      Carbon monoxide
      Chlorinated hydrocarbons
      Lead and its compounds
      Mercury and its compounds
      Nitrobenzol and other nitro compounds of benzol and its homologues
      Phosphorus
      Radioactive substances and x-rays
      Turpentine
      Other toxic substances that exert an injurious effect upon the blood-forming organs, the liver, or the kidneys

   Because these substances may exert a harmful influence upon the course of pregnancy, may lead to premature termination, or may injure the fetus, the maintenance of air concentrations within the so-called maximum permissible limits of state codes is not, in itself, sufficient assurance of a safe working condition for the pregnant woman. Pregnant women should be transferred from workrooms in which any of these substances are used or produced in any significant quantity.
6. A minimum of 6 weeks' leave *before* delivery should be granted with the presentation of a medical certificate of the expected date of delivery.
7. At any time during pregnancy, a woman should be granted a reasonable amount of additional leave with the presentation of a certificate from the attending physician to the effect that complications of pregnancy have made continuing employment prejudicial to her health or to the health of the child.

   To safeguard the mother's health she should be granted sufficient time off after delivery to return to normal and to regain her strength. The infant needs her care, especially during the first year of life. If it is essential that she return to work, the following recommendations are made:
   a. All women should be granted an extension of at least 2 months leave of absence after delivery.
   b. Should complications of delivery or of the postpartum period develop, a woman should be granted a reasonable amount of additional leave beyond 2 months following delivery with presentation of a certificate to this effect from the attending physician.

sit nor stand in one position for long periods. Activity is necessary to counter the usual sluggish, dependent circulation that potentiates development of varices and thrombophlebitis. The pregnant woman's chair should provide adequate back support. A footstool can prevent pressure on veins, relieve strain on varices, and minimize swelling of feet. Work breaks are best spent resting in the left lateral side-lying position. It is recommended that employers have an area where women can lie down. Standards for maternity care and employment of mothers in industry have been recommended by the United States Children's Bureau to safeguard the interests of expectant mothers employed in industry (box, p. 277).

The nurse can encourage each woman to consider the effects of working postnatally on herself and her newborn. Flexible scheduling of working hours, if possible, can allow for breast-feeding. Also, women who plan to return to work after giving birth may appreciate information about daycare centers.

Travel. If traveling for long distances, periods of activity and rest should be scheduled (see Employment, above). While sitting, the woman can practice deep breathing, foot circling, and alternating contracting and relaxing different muscle groups. Fatigue should be avoided.

Although travel in itself is not a cause of either abortion or premature labor, certain precautions are recommended. A woman who does not wear automobile restraints risks injury to herself and her fetus (Krozy et al. 1985) (see research highlight). Maternal death as a result of injury is the most common cause of fetal death (Crosby, 1983). The next most common cause is placental separation. Body contours change in reaction to the force of a collision. The uterus as a muscular organ can adapt its shape to that of the body. The placenta lacks the resiliency to change, and placental separation can occur (Crosby, 1983). A combination lap belt and shoulder harness is the most effective automobile restraint (Fig. 13-8) (Chang, 1985). Both shoulder and lap belts should be used. The lap belt should be worn low across the hip bones and as snug as is comfortable. The shoulder belt should be worn above the gravid uterus and below the neck to avoid chafing. The pregnant woman should sit upright. The headrest should be used to avoid a whiplash injury.

In high-altitude regions, lowered oxygen levels may cause fetal hypoxia. Women who travel extensively expose themselves to the risk of serious accident and may find themselves far removed from good maternity care. In addition, fatigue or tension, as well as altered regular personal habits and diet during arduous travel, may be detrimental. If long-distance travel is necessary, the trip should be made by air. Perhaps fortuitously, flight regulations do not permit pregnant women aboard during the last month without a statement from an obstetrician.

Many women experience a sense of uneasiness when traveling by any vehicle. They describe feelings of fear for the safety of their unborn baby. Guidelines for client teaching: safety, are found on p. 279.

Preparation for Feeding the Newborn. Pregnant women are usually eager to discuss their plans for feeding the newborn. Breast milk is the food of choice, and breast-feeding is associated with a decreased incidence in perinatal mor-

RESEARCH HIGHLIGHT

Automobile Seat Belt Practices of Pregnant Women

Purpose

This study by Arneson was conducted to examine the seat belt practices of pregnant women.

Sample/Methodology

A convenience sample of 87 women was obtained from the postpartum units of 3 hospitals. An interview schedule was used to collect data.

Findings

Less than 50% of the 87 women interviewed reporting using seat belts regularly during pregnancy. One third of the subjects reported always using seat belts, which is roughly twice the national average.

Many of the women who consistently used seat belts were not adjusting their belts properly. Almost one third of the women who used seat belts did not use a shoulder harness and did not position the lap-type belt low across the hips and under the abdomen. Less than 25% could recall having received any information about seat belt use during pregnancy. Posters and phamplets in the waiting rooms headed the list of sources of information. Few of the women recalled having a physician or nurse talk to them about seat belt use during their prenatal visits.

Implications

Health care professionals must devote more attention to this health practice beginning with the first prenatal visit. This information needs to be routinely incorporated into preparation for parenthood classes as well.

Arneson, S, et al: Automobile seat belt practices of pregnant women, JOGN Nurs 15(4):339, 1986.

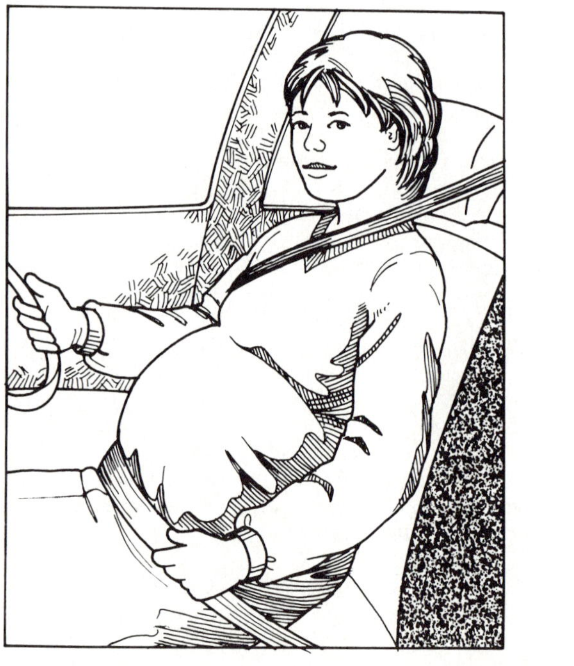

Fig. 13-8 Proper use of seat belt and head rest.

Guidelines For Client Teaching

SAFETY*

ASSESSMENT

1. Woman is pregnant.
2. Pregnant woman works within the home, in the yard, drives or rides in a car, and works as a hairdresser.

NURSING DIAGNOSES

Knowledge deficit related to source of safety hazards.
Knowledge deficit related to safety measures.
Potential for injury to mother and fetus related to possible hazards in the environment and workplace.

GOALS

Short-term

Woman is alerted to sources of safety hazards.
Woman is alerted to self-care related to safety measures.
Woman will use car safety belt and head rest consistently.
Woman will verbalize rationale for and consistently use gloves and good ventilation when using any chemicals, or avoid their use.

Intermediate

Woman will eliminate exposure to chemicals and fumes.

Long-term

Woman will persist in use of safety measures throughout life span.

REFERENCES AND TEACHING AIDS

Printed instructions and information from sources such as clinic, doctor, safety councils.
Copy of "Standards for Maternity Care and Employment" (U. S. Children's Bureau, box, p. 277).

CONTENT/RATIONALE	TEACHING ACTION
To identify factors that make safety awareness and measures critical during pregnancy:	
Maternal adaptations to pregnancy involve relaxation of joints, alteration in center of gravity, and neurologic changes responsible for faintness and discomforts. Problems with coordination and balance are common.	Encourage and answer questions regarding maternal changes—refer to guidelines for client teaching: body mechanics (p. 272) during pregnancy.
Embryonic and fetal development is vulnerable to environmental teratogens.	Exercise caution to avoid causing anxiety (see Chapter 2 for interview techniques).
To explore sources of safety hazards:	Review guidelines for client teaching: precautions for drug use, Chapter 12.
Many potentially dangerous chemicals are present in the home and yard. These include cleaning agents, paints, a variety of sprays, herbicides, and pesticides. The soil and water supply may be unsafe in some places.	Learn status of local area from community health agencies.
The work place often contain obvious and hidden hazards.	Review standards of maternity care and employment, p. 277, and guidelines for client teaching: body mechanics, p. 272.
Recent legislation specifies appropriate use of vehicular seat belts, but some people ignore it.	
Recreation requiring coordination and balance is best deferred.	Encourage and answer questions regarding which changes woman is able to implement.
High altitudes (not in pressurized aircraft) could jeopardize oxygen intake.	
Spouse's exhaled breath and clothes may contain contaminants.	
To increase self-care through consistent use of safety measures:	Present alternatives and problem-solve solutions together.
Read all labels for ingredients and proper use of product.	Explore with woman what she does during the course of a typical day. Make a list of potential/actual hazards and mutually problem-solve solutions (e.g., avoid use, provide substitutions, ensure ventilation and proper
Ensure adequate ventilation with "clean" air.	
Dispose of wastes appropriately.	

*Prevention of infection is covered in Chapter 30. Hazards to women's health care discussed in Chapter 43.

Continued.

Guidelines For Client Teaching—cont'd

CONTENT/RATIONALE	TEACHING ACTION
Wear gloves when handling chemicals. Change job assignments or work-place as necessary. Use good body mechanics. Use safety features on tools/vehicles; wear goggles, helmets, as specified. Avoid activities requiring coordination, balance, and concentration.	disposal, use safety equipment, make changes in sports and recreation, and schedule rest periods).
Take rest periods, reschedule daily activities to meet rest and relaxation needs. While traveling, use safety seat belts and head rests.	Show illustrations (Figs. 13-5 and 13-7) and discuss.

EVALUATION The nurse will know that teaching has been effective when all goals have been achieved. The woman can verbalize knowledge of hazards and problem-solve solutions. The woman consistently implements self-care safety measures. She and fetus experience no harm from safety-related causes.

bidity and mortality. However, immaturity of the infant, deep-seated aversion to breast-feeding by mother or father, and certain medical complications, such as pulmonary tuberculosis, are containdications to breast-feeding. The woman and her partner are encouraged to decide which method of feeding is suitable for them. Once the couple has been given information about the advantages and disadvantages of bottle- and breast-feeding, they are in a position to make an informed choice. Nurses need only to support their decisions.

The decision to breast-feed or bottle-feed the baby is most often made for psychological rather than physical reasons (Dawson et al., 1979). Nicholson (1985) notes that fears mothers may have about breast-feeding, such as inadequate milk supply, may influence their choice. A mother who is the sole supporting parent may find it impossible to breast-feed. In most traditional societies no alternative to breast feeding is perceived or practiced. Mothers from these societies require little or no encouragement to breast-feed.

Most women are motivated by the sixth or seventh month of pregnancy to learn about breast preparation and breast-feeding. Anticipatory guidance during pregnancy contributes to later success in breast-feeding (Nicholson, 1985). Teaching expectant mothers about nipple preparation for breast-feeding is an important nursing function. Guidelines for client teaching: nipple preparation are on p. 281.

The possibility of contaminants in breast milk concerns many women, both consumers and professionals (Doucette, 1978). Breast milk can be potentially hazardous as illustrated in the following examples. The mother harboring *Salmonella kottbus* transmits this organism through her milk. Environmental pollutants tend to concentrate in humans. The long-term effects of contamination of breast milk with pollutants such as polybrominated biphenyl (PBB) is as yet unknown. Medications that pass through the mother's milk are listed in Appendix I.

Evaluation

Maternal and fetal goals are continuously evaluated according to measurable, established criteria. The clinical findings that represent normal response are presented as outcome criteria in the general and specific nursing care plans that follow. These criteria are used as a basis for selecting appropriate nursing actions and evaluating their effectiveness.

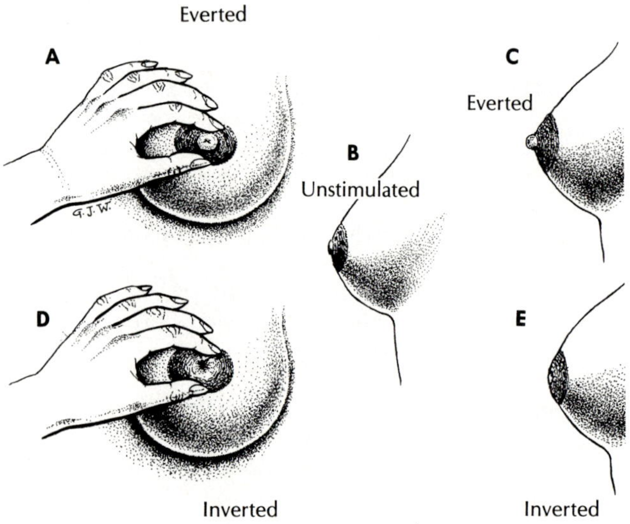

Fig. 13-9 **A** and **C**, When stimulated, nipples evert (protract or erect). **B**, Unstimulated, nipples look the same. **D** and **E**, When stimulated, nipples invert (retract).

Guidelines For Client Teaching

NIPPLE PREPARATION FOR BREAST-FEEDING

ASSESSMENT

1. Pregnant woman has decided to breast-feed.
2. Woman is motivated to learn about nipple preparation for breast-feeding.
3. Woman is in the sixth month of pregnancy.
4. Woman is not at risk for preterm labor.

NURSING DIAGNOSES

Knowledge deficit related to nipple preparation for breast-feeding.

Potential for nipple injury related to lack of prenatal preparation.

GOALS

Short-term

Woman learns her nipple formation and when to begin preparation techniques.

Intermediate

Woman performs those techniques needed to toughen and prepare her nipples for breast-feeding.

Long-term

Woman will be prepared psychologically for knowing and handling her breasts before initiating breast-feeding.

Woman has prepared her nipples adequately so that breast-feeding occurs with no injury to her nipples.

REFERENCES AND TEACHING AIDS

Books and pamphlets on breast-feeding from La Leche League, clinics.

Illustrations.

Variety of nipple shields.

List of references, or examples:

La Leche League International: The womanly art of breast feeding, Franklin Park, Ill, 1981, The League.

Riordan, JM: Breast feeding: a guide for nurses, St Louis, 1983, The CV Mosby Co.

CONTENT/RATIONALE	TEACHING ACTION
To determine nipple formation retractile or erectile (Fig. 13-9):	Instruct and demonstrate how to perform the *pinch test.* Use illustrations as necessary. Guide woman through pinch test. Encourage and answer questions.
Have woman place thumb and forefinger on her areola and press inward gently. This will cause her nipple to stand erect or to retract (invert). Most nipples erect.	
Inverted nipples need more preparation time. Nipple preparation for these women can start during the last 2 months of pregnancy.	
To provide information about actual techniques:	Discuss these procedures with the woman and provide time for her questions. Provide a chart to illustrate the anatomy of the breast.
Nipples are cleansed with warm water to prevent blocking of the ducts with dried colostrum. They are dried with a rough towel. Soap is not used because it removes protective oils that keep nipples supple. Soften dried precolostrum secretion with lanolin-based cream (e.g., Masse).	
Breasts are milked to remove colostrum and keep the milk ducts clear.	Demonstrate this procedure to the woman. If necessary ask for a return demonstration. Encourage discussion and questions. Provide pictures.
Western dress precludes natural toughening of nipples. Toughening of nipples can be accomplished in a variety of ways.	Provide options so woman can use method best suited to her, and to her spouse.
Following a bath or shower, towel dry nipples well, but not so hard as to cause irritation or soreness.	Demonstrate. Use illustrations.
Grasp nipple between thumb and forefinger. Roll nipples gently for short time each day. Since this procedure may cause uterine contractions, it may be contraindicated for those women at risk for premature labor.	Demonstrate. Use illustrations such as Fig. 13-10, *C.* Prepare the woman for and discuss the stimulation of uterine contractions.

Continued.

Guidelines For Client Teaching—cont'd

CONTENT/RATIONALE	TEACHING ACTION
Undress to bra, drop flaps over nipples. Expose nipples to air and sunlight for short periods of time each day. Avoid sunburn.	Discuss.
Incorporate oral stimulation of nipples by spouse during sexual intercourse.	Discuss. Recognize that this activity may be unacceptable to some people.
To encourage protraction of inverted nipples:	
Utilize one or more of the methods described above.	
Place forefingers close to inverted nipple, pressing firmly into breast tissue, and gradually pulling away from areola. Massage is done vertically and horizontally, about 5 times. Repeat each day.	Demonstrate. Use illustrations such as Fig. 13-10. Provide written instructions.
Obtain nipple cups designed specifically for correcting inverted nipples. Plastic doughnut-shaped cups are available for correcting inversions or retractions (Fig. 13-10, *D*). A continuous, gentle pressure exerted around the areola pushes the nipple through a central opening in the inner shield. Nipple cups should be worn during the last 2 trimesters of pregnancy for 1 to 2 hours daily. The time for wearing them should be increased gradually. Brand names for these cups include Woolwich, Netsy, La Leche League Cups, Nurse-Dri, Free and Dry, and Hobbit Shields.	Present displays of nipple cups. Encourage woman to handle cups and try them. Alert her to the fact that these cups can also be worn after childbirth. However, because body warmth can foster rapid bacterial growth and contamination, milk that collects in the cup should be discarded and not fed to the infant (Riordan, 1983).

EVALUATION The nurse will know that teaching was effective when woman correctly performs suggested techniques to prepare her breasts for breast-feeding. Evaluation of the long-term goals must be deferred until the postpartum period.

General Nursing Care Plan

SUBSEQUENT PRENATAL VISITS: SECOND TRIMESTER

ASSESSMENT	NURSING DIAGNOSIS (ND)/PLAN (P)/GOAL (G)	RATIONALE/ IMPLEMENTATION	EVALUATION
Woman making subsequent office or clinic visit.	ND: Knowledge deficit related to second trimester of pregnancy. P: Review schedule for care. G: The woman will become knowledgable about the second trimester of pregnancy.	*To determine woman's general well-being the nurse will:* Interview woman regarding events since previous visit. Inquire about any complaints or problems. Answer any questions woman may have. Identify personal and family needs. Assess learning needs.	Woman understands and verbalizes rationale for sharing any relevant information with the nurse. Woman exhibits a readiness to learn by verbalizing and asking appropriate questions.

General Nursing Care Plan—cont'd

ASSESSMENT	NURSING DIAGNOSIS (ND)/PLAN (P)/GOAL (G)	RATIONALE/ IMPLEMENTATION	EVALUATION
Physical evaluation of gravida.	ND: Altered body systems related to second trimester of pregnancy. P: Share findings from examination. G: The woman will maintain physical well-being during pregnancy by gaining knowledge about normal physical alterations during this time.	*To determine woman's physical well-being the nurse will*: Monitor the gravida's weight gain and blood pressure. Measure fundal height. Listen to fetal heart tones. Test urine for sugar and protein.	Woman understands and verbalizes rationale for observation of these parameters. Woman cooperates by bringing urine specimen with her.
Gravida needs education regarding self-care activities.	ND: Knowledge deficit related to self-care activities during second trimester of pregnancy. P: Review self-care activities. G: Woman will learn self-care activities.	*To educate the woman the nurse will*: Discuss importance of keeping scheduled appointments. Discuss good nutrition, eating habits, and a favorable weight gain. Explain importance of maintaining an exercise program. Discuss safety hazards relevant to work and travel. Explain importance of wearing nonrestrictive and flattering clothes to help woman with her self-image.	Woman keeps scheduled appointments. Woman reports eating habits and maintains a favorable weight gain. Woman verbalizes an understanding of a safe exercise program and safety hazards associated with work and travel. Woman refrains from wearing regular girdles, garters, or other restrictive clothes.
Lack of knowledge regarding danger signs.	ND: Knowledge deficit related to danger signs during second trimester. P: Teach danger signs. G: Woman will learn to recognize those signs and symptoms that signal danger for her and her fetus.	*To educate woman the nurse will discuss the following signs and symptoms with the client*: Absence of fetal movement or change in pattern of fetal movement. Swollen feet, ankles, hands, puffy eyes. Rapid gain in weight. Headaches, blurred vision, dizziness. Premature rupture of membranes. Vaginal bleeding. Sudden, sharp pains in abdomen. Provide gravida with phone numbers of doctor or hospital.	Woman verbalizes understanding of these danger signs and asks relevant questions. Woman knows where to call if she should experience any of these signs or symptoms.

Specific Nursing Care Plan

SECOND TRIMESTER

Mary Stewart, a 30-year-old lawyer is pregnant for the first time. She is in her second trimester and at the doctor's office for her monthly check-up. While the nurse is assessing her weight and vital signs, Mary reveals to the nurse that she is upset about the way she looks. "Nothing fits me any more, I'm as big as a house. My nipples have turned so dark, I feel funny about undressing in front of my husband. I also have a thick, white discharge from my vagina that makes me feel dirty all the time."

ASSESSMENT	NURSING DIAGNOSIS (ND)/PLAN (P)/GOAL (G)	RATIONALE/ IMPLEMENTATION	EVALUATION
Mary is experiencing anxiety and negative feelings toward her body.	ND: Body image disturbance related to the physiologic changes of pregnancy. P: Discuss Mary's feelings. G: Mary will accept and adapt to changing self-concept and body image.	*To help Mary accept changing self-image the nurse will*: Assess Mary's attitude toward her pregnancy. Discuss normal physiologic processes responsible for changes in body shape and pigmentation. Discuss maternity clothing that enhances Mary's professional image and self-concept. Discuss skin care. Suggest use of make-up to help disguise darkened areas of skin. Assess relationship of couple.	Mary verbalizes acceptance of changing body image. Mary verbalizes understanding of information presented. Couple can sit down and discuss these feelings openly.
Mary expresses problem with vaginal discharge.	ND: Knowledge deficit related to leukorrhea. P: Discuss vaginal discharge. G: Mary will become knowledgeable about the causes of leukorrhea and ways to deal with it comfortably.	*To help Mary deal with the problem of leukorrhea, the nurse will*: Define what leukorrhea is and what causes it. Describe signs to watch for that signal a change from normal leukorrhea (i.e., pruritis or blood stained). Discuss types of under garments to wear that aid in controlling problems with leukorrhea.	Mary verbalizes understanding of information presented. Mary asks appropriate questions. Mary verbalizes understanding and acceptance of information.

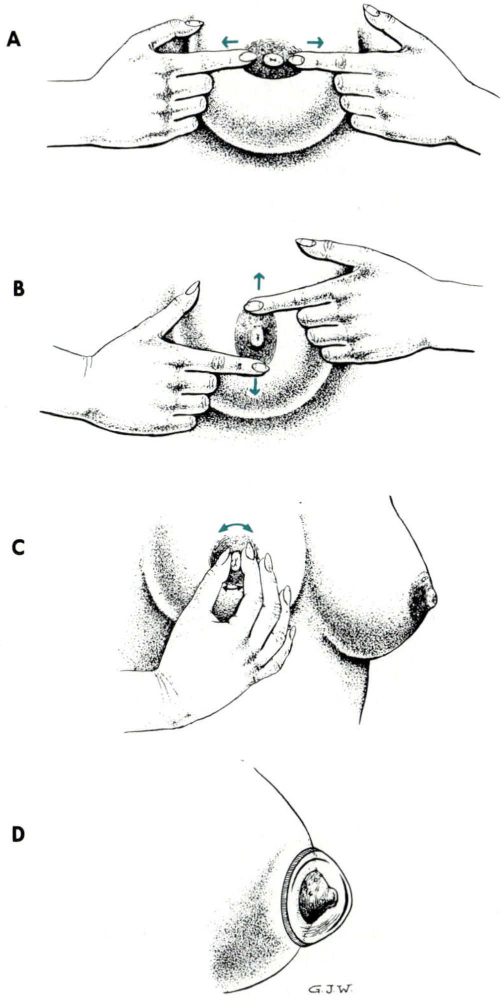

Fig. 13-10 A and B, Nipple stretching. C, Nipple rolling. D, Nipple cup in place. (Some concern has been expressed regarding nipple stimulation and potential for preterm labor.)

SUMMARY

Monthly prenatal visits during the second trimester are designed to monitor the individual gravida's pregnancy and responses to care. Diligent assessment during this period provides the basis for preventive care. A heightened readiness for learning is experienced by the gravida and her family. Counseling for self-care, fetal growth and development, and diagnostic tests is offered. Assessment findings of maternal and fetal physical well-being are evaluated for potential complications. The gravida and her family are alerted to danger signs that need immediate medical attention. Standards for maternity care and employment are shared with expectant parents. During this time, the relationship between the health-care team and the expectant parents progresses and the parents-to-be develop in their roles as active participants in their health care.

KEY CONCEPTS

- Blood pressure is evaluated on the basis of absolute values and length of gestation and interpreted in the light of modifying factors.
- Normal MAPs during the second trimester are <90 mm Hg.
- In the absence of factors that affect accuracy, measurement of fundal height is one of the indicators of the progress of fetal growth.
- Auscultation of fetal heart tones is another tool for assessing fetal health status.
- Discomforts and changes of pregnancy can cause anxiety to the gravida and her family.
- Education about healthy ways of using the body (e.g., exercise, body mechanics) is essential given maternal anatomic and physiologic responses to pregnancy.
- Appropriate use of auto seat belts is essential for the gravida.
- The gravida's readiness to learn is at a high level, making this an excellent time to help her expand her self-care skills.
- Standards for maternity care and employment have been developed by the U.S. Children's Bureau.
- Teaching expectant mothers about nipple preparation for breast-feeding is an important nursing function.

STUDY QUESTIONS AND ACTIVITIES

1. Observe and record the following in two contrasting settings, for example, a physician's office and a county welfare clinic.
   A. Did the tone and the information provided to the women and their families differ? If so, how?
   B. Did the women have rights and were they allowed to assert those rights? Did they?
   C. What questions were asked of the clients and what were the answers? Were those answers adequate?
   D. Compare the visits the student observed with the ideal text book description of client care.
   E. How did each clinical experience make you feel? Which approach would you use? What are your reasons?
2. Follow a home health nurse or public health nurse involved in prenatal care, classes, and case finding. Use the same questions as in activity 1.
3. Discuss with your peers and instructor the implication that the findings from activities 1 and 2 have for the following:
   A. The delivery of health care in our society
   B. The acceptance and use of health care in our society
4. For as many clients as possible, assess their learning needs and note their week of gestation.
5. What physical discomforts or problems might a 15-year-old primigravida in her twentieth week of pregnancy attending her local high school experience at this time? For one of these problems, role play how you would provide her with pertinent information.

6. What physical discomforts or problems might Mary P., age 36, a primigravida in her thirty-second week of pregnancy experience at this time? For one of these problems, role play how you would provide her with pertinent information.

References

Bryant, H: Antenatal counseling for women working outside the homes, Birth 12:4, Winter 1985

Chang A: Auto safety in pregnancy, a neglected area, Contemp OB/GYN 254:117, 1985

Cohen, A: Movement as a yardstick for fetal well-being, Contemp OB/GYN 26:61, Aug 1985

Crosby, WM: Traumatic injuries during pregnancy, Clin Obstet Gynecol 26(4):902, 1983

Dawson, KP, et al: Keeping abreast of the times: the Tauranga infant feeding survey, NZ Med J 89:75, 1979

Doucette, JS: Is breast-feeding still safe for babies? MCN 3:354, 1978

Krozy, RE, et al: Auto safety, pregnancy and the newborn, JOGN Nurs 14:1, Jan/Feb 1985

Nicholson, W: Midwives, mothers, and breastfeeding, Nursing Mothers Association of Australia, 5 Glendale St, Nunawading, Victoria 3131, 1985

Page, EW, Villee, CA, and Villee, DB: Human reproduction: essentials of reproductive and perinatal medicine, ed 3, Philadelphia, 1981, WB Saunders Co

Bibliography

Alexander, LL: The pregnant smoker: nursing implications, JOGN Nurs 16(3):167, 1987

Arneson, et al: Automobile seat belt practices of pregnant women, JOGN Nurs 15(4):330, 1986

Bentz, JM: Missed meanings in nurse/patient communication, MCN 5:55, Jan/Feb 1980

Bing, E, and Colman, L: Making love during pregnancy, New York, 1977, Bantam Books, Inc

Bond, MB: Reproductive hazards in the workplace, Contemp OB/GYN 28(3):57, 1986

Brown, MA: Marital support during pregnancy, JOGN Nurs 15(6):475, 1986

Brown, MA: How fathers and mothers perceive prenatal support, MCN 12(6):414, 1987

Brucker, MC, and Reedy, NJ: Maternity leaves and the Pregnancy Discrimination Act, JOGN Nurs 12:341, 1983

Bullard, JA: Exercise and pregnancy, Can Fam Physician 27:977, 1981

Chang, A, Magwene, K, and Frand, E: Increased safety belt use following education in childbirth classes, Birth 14(3):148, 1987

Chenger, P, and Kovacik, A: Dental hygiene during pregnancy: a review, MCN 12(5):342, 1987

Cooper, KH, Douglas, PS, and Solomon, HA: Exercise and cardiovascular health: 12 vital questions, Contemp OB/GYN 29:125, April 1987 (special issue)

Dameron, GW: Helping couples cope with sexual changes pregnancy brings, Contemp Obstet Gynecol 21:23, Feb 1983

Dean, J: Pregnancy and exercise: how much and what kind? On this the experts agree: more research is needed, Sportwest 1:30, Dec 1981

Droegemueller, W, et al: Comprehensive gynecology, St Louis, 1987, The CV Mosby Co

Fawcett, J, and York, R: Spouses' physical and psychological symptoms during pregnancy and the postpartum, Nurs Res 35(4):144, 1986

Foster, SD: MCN patient teaching, MCN 12(2):131, 1987

Hutchinson, PL, et al: Metabolic and circulatory responses to running during pregnancy, Phys Sportsmed 9:55, Aug 1981

Jopke, T: Pregnancy: a time to exercise judgement, Phys Sportsmed 11:139, July 1983

Lee, PA: Health beliefs of pregnant and postpartum Hmong women, West J Nurs Res 8(1):83, 1986

Leap, TL, et al: Equal employment opportunity and its implications for personnel practices in the 1980s, Labor Law J 31:669, 1980

Marbury, MC, et al: Work and pregnancy, Occup Med vol 26, 1984

Moore, L, et al: Self-assessment: a personalized approach to nursing during pregnancy, JOGN Nurs 15(4):311, 1986

Mueller, L: Pregnancy and sexuality, JOGN Nurs 14:4, July/Aug 1985

NAACOG: Reproductive health hazards: women in the workplace, vol 11, Feb 1985, NAACOG, 600 Maryland Ave, SW Suite 2000, Washington DC 20024

Parken, M: Culture and preventive health care, JOGN Nurs 7:40, 1978

Poland, M, Ager, J, and Olson, J: Barriers to receiving adequate prenatal care, Am J Obstet Gynecol 157(2):299, 1987

Pritchard, J, et al: Williams/obstetrics, ed 17, Norwalk, Conn, 1985, Appleton-Century-Crofts

Queenan, JT, moderator: Managing pregnancy in patients over 35, Contemp OB/GYN 29(5):180, 1987

Riordan, JM: A practical guide to breastfeeding, 1983, The CV Mosby Co

Sandberg, EC: Synopsis of obstetrics, ed 10, St Louis, 1978, The CV Mosby Co

Shanghold, M: Keeping fit during pregnancy, Fit 6:68, June 1982

Sherwen, LN: Psychosocial dimensions of the pregnant family, New York, 1987, Springer Publishing Co, Inc

Winslow, W: First pregnancy after 35: what is the experience? MCN 12(2):92, 1987

Zalar, MK: Sexual counseling for pregnant couples, MCN 1(3):176, 1976

CHAPTER

14

Third Trimester

Learning Objectives

Correctly define the key terms listed.

Discuss maternal and fetal assessment.

Formulate possible nursing diagnoses and the type of data base expected to support these diagnoses.

Review planning of care with gravidas and their families.

Evaluate emotional appraisal and marital support during pregnancy.

Discuss physiology and treatment of discomforts related to maternal adaptations.

Outline prebirth education for gravidas, siblings, and grandparents during this period.

Explain counseling for prenatal danger signs.

Discuss client teaching for recognizing preterm labor and identify six warning signs and symptoms of preterm labor.

Compare and contrast the childbirth preparation methods.

Assess birth setting choices in light of quality (of health care delivery) control and cost effectiveness.

Key Terms

alternative birth center
ankle edema
appraisal support
ASPO
birth-setting choices
Braxton Hicks' contractions
childbirth methods
consumer movement
control
cost effectiveness
dyspnea
emotional support
freestanding birth center
gate control theory
gingivitis and epulis
grandparent preparation
holistic health
home birth
ICEA
informational support
insomnia
instrumental support
Lamaze method
leg cramps
marital support
monitrices
parental competence
perineal discomfort
prenatal danger signs
preterm labor recognition
quality control
roll-over test
safe passage
sibling preparation
urinary frequency

The quiet period of the second trimester gives way to an active period, a trimester more oriented in reality for the expectant parents (see Chapter 11). Parental attachment to the fetus grows in the third trimester. Mixed among the daydreams about the "coming baby" are parental anxieties that focus on possible defects in mental and physical abilities of the child. The expectant mother's attention turns to thoughts of a "safe passage" for herself and her child. Fears of pain and mutilation and concerns about her behavior and possible loss of control during labor are important issues.

Physical discomforts and fetal movements often interrupt the expectant mother's rest. Dyspnea, return of urinary frequency, backache, constipation, and varicosities are experienced by most gravidas in late pregnancy. Increased bulkiness and awkwardness affect the gravida's ability to perform activities of daily living. Positions of comfort are more difficult to achieve. Increasingly, the gravida becomes more impatient to "get this over with."

For the expectant father, the moratorium phase of the second trimester passes into the focusing phase (see Chapter 11). Activity and energy to create and achieve characterize this phase. Styles of involvement differ according to the man's perception of the male and fathering roles within his social group. Many expectant fathers become more involved with the pregnancy. They begin to redefine their relationship to the fetus and themselves as fathers. Role playing through daydreaming is common. The expectant father feels some of the same concerns as the expectant mother. Often, however, he does not share these concerns with anyone.

Expectant families approaching childbirth have many needs. Siblings and grandparents must be considered, too. Clearly the nurse is in a pivotal position within the team of health care providers to assist parents with these needs during the third trimester of pregnancy. The schedule of care reflects the increased need. Starting with week 28, visits are scheduled every 2 weeks until week 36, and then every week until delivery.

Assessment

During the third trimester current family occurrences and their effect on the mother are assessed; for example, siblings' and grandparents' responses to the pregnancy and the coming child. In addition, the following questions are addressed:

- What anticipatory planning is in progress concerning new parenting responsibilities, sibling rivalry, recuperation from pregnancy and birth, and fertility management?
- What successes or frustrations is the mother experiencing with diet, rest and relaxation, sexuality, and emotional support?
- What is the mother's understanding of her family's needs in relation to the pregnancy and child?
- How well prepared are the parents in the event of emergency? That is, does the mother know and understand danger signs and how and to whom to report them?
- Does the mother know the signs of preterm and term labor?
- What is the mother's understanding of the labor process, expectations of herself and others during labor, and what to bring to the hospital?
- What plans has the mother and her family made for labor (see education for choice, p. 298)?
- What anxieties is the mother or her family experiencing regarding labor or child?
- What does the mother wish to know about control of discomfort during labor?
- Is the mother planning to attend any prebirth classes?
- Does the mother have questions about fetal development and methods to assess fetal well-being?

A checklist for third trimester assessment should be used to ensure that important areas are addressed (see box below).

Maternal Assessment

Interview. The initial question in the third-trimester interview is asked with the intent to identify the *gravida's*

THIRD TRIMESTER CHECKLIST

- Schedule and events of visits
- Counseling for self-care:
  - Adaptations/discomforts
    - Dyspnea
    - Insomnia
    - Psychosocial responses and family dynamics
    - Gingivitis and epulis
    - Urinary frequency
    - Perineal discomfort and pressure
    - Braxton Hicks' contractions
    - Leg cramps
    - Ankle edema
  - Safety (balance)
  - Exercise and rest
  - Relaxation
  - Nutrition
  - Sexuality
  - Danger signs-general
  - Danger signs-preterm labor
- Fetal growth and development
- Preparation for baby
  - Feeding method
  - Nipple preparation
- Preparation for labor
  - Recognition: false versus true
  - Prenatal classes
  - Control of discomfort
  - Hospital tour
  - Provision for other family members
  - Preparation for homecoming
- Diagnostic tests
  - Specify
- Other

ASSESSMENT OF MATERNAL PSYCHOLOGIC ADAPTATION TO PREGNANCY AND PARENTING AT 34 TO 36 WEEKS' GESTATION

Score

1. When did you first see a doctor about your pregnancy? Can you tell me why you chose to go at this particular time?
   - _____ Saw doctor after third missed menstruation; didn't realize was pregnant; thought lack of menstruation may be due to something else; went to see doctor to have this investigated (1 point)
   - _____ Saw doctor after second or third missed menstruation; went to see doctor because husband observed wife's irritability; went to have IUD checked (2 points)
   - _____ Vague about when visit to doctor was made; thinks she missed two menstruations; unplanned pregnancy; wanted to validate (3 points)
   - _____ Saw doctor about 1 week after second missed menstruation; knew she was already pregnant; planned; wanted to validate (4 points)
   - _____ Saw doctor about 1 week after first missed menstruation; wanted to have planned pregnancy validated (5 points)
2. As a child, was there someone in your immediate family that you saw as a loving kind of person? Who was the most loving person in your family? Your mother? Your father? What were your parents like?
   - _____ Did not have anyone in family that she saw as a loving person; expresses dislike and negative feelings about early childhood; may have been in numerous foster homes; parents very strict or very lenient (1 point)
   - _____ Defines problems in childhood: separations from parents; definite family problems (e.g., alcoholism); parents inconsistent (2 points)
   - _____ Vague about family; unable to give definite ideas re "a loving person"; ambivalent feelings expressed; unable to define characteristics (3 points)
   - _____ Describes relationship with a parent as being satisfactory; with warmth, but wants relationship with own child to be stronger (4 points)
   - _____ Mother or father seen as very positive, very warm person; expresses positive feelings (5 points)
3. What thoughts and ideas have you and your partner had on the changing of life-styles, working hours, or other adjustments pertaining to this pregnancy and new baby?
   - _____ Have thought about it but believe no changes or adjustments are necessary; state that they believe this is important, not to change things for the baby (1 point)
   - _____ Haven't thought about adjustments and changes; wonder if there will be a need to change; questioning possibility (2 points)
   - _____ Have had some thoughts about changes; think they want to wait to see what it will be like once baby arrives; think that it is easier to do after baby comes (3 points)
   - _____ Have already made a few changes; think that there will be a need for further changes; have spent time talking about it; have tentative plans (4 points)
   - _____ Have made changes to suit wife's needs for increased rest; have spent time thinking about the changes; have plans to help—baby-sitter, relatives visiting, etc. (5 points)
4. Do you think you will need help when you get home from the hospital? Have you made any plans for help? If so, what are they?
   - _____ No, doesn't want anyone interfering (2 points)
   - _____ No, believes can manage well by self (4 points)
   - _____ Ambivalent, doesn't know (6 points)
   - _____ No help available: has made definite plans on how to try to manage, or plan involves calling someone in case of emergency (8 points)
   - _____ Yes, has specific plans for husband or other person to be there for help (10 points)
5. Have you had any thoughts, ideas, or hunches about your baby's appearance and behavior after you bring him home from the hospital?
   - _____ Describes very unrealistic behaviors, such as regular sleeping or sleeping through the night; or describes three or four negative aspects (3 points)
   - _____ Describes one or two negative aspects along with two or three fears about not knowing what to do; or has no idea, gives it no thought (6 points)
   - _____ Unable to describe; can describe only in vague terms; describes fears relating to baby's crying (9 points)
   - _____ Can describe a few aspects (one or two) of baby's behavior (12 points)
   - _____ Describes realistically baby's sleeping, feeding, and crying behavior; has a few questions to have clarified (15 points)

Key:

8-20: very high, intervention needed
21-30: questionable, "at risk," further follow-up needed
31-33: low risk
34-40: no risk

Scoring:

Add points from each question
1. _____
2. _____
3. _____
4. _____
5. _____

TOTAL _____

Modified from Funke-Farber, J: Reliability and validity testing of maternal adaptive behavior, Edmonton, 1978, University of Alberta, Faculty of Nursing.

main concern for the moment. Focusing on the woman takes advantage of her readiness to learn and affirms the caregiver's interest in her as a person. Based on the client's expressed needs, her status to date, and generally accepted needs of most women in late pregnancy, the nurse's clinical judgment guides the content and direction of the interview.

A review of physical systems is appropriate at each meeting. Any suspicious signs or symptoms are assessed in depth. Discomforts reflecting pregnancy adaptations are identified. Special inquires are made about possible infections (e.g., genitourinary tract, respiratory tract). Knowledge of and success with self-care measures and prescribed therapy are assessed.

A variety of assessment tools have been devised to assess psychosocial responses to a variety of situations. One such tool (see box, p. 289) has been developed for the assessment of maternal psychologic adaptation to pregnancy and parenting at 34 to 36 weeks' gestation. Appropriate referral may be necessary.

The *roll-over test* is sometimes used as one predictor of a potential hypertensive problem in the third trimester. This test may be done at each visit after the twentieth week of gestation. The roll-over test can be done as follows (Zuspan and Quilligan, 1982; Fanaroff and Martin, 1987; Pritchard, MacDonald, and Gant, 1985): position the woman on her side. Determine the blood pressure (BP) level in the upper arm once it is stable. "Roll" her over onto her back, checking the pressure again. Wait 5 minutes and check the BP level once again. An increase of 20 mm Hg in diastolic blood pressure from the side position to the back position indicates a *positive roll test.* The significance of a roll test is that if negative, the chances are less than 1:100 that the gravida will develop preeclampsia. If the test is positive, even though the BP level is within normal limits and the gravida has no signs of fluid retention, full-blown pregnancy-induced hypertension (PIH) will develop at least 60% of the time. If the roll test is positive, it is imperative that home self-care measures be instituted. The woman should spend more time in bed in the lateral recumbent position, stress in the home should be reduced, and her diet should be reviewed (see Chapter 29).

Laboratory Tests. At each visit urine is tested for glucose (to assess for diabetes) and albumin protein (to assess for hypertension). A urine culture and sensitivity test is done as necessary. Hematocrit determination by finger stick is made at each visit in some facilities. Blood tests are repeated as necessary: Venereal Disease Research Laboratory (VDRL) test for syphilis; complete blood count (CBC) with hematocrit, hemoglobin, and differential values; antibody screen (Kell, Duffy, rubella, toxoplasmosis, anti-Rh, AIDS); sickle cell; and level of folacin when indicated. If not done earlier in pregnancy, a glucose screen for women over 25 years of age is performed. Cervical and vaginal smears are repeated at 32 weeks or as necessary: *Chlamydia* organisms; gonorrhea; and herpes simplex, types 1 and 2.

Fetal Assessment

Beginning at the thirty-second week, identification of fetal presentation, position, and station (engagement), with the aid of Leopold's maneuvers (see Chapter 18), is done weekly.

Fundal height is measured at each visit. The method described in Chapter 13 is used. Uterine measurements and size (weight) of fetus are compared with supposed duration of pregnancy. Although some clinicians can estimate fetal weight with unbelievable accuracy, estimations are generally inconsistent and unreliable. Accuracy in estimating fetal weight improves with ultrasound determination of biparietal diameter. Possible growth retardation of fetus, multiple pregnancy, or inaccuracy of the estimated date of delivery (EDD) may be disclosed by ultrasound (see Chapter 27).

Physical Examination. During the third-trimester physical examination, temperature, pulse, respirations, blood pressure, and weight are assessed and noted. Suspicious signs and symptoms uncovered during the interview are assessed. Presence, location, and degree of edema are documented carefully. Gestational age is confirmed. Weekly pelvic examinations are begun at weeks 36 to 38 and are continued until term, primarily to confirm presenting part, corroborate station, and determine cervical dilation and effacement. Risk assessment continues throughout pregnancy (see Chapter 27).

Fetal health status is evaluated at each visit. The mother is requested to describe fetal movements. She is asked if she has danger signs (see p. 293) to report, for example, change in fetal movements, rupture of membranes. (For a discussion of electronic monitoring, see Chapter 17; for other monitoring techniques, see Chapter 27.)

This period of rapid fetal growth is summarized in the box above.

FETAL DEVELOPMENT AT 40 WEEKS

1. Nutrients and maternal immunoglobulins are stored
2. Subcutaneous fat deposited
3. Dramatic storage of iron, nitrogen, and calcium
4. In male: testes are within well-wrinkled scrotum
5. In female: labia are well-developed and cover vestibule
6. Lanugo shed, except for shoulders, generally
7. Body contours plump
8. Decreased vernix
9. Scalp hair 2 to 3 cm (1 in) long
10. Cartilage in nose and ears well developed
11. 45 to 55 cm (18 to 22 in) in length
12. Weighs 3400 g (7½ lb) (average)
13. Fundal height below xiphoid after lightening

Nursing Diagnoses

Each gravida and her family respond to and are affected by pregnancy in different ways. Careful monitoring of the pregnancy and responses to care is of the utmost importance. The following are representative of nursing diagnoses that can be formulated in the third trimester from the data base of a "normal" pregnancy.

- Anxiety, potential, related to
  - Discomforts of pregnancy
  - Approaching labor
- Knowledge deficit related to
  - Assessment for risks such as preterm labor
  - Recognizing onset of true versus false labor
  - Preparation of sibling(s) and grandparents for labor and the newborn
  - Self-care measures
  - Emergency arrangements
- Altered family processes related to
  - Inadequate understanding of third trimester changes and needs
  - Increased concern about labor
  - Insomnia or sleep deficit
- Sleep pattern disturbance related to
  - Discomforts of late pregnancy
  - Anxiety about approaching labor
- Potential for injury to mother and fetus related to
  - Labor
  - Mother's altered balance and coordination
- Activity intolerance related to
  - Increased weight and change in center of gravity
  - Anxiety
  - Sleep disturbances

Planning

Planning care for clients and their families during the third trimester of pregnancy is given direction from identified nursing diagnoses and from a comprehensive view of the expectant family. A plan is developed mutually with the client to the extent possible. The plan is individualized, relating specifically to the client's needs and the needs of her family. The information in this chapter is general in nature; not all women will experience all problems discussed nor require all facets of care described. The nurse and client select those aspects of care that are relevant to the client and the client's family. The general and specific nursing care plans provide guidelines for students.

Implementation

Nurses assume many caregiving roles during the third trimester of pregnancy. The nurse-clinician's roles can be categorized as both supportive, and teacher/counselor/advocate. In these roles, the clinician is a consumer of nursing research and on the alert for potential research problems.

Supportive Activities

In this trimester, House's (1981) categorization of social support (see Chapter 11) serves as a guide in providing comprehensive support. This categorization of support includes emotional, appraisal, informational (see teacher/counselor/advocate section), and instrumental.

Esteem, affection, trust, concern, consideration of cultural and religious responses, and listening are components of emotional support. The woman's feelings of satisfaction with her relationships and support, and of competence and sense of being in control are important issues to address in the third trimester. A discussion of parental awareness of the unborn child's responses to stimuli, such as sound, light, maternal posture or tension, and patterns of sleeping and waking can be helpful. Opportunities are also provided to discuss probable emotional tensions related to the following: childbirth experience such as fear of pain, loss of control, and possible delivery of child before reaching hospital; responsibilities and tasks of parenthood; mutual parental concerns arising from anxiety for safety of mother and unborn child; mutual parental concerns related to siblings and their acceptance of new baby; mutual parental concerns about social and economic responsibilities; and mutual parental concerns for cognitive dissonance arising from conflicts in cultural, religious, or personal value systems.

The father's commitment to the pregnancy, the couple's relationship, and their concerns about sexuality and sexual expression emerge as concerns for many expectant parents. An important support measure is to validate normalcy of their responses (if they fall within normal limits). Validation, feedback, and social comparison characterize appraisal support.

Providing opportunity to discuss concerns, providing a listening ear, and validating the normalcy of responses will meet the gravida's needs to varying degrees. At other times, nurses need to implement specific "interventions targeted at improving expectant parents' partner support satisfaction, because this support constitutes the majority of their total support" (Brown, 1986).

Brown (1986) studied marital support in expectant couples in the latter half of pregnancy. Both women and men in the study stated that approximately four-fifths of their support came from their partner (Brown, 1986). In a satisfying marital relationship, women reported fewer symptoms during pregnancy. They also exhibited less anxiety and depression late in pregnancy and at 2 months and 1 year postpartum (Grossman, Eichler, and Winckoff, 1980). According to Lamb (1978), the ability of the husband to respond to his wife's increased expectations may well affect the whole course of the pregnancy, labor, and adjustment of the new family. Some people may intend to be supportive but may not be able to communicate their caring. One spouse may perceive as unsupportive, measures intended to be supportive by the other spouse. It is therefore important for the nurse to foster marital support during pregnancy.

Although many nurses feel that discussing marital relations is intrusive, sensitive and skilled practitioners can make an important difference in the way couples cope. Brown (1986) suggested several supportive nursing interventions. For example, nurses could help women assess their expectations for support, and their husbands' ability to meet these expectations, as well as devise strategies to facilitate meeting these needs from either their partner or significant others.

Nurses need to recognize the increased vulnerability of men during pregnancy and implement anticipatory guidance and health promotion strategies to help them with their concerns. Nursing intervention may directly help fathers with concerns such as the need to share intimate feelings or may do so indirectly by education of mothers. Health-care providers can stimulate and encourage open dialogue between the couple.

Nursing students especially are cautioned that, despite their knowledge, skill, concern, and caring, there will be clients who will be unable to benefit from their interventions. The discussion of models of helping and coping (see Chapter 2) assists in understanding nurse-client responses. It is equally important for the nurse to maintain self-esteem and a positive self-concept in the face of a less than optimum client outcome.

Teacher/Counselor/Advocate

Changes That are Normal for Pregnancy. Not only are some new discomforts seen in the third trimester, but others seen previously in the first trimester (e.g., fatigue) also recur. Women experiencing pregnancies later in life may experience an aggravation of varicose veins or severe backache from postural changes associated with a heavy, pendulous abdomen and relaxed jounts. Such symptoms are frightening and uncomfortable.

In Table 14-1, the physiology, prevention, and treatment of several discomforts are discussed. Flying exercise, conscious relaxation, exercises, body mechanics, safety, and employment issues are described and discussed in Chapters 12 and 13. Nutrition is covered in Chapter 15.

Table 14-1 *Problems Related to Maternal Adaptations During the Third Trimester*

Problem	Physiology	Treatment
Shortness of breath and dyspnea—occur in 60% of pregnant women	Expansion of diaphragm limited by enlarging uterus; diaphragm is elevated about 4 cm (1½ in); some relief after lightening	Good posture; flying exercise; sleep with extra pillows; avoid overloading stomach; stop smoking; refer to physician if symptoms worsen to rule out anemia, emphysema, and asthma
Insomnia (later weeks of pregnancy)	Fetal movements, muscular cramping, urinary frequency, shortness of breath, or other discomforts	Reassurance; conscious relaxation; back massage or effleurage (Fig. 14-1); support of body parts with pillows; warm milk or warm shower before retiring
Psychosocial responses (Chapter 11): mood swings, mixed feelings, increased anxiety	Hormonal and metabolic adaptations; feelings about impending labor, delivery, and parenthood	Reassurance and support from significant other and nurse; improved communication with partner, family, and others
Gingivitis and epulis (hyperemia, hypertrophy, bleeding, tenderness): condition will disappear spontaneously 1 to 2 months after delivery	Increased vascularity and proliferation of connective tissue from estrogen stimulation	Well-balanced diet with adequate protein and fresh fruits and vegetables; gentle brushing and good dental hygiene; avoid infection
Urinary frequency and urgency returns	Vascular engorgement and altered bladder function caused by hormones; bladder capacity reduced by enlarging uterus and fetal presenting part	Kegel's exercises; limit fluid intake before bedtime; reassurance; wear perineal pad; refer to physician for pain or burning sensation
Perineal discomfort and pressure	Pressure from enlarging uterus, especially when standing or walking; multiple gestation	Rest, conscious relaxation and good posture; maternity girdle; refer to physician for assessment and treatment if pain is present; rule out labor
Braxton Hicks' contractions	Intensification of uterine contractions in preparation for work of labor	Reassurance; rest; change of position; practice breathing techniques when contractions are bothersome; effleurage; rule out labor
Leg cramps (gastrocnemius spasm)—especially when reclining	Compression of nerves supplying lower extremities because of enlarging uterus; reduced level of diffusible serum calcium or elevation of serum phosphorus; aggravating factors: fatigue, poor peripheral circulation, pointing toes when stretching legs or when walking, drinking more than 1 L (1 qt) of milk per day	Rule out blood clot by checking for Homans' sign; use massage and heat over affected muscle; stretch affected muscle until spasm relaxes (Fig. 14-2); stand on cold surface; oral supplementation with calcium carbonate or calcium lactate tablets; aluminum hydroxide gel, 1 oz, with each meal removes phosphorus by absorbing it
Ankle edema (nonpitting) to lower extremities	Edema aggravated by prolonged standing, sitting, poor posture, lack of exercise, constrictive clothing (e.g., garters), or by hot weather	Ample fluid intake for "natural" diuretic effect; put on support stockings before arising; rest periodically with legs and hips elevated (Fig. 13-3), exercise moderately; refer to physician if generalized edema develops; *diuretics are contraindicated*

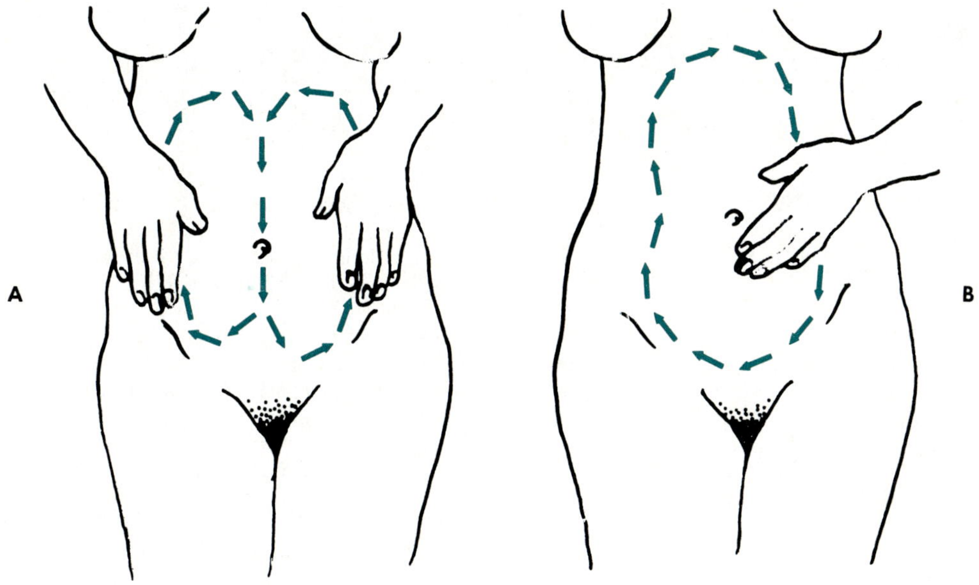

Fig. 14-1 Pattern for effleurage, a light, rhythmic stroking useful for inducing relaxation. **A**, Self-effleurage. **B**, Effleurage by another.

Review of Prenatal Danger Signs. The nurse needs to answer questions honestly as they arise during pregnancy. It is often difficult for the gravida to know when to report signs and symptoms. The mother is encouraged to refer to a printed list of danger signs (see p. 249) and to listen to her body. If she senses that "something is wrong," she should call her care provider. Several signs and symptoms need to be discussed more extensively. These include vaginal bleeding, alteration in fetal movements, symptoms of PIH, rupture of membranes, and preterm labor.

If **vaginal bleeding** occurs in the third trimester, it is important to rule out brownish spotting occurring 48 hours after vaginal examination and to rule out "show" of pinkish mucus. The woman is to come to the hospital's emergency area immediately for diagnosis and treatment if bleeding is other than one of the preceding types.

Should the gravida notice cessation, noticeable diminution, or acceleration in the amount of **fetal movement**, she is to come to the clinic or the physician's office for evaluation.

Appearance of *edema* of the hands and around the eyes, severe **headaches**, **visual changes**, or feelings of **jitteriness** require immediate professional evaluation for PIH.

A gush or trickle of clear **watery discharge** that appears to come from the vagina may indicate rupture of membranes. The diagnosis requires a visit to the clinic or hospital for evaluation.

Recognizing Preterm Labor. Teaching gravidas to recognize preterm labor is necessary for each woman. Hospitals have developed pamphlets to help mothers remember what they learn. Guidelines for client teaching: preterm labor recognition, p. 294, and signs of preterm labor, box, p. 295, follow.

Occasionally, birth occurs before the gravida has access to professional attendants. Emergency childbirth is outlined in Chapter 19.

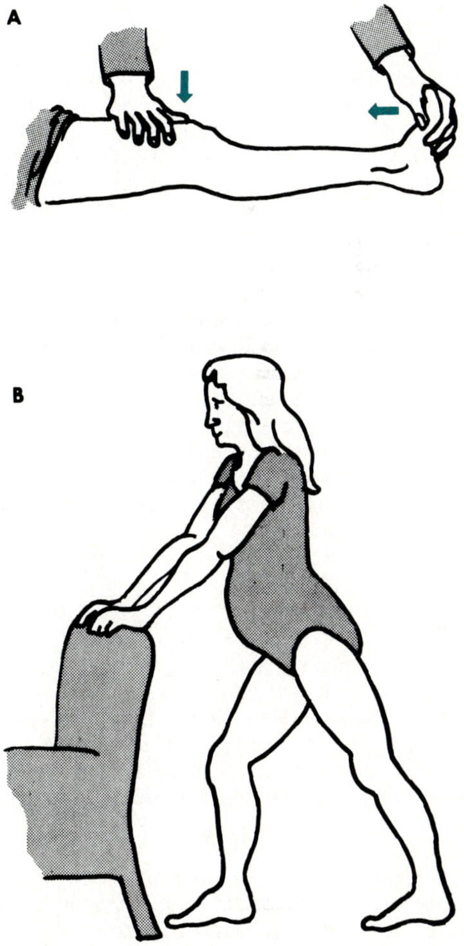

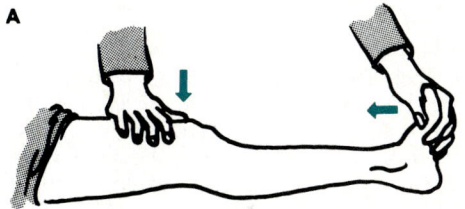

Fig. 14-2 Relief of muscle spasm (leg cramps). **A**, Another person dorsiflexes the foot with the knee extended. **B**, Woman stands and leans forward on affected leg.

Guidelines For Client Teaching

PRETERM LABOR RECOGNITION

ASSESSMENT

1. Pregnancy after the twentieth week but before the thirty-seventh week.
2. Gravida has no signs or symptoms of preterm labor at present.

NURSING DIAGNOSES

Knowledge deficit related to the warning signs of preterm labor.
Potential for injury to fetus related to preterm birth.
Potential for body image disturbance: situational low self-esteem related to preterm delivery.
Potential for spiritual distress related to preterm labor.

GOALS

Short-term

Woman begins to learn the warning signs and symptoms of preterm labor.

Intermediate

Woman remains alert for preterm labor without undue anxiety.
Woman definitely recognizes warning signs and symptoms and can self-detect uterine contractions.

Long-term

Woman knows what to do if she should exhibit any of the warning signs and symptoms of preterm labor.
Regardless of outcome of pregnancy, woman will maintain or enhance her self-concept and supportive family processes, and spiritual distress is avoided or minimized.

REFERENCES AND TEACHING AIDS

Printed instructions outlining warning signs and symptoms, steps to take if woman has problems, and the doctor's phone number.
Illustrations or charts.

CONTENT/RATIONALE	TEACHING ACTION
To understand the definition: Premature labor occurs after the twentieth week but before the thirty-seventh week of pregnancy. It is a condition in which uterine contractions (tightenings of the womb) cause the cervix (mouth of the womb) to open earlier than normal. It could result in the birth of a preterm baby. Babies born before 37 weeks may have problems breathing, eating, and keeping warm.	Read through pamphlet with woman or group of women. Women can use group for support.
To understand the cause: Although certain factors or reasons may increase a woman's chances of having preterm labor, such as carrying twins, the specific cause or causes of preterm labor are not known. Sometimes a woman may have preterm labor for no apparent reason.	Encourage discussion of this information and clarify or answer any questions woman may have. Discuss the woman's risk factors, if she has any.
To understand need for early recognition: It may be possible to prevent a preterm birth by knowing the warning signs and symptoms of preterm labor and by seeking care early if warning signs and symptoms should occur.	Reassure woman that she is not responsible if preterm labor proceeds despite her efforts.
To understand the difference between normal and preterm labor uterine contractions: It is *normal* to have some uterine contractions throughout the day. They usually occur when a woman changes positions, such as from sitting to lying down. These usually irregular and mild contractions are called Braxton-Hicks' contractions. They help with uterine tone and uteroplacental perfusion. It is *not normal* to have frequent uterine contractions (every ten minutes or more often for one hour). Contractions of labor are regular, frequent, and hard. They may also be felt as a tightening of the abdomen or a backache. This type of contraction causes the cervix to efface and dilate.	Instruct woman in self-detection of uterine contractions: Since the onset of premature labor is subtle and often hard to recognize, it is important to know how to feel your abdomen for uterine contractions. You can feel for contractions this way: While lying down, place your fingertips on the top of your uterus. A contraction is the periodic "tightening" or "hardening" of your uterus. If your uterus is contracting, you will actually feel your abdomen get tight or hard, and then feel it relax or soften when the contraction is over. Discuss and answer questions. Demonstrate. Watch return demonstration. Praise accomplishments appropriately.

Guidelines For Client Teaching—cont'd

CONTENT/RATIONALE	TEACHING ACTION
Warning signs and symptoms include: Uterine contractions that occur every 10 minutes or more with or without other signs. Menstrual-like cramps felt in lower abdomen constantly or intermittently. Low dull backache felt below the waistline constantly or intermittently. Pelvic pressure that feels like baby is pushing down constantly or intermittently. Abdominal cramping with or without diarrhea. Increase or change in vaginal discharge; more than usual or change in consistency or color.	Read through warning signs and symptoms with the client. Instruct the woman to begin assessment as follows: If you think you are having uterine contractions or any of the other signs and symptoms of premature labor: Lie down tilted toward your side. Place a pillow at your back for support. Sometimes lying down for an hour may slow down or stop the signs and symptoms. Do not lie flat on your back, because lying flat may cause contractions to occur more often or may result in supine hypotension syndrome. Do not turn completely on your side because you may not be able to feel the contractions. Check for contractions for 1 hour. To tell how often contractions are occurring, check the minutes that elapse from the beginning of one contraction to the beginning of the next.
To foster compliance and assist with decision-making: It is often difficult to identify preterm labor. Accurate diagnosis requires assessment by the care provider usually in the hospital or clinic.	Discuss and answer questions. Demonstrate positions. Suggest posting these instructions where they can be seen by everyone. Assist the woman with decision-making by providing written instructions such as the following: Call your doctor, clinic, or delivery room, or go to the hospital if: You have uterine contractions every 10 minutes or more often for 1 hour (more than 5 contractions in 1 hour) *or* You have any of the other signs and symptoms for 1 hour *or* You have any spotting or leaking of fluid from your vagina.

EVALUATION Teaching has been effective when all goals have been met. Woman verbalizes knowledge of the warning signs and symptoms and knows how to contact her physician. If preterm labor occurs, she recognizes it and informs her physician immediately. Regardless of the outcome of pregnancy, woman will maintain or enhance her self-concept and supportive family processes and spiritual distress is avoided or minimized.

SIGNS OF PRETERM LABOR

Uterine contractions—every 10 minutes or more often, with or without any other warning sign

Menstrual-like cramps—felt in lower abdomen: may come and go or be constant

Low dull backache—felt below waistline; may come and go or be constant

Pelvic pressure—feels like baby is pushing down: pressure comes and goes

Abdominal cramping—with or without diarrhea

Increase or change in vaginal discharge—more vaginal discharge than usual, or change into a mucousy, watery, or light bloody discharge

Childbirth Methods

Historical Overview. Since colonial times in America, women shared their information on childbirth with other women. Births occurred in the family's home with a midwife in attendance. However, in the nineteenth century, male physicians gradually came to be recognized as experts to whom women went for information about birth. By 1900 male physicians had usurped the age-old skills of women concerning childbirth and became for many the sole authorities.

In the United States the first formal classes in childbirth education were offered nationally in 1913 by the American Red Cross. The Maternity Center Association in New York City followed with classes for expectant parents as early as 1919. Literature on these early attempts at childbirth education revealed that the first classes for childbirth were developed out of a public health need to teach mothers basic hygiene.

An English physician, **Grantly Dick-Read,** published two books in which he theorized that pain in childbirth is socially conditioned and is caused by a fear-tension-pain syndrome. His first book, *Natural Childbirth,* was published in 1933. Dick-Read's second book, *Childbirth Without Fear,* was published in the United States in 1944. The work of Dick-Read became the foundation for organized programs of preparation for childbirth and teacher training throughout the United States, Canada, Great Britain, and South Africa. In 1960, the nurses prepared through such programs established the International Childbirth Education Association (ICEA).

During the 1960s the **Lamaze** method, also known as the psychoprophylactic method (PPM), gained popularity in the United States. PPM offered new perspectives on preparation for childbirth by emphasizing mind control. Marjorie Karmel introduced PPM to the United States in her book, *Thank You, Dr. Lamaze,* which was published in the United States in 1959. Others have written extensively on PPM. This system grew out of Pavlov's work on the higher nervous activity of humans and animals in which he proposed that every vital activity of an organism is a complex reflex process capable of conditioning.

In 1960 the American Society for Psychoprophylaxis in Obstetrics (ASPO) was formed in New York as a national organization to promote use of the Lamaze method and to prepare teachers of the method. The National Association of Childbirth Education, Inc. (NACE) (formerly the Childbirth Without Pain Education League, Inc [CWPL]), was formed in 1970 to teach the Lamaze method and prepare teachers. The Council of Childbirth Education Specialists, Inc. (CCES) was founded in New York City in 1971 and offered teacher training seminars throughout the United States.

A Denver obstetrician, Robert Bradley, published *Husband-Coached Childbirth* in 1965. In the book he advocates what he calls true 'natural' childbirth, without any form of anesthesia or analgesia and with a husband-coach and breathing techniques for labor. The American Academy of Husband-Coached Childbirth (AAHCC) was founded to make the **Bradley** method available and to prepare teachers.

Of the other techniques developed, the most widely known include the work of Kitzinger and Wright, developed in England. Wright's work is based on PPM and is described as "levels of breathing." Kitzinger's work is designed around a psychosexual approach, which proposes that birth is a sexual experience. As such, birth is perceived as a normal physiologic process in which the woman works in harmony with her body.

Hypnosis as a method of relieving pain in childbirth has been used since the 1800s. Through hypnosis the woman reaches a trancelike state, remaining awake but responsive to the hypnotist (**Johnson**, 1980). Hypnosis requires an extensive time commitment by the hypnotist. It is impractical for use with large numbers of women.

Components of Childbirth Methods. All preparation techniques have three components, which are (1) psychophysical, (2) psychologic, and (3) intellectual. The psychologic principles involved are suggestion and distraction. The confidence and assurance derived from participation in the classes help women (couples) cope with labor and delivery (Myles, 1981). Women benefit from learning the techniques for coping with pain and loss of control (Lederman, 1984).

Various studies have been undertaken to determine the physiologic effectiveness of prepared childbirth methods. These studies analyze data in terms of the amount of pain experienced during labor and birth, maternal and fetal complications, and the length of labor. Chertok (1967) and Velvovsky et al. (1960) reviewed many studies in which investigators demonstrated the effectiveness of preparation-for-birth approaches to pain relief during childbirth. Huttel et al. (1972) reported observations of less "complaint" and "tension" behaviors among women who were prepared for birth when compared with women who did not attend preparation classes. Huttel suggested that preparation for birth enables the mother to experience a shorter labor.

Although physiologic benefits of prepared childbirth are important, additional benefits have been claimed. A review of the literature by Buxton in 1962 concluded by emphasizing the critical importance of the psychologic benefits of preparation for birth. Unlike some of the contradictory material found on physiologic effects, research of psychologic effects on physiologic effects, research on psychologic effects continues to be overwhelmingly in agreement. Tanzer (1967) found the prepared women had a more positive subjective experience during delivery. It is particularly notable in this research how many of the women stressed the importance of having either their husband or another support person present during labor. Tanzer's results indicate that women experience a positive and highly desirable effect when their mates are present during birth. Other studies report that support and participation in labor and birth by the infant's father contribute to positive perceptions of the birth experience.

The intellectual components of preparation for childbirth are closely tied to the psychologic components. Research has indicated that the more knowledge a woman gains concerning pregnancy, labor, and birth as a result of childbirth preparation classes, the more favorable will be her attitude toward the pregnancy and the labor and delivery experience. A woman's perception of maintaining control is closely associated with satisfaction, according to studies by Willmuth (1975), Felton and Segelman (1978), Cronenwett (1980), and Cronenwett and Brickman (1983). Although the mechanisms by which preparation-for-childbirth classes affect the birth experience are not yet fully understood, it is clear that these classes affect the subjective experience in a positive manner.

Major methods taught in the United States are (1) the Dick-Read method, (2) the Lamaze method (PPM), and (3) the Bradley method. Each will be discussed, outlining the three components of prepared childbirth.

Dick-Read Method. This method, referred to as *childbirth without fear,* basically recommends three techniques: deep breathing both in abdominal respirations and thoracic respirations; shallow breathing; and breath holding for the second stage of labor.* The Dick-Read method also incorporates physical exercise to prepare the body for labor.

For most of labor the pattern of breathing is basically abdominal breathing. The woman is taught to force her abdominal muscles to rise during a contraction. In this way she lifts the abdominal muscles off the uterus as it rises forward during a contraction. Teachers of the Dick-Read method contend that the weight of the abdominal musculature on the contracting uterus increases pain.

Relaxation is an important part of the Dick-Read method. Women are taught to use conscious relaxation methods that involve progressive relaxation of the muscle groups in the entire body. Consequently, during labor the woman is able to relax completely between contractions. Using conscious relaxation techniques, some women are actually able to sleep between contractions.

According to Dick-Read (1959):

> Fear, tension and pain are three veils opposed to the natural design which have been concerned with preparation for and attendance at childbirth. If fear, tension, and pain go hand in hand, then it must be necessary to relieve tension and to overcome fear in order to eliminate pain. The implementation of my theory demonstrates the methods by which fear can be overcome, tension may be eliminated and replaced by physical and mental relaxation.

Dick-Read's program educated women to exchange understanding and confidence for fear of the unknown. Adequate prenatal education included information on nutrition and basic hygiene, as well as information on labor and birth.

In the Dick-Read method, support for the woman in labor was originally to be provided by nursing and medical attendants. However, in the adaptations of the Dick-Read method in use today, labor support is provided by the father or a support person chosen by the mother.

Lamaze Method. Known as the *Lamaze psychoprophylaxis method (PPM),* Lamaze combines controlled muscular relaxation and breathing techniques. Active relaxation is an integral part of the Lamaze method (Lamaze, 1970). The woman is taught to relax uninvolved muscle groups (neuromuscular control) while she contracts a specific muscle group (Fig. 14-3). By this process the woman can relax the uninvolved muscles in her body while her uterine musculature contracts. Women who attended Lamaze-type childbirth preparation classes maintained a significantly higher level of neuromuscular control during the first stage of labor than women who were self-prepared (Bernardini, Maloni, and Stegman, 1983).

The breathing techniques use the chest muscles. Lamaze teachers believe that chest breathing lifts the diaphragm off the contracting uterus, thus giving it more room to expand. These chest breathing patterns vary according to the intensity of the contractions and the progress of labor.

According to the Lamaze method, pain in labor is a conditioned response and women can be conditioned not to experience pain in labor. Instead of crying out and losing control during uterine contractions, women are taught to respond with conditioned relaxation and breathing patterns. The psychologic experience of maintaining control appears to be intimately related to the physiologic experience of maintaining control (Bernardini, Maloni, and Stegman, 1983).

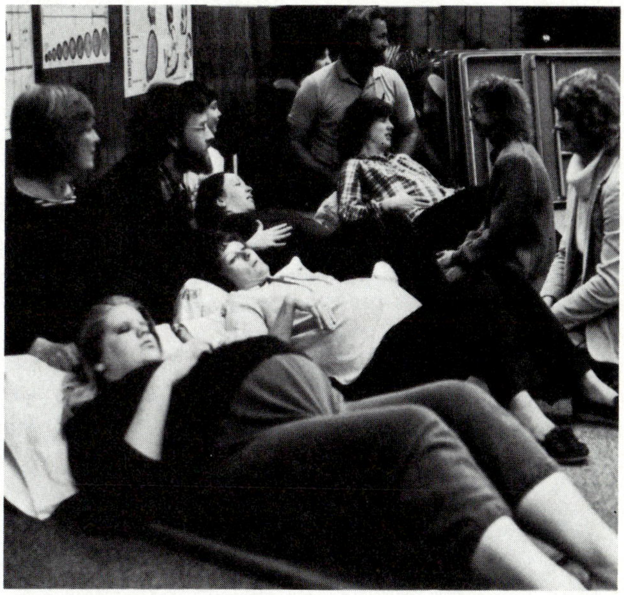

Fig. 14-3 Expectant parents attend classes to learn relaxation techniques.

Courtesy Lisa Livingston, Maternal Child Health Education, Community Birth Center, Community Hospital, Santa Cruz, Calif.

The Lamaze method emphasizes understanding the body and how it works. It offers a flexible but structured program to remove fear by education, thus eliminating distressing associations. This method finds its rationale in the neurophysiology of pain.

In the Lamaze method, support for the women in labor is provided by her husband or other support person. Specially trained labor attendants termed *monitrices* sometimes provide support for the laboring mother using the Lamaze method.

Bradley Method. This method of husband-coached childbirth uses breath control, abdominal breathing, and general body relaxation. Working in harmony with the body is emphasized (Bradley, 1965). Bradley based his method on observations of animal behavior during birth. His technique focuses on environmental variables such as darkness, solitude, and quiet to make childbirth a more natural experience. Women using the Bradley method often appear to be sleeping during labor. However, they are not asleep but simply in a state of deep mental relaxation. The importance of the husband's support is foremost in this method. Preparation-for-birth teaching concentrates on minimizing the need for analgesics or anesthetics for birth. There is also an emphasis on nutrition, omitting foods containing preservatives and added salt and sugar.

Each of these three methods just discussed emphasizes

*Breath holding is now discouraged

intellectual and physical components. However, the Dick-Read and Bradley methods emphasize the naturalness of childbirth, whereas Lamaze emphasizes active mental and physical conditioning. These methods have mutually influenced each other so that it is unusual to find classes in a pure "method" anymore. Different teachers develop their own methods, which may change with each group of expectant couples. Education in preparation for birth is continually evolving. The teachers themselves are being taught by the experiences of each expectant couple. Nursing research is needed to identify expectant parents priorities for childbirth preparation. One such study is presented in the research highlight, below. Books, journal articles, magazine articles, and audiovisual aids in childbirth education are proliferating. A list of some of the organizations involved in parent education can be found at the end of this chapter.

Recent trends. Childbirth education in the 1980s is at a crossroads. Once a small ***consumer movement,*** childbirth education gained momentum in the 1970s, paralleling the growth of the women's movement. Childbirth education has evolved into large professional organizations with significant influence on maternity care in the United States. Responding to this movement, health care professionals and hospitals are offering childbirth education programs in rapidly growing numbers. At the same time these hospital-sponsored programs are proliferating, there is a widening gap between the "medical" model of childbirth and the "physiologic" model. If the new programs are truly education and not indoctrination, they will present all known options for the birth experience and discuss both risks and benefits of obstetric procedures. Childbirth education must offer *choice* and not just hospital policy.

There also seems to be a gap forming ***within*** the original consumer-based childbirth education movement. Critics of methods to prepare for birth are presenting physiologic evidence that specific breathing techniques (such as breath holding while pushing) may be harmful to the fetus and have no influence on the progress of the second stage (see Chapter 19). Fresh approaches to old techniques are being proposed. These emphasize ***tuning into the laboring woman's body cues and encouraging her to do what feels natural.*** In this holistic approach to childbirth education the emphasis is on how the mind, body, and spirit are related and affect one another.

Women are encouraged to incorporate their natural responses into coping with the pain of labor and birth. Valuable tools to incorporate include vocalization or "sounding" to relieve tension in pregnancy and labor, massage with a light touch to encourage relaxation, visualization to guide women into positive spaces ("seeing" the vagina open up around the baby), hot compresses to the perineum, perineal massage, relaxing music and subdued lighting, and the use of warm water for showers or bathing during labor. In response to the critics, organizations also are adapting their teaching methods to changing times.

There are times when the woman or couple will choose not to cope with labor and request analgesia or anesthesia (total or partial). *Each woman has a right to labor and give birth in whatever way she chooses, provided the way is safe for both mother and baby.*

RESEARCH HIGHLIGHT

Identifying Priorities for Prepared Childbirth Research

Purpose

A Delphi study was conducted to identify priorities for research on prepared childbirth.

Sample/Methodology

Input from a panel of 22 Lamaze instructors and 22 maternity nurses resulted in the identification of four classes of categories: prenatal education/priorities, labor and delivery, postpartum, and complications.

Findings

The highest priority item for prenatal education/preparation was "What are the effects of (1) physical exercise during pregnancy, (2) relaxation practice, (3) practice of breathing techniques (different levels) on outcomes such as mother's perceived pain, use of analgesics/anesthetics, length of labor, postpartum comfort, and infant's health." The highest priority item for labor and delivery was, "Evaluate use of routine measures such as intravenous, enema, preparation, breath holding during pushing, episiotomy, circumcision. Are the advantages what they're reported to be? (For example, does the episiotomy decrease length of labor and "save" perineal muscles?)" The researchable idea about postpartum that received the highest rating was, "How effective would it be for the labor nurse to assist new mothers to 'reconstruct' their labor experiences, 'filling in the missing pieces' during the first few days postpartum?" For the final category, complications, the highest priority rating was, "What factors affect mothers' and fathers' responses to emergency cesarean birth?"

Implications

Impact evaluation of current practices was identified most commonly. In addition, other priorities related to needs of special populations, for example, pregnant adolescents or siblings, and also to improve health team functioning in childbirth were identified.

Thomas, BS: Identifying priorities for prepared childbirth research, JOGN Nurs 13(6):400, 1984.

Birth-setting Choices

The concept of family-centered maternity care is implemented in birth rooms or alternative birth centers (ABCs) in the hospital. Hospital ABCs, as well as freestanding birth centers, are intended to offer families an alternative to home birth, to be a compromise between hospital and home. More and more, consumers and professionals are accepting and using birth rooms and ABCs. These birth-setting choices have been shown to be safe alternatives to birth in a traditional delivery setting (Mann, 1981; Marieskind, 1980). In addition, they can be designed to ensure **quality control** and to be **cost effective**, two significant issues in the delivery of health care today.

Birth Rooms. In Manchester, Connecticut, an obstetrician, Philip Sumner, and his colleagues have had many years of experience with labor and birth in hospital birthing rooms. Unlike ABCs in hospitals, there is very little admission or risk criteria for the use of these rooms. The program at Manchester Memorial Hospital incorporates labor support by highly trained nurses, or **monitrices**. Prenatal education is stressed, and client feedback is overwhelmingly positive. Women labor, give birth, and spend the first bonding time with their families in birthing rooms. Transfer to a postpartum room is usually the only room change they have to make.

Birth rooms offer families a comfortable, private space for childbirth (Sumner and Phillips, 1981; Rosen, 1980). Fig. 14-4 shows one bed, which provides safe options for positioning of the mother in the event of labor or birth complications. The borning bed has the ability to "break," so the woman can quickly be put into stirrups. Generally, this option is not used unless an episiotomy is performed or laceration occurs. Even in the unbroken mode a simple push of a button will cause the upper half of the bed to raise approximately 25 cm (10 in) and allow the easy management of an unsuspected shoulder dystocia.

Giving birth in a birth room rather than moving from a labor room to a delivery room has the advantage of not interfering or disrupting the progress of labor. The woman is able to concentrate on pushing her baby out without expending energy moving to a stretcher and then moving again to the delivery table . Her vital signs may be taken continuously if necessary, and the fetal monitor may remain in place until the baby is born. The father is able to provide continuous support and does not have to be redirected to the new location. If rapid delivery is necessary, the woman's legs may be placed in the leg supports and the baby born quickly without time being wasted in transport to a delivery room. Other advantages of a birth room include the following:

1. The nursing staff no longer has to make decisions on when to move the mother to the delivery room.
2. There is no second room to be set up, so the nurses have ample time to prepare for an in situ delivery.
3. It may be possible to reduce costs, since fewer rooms are used, less laundry and equipment are involved, and there is better use of hospital space.

The concept underlying hospital birthing rooms is that of humanizing the birth experience, minimizing intervention, and affording continuity of care. Since these facilities are not a response to the home birth movement, they do not employ rigid screening criteria. Instead, they offer a two-tiered model of care (low risk and high risk) and emphasize individualizing the birth experience. When deemed necessary by the physician, nurse, or mother, local anesthesia, forceps, fetal monitoring, and so on are used to facilitate a safe but still joyous birth.

Alternative Birth Centers. Alternative birth centers (ABCs) usually are in hospital suites away from the traditional obstetrics department. They are located close to the delivery and operating rooms and medical or neonatal intensive care facilities for use when serious problems arise.

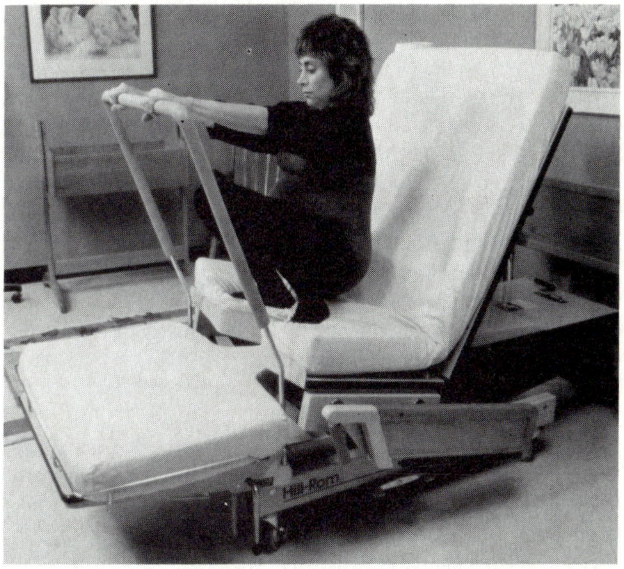

Fig. 14-4 Birth bed for single-room maternity care—labor, delivery, recovery, and postpartum care (LDRP).
Courtesy The Borning Corp, Spokane, Washington.

ABCs have homelike accommodations, including a double bed for the couple and a crib for the newborn. Emergency equipment and drugs are discreetly stored within cupboards, out of view, but easily accessible. Private bathroom facilities are incorporated into each birth center. There may be an early labor lounge or living room and small kitchen. There is careful screening of each applicant so that the ABC can rule out women with risk factors (see Chapter 27). Only low-risk and prepared women or couples are accepted.

The family is admitted to the ABC, labors there, and gives birth there. They may remain there until discharge if the time interval and requirements for room use permit. If the family has to remain in the hospital for more than 24 hours postpartum, the demand for use of the ABC by more prospective families may require transfer of the new family to a regular postpartum room.

Ideally the ABC becomes the private space for one childbearing family throughout their birth experience and until they are ready to go home. It is a warm, private, friendly space within a complex, fully equipped medical constellation. While emphasizing normalcy, self-help, and family participation, ABCs are fully supported by the presence of a maternity nurse or nurse-midwife and by the availability of obstetric and pediatric house staff at all times, with attending staff backup.

If a situation that could threaten the safety of the mother or baby should arise at any time in labor, the mother would be moved to the regular labor and delivery area. In such a situation the ABC nurse and the father of the baby would go with her.

Families who choose birth in the ABC may experience a warm, positive, family-centered, highly personalized, highly emotional birth within a structure offering safe and preventive perinatal care. Immediately outside the door of their alternative birth space, this family has available to them the sophistication of technical resources for management of complicated obstetric situations.

By agreement, medication and instrumentation (forceps, monitoring) are limited. Delivery can be accomplished in the woman's bed with skin-to-skin contact on the mother's abdomen after (usually) spontaneous birth. During labor and delivery, family, including older siblings, and friends of the mother's choosing may remain. Early discharge from the center, often during the day of delivery, must meet medical criteria. Many centers arrange for the mother and infant to be seen within 24 hours of discharge by a nurse midwife or neonatal nursing specialist.

Ideally, an ABC also offers childbearing couples alternative prices, in contrast to the high cost of obstetric care. Since alternative birth requires that the family occupy fewer spaces, less hospital time, and fewer supplies, linen, and staff, it is usually possible to reduce the overall cost of birth to the hospital and consumer.

The establishment of an ABC requires the hospital maternity personnel, childbirth educators, physicians, and parents to come together to develop a common philosophy from which can be elicited specific goals and objectives. The next step is to develop specific policies and procedures to provide uniform standards for quality control that will achieve the designated goals. An example of criteria relative to a couple's admission to an ABC follows*:

1. The program is designed for healthy pregnant women who expect a normal labor, birth, and postpartum course.
2. The expectant mother should discuss with her physician or midwife her desire to give birth in the alternative birth center as early as possible in pregnancy.
3. When an agreement has been reached that the alternative birth center will be used, the woman and her partner or support person should register for the alternative birth center orientation classes. All those who will be present during labor and birth are asked to attend the class series.
4. Attendance at childbirth preparation classes is important. If the expectant mother and her primary support person have attended classes during a previous pregnancy, a refresher class may be chosen by them.
5. A prenatal visit with the pediatrician or family physician of the parents' choice should be arranged so that plans can be made for the specific follow-up of the infant after birth and discharge from the alternative birth center.
6. A specific plan for family participation during labor and birth should be developed during pregnancy in consultation with the birth attendant.
7. Consent forms that must be signed before admission to the alternative birth center are Patient's Consent Form, Physician/Midwife's Agreement, Verification of Infant Care, and Consent for Sibling Participation.

*Hillcrest Medical Center, Tulsa, Oklahoma. From McKay, S, and Phillips, CR: Family-centered maternity care: implementation strategies, Rockville, Md, 1984. Reprinted with permission of Aspen Systems Corp.

Freestanding Birth Centers. Although most ABCs or birthing rooms are located in hospitals, there is a growing number of freestanding birth centers. These units are outside the hospital but are often close to a major hospital so that quick transfer to that institution is possible if necessary.

Most freestanding birth centers are staffed by physicians who have privileges at the local hospital, and certified nurse-midwives. Both groups are equipped to attend low-risk gravidas through the puerperium. Ambulance service and emergency procedures are readily available. Fees vary with the services provided and the ability of the family to pay (reduced-fee sliding scale). Several insurance companies, as well as Medicaid, recognize and reimburse these clinics.

Services provided by the freestanding birth centers include those necessary for safe management during the childbearing cycle. There are some significant additions, however:

1. Attendance at childbirth and parenting classes is required of all clients. Prenatal supervision of the woman in good nutritional and health status must begin in the first trimester. All clients must be familiar with situations requiring transfer to a hospital.
2. Each expectant family identifies their *"birth plan"* (Arms, 1978). This is an explanation of practices and procedures they would like to include in or exclude from their childbirth experience. Although the family is given a wide range of choices, they are asked to "assume that there will be no overriding medical or legal necessity for or against any of them in (their) individual case." A sampling of choices follows:
   a. *Preparation:* enema, "miniprep," hospital gown instead of own clothing?
   b. *Labor:* electronic monitor or fetoscope, freedom to choose positions and activity in labor (walking, squatting), analgesia, presence of siblings, translator?
   c. *Birth:* presence of mate or chosen person, presence of siblings, draping, mirror, dimmed lights, Leboyer bath?
   d. *Recovery:* recovery with or without baby or mate or chosen person?
   e. *After recovery:* rooming-in, sibling visitation, vitamin K for baby, circumcision, demand feeding—breast or bottle?

Birth centers usually have available a lending library, reference files on related topics, recycled maternity clothes and baby clothes and equipment, supplies and reference materials for childbirth educators. The centers have referral files for community resources that offer services relating to childbirth and early parenting, including support groups (such as single parents, postdelivery support group, parents of twins), genetic counseling, women's issues, and consumer action.

Home Birth. Home birth has always been popular in certain advanced countries, such as Great Britain, Sweden, and the Netherlands. In developing countries, hospitals or adequate lying-in facilities often are unavailable to most pregnant women, and home birth is a necessity. In North America home birth is gaining popularity.

National groups supporting home birth are HOME (Home Oriented Maternity Experience) and NAPSAC (National Association of Parents for Safe Alternatives in Childbirth). These groups support changes toward more humane childbearing practices at all levels, integrating the alternatives for childbirth to meet the needs of the total population.

The literature on childbirth contains excellent statistics on medically directed home birth services with skilled nurse-midwives and medical backup. Two examples of such services are the Chicago Maternity Center with 12,000 home births from 1950 to 1960 without a single maternal death and the home delivery statistics of the Frontier Nursing Service in Appalachia with 23 years without a single maternal death. In the United States there are reports of very low risk home delivery populations who have very low levels of difficulty and consequently have excellent statistics. However, there is danger in taking these data on very select populations and applying them to the total population. It must be recognized that even though labor and delivery are normal physiologic events, they do present potential hazards to the mother and fetus both before and after birth. These hazards require provisions for emergency intervention and medical backups that are available only in hospitals and some birthing homes or in independent birth centers.

Selective home birth in uncomplicated pregnancies is feasible, provided those women at high risk can be identified during the prenatal period and referred for hospital delivery and assuming that a transport system is available for transfer of women with suddenly complicated labors to a nearby adequate medical facility. Another acceptable plan provides for specialist care to be brought to the home by means of a so-called flying squad service, which is utilized in Great Britain, for example.

Collaboration with and supervision of midwives are the obstetrician's duty in many countries. Moreover, obstetric nursing practitioners or nurse-midwives have proved to be invaluable components of the health care team. Thus nurse specialists, general practitioners, and obstetric specialist consultants have become incorporated into home delivery units. A midwife or general practitioner can call on or refer women or infants to numerous essential backup services for study or specialty care during pregnancy and the early puerperium. When a woman is to be assisted by a midwife, it is the practice in most areas for the general practitioner to supervise her; meanwhile, both are under the direction of the obstetric specialist.

Although some physicians and nurses are proponents of home births that use good medical and emergency backup systems, many regard this practice as exposing the mother and the fetus to unnecessary danger.

Advantages. One advantage of home birth is that delivery may be more natural or physiologic in familiar surroundings. The mother may be more relaxed and less tense than she might be in the impersonal, sterile environment of a hospital. The family can assist in and be a part of the happy event, and mother-father-infant (and sibling-infant) contact is sustained and immediate. In addition, home birth may be less expensive than a hospital confinement. Serious infection may be less likely, assuming strict aseptic principles are followed. People generally are relatively immune to their own home bacteria.

Disadvantages. Because home births are not generally accepted by the medical community, a family may have difficulty finding a qualified health care professional to give prenatal care and to attend the delivery. Also, backup emergency care by a physician in a hospital may be difficult to arrange in advance. And, emergency transfer to a hospital could be life threatening if the hospital were more than a 10-minute distance from the home or if emergency care were not available during the transfer from home to hospital.

Contraindications. Hospital, not home, birth is indicated for the following:

1. High-risk women (fetal or maternal jeopardy) (see Chapter 27)
2. Women who cannot be transferred easily to a hospital should the need arise unexpectedly
3. Women who are opposed to home birth
4. Women with inadequate home facilities

Family Preparation. If a home birth is planned, it will usually be possible to obtain and store the necessary articles in advance. In contrast, if birth in the home or elsewhere is an emergency or is determined by circumstances beyond control, considerable improvisation may be necessary.

Facilities and supplies can approximate those available in hospitals. The family works closely with the physician, nurse, or midwife to complete preparations well in advance of delivery. Attendance by both parents-to-be at childbirth classes (prenatal classes for vaginal and abdominal births; instructions about the actual delivery of the child if this should occur before the midwife, physician, or other attendant arrives) adds to the competence and also to the pleasure of the parents and other family members. Classes for siblings and grandparents are recommended.

Detailed descriptions for preparation are required and may be obtained from either the physician's office or from local health agencies. The agencies may provide some of the equipment and supplies.

A visit to the home by the community health nurse is recommended well before the expected date of birth. At that time the process of birth can be discussed, so that all are aware of the characteristics of normal labor and birth and of the newborn, deviations from normal, and the plan of care for each stage.

Home birth is a selected alternative to hospital birth for some women and couples and a necessity for many. A physically and emotionally safe outcome can be anticipated for most women and couples and their infants, especially if they are prepared and have adequate health care support.

Prebirth Preparation

Not all gravidas and support persons attend formal classes in preparation for childbirth. For those who do attend, extensive preparation is possible (Fig. 14-3). Many do not take advantage of classes for a variety of reasons: employment; inaccessibility because of time, cultural/ethnic/religious orientation; cost; lack of knowledge regarding choices in prenatal education classes; lack of readiness. Therefore clinicians need to provide information that includes the following:

1. Process of labor: admission, examination, care in labor
2. Plans to get to hospital (when to go and where); care of other children
3. Methods to control pain (e.g., analgesia and anesthesia, breathing-relaxing techniques) (see Chapter 18)
4. Supplies to have in a suitcase ready for the trip to the hospital: personal items for grooming, items for labor as desired (i.e., warm socks, focal point), supportive bra, nightgowns, slippers
5. Responsibilities of the spouse, family member, or friend who will be accompanying the woman through labor and delivery
6. Care of the newborn (i.e., clothing, feeding, daily hygienic care), and postnatal care (see Chapter 22)
7. Emergency arrangements (e.g., precipitate delivery) (see Chapter 19)

A nurse needs to be ready to teach when the woman is ready to learn as shown by the following example. One nurse described her intervention with a gravid woman as follows:

> I tried to teach her about relaxation and breathing techniques during childbirth, but she was not interested. When she phoned to tell me she was at the hospital in labor, she said, "What was all that stuff you were saying about breathing?" In between the next few contractions I repeated the salient points.

Even if the woman (couple) has attended prebirth classes, the nurse discusses preparation for childbirth. The following topics are discussed:

- Symptoms of impending labor (see box below) and what information to report
- Breathing and relaxation techniques
- Involvement of husband or significant other
- Provision for needs of other children
- Plans to get to hospital
- Plans of labor, terminology, and what care to expect
- Preparation for baby
- Preparation of grandparents and siblings (see Chapter 11)

SYMPTOMS OF IMPENDING LABOR

1. Uterine contractions: The woman is instructed to report the frequency, duration, and intensity of uterine contractions. Nulliparas are usually counseled to remain at home until contractions are regular and 5 minutes apart. Parous women are counseled to remain at home until contractions are regular and 10 minutes apart. If the woman lives more than 20 minutes from the hospital or has a history of rapid labors, these instructions are modified accordingly.
2. Rupture of the membranes (see Chapter 18).
3. Bloody "show": The "show" is scant, pink in color, and sticky (contains mucus).

If a hospital delivery is planned, the woman is required to register at the hospital of choice. Most hospitals now provide pamphlets containing information such as where to report when labor begins and policies pertaining to visitors and visiting hours. Many facilities also conduct tours.

Counseling is provided to relieve emotional tensions. These tensions often relate directly to the childbirth experience (e.g., anxiety about pain or possible delivery of the child before reaching the hospital). Nursing strategies include providing an opportunity for discussing the woman's specific fears or anxieties, helping her make definite plans concerning what she will do when labor starts, repeating instructions willingly, and having "sharing sessions" with mothers who have recently delivered. If possible, involve significant others in preparation for the birth. Arrange to have them participate in a supportive way during labor and delivery. These techniques may be effective in allaying or diffusing anxiety.

Most men whose wives are approaching labor may have their anxieties decreased through intervention before the event. Fantasies can be replaced by knowledge gained through activities such as the following:

1. A hospital tour to enable visualization of the labor room and waiting areas (This will allow him to envision the environment, familiarize himself with the delivery room, and determine what his role will be)
2. A demonstration of helping and supportive measures to comfort his wife during labor
3. A brief review of what to expect from his wife during the labor process if she has medication or anesthesia or if she delivers without medication or anesthesia (e.g., irritability, breathing, grunting)
4. A description of what to expect of the staff during his wife's labor

A realistic discussion of all known factors helps the father problem-solve more rationally and plan for the event. Such discussions are ego strengthening because they help focus the father's energies toward more appropriate coping strategies by helping alleviate anxieties about the unknown. Today many men elect to participate actively during labor and the delivery of their child. However, some men through personal or cultural concepts of the father role neither wish to nor intend to participate. *The important concept is that the partners agree on the other's roles.* For nurses to advocate any changes in these roles may cause confusion or feelings of guilt.

Evaluation

Evaluation is a continuous process. To be effective, evaluation needs to be based on measurable outcome criteria. The criteria reflect the parameters used to measure the goals for care. The maternal and fetal areas consistently assessed as indicators of maternal and fetal well-being and the clinical findings that represent normal response are presented as outcome criteria in the general and specific nursing care plans, pp. 303–306. These criteria are used as a basis for selecting appropriate nursing actions and evaluating their effectiveness.

General Nursing Care Plan

THIRD TRIMESTER

ASSESSMENT	NURSING DIAGNOSIS (ND)/PLAN (P)/GOAL (G)	RATIONALE/ IMPLEMENTATION	EVALUATION
Woman in third trimester. Teaching needs: danger signs recognition of preterm labor.	ND: Knowledge deficit related to signs and symptoms of preterm labor. P: Provide information; discuss. G: Woman will learn signs and symptoms of preterm labor.	*To introduce the definition of preterm labor the nurse will:* Provide written materials defining signs and symptoms of preterm labor; nurse will read through this information with woman.	Woman verbalizes understanding of signs and symptoms of preterm labor.
	ND: Anxiety related to development of preterm labor. P: Provide information: discuss. G: Woman will remain calm and alert and report signs and symptoms promptly if they occur.	*To convey the need for early recognition the nurse will:* Discuss the causes of preterm labor. Inform gravida of warning signs and symptoms. Reassure woman.	Woman verbalizes understanding and asks appropriate questions.
	ND: Potential for injury to woman and fetus, related to preterm birth. P: Provide information: discuss. G: Injury to fetus and gravida will be averted	*To help gravida understand difference between normal and preterm uterine contractions the nurse will:* Discuss the differences. Supervise practice timing frequency of contractions.	Woman gives return demonstration.
Premature rupture of membranes (PROM).	ND: Potential for injury to fetus, related to PROM. P: Provide information; discuss. G: Injury to fetus from prolapsed cord or sepsis will be prevented or decreased.	*To teach woman how to recognize PROM the nurse will:* Describe rupture of membranes: a gush or trickle of clear watery discharge that seems to come from vagina. Tell woman that a positive diagnosis of PROM must be made at clinic or hospital.	Woman verbalizes understanding of information. Woman knows where to go if symptoms appear.
Absence or change in fetal movements.	ND: Knowledge deficit related to assessment of fetal movement, its change in character, or its absence. P: Provide information; discuss. G: Woman will learn to assess the character and frequency of fetal movement.	*To teach woman about fetal movement the nurse will:* Discuss fetal movements she is experiencing. Provide information on fetal activity. Discuss cessation, diminution, and acceleration of fetal movement.	Woman verbalizes understanding of information. Woman reports any change in fetal activity.
Teaching needs: discomforts. Diminished tolerance to activities of daily living (ADL).	ND: Activity intolerance related to maternal adaptations. P: Provide information; discuss.	*To help woman conserve energy the nurse will:* Discuss the importance of frequent rest periods during the day.	Woman (couple) verbalizes understanding of information.

Continued.

General Nursing Care Plan—cont'd

ASSESSMENT	NURSING DIAGNOSIS (ND)/PLAN (P)/GOAL (G)	RATIONALE/ IMPLEMENTATION	EVALUATION
	G: Woman (couple) will learn ways of conserving her energy.	Aid the woman in forming strategies to help her relax while on the job. Discuss ways in which the woman's partner can help her with household duties.	Woman (couple) verbalizes understanding of information.
Diminished sexual activity.	ND: Altered sexuality patterns related to discomforts of third trimester of pregnancy. P: Provide information; discuss. G: Woman (couple) will learn alternate ways of achieving sexual satisfaction during this time.	*To help the woman (couple) identify and accept changes in sexuality the nurse will*: Assess couple's sexual relationship. Encourage open discussion. Supply information on alternative methods, positions, etc. Encourage verbalization of fears and anxieties.	Sexual needs are met and are mutually satisfying. Couple verbalizes understanding and accepts changes in sexual patterns.
Problems sleeping.	ND: Sleep pattern disturbance related to late pregnancy. P: Provide information; discuss. G: Woman will learn ways to adjust sleep schedule and positions to aid in sleeping.	*To help woman develop strategies to rest and sleep the nurse will*: Assess the woman's "normal" requirement of sleep. Assess woman's level of fatigue and her response to decreased amount of sleep (decreased coping mechanisms, etc.) Suggest strategies such as relaxation techniques, warm bath/shower, reading, warm milk before bed, back rub. Suggest alternate positions for sleeping using more pillows.	Woman reports increased sleep/rest. Woman's fatigue reduced, coping mechanism increased.
Constipation.	ND: Constipation related to late pregnancy. P: Provide information; discuss. G: Woman will continue to eat fresh fruits, vegetables, and whole grain products and drink plenty of water to aid in bowel regularity.	*To help woman minimize problem the nurse will*: Dicuss high fiber diet. Discuss fluid intake. Discourage use of laxatives and cathartics: may cause premature labor. Discuss exercise.	Woman verbalizes understanding of information.
Urinary frequency.	ND: Altered patterns of urinary elimination related to late pregnancy. P: Provide information; discuss; review client teaching: prevention of urinary tract infection (UTI), Chapter 8. G: Woman understands information and infection does not occur.	*To teach woman about return of urinary frequency and edema the nurse will*: Provide information about third trimester physiologic changes. Advise woman to lie in left lateral position. Discuss adequate fluid intake. Discourage use of diuretics.	Woman verbalizes understanding of information.

General Nursing Care Plan—cont'd

ASSESSMENT	NURSING DIAGNOSIS (ND)/PLAN (P)/GOAL (G)	RATIONALE/ IMPLEMENTATION	EVALUATION
		Discourage sodium restriction in diet. Discuss ways to prevent UTI which is one of the leading causes of premature labor. Discourage long periods of standing or sitting. Suggest use of support hose.	Woman knows signs and symptoms of UTI to report to physician.
Expressed emotional anxiety.	ND: Ineffective family/individual coping, related to adaptations to pregnancy. P: Provide information; discuss. G: Woman (couple) will learn and demonstrate positive coping techniques.	*To help woman (couple) minimize anxiety and develop coping strategies the nurse will*: Assess level of anxiety Discuss those areas and situations that cause woman's (couple's) anxiety. Strongly suggest childbirth education classes (prenatal classes). Give reassurance	Resolution of problems through open discussion. Couple attends classes and works through those anxieties related to labor and delivery.
Backache.	ND: Pain: backache related to postural changes and relaxed joints. P: Provide information; discuss; demonstrate and observe return demonstration. Review client teaching: exercise, body mechanics, and relaxation, Chapter 13. G: Woman reports greater comfort.	*To help woman minimize discomfort of backache the nurse will*: Discuss causes. Teach woman relaxation techniques and exercises. Teach woman about proper body mechanics and good posture. Supply written materials on the above for woman's future reference. Discuss types of shoes and types of heels woman should be wearing.	Woman verbalizes understanding of information. Woman uses proper body mechanics and demonstrates good posture.
Shortness of breath.	ND: Ineffective breathing pattern related to limited diaphragmatic excursion in late pregnancy. P: Provide information; discuss. G: Woman will learn ways to cope with shortness of breath until lightening occurs.	*To teach woman ways of coping with shortness of breath the nurse will*: Discuss posture and exercises. Discuss positioning of body for sleep using extra pillows. Strongly suggest cessation of smoking. Discuss overeating.	Woman accepts information and utilizes suggestions given by nurse.
Leg cramps. Varicose veins.	ND: Pain related to maternal adaptations. P: Provide information, discuss, and demonstrate. G: Woman will learn self-care strategies to diminish discomfort.	*To minimize discomfort from leg cramps and varicose veins the nurse will*: Discuss diminution of fatigue, amount of milk ingested per day, and adequate calcium intake. Discuss use of maternity support hose. Suggest frequent rest periods and elevation of legs.	Woman verbalizes understanding of information given. Woman asks appropriate questions.

Specific Nursing Care Plan

THIRD TRIMESTER

Lynn G., a secundigravida, is in her thirty-fourth week of pregnancy. She has a 3-year-old son who goes to nursery school one-half day. For the past week Lynn has been busy getting the baby's room ready, shopping for the layette and attending to the normal household duties of a wife and mother. When the nurse at the obstetrician's office sees her, Lynn says she is concerned about how swollen her legs and feet get by dinner time. She also says her back "is going to break." The nurse observes Mrs. G. is wearing tight high heels and sheer stockings.

ASSESSMENT	NURSING DIAGNOSIS (ND)/PLAN (P)/GOAL (G)	RATIONALE/ IMPLEMENTATION	EVALUATION
Pregnant woman at 34-weeks gestation, complaining of leg edema.	ND: Pain: leg edema related to dependent stasis of fluid in tissues of lower limbs. ND: Knowledge deficit related to causes of dependent edema in third trimester. P: Provide information; discuss. G: Lynn will learn causes of dependent edema. G: Lynn will gain knowledge to help her minimize leg edema.	*To teach Lynn how to deal with dependent leg edema the nurse will:* Discuss third trimester physiologic changes in the body. Discuss what long periods of standing or sitting do for fluid shifts. Suggest the use of support hose or maternity support pantyhose. Discuss putting legs up for short rest periods during the day. Discourage use of diuretics. Discourage excessive sodium intake (Chapter 15). Discourage extremes in temperature.	Lynn verbalizes understanding of information presented. Lynn takes time during day to rest and elevate legs.
Pregnant woman has backache.	ND: Pain: backache, related to postural changes and relaxed joints. ND: Knowledge deficit related to causes of backache in late pregnancy. P: Provide information; discuss; demonstrate; and observe return demonstration. G: Lynn will learn causes of backache. G: Lynn will learn self-care strategies to diminish discomfort.	*To help Lynn minimize discomfort of backache the nurse will:* Discuss causes. Provide information about lordosis and muscle strain related to those causes. Discuss center of gravity and its shift as the pregnancy progresses. Teach proper body mechanics (Chapter 13). Discuss and demonstrate good posture. Discuss the shoes Lynn is wearing and why high heels cause problems for the pregnant woman. Teach Lynn relaxation techniques and exercises to help her back (Chapter 13).	Lynn verbalizes an understanding of information provided. Lynn uses proper body mechanics. Lynn uses good posture. Lynn wears low-heeled, wide-based shoes. Lynn uses exercises and relaxation techniques to decrease backache.

SUMMARY

Assessment for maternal and fetal risk factors continues throughout pregnancy. Prenatal danger signs and recognition of preterm labor are reviewed with each gravida and her family. During the last trimester, discomforts associated with advancing pregnancy and concerns about the approaching labor preoccupy expectant families. In addition to individual counseling, preparation for childbirth classes are available to assist expectant parents as they prepare for transition into parenthood.

Consumers learn about birth-setting choices from a variety of sources. Classes offered by community agencies, the media, newspapers, and advertisements alert consumers to available services. The knowledgeable nurse serves as a valuable resource for couples who want to individualize their childbirth experience.

KEY CONCEPTS

- The quiet period of the second trimester gives way to an active period more oriented to the reality of impending childbirth and parenting responsibilities.
- The psychosocial aspects of care are of paramount importance and may well affect the whole course of pregnancy, childbirth, and the adjustment of the new family.
- The discomforts of pregnancy require sensitive attention and a plan for teaching self-care measures.
- Regardless of the gravida's readiness to learn, attention to prebirth preparation is a necessary component of prenatal care.
- Each gravida needs to know how to recognize and report preterm labor and other danger signs and symptoms.

STUDY QUESTIONS AND ACTIVITIES

1. Complete the study questions and activities from Chapter 13 or repeat them with women in their third trimester.
2. Complete an assessment of a woman in her third trimester; record findings. With the woman, formulate at least one nursing diagnosis; plan and set goals; and implement, evaluate, and record the process and results.
3. Role-play one or more of the following; then critique the interactions in a group session:
   a. Marital support.
   b. Assisting an expectant couple in choosing a birth setting; that is, ABC or home birth.
   c. Teaching a gravida to recognize preterm labor.
4. In a simulated situation, teach self-care measures for the discomforts of pregnancy.
5. In a clinic or physician's office, measure fundal height and auscultate fetal heart rate.
6. Attend a prenatal education session and identify concerns of expectant parents.
7. Discuss pros and cons of sibling participation in pregnancy and labor.
8. Examine grandparental participation in pregnancy.
9. Attend a series of childbirth education classes as a participant observer:
   a. Describe teaching style in relation to parents' readiness to learn.
   b. Identify rationale for content taught.
   c. Choose one couple and describe the interaction between the pregnant woman and her coach.
10. Observe a client in labor with her coach. Describe the effectiveness of the support from both the coach and the nurse.
11. Discuss your own opinions concerning alternative birth settings. If possible, invite a woman who has experienced childbirth in one of the alternative settings and discuss her experience and her reactions to it.
12. Role-play a client who wishes to have a home birth interacting with a nurse who believes that home births are unsafe. Respond to the interaction with suggestions on how the nurse might attempt to understand the client's position.

Organizations Involved in Parent Education

The following organizations can provide information on parent education:

American Academy of Husband-Coached Childbirth (AAHCC)
P.O. Box 5224
Sherman Oaks, Calif. 91413

American Society for Psychoprophylaxis in Obstetrics (ASPO)
1411 K Street N.W., Suite 200
Washington, D.C. 20005

Council of Childbirth Education Specialists, Inc. (CCES)
168 West 86th Street
New York, N.Y. 10024

International Childbirth Education Association (ICEA)
P.O. Box 20048
Minneapolis, Minn. 55420

Maternity Center Association
48 East 92nd St
New York, N.Y. 10028

National Association of Childbirth Education, Inc. (NACE)
3940 11th Street
Riverside, Calif. 92501

Nurses' Association of the American College of Obstetricians and Gynecologists (NAACOG)
409 12th Street, S.W.
Washington, D.C. 20024-2191

Read Natural Childbirth Foundation, Inc.
1300 S. Elisco Drive, Suite 102
Greenbrae, Calif. 94904

References

Arms, S: Five women, five births, film, 1978, Davidson Films, Inc

Bernardini, JY, Maloni, JA, and Stegman, CE: Neuromuscular control of childbirth-prepared women during the first stage of labor, JOGN Nurs 2:105, March/April 1983

Bradley, R: Husband-coached childbirth, New York, 1965, Harper & Row, Publishers, Inc

Brown, MA: Marital support during pregnancy, JOGN Nurs 15(6):475, 1986

Buxton, CL: A study of psychological methods for relief of pain in childbirth, Philadelphia, 1962, WB Saunders Co

Chertok, L: Psychosomatic methods of preparation for birth, Am J Obstet Gynecol 98(5):698, 1967

Cronenwett, LR: Elements and outcomes of a postpartum support group program, Res Nurs Health 3(3):33, 1980

Cronenwett, LR, and Brickman, P: Models of helping and coping in childbirth, Nurs Res 32:84, March/April 1983

Dick-Read, G: Childbirth without fear, ed 2, New York, 1959, Harper & Row, Publishers, Inc

Fanaroff, AA, and Martin, RJ, editors: Neonatal-perinatal medicine: diseases of the fetus and infant, ed 4, St Louis, 1987, The CV Mosby Co

Felton, GS, and Segelman, FB: Lamaze childbirth training and changes in belief about personal control, Birth Fam J 5:141, Fall 1978

Grossman, FK, Eichler, LS, and Winckoff, SA: Pregnancy, birth and parenthood, San Francisco, 1980, Jossey-Bass, Inc, Publishers

House, JS: Work, stress and social support, Reading, Mass, 1981, Addison-Wesley Publishing Co, Inc

Huttel, FA, et al: A quantitative evaluation of psychoprophylaxis in childbirth, J Psychosom Res 16:81, 1972

Johnson, JM: Teaching self-hypnosis in pregnancy, labor, and delivery, MCN 5:98, 1980

Karmel, M: Thank you, Dr. Lamaze, New York, 1965, Doubleday & Co, Inc

Lamaze, F: Painless childbirth: the Lamaze method, Chicago, 1970, Regnery Books

Lamb, ME: Influence of the child on marital quality and family interaction during the prenatal, perinatal, and infancy periods. In: Lerner, R, and Spanier, G, editors: Child influences on marital and family interaction, New York, 1978, Academic Press, Inc

Lederman, RP: Psychosocial adaptation in pregnancy: assessment of seven dimensions of maternal development, Englewood Cliffs, NJ, 1984, Prentice-Hall, Inc

Mann, RJ: San Francisco General Hospital Nurse-midwifery practice: the first thousand births, Am J Obstet Gynecol 140:6, July 1981

Marieskind, HI: Women in the health system: patients, providers, and programs, St Louis, 1980, The CV Mosby Co

Myles, MF: Textbook for midwives, with modern concepts of obstetric neonatal care, ed 9, New York, 1981, Churchill Livingstone, Inc

Pritchard, JA and MacDonald, PC, and Gant, NF: Williams obstetrics, ed 17, Norwalk, 1985, Appleton-Century-Crofts

Rosen, EL: The birth room: implementation of an alternative, Can Nurse, p 30, March 1980

Sumner, P, and Phillips, C: Birthing rooms: concept and reality, St Louis, 1981, The CV Mosby Co

Tanzer, S: The psychology of pregnancy and childbirth: an investigation of natural childbirth, unpublished doctoral dissertation, Waltham, Mass, 1967, Brandeis University

Velvovsky, I, et al: Painless childbirth through psychoprophylaxis, Moscow, 1960, Foreign Languages Publishing House

Willmuth, LR: Prepared childbirth and the concept of control, JOGN Nurs 4(5):38, 1975

Zuspan, FP, and Quilligan, EJ, editors: Practical manual of obstetric care, St Louis, 1982, The CV Mosby Co

Bibliography

Anderson, SV: Siblings at birth: a survey and study, Birth Fam J 6:80, 1979

Anderson, SV, and Simken, P: Birth through children's eyes, Seattle, 1981, The Penny Press

Austin, SE: Childbirth classes for couples desiring VBAC (vaginal birth after cesarean), MCN 11(4):250, 1986

Barranti, C: The grandparent/grandchild relationship: family resource in an era of voluntary bonds, Fam Relations 34:3, July 1985

Bookmarks, ICEA Bookcenter, PO Box 20048, Minneapolis, MN 33420, Jan 1984 (A source of books on pregnancy and related topics.)

Brown, MA: Social support, stress and health: a comparison of expectant mothers and fathers, Nurs Res 35(2):72, 1986

Carter, ER: Quality maternity care for the medically indigent, MCN 11(2):85, 1986

Clinton, JF: Physical and emotional responses of expectant fathers throughout pregnancy and the early postpartum period, Int J Nurs Stud 24(1):59, 1987

Cohen, RL: A comparative study of women choosing wo different birth alternatives, Birth 9:1, Spring 1982

Cranley, MS: Roots of attachment: the relationship of parents with their unborn. In Raff, BS, editor: Perinatal parental behavior: nursing research and implications for newborn health, New York, 1981, Alan R Liss, Inc

Cronenwett, LR: Parental network structure and perceived support after birth of first child, Nurs Res 34(6):347, 1985

Cronenwett, LR: Network structure, social support, and psychological outcomes of pregnancy, Nurs Res 34(2):93, 1985

DelGiudice, GT: The relationship between sibling jealousy and presence at a sibling's birth, Birth 13(4):250, 1986

Durham, L, and Collins, M: The effect of music as a conditioning aid in prepared childbirth education, JOGN Nurs 15(3):268, 1986

Fawcett, J, and Henklein, JC: Antenatal education for cesarean birth: extension of a field test, JOGN Nurs 16(1):61, 1987

Fullerton, JDT: The choice of in-hospital or alternative birth environment as related to the concept of control, J Nurse Midwife, 27:2, March/April 1982

Gates, S: Children's literature: it can help children cope with sibling rivalry, MCN 5:351, 1980

Gill, PJ, and Katz, M: Early detection of preterm labor: ambulatory home monitoring of uterine activity, JOGN Nurs 15(6):439, 1986

Greene, R, and Polivka, J: The meaning of grandparent day cards: an analysis of the intergenerational network, Fam Relations 34:2, April 1985

Hart, G: Maternal attitudes in prepared and unprepared cesarean deliveries, JOGN Nurs 9:243, 1980

Hassid, P: Textbook for childbirth educators, ed 3, New York, 1984, JB Lippincott Co

Holt, JR: Best laid plans: pre- and postpartum comparison of self and spouse in primiparous Lamaze couples who share delivery and those who do not, Nurs Res 29:20, Jan/Feb 1980

Honig, JC: Preparing preschool-aged children to be siblings, MCN 11(1):37, 1986

Horn, M, and Manion, J: Creative grandparents: bonding the generations, JOGN Nurs 14:233, May/June 1985

Johnsen NM, and Gaspard, ME: Theoretical foundations of a prepared sibling class, JOGN Nurs 14:237, May/June 1985
Kemp, VH, and Page, CK: Maternal prenatal attachment in normal and high-risk pregnancies, JOGN Nurs 16(3):179, 1987
Kieffer, MJ: The birthing room concept at Phoenix Memorial Hospital. II. Consumer satisfaction during one year, JOGN Nurs 9:158, May/June 1980
Kitzinger, S: The experience of childbirth education, J Calif Perinatal Assoc 2(1):70, 1982
Kornhaber, A, and Woodward, KL: Grandparents/grandchildren: the vital connection, Garden City, NY, 1981, Anchor Press/Doubleday
Lumley, J: Preschool siblings at birth: short-term effects, Birth 10:11, Spring 1983
Maloni, JA, McIndoe, JE, and Rubenstein, G: Expectant grandparents class, JOGN Nurs 16(1):26, 1987
May, KA: Three phases of father involvement in pregnancy, Nurs Res 31:337, 1982
McKay, S, and Phillips, CR: Family-centered maternity care: implementation strategies, Rockville, Md, 1984, Aspen Systems Corp
Mercer, RT: She's a multip . . . she knows the ropes, MCN 4:301, Sept/Oct 1979
Miller, SJ: Prenatal nursing assessment of the expectant family, Nurse Pract 11(5):40, 1986
Milstein, JM: Alternative birthing sites: interference versus intervention, J Calif Perinatal Assoc 2(1):1982
Moore, D: Prepared childbirth and marital satisfaction during the antepartum and postpartum periods, Nurs Res 32:73, March/April 1983
Moore, L, et al: Self-assessment: a personalized approach to nursing during pregnancy, JOGN Nurs 15(4):311, 1986
Mueller, LS: Pregnancy and sexuality, JOGN Nurs 14(4):289, 1985
Newell, NJ: Grandparents: the overlooked support system for new parents during the fourth trimester, NAACOG Update Series, 1:lesson 21, 1984
Nicholas and the baby (16 mm film or ¾ inch videocassette), Centre Productions, Inc, Suite A, 1312 Pine St, Boulder, Colo 80302. (Film available for preparing older preschool and school-age children for participation in the birth experience)
Norton, SF, and Nichols, CW: Champions of choice, Am J Nurs 85(4):380, 1985
Oehler, J: The frog family books: color the pictures "sad" or "glad," MCN 6:281, 1981
Olson, ML: Fitting grandparents into new families, MCN 6(6):419, 1981
Periscope: Alternative birthing study publishes findings (the alternative birthing methods [ABM] study [Chapter 1645, Statutes of 1984 Vasconcellos]) Calif Perinatal Assoc, Winter 1987
Redman, BK: The process of patient education, ed 6, St Louis, 1988, The CV Mosby Co
Sherwen, LN: Psychosocial dimensions of the pregnant family, New York, 1987, Springer Publishing Co, Inc
Stainton, MC: The fetus: a growing member of the family, Fam Relations 34:321, 1985
Stephany, T: Supporting the mother of a patient in labor, JOGN Nurs 12(5):345, 1983
Sweet, PT: Prenatal classes especially for children, MCN 4:82, March/April 1979
Triolo, PK: Prepared childbirth, Clin Obstet Gynecol 30(3):487, 1987
Waller, MM: Siblings in the childbearing experience, NAACOG Update Series 1: lesson 17, 1984
Waryas, FS, and Luebbers, MG: A cluster system for maternity care, MCN 11(2):98, 1986
Winslow, W: First pregnancy after 35: what is the experience? MCN 12(2):92, 1987
Zalar, MK: Sexual counseling for pregnant couples, Matern Child Nurs J 1(3):176, 1976

CHAPTER

15

Maternal and Fetal Nutrition

Learning Objectives

Correctly define the key terms listed.

Explain optimum maternal weight gain during pregnancy focusing on nutritional values of foods eaten to achieve weight gain.

State recommended daily allowance (RDA) requirements for kcal, protein, vitamins, and minerals during pregnancy.

Give examples of food sources of the nutrients required for optimum maternal weight gain during pregnancy.

Examine the role of nutritional supplements during pregnancy.

List five nutritional risk factors during pregnancy.

Give examples of cultural food patterns and possible dietary problems for two ethnic groups.

Assess evaluative criteria for nutrition assessment.

Outline and give examples of nursing care related to maternal and fetal nutrition based on the 5-step nursing process.

Key Terms

anemia
anthropometry
blood-forming nutrients
calorie
fat-soluble vitamins
food craving
food taboo
hypervitaminosis
intrauterine growth retardation (IUGR)
iron supplementation
kcal
ketonemia
lactose intolerance
megaloblastic anemia
nutritional risk factor
pattern of weight gain
physiologic anemia of pregnancy
pica
recommended dietary allowance (RDA)
vegetarian diets
water-soluble vitamins

The Policy Statement on Nutrition and Pregnancy issued by the American College of Obstetricians and Gynecologists (ACOG) contains the following statement:

> A woman's nutritional status before, during and after pregnancy contributes to a significant degree to the well-being of both herself and her infant (Fig. 15-1). Therefore, what a woman consumes before she conceives and while she carries the fetus is of vital importance to the health of succeeding generations.

Considerable resources and information are available to assist a woman in selecting foods and dietary patterns associated with a healthy pregnancy and a healthy outcome. Pregnancy is an especially good time to promote good nutrition since expectant parents may be highly motivated to change poor eating habits.

NUTRITIONAL REQUIREMENTS

Weight Gain During Pregnancy

Optimum weight gain of the mother during pregnancy makes an important contribution to the pregnancy's successful course and outcome. The weight gained during a normal pregnancy will vary among individual women. The acceptable weight gain for most healthy women of normal weight for height carrying a single fetus is 12 kg (27 lb) (Naeye, 1979; Dohrmann and Lederman, 1986) with a range of 10 to 14.5 kg (22 to 32 lb).

Some of the maternal weight gain is caused by deposition of fat—maternal stores laid down for energy to sustain fetal growth during the latter part of pregnancy and energy for lactation to follow. About 2 to 4 kg (4 to 8 lb) of fat are commonly deposited for these stores, presumably as the result of stimulus by progesterone acting centrally to reset a "lipostat" in the hypothalamus. When the pregnancy is over, the lipostat reverts to its usual nonpregnant level, and the added fat is lost. The average weight of the products of a normal pregnancy are given below and illustrated in Fig. 15-2.

Products	*Weight*
Fetus	3400 g (7.5 lb)
Placenta	450 g (1 lb)
Amniotic fluid	900 g (2 lb)
Uterus (weight increase)	1100 g (2.5 lb)
Breast tissue (weight increase)	1400 g (3 lb)
Blood volume (weight increase)	1800 g (4 lb) (1500 ml)
Maternal stores	1800 to 3600 g (4 to 8 lb)
TOTAL	11,000 to 13,000 g (11 to 13 kg; 24 to 28 lb)

Pattern of Weight Gain. To monitor the desirable weight gain as compared with deviations in weight gain, a grid may be used for plotting the pregnant woman's weight throughout pregnancy. The weight gain should be the result of a well-balanced diet in appropriate amounts for age, height, weight, and activity level.

There is general agreement that the normal curve of weight gain should show little gain during the first trimester, a rapid increase during the second, and some slowing in the rate of increase during the third. During the first trimester, growth takes place almost entirely in maternal tissue, gain is primarily in maternal tissue during the second trimester and in fetal tissue in the third trimester. About 900 to 1800 g (2 to 4 lb) is an average gain during the first trimester. Thereafter, about 450 g (1 lb) a week during the remainder of the pregnancy is usual.

Deviations in Weight and Weight Gain. Deviations from usual values for either prepregnant weight or weight gain

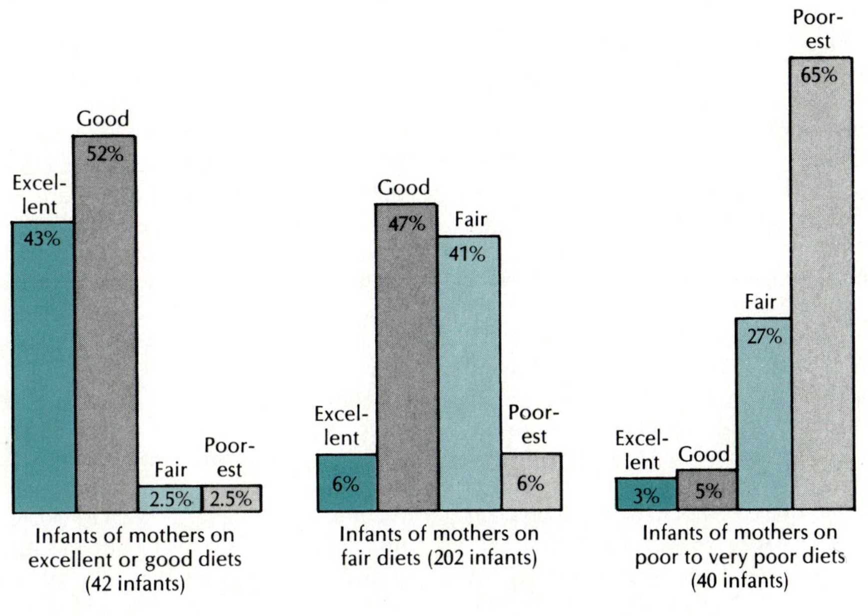

Fig. 15-1 Condition of infants at birth in relation to prenatal diet of mother.
From Mitchell, HS, et al: Nutrition in health and disease, ed 16, Philadelphia, 1976, JB Lippincott Co.

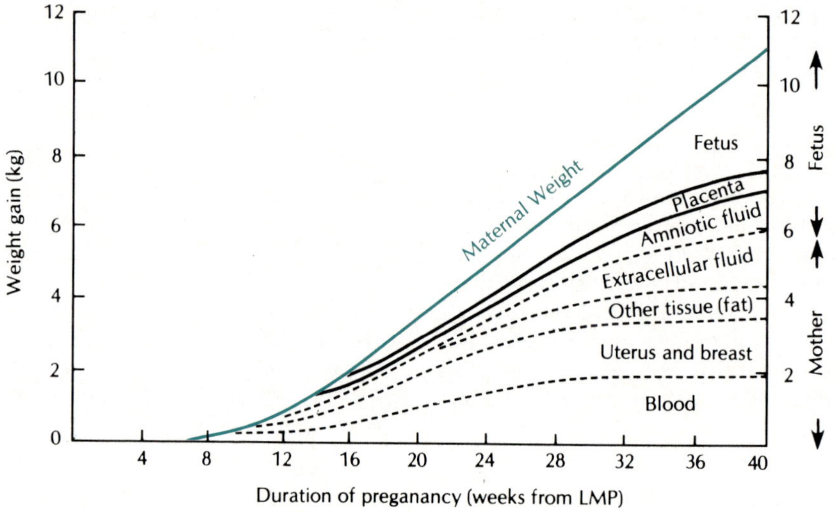

Fig. 15-2 Pattern and components of weight gain throughout course of pregnancy, assuming an 11 kg (24.5 lb) weight gain.

From Schneider, HA, et al: Nutritional support of medical practice, New York, 1977, Harper & Row, Publishers.

during pregnancy are relatively common. The following are considered to be deviations from the norm:

1. Underweight: prepregnant weight less than 85% of standard weight for age and height (see Appendix F).
2. Overweight: prepregnant weight more than 120% of standard weight for age and height (see Appendix F).
3. Inadequate gain: gain of 1 kg (2.2 lb) or less per month in the second or third trimester. Weight loss or failure to gain during pregnancy is a sign of nutritional difficulties.
4. Excessive gain: gain of 3 kg (6.6 lb) or more per month is likely to be caused by tissue fluid retention rather than by excessive caloric intake. A total weight gain of over 14.5 kg (32 lb) is associated with higher rates of perinatal mortality.

Hazards of Restricting Adequate Weight Gain. Young women in North America enter pregnancy already burdened by cultural obsession with thinness and "dieting." This conscious or unconscious pressure is difficult to dislodge. There are potential hazards, however, for both mother and infant from restricting weight gain during pregnancy. The mother's weight gain and prepregnancy weight are the two strongest influences (except gestational age) on birth weight. Infant birth weights, in turn, have been studied intensively with respect to infant mortality and morbidity, brain development, and learning disabilities in later life. Birth weights serve as practical indicators of the health and nutrition of a population.

The obese woman entering pregnancy faces an increased risk of severe complications notably hypertensive disorders and diabetes mellitus, which have adverse effects on pregnancy outcome. Obesity should not be equated with overall good nutrition; excessive caloric ingestion may mask other nutritional problems (e.g., anemia, inadequate protein intake). Some persons have advocated restriction of weight gain in such women so that they conclude pregnancy with a net loss. However, the advisability of such a course seems questionable on several grounds. First, dietary restrictions to limit calories may also result in displacement of other nutrients from the diet. Second, optimum protein utilization in pregnancy apparently requires a minimum of approximately 30 kcal/kg/24 hours. This weight gain may be excessive, however, if calculated on obese weight. Third, dietary restriction results in catabolism of fat stores, which in turn produces ketonemia. Ketonemia jeopardizes the development of the fetus. If the nutritional education focuses positively on the necessity for supplying fetal nutritional needs, the weight gain focus usually becomes secondary.

Nutrient Needs

What nutrients must the mother take to supply the fetus and her own changing body optimumly for this critical gestation period?

During the first trimester (the first 3 months), the fetus is small and undergoes differentiation, so that the mother's relative nutrient requirements are increased slowly from normal adult needs. These nutrients are essential during this vital period; only the *quantitative* need for them is not yet greatly increased. The importance of a diet that contains balanced portions of essential nutrients according to individually assessed quantities continues into the second trimester (Williams, 1988).

The last trimester of pregnancy is the period during which a greater *amount* of key nutrients is required by the fetus, as it lays down stores for growth. This need for increased amounts of certain nutrients is indicated by the recommended daily allowances (RDAs) outlined by the National Research Council (NRC) (Table 15-1). It should be remembered that although the recommended allowances provide a margin of safety above minimum requirements to allow for variations of need, some individuals require more for optimum nutrition. For example, the reference

Table 15-1 *Nutritional Requirements During Pregnancy*

Nutrient	Nonpregnant Female RDA (19-22 yr)	RDA for Pregnancy	RDA for Lactation	Reasons for Increased Need During Pregnancy	Food Sources
Calories	2400	2700	2600	Increased BMR,* energy needs; protein sparing	Carbohydrates; fats; proteins
Protein	44 g	74 g	64 g	Rapid fetal tissue growth; amniotic fluid; placental growth and development; maternal tissue growth; uterus, breasts; increased maternal circulating blood volume: hemoglobin increase, plasma protein increase; maternal storage reserves for labor, delivery, and lactation	Milk; cheese; egg; meat; grains; legumes; nuts
Minerals					
Calcium	800 mg	1200 mg	1200 mg	Fetal skeleton formation; fetal tooth bud formation; increased maternal calcium metabolism	Milk; cheese; whole grains; leafy vegetables; egg yolk; milk
Phosphorus	800 mg	1200 mg	1200 mg	Fetal skeletal formation; fetal tooth bud formation; increased maternal phosphorus metabolism	Milk; cheese; lean meats
Iron	18 mg	18+ mg (+30-60 mg supplement)	†	Increased maternal circulating blood volume, increased hemoglobin; fetal liver iron storage (primarily in third trimester); high iron cost of pregnancy	Liver; meats; egg; whole or enriched grain; leafy vegetables; nuts; legumes; dried fruits
Zinc	15 mg	20 mg	25 mg	Factor influencing growth	Wheat; bran; milk; liver; shellfish
Iodine	150 μg	175 μg	200 μg	Increased BMR—increased thyroxine production	Iodized salt
Magnesium	300 mg	450 mg	450 mg	Coenzyme in energy and protein metabolism; enzyme activator; tissue growth, cell metabolism; muscle action	Nuts; soybeans; cocoa; seafood; whole grains; dried beans and peas
Fat-soluble Vitamins					
A	800 RE‡ (4000 IU)	1000 RE (5000 IU)	1200 RE (6000 IU)	Essential for cell development, hence tissue growth; tooth bud formation (development of enamel-forming cells in gum tissue); bone growth	Butter; cream; fortified margarine; green and yellow vegetables
D	5 μg§ (200 IU)	10 μg (400 IU)	10 μg (400 IU)	Absorption of calcium and phosphorus, mineralization of bone tissue, tooth buds	Fortified milk; fortified margarine; fish liver oils; egg yolk; butter; liver

Adapted and revised from Williams, S: Handbook of maternal and infant nutrition, Berkeley, Calif, 1976, SRW Productions, Inc.

*Basal metabolic rate.

†Iron needs during lactation are not substantially different from those of nonpregnant women, but continued supplementation of the mother for 2 to 3 months after parturition is advisable to replenish stores depleted by pregnancy.

‡Retinol equivalents (RE) replace international units (IU).

§400 IU (international units) = 10 μg of pure crystalline vitamin D_3 (cholecalciferol).

Continued.

Table 15-1 *Nutritional Requirements During Pregnancy—cont'd*

Nutrient	Nonpregnant Female RDA (19-22 yr)	RDA for Pregnancy	RDA for Lactation	Reasons for Increased Need During Pregnancy	Food Sources
E	8 mg alpha-TE*	10 mg alpha-TE	11 mg alpha-TE	Tissue growth, cell wall integrity; red blood cell integrity	Vegetable oils; leafy vegetables; cereals; meat; egg; milk
C	60 mg	80 mg	100 mg	Tissue formation and integrity; cement substance in connective and vascular tissues; increases iron absorption	Citrus fruits; berries; melons; tomatoes; chili peppers; green peppers; green leafy vegetables; broccoli; potatoes
Folic acid (Folacin)	400 μg	800 μg (+200-400 μg supplement)	500 μg	Increased metabolic demand in pregnancy; prevention of megaloblastic anemia in high-risk women; increased heme production for hemoglobin; production of cell nucleus material; coenzyme in energy metabolism; coenzyme in protein metabolism	Meat; peanuts; beans and peas; enriched grains
B_1 (Thiamin)	1.1 mg	1.5 mg	1.6 mg	Coenzyme for energy metabolism	Pork, beef; liver; whole or enriched grains; legumes
B_2 (Riboflavin)	1.2 mg	1.5 mg	1.7 mg	Coenzyme in energy metabolism and protein metabolism	Milk; liver; enriched grains
B_6 (pyridoxine)	2.0 mg	2.6 mg	2.5 mg	Coenzyme in protein metabolism; increased fetal growth requirement	Wheat; corn; liver; meat
B_{12} (cobalamin)	3.0 μg	4.0 μg	4.0 μg	Coenzyme in protein metabolism, especially vital cell proteins such as nucleic acid; formation of red blood cells	Milk; egg; meat; liver; cheese
Niacin	14 mg	16 mg	19 mg	Coenzyme factor in metabolism	Meat; fish; poultry; liver; whole or enriched grains; peanuts

*Total vitamin E activity, estimated to be 80% as alpha-tocopherol and 20% as other tocopherols.

woman in the typical RDA table is aged 18 to 35 years, weighs 58 kg (128 lb), is 160 cm (64 in) tall, lives in a temperate climate, and is a normally active, healthy woman. Variations from this state would need to be considered when providing counseling. The increased quantitative need for nourishment by pregnant adolescents should be noted (see Chapter 35). The need for individual counseling and for therapeutic use of these recommendations as guidelines is clearly stated by the NRC:

> They are not called 'requirements' because they are not intended to represent merely literal (minimum) requirements of average individuals, but to cover substantially the individual variations in the requirements of normal people.

In considering the needs of the normal pregnant woman, therefore, the nutrient elements should be reviewed in terms of the general amount of increased intake indicated, and why this increase is recommended. Factors to be considered include the following:

1. *Uterine-placental-fetal unit.* Placentas of poorly nourished mothers often contain fewer and smaller cells. Poorly developed placentas have a reduced ability to synthesize substances needed by the fetus, to facilitate flow of needed nutrients, and to inhibit passage to potentially harmful substances. Therefore it is understandable that the infant of a poorly nourished mother would be poorly nourished and small for gestational age (SGA) (see Chapter 37). Maternal uterine adaptations are discussed in Chapter 10.

2. *Maternal blood volume and constituents.* Total blood volume is known to increase about 33% above normal during pregnancy. Plasma volume increases 50% in nulliparas and more in multiparas. Red blood cell (RBC) production is stimulated during pregnancy. The number of RBCs increases gradually; the expansion of plasma volume proceeds rapidly. This rapid increase in plasma volume results in hemodilution and is referred to as physiologic anemia of pregnancy. At the same time, a deficiency of iron or of folic acid may contribute to the development of true anemia.

Blood levels of many nutrients, for example, total protein, decrease during pregnancy secondary to hemodilution. Most plasma lipid fractions rise during pregnancy. For example, cholesterol increases from under 200 mg/dl to between 250 and 300 mg/dl.

3. *Maternal mammary changes.* Preparation of mammary glands for lactation is presented in Chapter 23.

4. *Metabolic needs.* Basal metabolic rates (BMRs), when expressed as kcal per minute, are about 20% higher in pregnant women than in nonpregnant women. This increase includes the energy cost for tissue synthesis. The increased basal energy need over the entire pregnancy period plus the energy needed for new tissue brings the total energy cost for pregnancy to about 80,000 kcal, or about 300 kcal/in 24 hours.

Water. Water as an essential nutrient is commonly overlooked during assessment. Among its many functions, water assists digestion by dissolving food and aiding its transport. Essential during the exchange of nutrients and wastes across cell membranes, water is the main substance of cells, blood, lymph, and other vital body fluids. It also aids in maintaining body temperature.

Drinking 6 to 8 glasses (1500 to 2000 ml) of water and juices every 24 hours is recommended. Other types of fluids may contain ingredients that are best used sparingly or omitted during pregnancy. For instance, fluids containing high levels of sodium, artificial sweeteners, and other additives are discouraged.

Protein. An additional daily allowance of 30 g of protein is recommended throughout pregnancy, raising the 44 g required by the normal nonpregnant woman to at least 74 g daily. This represents an increase of about 66% or two thirds. For a large number of high-risk or active women, however, as cited studies have shown, more protein is needed—closer to 100 g or about double their previous intake.

Protein, with its essential constituent, nitrogen, is the nutritional element that is basic to growth. Nitrogen balance studies give some indication of the large amounts of nitrogen and by the mother and child during pregnancy. Study of fetal tissue composition reveals that during the last half of gestation the amount of nitrogen stored by the embryo rises from approximately 0.9 to 55.9 g. The mature placenta at term has stored about 17 g of nitrogen; the amniotic fluid contains 1 g. An estimated 17 g of nitrogen is incorporated in the developing maternal breast tissue and nearly 40 g in the increased uterine tissue. In addition a maternal reserve of 200 to 350 g is stored for the approaching losses during labor and parturition (from 300 to 500 ml or more of blood may be lost during delivery) and in preparation for the physiologic demand of lactation.

In summary, more protein is essential to meet the demands posed by the rapid growth of the fetus; by the enlargement of the uterus, mammary glands, and placenta; by the increase in maternal circulating blood volume and the subsequent demand for increased plasma protein to maintain colloidal osmotic pressure; and by the formation of amniotic fluid and storage reserves for labor, delivery, and lactation (Williams, 1988).

Milk, meat, egg, and cheese are complete protein foods of high biologic value. Protein-rich foods also contribute other nutrients such as calcium, iron, and B vitamins. The amounts of these foods that would supply the quantities of protein needed are indicated in the recommended daily food plan (see Table 15-3). Additional protein may be obtained from legumes, whole grains, and nuts.

Recommended protein intake is adjusted to the body size of individuals. The following guidelines are suggested:

1. Mature women: 1.3 g protein per kg of pregnant weight
2. Adolescent girls (15 to 18 years of age): 1.5 g protein per kg of pregnant weight
3. Younger girls: 1.7 g protein per kg of pregnant weight

The greater protein intake recommended for adolescents and younger girls is needed to support possible continued maturation. If a multiple birth (e.g., twins) is expected, additional protein and other nutrients are also needed in the mother's diet.

Calories. Calories should be sufficient to meet energy and nutrient demands and to spare protein for tissue building. Classic studies indicate that a minimum of 36 calories per kg of body weight is required for efficient use of protein during pregnancy. Although only 300 calories additional to the amount ingested by the nonpregnant woman is recommended by the NRC, representing about a 10% to 15% increase over the usual previous intake, this amount is insufficient for many active or nutritionally deficient women, who may easily need as much as 2500 to 3000 calories. The emphasis should be a positive one on ample calories to ensure nutrient and energy needs, not a negative idea of restricting calories (Williams, 1988).

Minerals

Iron. The changes in maternal red blood volume and cell mass accompanying pregnancy represent a fundamental physiologic adjustment. Since full-term average-for-gestational-age (AGA) infants are born with high hemoglobin levels of 18 to 22 g/dl and with a supply of iron stored in the liver to last 3 to 6 months, the maternal organism must transfer about 300 mg of iron to the fetus during gestation.

If dietary iron is not available to meet the needs of the maternal-placental-fetal unit, fetal iron reserves will not be impaired but maternal iron stores will be depleted and maternal red cell mass will be reduced. If the mother has no iron reserves, which occurs commonly in young women, especially teenagers, maternal hemoglobin levels will drop more than usual and iron-deficiency anemia may be superimposed on the physiologic anemia of pregnancy. *Iron sup-*

plementation is usually started during the second trimester to maintain maternal reserves and to meet fetal requirements during pregnancy (see guidelines for client teaching: iron supplementation, p. 327).

Calcium. Almost all the additional calcium required during pregnancy is utilized by the fetus. Because it is virtually impossible to meet these requirements with foods other than dairy products, milk is considered by many to be particularly essential during pregnancy. One liter of milk contains 1200 mg of calcium, precisely the amount suggested in the RDAs. Individuals who do not consume milk or milk products—for example, persons with lactose intolerance or reduced intake of dairy foods—will require calcium supplementation.

Calcium and phosphorus are found in the same foods. If calcium needs are met, adequate phosphorus will be assured.

Sodium. During pregnancy there is a slight increase in the need for most nutrients, including sodium. Routine restriction of sodium is unphysiologic and unfounded. Diets low in calories and sodium place the normal mother and her fetus at unnecessary risk (Worthington-Roberts, Vermeersch and Williams, 1985; Williams, 1988). When sodium is restricted, the maternal organism undergoes a series of hormonal and biochemical changes in an effort to conserve sodium.

Sources of excessive sodium are discouraged, however. Excessive sodium is found in many canned and processed foods. Products devoid of nutritive value and excessively high in sodium include pretzels, potato chips, soft drinks, and bouillion cubes. Hidden sources of sodium occur in medications such as bicarbonate of soda. Some people are unaware that table salt contains sodium.

Zinc. The metal zine is a constituent of numerous enzymes involved in major metabolic pathways. It may be noteworthy that maternal zinc deficiency is highly teratogenic in rats. The incidence of malformations of the central nervous system (CNS) in humans appears to be increased in geographic areas where zinc deficiency is prevalent.

Fat-soluble Vitamins. *Because of the high potential for toxicity, gravidas are advised to take fat-soluble vitamin supplements only as prescribed.*

Vitamin A. The added allowance of vitamin A for pregnancy relates to fetal storage of the vitamin. The RDA can readily be provided by dietary sources. There appears to be no need for routine supplementation. Certain food faddists advocate massive amounts of vitamin A. Pregnant women should be cautioned against this practice. Toxicity related to *hypervitaminosis A* represents a potential danger to both the pregnant woman (liver damage) and to her unborn child (congenital malformations).

Vitamin D. Vitamin D plays an important role in promoting positive calcium balance in pregnancy. It is present naturally in only a few animal foods such as fish liver oils, eggs, butter, and liver. The main food sources are enriched or fortified foods. It is also produced in the skin by the action of ultraviolet light (irradiation) on dehydrocholesterol. Excessive amounts in the mother may cause *hypervitaminosis D* expressed as hypercalcemia in infants. Since most milk in the United States is fortified with vitamin D at a level of 10 μg per quart, the daily consumption of a quart of milk provides the full allowance of vitamin D and of calcium as well for most gravidas.

Water-soluble Vitamins. The water-soluble vitamins, in contrast to those soluble in fat, are readily excreted in urine. The daily diet must supply the RDA because storage is limited. Toxicity with overdosage is less likely than with fat-soluble vitamins.

Folic Acid. The augmented maternal erythropoiesis of pregnancy requires substantially increased amounts of folic acid (folacin). Moreover, because folic acid is intimately involved in DNA synthesis, requirements are particularly high in rapidly growing cells such as fetal and placental tissues. In view of the evidence indicating increased folic acid needs during pregnancy and dietary survey data suggesting that the usual American diet is marginal in folic acid content, authorities have advised routine folic acid supplementation for pregnant women.

B Vitamins. An important function of thiamin (vitamin B_1), riboflavin (B_2), pyridoxine (B_6), and cobalamin (vitamin B_{12}) is that of coenzyme in metabolism. Suggested increased RDAs during pregnancy can usually be provided by the diet. Low maternal levels of vitamin B_{12} are associated with prematurity and occur more often in smokers than in nonsmokers.

Ascorbic Acid (Vitamin C). The entire requirement of vitamin C may be readily provided by dietary sources. Some people do not think of vitamins as medications. Pregnant women should be cautioned against unprescribed use of any vitamin preparation, including vitamin C. The possibility of beneficial effects of extremely large ascorbic acid supplements for prevention of the common cold has created considerable interest. Aside from the controversial aspect of this type of pharmacologic treatment, its use in pregnancy is open to serious question.

Vitamin and Mineral Supplements. Nutrition counselors (nurses, nutritionists) must assess whether the woman has sufficient knowledge, motivation, and income to follow the nutrition guidance given. If needs can be met through diet, vitamin and mineral supplementation may not be necessary. For some gravidas a careful selection of vitamin and mineral supplements is of some value if problems are anticipated. It must be noted that supplementation cannot compensate for poor food habits. In some instances the prescriptions of supplements may give both the woman and the health care professional a false sense of security.

NUTRITION RISK FACTORS IN PREGNANCY

To assess effectively the nutritional status of the pregnant or lactating woman, the nutrition counselor needs to understand the major nutrition risk factors. Nutrition risk factors include those present at the onset of pregnancy and those that may occur during the course of pregnancy.

Risk Factors at the Onset of Pregnancy

See Chapter 35 for a discussion of the nutrition risk factors for pregnant adolescents.

The woman who has had three or more pregnancies

within 2 years, as well as the multiparous woman who has progressed from one pregnancy directly to another, is considered to be at increased risk. These women are prone to depleted nutrient stores. This situation can potentially compromise maternal and fetal health and well-being.

Special attention should be paid to the woman's obstetric history. Poor weight gain in pregnancy, pregnancy-induced hypertension (PIH), a previous stillbirth or delivery of a low-birth-weight infant, premature delivery, and perinatal infection are all common in women who are or have been poorly nourished in the past. As a result the woman with a poor reproductive history may need more than usual nutrition guidance.

For economically deprived women there are several programs that help with the purchase of food or that offer supplements, for example, the federal food stamp program and the supplemental food program for women, infants, and children, sometimes known as the WIC program.

A woman may enter pregnancy either having been or continuing to be on a faddish or otherwise nutritionally inadequate diet. The woman who practices pica may not consume adequate levels of nutrients. **Pica** is defined as regular and excessive ingestion of nonfood items (Argo starch or red clay) or of foods with limited nutritional value. The practice often relates to cultural or geographic factors or both (pp. 322, 325).

Recently megavitamin supplementation has become popular. Persons on a megavitamin regimen ingest massive amounts of vitamins far above the RDA levels. There is no documentation that these large amounts of vitamins are beneficial (Luke, 1985; Mirkin, 1985).

There are various types of vegetarian diets (see p. 327). The lactoovovegetarian eats no meat, fish, or poultry but will use either eggs (ovo) or dairy products (lacto) or both. Of particular concern is the strict vegetarian (vegan), who eliminates all products of animal origin, including meat, poultry, fish, cheese, eggs, and milk. The pregnant woman who practices strict vegetarianism may not receive adequate quantitites of complementary and complete proteins and may not obtain enough vitamin B_{12}. Thoughtful nutrition counseling will be required to work out a diet pattern for a strict vegetarian during the prenatal period.

The person who is a heavy smoker (more than 6 cigarettes per day), drug addict, or alcoholic (chronically using more than 150 ml [5 oz] of whiskey per day or its equivalent of beer or wine) is likely to have major physiologic problems. The effects of smoking during pregnancy include reduction in gestation length (with onset of premature labor) and infants who are SGA. In addition, there is always the possibility that women who indulge excessively in the use of cigarettes, drugs, or alcohol may not consume sufficient quantities of nutritious food. (For detailed discussion, see Chapter 39 and Appendix G.)

Medical problems such as anemia, thyroid dysfunction, and chronic medical or surgical gastrointestinal disorders may be associated with interference with the ingestion, absorption, or utilization of nutrients. Drugs utilized in treatment of these conditions may also affect nutrition by similar interference. Nutrition counseling should combine general nutrition guidelines for prenatal care *and* diet therapy recommended for a particular woman's medical condition.

Risk Factors During Pregnancy

The iron needs during pregnancy are obtained from maternal iron stores, diet, and supplementation. True anemia occurring during pregnancy is most often caused by iron deficiency. Many healthy American women do not have iron stores large enough to meet the demands of pregnancy. Iron supplementation will aid greatly in maintaining the hemoglobin at normal levels.

The cause of PIH is not known. It is characterized by an elevation in blood pressure, proteinuria, and rapid weight gain caused by edema. There is considerable controversy over the influence of nutrition (particularly sodium and protein) on the development of PIH (Worthington-Roberts, 1985; Zlatnik, 1983).

Normal pregnancy is a time of progressive maternal weight gain. The following are presumptive signs of maternal and fetal malnutrition: (1) failure to gain weight (less than 0.9 kg [2 lb] per month during the second and third trimesters), (2) actual weight loss, (3) significant nausea and vomiting during early pregnancy, and (4) poor or delayed uterine-fetal growth.

Inadequate maternal weight gain has been associated with lowered birth weight and evidence of intrauterine growth retardation (IUGR). It is therefore important to document the pattern of weight gain in pregnancy as well as the total amount gained.

Total maternal weight gain during the 40 weeks of pregnancy averages 11.5 kg (25 lb). This amounts to about 1.4 to 1.8 kg (3 to 4 lb) per month. Rapid accumulation of weight in a singleton pregnancy—that is, 0.9 to 2.3 kg (2 to 5 lb) per week results only from tissue fluid retention and may be associated with PIH. The woman must be assessed carefully for development of this condition.

Excessive weight gain associated with accumulation of fat is less dramatic and is best assessed by evaluating the woman's eating habits and by measuring subcutaneous fat stores by means of skinfold calipers. Sources of energy-rich but nutritionally poor food should be identified and eliminated. Weight reduction in pregnancy or lactation by dietary manipulation or drug administration or both is contraindicated because of potentially adverse and possibly toxic effects on fetal nutrition, growth, and development.

Demands of Lactation

Increased nutritional demands of lactation can also be a risk factor. Storage of 2 or 3 kg of fat during pregnancy provides the gravida with a reservoir of some 14,000 to 24,000 kcal for lactation needs. Ordinarily, fat stores will be gradually utilized for the first 4 to 6 months of lactation.

Without the demands of nursing, fat stores may remain a permanent addition to the maternal frame and increase the potential for obesity with advancing age and parity. A modest reduction in caloric intake after delivery is appropriate for the woman who does not breastfeed her infant. This is particularly true if she uses an oral contraceptive agent. For discussion of nutrition and oral hormone contraception refer to Chapter 42.

Assessment

Adequate nutrition is vital throughout the life span. During pregnancy, nutrition plays a key role in achieving an optimum outcome for the mother and her unborn baby. Motivation to learn about nutrition is usually higher during pregnancy, as parents strive to "do what's right for the baby." Optimum nutrition cannot eliminate all problems that may arise in pregnancy, but it establishes a good foundation for supporting the needs of the mother and her unborn child.

An individual assessment and evaluation of nutritional status must be made at the beginning of prenatal care and continued throughout the pregnancy (Brennan, 1979). The following methods of assessment provide the data necessary to determine need:

1. Interview (individual and family history, dietary assessment)
2. Physical examination, including assessment for skinfold thickness
3. Laboratory tests

Interview

Health History. Data from the pregnant woman's history are among the most important elements in nutrition assessment. These data must include basic information carefully taken from the prenatal record; data that have a bearing on nutritional status (see Chapter 8). From the obstetric history it is important to note the woman's age, number of pregnancies, and their outcomes, and the interval between pregnancies. Several medical problems have a nutritional base. These problems include diabetes mellitus, cystic fibrosis, PKU, anemia, and lactose intolerance (White and Owsley, 1983).

Social and Experiential History. Food habits and attitudes cannot be viewed in isolation: life situations and values, as well as physical and emotional factors, must also be considered. Thus if nutrition counseling is to be valid, it must be based on an individual plan of care.

A woman's living situation will have an influence on her eating behavior. Therefore the data on the home setting, housing, life-style, family members, occupation, socioeconomic status, food assistance needs, and family roles and attitudes concerning foods are important. What is her activity level? Is she a housewife, office worker, or farm laborer? Are there other "special" circumstances, for example, is she a model or dancer? How many people eat together for each meal? How many meals are taken per day?

Nutrition-related folklore and myths need to be identified. Some beliefs may prevent the gravida from complying with sound nutritional guidelines. A number of old wives' tales are given here: eating for two; a tooth for every pregnancy; if you eat green peppers, your baby will be hairy; eating prunes may cause the infant's face to be wrinkled; eating pickles could give the baby a sour disposition; eating carrots gives the baby red hair; eating a lot of eggs or chicken makes the baby an early riser; eating cheese causes the womb to rot. Cultural-ethnic food and religious practices need to be explored.

It is important to determine special diet practices such as faddish or unusual patterns. Strict vegetarian diets or various forms of pica may be nutritionally unsound. The use of *all* medications and vitamin and mineral supplements should be discussed with the woman.

Food allergies and milk or lactose intolerance need to be explored (White and Owsley, 1983). Lactose intolerance is a problem for certain ethnic groups and individuals. The nurse's help is often needed for the family to plan for protein and calcium intake from sources other than milk. One food, tofu (soybean cake), contains considerable calcium but no lactose. Of the cheeses, Swiss cheese contains the least amount of lactose.

Dietary Assessment. A *nutrition questionnaire* covering the background information is a useful tool in dietary assessment. The California Department of Health Services (1975) developed an excellent instrument be used specifically by the physician, nurse, or registered dietitian. The nutrition questionnaire on p. 319 groups questions into 11 sections that identify factors that may influence prenatal nutrition.

Additional information is gathered with the following questions. How many meals and snacks are served per day and how are these spaced? What is a typical menu? What quantities are served? How are foods selected and cooked? What is the woman's level of understanding of good nutrition? What does she consider to be "good nutrition"?

Since pregnancy is a time in the life cycle when nutrition is of special importance, it is essential to learn who the mother is, what her needs are, and how these needs can best be met. What does she perceive as nutritional problems and solutions? Only in this context can realistic guidance be provided.

Review of Systems. Several functional gastrointestinal problems are common during pregnancy. Nausea and vomiting, constipation and hemorrhoids, heartburn, or a full feeling may interfere with optimum nutrition. These complaints are highly individual in character. Their existence is usually uncovered during the review of the physical systems (see Chapters 12, 13, and 14).

Physical Examination

Two problems bear on the validity of the physical examination. First, the lack of standard definitions and the nonspecificity of most clinical manifestations of malnutrition result in considerable variation in interpretation of physical signs. Second, pregnancy may complicate specific interpretation of physical signs. Despite these shortcomings the physical assessment of nutritional status can be useful if it is utilized in conjunction with the biochemical analyses and dietary assessment (Table 15-2).

General screening for *dental health status* provides helpful information on nutritional status. The most com-

NUTRITION QUESTIONNAIRE

Name: ______________________________ Date: __________

Please answer the following by checking the appropriate box or filling in the blank. Answer only those questions that apply to you. All information is confidential.

1. a. Before this pregnancy, what was your usual weight?
   ______ kg (______________ lb)
   ☐ Don't know
   b. During your last pregnancy, how much weight did you gain? ______ kg (______________ lb)
   ☐ Don't know
   c. How much weight do you expect to gain during this pregnancy? ______ kg (______________ lb)
   ☐ Don't know
   d. Have you ever had any problems with your weight?
   ☐ Yes ☐ No If yes, what? ☐ Underweight
   ☐ Overweight ☐ Other ______
2. a. How would you describe your appetite?
   ☐ Hearty ☐ Moderate ☐ Poor
   b. With this pregnancy, have you experienced either of the following? ☐ Nausea ☐ Vomiting
3. How would you describe your regular eating habits?
   ☐ Regular ☐ Irregular
4. a. Indicate the person who does the following in your household:
   Plans the meals ______________
   Buys the food ______________
   Prepares the food ______________
   b. How much is spent on food each week for your household? ______ ☐ Don't know
   How many people does this feed? ______
   c. Indicate the type of kitchen equipment you have in your home:
   ☐ Refrigerator ☐ Hot plate ☐ Stove
5. a. Are you *now* taking any vitamin or mineral supplement?
   ☐ Yes ☐ No
   b. Do you take any pills to control your weight?
   ☐ Yes ☐ No
   c. Do you take diuretic (water) pills?
   ☐ Yes ☐ No
6. a. Are you now on a diet to lose weight?
   ☐ Yes ☐ No
   b. Are you *now* on a special diet (low salt, diabetic, gallbladder, etc.)?
   ☐ Yes ☐ No
   If yes, what kind of diet? ______________
   c. If you have been on a special diet in the past, indicate what kind and when. ______________
   ____
   ____
7. a. Is there any food you *cannot* eat?
   ☐ Yes ☐ No
   If yes, what food(s)? ______________
   ____
   What happens when you eat this food? ______________
   ____
   b. Do you have any cravings for things such as
   ☐ Cornstarch ☐ Plaster ☐ Dirt or clay
   ☐ Other ______________
8. Do you have either of the following problems?
   ☐ Constipation ☐ Diarrhea
9. a. Do you smoke? ☐ Yes ☐ No
   b. Do you drink any alcoholic beverages (liquor, wine, beer)? ☐ Yes ☐ No
10. Are you receiving either of the following?
   ☐ Food stamps ☐ WIC vouchers
11. How do you want to feed your baby? ☐ Breast milk ☐ Evaporated milk formula ☐ Commercial formula ☐ Undecided

Adapted from Nutrition during pregnancy and lactation, Sacramento, Calif, 1975, Maternal and Child Health Branch, California Department of Health Services.

mon clinical nutrition-related disorders that are likely to be encountered during the reproductive years are caries and periodontitis. These conditions cause mechanical and mastication difficulties that interfere with the ingestion of certain types of food.

Anthropometry, the study of human body measurements, provides both short- and long-term indications of the level of nutrition and is therefore a valuable component of the nutrition assessment profile. Assessment of height, weight, and skinfold thickness is performed. Care must be taken to ensure that proper equipment and techniques are used for anthropometric assessment; for example, the scale is calibrated to zero before a weight is taken.

Measurements of weight-for-age and weight-for-height are used in assessing obesity, but they do fail to distinguish muscular and skeletal tissue mass from fat. On the other hand, serial weight measurements give a reasonable indication of excessive weight gain and likely obesity.

Lean body mass can be estimated from the triceps fat-fold thickness and upper arm circumference. Measurement of skinfold thickness is the most convenient method of objectively assessing relative fatness. In general, two fat-fold measurements, one on a limb (left triceps) and one on the trunk (left subscapular), are advised to account for differing distributions of fat.

Erroneous information regarding specific indexes such as height and weight measurements can lead to inappropriate conclusions. An incomplete or inaccurate data base can result in poor decisions and client care management.

Laboratory Tests

Laboratory data provide vital baseline information for nutrition assessment at the beginning of pregnancy as well

Table 15-2 *Physical Assessment of Nutritional Status*

Signs of Good Nutrition	Signs of Poor Nutrition
General Appearance	
Alert, responsive	Listless, apathetic, cachectic
Weight	
Normal for height, age, body build	Overweight or underweight (special concern for underweight)
Posture	
Erect, arms and legs straight	Sagging shoulders, sunken chest, humped back
Muscles	
Well developed, firm, good tone, some fat under skin	Flaccid, poor tone, undeveloped, tender, "wasted" appearance, cannot walk properly
Nervous Control	
Good attention span, not irritable or restless, normal reflexes, psychologic stability	Inattentive, irritable, confused, burning and tingling of hands and feet (parasthesia), loss of position and vibratory sense, weakness and tenderness of muscles (may result in inability to walk), decrease or loss of ankle and knee reflexes
Gastrointestinal Function	
Good appetite and digestion, normal regular elimination, no palpable organs or masses	Anorexia, indigestion, constipation or diarrhea, liver or spleen enlargement
Cardiovascular Function	
Normal heart rate and rhythm, no murmurs, normal blood pressure for age	Rapid heart rate (above 100 beats/min: tachycardia), enlarged heart, abnormal rhythm, elevated blood pressure
General Vitality	
Endurance, energetic, sleeps well, vigorous	Easily fatigued, no energy, falls asleep easily, looks tired, apathetic
Hair	
Shiny, lustrous, firm, not easily plucked, healthy scalp	Stringy, dull, brittle, dry, thin and sparse, depigmented, can be easily plucked
Skin (General)	
Smooth, slightly moist, good color	Rough, dry, scaly, pale, pigmented, irritated, easily bruised, petechiae
Face and Neck	
Skin color uniform, smooth, pink, healthy appearance, not swollen	Greasy, discolored, scaly, swollen, skin dark over cheeks and under eyes, lumpiness or flakiness of skin around nose and mouth
Lips	
Smooth, good color, moist, not chapped or swollen	Dry, scaly, swollen, redness, angular lesions at corners of mouth, fissured, scarred (cheilosis, stomatitis)
Mouth, Oral Membranes	
Reddish pink mucous membranes in oral cavity	Swollen, boggy oral mucous membranes
Gums	
Reddish pink, healthy, no swelling or bleeding	Spongy, bleed easily, marginal redness, inflamed, gums receding
Tongue	
Healthy pink or deep reddish in appearance, not swollen or smooth, surface papillae present, no lesions	Swollen, scarlet and raw, magenta color, beefy (glossitis), hyperemic and hypertrophic papillae, atrophic papillae
Teeth	
No cavities, no pain, bright, straight, no crowding, well-shaped jaw, clean, no discoloration	Unfilled caries, absent teeth, worn surfaces, mottled (fluorosis), malpositioned
Eyes	
Bright, clear, shiny, no sores at corners of eyelids, membranes moist and healthy pink color, no prominent blood vessels or mound of tissue on sclera, no fatigue circles beneath	Eye membranes pale (pale conjunctiva), redness of membrane (conjunctival injection), dryness, signs of infection, Bitot's spots, redness and fissuring of eyelid corners (angular palpebritis), dryness of eye membrane (conjunctival xerosis), dull appearance of cornea (corneal xerosis), soft cornea (keratomalacia)
Neck (Glands)	
No enlargement	Thyroid enlarged
Nails	
Firm, pink	Spoon shaped (koilonychia), brittle, ridged
Legs, Feet	
No tenderness, weakness, or swelling; good color	Edema, tender calf, tingling, weakness
Skeleton	
No malformations	Bowlegs, knock-knees, chest deformity at diaphragm, beaded ribs, prominent scapulas

From Williams, SR: Nutritional guidance in prenatal case. In Worthington-Roberts, BS, Vermeersch, J, and Williams, SR: Nutrition in pregnancy and lactation, ed 3, St. Louis, 1985, The CV Mosby Co.

as a means of monitoring nutritional status throughout gestation. In general, laboratory tests provide a more objective and precise determination of nutritional status than do other assessment indexes.

Blood-forming Nutrients. Measures of the blood-forming nutrients—iron, folacin, and vitamins B_6 and B_{12}—are important guides for use in preventing and treating anemias often associated with pregnancy (see Chapter 34). The following can be measured in routine tests:

1. Hemoglobin levels
2. Hematocrit levels
3. Mean corpuscular volume (MCV)
4. Mean corpuscular hemoglobin concentration (MCHC)
5. Serum iron levels and percentage of concentration in saturation
6. Transferrin levels

Other tests include those for folic acid deficiency?

1. MCV
2. Hypersegmented polymorphonuclear leukocytes
3. Serum folic acid
4. RBC folic acid
5. Serum protein

Serum Albumin. An adequate level of serum albumin is important during pregnancy. Serum albumin helps maintain normal flow of tissue fluids from the circulating blood through the tissue for nourishment of cells and back into circulation by means of capillary fluid shift mechanisms. A protein deficit would contribute to a lowered plasma albumin level and in turn to an imbalance in the fluid shift mechanism, resulting in edema. An acceptable level of serum albumin during pregnancy is 3.5 g/dl or above.

Minerals and Vitamins. Depending on individual situations, tests for other vitamin and mineral levels may be performed, including determinations of the water-soluble vitamins (thiamin, riboflavin, niacin, and vitamin C), the fat-soluble vitamins (A, D, E, and K), and trace minerals.

Blood Lipids, Glucose, and Enzymes. Routine testing for urine sugar and ketone bodies is often done to screen for latent diabetes mellitus or gestational glycosuria. However, more definitive tests are necessary for accurate assessment for endocrine disturbances such as diabetes mellitus (Chapter 32). Other tests may be performed, if there is a complicating chronic disease, particularly cardiovascular or renal disease.

Nursing Diagnoses

Each gravida and her family will present the nurse with a unique set of nutritional needs. The nurse formulates appropriate nursing diagnoses based on the identified needs from the assessment data. Following are examples of nutrition-related nursing diagnoses arising from the course of prenatal period:

- Altered nutrition, less than body requirements, related to
  - Imbalance of intake versus activity expenditures
  - Inability to procure food (related to finances or cultural prescription)
  - Chewing difficulties secondary to poor dental hygiene
- Knowledge deficit, related to
  - Adequate nutrition or reliance on vitamin-mineral supplementation
  - Pica
  - Nutrition-related discomforts of pregnancy
  - Old wives' tales
  - Iron supplementation
- Potential for injury: fetus, related to
  - Overdoses of vitamins

See guidelines for client teaching, nursing care plan, and summary of nursing actions in this chapter.

Planning

The information in this chapter is general in nature. A plan is developed for each gravida utilizing content that relates specifically to her and her family's nutritional needs. Collaboration among the nurse, the registered dietitian, and the client is basic to the following step in the nursing process: setting the goals in client-centered terms, prioritizing the goals, and selecting nursing actions that will assist the client to meet the goals.

The Health Team Approach

The health team approach has been devised as an attempt to meet some of the problems brought about by the rapid increase in population and the equally rapid expansion of scientific knowledge, which has brought an increasing complexity to health care. The rapid advance of science requires the cooperation of a team of specialists who share their special knowledge and learn from each other for the welfare of the client.

Whether functioning in the hospital, the clinic, or the community, the registered dietitian (RD) and the nurse hold positions on the health team in a unique relation to the client. In certain respects they are closest to the client and the family and have the opportunity to help determine many of the client's needs, which include basic nutritional requirements. They must coordinate services and often are the only ones who can help the client understand and participate in her care. They have unparalleled opportunity to practice continuous client-centered care that treats the whole person. In carrying out the other aspect of this role, it will commonly be the RD or the nurse who reminds the entire health team that a person has emotional as well as physical needs, that she is part of a family whose members are also involved in her care, that she has responsibilities in or out of the home, and that she lives in a specific community environment.

Such practitioners are concerned not merely with the *how* but also with the *why*. More pointedly still, they are concerned with the *who* and realize that their most therapeutic contribution is their genuine involvement and concern.

Goals

General goals directed to the maternity population as a whole include the following:

1. To provide nutrition-related services for all pregnant women and their fetuses or newborns and families
2. To ensure optimum nutrition for women of childbearing age
3. To ensure optimum nutrition for the gravida and her fetus
4. To involve the woman as a participant in her own care

Implementation

Nurses assume many caregiving roles during the prenatal period including supportive and teacher/counselor/advocate.

Supportive Activities

The nurse-client relationship is important in setting the tone for further interactions (see Chapter 2). The techniques of listening with an attentive expression, touching, and using eye contact have their place, as does recognition of the client's feelings and her right to express them. One common complaint of gravidas is the weighing-in at the start of a prenatal visit. Weighing-in should be ego-building and psychologically unthreatening. Many women state that they "shake in their boots" while waiting to hear remarks of disgust and condemnation for gaining too much. To avoid this disapproval, some starve themselves the evening before the visit or take diuretics ("water pills"). Both alternatives are detrimental to the health of the mother and her unborn child (Dohrmann and Lederman, 1986).

Nutrition counseling provides the nurse with the opportunity to commend the gravida for her knowledge and use of good nutrition practices. The nurse can assist the woman to set her own goals and make her own decisions.

Teacher/Counselor/Advocate

There are several tools that are useful in providing nutrition information to the pregnant woman. The tools include a daily food guide, a sample meal pattern and sample menus, and information on ethnic preferences and vegetarian diets.

Daily Food Guide. A diet consisting of a variety of foods from all the basic food groups can supply needed nutrients (Table 15-3). The increased quantities of essential nutrients needed during pregnancy may be met by skillful planning around a daily food guide based on the RDAs.

It is necessary to show the woman how the daily food guide can be used. Table 15-4 provides a sample daily meal pattern and sample menus. A mutually developed plan is more likely to be followed by the client. Gravidas find a collaboratively written shopping list helpful in implementing the planned menus.

Ethnic and Cultural Influences. Consideration of a woman's cultural food preferences enhances the communication between her and her counselor, thus providing a greater opportunity to obtain compliance with a prescribed diet. However, within one cultural group there may occur several variations. Women in most cultures are encouraged to eat a normal diet. The nurse needs to know what constitutes a normal diet for each ethnic group. Thus careful exploration of individual preferences is needed (Table 15-5). The emphasis of counseling is to build an adequate diet utilizing the woman's usual foods and food preferences. To do otherwise is to waste time and energy for both the woman and the nurse.

Among Chinese-Americans, herbal teas, such as ginseng, may be used as a tonic in early pregnancy, and to strengthen the womb during the seventh and eighth months (Campbell and Change, 1973; Dunn, 1978). Chung (1977) refers to the use of ginseng tea as a dietary supplement by Chinese mothers, but these same women refuse

Table 15-3 *Daily Food Plan for Pregnancy and Lactation*

Food	Nonpregnant Woman	Pregnant Woman	Lactating Woman
Milk, cheese, ice cream, skimmed milk or buttermilk (food made with milk can supply part of requirement)	2 C	3-4 C	4-5 C
Meat (lean meat, fish, poultry, cheese, occasional dried beans or peas)	1 serving (3-4 oz)	2 servings (6-8 oz); include liver frequently	2½ servings (8 oz)
Eggs	1	1-2	1-2
Vegetable* (dark green or deep yellow)	1 serving	1 serving	1-2 servings
Vitamin C—rich food* Good source—citrus fruit, berries, cantaloupe Fair source—tomatoes, cabbage, greens, potatoes in skin	1 good source or 2 fair sources	1 good source and 1 fair source or 2 good sources	1 good source and 1 fair source or 2 good sources
Other vegetables and fruits	2 servings	4-6 servings	4-6 servings
Bread† and cereals (enriched or whole grain)	6 servings	10 servings	10 servings
Butter or fortified margarine	Moderate amount	Moderate amount	Moderate amount

Adapted from Williams, SR: Basic nutrition and diet therapy, ed 8, St Louis, 1988, The CV Mosby Co.

*Use some raw daily.

†One slice of bread equals 1 serving.

Table 15-4 *Sample Menus*

	Nonpregnant Woman	Pregnant Woman	Lactating Woman
Breakfast	120 ml (4 oz) orange juice ½ C oatmeal 240 ml (8 oz) milk Coffee or tea*	120 ml (4 oz) orange juice ½ C oatmeal 240 ml (8 oz) milk Coffee or tea*	120 ml (4 oz) orange juice ½ C oatmeal 240 ml (8 oz) milk Coffee or tea*
Morning snack		Fruit and/or cheese†	Fruit and/or cheese†
Lunch	1 tuna fish sandwich made with: 2 slices whole wheat bread ½ C tuna fish Diced celery and onion to taste, mayonnaise,* lettuce* 1 medium apple 240 ml (8 oz) milk	1 tuna fish sandwich made with: 2 slices whole wheat bread ½ C tuna fish, 1 hard-boiled egg Diced celery and onion to taste,* mayonnaise,* lettuce* 1 medium apple 240 ml (8 oz) milk	1 tuna fish sandwich made with: 2 slices whole wheat bread ½ C tuna fish, 1 hard-boiled egg Diced celery and onion to taste,* mayonnaise,* lettuce* 1 medium apple 240 ml (8 oz) milk
Afternoon snack		½ C salted peanuts 120 ml (4 oz) milk	½ C salted peanuts 240 ml (8 oz) milk
Dinner	3 oz roast beef ½ C egg noodles* with sautéed poppy seeds* ¾ C cut asparagus Salad made with: 1 C torn spinach Sliced mushrooms and radishes to taste* Oil and vinegar* Coffee or tea	6 oz roast beef ½ C egg noodles* with sautéed poppy seeds,* 1 pat butter ¾ C cut asparagus Salad made with: 1 C torn spinach Sliced mushrooms and radishes to taste,* tomato Oil and vinegar* 240 ml (8 oz) milk Coffee or tea	6-9 oz roast beef ½ C egg noodles* with sautéed poppy seeds,* 1 pat butter ¾ C cut asparagus Salad made with: 1 C torn spinach Sliced mushrooms and radishes to taste,* tomato Oil and vinegar* 240 ml (8 oz) milk Coffee or tea
Evening snack		1-2 oatmeal raisin cookies* 120 ml (4 oz) milk	2 oatmeal raisin cookies* 240 ml (8 oz) milk

Adapted from nutrition during pregnancy and lactation, Sacramento, 1975, Maternal and Child Health Branch, California Department of Health Services.
*This food is optional and is added to the basic diet.
†Serving size determined by caloric or dietary need.

Table 15-5 *Characteristic Food Patterns of Some Cultures*

Ethnic Group	Milk Group	Meat Group	Fruits and Vegetables	Breads and Cereals	Possible Dietary Problems
American Indian (many tribal variations; many "Americanized")	Fresh milk Evaporated milk for cooking Ice cream Cream pies	Pork, beef, lamb, rabbit Fowl, fish, eggs Legumes Sunflower seeds Nuts: walnut, acorn, pine, peanut butter Game meat	Green peas, beans Beets, turnips Leafy green and other vegetables Grapes, bananas, peaches, other fresh fruits Roots	Refined bread Whole wheat Cornmeal Rice Dry cereals "Fry" bread Tortillas	Obesity, diabetes, alcoholism, nutritional deficiencies expressed in dental problems and iron deficiency anemia Inadequate amounts of all nutrients Excessive use of sugar
Middle Eastern (Armenian, Greek, Syrian, Turkish)	Yogurt Little butter	Lamb Nuts Dried peas, beans, lentils	Peppers Tomatoes Cabbage Grape leaves Cucumbers Squash Dried apricots, raisins	Cracked wheat and dark bread	Fry many meats and vegetables Lack of fresh fruits Insufficient foods from milk group (use olive oil* in place of butter) Like sweetenings, lamb fat, and olive oil
Black	Milk Ice Cream Puddings	Pork: all cuts, plus organs, chitterlings	Leafy vegetables Green and yellow vegetables	Cornmeal and hominy grits Rice	Extensive use of frying, "smothering," or simmering

*Olive oil is all fat, with no other nutrient value.

Continued.

Table 15-5 *Characteristic Food Patterns of Some Cultures—cont'd*

Ethnic Group	Milk Group	Meat Group	Fruits and Vegetables	Breads and Cereals	Possible Dietary Problems
	Cheese: longhorn, American	Beef, lamb Chicken, giblets Eggs Nuts Legumes Fish, game	Potato: white, sweet Stewed fruit Bananas, and other fresh fruit	Biscuits, pancakes, white breads Puddings: bread rice Molasses*	Fats: salt pork, bacon drippings, lard, and gravies Like sweets Insufficient citrus and enriched breads Vegetables often boiled for long periods Limited amounts from milk group
Chinese (Cantonese most prevalent)	Cheese Milk: water buffalo	Pork sausage† Eggs and pigeon eggs Fish Lamb, beef, goat Fowl: chicken, duck Nuts Legumes	Many vegetables Radish leaves Bean, bamboo sprouts Soybean curd (tofu)‡	Rice/rice flour products Cereals, noodles Wheat, corn, millet seed	Tendency of northern China (Mandarin), coastal China (Shanghai), and inland China (Szechwan) immigrants to use more grease in cooking Limited use of milk and milk products Often low in protein, calories, or both May wash rice before cooking Soy sauce, ginger
Filipino (Spanish-Chinese influence)	Flavored milk Milk in coffee Cheese: gouda, cheddar	Pork, beef, goat, deer, rabbit Chicken Fish Eggs Nuts Legumes	Many vegetables and fruits	Rice, cooked cereals Noodles: rice, wheat	Limited use of milk and milk products Tend to prewash rice May have only small portions of protein foods
Italian	Cheese Some ice cream	Meat Eggs Dried beans	Leafy vegetables Potatoes Eggplant Spinach Fruits	Macaroni White breads, some whole wheat Farina Cereals	Prefer expensive imported cheeses; reluctant to substitute less expensive domestic varieties Tendency to overcook vegetables Limited use of whole grains Enjoys sweets Extensive use of olive oil Insufficient servings from milk group
Japanese (Isei, more Japanese influence; Nisei, more westernized)	Increasing amounts being used by younger generations	Pork, beef, chicken Fish Eggs Legumes: soya, red, lima beans Nuts	Many vegetables and fruits Seaweed Tofu	Rice, rice cakes Wheat noodles Refined bread, noodles	Excessive salt: pickles, salty crisp seaweed Insufficient servings from milk group May use refined or prewashed rice High intake of MSG and soy sauce

*Light molasses (first extraction): 1 tbsp = 50 calories, 33 mg of calcium, 0.9 mg of iron, 0.01 mg each of vitamins B_1 and B_2; dark molasses (third extraction): 1 tbsp = 45 calories, 137 mg of calcium, 3.2 mg of iron, 0.02 mg of vitamin B_1, 0.04 mg of vitamin B_2, 0.4 mg of niacin.

†Lower in fat content than Western sausage.

‡Good source of protein.

Table 15-5 *Characteristic Food Patterns of Some Cultures—cont'd*

Ethnic Group	Milk Group	Meat Group	Fruits and Vegetables	Breads and Cereals	Possible Dietary Problems
Mexican-Spanish, Mexican-American	Milk Cheese Flan Ice Cream	Beef, pork, lamb, chicken, tripe, hot sausage, beef intestines Fish Eggs Nuts Dry beans: pinto, chick-peas (often eaten more than once daily)	Spinach, wild greens, tomatoes, chilies, corn, cactus leaves, cabbage, avocado, potatoes Pumpkin, zapote, peaches, guava, papaya, citrus	Rice, oats, cornmeal Sweet bread Tortilla: corn, flour Biscuits Vermicelli *(fideo)*	Limited meats primarily due to economics Limited use of milk and milk products Some tendency toward increasing use of flour tortillas over more nutritious corn tortillas Large amounts of lard *(manteca)* Abundant use of sugar Tendency to boil vegetables for long periods
Polish	Milk Sour cream Cheese Butter	Pork (preferred) Chicken	Vegetables Cabbage Roots Fruits	Dark rye	Like sweets Tendency to over-cook vegetables Limited fruits (especially citrus), raw vegetables, and meats
Puerto Rican	Limited use of milk products Coffee with milk *(café con leche)*	Pork Poultry Eggs (Fridays) Dried codfish Beans (habichuelas)	Avacado, okra Eggplant Sweet yams Starchy vegetables and fruits *(viandas)*	Rice Cornmeal	Use small amounts of pork and poultry Use fat, lard, salt pork, and olive oil extensively Lack of butter and other milk products
Scandinavian: Danish, Finnish, Norwegian, Swedish	Cream Butter	Wild game Reindeer Fish Eggs	Fruit berries Dried fruit Vegetables: cole slaw, roots, avocado	Whole wheat, rye, barley, sweets (molasses for flavoring)	Insufficient fresh fruits and vegetables Like sweets, pickled salted meats, and fish
Southeast Asian: Vietnamese, Cambodian	Generally not taken Coffee with condensed cow's milk Plain yogurt Ice cream (rare) Soybean milk	Fish (daily): fresh, dried, salted Poultry/eggs: duck, chicken Pork Beef (seldom) Dry beans Bean curd	Seasonal variety: fresh or preserved Green, leafy Yams Corn Bean noodles	Rice: grains, flour, noodles, "cellophane" French bread	Fresh milk products generally not consumed Poultry/eggs: dependent on family wealth Meat considered "unclean" is avoided Pregnant women prefer a diet high in salt and pepper as well as rice and pork High intake of MSG and soy sauce
Jewish: orthodox	Milk Cheese	Meat (bloodless; Kosher prepared): beef, lamb, goat, deer, poultry (all types) Fish with fins and scales only No crustaceans	Wide variety	Wide variety	Milk and milk products not eaten with meat; milk may be taken before the meal or 6 hours following meal; different sets of dishes and silverware are used to serve milk and meat products

iron supplements supplied by Western medicine because they believe their bones will harden and they will have a difficult delivery.

Stern (1981) found that Filipino-Americans rarely attempt to explain their dietary beliefs to maternity nurses and obstetricians. They concur politely with dietary instructions and then return home to follow their traditional diet. However, nurses need to remember that dietary patterns, although ingrained, actually change rapidly, sometimes within one generation, and an individual food history is an important adjunct to knowledge of cultural food habits.

Food taboos are more common than food prescriptions. Vietnamese women are to avoid "unclean" foods such as beef, dog, rat, and snake meat (Hollingsworth et al., 1980). Japanese women are cautioned against hot, spicey, and salty food, as are Filipino women. Filipino women are to avoid sweet foods because they may cause a big baby and a difficult delivery (Affonso, 1978), whereas Japanese women are encouraged to gain as much weight as they are comfortable with, believing that a large weight gain is good for the baby (Bernstein and Kidd, 1982). Blacks in the southern United States, Guatemalans, Mexicans, and Mexican-Americans should not eat acid foods or fresh fruits and vegetables (Kay, 1982). According to Snow (1974), red meat should be avoided by blacks because it is too strong and virile a food.

Food taboos often follow the principles of imitative magic, in which physical characteristics of food eaten by the mother may be transmitted to the child. Filipinos avoid eating prunes (Affonso, 1978) and Chinese avoid eating soy sauce (Campbell and Change, 1973), in both instances to prevent a dark-skinned infant. Birthmarks and their pigmentation are often associated with the shape and color of the food eaten, such as the strawberry mark (Carrington, 1978). Campbell and Chang (1973) report that some Chinese mothers shun shellfish during the first trimester, believing it is responsible for allergies in the latter life of the child. Korean-American gravidas avoid duck, eggs, and peaches since these are some of the foods believed to affect the fetus adversely (Choi, 1986). The research highlight describes a study of Korean-American mothers.

Filipino mothers have said that they are not to eat squid during pregnancy for fear that the mother's insides will become tangled and the baby's cord will tie around its neck (Affonso, 1978).

Food cravings during pregnancy are considered normal by many cultures, but the specific kinds of cravings may be culturally specific (Carrington, 1978; Obeyesekere, 1963). In most cultures women crave acceptable foods, such as chicken, fish, and greens among blacks (Carrington, 1978). Affonso (1978) notes that the Filipinos believe cravings should be satisfied to prevent the premature arrival of the infant.

Women in some cultures desire nonnutritive substances such as laundry starch, clay, and dirt. Desiring or eating of these substances is called **pica.** Kay (1982) describes Mexican-American women eating clay. All of these nonnutritive substances are used by black women (Carrington, 1978). A longitudinal study indicated that 40% of pregnant women in Mississippi eat clay (Vermeer and Frate, 1975). One Canadian Ojibwa woman who had had five children stated that with each pregnancy she craved and ate large quantities of "clean" dirt.

RESEARCH HIGHLIGHT

Unique Aspects of Korean-American Mothers

Purpose

A descriptive study was conducted to explore Korean beliefs and attitudes toward pregnancy, birth, and postpartum practices.

Sample

The sample consisted of 21 healthy Korean-American mothers and their term infants.

Methodology

A questionnaire was developed specifically to assess Korean beliefs and attitudes.

Findings

Dietary strictures of Tae Kyo are (1) to rest and eat frequently, (2) to eschew certain foods, and (3) to avoid certain foods during pregnancy. Most of the mothers (81%) disagreed with the need to rest and eat frequently. As for abstention from certain foods, 43% complied. Finally, although 48% stated that they had avoided certain foods during pregnancy, 52% of the women did not.

Generally the Korean mothers chose to eat acceptable food by Tae Kyo practices and avoided taboo foods. They chose the best quality food in terms of appearance and shape so that they would not harm the unborn child. The most influential person regarding the food taboo was the expectant woman's mother.

Implications

The investigator stresses the importance of the effect of culture on mother-infant interaction and the importance of determining cultural practices and their meaning of health care to all expecting mothers, as well as to Korean mothers.

Choi, EC: Unique aspects of Korean-American mothers, J Obstet Gynecol Neonat Nurs 15(5):394, 1986.

Certain ethnic groups have been identified as having a greater incidence of pica than others. Lackey (1978) studied groups of black women and white women and found that women in both groups ate substances such as clay and starch, although the percentage of black women was higher. Causes of pica have been attributed to a variety of reasons and may be engaged in by children, as well as pregnant women. Pica may be a psychologic response of someone needing attention, a truly cultural phenomenon, a response to hunger, or the body's response to needed nutrients. Scientific controversy exists about whether the iron deficiency observed in persons with pica is the cause or the effect of the anemia. Whatever the reason, according to Leiderman et al. (1977), a documented sequela is increased iron deficiency anemia because of interference with absorption of necessary nutrients when clay is eaten.

Vegetarian Diet Practices. Vegetarianism has gained popularity in recent years. Foods basic to almost all vegetarian diets are vegetables, fruits, legumes, nuts, and grains.

Vegetarian diets may not satisfy all nutrient requirements for the pregnant and lactating woman. The use of eggs and of milk and milk products varies. There are four basic types of vegetarians:

1. *Lactoovovegetarian.* The vegetable diet is supplemented with milk, eggs, and cheese. There is no problem in securing adequate protein with this diet.
2. *Lactovegetarian.* The vegetable diet is supplemented with milk and cheese. Milk products add complete protein to this diet.
3. *Pure vegetarian, or vegan.* The all-vegetable diet includes vegetables, fruits, legumes, nuts, and grains but is not supplemented with any animal foods, dairy products, or eggs. More careful planning is required to achieve combinations providing the necessary amounts of the essential amino acids. Vitamin B_{12} deficiency is a potential problem.
4. *Fruitarian.* The fruitarian diet consists of raw or dried fruits, nuts, honey, and olive oil. Potential inadequacy is greater in this diet than in other diets.

In general, protein is not a problem for the vegetarian when caloric intake is adequate and a wide variety of plant proteins are selected. A modified food guide for vegetarians is presented in Table 15-6. It is necessary to eat certain combinations of plant foods to obtain complete proteins. These complete proteins contain the eight essential amino acids in amounts necessary for growth and maintenance. Unlike animal foods, most plant foods do not contain all the essential amino acids in these appropriate amounts. If one essential amino acid is missing, the protein is incomplete and cannot be utilized to build body tissues. The appropriate combination of two or more plant foods eaten at the same meal can make a "complete" protein.

Iron Supplementation and Nutrition Counseling. An important responsibility of the nurse is to teach women about meeting nutritional needs for themselves and their unborn babies. Guidelines for client teaching about iron supplementation are given below. Table 15-7 is another format that can be used for nutrition counseling during pregnancy.

Table 15-6 *Modified Food Guide for Vegetarian Diets*

	Recommended Number of Servings			
	Lactovegetarian		Lactoovovegetarian	
Food Group	Adult	Pregnant Adult	Adult	Pregnant Adult
Milk	4	5	4	5
Protein				
Eggs (2 = 1 serving)	0	0	½	1
Legumes	2	3	2	3
Nuts	1	1	1	1
Fruits and vegetables				
Vitamin C	3	3	3	3
Vitamin A	1½	2	1½	2
Other	3	4	3	3
Whole grain products	6	7	5	6
Others	0	1	0	1

Guidelines for Client Teaching

IRON SUPPLEMENTATION

ASSESSMENT

1. Gravida is in her second trimester. She mentions that she has been ingesting dry laundry starch because "all pregnant women crave it."
2. Woman is chewing ice from a paper cup while waiting to be seen by the physician.
3. Laboratory values: hemoglobin 10.2 g/dl; hematocrit, 34%.

NURSING DIAGNOSES

Altered nutrition: less than body requirements related to pica and the ingestion of nonnutritive substances.

Knowledge deficit related to pica and its possible significance.

Knowledge deficit related to proper nutrition, iron deficiency, and its effect on woman and her fetus.

GOALS

Short-term

Gravida starts taking iron supplement, as prescribed, immediately.

Gravida's laboratory data for hemoglobin and hematocrit indicate beginning improvement with the next test.

Gravida stops ingesting dry laundry starch.

Intermediate

Gravida continues to take iron supplements as long as prescribed.

Gravida understands anemia and its potential effects on her and her baby.

Gravida eats foods that are nutritionally sound.

Long-term

Woman and her baby do not suffer any adverse effects of anemia.

REFERENCES AND TEACHING AIDS

Printed instructions for using iron supplements.

Hospital-supplied pamphlets on nutrition, including information on food groups and supplements.

Laboratory slips showing woman's blood values.

Continued.

Guidelines For Client Teaching—cont'd

CONTENT/RATIONALE	TEACHING ACTION
To provide information about pica, share the following: Pica is a learned behavior. Cravings are not uncommon; if diet is well-balanced, occasional indulgence is probably not harmful. Many cultures have specific beliefs about cravings and "making the baby" or ease of delivery. Nonnutritive foods may provide unwanted calories, interfere with the absorption of iron, and contribute to iron-deficiency anemia.	Few women are willing to volunteer information on pica, so sensitive questioning is necessary to uncover the practice. Discuss the reasons for woman's cravings. Provide information on this practice without demeaning the woman's underlying cultural beliefs. Encourage discussion and questions.
To facilitate understanding of woman's condition: Discuss woman's laboratory report. Define hemoglobin, hematocrit, red blood cells, anemia; explain values and normal parameters.	Review, assess woman's level of understanding. Discuss clinical significance of the differences.
To increase woman's knowledge of nutrition: Discuss building blood through diet. Explain types and amounts of bloodforming nutrients. Explain that food sources of nutrients, such as liver and other red meats, dried beans, dried fruit, deep green vegetables, eggs, and enriched cereals, provide sources of iron.	Review; help woman identify food sources of nutrients in her current diet; praise her. Assist with menu selection to meet woman's preferences and her cultural prescriptions and proscriptions. Involve family members in planning dietary intake if possible.
To increase woman's knowledge of medical therapy for iron-deficienty anemia: Discuss building blood through iron supplementation (30 to 60 mg of elemental iron [150 to 300 mg of ferrous sulfate]). Explain that iron is absorbed most readily in the ferrous form in the presence of acid, before meals, but iron tablets on an empty stomach are highly irritating. Explain that enteric forms of iron supplementation are less effective because of poor absorption beyond the duodenum. Identify foods that decrease iron absorption: milk, cereal, and eggs.	Review this information Discuss and plan proper administration: Divide daily dose into 3 equal doses. Take tablets with a citrus fruit juice, which is a good source of vitamin C, or with vitamin C, 500 mg, orally, once daily. Take tablets after eating food that does not include cereal, eggs, or milk. Time medication to fit woman's (family's) mealtime and her convenience. After the first trimester and nausea has subsided, woman may be able to take the tablet with orange juice between meals.
To foster woman's compliance: Discuss side effects of iron supplementation: stools become dark-green to black in appearance; they may become more formed, contributing to constipation, or become loose; and gastric irritation and bad taste may occur.	Review side effects sensitively.
Monitor woman's progress—within 1 week there is an increase in the number of reticulocytes (immature red blood cells) and in the rate of hemoglobin synthesis.	Review woman's laboratory findings that confirm her improvement and provide her with tangible proof of her success; give appropriate praise.
To protect older children: Review need to secure medications from other children.	Review safety precautions against accidental ingestion of chemicals.

EVALUATION The nurse can be assured that teaching was effective when her laboratory report shows improvement in anemia (e.g., increase in reticulocyte count, mean corpuscular hemoglobin, hemoglobin, and hematocrit). The woman will indicate she has dark stools, can and does choose appropriate foods, and reduces or eliminates pica. The woman verbalizes her understanding of pica and anemia, and their potential effects on her and her fetus.

Table 15-7 *Examples of Nutrition Counseling During Pregnancy*

Client Knowledge Needs	Goals	Nursing Actions	Outcome Criteria
Why are nutrient needs increased during pregnancy?	Woman will know reason for increased nutrient and energy needs during pregnancy.	Explain that pregnancy is like building a house (the baby). You need materials (nutrients) and labor (energy). If you do not have enough materials or labor, the house will not be big or strong. This is also true for the baby.	Woman will explain why she needs more nutrients and energy while she is pregnant.
What are extra nutrients needed during pregnancy? How can they be obtained?	Woman will know additional nutrients needed during pregnancy and how to fulfill this need. Woman will meet her nutrient needs.	Explain that although all nutrient needs are increased during pregnancy, **seven** nutrients are particularly essential: **calories, protein, calcium, iron supplements, viamin A, vitamin C,** and **folic acid.** Use 24-hr recall to point out areas of concern. Discuss daily food guide (see Table 15-3).	Woman will identify which nutrients should be increased, including calories, protein, calcium, iron, vitamin A, vitamin C, and folic acid. Woman will suggest how she might fulfill these needs.
What is normal pattern of weight gain during pregnancy? What are components of normal weight gain in pregnancy?	Woman will know normal weight gain pattern and components of total weight gain during pregnancy.	Explain that normal weight gain pattern is about 1.4 kg (3 lb) in first trimester, 4.5 kg (10 lb) in second, and 4.5 kg (10 lb) in third. Discuss components of total weight gain as follows: 27%, fetus 12%, placenta and fluid in uterus 50%, increased maternal organs (uterus, fat, breasts) 10%, increased blood volume	Woman will explain what normal weight gain pattern is and will list following components that make up total weight gain: 27%, fetus 12%, placenta and fluid in uterus 50%, increase in maternal organs 10%, increased blood volume
What is relationship between good nutrition and normal weight gain in pregnancy?	Woman will know that good nutrition leads to normal weight gain in pregnancy.	Explain that monitoring weight is a way to measure whether fetus is receiving adequate supply of nutrients.	Woman will state that adequate supply of nutrients promotes normal development of infant and normal weight gain.
What is my weight gain?	Woman will achieve normal weight gain.	Explain that normal weight gain indicates that fetus is receiving adequate nutrients.	Woman will state how much she has gained.
How does it compare with average weight gain?	Woman will know how her weight gain compares with average weight gain.	Using pregnancy gain-in-weight grid, record weight gain at each visit. Discuss weight gain pattern.	Complete each time throughout second and third trimesters. Woman will state how her weight gain compares to average.
What are dangers of poor nutrition during pregnancy?	Woman will know that poor nutrition can lead to anemia, preeclampsia-eclampsia, obesity, or prematurity.	Explain that poor nutrition during pregnancy may lead to several problem conditions. Poor supply or iron, folic acid, protein, or vitamin C may lead to **anemia.** Generally poor nutrition may lead to **prematurity.** Poor selection of food may lead to **obesity.**	Woman will identify following problems that may result from poor nutrition in pregnancy: anemia, preeclampsia-eclampsia, obesity, and prematurity.

Adapted from Pregnancy protocol for nutrition counseling, Phoenix, 1978, Nutrition Services, Arizona Department of Health; and Detroit, 1979, Nutrition Division, City of Detroit Department of Health.

Specific Nursing Care Plan

MATERNAL/FETAL NUTRITION

Laura is a 22-year-old married woman who is 10 weeks pregnant with her second child. John, her first child, now a healthy 18 months of age, was born at term weighing 3500 g (7 lb 12 oz). Laura expressed concern that she would not have enough calcium because she "just had a baby 18 months ago and never could stand drinking milk." During the dietary assessment she reveals that she cannot drink orange juice. During her last pregnancy she drank caster oil in orange juice for "chronic constipation." History, physical examination, and laboratory results are not remarkable.

ASSESSMENT	NURSING DIAGNOSIS (ND)/ PLAN (P)/GOAL (G)	RATIONALE/ IMPLEMENTATION	EVALUATION
Laura is 10 weeks pregnant; first baby 18 months old. Laura does not drink milk. Laura cannot drink orange juice.	ND: Altered nutrition potential: less than body requirements related to inability to drink milk or orange juice. P: Explore alternate food sources. G: Laura will consume adequate intake of nutrients present in milk and orange juice.	*To ensure adequate intake of nutrients present in milk and orange juice, the nurse will:* Encourage her to choose sources she likes and can afford. Compose a list of foods specifying serving sizes.	Laura is able to choose alternate sources of nutrients. Laura ingests sufficient quantities of nutrients to meet RDA requirements and her own needs.
Laura is concerned because she is unable to use the usual food sources of nutrients.	ND: Self-esteem disturbance related to perceived lack of self-control in meeting nutritional needs. P: Mutually develop a nutrition guide. G: Laura will increase her perceived control of what happens to her and will enhance her self-concept.	*To increase Laura's perceived control of what happens to her and to enhance her self-concept, the nurse will:* Compliment her on her expressed concern and her knowledge of needed nutrients and on choosing equivalent alternatives. Discuss with her the four food groups and distribution of nutrients. Assist her to write out shopping list and sample menus including serving size.	Laura participates in her own care. Laura practices problem solving by exploring alternatives and making choices to meet changing needs. Laura indicates satisfaction in her new skills.
Laura states she had chronic constipation during her first pregnancy. Assess her understanding of constipation, and her usual methods of prevention and treatment. Assess usual bowel habits, daily fluid intake, dietary intake of roughage, exercise regime, if any.	ND: Knowledge deficit related to constipation during pregnancy, its prevention and treatment with nonpharmaceutical means. P: Fill in knowledge gaps. G: Knowledge deficit is removed. ND: Constipation related to knowledge deficit of self-help methods of prevention and treatment. P: Adjust maternal behaviors, teach self-help measures to prevent/relieve constipation. G: Augment coping skills using self-help measures without pharmaceuticals.	*To prevent constipation during this pregnancy or to treat constipation with nonpharmaceutic means the nurse will:* Review maternal adaptations to pregnancy that alter alimentary function. Teach methods of prevention and treatment. Help her incorporate knowledge into menu plan as necessary and set schedule for water intake, bowel elimination, exercise. Commend her on her participation in problem solving.	Laura is able to state physiologic basis of constipation. Laura learns methods of preventing/relieving constipation with nonpharmaceutical means. Laura does not experience constipation. Laura utilizes methods of preventing constipation.

Referral for Additional Services. Individuals with insufficient income to purchase foods may have a nutritionally inadequate diet. Nutrients such as protein and iron are among those more likely to be deficient in diets of low-income groups. To help improve the nutritional quality of the diet, the person with limited income should be encouraged to participate in federal food programs such as WIC and the food stamp program. Nutrition education and counseling are important to ensure the benefits of such programs.

The referral system has two functions. First, a comprehensive network of services can offer solutions to problems that a particular program may not have the resources to solve. Second, the referral system informs women about a program by making them aware of their needs for benefits from that service. Food assistance programs, such as the WIC program, are a particularly good example of resources that can be tapped for pregnant women.

A sample nursing care plan designed to meet the specific needs of a client is on p. 330.

Evaluation

Evaluation is a continuous process that begins during assessment. To be effective, evaluation is based on measurable outcome criteria. Nurses are accountable for measuring and documenting client outcomes. The criteria reflect the parameters used to measure the goals for care. The maternal and fetal areas consistently assessed as indicators of maternal and fetal well-being and the clinical findings that represent normal response are presented as outcome in Table 15-7. These criteria are used as a basis for selecting appropriate nursing actions and evaluating their effectiveness.

SUMMARY

Nutrition is an important component of care during the prenatal period. Scientific research has identified the nutrient needs for optimum body function, growth, development, maintenance and repair of body tissues, and prevention of disease. The nurse is in a strategic position to assist clients directly or through collaboration with a registered dietitian to meet their nutrition needs. Among the nurse's tools are a sound knowledge of maternal physiologic adjustments to pregnancy and nutritional needs and the nursing process.

KEY CONCEPTS

- A woman's nutritional status before, during, and after pregnancy contributes to a significant degree to the well-being of both herself and her infant, and is of vital importance to the health of succeeding generations.
- Many physiologic changes occurring during pregnancy influence the need for nutrients and the efficiency with which the body uses them.
- There are potential hazards for both mother and infant from restricting weight gain and salt during pregnancy.
- Water is an essential nutrient.
- Iron and folic acid supplementation are recommended during pregnancy.
- The nurse and the client are influenced by cultural and personal values and beliefs during nutrition counseling.
- Factors such as frequent pregnancies and insufficient income put the gravida at nutritional risk before and during pregnancy.

STUDY QUESTIONS AND ACTIVITIES

1. At the prenatal clinic, assess the nutritional status of a selected client utilizing your observational skills for physical signs and symptoms either during a physical examination or as the client is involved in other clinic routines.
2. Interview a client at the prenatal clinic utilizing the nutrition questionnaire and develop a daily food plan for her based on this formation.
3. Describe your own nutritional status and dietary strengths and weaknesses; your positive and negative eating habits; the influence of your culture, religion, and ethnic group on your dietary practices; your attitudes toward overweight and underweight persons; and how your views and beliefs about nutrition may influence women when providing care for prenatal clients.
4. Use the material compiled in activity 3 for discussion with peers about their views and beliefs. People of varying backgrounds may be able to offer additional insights into each others' problems with acceptance of clients' varying attitudes and practices.
5. Use the cultural preferences listed in Table 15-5 to develop sample menus for 1 day for clients coming from three of the backgrounds listed, taking into account the availability of ethnic and specialty foods and the constraints of an average income. (You may also want to take a research trip to several stores in the area to check for availability of special foods.)

References

Affonso, DD: The Filipino American. In Clark, AL, editors: Culture/childbearing/health professionals, Philadelphia, 1978, FA Davis Co

Bernstein, JL, and Kidd, YA: Childbearing in Japan, In Kay, MA, editor: Anthropology of human birth, Philadelphia, 1982, FA Davis Co

Brennan, RE, Caldwell, M, and Rickard, KA: Assessment of maternal nutrition, J Am Diet Assoc 75:152, Aug 1979

California Department of Health Services: Nutrition during pregnancy and lactation, Sacramento, Calif, 1975, Maternal and Child Health Branch, CDHS

Campbell, T, and Chang, B: Health care of the Chinese in America, Nurs Outlook 21:245, 1973

Carrington, BW: The Afro-American. In Clark, AL, editor: Culture/childbearing/health professionals, Philadelphia, 1978, FA Davis Co

Choi, EC: Unique aspects of Korean-American mothers, JOGN Nurs 15(5):394, 1986
Chung, JJ: Understanding the Oriental maternity patient, Nurs Clin North Am 12:67, 1977
Dohrmann, KR, and Lederman, SA: JOGN Nurs 15(6):446, 1986
Dunn, FL: Medical care in the Chinese communities of peninsular Malaysia. In Kleinman, A, et al, editors: Culture and healing in Asian societies, Cambridge, Mass, 1978, Schenkman Books, Inc
Hollingsworth, AO, et al: The refugees and childbearing: what to expect, RN 43:45, 1980
Kay, MA, editor: Anthropology of human birth, Philadelphia, 1982, FA Davis Co
Lackey, CJ: Pica—a nutritional anthropology concern. In Bauwens, EE: The anthropology of health, St Louis, 1978, The CV Mosby Co
Leiderman, PH, et al: Culture and infancy, New York, 1977, Academic Press, Inc
Luke, B: Megavitamins and pregnancy: a dangerous combination, MCN 10:18, Jan/Feb, 1985
Mirkin, G: Assailing vitamin abuse: facts about mega- and pseudo-vitamins, Contemp OB/GYN 25:86, May 1985 (special issue)
Naeye, RL: Weight gain and the outcome of pregnancy, Am J Obstet Gynecol 135:3, 1979
Obeyesekere, G: Pregnancy cravings (dola-duka) in relation to social structure and personality in a Sinhalese village, Am Anthropol 65:323, 1963
Snow, L: Folk medical beliefs and their implications for care of patients, Ann Intern Med 81:82, 1974
Stern, PN: Solving problems of cross-cultural health teaching: the Filipino childbearing family, Image 13:47, 1981
Vermeer, DE, and Frate, DA: Geophagy in a Mississippi county, Ann Assoc Am Geographers 65:414, 1975
White, JE, and Owsley, VB: Helping families cope with milk, wheat, and soy allergies, MCN 8:423, Nov/Dec 1983
Williams, SR: Nutrition and diet therapy, ed 8, St Louis, 1988, The CV Mosby Co
Worthington-Roberts, B: Nutrition deficiencies and excesses: impact on pregnancy, part 1, J Perinat 5:9, Summer 1985
Worthington-Roberts, BS, Vermeersch, J, and Williams, SR: Nutrition in pregnancy and lactation, ed 3, St Louis, 1985, The CV Mosby Co
Zlatnik, FJ, and Burmeister, LF: Dietary protein and preeclampsia, Am J Obstet Gynecol 147:345, 1983

Bibliography

Alexander, LL: The pregnant smoker: nursing implications, JOGN Nurs 16(3):167, 1987
Barnico, LM, and Cullinane, MM: Maternal phenylketonuria: an unexpected challenge, MCN 10:108, March/April 1985
Cagle, CS: Professionally speaking: access to care and prevention of low birth weight, MCN 12(4):235, 1987
Edwards, LE, et al: Pregnancy in the massively obese: course, outcome, and obesity prognosis of the infant, Am J Obstet Gynecol 131:479, 1978
Edwards, LE, et al: Pregnancy in the underweight woman: course, outcome and growth patterns of the infant, Am J Obstet Gynecol 135:297, 1979
Food and Nutrition Board: Recommended dietary allowances, rev ed, Washington, DC, 1980, National Academy of Sciences—National Research Council
Frank, DW, et al: Nutrition in adolescent pregnancy, J Calif Perinatal Assoc 1:21, 1983
Grosso, C, et al: The Vietnamese American family . . . and grandma makes three, MCN 6:177, 1981
Gulick, EE, Franklin, CM, and Elinson, M: Food beliefs and food behaviors among minority pregnant women, J Perinat 6(3):197, 1986
Hattner, J: Personal communication, Dietetics Department, Stanford University Hospital, Stanford, Calif
Haworth, JC, et al: Fetal growth retardation in cigarette-smoking mothers is not due to decreased maternal food intake, Am J Obstet Gynecol 137:719, 1980
Jacobson, HN: Diet therapy and the improvement of pregnancy outcome, birth 10:29, Spring, 1983
Laboratory indices of nutritional status in pregnancy, pub no F-427, Washington, DC, Sept 1977, National Academy of Sciences—National Research Council
Leininger, M: The Gadsup of New Guinea and early childcaring behaviors with nursing implications. In Leininger, M, editor: Transcultural nursing '79, New York, 1979, Masson Publishing USA, Inc
Lenke, RR, and Levy, HL: Maternal phenylketonuria and hyperphenylalaninemia, N Engl J Med 303:1202, 1980
Lipson, A, et al: Maternal hyperphenylalaninemia and fetal effects, J Pediatr 104:216, 1984
Leonard, LG: Pregnancy and the underweight woman, MCN 9(5):331, Sept/Oct 1984
Moore, L, et al: Self-assessment: a personalized approach to nursing during pregnancy, JOGN Nurs 15(4):311, 1986
Naeye, RL: Teenaged and pre-teenaged pregnancies: consequences of the fetal-maternal competition for nutrients, Pediatrics 67:146, 1981
Naeye, RL: Effects of maternal nutrition on fetal and neonatal survival, birth 10:109, Summer 1983
Orque, MS, Bloch, B, and Ahumada-Monrroy, LS: Ethnic nursing care: a multicultural approach, St Louis, 1983, The CV Mosby Co
Pritchard, JA, MacDonald, PC, and Gant, NF: Williams obstetrics, ed 17, Norwalk, Conn, 1985, Appleton-Century-Crofts
Queenan, JT, moderator: Managing pregnancy in patients over 35, Contemp OB/GYN 29(5):180, 1987
Seidel, HM, et al: Mosby's guide to physical examination, St Louis, 1987, The CV Mosby Co
Smith, N: Personal communication, San Francisco State University Department of Nursing, 1986
Truong, T: Personal communication, San Francisco State University, Department of Nursing, 1986
Willson, JR, Carrington, ER, and Ledger, WJ: Obstetrics and gynecology, ed 8, St Louis, 1987, The CV Mosby Co
Winslow, W: First pregnancy after 35: what is the experience? MCN 12(2):92, 1987
Worthington-Roberts, B: Nutrition deficiencies and excesses: impact on pregnancy, part 2, J Perinat 5:12, Fall 1985

UNIT

IV

Normal Childbirth

Birth is a time of physical and emotional crises for the woman, her child, and her family. It requires collaborative care between the obstetric team and the pregnant woman or couple. The goals of care are safe delivery of mother and child and promotion of emotional fulfillment for the entire family. Chapter 16 is concerned with labor—its essential factors, the process of labor, and the implications for nursing care. As the process of labor is described, its mechanism and duration are discussed. Chapter 17 focuses on the pharmacologic relief of pain and discomfort as an important part of skilled care of the maternity client. This chapter reviews the physiologic basis for pharmacologic care and accepted drugs and modalities used. The second part of this chapter presents a basis for understanding techniques associated with intermittant monitoring of clients during the prenatal period and continuous monitoring during labor. Chapters 18, 19, and 20 present in detail the care of clients during the first, second, third, and fourth stages of labor. The format of the process of nursing—assessment, formulation of nursing diagnoses, planning, implementation, and evaluation—is used throughout these chapters. The biologic and psychologic responses of woman, fetus, and newborn to the stress of labor are emphasized, and general and specific nursing care measures are presented. The care needed by other family members, such as father, siblings, and grandparents, is reviewed.

Nursing research highlights add support to the content. Abstracts of examples of published research follow.

Chapter 16: Progression of labor pain in primiparas and multiparas.

Chapter 18: The role of the nurse in labor and delivery as perceived by nurses and patients.

Chapter 19: Effect of the birth chair on duration of second stage of labor and maternal outcome.

Chapter 20: Measuring nurses' accuracy of estimating blood loss.

CHAPTER

16

Essential Factors and Processes and Maternal-Fetal Adaptations

Iris E. Campbell

Learning Objectives

Correctly define the key terms listed.

Explain the five essential factors that affect the labor process.

Describe the anatomical structure of the bony pelvis.

Differentiate the four types of pelves.

Determine the diameters of the pelvic inlet, cavity, and outlet and state the normal measurements.

Review the anatomy of the fetal skull and state the normal measurements.

Summarize the process of molding of the fetal head during labor.

Relate the mechanism of labor.

Assess the maternal anatomic and physiologic adaptations to labor.

Briefly explain the fetal adaptations to labor.

Key Terms

attitude
biparietal diameter
bloody show
breech presentation
bregma
cephalic presentation
denominator
descent
diagonal conjugate
engagement
expulsion
four stages of labor
gate-control theory
gynecoid pelvis
Leopold's maneuvers
lie
mechanism of labor
molding
pain threshold
partogram
position
powers
presentation
presenting part
restitution
station
suboccipitobregmatic diameter
vertex

During pregnancy, the mother and the fetus prepare to accomodate themselves to each other during the labor process. The fetal-placental unit has grown and developed in preparation for extrauterine life. The mother has undergone various physiologic adaptations during the period of gestation that prepare her for the birth process and role of mother. Labor and delivery is the culmination of the childbearing cycle and is an intense period during which the products of conception are expelled from the uterus. To implement nursing care in labor the nurse must use the nursing process. The essential factors and processes of labor must be understood along with the maternal and fetal adaptations to labor. The family's adaptations to childbirth are discussed in Chapter 11. In this chapter, essential terms are in **bold print**. Some of the important terms are defined below:

parturition Childbirth, birthing, the birth process

parturient A woman in labor

labor A coordinated sequence of involuntary uterine contractions that result in effacement and dilation of the cervix and voluntary bearing-down efforts that result in delivery; the actual expulsion of the products of conception—the fetus and placenta.

toko- and **toco-** (Greek) Combining forms meaning childbirth or labor

eutocia Normal labor

prodromal labor Early or premonitory manifestations of impending labor; events before the onset of true labor.

ESSENTIAL FACTORS IN LABOR: BASIS FOR ASSESSMENT

Five essential factors affect the process of labor and delivery. These factors are easily remembered as the five P's:

1. Passenger
   a. Fetus: gestational age, size, lie, presentation, position and attitude of the fetus; number of fetuses
   b. Placenta: type, sufficiency of, and site of insertion
2. Passage
   a. Configuration and diameters of the maternal pelvis
   b. Distensibility of the lower uterine segment, cervical dilation, and capacity for distension of pelvic floor, vaginal canal, and introitus
3. Powers
   a. Primary powers: intensity, duration, and frequency of uterine contractions
   b. Secondary powers: bearing-down efforts
4. Position of the mother: standing, walking, side-lying, squatting, hands and knees
5. Psychologic response: previous experiences, emotional readiness, preparation, cultural-ethnic heritage, support systems, and environment

Four of the five factors will be discussed in this chapter; the fifth factor, psychologic response, will be covered in Chapter 18.

Passenger

The passage of the fetus through the birth canal is a result of several interacting factors. It is influenced by the size of the fetal head and shoulders, the dimensions of the bony pelvis, and fetal presentation, position, and attitude.

Fetus. Because of its size and relative rigidity, the **fetal head** has a major effect on the birth process. The external cranial vault is composed of two parietal bones, two temporal bones, the frontal bone, and the occipital bone (Fig. 16-1, *A*). These bones are united by membranous **sutures:** the **sagittal**, lambdoidal, coronal, and frontal. The membrane-filled spaces called *fontanels* (Fig. 16-1, *B* and *C*), are located where the sutures intersect. The two most important fontanels are the anterior and posterior fontanels. During labor, vaginal palpation of fontanels and sutures identifies fetal presentation and position. Assessment of their size reveals information about the age and well-being of the newborn.

The larger of the two fontanels, the **anterior fontanel**, or **bregma** is diamond-shaped and is at the junction of the sagittal, coronal, and frontal sutures. It ossifies by 18 months of age. The **posterior fontanel** is at the junction of the sutures of the two parietal bones and the one occipital

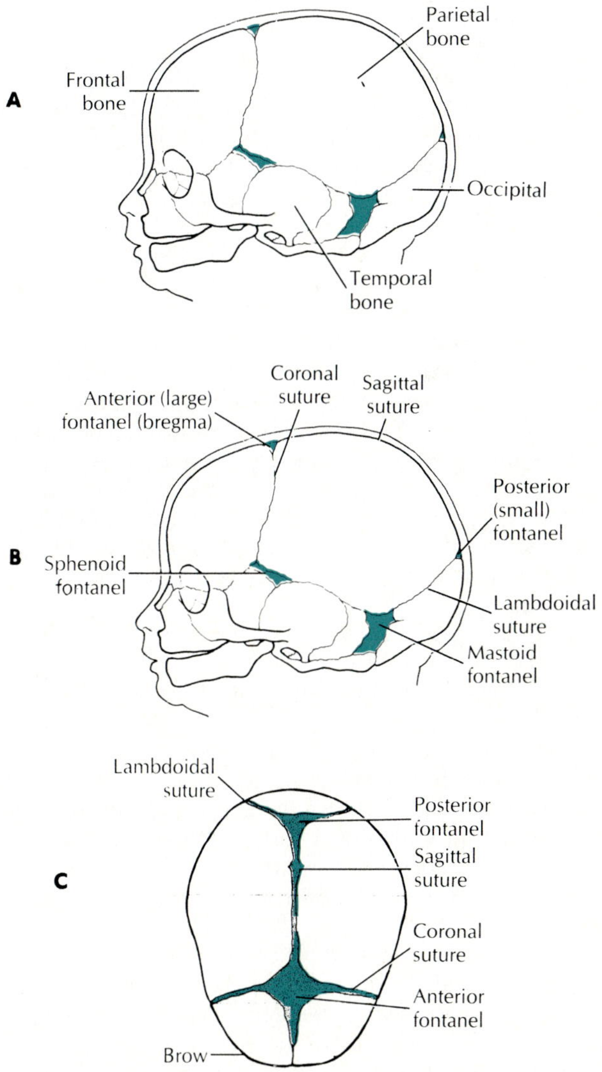

Fig. 16-1 Fetal head at term. **A**, Bones. **B** and **C**, Sutures and fontanels.

bone and is therefore triangular in shape. It is smaller than the anterior fontanel and closes 6 to 8 weeks after birth. The sutures and fontanels allow the brain to continue growing.

The bones of the cranial vault are not firmly united, and slight overlapping of the bones, or **molding** of the shape of the head, occurs during labor. This capacity of the bones to slide over one another permits adaptation to the various diameters of the maternal pelvis. Molding can be extensive, but with most newborns the head assumes its normal shape within 3 days of birth.

Principal measurements of the fetal skull are in centimeters (Fig. 16-2). The **biparietal diameter** is the largest transverse diameter. Of the anteroposterior diameters shown in Fig. 16-2, it can be seen that the attitudes of flexion or extension allow diameters of different sizes to enter the maternal pelvis. With the head in complete flexion, the smallest diameter, **suboccipitobregmatic**, presents and enters the true pelvis easily (Fig. 16-3).

Because of their mobility, the position of the **shoulders** (the shoulder girdle) can be altered during labor, so that one shoulder may occupy a lower level than the other. This permits a small shoulder diameter to negotiate the passage. The circumference of the hips, or pelvic girdle, is usually small enough not to create problems.

Lie is the relationship of the long axis (spine) of the fetus to the long axis (spine) of the mother. There are two lies: *longitudinal,* or vertical, in which the long axis of the fetus is parallel with the long axis of the mother, and *transverse,* or horizontal, in which the long axis of the fetus is at a right angle to that of the mother (Figs. 16-4 and 16-5). Longitudinal lies are either cephalic (head) or sacral (breech) presentations, depending on the fetal structure that first enters the mother's pelvis.

Presentation refers to the part of the fetus that enters the pelvic inlet first and leads through the birth canal during labor. The three main presentations are cephalic (head first), 96%; breech (buttocks first), 3%; and shoulders, 1%.

Presenting part refers to the leading, or most dependent portion of the fetus, lying over the internal os of the cervix. It is the part on which the caput succedaneum, a localized, easily identifiable edematous area of the scalp, forms and is the part first felt by the examining finger during a vaginal examination.

Attitude is the relationship of the fetal body parts to each other. The fetus assumes a characteristic posture (attitude) in utero partly because of the mode of fetal growth and partly because of accomodation to the shape of the uterine cavity. The shape of the fetus is roughly ovoid, the back is markedly flexed, the head is flexed on the chest, the thighs are flexed at the knee joints, and the arches of the feet rest on the anterior surface of the legs. This attitude is called *general flexion*. The arms are crossed over the thorax, and the umbilical cord lies between the arms and the legs.

Denominator refers to that part of the presentation that indicates or determines the position of the fetus in utero. In a cephalic presentation, the denominator is the occiput; in a breech presentation, it is the sacrum; in a face presentation, the mentum; and in a brow presentation, the denominator is the sinciput.

Position is the relationship of the denominator (occiput,

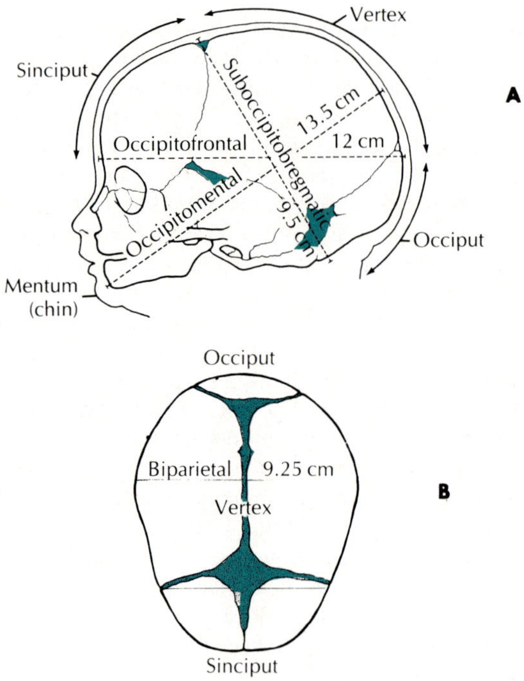

Fig. 16-2 Cephalic landmarks. **A,** Cephalic presentations: occiput, vertex, and sinciput; and cephalic diameters: suboccipitobregmatic, occipitofrontal, and occipitomental. **B,** Cephalic presentations and biparietal diameter.

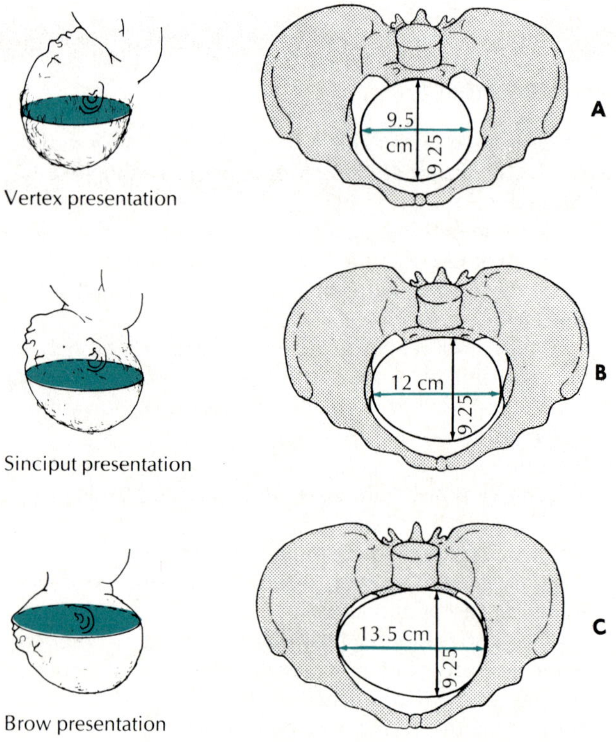

Fig. 16-3 Head entering pelvis. Biparietal diameter is indicated in black. **A,** Suboccipitobregmatic diameter: complete flexion of head on chest so that smallest diameter enters. **B,** Occipitofrontal diameter: moderate extension (military attitude) so that large diameter enters. **C,** Occipitomental diameter: marked extension (deflection) so that largest diameter, which is too large to permit head to enter pelvis, is presenting.

sacrum, mentus [chin], or sinciput) to the front, back, or sides of the mother's pelvis. The maternal pelvis has a 360-degree circumference. Eight points that are 45-degrees apart are the pelvic landmarks, and the position of the fetus is determined by the relationship of the denominator to one of these landmarks. Position is described in abbreviated form determined by the first letter of each key word. For example, right occipito-anterior position is written as ROA; right occipito-transverse is abbreviated as ROT. There are eight positions for each denominator (Table 16-1; Fig. 16-4).

Engagement indicates that the largest transverse diameter of the presentation has passed through the maternal pelvic inlet or brim. In a well-flexed cephalic presentation, the biparietal diameter (9.25 cm) is the widest (Fig. 16-3). Engagement can be determined by abdominal or vaginal examination.

Station is the relationship of the presenting part of the fetus to an imaginary line drawn between the maternal ischial spines. Station is expressed in terms of centimeters above or below the spines. For example, when the presenting part is 1 cm above the spines, it is noted as being minus one.

When the presenting part is 1 cm below the spines, however, the station is said to be plus one. At the level of the spines, the station is referred to as zero. The station of the presenting part should be determined when labor begins to keep accurate documentation of the rate of descent of the fetus during labor.

Placenta. Since the most common site for implantation of the fertilized ovum is the fundal part of the uterus, the developed placenta rarely impedes the process of labor. Placenta-related problems are included with content on hemorrhage in Chapter 31.

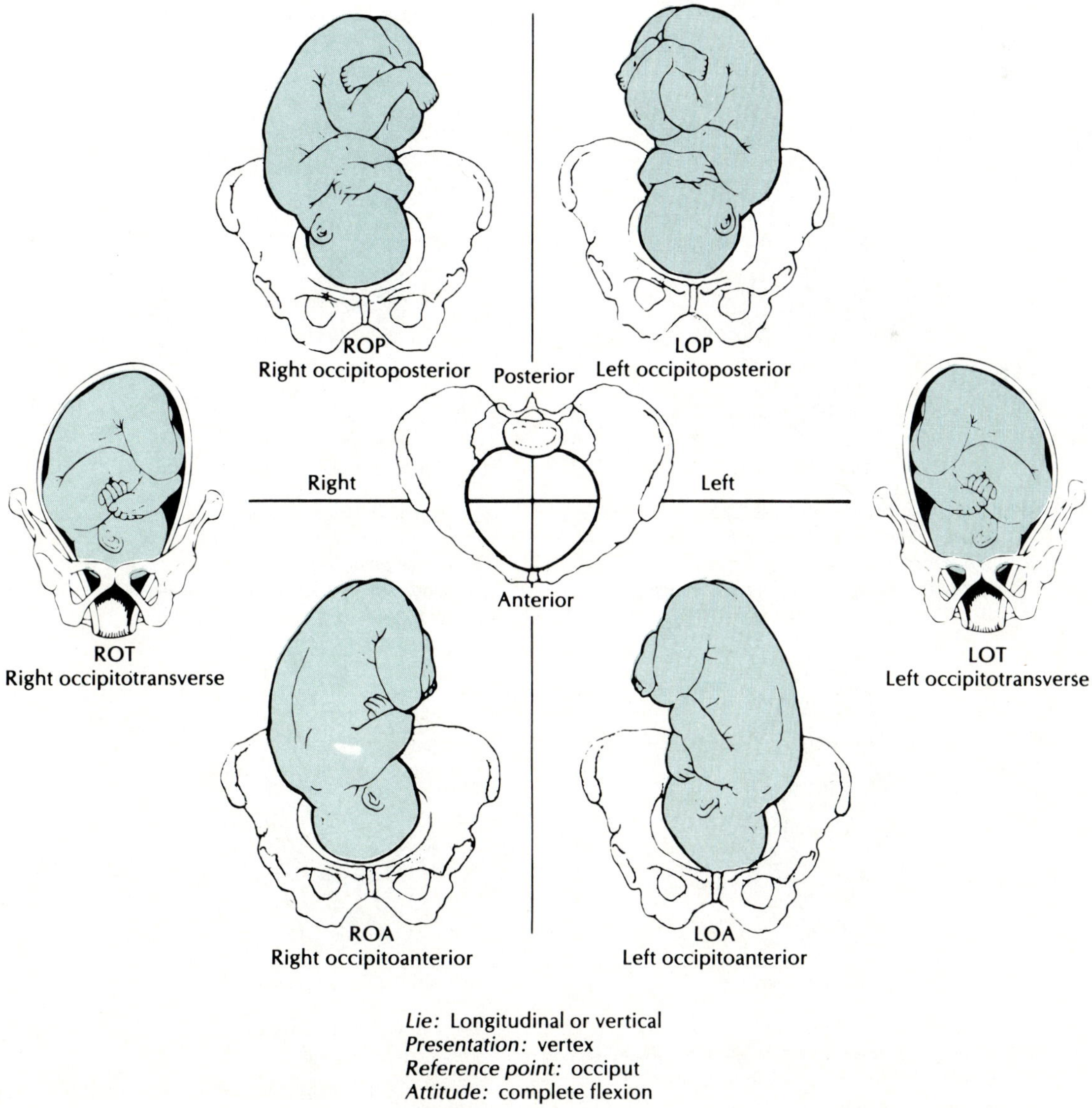

Fig. 16-4 Examples of fetal vertex (occiput) presentations in relation to front, back, or side of maternal pelvis.
Modified from Iorio, J: Childbirth: family-centered nursing, ed 3, St Louis, 1973, The CV Mosby Co.

Table 16-1 ***Fetal Lie, Presentation, and Position***

	Presenting Part	Example of Position
Longitudinal Lie		
Cephalic		
Vertex	Occiput	Left occipito-transverse (LOT)
Brow	Brow	Left brow anterior (LBA)
Face (chin) (rare)	Mentum	Right mento-posterior (RMP)
Pelvic		
Breech	Sacrum	Right sacro-anterior (RSA)
Transverse Lie		
Shoulder	Scapula	Right scapulo-anterior (RScA)

The Passage

The passage, or birth canal, is composed of the rigid bony pelvis and the soft tissues of the cervix, pelvic floor, vagina, and introitus.

Bony Pelvis. The anatomy of the bony pelvis was reviewed in Chapter 6. A further discussion of the importance of pelvic configurations as they relate to the labor process is necessary at this point.

Assessment of the bony pelvis may be performed during the first prenatal evaluation and need not be repeated if the pelvis is of adequate size and suitable shape. In the third trimester of pregnancy, the examination of the bony pelvis may be more thorough and the results more accurate because there is relaxation of pelvic joints and ligaments. The four pelvic joints are the symphysis pubis, the right and left sacroiliac joints, and the sacrococcygeal joint (Fig. 16-6). The hormones of pregnancy, especially the ovarian hormone progesterone, cause the development of considerable mobility. Widening of the symphyseal joint and instability may cause pain in any or all of the joints.

Because the examiner does not have direct access to the

A

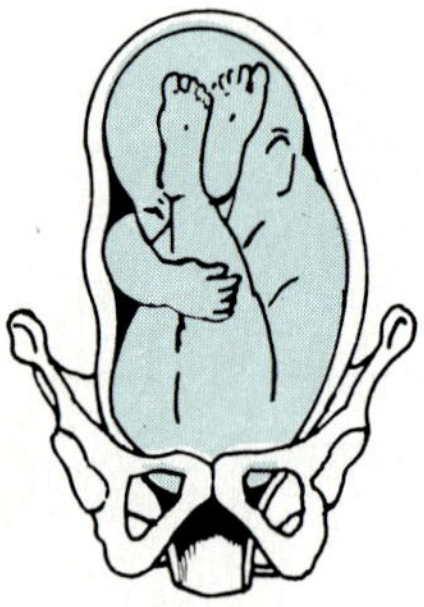

Frank breech

Lie: Longitudinal or vertical
Presentation: breech (incomplete)
Reference point: sacrum
Attitude: flexion, except for legs at knees

B

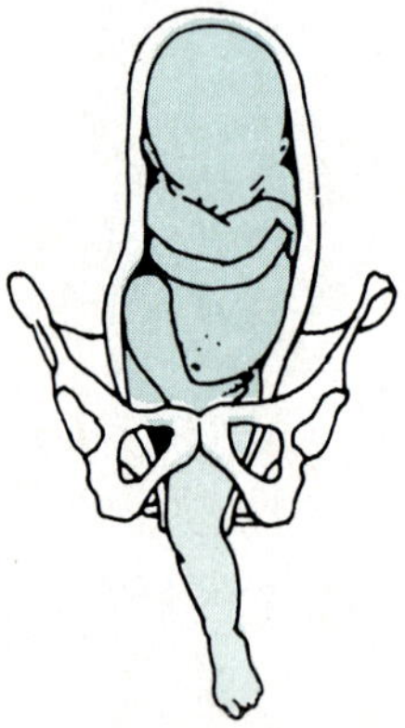

Single footling breech

Lie: Longitudinal or vertical
Presentation: breech (incomplete)
Reference point: sacrum
Attitude: flexion, except for one leg extended at hip and knee

C

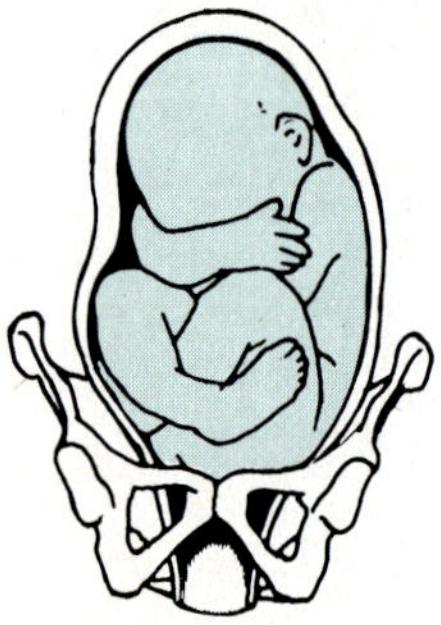

Complete breech

Lie: Longitudinal or vertical
Presentation: breech (sacrum and feet presenting)
Reference point: sacrum (with feet)
Attitude: general flexion

D

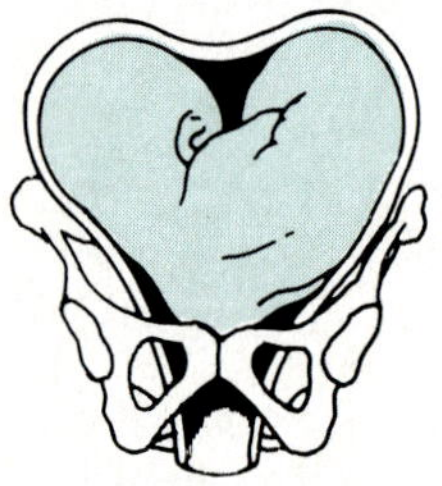

Shoulder presentation.

Lie: Transverse or horizontal
Presentation: shoulder
Reference point: scapula (Sc)
Attitude: flexion

Fig. 16-5 Fetal presentations. **A** to **C**, Breech (sacral) presentation. **D**, Shoulder presentation.

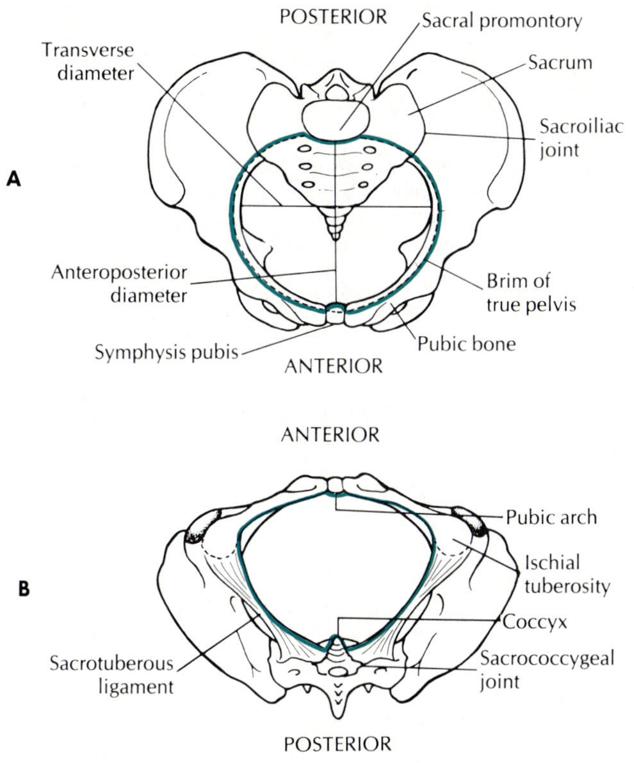

Fig. 16-6 Female pelvis. **A**, Pelvic brim (inlet, linea terminalis, or iliopectineal line) from above. **B**, Pelvic outlet from below.

bony structures and because the bones are covered with varying amounts of soft tissue, estimates of size and shape are approximate. Precise bony pelvis measurements can be determined using computed tomography and ultrasound, or x-ray films. However, x-ray examination is rarely done.

The bony pelvis is separated by the brim, or inlet, into two parts: the **false pelvis** and the **true pelvis** (see Fig. 6-19). The false pelvis is that part above the brim and is of no obstetric interest.

The true pelvis is divided into three planes: the inlet, or brim; the midpelvis, or cavity; and the outlet.

The **pelvic inlet**, or brim, of the pelvis, is formed anteriorly by the upper margins of the pubic bone, laterally by the iliopectineal lines along the innominate bones, and posteriorly by the anterior, upper margin of the sacrum, the sacral promontory (see Figs. 6-19 and 16-6, *A*).

The **pelvic cavity**, or midpelvis, is a curved passage having a short anterior wall and a much deeper concave posterior wall. It is bounded by the posterior aspect of the symphysis pubis, the ischium, a portion of the ilium, and the sacrum and coccyx (see Fig. 6-20).

The **pelvic outlet** when viewed from below is ovoid, somewhat diamond-shaped, bounded by the pubic arch anteriorly, the ischial tuberosities laterally, and the tip of the coccyx posteriorly (Fig. 16-6, *B*). In the latter part of pregnancy the coccyx is movable (unless it has been broken in a fall while skiing or skating, for example, and has fused to the sacrum during healing).

The pelvic canal varies in size and shape at various levels. The diameters at the plane of the pelvic inlet, midpelvis, and outlet, plus the axis of the birth canal (Fig. 16-7), determine whether vaginal delivery is possible and the manner by which the fetus may pass down the birth canal (mechanism of labor).

The **subpubic angle**, which indicates the type of pubic arch, together with the length of the pubic rami and the intertuberous diameter, is of great importance. Because the presenting part must pass beneath the pubic arch, a narrow subpubic angle will be less favorable than a rounded, wide arch. Measurement of the subpubic arch is shown in Fig. 16-8. A summary of obstetric measurements is given in Table 16-2. The most important measurements are depicted in Figs. 16-8 through 16-11.

The four basic types of pelves are classified as follows:

1. Gynecoid (the classical female type)
2. Android (resembling the male pelvis)
3. Anthropoid (resembling the pelvis of anthropoid apes)
4. Platypelloid (the flat pelvis)

Major gynecoid pelvic features are present in 50% of all women; significant anthropoid features are present in 24% of women; android configuration occurs in 23%; and the remaining 3% of women have platypelloid pelvic features. Examples of pelvic variations are given in Table 16-3 and Fig. 16-12. Female and male pelves are compared in Fig. 16-13.

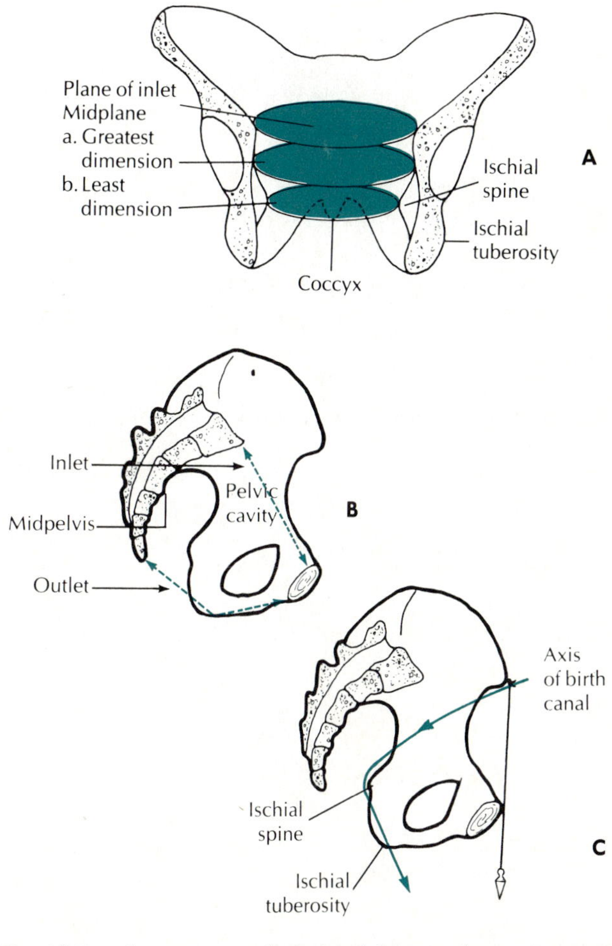

Fig. 16-7 Pelvic cavity. **A**, Inlet and midplane. Outlet not shown. **B**, Cavity of true pelvis. **C**, Note curve of sacrum and axis of birth canal.

Table 16-2 *Obstetric Measurements*

Plane of inlet (superior strait). The principal pelvic diameters of the plane of the inlet are as follows:

Conjugates		
Diagonal	12.5-13 cm	From *inferior border* of symphysis pubis to sacral promontory
Obstetric: measurement that determines whether presenting part can engage or enter superior strait	1.5-2 cm less than diagonal (radiographic)	From *posterior surface* of symphysis pubis to sacral promontory (normally ≥10 cm)
True (vera) (anteroposterior)	≥11 cm (12.5) (radiographic)	From *upper margin* of symphysis pubis to sacral promontory

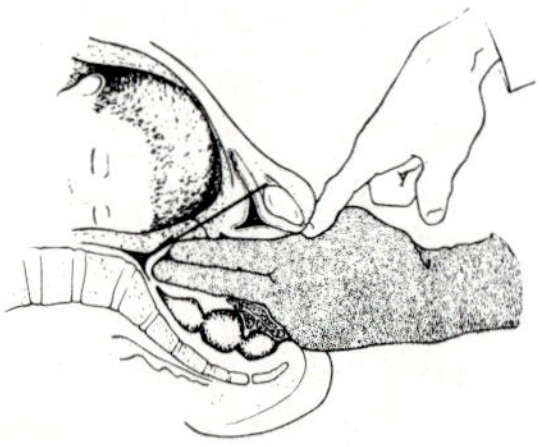

Fig. 16-9 Length of diagonal conjugate (solid colored line), obstetric conjugate (broken colored line), true conjugate (black line).

Transverse diameter	≥13 cm	Usually colon obscures this by filling left pelvis
Oblique diameter (R or L)	≥12.75 cm	From sacroiliac joint on one side to opposite iliopectineal prominence

Midplane of pelvis. The midplane of the pelvis normally is its largest plane and the one of greatest diameter.

Anteroposterior diameter	≥11.5 cm	From midsymphysis to sacrum (at fused second and third sacral vertebras)
Transverse diameter (interspinous diameter)	10.5 cm	Narrowest transverse diameter in the midplane

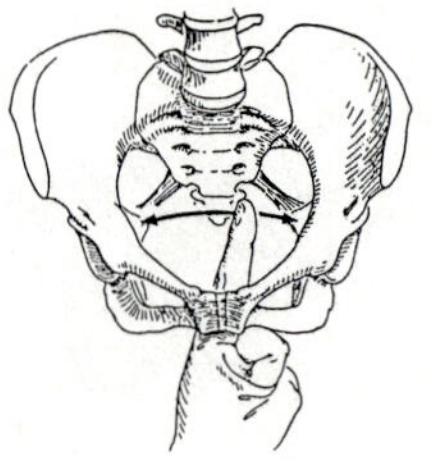

Fig. 16-10 Measurement of interspinous diameter.
From Malasanos, L, Barkauskas, V, Moss, M, and Stoltenberg-Allen K: Health assessment, ed 3, St Louis, 1986, The CV Mosby Co.

Posterior sagittal diameter	4.5 cm	Segment of anteroposterior diameter dorsal to line between ischial spines; although midplane is comparatively large, critical shortening of interspinous or posterior sagittal diameter of midplane may cause pelvic dystocia

Plane of pelvic outlet. The outlet presents the smallest plane of the pelvic canal. It encompasses an area including the lower portion of the symphysis pubis, the ischial tuberosities, and the tip of the sacrum. The significant diameters are as follows:

Anteroposterior diameter	11.9 cm	From lower border of symphysis pubis to tip of sacrum; coccyx may be displaced posteriorly during labor and is not considered to be a fixed bone
Transverse diameter (intertuberous diameter)	≥8 cm	From inner border of one ischial tuberosity to other

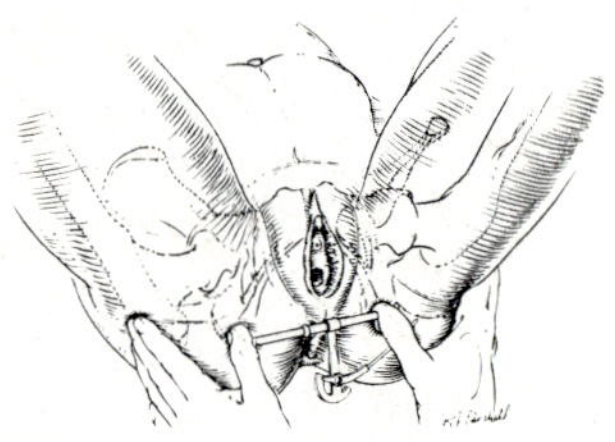

Fig. 16-11 Use of Thom's pelvimeter to measure intertuberous diameter.
From Malasanos, L, Barkauskas, V, Moss, M, and Stoltenberg-Allen, K: Health assessment, ed 3, St Louis, 1986, The CV Mosby Co.

Posterior sagittal diameter	9 cm	Projected from tip of sacrum to a point in space where intertuberous diameter transects anteroposterior projection

Soft Tissues. The soft tissues of the passage include the distensible lower uterine segment, cervix, pelvic floor muscles, vagina, and introitus.

Before labor begins, the uterus is composed of the uterine body (corpus) and cervix. After labor has begun, the uterine contractions cause the uterine body to differentiate into a thick and muscular upper segment and a thin-walled passive muscular lower segment tube. A physiologic retraction ring separates the two segments (Fig. 16-14). The lower uterine segment gradually distends to accomodate the intrauterine contents as the wall of the upper segment becomes thicker and its content is reduced.

The downward pressure caused by contraction of the fundus is transmitted to the cervix. The cervix then effaces (thins) (Fig. 16-14, *B* and *C*) and dilates (opens) (Fig. 16-14, *C* and *D*) sufficiently to allow descent of the presenting part into the vagina. Actually, the cervix is drawn upward and over the presenting part as the vertex or breech descends.

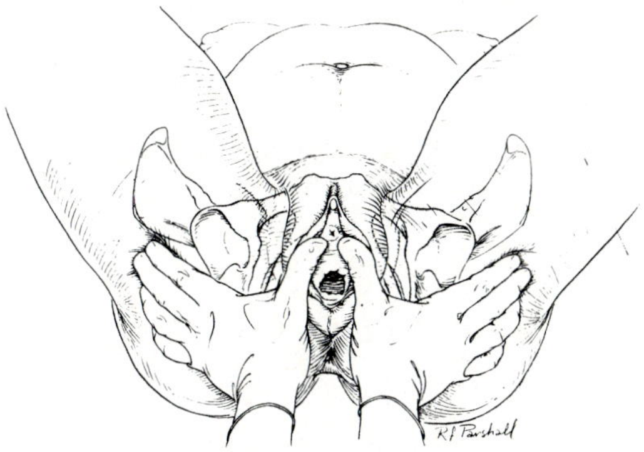

Fig. 16-8 Estimation of angle of subpubic arch. Using both thumbs, examiner externally traces descending rami down to tuberosities.
From Malasanos, L, Barkauskas, V, Moss, M, and Stoltenberg-Allen, K: Health assessment, ed 3, St Louis, 1986, The CV Mosby Co.

The pelvic floor is a muscular diaphragm that separates the pelvic cavity above from the perineal space below. This structure helps the presenting part of the fetus rotate anteriorly during the second stage of labor and directs it downward and forward along the lower straits of the birth canal. The vagina in turn distends to permit passage of the fetus into the external world. As noted earlier, the soft tissues of the vagina develop throughout pregnancy until at term the vagina can dilate to accomodate the fetus.

Powers

The forces acting to expel the fetus and placenta are derived from the **primary powers**, the involuntary uterine contractions. Following the first stage of labor, **secondary powers**, voluntary bearing-down efforts, augment the force of the involuntary contractions.

Primary Powers: Involuntary Uterine Contractions. Contractions originate at pacemaker points in the myometrium near the uterotubal junction. From the pacemaker points, contractions move over the uterus like a wave. Successive downward waves of contractions are separated by short rest periods. The following is a description of the primary forces from Willson, Carrington, and Ledger (1988).

> The ultimate effect . . . of a normal labor contraction . . . is a gradient of force directed from the fundus to the least active and weakest area of the uterus, the cervix. This is called *fundal dominance*. The force generated by each contraction is applied to the amniotic fluid and directly against the pole of the infant that

Table 16-3 *Comparison of Pelvic Types*

	Gynecoid (50% of Women)	Android (23% of Women)	Anthropoid (24% of Women)	Platypelloid (3% of Women)
Brim	Slightly ovoid or transversely rounded	Heart shaped, angulated	Oval, wider anteroposteriorly	Flattened anteroposteriorly, wide transversely
	Round	Heart	Oval	Flat
Depth	Moderate	Deep	Deep	Shallow
Side walls	Straight	Convergent	Straight	Straight
Ischial spines	Blunt, somewhat widely separated	Prominent, narrow interspinous diameter	Prominent, often with narrow interspinous diameter	Blunted, widely separated
Sacrum	Deep, curved	Slightly curved, terminal portion often beaked	Slightly curved	Slightly curved
Subpubic arch	Wide	Narrow	Narrow	Wide
Usual mode of delivery	Vaginal Spontaneous Occiput anterior position	Cesarean Vaginal Difficult with forceps	Vaginal Forceps/spontaneous occiput posterior or occiput anterior position	Vaginal Spontaneous

occupies the upper segment. Therefore each time the muscle contracts, the uterine cavity becomes smaller, and the presenting part of the infant or the forebag of waters lying ahead of it is pushed downward into the cervix. This tends to force it open, or *dilate* it.

A more potent factor in cervical dilatation, however, is the *retraction of the upper segment.* As this area of the uterus becomes shorter and thicker, it pulls the lower segment and the dilating cervix upward around the presenting part at the same time the uterus contracting directly against the infant tends to push it through the cervical opening (Fig. 16-15). The cervix opens or is dilated by a combinatin of these two factors but retraction is probably more important than the pressure of the presenting part, since dilatation will occur even though the presenting part does not descend into it. A *completely dilated cervix* that will permit a term infant to pass through it has a diameter of about 10 cm.

The primary powers are responsible for the effacement and dilation of the cervix and descent of the fetus. **Effacement** of the cervix means the shortening and thinning of the cervix during the first stage of labor. The cervix, normally 2 to 3 cm in length and about 1 cm thick, is obliterated or "taken up" by a shortening of the uterine muscle bundles during the thinning of the lower uterine segment

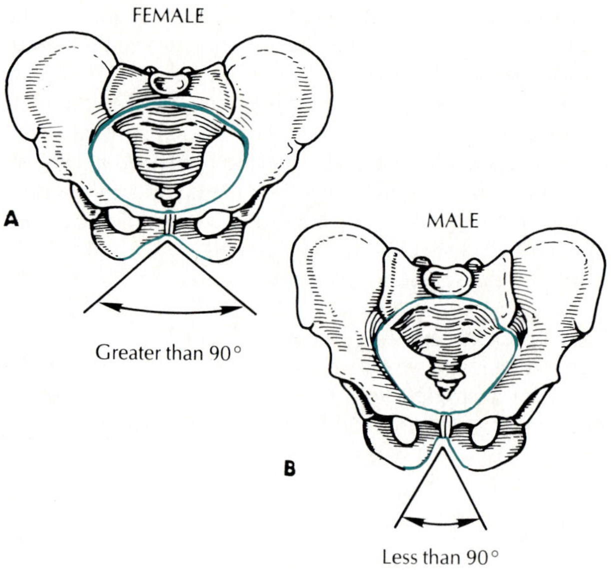

Fig. 16-13 Pelves. **A**, Gynecoid, female. **B**, Android, male. Compare shape of brim and angle of subpubic arch.

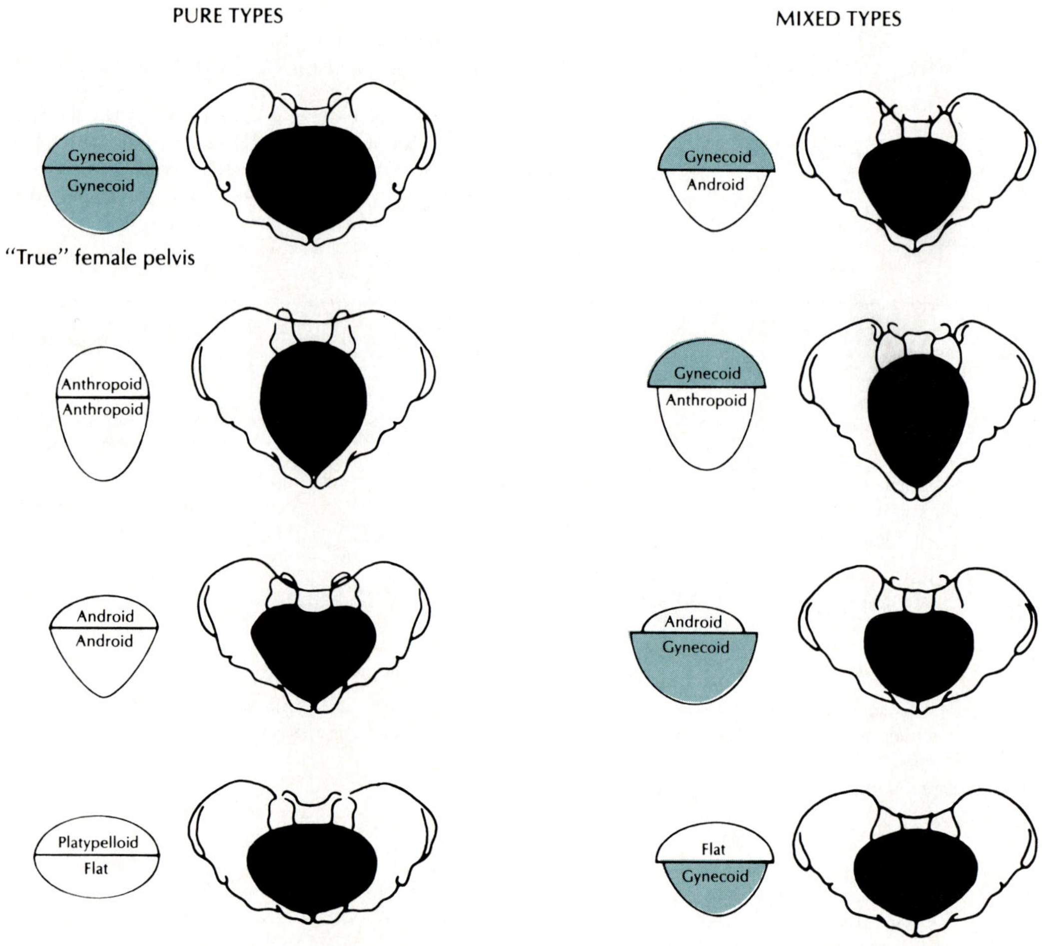

Fig. 16-12 Female pelves; pure and mixed types. Note differences in shape of inlets.

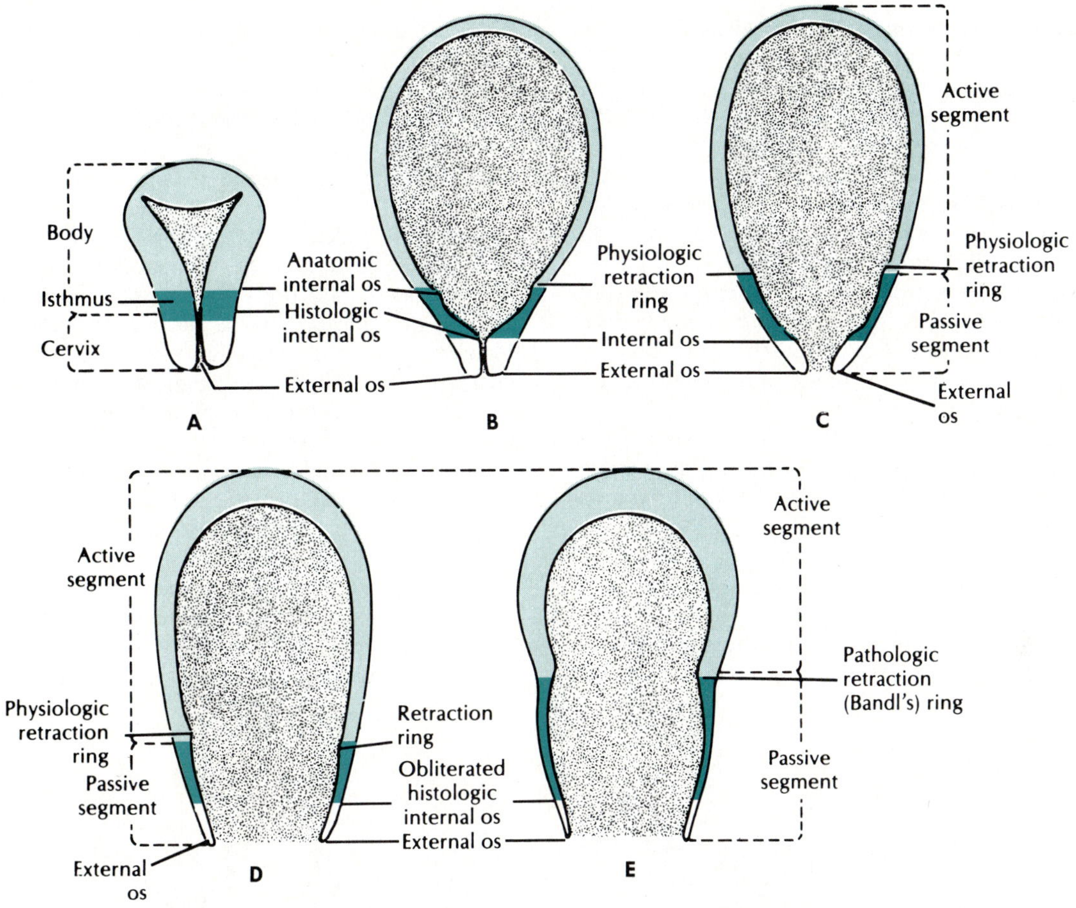

Fig. 16-14 Progressive development of segments and rings of uterus at term. Note comparison between **A**, nonpregnant uterus, **B**, uterus at term, and **C**, uterus in normal labor in early first stage, and **D**, second stage. Passive segment is derived from lower uterine segment (isthmus) and cervix, and physiologic retraction ring is derived from anatomic internal os. **E**, Uterus in abnormal labor in second-stage dystocia. Pathologic retraction (Bandl's) ring that forms under abnormal conditions develops from physiologic ring.

Modified from Willson, JR, Carrington, ER, and Ledger, WJ: Obstetrics and gynecology, ed 8, St Louis, 1988, The CV Mosby Co.

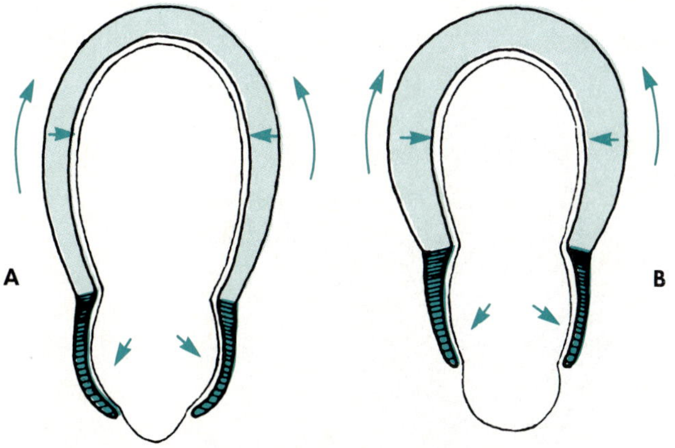

Fig. 16-15 Lower uterine segment and cervix are pulled up (retracted) as the fetus and amniotic sac are pushed downward. **A**, Cervix is effaced and partially dilated. **B**, Cervical dilation is complete. Cervix is being pulled upward as presenting part descends. Intrauterine space is decreasing.

From Willson, JR, and Carrington, ER: Obstetrics and gynecology, ed 8, St Louis, 1988, The CV Mosby Co.

in advancing labor. Eventually only a thin edge of the cervix can be palpated when effacement is complete. Effacement generally is advanced in nulliparas at term before more than slight dilation occurs. In multiparas, effacement and dilation of the cervix tend to progress together. Degree of effacement is expressed in percentages (e.g., a cervix is 50% effaced) (Fig. 16-16).

Dilation of the cervix is the enlargement or widening of the cervical os and the cervical canal during the first stage of labor. The diameter increases from perhaps less than 1 cm to approximately 10 cm to allow delivery of a term fetus. When the cervix is fully dilated (and completely retracted), it can no longer be palpated (Fig. 16-16).

Dilation of the cervix occurs by the drawing upward of the musculofibrous components of the cervix with strong uterine contractions. Pressure exerted by the amniotic fluid while the membranes are intact or force applied by the presenting part also encourages cervical dilation. Scarring of the cervix as a result of infection or surgery may retard cervical dilation.

Secondary Powers: Voluntary Bearing-down Efforts. As soon as the presenting part reaches the pelvic floor, the woman experiences an urge to push, a voluntary bearing-down effort (secondary power). The bearing-down effort is similar to that used in the process of defecation. However, a different set of muscles is used; the parturient contracts her diaphragm and abdominal muscles and pushes out the contents of the birth canal. Bearing-down results in increased intraabdominal pressure. The pressure compresses the uterus on all sides and adds to the power of the expulsive forces. The secondary forces have no effect on cervical dilation; they are of considerable importance in aiding the expulsion of the infant from the uterus and vagina after the cervix is fully dilated.

Any voluntary bearing-down efforts by the woman earlier in labor are counterproductive to cervical dilation. Straining will exhaust the woman and cause cervical trauma (p. 408).

Position of The Mother

The mother's position affects her anatomic and physiologic adaptations to labor. Her cardiac output normally increases during labor as uterine contractions return blood into the maternal vascular bed (see Table 16-4). The increase in cardiac output is possible if the maternal position prevents compression of the descending aorta and ascending vena cava. Increased cardiac output improves blood flow to the uterofetoplacental unit and the maternal kidneys.

Gravity is added to the psychologic benefits of various positions. In general, if the woman is in the upright position, uterine contractions are stronger and more efficient, and the duration of labor is shorter. The upright position includes standing, walking, and squatting. Frequent changes in position relieve fatigue and improve circulation to body parts. Maternal position changes enlist gravity to aid fetal descent through the birth canal.

Squatting during the second stage moves the uterus forward, thereby straightening the long axis of the birth canal (McKay, 1984). As the fetus descends in the birth canal, the pressure of the presenting part on stretch receptors of the pelvic floor stimulates the woman's bearing-down reflex. Stimulation of the stretch receptors in turn stimulates the release of oxytocin from the posterior pituitary (Ferguson's reflex). Oxytocin increases the intensity of the uterine con-

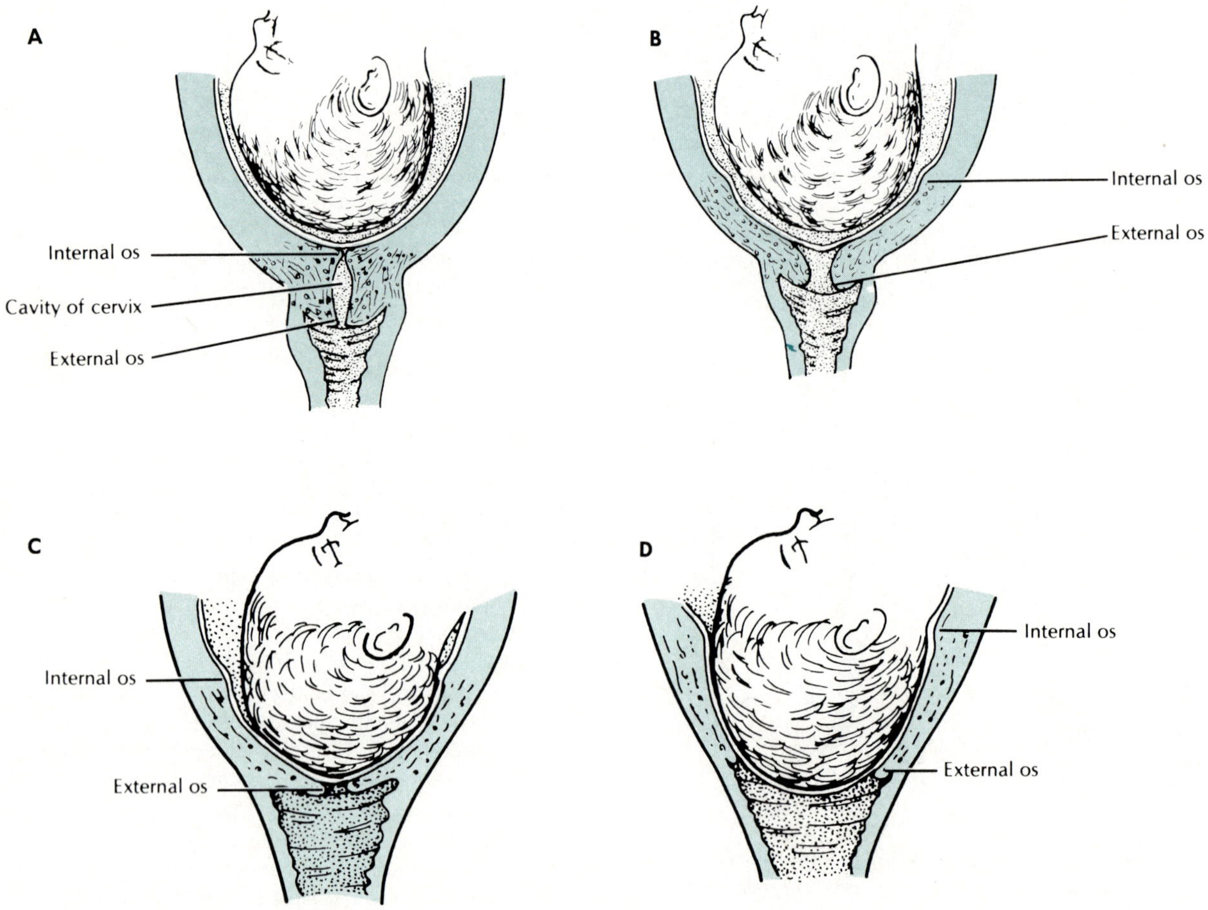

Fig. 16-16 Cervical effacement and dilation. Note how cervix is drawn up around presenting part (internal os). Membranes are intact, and head is not well applied to cervix. **A**, Before labor. **B**, Early effacement. **C**, Complete effacement (100%). Head is well applied to cervix. **D**, Complete dilation (10 cm). Some overlapping of cranial bones. Membranes still intact.

tractions. In a sitting position, such as squatting, abdominal muscles work in greater synchrony with uterine contractions during bearing-down efforts.

PROCESS OF LABOR

The phenomena of normal labor consist of the mechanism and stages of labor. The cardinal movements of the **mechanism of labor** are **descent**, **flexion**, **internal rotation**, **extension**, **external rotation**, and **expulsion** of the baby. There are three stages of labor. The **first stage** is the stage of dilation of the *cervix* from 0 to 10 cm, or full dilation. The **second stage**, expulsion, begins with complete cervical dilation and ends with the *birth of the baby*. The **third stage** begins with the delivery of the baby and ends with the *delivery of the placenta*. The first 1 to 2 hours after delivery constitute the period of recovery. This *recovery period* is referred to as the **fourth stage** of labor. Prodromal signs and symptoms are among the first indicators that the reproductive system is preparing for the childbirth.

Reproductive System Changes

Prodromes to Labor. In nulliparas the uterus gradually sinks downward and forward about 2 weeks before term, when the fetus's presenting part (usually the fetal head) descends into the true pelvis. This settling is called lightening or "dropping" and usually happens gradually (Fig. 16-17). After lightening, women feel less congested and breathe more easily. However, there is usually more bladder pressure as a result of this shift and consequently a return of urinary frequency. In multiparas, lightening may not take place until after uterine contractions are established and true labor is in progress.

Persistent low backache and sacroiliac distress as a result of relaxation of the pelvic joints may be described. Occasionally strong, frequent, but irregular uterine (Braxton Hicks') contractions may be identified by the gravida.

Before the onset of labor the vaginal mucus becomes more profuse in response to the extreme congestion of the vaginal mucous membranes. Brownish or blood-tinged cervical mucus may be passed (bloody show). The cervix becomes soft (ripens) and partially effaced and may begin to dilate. The membranes may rupture spontaneously.

Two other phenomena are common in the days preceding labor: (1) loss of 0.5 to 1.5 kg (1 to 3 lb) in weight, caused by water loss resulting from electrolyte shifts that in turn are produced by changes in estrogen and progesterone levels, and (2) a burst of energy. Women speak of a burst of energy that they often use to clean the house and put everything in order. This activity has been described as the "nesting instinct."

Onset of Labor. The onset of labor cannot be ascribed to a single cause. Many factors, including changes in the maternal uterus, cervix, and pituitary gland are involved. Hormones produced by the normal fetal hypothalamus, pituitary, and adrenal cortex probably contribute to the **initiation of labor.** Progressive uterine distension, increasing intrauterine pressure, and aging of the placenta seem to be associated with increasing myometrial irritability. This is a result of increased concentrations of estrogen and prostaglandins, and decreasing progesterone levels. In actuality, many factors may be responsible for initiating labor. The mutually coordinated effects of these factors result in strong, regular, rhythmic uterine contractions. Normally, these factors working in concert terminate in the birth of the fetus and the delivery of the placenta. It is still not completely understood how certain alterations trigger others and how proper checks and balances are maintained.

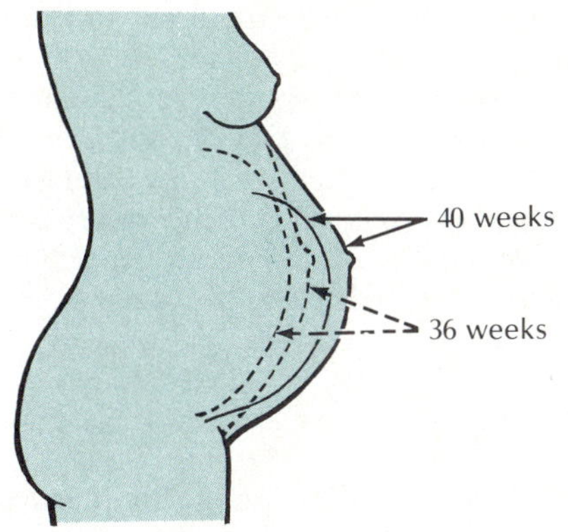

Fig. 16-17 Lightening.

Afferent and efferent nerve impulses to and from the uterus alter its contractility. Although nerve impulses to the uterus will stimulate contractions, the denervated uterus still contracts well during labor because oxytocin in the circulating blood is a regulator of labor. Therefore some women who are paralyzed can still give birth vaginally.

Mechanism of Labor: Vertex Presentation

The female pelvis has varied contours and diameters at different levels, and the presenting part of the passenger is large in proportion to the passage. For delivery to occur, the fetus must adapt to the birth canal during her or his descent. The turns and other adjustments necessary in the human birth process are termed the **mechanism of labor** (Fig. 16-18). The cardinal movements of the mechanisms of labor that occur in a vertex presentation are **engagement**, **descent**, **flexion**, **internal rotation**, **extension**, and **external rotation.** The fetus is born by expulsion. Although these phases will be discussed separately, a combination of movements is occurring simultaneously; for example, engagement involves both descent and flexion.

Engagement. When the biparietal diameter of the head passes the pelvic inlet, the head is said to be engaged in the pelvic inlet. In most nulliparous women this occurs before the onset of active labor because the firmer abdominal muscles direct the presenting part into the pelvis. In multiparous women with more relaxed musculature, the head often remains freely movable above the pelvic brim (**floating**) until labor is established. In the majority of cases the head of a normal-sized fetus enters the pelvis with the sagittal suture transverse to the pelvic inlet (Fig. 16-4).

Descent. Descent refers to the progress of the presenting part through the pelvis. As **partograms** (labor curves) (Figs. 18-7 and 18-8) indicate, there is little progress in descent during the latent phase of the first stage of labor. Descent becomes more rapid in the latter part of the active phase when the cervix has dilated to 5 to 7 cm. It is apparent especially when the membranes have ruptured.

Descent depends on three forces: (1) pressure of the amniotic fluid, (2) direct pressure of the contracting fundus on the fetus, and (3) contraction of the maternal diaphragm and abdominal muscles in the second stage. The effects of these forces are modified by the size and shape of the maternal pelvic planes and the size and capacity of the fetal head to mold.

The degree of descent is gauged by the station of the presenting part (Fig. 16-19). The speed of the descent increases in the second stage of labor. In nulliparas this descent is slow but steady; in multiparas the descent may be rapid. Progress in the descent of the presenting part is determined by vaginal examination until the presenting part can be seen at the introitus.

Flexion. As soon as the descending head meets resistance from the cervix, pelvic wall, or pelvic floor, flexion normally occurs, and the chin is brought into more intimate contact with the fetal chest (Fig. 16-18, *B*). Flexion permits the smaller suboccipitobregmatic diameter (9.5 cm) rather than the larger diameters to present to the outlet.

Internal Rotation. The maternal pelvic inlet is widest in the transverse diameter. Therefore the fetal head passes the inlet into the true pelvis in the occiput transverse position (Fig. 16-4). The outlet is widest in the anteroposterior diameter, however. To exit, the fetal head must rotate. Internal rotation begins at the level of the ischial spines but is not completed until the presenting part reaches the lower pelvis. As the occiput rotates anteriorly, the face rotates posteriorly. With each contraction the fetal head is guided by the bony pelvis and the muscles of the pelvic floor. Eventually the occiput will be in the midline beneath the pubic arch. The head is almost always rotated by the time it reaches the pelvic floor (Fig. 16-18, *C*). Both the levator muscles and the bony pelvis are important for anterior ro-

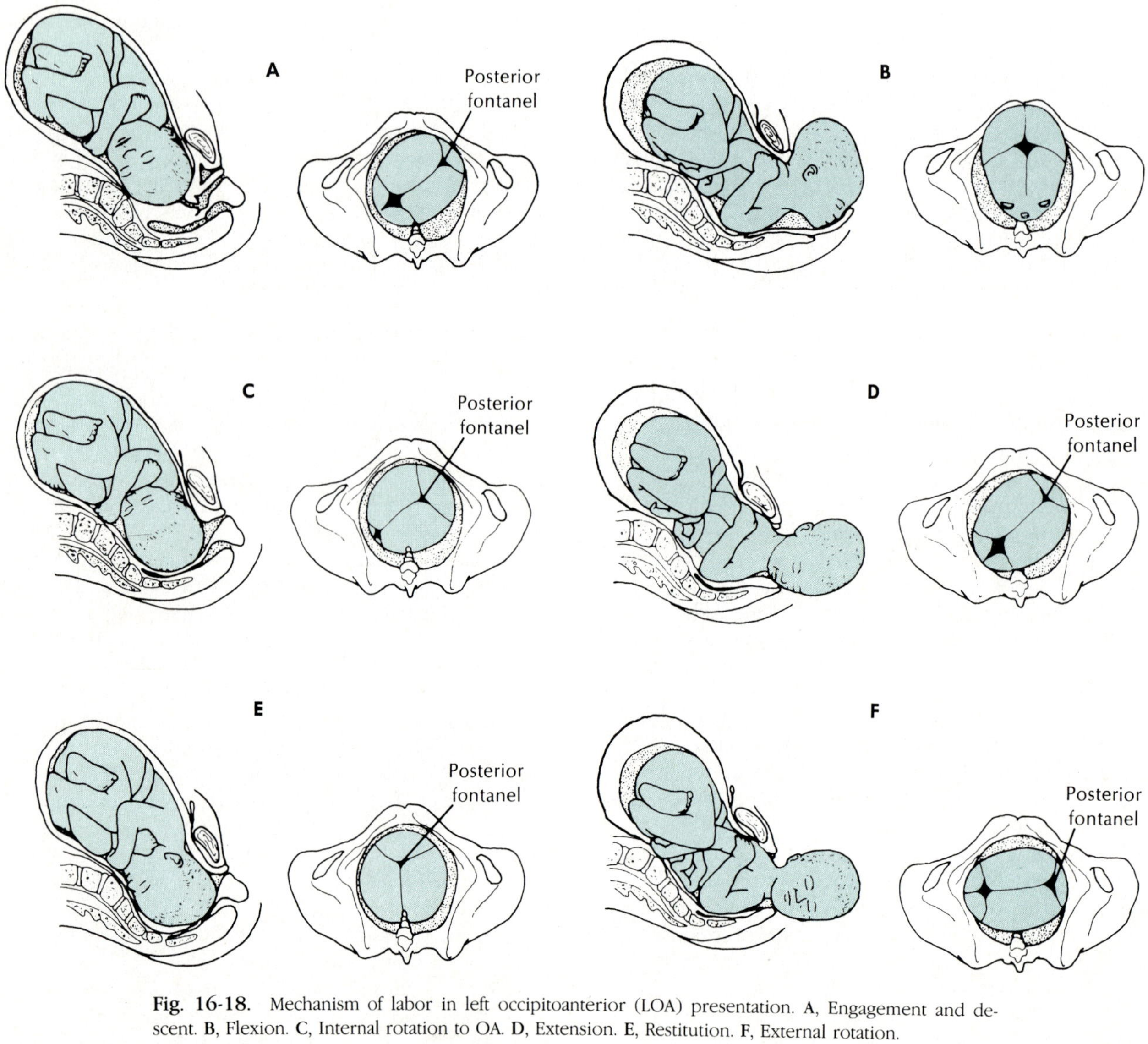

Fig. 16-18. Mechanism of labor in left occipitoanterior (LOA) presentation. **A**, Engagement and descent. **B**, Flexion. **C**, Internal rotation to OA. **D**, Extension. **E**, Restitution. **F**, External rotation.

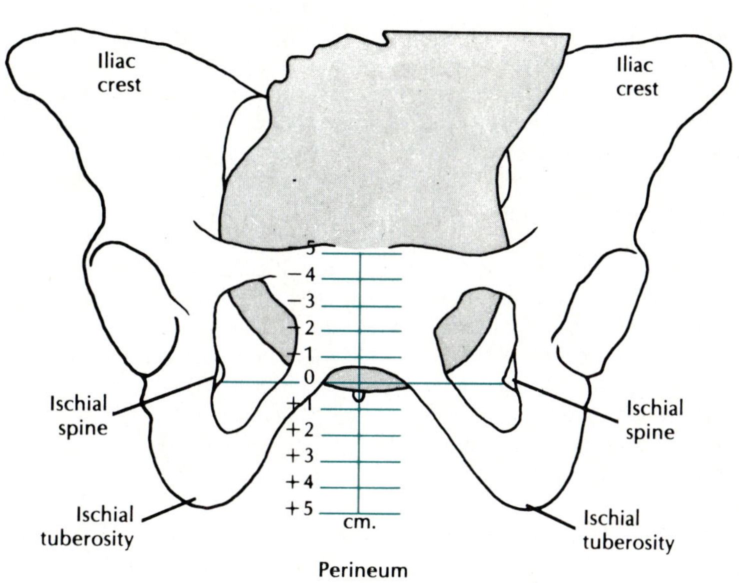

Fig. 16-19 Stations of presenting part, or degree of descent. Silhouette shows head of infant approaching station +1.
Courtesy Ross Laboratories, Columbus, Ohio.

tation. Previous childbirth injury or regional anesthesia compromises the function of the levator sling.

Extension. When the fetal head reaches the perineum to be born, it is deflected anteriorly by the perineum. The occiput acts as the fulcrum as it passes under the lower border of the symphysis pubis. As a result the head is born by extension: first the occiput, then the face, and finally the chin (Fig. 16-18, *D*).

Restitution and External Rotation. After delivery of the head, it rotates briefly to the position it occupied when it was engaged in the inlet. This movement is referred to as restitution (Fig. 16-18, *E*). The 45-degree turn realigns the infant's head with her or his back and shoulders. The head can then be seen to rotate further. External rotation occurs as the shoulders engage and descend in maneuvers similar to those of the head. As noted earlier, the anterior shoulder descends first. When it reaches the outlet, it rotates to the midline and is delivered from under the pubic arch. The posterior shoulder is guided over the perineum until it is free of the introitus.

Expulsion. After delivery of the shoulders, the head and shoulders are lifted up toward the mother's pubic bone and the trunk of the baby is delivered by a movement of lateral flexion in the direction of the symphysis pubis. When the baby is completely born, birth is complete. *This* is the end of the second stage of labor and *the time* is recorded on the records.

Stages of Labor

Normal labor (eutocia) is recorded when the woman is at or near term, without complications, when a single fetus presents by vertex, and when labor is complete within 24 hours.

The course of normal labor is remarkably constant and consists of three concomitant subprocesses: (1) regular progression of uterine contractions, (2) effacement and progressive dilation of the cervix, and (3) progress in descent of the presenting part. Four stages of labor are recognized.

First Stage of Labor. The first stage of labor is considered to last from the onset of regular uterine contractions to full dilation of the cervix. Commonly the onset of labor is difficult to establish; the woman may be admitted to the labor floor just before delivery so that the beginning of labor may be only an estimate. The first stage is much longer than the second and third combined. Great variability is the rule, however, depending on the essential factors discussed earlier. Some multiparas may reach full dilation in less than an hour, or, uncommonly a nullipara may reach complete dilation of the cervix in 24 hours.

The first stage of labor has been divided into two phases: a *latent phase* and an *active phase*.* During the latent phase there is more progress in effacement of the cervix and little increase in descent. During the active phase there is more rapid dilation of the cervix and descent of the presenting part. If the degree of dilation and descent is plotted in a graph, it forms an S curve. This curve can be used as a basis for assessment of progress in labor (Figs. 18-7 and 18-8).

Second Stage of Labor. The second stage of labor lasts from full dilation of the cervix to delivery of the fetus. Labor of up to 2 hours is considered within the normal range for the second stage.

Third Stage of Labor. The third stage of labor lasts from delivery of the fetus to delivery of the placenta. The placenta normally separates with the third or fourth strong

*Transition is a part of the active phase of the first stage of labor (see Chapters 17 and 33).

uterine contraction after the infant has been delivered. Then it should be delivered with the next uterine contraction after placental separation. Placental separation usually begins with the contraction that delivers the baby's trunk and is normally completed with the first contraction after the birth of the baby. However, delivery of the placenta within 45 to 60 minutes is generally considered within normal limits.

Fourth Stage of Labor. The fourth stage of labor arbitrarily lasts about 2 hours after delivery of the placenta. It is the period of immediate recovery, when homeostasis is reestablished. It serves as an important period of observation for complications, such as abnormal bleeding.

Duration of Labor. There are no absolute values for the normal length of the first stage of labor (Willson, Carrington, and Ledger, 1988). Variations may reflect differences in the client population or in clinical practice. Friedman (1978) provides statistical upper limits for the first and second stages of labor:

	Nulliparous	*Multiparous*
First stage		
Latent phase	20 hours	14 hours
Active phase	1.2 cm per hour	1.5 cm per hour
Second stage	2 hours	1.5 hours

The duration of the third stage will be 15 to 30 minutes or even longer if the physician waits for the mother to expel the placenta herself. When the placental stage is managed actively, its duration can be less than 5 minutes (Willson, Carrington, and Ledger, 1983).

A description of the labor experience of a significant number of parturients is given in Figs. 18-7 and 18-8. Friedman and Sachtleben (1965) used this information to predict the duration of normal labor for the first and second stages.

ANATOMIC AND PHYSIOLOGIC ADAPTATIONS

The mother and fetus must adapt anatomically and physiologically during the birth process. Accurate assessment of the parturient and fetus requires a knowledge of expected adaptations. Maternal and fetal responses are addressed below.

Maternal Adaptations

Body Systems. A thorough understanding of maternal adaptations to pregnancy (see Chapter 10) is fundamental to anticipating and meeting the parturient's needs. Table 16-4 summarizes normal adaptations by body systems, including objective and subjective symptomatology.

Discomfort During Labor

Origins. The discomfort experienced during labor has two origins. During the *first stage* of labor, uterine contractions cause (1) cervical dilation and effacement and (2) uterine ischemia (decreased blood flow and therefore local oxygen deficit) from contraction of the arteries to the myometrium.

The discomfort from cervical changes and uterine ischemia is *visceral.* The discomfort is located over the lower abdomen and radiates to the lumbar area of the back and down the thighs. Usually the woman experiences discomfort only during contractions and is free of pain between contractions.

During the *second stage* of labor, the stage of expulsion of the baby, the woman experiences perineal or *somatic* pain. Perineal discomfort results from traction on the peritoneum and uterocervical supports during contractions. It can also be produced by expulsive forces or from pressure by the presenting part on the bladder, bowel, or other sensitive pelvic structures.

Pain may be *local,* with cramplike pain and a tearing or bursting sensation because of distension and laceration of the cervix, vagina, or perineal tissues. It may also be *referred,* with the discomfort felt in the back, flanks, or thighs. Emotional tension from anxiety and fear may increase pain and perception of pain during labor.

Pain impulses during the first stage of labor are transmitted through the spinal nerve segment of T11-12 and accessory lower thoracic and upper lumbar sympathetic nerves. Pain impulses during the second stage of labor are carried through S1-4 and the parasympathetic system. Pain experienced during the third stage, as well as so-called afterpains, is uterine, similar to that experienced early in the first stage of labor. Areas of discomfort are illustrated in Fig. 16-20.

Symptomatology. Pain results in both psychic responses and reflex physical actions. The quality of physical pain has been described as pricking, burning, aching, throbbing, sharp, nauseating, or cramping. Pain in childbirth gives rise to symptoms that are identifiable. It may cause increased activity of the sympathetic nervous system. As a result there are changes in blood pressure, pulse, respirations, and skin color. Bouts of nausea and vomiting and excessive perspiration are also commonplace. Certain affective expressions of suffering are familiar to all. Affective changes include increasing anxiety with lessened perceptual field, writhing, crying, groaning, gesturing (hand clenching and wringing), and excessive muscular excitability throughout the body. Childbirth pain is of a limited duration (at most 2 to 3 days).

Perception of Pain

Pain Threshold. Although the pain threshold is remarkably similar in all people regardless of sexual, social, ethnic, or cultural differences, these differences play a definite role in the individual's perception of the pain experience. The reasons for the effects of such factors as culture, use of counterstimuli, or distraction in coping with pain are not fully understood. The meaning of pain and the verbal and nonverbal expressions given to pain are apparently learned from interactions within the primary social group. It is personalized for each individual. As pain is experienced, people develop various coping mechanisms to deal with it. Pain or the possibility of pain that has unknown qualities can induce fear in which anxiety borders on panic. Fatigue and sleep deprivation magnify pain. Parity may affect perception of labor pain (see research highlight, p. 350).

Table 16-4 *Maternal Anatomic and Physiologic Adaptation to Labor*

Body System	Normal Adaptation to Labor	Observable Findings
Cardiovascular		
Cardiac output	Increases; during each contraction 400 ml blood is emptied from uterus into maternal vascular system	Pulse slows BP increases No alteration in FHR
WBC	Mechanism unknown; possible WBC level changes secondary to physical/emotional stress	$\geq$25,000/mm^3
Peripheral vascular system	Response to cervical dilation; compression of vessels by fetus passing through birth canal	Malar flush Hot or cold feet Hemorrhoids
Respiratory		
Rate	Increased physical activity with increased oxygen consumption	Rate increases
Acid/base balance	Hyperventilation may be cause of increased pH early in labor; pH returns to normal by end of first stage	None if hyperventilation is controlled
Renal		
Fluids/electrolytes	Diaphoresis Increased insensible water loss through respirations Occasionally NPO	Possible temperature elevation Thirst
Bladder	Becomes an abdominal organ starting with the second trimester	When filling, palpable above symphysis pubis
	Deterrents to spontaneous voiding: tissue edema secondary to pressure from presenting part, discomfort, sedation, embarrassment	Possible inability to void spontaneously
Urine constituents	Breakdown of muscle tissue from the physical work of labor	1 + proteinuria
Integument	Great distensibility in area of vaginal introitus; degree of distensibility varies with the individual	Minute tears in skin around vagina
Musculoskeletal	Marked increase in muscle activity (in addition to uterine activity)	Diaphoresis Fatigue 1 + proteinuria ? Increased temperature
	Backache and joint ache (unrelated to fetal position) secondary to increased joint laxity at term	Verbal/nonverbal cues indicating back discomfort
	Leg cramps secondary to labor process and pointing of toes	Verbal/nonverbal cues
Neurologic	Sensorium alterations change as woman moves through phases of first stage of labor and as she moves from one stage to the next	Euphoria to increased seriousness to amnesia between contractions to elation or fatigue after delivery
	Discomfort (see discussion on pain during childbirth)	
	Endogenous endorphins and encephalins and physiologic anesthesia of perineal tissues with decreased perception of discomfort	Verbal/nonverbal cues absent or minimal
Gastrointestinal	Mouth breathing, dehydration, emotional response to labor	Verbal/nonverbal cues indicating dry mouth
	Decreased motility and absorption; delayed stomach emptying time	Nausea/vomiting of undigested foods eaten after onset of labor
	Nausea as a reflex response to full cervical dilation	Nausea/vomiting Belching
	History of diarrhea concurrent with onset of labor or	Verbal cue
	Presence of hard or impacted stool in rectum	Palpable on vaginal examination Fecal material extruded during delivery
Endocrine	Level of estrogen decreases; levels of progesterone, prostaglandins, and oxytocin increase	Labor is initiated and maintained
	Metabolism increases	Blood glucose may decrease

Gate-Control Theory. At times, pain stimuli that are particularly intense can be ignored. It may be that certain nerve cell groupings within the spinal cord, brain stem, and cerebral cortex have the ability to modulate the pain impulse through a blocking mechanism. This gate-control theory is helpful in understanding the approaches used in education-for-childbirth programs or the use of hypnosis in labor. According to this theory, local physical stimulation such as massage or stroking of the woman in labor can balance the pain stimuli. It is thought to work by closing down a hypothetical "gate" in the spinal cord, thus blocking pain signals from reaching the brain. Also, when the laboring woman performs neuromuscular and motor skills, activity within the spinal cord itself further modifies the transmission of pain. Cognitive activities of concentration on breathing and relaxation skills require selective and directed cortical activity, which activates and closes the gating mechanism as well. The gate-control theory emphasizes the need for a supportive setting for birth. In such an environ-

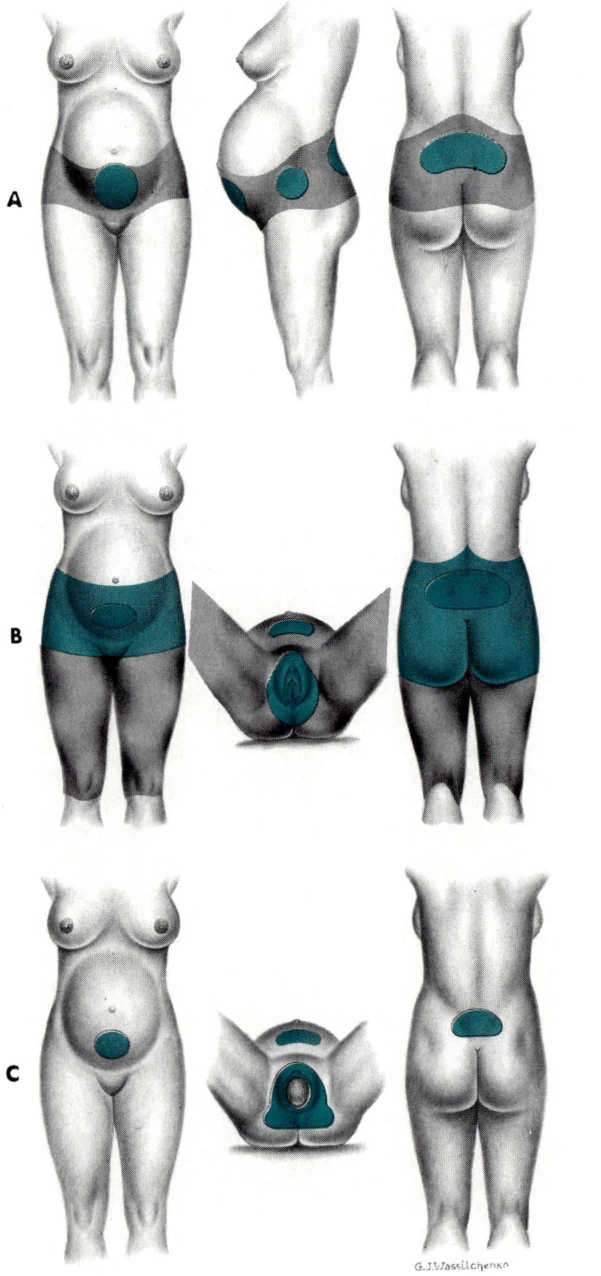

Fig. 16-20 Discomfort during labor. **A**, Distribution of labor pain during first stage. **B**, Distribution of labor pain during later phase of first stage and early phase of second stage. **C**, Distribution of labor pain during later phase of second stage and actual birth. (Gray shading indicates areas of mild discomfort; light colored shading indicates areas of moderate discomfort; dark colored areas indicate intense discomfort.)

RESEARCH HIGHLIGHT

Progression of Labor Pain in Primiparas and Multiparas

Purpose

Pain is a multidimensional subjective experience of discomfort composed of both sensory and affective components. This study was designed to systematically describe the different dimensions of pain during the progression of labor and delivery in primiparas and multiparas.

Sample

A sample of 138 Swedish women participated in the study. Pain was measured for the first three stages of labor. Data were collected at all three stages for only 84 of the women because the other women either did not arrive at the hospital until after the cervix was dilated 5 to 7 cm or because of the speed of delivery in Stage III.

Methodology

The Johansson Pain-o-meter and the Visual Analogue Scale were used to assess pain. The Pain-o-meter's allowance for assessment of the intensity of sensory and affective components of pain permits pain to be analyzed both quantitatively and qualitatively. The Visual Analogue Scale consists of a 10 cm straight line, which represents a continuum of intensity and has verbal anchors at opposite ends representing no pain, and pain as bad as it can be.

Findings

Primiparas reported higher affective pain in Stage III than multiparas. The sensory component of pain was the major pain intensity factor in both groups of subjects. Even though the primiparas received more medication, they reported much more affective pain than the multiparas during all three stages.

Implications

Pain had been discussed with the women in the sample during prepared child-birth courses. However, as a rule, laboring women experienced much more pain than they had anticipated. The investigators suggest the use of noninvasive pain-relief methods such as relaxation and music therapy as useful methods for reducing the affective component of pain.

Gaston-Johansson, F, Fridh, G, and Turner-Norvell, K: Progression of labor pain in primiparas and multiparas, Nurs Res 37(2):87, 1988.

ment the laboring woman can relax and allow the various higher mental activities to be implemented.

Fetal Adaptations

Fetal heart rate (FHR) monitoring provides reliable and predictive information about the condition of the fetus as it relates to oxygenation (Chapter 17). Stresses to the uterofetoplacental unit result in characteristic FHR patterns. It is important for the nurse to have a basic understanding of the factors involved in fetal oxygenation and of the fetal responses that reflect adequate fetal oxygenation.

Review of Uteroplacental Circulation. The placenta serves as a link between the fetal and maternal circulations. Uterine spiral arterioles must pass through the full thickness of the myometrium to reach the intervillous space. The maternal blood spurts through these arterioles into the intervillous space. Oxygen, nutrients, and inherent warmth are absorbed by the thin-walled fetal capillaries contained within the chorionic villi of the placenta. These are eventually carried to the fetus by the umbilical vein. Carbon dioxide and fetal waste products circulate back to the placenta through the umbilical arteries and fetal capillaries in the chorionic villi. Here they cross back through the intervillous space to the maternal circulation.

The average FHR at term is 140 beats per minute (bpm); the normal range is 120 to 160 bpm. Earlier in gestation the FHR is higher, with an average of approximately 160 bpm at 20 weeks' gestation. The rate decreases progressively as the maturing fetus reaches term. The normal range of pH in an adult is 7.35 to 7.45. The average fetal range is 7.30 to 7.35.

Origins of Fetal Stress. Uterofetoplacental circulation can be affected by many factors. These factors include maternal position, uterine contractions, blood pressure, and umbilical cord blood flow. Maternal position is discussed earlier in this chapter and in Chapter 18. Uterine contractions during labor tend to increase circulation through the spiral arteries and subsequent perfusion through the intervillous space. This stress seems to be well within the ability of the fetus to compensate for in most gestations. The fetus is exposed to increased pressure as she or he is moved passively through the birth canal during the mechanism of labor. Usually umbilical cord blood flow is undisturbed by uterine contractions or fetal position.

Normal Adaptations to Stress of Labor. A healthy fetus with an adequate uterofetoplacental circulation will respond in fairly predictable ways to stresses. Transitory accelerations and slight decelerations can be expected in response to spontaneous fetal movement, vaginal examination, fundal pressure, uterine contractions, and abdominal palpation. These changes prepare the fetus for initiating respirations after birth. During vaginal delivery, 7 to 42 ml of amniotic fluid is squeezed out of the fetal lungs. Normally, fetal Po_2 falls from 80 to 15 mm Hg, arterial Pco_2 rises from 40 to 70 mm Hg, and arterial pH falls below 7.35. These changes stimulate chemoreceptors in the aorta and carotid bodies to initiate respirations immediately after birth.

SUMMARY

A firm grasp of the theory of essential factors and processes in labor and maternal and fetal adaptations is only half of the preparation a nurse needs to implement the nursing process with parturients. Although anatomic and physiologic considerations are important, it is equally important to understand the family's adaptation to childbirth. Family responses and adaptation are discussed in Chapter 18.

KEY CONCEPTS

- Five essential factors affect the process of labor and delivery.
- Because of its size and relative rigidity, the fetal head has a major effect on the birth process.
- The diameters at the plane of the pelvic inlet, midpelvis, and outlet, plus the axis of the birth canal, determine whether vaginal delivery is possible and the manner by which the fetus may pass down the birth canal (mechanism of labor).
- The forces acting to expel the fetus and placenta are derived from involuntary uterine contractions during the first stage of labor, which are augmented by voluntary bearing-down efforts during the second stage.
- The mother's position affects her anatomic and physiologic adaptations to labor.
- The cardinal movements of the mechanism of labor are descent, flexion, internal rotation, extension, external rotation, and expulsion of the baby.
- Many factors, including changes in the maternal uterus, cervix, and pituitary gland, are involved in the initiation of labor.
- An understanding of maternal adaptations to pregnancy is fundamental to anticipating and meeting the parturient's needs.
- Discomfort during labor has two origins: visceral pain during the first stage and somatic pain during the second stage.
- A healthy fetus with an adequate uterofetoplacental circulation will respond in fairly predictable ways to stresses.

STUDY QUESTIONS AND ACTIVITIES

1. Use an anatomic model of the bony pelvis with a fetal doll to demonstrate maternal pelvic measurements and fetal head diameters.
2. Demonstrate fetopelvic relationships in the cardinal movements of the mechanism of normal (occiput anterior [OA] position) labor. Following this, practice various mechanisms and perform return demonstrations.
3. Assess each other as to type of pelvis using information presented in Table 16-3. Identify types of pelves when assessing women in prenatal clinic or physician's office.

4. Palpate sutures and anterior and posterior fontanels of newborns in the nursery.
5. Provide nursing care to women who are in false labor, as well as to those in established labor, to become skilled in assessing by fundal palpation the differences in the characteristics of uterine contractions.
6. Role play a primigravida who is 36-weeks pregnant and who is asking the nurse at the prenatal class how she will recognize signs that she is in labor. Explain the signs and symptoms of labor and encourage suggestions from other students.
7. Develop a nursing care plan for a woman in labor; discuss the differences in a plan for a woman in early labor and a woman in well-established labor.

References

Friedman, EA: Labor: clinical evaluation and management, ed 2, New York, 1978, Appleton-Century-Crofts
Friedman, EA, and Sachtleben, MR: Station of the fetal presenting part, Am J Obstet Gynecol 93:522, 1965
McKay, S: Squatting: an alternate position for the second stage of labor, MCN 9:181, May/June 1984
Willson, JR, Carrington, ER, and Ledger, WJ: Obstetrics and gynecology, ed 8, St Louis, 1988, The CV Mosby Co

Bibliography

Carlson, J, Diehl, J, Sachtleben-Murray, M, et al: Maternal position during parturition in normal labor, Obstet Gynecol 68:433, 1986
Curry, J: Pregnancy health fair, Can Nurse, p. 26, June 1988
Danforth, DN, editor: Obstetrics and gynecology, ed 4, Philadelphia, 1986, Harper & Row, Publishers, Inc
Dundes, L: The evolution of maternal birthing position, Am Public Health 77:5, 636, 1987
Feetham, SL: Acute and chronic pain in maternal-child health, MCN 9:249, July/Aug 1984
Jensen, MD, and Bobak, IM: Handbook of maternity care: a guide for nursing practice, St. Louis, 1980, The CV Mosby Co
Liggins, GC: New concepts of what triggers labor, Contemp OB/GYN 19(5):131, 1982
Malasanos, L, Barkauskas, V, Moss, M, and Stoltenberg-Allen, K: Health assessment, ed 3, St. Louis, 1986, the CV Mosby Co
McKay, S, and Roberts, J: Second stage labor: what is normal? JOGN Nurs 14:101, March/April 1985
Okita, JR, et al: Initiation of human parturition, Am J Obstet Gynecol 142:432, 1982
Pritchard, JA, MacDonald, PC, and Gant, NR: Williams obstetrics, ed 17, Norwalk, Conn, 1985, Appleton-Century-Crofts
Roberts, J, and Kriz, D: Delivery positions and perineal outcome, Nurse Midwife 29(3):186, 1984
Romond, JL, and Baker, IT: Squatting in childbirth: a new look at an old tradition, JOGN Nurs 14:406, Sept/Oct 1985

CHAPTER

17

Pharmacologic Control of Discomfort and Fetal Monitoring

Learning Objectives

Correctly define the key terms listed.

Discuss the types of analgesia and anesthesia used during labor.

Compare the types of pharmacologic control of discomfort by stage of labor and method of delivery.

Discuss the use of naloxone (Narcan).

Relate each stage of the nursing process in the management of labor discomfort.

Explain baseline fetal heart rate and evaluate its periodic changes.

Discuss fetal heart rate monitoring by periodic auscultation and electronic methods.

Describe fetal monitoring by blood sampling and assessment for meconium-stained amniotic fluid.

Review nursing standards for electronic fetal monitoring.

Key Terms

analgesia
anesthesia
ataractics
baseline fetal heart rate (FHR)
epidural blood patch
bradycardia
cricoid pressure
early neonatal neurobehavioral scale (ENNS)
electronic fetal monitoring (EFM)
hyperbaric
intrathecal
isobaric
local infiltration
meconium-stained amniotic fluid
meninges
narcotic agonist
narcotic antagonist
nonperiodic accelerations
paracervical block
peridural methods
periodic accelerations
periodic decelerations
pudendal
sedatives
smooth (flat) baseline
spinal (subarachnoid)
tachycardia
tocotransducer
ultrasound transducer
uteroplacental insufficiency
variability

Nursing care of the woman in labor may include pharmacologic control of discomfort and fetal monitoring. Medications for discomfort can be used throughout all stages of labor. Fetal monitoring may be used in both the first and second stages. The nurse must be knowledgeable in both of these areas to provide competent, comprehensive nursing care during labor.

ANALGESIA AND ANESTHESIA

The use of analgesia and anesthesia was not generally accepted as part of obstetric management until Queen Victoria used chloroform during the birth of her son in 1853. Much study has gone into the development of pharmacologic control of discomfort during the birth period. The goal of researchers is to develop methods that will provide adequate pain relief to women without adding to maternal or fetal risk.

Nursing management of obstetric analgesia and anesthesia combines the nurse's expertise in maternity care with a knowledge and understanding of anatomy and physiology, and of medications and their desired and undesired side effects and methods of administration.

Anesthesia encompasses analgesia, amnesia, relaxation, and reflex activity. It is the abolition of pain perception by interrupting the nerve impulses going to the brain. Analgesia is a component of anesthesia. The term *analgesia* is best reserved to describe only those states in which there is alleviation of the sensation of pain or the raising of one's threshold for pain perception. An *agonist* is an agent that does something; an *antagonist* is an agent that blocks something from happening.

Analgesia can be induced by (1) positive conditioning and (2) analgesic drugs (Table 17-1). A basic understanding of the normal course of labor and delivery and proper physical and psychologic preparation by the gravid woman will reduce pain during childbirth. Especially important is good antenatal care in its broadest sense; reassurance and suggestion are beneficial. Participation in childbirth preparation classes such as those proposed by Grantly Dick-Read or psychoprophylaxis by Lamaze (1972) or Bradley (1974) should do much to alleviate distress (see Chapter 14).

The type of analgesic or anesthetic to be used is chosen in part by the stage of labor and by the method of delivery (see box at right).

PHARMACOLOGIC CONTROL OF DISCOMFORT BY STAGE OF LABOR AND METHOD OF DELIVERY

First Stage	Second Stage
Systemic analgesia* Sedatives Narcotics Analgesic potentiators Paracervical block Peridural block (continuous) Lumbar epidural Caudal Subarachnoid spinal (continuous) Local Morphine	Local infiltration of perineum Pudendal nerve block Peridural block ("one shot") Lumbar epidural Caudal Subarachnoid spinal ("one shot," "saddle block") Inhalation Analgesia Anesthesia
Vaginal Birth	**Abdominal Birth**
Local infiltration Pudendal block Peridural block Subarachnoid spinal Inhalation analgesia	Subarachnoid spinal Peridural block Inhalation—general anesthesia

*Administered by labor nurse.

Systemic Analgesia

Sedatives. Sedatives such as barbiturates relieve anxiety and induce sleep only in prodromal or early latent labor and in the absence of pain. If the woman has pain, sedatives given without an analgesic may increase apprehension. Sedatives should not be employed late in the first stage or early in the second stage of labor if delivery is expected within 1 or 2 hours, because the newborn may exhibit severe central nervous system (CNS) depression. Undesirable side effects include respiratory and vasomotor depression of both mother and newborn. Sedatives do not cause amnesia but may confuse or distort recollection.

Sedative drugs may be short-acting (1 hour), for example, secobarbital (Seconal); intermediate (2 hours), for example, pentobarbital (Nembutal) sodium; or of long duration (3 hours), for example, phenobarbital (Luminal) sodium. Each of these drugs can be given orally or by intramuscular (IM) injection.

Narcotic Analgesic Compounds. Narcotic, opium-related drugs, for example, morphine and meperidine (Demerol), are especially effective for the relief of severe, persistent, or recurrent pain. They have no amnesic effect. These medications may be addictive if given regularly for a prolonged period, but labor does not fall into this category. Meperidine overcomes inhibitory factors in labor and may even relax the cervix (see medication cards at back of book). Narcotic-analgesic compounds, however, may have other undesirable side effects for the parturient; nausea and vomiting, respiratory depression, constipation, or urinary retention may develop. The fetus may be depressed. Resuscitation of the newborn may be difficult if sizable doses of narcotics are given within 1 or 2 hours of delivery. Narcotics should not be given after full dilation in a primigravida or after 7 or 8 cm dilation in a multipara, assuming a normal labor.

Mixed Narcotic Agonist-Antagonist Compounds. In the doses used during labor, compounds such as butorphanol tartrate (Stadol) and nalbuphine (Nubain) provide analgesia without causing respiratory depression. IM or intravenous (IV) routes are used for administration. If the woman has a preexisting narcotic dependency, the antagonist effect of these compounds will cause her to immediately exhibit symptoms of narcotic withdrawal.

Table 17-1 *Comparison of Modalities for Obstetric Analgesia*

Therapeutic Modality/Drug	Usual Parenteral Dose	Time of Administration	Advantages for Parturient	Disadvantages for Neonate	Nursing Concerns
Psychoprophylaxis		Late pregnancy Labor stages 1-3	No drugs Training in self-reliance	None	Pain controlled but not eliminated
Hypnosis		Late pregnancy Labor stages 1-3	No drugs In rare women, pain free	None	Suggestion reinforcement essential
Medications					
Sedatives					
Secobarbital sodium (Seconal) Pentobarbital (Nembutal) sodium	50-100 mg IM 50-100 mg IM	Early stage 1, midstage 1, or postdelivery	Disinhibition or somnolescence (no pain relief in usual doses)	Hypoactive "sleepy" neonate	Either subdued or excited; may become dehydrated
Narcotic Analgesics					
Morphine	8-15 mg IM or IV	Midstage 1	Analgesia excellent	Moderate to marked CNS depression if delivery <2 hr after administration	Emesis common
Meperidine	50-100 mg IM or IV	Midstage 1	Analgesia good	Slight CNS depression	Routine care
Narcotic Agonist-antagonist Compounds					
Butorphanol tartrate (Stadol) Nalbuphine (Nubain)	1-3 mg IM; 0.5-2 mg IV 0.2 mg/kg SC/IM; 0.1-0.2 mg/kg IV	Midstage 1	Analgesia without respiratory depression	None anticipated; monitor for CNS depression	If woman is dependent on narcotics, reversal of narcotic effect results in withdrawal symptoms
Narcotic Antagonist					
Naloxone (Narcan)	Adult—0.4 mg IM or IV; Neonate—0.01 mg/kg body weight, IV or SC	Stage 2 or to neonate	Reverses narcotic side effects (nausea, vomiting, tachycardia, hypertension, pruritus, respiratory depression)	None	Abrupt reversal of narcotic effect; withdrawal symptoms in narcotic addicts
Analgesic-potentiating Drugs (Ataractics, Tranquilizers)					
Promethazine (Phenergan) Hydroxyzine pamoate (Vistaril) Promazine (Sparine)	25-50 mg IM 25-50 mg IM or SC 50 mg IM	Early stage 1, midstage 1, and postdelivery	Apprehension, anxiety, depression relieved; narcotic effects potentiated; antiemetic	Drug enhances narcotic effect (CNS depression)	Closer supervision may be necessary because of mild pseudohypnotic state

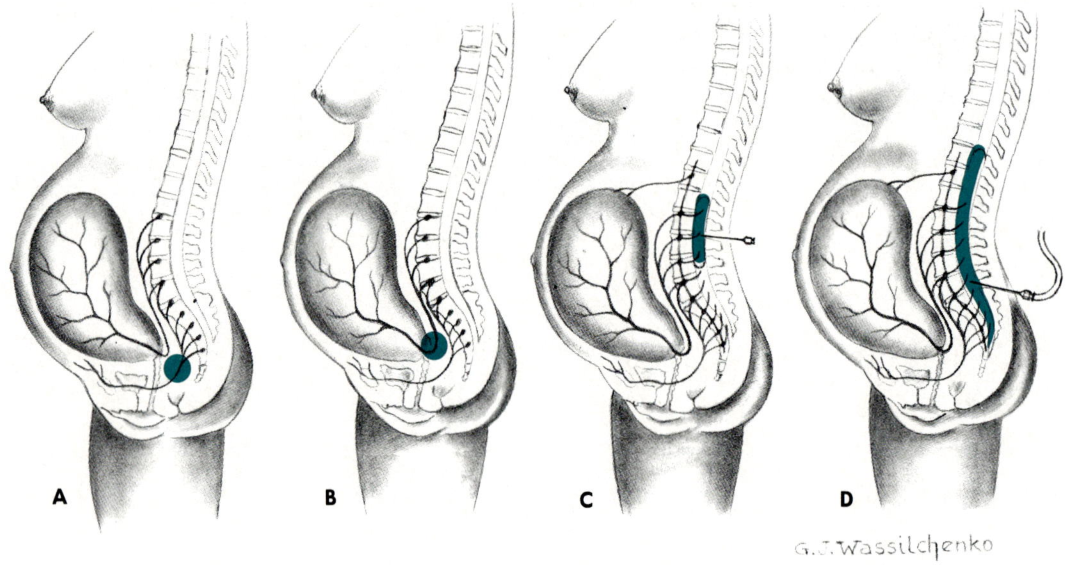

Fig. 17-1 Pain pathways and sites of pharmacologic nerve blocks. **A,** Pudendal block; suitable during second and third stages of labor and for repair of episiotomy. **B,** Paracervical (uterosacral) block: suitable during first stage of labor. **C,** Lumbar sympathetic block (one type of subarachnoid block): given as shown, suitable during first stage of labor (not usually method of choice; caudal is preferable). **D,** Epidural block: suitable during all stages of labor and for repair of episiotomy.

Narcotic Antagonists. If a traditional narcotic, such as morphine or meperidine, has been administered to a parturient, naloxone (Narcan), or the new narcotic antagonist naltrexone, promptly reverses the narcotic effects, including respiratory depression of the newborn. Therefore a narcotic antagonist is especially valuable if labor is more rapid than expected. If given to the mother approximately 10 to 15 minutes before delivery, the narcotic antagonist will counteract maternal and neonatal narcotic effects. If there is insufficient time for reversal of maternal-fetal effects of a narcotic drug, naloxone can be given, well diluted, into the umbilical vein of the newborn (see medication cards at back of book).

With the administration of naloxone, pain, of course, also returns. Naloxone also counters the effect or stress-induced elevated levels of endorphins (p. 739).

Analgesic-potentiators (Ataractics). Phenothiazines, so-called tranquilizer or antipsychotic drugs, have the property of augmenting most of the desirable but few of the undesirable effects of analgesics or general anesthetics. This category includes compounds such as promethazine (Phenergan), propiomazine (Largon), hydroxyzine pamoate (Vistaril), and promazine (Sparine).

As little as 50 mg of meperidine can be effective for the relief of pain during labor when given with, for example, 25 mg of hydroxyzine pamoate. Besides potentiating the effects of the analgesic, the ataractic (tranquilizer) also acts as an antiemetic. Fetal or neonatal problems rarely develop with these doses. The combination can be administered safely until the end of the first stage of labor.

Nerve Block Analgesia and Anesthesia

A variety of compounds are used in obstetrics to produce peripheral and regional analgesia and anesthesia. Most of these drugs are synthetically produced and are related chemically to cocaine and carry the suffix *-caine.* This helps identify a local anesthetic, but it does not distinguish the chemical group to which the drug belongs. Examples of common agents given in 0.5% to 1% solutions include lidocaine (Xylocaine) hydrochloride, bupivacaine (Marcaine), chloroprocaine* (Nesacaine), tetracaine (Pontocaine), and mepivacaine (Carbocaine).

The principal pharmacologic effect of local anesthetics is the temporary interruption of the conduction of nerve impulses, notably pain. Before the local anesthetic can act, it must reach the plasma membrane of the axon of the nerve to be blocked.

Rarely, individuals are sensitive (allergic) to one or more local anesthetics and develop tachycardia, syncope, or convulsions. Hypersensitivity does not depend on the route of administration. Non-allergy–related adverse effects, however, are often related to the route of administration. Testing with minute amounts of the drug to be used may determine such sensitivity. When excessive amounts of a regional anesthetic are injected, initially the CNS is stimulated. Stimulation may be followed by depression, hypotension, and other serious adverse effects. Atropine, antihistaminic drugs, oxygen, and supportive measures should bring relief. Adequate hydration is a prerequisite, so an IV line is placed before initiation of this type of anesthesia. All of these methods require sterile technique.

Local Infiltration Anesthesia. Infiltration anesthesia is

*Based on assessment using the Apgar score, blood gas analysis, drug concentration, and the assessment of newborn neurobehavioral response, it was found that bupivacaine and chloroprocaine offered some advantages over the other drugs: the newborns scored higher when these anesthetics were used than when the other agents were used (Lundberg, 1983).

produced by injecting dilute solutions (0.1%, i.e., 1% lidocaine hydrochloride in 10 to 20 ml) of the drug into the skin and then subcutaneously into the region to be anesthetized. Epinephrine often is added to the solution to intensify the anesthesia in a limited region and to prevent excessive bleeding and systemic effects (Hahn, Oestreich, and Barkin, 1986). Repeated injection will prolong the anesthesia as long as needed. The sensory nerve endings are anesthetized. This method of administration is used for minor surgery, such as incision (episiotomy) and repair of episiotomy and laceration.

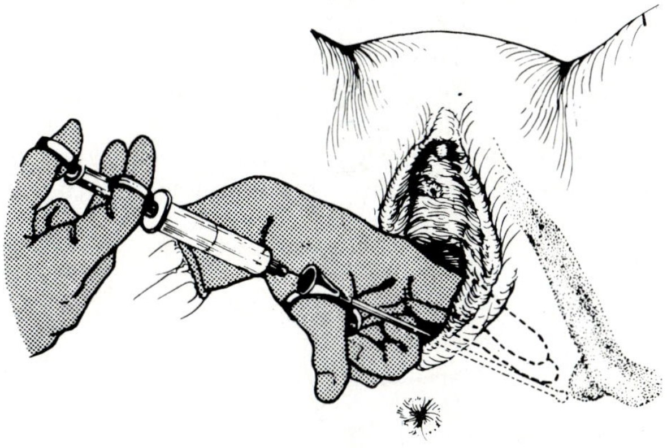

Fig. 17-2 Pudendal block. Use of needle guide ("Iowa trumpet") and Luer-Lok syringe to inject medication.
Modified from Benson, RC: Handbook of obstetrics and gynecology, ed 5, Los Altos, Calif, 1974, Lange Medical Publications.

Pudendal Block. Pudendal nerve block is administered 10 to 20 minutes before perineal anesthesia is needed. Once the presenting part descends through the cervix, vaginal and soon pudendal distension occur. Under these circumstances, vaginal and perineal pain can be eliminated by an anesthetic block of the pudendal and posterior cutaneous and hemorrhoidal nerves (Fig. 17-1, *A*).

The pudendal nerve, arising from S2 through S4 nerves, traverses the sacrosciatic notch just medial to the tip of the ischial spine on each side. Injection of an anesthetic solution at or near these points will anesthetize the pudendal nerves peripherally (Fig. 17-2). Anesthetic block of the posterior cutaneous nerves can be effected by depositing a small amount of the drug beneath the inferior median border of the ischial tuberosity. Infiltration of the anesthetic solution subcutaneously around the anus should block the hemorrhoidal nerves.

Pudendal block does not change maternal hemodynamic or respiratory functions nor does it affect the newborn adversely (Danforth and Scott, 1986). It does, however, have the same potential toxicity as all regional nerve blocks. Disadvantages therefore do exist. For example, the bearing-down reflex is lessened or lost completely. Anesthetic effect is insufficient to permit instrumental vaginal delivery except for low forceps; and it does not allow uterine exploration or manual removal of the placenta (Danforth and Scott, 1986).

Subarachnoid Spinal Anesthesia. Local anesthetic is injected through the third, fourth, or fifth lumbar interspace into the subarachnoid space (Figs. 17-3 and 17-4), where

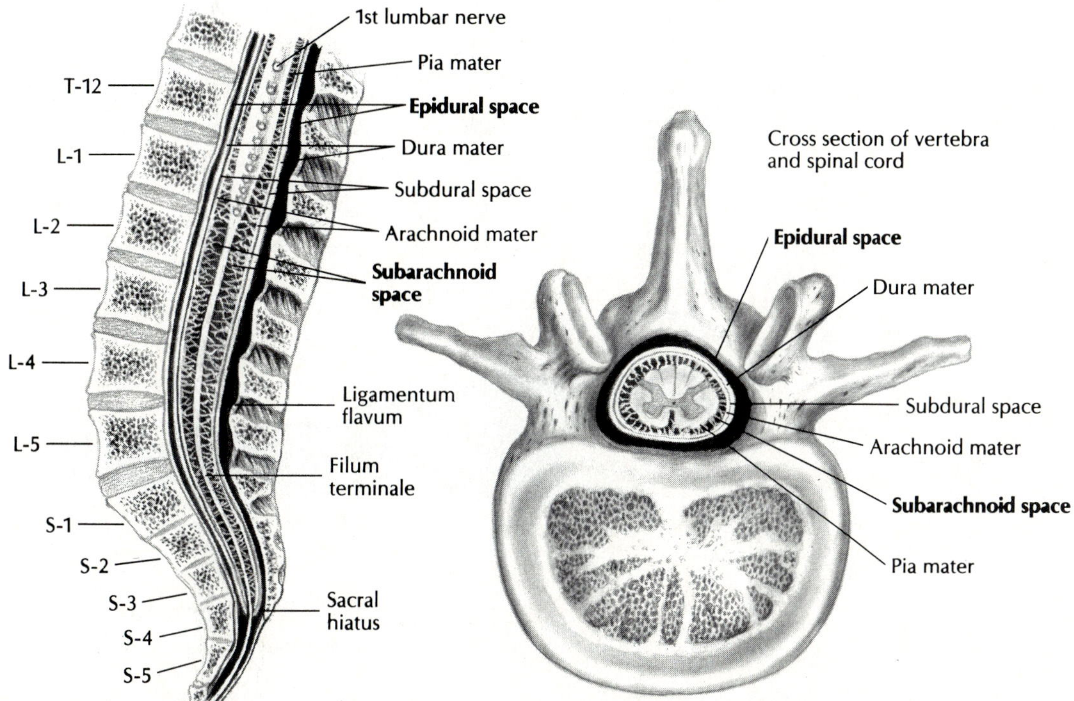

Fig. 17-3 Membranes and spaces of spinal cord.

the medication mixes with cerebrospinal fluid. The level and depth of the spinal sensory and motor blockade is regulated by the type of medication, the dosage, and the specific gravity of the solution. Solutions with the same specific gravity as spinal fluid (isobaric) act primarily at the site of injection. A solution with a specific gravity greater than that of spinal fluid (hyperbaric) is used, therefore, since it tends to diffuse downward. Dextrose solution added to the anesthetic increases its specific gravity. Therefore the spinal application can be used during the first (Fig. 17-1, *C*) or the second stage of labor or for abdominal surgery.

Low Spinal Block. The low spinal ("saddle") injection is made with the woman in a sitting position, her legs over the side of the delivery table, and her feet supported on a stool. The nurse stands in front of her. The woman rests her chin on her chest, arches her back "like a rainbow," and leans on the nurse for support. The nurse comforts and coaches her. This posture is assumed to widen the intervertebral space for ease in inserting the spinal needle and to allow the heavy anesthetic solution to gravitate downward. **The injection is made between contractions.** Once the anesthetic has been injected, the woman remains upright for about 30 seconds (as directed by the anesthesiologist) to permit downward diffusion. Then the woman is assisted to a supine position. She must remain supine with the head elevated slightly. The table can be tilted appropriately to "fix" the drug so that the level of dermal anesthesia is at or below the umbilicus. A very low spinal block anesthetizes the nerves L1-5 and S1-4, which supply the area over the low back, pudendum, and symphysis pubis, as well as the pelvic viscera. Onset of anesthesia usually occurs within 1 to 2 minutes after injection. Duration of anesthesia is 1 to 3 hours, depending on the anesthetic used.

Marked hypotension, decreased cardiac output, and respiratory inadequacy tend to occur during any spinal anes-

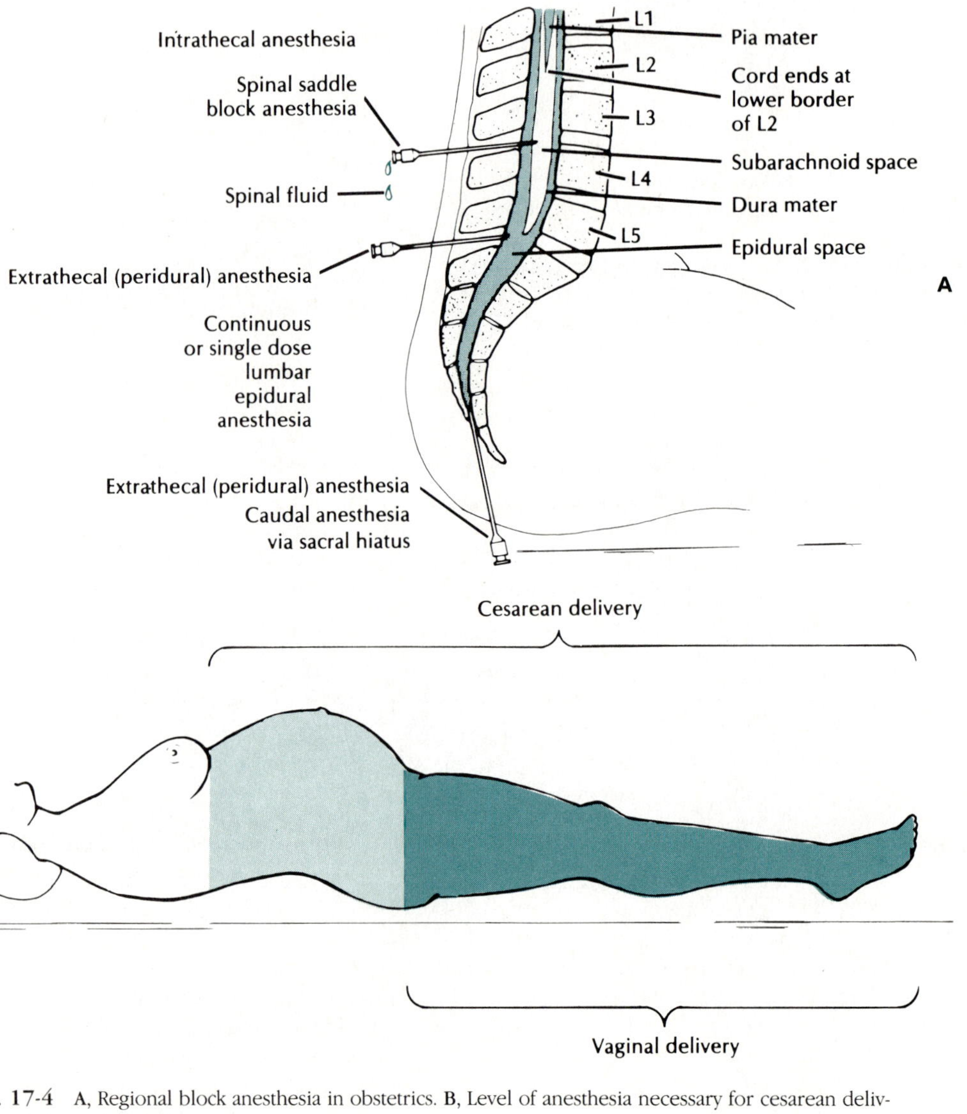

Fig. 17-4 **A**, Regional block anesthesia in obstetrics. **B**, Level of anesthesia necessary for cesarean delivery and for vaginal delivery.
Courtesy Ross Laboratories, Columbus, Ohio.

thesia. Therefore the blood pressure, pulse, respirations, and fetal heart rate (FHR) must be checked and recorded every 5 to 10 minutes. If signs of serious hypotension or fetal distress develop, oxygen should be given by mask. Vasopressors such as ephedrine are administered IV or IM. The rate of IV fluid infusion may be increased if marked hypotension develops. Since the mother is not able to sense her contractions, she must be instructed when to bear down. After delivery of the placenta the mother will need assistance to move back to her recovery bed. She must remain flat in bed for a minimum of 8 hours to prevent postlumbar (intrathecal) puncture (spinal) headache. A small, flat pillow may be used for her head.

Advantages of spinal anesthesia include ease of administration and absense of fetal hypoxia with maintenance of normotension. Maternal consciousness is maintained, excellent muscular relaxation is achieved, and blood loss is not excessive. Usually, no other anesthetic agents (e.g., inhalation drugs) are required. If stirrups are used for delivery, care must be taken to position them properly (Chapter 19). Spinal anesthesia may be the method of choice for women with severe respiratory problems or with liver, kidney, or metabolic disease.

Disadvantages of spinal anesthesia include drug reactions, rare chemical myelitis or infection, hypotension, and high spinal anesthesia with respiratory paralysis. There is an increased need for operative delivery (episiotomy, low forceps extraction) because of elimination of voluntary expulsive efforts. After delivery, there is an increased tendency for bladder and uterine atony, and spinal headache (see discussion below).

With *continuous spinal anesthesia,* an indwelling catheter, inserted in the subarachnoid space, allows the anesthetic to be delivered in fractional doses. This technique minimizes the likelihood of adverse effects. If anesthesia is needed over an extended period, the anesthetic can be replenished as needed. The size of the puncture hole into the subarachnoid space increases the potential for spinal headache.

Spinal Headache. Leakage of cerebrospinal fluid from the site of puncture of the meninges (membranous coverings of the spinal cord) is the major factor in the beginning of spinal headache. Headache may be postural and occur only in the head-up or sitting or standing position. Presumably, with postural changes, the diminished volume of cerebrospinal fluid allows traction on pain-sensitive CNS structures. Headache and auditory and visual problems may persist for days or weeks.

The likelihood of this unpleasant complication, however, can be reduced if the anesthesiologist uses a small-gauge spinal needle and avoids multiple punctures of the meninges. Positioning the woman absolutely flat in bed (with only a small, flat pillow for her head) for at least 8 hours has been recommended to prevent postspinal headache, but there is no definitive evidence that this procedure is effective. Positioning the woman on her abdomen is thought to decrease the loss of fluid through the puncture site. Hyperhydration has been claimed to be of value, but there is no compelling evidence to support its use (Pritchard, MacDonald, and Gant, 1985).

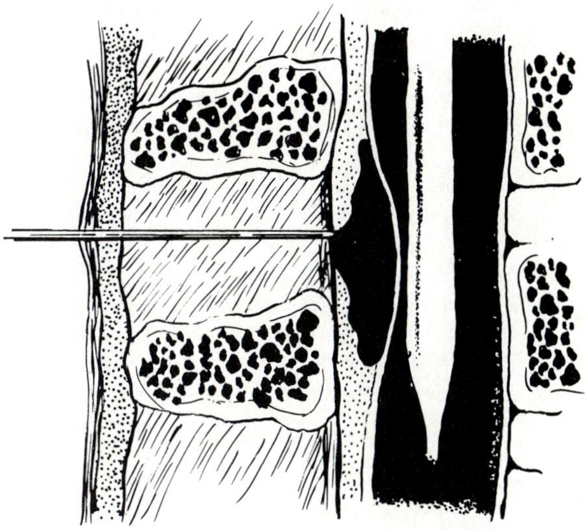

Fig. 17-5 Blood patch therapy for spinal headache.

Creation of an epidural blood patch (a patch repairing a tear or a hole in the dura mater around the spinal cord) has proven efficacious. To form a patch, a few milliliters of the woman's blood without anticoagulant is injected epidurally at the site of the spinal tap (Fig. 17-5), forming a clot that covers the hole and prevents further fluid loss. Saline similarly injected in larger volumes has also been claimed to provide relief. Abdominal support with a girdle or abdominal binder seems to afford relief and is worth trying. The headache may be remarkably improved by the third day and absent by the fifth day for some women.

Intrathecal Morphine Analgesia. A more recent method of administering narcotic drugs is by the intrathecal (IT) route (injection into subarachnoid space containing cerebrospinal fluid) (Danforth and Scott, 1986). This method is based on the existence of narcotic receptors along the pain pathway in the spinal cord, in the brain stem, and in the thalamus. Since these receptors are specific for narcotics, a small quantity (e.g., 0.5 mg morphine) produces marked analgesia lasting 12 to 24 hours. Comfort is achieved in 20 to 30 minutes and the effect lasts throughout labor, sometimes extending into the postpartum period. Since there is no associated sympathetic blockage, resultant maternal hypotension is not a problem. In addition, the motor power remains intact, preserving the woman's ability to bear down during the second stage of labor. Unfortunately, IT injection of morphine has considerable undesirable side effects, including respiratory depression, pruritus, nausea and vomiting, urinary retention, sleepiness, and the need for additional analgesia or anesthesia for forceps delivery or repair of episiotomy.

All of these side effects are related to the dose administered. With 0.5 mg morphine, analgesia is usually satisfactory, and the woman is alert. Naloxone 0.4 mg drawn in a syringe is kept in the woman's room. Equipment to support respiration should also be readily available.

Many obstetricians feel that the benefits of IT injection are not sufficient to warrant its routine use. However, the IT injection of morphine may lead to a more rational approach to pain control in which a drug is injected as close to the specific receptor as possible. Other narcotics, natural, synthetic, or agonist-antagonist, are being considered to maximize the beneficial effects and minimize the side effects of the IT narcotic technique (Danforth and Scott, 1986).

Peridural (Epidural) Block. Relief from the pain of uterine contractions and delivery, both vaginal and abdominal, can be accomplished by injecting a suitable local anesthetic into the peridural (epidural) space (see Figs. 17-3 and 17-4). The portal of entry into this space for obstetric analgesia and anesthesia is through either a lumbar intervertebral space or caudally through the sacral hiatus and sacral canal. A single injection or repeated doses through an indwelling plastic catheter results in excellent analgesia-anesthesia (Fig. 17-1, *D*).

Continuous Lumbar Epidural Block. Complete anesthesia for the discomfort of labor and vaginal delivery requires a block from T10 to S5. For abdominal delivery, a block is essential from at least T8 to S1. The diffusion of epidural anesthesia depends on the location of the catheter tip, the dose and volume of anesthetic agent used, and the woman's position (e.g., horizontal, or head-up position) (Pritchard, MacDonald, and Gant, 1985).

Continuous Caudal Block. The caudal space is the lowest extent of the epidural, or peridural, space (see Figs. 17-3 and 17-4). Emerging from the dural sac a few inches higher, a rich network of sacral nerves passes downward through the caudal space. A suitable anesthetic solution filling the caudal canal may eliminate the sensation of pain carried via the sacral nerves to produce anesthesia suitable for vaginal delivery. Higher levels with continuous caudal technique provide both analgesia in the first and second stages of labor and anesthesia for delivery.

Method of Administration. *The mother is hydrated with 500 ml to 1000 ml lactated Ringer's solution intravenously within 20 minutes before the block. Facilities for cardiopulmonary resuscitation, including oxygen and suction, must be immediately available.*

For introduction of epidural anesthesia, the woman is positioned as for a spinal injection or in a modified Sims' position (Fig. 17-6). For modified lateral Sims' position, the woman is placed on her left side, shoulders parallel, legs slightly flexed, and back arched.

For introduction of caudal anesthesia, the woman is placed in a modified knee-chest or Sims' position, with the upper leg well flexed at the hip and knee, and the lower leg extended. The injection site is cleansed and draped. Once the needle and fine plastic catheter have been inserted into the caudal canal (see Figs. 17-3 and 17-4), a test

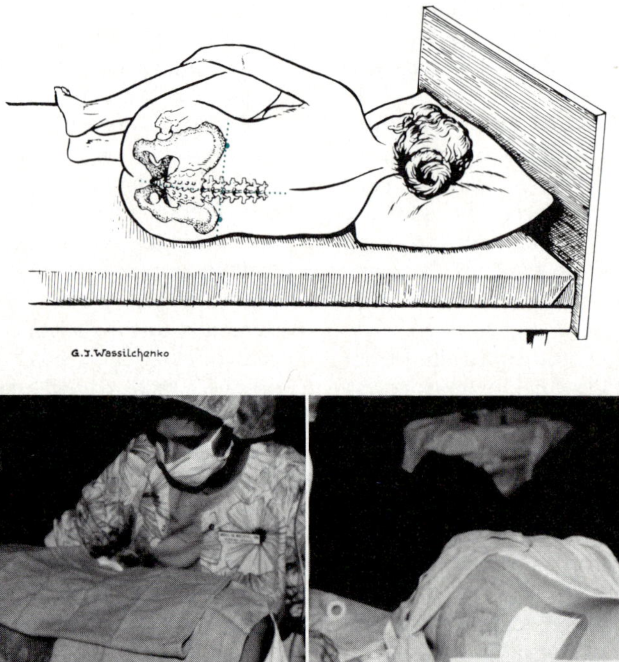

A

B

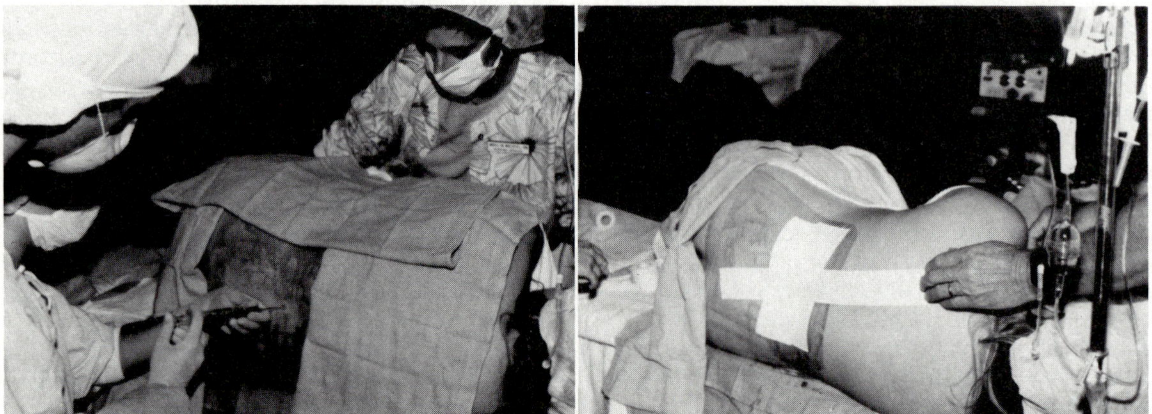

C

Fig. 17-6 **A,** Lateral decubitus position for epidural and subarachnoid block and anatomic landmarks to locate needle insertion site. **B,** Epidural anesthesia. Skin has been prepared with antiseptic solution (povidone-iodine) (Betadine). Area is draped with sterile towels. Nurse continues to support woman. **C,** Catheter is taped to woman's back; port segment is taped near her shoulder.

(**B** and **C** courtesy Stanford University Hospital, Stanford, California.)

dose is given. After 5 minutes the anesthesiologist checks the anal sphincter for relaxation and the temperature of the lower extremities. Relaxation of the anal sphincter and increased warmth of the feet indicate proper placement of the catheter in the caudal canal. The remainder of the dose is then given. Relief is experienced in a few minutes, and repeated doses may be administered as the effect wears off. The catheter and syringe are taped securely in position so that the woman is free to move about in bed. The blood pressure, pulse, respirations, and FHR must be measured and recorded every 15 minutes.

The woman is positioned to avoid weight of the uterus on abdominal vessels. Oxygen is available should hypotension occur despite maintenance of IV fluid and displacement of maternal uterus to the left. The anesthesiologist may need to inject ephedrine and accelerate IV fluid infusion.

As with a spinal anesthetic, the FHR and progress in labor must be monitored carefully. The parturient will not be aware of changes in strength of uterine contractions or descent of the presenting part. Occasionally depression of contractions may result, necessitating augmentation with oxytocin. She will need coaching to push, and low forceps will be required to complete delivery. After the third stage, she will need assistance to move to the recovery bed.

The *advantages* of continuous caudal block are numerous: fetal distress is rare, but it may occur with rapid absorption or marked hypotension; the mother remains alert and cooperative, and only partial motor paralysis develops; and good relaxation is achieved and blood loss is not excessive. Dose, volume, and type of anesthetic can be modified to allow the mother to push, to produce perineal anesthesia, and to permit forceps or even abdominal delivery if required (Pritchard, MacDonald, and Gant, 1985).

The *disadvantages* of continuous caudal block include the following: special training and experience are required by the anesthesiologist. Since a considerable amount of the drug must be used, reactions or rapid absorption of the anesthetic agent may result in hypotension, convulsions, or paresthesia. The incidence of operative delivery is increased because the woman cannot bear down effectively. Occasionally accidental high spinal anesthesia (and later, spinal headache) may follow inadvertent perforation of the dural (thecal) membrane.

For some women, the anesthetic selected is not effective, and a second form of anesthesia is required. Establishment of effective pain relief with maximum safety takes time. Consequently, in case of rapid labor, the potential for pain relief during labor and for delivery is not realized. Therefore epidural anesthesia for women of higher parity in active labor is likely to prove not worth the bother, risk, and expense (Pritchard, MacDonald, and Gant, 1985).

Epidural Narcotic Method. Epidural narcotic usage in obstetrics is being reported in the literature. There is a high concentration of opioid receptors in the spinal column that are open to the action of the opiates to block pain. These receptors are reached by a catheter placed in the epidural space. When used in labor, 1.5 mg morphine is administered through the epidural catheter. The women feel contractions, but no pain is noted by her or observers. Since the pushing reflex is not lost, the mother can cooperate during delivery. Maternal vital signs are normal during labor, and no motor or sympathetic block is noted. Women may experience itching of the face, mouth, and eyes. These symptoms are treated with promethazine (Phenergan) or metoclopramide (Reglan).

Women who deliver by the abdominal route are given epidural morphine 1 hour after surgery through the epidural catheter. The catheter is then removed, and the women are pain free for 24 hours. Ability to be up with ease and to care for the baby are two of the advantages to epidural morphine. The women cannot believe the effects of the morphine on pain. Early ambulation and freedom from pain facilitate bladder emptying. To women who have had a previous cesarean delivery with the usual postoperative pain, the effects of the epidural morphine seem miraculous. The nurse caring for the woman who has been given epidural morphine generally is amazed at the mother's ease in ambulation and relative freedom from pain.

The side effects of epidural morphine are nausea, vomiting, pruritus (itching), urinary retention, and delayed respiratory depression. The serious concern is for delayed respiratory depression. The woman is observed frequently and is placed on an apnea monitor for 24 hours (Fig. 17-7). Antiemetics, antipruritics, and naloxone (Narcan) are used to relieve the nausea, vomiting, pruritus, and respira-

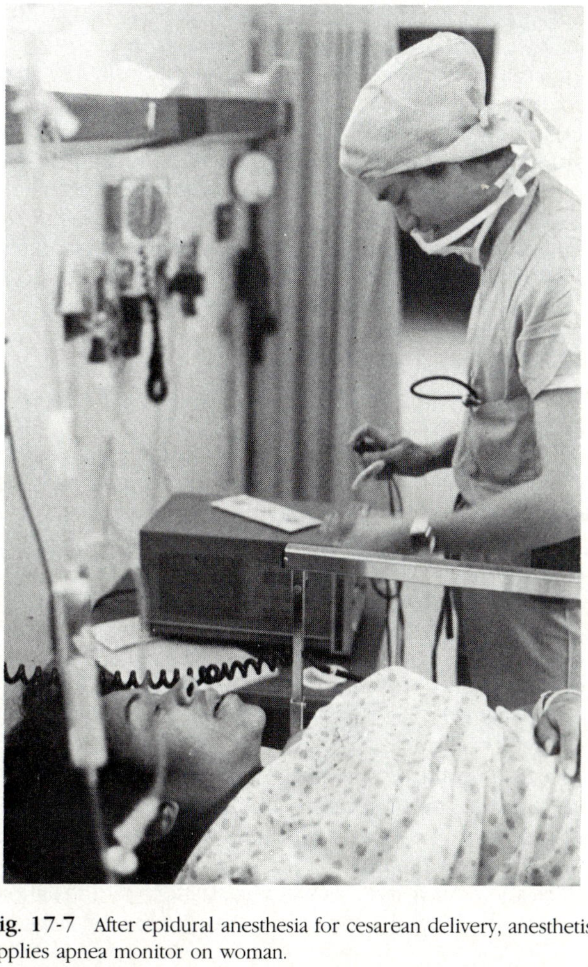

Fig. 17-7 After epidural anesthesia for cesarean delivery, anesthetist applies apnea monitor on woman.

tory depression. Hospital protocols provide specific directives for treatment for postepidural narcotic side effects.

Contraindications to Subarachnoid and Peridural Blocks. Some contraindications to epidural analgesia apply equally to caudal and subarachnoid blocks (Danforth and Scott, 1986):

1. *Antepartum hemorrhage.* Acute hypovolemia leads to increased sympathetic tone to maintain the blood pressure. Any anesthetic technique that blocks the sympathetic fibers can lead to significant hypotension that can endanger the mother and baby.
2. *Anticoagulant therapy or bleeding disorder.* If a woman is receiving anticoagulant therapy or has a bleeding disorder, injury to a blood vessel may result in a hematoma. The hematoma may compress the cauda equina or the spinal cord and lead to serious CNS sequelae.
3. *Infection at the injection site.* Infection can be spread through the peridural or subarachnoid spaces if the needle traverses an infected area. Amnionitis, on the other hand, is not a contraindication to these nerve blocks.
4. *Tumor at the injection site.* A tumor at the injection site is an unusual but definite contraindication.

Relative contraindications to intravertebral blocks include client refusal, extensive back surgery, morbid obesity or anatomic abnormality in which landmarks cannot be identified, and current or prior disease of the CNS (Danforth and Scott, 1986).

Paracervical (Uterosacral) Block. For paracervical anesthesia, a dilute local anesthetic drug (e.g., 5 ml of 1% procaine) is injected just beneath the mucosa in each fornix posterolateral to the cervix (9 and 3 o'clock positions) after the cervix is more than 5 cm dilated (see box, p 364). A needle guide (e.g., the "Iowa trumpet") is useful but not indispensable in facilitating the paracervical block (Fig. 17-8). Relief from discomfort is noticed within approximately 5 minutes. Excellent pain relief lasts for at least 1 hour.

Anesthesia extends from the lower uterine segment and cervix to the upper one third of the vagina (see Fig. 17-1, *B*); there is no perineal anesthesia. Although there may be a transient depression of contractions, there is little or no effect on the labor. Repeat injections may be given until the cervix is dilated to 8 cm, whereupon another method, such as pudendal block, will be necessary.

Paracervical block anesthesia may cause fetal intoxication because of rapid absorption of the drug. When the anesthetic is injected into the tissues lateral to the cervix, it is picked up by the circulation, which quickly involves the uterus and placenta. When overdosage occurs, the fetus may exhibit bradycardia because of the quinidine-like effect of the anesthetic on the myocardium or, as recent research indicates, because of a reduction in uterine blood flow. In addition, CNS medullary depression may develop, and the neonate may show vascular collapse and apnea at delivery.

Because of these potential complications, paracervical block may not be the method of choice for labor but remains an option for anesthesia during abortion or other gynecologic procedures.

Inhalation Analgesia. Self-administration of inhalation gases may be helpful, especially during the second stage of labor. The mother breathes subanesthetic concentrations of inhalation anesthetic; if given properly, the woman remains conscious but has profound pain relief. An example of this type of anesthetic is methoxyflurane (Penthrane). The route is usually self-administered from a capsule and mask strapped to the wrist. The physician sets the desired concentration and the woman inhales the drug during contractions. The goal of this method is for the woman to remain conscious while profound analgesia, as well as some amnesia for painful events, is achieved.

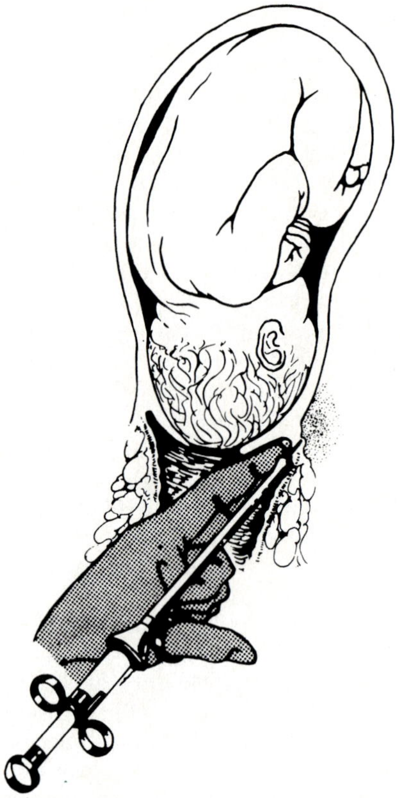

Fig. 17-8 Paracervical block. Note the position of the hand and fingers in relation to the cervix and fetal head and the shallow depth of the needle insertion. Note also that no undue pressure is applied at the vaginal fornix by the fingers or needle guide.
From Benson, RC: Handbook of obstetrics and gynecology, ed 7, Los Altos, Calif, 1980, Lange Medical Publications.

The nurse must stay with the woman and never administer the drug for her because overdose is a risk. The nurse must also monitor vital signs closely (be alert for cardiac arrhythmias) every 30 minutes and FHR every 15 minutes. The woman should remain conscious and not become delirious or excited. The nurse alerts the physician and removes the analgesic from the woman's hand if the mother has cardiac arrhythmia or loses consciousness or if FHR abnormalities occur. Today these inhalation analgesics are rarely used.

Inhalation analgesics such as nitrous oxide are nontoxic when administered with ample air or oxygen. Nitrous oxide is administered by trained personnel during contractions or continuously. The goal is analgesia. If the woman has used lysergic acid diethylamide (LSD) at some time in the past, she is not a candidate for this type of analgesia, since she will usually experience a "flashback" or "trip."

General Anesthesia. General anesthesia is rarely indicated for uncomplicated vaginal delivery. The woman is not awake with this method, and there is danger of aspiration and respiratory depression. It is safer than regional anesthesia for hypovolemic clients, however, and does not depress the newborn unless the mother is anesthetized deeply. An example is thiopental (Pentothal) sodium. Administered IV, thiopental sodium produces rapid induction of anesthesia but depresses the newborn. It is useful in controlling maternal convulsions. Halothane (fluothane) inhalation relaxes the uterus quickly and facilitates intrauterine manipulation, version, and extraction. The desired effect is general loss of sensitivity to touch, pain, and other stimulation.

If general anesthesia is being considered, the nurse gives the woman nothing by mouth and sees that an IV infusion is established. The nurse premedicates the woman with cimetidine or ranitidine to neutralize acid contents of the stomach. Sometimes the nurse is asked to assist with **cricoid pressure** before intubation. Priorities for recovery room care are to maintain open airway, maintain cardiopulmonary functions, and prevent postpartum hemorrhage. Routine postpartum care is organized to facilitate parent-child attachment as soon as possible and to answer the mother's questions. When appropriate, the nurse assesses the mother's readiness to see the baby and her response to the anesthesia and to the event that necessitated general anesthesia delivery (e.g., giving birth by cesarean delivery when vaginal delivery was anticipated).

Combination Anesthesia for Cesarean Birth. Light general anesthesia, considered by many to be ideal for cesarean delivery, is achieved with a combination of thiopental, nitrous oxide–oxygen, and succinylcholine. The woman is given oxygen for 3 minutes, followed by almost simultaneous rapid administration of thiopental and succinylcholine. During intubation, cricoid pressure is maintained to prevent aspiration of vomitus (Fig. 17-9). Cricoid pressure is often maintained by the nurse. When the woman is somnolent, a nitrous oxide–oxygen mixture is given. Excellent tolerance of the anesthetic is widely reported. Rapid resuscitation of the mother and even small-for-gestational-age (SGA) and growth-retarded infants can be achieved.

DRUG EFFECTS ON NEONATAL NEUROBEHAVIORAL RESPONSE

There is an ongoing debate concerning the effects of epidural anesthesia on the neonate's neurobehavioral responses. Studies of associations between neurobehavioral outcome and epidural anesthesia are far from consistent (Avard and Nimrod, 1985). One author found a beneficial effect (Hodgkinson et al., 1977). Some authors found that neonates did not score as well (Rosenblatt et al., 1981). Others found no difference (Marx, 1984; Abboud et al., 1982). However, the findings suggest a mild transient effect on newborn behavior.

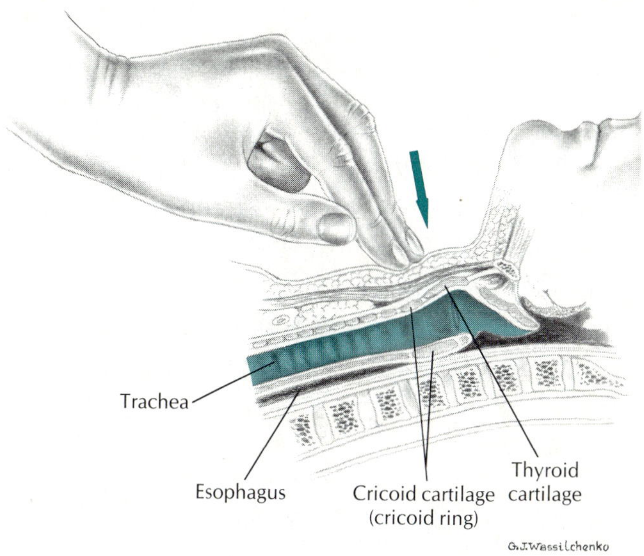

Fig. 17-9 Technique of applying pressure on cricoid cartilage to occlude esophagus prevents pulmonary aspiration of gastric contents during anesthesia induction.

Early Neonatal Neurobehavioral Scale

The value of the Apgar score is limited to detecting gross neonatal depression. Currently the early neonatal neurobehavioral scale (ENNS) is used most extensively. ENNS is used to evaluate the newborn at 1 hour and then at 4 and 8 hours after birth (Scanlon, 1974). The use of ENNS is similar to that of the Brazelton Neonatal Behavioral Assessment Scale (Chapter 21).

The ENNS bases evaluation on the Apgar score, specific tests, and general scores in light of the infant's state (see Table 21-4). Specific tests are scored from 0 for "absent" to 3 for "vigorous." These tests assess the infant's response to pinprick, response decrement to repeated pinprick, muscle tone evaluations, pull to sitting (head control), arm recoil (held to side), truncal tone, general body tone, rooting, sucking, Moro's reflex, response decrement to repeated Moro, response decrement to light, response to sound, and placing (standing up of infant).

The same scores are assigned for alertness, overall assessment, predominant state, and lability of state.

Amiel-Tison, Barrier, and Schnider Scale

A newer method than ENNS, the Amiel-Tison, Barrier, and Schnider (ABS) scale, is used for assessing neurologic and adaptive capacity (Bonica, 1980). The ABS scale emphasizes muscle tone and therefore may be more accurate in determining the effects of drugs. It can be performed any time after 15 minutes of birth. The measurement was 0 for "absent" and 2 for "vigorous" for each of 5 criteria.

Adaptive capacity considers response to sound, habituation to sound, response to light, habituation to light, and consolability. *Passive tone* is determined by assessing the scarf sign, recoil of elbows, popliteal angle, and recoil of lower limbs. *Active tone* rates the active contraction of neck flexors, active contraction of neck extensors (from leaning forward position), palmar grasp, response to traction (following palmar grasp), and supporting reaction (upright position). *Primary reflexes* include automatic walking, Moro's reflex, and sucking. *General assessment* involves alertness, crying, and motor activity.

Assessment

Before Administration of Medication

The assessment of the parturient, her fetus, and her labor is a joint effort of the nurse and the physician, who then consult with the woman. The needs of each woman are different. Many factors enter into the nursing assessment to determine choice of analgesia and anesthesia (see box, right). The choice of analgesia and anesthesia varies by phase and stage (see box, p. 354).

After Administration of Medication

The nurse monitors and records the woman's response to medication: level of pain relief, level of apprehension, return of sensations and perception of pain, and allergic or untoward reactions (e.g., hypotension, respiratory depression). The nurse continues to monitor maternal vital signs, blood pressure, strength and frequency of uterine contractions, changes in the cervix and station of the presenting part, presence of the bearing-down reflex, bladder filling, and state of hydration. Fetal response following administration of analgesia or anesthesia is vital. The woman is asked if she (or the family) has any questions. The nurse assesses the woman's and her family's understanding of the need for ensuring her safety (e.g., keeping side rails up, calling for assistance as needed).

The time between the administration of a narcotic and the time of the baby's birth is noted.

Nursing Diagnoses

Following are some examples of nursing diagnoses relevant to pharmacologic control of discomfort during the birth period:

- Pain, related to
  - The processes of labor
- Situational low self-esteem, related to
  - Negative perception of behavior
- Knowledge deficit, related to
  - Procedure for nerve block analgesia
  - Expected sensation during nerve block analegesia
  - Mother's role during nerve block analgesia
  - Options for analgesia and anesthesia
- Potential for dystocia or injury to bladder, related to
  - Loss of sensation after regional anesthesia
- Inability to bear down during second stage, related to
  - Loss of sensation after regional anesthesia
- Potential altered family processes, related to
  - Unmet expectations of labor and delivery

ASSESSMENT ON ADMISSION TO UNIT

History

The woman's prenatal chart is read for relevant information. In addition to identifying data, the woman's parity, estimated date of delivery, and complications and medications during pregnancy are noted. History of allergies are noted carefully and displayed prominently. History of smoking and neurologic and spinal disorders are noted.

Interview

Interview data establishes time and type of food taken at last meal; existing respiratory condition (cold, allergy); and unusual reactions to medications, cleansing agents, or tape. The woman is asked about childbirth preparation classes. Her preparation and preferences for management of discomfort are noted. Her knowledge of choices for management of discomfort is assessed.

The woman is asked about the onset of labor and status of membranes; or, the reason for this admission is determined—induction of labor, cesarean delivery. The events since the woman's last contact with the physician are reviewed (e.g., infections, diarrhea, change in fetal behavior). If verbal and physical signs are suggestive, the nurse inquires about substance abuse: type of drug used, time of last use, method of administration.

Physical Examination

The character and status of this labor and fetal response are assessed (Chapters 16 and 18). The nurse notes the degree of hydration by assessing intake and output, moisture of mucous membranes, and skin turgor. Evidence of skin infection near sites of possible needle insertion are recorded and reported. Signs of apprehension such as fist clenching and restlessness are noted.

If the woman is in labor, maternal and fetal vital signs; uterine contractions; and cervical effacement and dilation, station, and anticipated time until delivery are all considered. The gravida's perception of discomfort and her expressed need for medication add to the data base. Bladder distension is noted. Length of labor and degree of fatigue are important considerations.

Laboratory Tests

Laboratory tests are reviewed for anemia (hemoglobin and hematocrit), coagulopathy (bleeding disorder), and infection (white cell count and differential). The prenatal record is reviewed for a history of infection (blood test, urinalysis, culture and sensitivity) and other concurrent disorders (tests for substance abuse).

The types of antenatal diagnostic studies (contraction stress test [CST], amniocentesis [Chapter 27]) and findings are noted.

Planning

For each woman a plan is developed that relates specifically to her clinical and nursing problems. The plan involves the mother and family and incorporates their priorities and preferences. The nurse, in collaboration with the physician and parturient, selects those aspects of care relevant to the individual client.

Goals. The goals for nursing care related to pharmacologic control of discomfort include the following:

1. For the mother: To achieve adequate pain relief without adding to maternal risk (e.g., through appropriate medication, dosage, and timing and route of administration).
2. For the unborn and newborn: To maintain well-being and adjustment to extrauterine life.
3. For the family: To know of their needs and rights in relation to use of analgesia or anesthesia.

Implementation

Nurses assume many caregiving roles during the childbirth period. The nurse-clinician's roles can be categorized as supportive and teacher/counselor/advocate. In these roles the clinician is a consumer of nursing research and on the alert for potential research problems.

Supportive Activities

This brief discussion is probably one of the most significant in this text. The woman's *perception* of her behavior during labor is of utmost importance. If she had planned a nonmedicated birth, then needs and accepts medication, her self-esteem will falter. Verbal and nonverbal acceptance of her behavior is given as necessary and reinforced by visiting her the day after delivery if possible. Explanations about fetal response to maternal discomfort, the effects of maternal fatigue, and the medication itself are supportive measures. In some instances the husband needs support if he was planning on a nonmedicated delivery.

Parents may feel reassured somewhat by hearing that medication is sometimes indicated for the baby's benefit. A reasonable amount of stress is harmless to the mother and to labor progress, and actually benefits the fetus by promoting adaptation to labor and birth. Excessive stress (as yet undefined in perinatal medicine) however, causes increased maternal catecholamine production, which may be related to dysfunctional labor and fetal and neonatal distress and illness (Simkin, 1986a, b).

Teacher/Counselor/Advocate

Informed Consent. The anesthesiologist and obstetrician are responsible for informing gravidas of the alternative methods of pharmacologic pain relief available in the hospital setting. The description of the anesthetic techniques is essential to informed consent, even if the woman has received information about analgesia and anesthesia earlier in her pregnancy. This interview should take place just before or early in labor so the woman has time to consider the alternatives. The obstetric nurse plays a part in the informed consent by clarifying or describing the procedures or by acting as a client's advocate and asking the anesthesiologist for further explanations. The explanation of the procedure to be used for anesthesia must include maternal position for administering the anesthetic, skin preparation, degree of discomfort, time requirement, and interval before the anesthetic is effective. The woman must be informed that the anesthetic is not always effective and that there are potential side effects for both mother and fetus.

Timing of Administration. Many medication orders are written to be given on the nurse's judgment. These orders require clinical knowledge and expertise. To assist the nurse in decision making, a quick reference is provided in Table 17-1, which compares different modalities for relief of discomfort and gives usual parenteral dose, time of administration, advantages for the parturient, disadvantages for the neonate, and nursing concerns.

Other types of analgesia and anesthetics are the responsibility of the anesthesiologist. It is often the nurse who alerts the physician that a parturient is in need of pharmacologic relief of discomfort. The box on p. 354 lists pharmacologic control by stage of labor and method of delivery. A review of the origins of discomfort in Chapter 16 provides the basis for understanding the parturient's changing needs during labor.

Preparation for Procedures. The nurse reviews or validates the woman's choices for relief from discomfort and clarifies the mother's information, as necessary. The woman needs an explanation of the procedure and what will be asked of her (e.g., to maintain flexed position during insertion of epidural). The woman benefits from knowing how the medication is to be given, the degree of discomfort to expect from administration of the medication, sensations she can expect, skin preparation, time requirement for administration, and interval before medication "takes hold." The nurse explains the need for keeping the bladder empty. If an indwelling catheter is threaded and the woman feels a momentary twinge down her leg, hip, or back, she is assured that it is not a sign of injury.

For paracervical and pudendal blocks a long needle is used. The sight of this needle may be frightening. The woman can be reassured that only the tip of the needle will be inserted.

Instrumental Activities

Accuracy in monitoring the progress of labor is the basis for clinical judgment in the need for pharmacologic control of discomfort. Knowlege of medications used during childbirth is essential. The most effective route of administration for each woman is selected. The medication is prepared and administered correctly.

Intravenous Administration. The preferred route of administration is through IV tubing. The medication is given slowly in small doses at the *beginning* of three to five consecutive contractions (Petree, 1983). Since uterine blood vessels are constricted during contractions, the medication stays within the maternal vascular system for several seconds before the uterine blood vessels reopen. Through this method of injection, the amount of drug crossing the placenta to the fetus is minimized. With decreased placental transfer, the mother's degree of pain relief is maximized. The IV route has the following results:
1. Pain relief is obtained with small doses of the drug.
2. Onset of pain relief is more predictable.
3. Duration of effect is more predictable.

Intramuscular Administration. IM injections of analgesics, although still used, are no longer the preferred route of administration to the laboring woman. Identified disadvantages of the IM route include the following:
1. Onset of pain relief is delayed for several minutes.
2. Higher doses of medication are required.

3. Medication is released from the muscle tissue at an unpredictable rate and is available for transfer across the placenta to the fetus.

IM injections are given in the upper arm if regional anesthesia is planned later in the labor. This is because the autonomic blockage from the regional (e.g., epidural) anesthesia increases blood flow to the gluteal region and accelerates absorption of the drug. The maternal plasma level of the drug necessary to bring pain relief usually is reached 45 minutes after IM injection, followed by a decline in plasma levels. The maternal drug levels (after IM injectsions) are unequal because of uneven distribution (maternal uptake) and metabolism. The advantage of using the IM route is quick administration.

Assisting with Analgesia-anesthesia. An IV line is established before nerve blocks such as paracervical, peridural, and subarachnoid spinal and general anesthesia are introduced. Lactated Ringer's solution is often the infusate of choice. Infusion solutions without dextrose are preferred, especially when the solution needs to be infused rapidly (e.g., in the presence of severe dehydration or to maintain blood pressure). Solutions containing dextrose raise maternal blood glucose levels rapidly, necessitating the release of insulin; fetal or neonatal hypoglycemia may result. In addition, dextrose changes osmotic pressure so that fluid is excreted from the kidneys more rapidly. Therefore lactated Ringer's and normal saline solutions are the preferred infusates.

The woman needs assistance in assuming and maintaining the correct position for peridural and spinal anesthesia (see pp. 356-359).

Safety Measures. Following a nerve block the woman is protected by raised side rails, constant attendance, and a call bell within easy reach. She must be protected from prolonged pressure on an anesthetized part (e.g., lying on one side with weight on one leg; tight bedclothes on feet). If stirrups are used, the nurse pads them, adjusts both stirrups at the same level and angle, places both of the wom-

Specific Nursing Care Plan

ANALGESIA FOR PAIN DURING LABOR

Rose N. is a 31-year-old woman in active labor. At her last vaginal examination the physician found her to be 7 cm/90%/+2. Her contractions are coming every 2½ to 3 minutes and lasting 30 to 45 seconds. Rose and her husband attended childbirth education classes and are doing well with the breathing techniques. However, the pain of the contractions is getting too intense for Rose. The physician has ordered meperidine 50 mg and promethazine 25 mg to help her stay in control and decrease her anxiety.

ASSESSMENT	NURSING DIAGNOSIS (ND)/ PLAN (P)/ GOAL (G)	RATIONALE/ IMPLEMENTATION	EVALUATION
Rose is in active labor experiencing acute pain. Rose communicates verbally and nonverbally her anxiety and decreased coping mechanisms.	ND: Pain, related to increasing frequency and intensity of uterine contractions. P: Minimize pain and discomfort without jeopardizing mother or fetus. G: Rose will state she has the relief she wants and she and fetus remain well. ND: Ineffective individual coping related to increased intensity and frequency of labor contractions. P: Decrease anxiety and increase self control. G: Rose experiences minimum anxiety and remains in control.	*To help diminish pain of contractions and other labor-related effects the nurse will:* Provide comfort measures. Provide information about analgesics. Assist Rose and husband with relaxation techniques, breathing exercises, abdominal effleurage, and back rubs. Provide emotional support.	Rose is more calm and verbalizes less discomfort. Rose is lucid and in control.

an's legs into them simultaneously avoiding pressure to the popliteal angle, and applies restraints without restricting circulation.

The woman's record during childbirth serves as a documented means of communication among all members of the health care team. The record contains accurate and complete recordings of the history, physical examination, and laboratory tests; sequential observations; goals; interventions; and the fetus', and newborn's responses. The record should be readily accessible to the health care professionals caring for the mother and family. Documentation of the events is mandatory to meet legal requirements. Precise records also serve as a reservoir for research study.

Evaluation

Evaluation is a continuous process. To be effective, evaluation needs to be based on measurable outcome criteria. The criteria reflect the parameters used to measure the goals for care. The maternal and fetal areas consistently assessed as indicators of maternal and fetal well-being and the clinical findings that represent normal response are presented as outcome criteria in the nursing care plan below. These criteria are used as a basis for selecting appropriate nursing actions and evaluating their effectiveness.

Fetal Monitoring

Fetal Stress. Since labor represents a period of stress for the fetus, continuous monitoring of fetal health is instituted as part of the nursing care during labor. The fetal oxygen supply must be maintained during labor to prevent severe debilitating conditions after birth. Fetal stress can result in death in utero or shortly after birth. The fetal oxygen supply can be reduced in a number of ways:

1. Reduction of blood flow through the maternal vessels as a result of maternal hypertension or hypotension (sys-

ASSESSMENT	NURSING DIAGNOSIS (ND)/ PLAN (P)/ GOAL (G)	RATIONALE/ IMPLEMENTATION	EVALUATION
Assess vital signs, blood pressure, labor pattern, and FHR immediately after analgesia is given and at intervals indicated by hospital protocol.	ND: Potential for fetal and maternal compromise related to medication. ND: Potential for continued maternal discomfort related to medication. P: Observe for maternal and fetal response to medication and immediately intervene as necessary. G: Rose indicates she is more comfortable and she, her labor, and the fetus suffer no adverse sequelae.	*To be ready to intervene if necessary:* Observe Rose for comfort level. Observe Rose for side effects such as: hives, shortness of breath, and altered sensorium. Monitor for change in labor pattern. Monitor FHR for distress.	Rose's vital signs, blood pressure, and FHR remain within normal limits. Normal labor pattern continues. Rose experiences no adverse side effects.
Rose is apologetic for taking analgesic medication.	ND: Situational low self-esteem related to inability to cope with labor without medication. P: Provide information about advantages of analgesia during labor to prevent maternal fatigue, to facilitate labor, and to prevent fetal depression secondary to maternal response to pain. G: Rose and her husband do not feel as though they have failed because medication was needed.	*To help the couple accept the decision for medication the nurse will:* Assess Rose's (couple's) behavior. Support Rose's decision. Assist Rose through relaxation and breathing techniques to regain and maintain control. Provide verbal and nonverbal acceptance of her choice. Praise her (their) efforts.	Rose feels good about decision and maintains control during her labor.

tolic blood pressure of 100 mm Hg in brachial artery is necessary for placental perfusion).
2. Reduction of the oxygen content of the maternal blood as a result of hemorrhage or severe anemia.
3. Alterations in fetal circulation, occurring with compression of the cord, placental separation, or head compression (head compression causes increased intracranial pressure and vagal nerve stimulation with slowing of the heart rate.)

Fetal well-being during labor is measured by the *response of the FHR to uterine contractions.* In general, normal, active labor is characterized by:
1. A FHR between 120 and 160 beats/min with normal baseline variability and no ominous periodic changes.
2. Uterine contractions with the following characteristics (Tucker, 1978):
   a. Frequency of every 3 to 5 minutes.
   b. Duration of 30 to 60 seconds.
   c. Intensity resulting in a rise in intrauterine pressure to 50 to 70 mm Hg at the peak of a contraction.
   d. An average resting intrauterine pressure of between 8 and 15 mm Hg.

Baseline Fetal Heart Rate. The intrinsic rhythmicity of the fetal heart and the fetal autonomic nervous system control the FHR. An increase in sympathetic response results in acceleration of the FHR. An augmentation in parasympathetic response produces a slowing of the FHR. Usually there is a balanced increase of sympathetic and parasympathetic response during contractions, with no observable change in the FHR.

Baseline FHR is the average rate between contractions. At term this average is about 135 beats per minute (bpm), a decrease from 155 bpm early in pregnancy. The normal range at term is 120 to 160 bpm. Tachycardia refers to rates above 160 bpm, and bradycardia refers to rates below 120 bpm. (Bradycardia should be distinguished from prolonged deceleration patterns, which are *periodic changes* that are described later in this chapter.)

Tachycardia may result from maternal or fetal infection and maternal hyperthyroidism. It may also be an early response to fetal hypoxemia and can be produced by use of parasympathetic blocking drugs (e.g., atropine). **Bradycardia** is a later response to fetal hypoxemia and may occur for a brief period just before fetal demise. It may also result from placental transfer of drugs such as local anesthetics.

Another important aspect of the baseline FHR is the degree of **baseline variability** (beat-to-beat variations) (Fig. 17-10). Two types of variability have been described: long-term changes of 3 to 5 cycles/min and short-term changes of 120 to 180 cycles/min. These fluctuations correlate well with normal acid-base status and fetal health. Variability increases with gestation. Variability decreases with fetal sleep and the administration of certain drugs such as atropine, diazepam (Valium), promethazine (Phenergan), magnesium sulfate, and most sedatives and narcotic agents. Minimum baseline variability (3 to 5 bpm) indicates CNS depression and is associated with fetal hypoxemia. No variability (0 to 2 bpm) is described as a **smooth or flat baseline** and is considered to be an important warning sign of possible fetal jeopardy.

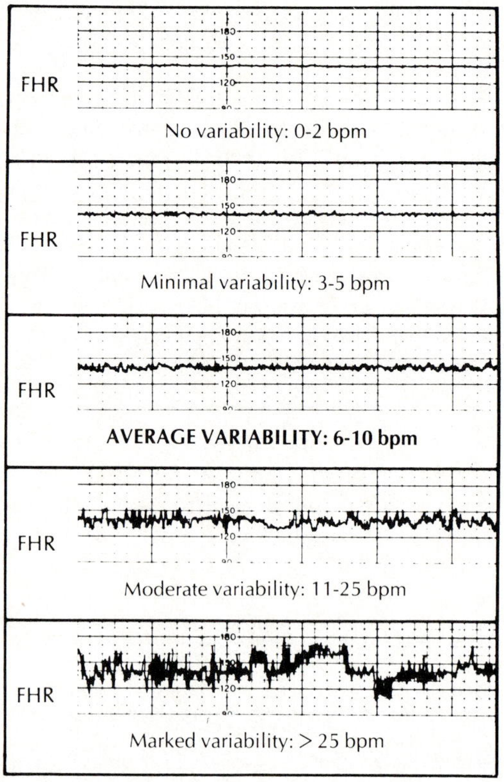

Fig. 17-10 Fetal heart rate variability. Short- and long-term variability tend to increase and decrease together.
From Tucker, SM: Fetal monitoring and fetal assessment in high-risk pregnancy, St Louis, 1978, The CV Mosby Co.

Periodic Changes in FHR. *Periodic changes* in the FHR are referred to as accelerations or decelerations, and the latter are described as early, late, or variable depending on their characteristics of timing, shape, and repetitiveness in relation to uterine contractions. **Periodic accelerations** (caused by dominance of the *sympathetic* response) are usually encountered with breech presentations (Fig. 17-11, *A*). Pressure applied to the infant's buttocks results in accelerations, whereas pressure applied to the head results in decelerations. Accelerations may occur, however, during the second stage of labor in cephalic presentations. **Nonperiodic accelerations** (Fig. 17-11 *B*) of the FHR occurring during fetal movement are indications of fetal well-being (nonstress test, Chapter 27).

Periodic decelerations (caused by dominance of *parasympathetic* response) may be benign or ominous. The three types of decelerations that are encountered during labor are early, late, and variable. Fetal decelerations are described by their relation to the onset and end of a contraction and by their shape. **Early** and **late** decelerations are described as uniform and bell shaped. **Variable** decelerations are U or V-shaped. Nursing actions for each type are described later in this chapter.

Early deceleration (slowing of heart rate) in response to compression of the fetal head is normal and usually does not indicate fetal distress (Fig. 17-12, *A*). Tracing is characterized by a uniform shape and an early onset correspond-

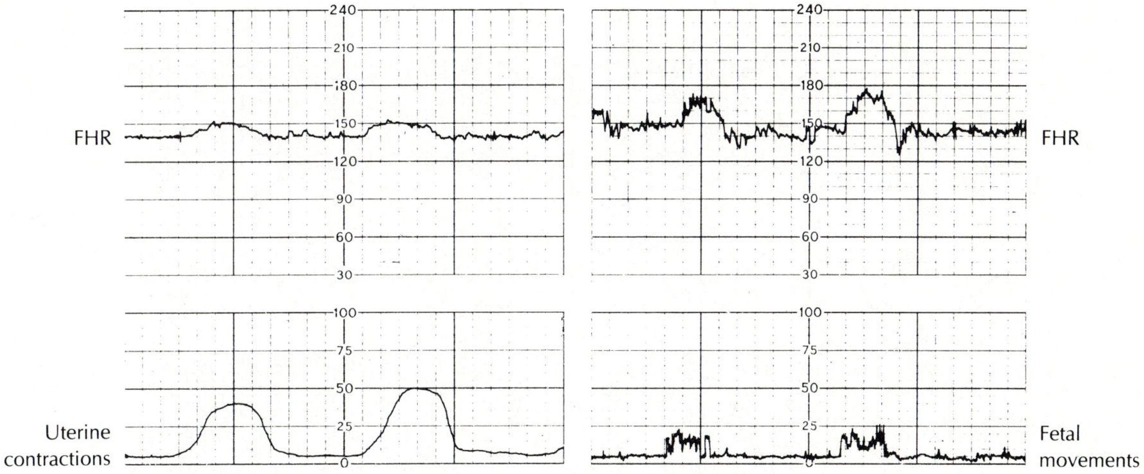

Fig. 17-11 **A**, Acceleration of fetal heart rate with uterine contractions. **B**, Acceleration of fetal heart rate with fetal movement.

From Tucker, SM: Fetal monitoring and fetal assessment in high-risk pregnancy, St Louis, 1978, The CV Mosby Co.

ing to the rise in intrauterine pressure as the uterus contracts. It is not a common occurrence. When present it usually occurs during the first stage of labor when the cervix is dilated 4 to 8 cm. Early deceleration is sometimes seen during the second stage when the parturient is pushing.

Late deceleration is also a smooth, curvilinear, uniform heart rate pattern that mirrors the pattern of intrauterine pressure during a contraction. However, the deceleration necessarily begins *after* the contraction has been established and consistently *persists into the interval after the contraction* (Fig. 17-12, *B*). **Late deceleration** when persistent or recurrent usually indicates fetal hypoxia because of deficient placental perfusion. Any drop in the FHR of more than 30 bpm is sufficient for the diagnosis of late deceleration. It is usually associated with maternal hypotension or excessive uterine activity (e.g., during induction of labor). However, it may result from any maternal, placental, umbilical cord, or fetal factors that limit effective oxygenation of the fetus. If associated with minimum baseline variability, it is increasingly significant as an indicator of fetal distress.

Variable deceleration indicates a transient drop in the FHR before, during, or after a uterine contraction (Fig. 17-12, *C*). There is no uniformity to the FHR pattern. Variable deceleratoin may be related to partial, brief compression of the cord. If encountered in the first stage of labor, it can usually be eliminated by changing the mother's position, such as from one side to the other. It is most commonly encountered during the second stage of labor as a result of cord compression during fetal descent. Variable deceleration is associated with neonatal depression only when cord compression is severe or prolonged (e.g., tight nuchal cord). Variable and late deceleration patterns then occur simultaneously or are replaced by persistent bradycardia.

Bradycardia that is persistent is an ominous sign, especially when it follows a uterine contraction. Bradycardia during several contractions may indicate cord compression or separation of the placenta. **Tachycardia,** when continued for an hour or more and accompanied by late deceleration, is an indication of fetal distress.

Monitoring Techniques. Following are methods of determining the degree of fetal distress throughout labor:

- Fetal heart rate monitoring
- Fetal blood sampling (pH and concentrations of oxygen and carbon dioxide [Po_2 and Pco_2])
- Noting the presence of meconium-stained amniotic fluid

Periodic Auscultation: FHR. Periodic auscultation of the fetal heart may reveal tachycardia, bradycardia, or arrhythmia that may occur during the brief examination (Fig. 17-13).

In the low-risk woman auscultation of the FHR may be done every 15 minutes in the first stage of labor and every 5 minutes during the second stage of labor. In both instances, auscultation is done for a period of 30 seconds immediately after a uterine contraction. However, ominous FHR patterns of a fetus in severe jeopardy may not occur during the periods of auscultation and may pass unrecognized by the examiner. Only marked degrees of fetal distress can be identified by listening to the FHR periodically (Pritchard, MacDonald, and Gant, 1985).

An improved method that is more likely to aid in diagnosing fetal compromise in the high-risk pregnancy is the counting of FHR during sequential contractions and for a full 3 minutes thereafter. Persistent, postcontraction bradycardia (e.g., FHR of 100 bpm, or a persistent drop of 30 bpm or more below baseline) or gross irregularity indicates fetal distress.

The woman becomes anxious if the examiner cannot count the FHR. For the inexperienced listener it often takes time to locate the heartbeat and find the area of maximum intensity. The mother can be told that the nurse is "finding the spot where the sounds are loudest." If it has taken considerable time to locate them, offer the mother an opportunity to hear them too, to reassure her. If the examiner cannot locate the FHR, an experienced nurse should be asked for assistance.

There are two modes of electronic monitoring. The ex-

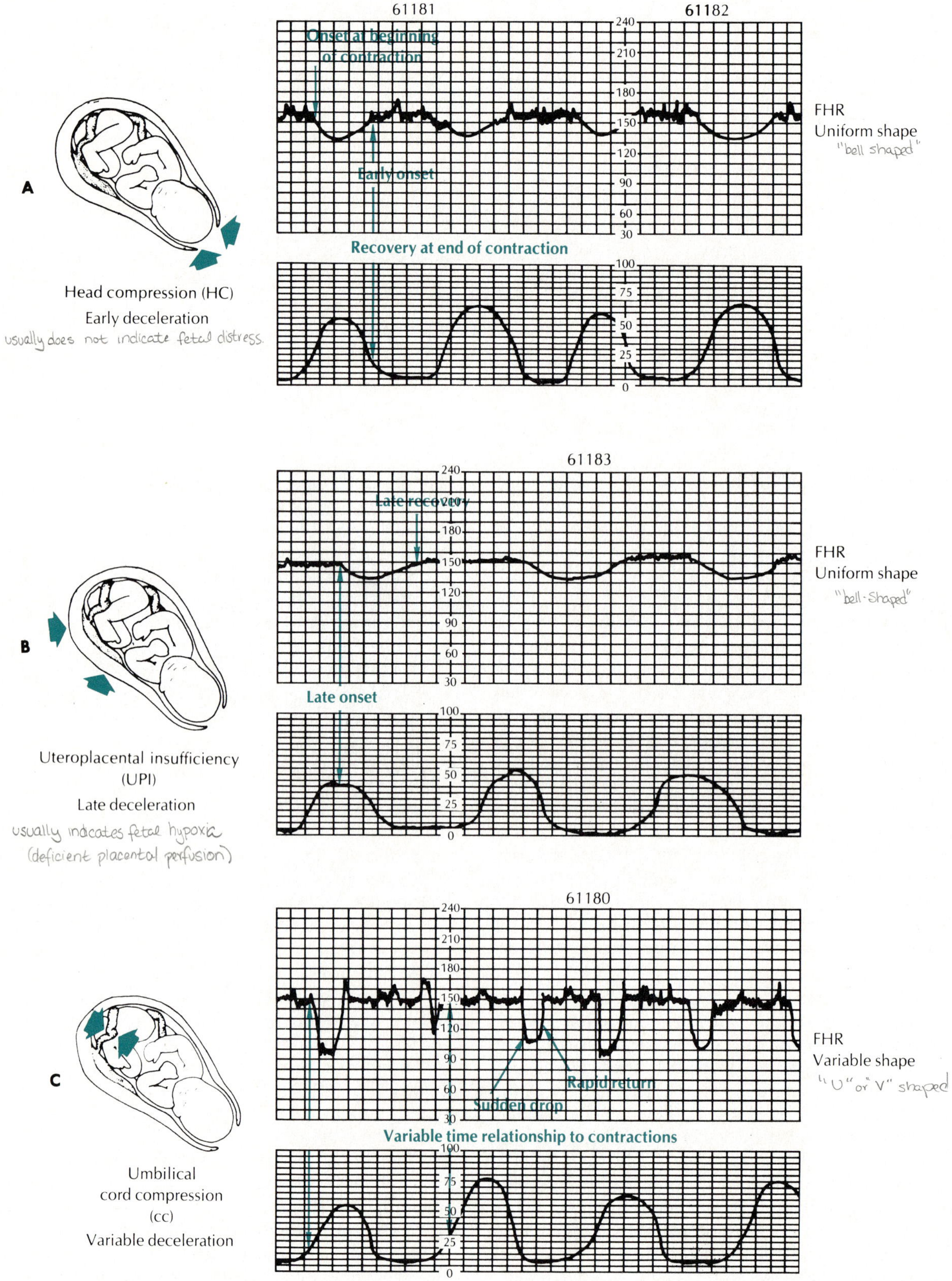

Fig. 17-12 **A,** Early decelerations caused by head compression. **B,** Late deceleration caused by uteroplacental insufficiency. **C,** Variable deceleration caused by cord compression.

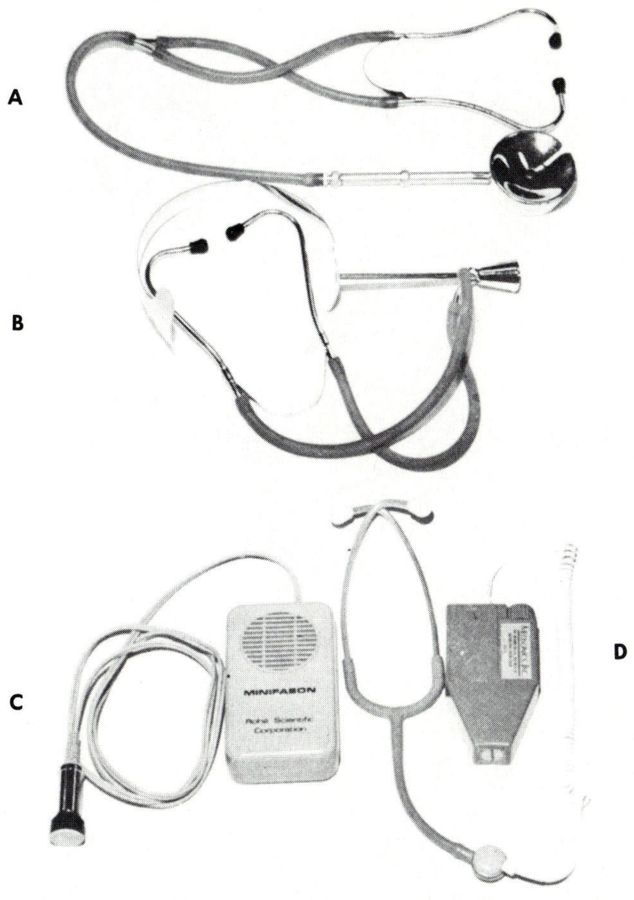

Fig. 17-13 A, Leffscope. B, DeLee-Hillis scope. C, Ultrasound fetoscope; amplifies sound to those in immediate area. D, Ultrasound stethoscope; amplifies mechanical movement of fetal heart to listener by means of ear pieces.

From Ingalls, AJ, and Salerno, MC: Maternal and child health nursing, ed 5, St Louis, 1983, The CV Mosby Co.

ternal mode employs the use of external transducers placed on the maternal abdomen to assess heart rate and uterine activity. The internal mode uses a spiral electrode applied to the fetal presenting part to assess the fetal electrocardiogram and the intrauterine catheter to assess uterine activity and pressure. A brief description contrasting the external and internal modes of electronic fetal monitoring (EFM) is provided in Table 17-2.

External EFM:FHR Continuous EFM has a lower false-normal rate than intermittent auscultation of the FHR (Quirk and Miller, 1986). Separate transducers monitor the FHR and uterine contractions (Fig. 17-14). The *ultrasound transducer* acts through the reflection of high-frequency sound waves from a moving interface, in this case the fetal heart and valves. Therefore short-term variability and beat-to-beat changes in the FHR cannot be assessed by this method. It is also difficult to reproduce a continuous and precise record of the FHR because of artifacts introduced by fetal and maternal movement. The FHR is transcribed to a strip chart, and a consistent waveform is observed on the oscilloscope. Once the *area of maximum intensity of FHR* has been located, conductive gel is applied to the crystals on the ultrasound transducer, and the transducer is then positioned below the umbilicus.

The *tocotransducer* (tocodynamometer) measures uterine activity transabdominally. A pressure-sensitive button on the side next to the abdomen is depressed by uterine contractions or fetal movement. The device is placed over the fundus above the umbilicus. The tocotransducer can measure and record the frequency, regularity, and duration of uterine contractions but not their intensity. This method is especially valuable during the first stage of labor in women with intact membranes or for use in the nonstress test (NST) or oxytocin challenge test (OCT).

The equipment is easily applied by the nurse but must be repositioned as the mother or fetus changes position.

Table 17-2 *External and Internal Modes of Monitoring*

External Mode	Internal Mode
Fetal Heart Rate (FHR)	
Ultrasound transducer: High-frequency sound waves reflect mechanical action of the fetal heart. Used during the antepartum and intrapartum period.	*Spiral electrode:* Electrode converts fetal ECG as obtained from the presenting part to FHR via a cardiotachometer. This method can only be used when membranes are ruptured and cervix sufficiently dilated during the intrapartum period. Electrode penetrates fetal presenting part 1.5 mm and must be on securely to ensure a good signal.
Phonotransducer: Microphone amplifies sound, reflects excessive noise when woman is in labor. Used infrequently for antepartum monitoring.	
Abdominal electrodes: Fetal ECG is obtained when electrodes are properly positioned. Used infrequently for antepartum monitoring because of ease and reliability of ultrasound transducer.	
Uterine Activity	
Tocotransducer: This instrument monitors frequency and duration of contractions by means of pressure-sensing device applied to the maternal abdomen. Used during both the antepartum and intrapartum periods.	*Intrauterine catheter:* This instrument monitors frequency, duration, and *intensity of contractions.* Catheter filled with sterile water is compressed during contractions, placing pressure on a strain gauge converting the pressure into millimeters of mercury on the uterine activity panel of the strip chart. It can be used when membranes are ruptured and cervix sufficiently dilated during the intrapartum period.

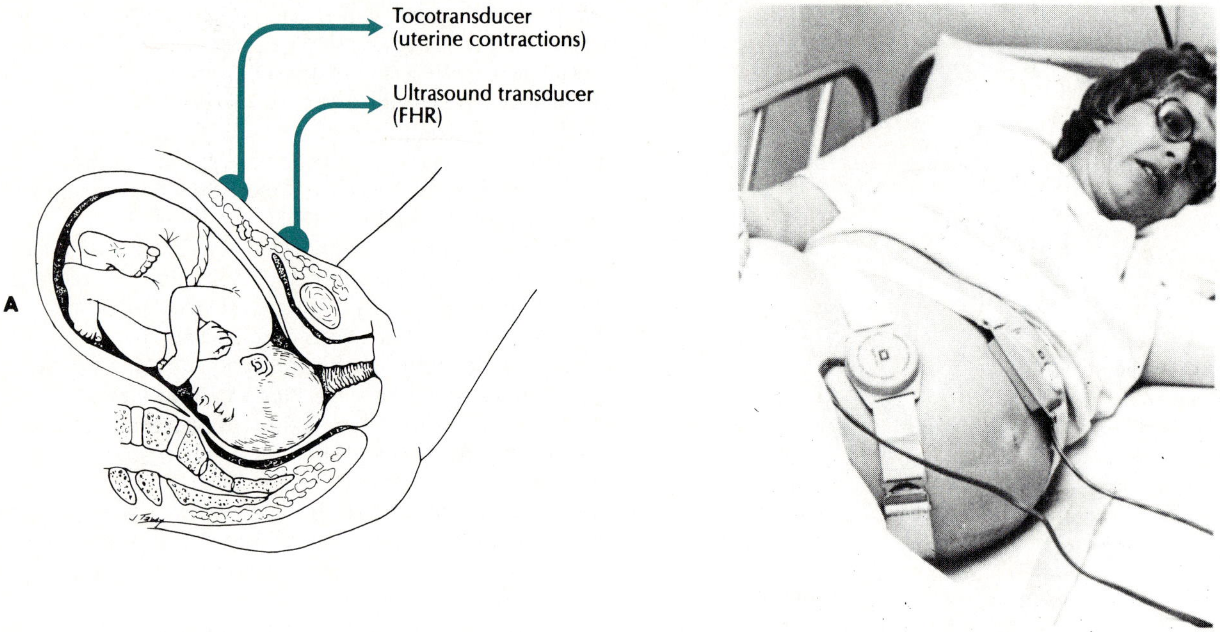

Fig. 17-14 Diagrammatic representation of external noninvasive fetal monitoring with tocotransducer and ultrasound transducer, **A**, with ultrasound transducer placed below umbilicus and tocotransducer placed on uterine fundus. **B**. Note that client is lying in left lateral position.
B from Tucker, SM: Fetal monitoring and fetal assessment in high-risk pregnancy, St Louis, 1978, The CV Mosby Co.

The woman is asked to assume a semi-sitting position or left-lateral position (Fig. 17-14, *B*). The equipment is removed periodically to permit washing of the applicator sites and giving of back rubs. This type of monitoring confines the woman to bed. Portable monitors allow observation of the FHR and uterine contraction patterns by means of centrally located electronic display units. These portable units permit ambulation during electronic monitoring (Fig. 1-2).

Internal EFM:FHR. The technique of continuous internal monitoring provides an accurate appraisal of fetal well-being during labor (Fig. 17-15). For this type of monitoring the membranes must be ruptured and the presenting part must be low enough for placement of the electrode. A small electrode attached to the presenting part yields a continuous rate on a graph and a visual report of the fetal cardiograph on the oscilloscope.* A catheter filled with sterile water is introduced into the uterine cavity. The fluid acts as a transmitter of changes in uterine pressure into millimeters of mercury. The normal range during a contraction is 50 to 75 mm Hg. The display of FHR and uterine activity on the chart paper differs for the two modes of electronic monitoring (Fig. 17-16). *Note that each small square represents 10 seconds; each larger box of 6 squares equals 1 minute.*

*Before this method is used, the possibility of hemophilia or other coagulation disorder in the infant must be ruled out by careful questioning of the mother. For example, "Have any of your relatives had trouble with bleeding?" Fetal death can be caused by exsanguination from the puncture wounds in the presenting part. (Note that in a vertex presentation, the electrode is placed over a bone—*not* over a suture or fontanel.)

Fetal Blood Sampling. The blood sample is obtained from the fetal scalp transcervically after rupture of membranes. The scalp is swabbed with a disinfecting solution before the puncture is made. Fetal acidosis follows fetal hypoxia, and some perinatologists insist that true fetal distress can be diagnosed only when serious FHR changes can be correlated with fetal blood acidosis ($pH \leq 7.20$).

Most infants who have low Apgar scores have scalp blood readings of pH 7.15 or less. If there are consecutive blood samples with a pH below 7.20, prompt delivery of the infant is imperative.

Meconium-stained Amniotic Fluid. The passage of meconium from the fetal bowel before birth may indicate fetal distress. Peristalsis of the bowel increases during hypoxia, and the contents are likely to be expelled. Although the presence of meconium-stained amniotic fluid is not always an indication of fetal difficulty, its presence requires immediate notification of the physician (see Chapter 18).

Pattern Recognition and Nursing Standards: EFM

Many factors must be evaluated to determine if an FHR pattern is reassuring or nonreassuring. This includes an assessment and evaluation of baseline rate, variability, accelerations, and decelerations, as well as consideration of the frequency and strength of uterine contractions. These factors must be evaluated based on other obstetric information, including parity, maternal and obstetric complications, progress in labor, and analgesia or anesthesia. The estimate of anticipated delivery time must also be considered. Intervention and interruption of labor are therefore based on medical judgment of a complex, integrated process.

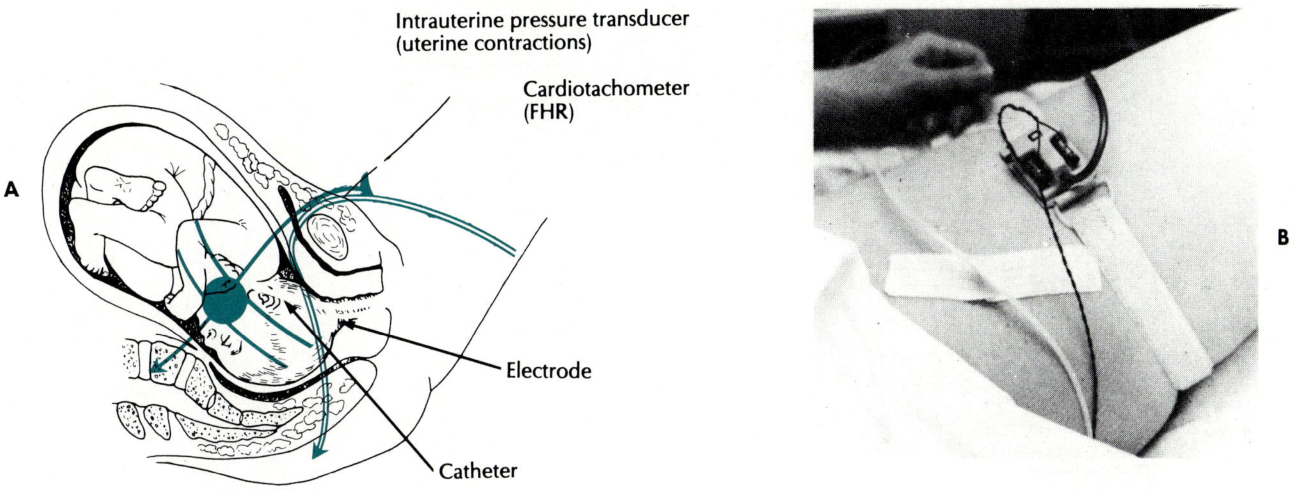

Fig. 17-15 **A**, Diagrammatic representation of internal invasive fetal monitoring with intrauterine catheter and spiral electrode in place (membranes ruptured and cervix dilated). **B**, Device secured to woman's thigh.

From Tucker, SM: Fetal monitoring and fetal assessment in high-risk pregnancy, St Louis, 1978, The CV Mosby Co.

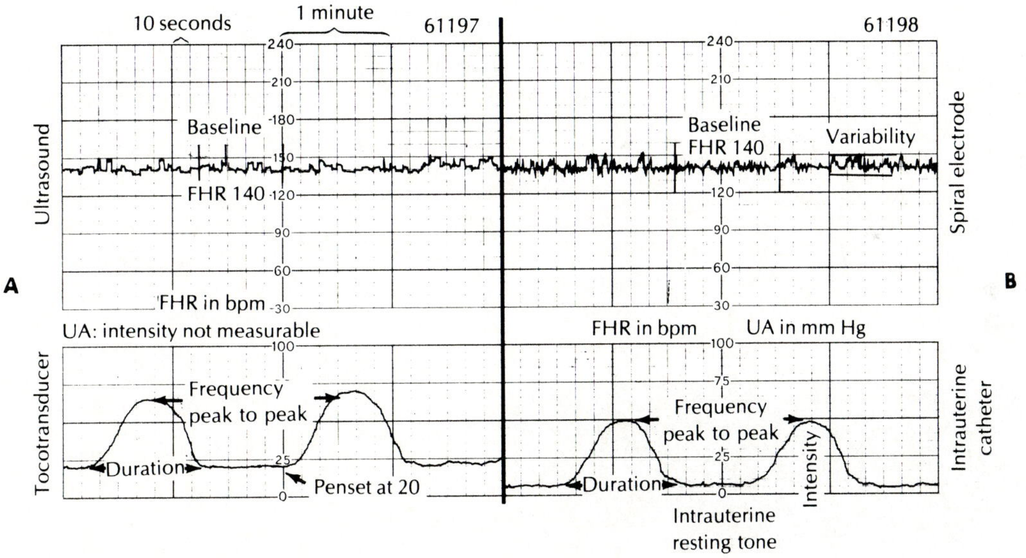

Fig. 17-16 Display of FHR and uterine activity on chart paper. **A**, External mode with ultrasound and tocotransducer as signal source. **B**, Internal mode with spiral electrode and intrauterine catheter as signal source.

From Tucker, SM: Fetal monitoring and fetal assessment in high-risk pregnancy, St Louis, 1978, The CV Mosby Co.

It is the responsibility of the labor and delivery room nurse to assess FHR patterns, perform independent nursing interventions, and report nonreassuring patterns to the physician.

Nurses planning to work with electronic monitors require additional education and training in their use. In addition to knowing how to apply the monitor and interpret tracings, the nurse needs to know how to trouble-shoot the monitor (see box, p. 377).

Review Chapter 4, for a clearer understanding of the legal responsibilities involved.

Table 17-3 presents nursing standards for fetal monitoring (Blank, 1985). FHR patterns and characteristics are described, clinical significance is indicated, and related nursing interventions are addressed in this reference table. Following Table 17-3 is the statement on EFM. The statement is jointly prepared by the American College of Obstetricians and Gynecologists and the NAACOG, the organization for obstetric, gynecologic, and neonatal nurses.

Text continued on p. 376.

Table 17-3 *Nursing Standards: Electronic Fetal Monitoring**

Fetal Heart Rate Patterns	Characteristics	Clinical Significance	Nursing Interventions
Baseline changes	Normal 120-160 bpm		
1. Tachycardia			
a. Moderate	160-180 bpm		None
b. Marked	Above 180 bpm	May be ominous when associated with late or variable decelerations and absence of variability.	Collaborate with physician in alleviating primary cause. Monitor maternal vital signs closely, change maternal position (left lateral preferred). Check hydration status and increase rate of maintenance intravenous until specific order can be obtained from physician. Administer oxygen at 5 L/min.† Observe for presence of meconium-stained fluid.
2. Bradycardia			
a. Moderate	100-120 bpm, transitory		Check maternal pulse.
b. Marked	Below 100 bpm	Ominous sign when associated with loss of variability or when preceded by or associated with late or variable decelerations.	Check maternal pulse. Change maternal position (left lateral preferred). Increase rate of maintenance intravenous until specific order can be obtained from physician. Discontinue Pitocin drip, if infusing. Administer oxygen at 5 L/min. Observe for presence of meconium-stained fluid. Notify physician.
3. Variability	Normal fluctuations of fetal baseline. Refers to the intervals between beats.		
a. Marked 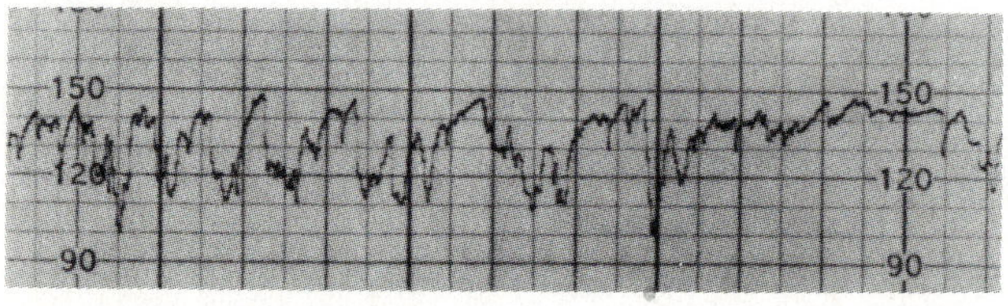			None
b. Average 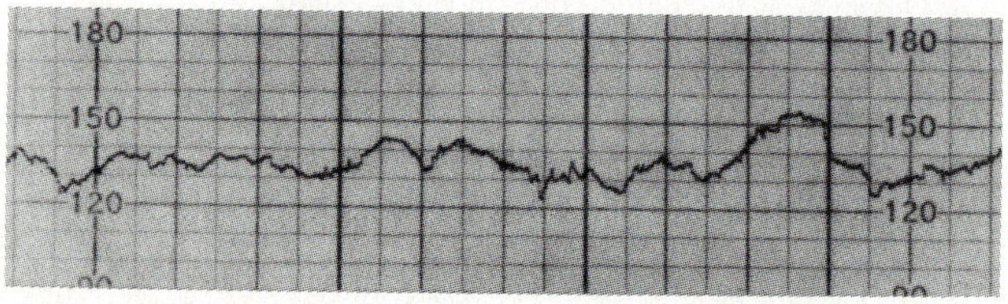			None
c. Minimal 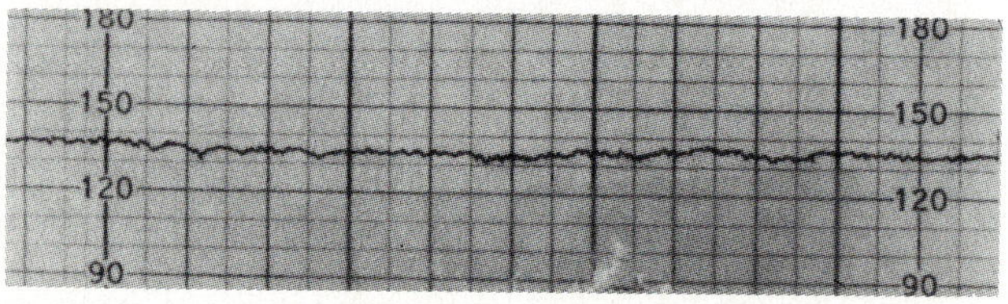		May be ominous if associated with changing baseline or decelerations	Observe closely for signs of decelerations and absence of variability. Optimize fetal blood flow by changing maternal position. Notify physician.

Table 17-3 *Nursing Standards: Electronic Fetal Monitoring*—cont'd*

Fetal Heart Rate Patterns	Characteristics	Clinical Significance	Nursing Interventions
d. Absent		Ominous sign of fetal distress when preceded by a period of acute insult.	Change maternal position (left lateral preferred). Increase rate of maintenance intravenous until specific order can be obtained from physician. Administer oxygen at 5 L/min. Observe for presence of meconium-stained fluid. Notify physician.
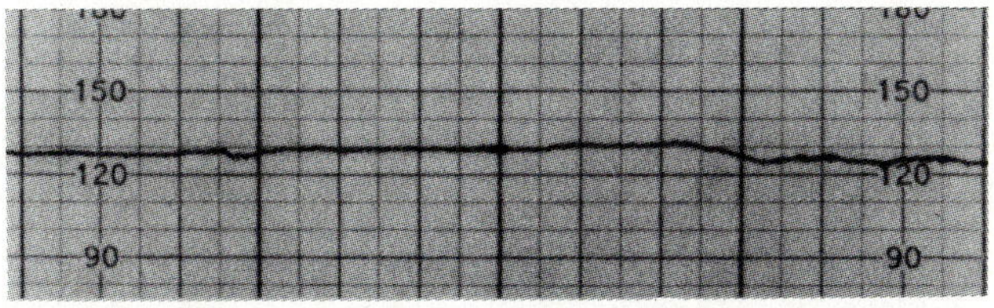			
4. Sinusoidal	Predominant pattern of rhythmic long-term variability with absence of beat-to-beat changes	When persistent, this pattern may be ominous.	Collaborate with physician in determining the significance and treatment of this pattern.
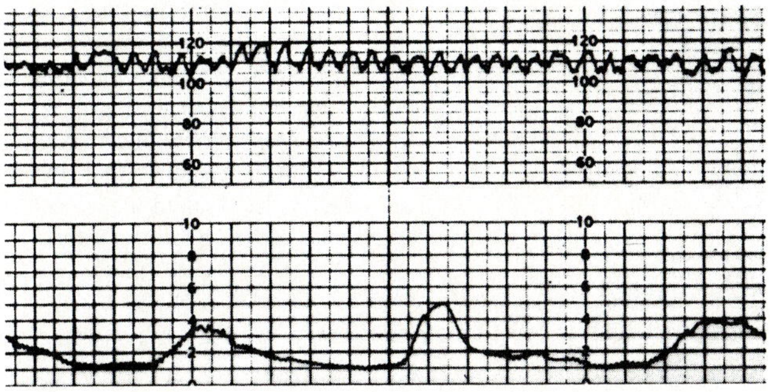			
Deceleration‡			
1. Early	Uniform shape, onset, and recovery correspond with contraction. Repetitive. Degree of deceleration usually does not exceed 110 bpm.		None
2. Late	Uniform shape with late onset (usually 20 sec after beginning of contraction). Depth of deceleration proportional to amplitude of contraction. Repetitive.	May be ominous sign, especially when associated with change in baseline and absence of variability.	Change maternal position, (left lateral preferred). Increase rate of maintenance intravenous until specific order can be obtained from physician. Discontinue Pitocin if infusing. Administer oxygen at 5 L/min. Observe for presence of meconium-stained fluid. Notify physician. Anticipate fetal scalp sampling.
3. Variable deceleration a. Mild	Variable shape with sudden drop not to go below 80, lasting less than 30 sec. Onset can be anytime. Recovery occurs rapidly. Baseline rate and variability remain unchanged.		Try alternate positions to minimize effects of cord compression. Notify physician.

From Blank, JJ: Electronic fetal monitoring: nursing management defined, JOGN Nurs 14:463, Nov/Dec, 1985.

*As part of fetal assessment and in keeping with NAACOG standards, the intrapartum nurse has the responsibility of observing, assessing, evaluating information received from the fetal monitor, and intervening appropriately. The ability to recognize and interpret FHR patterns and uterine activity is inherent in the nurse's role in EFM.

†Some hospital protocols specify 10-12 L/min.

‡See Fig. 17-13.

Continued.

Table 17-3 *Nursing Standards: Electronic Fetal Monitoring*—cont'd*

Fetal Heart Rate Patterns	Characteristics	Clinical Significance	Nursing Interventions
b. Deep	Variable shape with sudden drop below 80 lasting longer than 30 sec. Onset can be any time. Recovery slow, may be accompanied by overshoot of baseline. Associated with rising or falling baseline or decrease in variability.	May be ominous pattern when associated with changing baseline and loss of variability.	Try alternate position to minimize effects of cord compression. Increase rate of maintenance intravenous until order can be obtained from physician. Discontinue Pitocin if infusing. Administer oxygen at 5 L/min. Notify physician.
4. Prolonged deceleration	Drop in fetal heart rate at least 30 bpm, lasting 2½ min or more. Not necessarily in relation to contraction pattern.		Collaborate with physician in eliminating primary cause such as hyperstimulation. Alternate maternal position (left lateral preferred). Increase rate of maintenance intravenous until order can be obtained from physician. Discontinue Pitocin if infusing. Check maternal BP and pulse. Administer oxygen at 5 L/min. Observe for presence of meconium-stained fluid. Notify physician.

Joint ACOG/NAACOG Statement

The primary goal of obstetric and neonatal care is to ensure optimal maternal and fetal outcome. An important tool in attaining this goal is electronic monitoring of the fetal heart. Nurses and physicians who perform fetal monitoring are responsible for their actions and will be held to the established standard of care as defined by their professional organization, the standards of practice in their hospitals, and the laws governing practice in their respective states. Hospitals should have a policy for the use of electronic fetal monitoring (EFM) in their obstetric patients. It is recommended that high-risk patients be monitored with continuous EFM.

Recognition and documentation. Physicians and nurses who use EFM must be able to recognize fetal heart rate patterns, beat-to-beat variability, and uterine activity. Fetal monitoring patterns have been given descriptive names (e.g., accelerations and early, late, or variable decelerations). It is appropriate for physicians and nurses to use these terms in written chart documentation and verbal communication.* It is especially important that when a change in fetal heart rate patterns is noted that a subsequent return to normal patterns be documented as well.

The medical record should include observations and assessments of fetal heart rate and characteristics of uterine activity as well as specific actions taken when changes in fetal heart rate patterns are observed. The monitor tracing is a legal part of the medical record and should include identifying information about the patient as well as times and events related to the patient's ongoing care.

Nonreassuring patterns. After the identification of a nonreassuring pattern, the nurse is responsible for initiating appropriate nursing interventions, as indicated by the pattern identified, and for notifying a physician. Once the physician is notified of a nonreassuring pattern, the nurse can expect the physician to respond. There should be established hospital policy for the nurse to follow in the event the physician is unable to respond in a timely fashion.

Staffing. To implement adequate intrapartum care of the patient in labor, staffing should be adequate in the labor and delivery area. Appropriate recommendations can be found in AAP/ACOG *Guidelines for Perinatal Care.*

Education. Electronic fetal heart rate monitoring requires the presence of skilled individuals to recognize heart rate pattern changes and the availability of physicians capable of proper diagnosis. It is the responsibility of the hospital to verify the knowledge base of health professionals in the clinical application of electronic fetal monitoring and to encourage the continuous updating of their skills.

Monitoring in the delivery room. When continuous electronic fetal heart rate monitoring had been used during labor, the guidelines as recommended in *Standards for Obstetric-Gynecologic Services (Sixth Edition, page 36) should be followed.*

*In some hospitals, the nurse is directed to construct a narrative description of the FHR tracing, such as "V-shaped decelerations with rapid deceleration and acceleration phases, occurring during each contraction," instead of documenting "variable decelerations." The use of these narrative descriptions is thought to avoid potential legal liability by preventing the nurse from "interpreting" the tracing (Fields, 1987).

SUMMARY

Nursing care of the woman in labor may include pharmacologic control of discomfort, as well as fetal monitoring. The nurse's knowledge and competence in these areas

Checklist for Fetal Monitoring Equipment

Name: ______________________ Evaluator: ______________________

Date: ______________________

Items to be Checked

Preparation of Monitor

1. Is the paper inserted correctly?
2. Are transducer cables plugged into the appropriate outlet of the monitor?

Ultrasound Transducer

1. Has ultrasound transmission gel been applied to the crystals?
2. Was the FHR tested and noted on the chart paper?
3. Does a consistent wave form appear on the oscilloscope?
4. Is the strap secure and snug?

Tocotransducer

1. Is the tocotransducer firmly strapped where the least maternal tissue is in evidence?
2. Has it been applied without gel or paste?
3. Are there any accumulations of gel around the pressure button?
4. Was the pen-set knob adjusted between 20 and 25 mm marks and noted on chart paper?
5. Was this setting done between contractions?
6. Is the strap secure and snug?

Spiral Electrode

1. Are the wires attached firmly to the posts on the leg plate?
2. Is the spiral electrode attached to the presenting part of the fetus?
3. Is the inner surface of the leg plate covered with electrode paste?
4. Is the leg plate properly secured to the woman's thigh?

Internal Catheter/Strain Gauge

1. Is the strain gauge located about half the height of the uterus (approximately at maternal xiphoid)?
2. Is the catheter filled with sterile water?
3. Is the black line on the catheter visible at the introitus?

Items to be Checked

4. Is it noted on the chart paper that the stopcock was opened to room air (reading 0 on paper)?
5. Was the uterine activity (UA) tested at 50 for 10 seconds?
6. Is the stopcock turned off to the syringe during monitoring?

Charting

1. Are testings of FHR and UA written on chart paper at least every 4 hours?
2. Is the chart paper properly labeled with the following:
   a. Woman's name
   b. Identification number
   c. Date
   d. Time monitor attached and mode
   e. High-risk conditions (pregnancy-induced hypertension, diabetes, etc.)
   f. Membranes intact or ruptured
   g. Gestational age
   h. Dilation and station
3. Are the following noted?
   a. Maternal position and repositioning in bed
   b. Vaginal examinations
   c. Paracervical block
   d. Medication given
   e. BP and temperature, pulse, respiration (TPR)
   f. Voidings
   g. O_2 given
   h. Emesis
   i. Pushing
   j. Fetal movement
   k. Notations of baseline or periodic changes
   l. Any change in mode of monitoring
   m. Adjustments of equipment, i.e.
      (1) Relocation of transducers
      (2) Flushing catheter
      (3) Replacement of electrode
      (4) Replacement of catheter

From Tucker, SM: Fetal monitoring and fetal assessment in high-risk pregnancy, St Louis, 1978, The CV Mosby Co.

can have a significant impact on the woman's labor experience.

Nursing management of obstetric analgesia and anesthesia combines the nurse's expertise in obstetrics with knowledge and understanding of techniques, drugs, and their potential complications. A general knowledge of analgesia and anesthesia is basic to implementation of the nursing process in relation to use of medications during labor.

The physiologic requirements of the woman (e.g., adequate hydration, preventing hypotension) receiving pharmacologic control of discomfort have been presented. Effects on the unborn and newborn baby (e.g., uterine blood flow, oygenation, and glucose) have been discussed. The key is to provide the childbearing family with a choice in pain relief. It is then the duty of caring professionals to provide the safety in that choice by using their knowledge of drugs and techniques (Petree, 1983).

Normal FHR patterns correlate with high Apgar scores and low neonatal morbidity. An abnormal pattern is equated with fetal hypoxia, low Apgar scores, and high neonatal morbidity in many but by no means in all cases. Because FHR patterns suggesting hypoxia may occur in the absence of fetal distress, intermittent and continuous FHR assessments are screening rather than diagnostic devices. More investigation and clarification of the factors and findings involved will be necessary to perfect the interpretation of fetal monitoring.

KEY CONCEPTS

- The type of analgesic or anesthetic to be used is chosen in part by the stage of labor and the method of delivery.
- Narcotic effects can be potentiated with ataractics and reversed with an antagonist.
- Pharmacologic control of discomfort during labor required collaboration among the nurse, obstetrician, anesthesiologist, and parturient.
- The nurse must understand medications, their expected effect, potential side effects, and methods of administration.
- Placement of an IV line and maternal hydration are essential during regional nerve blocks.
- Maternal analgesia/anesthesia potentially affect neonatal neurobehavioral response.
- Fetal well being during labor is measured by the response of the FHR to uterine contractions.
- FHR characteristics include the baseline FHR and periodic changes in FHR.
- Monitoring techniques of fetal well-being include FHR assessment, blood sampling, and watching for presence of meconium-stained amniotic fluid.
- It is the responsibility of the labor and delivery room nurse to assess FHR patterns, perform independent nursing interventions, and report nonreassuring patterns to the physician.
- The ACOG and NAACOG have established nursing standards for EFM.

STUDY QUESTIONS AND ACTIVITIES

1. Prepare a teaching project for a prenatal class covering pharmacologic control of discomfort during the birth period. Use visual aids when possible. Develop an evaluation tool for the project for use by clients, peers, and instructor.
2. Arrange a group discussion on individual reactions to pain and culturally determined behaviors, with extension of the discussion of how the atmosphere of the childbirth setting and the attitudes of health care personnel might interact with these factors in the client's perception of pain during childbirth.
3. Study at least 10 actual or sample fetal monitor strips and determine:
   a. FHR baseline
   b. Variability
   c. Contraction interval, duration, intensity, and resting tone
   d. Periodic changes, if any
4. For activity 3, describe the appropriate nursing actions for each sample in writing; exchange and compare their descriptions with those developed by other students.
5. Role-play a mother in the first stage of labor who is upset and unknowledgeable of the uses of the fetal monitor and a nurse who is using the equipment in an actual case for the first time. Make suggestions concerning actions that would be supportive and reassuring.
6. Role-play an interaction of a woman who had expected to avoid all pharmacologic treatment for discomfort but who now must have some relief with a nurse who is convinced that discomfort should be avoided if at all possible. Analyze the verbal and nonverbal behaviors of both role players.

References:

Abboud, TK, et al: Maternal, fetal and neonatal responses after epidural anesthesia with bupivacaine, 2-chloroprocaine or lidocaine, Anesth Analg 61:638, 1982

American Academy of Pediatrics/American College of Obstetricians and Gynecologists: Guidelines for Perinatal Care, Elk Grove Village, IL, AAP/ACOG, 1983

American College of Obstetricians and Gynecologists: Standard for Obstetric-Gynecologic Services, ed 6, Washington, DC, ACOG, 1985

Avard, DM, and Nimrod, CM: Risks and benefits of obstetric epidural analgesia: a review, Birth 12:215, Winter 1985

Blank, JJ: Electronic fetal monitoring, JOGN Nurs 14:463, Nov/Dec 1985

Bonica, JJ: Obstetric analgesia and anesthesia, ed 2, Amsterdam, 1980, World Federation of Societies of Anaesthesiologists

Bradley, RA: Husband-coached childbirth, New York, 1974, Harper & Row Publishers, Inc

Danforth, DN, and Scott, JR (editors): Obstetrics and gynecology, ed 5, Philadelphia, 1986, JB Lippincott Co

Fields, LM: Electronic fetal monitoring: practices and protocols for the intrapatum patient, J Perinat Neonat Nurs, 1(1):5, 1987

Hahn, AB, Oestreich, DJ, and Barkin, RL: Mosby's pharmacology in nursing, ed 16, St Louis, 1986, The CV Mosby Co

Hodgkinson, R et al: Neonatal neurobehavioral tests following vaginal delivery under ketamine, thiopental, and extradural anesthesia, Anesth Analg 56:548, 1977

Lamaze, F: Painless childbirth, New York, 1972, Pocket Books

Lundberg, GD, editor: Anesthetics and neonatal response, JAMA 250:2133, 1983

Marx, GF: Pain relief during labor—more than comfort, J Calif Perinat Assn 4:36, Winter 1984

Nurses Association of the American College of Obstetricians and Gynecologists: Statement: electronic fetal monitoring, joint ACOG-NAACOG statement, Washington, DC, 1986, The Association

Petree, B: A nursing perspective of obstetrical analgesia/anesthesia, NAACOG update series, 1:lesson 12, 1983

Pritchard, JA, MacDonald, PC, and Gant, NF, editors: Williams' obstetrics, ed 17, Norwalk, Conn, 1985, Appleton-Century-Crofts

Quirk, JG, and Miller, FC: FHR tracing characteristics that jeopardize the diagnosis of fetal well-being, Clin Obstet Gynecol 29(1):12, 1986

Rosenblatt, DB, et al: The influence of maternal analgesia on neonatal behavior. II. Epidural bupivacaine. Br J Obstet Gynaecol 88:407, 1981

Scanlon, JW, et al: Anesthesiology 40:121, 1974

Simkin, P: Stress, pain, and catecholamines in labor. I. A review, Birth 13(4):227, 1986a

Simkin, P: Stress, pain, and catecholamines in labor. II. A pilot survey of new mothers, Birth 13(4):234, 1986b

Bibliography

Albright, GA: Neurobehavior assessment—a prospective, J Calif Perinatal Assoc 1:60, 1981
Amiel-Tison, C, et al: A new neurologic and adaptive capacity scoring system for evaluation obstetric medications in full-term newborns, Anesthesiology 56:340, 1982
Boesel, RR, Olson, AE, and Johnson, JW: Umbilical cord blood studies help assess fetal status, Contemp OB/GYN, 28(5):63, 1986
Booth, T: Relaxation for childbirth, Int Childbirth Educ, 2(2):43, 1987
Bromage, RP, et al: Epidural narcotics for postoperative analgesia, Anesth Analg 59:473, 1980
Cheek, TG, and Gutsche, BB: Epidural analgesia for labor and vaginal delivery, Clin Obstet Gynecol 30(3):515, 1987
Chestnut, DH: Regional anesthesia, other than epidural, for labor and vaginal delivery, Clin Obstet Gynecol 30(3):530, 1987
Clark, PE, and Clark, MJ: Therapeutic touch: is there a scientific basis for the practice? Nurs Res 33:37, Jan Feb, 1984
Collins, BA: The role of the nurse in labor and delivery as perceived by nurses and patients, JOGN Nurs 15(5):412, 1986
Dailey, P, et al: Neurobehavioral testing of the newborn infant, Clin Perinatal 9:1, Feb 1982
Datta, S, et al: Neonatal effect of prolonged anesthetic induction for cesarean section, Am J Obstet Gynecol 58:331, 1981
Dewan, DM: Anesthesia for preterm delivery, breech presentation, and multiple gestation, Clin Obstet Gynecol 30(3):566, 1987
Donovan, M, editor: Pain control, Nurs Clin North Am, September 1987
Fishburne, JI: Systemic analgesia during labor, Clin Perinatol 9:29, 1982
Freeman, RK, and Garite, TJ: Fetal heart rate monitoring, Baltimore, 1982, Williams & Wilkins
Funk, M, and Buerkle, L: Intrauterine treatment of fetal tachycardia, JOGN Nurs 15(4):298, 1986
Garite, TJ, and Ray, D: Intrauterine resuscitation with tocolysis, Contemp OB/GYN 31(3):24, 1988
Garite, TJ, and Towers, C: Seeking the cause of transient bradycardia, Contemp OB/GYN 28(3):36, 1986
Gibbs, RF, editor: Legal perspectives on anesthesia, vol 4, Jan Feb 1984 (Entire issue; McMahon Publishing Co Georgetown, Conn 06829)
Haight, K: What you should know about epidural analgesia, Nursing '87 17(9):58, 1987
Hughes, SC: Intraspinal narcotics in obstetrics, Clin Perinatol 9:167, 1982
Huhman, M: Endogenous opiates and pain, Adv Nurs Sci 4(4):62, 1982
Inturrisi, M, Camenga, CF, and Rosen, M: Epidural morphine for relief of postpartum, postsurgical pain, JOGN Nurs 17(4):238, 1988
Investigators: a look at endorphins in reproductive medicine, Contemp Obstet Gynecol 20(3): 117, 1982
James, FM: Anesthesia for nonobstetric surgery during pregnancy, Clin Obstet Gynecol 30(3):621, 1987
Jankowski, H, and Wells, S: Self-administered medications for obstetric patients, MCN 12(3):199, 1987
Jones, MM, and Joyce, TH: Anesthesia for the parturient with pregnancy-induced hypertension, Clin Obstet Gynecol 30(3):591, 1987
Kirshon, B, and Cotton, DB: Invasive hemodynamic monitoring in the obstetric patient, Clin Obstet Gynecol 30(3):579, 1987
Lowe, NK: Parity and pain during parturition, JOGN Nurs 16(5):340, 1987
Lynn, N: ICEA review: pain theory and childbirth, Int Childbirth Educ 2(2):21, 1987
McCaffery, M: Patient-controlled analgesia: more than a machine, Nursing '87 17(11):62, 1987
McGilvray, R: Over the counter drugs in pregnancy, Int Childbirth Educ 2(2):37, 1987
McKlveen, RE, and Ostheimer, GW: Resuscitation of the newborn, Clin Obset Gynecol 30(3):611, 1987
Nursing photobook. Using monitors. Nursing '81 books, Horsham, Pa., Intermed Communications, Inc.
Pearson, J: Some women's experiences of epidurals, Int Childbirth Educ 2(2):19, 1987
Pedersen, H, and Finster, M: Selection and use of local anesthetics, Clin Obstet Gynecol 30(3):505, 1987
Redick, LF: Epidural anesthesia, Clin Perinatol 9:63, 1982
Reisner, LS: Anesthesia for cesarean delivery, Clin Obstet Gynecol 30(3):539, 1987
Rimar, JM: Epidural morphine for analgesia following a cesarean, MCN 11(5):345, 1986
Roberts, S and Chestnut, DH: Anesthesia for the obstetric patient with cardiac disease, Clin Obstet Gynecol 30(36):601, 1987
Roberts, WE, et al: Pros and cons of meperidine for intrapartum analgesia, Contemp OB/GYN 23:69, April 1984
Ross, BK, and Hughes, SC: Epidural and spinal narcotic analgesia, Clin Obstet Gynecol 30(3):552, 1987
Sarno, AP, and Phelan, JP: Intrauterine resuscitation of the fetus, Contemp OB/GYN 32(1):143, 1988
Schifrin, BS: Polemics in perinatology: the future of fetal monitoring, J Perinatol 6(4):331, 1986
Schwarz, T: Prolong regional analgesia with morphine—epidurally, RN 45(5): 32, 1982
Simkin, P: Comfort measures for labor, Int Childbirth Educ 2(2):5, 1987
Smith, CM: Epidural anesthesia in labor: various agents employed, JOGN Nurs 13(1):17, 1984
Spielman, FJ: Systemic analgesics during labor, Clin Obstet Gynecol 30(3):495, 1987
Triolo, PK: Prepared childbirth, Clin Obstet Gynecol 30(3):487, 1987
Tucker, SM: Pocket guide to fetal monitoring, St Louis, 1988, The CV Mosby Co
Yurth, DA: Placental transfer of local anesthetics, Clin Perinatol 9:13, 1982

CHAPTER 18

The First Stage of Labor

Iris E. Campbell

Learning Objectives

Correctly define the key terms listed.

Review the factors involved in the initial assessment of the woman in labor.

List the information that can be obtained from the woman's prenatal record.

Summarize the subsequent assessment of progress during labor.

Identify nursing diagnoses and develop an appropriate plan of care.

Evaluate the role of supportive persons in relation to the phases of the first stage of labor.

Explain the ways in which the nurse can assist support persons.

Outline the preparation for giving birth in the delivery room.

Key Terms

active phase
area of maximum intensity
cervical dilation
descent
duration (of contractions)
effacement
effleurage
fetal heart rate (FHR)
frequency of contractions
hyperventilation
Hawthorne effect
inadequate uterine relaxation
intensity (of contractions)
latent phase
mini-prep
partogram
regularity of contractions
show
slow breathing
transcutaneous electrical nerve stimulation (TENS)
transitional phase

Nursing care of the woman during the first stage of labor is directed toward safe delivery of a live, healthy baby to a couple who have had a happy and fulfilling childbirth experience. If a hospital delivery has been elected, the woman is admitted to the labor unit (Fig. 18-1). If an alternative birth setting, such as home or birthing center has been chosen, the family follows the birth plan instructions previously agreed on. The ongoing care should be based on valid research rather than on unvalidated tradition. Many families now have high expectations of childbirth and are seeking more autonomy in labor. The first stage of labor is characterized by the onset of symptoms the expectant mother has been prepared to recognize during the prenatal period. The months of waiting are at an end. The time has arrived for the birth of the baby. The woman and her family are about to experience the miracle of birth, one of the most meaningful events of their lives.

The first stage of labor begins with the onset of regular uterine contractions and culminates when the cervix has reached full dilation. Care of the woman in labor begins with the woman's report of the following:

1. Onset of progressive, regular uterine contractions that increase in strength and frequency
2. Rupture of the membranes
3. Bloody vaginal discharge (bloody show)

When the woman and her partner arrive at the labor unit, greet them warmly, call them by name, and extend a welcome to them. Welcoming the family will be discussed in more detail under the implementation phase of the nursing process. On admission to the unit, assessment of the woman is the most important priority.

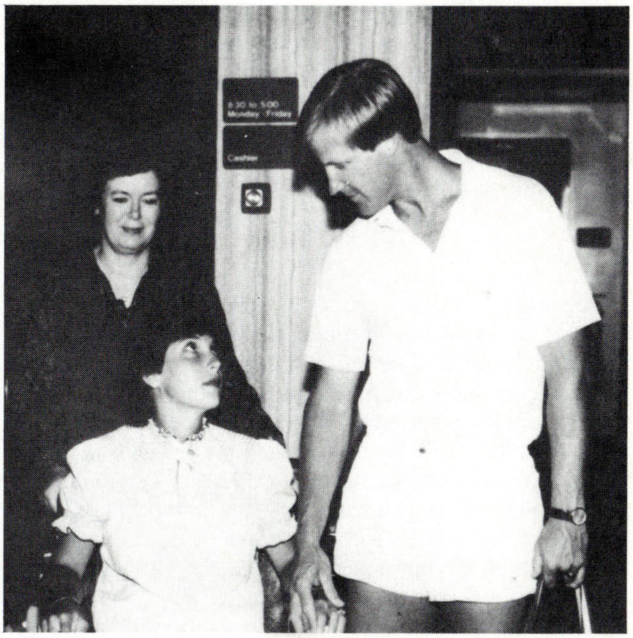

Fig. 18-1 Couple arrives on labor/birth unit accompanied by maternal grandmother.
Courtesy Marjorie Pyle, RNC, Lifecircle, Costa Mesa, Calif.

INITIAL ASSESSMENT

The admission form can be used to guide the nurse's assessment of the woman in labor. The data for the admission record is obtained from several sources and includes review of the prenatal record; interview information; obtaining baseline physiologic parameters; laboratory results; psychological, social, and cultural factors; and assessment of the woman's current clinical status.

Prenatal Record

Before the nurse's first meeting with the woman who is in labor, a review of the woman's prenatal record is made. Significant items are noted. If the woman has not had any prenatal care, the needed information must be obtained on admission. It is best to complete her data base before active labor begins.

General Information. **Age** is important. The needs of a 12-year-old girl and those of a 42-year-old woman vary in some respects. **Height and weight** are also significant. A woman who stands 145 cm (4 ft 10 in) and weighs 77 kg (170 lb) may require interventions different from those needed by the woman who also weights 77 kg but is 177.5 cm (5 ft 11 in) tall. **General health**, any **medical conditions**, and history of **surgical interventions** are carefully noted.

Past Obstetric History. **Parity and gravidity** are recorded (Chapter 10). Previous obstetric experience is reviewed for the following:

1. Problems: spontaneous abortions, preterm labors, stillbirths, premature rupture of membranes, bleeding, hypertension, anemia, gestational diabetes, infections (especially sexually transmitted diseases)
2. Type of labors: duration of labors, anesthesia used
3. Type of deliveries: normal spontaneous vaginal delivery (NSVD), forceps assisted, cesarean
4. Condition of babies at birth: weight, Apgar scores, singleton (one baby) or multiple (twins, triplets) births

History of Present Pregnancy. Pertinent information includes the date of the last normal menstrual period (LNMP), date of quickening, growth of height of the fundus, and estimated weight of the fetus. These data are used to confirm the expected date of delivery (EDD) (EDD is gradually replacing the older term, expected date of confinement [EDC]). The woman's vital signs, blood pressure, weight and pattern of weight gain, and results of urinalysis help confirm the normalcy of this pregnancy. The FHR and its location provide a baseline against which the nurse can compare findings of initial assessment.

Data noted include the gestational week of initial visit, diagnostic studies done, and problems encountered. The medications used during this pregnancy are carefully documented. Commonly, prenatal records indicate the woman's preferences for anesthesia, feeding her newborn, and the name of her pediatrician.

Laboratory tests performed during this pregnancy and the findings are recorded. These tests include the initial blood test for blood group and Rh factor, hemoglobin and hematocrit, and sickle cell trait, if indicated. Antibody titers are determined. As necessary, throughout the pregnancy, tests are repeated for hematocrit and hemoglobin and antibody titers. Urinalysis is usually recorded for each visit. Urine is assessed for protein, acetone, and glucose.

To complete the admission form, the nurse uses the assessment techniques of interviewing, physical examination, and laboratory tests. Each of these techniques will be discussed individually.

Interview

Any information not found in the prenatal record is requested on admission. Pertinent data include choice of infant feeding method, anesthesia, and pediatrician. A client profile is obtained; this profile indicates the woman's preparation for childbirth, supportive persons desired and available, and ethnic or cultural expectations or needs.

The woman's chief complaint or reason for coming to the hospital is determined. The chief complaint may be rupture of membranes with or without contractions. In this case she is in for an **obstetric check**. The obstetric check is reserved for women who are unsure about onset of labor. This designation allows time on the unit for diagnosis of labor without official admission, and minimizes or avoids cost to the client.

The woman may have been scheduled for induction of labor (see Chapter 33). Induction of labor and other complications of labor, such as premature rupture of membranes, require special alterations in the nursing care plan. However, even in those instances some nursing care remains the same.

The onset of labor may be difficult to determine even for the experienced gravida. The woman is asked to recall the events of the previous days. She is assessed for the prodromal signs of labor (Chapter 16) and for the onset of regular contractions. She is asked to describe the following:

1. Frequency and duration of contractions.
2. Location and character of discomfort from contractions.
3. Persistence of contractions despite changes in maternal position, when walking or lying down.
4. Presence and character of vaginal discharge or show.
5. Status of amniotic membranes, such as gush or seepage of fluid. If there is a discharge that may be amniotic fluid, she is asked the date and time the fluid was first noted. This information is recorded and followed by physical examination to confirm rupture of membranes.

In case general anesthesia may be required at a moment's notice, it is important to know about the woman's respiratory status. The nurse asks if the woman has a "cold" or related symptoms, "stuffy nose," sore throat, or cough. Allergies are rechecked, including allergies to drugs routinely used, such as meperidine (Demerol) or mepivacaine (Carbocaine). Some allergic responses cause swelling of mucous membranes of the respiratory system. Because vomiting and subsequent aspiration into the respiratory tract can complicate an otherwise normal labor, the nurse records the type and time of the woman's last meal.

This initial assessment confirms the onset of true labor and provides information on the woman's current clinical condition. The questions to be answered are:

1. Has labor begun?
2. How far has labor progressed?
3. Have the membranes ruptured?
4. What is the woman's psychologic response to the onset of labor?
5. Are there any complications that may require intervention?

Has Labor Begun?

False labor may be experienced from the thirty-eighth week of pregnancy onward. It can be disheartening for the woman and her partner to find that the contractions she is having are not true labor contractions and that she must return home to await the onset of true labor. (For a comparison of true and false labor, see guidelines for client teaching, p. 383).

How Far has Labor Progressed?

The nullipara, because of eagerness to complete labor, may come to the hospital early in the first stage. If she lives near the hospital, she may be asked to return home to wait for further progress either in frequency and strength of contractions or in amount of show. She is encouraged to walk about but is asked to restrict ingestion to clear fluids. Clear fluids are those fluids one can see through, for example, tea with honey and lemon, homemade broth (not salt-loaded bouillon), and apple juice. If the woman lives a considerable distance from the hospital, she may be admitted and the same care given. (For minimum schedule for assessments, see Table 18-1; for progression of labor, see Table 18-2.)

Determine the degree of progress as follows:

1. Assess the character of the contractions.
   a. Have the woman describe when the contractions began and what they are like now.
   b. Assess their duration, intensity (in some parts of the United States, the terms *strength* or *magnitude* are used instead), frequency, and regularity (see discussion that follows).
2. Assess the nature of the vaginal discharge and its amount, color, and character. Bloody show must be distinguished from bleeding. Show is pink in color and feels sticky from the mucus it contains. It is scant to begin with and increases with effacement and dilation of the cervix. A woman may report a scant brownish discharge. This may be attributable to trauma to the cervix as a result of vaginal examination or coitus within the last 48 hours.
3. Perform a vaginal examination (see Procedure 18-1 and Fig. 18-2) or assist the physician in assessing the following:
   a. Effacement and dilation of the cervix.
   b. Presentation and position of the fetus.
   c. Station of the presenting part.
   d. Degree of molding of the fetal head.
   e. Presence and amount of stool in the rectum.

Text continued on p. 386.

Guidelines For Client Teaching

DISTINGUISHING TRUE LABOR FROM FALSE LABOR

ASSESSMENT

1. Woman pregnant for first time.
2. Woman expresses a desire to learn the difference between true and false labor.

NURSING DIAGNOSES

Knowledge deficit related to the difference between true and false labor.

Anxiety related to lack of knowledge.

GOALS

Short-term

Woman will learn about Braxton-Hicks' contractions.

Woman will be instructed on the signs and symptoms of true labor.

Intermediate

Woman can time Braxton-Hicks' contractions for practice.

Long-term

Woman feels confident and can apply those things learned when true labor begins.

REFERENCES AND TEACHING AIDS

Printed materials containing comparison between true and false labor and the doctor/clinic/hospital's number.

CONTENT/RATIONALE	TEACHING ACTIONS
To teach woman about Braxton-Hicks' contractions: Define Braxton-Hicks' contractions as mild, intermittent, painless contractions that occur during pregnancy and aid in keeping uterine tone and facilitate placental perfusion.	Discuss this with the woman/couple. Encourage questions.
As pregnancy progresses these contractions become more frequent and are felt as a tightening of the abdomen. Woman may obtain relief with walking or lying down. Braxton-Hicks' contractions do not increase in intensity over time, nor is there a change in interval time between each contraction.	Have woman/couple place hands on her abdomen to try and feel for this tightening.
Contractions of true labor occur regularly, with intensity increasing and intervals between them shortening. May be located in lower back or feel like GI upset, may be accompanied by diarrhea.	Explain how true labor works to dilate and efface the cervix. Use available illustrations or audiovisual materials.
To teach other signs and symptoms of labor: Discuss show—in true labor this is usually present as a pinkish mucus that may contain mucous plug from cervix.	Discuss the mucous plug and its purpose. Show the woman a picture or illustration of what a bloody show would look like.
There is no show in false labor unless woman has had a vaginal exam within last 48 hours; mucus may be brownish stained.	
Discuss cervix—becomes effaced and dilated as time progresses. No change with false labor.	
Discuss descent of fetus—progressive as labor continues. No descent of fetus in false labor.	Explain how fetus moves down into the true pelvis.
Discuss fetal movement—no significant change in true labor. May intensify for a short time or remain the same with false labor.	Encourage discussion and questions.

EVALUATION Teaching has been effective when all goals have been obtained. Woman is able to feel, time, and describe Braxton-Hicks' contractions. Woman is able to verbalize the difference between false and true labor. Woman recognizes when true labor begins.

Table 18-1 *Minimum Assessment of Progress of First Stage of Labor*

	Cervical Dilation		
	0-5 cm	6-7 cm	8-10 cm
Vital signs*	Every 4 hr	Every 4 hr	Every 4 hr
Blood pressure	Every 60 min	Every 30 min	Every 30 min
Contractions	Every 30 min to 1 hr	Every 15 min	Every 5-10 min
Fetal heart rate (FHR)	Every 15 min†	Every 15 min†	Every 15 min†
Show	Every 60 min	Every 30 min	Every 10-15 min
Behavior, appearance, energy level	Every 30 min	Every 15 min	Every 5 min
Vaginal examination‡	To be done only for following reasons: 1. To confirm diagnosis when symptoms indicate change (e.g., strength, duration, or frequency of contractions; increase in amount of bloody show; membranes rupture; or woman feels pressure on her rectum) 2. To determine whether dilation and descent are sufficient for administration of anesthetic 3. To reassess progress if labor takes longer than expected 4. To determine station of presenting part		

*If membranes have ruptured, check temperature every 2 hours.

†For a period of 30 seconds immediately after a uterine contraction (Zuspan and Quilligan, 1982).

‡In presence of vaginal bleeding, physician performs vaginal examination, usually under double setup.

Table 18-2 *Maternal Progress in First Stage of Labor Within Normal Limits*

	Phases Marked by Cervical Dilation*		
Criterion	0-3 cm	4-7 cm	8-10 cm Transition
Duration	About 8-10 hr	About 3 hr	About 1-2 hr
Contractions			
Magnitude (strength)	Mild	Moderate	Strong to expulsive
Rhythm	Irregular	More regular	Regular
Frequency	5-30 min apart	3-5 min apart	2-3 min apart
Duration	10-30 sec	30-45 sec	45-60 (few to 90) sec
Descent			
Station of presenting part	Nulliparous: 0 Multiparous: 0 to −2 cm	About +1 to +2 cm About +1 to +2 cm	+2 to +3 cm +2 to +3 cm
Show			
Color	Brownish discharge, mucous plug or pale, pink mucus	Pink to bloody mucus	Bloody mucus
Amount	Scant	Scant to moderate	Copious
Behavior and appearance	Excited; thoughts center on self, labor, and baby; may be talkative or mute, calm or tense; some apprehension; pain controlled fairly well; alert, follows directions readily; open to instructions	Becoming more serious, doubtful of control of pain, more apprehensive; desires companionship and encouragement; attention more inner directed; fatigue evidenced; malar flush; has some difficulty following directions	Pain described as severe; backache common; feelings of frustration, fear of loss of control, and irritability surface; vague in communications; amnesia between contractions; writhing with contractions; nausea and vomiting, especially if hyperventilating; hyperesthesia; circumoral pallor, perspiration on forehead and upper lips; shaking tremor of thighs; feeling of need to defecate, pressure on anus

*The pace of progress in cervical dilation (according to Friedman and Sachtleben, 1965) varies as follows: from 0 to 2 cm **(latent phase)**, progress is slow; from 2 to 4 cm **(phase of acceleration)**, pace quickens; from 4 to 9 cm **(phase of maximal acceleration)**, pace is most rapid; and from 9 to 10 cm **(phase of deceleration)**, pace slows again (Figs. 18-7 and 18-8).

In the nullipara, effacement is often complete before dilation begins; in the multipara, it occurs simultaneously with dilation.

Procedure 18-1

PERFORMING OR ASSISTING WITH A VAGINAL EXAMINATION

DEFINITION

The periodic assessment of the condition of the cervix, membranes, and fetus before and during labor.

PURPOSE

To assess the cervix: degree of softness (readiness for labor), effacement, and dilation.
To assess fetal presentation and position.
To assess degree of fetal descent or station.
To assess degree of molding of the fetal head; if presenting.
To assess the membranes: intact, bulging, or ruptured.
To assess how well the presenting part is applied to the cervix.
To assess the presence and amount of stool in the maternal rectum.
To apply internal fetal monitor (scalp clip).
To insert intrauterine pressure catheter for internal monitoring of uterine contractions.

EQUIPMENT

Sterile gloves.
Antiseptic solution, sterile water, or water-soluble gel.
Drapes.
Light source.
Nitrazine (Litmus) paper.
Intrauterine pressure catheter (optional).
Scalp clip (optional).

NURSING ACTIONS	RATIONALE
Assess for vaginal bleeding, one indication of placenta previa, a cause of life-threatening hemorrhage (see Chapter 31).	To prevent hemorrhage should a placenta previa exist.
If no bleeding is present, ask woman to empty her bladder.	To increase maternal comfort and facilitate accurate assessment.
Drape appropriately.	To respect woman's modesty and to protect privacy.
Position light source.	To permit visualization of vulva.
Assist woman to a supine position with one pillow under her head and her knees flexed and separated.	To facilitate examination. To relax abdominal musculature and increase comfort.
Place small rolled towel under woman's right hip.	To displace uterus to the left, off major blood vessels to prevent supine hypotension syndrome.
Wash hands, apply gloves, or help examiner put on gloves.	To maintain asepsis for the mother and the examiner.
Lubricate examining fingers with sterile water, antiseptic solution or water-soluble gel (see assessment for rupture of membranes, pp. 392-394).	To facilitate examination; maintain asepsis; prevent interference with reading of Nitrazine (Litmus) paper when water is used.
Separate labia with one gloved hand, introduce middle and index finger of examining hand into vagina with palmar surface downward. Maintain downward pressure toward less sensitive posterior vaginal wall.	To prevent rolling of labia into vagina as fingers of examining hand enter vagina and to aid in preventing infection. To lessen discomfort by directing pressure toward less sensitive posterior vaginal wall.
Curl last two fingers (Fig. 18-2, *A*)	To lessen chance of contamination or infection from anal area.
Place other hand on uterine fundus and exert a gentle downward pressure.	To facilitate assessment by steadying the fetus and applying the presenting part to the cervix.
Rotate fingers as necessary to complete assessment of fetus, station, cervix, status of amniotic membrances, and rectal fullness.	To perform assessment. To assess need for enema, if physician deems necessary.
Coach woman with breathing and focusing.	To assist with perineal relaxation.
Remind woman to keep her eyes open and her hands relaxed.	To assist woman to relax perineum and "stay in control."
If woman shows signs of supine hypotension or vasovagal syncope (see Emergency, Chapter 8) (i.e., she becomes pale, breathless, and faint, with clammy skin), turn her on her left side.	To relieve the signs and symptoms (see Emergency, Chapter 8).

Continued.

Procedure 18-1—cont'd

NURSING ACTIONS		RATIONALE
After completing the examination, clean the woman's vulva and place a clean pad on bed under her; Dispose of soiled articles per hospital protocol, remove and discard gloves, and wash hands, reposition bed covers according to woman's preference.		To increase comfort, both physical and emotional. To implement universal precautions when handling body fluids (see Chapter 30). To maintain cleanliness and decrease possibility of infection. To respect woman's dignity.
Answer any questions about the findings.		To help decrease anxiety and increase woman's (couple's) sense of control over the situation.
Enter initial findings on admission form:		To establish data base to compare future findings. To provide data base for next steps in the nursing process.
Cervix		
Dilation	0 to 10 cm	
Effacement	0 to 100%	
Consistency	Thick/firm to soft ("ripe")	
Position	Anterior/posterior	To promote collaboration with other members of the health care team.
Fetus		
Presentation and position	Vertex, left occipitoanterior	
Station	Floating to 0 to +4	

Have the Membranes Ruptured?

Labor is initiated by spontaneous rupture of the membranes (SROM) in almost 25% of gravidas. The lag period, rarely exceeding 24 hours, precedes the onset of labor. The length of uterine inactivity is directly related to the duration of pregnancy. If the woman is only 32 weeks pregnant, for example, several days may pass before labor begins. If she is at term, labor usually ensues within 12 hours of rupture of the membranes. After a delay of 24 hours, the woman is said to have premature or prolonged rupture of the membranes (PROM). If they are ruptured, note the color and character of the amniotic fluid, ask for the time of rupture, and check the vaginal discharge with phenaphthazine (Nitrazine paper) for pH (positive = dark blue) because pH is weakly basic at 7.2.

What is the Woman's Psychologic Response to the Onset of Labor?

The woman's general appearance and behavior (and that of her partner) provide valuable clues as to the type of supportive care she will need. The nurse notes the following:

1. *Verbal interaction.* Is the woman talkative or mute? Does she talk to staff members freely or only in response to questions? How does she talk to her support person? Does that person do all the talking?

2. *Body posture and set.* Is the woman relaxed or tense? What is her anxiety level? Does she lie rigidly on her back or sit up tailor fashion? Where does her partner sit?

3. *Perceptual acuity.* Does the woman have any helpful or harmful background knowledge? Does her anxiety level require repeated explanations? Does she understand what the nurse says? Can she repeat what has been said or demonstrate that she understands (e.g., use the call bell correctly)?

4. *Energy level.* Does the woman look tired? How much rest has she had in the previous few days? Does excitement mask a depleted energy reserve?

5. *Discomfort or pain.* How much does the woman relate what she is experiencing? How does she react to a contraction?

6. *Cultural background.* Does the woman's ethnic/cultural heritage define any prescriptions or proscriptions for her behavior or the care she receives during labor? What are her expectations of the hospital and the staff?

Are There Any Complications That May Require Intervention?

Although some complications of labor are anticipated, others appear only in the clinical course of labor. Knowledge of pregnancy, careful initial assessment, and follow-up of progress are necessary during normal labor, as well as during an abnormal labor (see danger signs box).

DANGER SIGNS

During Labor

1. Intrauterine pressure above 75 mm Hg
2. Contractions lasting longer than 60 seconds
3. Contractions occuring more than every 2 minutes
4. Fetal bradycardia, tachycardia
5. Irregular fetal heart rate
6. Absence of fetal heart beat

A

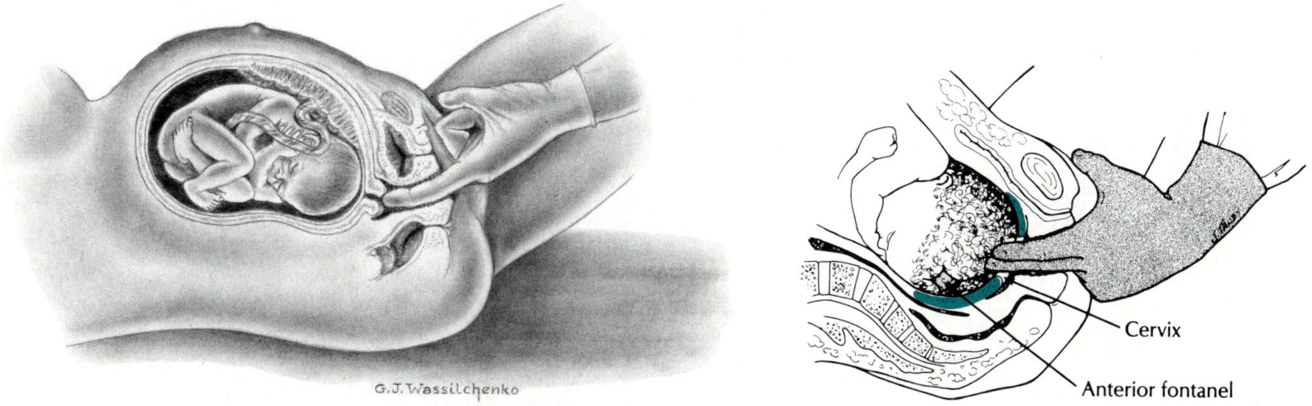

B

Fig. 18-2 Vaginal examination. **A**, Undilated, uneffaced cervix. Membranes intact. **B**, Palpation of sagittal suture line. Cervix effaced and partially dilated.

Physical Examination

The initial examinations confirm the onset of true labor. The findings serve as a baseline for assessing the woman's progress from that point in time. Physical examinations performed include the following:

1. Vital signs and blood pressure
2. Brief physical assessment: heart, lungs; presence of edema of the legs, face, hands, or sacrum (see Chapters 8 and 29).
3. Abdominal palpation: Leopold's maneuvers
4. Fetal heart rate (FHR), rhythm, area of maximum intensity (MI)
5. Uterine contractions

The assessment procedures that follow can be used as a basis for teaching women and their families. The purpose, equipment needed, and nursing actions and rationale of each procedure can be shared with the woman. All procedures are preceded by thorough handwashing. The procedures and findings are explained to the woman whenever possible. Universal precautions and precautions for invasive procedures are taken as needed (Chapter 30). Findings and the time the procedure is performed are carefully noted and initialed on the chart. Handwashing is also important *after* the examinations. Accurate charting is done as soon after interaction with a client as possible.

Vital Signs and Blood Pressure. Vital signs and blood pressure (BP) are assessed on admission of the client to the hospital. Findings are assessed for normalcy and are used for comparison with future values. If the BP is elevated, it should first be determined whether the correct BP cuff has been used, and BP should then be reassessed 30 minutes later to obtain a true reading after the woman has relaxed. An appropriate sized cuff is one that is 20% wider than the diameter of the extremity around which it is wrapped; usually about 12 to 14 cm (about 6 in) for average-size individuals and 18 to 20 cm (about 8 in) for obese individuals. Too small a cuff gives a false high BP; too large a cuff results in a false low BP.

Abdominal Palpation: Leopold's Maneuvers. Leopold's maneuvers are performed to determine fetal presentation, lie, position, and engagement. The four maneuvers provide a systematic examination. Proficiency in determining presentation and position by abdominal palpation requires considerable practice, so every opportunity to learn must be used to perform the technique. Gross maternal obesity, excessive amniotic fluid (hydramnios), or tumors may make it difficult to feel the fetal contours (see Procedure 18-2, and Fig. 18-3).

Auscultation of FHR. The area of MI of the FHR is the location of the maternal abdomen where the FHR is heard the loudest. The MI is also an aid in determining the fetal position (Figs. 18-4 and 18-5). In vertex and breech presentations, with the head well flexed on the fetal chest, the FHR is heard loudest through the fetal back. In vertex presentations the FHRs commonly are heard below the mother's umbilicus in a lower quadrant of the abdomen (Fig. 18-4,*A* and 18-5,*B*). In breech presentations the FHRs are usually heard loudest above the level of the umbilicus (Fig. 18-4,*C* and 18-5,*A*). As the fetus undergoes descent and internal rotation, the MI changes and is found to move downward and to the midline. In Fig. 18-4,*B*, the MI of the fetus in the right occipito-anterior (ROA) position is seen to move to the midline just over the symphysis pubis. Just before delivery the fetal position is occipito-anterior (OA) and the fetal back is directly above the symphysis pubis. (See also Chapter 17 for fetal monitoring).

Uterine Contractions. The primary powers, the uterine contractions, and their functions are described in detail in Chapter 16. There are three methods of assessing contractions: by the subjective description given by the woman, by palpation and timing by a nurse or physician, and by electronic monitoring devices (see Chapter 17).

Each contraction exhibits a wavelike pattern; it begins with a slow increment, gradually reaches an acme, and then diminishes rather rapidly (decrement). This is followed by an interval of rest (intrauterine pressure is 8 to 15 mm Hg), which is broken when the next contraction begins (Fig. 18-6).

In describing a uterine contraction, reference is made to the following characteristics:

1. **Frequency**. Contractions occur intermittently throughout labor. They begin at about 20 to 30 minutes apart and become closer together until, at the height of the

Procedure 18-2

ABDOMINAL PALPATION: LEOPOLD'S MANEUVERS

DEFINITION

Four maneuvers for assessing fetal position by external palpation of the mother's abdomen.

PURPOSE

To identify number of fetuses.
To identify fetal presentation, lie, presenting part, degree of descent, and fetal attitude.
To identify point of maximum intensity (PMI) of FHR in relation to the woman's abdomen.
To monitor the descent and internal rotation of the fetus.

EQUIPMENT

Fetal monitoring device.

NURSING ACTIONS	RATIONALE
Wash hands	To prevent nosocomial infection.
Ask woman to empty bladder.	To increase maternal comfort during examination. To facilitate accurate assessment.
Position woman supine with one pillow under her head and with her knees slightly flexed.	To ensure comfort. To relieve tension of abdominal musculature.
Place small rolled towel under woman's right hip.	To displace uterus to left off of major blood vessels. (Avoids supine hypotensive syndrome, p. 152).
If right-handed, stand at woman's right, facing her:	To facilitate examination by using dominant hand.
1. Identify fetal part that occupies the fundus. The head feels round, firm, freely movable, and palpable by ballottement; the breech feels less regular and softer (Fig. 18-3, *A*).	To identify fetal lie (vertical or horizontal) and presentation (vertex or breech).
2. Using palmar surface of one hand, locate and palpate the smooth convex contour of the fetal back and the irregularities that identify the small parts (feet, hands, elbows) (Fig. 18-3, *B*).	To assist in identifying fetal presentation.
3. With the right hand, determine which fetal part is presenting over the inlet to the true pelvis. Gently grasp the lower pole of the uterus between the thumb and fingers, pressing in slightly (Fig. 18-3, *C*). If the head is presenting and not engaged, determine the attitude of the head.	Confirms presenting part. Helps identify degree of descent. If the presenting part is not engaged, it can be rocked from side to side; if engaged, it cannot be rocked.
4. Turn to face gravida's feet. Using two hands, outline the fetal head (Fig. 18-3, *D*).	When presenting part has descended deeply, only a small portion of it may be outlined. Palpation of cephalic prominence assists in identifying attitude of head. If the cephalic prominence is found on the same side as the small parts, the head must be flexed, and the vertex is presenting (Fig. 18-3, *D*). If the cephalic prominence is on the same side as the back, the presenting head is extended (Fig. 16-3, *C*).
Determination of PMI of FHR	
Wash hands	To prevent nosocomial infection.
Perform Leopold's maneuvers.	To locate fetal back, presentation, and position.
Auscultate FHR (Figs. 18-4, 18-5, and 17-13).	To assist in estimating PMI.
Apply monitor prn (see Chapter 17).	To assist in assessing fetal well-being.
Wash hands.	To implement universal precautions (Chapter 30) when handling body fluids.
Chart fetal presentation, position, and lie; whether presenting part is flexed or extended, engaged or free floating.	To provide data base for future findings. To provide data base for next steps in the nursing process.
Use hospital's protocol for charting (e.g., "Vtx, LOA, floating")	To promote collaboration with other members of the health care team.

Procedure 18-2—cont'd

NURSING ACTIONS	RATIONALE
Chart PMI of FHR using a two-line figure to indicate the four quadrants of the maternal abdomen, right upper quadrant (RUQ), left upper quadrant (LUQ), left lower quadrant (LLQ), and right lower quadrant (RLQ):	To provide data base for future comparison. To provide data base for nursing process.

RUQ	LUQ
RLQ	LLQ

NURSING ACTIONS	RATIONALE
The umbilicus is the point where the lines cross. The PMI for the fetus in vertex presentation, in general flexion with the back on the mother's right side, is commonly found in the mother's right lower quadrant, and is recorded with an "x" or with the FHR as follows:	To assist other examiners.

x	

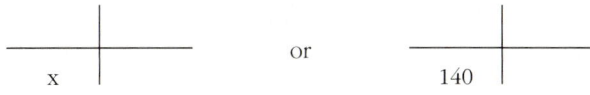

or

140	

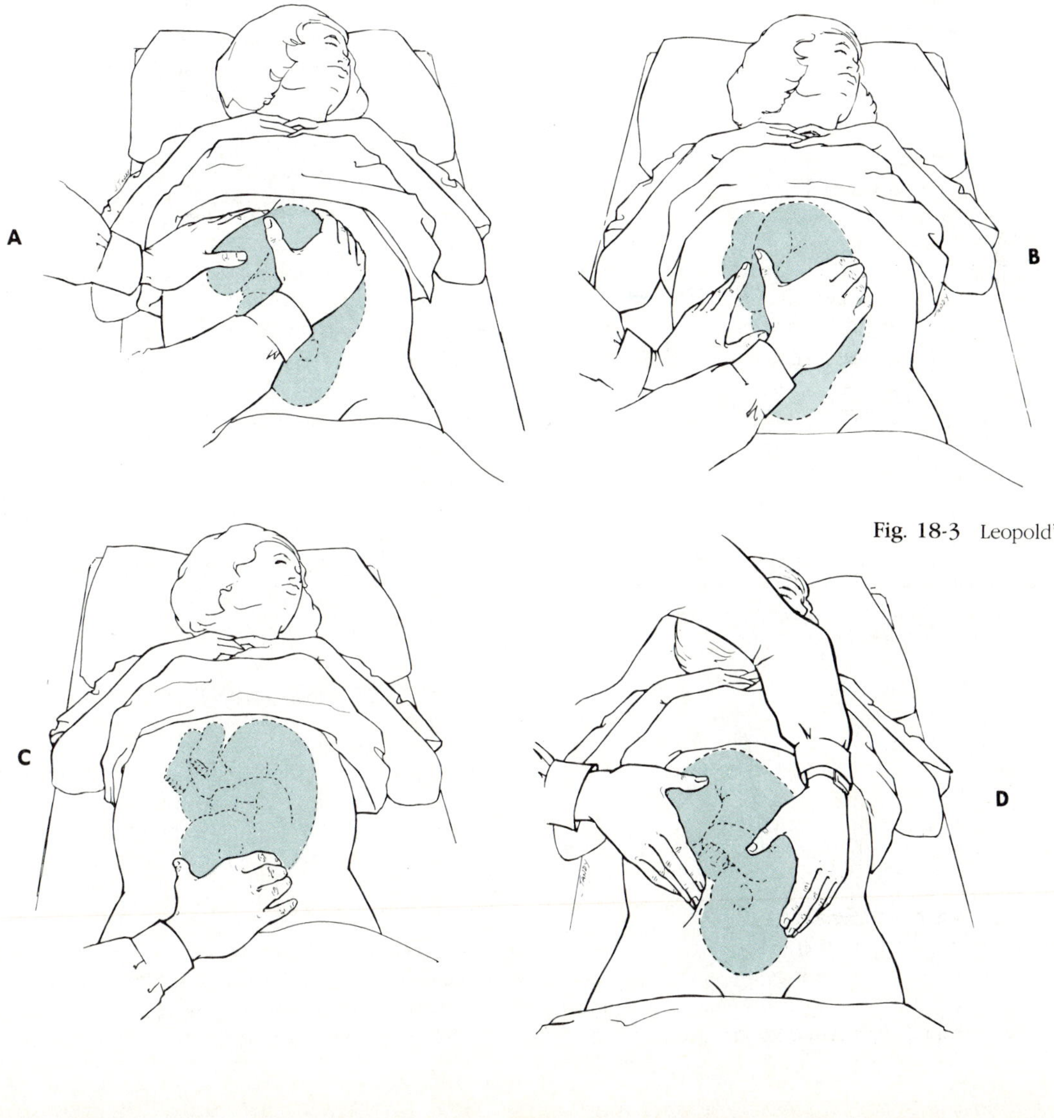

Fig. 18-3 Leopold's maneuvers.

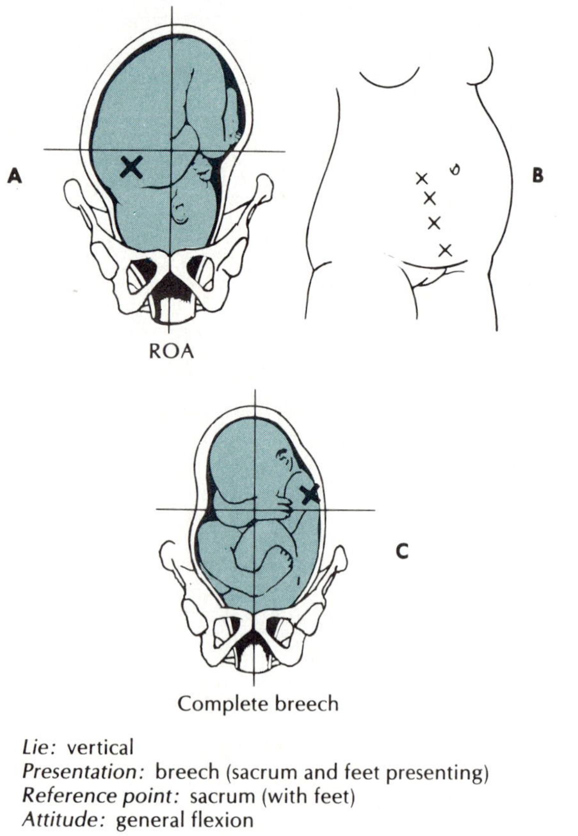

Fig. 18-4 The area of the FHR. **A**, With fetus in ROA position. **B**, Changes in area of MI as fetus undergoes internal rotation from ROA to OA for delivery. **C**, With fetus in LSP (left sacrum posterior) position.
A and C courtesy Ross Laboratories, Columbus, Ohio.

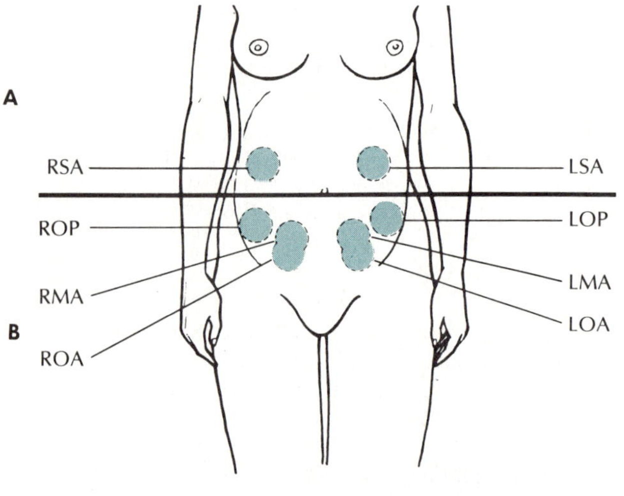

Fig. 18-5 Areas of maximum intensity of FHR for differing positions: *RSA,* right sacrum anterior; *ROP,* right occipitoposterior; *RMA,* right mentum anterior; *ROA,* right occipitoanterior; *LSA,* left sacrum anterior; *LOP,* left occipitoposterior; *LMA,* left mentum anterior; and *LOA,* left occipitoanterior. **A**, Presentation is *breech* if FHR is heard *above* umbilicus. **B**, Presentation is *vertex* if FHR is heard *below* umbilicus.

expulsive efforts, they are as frequent as every 2 to 3 minutes.

2. **Regularity.** Contractions occur more and more regularly as labor becomes well established.
3. **Duration.** The length of time a contraction lasts increases from 30 seconds to between 60 and 90 seconds near full dilation of the cervix. Then the duration becomes about 60 seconds until delivery of the fetus is accomplished.
4. **Intensity.** The strength of the contraction also increases as labor progresses; from weak contractions noted early in labor to strong expulsive contractions (intrauterine pressure measured at 50 to 75 mm Hg) near the time of delivery.

Uterine contractions are measured in **Montevideo units (MUs)** in some parts of the United States. The intensity of the contractions is measured in total millimeters of mercury per 10 minutes, using an intrauterine pressure catheter. Until the thirtieth week of pregnancy, the intensity of contractions measures fewer than 20 MUs. Contraction intensity increases thereafter from 30 to 80 MUs as pregnancy approaches term. During early labor, contraction intensity averages 80 to 120 MUs. Near the end of labor (5 contractions per 10 minutes) the average of 250 MUs is reached. This method cannot be used, however, to determine the duration of a contraction (Pernoll and Benson, 1987).

Palpation of uterine contractions is a less precise method of determining the intensity of uterine contractions. Practice is required to discern between mild, moderate, and strong contractions. The definitions of these descriptive terms are as follows:

mild contractions: Slightly tense fundus that is easy to indent with fingertips
moderate contractions: Firm fundus that is difficult to indent with fingertips
strong contractions: Rigid, boardlike fundus that is almost impossible to indent

In most cases the woman is not aware of the sensation of the contracting of the uterus until each contraction is fairly well established. Commonly, her description of the end of a contraction is related to the end of pain sensation (felt in the lower part of the uterus, not in the fundus). This sensation may persist after the cessation of the actual contraction. Therefore the woman's description of each contraction may not be as accurate as that obtained by the nurse by abdominal assessment.

SUBSEQUENT ASSESSMENT OF PROGRESS DURING LABOR

Findings from initial assessments serve as a basis for comparison with expected symptomatology of labor (Table 18-2, guidelines for client teaching, p. 383). Assessment is continuous throughout labor. The routine for assessment of progress and of the continued well-being of the mother and fetus is usually set on a minimum level by hospital policy (Table 18-1). Any unusual findings would prompt an increase in the timing of assessment procedures.

The symptomatology of progress in labor is well defined (Table 18-2). The character of the woman's uterine contrac-

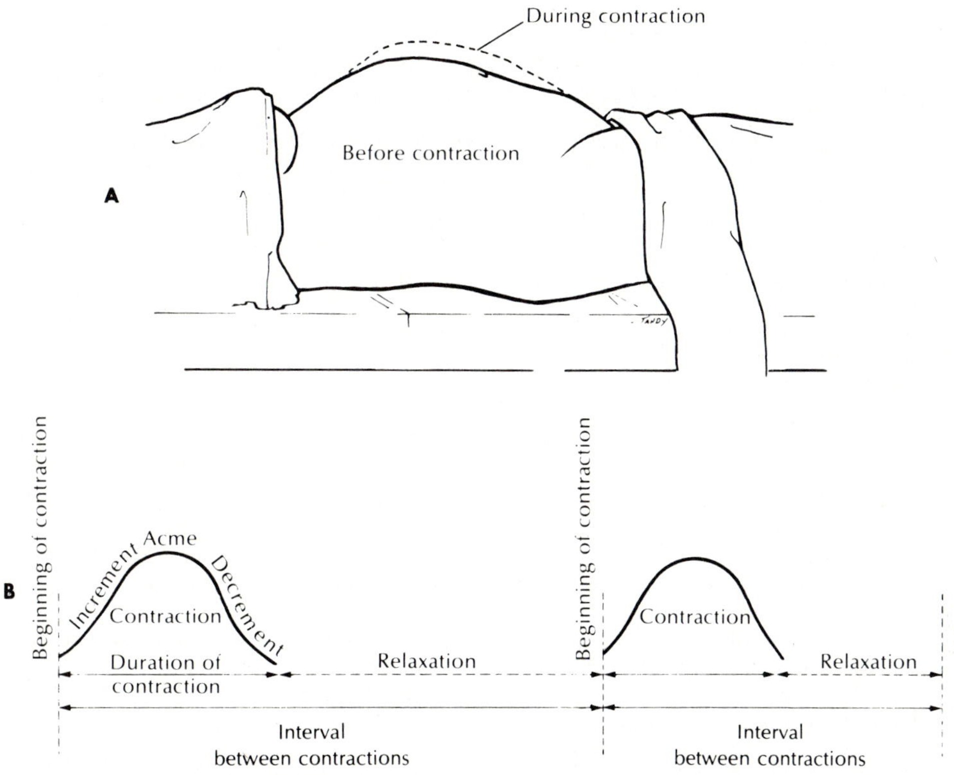

Fig. 18-6 Assessment of uterine contractions. **A**, Abdominal contour before and during uterine contraction. **B**, Wavelike pattern of contractile activity.

tions and her behavior and appearance correlate with the phase of labor she is experiencing.

The woman's response to labor may also be reflected in vital signs and BP. Fear, anxiety, and fatigue can cause alterations in the baseline findings. Continued fetal well-being is monitored through assessment of the FHR and of the character of the amniotic fluid discharge.

Careful assessment provides the cues for selection and implementation of nursing actions. *The nurse assumes much of the responsibility for making the assessment of progress. It is the nurse's responsibility to keep the physician informed about progress and any deviations from normal findings.*

Uterine Contractions, Cervical Dilation, and Descent

A general characteristic of effective labor is regular uterine activity. Uterine activity is not directly related to labor progress. Minimum activity may cause rapid progress in some women. For other women a large amount of uterine activity may produce slow progress or no progress.

Several methods are available for evaluation of uterine contractions. To assess uterine contractions, palpate using the sensitive fingertips, not the palmar surface of the hand. The fingers are kept moving over the uterus as the contraction proceeds from increment, to acme, through decrement to relaxation. The nurse assesses the *strength* of contractions as mild, moderate, or strong. *Duration* is assessed in seconds (e.g., 30 to 45 sec) from onset to relaxation. *Frequency* is usually assessed in minutes from the beginning of one contraction to the beginning of the next. Frequencies of contractions are assessed for *regularity* (e.g., every 5 to 10 minutes, every 2 minutes). Maternal response is related to the sensation of discomfort. Therefore maternal subjective description may not be as accurate as the nurse's objective assessment. For electronic monitoring of uterine activity, see Chapter 17. Placement of an intrauterine pressure catheter is described in Procedure 18-3.

When uterine activity is discussed it must be related to (1) its effect on progress in cervical effacement and dilation and descent of the presenting part and (2) its effect on the fetus (see fetal monitoring). Graphing labor progress with both cervical dilation and station (descent) of the presenting part validates the normal progress of labor. It also facilitates early identification of deviations from normal patterns. The normal pattern of cervical dilation and descent in a nulliparous labor is shown in Fig. 18-7, *A*. The pattern in a parous labor is shown in Fig. 18-7, *B*.

Each time an assessment is made, the findings are plotted on a partogram (a graphic chart) and a pattern emerges (Fig. 18-8). In addition to recording the findings on the partogram, nurses are responsible for notifying the physician should an abnormal pattern emerge. Therefore an understanding of the partogram is necessary. As a result of the clinical research of Friedman and Sachtleben (1965) a standardized graph was developed, thereby facilitating the early recognition of normal and abnormal labor patterns.

Cervical Effacement

Effacement precedes cervical dilation in the nullipara and it often accompanies dilation in the multipara. The pro-

Procedure 18-3

PLACEMENT OF AN INTRAUTERINE PRESSURE CATHETER (IUPC)

DEFINITION

The use of an internal pressure catheter and transducer to monitor labor contractions.

PURPOSE

To assess contractions more accurately.
To monitor dysfunctional labor patterns.
To titrate oxytocin more accurately.

EQUIPMENT

Sterile IUPC kit.
Sterile water for injection.
10 ml syringe.
19-gauge needle.
Strain gauge apparatus, transducer, and sterile dome.

NURSING ACTIONS	RATIONALE
Wash hands before and after touching woman or equipment.	To prevent nosocomial infection and implement universal precautions.
Explain procedure to woman/couple.	To decrease anxiety and gain cooperation.
Assist woman into dorsal lithotomy position with sterile drapes under buttocks.	To assist in passage of catheter and provide a clean environment.
Using aseptic technique, open sterile kit. Attach dome to transducer and fill with sterile water; keep air bubbles out of dome.	To avoid contamination of equipment. To prepare equipment for use. To ensure accurate measurement.
While physician is placing catheter, provide support to the woman.	To help facilitate catheter insertion.
Stand by and observe while physician calibrates machine.	To ensure correct interpretation of monitor strip.
Flush catheter every hour with sterile water while monitoring.	To remove vernix or air bubbles that may enter the catheter and cause a false reading.
Ask woman to cough or apply fundal pressure periodically while observing graph.	To check functioning of catheter.
Chart insertion and functioning of catheter.	To aid in collaboration of health care team.
Apply gentle traction to remove catheter before delivery.	To allow delivery of baby without obstruction.

cess of effacement plays a role in dilation. As the cervix is retracted upward, it becomes a part of the lower uterine segment. The "taking up" of the cervix reduces the length of the cervix from about 2 cm to a few millimeters when it is 100% effaced. This upward pull on fibers of the lower uterus and downward push on the fetus presses the presenting part onto the cervix. As uterine contraction and retraction continue, the cervical os dilates (opens) progressively. Effacement does not appear on the partogram.

Cervical Dilation

On the partogram the phases of cervical dilation are identified by the letters L, A, M, and D. A number, for example, "2," refers to the stage of labor. The **latent phase** (L) of the first stage of labor is that time between the onset of labor and onset of acceleration. The **active phase** begins with the **acceleration phase** (A) and spans the time between the onset of the upward curve of cervical dilation and full dilation of the cervix. Friedman (1978) divides the active phase into three parts: (1) *acceleration phase* (A), (2) *phase of maximum slope* (M), and (3) *deceleration phase* (D). The dotted line in Fig. 18-7 denotes cervical dilation. The rate of cervical dilation is indicated by the symbol "O" in Fig. 18-8. A line drawn through the symbols depicts the slope of the curve.

Descent

Located over the graph are the letters L, A, and M. The L refers to the latent phase of minimum descent. **Active descent** (A) generally begins when the cervical dilation curve reaches its phase of maximum slope. The rate of descent reaches its maximum at the beginning of the deceleration phase of cervical dilation. **Maximum descent** (M) continues in a linear manner until the perineum is reached (Zuspan and Quilligan, 1982). In Fig. 18-7 the solid line shows the rate of descent. In Fig. 18-8, station is indicated with an "X." A line drawn through the Xs reveals the pattern of descent.

Rupture of Membranes and Amniotic Fluid

SROM may occur at any time during labor. Rupture of membranes must be noted and confirmed, and amniotic fluid assessed when it does occur. Tests for assessing rupture of membranes are discussed in Procedure 18-4. See nursing care plan: hyperventilation and SROM, p. 409. The routine for assessment of amniotic fluid includes the following (see danger signs: rupture of membranes).

Color. Amniotic fluid is normally pale straw colored. If it is greenish brown, the fetus has probably undergone a hypoxic episode resulting in relaxation of the anal sphincter. Passage of meconium from the bowel is a sequel to

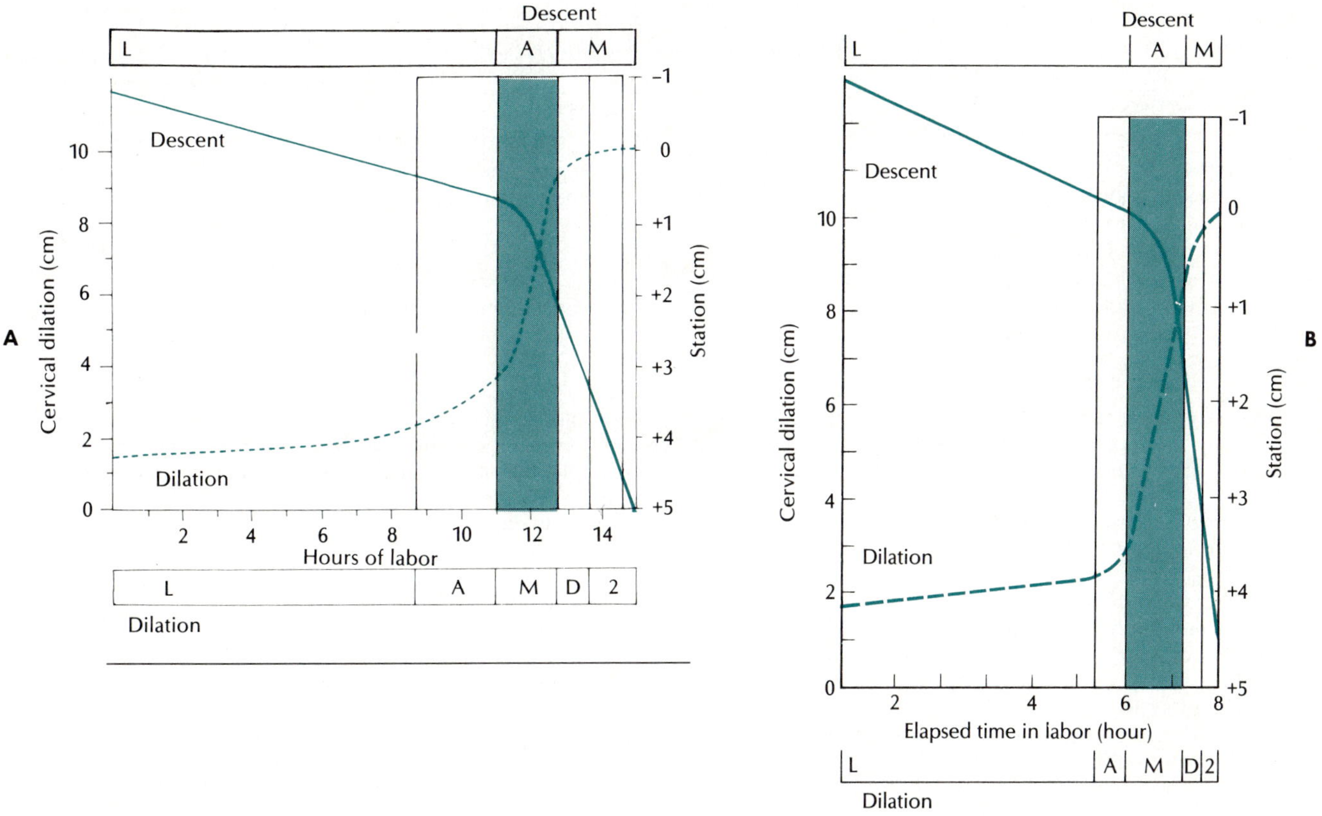

Fig. 18-7 Partogram showing relationship between dilation and descent of presenting part. **A**, Nulliparous labor. **B**, Multiparous labor.

B adapted from Friedman, EA, and Sachtleben, MR: Am J Obstet Gynecol 93:522, 1965.

Procedure 18-4

TESTS FOR RUPTURE OF MEMBRANES

DEFINITION

Affirmation of rupture of membranes or leakage of amniotic fluid by using definitive diagnostic measures.

PURPOSE

To determine if membranes have ruptured. To determine if fluid leakage is urine or amniotic fluid.

EQUIPMENT

Nitrazine paper.
Sterile glove, water, swab.
Microscope, clean glass slide.
Nile blue stain.

NURSING ACTIONS	RATIONALE
Nitrazine Test for pH	
Explain procedure to woman (couple).	To diminish anxiety and assist her (them) to maintain sense of control.
Procedure	
Use Nitrazine paper, a dye 1-1 impregnated test paper for pH.	To differentiate amniotic fluid, which is slightly alkaline, from urine and purulent material (pus), which are acidic.
Wearing a sterile glove lubricated with water, place a piece of test paper at the cervical os.	To maintain asepsis. To avoid affecting pH. To ensure testing for amniotic fluid.
OR	
Use a sterile, cotton-tipped applicator to dip deep into vagina to pick up fluid; touch applicator to test paper.	To maintain asepsis. To ensure testing for amniotic fluid.

Continued.

Procedure 18-4—cont'd

NURSING ACTIONS	RATIONALE
Read results:	To complete the test.
Membranes probably intact: Yellow pH 5.0; Olive yellow pH 5.5; Olive green pH 6.0	To identify vaginal and most body fluids that are acidic.
Membranes probably ruptured: Blue-green pH 6.5; Blue-gray pH 7.0; Deep blue pH 7.5	To identify amniotic fluid that is alkaline.
Realize that false tests are possible because of presence of bloody show or insufficient amniotic fluid.	To minimize misdiagnosis.
Remove gloves and wash hands.	To implement universal precautions while handling body fluids (Chapter 30).
Chart results: positive or negative.	To provide data base.
Test for Ferning or Fern Pattern (usually performed by physician)	
Explain procedure to client/couple	To reduce anxiety.
Wash hands, apply gloves, obtain specimen of fluid.	To minimize nosocomial infection.
Spread a drop of fluid from vagina on a clean glass slide with a sterile, cotton-tipped applicator.	To prepare specimen for assessment. To maintain asepsis.
Allow fluid to dry.	To prepare specimen.
Assess slide under microscope: observe for appearance of ferning (a frondlike crystalline pattern) (do not confuse with cervical mucus test, when high levels of estrogen are responsible for the ferning).	To support finding of ruptured membranes.
Observe for absence of ferning.	To alert staff to possibility that specimen was inadequate or that specimen was urine, vaginal discharge, or blood.
Remove gloves and wash hands.	To implement universal precautions when handling body fluids (Chapter 30).
Chart results: either a positive or negative fern test.	To provide a data base.
Test for Lanugo Hairs or Fetal Squamous Cells (usually performed by physician)	
Explain procedure to client/couple.	To reduce anxiety.
Wash hands and apply gloves.	To prevent nosocomial infection.
Aspirate fluid from posterior vaginal vault with sterile aspiration syringe.	To obtain specimen. To maintain asepsis.
Place on clean glass slide.	To prepare specimen for assessment.
Observe under microscope for presence of fetal lanugo hairs or fetal squamous cells.	To support finding of ruptured membranes.
Stain with Nile blue stain to identify fetal cells because some squamous cells that contain lipids stain yellow; other squamous cells and hairs stain blue.	To support finding of ruptured membranes.
Assess findings.	To provide data for analysis.
Remove gloves and wash hands.	To implement universal precautions when handling body fluids (Chapter 30).
Chart results: Nile blue stain shows some squamous cells and some blue squamous cells and hair.	To provide data base.

hypoxia.* Yellow-stained fluid may indicate (1) fetal hypoxia that occurred 36 hours or more before rupture of the membranes or (2) fetal hemolytic disease (Rh or ABO incompatibility, intrauterine infection).

Meconium-stained amniotic fluid may be a normal finding in breech presentation. Frank meconium may often be seen exuding into the birth canal. However, even in the case of a breech presentation the passage of meconium may indicate fetal distress and not just pressure on the fetal rectum. Although meconium-stained fluid may be noted with fetal asphyxia, *its presence is not always diagnostic of prospective fetal distress.* However, it should be promptly reported and recorded, and the FHR monitored closely. Port wine-colored amniotic fluid is one indicator of pre-

*May also be seen in response to maternal marijuana use (Chapter 39).

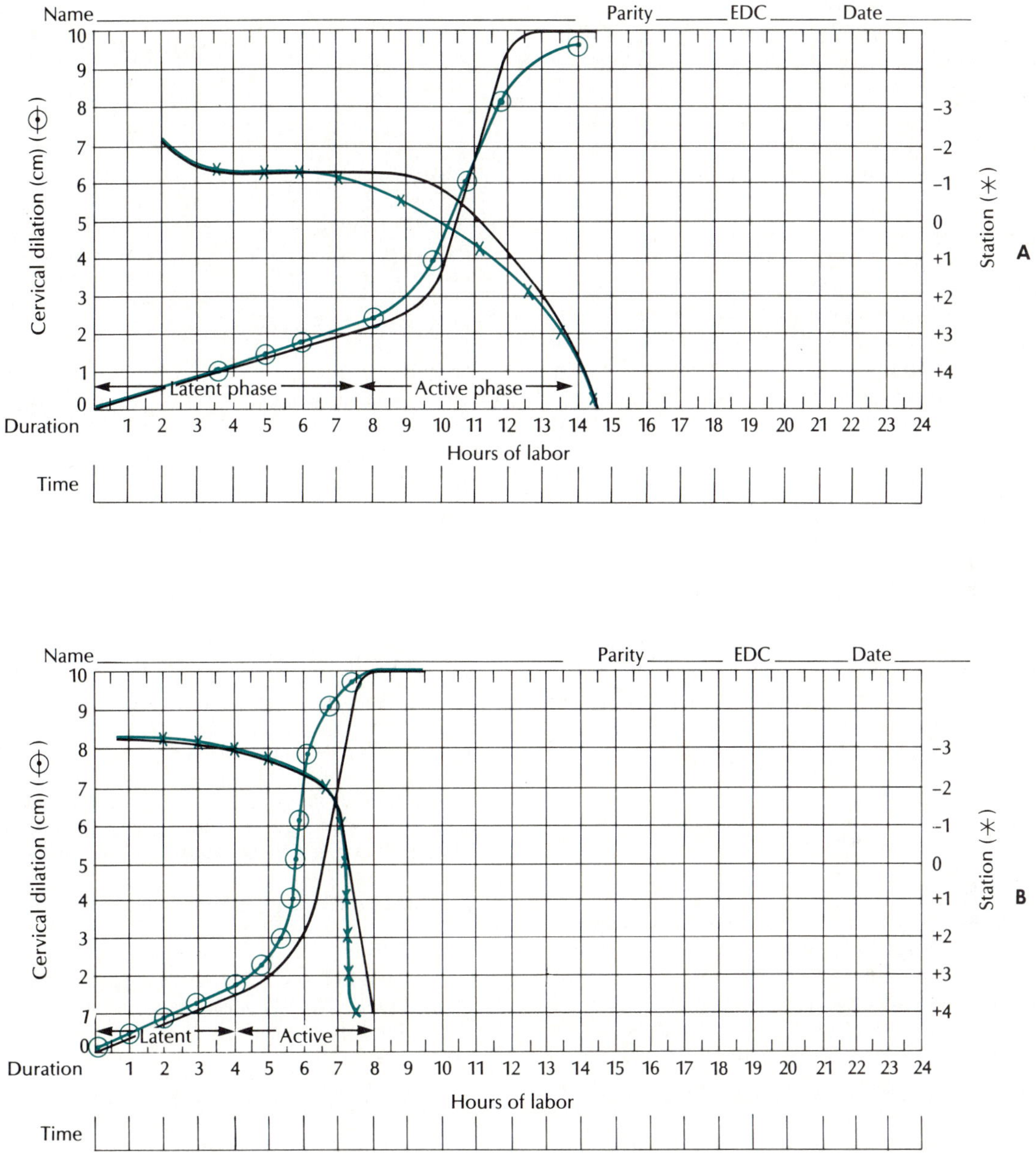

Fig. 18-8 Partogram for assessment of patterns of cervical dilation and descent. Individual woman's labor patterns *(colored)* superimposed on prepared labor graph *(black)* for comparison. **A**, Nulliparous labor. **B**, Multiparous labor.

mature separation of the placenta (abruptio placentae) (see Chapter 31).

Character. Amniotic fluid normally looks like water and has a characteristic odor. Thick consistency and unpleasant odor are associated with infection.

Amount. A normal range for the amount of amniotic fluid is 500 to 1200 ml. *Hydramnios,* an excessive amount of amniotic fluid (more than 2000 ml), is commonly associated with congenital anomalies in the neonate (see Chapter 40).

Oligohydramnios, an abnormally small amount or virtual absence of amniotic fluid (less than 500 ml) may be accompanied by such abnormalities as agenesis or malformation of the ears. In the presence of oligohydramnios, genitourinary tract anomalies, particularly renal agenesis may be seen (see Chapter 40).

Infection. Complications associated with ruptured membranes may include infection and prolapsed cord. Once the membranes have ruptured, the "clock of infection" begins to tick.* Prophylactic antibiotic therapy rarely will protect against chorioamnionitis. In most cases such

*Ascending infection may involve intact membranes and may be the direct cause of premature rupture of membranes (Chapter 39).

treatment results in the development of antibiotic-resistant strains of many pathogenic organisms. The maternal temperature and vaginal discharge are assessed frequently for early identification of developing infection. For a discussion of herpetic vaginal or perineal lesions and mode of delivery, see Chapter 30.

Prolapsed Cord. See discussion of emergencies, p. 400.

Stress in Labor

Fetal Stress. Since labor represents a period of stress for the fetus, continuous monitoring of fetal health is instituted as part of the nursing care during labor (Chapter 17). The procedure for determining the area of MI of the FHR is given in Procedure 18-2.

Maternal stress. Women and their families approach labor with a feeling of satisfaction that the preparatory phase of pregnancy is now at an end; within a relatively short time their child will be born. However, most women have two major concerns. First a woman may ask, "Will my child be all right?" Second, she may ask, "Will my labor be as expected? How will I act? Will I be okay?"

Further assessment of the woman's first question by asking her why she is so worried is probably not appropriate at this time. Her second question needs to be assessed further now. Her (or the couple's) goals for this labor may be noted in her prenatal record. For example, she (or they) may have indicated preferences for the following:

1. Medicated or unmedicated labor
2. Support person she wants with her—husband, mother, coach, other
3. Electronic monitor or not
4. Episiotomy or not

Some women and couples want an active role in decision making; others want to leave it all in the hands of the physicians and nurses. Each individual has her or his own self-expectations and expectations of others. Regardless of the actual labor and delivery experience, the woman's or couple's *perception of the birth experience* is most positive if she or they evaluate the events and performance as meeting expectations. It is also important for the nurse to meet their expectations and assure that there is a fit between the woman's or couple's perceptions and the nurse's perception of the nursing role (see research highlight).

Women from various cultures are taught from childhood the "right" way to behave during labor. They are taught that they should moan, scream, remain silent, or be totally anesthetized, depending on the culture. If a woman can follow through with the social expectations of her culture, she perceives herself as having mastery, as having had control over her labor. Her self-esteeem receives a boost.

The woman's level of anxiety may rise when she does not understand what is being said. Observe the facial expression and body language of the woman who has just been examined vaginally when the physician, within the parturient's hearing, tells the nurse, "She's a primigravida, EDD 2 weeks from now. She's 50% effaced but I can barely get a fingertip in there. She had bloody show but she'll have to drop the head some yet. If her membranes don't break by themselves, I'll pop them myself. The contractions are weak now; they'll have to get a lot harder to get the job done. Do a mini-prep on her." Understandably the woman who is unfamiliar with these terms could panic. Many of the terms—bloody show, drop the head, membranes break—sound violent and could conjure up thoughts of injury or pain. If the woman thought that her "weak" contractions were uncomfortable, she may become tense anticipating the more intense uterine contractions that are needed "to get the job done."

Paternal Stress. The father's behavior is also assessed. Is he hesitant to go into the labor room? Does he appear confident? Does he appear aggressive or hostile as he strides into the labor room? (He may be asserting his felt need to be with his wife or just covering up his anxieties.)

RESEARCH HIGHLIGHT

The Role of the Nurse in Labor and Delivery as Perceived by Nurses and Patients

Purpose

This study was performed to learn if there were differences in the perception of the role of the labor and delivery nurse as perceived by the nurses, expectant mothers who received Lamaze and Red Cross (L/RC) preparation for childbirth, and expectant mothers who received only Red Cross (RC) preparation.

Sample

A convenient sample of 10 L/RC expectant mothers, 11 RC expectant mothers, and 27 labor and delivery nurses participated in the study.

Methodology

A Q-sort methodology was used. A series of 50 statements was developed from a pilot Q-sort of 85 items. Two subdomains were identified: physical support and nurse control (PS-NC scale), and emotional support and mother control (ES-MC scale).

Findings

Major findings from the study showed that there were no statistically significant differences between the expectations of the nurse's role in labor and delivery as perceived by expectant mothers and labor and delivery room nurses. RC-expectant mothers did not perceive the role of the nurse to relate more to physical support and a controlling influence of the nurse. Finally, L/RC-expectant mothers did not perceive the role of the nurse to relate more to emotional support and a controlling influence by the mother.

Implications

Labor and delivery nurses are meeting the expectations of parturients. However, there are slight differences in perceptions so that individualization of care remains the priority.

Collins, BA: The role of the nurse in labor and delivery as perceived by nurses and patients, JOGN Nurs 15:412, Sept/Oct 1986.

Is he hungry? (He could faint from low blood sugar.) Is he sleepy, red eyed, or glassy eyed from fatigue? Does he look worried? Does he pull back and say that he is "just an onlooker" (observer)?

The nurse assesses the father's and mother's perception and preference as to the type and amount of participation he is to have. Is he prepared through classes? Which kind? How does the couple interpret information given them in classes (for example, does natural childbirth mean the woman is not to receive medication)? Does the father want to provide comfort measures? Which comfort measures does he need to learn? Is he considering accompanying her at the birth?

Has the father been on a hospital tour? Does he want a tour? Is he oriented to the unit? To this hospital? Does he have questions regarding the delivery room, the nursery, the postdelivery area, and subsequent care?

Nursing Diagnoses

Nursing diagnoses lend direction to types of nursing actions needed to implement a plan of care. Before establishing nursing diagnoses, the nurse analyzes the significance of findings collected during assessment.

Initial assessment
- *Prenatal record:* Impaired verbal communication related to foreign language barrier
- *Interview:* Knowledge deficit related to lack of previous experience or preparation-for-parenthood classes
- *Physical examination:* Anxiety related to knowledge deficit regarding physical examination procedures
- *Laboratory tests:* Potential for injury related to lack of prenatal testing of blood and urine

Subsequent assessments
- Pain related to bed rest
- Fluid volume deficit related to decreased fluid intake
- Impaired gas exchange related to hyperventilation
- Impaired physical mobility related to station of fetal presenting part, status of fetal membranes, or fetal monitoring
- Altered patterns of urinary elimination related to bed rest, lack of privacy, analgesia, or anesthesia

Assessment of stress during labor
- Impaired gas exchange, fetal, related to maternal position
- Spiritual distress, maternal, related to inability to meet expectations of self
- Ineffective family coping: compromised, related to knowledge deficit of comfort measures that can be used for parturient

Planning

During this important step, goals are set in client-centered terms, and the goals are prioritized. Nursing actions are selected, with the client where appropriate, to meet the goals. Planning with the client is essential for the implementation of goals.

Goals

1. Labor is confirmed
2. Normal progress of labor and well-being of the mother and fetus are supported
3. Deviations in progress in labor or alterations in maternal or fetal well-being are identified and managed appropriately
4. The mother's and family's wishes regarding the extent of their pariticipation in labor are respected and supported
5. The mother's and family's perception of the events of the first stage of labor meet their expectations

Implementation

Procedures

Standards of care guide the nurse in preparing for and implementing procedures with the expectant mother (Chapter 2). The experienced nurse is expected to be familiar with and carry out hospital protocols and policies. The nursing student (depending on skill level) can gain competency and beginning expertise by reviewing nursing techniques, practicing nursing skills in simulated laboratory settings, performing "hands-on care," reviewing hospital protocols and policies, and requesting anticipatory guidance as needed. Protocols for care include the following:

1. Check the physician's orders
2. Assess the physician's orders for appropriateness and correctness; for example, perineal shave, enema (when not to carry out these procedures)
3. Check labels on intravenous (IV) solutions, drugs or any other materials used for nursing care
4. Check expiration date on any packs of supplies used for ordered procedures
5. Ensure that information on the woman's identification band is correct (also check that identification band is accurate, for example, if she has allergies, the band is the appropriate color)
6. Employ an empathic approach when giving care:
   a. Use words the woman can understand when explaining procedures
   b. Establish a rapport with the woman and her support person(s)
   c. Be kind and caring when performing necessary procedures
   d. Be aware that pain and discomfort is as the woman describes
   e. Repeat instructions as necessary and ensure that they are understood by the woman
   f. Carry out appropriate comfort measures, for example, mouth care and back care, and ensure support person is coping
   g. Always wash hands on completion of nursing care
7. Complete procedures, for example, label specimens, record procedures on chart regarding maternal and fetal well being
8. Facilitate uterine perfusion by preventing supine hypotension (Fig. 18-9).

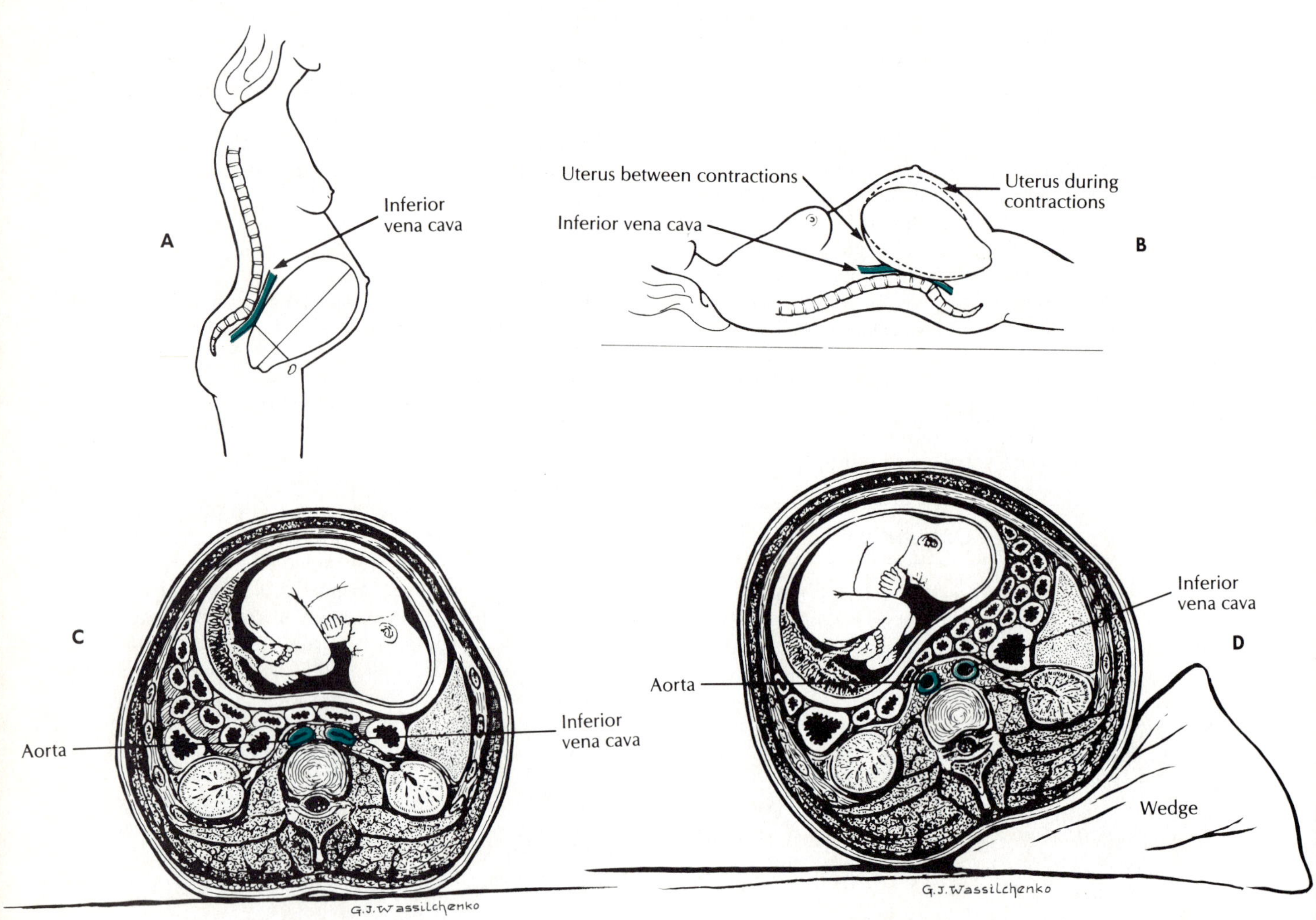

Fig. 18-9 Supine hypotension. Note relationship of gravid uterus to ascending vena cava in standing posture, **A**, and in supine posture, **B**. **C**, Compression of aorta and inferior vena cava with woman in supine position, **D**, Relieved by use of a wedge pillow placed under woman's right side.

These procedures can be used for instructing clients and their families. Procedure 18-5 (mini-prep) may be categorized under protective nursing interventions (Chapter 2).

Emergency Interventions

Prolapsed Umbilical Cord. Prolapse of the umbilical cord occurs when the cord lies below the presenting part of the fetus when the membranes are ruptured (prolapse of the cord means that a loop of cord is displaced below the presenting part with the membrane intact). Prolapsed cord occurs in about one in 400 deliveries (Fig. 18-10). Two factors contribute to this situation: a long cord and an unengaged presentation or malpresentation, for example, a breech presentation or shoulder presentation. When the presenting part does not fit into the lower uterine segment, as in polyhydramnios or when the membranes rupture, a sudden gush of amniotic fluid may cause the cord to be displaced downward. Similarly the cord may prolapse during artificial rupture of the membranes (AROM) if the presenting part is high. A small fetus also may not fit into the lower uterine segment and as a result, cord prolapse is more likely to occur. Other factors predisposing to cord prolapse and associated with a high presenting part are multiparity, cephalopelvic disproportion, and placenta previa. Prolapse of the cord is difficult to diagnose; however, an alert nurse or physician may make the diagnosis on vaginal examination after a sudden gush of fluid (see danger signs: rupture of membranes). Prompt recognition is important, since fetal hypoxia from prolonged cord compression (more than 5 minutes) usually results in central nervous system (CNS) damage or demise of the fetus (see danger signs: prolapsed cord).

Pressure on the cord is relieved by applying direct pressure on the presenting part by the examiner's fingers and by having the woman assume Trendelenburg's position until delivery is accomplished (see emergency procedure, p. 400, and Fig. 18-11). Cesarean birth is essential unless the cervix is fully dilated. If the cervix is completely dilated, rapid forceps delivery or vacuum extraction of the head or extraction of a breech presentation may be possible. Prompt delivery in the most appropriate manner is imperative for the safety of the mother and fetus.

Procedure 18-5

PREPARATION OF THE VULVA AND THE MINI-PREP

DEFINITION

The act of cutting and or shaving the pubic and perineal hairs before delivery of the baby.

PURPOSE

To cleanse the vulva.
To facilitate cutting and repairing of episiotomy.
To curtail infection.

EQUIPMENT

Soap.
Warm water.
Bedpan prn.
Underpads.
Razor (sterile, disposable) or scissors or Prep Kit.
Examination gloves.
Drape.

NURSING ACTIONS	RATIONALE
Check physician's orders.	To confirm physician's orders.
Explain procedure to woman.	To reduce anxiety.
Explain to woman that she may experience itching as the hair grows back.	To prepare woman.
Put on gloves.	To prevent nosocomial infection and to implement universal precautions while handling body fluids, (Chapter 30).
Cleanse vulvar area with soap solution or nonirritating detergent preparation: on admission, after elimination, after vaginal examination, and for vaginal discharge.	To maintain cleanliness. To curtail infection. To promote comfort.
If voided urine specimen is indicated, obtain after cleansing vulva.	To minimize potential for contamination with vaginal discharge.
Proceed with mini-prep after checking hospital protocol. A mini-prep varies with the institution and physician. It is the clipping of vulvar hair with scissors or shaving of a small area between the vagina and the anus, the site used for episiotomies.	
Use extreme care in shaving because even in expert hands the razor leaves nicks and scrapes that serve as portals of entry for infection.	To minimize danger of opening portals for infection and of inadvertently cutting off small warts or moles.
Accomplish prep quickly between contractions.	To promote comfort and minimize danger of nicking.
Following the prep, pat the area dry with a dry towel. Change to a dry underpad.	To promote comfort.

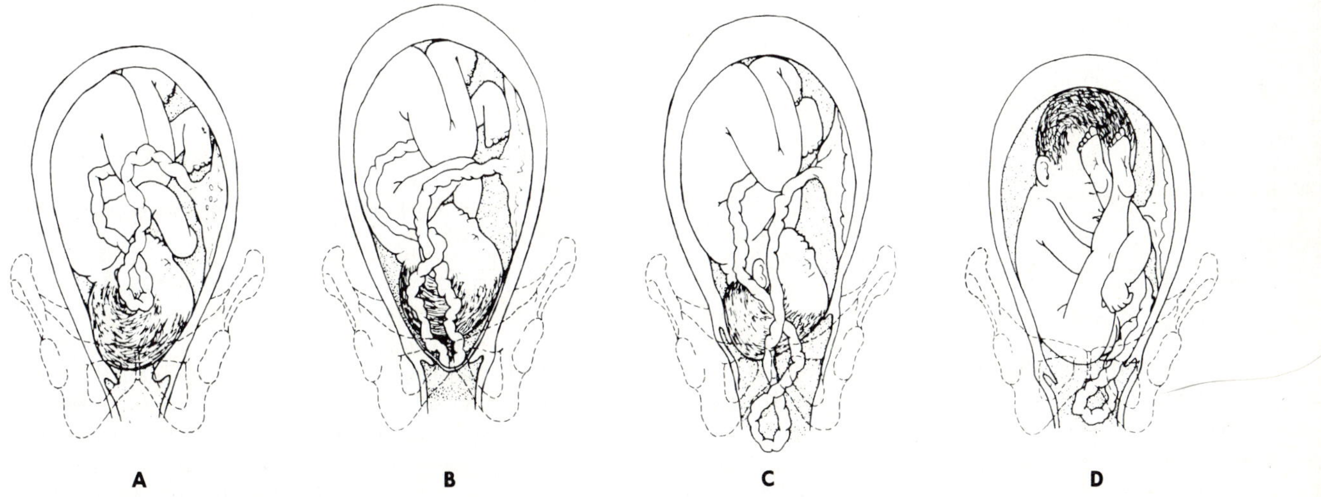

Fig. 18-10 Prolapse of umbilical cord. Note pressure of presenting part on umbilical cord, which endangers fetal circulation. **A**, Occult (hidden) prolapse of cord. **B**, Complete prolapse of cord. Note membranes are intact. **C**, Cord presenting in front of fetal head and may be seen within vagina. **D**, Frank breech presentation with prolapsed cord.

EMERGENCY PROCEDURE

PROLAPSE OF CORD

DEFINITION

Protrusion of the umbilical cord in advance of the presenting part.

PURPOSE

To stop compression of the umbilical cord.
To stop umbilical cord from drying out.
To facilitate a delivery that will be the least harmful to mother and fetus.

EQUIPMENT

Fetoscope or doppler; sterile gloves; towels; oxygen equipment; IV fluid and equipment; sterile, normal saline.

NURSING ACTIONS	RATIONALE
Preprocedure	
Explain what is happening to woman (couple). Explain procedure.	To reduce anxiety and elicit cooperation of woman (couple).
Procedure	
Glove the examining hand quickly and insert two fingers into the vagina to the cervix. With one finger on either side of the cord or both fingers to one side, exert upward pressure against the presenting part to relieve compression of the cord (Fig. 18-11). Apply a rolled towel under the woman's right hip.	To maintain asepsis. To reinsert cord without compressing it. To stop compression from the presenting part. To stop supine hypotensive syndrome.
Place woman into extreme Trendelenburg's or modified Sims' position.	To allow gravity to pull presenting part down and relieve compression of the cord.
Notify physician immediately.	Delivery must be done at once.
If cord is protruding from vagina, wrap loosely in a sterile towel wet with sterile normal saline.	To stop cord from drying out and becoming nonfunctioning.
Administer oxygen by mask 10 to 12 L/min to the woman until delivery is accomplished.	To increase oxygen to fetus. To increase placental perfusion.
Start IV fluids or increase existing drip rate.	To increase circulating fluid volume to fetus. To maintain maternal blood pressure and hydration.
Deliver fetus immediately. If cervix completely dilated, vaginal delivery is possible.	To allow for a favorable outcome and good prognosis for mother and baby.
If cervical dilation incomplete, cesarean delivery is the method of choice.	To decrease trauma to mother and baby.
Postprocedure	
Vaginal delivery: assess mother and baby for trauma or untoward effects. Pediatrician should examine infant in nursery. Assess mother for emotional stress and trauma.	Stressful situation may have physical or emotional sequela following. Be alert for any problems. Any high-risk delivery should have a pediatrician or neonatologist in attendance to care for the infant.
Cesarean delivery: same as above, add postoperative assessment and observation of postanesthesia problems.	
Chart incident and results of treatment.	To provide data base for future comparison. To provide information for implementation of nursing process. To promote collaboration between members of health care team.

Fetal Distress or Abnormal FHR Patterns. Fetal distress may occur in the absence of prolapsed cord. The physician must be informed immediately. The nurse reports the nursing measures implemented, and the fetal response to the interventions instituted. For further discussion, see Chapter 17.

Inadequate Uterine Relaxation. Uterine contractions can be stressful to both the mother and the fetus. To prevent possible damage to the fetus and unnecessary stress to the mother, the nurse assesses the strength, duration, and frequency of contractions to identify abnormal contraction patterns. If the nurse identifies inadequate relaxation of the uterus, for example, contractions lasting longer than 90 seconds, relaxation between contractions inadequate or less than 30 seconds, the nursing actions in the emergency procedure on p. 402 must be implemented without delay.

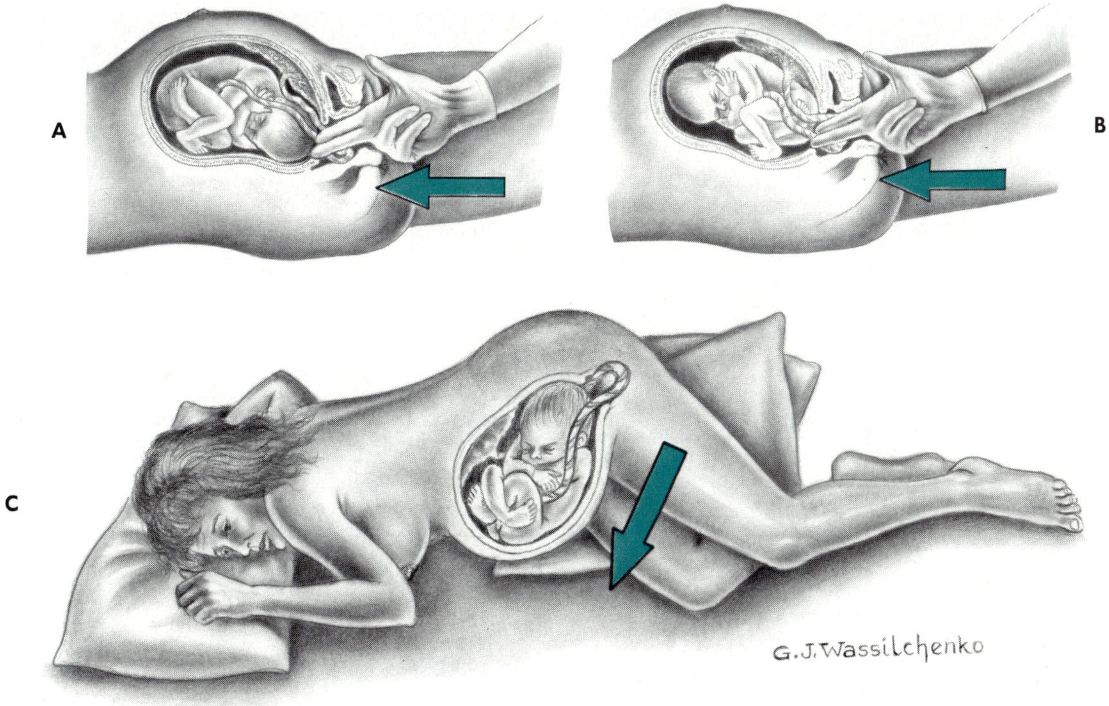

Fig. 18-11 Arrows indicate direction of pressure against presenting part to relieve compression of prolapsed umbilical cord. Pressure exerted by examiner's fingers in **A**, vertex presentation, and **B**, in breech position. **C**, Gravity relieves pressure with woman in modified Sims' position with hips elevated as high as possible with pillows.

DANGER SIGNS

RUPTURE OF MEMBRANES

1. Premature rupture of membranes
2. Bloody, foul-smelling, or meconium stained fluid
3. Change in fetal heart rate pattern
4. Signs of fetal distress
5. Premature labor contractions

DANGER SIGNS

PROLAPSED CORD

1. Premature rupture of membranes
2. Presenting part not engaged
3. Fetal distress or abnormal fetal heart rate pattern
4. Protruding cord from vagina

Motherhood with Dignity

Admission to the Labor Unit. First impressions are vivid. The woman and her partner or family need to feel welcome. The nurse addresses them by name and introduces herself. The nurse then determines whether the woman wishes her partner or family member to stay throughout assessment and other admission procedures. If not, the partner may be directed to the waiting area. The woman is asked to undress and get into bed. Her personal belongings are put away safely. For legal reasons, most hospitals have a checklist or other method of recording the woman's belongings that becomes part of her permanent record. If the woman prefers to wear some items of her own (such as knee socks), these are noted on her chart.

The woman's understanding of the use of the call bell (or light) is checked. She is told the reasons that bathroom privileges are permitted or not. If the membranes have ruptured, have her remain in bed until assessment for potential prolapse of the umbilical cord is completed. The routine of care is reviewed, that is, which techniques will be used to assess progress, the reasons for using them, and how the woman or couple may assist in reporting her progress. For the minimum schedule for assessment of

EMERGENCY PROCEDURE

INADEQUATE UTERINE RELAXATION

DEFINITION

Inadequate resting tone between uterine contractions. May cause fetal distress caused by poor delivery of oxygen to the placenta and fetus.

PURPOSE

To increase uterine muscle relaxation. To increase placental perfusion.

EQUIPMENT

Oxygen mask or cannula; mechanical oxygen source; IV fluid without oxytocin added.

NURSING ACTIONS	RATIONALE
Preparation	
Assess problem by monitoring labor and its effects on the fetus.	Uterine contractions are monitored continuously during labor. FHR observed for unusual patterns.
Explain procedure to client.	Elicits cooperation through understanding.
Procedure	
Change maternal position. Turn woman to her left side, if that is ineffectual, put woman in modified Sim's position.	Increases placental perfusion and increases oxygen delivered to the fetus.
Stop oxytocin infusion (if there is one running) and replace it with a plain IV.	Stops stimulation of the uterine muscle. Allows muscle to relax.
Notify physician.	Allows collaboration in decision-making and informs him/her of possible problems.
Administer oxygen by face mask or nasal cannula at 10 to 12 L per min until physician arrives and decides course of action.	Increases amounts of oxygen available to the muscle and the fetus.
Record problems observed and actions taken by medical/nursing personnel.	Provides information for future care and collaboration.

progress during the first stage of labor, see Table 18-2.

If the woman has not already done so, she signs the necessary papers giving permission for care for herself and her newborn. Her identification bracelet is secured. Legally a permit for care must be signed before the woman receives any medication for discomfort or any procedures are done to her.

If parking is a problem at the facility, the nurse inquires if the woman came by car and where the car is parked. The nurse may need to advise a family member to repark the car, or, as in a recent case where the woman drove in herself and therefore could not repark the car, the nurse must inform the hospital's security forces. Some women, especially those who arrive in labor unexpectedly (for example, directly from the physician's office), welcome the offer of a telephone to notify their families. In some instances the nurse may have to make the calls to the family.

Do not increase the woman's anxiety by quizzing her about her understanding of terms commonly used during labor. As the nurse reviews the woman's prenatal record, the nurse can add short definitions or explanations for technical terms and abbreviations. The woman's interest and response guide the nurse in choosing the depth and breadth of the explanations. The nurse's openness and willingness to explain can be reassurance in itself—it indicates to the woman and her family that there need be no "secrets." A general nursing care plan for admission of a woman in labor follows.

Fluid Intake, Voiding, Bowel Elimination, and General Hygiene. Intake, elimination, and general hygiene are basic human needs. The parturient also has these same needs. However, nursing care of the parturient is modified somewhat. A summary of nursing actions and rationales is presented in Table 18-3.

Maternal Position During Labor. A great deal of discussion both within the nursing profession and among consumers of maternity care now rages around the way a woman should behave in labor. Should she be kept in bed, or should she be allowed to walk about, stand, sit, squat, or kneel (Fig. 18-12, *A*)? There is no "right" position. Should she deliver in the dorsal or semirecumbent position where most medical techniques and procedures can be best applied, or should she be allowed to adopt the position that she finds most comfortable without regard for the convenience of conventional obstetrical practices (Romney and White, 1984)? Research has shown that women in the upright position (Fig. 18-12, *B*) during labor and birth have stronger and more effective uterine contractions. This results in shorter labor duration and increased comfort. Variation in the positions that women assume during the birth process has not been dictated as much by physiology as by culturally oriented patterned behavior.

General Nursing Care Plan

FIRST STAGE OF LABOR

ASSESSMENT	NURSING DIAGNOSES (ND)/ PLAN (P)/GOAL (G)	RATIONALE/ IMPLEMENTATION	EVALUATION
Term pregnancy. Admission to labor unit in labor. Latent phase of labor. Assess level of knowledge.	ND: Anxiety, mild, related to excitement of onset of labor and fear of unknown. ND: Knowledge deficit related to latent phase of first stage of labor. P: Reduce anxiety by providing adequate and relevant teaching and relaxation techniques. G: Woman (and her family) verbally and nonverbally communicates less anxiety, more comfort, and ability to collaborate with her care.	*To provide reassurance and help woman relax, the nurse will:* Support woman's knowledge of labor. Explain all procedures. Answer all questions and provide information as needed. Orient women and support person to environment. Support woman's preference for breathing and relaxation techniques to be used at this time. Provide comfort measures. Monitor vital signs, FHR, and progress of labor. Provide privacy.	Woman remains calm and retains psychologic and physiologic control.
Diminished oral intake. Monitor intake and output; vital signs, FHR, blood pressure, and respirations, and amount of diaphoresis.	ND: Fluid volume deficit related to decreased intake and increased loss of fluid with the work of labor. P: Provide and maintain adequate fluid intake. G: Woman remains appropriately hydrated.	*To maintain adequate hydration the nurse will:* Explain to woman and support person why oral fluids are restricted or stopped at this time. Start and maintain an IV infusion. Provide ice chips or sips of clear fluids if allowed. Provide mouth care as needed.	Woman's temperature, skin turgor, and moisture of mucous membranes remain normal. Specific gravity of urine remains within normal limits. Woman verbalizes understanding of procedures and information given. Woman does not suffer the fatigue associated with dehydration.
Rupture of membranes: baseline data of maternal vital signs and FHR; fetal lie, station, presentation, and position; status of membranes (bulging?); character of vaginal discharge.	ND: Potential for injury, maternal and fetal, related to contamination, infection, prolapsed cord, abnormal fetal position. P: Decrease or prevent potential complications related to rupture of membranes. G: Woman and fetus are not compromised as a result of rupture of membranes.	*To prevent potential problems the nurse will:* Maintain asepsis during vaginal examinations. Change dirty linen or underpads frequently. Continue to monitor: maternal vital signs (especially temperature and pulse); FHR for tachycardia; vaginal secretions; fetal lie and position, using Leopold's maneuvers. Observe for physical signs of umbilical cord prolapse, and implement emergency procedure, prn (p 400): Reposition client to left lateral position or other positions as necessary.	Woman verbalizes understanding of procedures and information. Woman reports subjective symptoms as necessary. Woman and infant are not compromised as a result of rupture of membranes. FHR indicates continued fetal well-being. Fetal scalp pH indicates continued fetal well-being. Cesarean delivery is accomplished in a timely fashion; mother and infant are in good condition.

Continued.

General Nursing Care Plan—cont'd

ASSESSMENT	NURSING DIAGNOSES (ND)/ PLAN (P)/GOAL (G)	RATIONALE/ IMPLEMENTATION	EVALUATION
		Provide oxygen by nasal cannula or face mask as necessary. Increase rate of infusion of maintence intravenous fluid. Assist with fetal scalp blood sampling as necessary. Assist with preparation for surgery as necessary.	
First stage of labor. Woman in active phase. Baseline data: maternal vital signs; FHR; labor pattern. Degree of perceived discomfort.	ND: Pain, related to increasing frequency and intensity of uterine contractions. P: Decrease maternal discomfort without compromising mother or fetus. G: Mother perceives decreased discomfort; FHR remains within normal limits.	*To provide pain relief the nurse will:* Assess woman's verbal and nonverbal communication. Promote the use of psychoprophylactic breathing techniques. Provide comfort measures. Assess vital signs, including blood pressure, FHR, frequency, and intensity of uterine contractions.	Woman verbalizes understanding of information presented. Woman participates in her care as much as possible and within her personal preferences. Baseline data remains within normal limits.
Bladder fullness.	ND: Altered patterns of urinary elimination related to discomfort, effects of analgesia, or fetal position. P: Monitor degree of bladder fullness and ensure bladder emptying. G: Bladder will be emptied periodically.	Administer analgesics as ordered. Offer bedpan frequently to avoid bladder distension; catheterize prn. Assess vaginal discharge. Assess for side effects from analgesics or anesthetics. Administer oxygen as needed. Monitor IV or po fluids.	Bladder fullness is prevented.
Woman in stressful and threatening situation.	ND: Ineffective individual coping related to anxiety, fear, and decreased problem-solving capability. P: Support woman's (family's) coping and self-esteem. G: Woman's self-esteem is maintained or increased as her perception of her behavior during labor matches her self-expectations.	*To help woman cope with increasing pain and anxiety of active labor the nurse will:* Assess anxiety level. Assess behavior of support person and its effect on the woman. Provide information. Provide comfort measures. Assist woman and support person in focusing on breathing and relaxation techniques to maintain control. Give quiet reassurance. Support woman's decisions for pain medications.	Woman remains calm and in control. Support person providing necessary help and reassurance to woman. Woman and support person express satisfaction with their behavior during labor and with the management of their labor.

Table 18-3 *Fluid Intake, Voiding, Bowel Elimination, and General Hygiene: Nursing Actions and Rationales*

Need	Nursing Actions	Rationale
Fluid Intake		
Oral	Per physician's orders: Offer clear fluids, which are fluids you can see through; tea with honey and lemon, homemade broth (not salt-loaded bouillon), apple juice, and lollipops are examples of clear fluids.	Meets standard of care; provides hydration; provides calories; warm teas are used by many cultural groups to counteract the effects of heat loss during labor and delivery; absorb quickly and are less likely to be vomited; provides positive emotional experience.
	Offer small amounts of ice chips, if ordered.	Deters vomiting and its potential sequelae, aspiration and tracheal irritation.
IV	Establish and maintain IV	Maintain hydration.
Nothing by mouth (NPO)	Inform family of NPO and rationale.	A precautionary measure if anesthesia is a possibility; deters vomiting and its possible sequelae.
	Provide mouth care.	Promotes comfort.
Voiding	Encourage voiding at least every 2 hours.	A full bladder may impede descent of presenting part; overdistension may cause bladder atony and injury and difficulty in voiding postnatally.
Ambulatory	Ambulate to bathroom per physician's orders, *if*:	Reinforces normal process of labor.
	The presenting part is engaged, or The membranes are not ruptured, and	Precautionary measure against prolapse of umbilical cord.
	The woman is not medicated.	Precautionary measure against injury.
Bedrest	Offer bedpan.	Prevents hazards of bladder distension and ambulation.
	Turn on the tap water to run; pour warm water over the vulva; and give positive suggestion.	Encourages voiding.
	Provide privacy.	Shows respect for gravida.
	Put up side rails on bed. Place call bell within reach.	Prevents injury from fall.
	Offer washcloth for hands.	Maintains cleanliness and comfort.
	Wash vulvar area.	Maintains standard of care.
Catheterization	Catheterize per physician's order per hospital protocols.	Prevents hazards of bladder distension.
	Insert catheter between contractions.	Minimizes discomfort.
	Avoid force if obstacle to insertion is noted.	"Obstacle" may be caused by compression of urethra by presenting part.
	If presenting part is low, introduce 2 fingers of free hand into introitus to apply upward pressure on presenting part while other hand inserts the catheter.	Minimizes potential for injury and subsequent infection to urethra.
Bowel Elimination	After careful assessment *experienced* nurse ambulates woman to bathroom or offers bedpan.	Women often misinterpret rectal pressure from the presenting part as the need to defecate.
General Hygiene		Improves woman's morale and comfort. Maintains cleanliness.
Showers/bed baths	Assess for progress in labor.	Determines appropriateness for the activity.
	Supervise showers closely if gravida is in true labor.	Prevents injury from fall; labor may accelerate.
	Suggest allowing warm water to strike lower back.	Aids relaxation; increases comfort.
Vulva	See Procedure 18-5	
Oral hygiene	Offer toothbrush, mouthwash, or wash the teeth with an ice-cold wet washcloth every hour.	Refreshes mouth; improves morale; helps counteract dry, thirsty feeling.
Hair	Comb, braid per gravida's wishes	Improves morale; helps maintain a "nonsick" attitude.
Hand-washing	Offer washcloths before and after voiding and prn.	Maintains cleanliness; improves morale and comfort.
Gowns/linens	Change prn; fluff pillows.	

A 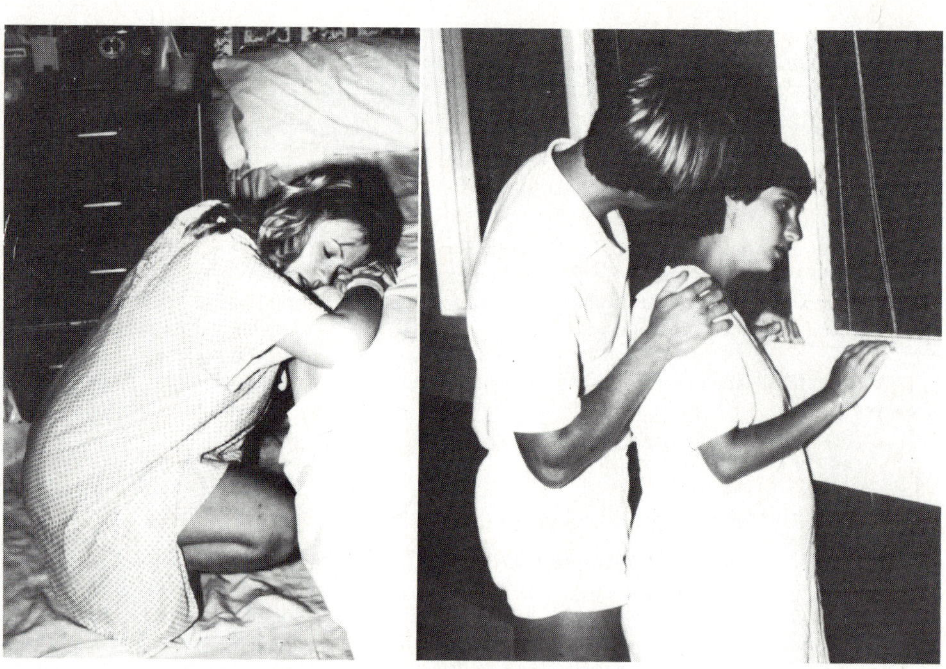 B

Fig. 18-12 Maternal positions for labor. A, Squatting. B, Walking with husband.

Much research is being directed toward a better understanding of the physiologic and psychic effects of maternal position in labor. It is important to appreciate that clinical entities such as fetal presentations or mechanisms of labor may be helped or hindered by maternal posture.

Support Measures. Important components of the nursing care of the woman in labor relate to (1) helping the parturient participate to the extent she wishes in the delivery of her infant, (2) meeting the woman's goals for herself, (3) helping the parturient conserve her energy, and (4) helping control the woman's discomfort.

The nurse acts as an advocate for the woman and her family. Couples who have attended childbirth education programs using the psychoprophylactic approach will know something about the labor process, coaching techniques, and comfort measures (see Chapter 14). However, the staff's role is to be supportive and keep them informed of progress. Even if the couple has not attended such classes, the various techniques may be taught to a degree during the early phase of labor. The nurse will be expected to do more of the coaching and give supportive care. If the woman is alone, the nursing staff acts as the substitute family. Staff members coach and support her. They help the woman use her energy constructively in relaxing and working with the contractions.

Comfort measures vary with the situation (Fig. 18-13). The nurse can draw on the couple's repertoire of comfort measures learned during the pregnancy. The comfort measures to be discussed below include maintaining a comfortable, supportive atmosphere in the labor and delivery area; using touch therapeutically; providing nonpharmacologic management of discomfort; and administering analgesics when necessary; but, most of all, just *being there.*

Atmosphere of the Labor and Delivery Area. Labor rooms need to be light and airy. However, the bright overhead lights are turned off when not needed. The area should be large enough to accommodate the woman's partner in a comfortable chair, as well as the monitoring equipment and hospital personnel. In some hospitals, couples are urged to bring extra pillows to help make the hospital surrounding more homelike. Labor areas *should be constructed with windows* that can be hung with colorful curtains. When people stay in any area for a period of time and do not have access to a view of the outside world, it is

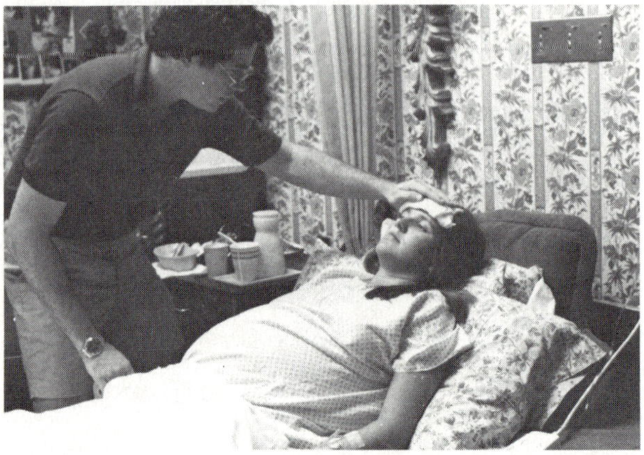

Fig. 18-13 Father providing comfort with a cool cloth to forehead.

easy to become disoriented in time and to focus unnaturally on whatever is happening to them.

The room temperature is kept at a comfortable level—between 20° and 22.2° C (68° and 72° F). Although most women feel warm during labor, a number complain of feeling cold. A warm blanket placed over the woman and one wrapped around her feet are comforting. Many women wish to wear socks. For those who feel too warm, a cool moist cloth placed on the forehead can be soothing, as can ice chips given for sucking (where permissible) (Fig. 18-13).

Touch. Most women respond positively to touch in labor. They appreciate gentle handling by the staff. **Effleurage** (a light rhythmic stroking over the woman's abdomen in rhythm with breathing during contractions) (Fig. 14-1) may be effective in helping them relax between contractions. Counterpressure against the sacrum during a contraction results in relief from discomfort (Fig. 18-14). Back rubs, including over the sacral area and the buttocks (especially for women who have been in labor a long time), every hour or two and as necessary between contractions help ease tension. If possible, warm foot baths followed by foot massage can result in general body relaxation.

The woman's awareness of the soothing qualities of touch changes as labor progresses. Many women develop hyperesthesia (increased sensitivity, especially in the skin) as labor progresses. They may tell their coach to "leave me alone," or they may say, "Don't touch me." The partner who is unprepared for this normal response may feel rejected and may react by withdrawing active support. The nurse can point out that this response on the part of the woman is a positive indication that the first stage is ending and that the transition stage is approaching. The woman's aggressive behavior is accepted; negative comments toward the woman are unwarranted and inappropriate.

Sound is the touching of sound waves against the tympanic membrane of the ear. The nurse can use soft tones

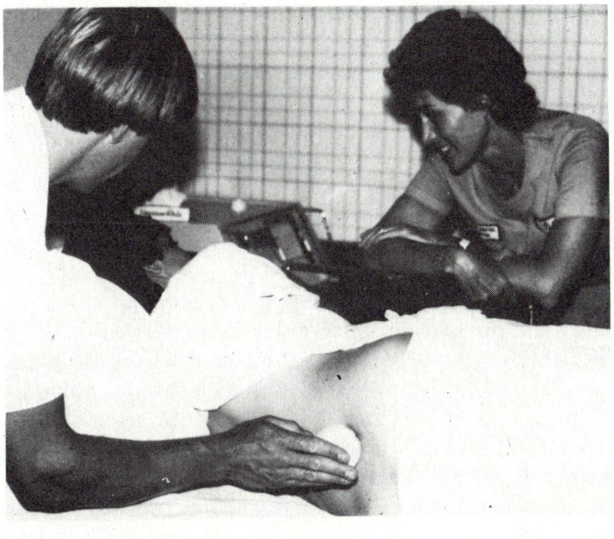

Fig. 18-14 Father applies sacral pressure with a tennis ball while nurse provides verbal encouragement.

in speaking to the woman. Even firm commands to breathe a certain way or to pant-breathe to avoid pushing at the wrong time can be done without resorting to harsh, vibrant speech.

The manner in which a woman is touched during her labor is often reflected in the manner in which she touches others. This may influence her response toward her infant after birth. She must be mothered in order to mother.

Nonpharmacologic Management of Discomfort. The alleviation of pain is important. Commonly it is not the amount of pain the woman experiences, but *whether she meets her goals for herself in coping with the pain* that influences her perception of the birth experience as "good" or "bad." The observant nurse looks for cues to identify the woman's desired level of control in the management of pain and its relief.

The origins of discomfort during labor, the symptomatology of pain, pain threshold, and the gate-control theory of pain and pharmacologic control of discomfort are discussed in Chapter 17. The pain associated with parturition was accepted as a necessary part of childbirth until the discovery of the first anesthetics, nitrous oxide and ethyl ether. Since that time much research has gone into the development of methods of pain control that can bring effective relief for the mother without harm to the child. The perfect solution is yet to be found; therefore at times the safety of the child must take precedence over the comfort of the mother.

Nonmedicated methods of relief of discomfort are taught in many different types of prenatal preparation classes. In Chapter 11, three methods are described: Dick-Read, Lamaze, and Bradley. Whether or not a woman or couple has attended these classes or read from the various books and magazines on the subject, the nurse can teach techniques to relieve discomfort during labor. Following are some nonmedicated methods of managing discomfort during labor.

Focusing and Feedback Relaxation. Some women bring a favorite device for use in focusing attention. Others choose some fixed object in the labor room. As the contraction begins, they may focus on this object to reduce their perception of pain. This technique, coupled with feedback relaxation, helps the woman work with her contractions rather than against them. The coach monitors this process, giving the woman cues as to when to begin the breathing techniques. After the degree of relaxation has been assessed, the woman can be reminded to use relaxation techniques practiced in the prenatal period. The coach also keeps her from being disturbed by routine examination for progress of checking of FHR. These procedures are postponed until the contraction is completed.

Breathing Techniques. Different approaches to childbirth preparation stress varying techniques for using breathing as a "tool" to help the woman maintain control through contractions. In the first stage, breathing techniques can promote relaxation of abdominal muscles and thereby increase the size of the abdominal cavity. This lessens friction and discomfort between the uterus and the abdominal wall. Since the muscles of the genital area also become more relaxed, they do not interfere with descent. In the second stage, breathing is used to increase abdominal pressure and thereby assist in expelling the fetus. It is also used to relax the pudendal muscles to prevent precipitate expulsion of the head.

For those couples who have prepared for labor by practicing such techniques, occasional reminders to the couple may be all that is necessary. For those who have had no preparation, instruction in simple breathing and relaxation can be given early in labor and is often surprisingly successful. Motivation is high, and learning readiness is enhanced by the reality of labor.

1. *Cervical dilation to 3 cm.* As the woman feels the onset of a contraction, she takes a deep, cleansing breath in through the nose and out through pursed lips. Then she is encouraged to concentrate on slow, rhythmic chest breathing (6 to 9 breaths per minute) through the contraction (Fig. 18-15). When the contraction is over, she takes a final deep breath in and then "blows the contraction away" through pursed lips. She may focus on a chosen fixed point or simply close her eyes.

2. *Cervical dilation of 4 to 7 cm.* Breathing during this phase is similar to that advocated in the early phase. When cervical dilation reaches 5 cm, some women begin to concentrate seriously on the strength of the contractions and the discomfort accompanying them. At this time a change to a shallower, lighter breathing can be suggested (no more than 16 breaths per minute to prevent hyperventilation). Other women can be helped by changing to slow abdominal breathing. Another technique that is often successful is to have the woman slowly raise her abdomen as she breathes in, following the support person's hand "up to the ceiling" or "out to the side of the bed" (if she is in side-lying position). This focusing mechanism results in the lifting of the abdominal wall away from the contracting uterus.

3. *Cervical dilation of 8 to 10 cm: transition.* The most difficult time to maintain control during contractions comes when the cervical dilation reaches 8 to 10 cm. This period is also called the **transition period**. Even for the woman who has prepared for labor, concentration on breathing techniques is difficult to maintain. The type used may be the 4:1 pattern: breath, breath, breath, breath, puff (as though blowing out a candle). This ratio may increase to 6:1 or 8:1. These patterns begin with the routine cleansing breath and end with a deep breath exhaled to "blow the contraction away". An undesirable side effect of this type of breathing may be **hyperventilation**. The woman must be aware of the accompanying symptoms of the resultant **respiratory alkalosis**: lightheadedness, dizziness, tingling of fingers, or circumoral numbness. Alkalosis may be overcome by having the woman breathe into a paper bag that is tightly held around the mouth and nose. This enables her to rebreathe carbon dioxide and replace the bicarbonate ion. She can breathe into her cupped hands if no bag is available.

As the fetal head reaches the pelvic floor, the woman will experience the urge to push and will automatically begin to exert downward pressure by contracting her abdominal muscles. Descent cannot continue until the cervix is

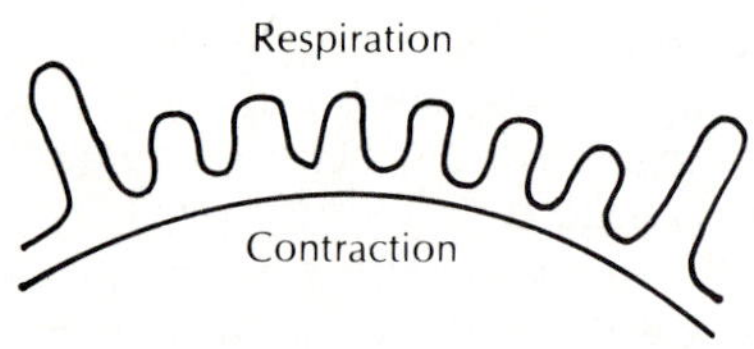

Fig. 18-15 Slow chest breathing.
From Phillips, CR: Family-centered maternity/newborn care, ed 2, St Louis, 1987, The CV Mosby Co.

fully dilated and the presenting part is free to move down the birth canal. *Pushing before full dilation* is reached compresses the cervix between the fetal head and the pubic bone. This compression *may result in fetal distress or in cervical edema.* It may even slow the dilation process. The woman can control the urge to push by taking panting breaths or by slowly exhaling through pursed lips. This is good practice for the type of breathing to be used as the fetal head is slowly delivered. See nursing care plan: hyperventilation and SROM, p. 409.

Transcutaneous Electrical Nerve Stimulation. The application of pressure to or rubbing of a part of the body that is sore is an age-old remedy to relieve discomfort. Effleurage and sacral pressure or massage are two methods that have brought relief to many women during the first stage of labor. The gate-control theory may supply the reason for the effectiveness of these measures (Chapter 17). Transcutaneous electrical nerve stimulation (TENS) may operate on the same principle. TENS may also be effective because of the "placebo effect"; that is, confidence in TENS may stimulate the release of endogenous opiates (enkephalins) in the woman's body and thus alleviate the discomfort.

Two pairs of electrodes are taped on either side of the thoracic and sacral spine. Continuous mild electrical currents are applied from a battery-operated device. During a contraction the woman increases the stimulation by turning control knobs on the device. Women describe the sensation as a tingling or buzzing and pain relief as good or very good. The use of TENS poses no risk to the mother or fetus. TENS is credited with reducing or eliminating the need for analgesia and with increasing the woman's perception of control over the experience.

The nurse assists the mother who is using TENS by explaining the device and its use, by carefully placing and securing the electrodes, and by closely evaluating its effectiveness.

Sociocultural Aspects of Coping and Helping. The quality of the nurse-client relationship is a factor in the woman's ability to cope with the discomfort of the labor process. The nurse who is aware of sociocultural aspects of helping and coping acts as a protective agent for the woman. The responsibility for initiating and maintaining such a therapeutic relationship rests with the nurse.

An area in which the nurse and the pregnant woman from different cultures could misunderstand each other is pain (Table 18-4).

A study of nurses from the United States, Japan, Puerto Rico, Korea, Thailand, and Taiwan revealed that nurses

Specific Nursing Care Plan

HYPERVENTILATION AND SPONTANEOUS RUPTURE OF MEMBRANES

Judy S. is a 30-year-old multipara in labor. She is assessed at being 8 cm dilated, station +2, membranes intact when her husband brings her to the labor and delivery area. Judy and her husband have been through prepared childbirth classes and she is doing her breathing exercises with each contraction. As the nurse is helping Judy into the bed, her membranes rupture with a gush of clear fluid. The nurse immediately assesses the FHR and the fluid that was lost.

The contractions are now coming faster and harder and Judy is starting to hyperventilate. She starts complaining of numbness of her fingers and around her mouth and lightheadedness. The nurse tries to calm her breathing pattern down and gives her a bag to breathe into.

ASSESSMENT	NURSING DIAGNOSIS (ND)/ PLAN (P)/GOAL (G)	RATIONALE/ IMPLEMENTATION	EVALUATION
Spontaneous rupture of membranes (SROM) Station +2 8 cm dilated Multipara	ND: Potential for injury to mother or newborn related to rapid delivery. ND: Potential for infection related to delayed delivery after SROM. P: Confirm fetal status, SROM, and progress of labor; notify physician or midwife. G: Fetal status, amniotic fluid, and progress of labor are within normal limits; infection does not occur; physician or midwife is present for birth.	*To confirm and assess fetal status and rupture of membranes, the nurse will:* Assess FHR and progress of labor. Assess the color of the fluid—normally straw-colored. Assess character of the fluid—normally looks like water and has a characteristic odor. Assess amount of fluid lost—an excessive amount, polyhydramnios, or an abnormally small amount, oligohydramnios, signals congenital anomalies. Record findings and notify physician or midwife.	Fetal status remains within normal limits. Progress of labor continues within normal limits. Woman understands reasons for procedures.
Numbness in fingers and around mouth Lightheadedness Rapid respiratory rate	ND: Impaired gas exchange related to respiratory alkalosis. ND: Altered cardiopulmonary tissue perfusion related to hyperventilation and respiratory alkalosis. P: Correct alkalosis and breathing pattern to reestablish adequate perfussion for mother and fetus. G: Mother resumes normal breathing pattern with no signs or symptoms of alkalosis. G: FHR stays within normal limits.	*To assist woman in treating hyperventilation, the nurse will:* Provide a paper bag for the woman to breathe into. She may also breathe into cupped hands, if no bag is available. Explain to woman what is happening and how rebreathing her own air is therapeutic. Coach woman to breathe without hyperventilation. Identify stress (e.g., anxiety, knowledge deficit, or discomfort) that may underlie woman's hyperventilation; relieve the identified stress.	Woman ceases to hyperventilate and signs and symptoms are relieved. FHR remains within normal limits. Concurrent stress is relieved.

Table 18-4 *Sociocultural Basis of Pain Experience*

	Woman in Labor	Nurse
Perception of meaning	Origin: Cultural concept of and personal experience with pain; for example: Pain in childbirth is inevitable, something to be borne Pain in childbirth can be avoided completely Pain in childbirth is punishment for sin Pain in childbirth can be controlled	Origin: Cultural concept of and personal experience with pain; in addition, nurse becomes accustomed to working with certain "expected" pain trajectories. For example, in obstetrics, pain is expected to increase as labor progresses, be intermittent in character, and have end point; relief can be derived from drugs once labor is well established and fetus or newborn can cope with amount and elimination of drug; relief can also come from woman's knowledge and attitude and support from family or friends
Coping mechanisms	Woman may do the following: Be traditionally vocal or nonvocal; crying out or groaning or both may be part of ritual of her response to pain Use counterstimulation to minimize pain; for example, rubbing, applying heat, or counterpressure Have learned to use relaxation, distraction, autosuggestion as pain-countering techniques Resist any use of "needles" as modes of administering pain relief	Nurse may do the following: Have learned to use self effectively; for example, tone of voice, closeness in space, touch, as media for message of interest and caring Use avoidance, belittling, or other distancing actions as protective device for self Use pharmacologic resources at hand judiciously Be skilled in use of comfort measures Assume accountability for control and management of pain
Expectations of others	Nurse may be seen as someone who will accept woman's statement of pain and act as her advocate Medical personnel may be expected to relieve woman of all pain sensations Nurse may be expected to be interested, gentle, kindly, and accepting of behavior exhibited	Nurse may accept only certain verbal or nonverbal behaviors as responses to pain Nurse may expect couple who are prepared for childbirth to refuse medication and to wish to "do everything on their own" Nurse may find it difficult to accept woman's definition of pain; that is, woman may wish to experience and participate in controlling pain or may not be able to accept any pain as reasonable

from diverse cultures make different inferences about physical pain and psychologic distress (Davitz, Davitz, and Higuchi, 1977). Reviewing these nurses' responses to a questionnaire composed of vignettes describing different client situations, it was found that Korean and Japanese nurses in this sample made the highest inferences of physical pain. Taiwanese nurses inferred a moderate degree of physical pain with the smallest variability in ratings. Regarding psychologic distress, Korean and Puerto Rican nurses inferred the greatest degree of psychologic discomfort. Nurses sampled from the United States were midway between the other national groups and showed the smallest variability. Taiwanese nurses inferred the least suffering of all the groups.

An important implication of these findings is that Oriental national groups differ among themselves in terms of response to pain, just as one would expect groups from various Western societies to differ. A Puerto Rican nurse interestingly interpreted these findings to indicate that the amount of physical pain cannot always be judged by the woman's behavior. This nurse stated that pregnant Puerto Rican women might be very emotional despite the absence of unusual labor pains (Davitz, Davitz, and Higuchi, 1977).

Indochinese women walk around during labor and do not ask for medications. These women and others exert great self-control, to the point that the nurse may not recognize an impending delivery (Hollingsworth, 1980). Black women commonly find comfort in having another woman such as a mother or sister pray with them during the discomfort of labor. Based on these data, the nurse need not label clients from the same cultural group as alike in their responses to pain. Not all Orientals are stoic, nor do all Western people respond to pain in the same manner. Zborowski (1952) found that people of Irish, Jewish, Italian, and "old American" descent respond to pain differently. Although Irish clients may admit that they are suffering to relatives and friends, when in pain, these clients tended to prefer to suffer in physical isolation. Old Americans of Anglo-Saxon origin, usually of Protestant faith, and whose ancestors came to the United States more than three generations ago, did not express their pain. However, when their pain became very severe, they withdrew from people and cried only when alone.

Zborowski reported that Italian and Jewish people had a low tolerance for pain and were emotional in expressing pain. People from these two groups demanded instant relief and gave an impression of having extraordinary sensitivity. Apparently, Jewish clients' intense reactions to pain were intended to mobilize others (doctors, family members) to give them the best possible care. This purpose did not seem to be a major concern to Italian clients, who were reluctant to complain for fear that this would drive family members and friends away. When compared with Jewish clients, Italians were more concerned with the immediate amelioration of pain and its effects rather than with any future-oriented reason.

General Nursing Actions. Even if the laboring woman and her partner (or family or support persons) are well prepared, the nurse remains an important member of the childbirth team. Labor is a crisis time, and all people, no matter how well prepared, enter labor with some level of anxiety. The following are some helpful actions that the nurse as a support person can use to offer both verbal and practical support during labor:

1. Remember that labor is stressful, even if the couple is prepared. Continually encourage relaxation. They need you. Do not leave them totally alone. Provide company when they need it—and privacy when they need it.
2. Minimize adverse environmental stimuli. Control glaring lights. Decrease traffic flow and noise in the birth setting.
3. Remind the mother that she is to select the *position* in which she feels most comfortable during labor and to change her position whenever she wishes. Encourage walking in early labor.
4. Provide privacy and a space with adequate room temperature and ventilation.
5. Talk of contractions, not pains. Remember, the woman is having "contractions!"
6. Relax and get as near to the woman's level as possible. Sit by the bedside. Do not tower over her. Touch!
7. Adjust the labor bed to provide a comfortable position (usually elevating the top of the bed to 45 degrees). The woman should never be flat on her back because the weight of the uterine contents puts too much pressure on major blood vessels, thus reducing the blood flow back to the brain. Use pillows to support all dependent body parts.
8. Use comfort measures such as cold cloths, backrubs, and ice chips. Showers or tub baths may be taken depending on the progress of labor. Allowing warm water to strike the lower part of the back may be relaxing.
9. Try effleurage. It is best done by the woman herself, although it may be done for her.
10. Carry on a conversation if necessary only between contractions.
11. Talk with the father or other support person. Give reassurance and remember that the father also has needs for nourishment, rest, and elimination. Let him know where the bathroom is and where he may purchase food. Also, reassure him that you will stay with the laboring woman if he needs to leave for a while to tend to his own needs.
12. Do not ask irrelevant questions. Keep talk to a minimum. It uses energy needed to cope. Be aware of attitudinal changes as labor progresses.
13. Keep your voice well modulated at all times.
14. Remind the mother to urinate frequently. A full bladder can slow down the descent of the baby.
15. Encourage rest between contractions.
16. Keep the couple informed of what is happening: how many centimeters dilated, station, effacement, and fetal position.
17. Assure the mother she is doing well, offer encouragement, agree with her if she says it hurts but offer positive comments, too.
18. Do not distract the woman during conractions. Wait until a contraction is over to do a nursing procedure.
19. Remember that transition (8 to 10 cm) may be the most intense time during labor. Because the woman may fall asleep between contractions, they may get ahead of her. She may become very irritable.
20. During the actual birth stage, trust the woman and work with her body. This is not an athletic contest; the goal is pelvic floor release and relaxation. Encourage a series of quick breaths, holding one for 5 seconds while pushing and then taking another breath. Give verbal support such as, "Beautiful! Go with it! Let it flow! Open up below! Soft and loose! Open the door!" You might even give the woman a mirror so that she can watch her own progress as she pushes the baby out.
21. If the couple is giving birth in the delivery room, give the father or other support person the clothes to wear in the delivery room well in advance so that there is no last-minute rush.
22. As you encourage relaxation, encourage *release* toward your touching hand on her body. This will help the woman increase her body awareness.
23. Always encourage the breathing that *feels* right for each woman. She may have practiced one type of breathing before labor only to find that it is not helpful during a certain part of labor. If this happens, be flexible. Encourage her to find what is working for her and stick with it.
24. There is no failure! Some people who have prepared faithfully for a "natural" childbirth will not be able to achieve that goal because of circumstances beyond their control. They may need analgesia, anesthesia, or a cesarean birth. If they are disappointed, encourage them to talk about their disappointment and then help them work through it by emphasizing that there is no failure. When they have achieved a meaningful and safe birth experience, they have achieved their goal.
25. Throughout the entire labor process be constantly and consistently aware of the needs of the fetus. When the couple has prepared diligently for labor and are extremely intent on what they are doing, it is often easy for the support person to get caught up in that intensity and feel reluctant to do any procedure that might "spoil" their experience. Continually think of yourself as a fetal advocate and use your knowledge and skills to make sound judgments that will lead to a meaningful and safe birth experience for all family members.
26. Share in the couple's joy (or their grief).

The helpful actions for labor support given in this unit are useful for all laboring women (Table 18-5). However, if there is no family or friend to support the laboring woman, then the nurse's role becomes even more crucial. A woman should never have to labor alone! If the realities of staffing shortages prevent constant attendance to women laboring alone, seek labor support persons from commu-

Table 18-5 *Summary of Woman's Expected Responses and Support Person's Actions by Phase of Cervical Dilation*

	Woman	Support Person
Dilation of Cervix 0-3 cm		
Contractions 10-30 sec long, 5-30 min apart, mild to moderate Mood: alert, happy, excited, mild anxiety	Settles into labor room; selects focal point Rests or sleeps if possible Uses breathing techniques: begin contraction with deep breath in through nose and out through pursed lips; slow chest breathing, 6-9/min through contraction; end contraction with deep breath in and out Uses effleurage; focusing and relaxation techniques	Provides encouragement, feedback for relaxation, companionship Assists with contractions Alerts woman to the following: beginning of contraction; time called out at 15 sec, 30, etc.; ending of contraction Uses focusing techniques: concentration on fixed point in room; "Listen to me and follow my breathing"; "Watch my face" Concentration on breathing technique Uses comfort measures Position most comfortable for woman Keeps woman aware of progress, explains procedures and routines Gives praise Offers ataractics as ordered (Chapter 17)
Dilation of Cervix 4-7 cm		
Contractions 30-40 sec long, 3-5 min apart, moderate to strong Mood: seriously labor oriented, concentration and energy needed for contractions, alert, more demanding	Continues relaxation, focusing techniques Uses breathing techniques Begin contraction with deep breath in and out, then slow chest breathing until contraction intensifies, then shallow, effortless breathing, moderate pace, high in chest through peaking of contraction; slow chest breathing as contraction subsides OR Use abdominal breathing to raise abdominal wall away from uterus; end contraction with deep breathing in and out	Acts as buffer, limits assessment techniques to between contractions Assists with contractions May need to encourage woman to help her maintain breathing techniques Uses same instructions Uses same focusing devices as in early phase Uses comfort measures Positions woman on side to minimize pressure of uterus on vena cava and aorta Encourages voluntary relaxation of muscles of back, buttocks, thighs, and perineum; effleurage Uses counterpressure to sacrococcygeal area Encourages and praises Keeps woman aware of progress Offers analgesics and anesthetics as ordered Checks bladder, encourages to void Gives mouth care, ice chips
Dilation of Cervix 8-10 cm (transition)		
Contractions 45-60-90 sec long, 2-3 min apart, strong Mood: irritable, intense concentration, symptoms of transition	Continues relaxation, needs greater concentration to do this Breathing techniques Uses 4:1 pattern if possible Uses panting to overcome response to urge to push	Stays with woman, provides constant support Assists with contractions Probably will need to remind, reassure, and encourage to reestablish breathing pattern and concentration If sedated or drowsy, woman needs warning to begin breathing pattern before contraction becomes too intense If woman begins to push, institutes panting respirations Uses comfort measures Accepts woman's inability to comply with instructions Accepts irritable response to helping, such as counterpressure Supports woman who has nausea and vomiting, gives mouth care as needed, gives reassurance regarding symptomatology of end point of first stage Uses countertension techniques (effleurage and voluntary relaxation) Keeps woman aware of progress, tells woman when time to push

nity volunteer groups. A few days spent in teaching and preparation of these volunteers could provide countless hours of labor support for women alone at this crisis time in their lives. Until labor support groups can be formed, you can communicate openly and honestly with women laboring alone. Inform them of the constraints on your time. Let them know where you will be when you leave their side, how they can communicate with you, and when you will be back.

Women alone or couples who have not attended preparation-for-birth classes can learn relaxation and slow chest breathing techniques with your help during labor. Inform them that there are ways to cope with labor and that you can help them learn these techniques right then and there. A motivated learner is the best learner, and most laboring women are highly motivated for relief of discomfort.

Fatherhood with Dignity

Miller (1966) remarked, "There is joy in having a baby, and joy is an experience worth sharing." Conception is a psychologic, as well as a physiologic, experience of a man and woman creating a new life; birth can be no less. Conception is the experience of two people; birth, the experience of three (or more) people.

Involving the father in the birth of his child dispels feelings of alienation, isolation, impotence, helpless inaction, and insignificance. *Ethnic definition and role expectations govern the type and degree of the individual's involvement.*

Individual preference for the kind of involvement spans a full spectrum of possibilities. One family, recent arrivals from Italy, is a case in point. The father absented himself to the waiting room while the female relatives took turns attending his wife and reporting her progress to him at intervals. After delivery, wife and son were wheeled back to the labor area. The father entered proudly as the female relatives stepped aside. He made what sounded like endearing comments to wife and son and kissed them both; then all the relatives left. The new mother beamed. The students present expressed negative reactions about this father, whose participation in this event was perceived as tangential and unsupportive. One student was assigned to this mother's postdelivery care and to make a home visit. Her report and discussion of her experience with the group clarified the situation as "right" for this family.

Other men seek a different type of involvement. What are their hopes and expectations for this experience for themselves and their wives? What is the nurse's role in relation to their decisions? These questions will be discussed in the following sections.

Birth Process as Seen Through Father's Eyes. The nurse should recall her feelings the first time she witnessed a woman in active labor. The father's experience can be no less intense. In addition, the woman in labor is not a client to him; she is birthing their baby.

During the delivery he may see the following:

1. Her facial and physical expression of pain; grimace and effort written on her face while pushing
2. Blood, mucus, and watery drainage from her vagina
3. Fecal discharge
4. Bulging perineum just before birth
5. Episiotomy, if done, and repair
6. Delivery by forceps, if used
7. Her postures for vaginal examinations, for observations of the perineum, and for delivery
8. Dry heaves or vomiting

He may hear the following:

1. Her moans and grunts (especially while pushing)
2. Dry heaves or efforts at vomiting
3. Hospital noises (such as call lights, page systems, clanging, sterilizer buzzers, fetal monitoring devices)
4. Protests about fathers who "belong in a waiting room" and who "should leave this to us"
5. Extraneous, irrelevant social or business chatter among staff

He may smell the following:

1. Vaginal drainage
2. Fecal drainage
3. Vomitus (occasionally)
4. Cleaning solutions

With the emergence of the infant, the father will see and hear the following:

1. Small patch of scalp and hair at the introitus
2. Prolonged (usually) emergence of the molded fetal head (one father commented, "and then when all that kept coming out was head and more head and no eyes or ears, I wondered when they would come")
3. Blue-purple coloration of the fetal scalp and body along with blood, amniotic fluid, vernix, and occasionally meconium
4. Cord being loosened around the child's neck or being eased over his head and shoulders
5. Mucus draining from nose and mouth and the physician or nurse suctioning the infant
6. Sounds of suctioning
7. Cutting the cord
8. Verbal communications between physician and nurse regarding position, cord, placement of episiotomy, and similar medical matters in terms often unfamiliar to him

Father in Labor Suite. "He'll just be underfoot." "He'll add confusion and increase the chance of infections and the number of lawsuits." These typical statements for years kept the father apart from his wife and child. These fears proved largely unfounded when fathers were reunited with their laboring wives. Fathers proved helpful, comforting, and reassuring to their wives. There was no change in the incidence of infection or lawsuits. Furthermore, it was found that it was easier for the physician and parents to cope with the birth of a child with a defect when both parents were active participants on an adult-to-adult level with the physician.

The father may be an adjunct to the nurse-physician team in several ways. For example, he may assist with comfort measures such as pillows, ice chips, washcloths to forehead, and back rubs. He may provide almost constant companionship to offset the aloneness of labor and the anxiety it can foster. Should something occur when the nurse or physician is out of the room, the father can call for help. In addition, he is usually better equipped to interpret the mother's wishes and needs to the staff.

Participation in the birth is ego building. The father *can* be of assistance; his presence *is* important. It is commonly observed that a caring person can be worth his or her weight in Demerol (meperidine). Recently a 16-year-old unwed mother in labor with her first child thrashed about, moaning and screaming with each contraction. A nurse remained at her bedside, coaching and comforting to no avail. The unwed adolescent father arrived and was immediately escorted into her room. The young woman continued her labor calmly and unmedicated through delivery.

When the father is active and supportive, the mother turns to him. The physician remains the medical-surgical expert, without taking on the father or husband-surrogate role as well. The couple's future relationship and their relationship with their child may be positively influenced. Mutuality is fostered when the mother can turn to the father and say, "I could never have done it without you. You were my pillar of strength."

Supporting the Father During Labor. Supporting the father, as well as the mother, in labor elevates the nurse's role. It is another step forward from merely providing custodial care to enacting a therapeutic role. Supporting the father reflects the nurse's orientation and commitment to the person, the family, and the community. Therapeutic nursing actions convey to the father several important concepts.

First, he is of value as a person. He is not a comic strip character, inept and bungling or idle, nervous, and inconsequential. Second, he can learn to be a partner in the mother's care. Finally, childbearing is a partnership.

Even if the father enters the labor unit without any parent education classes, he can be taught "on the job," and his choices can be supported. The nurse can support the father in the following ways:

1. Regardless of the degree of involvement desired, orient him to the maternity unit, including wife's labor room and what he can do there (sleep, telephone, smoke or not), restroom, cafeteria, Dads' Room, nursery, visiting hours, and names and functions of personnel present.
2. Respect his or their decisions as to his degree of involvement, whether the decision is active participation in the delivery room or just being kept informed. When appropriate, provide data on which he or they can base decisions; offer freedom of choice as opposed to coercion one way or another. This is *their* experience and *their* baby.
3. Indicate to him when his presence has been helpful.
4. Offer to teach him comfort measures to the degree he wants to know them. Reassure him that he is not assuming the responsibility for observation and management of his wife's labor. Supportive behaviors can be classified into three categories:
   a. Physical care
   b. Nonverbal care (such as holding her hand, smiling, kissing)
   c. Verbal care (coaching breathing and relaxation techniques, complimenting)
5. Communicate with him frequently regarding her progress and his needs. Keep father or couple informed of procedures to be done, what to expect from procedures, and what is expected of him.
6. Prepare him for changes in her behavior and physical appearance.
7. Remind him to eat; offer snacks and fluids if possible.
8. Relieve him as necessary; offer blankets if he is to sleep in a chair by the bedside. Acknowledge the stress of the situation on each partner and identify normal responses. The nonjudgmental attitude of staff helps the father and mother accept their own and the other parent's behavior.
9. Attempt to modify or eliminate unsettling stimuli (such as extra noise, extra light, chatter); keep the woman clean and dry.

A well-informed father can make a significant contribution to the health and well-being of the mother and child, their family interrelationship, and his self-esteem. It has been found that a significantly lower percentage of women suffered postdelivery emotional upsets when their partners received support and assistance from prenatal classes, physicians, and nurses throughout the childbearing cycle. This is continued by the care from community health nurses in the home.

Culture and Father Participation. Many hospitals encourage the father's presence during labor and delivery. If he is not able to be there, another significant person may be present. In several cultures the father may be available, but his presence with the mother may not be appropriate and he may resist involvement at this time. His behavior could be misconstrued by the nursing staff as lack of concern, caring, or interest. Griffith (1982) identifies the importance of the affectional bond between a Mexican woman and her mother and sisters or other female relatives in regard to home-related activities such as childbearing. This is also true for many other groups, and the presence of another woman or women is highly desired. If childbearing occurs in the hospital, at least one woman must be present for assistance. Southeast Asians (Hollingsworth and others, 1980), blacks (Carrington, 1978; Johnson and Snow, 1978), and American Indians (Farris, 1978; Horn, 1982) are some of the major cultural groups indicating a preference for a woman's assistance during childbearing.

According to Pillsbury (1978), the Chinese husband is not allowed in the delivery room, lest he become polluted by the woman's blood. A nurse from a different culture might think it odd that a Chinese husband did not seem to have given any emotional support to his wife during labor and delivery. There are various reasons for the husband's behavior: (1) Oriental men are usually embarrassed to show their emotions in public, (2) Oriental men consider childbirth as solely the woman's work, and (3) Oriental women feel embarrassed and uncomfortable about their husbands' involvement with a function that they consider their prerogative (Chung, 1977). Nevertheless, Oriental men have as much emotion as Western men. However, Oriental women have significant others who can provide emotional support—mothers, inlaws, cousins, other members of the extended family, or close friends. In the absence of these significant others the husband provides the wife with as much emotional support as possible (such as interpreting for a wife who doesn't speak English).

In India all attendants at birth are women; men are totally excluded (Flint, 1982). On the other hand, in Guatemala, a husband may assist his wife and the midwife during delivery (Cosminsky, 1982). During the labor process of the Navajo in the Southwestern United States, people passing by the hogan (home) are encouraged to enter and provide support for the mother (Newton, 1972). Because of the wide variation in who comprises the preferred person or persons, it is critical for the nurse to determine from the woman and her family what persons are wanted during labor and delivery.

Grandparenthood with Dignity

Support of grandparents is similar to that provided the father as discussed in the preceding pages. The nurse acts as a role model for parents by treating grandparents with dignity and respect, by acknowledging the value of their contributions to parental support, and by recognizing the difficulty parents have in witnessing their child's discomfort or crisis, regardless of the child's age.

Of particular value is the availability of another person or persons to relieve the father or coach. This may be necessary to assist the parturient with walking, especially if IV poles are to be pushed; and to help the parturient when she needs two tasks performed simultaneously.

Whenever possible the nurse offers the grandparent emotional support. This can be done by providing liquid refreshment even if unsolicited and by initiating discussion with open-ended questions or statements, such as "It is sometimes hard to watch a daughter in labor. . . ."

These nursing actions are therapeutic for the entire family unit. According to Barnard (1978), "Rather than compete with family members, we can use them, provide support to them, and teach them. The family's influence will far outlast our contact with the client. If we can improve this social unit's ability to care, we will have a powerful health care system indeed." Support for the mother of a laboring woman—mothering *her* mother—is an important place to begin (Stephany, 1983).

Siblings During Labor

Preparation for acceptance of the new child helps with the attachment process. Parents, brothers and sisters, and other extended family members benefit from *cognitive rehearsal* for the new addition to the family. Preparation for and participation during pregnancy and labor may help the older children accept this change. The older child or children become *active* participants who are important to the family (Bliss, 1980). Rehearsal for the event before labor is essential. Preparation for the entire family includes the additional support person who is to be responsible for the older children during the entire childbirth process.

The age and developmental level of the children influence their responses. The child under 2 years of age shows little interest in pregnancy and labor; for the older child the experience may reduce fears and misconceptions. Preparation is adjusted to the age and developmental level of the child. Most parents have a "feel" for the maturational level and ability to cope of their children. Preparation includes description of anticipated sights and sounds. The children must learn that their mother will be working hard. She will not be able to talk to them during contractions. She may groan and pant at times. Labor is uncomfortable, but their mother's body is made for the job. The sights, sounds, smells, and behavior of participants will be similar to those for which fathers are prepared (p. 413). The film *Nicholas and the baby* is available for preparing older preschool and school-age children for participating in the birth experience.

Leonard et al. (1979) observed the behavior of children present during labor, delivery, and the postpartum period. In general the preschool-age children tended to interact eagerly with their parents during early labor. They were seen to withdraw from the happenings as labor progressed. None of the children seemed to become acutely distressed during the experience. However, children need to feel free to ask questions and express personal feelings (Daniels, 1983).

Preparation for Giving Birth in the Delivery Room

If any woman in labor, be she a nullipara or multipara, states: *"The baby is coming!"* it is too late for transfer to the delivery room (or if in a birthing room, it may be too late to have the physician present). The birth is imminent. Prepare to assist with the delivery until the physician arrives. (See When the Nurse Must Assist the Mother to Give Birth, p. 438).

The delivery room nurse is responsible for ensuring that the facility is properly prepared and that all supplies and equipment are in working order at all times. The role of the woman's partner is reviewed and suitable operating room clothing provided. It is essential that the woman's record be up-to-date, because her condition can change quickly.

All nursing care and the woman's or couple's responses must be recorded to (1) ensure continuity of care, (2) ensure appropriate assessment of the woman's progress, and (3) document the nursing and other care given. Courts of law insist that the nursing and medical care that is not documented on the client's record has not been given.

The following are suggestions for preparation for delivery. These items may vary among different facilities so that the protocols from each facility's procedure manual should be consulted.

1. Scrubbing facilities, scrub brushes, cuticle sticks, cleaning agent, and masks are available.
2. The following have been done:
   a. Sterile gowns and gloves for physician or nurse-midwife, sterile drapes and towels for draping the woman, and sterile instruments and other supplies (such as bulb syringes, sutures, and anesthetic solutions) are arranged for convenience in use on sterile table.
   b. Sterile basin and water for hand washing during delivery process are readied for use.
   c. Supplies for cleansing vulva are available (sterile basin, sterile water, and cleaning solution).
   d. Delivery area is warmed and free of drafts.
   e. Infant receiving blankets and heated crib are readied. Material for prophylactic care of infant's eyes is available (see p. 438).

3. Equipment is in working order: delivery table (bed or chair), overhead lights, and mirror.
4. Emergency equipment, anesthesia, cardioscope, and supplies are available and in working order if needed for emergency situations such as control of maternal hemorrhage or fetal respiratory distress.
5. Additional supplies (anesthetics, oxytocics for injection, and obstetric forceps) are available.
6. Woman's record is up-to-date and ready for use in delivery area. In areas such as labor unit, recordings are made concomitantly as symptoms are noted, assessments are made, and care is given. Since woman's condition can change quickly, it is imperative to have recordings complete at all times.

Transfer to the Delivery Room*

Nullipara:	when the presenting part begins to distend the perineum
Multipara:	when the cervix is 8 to 9 cm dilated

Evaluation

Evaluation of progress and outcomes is a continuous activity during the first stage of labor. Each interaction with the mother-to-be and her family must be carefully evaluated by the nurse; the degree to which formulated goals for care are being met must be critically appraised. If the evaluation process identifies that results fall short of achieving any goal, further assessment, planning, and implementation are imperative to attain the correct nursing care for the woman and her family.

SUMMARY

The childbearing family has many special needs and concerns during the first stage of labor. Parents are requesting and occasionally demanding alternatives to traditional care. Hospitals must now provide a variety of birthing experiences, for example, labor and delivery in the same setting (birthing rooms), different methods of delivery, for example, the Leboyer Method (1976). These needs can only be met by a skillful, knowledgeable, caring nurse. The nurse who uses the nursing process as a systematic approach can provide comprehensive, empathic nursing care. All members of the family unit are given an opportunity to participate in this meaningful event if they so desire. Consideration of the family's cultural orientation allows the nurse to provide care that is acceptable to the family.

With knowledgeable nursing and medical care, consumers of care in the childbearing phase are best served by allowing the family to participate in the birth option of their choice. In this manner, the family has its best chance of experiencing a safe and satisfying culmination of the birth of a new family member.

*In many facilities, it is now common practice to have the woman labor, deliver, and recover in the LDR (Labor, Delivery, and Recovery) room, thus alleviating the added stress of transfer to a new and often strange environment at a critical time in the childbirth process.

KEY CONCEPTS

- The onset of labor may be difficult to determine even for the experienced gravida.
- Although some complications of labor are anticipated, others appear only in the clinical course of labor.
- The nurse assumes much of the responsibility for making the assessment of progress and keeping the physician informed about that progress and any deviations from normal findings.
- Although meconium-stained fluid may be noted with fetal asphyxia, its presence is not always diagnostic of prospective fetal distress.
- Regardless of the actual labor and delivery experience, the woman's or couple's perception of the birth experience is most positive if she or they evaluate the events and performances as meeting expectations.
- The woman's level of anxiety may rise when she does not understand what is being said to her and about her labor because of the medical terminology used or because of a language barrier.
- Prolapsed umbilical cord occurs in about 1 in 400 deliveries and requires prompt recognition and therapy to prevent fetal hypoxia.
- Coaching, support, and comfort measures assist the woman to use her energy constructively in relaxing and working with the contractions.
- Pushing before full cervical dilation is reached compresses the cervix and may result in fetal distress or cervical edema.
- The nurse who is aware of sociocultural aspects of helping and coping acts as a protective agent for the parturient.
- The quality of the nurse-client relationship is a factor in the woman's ability to cope with the discomfort of the labor process.

STUDY QUESTIONS AND ACTIVITIES

1. Admit clients to the labor suite, collect data for assessment, and prepare a plan for care based on the nursing diagnoses you have developed. Review the standards of nursing care in the labor suite as established by the clinical agency and compare these with your nursing care plans.
2. Diagram on partograms the cervical dilations and stations of the fetal presenting part of both nulliparous and multiparous women during labor and compare findings. Discuss how results differ, whether they follow the normal labor curve, and how you account for any deviations from normal.
3. Using the records of women in uncomplicated labor, role-play appropriate nursing actions. Examples of situations to explore are the following: woman in early labor with severe backache; woman and her partner have agreed to have no medication for relief of pain in labor; woman is asking for explanation of breathing practices that she was taught in prenatal classes; woman is requesting information on why she is leaking fluid from the vagina; woman and her partner are concerned about recognizing the onset of the second stage of labor.

4. Research various cultures' attitudes, perceptions, and beliefs in relation to childbirth and compare with your own. Explain to group how these factors might affect the behavior of parents and grandparents and nurses during the first stage of labor.
5. During the first stage of labor, prepare the woman for and assist with monitoring vital signs and vaginal examination, assessing uterine contractions, and providing support to the woman and her partner.

References

Barnard, R: The family and you, MCN 3:83, 1978
Bliss, J: New baby in the family, Can Nurse 76:42, 1980
Carrington, BW: The Afro-American. In Clark, AL: editor: Culture/childbearing/health professionals, Philadelphia, 1978, FA Davis Co
Chung, JJ: Understanding the Oriental maternity patient, Nurs Clin North Am 12:67, 1977
Cosminsky, S: Knowledge and body concepts of Guatemalan midwives, In Kay, MA, editor: Anthropology of human birth, Philadelphia, 1982, FA Davis Co
Daniels, MB: The birth experience for the sibling: Description and evaluation of a program, J Nurs Midwife 28(5):15, 1983
Davitz, LL, Davitz, JR, and Higuchi, Y: Cross-cultural inferences of physical pain and psychological distress, Nurs Times 73:556, 1977
Farris, L: The American Indian. In Clark, AL, editor: Culture/childbearing/health professionals, Philadelphia, 1978, FA Davis Co
Flint, M: Lockmi: an Indian midwife. In Kay, MA, editor: Anthropology of human birth, Philadelphia, 1982, FA Davis Co
Friedman, FA: Labor: clinical evaluation and management, ed 2, New York, 1978, Appleton-Century-Crofts
Friedman, EA, and Sachtleben, MR: Station of the presenting part, Am J Obstet Gynecol 93:522, 1965
Griffith, S: Childbearing and the concept of children, JOGN Nurs 11:181, 1982
Hollingsworth, AO, et al: The refugees and childbearing: what to expect, RN 43:45, 1980
Horn, BM: Northwest coast Indians: the Muckleshoot. In Kay, MA, editor: Anthropology of human birth, Philadelphia, 1982, FA Davis Co
Jimenez, SL: Application of the body's natural pain relief mechanisms to reduce discomfort in labor and delivery, NAACOG Update Series, lesson 1, vol 1, 1983
Johnson, SM, and Snow, LF: The profile of some unplanned pregnancies. In Bauwens, EE, editor: The anthropology of health, St Louis, 1978, The CV Mosby Co
Leboyer, F: Birth without violence, New York, 1976, Alfred A Knopf, Inc
Leonard, CH, Irvin, N, Ballard, RA, et al: Preliminary observations on the behavior of children present at the birth of a sibling, Pediatrics 64:949, 1979
Miller, JS: Return the joy of home delivery with fathers in the delivery room, Hosp Top 44:105, Jan 1966
Mitchell, PH, and Loustan, A: Concepts basic to nursing, New York, 1981, McGraw-Hill Book Co
Newton, N: Childbearing in broad perspective: pregnancy, birth and the newborn baby, Boston, 1972, Delacorte Press
Nicholas and the baby (16 mm film or ¾ inch videocassette), Centre Productions, Inc, 1312 Pine St, Suite A, Boulder Colo 80302
Pernoll, ML, and Benson, RC, editor: Current obstetric and gynecologic diagnosis and treatment 1987, ed 6, Los Altos, 1987, Appleton & Lange
Pillsbury, BLK: "Doing the month": confinement and convalescence of Chinese women after birth, Soc Sci Med 12:11, 1978
Romney, ML, and White, VGL: Current practices in labor. In Field, PA, editor: Perinatal nursing, Edinburgh, 1984, Churchill Livingstone, Inc
Stephany, T: Supporting the mother of a patient in labor, JOGN Nurs 12(5):345, 1983
Zborowski, M: Cultural components in responses to pain, J Soc Issues 3:16, 1952
Zuspan, FF, and Quilligan, EJ, editors: Practical manual of obstetric care, St Louis, 1982, The CV Mosby Co

Bibliography

Bates, B, and Turner, AN: Imagery and symbolism in the birth practices of traditional cultures, Birth 12:29, Spring 1985
Bauwens, E, and Anderson, S: Home births: a reaction to hospital environmental stressors. In Bauwens, EE, editor: The anthropology of health, St Lous, 1978, The CV Mosby Co
Benner, P: From novice to expert—excellence and power in clinical practice, Menlo Park, Calif, 1984, Addison-Wesley Publishing Co
Bentz, JM: Missed meanings in nurse/patient communications, MCN 5(1):55, 1980
Bjorkman LA Du, E: Childbirth care for Hmong families, MCN 10(6):382, 1985
Bloom, KC: Assisting the unprepared woman during labor, JOGN Nurs 13:303, Sept/Oct 1984
Campbell, A, and Worthington, EL: Teaching expectant fathers how to be better childbirth coaches, MCN 7(1):28, 1982
Chute, GE: Expectation and experience in alternative and conventional birth, JOGN Nurs 14:61, Jan/Feb 1985
Collins, BA: The role of the nurse in labor and delivery as perceived by nurses and patients, JOGN Nurs 15(5):412, 1986
Craig, J: Birth of a grandchild brings time of reflection, Menninger Perspect 23, 1980
Danforth, DN, and Scott, JR, editors: Obstetrics and gynecology ed 5 Philadelphia, 1986, JB Lippincott Co
Erikson, EH: Childhood and society, New York, 1964, WW Norton & Co, Inc
Fullerton, JD: The choice of in-hospital or alternative birth environment as related to the concept of control, J Nurse Midwife 27(2):17, 1982
Grosso, C, et al: The Vietnamese American family . . . and grandma makes three, MCN 6:177, 1981
Hageman, JR, et al: Delivery room management of meconium staining of the amniotic fluid and the development of meconium aspiration syndrome, J Perinatol 8(2):127, 1988
Hassid, P: Textbook for child educators, ed 2, Philadelphia, 1984, JB Lippincott Co
Haun, N: Nursing care during labor, Can Nurse 80:26, Oct 1984
Horn, M, and Manion, J: Creative grandparenting: bonding the generations, JOGN Nurs 14:233, May/June 1985
Howe,CL: Physiologic and psychosocial assessment in labor, Nurs Clin North Am 17(1):49, 1982
Howley, C: The older primipara: implications for nurses, JOGN Nurs 10(3):182, 1981
Investigators: A look at endorphins in reproductive medicine, Contemp OB/GYN 20(3):117, 1982

Jimenez, SL: The pregnant woman's comfort guide, Englewood Cliffs, NJ, 1983, Prentice-Hall, Inc

Johnsen, NM, and Gaspard, ME: Theoretical foundations for a prepared sibling class, JOGN Nurs 14:237, May/June 1985

Kintz, DL: Nursing support in labor, JOGN Nurs 16:126, March/April 1987

Kitzinger S: Pregnancy and childbirth, London, 1980, Michael Joseph

Kowba, MD, and Schwirian, PM: Direct sibling contact and bacterial colonization of newborns, JOGN Nurs 14:412, Sept/Oct 1985

Leininger, M: Transcultural nursing: an essential knowledge and practice field for today, Can Nurs 80:41, Dec 1984

MacDonald, J: Birth attendants: another choice, Can Nurse 80:22, Oct 1984

Maloney, R: Childbirth education classes: expectant parents' expectations, JOGN Nurs 14:245, May/June 1985

Marecki, M, et al: Early sibling attachment, JOGN Nurs 14:418, Sept/Oct 1985

May, KA: The father as observer, MCN 7(5):319, 1982

McKay, S, and Phillips, CR: Family-centered maternity care: implementation strategies, Rockville, Md, 1984, Aspen Systems Corp

Miller, FC, et al: Effects of position change during labor on intrauterine resting pressure, J Calif Perinat Assoc 2(2):50, 1982

Namikoshi, T: The complete book of shiatsu therapy, Tokyo, 1981, Japan Publications

Olson, ML: Fitting grandparents into new families, MCN 6(6):419, 1981

Orque, MS, et al: Ethnic nursing care: a multicultural approach, St Louis, 1983, The CV Mosby Co

Poole, C: Educating new labor and delivery room nurses, JOGN Nurs 14:459, Nov/Dec 1985

Powers, BA: The use of orthodox and Black-American folk medicine, Adv Nurs Sci 4:35, 1982

Roberts, J: Alternative positions for childbirth: first stage, J Nurse Midwife 25:11, 1980

Robertson, JF: Grandmotherhood: a study of role conception, J Marriage Fam 39:165, 1977

Romond, JL, and Baker, IT: Squatting in childbirth: a new look at an old tradition, JOGN Nurs 14:406, Sept/Oct 1985

SantoPietro, MC: How to get through to a refugee patient, RN 44:43, 1981

Satir, V: Peoplemaking, Palo Alto, Calif, 1972, Science & Behavior Books

Stanton, ME: The myth of "natural" childirth: the practices of people in traditional cultures, J Nurs Midwife 24(2):25, 1979

Sweet, PT: Prenatal classes especially for children, MCN 4:82, 1979

Trause, MA, and Irvin, NA: Care of the sibling. In Klaus, MH, and Kennell, JH, editors: Parent-infant bonding, St Louis, 1982, the CV Mosby Co

Waller, MM: Siblings in the childbearing experience, NAACOG Update Series, lesson 17, vol 1, 1984

Whaley, LF, and Wong, DL: Nursing care of infants and children, ed 3, St Louis, 1987, The CV Mosby Co

Willson, JR, Carrington, ER, and Ledger, WJ: Obstetrics and gynecology, ed 8, St Louis, 1988, The CV Mosby Co

Winslow, W: Perinatal nursing education, Can Nurse, p 31, June 1988

Zepeda, M: Selected maternal infant care practices of Spanish-speaking people, JOGN Nurs 11:371, 1982

CHAPTER

19

Second and Third Stages of Labor

Iris E. Campbell

Learning Objectives

Correctly define the key terms listed.

Describe assessment of the mother during the second stage of labor.

Summarize the nurse's role with the parturient and her family during the second stage of labor.

Discuss assessment of the mother during the third stage of labor.

Review the nurse's role with the new mother and her family during the third stage of labor.

Discuss assessment of the neonate during the third stage of labor.

Summarize the nurse's role with the neonate during the third stage of the mother's labor.

Describe in detail and state in logical order, emergency childbirth.

Outline the nurse's role in the care of the new mother who experienced an episiotomy or a laceration.

Develop a complete nursing care plan for a woman and her family through the second and third stages of labor.

Key Terms

active birth
Apgar score
bearing down
caput succedaneum
caul
crowning
descent phase
episiotomy
eye prophylaxis
Ferguson's reflex
final/transition
laceration
lithotomy
nuchal cord
ophthalmia neonatorum
placental separation
ring of fire
Ritgen's maneuvers
Sims' position
Valsalva maneuver
vocalization
Wharton's jelly

In this chapter the physiologic and psychosocial processes of the second and third stages of labor are presented. Nursing care of the woman who experiences the rhythmic nature of the second stage of labor and birth will be discussed. Nursing responsibilities for the woman who delivers in a traditional setting are addressed. Nursing care of the newborn during the mother's third stage of labor is covered. Whereas the third stage is primarily the focus of the physician or nurse-midwife, most responsibility for the normal newborn rests with the nurse.

SECOND STAGE OF LABOR

The second stage of labor is the stage of expulsion of the fetus. It extends from full cervical dilation (10 cm) through the birth of the baby. The three phases of the second stage are **latency/resting, descent**, and **final transition**. There is a rhythmic nature to the second stage of labor (Carr, 1983). The rhythm and movement emerge for the woman encouraged to listen to her body as she progresses through this stage. A woman will normally respond by changing body positions, pushing when she has an urge to push, and vocalizing as she bears down. If a woman is confined to bed in a recumbent position this rhythmic urge to push is lost. The rhythm is also lost if she is moved to another room and placed on a delivery table in the lithotomy position, as has been the custom in North America for the past 30 years. In most societies labor and delivery occur in the same room. In most nonWestern societies women use a variety of positions for labor such as kneeling, sitting, standing, or squatting. In Western society we are seeing an active birth movement developing in which women are asking for freedom of choice in relation to the position selected for both labor and birth.

"In the majority of cases, labor and delivery are physiologic processes, and do not, in the true sense, require 'management'" (Danforth and Scott, 1986). In response to the question of whether the obstetrician should interfere with the process of labor during the second stage, Warrington (1842) replied, "He should let it alone if he has ascertained the position is correct."

Assessment

Identification of Second Stage. The only positive objective sign that the second stage of labor has begun is when no cervix can be felt on vaginal examination (Myles, 1985). Other signs that suggest the onset of the second stage include the following:

1. Sudden appearance of sweat on upper lip
2. An episode of vomiting
3. An increased bloody show
4. Shaking of extremities
5. Increased restlessness; verbalization that "I can't go on"
6. Involuntary bearing-down efforts

These signs commonly appear at the time the cervix reaches full dilation (Danforth and Scott, 1986; Myles, 1985). Other indicators for assessing progress during each phase of the second stage can be found in Table 19-1.

Schedule of Assessments. Assessment is continuous during the second stage of labor. The specific type and timing of assessments are determined by hospital protocol. These may include the following types of assessments (see Chapter 18 for assessment procedures).

In the second stage *each* contraction is monitored for frequency, strength, duration, intensity, and fetal response. Descent of the presenting part is confirmed by vaginal examination until the presenting part can be seen at the introitus. The degree of bladder filling is assessed, since a full bladder can impede descent of the head and affect uterine contractions.

Maternal pulse and blood pressure (BP) are checked every 30 minutes. The BP is obtained between contractions. The presence of amnesia between contractions is noted. The partner's or father's response is assessed.

If the fetal heart rate (FHR) is monitored intermittently with a fetoscope, it is checked after every contraction or every 5 minutes. If continuous FHR monitoring is used (Chapter 17), the nurse checks the tracings on the monitor with each contraction. Mild, brief bradycardia and decelerations can occur in 90% or more of women during the second stage of labor (Mahan and McKay, 1984). If recovery of the FHR from the deceleration is prompt after the contraction and expulsive forces cease, these episodes are not of major concern. (Pritchard, MacDonald, and Gant, 1985).

All protocols include assessment of show and amniotic fluid. Show is checked for evidence of excessive bleeding. Amniotic fluid is checked for meconium staining, odor, and amount (Procedure 18-4). Amniotic fluid is normally odorless but an odor can be detected when intrauterine infection (amnionitis) is present. Vaginal examinations are avoided or the number restricted whenever possible.

Duration of Second Stage. There is considerable controversy over the precise duration of the second stage and the time limits that should be regarded as normal. Friedman's curves for nulliparous and multiparous women are commonly used to assess the progress of the second stage. A second stage of more than 2 hours for a nullipara and 1 hour for a multipara is considered abnormal and must be reported to a physician. Other factors that must be considered are the FHR pattern, the descent of the presenting part, the quality of the uterine contractions, and the fetal blood pH. (Mahan and McKay, 1984). The range and average duration of the second stage of labor based on Friedman's data vary with parity:

Parity	*Range (min)*	*Average (min)*
Nulliparas	25 to 75	57
Multiparas	13 to 17	14.4

The nurse should be aware of the danger signs during labor (Chapter 18, p. 386).

Yeates and Roberts (1984) compared the duration of the second stage when women engage in coached pushing or are allowed to push spontaneously when they feel the urge. Their findings are based on a small sample but suggest that spontaneous pushing may be the most effective in aiding in the descent and rotation of the newborn.

Timing of Transfer to Delivery Room. Whereas labor

Table 19-1 *Maternal Progress in Second Stage of Labor*

Criterion	Latent/Resting (10-20 min)	Descent	Final/Transition
Contractions Magnitude (intensity) Frequency Duration	Period of physiologic lull for all criteria Period of peace and rest (Carr, 1983; Mahan and McKay, 1984)	Significant increase $2\frac{1}{2}$ min 90 sec	Overwhelmingly strong Expulsive $2\frac{1}{2}$ min 90 sec
Descent		Increases and **Ferguson's reflex*** activated	Rapid
Show: color and amount		Significant increase in dark red bloody show	Fetal head visible at introitus; bloody show accompanies birth of head
Spontaneous bearing-down efforts	Slight to absent except with peaks of strongest contractions (Carr, 1983)	Increased urgency to bear down	Greatly increased
Vocalization		Grunting sounds or expiratory vocalization (Carr, 1983; Mahan and McKay, 1984)	Grunting sounds and expiratory vocalizations continue
Maternal behavior (Carr, 1983)	Experiences sense of relief that transition to second stage is finished Feels fatigued and sleepy Feels a sense of accomplishment and optimism, since the "worst is over" Feels in control	Senses increased urgency Alters respiratory pattern: has short 4 to 5 sec breath-holds with regular breaths in between, 5-7 times per contraction Makes grunting sounds or expiratory vocalizations	Expresses sense of extreme pain Expresses feelings of powerlessness Shows decreased ability to listen or concentrate on anything but giving birth Describes the **"ring of fire"**† Often shows excitement immediately following delivery of head

*Ferguson's reflex. Pressure of presenting part on stretch receptors of pelvic floor stimulates release of oxytocin from posterior pituitary, resulting in more intense uterine contractions.
†Ring of fire. Burning sensation of acute pain as vagina stretches and fetal head crowns.

and delivery in the same room is ideal, many hospitals lack birthing rooms and therefore transfer during second stage is required. If birth is to occur in the delivery room, it is best to transfer the woman early enough to avoid a last minute rush. For nulliparas transfer can take place when the presenting part begins to distend the perineum. For multiparas transfer should take place in the first stage, when the cervix is dilated 8 to 9 cm (see box below).

See also Table 19-2 for expected maternal behaviors during the descent phase of the second stage of labor.

If any parturient, nullipara or multipara, states, "The baby is coming!" the baby *is* coming, and it is too late for the transfer. The baby is coming *now*—prepare to assist her if the physician is not yet present. See When the Nurse must Assist the Mother to Give Birth, pp. 438 to pp. 440.

TRANSFER TO DELIVERY ROOM

Parity	Stage	Characteristic
Nulliparas	Second	When the presenting part begins to distend the perineum
Multiparas	First	When the cervix is dilated to 8 to 9 cm

Recording of all vital signs and of labor progress must be done concurrently with care. The course of labor and maternal-fetal response may change without warning. It is of legal importance that all charting be accurate and complete.

Nursing Diagnoses

Nursing diagnoses lend direction to the nursing action needed to implement care. Before establishing diagnoses the nurse analyzes the significance of the findings collected during assessment. Following are some nursing diagnoses indicating potential areas for concern during the second stage.

- Potential for injury to mother and fetus related to
  - Persistent use of Valsalva maneuver
- Situational low self-esteem, related to
  - Knowledge deficit of normal, beneficial effects of vocalizations during bearing-down efforts
- Ineffective individual coping, related to
  - Coaching that contradicts woman's physiological urge to push
- Pain, related to

  - Knowledge deficit of underlying reasons for perineal sensations
- Situational low self-esteem of mother because of
  - Inability to carry out plan for unmedicated childbirth
- Potential for injury because of
  - Inappropriate positioning of mother's legs in stirrups, when these are used
- Situational low self-esteem of father because of
  - Inability to support mother during final stage of labor

Planning

In both the second and third stages of labor planning must be completed with speed and accuracy. Goals must be set and prioritized and may change as the second stage progresses. The nurse's ability and adaptability in relation to planning care will depend on her experience, which will influence her competence (Chapter 2). A specific nursing care plan for a woman in the second stage of labor is provided on p. 423.

Goals

1. A second stage that is physically and emotionally satisfying for the woman and her family
2. A cheerful, comfortable, and supportive environment
3. Participation of the woman in the process of birth
4. Inclusion of family members of woman's choice

Implementation

The nurse implements plans to monitor constantly (1) the events of the second stage and mechanism of delivery, (2) maternal physiologic and emotional responses to the second stage, (3) paternal response to the second stage, and (4) fetal response to the stress of the second stage.

The nurse continues to provide comfort measures for the mother such as positioning, mouth care, maintaining clean, dry bedding, and avoiding extraneous noise, conversation, or other distractions (e.g., laughing, talking of attending personnel in or outside the labor area). The woman is encouraged to indicate other support measures she would like. Some options are not universally available, for example, the warm tub at Pithiviers, France, or a warm shower.

If the mother is to be transferred to another area for delivery, the nurse makes the transfer early enough to avoid rushing the client. The delivery area is also readied for the birth (see Chapter 18). Fig. 19-1 illustrates a typical delivery room, and Fig. 18-13 shows a couple in a birthing room.

Maternal Position. The woman may want to assume various positions such as squatting. For this position a firm surface (not the mattress or a bed) is required, and the woman will need side support. Another position is the side-lying position with the upper leg held by the nurse or coach or placed on a pillow. Some women prefer Fowler's position (can be attained with the support of a wedged pillow or with the father supporting the woman). Others prefer the hands and knees or standing position when bearing down. When a woman is in the standing position, with weight being borne on both femoral heads, the pressure in the acetabulum will increase the transverse diameter of the pelvic outlet by up to 1 cm. This can be helpful if descent of the head is delayed as a result of failure of the occiput to rotate from the lateral (transverse diameter of pelvis) to the anterior position.

Bearing-down Efforts. As the fetal head reaches the pelvic floor most women experience the urge to push. Automatically the woman will begin to exert downward pressure by contracting her abdominal muscles while relaxing her pelvic floor. It is an involuntary reflex response to the pressure of the presenting part on stretch receptors of pelvic musculature. A strong expiratory grunt may accompany the push. When coaching women to push, the nurse encourages them to push as *they* feel like pushing rather than giving a prolonged push on command. The nurse monitors the woman's breathing so that the woman does not hold her breath more than 5 seconds at a time. Prolonged breath holding may trigger the **Valsalva maneuver**, which results from the woman's closing the glottis, thereby increasing intrathoracic and cardiovascular pressure. In addition, holding the breath for more than 5 seconds diminishes the perfusion of oxygen across the placenta and results in fetal hypoxia. The nurse reminds the woman to take deep breaths to refill her lungs following each contraction.

To ensure slow delivery of the fetal head, the nurse encourages the woman to control the urge to push. The urge to push is controlled by coaching the woman to take panting breaths or to exhale slowly through pursed lips as the baby's head crowns. The woman needs simple, clear directions from *one* coach (see also Chapter 18).

Amnesia between contractions is often pronounced in the second stage, and the woman may have to be roused to cooperate in the bearing-down process. Parents who have attended childbirth classes may have devised a set of verbal cues for the parturient to follow. It is helpful if they print these on a card that may be attached to the head of the bed so that the nurse can better substitute as coach if the partner has to leave.

Fetal Heart Rate. FHR must be checked as noted previously. If the rate begins to drop or if there is a loss of variability, then prompt treatment will need to be initiated. The woman can be turned on her left side to reduce the pressure of the uterus against the ascending vena cava and descending aorta (Fig. 18-9), and oxygen can be administered by mask at 10 to 12 L/min. This is often all that is required to restore the normal rate. If the FHR does not return to normal immediately, quickly notify the physician as medical intervention to hasten the birth may be indicated.

Support of the Father/Coach. During the second stage the woman needs continuous support and coaching. The coaching process can be physically and emotionally tiring for the father/coach. The nurse can offer him nourishment, fluids, and short breaks. If the father is to attend the delivery, he is given instructions as to donning cover gown, mask, hat, and shoes and he is advised as to areas in which he has freedom to move and what support he can give to his wife (some are prepared to do coaching for pushing and panting) (Table 19-2).

Birth Beds and Chairs. There is no single position for childbirth. Labor is a dynamic, interactive process between the mother's uterus, pelvis, and voluntary muscles. Angles between the baby and mother's pelvis constantly change as the infant turns and flexes down the birth canal. If able to, a mother will constantly change position in labor. The birth bed (see Chapter 11 [Fig. 11-11]) changes shape according to the mother's needs. She can squat, kneel, recline, or sit, choosing the position most comfortable for her. At the same time, there is excellent exposure for examination, electrode placement, fetal scalp sampling, and delivery. With the birth bed the mother has full control of both seat and back functions and can adjust her position for maxi-

Specific Nursing Care Plan

MULTIPARA IN SECOND STAGE OF LABOR

Martha, a multipara, has been in labor for 4 hours and is now fully dilated. She is to give birth in the labor room. Every time she has a contraction she stiffens up and holds her breath. She looks anxious. She moaned during one contraction and apologized profusely, stating, "I'm such a baby."

ASSESSMENT	NURSING DIAGNOSIS (ND)/ PLAN (P)/GOAL (G)	RATIONALE/ IMPLEMENTATION	EVALUATION
Martha is holding her breath during contractions. Martha exhibits fear and anxiety.	ND: Impaired gas exchange, maternal and fetal, related to maternal breath holding. ND: Ineffective breathing pattern related to anxiety. ND: Decreased cardiac output related to breath holding and performance of Valsalva maneuver (see p. 422). P: Encourage normal breathing pattern and avoidance of Valsalva maneuver. G: Woman will establish and maintain normal breathing pattern.	*To improve breathing and increase gas exchange the nurse will:* Coach Martha to reestablish appropriate breathing pattern. Help Martha focus attention by doing the breathing with her and making eye contact with her. Encourage Martha to use open glottis technique when pushing.	Martha's breathing pattern improves and controlled respirations return; Valsalva maneuver is avoided.
Martha is reluctant or feels ashamed if she vocalizes during a contraction.	ND: Knowledge deficit related to physiologic response to contractions. ND: Situational low self-esteem, related to misperception of accepted behavior during labor. P: Inform Martha about benefit of vocalization during contractions (i.e., prevents valsalva maneuver). Encourage Martha to vocalize prn. G: Martha accepts as normal her need to vocalize; breath holding and valsalva maneuver are avoided.	*To encourage Martha to vocalize during contractions the nurse will:* Provide information (Table 19-2). Coach Martha through contractions giving her verbal and nonverbal approval and reassurance.	Martha uses vocalization prn during contractions. Martha expresses her understanding of use of vocalization. Martha maintains her self-esteem.

mum comfort. The mother and fetus can maintain a close personal contact and a new degree of involvement in the birth process if they desire. The bed can be positioned for administering anesthesia, the V-shaped perineal cut-out is adaptable to both spontaneous birth and forceps and the bed can be used to transport to surgery in the event of a cesarean birth.

Birth chairs may also be used and may provide women with a better physiological position during childbirth, although some women feel restricted by a chair. Potentially there is both a physiologic and psychological advantage to the upright position. The mother can see the birth as it occurs and also maintain *en face* contact with the attendant (Balaskis, 1983). Most chairs are designed so if an emergency occurs the chair can be adjusted to the horizontal or Trendelenburg's position. However, some evidence is offered for a higher incidence of postpartum hemorrhage when a chair is used. There is also an increased risk of perineal edema caused by the pressure of the rim of the chair, which may obstruct venous return from the perineal region (see research highlight, p. 426).

In some hospitals oversize beanbag chairs are being used for both labor and delivery. These chairs mold around and support the mother in whatever position she selects. These chairs are of particular value for mothers who seek active involvement in the birth process. The chairs are covered in washable, fire-retardant material and filled with nonflammable Styrofoam beads.

Preparation for Birth in a Delivery Room. If the woman is to be transferred to a delivery area for completion of the birth process, the nurse uses the guidelines for transfer to the delivery room stated earlier on p. 420-421.

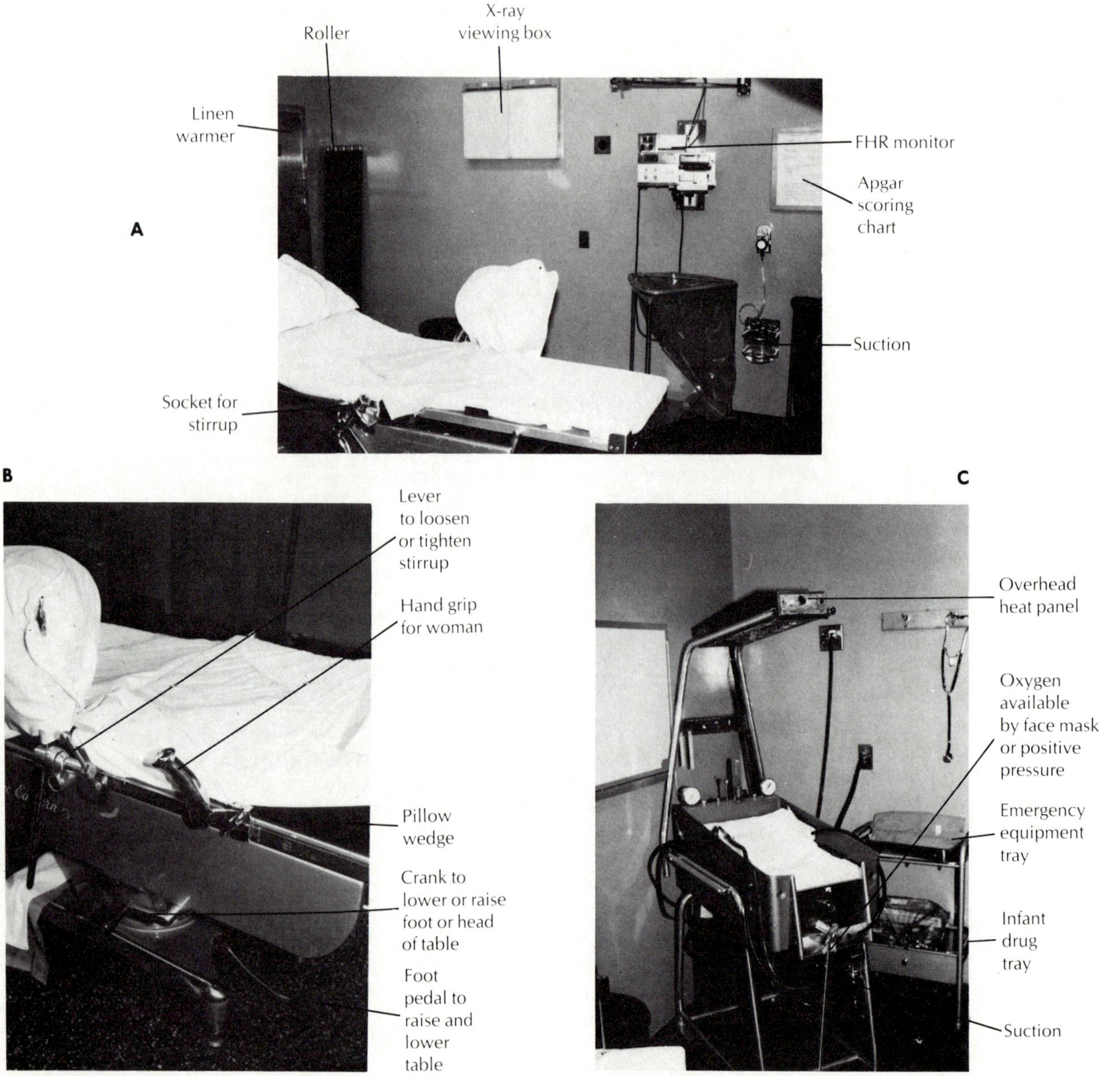

Fig. 19-1 Delivery room.

The Delivery Room Birth Table. Delivery rooms are specifically designed to facilitate care during delivery (Fig. 19-1). The delivery table is designed with many features: the entire table can be raised or lowered, and the head or foot may be raised or lowered. A wedge pillow or bolster can be inserted under the top of the mattress to raise it slightly, or the head of the table can be raised to prevent supine hypotension and to facilitate pushing. The table is equipped with stirrups for supporting the legs and handle grips to aid in bearing down. If stirrups are used, the bed can be "broken"; that is, the lower half of the bed can be lowered and rolled back to fit under the top half.

Supplies, Instruments, and Equipment. The delivery table is prepared and instruments are arranged on the instrument table (Fig. 19-2). Standard procedures are followed for gloving, identifying and opening sterile packages, adding sterile supplies to the instrument table, and unwrapping and handing sterile instruments to the physician or nurse-midwife. Fig. 19-3 illustrates the proper sequence for perineal cleansing. The crib and equipment are readied for the arrival of the infant (Fig. 19-1, *C*).

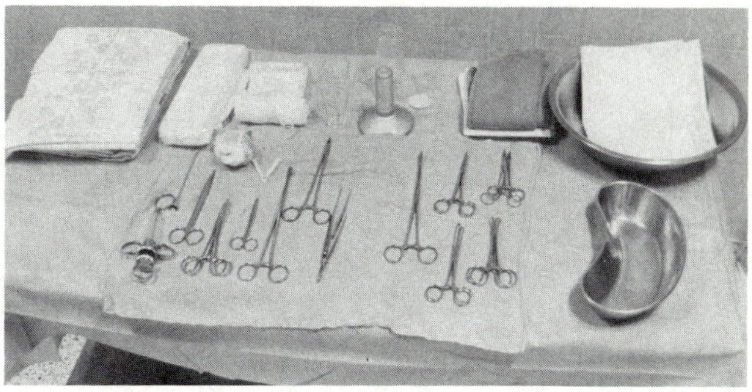

Fig. 19-2 Instrument table (all equipment sterile). *Top, left to right:* receiving blanket, perineal pad, vaginal roll, medicine glasses (for anesthetic agent), hand cover for spotlight, urine specimen bottle, towels, and placenta bowl and paper towel for covering scales. *Bottom, left to right:* syringe (anesthetic) needle guard, episiotomy scissors, bulb syringe (covered with gauze for aspirating newborn), two artery forceps, scissors, cord clamp, ring forceps, needle holder, thumb forceps (for repair of episiotomy), extra instruments (ring forceps, small artery forceps, toothed forceps, Allis clamps and sharp hook forceps for holding drapes in place), and kidney basin.

Table 19-2 *Summary of Woman's Expected Responses and Support Person's Actions by Phase of Second Stage of Labor*

Phase	Woman	Nurse/Support Person
Latent/resting	Experiences a short period (10-20 min) of peace and rest	Encourages woman to listen to her body (Carr, 1983) Continues support measures (Chapter 18, Implementation) If descent phase does not begin after 20 min, suggests upright position to encourage progression of descent
Descent	Senses increased urgency to bear down as Ferguson's reflex is elicted Notes increase in intensity of uterine contractions Demonstrates change in respiratory pattern, e.g., 5-second breath-holds, 5 to 7 per contraction Makes grunting sounds or expiratory vocalizations	Endorses respiratory pattern (short breath-holds with glottis closed) Stresses normalcy and benefits of grunting sounds and expiratory vocalizations Encourages pushing *with* urge to push Encourages/suggests maternal movement and position changes (upright, if descent is not occurring) If descent is occurring, encourages woman to listen to her body regarding movement and position change Discourages long breath holding If transfer to a delivery room (DR) cannot be avoided, nurse transfers her early to avoid rushing or offers her option of walking to DR if permitted If descent is too fast, places woman in lateral recumbent position to slow descent (Carr, 1983)
Final/transitional	Behaves in manner similar to transition during first stage (8-10 cm) Experiences a sense of severe pain and powerlessness (Carr, 1983) Shows decreased ability to listen Concentrates on delivery of baby until head is born Experiences contractions as overwhelming in intensity Reports "ring of fire" as head crowns Maintains respiratory pattern of 3 to 5, 5-second breath-holds per contraction followed by forced expiration Eases head out with short expirations Responds with excitement and relief after head is born	Encourages slow, gentle pushing (Carr, 1983) Explains that "blowing away the contraction" facilitates a slower birth of the head Provides mirror or guides woman to see/touch emerging fetal head (best to extend over 2 to 3 contractions) to help her understand the perineal sensations Coaches relaxation of mouth, throat, and neck to relax pelvic floor Applies warm compresses to perineum to aid relaxation

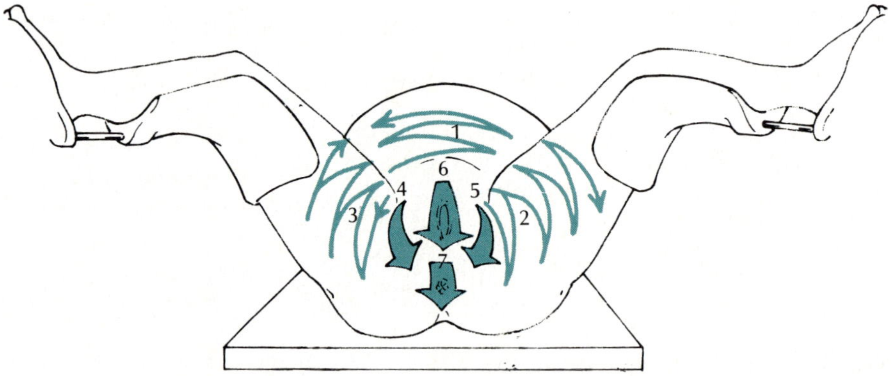

Fig. 19-3 Perineal cleansing. Use cotton swabs or gauze squares well moistened with disinfectant solution. Begin cleansing at number 1 and proceed in order through number 7. Discard swab after each step. Finish cleansing with wash of sterile water.

RESEARCH HIGHLIGHT

Effect of the Birth Chair on Duration of Second Stage Labor and Maternal Outcome

Purpose

To determine the effect of delivering in a birth chair on duration of second stage of labor, perineal swelling, incidence of episiotomies, lacerations, hemorrhoids, and maternal blood loss.

Sample/Methodology

A prospective, quasi-experimental design was used to compare 33 primiparous women who delivered in a birth chair and 22 women who delivered on a delivery table. For this study the angle of the birth chair was tilted to a more horizontal position during or immediately after delivery in 88% of the cases.

Findings

There were no statistically significant differences between groups for mean duration of second stage or mean time bearing-down. There was a higher, but not significant incidence of episiotomies, lacerations, and hemorrhoids in the birth chair group. No difference was found in pre- and postdelivery hemoglobin and hemotocrit levels between the groups. The incidence of perineal swelling was significantly higher in the birth chair group.

Implications

Nurses caring for women who plan to deliver in a birth chair are encouraged to avoid transferring women to the chair until there is good fetal descent and presence of involuntary bearing-down.

Cattrell, BH, and Shannahan, MD: Effect of the birth chair on duration of second stage labor and maternal outcome, Nurs Res 35:364, 1986.

Birth in a Delivery Room. The woman will need assistance to move from the labor bed to the delivery table. If this is done between contractions, the mother can help, but because of her awkwardness, she cannot be rushed.

The position assumed for delivery may be (1) modified Sims' position (if this is the case, the attendant will need to support the upper leg), (2) dorsal position, or (3) lithotomy position.

The lithotomy position has been the position most commonly used for delivery in Western cultures although this is changing slowly. The lithotomy position makes it more convenient for the physician to deal with any complications that arise. For this position the buttocks are brought to the edge of the table, and the legs are placed in stirrups. Care must be taken to pad the stirrups, raise and place both legs simultaneously, and adjust the shanks of the stirrups so that the calfs of the legs are supported. There should be no pressure on the popliteal space. If the stirrups are uneven in height, the woman can develop strained ligaments in her back as she bears down. This strain causes considerable discomfort in the postdelivery period. The lower portion of the table may be dropped down and rolled back under the table.

Once the woman is positioned for delivery, the vulva is washed thoroughly with soap and water or a surgical disinfectant (Fig. 19-3). The physician or midwife dons cap and mask, scrubs hands, and puts on the sterile gown and gloves. The woman may then be draped with sterile towels and sheets. The husband or coach helps the mother remember not to touch the sterile drapes.

The circulating nurse will continue to coach and encourage the parturient. Once the woman's legs are in the stirrups, the handle grips can be used to exert counter pressure. The nurse will check FHR after every contraction and notify the physician as to the rate and regularity. The equipment for taking the BP should be readied for instant use if signs of shock develop. However, the readings are distorted (increased) by the increase in thoracic and abdominal pressures as the woman pushes. A reading will be taken after delivery before transferring the woman to the recovery room. An oxytocic medication such as Syntocinon may be prepared for administration after delivery. Observations and procedures are recorded on the chart.

Fathers are encouraged to be present at the birth of their infants if this is in keeping with their cultural expectations. The psychologic closeness of the family unit is maintained, and the father can continue the supportive care given in labor. The father needs as much opportunity as does the mother to initiate the attachment process with the baby. Studies indicate, however, that it is the continuous long-term contact between father and child that acts to cement the bonds and that there is no immediate "magic moment" of bonding.

The father is usually gowned in a clean scrub outfit and wears a cap and a mask. These supplies need to be provided in ample time for him to don them before the delivery. If the couple has decided that the father is not to be present, their decision should be respected.

Contact with parents is maintained by touch, verbal comforting instructions as to reasons for care, and sharing in parents' joy at birth of their child. The nurse notes and records the time of birth (i.e., when infant is born completely).

Mechanism of Delivery: Vertex Presentation. The nurse who is knowledgeable about the mechanism of delivery has increased skills as support person and teacher/counselor/advocate. While most of the time the delivery remains in the hands of the obstetrician or nurse-midwife, there may be a time when the nurse must assist the woman to give birth (p. 438). The nurse's knowledge of the birth process provides a basis for client preparation before and during pregnancy.

A brief review of the mechanisms of labor (see Chapter 16 and Fig. 16-18) is given to the woman. Once the cervix is fully dilated, descent occurs. The vertex advances with each contraction and recedes slightly as the contraction wanes; descent is constant, and late in the second stage the head reaches the pelvic floor. *Bulging of the perineum* occurs during the phase of descent when the fetal presenting part is distending the perineum but is not yet visible at the introitus. The occiput generally rotates anteriorly, and with voluntary bearing-down efforts, the head appears at the introitus (Fig. 19-4). Although more and more head may be seen with each push, the head "crowns" when its widest part (the biparietal diameter) distends the vulva just before birth. Immediately before delivery, the perineal musculature becomes greatly distended. If an **episiotomy** is necessary, it is done at this time to minimize soft tissue damage (p. 440). The head delivers by extension and following delivery restitutes in line with the shoulders. Interiorly the shoulders rotate into the antero-posterior diameter of the pelvis; external rotation of the head is observed. The body is born by lateral flexion.

The three phases of a spontaneous delivery of the fetus in a vertex presentation are (1) delivery of the head, (2) delivery of the shoulders, and (3) delivery of the body and extremities.

Delivery of Head. The vertex first appears, followed by the forehead, face, chin, and neck. The speed of delivery of the head must be controlled, or sudden birth of the head may cause severe lacerations through the anal sphincter or even into the rectum (p. 441). The physician or nurse-midwife controls the birth of the head by (1) applying pressure against the rectum, drawing it downward to aid in flexing the head as the back of the neck catches under the symphysis pubis; (2) then applying upward pressure from the coccygeal region (modified Ritgen's maneuver) (Fig. 19-5), to extend the head during the actual delivery, thereby protecting the musculature of the perineum; and (3) assisting the mother with voluntary control of the bearing-down efforts by coaching her to pant. In addition to protecting the maternal tissues, gradual delivery is imperative to prevent fetal intracranial injury.

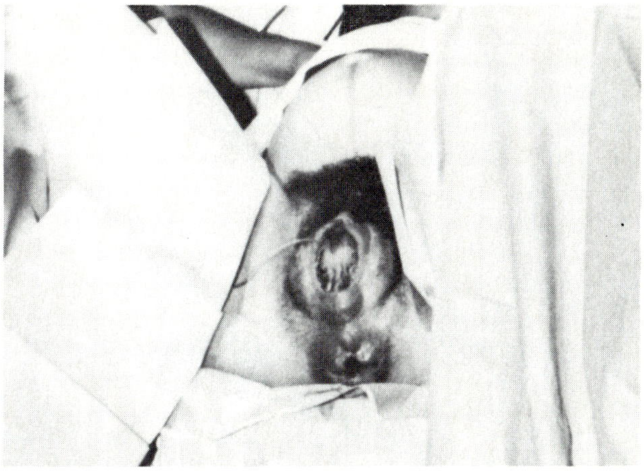

Fig. 19-4 Oval-shaped appearance of introitus. Note prominent anal hemorrhoids as head distends perineum.
Courtesy Marjorie Pyle, RNC, Lifecircle, Costa Mesa, Calif.

The membranes may not be ruptured before delivery. During birth of the head these membranes look like a hood covering the head. This hood of intact amniotic membranes covering the head during birth is known as a *caul.* In Scotland a child born with a caul is thought to be gifted with "second sight."

The umbilical cord often encircles the neck (nuchal cord) but rarely so tightly as to cause hypoxia. The cord should be slipped gently over the head (Fig. 19-6, *A*). If the loop is tight or if there is a second loop, the cord is clamped twice, severed between the clamps, and unwound from around the neck before the delivery is continued. Mucus, blood, or meconium in the nasal or oral passages may prevent the newborn from breathing. Moist gauze sponges are used to wipe the nose and mouth. A bulb syringe is inserted into the mouth and oropharynx first to aspirate contents. Next, the nares are cleared while the head is being supported (see discussion of suctioning the neonate, Chapter 22).

Delivery of Shoulders. Before the shoulders can deliver they must engage in the pelvic inlet. Internal rotation of the shoulders, accompanied by restitution (Fig. 19-7, *A*) and external rotation of the head, occurs (Fig. 19-7, *B*) the

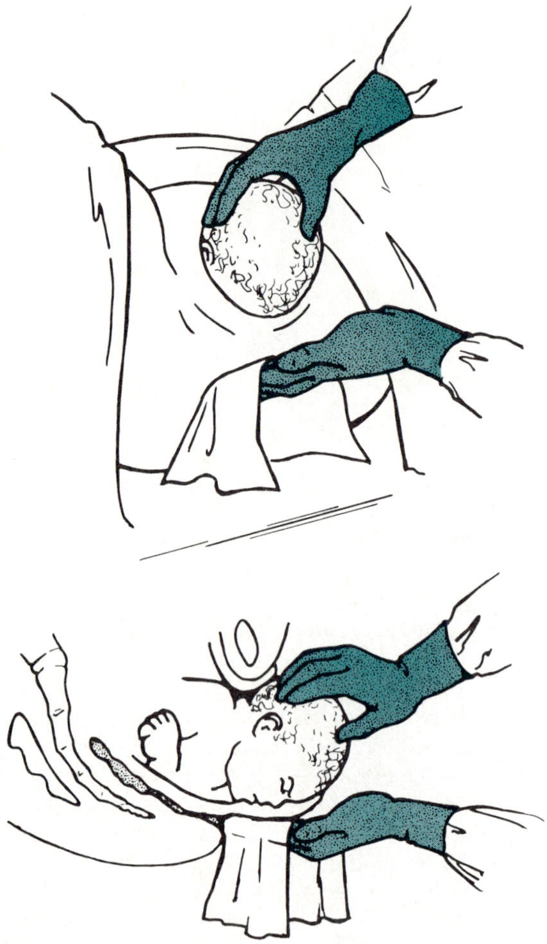

Fig. 19-5 Delivery of head by modified Ritgen maneuver. Note control to prevent rapid delivery of head.

shoulders now lie in the anterio-posterior diameter of the inlet (see also Fig. 16-18, *E, F*). The shoulders can now pass through the pelvic cavity. While awaiting rotation, the physician wipes the baby's face with sterile gauze squares and uses the bulb syringe to clear the nose of mucus, ready for the baby's first breath.

The head is drawn downward and backward by the obstetrician or midwife to help the anterior shoulder impinge beneath the arch of the symphysis and slide beneath the pubic arch. Normally the anterior shoulder is delivered with this slight downward traction toward the perineum. The posterior shoulder distends the perineum, and to prevent perineal trauma, the head is lifted toward the symphysis pubis, the shoulder being delivered over the perineum (Fig. 19-6, *B*) (Myles, 1985).

Delivery of Body and Extremities. Expulsion (Fig. 19-7, *C*) is controlled so that it occurs slowly. Lateral flexion is continued, the weight of the baby is supported by the doctor's or midwife's lower hand (Fig. 19-7, *C*), again to prevent perineal trauma. Slight rotation of the body to right or left may be used to facilitate the birth. The time of birth is considered the precise time when the whole body is out of the mother. This must be recorded on the record.

Preparation for Birth in a Birthing Room. In some hospitals, parents have the option to give birth in one room without changing rooms or beds. Expectant parents and siblings usually attend classes to prepare for the experience. The mother in Fig. 19-8 noted her progress by feeling the baby's head distend the perineum. She had chosen the side-lying position for bearing down and giving birth. Local anesthesia with episiotomy (Chapter 17) is an option in many birth rooms (Fig. 19-9).

Siblings During the Second Stage. A young child may become frightened by the intensity of the second stage. Sights such as rupture of the membranes and sounds such as their mother's moans, screams, and grunts can be unset-

A

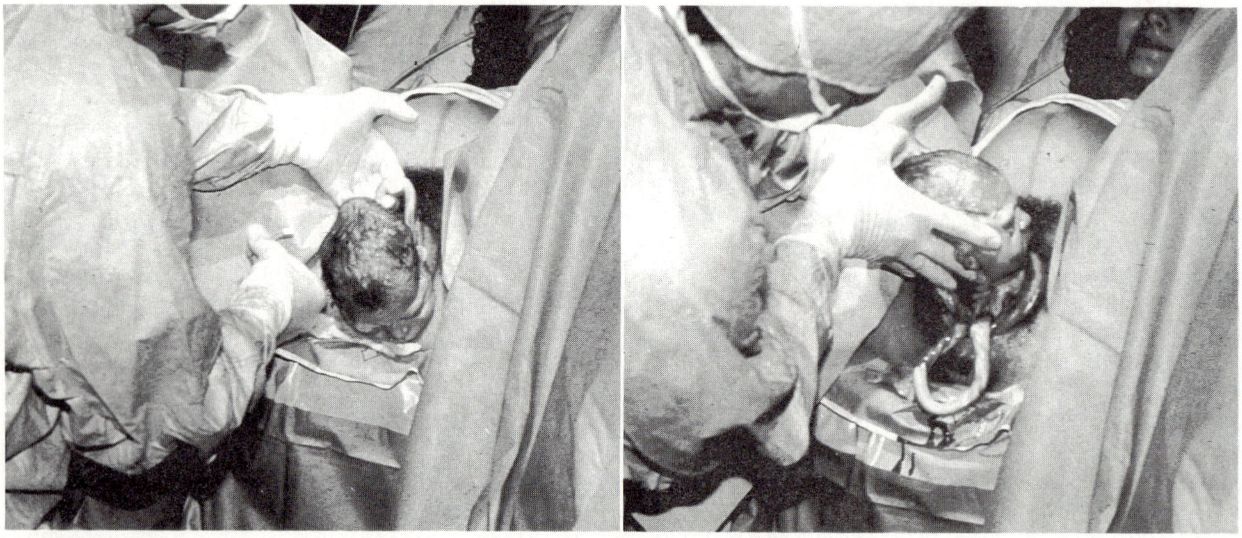

B

Fig. 19-6 A, Loosening nuchal cord. B, Birth of posterior shoulder.
Courtesy of Marjorie Pyle, RNC, Lifecircle, Costa, Mesa, Calif.

A

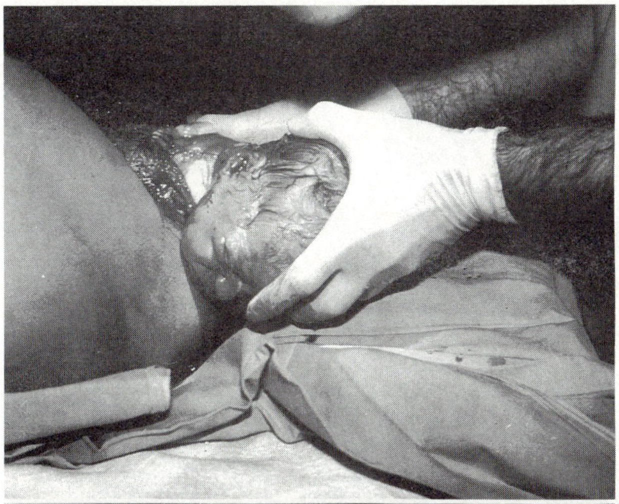

B C

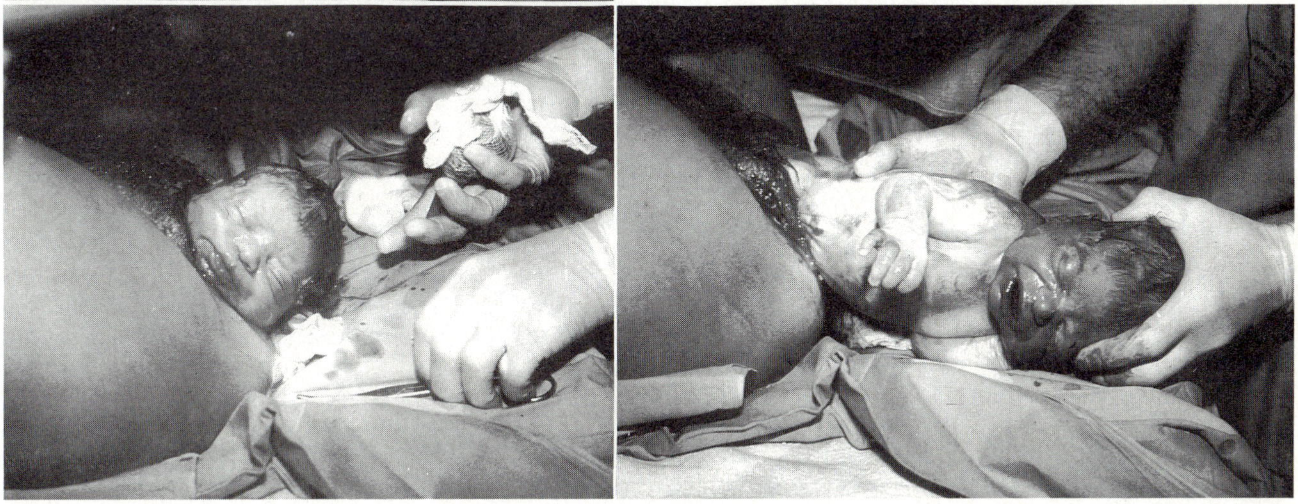

Fig. 19-7 Mechanism of labor. **A**, Restitution. **B**, External rotation. **C**, Slow expulsion of fetus/newborn. Note bulb syringe in hand in **B**.
Courtesy of Marjorie Pyle, RNC, Lifecircle, Costa Mesa, Calif.

A B

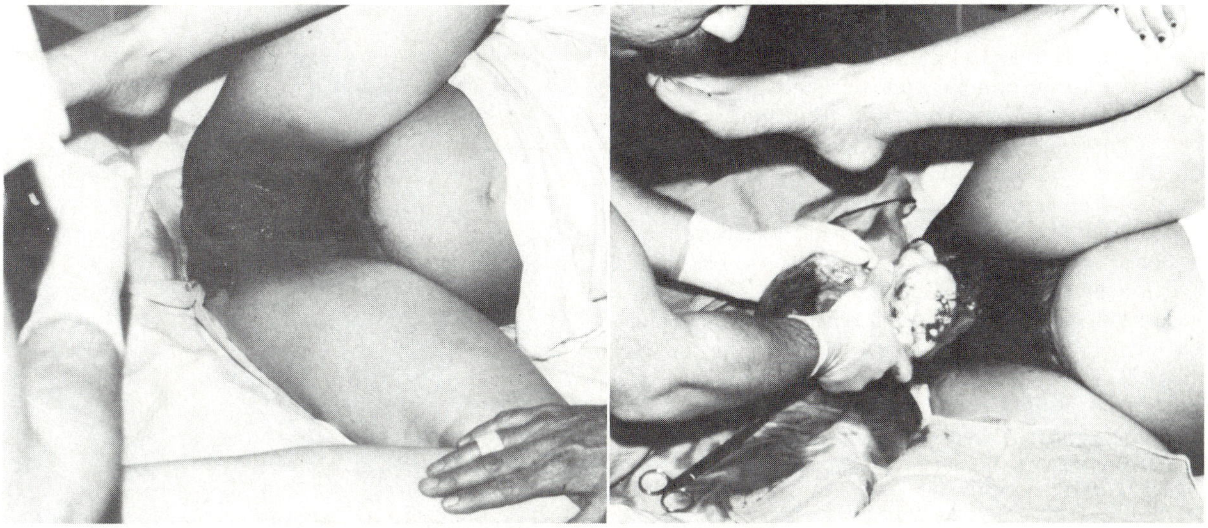

Fig. 19-8 Side-lying position. **A**, Perineal bulging. **B**, Slow expulsion of fetus/newborn.
Courtesy of Marjorie Pyle, RNC, Lifecircle, Costa Mesa, Calif.

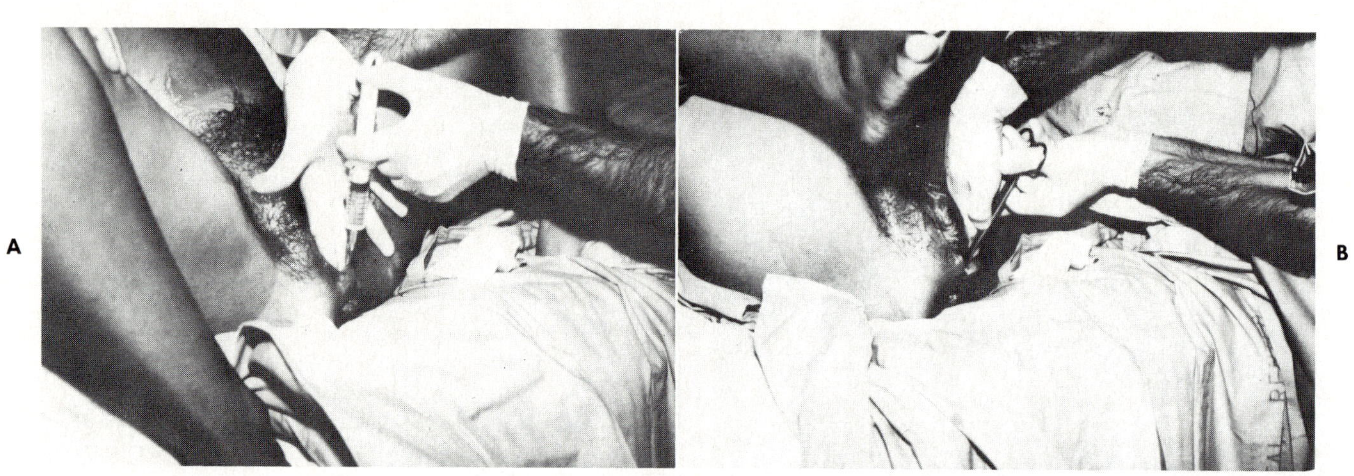

Fig. 19-9 A, Local infiltration anesthesia. B, Episiotomy.
Courtesy of Marjorie Pyle, RNC, Lifecircle, Costa Mesa, Calif.

tling (Quinlan, 1983). The child needs someone to be close and to give explanations simply and calmly. The child may want to be held. Long-term effects on young children witnessing birth are not yet known.

Evaluation

Evaluation of outcomes is an ongoing activity. During each encounter with the woman and her family during the second stage of labor the nurse evaluates the degree to which goals for care are being met. If the evaluation shows that results fall short of achieving any goal, further assessment, planning, and implementation are warranted.

THIRD STAGE OF LABOR: THE MOTHER

Separation and Delivery of Placenta. The third stage of labor extends from the birth of the baby until the delivery of the placenta. The goal in the management of the third stage of labor is the prompt separation and expulsion of the placenta, achieved in the easiest, safest manner.

The placenta is attached to the decidual layer of the thin endometrium of the basal plate by numerous, randomized, fibrous anchor villi—much like a postage stamp is attached to a sheet of postage stamps. After the fetus is delivered, in the presence of strong uterine contractions, the placental site is markedly reduced in size. This reduced size causes the anchor villi to break and the placenta to separate from its attachments. Normally the first few strong contractions 5 to 7 minutes after the birth of the baby shear the placenta from the basal plate. A placenta will not be easily freed from a flaccid (relaxed) uterus because the placental site is not reduced in size.

Assessment

Identification of the Third Stage. Placental separation is indicated by the following (Fig. 19-10):

1. A firmly contracting fundus
2. A change in the uterus from a discoid to a globular ovoid shape, as the placenta moves to the lower segment
3. A sudden gush of dark blood from the introitus
4. Apparent lengthening of the umbilical cord as the placenta gets closer to the introitus
5. A vaginal fullness (the placenta) noted on vaginal or rectal examination, or fetal membranes seen at the introitus

Whether the placenta presents by the shiny fetal surface (Schultze mechanism) or whether it turns to show first its dark roughened maternal surface (Duncan's mechanism) is of no clinical importance. At one time it was believed that Duncan's mechanism was associated with a significantly greater blood loss, but this has been disproved. After the placenta with its membranes is born, it is examined for intactness to be certain that no portion of it remains in the uterine cavity (that is, no retained fragments of the placenta or membranes) (Fig. 19-11).

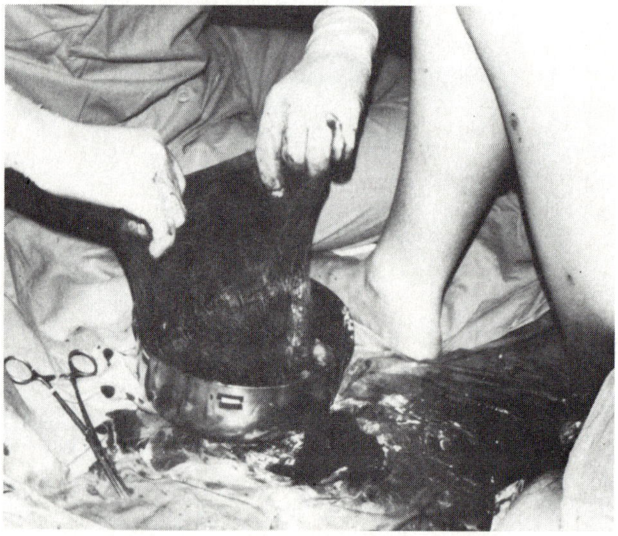

Fig. 19-11 Examination of the placenta.
Courtesy of Marjorie Pyle, RNC, Lifecircle, Costa Mesa, Calif.

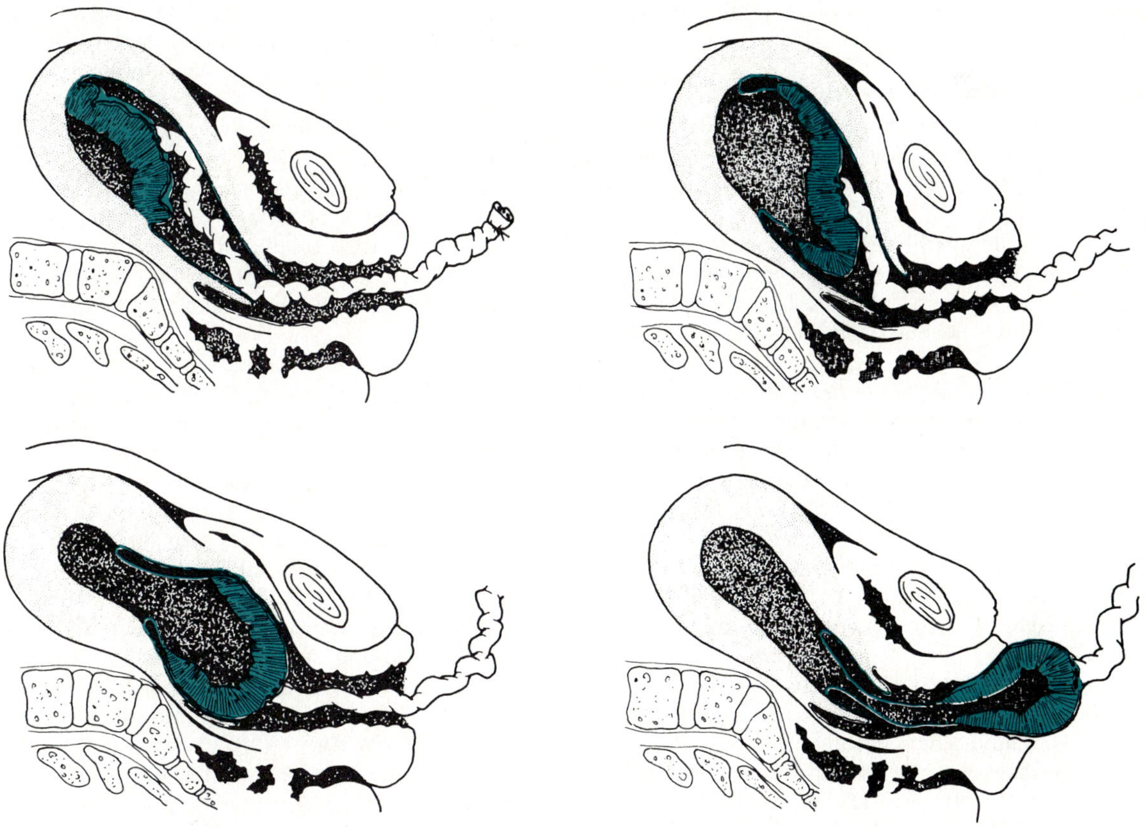

Fig. 19-10 Third stage of labor. **A**, Placenta begins by separating in central portion with retroplacental bleeding. Uterus changes from discoid to globular shape. **B**, Placenta completes separation and enters lower uterine segment. Uterus is globular in shape. **C**, Placenta enters vagina, cord is seen to lengthen, and there may be increase in bleeding. **D**, Expression (birth) of placenta and completion of third stage.

Maternal Physical Status. Physiologic changes following delivery are profound. The cardiac output is increased rapidly as maternal circulation to the placenta ceases and the pooled blood from the lower extremities is mobilized. The pulse rate slows in response to the change in cardiac output. Pulse rates tend to remain slightly slower than before pregnancy during the first 7 to 10 days after delivery.

The blood pressure usually returns to the woman's usual nonpregnant levels shortly after delivery. Several factors contribute to an elevated blood pressure: the excitement of the second stage, certain medications, and the time of day (blood pressure is highest during the late afternoon). Analgesics and anesthetics may lead to hypotension in the hour following birth.

Even as the physician or nurse-midwife is completing the third stage of labor, the nurse observes the mother for signs of an altered level of consciousness (LOC) or alteration in respirations. Because of the rapid cardiovascular changes (e.g., the increased intracranial pressure during pushing and the rapid increase in cardiac output), this period represents the risk of *rupture of a preexisting cerebral aneurysm* and of pulmonary emboli. The risk of *pulmonary amniotic fluid emboli* arises from another source as well. As the placenta separates, there is a possibility of amniotic fluid entering the maternal circulation if the uterine musculature does not contract rapidly and well. The incidence of these possible complications is small; however, the alert nurse can contribute to their immediate recognition and the prompt initiation of therapy.

Nursing Diagnoses

Before establishing nursing diagnoses, the nurse correlates the events of the third stage and the mother's physical and emotional responses to the third stage of labor. The following is an example of a nursing diagnosis: ineffective individual (mother) coping related to knowledge deficit of sensations to expect during the third stage of labor.

Planning

Planning for this stage focuses on the woman's rapid physiologic changes and timely intact delivery of the placenta. Concomitantly, the emotional environment of the family is maintained.

Goals

1. A third stage that is physically safe for the mother and newborn
2. A cheerful, comfortable, and supportive environment

3. The presence of family members of the mother's choice

Implementation

In the Delivery Area. To assist the mother in delivery of the placenta, the nurse or physician instructs the woman to push when signs of separation have occurred. If an oxytocin medication is ordered, the nurse administers the medication in the dosage and by the route indicated by the physician (or nurse-midwife). If possible, the placenta should be expelled by maternal effort during a uterine contraction but assistance such as *alternative compression* and *elevation of the fundus,* plus *minimum,* controlled traction of the umbilical cord may be employed to facilitate delivery of the placenta and membranes. When the third stage is complete and tears or episiotomy are sutured (p. 440), the vulval area is gently cleansed with sterile water by the physician (or nurse-midwife). The circulating nurse (or the physician) performs the following:

1. Applies a sterile perineal pad
2. Removes the drapes if used, or places dry linen under the buttocks
3. Repositions the delivery table or bed
4. Lowers the mother's legs simultaneously from the stirrups if she is in lithotomy position
5. Assists the woman onto her bed if she is to be transferred from the delivery area to the recovery area (the nurse will need assistance to move the woman from a delivery table onto a bed if the woman has had anesthesia and does not have full use of her lower extremities)
6. Dresses the woman in a clean gown and covers her with a warmed blanket
7. Raises the side rails of the bed during the transfer (in some hospitals, the mother is given the baby to hold during the transfer; in some hospitals, the father carries the baby; in other hospitals, the nurse carries the baby either to the nursery or to the recovery area for the duration of the mother's recovery period)

NOTE: The nurse is to observe excellent body mechanics to avoid injury to own back or other body structure.

If the woman labors, gives birth, and recovers in the same bed and room, she is refreshed as described above. After the woman is discharged, the delivery area is cleaned as necessary.

The Family During the Third Stage. Most parents enjoy being able to handle, hold, explore, and examine the baby right after birth. The newborn is placed on the mother's abdomen, which has been draped with a warm receiving blanket. Both parents can assist with the thorough drying of the infant.

The mother may cut the cord or the cord may be left long enough so that the father can clamp it and cut off the extra portion. The mother can hold the infant next to her skin to maintain the baby's body heat and provide skin contact; care must be taken to keep the head warm as well. It is the nurse's responsibility to make sure the baby is kept warm and is in no danger of slipping from the parent's grasp.

Many women wish to begin to breast-feed their infants at this time to take advantage of the infant's alert state and to stimulate the production of oxytocin that promotes contraction of the uterus. Others wish to wait until the infant, mother, father, and older siblings are together in the recovery room.

While the physician carries out the postdelivery vaginal examination and, if necessary, repairs the episiotomy, the mother usually feels discomfort. Therefore, while the process is being completed, the infant can be weighed and measured, wrapped in warm blankets, and given to the father to hold.

Parent-newborn Relationships. The mother's reaction to the sight of her newborn may range from excited outbursts of laughing, talking, and even crying to apparent apathy. A polite smile and nod may acknowledge the comments of nurses and physicians. Occasionally the reaction is one of anger or indifference; the mother turns away from the baby, concentrates on her own pain, and sometimes makes hostile comments. These varying reactions can arise from pleasure, exhaustion, or deep disappointment. Whatever the reaction and cause may be, the mother needs continuing acceptance and support from all the staff. A written form accompanying the baby's chart should record the parents' reaction at birth. How do parents *look?* What do they *say?* What do they *do?*

Some warning signs in parent-child relationships apparent immediately following delivery are listed in the box below.

Siblings, who may have appeared only remotely interested in the final phases of the second stage, experience renewed interest and excitement and should be encouraged to hold the new family member (Fig. 19-12).

Parents are responsive to praise of their newborn. Many require reassurance that the blue appearance of the baby after delivery is normal until respirations are well established. The reason for the molding of the baby's head must be reviewed with parents. Information about hospital routine as to future parent-child contacts can be repeated. The hospital staff, by their interest and concern, can do much

WARNING SIGNS: PARENT-NEWBORN RELATIONSHIPS IMMEDIATELY FOLLOWING DELIVERY

1. Passive reaction, either verbal or nonverbal (parents do not touch, hold, or examine baby or talk in affectionate terms or tones about baby)
2. Hostile reaction, either verbal or nonverbal (parents make inappropriate verbalization, glances, or disparaging remarks about physical characteristics of child)
3. Disappointment over sex of baby
4. No eye contact
5. Nonsupportive interaction between parents (if intereaction seems dubious, talk to nurse and physician involved with delivery for further information)

Reproduced by permission from Gray, JD, Christy, AC, Dean, GD, and Kempe, CH: Prediction and prevention of child abuse, Semin Perinatol 3:95 Jan 1979

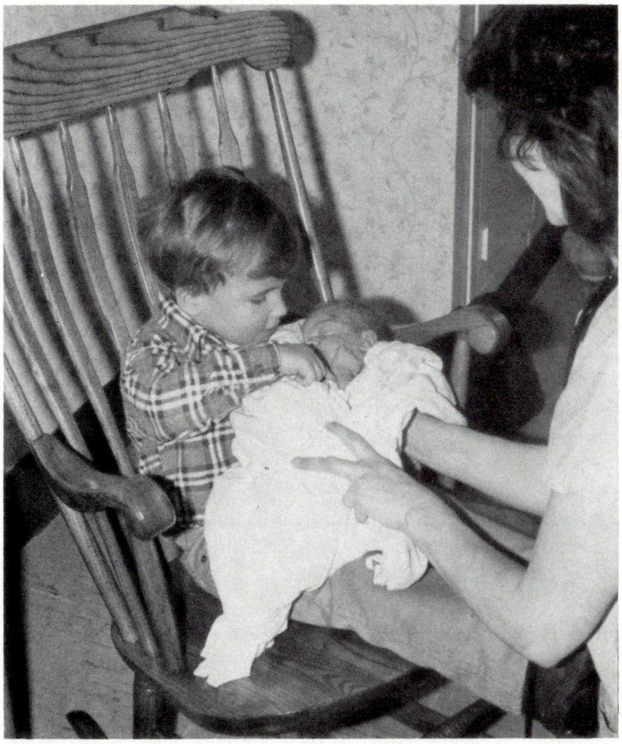

Fig. 19-12 Nurse helps big brother become acquainted with new baby sister.

to make this a satisfying experience for both parents.

Evaluation

Evaluation of outcomes is an ongoing activity. During each encounter with the new mother during the third stage of labor, the nurse evaluates the degree to which goals for care are being met. If the evaluation shows that results fall short of achieving any goal, further assessment, planning, and implementation are warranted.

THIRD STAGE OF LABOR: THE NEWBORN

Assessment

Before birth, the nurse evaluates the maternal history, including labor, to identify potential problems for the neonate. Although an extensive examination will be performed later, a minimum examination of the neonate is completed immediately following birth. The physician or nurse performs the following assessments and records findings (Fig. 19-13):

1. Assesses respirations and neonate's ability to keep airway clear
2. Estimates infant's health status using Apgar rating at 1 and 5 minutes of age (Fig. 19-13)
3. Examines the cord for anomalies and verifies the presence of two arteries and one vein (Fig. 19-14), checks cord clamp is in place (Figs. 19-15 and 19-16)

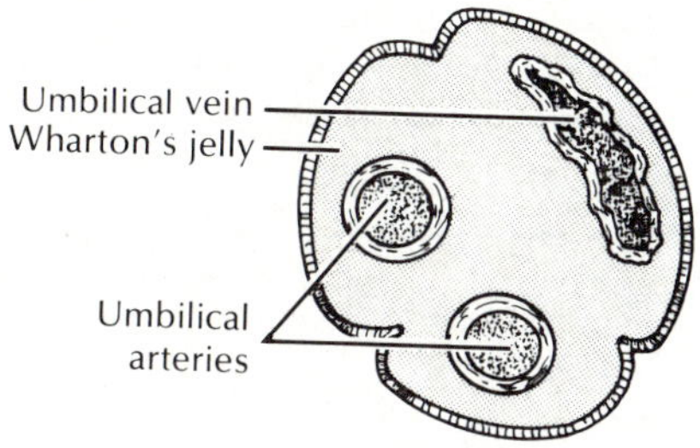

Fig. 19-14 Cross section of umbilical cord. Note collapsed appearance of thin-walled umbilical vein and contour of thicker, muscular-walled arteries.

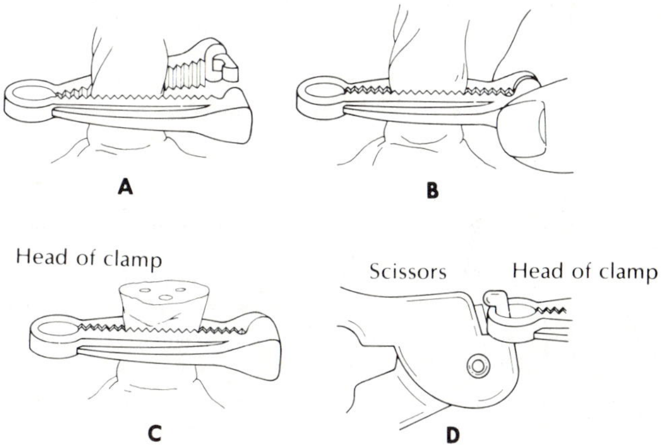

Fig. 19-15 Hollister cord clamp. **A**, Position clamp close to umbilicus. **B**, Secure cord. **C**, Cut cord. **D**, Remove clamp, using scissors, after cord dries (about 24 hours).

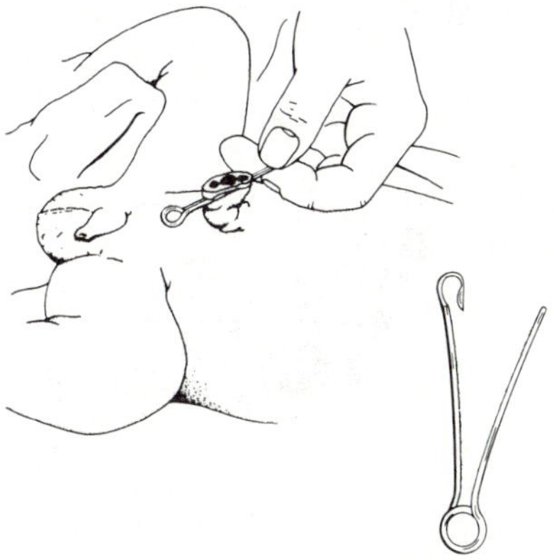

Fig. 19-16 Hesseltine cord clamp.

4. Collects cord blood from placenta for analysis (Rh factor, blood grouping, and hematocrit)
5. Assesses weight, length, and gestational age
6. Notes passage of meconium or urine
7. Performs minimum physical examination and assessment of neonate such as the following (see Chapter 21 for more in-depth discussion and techniques):
   a. *External:* notes skin color, staining, peeling, or wast-

Fig. 19-13 Physical assessment of the newborn.
Modified from form used by Kaiser-Permanente Hospital, Santa Clara, Calif.

Addressograph

Mother's room number ______

Date ______

Antepartum

(1) G ______ ______
(2) EDC ______
(3) ABO ______ ______
(4) Titre ______
(5) VDRL ______
(6) Br ______ Bottle ______

(7) RI* ______ NRI ______
(8) PPTL† ______
(9) Adoption ______
Comments ______

Complications

(1) Family history of bleeding ______
(2) Preeclamptic ______
(3) Gestational diabetic ______
(4) Prenatal meds ______
(5) Pertinent history ______

Intrapartum

(1) Induction or augmentation
(2) Amniotic fluid
(A) PROM § ______ hr.
(B) Hydramnios ______
(C) Mec. stained ______ Heavy ______ Light ______ Terminal ______

(3) Monitored‡ ______ ED ______ V ______ LD ______ Baseline ______
(4) Fetal blood sample X ______ Reason ______
(5) Maternal problems ______
(6) Pertinent meds & time ______
(7) Comments ______

Postnatal

(1) Sex: M ______ F ______
(2) Del. date ______
(3) Time ______ AM ______ ______
(4) Weight ______ g
______ lb ______ oz
(5) Length ______ cm ______ in
(6) ID band # ______
(7) Void ______ Stool ______
(8) Eye prophylaxis: erythromycin ______
(9) Cord around neck X
1 2 3
(10) # vessels 2 3
(11) Method of delivery
(A) Spontaneous
Mid ______ Low ______
(B) Forceps
(C) Breech ______
(D) C/B ______
(why)

Apgar score

	0	1	2	1 min	5 min
Heart rate	Absent	Less than 100	Over 100		
Resp. effort	Absent	Slow irreg.	Good cry		
Muscle tone	Limp	Some flexion	Active motion		
Reflex irritability	No response	Grimace	Cry		
Color	Pale	Body pink, ext. blue	All pink		

(12) Placenta
(A) Normal ______
(B) Small ______
(C) Abruptio ______ Previa ______
(D) Other ______

(13) Comments ______

Signature ______

* RI, rooming in; NRI, not rooming in.
† PPTL, postpartum tubal ligation (or occlusion).
‡ Monitored (electronic): ED, early deceleration; V, variable deceleration; LD, late deceleration.
§ *PROM*, premature rupture of membranes; *G*, gravida; *P*, para; *BR*, breast; *Mec.*, meconium; *C/B*, cesarean birth

Fig. 19-13—cont'd Physical assessment of the newborn.
Modified from form used by Kaiser-Permanente Hospital, Santa Clara, Calif.

Postnatal resuscitation

(1) Pediatrician: Notified ____ AM ____ PM ____
In attendance ____
(2) O_2 ____ Mask ____ Bag ____
(3) Oral suction ____ Mec ____ Mucus ____
(4) Delees suction ____
(5) Intubation: Successful ____ Unsuccessful ____
(A) Suctioned: Clear ____
Thick ____
Mec. ____ Thin ____
(B) Lavaged ____
(6) Cardiac massage ____
(7) Med and route ____
(8) Comments ____

Nursery

(1) Admit to nsy* ____ @ ____ (AM/PM or military time)
(2) Admit to ICN ____ @ ____ AM ____ PM
(or transferred via ____
to regional center) ____
(3) MD notified, i.e. problem/client ____
____ AM ____
____ PM ____
(4) Admission v.s.: T ____ P ____ R ____
(5) Est. gest. age ____ wk
(6) Color ____
(7) Cry ____
(8) O_2 ____
(9) Suctioned ____
(10) Head ____ Chest ____
(11) Comments ____

Signature

Item	Findings	Clinical significance
Posture		
Measurements Weight		
Length		
Head circumference		
Chest circumference		
Vital signs Blood pressure		

**nsy*, nursery; *ICN*, intensive care nursery

ing (dysmaturity); considers length of nails and development of creases on soles of feet; checks for presence or absence of breast tissue; assesses nasal patency by closing one nostril at a time while observing the infant's respirations and color; notes meconium staining of cord, skin, fingernails, or amniotic fluid (may indicate fetal hypoxia; offensive odor may indicate intrauterine infection)

   b. *Chest:* palpates for site of maximum cardiac impulse and auscultates for rate and quality of heart tones, compares and notes character of respirations and presence of rales or rhonchi by holding stethoscope in each axilla
   c. *Abdomen:* verifies presence of a domed abdomen and absence of anomalies (Chapter 21)
   d. *Neurologic:* checks muscle tone and reflex reaction and appraises Moro's reflex (at 1 and 5 minutes); palpates large fontanel for fullness or bulge; notes by palpation the presence and sizes of the sutures and fontanels
   e. *Other observations:* notes gross structural malformations obvious at birth (described in general terms and recorded on delivery record)

8. Assesses parents' response to newborn and to each other; assessment of the parent-child relationship is discussed under the nursing care of the mother during the fourth stage of labor

Nursing Diagnoses

Nursing diagnoses lend direction to the type of nursing actions needed to implement a plan of care. Before establishing nursing diagnoses, the nurse analyzes the significance of findings collected during assessment. Following are some examples of nursing diagnoses:

- Ineffective airway clearance related to
  - Airway obstruction with mucus and amniotic fluid
- Ineffective thermoregulation related to
  - Environmental factors
- Altered health maintenance related to
  - Congenital disorders

Planning

During this important step, goals are set in client-centered terms. The goals are prioritized. Nursing actions are selected, with the client where appropriate, to meet the goals. The speed and accuracy with which planning is accomplished depends on the nurse's level of competence (Chapter 2).

Goals

1. A clear airway is maintained
2. Cold stress is prevented
3. A safe environment is maintained
4. Any potential or actual problem that may require immediate medical intervention is identified
5. The parents' attachment to or acquaintance with the neonate is facilitated

Implementation

Events move rapidly during this time period. Assessment must be followed quickly by appropriate implementation. The physician/midwife may be concentrating on the progress of the third stage for the mother. The nurse assumes responsibility and accountability for accurate assessment of and timely intervention for the newborn. A summary of nursing interventions with the rationales is provided in Table 19-3.

Abnormal Neonatal Breathing. Initiation and maintenance of respiration is the top priority. Abnormal breathing must be recognized and treated (see danger signs box, p. 517, and emergency procedure, p. 523, Chapter 22).

General Nursing Actions. Nursing actions that usually apply to this period include a variety of activities. Among them are actions relevant to the care of the **airway, cord clamping, attachment and warmth, Apgar score, eye prophylaxis, measurement of weight and length,** and **identification.** A summary of these nursing actions and the rationale for each are given in Table 19-3.

Eye Prophylaxis. Instillation of a prophylactic agent in the eyes of all newborns is mandatory in the United States. In some Canadian institutions the parents may sign a form refusing eye treatment. Wahlberg's (1985) research in Sweden has shown that eye prophylaxis is unnecessary except for infants deemed "at risk" for venereally transmitted eye infection. The agent used for prophylaxis varies according to hospital protocols. The medication and the method of instillation into the conjunctival sacs is outlined in the box on p. 438, and depicted in Fig. 19-17.

Evaluation

Evaluation of nursing care and outcomes is an ongoing activity in the care of both mother and baby. During each encounter with the new mother the neonate, and the fam-

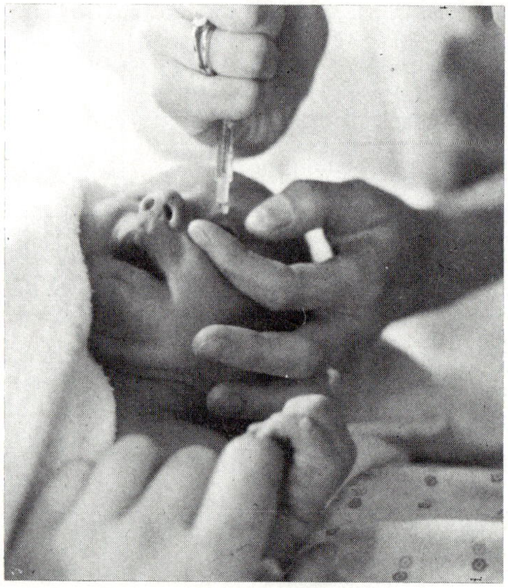

Fig. 19-17 Instillation of ophthalmic erythromycin drops using needleless syringe. Drops are instilled into conjunctival sac.

Table 19-3 *Nursing Care of the Neonate: Implementation and Rationales*

Implementation	Rationale
Airway	
Hold baby with head lowered (10 to 15 degrees).	Uses gravity to help remove fluids.
Suction oral pharynx with a small bulb syringe as soon as head is born.	Expedites drainage and prevents aspiration of amniotic fluid, mucus, and blood (maternal).
Suction nares next.	Prevents inspiration following stimulation of nares before mouth is clear.
Avoid deep suctioning with a catheter, if possible.	May cause bradycardia or laryngospasm or both.
Avoid suspending neonate by the ankles.	Results in hyperextension of baby whose entire development occurred in the flexed position (may be detrimental or painful).
Cord Clamping	
Immediately following birth, neonate is kept at about the same level as the uterus, until cord clamp is applied or until cord has stopped pulsating. Cord pulsations usually cease within seconds after respiration is initiated.	If neonate is held above level of uterus, allows gravity to drain blood to the placenta. If neonate is held below level of uterus, allows gravity to drain blood from placenta to neonate.
Without "stripping" ("milking") it, the cord is clamped close to the umbilicus approximately 30 seconds after birth if neonate appears normal and mature (Figs. 19-15 and 19-16).	Some parents want the baby to receive an extra supply of blood and advocate "stripping" the cord toward the baby. Ordinarily it is unwise to strip the cord before clamping and cutting because postdelivery red blood cell destruction, which normally occurs neonatally, will be increased and hyperbilirubinemia (see Chapter 40) may ensue. In addition, polycythemia (increased number of red blood cells) increases blood viscosity, leading to cardiopulmonary problems in the neonate.
The cord is clamped 8 to 10 cm from the umbilicus if there is a possibility for exchange transfusion (see erythroblastosis, Chapter 40).	Permits access to umbilical vessels.
Assess cord for two arteries and one vein (Fig. 19-14).	Alerts physician for need of further assessment if there is only one artery (Chapter 40)
Attachment and Warmth	
If neonate is full term, of adequate weight for gestational age, and in good condition, dry quickly and place her or him on mother's abdomen and cover both of them with a warm blanket. Or wrap neonate in warm blanket first.	Facilitates attachment, especially if there is skin-to-skin contact. Assures and relaxes mother. Prevents cold stress to neonate.
Caution parents to keep neonate's head covered.	Prevents cold stress to neonate (Chapter 22).
Apgar Score	
Appraise neonate at 1 minute and again at 5 minutes. Use the Apgar scoring method (Fig. 19-13).	Permits a rapid and semiquantitative assessment based on five signs indicative of the physiologic state of the neonate (Fig. 19-13): heart rate, based on auscultation with stethoscope; respiration, based on observed movement of chest wall, muscle tone, based on degree of flexion and movement of the extremities; reflex ability, based on response to gentle slaps on the soles of the feet; and color (pallid, cyanotic, or pink). The 5-minute score correlates with neonatal mortality and morbidity.
Eye Prophylaxis	
Instill medication in conjunctival sacs (Fig. 19-17). OR If family objects to eye prophylaxis, physician requests parent(s) to sign an informed consent. Note parents' refusal in neonate's record. May delay instillation safely until the fourth stage (about 2 hours after birth).	Meets the legal requirement for all newborns to have treatment to prevent conjunctival infections: gonococcal, pneumococcal, or chlamydial. Such infections, known as ophthalmia neonatorum, can lead to varying degrees of blindness. Recommendations of the National Society to Prevent Blindness, Committee on Ophthalmia Neonatorum, June 15, 1981, are given on p. 438.
Newborn Weight and Length	
Weigh and measure the neonate. This may be delayed until the fourth stage.	Pleases parents who are anxious to know and who want to spread the word to relatives and friends.
Identification	
Identify the neonate by one of a number of techniques *before mother or baby leaves the delivery area.*	Although rare, an occasional mix-up in the identity of newborns occurs. Identification and care to check both mother's and baby's ID numbers prevent unnecessary anxiety and legal complications.

RECOMMENDATIONS FOR NEONATAL TREATMENT OF CONJUNCTIVA

1. Instillation of a prophylactic agent in the eyes of all newborn infants.
2. Acceptable prophylactic agents that prevent **gonococcal ophthalmia neonatorum** include the following:
   a. Silver nitrate solution (1%) in single-dose ampules (this substance may cause chemical conjunctivitis)
   b. Erythromycin (0.5%) ophthalmic ointment or drops in single-use tubes or ampules
   c. Tetracycline (1%) ophthalmic ointment or drops in single-use tubes or ampules
3. Acceptable prophylactic agents that prevent **chlamydial ophthalmia neonatorum** include the following:
   a. Erythromycin (0.5%) ophthalmic ointment or drops in single-use tubes or ampules
   b. Tetracycline (1%) ophthalmic ointment or drops in single-use tubes or ampules
   Silver nitrate does not prevent chlamydial infections.
4. Prophylactic agents should be given shortly after birth. A delay of up to 1 hour* is probably acceptable and may facilitate initial maternal-infant bonding.
5. The importance of performing the instillation so the agent reaches all parts of the conjunctival surface is stressed. This can be accomplished by careful manipulation of the lids with fingers to ensure spreading of the agent. If medication strikes only the eyelids and lid margins but fails to reach the cornea, the instillation should be repeated. Prophylaxis should be applied as follows:
   a. **Silver nitrate†**
      (1) Carefully clean eyelids and surrounding skin with sterile cotton, which may be moistened with sterile water.
      (2) Gently open baby's eyelids and instill two drops of silver nitrate on the conjunctival sac. Allow the silver nitrate to run across the whole conjunctival sac. Carefully manipulate lids to ensure spread of the drops. Repeat in the other eye. Use two ampules, one for each eye.
      (3) After 1 minute, gently wipe excess silver nitrate from eyelids and surrounding skin with sterile water. *Do not irrigate eyes.*
   b. **Ophthalmic ointment (erythromycin or tetracycline)**
      (1) Carefully clean eyelids and surrounding skin with sterile cotton, which may be moistened with sterile water.
      (2) Gently open baby's eyelids and place a thin line of ointment, at least 1 to 2 cm (½ in), along the junction of the bulbar and palpebral conjunctiva of the lower lid. Try to cover the whole lower conjunctival area. Carefully manipulate lids to ensure spread of the ointment. *Be careful not to touch the eyelid or eyeball with the tip of the tube.* Repeat in other eye. Use one tube per baby.
      (3) After 1 minute, gently wipe excess ointment from eyelids and surrounding skin with sterile water. *Do not irrigate eyes.*
   c. **Ophthalmic drops (erythromycin or tetracycline)**
      (1) Apply as for silver nitrate.
6. The eye should not be irrigated after instillation of a prophylactic agent. Irrigation may reduce the efficacy of prophylaxis and probably does not decrease the incidence of chemical conjunctivitis.
7. Infants born to mothers infected with agents that cause ophthalmia neonatorum may require special attention and systemic therapy as well as prophylaxis. A single dose of aqueous crystalline pencillin G, 50,000 units/kg body weight for term and 20,000 units for low-birth-weight infants should be administered intravenously to infants born to mothers with gonorrhea.
8. The detection and appropriate treatment of infections in pregnant women, which may result in ophthalmia neonatorum, are encouraged.
9. All physicians and hospitals should be required to report cases of ophthalmia neonatorum and etiologic agents to state and local health departments so that incidence data may be obtained to determine the effectiveness of the control measures.

From National Society to Prevent Blindness, NSPB Committee on Ophthalmia Neonatorum, June 15, 1981.
*Centers for Disease Control, Atlanta, specifies up to 2 hours' delay is safe.
†Since June 1986, Canadian Hospitals have not recommended the use of silver nitrate.

ily. During the third stage of labor, the nurse evaluates the degree to which goals for care are being met. If the evaluation shows that results fall short of achieving any goal, further assessment, planning, and implementation are warranted.

EMERGENCY CHILDBIRTH: WHEN THE NURSE MUST ASSIST THE MOTHER TO GIVE BIRTH

Even under the best of circumstances there will probably come a time when the maternity nurse will be required to deliver an infant without medical assistance. Consider the precipitous multipara who arrives at the community hospital fully dilated in the middle of the night. As it is impossible to prevent an impending delivery, the maternity nurse needs to be able to function independently and to be skilled in safely delivering a vertex fetus.

Emergency Birth of Fetus in Vertex Presentation

The following measures are necessary for the emergency birth of a fetus in the vertex position:

1. The woman will usually assume the position most suitable for her. If she is in a bed and there is time, elevate the head of the bed about 45 degrees. This position, in addition to facilitating perfusion of the uterus, allows you to maintain eye-to-eye contact with the woman. Occasionally the woman will assume the crawling position, on hands and knees. Some women will stand and lean over a bed or their support person's shoulder. Others will assume a side-lying position.
2. Reassure the woman verbally with eye-to-eye contact and a calm, relaxed manner. If there is someone else available (e.g., the father), that person could help support her in position, assist with coaching, and compliment her on her efforts.

3. Wash your hands with soap and water or wash-and-dry pledgets if possible.
4. Place under woman's buttocks whatever clean material or clean newspapers are available.
5. Avoid touching the vaginal area to decrease the possibility of infection. (If there is time, scrub your hands and fingernails for 5 minutes before touching the parturient.) If hands are clean or sterile gloves are available, massage or support perineum as needed.
6. The perineum thins and distends. As the head begins to crown, the birth attendant should do the following:
   a. Tear the amniotic membrane (caul) if it is still intact.
   b. Instruct the woman to pant or pant-blow, thus avoiding the urge to push.
   c. Place the flat side of the hand on the exposed fetal head and apply *gentle* pressure toward the vagina to prevent the head from "popping out" (see Fig. 19-5). The mother may participate by placing her hand under yours on the emerging head.
   NOTE: Rapid delivery of the fetal head must be prevented because (1) it is followed by a rapid change of pressure within the molded fetal skull, which may result in dural or subdural tears, and (2) it may cause vaginal or perineal lacerations.
7. Instruct the mother to pant or pant-blow as you check for an umbilical cord. If the cord is around the neck, try to slip it up over the baby's head or pull *gently* to get some slack so that it can slip down over the shoulders.
8. Support the fetal head as restitution (external rotation) occurs. After restitution, with one hand on each side of the baby's head, exert *gentle* pressure downward so that the anterior shoulder emerges under the symphysis pubis and acts as a fulcrum; then as *gentle* pressure is exerted in the opposite direction, the posterior shoulder, which has passed over the sacrum and coccyx, is delivered.
9. Be alert! Hold the baby securely because the rest of the body may deliver quickly. The baby will be slippery!
10. Cradle the baby's head and back in one hand and the buttocks in the other, keeping the head down to drain away the mucus. Use a bulb syringe to remove mucus if one is available.
   NOTE: Do not hold the baby upside down by the ankles because to do so (1) hyperextends the spine, which has been flexed since conception; (2) increases intracranial pressure and the danger of capillary rupture; (3) may cause direct tissue trauma to the ankles; and (4) increases the possibility of dropping a wet, slippery baby.
11. Dry the baby rapidly (to prevent rapid heat loss), keeping the baby at the same level as the mother's uterus.
   NOTE: Keep the baby at the same level to prevent gravity flow of baby's blood to or from the placenta and the resultant hypovolemia or hypervolemia. Also, do not "milk" the cord: hypervolemia can cause respiratory distress initially or hyperbilirubinemia subsequently (Chapter 40); and if isoimmunization has occurred, the baby may receive an additional inoculation of harmful antibodies (e.g., anti-Rh positive or anti-A or anti-B antibodies).
12. As soon as the infant is crying, place the baby on mother's abdomen, cover baby (remember to keep head warm too) with her clothing, and have her cuddle baby. Compliment her (them) on a job well done and on the baby if appropriate. (If something appears to be the matter with the baby, do not lie!) She may wish to expose the part of the baby that will be touching her skin for skin-to-skin contact.
   NOTE: Soon after the Wharton's jelly in the cord is exposed to cool air and shrinks and the infant cries, the umbilical vessels stop pulsating and the blood flow ceases. The baby's presence on the mother's abdomen stimulates the release of oxytocin from the posterior pituitary and thus stimulates uterine contractions, which aid in placental separation.
13. *Wait* for the placenta to separate; *do not* tug on the cord.
   NOTE: Injudicious traction may tear the cord, separate the placenta, or invert the uterus. Signs of placental separation include (1) a slight gush of dark blood from the introitus, (2) lengthening of the cord, and (3) change in uterine contour from discoid to globular shape.
14. Instruct the mother to push to deliver the separated placenta. Gently ease out the placental membranes, using an up-and-down motion until membranes are removed. To minimize complications do not cut the cord without proper clamps or ties and a sterile cutting tool and inspect the placenta for intactness. Place the baby on the placenta and wrap the two together for additional warmth.
   NOTE: There is no hurry to cut the cord. The infant will not lose blood through the placenta because the cord circulation ceases (clots) within minutes of birth. If a cord tie is needed, use technique in Fig. 19-18.
15. Check the firmness of the uterus. Gently massage the uterus and demonstrate to the mother how she can massage her own uterus properly.
16. Clean the area under the mother's buttocks.
17. Prevent or minimize hemorrhage.

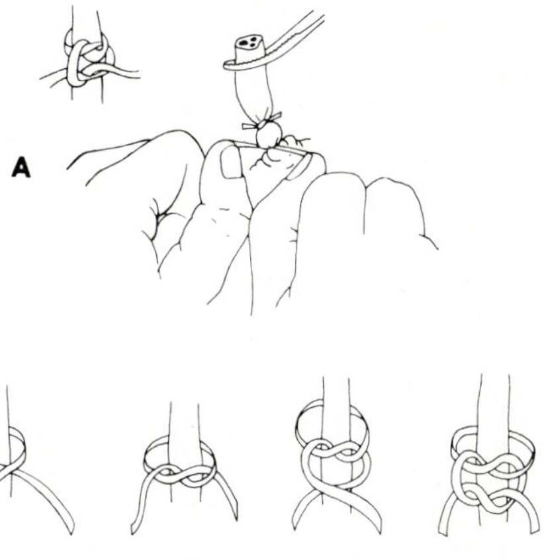

Fig. 19-18 Technique of tying off umbilical cord using, **A**, soft flat tape to prevent cutting through cord as it is drawn tight and, **B**, square knot to prevent slippage.

a. Hemorrhage from uterine atony.
   (1) *Gently* massage fundus to stimulate uterine musculature to contract.
   NOTE: Overstimulation may fatigue the myometrium and cause atony.
   (2) Put the baby to the breast as soon as possible. Sucking or nuzzling and licking the breast stimulate the release of oxytocin from the posterior pituitary.
   NOTE: If the baby does not nurse, manually stimulate the mother's breasts.
   (3) If medical assistance is delayed, do not allow the mother's bladder to become distended.
   (4) Expel any clots from her uterus.
   NOTE: The fundus should be firm to prevent accidental inversion during this procedure. While holding the bottom of the uterus just above the symphysis pubis, apply gentle pressure on the firm fundus downward toward the vagina.

b. Hemorrhage from perineal lacerations.
   (1) Apply a clean pad to the perineum.
   (2) Instruct the mother to press her thighs together.

18. Comfort or reassure the mother and her family or friends. Keep her and the baby warm. Give her fluids if available and tolerated.
19. If this is a multiple birth, identify the infants in order of birth.
20. Make notations on the birth.
    a. Fetal presentation and position.
    b. Presence of cord around neck or other parts and number of times cord encircles part.
    c. Color, character, and amount of amniotic fluid.
    d. Time of delivery.
    e. Estimated time of Apgar score, resuscitation, and ultimate condition of baby.
    f. Sex of baby.
    g. Approximate time of placental expulsion, its appearance, and completeness.
    h. Maternal condition: affect, amount of bleeding, and status of uterine contractions.
    i. Any unusual occurrences during the delivery.

Lateral Sims' Position for Delivery

A lateral Sims' posture may be the position of choice for delivery when (1) the delivery is progressing rapidly and there is insufficient time for slow distension of the perineum; (2) the fetal head seems too large to pass through the introitus without laceration, and episiotomy is not possible; or (3) the apparent size of the fetus is consistent with possible shoulder dystocia.

In the lateral Sims' position, less stress is placed on the perineum and better visualization of the perineum is possible. In the event of shoulder dystocia, lateral Sims' posture increases the space needed for delivery.

Birth and Management of Preterm Infant

The actual process of birthing the preterm infant does not vary from that of the term infant. However, the care of the infant after birth requires some modification as follows:

1. Warmth is essential.
2. Minimize handling, maintain a clean airway, and feed and change the infant.
3. Nutrition may be a problem if a medical facility is not available. Although the infant may be unable to nurse at the breast, slow feeding is important, using a medicine dropper, for example.
4. Urge the preterm infant to breathe by stimulating her or him *gently* when she or he "forgets," for example, rub her or his back or the soles of the feet.
5. Transport the infant to a medical facility equipped to handle preterm infants as early as possible (see Chapter 36).

CHILDBIRTH TRAUMA

Episiotomy

An episiotomy is an incision made in the perineum to enlarge the vaginal outlet. Episiotomies are performed more commonly in the United States and Canada than in Europe. The use of the side-lying position for delivery is routinely used in Europe while the position with legs in stirrups is more commonly used in the United States and Canada. With the side-lying position there is less tension on the perineum and a gradual stretching of the perineum is possible. As a result the indications for use of episiotomies are less.

The proponents of use of the episiotomy maintain it serves the following purposes:

1. Prevents tearing of the perineum: The clean and properly placed incision heals more promptly than does a ragged tear. Some conditions that predispose a woman to perineal tearing and are therefore indications for episiotomy are a large infant, rapid labor in which there is not sufficient time for stretching of the perineum to take place, a narrow subpubic arch with a constricted outlet, and malpresentations of the fetus (e.g., face).
2. May minimize prolonged and severe stretching of the muscles supporting the bladder or rectum, which may later lead to stress incontinence or to vaginal prolapse.
3. Reduces duration of the second stage, which may be important for maternal reasons (e.g., a hypertensive state) or fetal reasons (e.g., persistent bradycardia).
4. Enlarges the vagina in case manipulation is needed to deliver an infant, for example, in a breech presentation or for application of forceps.

Those who are opposed to the *routine* use of episiotomies maintain that:

1. The perineum can be prepared for delivery through use of the Kegel's exercises and use of the exercises in the postpartum period improves and restores the tone of the perineal muscles.
2. Lacerations may occur even with the use of an episiotomy (Chapter 31).
3. Pain and discomfort from episiotomies can interfere with mother-infant interactions and the reestablishment of parental sexual intercourse.

4. Episiotomies *are indicated* (a) if the well-being of the mother or fetus is in jeopardy to shorten the second stage of labor, (b) if the infant is preterm and cerebral hemorrhage is a possibility because of capillary fragility, (c) if the infant is large (greater than 4000 g [9 lb]), or (d) in most forceps and breech deliveries (Pernoll and Benson, 1987).

The type of episiotomy is designated by site and direction of the incision (Fig. 19-19).

Median episiotomy is the one most commonly employed. It is effective, easily repaired, and generally the least painful. Occasionally there may be an extension through the rectal sphincter (third-degree laceration) or even into the anal canal (fourth-degree laceration). Fortunately primary healing and a good repair usually will be followed by good sphincter tone.

Mediolateral episiotomy commonly is employed in operative delivery when posterior extension is likely. Although a fourth-degree laceration may thus be avoided, a third-degree laceration may occur. Moreover, as compared with a median episiotomy, blood loss is greater and the repair more difficult and painful. Repair of left mediolateral episotomy is shown in Fig. 19-20.

Lateral episiotomy affords very little relaxation of the introitus, is associated with profuse bleeding, and is difficult to repair. This incision should not be used (Pernoll and Benson, 1987), and for nursing care related to episiotomies, see Chapters 20 and 26.

Lacerations

Most acute injuries and lacerations of the perineum, vagina, uterus, and their support tissues occur at parturition, and their management is an obstetric problem. Some childbirth injuries to the supporting tissues, whether they were acute or nonacute and whether they were repaired or not, may become gynecologic problems later in life (Chapter 41).

The soft tissues of the birth canal and adjacent structures suffer some damage during every delivery. Damage is usually more pronounced in nulliparas because the tissues are firmer and more resistant than in multiparas. Perineal skin and vaginal mucosa may appear intact, obscuring numerous small lacerations in underlying muscle and its fascia. Damage to pelvic supports is usually easily apparent and thus is repaired after delivery.

The individual woman's tendency to sustain lacerations varies; for example, the soft tissue in some women may be less capable of distension. Heredity may be a factor for example, the tissue of very light-skinned women, especially those with reddish hair, is not as readily distensible as that of a darker-skinned woman. Women whose tissues show a tendency to lacerate may also exhibit varicose veins and diastasis recti abdominis (Fig. 10-11). These women may also heal less efficiently.

Immediate repair promotes healing and limits residual damage, as well as decreases the possibility of infection. After every delivery the cervix, vagina, and perineum are inspected immediately. During the early days post delivery, the nurse and physician carefully inspect the perineum and

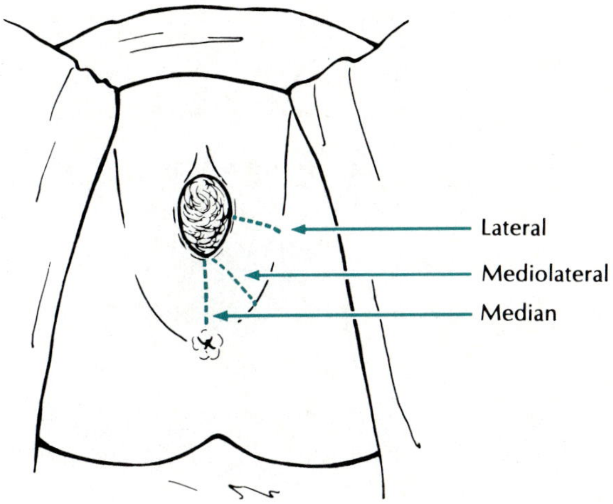

Fig. 19-19 Types of episiotomies.

evaluate lochia and symptoms to identify any previously missed damage (Chapters 20, 24, and 31).

Perineal Lacerations. Perineal lacerations usually occur as the fetal head is being born. The extent of the laceration is defined on the basis of depth (Chapter 31).

1. *First degree.* Laceration extends through the skin and structures superficial to muscles.
2. *Second degree.* Laceration extends through muscles of perineal body.
3. *Third degree.* Laceration continues through anal sphincter muscle.
4. *Fourth degree.* Laceration also involves the anterior rectal wall.

Lacerations in the lower vagina occur along one or both lateral walls (sulci), rather than up the midline. At least the fascia of the elevator ani muscle is injured in all but the most superficial perineal tears. Perineal injury is often accompanied by small lacerations in the medial surfaces of the labia minora below the pubic rami and to the sides of the urethra and clitoris. Lacerations in this greatly vascular area result in profuse bleeding (Chapter 31).

Immediate repair with absorbable suture (Fig. 19-21) is indicated. Third- and fourth-degree lacerations require special attention so that the woman retains fecal continence. Postdelivery nursing care is discussed in Chapters 20 and 26. The woman's comfort is increased and healing is promoted by measures taken to ensure soft stools for a few days. Antimicrobial therapy is not deemed necessary.

When the levator ani (including the iliococcygeus and pubococcygeus muscles, which form the slinglike support of pelvic viscera [Fig. 6-15]) is not involved, simple perineal injuries usually heal without permanent disability whether or not they were repaired. However, the *vaginal introitus may gape* if torn or severed (episiotomy) ends of superficial perineal muscles (e.g., bulbocavernosus [Fig. 6-16]) are not well approximated during repair.

The ends of the torn or severed anal sphincter muscles must be repaired adequately to avoid *fecal incontinence* (Fig. 19-22). It is easier to repair a new perineal injury to prevent sequelae than it is to correct long-term damage.

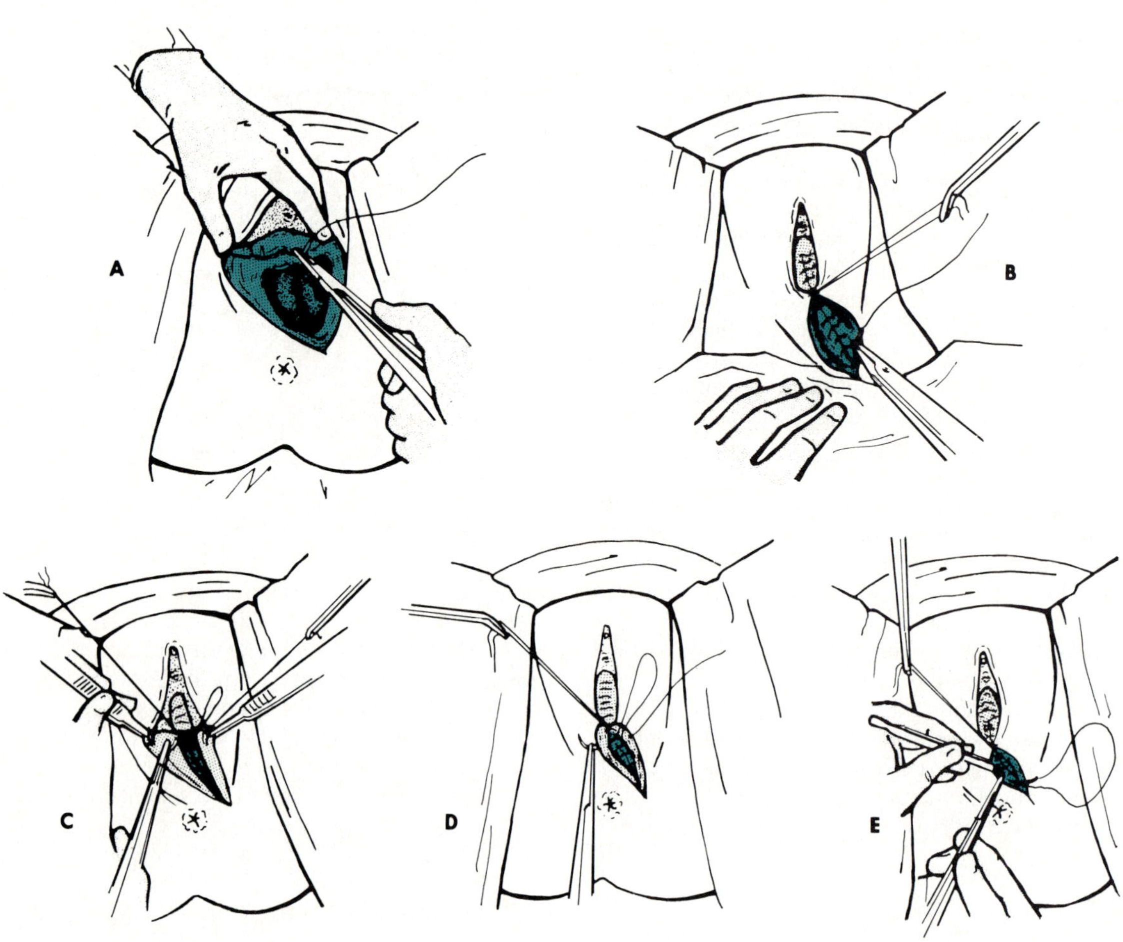

Fig. 19-20 Repair of left mediolateral episiotomy. **A** and **B**, Repair of levator muscle and its severed fascia. Attendant approximates cut edges of vaginal orifice, using forceps to exert traction on suture of bulbocavernosus muscles. **C**, Repair of cut ends. **D**, Repair of muscle and fascial components of urogenital diaphragm. **E**, Closure of skin edges. Sutures are placed just under dermis so that no sutures are visible when skin edges are approximated.

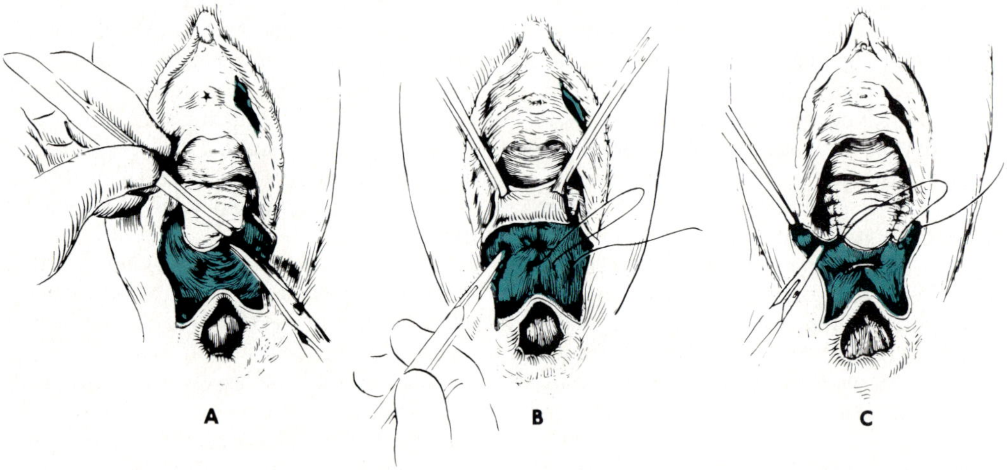

Fig. 19-21 Perineal lacerations. **A**, Bilateral sulcus tears, periurethral tear, and separation of anal sphincter. **B**, Exposure and approximation of levator ani structures. **C**, Approximation of torn bulbocavernosus muscle.

From Willson, JR: Atlas of obstetric technic, ed 2, St Louis, 1969, The CV Mosby Co.

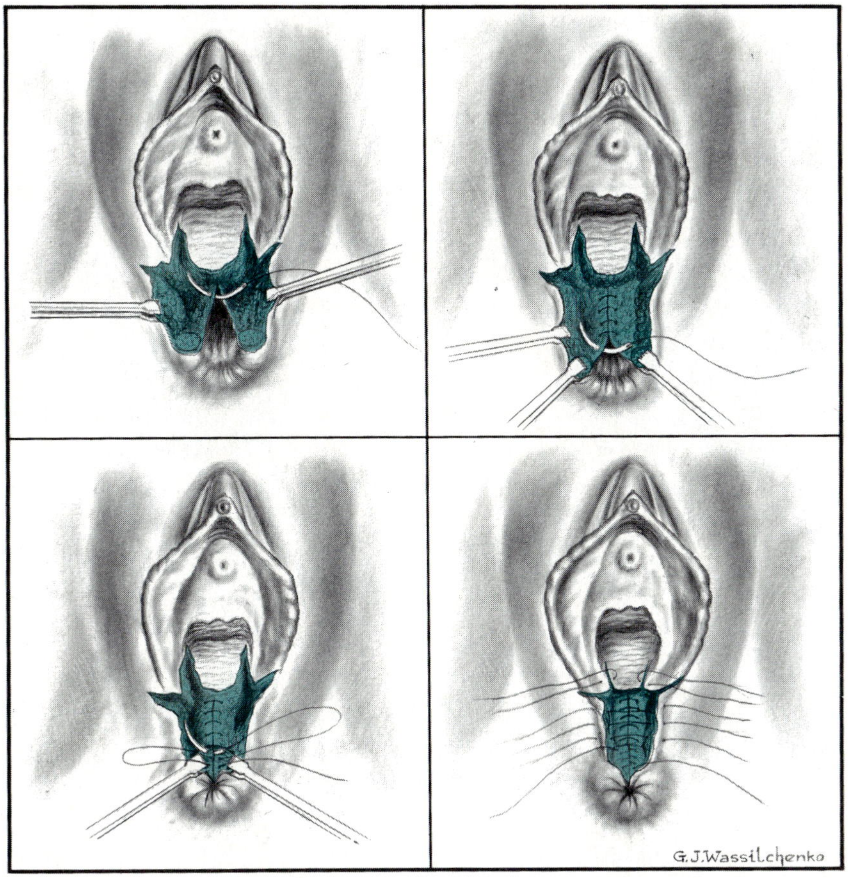

Fig. 19-22 Repair of fourth-degree laceration. **A,** Repair of rectal mucosa, with inverted sutures buried in muscles of rectal wall. **B,** Sutures of levator muscles to be buried; ends of sphincter drawn forward—first step of sphincter suture. **C,** Second step of sphincter suture—beginning figure-of-eight sutures. **D,** Sphincter suture completed and ready for tying. Remainder of perineal repair in usual manner.

Vaginal Lacerations. Vaginal lacerations often accompany perineal lacerations. Vaginal lacerations tend to extend up the lateral walls (sulci) and, if deep enough, to involve the levator ani. Additional injury may occur high in the vaginal vault near the level of the ischial spines. Vaginal vault lacerations may be circular and may result from forceps rotation, especially in the presence of cephalopelvic disproportion (CPD) (Chapter 33).

A cervical or vaginal laceration extending into the broad ligament should *not* be repaired vaginally. Laparotomy with evacuation of the resultant hematoma and hemostatic repair or hysterectomy will be required (Pernoll and Benson, 1987).

The location of the lacerations and the rapid and profuse bleeding make it difficult to expose and repair these tears. Late sequelae and management depend on the injury and the results of subsequent repair of injuries to the levator ani (Chapter 41).

Cervical Injuries. The greatest percentage of cervical injuries are obstetric in origin and occur when the cervix is being retracted over the advancing fetal head. Obstetrically acquired *cervical lacerations* usually occur at the lateral angles of the external os; most are shallow and bleed little (Fig. 19-23). More extensive lacerations may extend to the vaginal vault or beyond the vault into the lower uterine segment; serious bleeding may occur. Serious lacerations may follow injudicious attempts to enlarge the cervical opening artificially or to deliver the fetus before full cervical dilation is achieved.

Anterior lip incarceration can occur. Occasionally the cervix is injured if the anterior lip is trapped between the fetal head and the pubic bone, an event that occurs most often when there is some degree of cephalopelvic disproportion (Chapter 33). Since the trapped (incarcerated) cervix cannot be retracted upward around the descending head, the lower uterine segment above it thins excessively and may rupture. The anterior lip becomes edematous, bruised and almost black in color, and diffused with blood. The condition is exacerbated by women pushing before full dilation of the cervix (p. 408). Unless the anterior lip is freed by pushing the head upward and easing the cervix over the head, the entire cervix may be torn loose; this condition is called *annular amputation.*

Uterine Rupture. The most serious of childbirth injuries, rupture of the uterus, occurs approximately once in 1500 to 2000 deliveries. Although the uterus may rupture

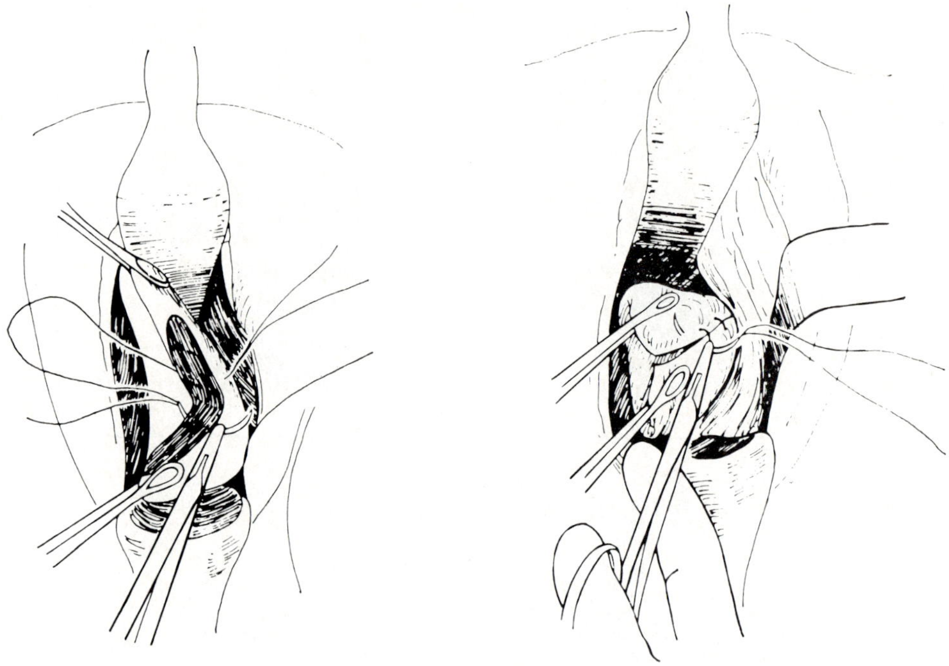

Fig. 19-23 Exposure and repair of cervical laceration. Interrupted sutures are placed through entire thickness of cervix.
From Willson, JR, et al: Obstetrics and gynecology, ed 7, St Louis, 1983, The CV Mosby Co.

during pregnancy, the uterine wall usually gives way during the stresses of labor. Hysterectomy may be indicated if the uterus is severely damaged. Uterine rupture is discussed in Chapter 33 (dystocia).

SUMMARY

Nursing care during the second and third stages of labor considers all members of the childbearing family. The new mother has now completed what in most instances is an exhilarating and rewarding experience. The maternity nurse is in an ideal position to encourage and promote early family participation and attachment and to focus on the individual health care needs of each member of the childbearing family. The nurse's expertise takes into consideration the management of a challenging emergency vertex childbirth in a calm, supportive, and professional manner. The maternity nurse uses specialized skills to provide safe, quality nursing care during the second and third stages of labor.

KEY CONCEPTS

- When allowed to respond to the rhythmic nature of the second stage of labor, the woman will normally change body positions, push when she has an urge, and vocalize as she bears down.
- The only positive objective sign that the second stage has begun is when no cervix can be palpated on vaginal examination.
- If any parturient, nullipara, or multipara states, "The baby is coming!' the baby *is* coming, and it is too late for transfer to a delivery room.
- During the second stage, the woman needs continuous monitoring, support, and coaching.
- There are five signs that placental separation has occurred and the placenta is ready to be expelled; before placental separation, excessive traction can result in immediate or delayed injury to the mother.
- Most parents (families) enjoy being able to handle, hold, explore, and examine the baby immediately after birth.
- Nurses must be alert to the appearance of warning signs in parent-child relationships during the post delivery period.
- As the neonate makes the transition from intrauterine to extrauterine life, initiation and maintenance of respiration and prevention of cold stress are top priorities.
- In a situation such as emergency childbirth out of the hospital, in the absence of injectable oxytocin, the neonate's sucking or nuzzling and licking the breast stimulate the release of natural oxytocin from the mother's posterior pituitary.
- Episiotomies and lacerations may be seen even with "normal" childbirth and their appropriate and prompt repair is essential.

STUDY QUESTIONS AND ACTIVITIES

1. Interview at least three new mothers about their response to the first sight of the newborn and report their answers to the group. Identify possible reasons for variations in response and discuss, in a group, why these responses could be warning signs for future parenting problems.
2. Evaluate the birth settings available and the procedures followed in the institution you are in and assess their potential effect on parent-newborn bonding.
3. Observe several clients in the second stage of labor and develop generalizations about the behaviors observed.
4. In a group, discuss responses to the first delivery you have observed. Express negative feelings and explore their cause.
5. Monitor a mother during the third stage of labor and make a list of the potential problems that can occur during this stage.
6. Watch parents interact with their new baby. Identify behaviors that make you uncomfortable. In a group, explore behaviors, the parents and your own feelings.

References

Balaskis, J: Active birth, London, 1983, Unicorn
Carr, KG: Management of the second stage of labor, NAACOG Update series, lesson 9, vol 1, 1983
Danforth, DN, and Scott, JR, editors: Obstetrics and gynecology, ed 5, Philadelphia, 1986, JB Lippincott Co
Mahan, CS, and McKay, S: Are we overmanaging second stage labor? Contemp OB/GYN 24:37, Dec 1984
Myles, M: Textbook for midwives, ed 10, Edinburgh, 1985, Churchill Livingstone, Inc
Wahlberg, V: Newborn care: an evaluation of silver nitrate prophylaxis. In Field, PA, editor: Perinatal nursing, London, 1985, Churchill Livingstone, Inc
Warrington, J: The obstetric catechism, Philadelphia, 1842, Crolius and Clading
Yeates, J, and Robers, J: A comparison of 2 bearing down techniques during the second stage of labor, J Nurse 29:3, 1984
Pernoll, ML, and Benson, RC, editors: Current obstetric and gynecologic diagnosis and treatment, ed 6, Los Altos, Calif, 1987, Appleton & Lange
Pritchard, JA, MacDonald, PC, and Gant, NF: Williams obstetrics, ed 17, Norwalk, Conn, 1985, Appleton-Century-Crofts
Quinlan, P: Genevieve's birth at Pithiviers, Birth 10:187, Fall 1983

Bibliography

Amderberg, GJ: Initial acquaintance and attachment behavior of siblings with the newborn, JOGN Nurs 17(1):49, 1988
Andrews, CM, and Andrews, EC: Nursing, maternal postures, and fetal position, Nurs Res 32:336, Nov/Dec 1983
Bates, B, and Turner, AN: Imagery and symbolism in the birth practices of traditional cultures, Birth 12:29, Spring 1985
Carlson, J, Diehl, J, Sachtleben-Murray, M, et al: Maternal position during parturition in normal labor, Obstet Gynecol 68:443, 1986
Coltrell, BH, and Shannahan, MD: Effect of the birth chair duration of second stage labor and maternal outcome, Nurs Res 35:364, 1986
Dundes, L: The evolution of maternal birthing positions, Am J Public Health 77:636, Sept/Oct 1987
Griffith, R, and Hare, M: Do women really want natural childbirth, Midwives Chronicle 98(1167):92, 1985
Hageman, JR, et al: Delivery room management of meconium staining of the amniotic fluid and the development of meconium aspiration syndrome, J Perinatol 8(2):127, 1988
Hansen, J, and Ueland, K: Maternal cardiovascular dynamics during pregnancy and parturition. In Marx, F, editor: Parturition and perinatology, Philadelphia, 1974, FA Davis Co
Haun, N: Nursing care during labor, Can Nurse, 80:26 Oct 1984
Horn, M, and Manion, J: Creative grandparenting: bonding the generations, JOGN Nurs 14:233, May/June 1985
ICEA Review: Maternal position during labor and birth, Milwaukee, 1978, International Childbirth Education Association, Inc
Johnsen, NM, and Gaspard, ME: Theoretical foundations of a prepared sibling class, JOGN Nurs 14:237, May/June 1985
Kowba, MD, and Schwirian, PM: Direct sibling contact and bacterial colonization in newborns, JOGN Nurs 14:412, Sept/Oct 1985
Lehrman, E: Birth in the left lateral position: an alternative to the traditional delivery position, J Nurse Midwife 30:193, July/Aug 1985
Mercer, R, and Slainlan, CM: Perceptions of the birth experience: a cross-cultural comparison, Health Care for Women International 5:29, 1984
McKay, S: Squatting: an alternative position for the second stage of labor, MCN 9:181, May/June 1984
McKay, S, and Roberts, J: Second stage labor: what is normal, JOGN Nurs 14:101, March/April 1985
Ramona, J, and Baker, I: Squatting in childbirth: a new look at an old tradition, JOGN Nurs 14:406, Sept/Oct 1985
Roberts, J, and Kniz, D: Delivery positions and perineal outcomes, J Nurse Midwife 29:186, May/June 1984
Roberts, JE, Goldstein, SA, and Griener, JS, et al: A descriptive analysis of involuntary bearing-down efforts during the expulsive phase of labor, JOGN Nurs 16:48, Jan/Feb 1987
Rosse, MA, and Lindell, SG: Maternal positions and pushing techniques in a nonprescriptive environment, JOGN Nurs 15:203, May/June 1986
Stewart, P, Hillan E, and Calder, A: A randomized trial to evaluate the use of the birthing chair for delivery, Lancet 1(8337):1296, 1983
Turner, M, Romney, M, Webb, J, and Gordon, HL: The birth chair: an obstetric hazard, J Obstet Gynecol 6:232, April 1986
Shannon-Babitz, M: Addressing the needs of fathers during labor and delivery, MCN 4(6):378, 1979
Simkin, P: Preparing parents for second stage, Birth Fam J 9:229, Winter 1982
Sumner, PE, and Phillips, CR: Birthing rooms: concept and reality, St Louis, 1981, The CV Mosby Co
Winslow, W: Perinatal nursing education, Can Nurse, p 31, June 1988

CHAPTER

20

The Fourth Stage of Labor

Iris E. Campbell

Learning Objectives

Correctly define the key terms listed.

Review the immediate care of the mother following delivery.

Identify priorities of maternal care immediately after delivery.

Discuss the maternal fluid balance and nutritional needs.

List measures to prevent hemorrhage.

Formulate measures to prevent bladder distension.

Develop measures to support parental emotional needs.

Explain measures to facilitate parent-infant interaction.

Summarize measures to promote comfort.

Review transfer of mother and newborn to postdelivery area.

Key Terms

afterpains
atony
bladder distension
bonding
comfort
emotional needs
fluid balance
hemorrhage
hemorrhoids
hypovolemic shock
involution
living ligatures
lochia
orthostatic hypotension
pharmacologic control of postdelivery hemorrhage
retained placental fragments
splanchnic engorgement
uterine hypotonia

The fourth stage of labor, the stage of recovery, is a critical period for the mother and newborn, who are not only recovering from the physical process of birth, but are also initiating new relationships.

During the 2 hours after the birth, the maternal organism makes its initial readjustment to the nonpregnant state, and body systems begin to stabilize. The newborn continues with the transition from intrauterine to extrauterine existence. Since many parents are opting for early discharge from the hospital, and others must leave because of diagnosis related group (DRG) and insurance requirements, the health care team must be reasonably assured that there is no potential for disruption in these normal processes for the mother or newborn. The nurse's skills as a technician, teacher/counselor/advocate, and support person can make a critical difference during the fourth stage. The focus of this chapter is the application of the nursing process during this period of readjustment. Some important terms are defined below:

puerperium: Variable period, usually 6 to 8 weeks, that begins with the delivery of the placenta and ends either with the resumption of ovulatory menstrual periods or when involuntary changes that result in the nonparous state are complete (e.g., after postdelivery hysterectomy); the postpartum period; the postnatal period; the postdelivery period.

p. immediate: The first 24 hours after delivery.

involution: Process that results in the healing of the birth canal and the return of the uterus and all systems to or almost to the prepregnant state. Generally, changes reflect reversals of the anatomic and physiologic adaptations to pregnancy.

lochia: Uterine discharge after delivery.

atonic uterus: A lack of tone in the uterine muscle caused by interference with the ability of the muscle to contract and retract.

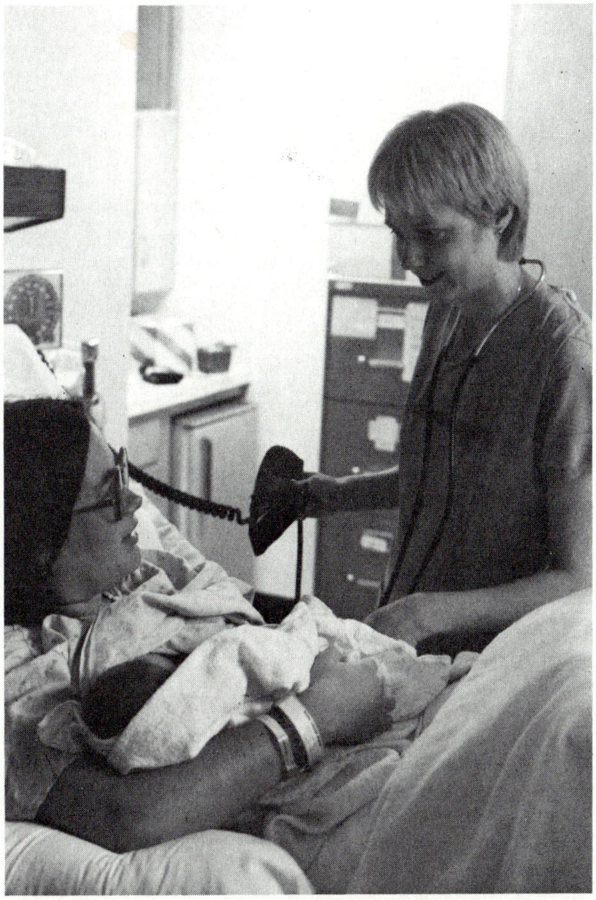

Fig. 20-1 Nurse prepares to assess for blood pressure, pulse, and temperature. As she interacts with new mother, nurse also assesses for alertness, signs of discomfort, and cues to her reaction to birth experience and newborn.

Assessment

If the nurse is unfamiliar with the new mother, assessment begins with review of the prenatal and labor record. Of primary importance are conditions that could predispose the mother to hemorrhage, which is a potential danger during the fourth stage of labor for any woman.

To assist the nurse to provide comprehensive care, a worksheet is suggested (see p. 448). On a busy unit even experienced nurses appreciate a checklist. During the first hour in the recovery room, physical assessment of the mother is frequent. All factors except temperature are assessed every 15 minutes for 1 hour (Table 20-1). After the fourth 15-minute assessment, if all parameters have stabilized within the normal range, assessment is repeated twice more at 30-minute intervals (see Fig. 20-1). The physical assessment of the mother during the fourth stage of labor is given in Procedure 20-1. The area of examination and purpose, the method of assessment, and findings within normal limits are discussed briefly.

Nursing Diagnoses

Nursing diagnoses lend direction to the type of nursing action needed to implement a plan of care. Before establishing nursing diagnoses, the nurse analyzes the significance of findings collected during assessment. Examples of nursing diagnoses include the following:

- Potential for hemorrhage, related to
  - Uterine atony
- Urinary retention related to
  - Effects of labor and delivery on urinary tract sensation
- Pain, related to
  - Childbirth trauma
- Potential for injury, related to
  - Ambulating the first time without assistance
- Potential for altered parenting, related to
  - Postpartum pain or fatigue
- Potential for altered parenting, related to
  - Breast-feeding difficulties
- Altered family process, related to
  - Addition of new member

WORKSHEET: FOURTH STAGE OF LABOR

G ________ P ________ AB ________ Analgesia/anesthesia ________
Type of delivery ________ Sex ________ Apgar ________ Episiotomy ________ Lac ________

Time	Admit	15 min	30 min	45 min	1 hr	1 hr 15 min	1 hr 30 min	1 hr 45 min	2 hr
Fundus									
Lochia: color and amount									
Blood pressure									
Temperature, pulse, and respirations									
Perineum									
Pain: type and location									
Intake and output									
Parent-child interactions									
Medications									
Comments:									

Table 20-1 *Physical Assessment of the Mother During Fourth Stage of Labor*

Factors	Minimum Assessment	Findings and Comments
Blood pressure	Every 15 min for 1 hr or until stable, then every 30 min times 2	Slightly elevated from excitement and effort of delivery; returns to normal within 1 hr
Pulse	Every 15 min for 1 hr or until stable; then every 30 min times 2	Normal rate for individual within 1 hr; slight bradycardia may occur (50-70 bpm)
Temperature	Once, at 1 hr; then as per hospital protocol	May be elevated if dehydrated or fatigued
Fundus	Every 15 min for 1 hr or until stable; then every 30 min times 2	Firm: midline, 2 cm below or at umbilicus Soft: massage until firm and express clots until contracted to midlevel Right of midline: check bladder for distension
Bladder	Every time fundus is assessed	Fills quickly because of postdelivery diuresis and intravenous fluids.
Lochia	Every 15 min (in conjunction with assessment of fundus)	Moderate flow: normal; if flow comes in spurts, suspect cervical tear Heavy flow: recheck in 3-5 min and report
Perineum	Check in conjunction with assessment of lochia	Condition of episiotomy and perineum: clean, edematous, discolored, stitches intact

Procedure 20-1

POSTPARTUM ASSESSMENT DURING FOURTH STAGE OF LABOR

DEFINITION

Physical assessment of woman in the immediate postpartum period.

PURPOSE

To monitor the new mother's physical recovery from childbirth through accurate assessment of vital signs and blood pressure, uterine involution and lochial discharge, bladder function, and condition of perineum.

EQUIPMENT

Blood pressure cuff and sphygmomanometer; thermometer; light source; prn supplies: gloves, perineal pads, wash cloth, soap, warm water, towels, ice bags.

NURSING ACTIONS	RATIONALE
Assemble equipment.	Saves time and avoids leaving woman until assessment is completed.
Explain procedure.	Reduces anxiety and elicits woman's (and family's) cooperation.
Wash hands.	Prevents nosocomial infection.
Blood pressure	
Measure per assessment schedule (Table 20-1) using appropriate size cuff (p. 387).	Provides data base for diagnosis of complications (e.g., hemorrhage); usually stabilizes at prelabor values during first hour.
Pulse	
Count pulse, assess rate, amplitude (indicating volume), rhythm and symmetry, regularity.	Provides data base for diagnosis of complications; usually stabilizes at prelabor levels during first hour; bradycardia, 50-70 beats/min.
Temperature	
Determine temperature.	Provides data base for diagnosis of complications; usually stabilizes within normal range during first hour, or slight elevation to 38° C (100.4° F) related to dehydration.
Fundus (Fig. 20-2)	
Apply gloves, prn.	Implements universal precautions.
Position woman with knees flexed.	Relieves tension on abdomen and facilitates palpation.
Just below umbilicus, cup hand, press firmly into abdomen.	Locates fundus.
If fundus is firm (and bladder is empty), with uterus in midline, measure its position relative to woman's umbilicus. Lay fingers flat on abdomen under umbilicus; measure how many fingerbreadths fit between umbilicus and top of fundus.	Monitors uterine involution. Provides data base for possible deviations from normal (e.g., atonic uterus, retained placental fragments, Chapter 30). Most authers identify a level below the umbilicus.*
If fundus is *not* firm, stimulate "living ligature" to regain tone and expel any clots before measuring distance from umbilicus.	Facilitates more accuracy in assessment and assists in prevention of hemorrhage.
Place hands appropriately, massage gently only until firm.	Avoids overstimulation, which causes muscle fatigue and relaxation.
Expel clots while keeping hands placed as in Fig. 20-2. With upper hand, firmly apply pressure downward toward vagina; observe perineum for amount/size of expelled clots. Measure height of firm fundus.	Removes clots, which prevent uterus from retaining tone. Support of uterus during expulsion of clots prevents its inversion. Allows nurse to assess expelled clots.
Bladder	
Assess distension by noting location and firmness of uterine fundus and by observation and palpation of bladder. If bladder is distended, it is seen as a suprapubic rounded bulge that is dull to percussion and fluctuates like a water-filled balloon. When the bladder is distended, the uterus may be boggy, well above umbilicus, and usually to woman's right side.	Identifies bladder fullness. Overdistension displaces uterus upward and usually to the right of the midline and prevents efficient uterine contractions, which may lead to hemorrhage.
Assess bladder function. Ask woman to void; measure amount of urine voided.	Identifies degree of return of normal bladder function.
Catheterize prn.	Identifies possible need for intervention (e.g., catheterization). Overdistension causes maternal discomfort, is a significant factor in uterine hemorrhage (Chapter 31) and can result in bladder atony.
Reassess and compare findings with signs of an empty bladder: fundus firm, in midline; bladder nonpalpable.	

*Level of contracted fundus immediately after expulsion of placenta: Midway between umbilicus and symphysis, or slightly higher (Pritchard, MacDonald, and Gant, 1985, p. 367). At a level below umbilicus, size of 15- to 16-week gestation (Danforth, 1982, p. 787). Superior surface can be felt below the umbilicus (Willson, Carrington, and Ledger, 1983, p. 584). At 2 cm (about 2 fingerbreadths) above level of umbilicus descending by 1 cm in 12 hours (Quistad, 1984, p. 40). Midway between symphysis and umbilicus. Rises to level of umbilicus within a few hours. Remains at level of umbilicus or 1 fingerbreadth below for a day or two (Varney, 1980, p. 348).

Procedure 20-1—cont'd

NURSING ACTIONS	RATIONALE
Lochia (Fig. 20-3)	
Observe lochia on perineal pads and on linen under mother's buttocks. Determine amount and color; note size and number of clots.	Provides data base to differentiate between lochia of normal involution and discharge signaling complication such as infection (Chapter 30) or hemorrhage (Chapter 31).
Note odor. Observe perineum for source of bleeding (e.g., episiotomy, lacerations)	Allows for comparison with normal findings: lochia rubra is moderate and may contain some small clots. Odor of normal menstrual flow. Lochia does not come out in a continuous trickle or in spurts.
Perineum	
Ask or assist woman to turn on her side and flex upper leg on hip. Lift upper buttock. Observe perineum in good lighting.	Provides data base to differentiate between birth trauma within normal limits and possible complications (e.g., hidden lacerations, separation of repaired episiotomy). Allows comparison with normal findings: vaginal birth: mild edema or labial swelling; slight bruising. Episiotomy or laceration repair is intact, dry, mildly edematous but not inflamed.

Planning

During the planning step, goals are set in client-centered terms. The goals are prioritized. Nursing actions are selected, with the client where appropriate, to meet the goals. The speed and accuracy with which planning is accomplished depends on the nurse's level of competence (Chapter 2).

Goals

1. Hemorrhage is prevented.
2. Basic needs of physical comfort, nutrition, hydration, elimination, and safety are met.
3. The woman (couple) begins to integrate and come to terms with the labor and delivery experience she (they) just had.
4. Family members initiate the attachment process to the newborn.
5. Family members are satisfied by the degree of involvement each had during the fourth stage.

Implementation

During the fourth stage of labor, the nurse must organize care to include observation of vital signs, provision of comfort measures, and education of the mother. Nursing concerns include prevention of hemorrhage, prevention of urinary bladder distention, the maintenance of comfort, the maintenance of cleanliness, the maintenance of fluid balance and nutrition, and the support of parental emotional needs. The guidelines for client teaching that follow include assessment, findings, nursing actions, teaching, and evaluation for emotional and physical factors during the fourth stage of labor.

Prevent Hemorrhage

The assessments presented in Table 20-1 are designed for early identification of events that may lead to hemorrhage. The mother's temperature, pulse, and blood pressure (BP) are assessed and recorded and should be within normal limits. The pulse rate will generally be between 60 and 70 bpm. If the pulse rate is over 90 bpm, investigation and continued supervision are necessary. The temperature may be below normal because of loss of body heat. On occasion it may be over 37.2° C (99° F.). After a difficult labor, systolic BP less than 110 mm Hg and accompanied by a pulse over 100 bpm, is usually the result of hemorrhage or shock.

The uterus must be palpated at frequent intervals to make sure that it is not filling with blood (Fig. 20-2). The pad must be checked frequently to ensure that blood is not excessive (Fig. 20-3). Lochia may be described as scant, light, moderate, or heavy (profuse) (See research highlight). Normally, the fundus is firm or may be returned to a state of firmness with intermittent gentle massage. As noted earlier, *atony (relaxation) of the uterine musculature* may occur. As the relaxed uterus distends with blood and clots, blood vessels in the placental site are not clamped off by the "living ligature," and bleeding results.

NOTE: To express clots it is necessary to express gently the accumulated blood and clots before the uterus will contract again. First, make certain the fundus is firm, then press gently on the uterus in the direction of the vagina. If atony is not controlled by this treatment, medical intervention must be instituted (see Chapter 31).

As the effect of the oxytocic medication administered after delivery wears off, the amount of lochia will increase because the myometrium relaxes somewhat. The nurse always checks under the mother's buttocks, as well as on the perineal pad. Bleeding may flow between the buttocks onto

Guidelines For Client Teaching

EMOTIONAL FACTORS DURING THE FOURTH STAGE OF LABOR

ASSESSMENT

1. Woman has completed labor and given birth within previous 2 hours.
2. Woman gives verbal cues that suggest failure, loss of self-esteem (e.g., "I was such a baby").
3. Woman embarrassed about behavior during labor and delivery (e.g., "I'm sorry for screaming").
4. Woman indicates desire to hold newborn; other family members desire to hold newborn.
5. Woman indicates desire to breast-feed.
6. Woman (couple) talks about met and unmet expectations.
7. Woman (couple) reacts to newborn.

NURSING DIAGNOSES

Situational low self-esteem related to labor and delivery experience.

Potential altered parenting related to care of newborn.

Potential short-term memory deficit related to events of labor and delivery and body's potential for natural amnesia.

Knowledge deficit related to care of newborn, breast-feeding, and process of integration of the birth experience.

Potential altered thought processes related to sensory overload during labor and delivery.

GOALS

Short-term

Woman (couple) will relive and replay birth experience.

Woman will begin to feel comfortable with her behavior.

Woman will begin to breast-feed.

Woman will begin to bond with her newborn.

Intermediate

Woman (couple) will resolve feelings of birth experience and begin to feel satisfaction from the process.

Woman will gain satisfaction from breast-feeding.

Woman (couple) and family will become attached to newborn.

Long-term

Woman (couple) will have joyous memories of the birth experience.

Woman will continue to derive satisfaction from breast-feeding.

Woman (couple) will cherish her new infant and provide love and care for her/him.

REFERENCES AND TEACHING AIDS

Printed material explaining normal reactions to labor and delivery processes.

Breast-feeding information (see client teaching: breast-feeding, Chapter 23).

Pamphlets and booklets describing newborn care.

CONTENT/RATIONALE	TEACHING ACTIONS
To foster self-esteem and facilitate integration of experience, the nurse is aware that: Women approach labor with certain self-expectations. "Normal" behavior during labor includes behaviors that are unacceptable to many people, such as loss of control, moaning, belching, grunting. Normal amnesia, medications, and labor preclude a clear recall of events; gaps in recall or misinterpretations prevent positive coping and self-esteem.	Implement communication techniques (Chapter 2). Listen to mother's replay of her experience. Phrase questions and answers in manner that indicates that her responses during all stages of labor were within expected range.
To foster parent-child attachment, the nurse is aware that: Attachment to newborn is a continuous process. Fatigue of either mother or baby may delay but will not adversely influence attachment response.	Assess woman's readiness (absence of sedation or fatigue) and newborn's condition. Wrap baby warmly. Position baby in woman's arms for maximum safety. Ensure woman's comfort. Point out newborn's individual characteristics. Help the mother put baby to breast if she wishes to.
To foster individual and family satisfaction, the nurse is aware that: Each ethnic and cultural group and individual couple have developed workable ways for family interactions. There is no one "right" way.	*Meet family's ethnic and cultural and couple's expectations for care:* Accept degree of involvement of individuals regarding overt expression of joy or love. Accept family's desires regarding neonate (e.g., some may want newborn to be cared for in nursery).

EVALUATION Woman gives nonverbal cues that she is beginning to accept her behavior and the experience. Woman (couple) begins attachment process. Family indicates satisfaction with the experience.

Guidelines For Client Teaching

PHYSICAL FACTORS DURING THE FOURTH STAGE OF LABOR

ASSESSMENT

1. Woman has given birth within the last 2 hours.
2. Physical parameters must be observed to avoid harm to postpartum woman.
3. Uterus must remain firm to prevent hemorrhage.
4. Urinary bladder must be emptied periodically to prevent distension and boggy, or atonic uterus.
5. Interest in breast-feeding established.
6. Breast-feeding may begin in recovery room if all parameters are normal.
7. Watch for verbal and nonverbal cues of pain and discomfort.
8. Woman complains of fatigue.
9. Woman has elevated temperature.
10. Woman's fluid intake (oral and intravenous) limited.
11. Woman states she is hungry.
12. Effects of analgesia or anesthesia given for later part of labor and the delivery wearing off.

NURSING DIAGNOSES

Pain, related to episiotomy, hemorrhoids, involution of the uterus, full bladder

Knowledge deficit related to the fourth stage of labor.

Potential fluid volume deficit related to decreased oral fluid intake and IV administration.

Altered nutrition: potential for less than body requirements, related to having nothing by mouth during labor and delivery.

Impaired skin integrity related to lacerations of the perineum or episiotomy.

Sleep pattern disturbance related to labor and delivery.

Activity intolerance related to fatigue.

Potential for infection related to alteration in skin integrity.

GOALS

Short-term

Woman will get rest and sleep.

Woman's hunger and thirst will be satisfied.

Woman's bladder will be emptied periodically.

Woman's pain and discomfort will be diminished.

Anesthesia from delivery will wear off.

Intermediate

Woman's perineal swelling will start to subside and healing will begin.

Woman's fundus will remain firm and lochia rubra will remain within normal limits.

Woman will begin to breast-feed.

Woman will ambulate with assistance to the bathroom to void.

Long-term

Woman will ambulate to bathroom by herself to void.

Woman will begin self-care activities.

Woman will continue to breast-feed.

Uterus will begin to involute.

REFERENCES AND TEACHING AIDS

Prelabor and delivery counseling using pamphlets and booklets explaining the physiologic changes that take place during the fourth stage of labor.

CONTENT/RATIONALE	TEACHING ACTIONS
To **prevent hemorrhage** *through direct care and through teaching woman self-care, the nurse shares the following:* Uterus must remain firm to become the **living ligature**.	Identify for woman the location and size of the uterus.
When uterus becomes boggy, or atonic, living ligature is no longer working to stop excessive bleeding. If gentle massage does not work, further assessment must be performed.	Show mother how to massage uterus gently to firm up uterine fundus. Explain what the term *involution* means. Discuss lochia and clot formation.
When lochia is heavy, reassessment of source of bleeding, uterine tone, and bladder distension must be made. Clots should be expelled. Note size and amount.	Give rationale for assessing, discuss meaning of terms. Teach woman about expected regression (color and amount) during involution. Explain that atony and subsequent hemorrhage can be the result of a distended bladder. Bleeding may be from another source. Clots prevent the living ligature from working.
To prevent hemorrhage by averting bladder problems: Assess woman's intake of fluids, oral and intravenous.	Discuss rationale for keeping bladder empty: prevent uterine atony and trauma to bladder.

Guidelines for Client Teaching—cont'd

CONTENT	RATIONALE
Assess rate of diuresis as evidenced by bladder filling. Assess woman's ability to void. Share information related to diuresis and postdelivery bladder function	Provide privacy, sound of running water, fluids to drink. If available, expose urinary meatus to vapors from spirits of peppermint. Offer analgesia to assist woman to relax urinary meatus. Suggest she void while in sitz bath or while using surgigator. Discuss possible catheterization if trauma and edema to tissues or anesthesia impairs normal urination pattern.
To prevent hemorrhage through stimulation of endogenous oxytocin and help woman meet her goal to breast-feed: Review the benefits to the newborn (who is healthy and ready to nurse) and to her. See guidelines for client teaching: breast-feeding, Chapter 23.	Show woman how to put the infant to breast and explain that nipple stimulation results in the release of oxytocin, which causes the uterus to contract and assists involution.
To foster **comfort:** Reassure woman that discomfort is "normal." Episiotomy: positioning, icepacks, medication (local or systemic). Afterpains: warm blanket, empty bladder, medication.	Validate that woman's discomfort is expected and interventions are available to help. Implement care (icepacks, medications); show rationale and expected outcomes.
To maintain **hydration**, the nurse is aware that: Drinking small amounts of fluids slowly prevents nausea and vomiting. There is a relationship between fluid deficit and temperature rise and fatigue.	Provide explanations. Maintain intravenous fluids or provide oral fluids, as ordered. Caution against drinking large amounts at one time or rapidly.
To maintain **nutrition**, *the nurse is aware that:* Giving birth consumes considerable energy. There is a relationship between food deficit and fatigue and rate of recovery.	Provide rationale. Provide foods as ordered. Begin postpartum nutrition counseling.
To prevent dysfunction in **bladder elimination**, *the nurse is aware that:* Overdistension can lead to bladder atony and delayed recovery. Urine retention can predispose to bladder infection.	Provide rationale for need to prevent bladder distension. Encourage woman to void. Catheterize as needed, per physician's order.
To maintain **safety**, *the nurse is aware that:* Postdelivery splanchnic engorgement predisposes the woman to orthostatic hypotension. Recovery from effects of analgesia/anesthesia varies: Some analgesics affect the woman's balance. Spinal anesthesia requires a period of bed rest with only a small flat pillow under the woman's head Childbirth increases the woman's vulnerability to infection because of a variety of reasons, including fluid and calorie deficit and tissue trauma.	Request that woman ask for assistance to ambulate. Put side rails up and call bell within reach, and provide rationale Help woman maintain flat position for specified time after spinal anesthesia, and provide rationale Explain rationale to promote comfort and healing and to prevent infection. Demonstrate perineal care. Teach woman signs and symptoms to report after discharge home.

EVALUATION The nurse can be reasonably assured that teaching and care were effective when all goals for care have been achieved. The uterus retains tone. Mother locates and massages uterus. The lochia is moderate or less with no clots or just a few small clots. The mother voids completely so that uterus is firm, in midline, and below umbilicus; her bladder is emptied without additional trauma and by using strict aseptic technique. Mother understands cause of possible sensation of afterpains during breast-feeding. Woman's nonverbal and verbal responses validate that she is comfortable, and she is able to rest comfortably. Woman is well hydrated (elevated temperature and fatigue take time to resolve). Her hunger is satisfied. She takes oral fluids and foods without difficulty. Before ambulating, woman requests assistance, ambulates without difficulty, and incurs no injury. Woman understands rationale for all care provided her.

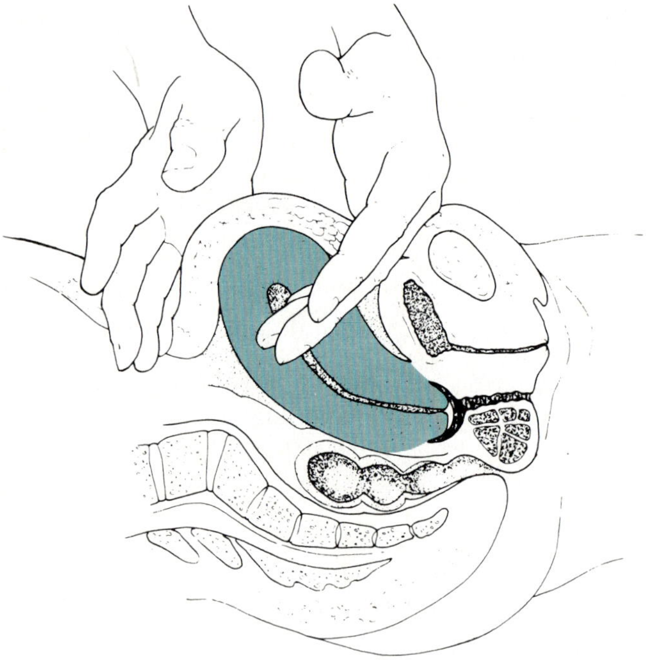

Fig. 20-2 Palpating fundus of uterus during first hour after delivery. Note that upper hand is cupped over fundus; lower hand dips in above symphysis pubis and supports uterus while it is massaged gently.

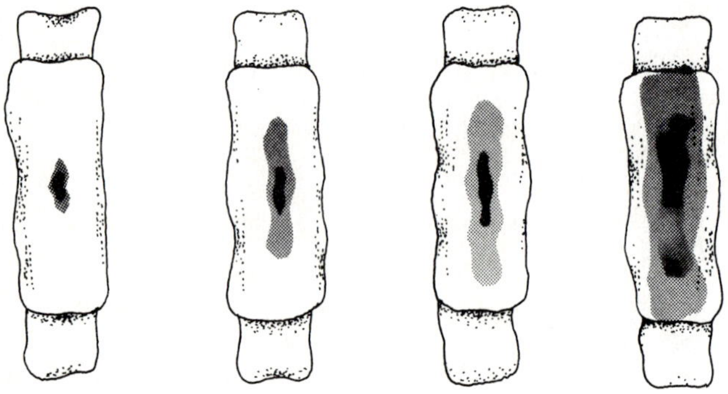

Fig. 20-3 Peripad-saturation volumes.

the linens under the mother while the amount on the perineal pad is slight. A perineal pad that is soaked through from tail to tail contains approximately 100 ml of blood. If a pad is found to be soaked through in 15 minutes, or if blood is seen pooled under the buttocks, continuous observation of blood loss, vital signs, and maternal color and behavior is indicated.

If bleeding is in the form of a continuous trickle or is seen to come in spurts, lacerations of the vagina or cervix or the presence of an unligated vessel in the episiotomy are suspected. The woman will most likely be returned to the delivery area to permit visualization of the site and surgical correction.

Danger Signs: Hypovolemic Shock. Hemorrhage and early hemorrhagic shock may occur in an otherwise normal fourth stage of labor. Prompt identification and inter-

RESEARCH HIGHLIGHT

Measuring Nurses' Accuracy of Estimating Blood Loss

Purpose

Nurses have the responsibility of assessing blood loss of women during the postpartum period. There is no accurate method or tool to measure the amount of blood loss other than the accepted practice of assigning a subjective evaluation term such as *heavy, moderate,* or *slight.* The purpose of this study was to identify whether there were differences between the actual amount and estimated amounts of blood on peripads.

Sample

A convenient sample of 42 registered nurses was used. The subjects worked in labor, delivery, postpartum, the operating room, and emergency room.

Methodology

The nurses were asked to note for each of 20 prestained peripads, their estimate of blood in centimeters and whether they considered the drainage heavy, moderate, or slight.

Findings

The greatest percentage (71%) of the subjects overestimated blood loss. Blood loss was underestimated by 25% of the subjects. There were no differences in accuracy among variables of education, years of experience, specialty area, or when and how nurses learned to estimate blood loss. Subjects also had difficulty in estimating small and large amounts of blood. Although in error, they were consistent in estimating repeated samples with the same amounts of blood.

Implications

Nurses in each service setting need to develop an inservice protocol to achieve a comparable degree of agreement among the staff. Protocols for care need to be developed based on this standardized method of estimating blood loss.

Higgins, PG: Measuring nurses' accuracy of estimating blood loss, J Adv Nurs 7:175, 1982.

DANGER SIGNS

Hypovolemic Shock

1. **Persistent significant bleeding—perineal pad soaked within 15 minutes; *may not be accompanied by a change in vital signs or maternal color or behavior***
2. **Mother states she feels light-headed, "funny," "sick to my stomach," or sees "stars"**
3. **Mother begins to act anxious, or exhibits air hunger**
4. **Woman's color turns ashen or grayish**
5. **Temperature of skin feels cool and clammy**
6. **Increasing pulse rate**
7. **Falling BP**

EMERGENCY PROCEDURE

HYPOVOLEMIC SHOCK

DEFINITION

State of physical collapse and prostration caused by massive blood loss, circulatory malfunction, and inadequate tissue perfusion.

PURPOSE

To identify and control bleeding.
Prompt replacement of blood and fluid volumes.
Prevention of total collapse and death.

EQUIPMENT

IV fluid; IV tubing, needles, angiocaths; aromatic spirits of ammonia; oxytoxic medication; oxygen with nasal prongs or mask.

NURSING ACTIONS	RATIONALE
Preprocedure	
Observe mother for persistent heavy bleeding: the soaking of a second perineal pad in 15 minutes, may or may not be accompanied by a change in vital signs, skin color, or behavior.	Fast diagnosis leads to quick action and a favorable prognosis. Blood volume still sufficient for body to compensate for loss.
Assess mother for signs of shock (i.e., feels light-headed, sick feeling in stomach, sees "stars," starts to act anxious, ashen or grayish color appears, skin feels cool and clammy, exhibits air hunger). Pulse rate increases as blood pressure falls.	Compensatory mechanisms becoming ineffective. Sympathetic nervous system stimulated. Hypoxia of brain cells. Hypoxia of tissue cells. β-adrenergic receptor stimulation. Attempt made to compensate for tissue hypoxia and metabolic acidosis.
Procedure	
Call for help immediately-bring help **to you**	**Do not leave** the woman.
Tilt woman onto her side and raise her legs **high.** Increase flow of IV drip.	To increase circulating blood volume; prevent supine hypotension.
If uterus is atonic, massage gently and expel clots to allow uterus to contract; compress uterus manually, as needed, using two hands. Add oxytocic to IV drip, as ordered.	To prevent further loss of blood by stimulating uterine contractions. To stimulate uterine contractions.
Break ampule of aromatic amonia, a respiratory stimulant; give oxygen by face mask or nasal prongs at 8 to 10 L/min.	To facilitate oxygen by stimulating respirations and increasing available oxygen.
Postprocedure	
Chart incident and medical and nursing interventions employed. Chart results of treatments.	To provide data base for future comparison. To provide information for implementation of nursing process.
Reassure woman (couple).	To decrease anxiety.

vention usually result in rapid stabilization of the woman's pulse, BP, and other signs. The box on p. 454 is a quick reference for signs and symptoms. Interventions are presented in the emergency procedure for hypovolemic shock.

Prevent Bladder Distension

Palpation to determine the amount of *bladder distension* should accompany palpation of the fundus. The full bladder forces the uterus upward and to the right of the midline. Such a position interferes with the contractility of the uterine muscles, and hemorrhage results. In addition to the possibility of causing uterine relaxation, distension of the urinary bladder can result in atony of the bladder wall. Atony leads to urinary retention, which provides a favorable environment for infection. A specific nursing care plan for a client with bladder distension is on p. 456.

A nurse encourages the woman to void naturally, employing one or more of the following: placing a bedpan under the mother, giving her water to drink if the physician has ordered oral fluids, turning on the water faucet, helping her walk to the bathroom (if ordered), and providing privacy. If after these measures the woman cannot void, most physicians write an order for catheterization.

Spirits of peppermint are sometimes used to aid the woman to void naturally. "Spirits" are concentrated alcohol solutions of volatile substances; they are also known as essences. Spirits of peppermint give off vapors. These vapors have an external, local relaxing effect on the sphincter muscle of the urinary meatus. Use of peppermint spirits may make it unnecessary to catheterize. The nurse places a bed-

Specific Nursing Care Plan

NEW MOTHER WITH BLADDER DISTENSION

Stacey L., a 25-year-old first-time mother is 12 hours postdelivery. She is complaining of pain in her abdomen and inability to void. On examination you find her fundus firm above the umbilicus and off to the right. Lochia is moderate and rubra. Urinary bladder is full and palpable at the symphysis pubis. Stacey has asked that her baby stay in the nursery because she "can't deal with her right now; she hasn't let me sleep for the last month!"

ASSESSMENT	NURSING DIAGNOSIS (ND)/ PLAN (P)/ GOAL (G)	RATIONALE/ IMPLEMENTATION	EVALUATION
New mother—12 hours postpartum. Pain in abdomen. Bladder distension. Adequate intake and output. Fundus firm, above umbilicus, and not in midline. Lochia not excessive. Episiotomy.	ND: Pain, related to distended bladder. ND: Altered patterns of urinary elimination: distension, related to increased bladder filling and retention of urine from birth trauma, edema, or regional anesthesia. P: Empty bladder and relieve discomfort. G: Stacey empties bladder without assistance and relieves pain of distension.	*To assist Stacey in voiding the nurse will:* If able, assist Stacey to bathroom, or assist her on bedpan. a. Run water from faucet. b. Pour warm water over perineum. c. Use sitz bath. d. Use spirits of peppermint (p. 455). Administer analgesic if inability to void is caused by perineal discomfort. If all nursing measures fail, obtain doctor's order to catheterize.	Stacey voids and empties bladder unassisted. Stacey verbalizes discomfort and pain are relieved. If catheterization is necessary, Stacey suffers no adverse sequelae, (e.g., infection).
Stacey not interested in interaction with newborn. Lack of appropriate parental behaviors. Stacey states she is fatigued. Assess maternal physical discomfort.	ND: Altered parenting related to mother's physical condition and emotional lability. P: Increase mother's comfort, facilitate rest, provide care to *her,* allow time for her to be "ready" for the baby and provide information as necessary. G: Stacey's physical problems will be resolved and maternal-infant attachment will be initiated.	*To promote mother-infant attachment the nurse will:* Increase woman's comfort through rest, relaxation techniques, local medication to perineum, analgesia, and food; acknowledge that she has just accomplished a significant event. When woman indicates readiness: Introduce her to newborn, pointing out special qualities. Demonstrate care of newborn. Assist her in newborn care. Provide opportunities for teaching mother about infant and for spending time with infant. Provide information on the process and time that can be involved in the development of attachment.	Stacey's comfort will improve and mother-infant attachment is observed by health care providers.

pan under the woman and pours a few drops of peppermint spirits *into the bedpan.* The vapors rise to flow over the vulvar area, the urinary meatus relaxes, and urine is released. Nothing touches the woman except the vapors; the woman feels no sensation, only notices the aroma of peppermint. Most hospitals do not require a physician's order for this technique.

Maintain Comfort

The mother is settled comfortably in bed. A new mother needs to remain in bed for at least 2 hours even if she has an unmedicated delivery. The rapid decrease in intraabdominal pressure after birth results in a dilation of blood vessels supplying the intestines (known as splanchnic engorgement). **Splanchnic engorgement** pools blood in the viscera. Therefore when the woman stands up, she may feel faint (orthostatic hypotension). Women and their families need to be forewarned so that they know to call for assistance, especially the first time or two that the woman gets out of bed.

The woman who has received analgesics needs to be watched until she is fully recovered from the medication (i.e., vital signs are stable within her normal range, and she is fully awake). A woman who has had saddle block anesthesia will need to remain flat in bed. She must remain on her side, abdomen, or back with her head raised not more than 15 to 20 cm (6 to 8 in) for 8 to 12 hours to prevent development of a spinal headache (see Chapter 17).

Maintain Cleanliness

Cleanliness is one measure that increases the mother's comfort. The vulva is swabbed and a sterile pad placed in position, buttocks dried, and any wet linen removed so that the woman will be warm and comfortable. While demonstrating good handwashing technique before touching the mother's perineal area, the nurse verbally emphasizes the action. The nurse reminds the mother to cleanse the vulval area using a separate tissue for one wipe from front to back and then to re-wash her hands. Some hospitals routinely offer a bed bath during this period.

The nurse's attention to the mother's needs demonstrates a sense of caring. The woman feels more comfortable even if the same amount of discomfort is still present.

Prevent Discomfort

Uterine contractions may result in discomfort known as *afterpains.* The volume within the uterus is decreased after delivery. The force of the myometrial contractions is considerable; the intrauterine pressure is much greater than that during labor, reaching 150 mm Hg or more.

During the first 2 hours after delivery, uterine contractions are regular and strong, especially in multiparas. The nurse adds to the woman's comfort by performing the following measures:

1. Explaining the normal physiology of afterpains
2. Helping the mother keep her urinary bladder empty
3. Providing a warmed blanket to the mother's abdomen
4. Administering analgesics ordered by the physician
5. Encouraging relaxation and breathing exercises

As the bladder fills it presses against the uterus causing it to relax. The uterus attempts to stay firm by increasing the force of contractions, thereby increasing the discomfort of afterpains. Gentle massage of the fundus increases uterine contractions, thereby intensifying afterpains. To help the new mother cope with the discomforts of assessment measures, the nurse explains what is being done and why.

The *episiotomy* area or *hemorrhoids* may contribute to the new mother's discomfort. Ice packs wrapped in gauze or other protective cloth may be placed over the episiotomy. Cold therapy is used to numb the area and to minimize the amount of edema that occurs, thus reducing discomfort. The ice pack is most effective in minimizing edema if it is used for the first hour or two after delivery. The physician may order any one of several antiseptic or anesthetic ointments or sprays to ease discomfort in the perineal area. A side-lying position relieves direct pressure on the area.

If the woman has had a saddle block or other regional anesthetic, the nurse's description of sensations to expect as the anesthetic wears off can be reassuring. Women describe the sensation as tingling or prickly, much like that experienced by people after they have been sitting cross-legged for a long time and the legs have "gone to sleep."

Some women experience intense *tremors* after delivery that resemble the shivering of a chill. This chilling may be related to the sudden release of pressure on pelvic nerves. According to another theory, chilling may be symptomatic of a fetus-to-mother transfusion that sometimes occurs during placental separation. The feeling of a chill may be a reaction to epinephrine (adrenaline) production during delivery. The nurse can help the woman relax or feel comforted by providing her with warm blankets and an explanation that the tremors are commonly seen after delivery and are not related to infection. The warm blanket also provides a means of "mothering the mother." This helps restore her energy so she can move from a focus on herself to a focus on her baby.

If the nurse administers analgesics, the sedating effect of these analgesics necessitates such protective care as raising side rails, placing call bell within reach, and cautioning about remaining in bed. The woman must be warned about the "head-spinning" effect of the medications.

Maintain Fluid Balance (Hydration) and Meet Nutritional Needs

Because of the restrictions on fluid intake and the loss of fluids (blood, perspiration, or emesis) during labor, many women are thirsty and request fluids soon after giving birth. Clear fluids, such as apple juice or tea, and toast can be given unless the mother's condition does not allow this (Fig. 20-4). The nurse records the type of fluids and foods taken, the time, the amount, and the mother's tolerance of the fluids or foods ingested. The physician may order continued parenteral fluids at a "keep open" rate in

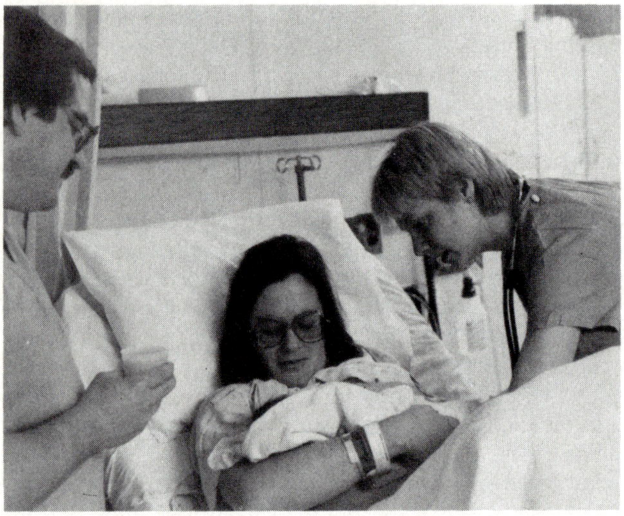

Fig. 20-4 Husband offers his wife orange juice while she breast-feeds their baby. Nurse is explaining technique of breast-feeding.
Courtesy Stanford University Medical Center, Stanford, Calif.

the event of hemorrhage or need for intravenous (IV) medications.

Support Parental Emotional Needs

It is acceptable for the nurse openly to share in the excitement and joy of birth. The nurse assists the parents by accepting any expressions of disappointment (about the child's sex or appearance) and reassures them that these feelings are within normal limits. The nurse may reassure the mother that her behavior during labor was acceptable if the mother appears worried about this. The new mother may need to talk about her labor and may endeavor to fill-in gaps that she cannot remember, particularly if the delivery was hurried (Affonso, 1977).

Psychic states of new mothers range from euphoria, a feeling of well-being, to a sleepy state marked by an unawareness of surroundings. As noted earlier, first reactions of new mothers and fathers to their newborns vary widely. These reactions give the obstetric team cues to use in individualizing plans of care. Women who have experienced long, difficult labors or who are in pain are commonly too exhausted to extend interest to the child. The nurse can offer to take the baby to the nursery until the mother is rested. The father can be invited to accompany the nurse to the nursery at this stage (Fig. 20-5). After sufficient rest a mother's attitude can be surprisingly different. The child unwanted for diverse reasons may continue to be rejected or given only mild interest. The attitude of the husband is often reflected in the mother. His pleasure arouses a responsive pleasure, or his disappointment arouses corresponding disappointment.

Ethnic or cultural origins dictate behaviors that are deemed appropriate for special occasions. Some parents may not be able to express their delight openly; others wish to welcome the newcomer noisily.

The single mother may think she is not expected to ex-

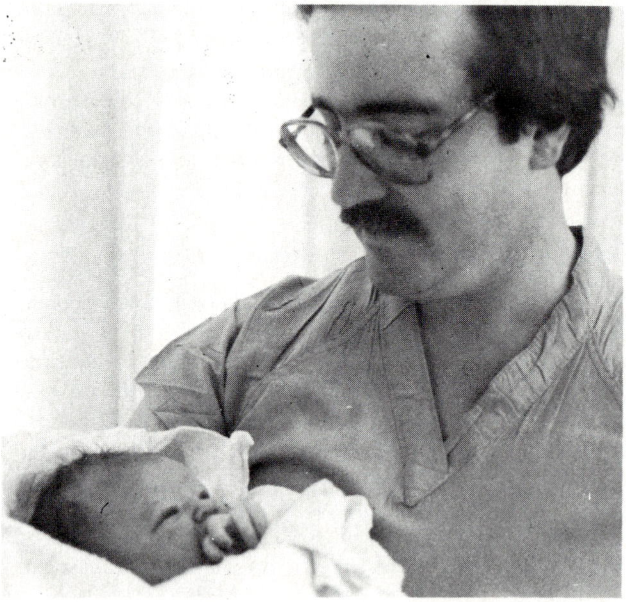

Fig. 20-5 A proud father's pensive moment with his son.
Courtesy Stanford University Medical Center, Stanford, Calif.

press joy or pleasure in her baby. The nurse can encourage the woman to express her feelings of pleasure. If the single mother does not wish to see or touch the child, the nurse, verbally or nonverbally, can indicate to the mother that her decision is acceptable.

Some mothers, particularly with their firstborn, are surprised and disturbed by the passivity or disinterest they experience on seeing their long-awaited infant. The nurse can reassure the mother of the normalcy of these feelings. The idealized "mother love" does not necessarily come into being right after delivery. The gradual growth of such love comes to some as they assume the care and responsibility for their child.

The nurse can facilitate parent-child attachment or acquaintance by providing a warm, quiet, darkened environment. An infant responds by opening the eyes. Parents are encouraged to hold the infant *en face.* In the *en face* position, parents and newborns gaze into each other's eyes. Newborns focus best at about 20.3 cm (8 in) distance. Body odor can be noticed (mothers have remarked that each child smells different). Skin contact between mother and baby should be encouraged during this time. Newborn temperatures remain stable if mother and newborn are covered by a flannelette blanket. The mother is encouraged to explore her baby and put her baby to the breast, if she plans to breast-feed. Immediately after birth the baby has a strong desire to suck, so this early feed is most encouraging for the mother and bonding is promoted. There is also evidence to suggest that women who breast-feed their babies soon after delivery breast-feed longer (Houston, 1984). In addition, when the baby sucks at the breast, oxytocin is released from the posterior lobe of the pituitary gland and stimulates the uterus to contract.

During the fourth stage of labor, the nurse uses every opportunity to teach the new mother. Regardless of parity,

Table 20-2 *Recovery Nurse's Report to Postpartum Nurse*

Item	Example
Type of labor and delivery; unusual observations, if any, of the placenta	Spontaneous or assisted (forceps) vaginal delivery; vertex presentation
Gravidity and parity, age	GI, PI, 22 years old
Anesthesia and analgesia used	None; epidural, low spinal, local
Condition of perineum	Episiotomy; repair of lacerations
Events since delivery	Vital signs, BP, fundus, lochia, intake and output, medications (dosage, time of administration, and results), response to newborn, observation of family interactions, including siblings, if present
Condition and sex of newborn; other information	Apgar at 1 and 5 min; time of birth; eye prophylaxis given; weight; whether breast- or bottle-feeding; if breast-feeding, whether newborn was at breast; name of pediatrician
Relevant information from prenatal record	Need for rubella vaccination
Miscellaneous information	
Intravenous drip	If IV drip is infusing, rate of infusion, medications added (e.g., Pitocin), whether to keep open or discontinue after completion of bag that is hung
Social factors	If woman is giving baby up for adoption, whether she wants to see baby, breast-feed, allow visitors, or other preferences she may have

new mothers can benefit from explanations for the various nursing actions during the immediate puerperium (Mercer, 1979). Examples of teaching are correlated with goals, assessment findings, nursing actions, and evaluation in the guidelines for client teaching in this chapter.

Transfer of Mother and Newborn to Postdelivery Area

At the end of the second hour after delivery the nurse carries out a final assessment. If the new mother's physical state has stabilized, the mother has completed the fourth stage of labor and is ready for transfer to the postdelivery area. The nurse checks the mother's record for completeness before transfer to the postpartum unit. On arrival the delivery nurse assists the mother into bed and introduces her to the nurse on the postpartum unit and to other women who may be sharing her room. The delivery nurse gives a report to the postpartum nurse (Table 20-2).

The newborn is transferred to either the postpartum unit to room-in with the mother or to the newborn nursery. The recovery nurse gives a report on the newborn to the appropriate nurse. An example of pertinent information to relay is given in Table 20-3.

Evaluation

Ongoing evaluation and moment-to-moment adjustment of the nursing care plan are common during the fourth stage of labor. The nurse uses the goals of care as guides to nursing actions. Care is evaluated as effective if the goals have been achieved.

Table 20-3 *Recovery Nurse's Report on Newborn*

Item	Example
Type of labor and delivery; unusual events (e.g., cord around neck)	Spontaneous or assisted (forceps, vacuum extractor) vaginal birth in vertex presentation
Gravidity and parity, age of mother	GI, PI, 22 years old
Analgesia and anesthesia	None; epidural, low spinal, or local
Condition at birth	Apgar scores at 1 and 5 min
Sex and weight	Male; 3400 g (7 lb, 8 oz)
Events since birth*	Nursed at breast; took nipple well
	Voided ×1; meconium ×1
	Eye prophylaxis
	Vitamin K injection
	Held by siblings who are happy (or have other response) to newborn
Relevant information from prenatal record	Unremarkable pregnancy

*Neonatal adjustment to extrauterine existence and recovery of the neonate are discussed in detail in Chapter 21 and Unit 5.

SUMMARY

During the fourth stage of labor the new mother's recovery from childbirth is monitored closely. Her basic needs for comfort, fluids, nutrients, elimination, cleanliness, and safety are met. She and her family begin to integrate the experience and the newborn into their lives. A data base is prepared for use in continuing care on the postpartum unit or after return to the home.

KEY CONCEPTS

- The fourth stage of labor, the stage of recovery, is a critical period for the mother and newborn.
- A primary nursing concern during this period is the prevention of hemorrhage.
- Other physical nursing concerns include the prevention of urinary bladder distension and the maintenance of comfort, cleanliness, fluid balance, and nutrition.
- Safety for the mother is an issue until she is fully recovered from analgesia or anesthesia, splanchnic engorgement, and fatigue.
- The mother needs to fill in the "missing pieces" to begin to integrate the experience of labor and delivery.
- The nurse can facilitate mother-infant attachment by meeting the new mother's physical, support, and teaching needs.
- Meeting the family's ethnic and cultural expectations for care is an important component of the nursing care plan.
- Regardless of parity, marital status, or age, new mothers can benefit from explanations for the various nursing actions during the immediate puerperium.

STUDY QUESTIONS AND ACTIVITIES

1. Care for at least one client in the fourth stage of labor. Meet in small groups and discuss nursing assessments, diagnoses, plans, and evaluation. Compare and contrast both physical and psychologic aspects of the fourth stage of labor and suggest reasons for any differences.
2. Role-play the following situations:
   a. The nurse interacting with mother and father who are expressing disappointment over the sex of the child; with the husband hinting that this is his wife's fault.
   b. The nurse interacting with a single mother who expresses no interest in seeing her child.
   c. The nurse interacting with parents who express avoidance behaviors toward the child.

   In each situation the group should evaluate the responses of all participants and suggest alternative actions, responses and reasons for responses.
3. Rehearse appropriate nursing actions for a client who may be experiencing hemorrhage.
4. Write explanations, in effective language, for the reasons for gentle massage of the fundus; these explanations should be suitable for educating a client with limited understanding of physiology.

References

Affonso, D: Missing pieces: a study of postpartum feelings, Birth Fam J 4:159, Winter 1977

Houston, MJ: Home support for the breastfeeding mother. In Houston, M, editor: Maternal and infant health care, Edinburgh, 1984, Churchill Livingstone, Inc

Mercer, RT: "She's a multip . . . she knows the ropes," MCN 4:30, Sept/Oct 1979

Pritchard, JA, MacDonald, PC, and Gant, NF: Williams obstetrics, ed 17, Norwalk, Conn, 1985, Appleton-Century-Crofts

Bibliography

Anderberg, GJ: Initial acquaintance and attachment behavior of siblings with the newborn, JOGN Nurs 17(1):49, 1988

Bentz, JM: Missed meanings in nurse/patient communications, MCN 5(1):55, 1980

Brucker, MC: Pain control of the fourth stage, NAACOG Newsletter 14(8):1, 1987

Chute, GE: Expectation and experience in alternative and conventional birth, JOGN Nurs 14(1):61, 1985

Ellison, SL, et al: Sucking in the newborn infant during the first hour of life, J Nurse Midwife 24:6, 1979

Elliott, R: Maternal-infant bonding: taking stock, Can Nurse 79(8):28, 1973

Field, PA: Maternity nurses: how parents see us, Int J Nurs Stud 24(3):1981, 1987

Gorrie, TM: Postpartal nursing diagnosis, JOGN Nurs 15(1):52, 1986

Hans, A: Postpartum assessment: the psychological component, JOGN Nurs 15(1):49, 1986

Haun, N: Nursing care during labor, Can Nurse 80(9):26, 1984

Honig, JC: Preparing school-aged children to be siblings, MCN 11(1):37, 1986

Horn, M, and Manion, J: Creative grandparenting: bonding the generations, JOGN Nurs 14(3):233, 1985

Johnsen, NM, and Gaspard, ME: Theoretical foundations of a prepared sibling class, JOGN Nurs 14(3):237, 1985

Konrad, CJ: Helping mothers integrate the birth experience, MCN 12(4):268, 1987

Kowba, MD, and Schwirian, PM: Direct sibling contact and bacterial colonization in newborns, JOGN Nurs 14:412, Sept/Oct 1985

Leininger, M: Transcultural nursing: an essential knowledge and practice field for today, Can Nurse 80:41, Dec 1984

Macdonald, J: Birth attendants: another choice, Can Nurse 80:22, Oct 1984

Maloney, R: Childbirth education classes: expectant parent's expectations, JOGN Nurs 14:245, May/June 1985

Maloni, J: The birthing room: some insights into parents, MCN 5(5):314, 1980

Marecki, M, et al: Early sibling attachment, JOGN Nurs 14:418, Sept/Oct 1985

McKay, S, and Mahan, CS: Ways to upgrade postpartal care, Contemp OB/GYN 27:63, Nov 1985

Myles, MF: Textbook for midwives with modern concepts of obstetric and neonatal care, ed 10, New York, 1985, Churchill Livingstone, Inc

Phillips, CR, and Anzalone, JT: Fathering: participation in labor and birth, ed 2, St Louis, 1982, The CV Mosby Co

Stolte, KM: Nursing diagnosis and the childbearing woman, MCN 11:13, Jan/Feb 1986

Taubenheim, AM: Paternal-infant bonding in the first-time father, JOGN Nurs 10:261, 1981

Wieser, MA, and Castiglia, PT: Assessing early father-infant attachment, MCN 9:104, March/April 1984

Wiggins, JD: Childbearing: physiology, experiences, needs, St Louis, 1979, The CV Mosby Co

Wilcox, KS: "We're the world's highest-paid babysitters," RN 40: April 1985

Winslow, W: Perinatal nursing education, Can Nurse, p 31, June 1988

UNIT

V

Normal Newborn

Newborns face a critical period of adjustment to extrauterine existence. Their ability to make the requisite adjustments depends in part on their biologic and behavioral readiness and the care afforded them by family and professional workers.

Chapter 21 reviews basic knowledge of the biologic and behavioral characteristics of the newborn that nurses need for understanding, initiating, and teaching care of the newborn. Chapter 22 focuses on the nursing process as applied to care for the dependent infant. The necessary information and techniques for accurate assessment are presented. The care of the newborn is shared by the nurse and the family. Consistent physical care and enriching social contacts promote the newborn's growth and development. This chapter contains descriptions of child care activities used by the nurse and taught by the professional to the parents. Chapter 23 centers on the nutritional needs of the newborn, which must be met if there is to be optimum growth and development. The nurse needs knowledge of nutritional requirements and skills in supporting and teaching parents. This chapter presents content basic to breast-feeding or bottle-feeding of newborns and material to be used for anticipatory guidance during the infant's early months. Techniques for assessing the nutritional status of the infant and for community teaching are included.

Nursing reasearch highlights are included. Abstracts of examples of nursing research follow.

Chapter 21: Parents' perceptions of their newborn after structured interactions.

Chapter 22: Serum indirect bilirubin levels and meconium passage in early fed normal newborns; and, neonatal jaundice in the home: assessment with a noninvasive device.

Chapter 23: Minimum breast-feeding.

CHAPTER

21

Biologic and Behavioral Characteristics of the Newborn

Learning Objectives

Correctly define the key terms listed.

List biologic characteristics for the following systems: cardiovascular, hematopoietic, respiratory, renal, gastrointestinal, hepatic, immune, integumentary, reproductive, skeletal, neuromuscular, thermogenetic.

Compare and contrast these systems with those of the adult.

Describe the behavioral characteristics of the newborn.

Summarize the newborn's biologic and behavioral characteristics in a manner easily understood by parents.

Key Terms

Brazelton neonatal behavioral assessment scale
cardiovascular characteristics
cold stress
fluid and electrolyte balance
hematopoietic characteristics
hyperbilirubinemia
immune system status
integumentary characteristics
newborn stools
neuromuscular-skeletal characteristics
newborn reflexes
reproductive system characteristics
respiratory patterns
responses to environmental stimuli
sensory behaviors
sleep-wake cycles
state-related behaviors
thermogenesis
transition period

The newborn infant must accomplish a number of developmental tasks to achieve autonomy. The biologic tasks involve (1) establishing and maintaining respirations, (2) ingesting, retaining, and digesting nutrients, a transition from maternal parenteral to infant enteral nutrition, (3) elimination of waste, (4) regulation of temperature, and (5) regulation of weight. The *behavioral tasks* include (1) establishing a regulated behavioral tempo independent of the mother, which involves self-regulation of arousal, self-monitoring of changes in her or his state, and patterning of sleep, (2) processing, storing, and organizing the multiple stimuli to which she or he is exposed, which is cognitive in nature, and (3) establishing a relationship with her or his caregivers and with the environment (Lewis and Zarin-Ackerman, 1977) (see also Chapter 22).

By term the infant's various anatomic and physiologic systems have reached a level of development and functioning that permits a physical existence apart from the mother and a readiness for social interaction.

Desmond et al. (1966) noted that infants pass through phases of instability in the first 6 to 8 hours after birth; these phases collectively are termed the *transition period* between intrauterine and extrauterine existence (Fig. 21-1). The first phase lasts up to 30 minutes after birth and is called the **first period of reactivity**. The **second period of reactivity** occurs roughly between the fourth and eighth hours after birth. This sequence occurs in all newborns, regardless of gestational age or type of delivery (vaginal or cesarean). There will be variations, however, in the length of time the periods last, depending on amount and kind of stress experienced by the fetus.

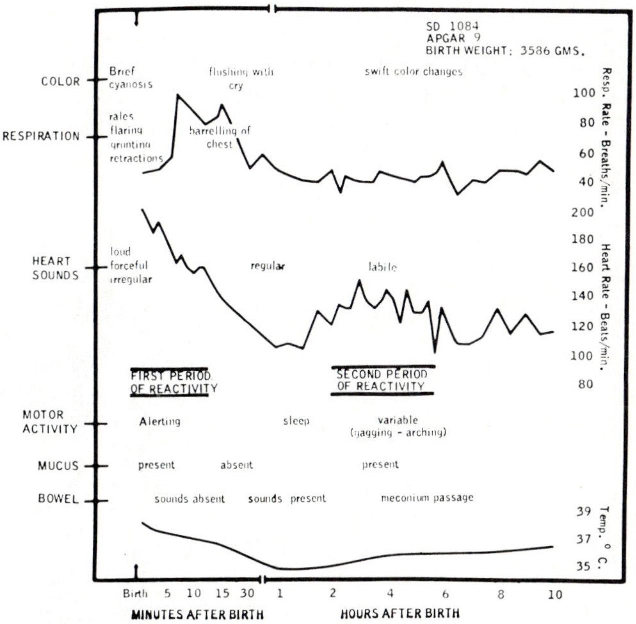

Fig. 21-1 Normal transition period.
From Desmond, M, Rudolph, A, and Phitakspharaiwan, P: Pediatr Clin North Am 13:651, 1966.

BIOLOGIC CHARACTERISTICS

The profound biologic adaptations that occur at birth make possible the infant's transition from intrauterine fetal circulation (Fig. 21-2) to extrauterine life. These adaptations set the stage for future growth and development. The **neonatal period**, from birth through day 28, represents a time of dramatic physical change for the newborn.

Cardiovascular System

The cardiovascular system changes markedly after birth. There is closure of the foramen ovale, ductus arteriosus, and ductus venosus. The umbilical arteries and vein and the hepatic arteries become ligaments.

The infant's first breath inflates the lungs and thereby reduces pulmonary vascular resistance to the pulmonary blood flow. As a result there is a drop in pulmonary artery pressure. This sequence is the major mechanism by which pressure in the *right atrium declines*. The increased pulmonary blood flow returned to the left side of the heart *increases* the pressure in the *left atrium*. This change in pressures causes a functional closure of the foramen ovale. Temporary reversal of flow through the foramen ovale may occur with crying and lead to mild cyanosis during the first few days of life.

The ductus arteriosus constricts in response to the establishment of a high oxygen level in the arterial blood. Eventually it occludes and becomes a ligament. With the clamping and severing of the cord, the umbilical arteries and vein and the ductus venosus close immediately and are converted into ligaments. The umbilical arteries also occlude and become ligaments. The changes in blood flow with birth of the infant have the effect of transforming the circulatory system. Before birth the two ventricles act in parallel (simultaneously), with shunts (foramen ovale and ductus arteriosus) adjusting possible unequal outputs. After birth the two pumps act in series (one following the other), which requires that the outputs of the right and left sides of the heart be equal (Vaughan, McKay, and Behrman, 1979). Table 21-1 summarizes the cardiovascular changes at birth.

Heart Rate and Sounds. The heart rate averages 140 beats per minute (bpm) at birth with variations noted during sleeping and waking states. At 1 week of age the mean heart rate is 128 bpm asleep and 163 bpm awake; at 1 month of age it is 138 bpm asleep and 167 bpm awake. Sinus arrhythmia (irregular heart rate) may be considered a physiologic phenomenon in infancy and an indication of good heart function (Lowrey, 1986).

Heart sounds after birth reflect the series action of the heart pump. They are described as the familiar "lub, dub, lub, dub" sound. The "lub" is associated with closure of the mitral and tricuspid valves at the beginning of systole and the "dub" with closure of the aortic and pulmonic valves at the end of systole. The "lub" sound is called the *first heart sound* and the "dub" the *second heart sound* because the normal cycle of the heart is considered to start with the beginning of systole (Guyton, 1985). Heart sounds during the neonatal period are of higher pitch, shorter duration, and greater intensity than during adult life. The first sound is typically louder and duller than the second sound, which is sharp in quality. Most heart murmurs heard during the neonatal period have no pathologic significance, and more than half disappear by 6 months. By term the infant's heart lies midway between the crown of the head and the buttocks, and the axis is more transverse than that of the adult.

The apical impulse (point of maximal impulse [PMI]) in the newborn is at the fourth intercostal space and to the left of the midclavicular line (Fig. 21-3). The PMI is often

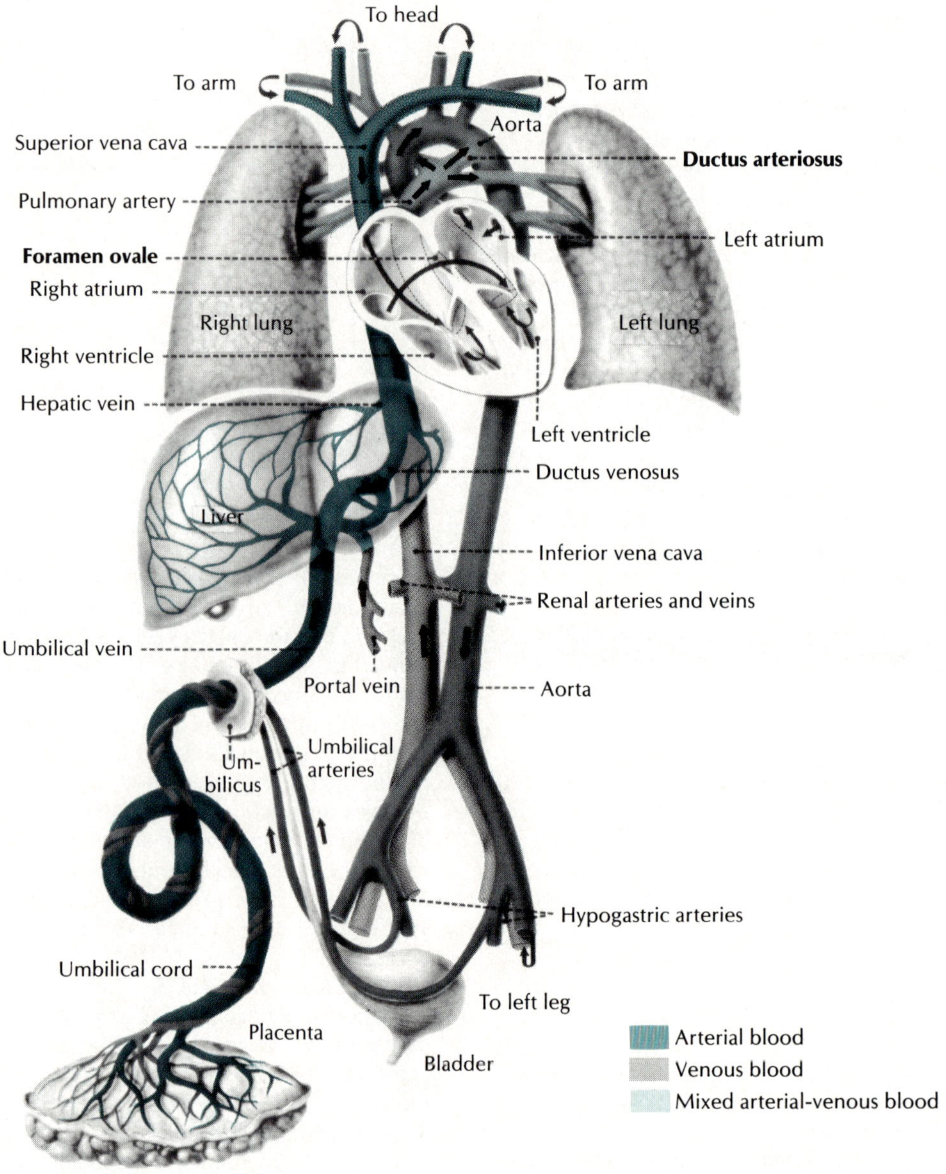

Fig. 21-2 Fetal circulation. *Before birth.* Arterialized blood from the placenta flows into the fetus through the umbilical vein and passes rapidly through the liver into the inferior vena cava; from there it flows through the foramen ovale into the left atrium, soon to appear in the aorta and arteries of the head. A portion bypasses the liver through the ductus venosus. Venous blood from the lower extremities and head passes predominantly into the right atrium, the right ventricle, and then into the descending pulmonary artery and ductus arteriosus. **Thus the foramen ovale and the ductus arteriosus act as bypass channels,** allowing a large part of the combined cardiac output to return to the placenta without flowing through the lungs. Approximately 55% of the combined ventricular output flows to the placenta; 35% perfuses body tissues; and the remaining 10% flows through the lungs (Fanaroff, 1987). *After birth.* The foramen ovale closes; the ductus arteriosus closes and becomes a ligament; the ductus venosus closes and becomes a ligament; and the umbilical vein and arteries close and become ligaments.
Courtesy Ross Laboratories, Columbus, Ohio.

visible. The apical impulse in the adult is at the fifth intercostal space at or just medial to (to the right of) the midclavicular line.

Blood Pressure. Blood pressure (BP) in infants varies from day to day. A drop in systolic BP (about 15 mm Hg) the first hour after birth is common. Values from several hours after delivery through the neonatal period average a systolic pressure of 78 and a diastolic pressure of 42 (see discussion of Doppler technique, Chapter 36). Crying and movement result in changes in BP, especially systolic.

Blood Volume. Blood volume in the newborn ranges from 80 to 110 ml/kg during the first several days and doubles by the end of the first year. The newborn has approximately 10% greater blood volume and nearly 20% greater red blood cell mass than the adult. However, the newborn's blood is about 20% less plasma volume when compared by kilogram of body weight with the adult. The infant born prematurely will have a greater blood volume than the term newborn. This is because the baby has a greater plasma volume, not a greater red blood cell mass.

A number of differences in the circulatory dynamics of the newborn result from early or late clamping of the cord. Late clamping results in an expansion of blood volume from the so-called placental transfusion, an increase of close to 60%. This in turn causes an increase in heart size, higher systolic BP, and an increased respiratory rate. Pulmonary rales and transient cyanosis are also encountered more commonly. To date the value of early or late clamping of the cord has not been determined (Pritchard, MacDonald, and Gant, 1985).

Hematopoietic System

The hematopoietic system of the newborn exhibits certain variations from that of the adult. There are differences in red blood cells and leukocytes and relatively few differences in platelets.

Red Blood Cells and Hemoglobin. At birth the average values of red blood cells (RBCs) and hemoglobin are higher than those values in the adult. These fall and reach

Table 21-1 *Cardiovascular Changes at Birth*

Prenatal Status	Postdelivery Status	Associated Factors
Primary Changes		
Pulmonary circulation: high pulmonary vascular resistance; increased pressure in right ventricle and pulmonary arteries	Low pulmonary vascular resistance; decreased pressure in right atrium, ventricle, and pulmonary arteries	Expansion of collapsed fetal lung with air
Systemic circulation: low pressures in left atrium, ventricle, and aorta	High systemic vascular resistance; increased pressure in left atrium, ventricle, and aorta	Loss of placental blood flow
Secondary Changes		
Umbilical arteries: patent; carry blood from hypogastric arteries to placenta	Functionally closed at birth; obliteration by fibrous proliferation may take 2-3 months; distal portions become lateral vesicoumbilical ligaments; proximal portions remain open as superior vesicle arteries	Closure precedes that of umbilical vein; probably accomplished by smooth muscle contraction in response to thermal and mechanical stimuli and alteration in oxygen tension; mechanically severed with cord at birth
Umbilical vein: patent; carries blood from placenta to ductus venosus and liver	Closed; after obliteration it becomes *ligamentum teres hepatis*	Closure shortly after umbilical arteries; hence blood from placenta may enter neonate for short period after birth; mechanically severed with cord at birth
Ductus venosus: patent; connects umbilical vein to inferior vena cava	Closed, after obliteration it becomes *ligamentum venosum*	Loss of blood flow from umbilical vein
Ductus arteriosus: patent; shunts blood from pulmonary artery to descending aorta	Functionally closed almost immediately after birth; anatomic obliteration of lumen by fibrous proliferation requires 1-3 months; becomes *ligamentum arteriosum*	High systemic resistance increases aortic pressure; low pulmonary resistance reduces pulmonary arterial pressure Increased oxygen content of blood in ductus arteriosus creates vasospasm of its muscular wall
Foramen ovale: forms a valve opening that allows blood to flow directly to left atrium	Functionally closes at birth; constant apposition gradually leads to fusion and permanent closure within a few months or years in majority of persons	Increased pressures in left atrium together with decreased pressure in right atrium cause closure of valve over foramen

From Whaley, LF, and Wong, DL: Nursing care of infants and children, ed 3, St Louis, 1987, The CV Mosby Co

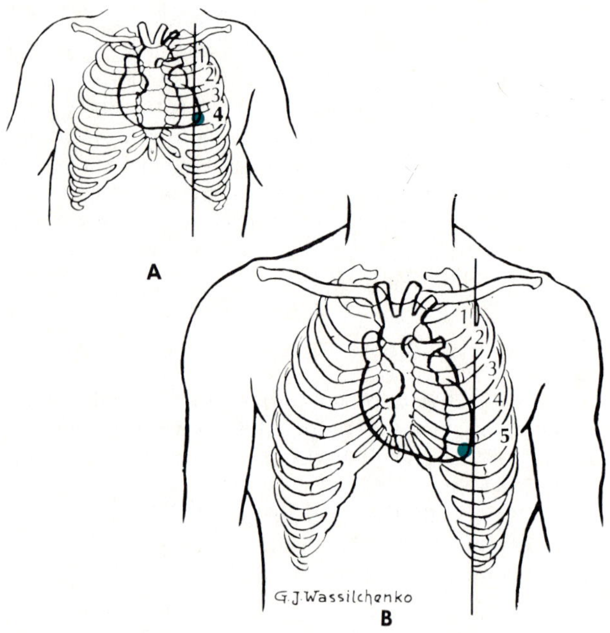

Fig. 21-3 Differences in location of apical pulse in newborn from that of adult. **A**, Neonate. **B**, Adult.

From Whaley, LF, and Wong, DL: Nursing care of infants and children, ed 3, St Louis, 1987, The CV Mosby Co.

the average levels of 11 to 17 g/dl and 4.2 to 5.2/mm,^{3} respectively, by the end of the first month. The blood values may be affected by delayed clamping of the cord, which results in a rise in hemoglobin, RBCs, and hematocrit. The source of the sample is another significant factor, since capillary blood will give higher values than venous blood. Also, the time after birth when the blood sample was obtained is significant, since the slight rise in RBCs after birth is followed by a substantial drop. At birth the infant's blood contains about 80% fetal hemoglobin, but because of the shorter life span of the cells containing fetal hemoglobin, the percentage falls to 55% by 5 weeks and 5% by 20 weeks. Fortunately iron stores generally are sufficient to sustain normal RBC production for 6 months, and thus the slight brief anemia is not serious.

Leukocytes. Leukocytosis, with the white blood cell count (WBC) approximately 18,000/mm,^{3} is normal at birth. The number, largely polymorphs, increases to about 23,000 to 24,000/mm^3 during the first day after birth. A resting level of 11,500/mm^3 normally is maintained during the neonatal period. Serious infection is not well tolerated by the newborn, and a marked increase in the WBC is unlikely even in critical sepsis. In most instances sepsis is accompanied by a decline in white cells, particularly in neutrophils. The activity of the marrow is accurately reflected by the number of circulating cells—both erythrocytes and leukocytes. The early high WBC of the newborn decreases rapidly. A relative leukopenia found in black children and adults is apparent by 1 year of age and is primarily caused by a decreased number of neutrophils. By 6 years of age the peripheral blood picture is approximately the same as that of an adult (see Appendixes E and H).

Platelets. Platelet count and aggregation are essentially the same in newborns as in adults. One exception is the infant of a mother who has taken acetylsalicylic acid (aspirin) or chlorpromazine, both of which interfere with the release of adenosine diphosphate (ADP). Otherwise bleeding tendencies in the newborn are rare, and unless there has been a marked vitamin K deficiency, clotting is sufficient to prevent hemorrhage.

Blood Groups. The infant's group is established early in fetal life. However, during the neonatal period there is a gradual increase in the strength of the agglutinogens present in the RBC membrane.

Respiratory System

At birth, air must be substituted for fluid that has filled the respiratory tract to the alveoli. During the course of normal vaginal delivery, between 7 and 24 ml of lung fluid is squeezed or drained from the newborn's lungs (Aladjem et al., 1980). After delivery the major portion of the fetal lung fluid is absorbed across the alveolar membrane into the blood capillaries. This is largely a result of the pressure gradient from alveoli to interstitial tissue to blood capillary. Reduced vascular resistance also accommodates this flow of lung fluid; however, it is the diminished intravascular pressure that is ultimately responsible.

Initial Breathing. Abnormal respiration and failure to completely expand the lungs retard the egress of fetal lung fluid from alveoli and interstices into the pulmonary circulation. Retention of fluid in turn alters pulmonary function.

Initial breathing is probably the result of a reflex triggered by pressure changes, chilling, noise, light, and other sensations related to the birth process. In addition the chemoreceptors in the aorta and carotid bodies initiate neurologic reflexes when the arterial Po_2 falls from 80 to 15 mm Hg, arterial Pco_2 rises from 40 to 70 mm Hg, and arterial pH falls below 7.35. (When these changes are extreme, however, depression ensues.) In most cases an exaggerated respiratory reaction follows within 1 minute of birth, and the infant takes a first gasping breath and cries.

With the first breath the infant develops a considerable negative intrathoracic pressure. Air is drawn in, and about half of this remains as residual pulmonary volume. Normally only a few breaths are required to expand the lungs well; subsequently the pressure will be lower than at the onset of respiration.

Respirations. After respirations are established, they are shallow and irregular, ranging from 30 to 60 breaths per minute, with short periods of apnea (less than 15 seconds). Apnea (periodic breathing) is characteristic of the newborn. It occurs most often during the active (rapid eye movement [REM]) sleep cycle and decreases in frequency and duration with age. However, any apneic period should be evaluated.

Infants are obligatory nose breathers. The reflex response to nasal obstruction is opening the mouth to maintain an airway. This response is not present in most babies until 3 weeks after birth but may occur earlier in certain races (Freedman, 1979). Therefore cyanosis or asphyxia may occur with nasal blockage.

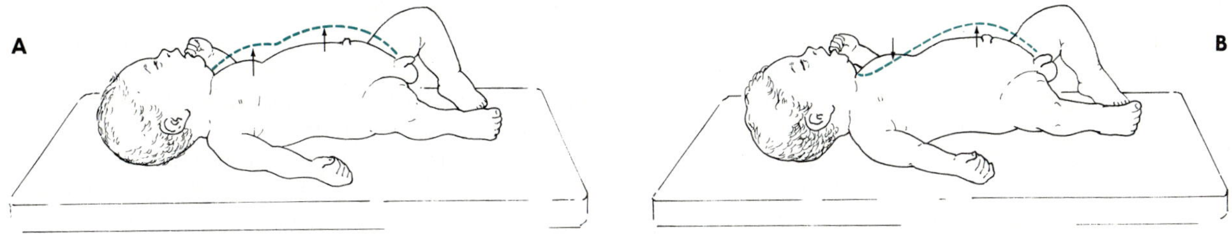

Fig. 21-4 A, Normal respiration. Chest and abdomen rise with inspiration. B, Seesaw respiration. Chest wall retracts and abdomen rises with inspiration.
Courtesy Mead Johnson & Co, Evansville, Indiana.

The chest circumference is approximately 30 to 33 cm (12 to 13 in) at birth. The ribs of the infant articulate with the spine at a horizontal rather than a downward slope; consequently the rib cage cannot expand as readily as does the adult's with inspiration. Neonatal respiratory function is largely a matter of diaphragmatic contraction. The negative intrathoracic pressure is created by the descent of the diaphragm, much like negative pressure is created in the barrel of a syringe when medication is drawn up by retracting the plunger. The infant's chest and abdomen rise simultaneously with inspiration (Fig. 21-4, *A*). *Seesaw respirations are not normal* (Fig. 21-4, *B*).

Auscultation of the chest of an infant reveals loud, clear breath sounds that seem very near, because little chest tissue intervenes. Several significant differences exist between the respiratory system of the infant and the adult:

1. Infants are obligate nose breathers.
2. The infant's tongue is relatively large whereas the glottis and trachea are small.
3. All lumens of the infant are narrower and more easily collapsed.
4. Respiratory tract secretions of the infant are more abundant than those of the adult.
5. The mucous membranes of the infant are more delicate and therefore more susceptible to trauma. The ciliated columnar epithelium just below the vocal cords is especially prone to edema.
6. The alveoli of the infant are more sensitive to changes in pressures.
7. The capillary network of the infant is less well developed. Capillaries are more friable and have less well developed vasoconstrictive and dilative abilities.
8. The infant's bony rib cage and respiratory muscles are not as well developed.

Renal System

At term the kidneys occupy a large portion of the posterior abdominal wall. The bladder lies close to the anterior abdominal wall and is partially an abdominal, as well as a pelvic organ. In the newborn almost all palpable masses in the abdomen are renal in origin.

Kidney function comparable to that of the adult is not approached until the second year of life. The newborn has a minimal range of chemical balance and safety. Diarrhea, infection, or improper feeding can lead rapidly to acidosis and fluid imbalances—dehydration or edema. Renal immaturity also limits the neonate's ability to excrete drugs.

Small amounts of urine are usually present in the bladder at birth, however, the newborn may not void for 12 to 24 hours. Voiding after this period is frequent. Six to ten voidings of pale, straw-colored urine are indicative of adequate fluid intake. The usual urinary output by 10 days is 50 to 300 ml/24 hours.

Fluid and Electrolyte Balance. Differences between the newborn and adult physiologic response include:

1. The distribution of extracellular and intracellular fluid differs from that of the adult. About 40% of the body weight of the newborn is extracellular fluid, whereas in the adult it is 20%.

2. The rate of exchange of extracellular fluid is different. The newborn daily takes in and excretes 600 to 700 ml of water, which is 20% of the total body fluid, or 50% of the extracellular fluid. In contrast, the adult exchanges 2000 ml of water, which is 5% of the total body fluid and 14% of the extracellular fluid.

3. The composition of body fluids shows variations. There is a higher concentration of sodium, phosphates, chloride, and organic acids and a lower concentration of bicarbonate ions. These findings mean that the newborn is in a compensated acidotic state and in a state of potential manifest edema.

4. The glomerular filtration rate is about 30% to 50% of that of the adult. This results in a decreased ability to remove nitrogenous and other waste products from the blood. However, the newborn's ingested protein is almost totally metabolized for growth.

5. The decreased ability to excrete excessive sodium results in hypotonic urine compared to plasma.

6. The sodium reabsorption is decreased as a result of a lowered sodium-potassium-activated adenosine triphosphatase (ATPase) activity.

7. The newborn can dilute urine down to 50 milliosmols (mOsm). An osmol is a measure of total number of particles. One gram molecular weight (mole) of nondiffusible and nonionizable substance is equal to 1 osmole. Capacity to dilute urine exceeds capacity to concentrate it. There is some limitation in the ability to increase urinary volume.

8. The newborn can concentrate urine to 600 to 700 mOsm compared with the adult's capacity of 1400 mOsm. The inability to concentrate urine is not absolute, but in terms of adult function, it is somewhat limited.

9. The infant has a higher renal threshold for glucose.

Gastrointestinal System

In the adequately hydrated infant the mucous membrane of the mouth is moist and pink. Pallor and cyanosis of the mucous membrane are normally not present. Drooling of mucus is common in the first few hours after birth. There are no clefts in the palate. Retention cysts, small whitish areas, may be found on the gum margins and at the juncture of the hard and soft palate. The cheeks are full because of well-developed sucking pads. These, like the labial tubercles (sucking calluses) on the upper lip, disappear when the sucking period is over.

A special mechanism present in normal newborns weighing more than 1500 g coordinates the breathing, sucking, and swallowing reflexes necessary for oral feeding. Sucking in the newborn takes place in small bursts of three or four sucks at a time. In the term newborn, longer and more efficient sucking attempts occur in only a few hours. The infant is unable to move food from the lips to the pharynx; therefore it is necessary to place the nipple (breast or bottle) well inside the baby's mouth. Peristaltic activity in the esophagus is uncoordinated in the first few days of life. It quickly becomes a coordinated pattern in normal infants, and they swallow easily.

Bacteria are not present in the infant's gastrointestinal tract at birth. Soon after birth, oral and anal orifices permit entrance of bacteria and air. Bowel sounds can be heard 1 hour after birth. Generally the highest bacterial concentration is found in the lower portion of the intestine, particularly in the large intestine. The normal intestinal flora help synthesize vitamin K, folic acid, and biotin.

The capacity of the stomach varies from 30 to 90 ml depending on the size of the infant. Emptying time for the stomach is highly variable. Several factors, such as time and volume of feedings, type and temperature of food, and psychic stress, may affect the emptying time. This can range from 1 to 24 hours. Regurgitation may be noted in the neonatal period. The cardiac sphincter and nervous control of the stomach are still immature.

Digestion. Two principal types of cells make up the lining of the stomach. The first type, chief cells, synthesizes and secretes pepsinogen, which aids protein digestion. The second type, parietal cells, secrete hydrochloric acid, which forms the gastric acidity. The enzyme pepsin and gastric acidity are necessary for preliminary digestion of milk before its entrance into the small intestine. The infant's gastric acidity at birth normally equals the adult level but is reduced within a week and may remain reduced for 2 to 3 months. The reduction in gastric acidity may lead to "colic." Infants with colic usually remain awake, crying in apparent distress between 2 feedings, often the same ones every day. Nothing seems to appease them. Infant massage (Chapter 26) may help. They appear to "grow out" of this behavior by age 3 months.

Further digestion and absorption of nutrients occur in the small intestine. This complex process is made possible by pancreatic secretions, secretions from the liver through the common bile duct, and secretions from the duodenal portion of the small intestine.

The infant's ability to digest carbohydrates, fats, and proteins is regulated by the presence of certain enzymes. Most of these are functional at birth. One exception is *amylase,* produced by the salivary glands after about 3 months and by the pancreas at about 6 months of age. This enzyme is necessary to convert starch into maltose. The other exception is *lipase,* also secreted by the pancreas; it is necessary for the digestion of fat. Thus the normal newborn is capable of digesting simple carbohydrates and proteins but has a limited ability to digest fats (see Chapter 23 for more detail).

Stools. At birth the lower intestine is filled with meconium. **Meconium** is formed during fetal life from the amniotic fluid and its constituents, intestinal secretions and shed mucosal cells. Meconium is greenish black and viscous and contains occult blood. The first meconium passed is sterile, but within hours all meconium passed contains bacteria. The first passage of meconium occurs within 24 hours in 90% of normal infants. Most of the rest do so within 36 hours (Pritchard, MacDonald, and Gant, 1985).

The number of stools varies considerably during the first week, being most numerous between the third and sixth days. **Transitional stools** (thin, slimy, and brown to green because of the continued presence of meconium) are passed from the third to sixth day. The stools of breast-fed babies and formula-fed babies differ. The stools of the breast-fed baby are loose, golden yellow in color, and nonirritating to the infant's skin. It is normal for the baby to have a bowel movement with each feeding or a bowel movement every 3 to 4 days. Even if the latter is the case, the stools remain loose and unformed. The stools of the formula-fed baby are formed but soft, are pale yellow, and have a typical stool odor. They tend to be irritating to the infant's skin. The number of stools decreases in the first 2 weeks from five or six each day (after every feeding) to one to two per day.

Distension of the stomach muscles cause a corresponding relaxation and contraction of the muscles of the colon. As a result, infants often have bowel movements during or just after a feeding. Breast-fed babies are more likely to stool during a feeding than formula-fed babies. Stooling at these times has been attributed to the gastrocolic reflex.

The infant develops an elimination pattern by the second week of life. With the addition of solid food the baby's stool gradually assumes the characteristics of an adult's stool.

Feeding Behaviors. Variations occur among infants regarding interest in food, symptoms of hunger, and amount ingested at any one time. The amount that the infant takes at any one formula-feeding depends, of course, on the size of the infant; but other factors seem to play a part: if put to breast, some infants feed immediately, whereas others require a learning period of up to 48 hours before breast-feeding can be said to be effective. Random hand-to-mouth movement and sucking of fingers have been seen in utero. These actions are well developed at birth and are intensified with hunger.

Hepatic System

The liver performs a number of functions, one of which is to control the amount of circulating unbound bilirubin.

The pigment bilirubin is derived from the hemoglobin released with the breakdown of RBCs (90% to 95%). The remaining pigment is derived from the myoglobin in muscle cells. The hemoglobin is phagocytized by the reticuloendothelial cells, converted to bilirubin, and released in an unconjugated form. Unconjugated bilirubin, termed *indirect bilirubin,* is relatively insoluble and is almost entirely bound to circulating albumin, a plasma protein. The unbound bilirubin can leave the vascular system and permeate other extravascular tissues (e.g., the skin, sclera, oral mucous membranes). The resultant yellow coloring is termed **jaundice**.

In the liver the unbound bilirubin is conjugated with glucuronide in the presence of the enzyme glucuronyl transferase. The conjugated form of bilirubin is excreted from liver cells as a constituent of bile. It is termed *direct bilirubin* and is soluble. Along with other components of bile, direct bilirubin is excreted into the biliary tract system that carries the bile into the duodenum. Bilirubin is converted to urobilinogen and stercobilin within the duodenum through the action of the bacterial flora. Urobilinogen is excreted in urine and feces; stercobilin is excreted in the feces (Fig. 21-5). Total serum bilirubin is the sum of conjugated (direct) and unconjugated (indirect) bilirubin.

The full-term newborn's liver is usually sufficiently mature and the production of glucuronyl transferase great enough to conjugate the circulating unconjugated bilirubin. Adequate serum albumin–binding sites are also available

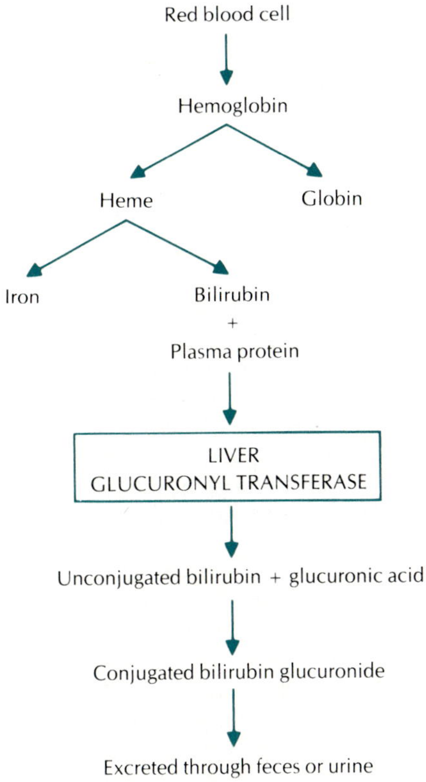

Fig. 21-5 Formation and excretion of bilirubin.
From Whaley, L, and Wong, DL: Nursing care of infants and children, ed 3, St Louis, 1987, The CV Mosby Co.

unless the infant experiences asphyxia neonatorum, cold stress, or hypoglycemia. Maternal prebirth ingestion of drugs such as sulfa drugs and aspirin can reduce the amount of serum albumin–binding sites in the newly born. Although the neonate has the functional capacity to convert bilirubin, physiologic hyperbilirubinemia occurs in most infants.

Physiologic Hyperbilirubinemia. Physiologic hyperbilirubinemia or neonatal jaundice is a normal occurrence in 50% of full-term and 80% of preterm newborns. Korones (1986) notes that neonatal jaundice occurs because:

1. The newborn has a higher rate of bilirubin production. The number of fetal red blood cells per kilogram of weight is greater than the adult. The fetal red blood cells have a shorter survival time, 40-90 days compared to 120 days in the adult.
2. There is considerable reabsorption of bilirubin from the neonatal small intestine.

Although neonatal jaundice is considered benign, bilirubin may accumulate to hazardous levels and become pathologic (Chapter 40). Physiologic jaundice fulfills the following specific criteria (Korones 1986):

> (1) the infant is otherwise well: (2) in term infants, jaundice first appears after 24 hours and disappears by the end of the seventh day; (3) in premature infants, jaundice is first evident after 48 hours and disappears by the ninth or tenth day; (4) serum unconjugated bilirubin concentration does not exceed 12 mg/100 ml, either in term or preterm infants, (5) hyperbilirubinemia is almost exclusively of the unconjugated variety, and conjugated (direct) bilirubin should not exceed 1 to 1.5 mg/100 ml; (6) daily increments of bilirubin concentration should not surpass 5 mg/100 ml. Bilirubin levels in excess of 12 mg/100 ml may indicate either an exaggeration of the physiologic handicap or the presence of disease. *At any serum bilirubin level, the appearance of jaundice during the first day of life or persistence beyond the ages previously delineated usually indicates a pathologic process.*

Jaundice is noticeable first in the head and then progresses gradually toward the abdomen and extremities because of the neonate's circulatory pattern (cephalocaudal developmental progression). The appearance of jaundice in the various body locations gives a rough estimate of the circulating levels of unbound bilirubin. For example, when jaundice appears over the nose, the circulating level of unbound bilirubin is approximately 3 mg; levels at which other body areas appear jaundiced are as follows:

Approximate Level of Hyperbilirubinemia by Cephalocaudal Distribution

Nose: 3 mg/dl	Abdomen: 10 mg/dl
Face: 5 mg/dl	Legs: 12 mg/dl
Chest: 7 mg/dl	Palms: 20 mg/dl

Several nursery practices may influence the appearance and degree of physiologic hyperbilirubinemia. *Early feeding* tends to keep the serum bilirubin level low by stimulating intestinal activity and the passage of meconium and stool. Removal of intestinal contents prevents the reabsorption (and recycling) of bilirubin from the gut, a residual mechanism left over from fetal life (De Carvalho et al., 1982; Ostler, 1980).

Chilling of the newborn may result in acidosis and raise the level of free fatty acids. In the presence of acidosis, albumin binding of bilirubin is weakened and biluribin is freed. Bilirubin is displaced from its serum albumin–binding sites by the free fatty acids and as unbound bilirubin can be deposited in body tissues. **Kernicterus,** the most serious complication of neonatal hyperbilirubinemia, is caused by the precipitation of bilirubin in neuronal cells, resulting in their destruction (see Chapter 40). Cerebral palsy, epilepsy, and mental retardation are expected in survivors.

There is an increase in the number of mothers and infants being discharged from the hospital between 2 and 48 hours after birth and others who have elected to give birth at home. As a result the professional attendant may not be available to assess pathologic rises in circulating unbound bilirubin. *Therefore all parents need instruction in how to assess jaundice and to whom to report the findings* (see Chapter 22).

Breast Milk Jaundice. Breast milk jaundice (BMJ) has been defined as progressive indirect hyperbilirubinemia beyond the first week of life. Jaundice from ingestion of breast milk occurs in 0.5% to 2% of fullterm neonates (Saul and Warburton, 1984). It is thought that an enzyme present in the milk of some women inhibits the enzyme glucuronyl transferase, which is necessary for the conjugation of bilirubin. Although breast milk jaundice is a form of physiologic jaundice, it occurs after the mature milk has come in, usually about the **fifth or sixth day of life** in a thriving infant whose mother is lactating well. This type of jaundice usually persists longer—up to 6 weeks. Unconjugated bilirubin rises beyond physiologic limits (15 to 20 mg/dl) by the seventh day. The levels subside by 5 to 10 mg if breastfeeding is discontinued for 12 to 24 hours; then usually 3 to 5 days pass before the previous high level is again reached. Mothers are encouraged to maintain their milk supply during this test period by pumping or manually expressing the milk. Mothers need reassurance that nothing is wrong with their milk (Brovten et al., 1985; Lascari, 1986; Locklin, 1987).

Although the indirect bilirubin level may range from 10 mg/dl to 30 mg/dl during this time, no cases of bilirubin encephalopathy related to BMJ have been reported (Brovten and others, 1985). It is unfortunate that many breastfeeding women have been made to feel their milk is pathogenic for their offspring.

Breast-feeding Jaundice. Breast-feeding jaundice usually becomes apparent about the **third day of life.** There is no other apparent clinical cause. Dehydration, lack of fluid, and weight loss are not causes (DeCarvalho, Hall, and Harvey, 1981). Recent research has documented that the number of breast-feedings during the first 3 days of life are related to bilirubin levels and display a significant relationship (Lascari, 1986; Ostler, 1980). The greater the number of feedings, the lower the bilirubin level (DeCarvalho et al., 1982; Lascari, 1986; Ostler, 1980). The number of feedings per day should be eight or more. The mother is encouraged to feed around the clock. Early breastmilk colostrum is a natural laxative that helps promote passage of meconium. Consequently early, frequent nursings will enhance meconium excretion and decrease bilirubin levels (Ostler, 1980).

Immune System

All newborns and especially preterm newborns are at high risk for infection during the first several months of life. During this period, infection represents one of the leading causes of morbidity and mortality. The newborn is unable to limit the invading pathogen to the portal of entry because of a generalized hypofunction of the inflammatory and immune mechanisms (Medici, 1983).

Resistance to infection (immunity) includes both nonspecific and specific protective mechanisms (see Chapter 6). Medici (1983) summarizes the newborn's defense mechanisms as follows:

> The term and preterm neonate has an increased incidence of infection for the first 4 to 6 weeks of life. This reflects the immaturity of a number of protective systems which significantly increases the risk of infection in this patient population. Natural barriers such as the acidity of the stomach or the production of pepsin and trypsin which maintain sterility of the small intestine are not fully developed until 3 to 4 weeks. The membrane protective IgA is missing from the respiratory and urinary tracts, and unless the newborn is breast-fed, it is absent from the gastrointestinal tract as well. The immune system is in great part suppressed; possibly this is a mechanism for preventing maternal recognition of paternal antigens with subsequent rejection of the fetus. Finally, the qualitative and quantitative response of the inflammatory factors and sluggish responses of the phagocytic cells.

Integumentary System

The epidermis (skin) of the term newborn possesses the characteristic five layers (strata) of the adult: germinativum, spinosum, granulosum, corneum, and on the palmar and plantar surfaces, stratum lucidum underneath the stratum corneum. In the neonate the *stratum corneum is thin and fused with the vernix caseosa* (a reason for not removing the vernix at birth). The stratum corneum later becomes the effective skin barrier.

The term infant has an erythematous skin (beefy red) for a few hours after birth, after which it fades to its normal color. It often appears blotchy or mottled, especially over the extremities. The hands and feet appear slightly cyanotic. This bluish discoloration, **acrocyanosis,** is caused by vasomotor instability, capillary stasis, and a high hemoglobin level; it is normal, appearing intermittently over the first 7 to 10 days, especially with exposure to cold.

The healthy term newborn is plump. Subcutaneous fat accumulated during the last trimester acts to insulate the newborn. The preterm infant has difficulty maintaining an even body temperature because of the lack of this fat. The skin may be slightly tight, suggesting fluid retention. Fine **lanugo hair** may be noted over the face, shoulders, and back. Actual edema of the face and **ecchymosis** (bruising) may be noted as a result of face presentation or forceps delivery.

Caput Succedaneum. Caput succedaneum is a localized,

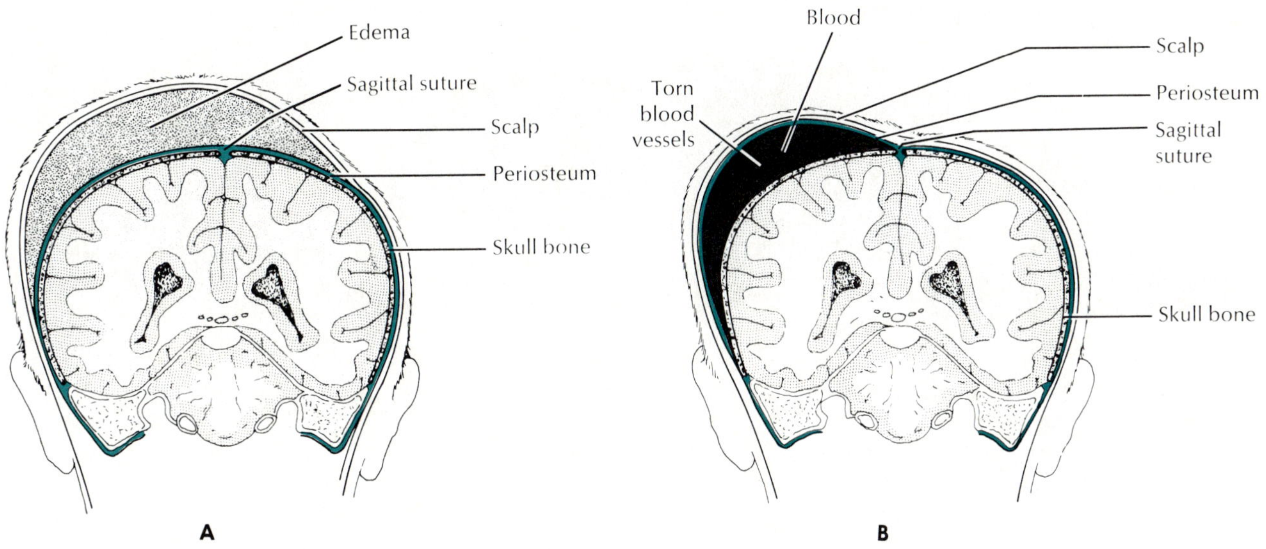

Fig. 21-6 Differences between caput succedaneum and cephalhematoma. **A**, Caput succedaneum: edema of scalp noted at birth; crosses suture line. **B**, Cephalhematoma: bleeding between periosteum and skull bone appearing within first 2 days; does not cross suture lines.

easily identifiable edematous area of the scalp (Fig. 21-6, *A*). The sustained pressure of the presenting vertex against the cervix results in compression of local vessels, thus slowing venous return. The slower venous return causes an increase in tissue fluids within the skin of the scalp, and an edematous swelling develops. This boggy edematous swelling present at birth extends across suture lines of the fetal skull and disappears spontaneously within 3 to 4 days. Excessive pressure to the presenting vertex as it passes over the bony maternal pelvis may cause a cephalhematoma to develop.

Cephalhematoma. Cephalhematoma is a collection of blood between a skull bone and its periosteum. Therefore a cephalhematoma never crosses a cranial suture line (Fig. 21-6, *B*). Cephalhematoma is caused by pressure during delivery. Bleeding may occur with spontaneous delivery from pressure against the maternal bony pelvis. Low forceps delivery, as well as difficult forceps rotation and extraction, may also cause bleeding. This soft, fluctuating, irreducible fullness does not pulsate or bulge when the infant cries. It appears several hours after birth or the day after delivery or becomes apparent following absorption of a caput succedaneum (Fig. 21-6, *A*). It is usually largest on the second or third day, by which time the bleeding stops. The fullness of cephalhematoma spontaneously resolves in 3 to 6 weeks. It is not aspirated because infection may develop if the skin is punctured.

As the hematoma resolves, the hemolysis of RBCs occurs. Hyperbilirubinemia (jaundice) may result after the newborn is home. Therefore the parents are instructed to observe the newborn for jaundice and may be asked to bring the infant in to be rechecked before the usual 4-week visit.

Desquamation. Desquamation of the skin of the term infant does not occur until a few days after birth. Its presence at birth is an indication of postmaturity.

Sweat and Oil Glands. Sweat glands are present at birth but do not function effectively (i.e., do not respond to increases in ambient or body temperature), perhaps because the neurogenic stimuli are still immature. There is some fetal sebaceous (oil) gland hyperplasia and secretion of sebum as a result of the hormonal influences of pregnancy. **Vernix caseosa**, a cheeselike substance, is a product of the sebaceous glands. Distended sebaceous glands, noticeable in the newborn, particularly on the checks and nose, are known as **milia**. Although sebaceous glands are well developed at birth, they are only minimally active during childhood. They become more active as androgen production increases before puberty.

Mongolian Spots. Mongolian spots, bluish-black areas of pigmentation, may appear over any part of the extensor surface of the body, including the extremities. They are more commonly noted on the back and buttocks. The occurrence of Mongolian spots is not primarily related to race. Thus these pigmented areas are noted in babies whose origins are from the shores of the Mediterranean, Latin America, Asia, or a number of other areas in the world. They are more common in dark-skinned individuals regardless of race. They fade gradually over a period of months or years.

Nevi. Known as "stork bites," **telangiectatic nevi** are pink and easily blanched (Fig. 21-7, *A*). They appear on the upper eyelids, nose, upper lip, lower occiput bone, and nape of the neck. They have no clinical significance and fade between the first and second years.

The **strawberry mark**, or nevus vasculosus, is the second most common type of capillary hemangioma (Fig. 21-7, *B*). It consists of dilated, newly formed capillaries occupying the entire dermal and subdermal layers with associated connective tissue hypertrophy. The typical lesion is a raised, sharply demarcated, and bright or dark red, rough-surfaced swelling that resembles a strawberry. Lesions are

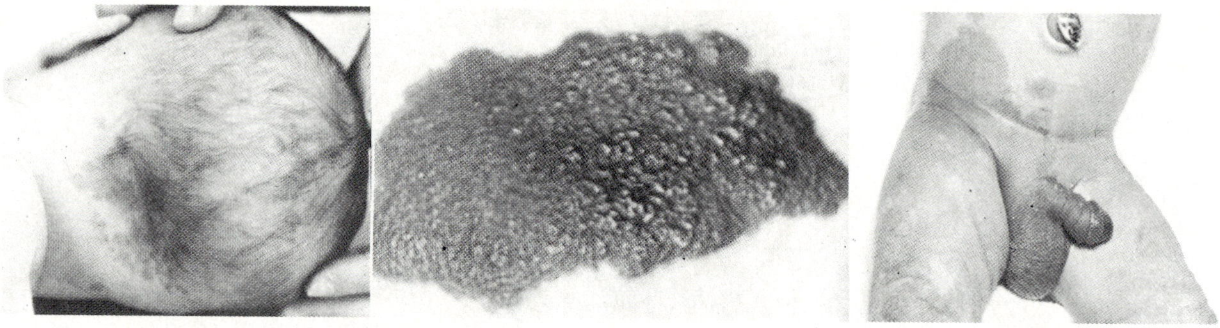

A B C

Fig. 21-7 **A**, Telangiectatic nevi (stork bite). **B**, Strawberry mark, or nevus vasculosus. **C**, Port-wine stain, or nevus flammeus.
Courtesy Mead Johnson & Co, Evansville, Indiana.

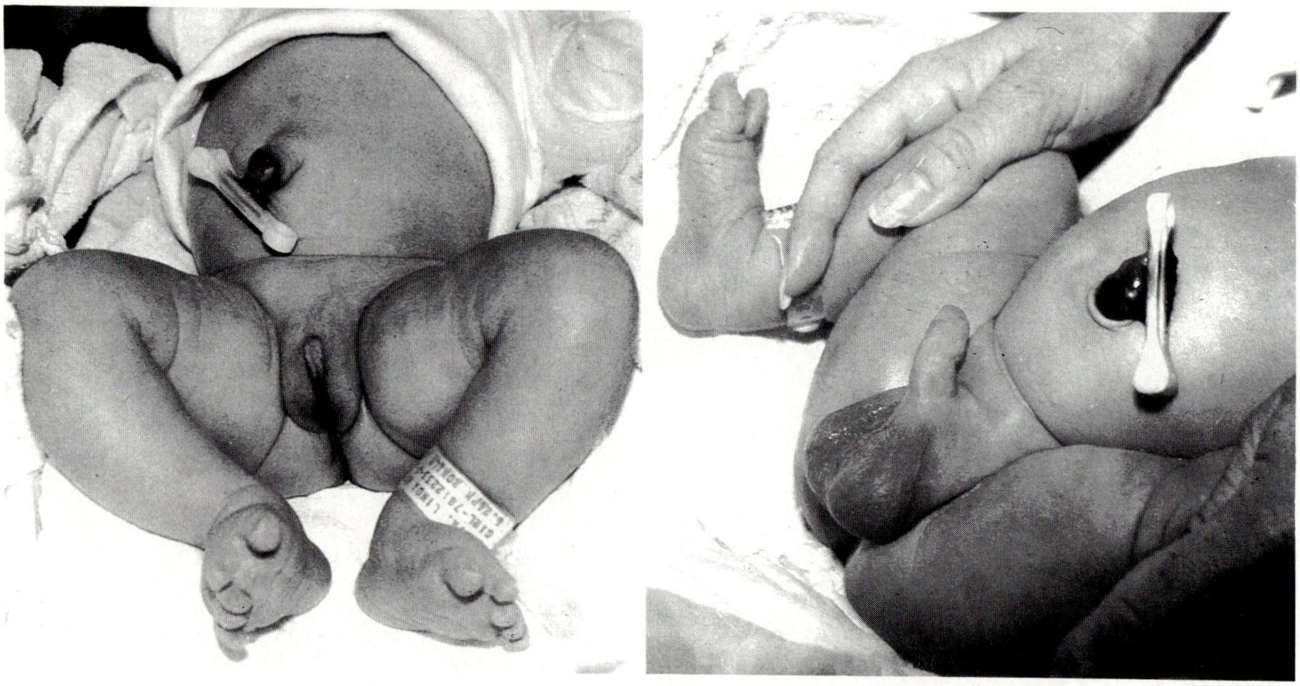

A B

Fig. 21-8 **A**, Genitals in female term infant. Note mucoid vaginal discharge. **B**, Genitals in male infant. Uncircumcised penis. Rugae cover scrotum, indicating term gestation. Cord has been swabbed with ethylene blue to prevent infection.

usually single but may be multiple; 75% occur in the head region. These lesions can remain until the child is of school age or sometimes even longer.

A **port-wine stain**, or nevus flammeus, is usually observed at birth and is composed of a plexus of newly formed capillaries in the papillary layer of the corium. It is red to purple, varies in size, shape, and location, and is not elevated (Fig. 21-7, *C*). True port-wine stains do not blanch on pressure and do not disappear spontaneously.

Erythema toxicum. An evanescent rash, erythema toxicum is also called **erythema neonatorum**, or "fleabite" dermatitis. It has lesions in different stages, erythematous macules, papules, or small vesicles, and may appear suddenly anywhere on the body. The rash is thought to be an inflammatory response. Eosinophils, which help decrease inflammation, are found in the vesicles. The rash is found only in term neonates (36 or more weeks gestational age) during the first 3 weeks of age (Medici, 1983). Although the appearance is alarming, it has no clinical significance and requires no treatment.

The intact skin of the infant acts as an effective barrier to infection; however, the fragility of the skin makes it more vulnerable to disruption of the surface when traumatized by too vigorous handling, rubbing, or excoriation.

Reproductive System

Female. At birth the ovaries contain thousands of primitive germ cells. These represent the full complement of potential ova, since no oogonia form after delivery in term infants. The ovarian cortex, which is made up primarily of primordial follicles, forms a thicker portion of the ovary in the female newborn than in the adult. The number of ova decreases from birth to maturity by approximately 90%.

The infant's uterus, enlarged during pregnancy because of maternal estrogen, undergoes involution in the first weeks of life and decreases in size and weight.

Hyperestrogenism of pregnancy followed by a drop after delivery results in a mucoid vaginal discharge and even some slight bloody spotting. Vaginal tags are common findings and have no clinical significance. External genitals are usually edematous with increased pigmentation. In term neonates, labia majora and minora obscure the vestibule (Fig. 21-8, *A*).

Male. The testes have descended into the scrotum in 90% of newborn boys. Although this percentage drops with premature birth, by 1 year of age the incidence of undescended testes in all boys is less than 1%. Spermatogenesis does not occur until puberty (see Chapter 6).

Adhesions of the foreskin (prepuce) are almost universally present in newborn boys. During prenatal development the tissue of the prepuce is continuous with the epidermis that covers the glans. Gradually the preputial space between the prepuce and glans forms. The complete separation of the two tissue areas is generally not complete at birth. For this reason the prepuce of the newborn is usually not retractable.

External genitals in the term neonate are increased in size and pigmentation in response to maternal estrogen. The scrotal sac is covered with rugae (Fig. 21-8, *B*).

Swelling of Breast Tissue. Swelling of the breast tissue in infants of both sexes is caused by the hyperestrogenism of pregnancy. In a few infants a thin discharge (witch's milk) can be seen. The finding has no clinical significance, requires no treatment, and will subside as the maternal hormones are eliminated from the infant's body.

Skeletal System

The cephalocaudal direction of development is evident in total body growth seen in significant changes in body proportions by term gestation (Fig. 21-9). The head at term is one fourth of the total body length. The arms are slightly longer than the legs. In the newborn the lower limbs are one third of the total body length but only 15% of the total body weight; in the adult the lower limbs comprise one half of the total body height and 30% of total body weight. As growth proceeds, the midpoint in head-to-toe measurements gradually descends from a level even with the umbilicus at birth to the level of the symphysis pubis at maturity (Whaley and Wong, 1987).

The face is small in relation to the skull. The skull is large and heavy in comparison. Cranial size and shape can be distorted by molding (Fig. 21-10). The bones in the vertebral column of the newborn form two primary curvatures, one in the thoracic region and one in the sacral region (Fig. 21-11, *A*). Both are forward, concave curvatures. As the infant gains control of his head, at approximately 3 months of age, a secondary curvature appears in the cervical region (Fig. 21-11, *B*).

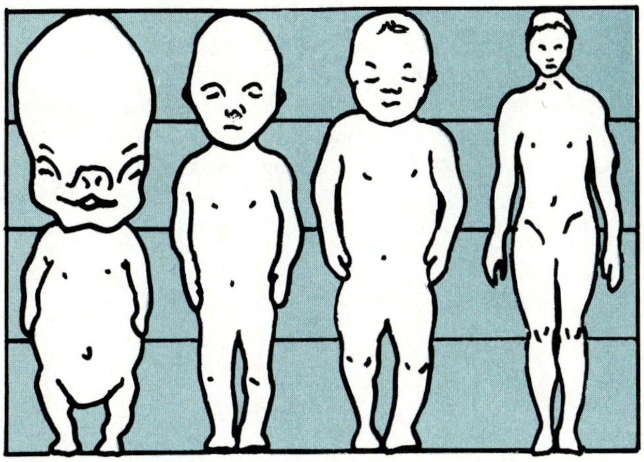

Fig. 21-9 Changes in body proportions from before birth to adulthood.

In some newborn infants there is a significant separation of the knees when the ankles are held together resulting in an appearance of bowlegs (Fig. 21-12, *A*). Muscle development gives bowed appearance; leg bones are straight. Before the child begins to walk, there is no clearly apparent arch to the foot (Fig. 21-12, *B*).

Neuromuscular System

Until the late 1950s the human newborn was considered to be immature, disorganized, and able to function only at a brainstem level. Neurobehavioral assessment of the neonate was therefore based mainly on evaluation of muscle tone and primitive reflexes (Table 21-2). Recent studies have recognized the term newborn to be a vital, responsive, and reactive being (Table 21-2). The newborn shows remarkable sensory development and an amazing ability for self-organization and social interaction (Fanaroff, 1987).

Postdelivery growth of the *brain* follows a predictable pattern: rapid during infancy and early childhood, more gradual during the remainder of the first decade, and minimal during adolescence. The cerebellum ends its growth spurt, which began at about 30 gestational weeks, by the end of the first year. This is perhaps why it is vulnerable to nutritional or other trauma in early infancy (see discussion of newborn nutrition, Chapter 23, and kernicterus, Chapter 40).

The brain requires glucose as a source of energy and a relatively large supply of oxygen for adequate metabolism. Oxygen requirements range from 5 to 8 ml/100 g. Such requirements signal a need for careful assessment of the infant's ability to maintain an open airway and of respiratory conditions requiring oxygen therapy. The necessity for glucose requires an awareness of those neonates who may have hypoglycemic episodes.

Spontaneous motor activity may be seen in transient tremors of mouth and chin, especially when crying, and of extremities, notably the arms and hands. Persistent tremors or tremors involving the total body may be indicative of pathologic conditions. Marked tonicity, clonicity, and twitching of facial muscles are signs of convulsions. There is a need for the physician to differentiate among normal tremors, tremors of hypoglycemia, and central nervous system (CNS) disorders so that corrective care can be instituted, as necessary.

Neuromuscular control in the newborn, although still very limited, can be noted. If newborns are placed facedown on a firm surface, they will turn their heads to the

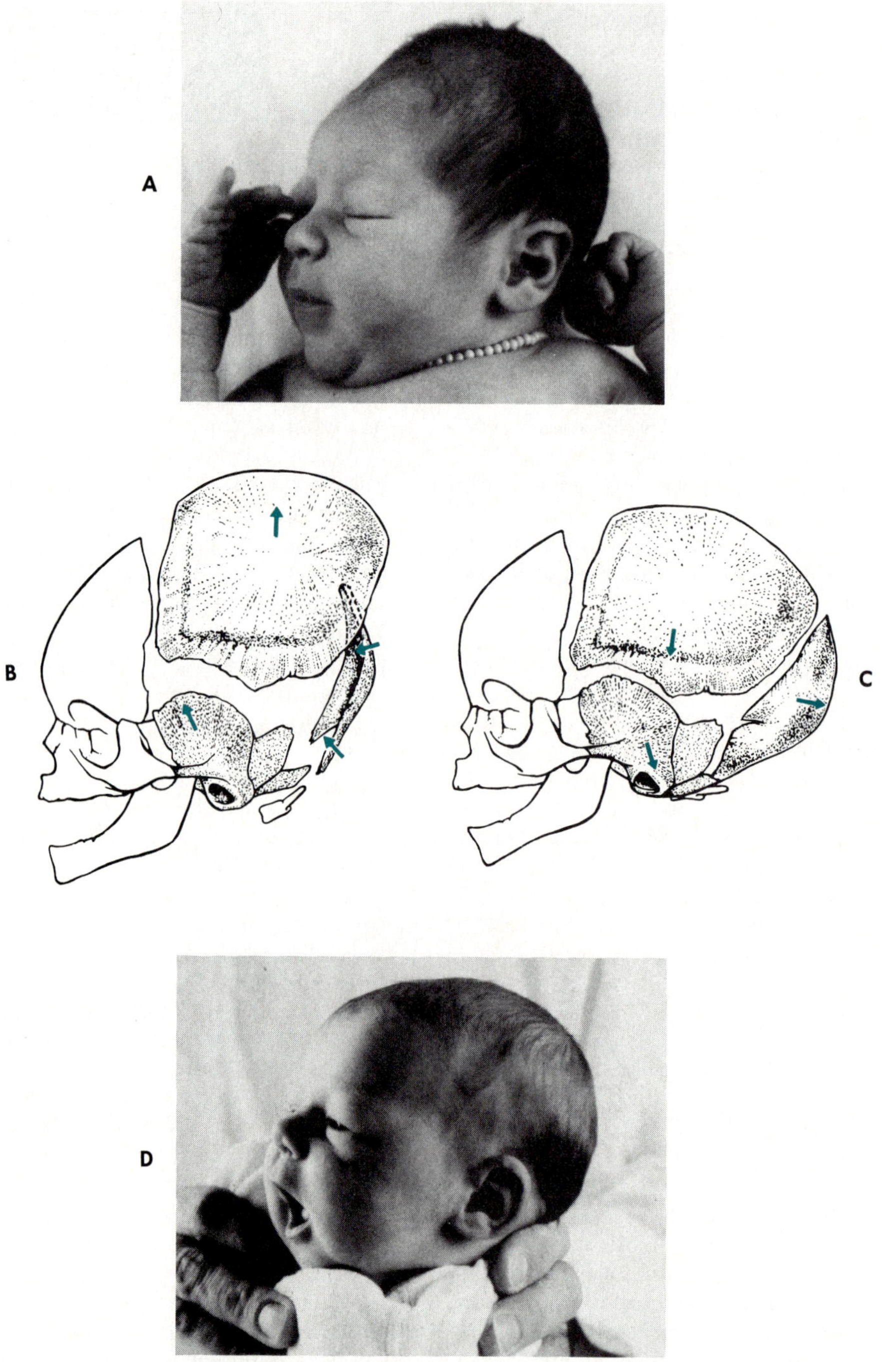

Fig. 21-10 A, Molding after vaginal birth. B, Movement of cranial bones during molding. C, Return of cranial bones to alignment. D, Absence of molding.

side to maintain an airway. They attempt to hold their heads in line with their bodies if they are raised by their arms. Various reflexes serve to promote their safety and an adequate food intake. This is described further in this chapter under behavioral characteristics of the newborn.

Thermogenetic System

Thermogenesis means the production of heat (thermo = heat, genesis = origin). Effective neonatal care is based on the maintenance of an optimum thermal environment. In homoiothermic individuals the narrow limits of normal body temperature are maintained by producing heat in response to its dissipation. Hypothermia from excessive heat loss is a prevalent and dangerous problem in neonates. The newborn infant's ability to produce heat often approaches the capacity of the adult. However, the tendency toward rapid heat loss in a suboptimum thermal environment is increased in the newborn and is often hazardous to well-being.

Heat Production. The shivering mechanism of heat production is rarely functioning in the newborn. Non-shivering thermogenesis is accomplished primarily by **brown fat** and secondarily by increased metabolic activity in the brain, heart, and liver. Brown fat is unique to the newborn (Davis, 1980; Korones, 1986). It is located in superficial deposits in the interscapular region and axillas, as well as in deep deposits at the thoracic inlet, along the vertebral column, and around the kidneys. Brown fat has a richer vascular and nerve supply than does ordinary fat. Heat produced by intense lipid metabolic activity in brown fat can warm the neonate by increasing heat production as much as 100%. Reserves of brown fat, usually present for several weeks after birth, are rapidly depleted with cold stress. The less mature the infant, the less reserve of this essential fat is available at birth.

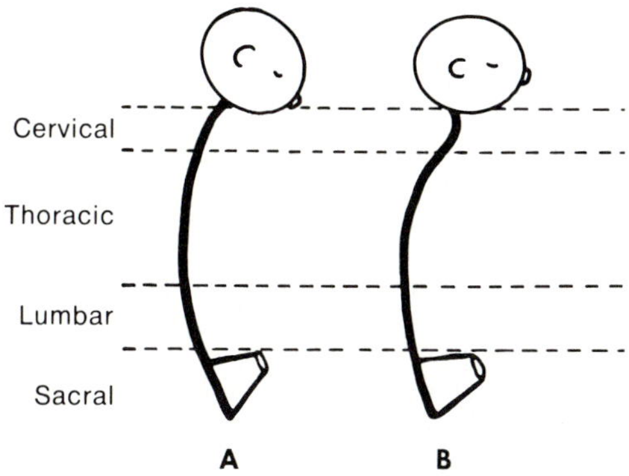

Fig. 21-11 Development of spinal curvatures. **A**, Newborn infant. **B**, Cervical secondary curvature.

From Whaley, LF, and Wong, DL: Nursing care of infants and children, ed 3, St Louis, 1987, The CV Mosby Co.

Heat Loss. Heat loss occurs in four ways:

1. *Convection:* the flow of heat from the body surface to cooler ambient air. For this reason nursery ambient temperatures are kept at 24° C (75° F), and newborns are wrapped to protect them from the cold.
2. *Radiation:* the loss of heat from the body surface to cooler solid surfaces not in direct contact but in relative proximity to each other. Nursery cribs and examining tables are placed away from outside windows.
3. *Evaporation:* the loss of heat that occurs when a liquid is converted to a vapor. In the newborn, heat loss by evaporation occurs as a result of vaporization of moisture from the skin. This process is invisible and is known as *insensible water loss* (IWL). This heat loss can be intensified by not drying the newborn directly after birth or by bathing and drying the infant too slowly.
4. *Conduction:* the loss of heat from the body surface to cooler surfaces in direct contact. The newborn when admitted to the nursery is placed in a warmed cot to minimize heat loss. Loss of heat must be controlled to protect the infant. As noted above, control of such modes of heat loss is the basis for caregiving policies and techniques.

Temperature Regulation. Anatomic and physiologic differences among the newborn, child, and adult are notable:

1. The newborn's thermal insulation is less than an adult's. Blood vessels are closer to the surface of the skin.

Text continued on p. 489.

A
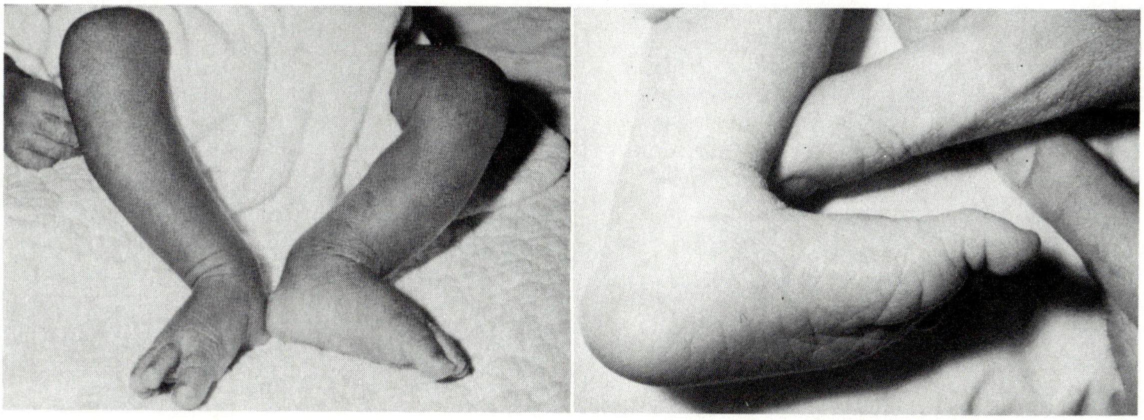
B

Fig. 21-12 Extremities. **A**, Bowed appearance of legs. **B**, Normal absence of arch in newborn.

Table 21-2 ***Physical Assessment of Newborn***

Area Assessed and Appraisal Procedure	Normal Findings: Average Findings	Normal Findings: Normal Variations	Deviations from Normal Range (Possible Causes)
Posture			
Inspect newborn before disturbing for assessment Refer to maternal chart for fetal presentation, position, and type of birth (vaginal, surgical), since newborn readily assumes prenatal position	Vertex: arms, legs in moderate flexion; fists are clenched Newborn resists having extremities extended for examination or measurement and will cry when this is attempted Crying ceases when allowed to reassume curled-up fetal position Normal spontaneous movement is bilaterally asynchronous (legs move in bicycle fashion) but equally extensive in all extremities	Frank breech: more straight and stiff, so that newborn will assume intrauterine position in repose for a few days Prenatal pressure of limb or shoulder may cause temporary facial asymmetry (Fig. 21-13) or resistance to extension of extremities	Lack of muscle tone, relaxed posture while awake: prematurity or hypoxia in utero Hypertonia: drug dependence, CNS disorder Opisthotonos: CNS disturbance Limitation of motion in any of extremities: see Extremities, below

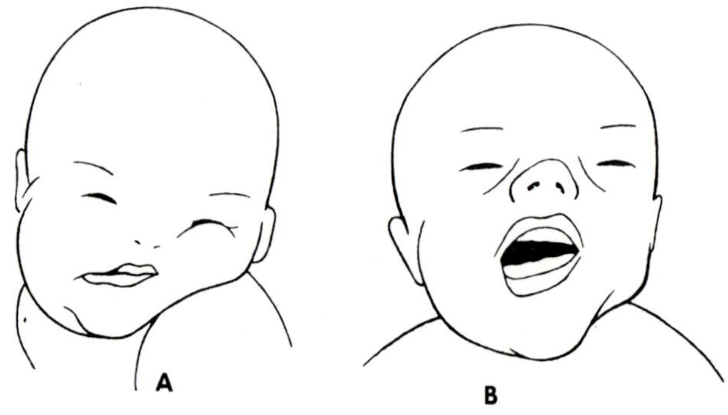

Fig. 21-13 **A**, Facial asymmetry from prenatal pressure. **B**, Lopsided appearance disappears spontaneously in time.
Courtesy Mead Johnson & Co, Evansville, Indiana.

Vital Signs			
Blood pressure (BP) Electronic monitor BP cuff: BP cuff width affects readings; use cuff 2.5 cm (1 in) wide and palpate radial pulse (see Chapter 36)	75/42 (approximately) At birth Systolic: 60-80 mm Hg Diastolic: 40-50 mm Hg At 10 days Systolic: 95-100 mm Hg Diastolic: slight increase	Varies with change in activity level: awake, crying, sleeping	Difference between upper and lower extremity pressures may provide early clue to coarctation of aorta Hypotension Hypertension: coarctation of aorta
Heart rate and pulses Thorax Inspection Palpation Auscultation Apex: mitral valve Second interspace, left of sternum: pulmonic valve Second interspace, right of sternum: aortic valve Junction of xiphoid process and sternum: tricuspid valve	Pulsations visible in left midclavicular line; fifth intercostal space Apical pulse; fourth intercostal space 120-140/min Quality: *first sound* (closure of mitral valves) and *second sound* (closure of aortic and pulmonic valves) should be sharp and clear	100 (sleeping) to 160 (crying); may be irregular for brief periods, especially after crying Murmurs, especially over base or at left sternal border in interspace 3 or 4 (foramen ovale anatomically closes at about 1 year) Average pulses (slightly faster for girls) 2 yr: 105 6 yr: 100 8-12 yr: 85-90 16 yr: 80 18 yr: 70	Tachycardia (persistent; ≥170): RDS Bradycardia (persistent; ≤120): congenital heart block Murmurs: may be functional Arrhythmias: irregular rate Sounds Distant: pneumomediastinum Poor quality Extra Heard on right side of chest: dextrocardia (often accompanied by reversal of intestines)

Table 21-2 *Physical Assessment of Newborn—cont'd*

Area Assessed and Appraisal Procedure	Normal Findings: Average Findings	Normal Findings: Normal Variations	Deviations from Normal Range (Possible Causes)
Femoral pulse palpation: flex thighs on hips; place fingers along inguinal ligament about midway between symphysis pubis and iliac crest; feel bilaterally at same time (Fig. 21-14)	Femoral pulses should be equal and strong		Weak or absent femoral pulses Hip dysplasia Coarctation of aorta Thrombophlebitis

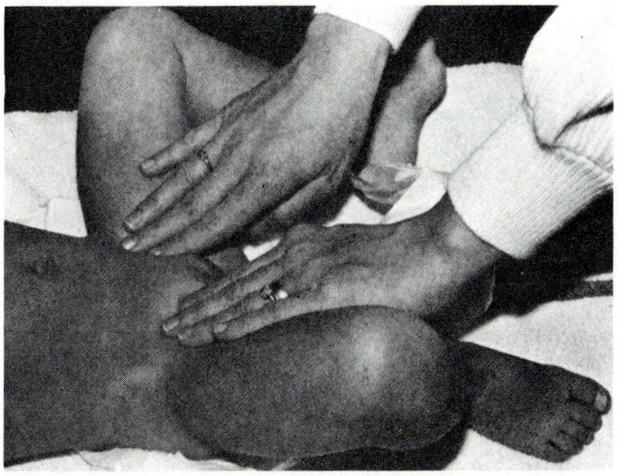

Fig. 21-14 Pulses are palpated simultaneously with tips of fingers along inguinal ligament about midway between iliac crest and pubic symphysis.
From Whaley, LF, and Wong, DL: Nursing care of infants and children, ed 3, St Louis, 1987, The CV Mosby Co.

Area Assessed and Appraisal Procedure	Normal Findings: Average Findings	Normal Findings: Normal Variations	Deviations from Normal Range (Possible Causes)
Temperature Axillary: method of choice until 6 yr of age; hold in axillary fold for 5 min Rectal: before passage of meconium check for patent anus; insert thermometer with great caution no further than 1 to 2 cm (¼ to ½ in) into rectum, gently; hold in place for 5 min, keeping legs immobilized to prevent thermometer from being dislodged or broken (there is a risk of traumatizing or perforating rectal mucosa) Electronic: thermistor probe (avoid taping over bony area) (see Chapter 36)	Axillary: 36.5°-37° C (97.6°-98.6° F) Rectal: may be misleading—even in cold stress may remain unchanged until metabolic activity can no longer maintain core temperature Temperature stabilization by 8-10 hr of age Shivering mechanism undeveloped	36.4° to 37.2° C (97.5° to 99° F) Heat loss: 200 kcal/kg/min from evaporation, conduction, convection, radiation	Subnormal—may reflect the following: Prematurity, infection, low environmental temperature, inadequate clothing; and dehydration Increased (pyrexia)—may reflect the following: Infection, high environmental temperature, excessive clothing, proximity to heating unit or in direct sunshine, drug addiction (following increased activity level of infant), and diarrhea and dehydration Temperature not stabilized by 10 hr after birth If mother received magnesium sulfate, newborn is less able to conserve heat by vasoconstriction; maternal analgesics may reduce thermal stability in newborn
Respiratory rate and effort Observe respirations when infant is at rest Count respirations for full minute Apnea monitor Listen for sounds audible without stethoscope	40/min Tend to be shallow, and when infant is awake, irregular in rate, rhythm, and depth No sounds should be audible on inspiration or expiration Breath sounds: bronchial; loud, clear, near	30-60/min May appear to be Cheyne-Stokes with short periods of apnea and with no evidence of respiratory distress First period (reactivity): 50-60/min	Apneic episodes: ≥15/sec Preterm or premature infant: "periodic breathing" Rapid warming or cooling of infant Bradypnea: ≤25/min Maternal narcosis from anal-

Continued.

Table 21-2 *Physical Assessment of Newborn—cont'd*

Area Assessed and Appraisal Procedure	Normal Findings: Average Findings	Normal Findings: Normal Variations	Deviations from Normal Range (Possible Causes)
Observe respiratory effort		Second period: 50-70/min Stabilization (1-2 days): 30-40/min	gesics or anesthetics Birth trauma Tachypnea: ≥60/min RDS Aspiration syndrome Diaphragmatic hernia Sounds Rales, rhonchi, wheezes Expiratory grunt Distress: Nasal flaring, retractions, chin tug, labored breathing
Weight*			
Put protective liner in place and adjust scale to 0 (Fig. 21-15) Take weight at same time each day Protect newborn from heat loss	3400 g (7 lb 8 oz) Regains birth weight within first 2 weeks	2500-4000 g (5 lb 8 oz to 8 lb 13 oz) (Fig. 37-1) Acceptable weight loss: 10% or less (to estimate percent of weight loss, see Chapter 36)	Weight ≤2500 g Prematurity Small for gestational age Rubella syndrome Weight ≥4000 g Large for gestational age (LGA): maternal diabetes Hereditary: normal for these parents Weight loss over 10%: dehydration?
Head Circumference			
Measure head at greatest diameter: occipitofrontal circumference (Fig. 21-16, *A*) May need to remeasure on second or third day after resolution of molding and caput succedaneum	33-35.5 cm (13-14 in) Circumferences of head and chest may be about the same for first 1 or 2 days after birth	32-37 cm (12½-14½ in)	Microcephaly (under 32 cm) Rubella Toxoplasmosis Cytomegalic inclusion disease (CMV) Hydrocephaly (≥4 cm more than chest) Increased intracranial pressure Hemorrhage Space-occupying lesion
Chest Circumference			
Measure at nipple line (Fig. 21-16, *B*)	2 cm (¾ in) less than head circumference; averages between 30-33 cm (12-13 in)		Prematurity: ≤30 cm Postmaturity: some SGA and some LGA

*NOTE: Weight, length, and head circumference should all be close to same percentile for any child.

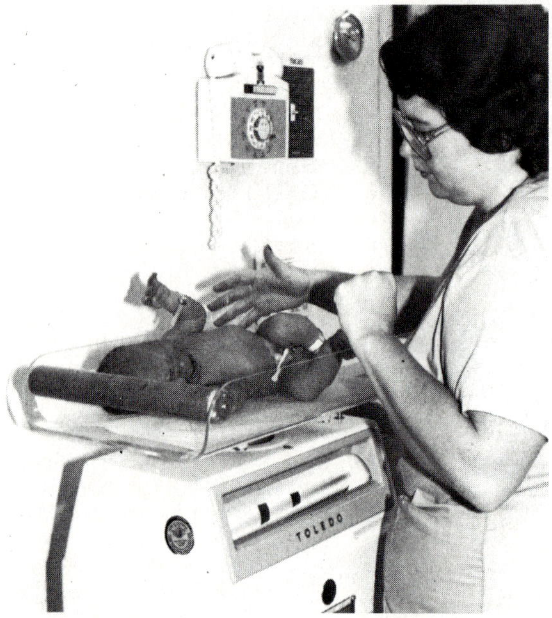

Fig. 21-15 Weighing infant. Note hand is held over infant as safety measure. Scale is covered to provide warmth and protection against cross infection.

Table 21-2 *Physical Assessment of Newborn—cont'd*

Area Assessed and Appraisal Procedure	Normal Findings: Average Findings	Normal Findings: Normal Variations	Deviations from Normal Range (Possible Causes)
Abdominal Circumference			
Measure below umbilicus (Fig. 21-16, *C*)	Abdomen enlarges after feeding because of lax abdominal muscles		Enlarging abdomen between feedings may indicate abdominal mass or blockage in intestinal tract
Length			
Measure recumbent length from top of head to heel; difficult to measure in full-term infant because of presence of molding, incomplete extension of knees (Fig. 21-16, *D*)	50 cm (20 in)	45-55 cm (18-22 in)	Chromosomal aberration Heredity: normal for these parents

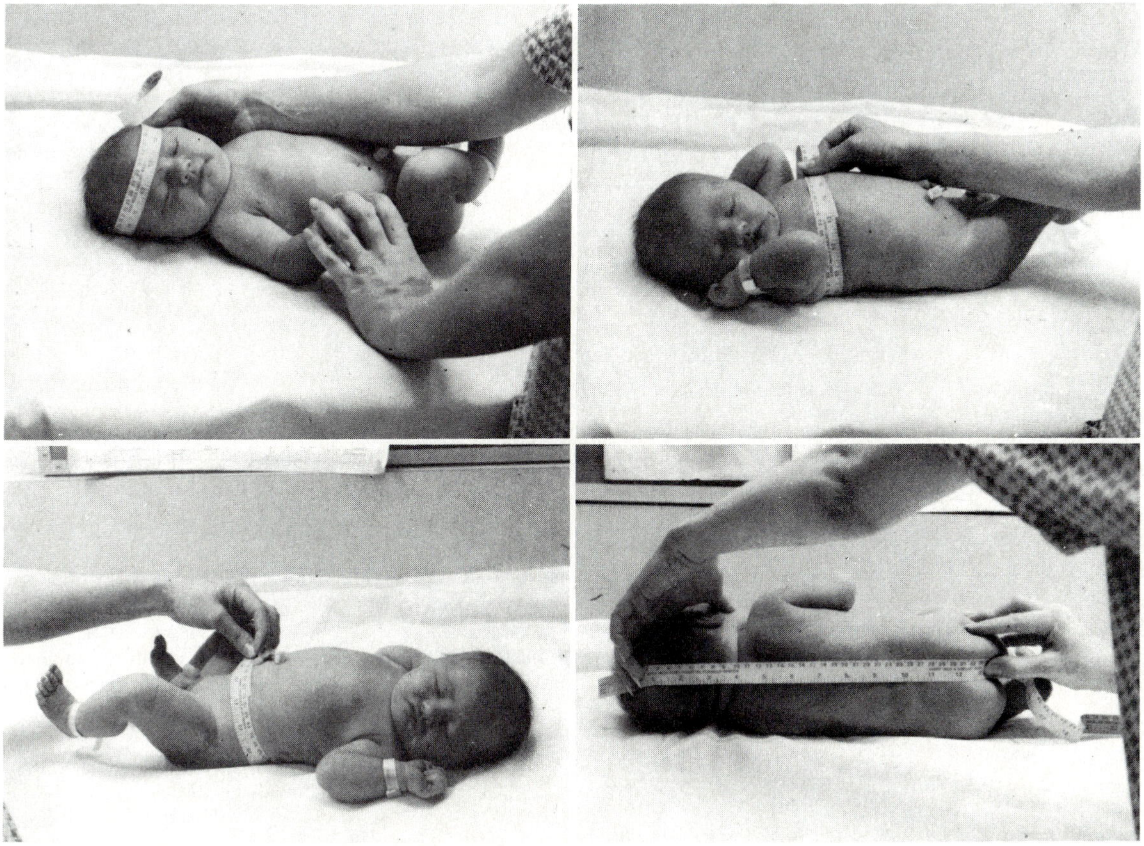

Fig. 21-16 Measurements. **A**, Circumference of head. **B**, Circumference of chest. **C**, Abdominal circumference. **D**, Length, crown to rump. To determine total length, length of legs is included.

Continued.

Table 21-2 *Physical Assessment of Newborn—cont'd*

Area Assessed and Appraisal Procedure	Normal Findings: Average Findings	Normal Findings: Normal Variations	Deviations from Normal Range (Possible Causes)
Integument			
Color Inspection and palpation Inspect naked newborn in well-lit, warm area without drafts; natural daylight provides best lighting Inspect newborn when quiet and when active	Varies with ethnic origin; skin pigmentation begins to deepen right after birth in basal layer of epidermis Generally pink Acrocyanosis, especially if chilled	Mottling Harlequin sign Plethora Telangiectases ("stork bites" or capillary hemangiomas) Erythema toxicum neonatorum ("newborn rash")	Dark red: prematurity Pallor Cardiovascular problem CNS damage Blood dyscrasia; blood loss; twin transfusion Nosocomial problem (e.g., infection)
			Cyanosis Hypothermia Infection Hypoglycemia Cardiopulmonary diseases Malformations: cardiac, neurologic, or respiratory
Check for jaundice			Jaundice Gray: hypotension, poor perfusion
		Petechiae over presenting part	Petechiae over any other area may be caused by the following: Clotting factor deficiency Infection
		Ecchymoses from forceps in vertex births or over buttocks and legs in breech births	Ecchymoses in any other area: hemorrhagic disease
Birthmarks Inspect and palpate for location, size, distribution, characteristics, color	Transient hyperpigmentation Areolae Genitals Linea nigra	Mongolian spotting Infants of black, Oriental, and American Indian origin; 70% Infants of white origin: 9%	Hemangiomas (vascular tumors) Nevus flammeus (port-wine stain) Strawberry mark Cavernous hemangiomas
Condition Inspect and palpate for intactness, smoothness, texture, edema	No skin edema Texture: thick; superficial or deep cracking Opacity: few large blood vessels seen indistinctly over abdomen	Slightly thick; superficial cracking, peeling, especially of hands, feet No blood vessels seen; a few large vessels clearly seen over abdomen Some fingernail scratches	Prematurity Edema on hands, feet; pitting over tibia Texture thin, smooth, or of medium thickness; rash or superficial peeling seen Numerous vessels easily seen over abdomen Postmaturity Texture thick, parchmentlike Skin tags; webbing Papules, pustules, vesicles, ulcers, maceration: impetigo, candidiasis, herpes Diaper rash

Table 21-2 *Physical Assessment of Newborn—cont'd*

Area Assessed and Appraisal Procedure	Normal Findings: Average Findings	Normal Findings: Normal Variations	Deviations from Normal Range (Possible Causes)
Hydration and consistency			
Weigh infant routinely Inspection and palpation Gently pinch skin between thumb and forefinger over abdomen and inner thigh to check for turgor Check subcutaneous fat deposits (adipose pads) over cheeks, buttocks	Dehydration: best indicator is loss of weight After pinch is released, skin returns to original state immediately	Normal weight loss after birth is up to 10% of birth weight May feel puffy Amount of subcutaneous fat varies	Loose, wrinkled skin Prematurity Postmaturity Dehydration: fold of skin persists after release of pinch Tense, tight, shiny skin: edema, extreme cold, shock, infection Lack of subcutaneous fat (e.g., clavicle or ribs prominent): prematurity, malnutrition
Check voiding	Voids 6-10 times per day		
Vernix caseosa			
Observe amount		Amount varies; usually more is found in creases, folds	Absent or minimal: postmaturity Excessive: prematurity
Observe its color and odor before bath or wiping If not readily apparent over total body, check in folds of axilla and groin	Whitish, cheesy, odorless		Yellow color Possible fetal anoxia 36 hours or more before birth Rh or ABO incompatibility (see Chapter 40) Green color: possible in utero release of meconium because of fetal anoxia less than 36 hr before birth or presence of bilirubin Odor; possible intrauterine infection (e.g., amnionitis)
Lanugo			
Inspect for this fine, downy hair: amount, distribution	Over shoulders, pinnae of ears, forehead	Amount varies	Absent: postmaturity Excessive: prematurity, especially if lanugo is abundant and long and thick over back
Head			
Palpate skin	See Integument, p. 470	Caput succedaneum; may show some ecchymosis	Cephalhematoma
Palpate, inspect, measure fontanels	Anterior fontanel 5 cm diamond; increases as molding resolves Posterior fontanel triangle; smaller than anterior	Fontanel size varies with degree of molding Fontanels may be difficult to feel because of molding	Fontanels (Fig. 16-2) Full, bulging: possible intracranial lesion (e.g., tumor, hemorrhage, infection) Large, flat, soft: malnutrition, hydrocephaly, retarded bone age (hypothyroidism) Depressed: dehydration Large mastoid and sphenoid fontanels: hydrocephaly
Palpate sutures	Sutures palpable and not joined	Sutures may overlap with molding (Fig. 21-10)	Sutures Widely spaced: hydrocephaly Premature synostosis (closure)

Table 21-2 *Physical Assessment of Newborn—cont'd*

Area Assessed and Appraisal Procedure	Normal Findings: Average Findings	Normal Findings: Normal Variations	Deviations from Normal Range (Possible Causes)
Inspect pattern, distribution, amount of hair; feel texture	Silky, single strands, lies flat; growth pattern is toward face and neck	Amount varies	Fine, wooly: prematurity Unusual swirls, patterns, hairline or coarse, brittle: endocrine or genetic disorder
Inspect shape and size	Makes up one fourth of body length Molding	Slight asymmetry from intrauterine position	Molding (Fig. 21-10) Severe molding may result from birth trauma Lack of molding: prematurity, breech presentation, cesarean birth Circumference ≥4 cm larger than chest circumference: hydrocephaly; ≤32 cm: prematurity, microcephaly

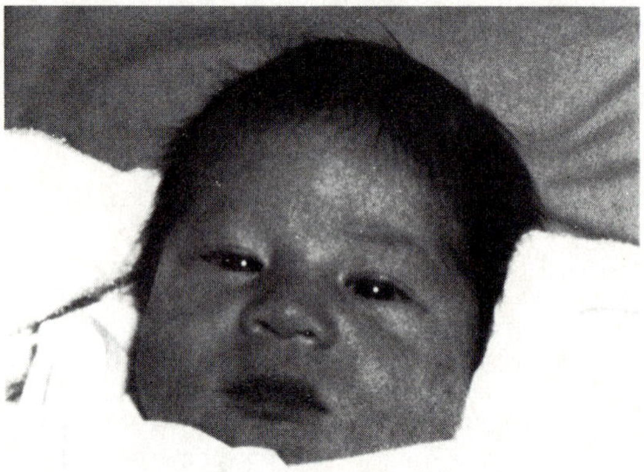

Fig. 21-17 Eyes. Pseudostrabismus. Inner epicanthal folds cause eyes to appear malaligned; however, corneal light reflexes fall perfectly symmetric. Eyes are symmetric in size and shape and well placed.

Area Assessed and Appraisal Procedure	Average Findings	Normal Variations	Deviations from Normal Range (Possible Causes)
Eyes (Fig. 21-17)			
Placement on face			
Symmetry in size, shape	Symmetric in size, shape		
Eyelids: size, movement, blink	Blink reflex	Edema from instilling silver nitrate	
	Epicanthal folds: normal racial characteristic		Epicanthal folds when present with other signs, may be caused by chromosomal disorders (e.g., Down's syndrome, cri-du-chat syndrome)
Discharge	None	Some discharge from silver nitrate	
Eyeballs: presence, size, shape	No tears Both present and of equal size; both round, firm	Occasionally has some tears Subconjunctival hemorrhage	Agenesis or absence of one or both eyeballs Small eyeball size: rubella syndrome Lens opacity or absence of red reflex: congenital cataracts, possibly from rubella Lesions: coloboma (absence of part of iris) Pink color of iris: albinism Jaundiced sclera Discharge: purulent Pupils: unequal, constricted, dilated, fixed
Eyeball movement	Random, jerky, uneven, can focus momentarily, can follow to midline	Transient strabismus or nystagmus until third or fourth month	Persistent strabismus
Eyebrows: amount, pattern	Distinct		

Table 21-2 *Physical Assessment of Newborn—cont'd*

Area Assessed and Appraisal Procedure	Normal Findings: Average Findings	Normal Findings: Normal Variations	Deviations from Normal Range (Possible Causes)
Nose			
Observe shape, placement, patency, configuration of bridge of nose	Midline Apparent lack of bridge, flat, broad Some mucus but no drainage Obligatory nose breathers Sneezes to clear nose	Slight deformity from passage through birth canal	Copious drainage, with or without regular periods of cyanosis at rest and return of pink color with crying: choanal atresia, congenital syphilis Malformed: congenital syphilis, chromosomal disorder Flaring of nares
Ears			
Observe size, placement on head, amount of cartilage, open auditory canal Hearing	Correct placement: line drawn through inner and outer canthi of eye should come to top notch of ear (at junction with scalp) (Fig. 21-18) Well-formed, firm cartilage	Size: small, large, floppy Darwin's tubercle (nodule on posterior helix)	Agenesis Lack of cartilage: possible prematurity Low placement: possible chromosomal disorder, mental retardation, kidney disorder Preauricular tags Size: may have overly prominent or protruding ears
Facies			
Observe overall appearance of face	Infant looks "normal"; features are well placed, proportionate to face	"Positional" deformities (Fig. 21-13)	Infant looks "odd" or "funny" Usually accompanied by other features, such as low-set ears and other structural disorders

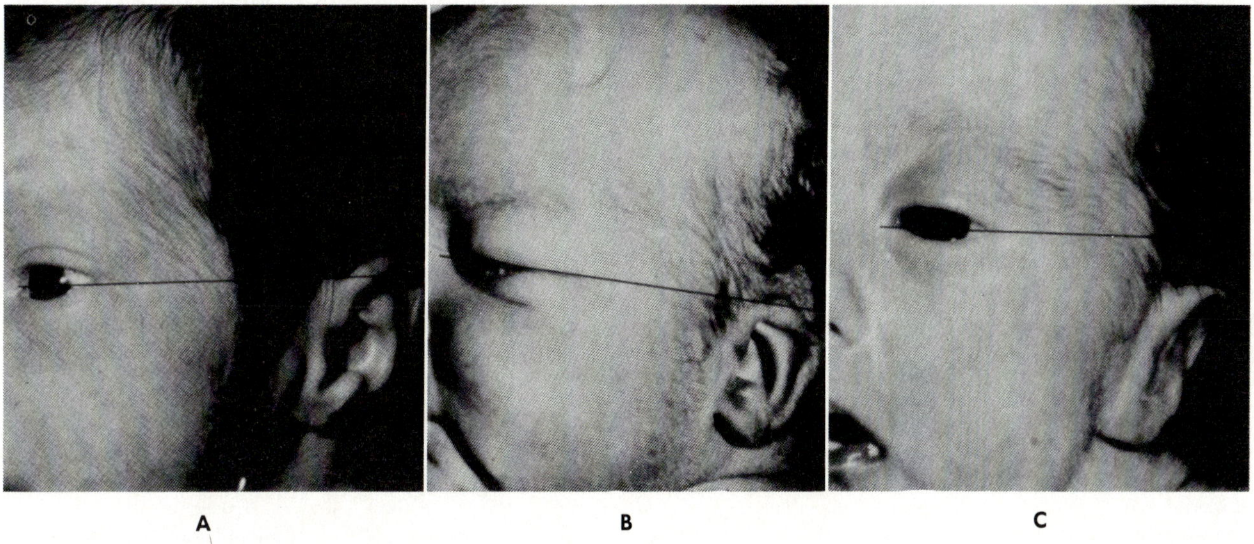

Fig. 21-18 Placement of ear insertion on head in relation to line drawn from inner to outer canthus of eye. **A**, Normal position. **B**, Abnormally angled ear. **C**, True low-set ear.
Courtesy Mead Johnson & Co, Evansville, Indiana.

Continued.

Table 21-2 *Physical Assessment of Newborn—cont'd*

Area Assessed and Appraisal Procedure	Normal Findings		Deviations from Normal Range (Possible Causes)
	Average Findings	Normal Variations	
Mouth			
Inspection and palpation Placement on face Lips: color, configuration, movement, rooting reflex, sucking Gums Tongue: attachment, mobility, movement, size Cheeks Palate (soft, hard) Arch Ulva Saliva: amount, character Chin Reflexes	Pink gums Symmetry of lip movement Tongue does not protrude, is freely movable; symmetric in shape, movement Sucking pads inside cheeks Soft and hard palates intact Uvula in midline Reflexes present	Transient circumoral cyanosis Short frenulum Anatomic groove in palate to accommodate nipple; disappears by 3-4 yr of age Epsteins pearls (Bohn's nodules): whitish, hard nodules on gums Reflex response dependent on state of wakefulness and hunger	Gross anomalies Placement, size, shape Cleft lip and/or palate, gums Cyanosis; circumoral pallor Asymmetry in movement of lips: seventh cranial nerve paralysis Macroglossia Prematurity Chromosomal disorder Excessive saliva Esophageal atresia Tracheoesophageal fistula Micrognathia: Pierre Robin or other syndrome Teeth: predeciduous or deciduous Thrush: white plaques on cheeks or tongue that bleed if touched
Neck			
Inspection and palpation Length Movement of head Sternocleidomastoid muscles; position of head Trachea: position; thyroid gland Reflex response	Short, thick, surrounded by skinfolds; no webbing Head held in midline, i.e., sternocleidomastoid muscles are equal; no masses Freedom of movement from side to side and flexion and extension; cannot move chin past shoulder Thyroid not palpable	Transient positional deformity apparent when neonate is at rest: head can be moved passively	Webbing Restricted movement; head held at angle; possible torticollis (wryneck), opisthotonos Masses: enlarged thyroid Distended veins: cardiopulmonary disorder Skin tags Positive owl's sign: prematurity Absence of head control: prematurity; Down's syndrome
Chest			
Inspection and palpation Shape Clavicles Ribs Nipples: size, placement, number Breast tissue Respiratory movements Amount of cartilage in rib cage Auscultation Heart tones and rate and breath sounds (see Vital signs, above)	Almost circular; barrel shaped Symmetric chest movements; chest and abdominal movements synchronized during respirations Breast nodule: approximately 6 mm Nipples prominent, well formed; symmetrically placed	Occasional retractions, especially when crying Breast nodule: 3-10 mm Secretion of witch's milk	Bulging of chest Pneumothorax Pneumomediastinum Malformation: funnel chest (pectus excavatum) Fracture of clavicle Nipples Supernumerary, along nipple line Malpositioned or widely spaced Lack of breast tissue: possible prematurity Poor development of rib cage and musculature: possible prematurity

Table 21-2 *Physical Assessment of Newborn—cont'd*

Area Assessed and Appraisal Procedure	Normal Findings: Average Findings	Normal Findings: Normal Variations	Deviations from Normal Range (Possible Causes)
			Sounds: bowel sounds (see Abdomen, below) Retractions with or without respiratory distress
Abdomen			
Inspect, palpate, and smell umbilical cord	Two arteries, one vein (AVA) Whitish gray Definite demarcation between cord and skin; no intestinal structures within cord Dry around base; drying Odorless	Reducible umbilical herniation	One artery: internal anomalies Bleeding or oozing around cord: hemorrhagic disease Redness or drainage around cord: infection, possible persistence of urachus Hernia: herniation of abdominal contents into area of cord (e.g., omphalocele); defect covered with thin, friable membrane, may be extensive Gastroschisis: congenital fissure of abdominal cavity Meconium stained: intrauterine distress
Inspect size of abdomen (Fig. 21-16, *C*) and palpate contour Auscultate for bowel sounds	Rounded, prominent, dome shaped because abdominal musculature is not fully developed No distension Bowel sounds heard 1 hr after birth	Some diastasis of abdominal musculature	Distension At birth Ruptured viscus Genitourinary masses or malformations: hydronephrosis; teratomas Abdominal tumors Mild Aerophagia Overfeeding High gastrointestinal tract obstruction Marked Lower gastrointestinal tract obstruction Imperforate anus Intermittent or transient Aerophagia Overfeeding Partial intestinal obstruction from stenosis of bowel Annular pancreas Malrotation of bowel or adhesions Sepsis
Auscultate bowel sounds and note number, amount, and character of stools, and behavior—crying, fussiness—before or during elimination	Sounds present within 1-2 hr after birth Meconium stool passes within 24-48 hr after birth		Scaphoid, with bowel sounds in chest and respiratory distress: diaphragmatic hernia
Color		Linea nigra may be apparent; possibly caused by hormone influence during pregnancy	

Continued.

Table 21-2 *Physical Assessment of Newborn—cont'd*

Area Assessed and Appraisal Procedure	Normal Findings: Average Findings	Normal Findings: Normal Variations	Deviations from Normal Range (Possible Causes)
Movement with respiration	Respirations primarily diaphragmatic; abdominal and chest movements synchronous		Decreased abdominal breathing Intrathoracic disease Diaphragmatic hernia
Genitals			
Girl			
Inspection and palpation			
General appearance	Female genitals	Increased pigmentation caused by pregnancy hormones	Ambiguous genitals—enlarged clitoris with urinary meatus on tip; fused labia: chromosomal disorder; maternal drug ingestions
Clitoris	Usually edematous		
Labia majora	Usually edematous; cover labia minora in term neonates	Edema and ecchymosis following breech birth	
Labia minora	May protrude over labia majora	Vaginal tag	Stenosed meatus
Discharge	Smegma	Blood-tinged discharge from pseudomenstruation caused by pregnancy hormones	Labia majora widely separated and labia minora prominent: prematurity
Vagina	Orifice open Mucoid discharge	Some vernix caseosa may be between labia	Absence of vaginal orifice or imperforate hymen Fecal discharge: fistula
Urinary meatus	Beneath clitoris; hard to see—watch for voiding	Rust-stained urine (uric acid crystals) (To determine whether rust color is caused by uric acid or blood, wash under running warm tap water. Uric acid washes out, blood does not)	
Boy			
Inspection and palpation			
General appearance	Male genitals	Increased size and pigmentation caused by pregnancy hormones	Ambiguous genitals
Penis	Meatus at tip of penis		Urinary meatus not on tip of glans penis
Urinary meatus seen as slit			Hypospadias, Epispadias } may be associated with other anomalies
Prepuce	Prepuce (foreskin) covers glans penis and is not easily retractable	Prepuce removed at circumcision Size of genitals varies widely	
Scrotum	Large, edematous, pendulous; covered with rugae	Scrotal edema and ecchymosis if breech birth	Adherent or tight prepuce: phimosis
Rugae (wrinkles)		Hydrocele, small, noncommunicating	Scrotum smooth and testes undescended: prematurity, cryptorchidism Hydrocele Inguinal hernia Round meatal opening
Testes	Palpable on each side	Bulge palpable in inguinal canal	If not palpable may be in abdomen
Urination	Voiding before 24-48 hr, stream adequate, amount adequate	Rust-stained urine (uric acid crystals)	
Reflexes			
Erection	Erection may occur when genitals are touched		
Cremasteric	Testes are retracted, especially when neonate is chilled		

Table 21-2 *Physical Assessment of Newborn—cont'd*

Area Assessed and Appraisal Procedure	Normal Findings: Average Findings	Normal Findings: Normal Variations	Deviations from Normal Range (Possible Causes)
Extremities			
Clavicles	Intact		Fracture (see Chapter 38)
General Inspection and palpation Degree of flexion Range of motion Symmetry of motion Muscle tone	Assumes position maintained in utero Attitude of general flexion Full range of motion, spontaneous movements	Transient (positional) deformities	Limited motion: malformations Poor muscle tone Positive scarf design (see Chapter 37)
Arms Inspection and palpation Color Intactness Appropriate placement Number of fingers Palpate humerus Joints Shoulder Elbow Wrist Fingers Reflex: grasp	Longer than legs in newborn period Contours and movement are symmetric Should be intact Fist often clenched with thumb under fingers Full range of motion; symmetric contour	Slight tremors may be seen at times Some acrocyanosis, especially when chilled	Assymmetry of movement Fracture Brachial nerve trauma Malformations Asymmetry of contour Malformations Fracture Amelia or phocomelia Webbing of fingers: syndactyly Absence or excess of fingers Palmar creases Simian line (commonly seen in Down's syndrome) seen with short, incurved little fingers Strong, rigid flexion; persistent fists; fists held in front of mouth constantly: CNS disorder Increased tonicity, clonicity, prolonged tremors (especially if whole body is involved): CNS disorder
Legs Inspection and palpation Intactness Length—in relation to arms and body and to each other Major gluteal folds Number of toes Femur Head of femur as legs are flexed on hips and abducted; placement in acetabulum; femoral pulses Color	Appear bowed since lateral muscles more developed than medial muscles Major gluteal folds even Femur should be intact No click should be heard; femoral head should not override acetabulum (Fig. 21-19) Feet flat; soles well lined (or wrinkled) over two-thirds Plantar fat pad gives flat-footed effect Inspection and palpation Joints Hip Knee Ankle Toes Reflexes	Feet appear to turn in but can be easily rotated externally, also positional defects tend to correct while infant is crying Acrocyanosis	Amelia, phocomelia Chromosomal defect Teratogenic effect Webbing, syndactyly: chromosomal defect Absence or excess of digits Chromosomal defect Familial trait Femoral fracture: after difficult breech delivery Congenital hip dysplasia Absent femoral pulses Soles of feet Poorly lined: prematurity Covered with lines: postmaturity Simian line: Down's syndrome Congenital clubfoot Hypermobility of joints: Down's syndrome Yellowed nail beds Temperature of one leg differs from that of the other

Continued.

Table 21-2 *Physical Assessment of Newborn—cont'd*

Area Assessed and Appraisal Procedure	Normal Findings: Average Findings	Normal Findings: Normal Variations	Deviations from Normal Range (Possible Causes)
Back			
Anatomy (Fig. 21-20) Inspection and palpation Spine Shoulders Scapulae Iliac crests Base of spine—pilonidal area	Spine straight and easily flexed Infant can raise and support head momentarily when prone Shoulders, scapulae, and iliac crests should line up in same plane	Temporary minor positional deformities, which can be corrected with passive manipulation	Limitation of movement: fusion of deformity of vertebras Pigmented nevus with tuft of hair when located anywhere along the spine is often associated with spina bifida occulta Spina bifida cystica Meningocele Myelomeningocele
Reflexes (spinal related) Test reflexes			
Anus			
Inspection and palpation Placement Number Patency Test for patency and sphincter response (active "wink" reflex) Observe for following: Abdominal distension Passage of meconium Passage of fecal drainage from surrounding orifices	One anus with good sphincter tone Passage of meconium within 24 hours after birth Good "wink" reflex of anal sphincter	Passage of meconium within 48 hr after birth	Low obstruction: anal membrane (thermometer cannot be inserted) High obstruction: anal or rectal atresia (thermometer may be inserted, but there is no passage of meconium) Drainage of fecal material from vagina in female or urinary meatus in male: possible rectal fistula
Stools	See p. 468		

A

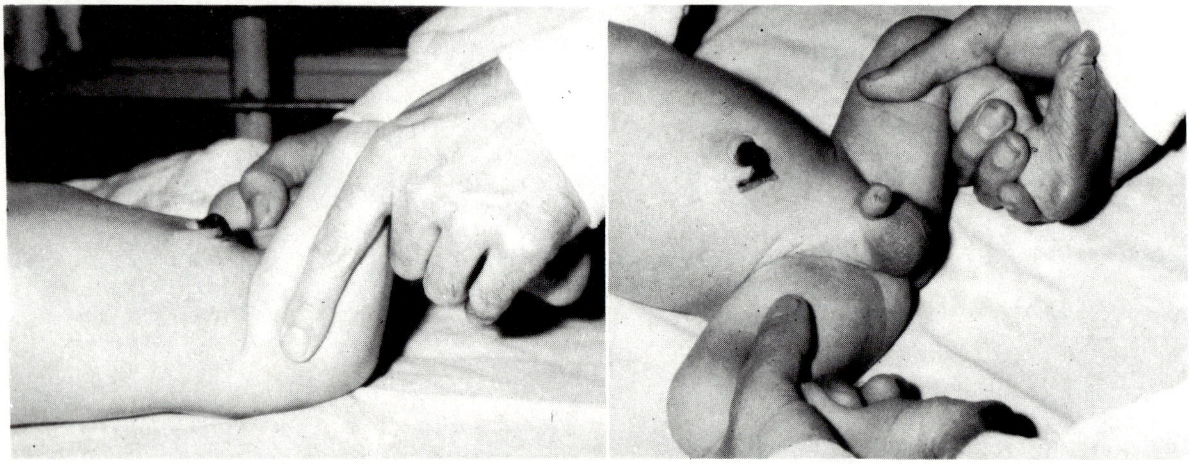

B

Fig. 21-19 Method of assessing for hip dysplasia using Ortolani's maneuver. **A**, Examiner's middle fingers are placed over greater trochanter and thumbs over inner thigh opposite lesser trochanter. **B**, Gentle pressure is exerted to further flex thigh on hip, and thighs are rotated outward. If hip dysplasia is present head of femur can be felt to slip forward in acetabulum and slip back when pressure is released and legs returned to their original position. A click is sometimes heard (Ortolani's sign).

Changes in environmental temperature alter that of blood, thereby influencing temperature-regulating centers in the hypothalamus.
2. The newborn has a larger body surface to body weight (mass) ratio. The flexed position that the newborn assumes is a safeguard against heat loss because it substantially diminishes the amount of body surface exposed to the hostile thermal environment.
3. The neonate's vasomotor control is less well developed. However, the ability to constrict subcutaneous and skin vessels is as efficient in premature infants as it is in adults.
4. The newborn produces heat primarily by nonshivering thermogenesis.
5. The neonate's sweat glands have little homoiothermic function until the fourth week or later of extrauterine life.

In response to the discomfort of lower environmental temperature, the normal term infant may try to increase body temperature by crying or by increased motion activity. Crying increases the work load, and the cost of energy (calories) may be expensive, particularly in a compromised infant.

Cold Stress. Cold stress imposes metabolic and physiologic problems on all infants, regardless of gestational age and condition. The respiratory rate is increased as a response to the increased need for oxygen when the oxygen consumption increases significantly in cold stress. Oxygen consumption and energy in the cold-stressed infant are diverted from maintaining normal brain cell and cardiac function and growth to thermogenesis for survival.

If the infant cannot maintain an adequate oxygen tension, vasoconstriction follows and jeopardizes pulmonary perfusion. As a consequence, arterial blood gas levels of Po_2 are decreased, and the blood pH drops. These changes aggravate existing respiratory distress syndrome (RDS), also known as hyaline membrane disease (HMD) (Chapter 37). Moreover, decreased pulmonary perfusion and oxygen tension may maintain or reopen the right-to-left shunt across the patent ductus arteriosus (Table 21-1).

The basal metabolic rate will be increased with cold stress. If cold stress is protracted, anaerobic glycolysis occurs, resulting in increased production of acids. Metabolic acidosis develops, and if there is a defect in respiratory function, respiratory acidosis also develops. Excessive fatty acids displace the bilirubin from the albumin-binding sites. The increased level of circulating unbound bilirubin that results increases the risk of kernicterus even at serum bilirubin levels of 10 mg/dl or less.

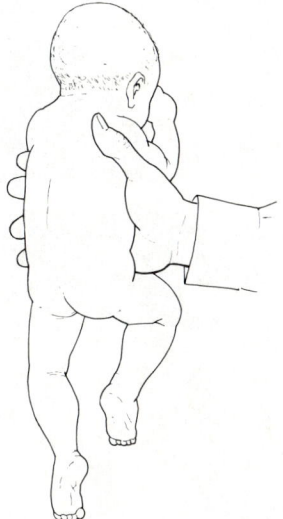

Fig. 21-20 Examining back. Infant's back should be slightly flexed, freely movable, and free of defects. Infant should kick both legs.

Physical Assessment

Biologic characteristics are demonstrated through physical assessment. Average findings, normal variations, and deviations from normal range are displayed in Table 21-2. These findings provide a data base for implementing the nursing process with newborns (and their families) discussed in Chapter 22.

Neurologic Assessment. The physical assessment includes a neurologic assessment of the newborn's reflexes. This provides useful information about the infant's nervous system and state of neurologic maturation. Many of the reflex behaviors are important for survival, for example, sucking and rooting. Others act as safety mechanisms, for instance, gagging, coughing, and sneezing. The assessment needs to be carried out as early as possible because abnormal signs present in the early neonatal period may disappear. They may reappear months or years later as abnormal functions. Table 21-3 gives the techniques for eliciting significant reflexes and characteristic responses.

BEHAVIORAL CHARACTERISTICS

The healthy infant must achieve behavioral as well as biologic tasks to develop normally. Behavioral characteristics form the basis of the social capabilities of the infant. Through the first half of this century the focus of developmental research was on how the infant was affected by the environment. Infants were considered to have been born with neither personality nor ability to interact.

Today it is recognized that newborns are well equipped to begin social interactions with their parents. The behavioral characteristics of the newborn represent a second phase in human development. The first phase, fetal phase, of development was discussed in Chapter 9. Research now indicates that the individual personalities and behavioral characteristics of infants play a major role in the ultimate relationship between infants and their parents.

Brazelton (1973) and others have brought the behavioral states of the newborn into prominence. The behavioral assessment scale developed by Brazelton (1977) (known as the Brazelton Neonatal Behavioral Assessment

Fig. 21-21 **A**, Sucking. Also note hand-to-mouth facility with prolonged sucking. **B**, Rooting reflex is apparent when corner of newborn's mouth is touched. Bottom lip lowers on same side; tongue moves toward stimulation.
Courtesy Joan Edelstein and Ralph Levy, San Jose, Calif.

A

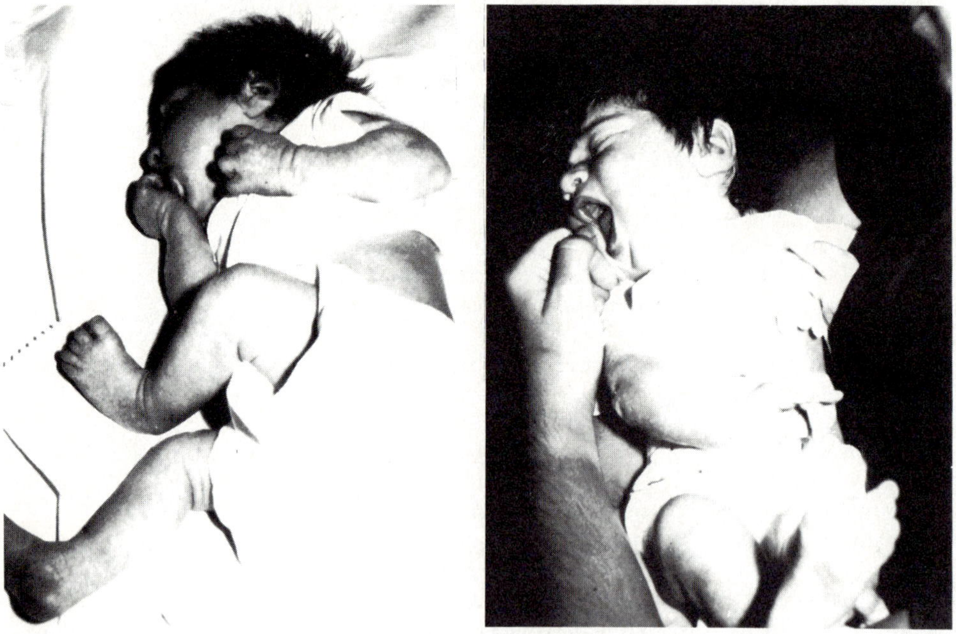

B

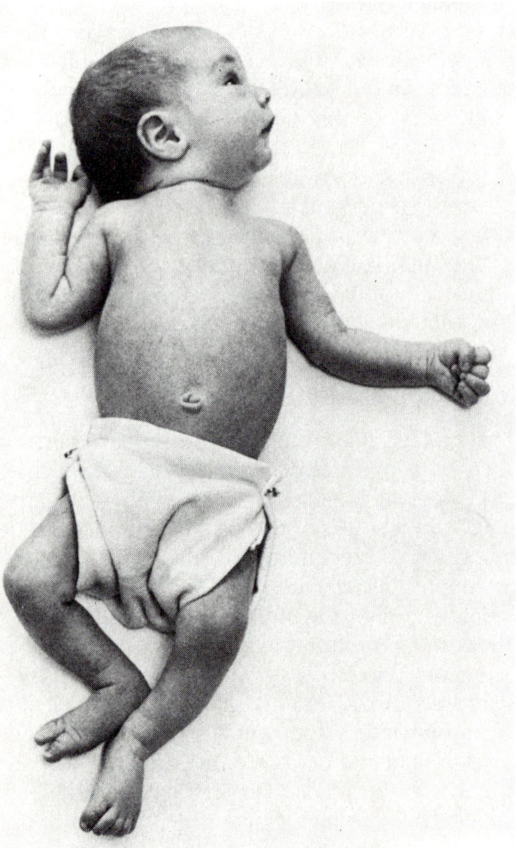

Fig. 21-22 Classic pose in spontaneous tonic neck reflex.
Courtesy Mead Johnson & Co, Evansville, Indiana.

A

B

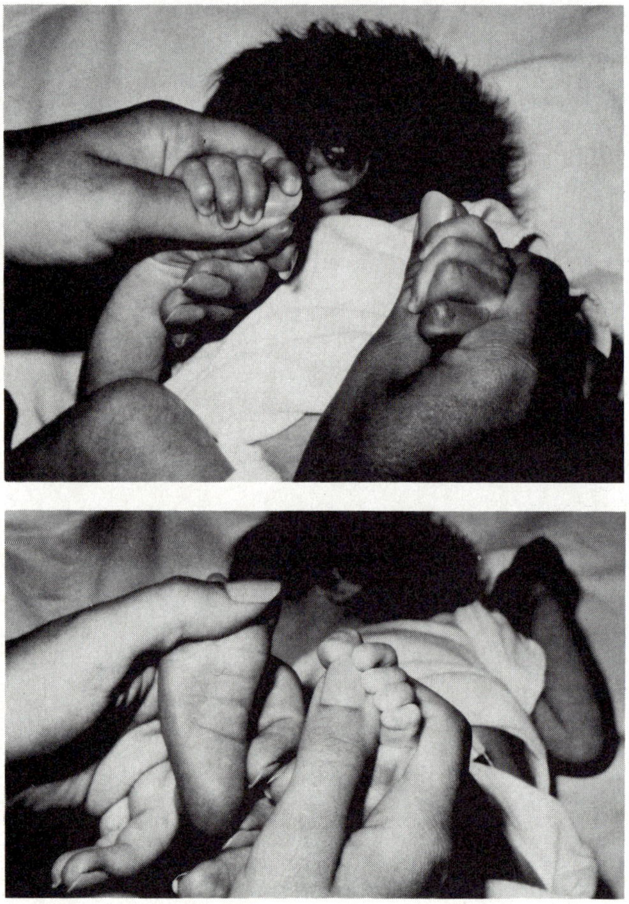

Fig. 21-23 **A**, Palmar (hand) grasp. **B**, Plantar grasp.
Courtesy Joan Edelstein and Ralph Levy, San Jose, Calif.

Table 21-3 *Assessment of Newborn's Reflexes*

Reflex	Eliciting the Reflex	Characteristic Response	Comments
Sucking and rooting (Fig. 21-21)	Touch infant's lip, cheek, or corner of mouth with nipple	Infant turns head toward stimulus, opens mouth, takes hold, and sucks	Difficult if not impossible to elicit after infant has been fed; if weak or absent, consider prematurity or neurologic defect Parental guidance Avoid trying to turn head toward breast or nipple; allow infant to root. Disappears after 3-4 mo but may persist up to 1 yr
Swallowing	Swallowing usually follows sucking and obtaining fluids, suck and swallow are often uncoordinated in early-born infant and may also occur during first few hours of term (normal) infant's life	Swallowing is usually coordinated with sucking and usually occurs without gagging, coughing, or vomiting	If weak or absent, may indicate prematurity or neurologic defect
Extrusion	Touch or depress tongue	Newborn forces tongue outward	Disappears at about fourth mo
Glabellar (Myerson's)	Tap over forehead, bridge of nose, or maxilla of neonate whose eyes are open	Newborn blinks for first 4 or 5 taps	Continued blinking with repeated taps is consistent with extrapyramidal disorder
Tonic neck or "fencing" (Fig. 21-22)	With infant falling asleep or sleeping, turn head quickly to one side	With infant facing left side, arm and leg on that side extend; opposite arm and leg flex (turn head to right, and extremities assume opposite postures)	Responses in legs are more consistent Complete response disappears by 3-4 months; incomplete response may be seen until third or fourth year After 6 weeks persistent response is sign of possible cerebral palsy
Grasp (Fig. 21-23) Palmar Plantar	 Place finger in palm of hand Place finger at base of toes	Infant's fingers curl around examiner's fingers; toes curl downward	Palmar response lessens by 3-4 months; parents enjoy this contact with infant; plantar response lessens by 8 months
Moro's (Fig. 21-24)	Hold infant in semisitting position; allow head and trunk to fall backward to an angle of at least 30 degrees Place infant on flat surface; strike surface to startle infant	Symmetric abduction and extension of arms; fingers fan out and form a C with thumb and forefinger; slight tremor may be noted; arms are adducted in embracing motion and return to relaxed flexion and movement Legs may follow similar pattern of response Premature infant does not complete "embrace," instead, arms fall backward because of weakness	Present at birth; complete response may be seen until 8 weeks* of age; body jerk only, between 8-18 wk; absent by 6 mo if neurologic maturation is not delayed; may be incomplete if infant is deeply asleep; give parental guidance about normal response Asymmetric response; possible injury to brachial plexus, clavicle, or humerus Persistent response after 6 mos: possible brain damage
Startle	Loud noise of sharp hand clap elicits response; best elicited if newborn is 24-36 hours old or older	Arms abduct with flexion of elbows; hands stay clenched	Should disappear by 4 mo Elicited more readily in premature newborn (inform parents of this characteristic)
Pull-to-sit (traction) (Fig. 21-25)	Pull infant up by wrists from supine position	Head will lag until infant is in upright position; then head will be held in same plane with chest and shoulder momentarily before falling forward; head will right itself spontaneously for a few moments	Depends on general muscle tone and maturity and condition of infant

*All durations for persistance of reflexes are based on time elapsed since 40 weeks' gestation, that is, if this newborn was born at 36 weeks' gestation, add 1 month to all time limits given.

Continued.

Table 21-3 *Assessment of Newborn's Reflexes—cont'd*

Reflex	Eliciting the Reflex	Characteristic Response	Comments
Trunk incurvation (Galant) (Fig. 21-26)	Infant should be prone on flat surface; run finger down back about 4-5 cm (1½-2 in) lateral to spine, first on one side, and then down other	Trunk is flexed and pelvis is swung toward stimulated side	Response disappears by fourth wk
Magnet (Fig. 21-27)	Infant should be supine; partially flex both lower extremities and apply pressure to soles of feet	Both lower limbs should extend against examiner's pressure	
Crossed extension (Fig. 21-28)	Infant should be supine; extend one leg, press knee downward, stimulate bottom of foot; observe opposite leg	Opposite leg flexes, adducts, and then extends	
Babinski's sign (plantar) (Fig. 21-29)	On sole of foot, beginning at heel, stroke upward along lateral aspect of sole, then move finger across ball of foot	All toes hyperextend, with dorsiflexion of big toe	Absence requires neurologic evaluation; should disappear after 1 yr of age
Stepping or "walking" (Fig. 21-30)	Hold infant vertically, allowing one foot to touch table surface	Infant will simulate walking, alternating flexion and extension of feet; term infants walk on soles of their feet, and premature infants walk on their toes	Normally present for 3-4 wks
Neck righting	Place newborn in supine position and turn head to one side	Shoulder and trunk and then pelvis will turn to be in alignment with head	Disappears at 10 mo of age; absence: implications same as for absent tonic neck reflex
Otolith righting	Hold newborn erect and tilt body	Head returns to erect, upright position	Absence: implications same as for absent tonic neck reflex
Crawling (Fig. 21-31)	Place newborn on abdomen	Newborn makes crawling movements with arms and legs	Should disappear about 6 wk of age
Deep tendon	Use finger instead of percussion hammer to elicit patellar, or knee jerk, reflex; newborn must be relaxed	Reflex jerk is present; even with newborn relaxed, nonselective overall reaction may occur	
Landau	Over a crib or a table, using two hands, suspend infant in prone position	Infant attempts to hold spine in horizontal plane	Absence suggests need for neurologic examination
Yawn, stretch, burp, hiccup, sneeze	Spontaneous behaviors	May be slightly depressed temporarily because of maternal analgesia or anesthesia, fetal hypoxia, or infection	Parental guidance Most of these behaviors are pleasurable to parents Parents need to be assured that behaviors are normal Sneeze is response to lint, etc., in nose and (usually) not an indicator of a cold
Sweat	Usually not present in term newborn	Sweat response usually not present in term infant; may be seen in infants with cardiac response	Parental guidance Amount of clothing for infant: indoors, outside Room temperature
Shiver	Usually not present in term newborn	Shiver response usually not present in term infant; if seen, check infant for postmaturity	See above
Kernig's sign	Flex thigh on hip and extend leg at knee	Procedure should be accomplished easily and without inflicting pain	Pain and resistance to extension of knee suggest meningeal irritability
Brudzinski's sign	Place infant in supine position; flex neck and observe knees	Infant does not move legs when neck is flexed	Spontaneous flexion of knees suggest meningeal irritability
Paradoxic irritability	Ascertain that infant is not hungry; hold and cuddle infant	Infant usually responds by quieting down	Infant cries when touched and held; response suggests meningeal irritability

A

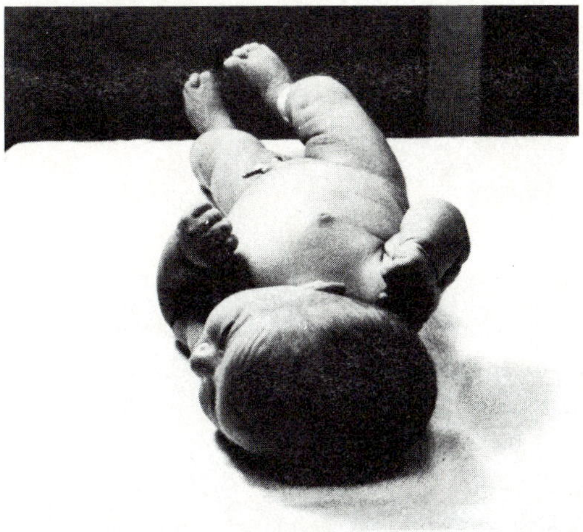

Fig. 21-24 A, Position of rest. B, Moro's reflex consists predominantly of abduction and extension of arms. C, Interesting subtlety of Moro's response in newborn infants is C position of fingers.
Courtesy Mead Johnson & Co, Evansville, Indiana.

B

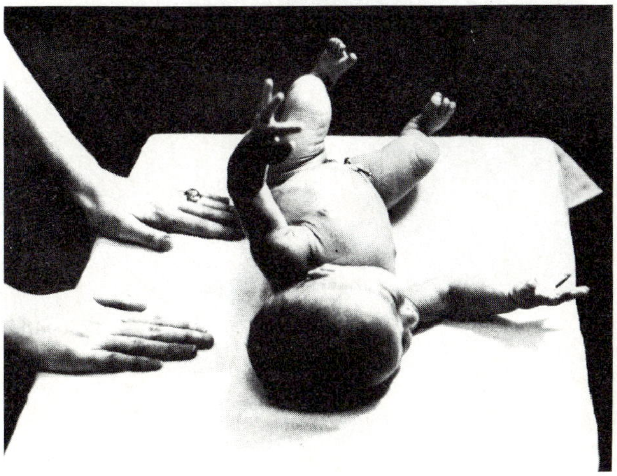

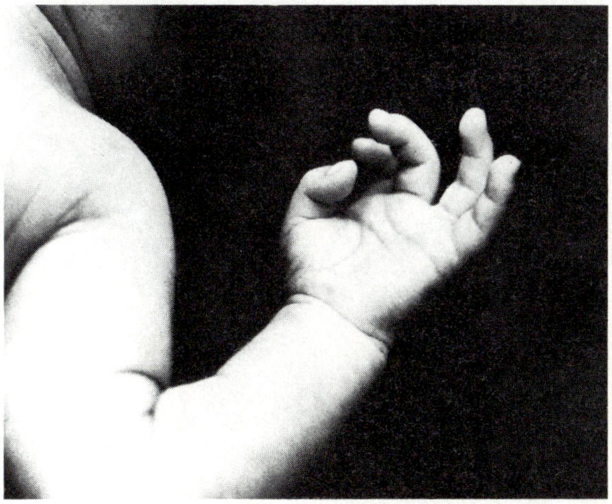

C

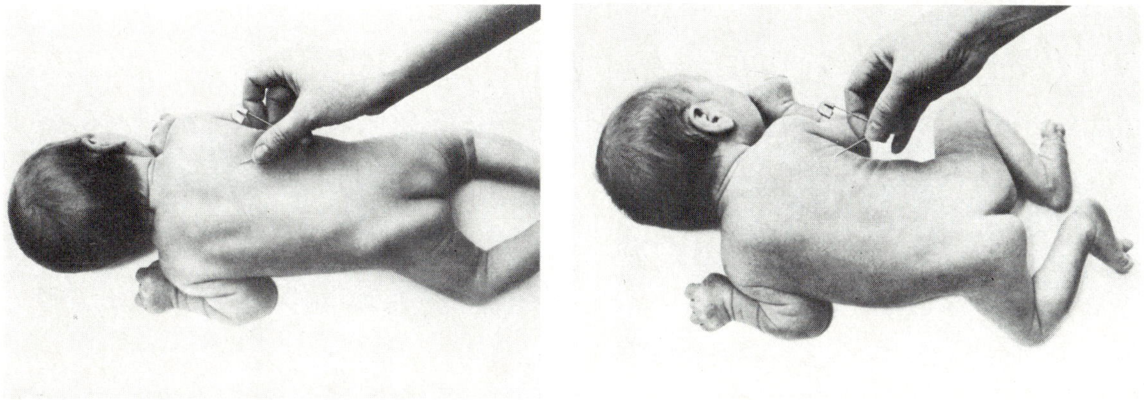

Fig. 21-26 Trunk incurvation reflex. In prone position, infant responds to linear skin stimulus (pin or finger) along paravertebral area by flexing trunk and swinging pelvis toward stimulus. With transverse lesions of cord, there will be no response below that level. Complete absence of response suggests general depression or nervous system abnormality. Response may vary but should be obtainable in all infants, including premature ones. If not seen in the first few days, it is usually apparent by 5 to 6 days.
Courtesy Mead Johnson & Co, Evansville, Indiana.

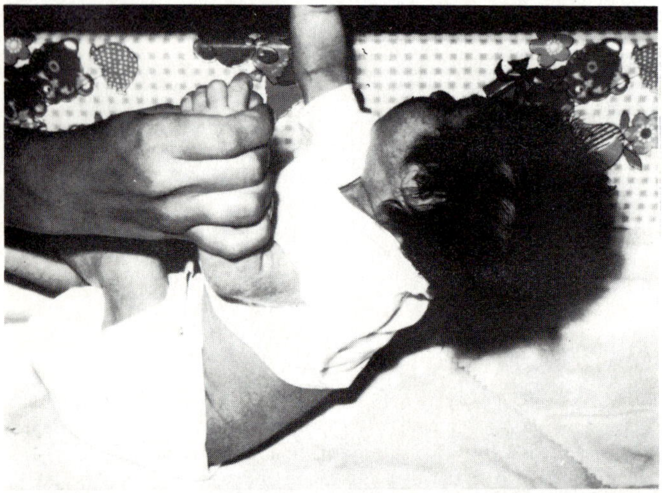

A

Fig. 21-25 Pull-to-sit (or traction reflex). **A**, Head falls backward. **B**, Infant attempts to right head. **C**, Infant unable to maintain head up.
Courtesy Joan Edelstein and Ralph Levy, San Jose, Calif.

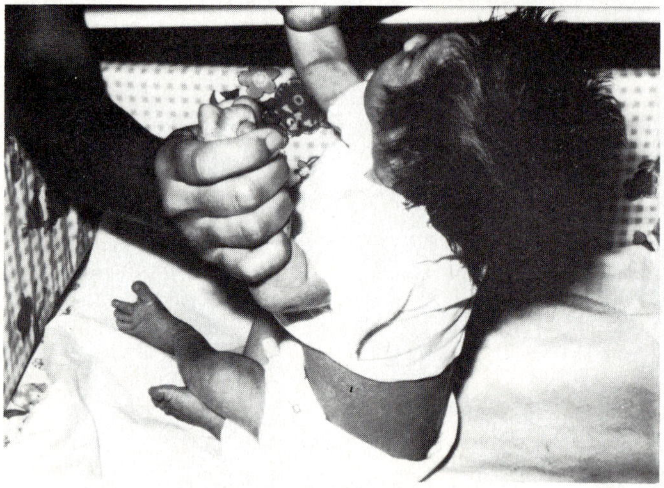

B

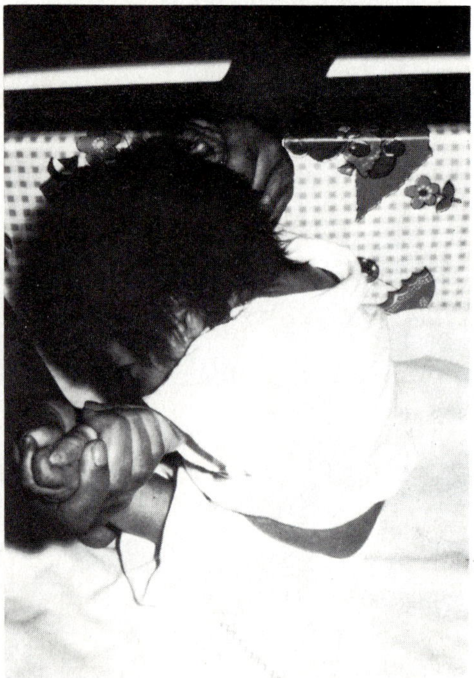

C

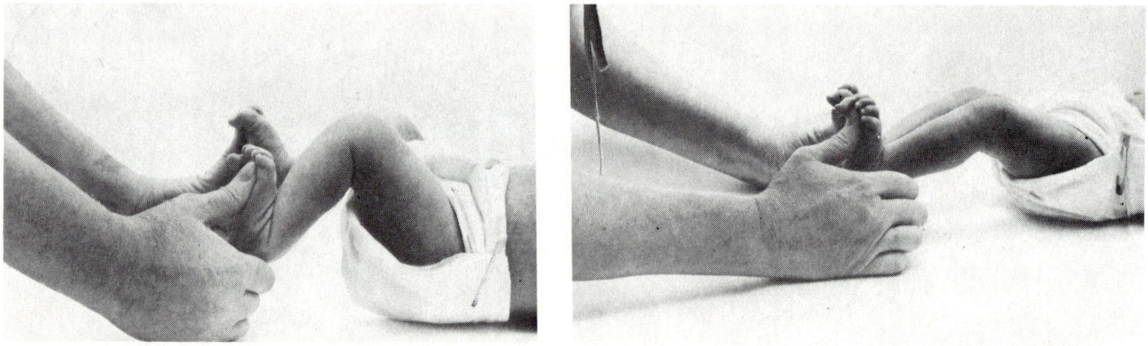

Fig. 21-27 Magnet reflex. With child in supine position and lower limbs semiflexed, light pressure is applied with fingers to both feet. Normally, while examiner's fingers maintain contact with soles of feet, lower limbs extend. Absence of this reflex suggests damage to spinal cord or malformation. Weak reflex may be seen following breech presentation *without* extended legs or may indicate sciatic nerve stretch syndrome. Breech presentation *with* extended legs may evoke an exaggerated response.
Courtesy Mead Johnson & Co, Evansville, Indiana.

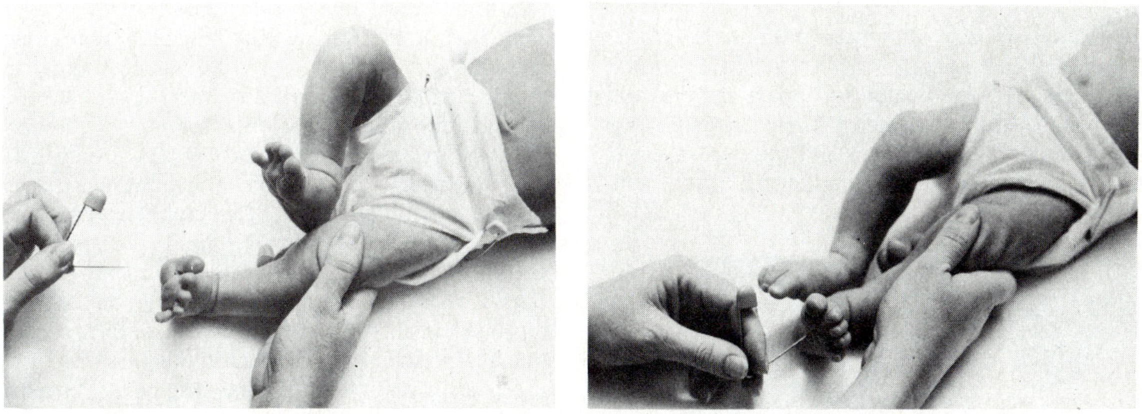

Fig. 21-28 Crossed extension reflex. With child in supine position, examiner extends one of infant's legs and presses knee down. Stimulation of sole of foot of fixated limb should cause *free* leg to flex, adduct, and extend as if attempting to push away stimulating agent. This reflex should be present during newborn period. Absence of response suggests a spinal cord lesion; weak response suggests peripheral nerve damage.
Courtesy Mead Johnson & Co, Evansville, Indiana.

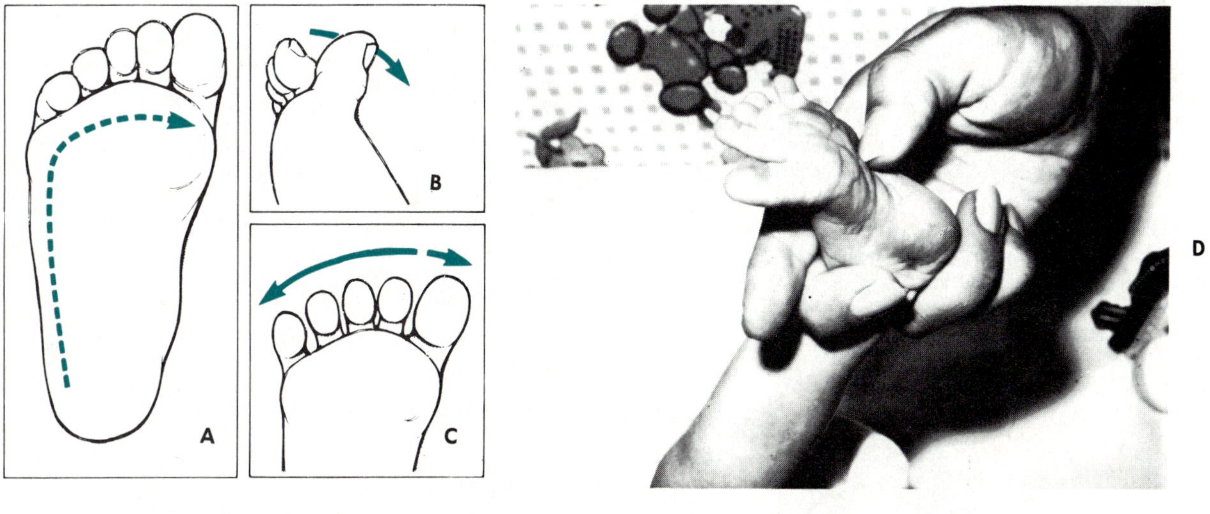

Fig. 21-29 Babinski's reflex. **A**, Direction of stroke. **B**, Dorsiflexion of big toe. **C**, Fanning of toes. **D**, Babinski's reflex in newborn.
From Whaley, LF, and Wong, DL: Nursing care of infants and children, ed 3, St Louis, 1987, The C V Mosby Co.

Scale [BNBAS]) and the Mother's Assessment of the Behavior of her Infant (MABI) developed by Field et al. (1978) provide a psychologic assessment of a newborn's capabilities. These capabilities are relevant to later personality development. It is their contention that the behavioral responses of infants are indicative of cortical control, responsiveness, and eventual ability to manage her or his environment. They emphasize the importance of infant-parent interaction. By their responses infants act to either consolidate relationships or alienate the persons in their immediate environment. By their actions they encourage or discourage attachment and care-taking activities. The development of parent-child love does not occur without feedback. The absence of feedback because of separation or incorrectly interpreted feedback can impair the growth of parental love (Chapter 25).

One of the first tasks parents must accomplish is to become aware of the unique behavioral responses of their child. Brazelton (1969) demonstrated that normal babies differ in such things as activity (active, average, quiet), feeding patterns, sleeping patterns, and responsiveness from the moment of birth. He suggests that the parents' reactions to their infants are determined in part by these differences. Perry (1983) used Brazelton's NBAS to study parent's perceptions of their infant's behaviors (See research highlight).

Sleep-wake Cycles

Infant variations in *state of consciousness* are called the sleep-wake cycles (Brazelton, 1973). They form a continuum with deep sleep, narcosis, or lethargy at one end and extreme irritability at the other end. There are two sleep states, deep sleep and light sleep, and four wake states, drowsiness, quiet alert, active alert, and crying. Infants' abilities to control their responses vary as they move from the sleep state to the waking state. Brazelton notes that infants' uses of a particular sleep or wake state to control or modify their reactions to external and internal stimuli reflect their potential for organization of behavior.

As shown in Table 21-4 and Fig. 21-32, each state has its distinguishing characteristics. The quiet alert state is also termed the optimum state of arousal. This state "allows sustained attention to external stimuli, purposeful hand-eye coordinated movements and active manipulation of the outside world" (Lewis and Zarin-Ackerman, 1977). During this state infants may be observed smiling, vocalizing, or moving in synchrony. Even during the first day of life, smiling is evident in a surprising number of infants (Wolff, 1969). They seem to watch their parents' faces carefully and respond to other persons talking to them. Many infants be-

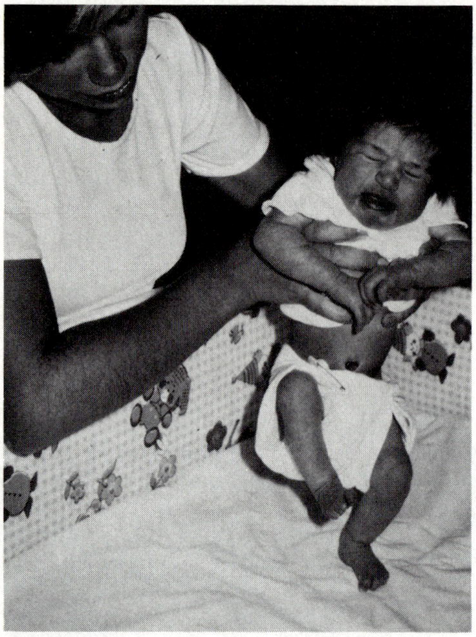

Fig. 21-30 Automatic walking reflex is phase of neuromuscular maturity from which infant normally graduates after 3 to 5 weeks. If infant is held so that sole of his foot touches table, reciprocal flexion and extension of leg occur, simulating walking.
Courtesy Joan Edelstein and Ralph Levy, San Jose, Calif.

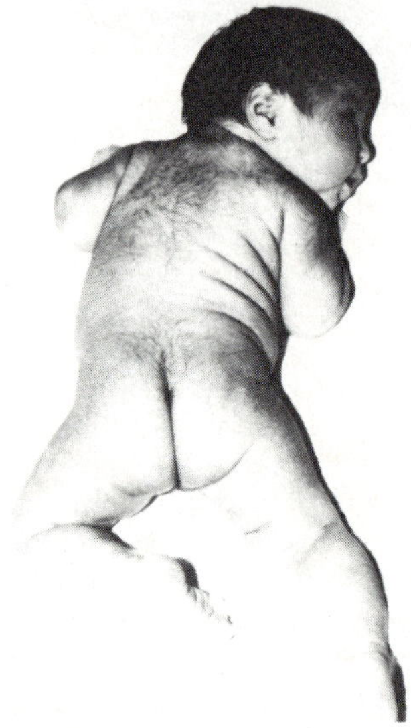

Fig. 21-31 Crawling.
Courtesy Marjorie Pyle, RNC, Life circle, Costa Mesa, Calif.

RESEARCH HIGHLIGHT

Parents' Perceptions of Their Newborn Following Structured Interactions

Purpose

To investigate whether infant behavior is related to parents' perceptions and whether parents' perceptions could be influenced.

Sample

Fifty-seven first-time parents comprised three experimental groups that participated in structured interactions with their infants. A control group did not participate in a structured interaction.

Methodology

The structured interaction was an assessment of the infant by the parents using the MABI. Behavior of the infants was assessed using the NBAS. Perceptions of the parents were measured three times using the Neonatal Perception Inventories.

Findings

No relation was found between parents' perceptions and infant behavior. Mothers' perceptions increased at the second time but not at other times. Fathers' perceptions were not influenced. The congruency of maternal and paternal perception increased over time. Seven additional variables influenced mothers' but not fathers' perceptions. Fathers were more intrigued with infant capabilities than were mothers.

Implications

The nurse may facilitate a positive parent/infant relationship by providing opportunities for interaction with infants in the early newborn period. Other variables affect perception. Nurses need to be alert to factors that may interfere with positive perceptions of infants and minimize negative effects of these factors.

Perry, SE: Parents' perceptions of their newborn following structured interactions, Nurs Res 32:208, 1983.

Table 21-4 *Behavioral States and State Behavior*

State	Characteristics of State: Body Activity	Eye Movements	Facial Movements	Breathing Pattern	Level of Response
Sleep States					
Deep sleep	Nearly still, except for occasional startle or twitch	None	Without facial movements, except for occasional sucking movement at regular intervals	Smooth and regular	Threshold to stimuli is very high so that only very intense and disturbing stimuli will arouse infants
Light sleep	Some body movements	Rapid eye movements (REMS), fluttering of eyes beneath closed eyelids	May smile and make brief fussy or crying sounds	Irregular	More responsive to internal and external stimuli; when these stimuli occur, infants may remain in light sleep, return to deep sleep, or arouse to drowsy
Awake States					
Drowsy	Activity level variable, with mild startles interspersed from time to time; movements usually smooth	Eyes open and close occasionally, are heavy-lidded with dull, glazed appearance	May have some facial movements; often there are none, and face appears still	Irregular	Infants react to sensory stimuli although responses are delayed; state change after stimulation commonly noted
Quiet alert	Minimum	Brightening and widening of eyes	Faces have bright, shining, sparkling looks	Regular	Infants attend most to environment, focusing attention on any stimuli that are present; optimum state of arousal
Active alert	Much body activity; may have periods of fussiness	Eyes open with less brightening	Much facial movement; faces not as bright as quiet alert state	Irregular	Increasingly sensitive to disturbing stimuli (hunger, fatigue, noise, excessive handling)
Crying	Increased motor activity, with color changes	Eyes may be tightly closed or open	Grimaces	More irregular	Extreme response to unpleasant external or internal stimuli

From Barnard, KE, et al: Behavioral states and state behaviors. In Early parent-infant relationships, copyright 1978 by the March of Dimes Birth Defects Foundation, White Plains, NY., Reprinted by permission.

gin a type of vocalizing by the time they are 2 weeks of age, making cooing, small, throaty noises while feeding.

The infant employs purposeful behavior to maintain the optimum arousal state: (1) active withdrawal by increasing physical distance, (2) a rejecting motion of pushing away with hands and feet, (3) decreasing sensitivity by falling asleep or breaking eye contact by turning the head, or (4) use of signaling behavior, such as fussing, or crying (Brazelton, 1973). Use of such behaviors permits infants to quiet themselves and reinstate readiness to interact again.

The first 6 weeks of life involve a steady decrease in the proportion of active REM sleep to total sleep. A steady increase in the proportion of quiet sleep to total sleep time also occurs. There is a 25% increase in wakefulness over the first 3 or 4 weeks. For the first few weeks the wakeful periods seem dictated by hunger, but soon thereafter a need for socializing appears to function as well. The newborn sleeps a total of about 17 hours a day, with the periods of wakefulness gradually increasing. By the fourth week of life, some infants are staying awake from one feeding session to the next. It is not until 4 or 5 years of age that children achieve the adult pattern of sleeping.

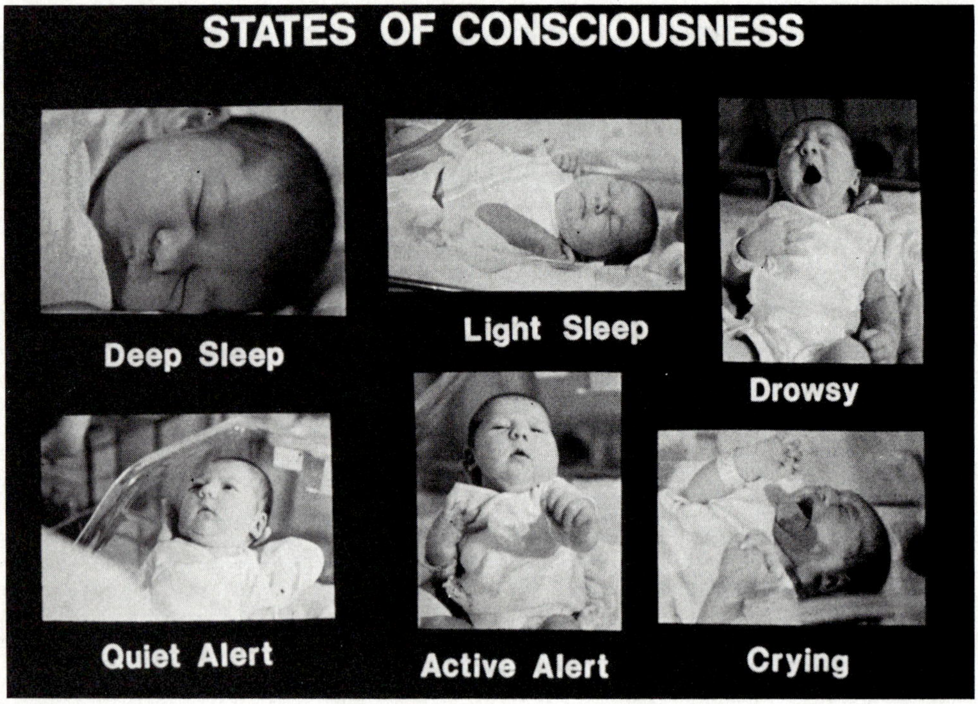

Fig. 21-32 Summary of sleep-wake states of newborn. States of consciousness: deep sleep, light sleep, drowsy, quiet alert, active alert, crying.
Courtesy March of Dimes.

Other Factors Influencing Newborn's Behavior

Several other variables, in addition to sleep-wake state, affect the newborn's responses. Several factors are discussed below.

Gestational Age. The gestational age of the infant and level of CNS maturity will affect observed behavior. An infant with an immature CNS will have an entire body response to a pinprick of the foot. The mature infant will withdraw the foot. CNS immaturity will also be reflected in reflex development and sleep-wake cycles.

Time. Length of time to recuperate from labor and birth will affect the behavior of infants as they attempt to become initially organized. Time since the last feeding and time of day may influence infants' responses.

Stimuli. Environmental events and stimuli will have an effect on the behavioral responses of infants. Nurses in intensive care nurseries observe that infants respond to loud noises, bright lights, monitor alarms, and tension in the unit. It has been well documented that infants are affected by nonverbal behavior in the environment. Infants of mothers who are tense have more muscle activity and their heart rates change parallel to their mothers during feeding. In addition, the newborn responds differently to animate and inanimate stimulation.

Medication. There is controversy concerning the effects on infant behavior of maternal medication (analgesia, anesthesia) during labor. Some researchers have noted that infants of mothers who were given medications may continue to demonstrate poor state organization beyond the fifth day (Murray, 1981). Others maintain that the effect can be beneficial or that there is no effect (Chapter 17).

Culture. Some of the most interesting research findings have been the differences in infant behavior across cultures (Freedman, 1979). Freedman and Freedman (1969) found that Chinese-American infants had more self-quieting activities, fewer state changes, and more rapid responses to consoling activities than white American infants did. The Zinacanteco Indians in southern Mexico demonstrated greater motor maturity and increased ability to maintain quiet alert states for longer times than American infants (Brazelton, 1969).

Sensory Behaviors

From birth, infants possess sensory capabilities that indicate a state of readiness for social interaction. Infants are able to use behavioral responses effectively in establishing their first dialogues. These responses, coupled with the newborns' "baby appearance" (the face is proportioned so that the forehead and eyes are larger than the lower portion of the face) and their smallness and helplessness, rouse feelings of wanting to hold, protect, and interact with them.

Vision. The infant's eyes drift off target because muscle control and coordination are immature. This glancing away permits the image being viewed to fall on the fovea (retinal area of clearest vision) more directly. The clearest visual distance is 17 to 20 cm (7 to 8 in), which is about the distance the infant's face is from the mother's face as she breast feeds or cuddles. Infants are sensitive to light. They will frown if a bright light is flashed in their eyes and will turn toward a soft red light. If the room is darkened, they will open their eyes widely and look about. This is noticeable when the delivery area is darkened after birth. By 2 months of age they can detect color, but under 5 days of age they seem more attracted by black-and-white patterns (Frantz, 1966).

Response to movement is noticeable. If a bright object is shown to newborns (even at 15 minutes of age), they will visually follow it, and some will even turn their heads to do so. Because human eyes are bright, shiny objects, newborns will track their parents' eyes. Parents will comment on how exciting this behavior is.

Visual acuity is surprising; even at 2 weeks of age infants can distinguish patterns with stripes 3 mm (⅛ in) apart. By 6 months their vision is as acute as that of an adult (Frantz and Miranda, 1975). They prefer to look at patterns rather than plain surfaces, even if the latter are brightly colored. They also prefer more complex patterns to simple ones. They prefer novelty (changes in pattern) by 2 months of age. This is significant knowledge, since it means the infant of a few weeks of age is capable of responding actively to an enriched environment.

From birth onward, infants are able to fix their eyes and gaze intently at objects. They gaze at their parents' faces and respond to changes in them with apparent imitative effect. This ability permits parents and children to gaze into each other's eyes, and a subtle communication pattern is thereby set up. Some researchers have indicated that there may be an ethnic component to this pattern. Freedman (1979) reported a study comparing Navaho and Anglo mothers in their efforts to get their babies' attention. The Anglo mothers became animated, smiled, and used gestures and high-pitched vocal sounds. The Navaho mothers gazed quietly at their babies until their eyes met and the infant gazed quietly back. Such responses may persist over time and influence behavior, as indicated by the following example:

> A 7-month-old Indian infant admitted for treatment of an ear infection seemed lonely and depressed. He would stare solemnly at me with his big brown eyes. I tried to cheer him by talking and shaking toys at him, but he would lie stiffly in my arms and gave no indication of noticing me. One evening when giving him his bottle I did not respond to his look by talking (I don't know why) but just looked back at him. After a bit he seemed to give a sigh, I could feel his little body relax against mine, and he reached up and patted the bottle.

The need to have eye contact is a compelling one (Robson, 1967). Children of blind parents and parents who have blind children must circumvent this obstacle for the formation of a relationship (see Chapter 25).

Hearing. It has been demonstrated that newborns, at 1 minute of age, can correctly look toward sound presented alternately to them on the right and the left side. They were especially good at detecting sound directly in front of them. The newborns were also able to discriminate frequencies of sound in the range of the human voice (500 to 900 decibels) (Wertheimer, 1961; Clifton et al., 1981).

Even more discrete differentiation of sound can be demonstrated by a newborn's consistent, preferential turning toward the sound of his mother's voice immediately after birth (Brazelton, 1977). This occurs even when another female voice has previously captured the neonate's attention. The phenomenon can be demonstrated to mothers with consistent success. The origins of this behavior have been discovered by Truby, a linguist, who with a Swedish pediatrician and an American dentist developed highly sophisticated measuring devices to record and analyze the cry of newborns. They discovered that cry imprints produced for each newborn had, like footprints and fingerprints, and individual uniqueness (Truby and Lind, 1965). When a newborn's cry print was compared with the mother's speech patterns, unmistakable similarities were present. Later studies of the cries of very young premature babies, as small as 900 g (2 lb), corresponded to the mother's speech patterns (Truby, 1975). Infants of mute mothers did not cry or cried strangely. It was hypothesized that the fetus receives and stores speech features from the mother through hearing and listening while in utero.

All these studies indicate a selective listening to the maternal voice sounds and rhythms during intrauterine life that prepare newborns for recognition and interaction with their primary caregivers—their mothers. Newborns are accustomed in the uterus to hearing the regular rhythm of the mother's heartbeat. As a result they respond by relaxing and ceasing to fuss and cry if a regular heartbeat simulator is placed in their cribs.

The acute sensitivity to the human voice has been tested experientially. In observations of the responses of quiet, alert newborns to computer-simulated cries and the cries of human newborns, more restlessness and crying occurred in response to the genuine cry. Newborns less than 35 hours old typically began to cry when submitted to the cry of other newborns but quieted at the sound of their own cry (Martin, 1981).

Condon and Sander (1974) describe normal patterns of response to speech sounds. In these patterns the listener's body motions are synchronous with those of the speaker. The researcher termed these patterns **interactional synchrony.** Condon and Sander found that alert, moving newborns coordinated their movements to the sounds of adult speech patterns and continued to do so when tested again the following day. Brazelton (1969) notes that this "dancing in tune" gives feedback to the speaker and encourages more interaction. Infants have been shown to imitate parents' actions by 2 weeks of age (Meltzoff and Moore, 1977).

Movement of head, shoulders, elbows, hips, and feet occurred without eye contact with the speaker (an adult male voice). Some newborns received recorded voices and other direct voice contact. The results were the same—sustained, coordinated movement. No change in the findings occurred when the language was changed to Chinese nor when infant posture was changed from being held to being supine in their cribs. However, when disconnected vowel and tapping sounds were made, the degree of correspondence of body movement with the sound disappeared. The human infant appears to be particularly *tuned in* to the rhythms of human speech in preference to all other sounds.

Touch. Sensory pathways for kinesthetic (movement) and tactile (touch) activities are the first to complete myelinization in the infant (Kolb, 1959; Purpura, 1975). The newborn's responses to touch suggest this sensory system is well prepared to receive and process tactile messages. Many of the reflexes of the newborn demonstrated a response to tactile stimulation (Table 21-3).

The new mother uses touch as one of the first interaction behaviors: fingertip touch, soft stroking of the face, and gentle massage of the back. Since touch between strangers is avoided in some cultures, it would seem that this automatic maternal touching behavior evidences an already intimate relationship. Birth trauma or stress and depressant drugs taken by the mother decrease the infant's sensitivity to touch or painful stimuli.

Taste. Newborns have repeatedly demonstrated a preference for sweet fluids over sour or bitter ones. Facial expressions indicating newborn response to taste have been recorded in a series of studies. The facial expressions of a selected variety of people were photographed as various tastes were presented (Steinner, 1973, 1979). Premature and normal newborns; anencephalic newborns; mentally retarded, facially deformed, or congenitally blind adolescents; and normal adults showed the same responses. Sour fluids precipitated puckering of the lips; bitter fluids caused retching or spitting, and sweet tastes resulted in relaxed expressions interpreted as enjoyment and satisfaction. These studies demonstrate not only the newborn's response to various tastes but also the strength of the taste response and its independence from cortical levels of the nervous system.

It is generally accepted that young infants are particularly oriented toward the *use of their mouths* both for meeting their nutritional needs for rapid growth and for releasing tension through sucking. The early development of circumoral sensation and muscle activity as well as taste would seem to be preparation for survival in the extrauterine environment.

Smell. Several studies have tested newborn response to odors. The findings demonstrate not only a preference for smells deemed pleasant by adults but also that newborns have the ability to learn and remember.

Steiner (1979) experimented with newborns' responses to smell. Using photographic recordings of facial expressions, Steiner found that newborns, some of whom were only hours old and inexperienced with food odors, showed a preference for the odors of banana, vanilla, and strawberry. The newborns rejected smells of fish or rotten eggs. These odors were presented to the newborns on cotton swabs held under their noses.

One of the most well-known studies of infant learning through the olfactory tract was done by Macfarlane (1975). Newborns were tested for recognition of their mother's breast pads. By age 2 to 7 days, infants turned more often toward their mother's used breast pad than an unused one when both were placed above them. Within another few days these infants turned preferentially toward their own mother's used breast pad than that of another nursing mother.

The significance of smell in maternal identification of offspring and vice versa in the animal world is well documented. Maternal identification of the human newborn by smell has not been studied extensively. Stainton (1985) noted that mothers reported their infants smell differently from birth onward.

Response to Environmental Stimuli

Each newborn has a predisposed capacity to handle the multitudinous stimuli in the external world (Brazelton, 1961). Individual variations in the primary reaction pattern of newborns have been described and termed *temperament* (Thomas, 1961, 1970). The style of behavioral response to stimuli is guided by the temperament that affects the newborn's sensory threshold, ability to habituate, and response to maternal behaviors.

Habituation. The newborn is able to control the type and amount of incoming stimuli processed with the ability to *habituate.* Habituation is a psychologic and physiologic phenomenon whereby the response to a constant or repetitive stimuli is decreased (Bridger, 1975; Ornstein, 1972). In the term newborn this can be demonstrated in several ways. Shining a bright light into a newborn's eyes will cause a startle or squinting the first two to three times and possibly a hand or arm will be brought up over the eyes. The third or fourth flash will elicit a diminished response and by the fifth or sixth flash, the infant ceases to respond (Brazelton, 1973, 1977). The same response pattern holds true for the sounds of a rattle, a bell, or a pinprick to a heel. A newborn presented with new stimuli will become wide-eyed and alert, gaze for a time, but eventually show a diminished interest.

As well as shutting out repetitive stimuli, the ability to habituate enables the newborn to select stimuli that potentiate continued learning about the social world, avoiding overload. The intrauterine experiences seem to have programmed the newborn to be especially responsive to human voices, soft lights, soft sounds, sweet tastes, and perhaps patting and rubbing.

Habituation is an early form of learning (Stone et al., 1973). The newborn quickly learns the constant sounds in a newborn nursery and in the home environment and is able to sleep in their midst. The selective responses of the newborn indicate cerebral organization capable of remembering and making choices. The ability to habituate depends on state of consciousness, hunger, fatigue, and temperament. These factors also affect consolability, cuddliness, irritability, and crying.

Consolability. Korner (1971) reports on studies conducted over several years that describe variations in the ability of newborns to console themselves or to be consoled. In the crying state, most newborns will initiate one of several ways to reduce their distress and move to a lower state. hand-to-mouth movements are common with or without sucking, as well as alerting to voices, noises, or visual stimuli in the environment.

Cuddliness. The degree to which a newborn will mold into the contours of the person holding them varies. Korner and Thoman (1970) tested the effect of body contact and vestibular stimulation in both soothing babies and creating alertness. The vestibular stimulation of being picked up and moved had the greater effect. Schaffer and Emerson (1964) classified newborns into "cuddlers," "noncuddlers," and an "intermediate group."

Irritability. Some newborns cry longer and harder than others. For some the sensory threshold seems low. They are readily upset by unusual noises, hunger, wetness, or new experiences and respond intensively. Others with a high sensory threshold require a great deal more stimulation and variation to reach the active, alert state (Korner, 1971).

Crying. Crying in an infant may signal hunger, pain, desire for attention, or fussiness (see Chapter 25). As mother and infant become more adept at interpreting each other's behavior, some mothers state that they are able to distinguish the reasons for crying.

> I can tell when she's hungry. Crying starts in a plaintive way and then becomes more and more demanding. When she is hurt, she lets out a startled yell as though she couldn't believe it was happening to her. Sometimes when she is put down to sleep, she starts a kind of talking cry, jerky and demanding; it gets louder, and if nothing happens, fades away in little spurts. The fussy cry is the hardest to take—nothing seems to work; like a complaining sound it goes on and on.

A report such as this means that the mother and baby are communicating effectively.

Temperament. The behavioral styles of infants and children "show distinct individuality in temperament in the first weeks of life, independently of their parents' handling or personality style"; "the original characteristics of temperament tend to persist in most children over the years" (Chess, 1969; Chess and Thomas, 1977).

Chess (1969) developed nine categories of primary reactivity to evaluate behavioral style:

1. Activity level: the diurnal proportion of diurnal active to inactive periods.
2. Rhythmicity: the regularity and predictability of bodily functions and sleep-wake cycle.
3. Approach or withdrawal: the response to a new stimulus.
4. Adaptability: the speed and ease with which current behavior is modified in response to environmental changes.
5. Intensity of reaction: the energy in a response regardless of its quality or direction.
6. Threshold of responsiveness: the intensity of stimuli required to evoke a response.
7. Quality of mood: the proportion of happy behavior to unhappy behavior.
8. Distractibility: the efficacy of external stimuli in changing the direction of ongoing behavior.
9. Attention span and persistence: the length of time one activity is pursued and the effect of distraction.

These nine categories were then grouped into three major patterns of behavioral style or temperament:

1. The easy child who demonstrates regularity in bodily functions, readily adapts to change, has a predominantly positive mood, a moderate sensory threshold, and approaches new situations or objects with a response of moderate intensity.
2. The slow-to-warm-up child who has a low activity level, withdraws on first exposure to new stimuli, is slow to adapt, low in intensity of response, and is somewhat negative in mood.
3. The difficult child who is irregular in bodily functions, intense in reactions, generally negative in mood, resistant to change or new stimuli, and often cries loudly for long periods.

The human newborn possesses sensory receptors capable of responding selectively to various stimuli present in the internal and external environment. The infant also possesses individual characteristics that define her or him as a unique personality. The range of the infant's responses may impress the parent with the newborn's formidable neurologic capacity. The newborn's innate ability is truly amazing (Tables 21-5 and 21-6).

Text continued on p. 504.

Table 21-5 *Infant State-Related Behavior*

Behavior	Description of Behavior	Infant State Consideration	Implications for Caregiving
Alerting	Widening and brightening of the eyes. Infants focus attention on stimuli, whether visual, auditory, or objects to be sucked.	From drowsy to active alert to quiet alert	Infant state and timing are important. When trying to alert infants, one may try to: 1. Unwrap infants (arms out at least). 2. Place infants in upright position. 3. Talk to infants, putting variation in your pitch and tempo. 4. Show your face to infants. 5. Elicit the rooting, sucking, or grasp reflexes. Being able to alert infants is important for caregivers, as alert infants offer increased feedback to adults.
Visual response	Newborns have pupillary responses to differences in brightness. Infants can focus on objects or faces about 7-8 inches away. Newborns have preferences for more complex patterns, human faces, and moving objects.	Quiet alert	Newborn's visual alertness provides opportunities for eye-to-eye contact with caregivers, an important source of beginning caregiver-infant interaction.
Auditory response	Reaction to a variety of sounds, especially in the human voice range. Infants can hear sounds and locate the general direction of the sound, if the source is constant and remains coming from the same direction.	Drowsy, quiet alert, active alert	Enhances communication between infants and caregivers. The fact that crying infants can often be consoled by voice demonstrates the value this stimulus has to infants.
Irritability	How easily infants are upset by loud noises, handling by caregivers, temperature changes, removal of blankets or clothes, etc.	From deep sleep, light sleep, drowsy, quiet alert, or active alert to fussing or crying	Irritable infants need more frequent consoling and more subdued external environments. Parents can be helped to cope with more irritable infants through the items listed under "Consoling by caregivers."
Readability	The cues infants give through motor behavior and activity, looking, listening, and behavior patterns.	All states	Parents need to learn that newborns' behaviors are part of their individual temperaments and not reflections on their parenting abilities or because their infants do not like them. By observing and understanding an infant's characteristic pattern, parents can respond more appropriately to their infant as an individual.
Smile	Ranging from a faint grimace to a full-fledged smile. Reflexive.	Drowsy, active alert, quiet alert, light sleep	Initial smile in the neonatal period is the forerunner of the social smile at 3-4 weeks of age. Important for caregivers to respond to it.
Habituation	The ability to lessen one's response to repeated stimuli. For instance, this is seen where the Moro's response is repeatedly elicited. If a noise is continually repeated, infants will no longer respond to it in most cases.	Deep sleep, light sleep, also seen in drowsy	Because of this ability families can carry out their normal activities without disturbing infants. Infants are not victims of their environments. Infants can shut out most stimuli, similar to adults not hearing a dripping faucet after a period of time. Infants who have more difficulty with this will probably not sleep well in active environments.

Table 21-5 *Infant State-Related Behavior—cont'd*

Behavior	Description of Behavior	Infant State Consideration	Implications for Caregiving
Cuddliness	Infant's response to being held. Infants nestle and work themselves into the contours of caregiver's bodies versus resist being held.	Primarily in awake states	Cuddliness is usually rewarding behavior for the caregivers. It seems to convey a message of affection. If infants do not nestle and mold, it would be wise to discuss this tendency and show the caregivers how to position infants to maximize this response.
Consolability	Measured when infants have been crying for at least 15 seconds. The ability of infants to bring themselves or to be brought by others to a lower state.	From crying to active alert, quiet alert, drowsy, or sleep states	Crying is the infant behavior that presents the greatest challenge to caregivers. Parents' success or failure in consoling their infants has a significant impact on their feelings of competence as parents.
Self-consoling	Maneuvers used by infants to console themselves and move to a lower state: 1. Hand-to-mouth movement. 2. Sucking on fingers, fist, or tongue. 3. Paying attention to voices or faces around them. 4. Changes in position.	From crying to active alert, quiet alert, drowsy, or sleep states	If caregivers are aware of these behaviors, they may allow infants the opportunity to gain control of themselves instead of immediately responding to their cues. This does not imply that newborns should be left to cry. Once newborns are crying and do not initiate self-consoling activities, they may need attention from caregivers.
Consoling by caregivers	After crying for longer than 15 seconds, the caregivers may try to: 1. Show face to infant. 2. Talk to infant in a steady, soft voice. 3. Hold both infant's arms close to body. 4. Swaddle infant. 5. Pick up infant. 6. Rock infant. 7. Give a pacifier or feed.	From crying to active alert, quiet alert, drowsy, or sleep states	Often parental initial reaction is to pick up infants or feed them when they cry. Parents could be taught to try other soothing maneuvers.
Motor behavior and activity	Spontaneous movements of extremities and body when stimulated versus when left alone. Smooth, rhythmical movements versus jerky ones.	Quiet alert, active alert	Smooth, nonjerky movements with periods of inactivity seem most natural. Some parents see jerky movements and startles as negative response to their caregiving and are frightened.

From Barnard, KE, et al: Infant state-related behavior chart. In Early parent-infant relationships, copyright 1978 by the March of Dime Birth Defects Foundation, White Plains, NY. Reprinted with permission.

Table 21-6 *Infant Behavioral Patterns and Sensory Capabilities*

Pattern/Capability	Parameters of Normal	Deviations From Normal/Probable Conditions
Behavioral Patterns	Cortical control and responsiveness	CNS disorders
Feeding	Variations in interest, hunger; usually feeds well within 24 hours of birth	Lethargic, tires easily or may perspire while attempting to feed; poor suck, poor coordination with swallow, cyanosis, choking
Social	Cry is lusty, strong; soon indicative of hunger, pain, attention seeking	Weak or absent; high pitched
	Smiling, focusing evident within first week	Absence; no focusing on person holding him; unconsolable
	Responds by quietness and increased alertness to cuddling, voice	

Continued.

Table 21-6 *Infant Behavioral Patterns and Sensory Capabilities—cont'd*

Pattern/Capability	Parameters of Normal	Deviations From Normal/Probable Conditions
Sleep-wakefulness	Transitional period with 2 periods of reactivity: at birth and 6-8 hours later	Lethargy; drowsiness
	Stabilization with wakeful periods about every 3-4 hours	Disorganized pattern
Elimination	Develops own pattern within first 2 weeks:	
	Stooling: see "Elimination behaviors"	See "Elimination behaviors"
	Urination:	Diminished number: dehydration
	First few days: 3-4 times daily	
	End of first week: 5-6 times daily	
	Later: 6-10 times daily with adequate hydration	
Reflex response	Brainstem development and musculoskeletal intactness	Present in anencephalic neonates also
	See "Assessment of newborn's reflexes"	Absence; hyperreactive; incomplete; asynchronous
Sensory Capabilities		
Vision	Limited accommodation with clearest vision within 18-20 cm (7-8 in)	Absence of these responses may be caused by absence of or diminished acuity or by sensory deprivation
	Detects color by 2 months but attracted by black-white pattern at 5 days or less	
	Focuses and follows by 15 min of age	
	Prefers patterns to plain surfaces	
	Prefers changes in patterns by 2 months	
	At birth, can gaze intently	
Hearing	By 2 min of age, moves eyes in direction of sound	Absence of response: deafness
	Responds to high pitch by "freezing," followed by agitation; to low pitch (crooning) by relaxation	
	Can hear beginning in last trimester of fetal life	
Touch	Sensitivity to pain may be diminished (because of β-endorphins present prenatally)	
	Soothed by massaging, warmth, weightlessness (as in warm water bath)	Unable to be comforted; possible drug dependence
Smell	By days 2 to 7 can distinguish between own mother's used breast pads and those of another woman	
Taste	By 3 days of age, can distinguish between sucrose and glucose and grimaces in response to drop of lemon juice on tongue	
Motor	Coordinates body movement to parent's voice and body movement; imitates parent's actions by 2 weeks of age	Absence

SUMMARY

During the period of infancy the infant within the "protective envelope of nurturing adults" (Brazelton, 1982) can learn complex coping mechanisms and control systems. These in turn help the infant be alert, pay attention, and master rules of communication. The newborn and adult learn about each other and about themselves—a feeling of mutuality, of identification with the "other" is accomplished. The nurse uses knowledge of the biologic and behavioral characteristics of the newborn as a basis for the care of the infant and the teaching and counseling of the parents.

KEY CONCEPTS

- By term the infant's various anatomic and physiologic systems have reached a level of development and functioning that permits a physical existence apart from the mother and sensory capabilities that indicate a state of readiness for social interaction.
- There are several significant differences between the respiratory, renal, and thermogenetic systems in the newborn and those of the adult that have import for nursing care.
- At any serum bilirubin level, the appearance of jaundice during the first day of life or persistence of jaundice usually indicates a pathologic process.
- Chilling of a newborn, even a healthy term newborn, may result in acidosis and raise the level of free fatty acids.
- Many reflex behaviors are important for the newborn's survival.
- The individual personalities and behavioral characteristics of infants play a major role in the ultimate relationship between infants and their parents.
- Behavioral responses of infants are indicative of corti-

cal control, responsiveness, and eventual ability to manage her or his environment.

- The development of parent-child love does not occur without feedback.
- Sleep-wake cycles and other factors influence the newborn's behavior.
- Each newborn has a predisposed capacity to handle the multitude of stimuli in the external world.

STUDY QUESTIONS AND ACTIVITIES

1. Observe a normal newborn immediately after birth and in follow-up periods for several days thereafter. Write reports on daily observations, including both physiologic and behavioral data; compare and contrast data, and identify questions for further research.
2. Prepare teaching materials on changes and challenges to one of the newborn's body systems that could be used for educating a new-parent class. Present the material prepared to the group for discussion and additional suggestions.
3. For those who have baby books of themselves, share these with the class. In group discussion, discuss what items were considered important when the data were recorded, and what changes you might suggest for a baby book to be kept today.
4. Research theories of newborn behavior and sensory abilities before 20 years ago and over the last 10 years. Discuss changes in attitude and expectations toward the newborn and how these might affect treatment and care of the newborn.
5. Use research on newborns' sensory abilities and social responses to design a nursery for the new baby that incorporates these findings, together with a list of suggestions of parent-child interactions appropriate to these findings.

References

Aladjem, SA, et al: Clinical perinatology, ed 2, St Louis, 1980, The CV Mosby Co

Brazelton, TB: Infants and mothers, ed 1, New York, 1969, Dell Publishing Co, Inc

Brazelton, TB: Effect of maternal expectations on early infant behavior, Early Child Dev Care 2:259, 1973

Brazelton, TB: The remarkable talents of the newborn, Paper presented at Parent to Infant Attachment Conference, Cleveland, November 6, 1977

Bridger, WH: Sensory discrimination and autonomic function in the newborn, Am Acad Child Psychiatry 15:257, 1975

Brovten, D, et al: Breastmilk Jaundice, JOGN Nurs 14(3):220, 1985

Chess, S: Individuality and baby care, Dev Med Child Neurol 11:749, 1969

Chess, S, and Thomas, A: Temperament and the parent-child interaction, Pediatr Ann 6(9):26, 1977

Clifton, RK, et al: Newborns' orientation toward sound: possible implications for cortical development, Child Dev 52:833, 1981

Condon, WS, and Sander, LW: Neonate movement is synchronized with adult speech: interactional participation and language acquisition, Science 183:99, 1974

Davis, V: The structure and function of brown adipose tissue in the neonate, JOGN Nurs 9(6):368, 1980

DeCarvalho, M, Hall, M, and Harvey, D: Effects of water supplementation on physiological jaundice, Arch Dis Child 56:568, 1981

De Carvalho, M, et al: Frequency of breast-feeding and serum bilirubin concentration, J Dis Child 136:737, 1982

Desmond, MM, et al: The transitional care nursery, Pediatr Clin North Am 13:651, 1966

Fanaroff, A, and Martin, R: Behrman's neonatal-prenatal medicine, St Louis, ed 2, 1987, The CV Mosby Co

Field, R, et al: Mothers' assessments of the behavior of their infants, Infant Beh Dev 1:156, 1978

Frantz, RL: Pattern discrimination and selective attention as determinants of perceptual development from birth. In Kidd, AJ, and Rivaire, JL, editors: Perceptual development in children, New York, 1966, International Universities Press, Inc

Frantz, RL, and Miranda, SB: Newborn infant attention to form and contour, Child Dev 46:224, 1975

Freedman, DG: Ethnic differences in babies, Hum Nature, p 4, Jan 1979

Freedman, DG, and Freedman, N: Behavioral differences between Chinese-American and European-American newborns, Nature 224:1227, 1969

Guyton, A: Textbook of medical physiology, Philadelphia, 1985, WB Saunders Co

Kolb, L: Disturbances of the body image. In Arieti, S, editor: American handbook of psychiatry, vol 1, New York, 1959, Basic Books, Inc, Publishers

Korner, AF: Individual differences at birth: implications for early experiences and later development, Am J Orthopsychiatry 41:608, 1971

Korner, AF, and Thoman, EB: Visual alertness in neonates as evoked by maternal care, J Exp Child Psychol 10:67, 1970

Korones, SB: High-risk newborn infants: the basis for intensive nursing care, ed 4, St Louis, 1986, The CV Mosby Co

Lewis, M, and Zarin-Ackerman, J: Early infant development. In Behrman, RE, et al, editors: Neonatal-perinatal medicine: diseases of the fetus and infant, ed 2, St Louis, 1977, The CV Mosby Co

Locklin, M: Assessing jaundice in full-term newborns, Pediatr Nurs 13(1):15, 1987

Lowrey, G: Growth and development of children, ed 8, Chicago, 1986, Year Book Medical Pulishers, Inc

Macfarlane, A: Olfaction in the development of social preferences in the human neonate. In Parent-infant interaction: CIBA Symposium, 1975

Martin, C: Newborns pacified by tapes of their own crying, Brain/Mind Bulletin 10:2, 1981

Medici, M: The fight against infection: the neonates' defense mechanisms, J Calif Perinat Assoc 3(2):25, 1983

Meltzoff, A, and Moore, M: Imitation of facial and manual gestures by human neonates, Science 198:75, 1977

Murray, AD, et al: Effects of epidural anesthesia on newborns and their mothers, Child Dev 52(1):71, 1981

Ornstein, RE: The psychology of consciousness, San Francisco, 1972, WH Freeman & Co, Publishers

Ostler, CW: Initial feeding time of newborn infants: effect upon first meconium passage and serum indirect bilirubin levels, Issues Health Care Wom p 3, 1980

Perry, SE: Parents' perceptions of their newborn following structural interactions, Nurs Res 32:208, 1983

Pritchard, J, McDonald, P, and Gant, N: Williams' obstetrics, ed 17, East Norwalk, Conn, 1985, Appleton-Century-Crofts

Purpura, D: Dendrite differentiation in human cerebral cortex: normal and aberrant developmental patterns, Adv Neurol 12:91, 1975
Robson, KS: The role of eye-to-eye contact in maternal-infant attachment, J Child Psychol Psychiatry 8:13, 1967
Saul, K, and Warburton, D: Increased incidence of early-onset hyperbilirubinemia in breast-fed versus bottle-fed infants, J Perinatol 4(3):36, 1984
Schaffer, H, and Emerson, P: Patterns of response to physical contact in early human development, J Child Psychol Psychiatry 5:1, 1964
Stainton, MC: Origins of attachment: culture and cue sensitivity. Dissertation Abstracts International, *46,* 3786-B. (University Microfilms No. 8600606), 1985
Steiner, JE: The gustofacial response: observation on normal and anencephalic newborn infants. In Bosma, JF, editor: Fourth symposium on oral sensation and perception: development in the fetus and infant, Bethesda, MD, 1973, US Department of Health, Education and Welfare
Steiner, JE: Human facial expressions in response to taste and smell stimulation, Adv Child Dev Behav 13:257, 1979
Stone, LJ, et al: The competent infant: research and commentary, New York, 1973, Basic Books, Inc, Publishers
Thomas, A, et al: Individuality in responses of children to similar environmental situations, Am J Psychiatry 117:798, 1961
Thomas, A, et al: The origin of personality, Sci Am 223:102, 1970
Truby, HM: Prenatal and neonatal speech, prespeech and an infantile speech lexicon. In Child language—1975, Word 27 (special issue):1, 1975
Truby, H, and Lind, J: Cry sounds of the newborn infant. In Lind, J, editor: Newborn infant cry, Acta Pediatr Scand 163(suppl):7, 1965
Vaughan, VC, McKay, R, and Behrman, R: Nelson's textbook of pediatrics, Philadelphia, 1979, WB Saunders Co
Wertheimer, M: Psychomotor coordination of auditory and visual space at birth, Science 134:1962, 1961
Whaley, LF, and Wong, DL: Nursing care of infants and children, ed 3, St Louis, 1987, The CV Mosby Co
Wolff, PH: Observations on newborn infants, Psychosom Med 21:110, 1969

Bibliography

Anderson, CJ: Enhancing reciprocity between mother and neonate, Nurs Res 30(2):89, 1981
Apostolakis, E: Visual preferences of preterm and term infants, J Calif Perinat Assoc 11:61, Spring 1982
Brazelton, TB: Joint regulation of neonate-parent behavior. In Tronick, EZ, editor: Social interchange in infancy: affect, cognition, and communication, Baltimore, 1982, University Park Press
Brazelton, T: Infants and mothers, ed 2, New York, 1983, Dell Publishing Co, Inc
Bushnell, IWR: Discrimination of faces by young infants, J Exp Child Psychol 33:298, 1982
Censullo, M, et al: An instrument for the measurement of infant-adult syncrony, Nurs Res 36(4):244, 1987
Crockenberg, SB: Infant irritability, mother responsiveness and social support influences on the security of infant-mother attachment, Child Dev 52(3):857, 1981
Davis, V: The structure and function of brown adipose tissue in the neonate, JOGN Nurs 9(6):368, 1980
Färdig, J: A comparison of skin-to-skin contact and radiant heaters in promoting neonatal thermoregulation, J Nurse Midwife 25(1):19, 1980
Judd, JM: Assessing the newborn from head to toe, Nurs '85 15(12):34, 1985
Krantz, DH, Human color vision, Contemp Psychol 27:88, 1982
Ludington-Hoe, S: What can newborns really see? Am J Nurs 83:1286, 1983
Reid, T: Newborn cyanosis, Am J Nurs 82(8):1230, 1982
Rosner, BS, and Doherty, NE: The response of neonates to intrauterine sounds, Dev Med Child Neurol 21(6):723, 1979
Tedder, JL: Newborn circumcision, JOGN Nurs 16(1):42, 1987

CHAPTER 22

Nursing Care of the Normal Newborn

Learning Objectives

Correctly define the key terms listed.

Discuss the components of assessment of the newborn from the antenatal, intranatal, and postnatal periods.

Explain what is meant by a safe environment.

Review procedures for heel stick, assisting with venipuncture, collection of urine specimen, and restraining the infant.

Compare methods of maintaining an adequate oxygen supply.

Outline in detail the emergency procedure for cardiopulmonary resuscitation and relieving airway obstruction.

Discuss methods to maintain the infant's temperature.

Describe precautions in administering an intramuscular injection to a newborn.

Discuss phototherapy and guidelines for teaching parents about it.

Explain circumcision: purposes, methods, postoperative care, and parent teaching.

Determine each daily care activity.

Review anticipatory guidance for parents.

Key Terms

acid mantle
anticipatory guidance
apnea
bulb syringe
cardiopulmonary resuscitation (CPR)
clovehitch restraint
cradle cap
DeLee mucus-trap catheter
excoriations
hyperbilirubinemia
hypothermia
mummy technique
perinatology
phenylketonuria (PKU)
phototherapy
tachypnea
thermistor probe

During the neonatal period the prenatal and postnatal characteristics of the infant merge. Gradually the former disappear as the infant grows and matures outside the womb. Although most infants make the necessary biopsychosocial adjustment to extrauterine existence without undue difficulty, their well-being depends on the care they receive from others. The nursing care described in this chapter is based on careful assessment of biologic and behavioral responses and formulation of nursing diagnoses. It includes planning and implementing appropriate nursing actions and evaluating their effectiveness.

Assessment

Routine assessment of the infant is a continuous process. Whenever any care is given to a newborn, observations and recordings of the child's progress are made. At the beginning of each 8-hour shift the following assessments are made, compared with the norm, and recorded:

1. Respiratory rate, rhythm, and effort
2. Breath sounds
3. Heart rate and rhythm
4. Skin color
5. Activity level and muscle tone
6. Feeding and elimination behavior

The first *assessment* of the infant is done at birth, using the Apgar scoring technique and a brief *physical assessment* (see Chapter 19). The assessment for gestational age, if considered necessary, is done within the first 2 hours after birth (see Chapter 37).

Admission to the Nursery

Having verified the infant's identification with the transfer nurse from the delivery unit, the nursery nurse places the baby in a warm environment and begins the admission assessment, which includes pertinent information from the mother's prenatal record and the record of events during the mother's labor and the newborn's birth. Often a form such as the one in Fig. 22-1 is used to record findings. This form shows at a glance, significant data from the antenatal period through nursery admission. An example of newborn nursery routine orders is shown in the box below.

ROUTINE NURSERY ORDERS

1. Vital signs: on admission, q4h × 2, and q8h until discharge
   a. Respirations, color, and tone q15min × 2h
   b. Temperature, pulse q30min × 2
2. Measure and record weight, height, head and chest circumferences; weigh q8h
3. Hematocrit, prn; note if ≥ 65%
4. Blood sugar, prn; note if ≤ 40 mg/dl
5. Inquire if baby is to be breast-fed or formula-fed
6. Inquire if male child is to be circumcised
7. Have blood drawn for phenylketonuria (PKU), thyroxine (T_4), and galactosemia screening on day of dismissal or third day

Extensive Physical Examination

A second more thorough physical examination is done within 24 hours after delivery, when the newborn's temperature is stabilized. The *goal* of this examination is to compile a complete record of the newborn that will act as a data base for subsequent assessment and care. Having the parents present during this extensive examination permits prompt discussion of parental concerns, and involves the parents actively in the health care of their child from birth. At the same time, *parental interactions with the child* can be observed; this aids in early diagnosis of concerns in parent-child relationships and learning needs.

The area used for the examination should be well lighted, warm, and free of drafts. The child is undressed as needed and placed on a firm, flat surface. The infant may need to be picked up and cuddled at times for reassurance. The examination is carried out in a systematic manner. It begins with a general evaluation of such characteristics as appearance, maturity, nutritional status, activity, and state of well-being. This general evaluation is followed by more specific observations (see Tables 21-2 and 21-3).

Data is recorded as descriptive notes or is summarized on standard forms. Identifying data is entered first: addressograph; birthdate; weight; length; chest, head, and abdominal circumferences; race; sex; mother's and infant's blood type and Rh; Coombs' test results; and time of examination.

The *general appearance* (posture, maturity, activity, tone, cry, color, edema) and *sleep-wake state* (see Table 21-4) are assessed before disturbing the infant. These observations aid in the interpretations of the findings. Each examiner has a preferred pattern for assessment. One pattern is shown in Tables 21-2 and 21-3. Blood pressure (BP) is not assessed routinely. *Heart and respiratory rates* are easiest to assess when the newborn is quiet. Count respirations by observing the chest wall. Note whether the sternum retracts or nares flare and chin lags on inspiration. Note whether the infant is a normal nose breather (i.e., sleeps with mouth closed, does not have to interrupt feedings to breathe). Assess breath sounds. Note abnormal sounds—grunting or wheezing—during inspiration or expiration.

Note the efficiency of the gagging, sneezing, and swallowing reflexes related to maintaining a clear airway.

Watch for bouts of rapid and irregular respirations, gagging, and regurgitation of mucus during "reactivity" periods following birth and after 4 to 6 hours of life.

Assess infant's *color* for cyanosis. Color over head and trunk and mucous membrane is indicative of adequate oxygenation. Feet and hands may remain slightly cyanotic for 48 hours, especially when they are cold.

On admission and each time the *skin* is exposed while giving care, assess the infant's skin for rashes, excoriations (e.g., from fingernails), color (e.g., petechiae, ecchymosis, jaundice, general color, mottling), wounds (e.g., internal fetal monitoring, forceps, scalpel during cesarean birth, circumcision, cord, heel sticks, injections), vernix caseosa, and lanugo. The *temperature* is measured.

Assess the baby's *head:* skin, hair pattern and distribution, molding, fontanels and sutures, size, shape, symmetry, eyes, nose, mouth, ears, and facies. Inspect and palpate the neck. *Chest assessment* includes measuring the chest cir-

Physical Assessment of the Newborn

Antenatal

(1) G ____ P ____
(2) EDD ____
(3) ABO ____ RH ____
(4) TITRE ____
(5) VDRL ____
(6) BR ____ Formula ____

(7) Room ____
(8) PPTL ____
(9) Adoption ____
Comments: ____

Complications

(1) Family history of bleeding ____
(2) Preeclamptic ____
(3) Gestational diabetic ____
(4) Prenatal meds ____
(5) Pertinent history ____

Intranatal

(1) Induction or augmentation
(2) Amniotic fluid
(A) PROM ____ Hrs.
(B) Hydramnios ____
(C) Mec. stained ____ Heavy ____ Light ____ Terminal ____

(3) Monitored ____ ED ____ V ____ LD ____ Baseline ____
(4) Fetal blood sample X ____ Reason ____
(5) Maternal problems ____
(6) Pertinent meds & time ____
(7) Comments ____

Postnatal

(1) Sex—M ____ F ____
(2) Del. date ____
(3) Time ____ AM ____ PM ____
(4) Weight ____ g ____ lb ____ oz
(5) Length ____ cm ____ in
(6) ID Band # ____
(7) Void ____ Stool ____
(8) Eryth. Soln. ____
(9) Cord around neck X 1 2 3
(10) # Vessels 2 3
(11) Method of delivery
(A) Spontaneous
(B) Forceps Mid ____ Low ____
(C) Breech ____
(D) C/B ____ (WHY)
(12) Placenta
(A) Normal ____
(B) Small ____
(C) Abruptio ____ Previa ____
(D) Other ____

Apgar score

Apgar score	0	1	2	1 Min	5 Min
Heart rate	Absent	Less than 100	Over 100		
Resp effort	Absent	Slow irreg	Good cry		
Muscle tone	Limp	Some flexion	Active motion		
Reflex irritability	No response	Grimace	Cry		
Color	Pale	Body pink ext. blue	All pink		
Total score					

(13) Vitamin K ____
(14) Comments ____

Postnatal resuscitation

(1) Pediatrician-notified ____ AM ____ PM ____
—in attendance ____
(2) O_2 ____ Mask ____ Bag ____
(3) Oral suction ____ Mec ____ Mucus ____
(4) Delees suction ____
(5) Intubation—Successful ____
Unsuccessful ____
(A) Suctioned-Clear ____
-Mec. ____ Thick ____ Thin ____
(B) Lavaged ____
(6) Cardiac massage ____
(7) Med and route ____
(8) Comments ____

Nursery

(1) Admit to nsy @ ____ AM ____ PM ____
(2) Admit to: Armstrong ____ Isolette ____ Crib ____
(3) MD notified, i.e. problem/client ____ AM ____ PM ____
(4) Admission v.s.: T ____ P ____ R ____
(5) Est. gest. age ____ Weeks
(6) Color ____
(7) Cry ____
(8) O_2 ____
(9) Suctioned ____
(10) Head ____ Chest ____
(11) Comments ____

____
Signature

Fig. 22-1 Physical assessment of the newborn.

cumference and noting the shape of the thorax, the breasts and nipples, and chest movement with respirations (Figs. 21-3 and 21-4). The shape of the *abdomen* and the condition of the umbilical cord are assessed. Abdominal circumference is measured. Bowel sounds and record of stooling behavior are noted. The newborn's *genitals, urinary meatus,* and *anus* are assessed carefully. The *skeletal system* is also inspected.

Neonatal *reflexes* are assessed. The responses reveal the status of the neuromuscular and skeletal systems. The baby's state-related behaviors (see Table 21-5) and behavioral patterns and sensory capabilities (see Table 21-6) are assessed and documented.

Nursing Diagnoses

Analysis of the significance of findings collected during assessment leads to the establishment of nursing diagnoses. Possible nursing diagnoses *for the newborn* are as follows:

- Ineffective breathing pattern related to
  - Obstructed airway
- Pain related to
  - Circumcision
- Impaired gas exchange related to
  - Hypothermia (cold stress)
- Potential for ineffective thermoregulation related to
  - Heat loss to environment
- Potential for infection related to
  - Environmental factors

Possible nursing diagnoses *for the parent or parents* are as follows:

- Altered parenting related to
  - Knowledge deficit of newborn's social capabilities
  - Knowledge deficit of newborn's dependency needs
- Knowledge deficit related to
  - Biologic and behavioral characteristics of the newborn
- Situational low self esteem related to
  - Misinterpretation of newborn's responses

See the nursing care plan on p. 542.

Planning

Plans for care of the newborn reflect the rapid growth and development during the neonatal period. Changes in biologic and behavioral states are measured in minutes and hours since birth. The neonatal period extends through the first 28 days after birth. By that time the rate of change has slowed enough so that the child's appearance and needs can be referred to in terms of weeks and months.

The focus of care changes between birth and 28 days. During the first 2 hours of life (HOL) the main focus is on the infant's physiologic adaptation. By the end of the neonatal period the infant's socialization needs assume equal importance with physiologic needs.

The care given the neonate during the *first 2 HOL* is part of the care given parents and newborns in the fourth stage of labor (Chapter 20). Care related to *nutritional needs* of infants, including techniques of feeding, is presented in Chapter 23. *Parent-child interactions* are discussed in detail in Chapters 25 and 26.

The information in this section pertains to the maintenance of vital functions, the daily care of infants, and the forms of general therapy carried out routinely in newborn nurseries. Parental education before discharge from the hospital and at the well-baby visit is outlined. An example of an individualized care plan is presented on p 542.

Goals. The goals for newborn care relate to the infant and to the caregiver. The *goals for the infant* include the following:

1. To support the infant's transition from intrauterine to extrauterine life
2. To provide freedom from trauma such as injury and infection
3. To provide opportunities to continue the relationship with the primary caregivers begun in the prenatal period

Goals for the parents include the following:

1. To provide the client with knowledge, skill, and confidence relevant to child care activities
2. To provide opportunities that help parents recognize their knowledge of the infant's behavior begun prenatally
3. To provide opportunities for the parents to reorganize and intensify relationships with their newborn

Implementation

The technical aspects of neonatal care include techniques for health maintenance, detection of disability, and institution of remedial measures. These techniques can be used for teaching purposes. Careful and concise recording of client responses or laboratory results contributes to the continuous supervision vital to mother, newborn, and family.

Protective Environment

The provision of a protective environment is basic to the care of the newborn. The construction, maintenance, and operation of nurseries in accredited hospitals are directed by national professional organizations such as the American Academy of Pediatrics and local or state governing bodies. Detailed information concerning standards of care for newborn nurseries may be obtained from a number of sources (see Appendixes B and K). Prescribed standards cover areas such as the following:

1. *Environmental factors:* provision of adequate lighting, elimination of potential fire hazards, safety of electric appliances, adequate ventilation, controlled temperature (warm and free of drafts) and humidity (lower than 50%).

2. *Measures to control infection:* adequate floor space to permit positioning bassinets at least 60 cm (24 in) apart, hand-washing facilities, techniques for safe formula preparation and storage, and cleaning and sterilizing of equipment and supplies.

In addition, hospital personnel develop their own policies and procedures directed toward protecting the newborns under their care. For instance:

1. Nursery personnel are restricted to those directly involved in the care of mothers and infants, thereby reducing the opportunities for the introduction of pathogenic organisms. In this respect children born at home are at an advantage because they usually come in contact only with family members. This home environment is somewhat duplicated in hospitals when the infant and mother "room together." The mother and father are active in the care, thereby reducing the number of nursing personnel involved. In many hospitals, nurseries are constructed with anterooms. Physicians carry out examinations here and procedures such as circumcisions. Parents may also come here to feed and hold their infants when the newborn must remain in the hospital for care.

2. Personnel assigned to the nursery wear special uniforms or cover gowns, and before beginning the care of infants, they carry out a *hand-washing technique.* In light of the AIDS issue the Centers for Disease Control (CDC) in Atlanta recommends the following practice (NAACOG, 1986): *health care workers must wear gloves when touching mucous membranes or nonintact skin of all patients.* In addition, masks, eye coverings, and gowns must be used when indicated. Health-care personnel *must wear gloves and gowns when handling the infant until blood and amniotic fluid have been removed from the infant's skin, when drawing blood (e.g., heel stick), and when caring for a fresh wound (e.g., circumcision).*

3. Anyone coming from "outside" is expected to gown and *wash her or his hands* before coming in contact with infants or equipment. Such people include nurses, physicians, parents, brother and sisters, department supervisors, electricians, and housekeepers.

4. Individuals with infectious conditions are excluded from contact or must take special precautions when working with newborns; this includes people with upper respiratory tract infections, gastrointestinal tract infections, and infectious skin conditions. Most agencies have now coupled this day-to-day self-screening of personnel with yearly health examinations.

Restraining the Infant

Reasons for restraining an infant include (1) protecting the infant from injury, (2) facilitating examinations, and (3) limiting discomfort during tests, procedures, and specimen collections. When restraining an infant, one must keep in mind special considerations:

1. Check the infant frequently.
2. Apply restraints and check them frequently to prevent skin irritation and circulatory impairment.
3. Maintain proper body alignment.
4. Apply restraints without use of knots or pins if possible. If knots are necessary, make the kind that can be released quickly. Use pins with care to prevent puncture wounds and pressure areas—and to prevent the infant's swallowing one of them.
5. If the child is in an incubator, secure her or him to the mattress to protect the extremities, especially when the lid is raised or the mattress moved.

Mummy Technique. The mummy technique is used with the stronger, more vigorous newborn. It is used during examinations, treatments, or specimen collections that involve the head and neck.

Equipment includes a blanket and one or two large safety pins (Fig. 22-2, *A*).

The procedure is as follows:

1. Spread blanket on flat surface; crib should suffice.
2. Fold over one corner (12 o'clock position).
3. Lay newborn on blanket so that neck is at fold.
4. Fold corner at 9 o'clock position over right shoulder, tuck this corner securely under infant's left side.
5. Bring corner at 6 o'clock position up over feet and tuck it either under infant's left side or, if long enough, fold it over blanket, crossing it under infant's chin.
6. Swing corner of 3 o'clock position snugly over infant and fold under infant's right side. Pin this corner into place.

Extremity Restraints. This type of restraint is used to control movements of the infant's arms or legs. It is used during many procedures, such as intubating or gavage feedings.

Equipment includes gauze strips or wide strips of soft material and cotton wadding; pins are optional.

The procedure depends on which type of extremity restraints is used. Following are examples:

1. *Pad extremity with cotton wadding.* Fold one end of gauze strip over extremity and pin. Pin other end to mattress.
2. *Clove-hitch restraint.* Arrange a long strip of material that is 5 cm (2 in) wide as shown in Fig. 22-2, *B.* Loop device over extremity, which has been padded with cotton; pin loose ends to mattress (Fig. 22-2, *C*). Clove-hitch does not tighten even if infant's movements tug on restraint.

Towel Support. Although the towel support is not a true restraint, it controls the infant's position and movement. The towel may be rolled and placed at the infant's back or sides or folded and placed under the neck or upper back. A towel support has the following advantages:

1. It provides comfort and security by stabilizing the infant's position.
2. It maintains positioning to assist respiratory effort and gastrointestinal functions and prevent skin breakdown.
3. It prevents the infant from rolling against the incubator wall, where the child may lose heat by convection.
4. It prevents the infant from falling out of the incubator when the lid is lifted.

Restraint Without Appliance. The nurse may restrain the infant by using the hands and body. Fig. 22-2, *D,* illustrates restraint of the infant in position for lumbar puncture.

Collection of Specimens

Ongoing evaluation of a newborn requires obtaining blood and urine specimens. The following procedures are used for collecting those specimens: heel stick, p. 513; assisting with venipuncture, p. 514; and collection of urine specimen, p. 515.

Fig. 22-2 **A**, Mummy technique to restrain infant. **B**, Clovehitch device. This restraint does not tighten after its application. Apply padding before applying device. **C**, Clovehitch restraints in place. **D**, Position for lumbar puncture.

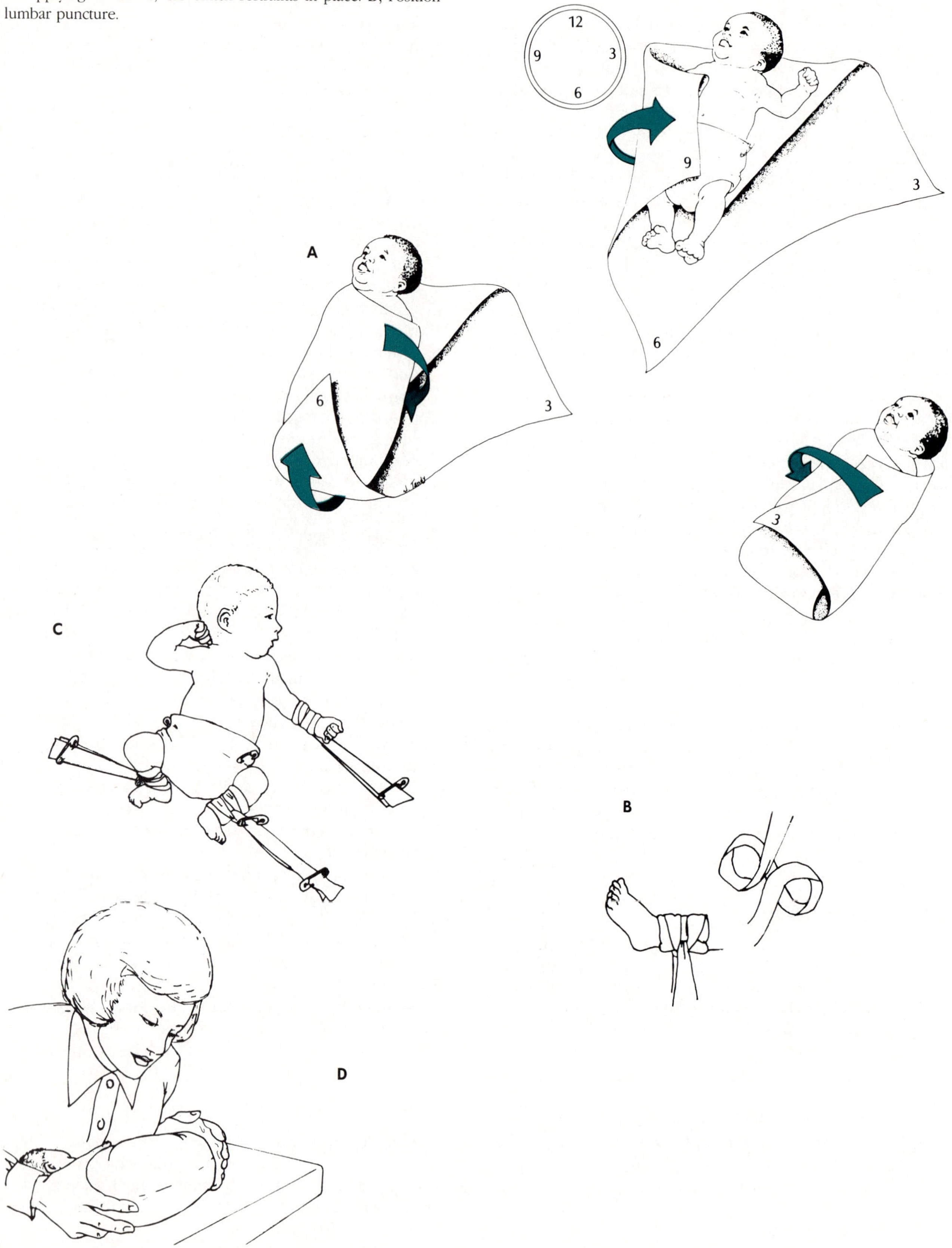

Procedure 22-1

HEEL STICK

DEFINITION

Collection of a capillary sample of blood by puncturing the outer aspect of the infant's heel.

PURPOSE

To obtain blood for the determination of the infant's blood glucose level and hematocrit.

To test for phenylketonuria (PKU), galactosemia, and hypothyroidism.

EQUIPMENT

Bard-Parker Number 11 or Redi-Lance blade; 70% alcohol; sterile cotton pledget or gauze square; capillary tube; plastic bandage; lab slip and label.

NURSING ACTIONS	RATIONALE
Wash hands before and after touching infant and equipment.	To prevent nosocomial infection and implement universal precautions and precautions for invasive procedures.
Apply gloves.	
Identify infant.	To ensure procedure is done on correct infant.
Wrap foot selected for heel stick (Fig. 22-3, *A*).	To increase blood flow to extremity.
Select correct site on heel, (Fig. 22-3, *B*).	To avoid residual scars and corn formation that may result if procedure is not done in proper area of heel.
Cleanse heel by rubbing with 70% alcohol.	To prevent infection.
Dry with sterile cotton pledget or gauze square.	To avoid introduction of contaminants into puncture.
Use blade to puncture heel deep enough to obtain free flow of blood.	To obtain sufficient blood for test.
Discard first drop.	To minimize contamination.
Quickly collect blood in appropriate capillary tubes.	To prevent coagulation of blood.
Cover puncture site with plastic bandage.	To prevent further bleeding and infection.
Send specimen with completed laboratory slip for analysis.	To allow ongoing evaluation and adjustment of care plans.
Record time, site of puncture, infant response.	To ensure communication with other caregivers.
Cuddle and comfort infant when procedure is completed.	To promote feelings of safety.

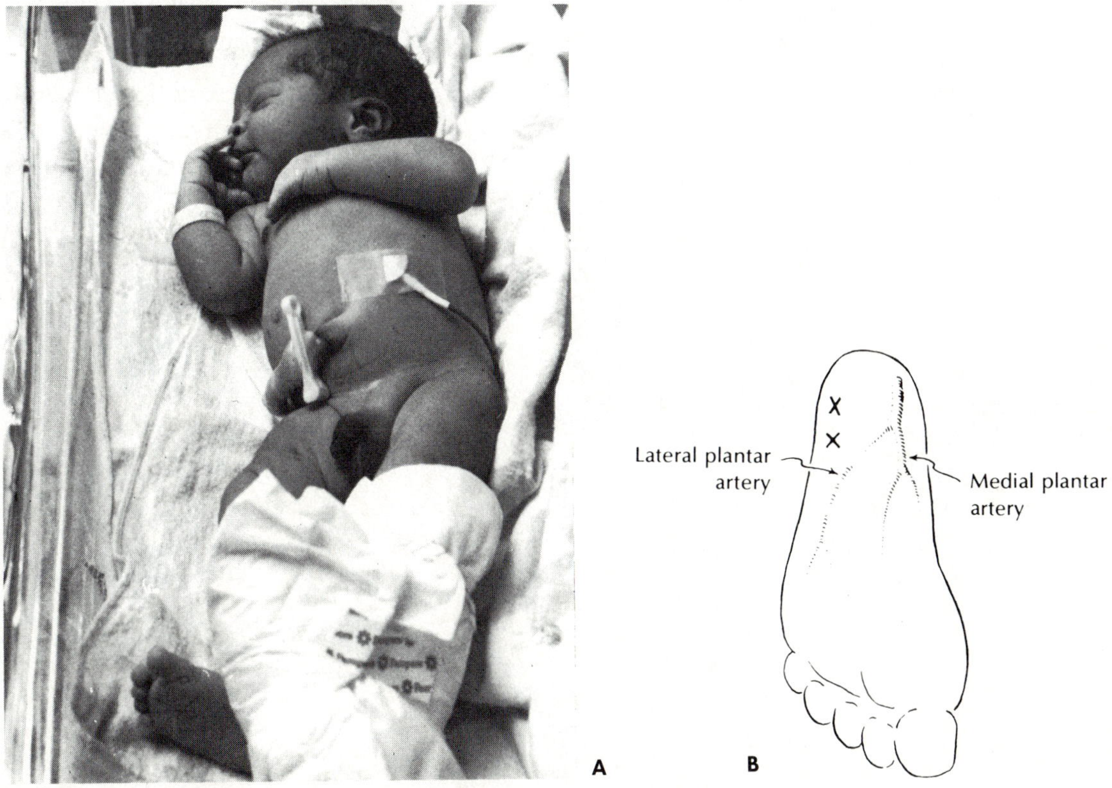

Fig. 22-3 **A**, Newborn with foot wrapped for warmth to increase blood flow to extremity before heel stick. **B**, Puncture sites (x) on sole of infant's foot for heel-stick samples of capillary blood.

Procedure 22-2

ASSISTING WITH VENIPUNCTURE

DEFINITION

Collection of venous blood.

PURPOSE

To obtain sample of venous blood for laboratory analysis.

EQUIPMENT

Restraint blanket; sterile syringe and needles; labeled specimen tubes; laboratory slips; sterile alcohol wipes.

NURSING ACTIONS	RATIONALE
Wash hands before and after touching infant and equipment.	To prevent nosocomial infection and implement universal precautions and precautions for invasive procedures.
Identify infant.	To ensure procedure is done on correct infant.
For *external jugular venipuncture:* "Mummy" the infant as necessary. Lower the infant's head over rolled towel, edge of table, or your knee, and stabilize.	To ensure safety and expose insertion site.
For *femoral venipuncture:* Position the infant in frog posture. Place hands over infant's knees. Avoid pressure of fingers over inner aspect of thigh.	To ensure safety and expose insertion site. To prevent occlusion of vein in this area.
Handle the infant gently and talk quietly to her or him during the procedure.	
When procedure is completed, apply pressure over the area with sterile gauze for 1 to 3 minutes.	To prevent leakage of additional blood into tissues or formation of hematoma, which may result in hyperbilirubinemia when the trapped RBCs break down.
Observe infant for 1 hour.	To detect further bleeding (oozing, hematoma). Any enclosed bleeding could lead to hypovolemic shock, hyperbilirubinemia, or both.
Send specimen with completed laboratory slip for analysis.	To allow ongoing evaluation and adjustment of care plans.
Record time, site of puncture, amount of blood taken, reason for specimen, and infant's response.	To ensure communication with other caregivers.
Cuddle and comfort infant when procedure is completed.	To promote feelings of safety.

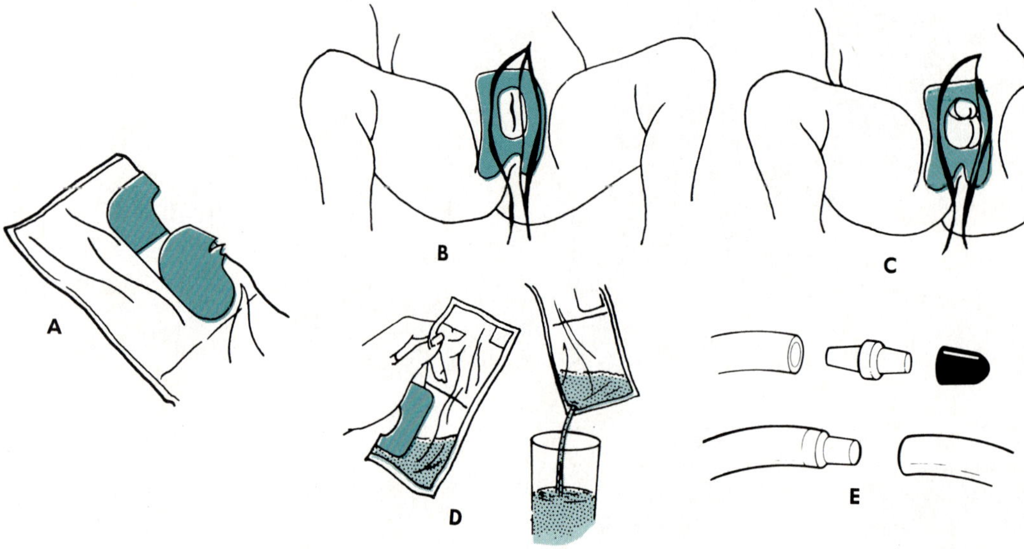

Fig. 22-4 Hollister U-Bag (see Procedure 22-3). Courtesy Hollister, Inc, Chicago.

Procedure 22-3

OBTAINING URINE SPECIMEN

DEFINITION

Collection of urine from infant.

PURPOSE

To obtain urine specimen for analysis.

EQUIPMENT

A variety of urine collection bags are available, including the Hollister U-Bag.

NURSING ACTIONS	RATIONALE
Wash hands before and after touching infant or equipment	To prevent nosocomial infection and to implement universal precautions.
Identify infant.	To ensure procedure is done on correct infant.
Separate infant's legs. Make sure pubic and perineal area is clean, dry, and free of mucus. Do not apply powders, oils, or lotions to skin.	To ensure leak-proof seal. To decrease chance of contamination.
Remove protective paper, exposing hypoallergenic adhesive (Fig. 22-4, *A*).	To expose adhesive and decrease chance of allergic reaction.
For girls, stretch perineum to flatten skin folds. Press adhesive firmly to skin all around urinary meatus and vagina. (NOTE: start with narrow portion of butterfly-shaped adhesive patch.) *Be sure to start at bridge of skin separating rectum from vagina and work upward* (Fig. 22-4, *B*).	To ensure leak-proof seal. To decrease chance of contamination from urine and stool.
For boys, tuck penis and scrotum through aperture of collector before removing protective paper from adhesive. Fit bag over penis, and press flaps firmly to perineum, making sure entire adhesive coating is firmly attached to skin with no puckering of adhesive (Fig. 22-4, *C*).	To ensure leak-proof seal.
To drain, hold bag in left hand. Tilt bag so urine is away from tab. Remove tab and drain into clean receptacle (Fig. 22-4, *D*).	To facilitate emptying without use of scissors, which can contaminate or be contaminated.
OR	
Apply the 24-hour U-Bag in the manner just described and: Direct the drainage into a receptacle. The collection tube can be shortened or capped (Fig. 22-4, *E*).	
See directions accompanying the bag.	
Send specimen with completed laboratory slip for analysis.	To allow ongoing evaluation.
Record time, reason for specimen.	To ensure communication with other caregivers.

Maintenance of an Adequate Oxygen Supply

Four conditions are essential for maintenance of an adequate oxygen supply:

1. A clear airway, fundamental to adequate ventilation
2. Respiratory efforts, necessary to ensure continued ventilation
3. A functioning cardiopulmonary system, essential to maintain oxygen
4. Heat support, necessary because exposure to cold stress increases oxygen needs

Maintenance of Clear Airway. Generally the normal full-term infant born vaginally has little difficulty clearing the air passages. Most secretions are drained by gravity, propelled to the oropharynx by the cough reflex, to be drained or swallowed. The infant is maintained in a side-lying position with a rolled blanket at the back to facilitate drainage (Fig. 22-5). If excessive mucus is present, the foot

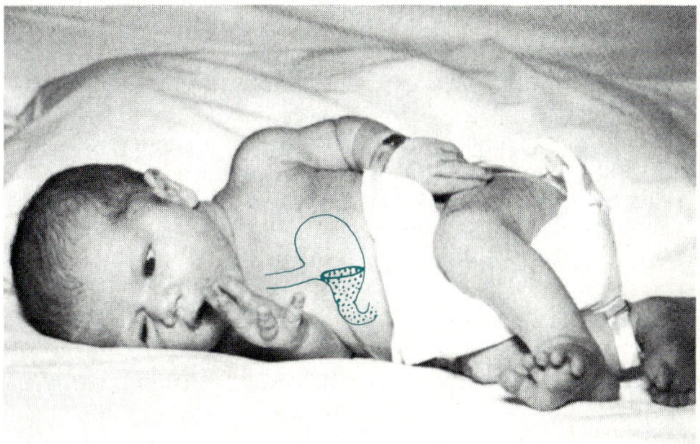

Fig. 22-5 Infant is turned to right side and supported in this position to facilitate drainage from mouth.

of the crib is elevated and the oropharynx is suctioned with a bulb syringe (Fig. 22-6) or a DeLee mucus-trap catheter (Fig. 22-7). The nurse's knowledge and skill in suctioning may be critical in helping both normal and distressed infants establish or maintain adequate respirations. "Milking" the trachea is ineffective. This procedure may injure cartilage and will often delay effective suctioning.

Relieving Airway Obstruction. A choking infant is placed face down over the rescuer's arm with the head lower than the trunk and the head supported (Fig. 22-8, Whaley and Wong, 1987). Additional support can be achieved if the rescuer supports own arm firmly against own thigh (Committee on Accidents and Poison Prevention, 1986). Four quick, sharp back blows are delivered between the infant's shoulder blades with the heel of the rescuer's hand. Less force is required than would be applied to an adult. After delivery of the back blows, the rescuer's free hand is placed flat on the infant's back so that the infant is "sandwiched" between the two hands, with the neck and chin well supported. While the rescuer maintains support with the infant's head lower than the trunk, the infant is turned and placed supine on the rescuer's thigh, where four chest thrusts are applied in rapid succession in the same manner as external chest compressions described for CPR (see Fig. 22-9 and emergency procedure p. 520).

Maintenance of Respiratory Efforts. The normal term infant establishes respirations within minutes of birth, usually without undue difficulty. However, nursery personnel need to be skilled in the techniques for reestablishing respirations and providing increased oxygen in case the need arises (see danger signs box, p. 517). A humidified oxygen source and equipment for the administration of oxygen must be readily available.

Procedure 22-4

SUCTIONING OF UPPER AIRWAY: ASPIRATION OF MOUTH AND NOSE (Fig. 22-6, *A-C*)

DEFINITION

Use of a blunt-tipped, flexible rubber syringe for removal of secretions from mouth and nose.

PURPOSE

To remove mucus from mouth and nose.

EQUIPMENT

Sterile bulb syringe (intact and fairly firm).

NURSING ACTIONS	RATIONALE
Wash hands before and after touching baby and equipment.	To prevent nosocomial infection and to implement universal precautions.
Position infant:	
Support the wrapped infant on the arm or on the hip (in a football hold), positioning the child's head downward.	To assist gravity drainage.
NOTE: *Never* suspend infant by ankles in head-down position	To avoid raising cerebral venous pressure, increasing the risk of accidently dropping the infant, hyperextending and stretching the spine, and causing pain to the baby.
Suction mouth first.	To avoid stimulation of sensitive receptors around the nares that respond to stimuli by initiating gasp. Any mucus present could be pulled into lower airway.
NOTE: Compress the bulb *before* insertion, expelling air (Fig. 22-6, A).	To prevent blowing secretions deeper into mouth and nose.
Insert syringe into space between cheek and gums, release compression gradually, and create suction (to suck out mucus).	To prevent tissue trauma and remove secretions.
Remove syringe from mouth. Compress syringe to empty it and to create new vacuum to repeat procedure.	To prevent secretions from being forced into respiratory tract.
Repeat these last two steps as needed in mouth, then in nose. Stop suctioning when cry is clear (infant cry does not sound as though there were mucus or a bubble in the mouth).	To assess for patent airway. If cry is clear, infant's airway is patent.
Cuddle and reassure infant once episode is over.	To comfort infant since discomfort and fear and subsequent crying increases need for oxygen.
Demonstrate care of gagging or choking infant to parents.	To teach procedure since learning to meet this emergency in the hospital increases parental self-confidence and self-esteem and prepares parents for this activity at home.
Supervise parents in this technique.	To permit correction of any parental errors.

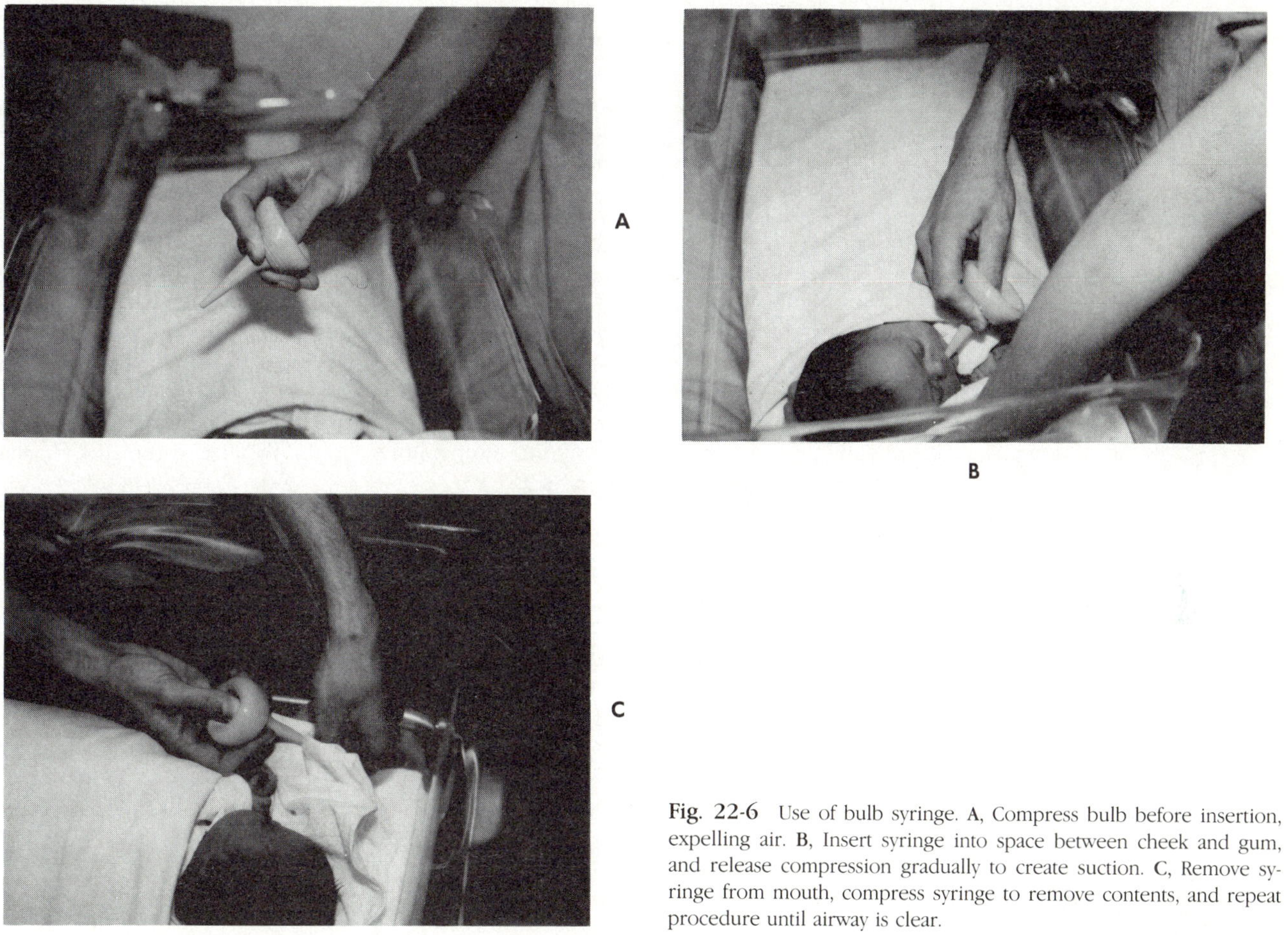

Fig. 22-6 Use of bulb syringe. **A**, Compress bulb before insertion, expelling air. **B**, Insert syringe into space between cheek and gum, and release compression gradually to create suction. **C**, Remove syringe from mouth, compress syringe to remove contents, and repeat procedure until airway is clear.

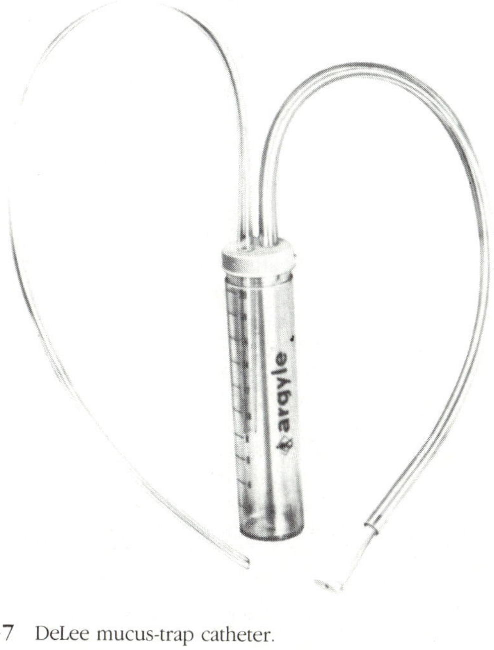

Fig. 22-7 DeLee mucus-trap catheter.

DANGER SIGNS

Abnormal Newborn Breathing

1. Bradypnea—respirations $\leq$ 25 per min
2. Tachypnea—respirations $\geq$ 60 per min
3. Abnormal breath sounds—rales, rhonchi, wheezes, expiratory grunt
4. Respiratory distress—nasal flaring, retractions, chin tug, labored breathing

Maintenance of Cardiopulmonary Function. Cardiac arrest can occur in term newborns who have experienced stress. Careful monitoring of infants is essential if treatment is to be instituted rapidly.

Cardiopulmonary Resuscitation. Complete apnea signals the need for rapid and vigorous action to maintain cardiac function. The nurse must be alert and ready to initiate immediate action. The newborn's prompt response is necessary for intact neurologic survival. The actions in the emergency procedure on p. 520 are based on standards and guidelines for cardiopulmonary resuscitation (CPR)

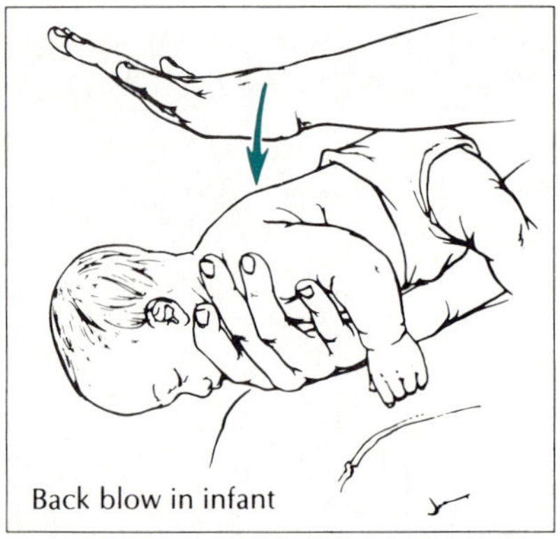

Fig. 22-8 Back blow in infant for clearing airway obstruction.
From Standards for Cardiopulmonary Resuscitation (CPR) and Emergency Cardiac Care (ECC): Part IV. Pediatric basic life support, JAMA 225 (21):2954, 1986.

and emergency cardiac care published by the American Medical Association in Nursing '87 Books (1987) and Standards for Cardiopulmonary Resuscitation (CPR) and Emergency Cardiac Care (ECC) (1986). Emergency procedures for mouth-to-mouth resuscitation, p. 522, and abnormal newborn breathing, p. 523, are also provided.

Heat Support. During all procedures heat loss must be avoided or minimized for the infant. Placing the infant in a warmed Kreisselmann or comparable crib or under overhead radiant heat or another source of heat will accomplish this. Cold stress is detrimental to the newborn. It increases the need for oxygen and can upset the acid/base balance. The temperature may be taken either by axilla or rectum every hour until stabilized (Fig. 21-16). Initial temperatures as low as 36° C (96.8° F) are not uncommon. By the twelfth hour the temperature should stabilize within the normal

Text continued on p. 523.

Procedure 22-5

SUCTIONING OF MIDAIRWAY (NASOPHARYNX AND OROPHARYNX) AND STOMACH ASPIRATION USING THE DeLee MUCUS TRAP (Fig. 22-7)

DEFINITION

Use of a mucus-trap catheter for removal of secretions.

PURPOSE

To remove mucus or meconium from the nasopharynx and oropharynx.
To remove amniotic fluid from the stomach.

EQUIPMENT

Sterile DeLee mucus-trap catheter (available in reusable glass or disposable plastic) with two-hole tip.
Sterile water. A 120 ml (4 oz) bottle of sterile water for feeding is convenient, already in a sterile container, and decreases risk of contamination possible with large stock bottles.

NURSING ACTIONS	RATIONALE
Wash hands before and after touching baby and equipment. Apply gloves.	To prevent nosocomial infection and to implememt universal precautions, and precautions for intrusive procedures.
Place infant in supine position.	To facilitate suctioning.
Lubricate catheter in sterile water.	To facilitate passage of tube and prevent infection.
Aspirate mouth and throat first, then the nose.	To prevent infant's inhalation of pharyngeal secretions.
Insert catheter:	To decrease risk of laryngeal spasm and reflex.
Orally along base of tongue.	
Nasally horizontally into nares, then raising it to advance it beyond bend at back of nares.	
Avoid forcing catheter.	**Hazard:** To prevent direct tissue trauma or perforation in presence of congenital anomalies such as choanal, esophageal, or intestinal atresia.
Suction is applied by user.	To provide sufficient negative pressure to withdraw mucus or other substances.
Limit suctioning to 10 times or less.	To avoid prolonged suctioning that stimulates laryngospasm and reduces oxygen (0_2) content in airway.
Apply suction only as tube is withdrawn.	To prevent direct tissue trauma.
Rotate catheter when suctioning.	To prevent tissue trauma consequent to tissue's being drawn into eye of catheter.
Discontinue suctioning when:	To pass the catheter correctly: Gagging indicates entrance into esophagus; coughing indicates entrance into trachea.
The cry is clear.	
Air entry into lungs is heard by stethoscope.	
Cuddle infant.	To reassure infant.
Detach mucus trap and send the enclosed specimen to the laboratory for examination and culture as necessary.	To allow ongoing evaluation of infant's condition.
Record the amount of mucus or amniotic fluid removed.	To ensure communication with other caregivers.

Procedure 22-6

SUCTIONING OF MIDAIRWAY (NASOPHARYNX AND OROPHARYNX) USING A NASOPHARYNGEAL CATHETER WITH MECHANICAL SUCTION APPARATUS

DEFINITION

Use of mechanical suction apparatus and external suction source for removal of secretions.

PURPOSE

To remove excessive or tenacious mucus from the nasopharynx and oropharynx in resuscitating an infant.

EQUIPMENT

Catheters:

French, rubber (moderately firm); sizes 10, 12, and 14; whistle tip; two-hole tip French; plastic disposable: sizes 8, 10, and 12; finger control; two-hole tip.

External suction source.

Sterile water. A 120 m1 (4 oz) bottle of sterile water for feeding is convenient, is already in sterile container, and reduces risk of contamination possible with large stock bottles.

NURSING ACTIONS	RATIONALE
Wash hands before and after touching baby and equipment. Glove.	To prevent nosocomial infection and to implement universal precautions.
Position the infant: Place the infant in supine position. Place a folded towel under the head to move it slightly forward from the neck (as in sniffing).	To (1) separate tongue from pharyngeal wall and (2) to prevent obstruction of newborn's normally low palate and macroglossia. (Some physicians prefer to work with the baby on a flat surface with no towel.)
Adjust negative pressure on portable or wall gauges.	To prevent excessive suctioning.
Keep deep suctioning to a minimum.	**Hazard:** To prevent direct trauma to mucosa with edema formation, bleeding, or increased secretions. To prevent stimulation of vagal reflex: bradycardia, cardiac arhythmias, laryngospasm, and apnea, especially if this type of suctioning is done within a few minutes of infant's birth.
Limit each suctioning to 10 seconds or less.	To prevent laryngospasm and oxygen depletion.
If infant is active, an attendant may be needed to stabilize infant's head. Or if there is time, restrain infant by mummy technique before this procedure.	To prevent trauma and facilitate suctioning. Both hands are needed to manipulate catheter and finger control of suction pressure.
Lubricate catheter in sterile water.	To facilitate passage of tube and prevent infection.
Turn suction **off** as tube is put into position.	To prevent direct tissue trauma.
Avoid forcing catheter.	**Hazard:** To prevent direct tissue trauma or perforation in presence of congenital anomalies such as choanal, esophageal, or intestinal atresia.
Insert catheter: Orally along base of tongue. Nasally horizontally into nares, then raising it to advance it beyond bend at back of nares.	To decrease risk of laryngeal spasm and reflex apnea.
With catheter in place, put thumb over finger control to create suction. Rotate tubing between fingers while withdrawing catheter.	To prevent direct trauma caused by drawing mucosa into eye of catheter.
Apply suction only as tube is withdrawn.	To prevent direct tissue trauma.
Rotate catheter when suctioning.	To prevent tissue trauma consequent to tissues being drawn into eye of catheter.
Observe infant's response. Withdraw tube to suction posterior nasopharynx.	To prevent gagging, which indicates entrance into esophagus; coughing indicates entrance into trachea.
Comfort infant.	To prompt feelings of safety.
Record procedure.	To ensure communication with other caregivers.

EMERGENCY PROCEDURE

CARDIOPULMONARY RESUSCITATION (CPR) (Fig. 22-9)

DEFINITION

A basic emergency procedure for life support consisting of artificial respiration and manual external cardiac massage.

PURPOSE

To prevent cardiac arrest following cessation of respirations (apnea extending beyond 15 sec).
To restore cardiac function.
To restore respiratory function.

EQUIPMENT

Resuscitation equipment should be readily available in areas in which respiratory arrest might take place, and the status of this equipment should be checked regularly, at least once a day.

NURSING ACTIONS	RATIONALE
Wash hands before and after touching infant and equipment. Glove.	To prevent nosocomial infection and to implement universal precautions.
Resuscitation	
Observe color; tap, or gently shake shoulders.	To determine unresponsiveness or respiratory difficulty.
Yell for help; if alone, perform CPR for 1 min before calling for help again.	To bring help.
Turn infant to back, supporting head and neck	To protect neck.
Place on firm, flat surface.	To support infant's spine; prevents injury during compression of sternum.
Clear airway, prn (see below).	To provide unobstructed ventilation.
Tilt head back gently to "sniffing" or neutral position; use head-tilt/chin-lift maneuver (Fig. 22-9, *A*).	To open airway.
Do not hyperextend neck.	To prevent kinking of airway.
Assess for evidence of breathing:	To avoid unnecessary intervention.
Observe for chest movement.	
Listen for exhaled air.	
Feel for exhaled air flow.	
Breathe for infant (Fig. 22-9, *B*):	To assist ventilation.
Take a breath.	
Open mouth wide and place over mouth and nose of infant to create seal. (See emergency procedure, mouth-to-mouth resuscitation, p. 522).	To provide mouth-to-mouth and mouth-to-nose resuscitation.
NOTE: Repeat the word *ho* as you gently puff volume of air *in your* cheeks into infant. *Do not* force air.	To permit insufflation under pressure. To reduce risk of gastric distension, regurgitation, and subsequent aspiration.
Infant's chest should rise slightly with each puff; keep fingers on chest wall to sense air entry.	
Give two slow breaths (1.0 to 1.5 seconds per breath) pausing to inhale between breaths.	
Check pulse of brachial artery (Fig. 22-9, *C*) while maintaining head tilt.	To determine need for intervention.
If pulse is present, initiate rescue breathing. Continue until spontaneous breathing resumes at rate of every 3 seconds or 20 times per minute.	To avoid unnecessary intervention.
If pulse is not present, initiate chest compressions and coordinate with breathing.	To restore cardiac function.
NOTE: When two people are present, breathing and compressions are shared.	To prevent fatigue!
Provide compressions/breathing:	To coordinate compressions/breathing.
Pause at end of every fifth compression to allow chest to fall by passive recoil.	To allow removal of insufflated air.
Maintain 5:1 ratio for 1 or 2 rescuers.	To maintain arterial Po_2 level.
Reassess after 10 cycles, and every few minutes thereafter.	

EMERGENCY PROCEDURE—cont'd

NURSING ACTIONS	RATIONALE
Chest compressions:	
Maintain head tilt. With other hand, position fingers for chest compressions.	To restore cardiac function.
Place index finger of hand farthest from infant's head just under imaginary line drawn between nipples (Fig. 22-9, *D*).	
Move index finger to a position one fingerbreadth below this intersection.	To identify compression area.
Using 2 or 3 fingers, compress sternum to depth of ½ or ¾ inch.	To minimize the chance of damage that might occur to the liver or spleen.
Release pressure without moving fingers from the position.	
Repeat at a rate of at least 100 times per minute; 5 compressions in 3 seconds or less.	To approximate normal neonatal rate.
Perform 10 cycles of 5 compressions and 1 ventilation. (If possible, compressions are accompanied by positive-pressure ventilation at a rate of 40 to 60 per minute). Use this mnemonic: one-two-three-four-five-pause-head tilt-chin lift-ventilate- continue compressions. After cycles, check the brachial pulse to determine pulselessness (Nursing '87 Books).	To assist recall of correct ratio and timing.
Discontinue compressions if the infant's spontaneous heart rate reaches or exceeds 80 beats per minute (Hazinski, 1987).	To prevent disrupting cardiac rhythm that has resumed.
Relieving airway obstruction	
Use no blind finger sweeps.	To avoid pushing obstruction deeper.
Initiate back blows and chest thrusts (Fig. 22-8).	**Hazard:** To avoid the risk of injury to abdominal organs, Heimlich maneuver (abdominal thrusts) should not be used for infants of 1 year of age or less.
Position child prone over forearm with head down and with infant's jaw firmly supported.	To employ gravity to help remove obstruction.
Rest supporting arm on thigh.	To prevent rescuer's fatigue.
Deliver four back blows forcefully between infant's shoulder blades with heel of free hand.	To move obstructive materials outward.
Place free hand on infant's back to sandwich her/him between both hands: one hand supports the neck, jaw, and chest; the other supports the back.	To avoid injury to infant while turning infant.
Turn infant over and place head down, supporting head and neck. Apply four chest thrusts to same location as chest compressions but use a slower rate.	To force obstruction outward.
Open the airway with a head-tilt chin-lift maneuver and attempt to ventilate.	To ventilate infant.
Repeat the sequence until it is effective.	
ALTERNATIVE POSITION: Place infant face down on your lap with head lower than trunk and head firmly supported. Apply back blows, turn infant, and apply chest thrusts as above.	To employ gravity to remove obstruction.
Continue emergency procedures until signs of recovery occur, as indicated by palpable peripheral pulses, return of pupils to normal size and responsiveness, and the disappearance of mottling and cyanosis.	To continue ventilation. To meet standards of care.
Record time and duration of procedure and effects of intervention.	To ensure communication with other caregivers.
Teach procedure to parents or other caregivers.	To increase parents' knowledge and skill in self-care measure.

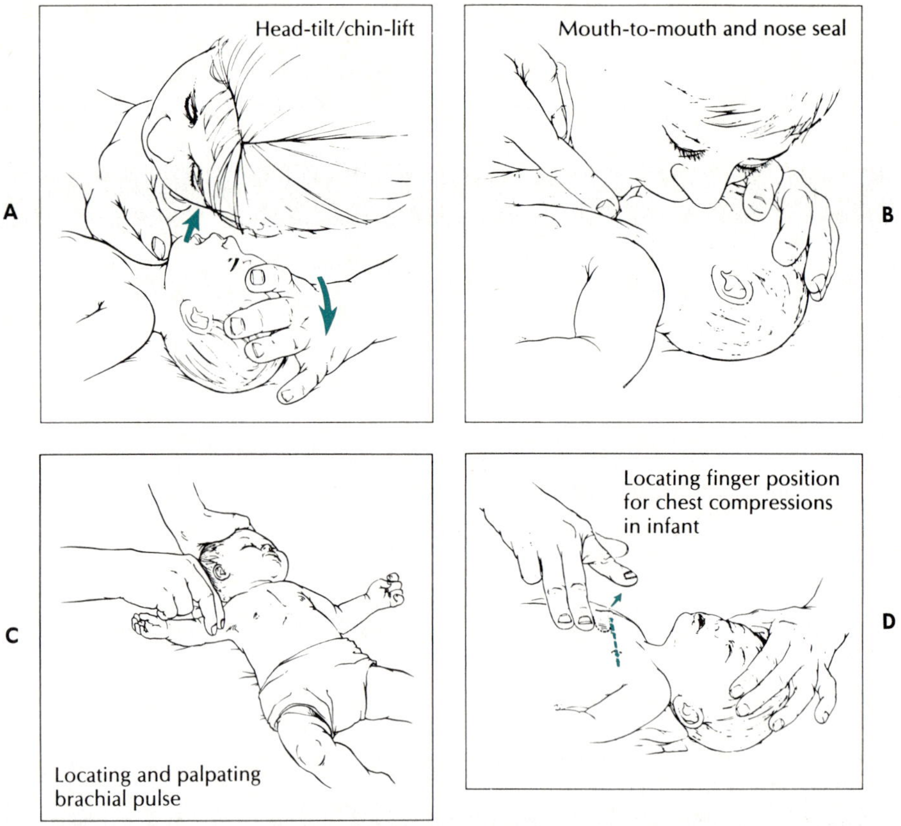

Fig. 22-9 Procedures for cardiopulmonary resuscitation.
From Standards for Cardiopulmonary Resuscitation (CPR) and Emergency Cardiac Care (ECC): Part IV. Pediatric basic life support, JAMA 225 (21):2954, 1986.

EMERGENCY PROCEDURE

MOUTH-TO-MOUTH AND MOUTH-TO-NOSE RESUSCITATION

DEFINITION

Artificial resuscitation performed when respirations have ceased.

PURPOSE

To reestablish respiration.

EQUIPMENT

None needed. If available: rolled towel, plastic airway, oxygen, suction.

NURSING ACTIONS	RATIONALE
Wash hands before and after touching infant and equipment. Glove.	To prevent nosocomial infection and to implement universal precautions.
Clear airway of any mucus or debris.	To prevent blowing debris down airway.
Position infant in "sniffing" position by putting rolled towel under head to move it slightly forward from neck, or leave infant on flat surface.	To open airway by straightening trachea and permitting back of tongue to fall away from posterior pharynx.
Insert plastic airway if available.	To provide unobstructed airway (especially from tongue if infant is flaccid).
Place your mouth over infant's nose and mouth to create seal.	To permit insufflation under pressure.
Repeat the word *ho* as you gently *puff* volume of air *in your cheeks* into infant. *Do not* force air.	To prevent injury to lung tissue (e.g., pneumothorax, pneumomediastinum).
Repeat puffs at rate of 30/per min.	To approximate normal respiratory rate.
Infant's chest should rise slightly with each puff; keep fingers on chest wall to sense air entry.	To determine if air is reaching alveolar level.
Allow chest to fall by passive recoil.	To allow removal of insufflated air.
If available, place tubing of oxygen in your mouth as you inhale quickly between puffs.	To increase O_2 content in insufflated air.
Consider airway obstruction. Prepare for laryngoscopy and endotracheal intubation aspiration. See your hospital procedure manual.	To assess for obstruction; note if chest wall does not rise and the infant's vital responses do not improve in 30 sec.
Record procedure.	To ensure communication with other caregivers.

EMERGENCY PROCEDURE

ABNORMAL NEWBORN BREATHING

DEFINITION

The assessment and treatment of abnormal or difficult breathing patterns in the newborn infant.

PURPOSE

To recognize difficult respiratory effort in the newborn.
To clear mucus and secretion from infant's airway.
To resuscitate infant if respirations have stopped.
To prevent cardiac arrest.
To provide more available oxygen to the infant.

EQUIPMENT

Bulb syringe, sterile DeLee catheter, oxygen source, stethoscope, external suction source, sterile water.

NURSING ACTIONS	RATIONALE
Wash hands before and after touching newborn or equipment.	To prevent nosocomial infection and implement universal precautions.
Assess infant's skin color.	*To identify abnormal newborn breathing:* pallor and cyanosis signal poor tissue perfusion.
Observe infant's respiratory effort.	Flaring of the nares and expiratory grunt are early signs of respiratory distress.
Watch for retractions: subcostal, xiphoid, intercostal, suprasternal, or clavicular.	Infant is using secondary muscles to breathe; using maximum effort to overcome respiratory distress.
Listen to respirations and lung sounds with a stethoscope.	Rales, rhonchi, and wheezes can be heard if they are present.
Position infant with head down.	To allow for gravity drainage.
If lung sounds are clear, use a bulb syringe to clear mouth and nose of secretions. (See Procedure 22-4.)	*To identify obstruction:* When lung sounds are clear, obstruction may be in nares or mouth.
When bulb syringe doesn't work, employ a DeLee mucus-trap catheter to clear midairway (see Procedure 22-5) or a mechanical suction apparatus (see Procedure 22-6).	Mucus may be obstructing nasopharynx and oropharynx. *To apply suction:* Mechanical suction apparatus may be more easily available than a DeLee mucus-trap catheter.
If respirations have ceased, start mouth-to-mouth resuscitation after suctioning is complete. (See emergency procedure: mouth-to-mouth resuscitation, p. 522).	To prevent pushing mucus and debris farther down the airway.
When respirations are reestablished and fairly regular, start oxygen therapy.	To increase level of available oxygen to the infant to aid tissue perfusion.

range. The nurse can help stabilize the infant's body temperature in one of the following ways:

1. Check the temperature in the nursery. (The ambient temperature of the nursery unit should be 24° C [75° F].)
2. Keep the baby dry and wrapped in warmed blankets, taking care to keep the head well covered while the parent is holding the infant. (Check the baby's body temperature at least every hour until it is stabilized; this also helps prevent hyperthermia.)
3. Place the thoroughly dried, unclothed baby under a radiant heat panel until the body temperature is stabilized (Procedure 22-7).
4. Perform examinations or other activities with the baby under a heat panel and postpone the initial bath until the newborn's skin temperature reaches 36.5° C (97.6° F) or core temperature is within the normal range. Minimize the heat loss.

Warming Infant with Hypothermia. Even a normal full-term baby in good health can become hypothermic. Birth in a car on the way to the hospital, a cold delivery room, or inadequate drying and wrapping immediately after birth may cause the infant's temperature to fall. Warming the hypothermic baby is accomplished with care. Rapid warming or cooling may cause apneic spells and acidosis in an infant. Therefore the warming process is monitored to progress slowly over a period of 2 to 4 hours (Procedure 22-8).

Certain techniques, such as administering vitamin K intramuscularly, are routine in newborn nurseries (Procedure 22-9). Others, such as the therapy for treatment of hyperbilirubinemia and circumcision, are performed frequently. Nurses must become skilled in the use of therapies to ensure infant safety and therapeutic effectiveness. Parents expect to be told the reasons for the particular therapy and what results to expect.

Procedure 22-7

WARMING INFANT USING SERVO-CONTROL INCUBATOR

DEFINITION

Use of infant's skin temperature, rather than circulating air to provide point of control.

PURPOSE

To maintain or restore infant's body temperature if it has not returned to normal within 2 hours using a radiant overhead heater.

EQUIPMENT

Servo-Control incubators or their equivalents employ the same principle as the thermostat in maintaining an even temperature in an oven or a room.

NURSING ACTIONS	RATIONALE
Wash hands before and after touching infant and equipment. Glove, prn.	To prevent nosocomial infection and to implement universal precautions.
Set the incubator control panel at the predetermined physician-ordered level, usually between 36° and 37° C (96.8° and 98.6° F).	To maintain a skin temperature of 36.5° C (97.6° F)
Tape a thermistor probe (automatic sensor) from the control panel to the right upper quadrant of the abdomen immediately below the right intracostal margin, never over a bone.	To ensure detection of even minor changes resulting from peripheral vasoconstriction, dilation, or increased metabolism long before a change in deep (core) body temperature develops.
Check the sensor periodically for its continued firm application to skin; check and record the core temperature with a clinical thermometer; record incubator temperature readings.	To ensure proper functioning of the equipment.
Record skin temperature reading and ambient temperature inside the incubator every 2 to 4 hours after the infant's temperature is stabilized.	To help in assessing the maintenance of adequate body temperature.
Record the infant's general appearance and behavior.	To ensure communication with other health care workers.

Procedure 22-8

WARMING INFANT USING OVERHEAD RADIANT HEATER

DEFINITION

Use of an overhead radiant heat source to prevent cold stress in an infant.

PURPOSE

To maintain or restore infant's body temperature.

EQUIPMENT

Overhead radiant heater. The heater thermostat must be kept plugged into an electrical outlet at all times. It is set to maintain an abdominal skin temperature of 36.5° C (97.6° F). The set point of 36.4° C (97.5° F) is usually chosen for activation of the heater. A probe may be attached to the infant's skin by a heat-deflector sticker.

NURSING ACTIONS	RATIONALE
Wash hands before and after touching infant and equipment. Glove, prn.	To prevent nosocomial infection and to implement universal precautions.
Turn radiant heater on.	To allow a few minutes for heater to warm up.
With warm, absorbent blanket, dry and place newborn under radiant heat shield.	To reduce heat loss by evaporation, conduction, convection, and radiation.
Adjust bassinet in head-down position (about 10 degrees).	To allow for gravity drainage of mucus in respiratory tract. If infant is suspected of having intracranial hemorrhage, keep head on same level as body or slightly elevated if mucus is not excessive.
Remove gross soiling (e.g., meconium, blood).	To facilitate observation of skin coloring and any changes.
Check thermostat setting for accuracy.	To prevent overheating or underheating.
Apply thermistor probe (metal side next to the infant) with paper tape or nonirritating plastic tape to anterior ab-	To improve accuracy of skin temperature reading. Sensors respond more quickly to change.

Procedure 22-8—cont'd

NURSING ACTIONS	RATIONALE
dominal wall between navel and ziphoid process; do not place over bony rib cage. Thermistor, after it is taped to abdominal wall, must be covered by small plastic-foam square insulator. Optimumly, it has a cover of aluminum foil.	To provide foam insulation to thermistor. To prevent warming thermistor more quickly than baby is warmed (mechanism would respond to heated probe rather than to warmed baby).
Check frequently to ensure that probe retains skin contact.	To prevent overheating or underheating.
Observe infant for color change; crying and restlessness; increased respiratory rate.	To determine if abnormal behavior is caused by cold stress or other factors (e.g., debility, sepsis).
Note previous symptoms; recheck probe, thermostat setting, and heater contact.	Rules out equipment malfunction.
Record findings. Note time and duration of procedure.	To ensure communication with other health care workers.

Procedure 22-9

INTRAMUSCULAR INJECTION

DEFINITION

Placement of medication within muscle tissue.

PURPOSE

To administer medication to the newborn.

EQUIPMENT

Syringe and needle, alcohol swab, medication, bandage.

NURSING ACTIONS	RATIONALE
Wash hands before and after touching infant and equipment. Glove, prn.	To prevent nosocomial infections and to implement universal precautions.
Recheck physician's order. Identify infant.	To ensure procedure is done on correct infant.
Restrain infant if necessary.	Newborn infants offer little, if any resistance to injections. Although they squirm and may be difficult to hold in position if they are awake, they can usually be restrained without assistance from a second person if the nurse is skilled.
Use filter needle to withdraw medication. Replace filter needle with short, small-gauge tuberculin needle.	To avoid drawing small glass shards into the syringe, which could cause injury to the infant.
Select site for injection. NOTE: The posterior gluteal muscle is very small, poorly developed, and dangerously close to the sciatic nerve, which occupies a larger proportion of space in infants than in older children. Therefore it is not recommended as an injection site until the child has been walking for at least one year.	Selection of the site for injection is important. Injections must be placed in muscles large enough to accommodate the medication, yet major nerves and blood vessels must be avoided. The muscles of newborns may not tolerate more than 0.5 ml. The preferred site for newborns is the vastus lateralis (Fig. 22-10, *A*), although the rectus femoris muscle can also be used. These two muscles, except for the femoral artery on the medial aspect of the thigh, are free of important nerves and blood vessels. The vastus lateralis muscle is the larger of the two and is well developed in the newborn.
Prepare injection site with alcohol cleansing.	To prevent infection.
Grasp the muscle mass of the thigh to be injected firmly in one hand and compress the muscle mass for injection with the other hand (Fig. 22-10, *B*).	To stabilize the limb.
Inject the medication: Poise the needle just over the site (without touching the skin) and insert the needle with quick flexion of the wrist.	The dart method for injection is inappropriate when aiming at such a small target.
Comfort the infant and settle in crib.	To allay tension.
Discard equipment	
Record medication, amount, route, and site of injection.	To ensure communication with other caregivers.

Therapy for Hyperbilirubinemia

The best therapy for hyperbilirubinemia is prevention. Feeding of the newborn soon after birth stimulates the passage of meconium. Serum indirect bilirubin levels have been studied in relation to meconium passage in early fed normal newborns (see research highlight). The goal of hyperbilirubinemia treatment is to help the newborn's body reduce serum levels of unconjugated bilirubin. The term infant may have trouble conjugating the increased amount of bilirubin derived from disintegrating fetal red blood cells; the serum levels of unconjugated bilirubin rise beyond the limits of normal 12 mg/dl. If untreated the levels can continue to rise and the risk of kernicterus increases (Chapter 40).

There are two principal methods for reducing serum bilirubin levels: exchange blood transfusion and phototherapy. Exchange transfusion is used to treat infants whose levels of bilirubin cannot be controlled by phototherapy (Chapter 40).

Phototherapy. Recent research (Speck, 1985) indicates that phototherapy (Procedure 22-10) causes a structural isomerization of bilirubin in the skin. During phototherapy infants form a substance called lumirubin, a watersoluble product. Lumirubin is formed slowly and excreted rapidly. Lumirubin is excreted both in the urine and feces. Since lumirubin is excreted efficiently by infants, increasing the formation of lumirubin improves the efficacy of phototherapy in the treatment of neonatal jaundice.

RESEARCH HIGHLIGHT

Serum Indirect Bilirubin Levels and Meconium Passage in Early Fed Normal Newborns

Purpose

To investigate the effect of early feeding with formula and sterile water: on time of initial meconium passage, serum indirect bilirubin levels at 48 hours of life (HOL), observed jaundice at 48 HOL, and percentage of weight change at 48 HOL.

Sample

A nonprobability sample of 30 normal newborns was studied. Subjects were sequentially assigned to a control and two experimental groups.

Methodology

The control group received routine nursery feeding of sterile water at 4 HOL and formula at 8 HOL. The water-fed group was held and given sterile water at 1, 2, and 3 HOL. The formula-fed group was held and given Enfamil (2 kcal/30 ml) at 1, 2, and 3 HOL.

Findings

Mean time of first meconium passage was 1.7 hours earlier in formula-fed infants, but the difference between the two experimental groups was not statistically significant. There was no significant difference between groups on serum indirect bilirubin levels at 48 HOL, however, the mean for the formula-fed group was lower. The differences among the means of weight loss were not statistically significant. There was a weak positive linear relationship between initial meconium passage and serum indirect bilirubin at 48 HOL.

Implications

The investigators recommended replicating the study. A larger number of infants is needed for more conclusive results. Because physiologic jaundice peaks at about 72 hours in normal-term infants, it is recommended that serum indirect bilirubin be drawn 72 hours rather than 48 HOL. In addition, because of the theoretical relationship between meconium passage and serum bilirubin levels, a more important measure might be time of passage of the first yellow stool.

Boyer, DB, and Vidyasager, D: Serum indirect bilirubin levels and meconium passage in early fed normal newborns, Nurs Res 36(3):174, 1987.

RESEARCH HIGHLIGHT

Neonatal Jaundice in the Home

Purpose

To determine the effectiveness of a battery-operated portable bilirubinometer for home testing of neonatal jaundice for infants discharged at 48 hours or less.

Sample

A convenience sample of 20 normal neonates (18 to 78 hours old) were simultaneously screened for jaundice with both a single reading from the noninvasive bilirubinometer and a serum bilirubin level. The procedures were done as part of a mother-infant assessment during a home visit.

Methodology

A Pearson r-correlation coefficient was calculated to establish the relationship between total bilirubin serum levels and bilirubinometer readings.

Findings

The total serum bilirubin level averaged 11.73 with a range of 3.5 to 17.5. The average meter reading was 17, with a range of 11 to 24. No instances of false negatives and three instances of false positives were identified. Therefore in this sample, no infants with hyperbilirubinemia would have been missed.

The Pearson r-correlation coefficient for Caucasian infants only, was 0.77.

Implications

These findings suggest that the bilirubinometer can be of great value to the health professional caring for an ethnically homogeneous population. Further study to measure infants-of-color is needed to establish norms for those populations. In addition, the authors suggest that the noninvasive device can help nurses refine their skills in visual assessment.

Brucker, MC, et al: Neonatal jaundice in the home: assessment with a noninvasive device, JOGN Nurs 16(5):355, 1987.

VASTUS LATERALIS MUSCLE

Landmarks

1 Greater trochanter

2 Knee

Injection site: lateral aspect of muscle mass in middle third of distance between landmarks; injected at 45 degree angle in direction of knee

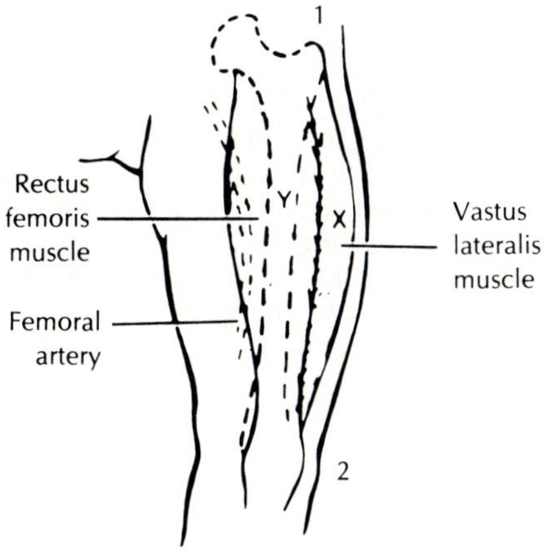

A

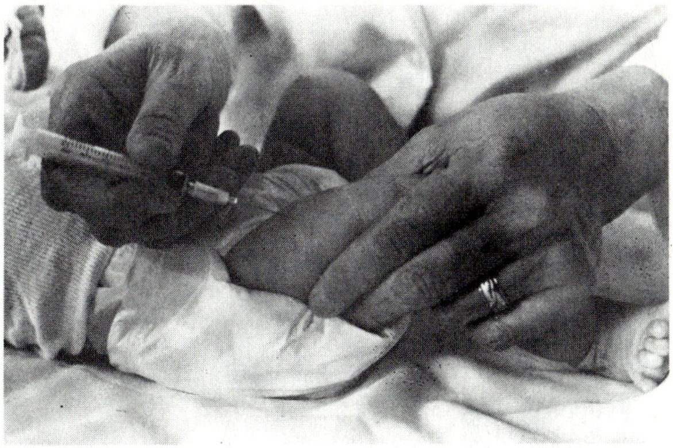

B

Fig. 22-10 **A**, Acceptable intramuscular injection sites for children, X, preferred injection site; Y, alternate injection site. **B**, Infant's leg stabilized for intramuscular injection.

From Whaley, LF, and Wong, DL: Nursing care of infants and children, ed 3, St Louis, 1987, The CV Mosby Co.

Procedure 22-10

PHOTOTHERAPY

DEFINITION

The treatment of neonatal hyperbilirubinemia and jaundice by exposing infant's bare skin to intense fluorescent light. The blue range of light accelerates the removal of bilirubin in the skin.

PURPOSE

To reduce levels of unconjugated bilirubin and prevent kernicterus.

EQUIPMENT

Phototherapy unit, eye patches (Fig. 22-11, *A*) diaper—a face mask with wire support removed works effectively (Fig. 22-11, B) (some institutions use disposable diapers).

NURSING ACTIONS	RATIONALE
Wash hands before and after touching infant and equipment. Glove.	To prevent nosocomial infection and to implement universal precautions.
Identify infant.	To ensure procedure is done on correct infant.
Undress infant.	To expose as much skin area as possible to light.
Protect infant's eyes with eye patches (Fig. 22-11).	To prevent possible injury to conjunctiva or retina.
Be sure eyes are closed.	To prevent corneal abrasions.
Check eyes for drainage each shift.	To prevent or allow prompt treatment of purulent conjunctivitis, should it occur. Research evidence suggests that exposure of the eyes to the phototherapy light units may injure the retina.
Diapering may be accomplished by using a "string bikini", paper face mask with the metal strip removed (Fig. 22-11, *B*); or a disposable diaper.	To allow optimum skin exposure, yet sufficient to protect genitals and bedding. Metal strip is heated by light and can burn baby's skin.
After placing baby under light, monitor skin temperature. If infant is in incubator, temperature dial on control panel may need to be turned to maintain proper temperature.	To prevent hyperthermia or hypothermia. To prevent serious injury, all electric equipment should be grounded, free of defects, and operationally sound to maximize therapeutic effectiveness and to prevent electric shock or burn to the infant or the nurse.

Continued.

Procedure 22-10—cont'd

NURSING ACTIONS	RATIONALE
For feeding and especially for parents' visits, discontinue phototherapy and unwrap baby's eyes. Hold for feedings.	To meet need for psychosocial contact and bonding. Parent has opportunity to make eye contact, a necessary activity to develop attachment.
Observe infant's behavior:	To continue surveillance.
Eating and sleeping patterns. Loose greenish stools, green urine.	Effect of phototherapy on biologic rhythms uncertain. Data base is needed to differentiate common side effects (loose greenish stools or green urine) from other problems that need treatment. Green color comes from end products of bilirubin.
Replace fluid losses by increasing fluid volume offered to infant by 10 to 20 ml/kg/day.	To prevent dehydration: insensible and intestinal water loss is increased during phototherapy.
Protect skin from excoriation (includes diaper rash).	To prevent infection of broken-down skin areas.
Clean urine and stool off of skin during diaper change.	To prevent harming of skin by chemicals in excreta.
Send serial bilirubins for analysis.	To evaluate level of bilirubin and effectiveness of treatment.
Record time therapy began, note time removed for care, and if therapy discontinued. Record infant response (e.g., temperature, stools).	To ensure communication with other caregivers.

The effectiveness of phototherapy is increased by increasing the intensity of the light. An alternative method is to use *green* fluorescent light in place of *blue or white* light. Green fluorescent light does not appear to produce undesirable side effects (Speck, 1985). *Bronze baby syndrome* has occurred in some newborns receiving phototherapy. The serum, urine, and skin turn bronze (brown-black). The cause is unclear. Almost all newborns recover from bronze baby syndrome without sequelae.

Parent Education. Serum levels of bilirubin in the newborn continue to rise until the fifth day of life. Most parents leave the hospital by the third or fourth day and some as early as two hours after delivery. Therefore parents must be able to assess the degree of jaundice the newborn exhibits. They should have written instructions as to whom they should report the infant's condition. Some hospitals have a nurse make a home visit to evaluate the infant's responses. Assessment with a noninvasive device has been studied. (See research highlight p. 526, bottom right). The guidelines for client teaching (p. 529) provide a teaching tool to acquaint parents with the problem of hyperbilirubinemia and its treatment if it should arise.

A

B

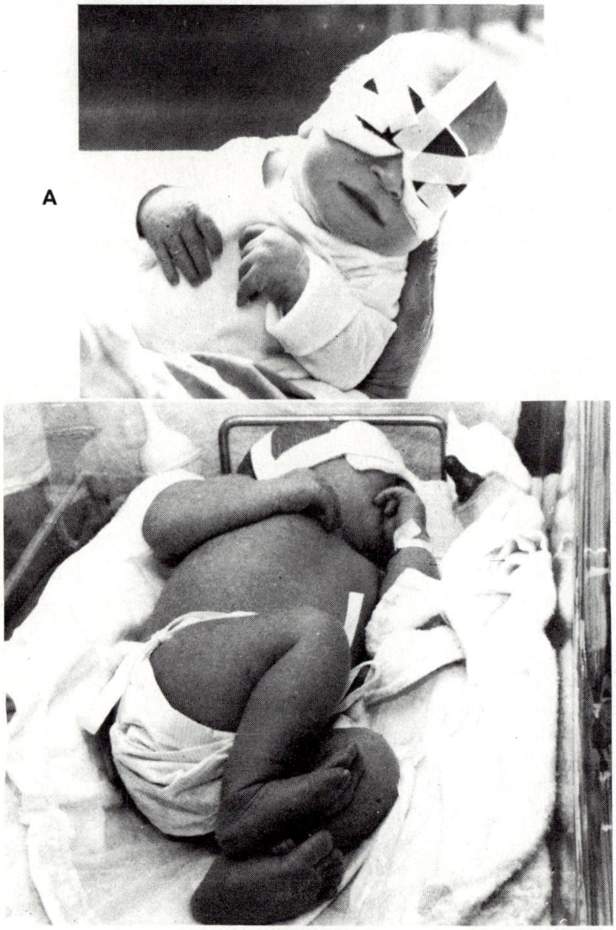

Fig. 22-11 A, Placement of eye patches for protection of eyes when infant is receiving phototherapy. Infant is undressed before being put under light. B, Under Bililite newborn wears surgical face mask in place of a diaper.
Courtesy Olympic Medical Corp, Seattle.

Guidelines For Client Teaching

HYPERBILIRUBINEMIA

ASSESSMENT

1. Infant, female term newborn, 8 lb 4 oz, 3 days old.
2. Infant bilirubin level is 13.5 mg/dl.
3. Infant breast-feeding.
4. Physician's orders: serial total bilirubin levels; phototherapy.
5. Parents unaware of causes of jaundice and what phototherapy is.

NURSING DIAGNOSIS

Knowledge deficit (parental) related to hyperbilirubinemia and phototherapy.

GOALS

Short-term

To teach parents what hyperbilirubinemia is and why phototherapy is ordered.

Intermediate

To increase parents' ability to evaluate their newborn at home for hyperbilirubinemia.

To reduce parents' anxiety.

Long term

To provide knowledge of hyperbilirubinemia that can be used to prompt treatment for older infants, subsequent infants, and other family members.

REFERENCES AND TEACHING AIDS

Charts, phototherapy equipment, eye mask, paper diaper (or face mask with wire support removed), and printed pamphlets provided by hospital or formula companies for parents to take home and refer to later.

CONTENT/RATIONALE	TEACHING ACTIONS
To review meaning of terms parents will hear: Hyperbilirubinemia: higher levels of bilirubin than normal. Bilirubin: end product of red blood cells when they mature and break down. Jaundice: yellow color of whites of eyes, skin, and mucous membranes caused by circulating bilirubin. Phototherapy: the use of fluorescent light to break down bilirubin in the skin into substances that can be excreted in the feces (stool) or urine.	Seat parents in a quiet place, where they can see charts and talk easily to the nurse. Have chart made with terms spelled out. If possible, have parents hold their wrapped infant for this part of the class.
To review process of excreting bilirubin: When red blood cells (RBCs) break down they release bilirubin. Bilirubin circulates in the blood. In the liver it is combined with another substance. In the combined form it goes by way of the blood to the kidneys and the intestines. It gives the yellow color to urine and the brown color to the stool.	Point to chart depicting process as you explain. Ask for questions. Remind parents this is a process difficult for nurses and physicians to learn, so therefore many questions and repeated explanations are expected.
Before the baby was born, her RBCs were more numerous than ours. They also had a shorter life span, 70 to 90 days instead of 120 days. When the RBCs broke down, the baby's blood carried most of the bilirubin by way of the placenta to the mother's liver to be excreted.	Show picture of baby in utero. Trace route of blood from baby to mother's liver.
After the baby was born, her liver began to take care of all the bilirubin. Even though the baby's liver functions well, it cannot handle the whole load. Bilirubin seeps out of the blood and into the tissues, staining them yellow. The blood level of bilirubin rises quickly up to the fifth day, and then goes down; the jaundice usually clears up by the end of the week.	Point out yellowness of baby's skin. Show chart with approximate amounts of bilirubin and location. Prepare graph illustrating rise and fall of bilirubin over the first week of life.
If the baby is breast-feeding, a certain amount of the jaundice may be caused by the free fatty acids, which interfere with the conjugation of bilirubin.	Show chart with contents of breast milk and point out the level of free fatty acids. Refer back to chart depicting process of conjugation.

Continued.

Guidelines For Client Teaching—cont'd

CONTENT/RATIONALE	TEACHING ACTIONS
Some babies seem to have extra bilirubin to excrete. The amount in the tissues becomes too great when the blood level reaches 12 mg/dl. There is a danger that the bilirubin at high levels will cause damage to the brain. So your doctor wants the baby to be placed under the Bililight for phototherapy. This will help the baby handle the extra bilirubin and prevent damage to the baby's brain.	Show Bililight equipment. Let parents feel warmth of the light.
We put eye masks on the baby to keep the light from her eyes.	Demonstrate use of eye mask. Bring infant and place in crib away from Bililight. Apply the eye mask.
We keep the baby undressed so as much light as possible can reach her skin.	Undress baby. Place under Bililight.
We use a paper diaper or the face mask as a small diaper (a "string bikini").	Diaper the infant.
We will take her temperature often so she will not become too hot or too cold.	Take and record temperature. Settle baby comfortably.
We will give her extra water to drink because she will have watery, green stools from the extra bilirubin being excreted.	Return to seats and review care. Distribute pamphlets.
We will be taking her out of the Bililight for feedings and cuddling. We will let you know when to come for feedings and to hold her.	
We will be taking blood tests to check the amount of bilirubin and we will let you know the results.	
To reassure parents that they can have questions answered after discharge.	Leave parents with infant. Tell them they can touch her, but not shield her skin from the light.
If you have any questions, ask us any time. We will give you our phone number and you can call at any hour. It is hard not being able to take her home with you.	Demonstrate stroking baby's hand. Return in about 10 minutes to see if there are any questions. Arrange feeding schedule with mother. Mother can continue to breast-feed or bring breast milk for feedings she will miss (Chapter 23).

EVALUATION Woman (couple) verbalizes understanding of what has been taught and asks appropriate questions.

Circumcision

Historical Perspective. Circumcision has been a rite in many cultures for centuries. It continues to be a ritual in religion, for example, the Jewish faith. Circumcision became a common practice in the United States in the early 1870s. From that time until the 1930s people thought masturbation was harmful and that removal of the foreskin would discourage it by making it less pleasurable. Circumcision was also credited with preventing or curing a number of conditions such as epilepsy, syphilis, asthma, mental illness, and tuberculosis. About 25% of the world's population circumcise their males sometime between birth and young adulthood.

Current Views. Recent studies (Pritchard, MacDonald, and Gant, 1985; Witchell, 1985) do not support the connection between circumcision and penile or prostatic cancer and cervical cancer in the female partner.

No evidence supports the claim that circumcision decreases the risk to the male for sexually transmitted diseases. Claims that circumcision facilitates hygiene can be refuted by teaching the young child daily cleansing of the penis. The use of circumcision for all males to prevent phimosis is unwarranted. *Phimosis* is a *rare* condition that can interfere with or impede the flow of urine (if the foreskin opening is tiny) and predispose to infection between the foreskin and glans.

It was thought that eliminating the foreskin would cure premature ejaculation because the foreskin contains numerous nerve endings that respond rapidly and intensely to sexual arousal. Premature ejaculation is now known to be primarily caused by emotional problems and not physical conditions.

Complications can occur with newborn circumcision. Possible difficulties include urethral fistulas and excessive removal of penile skin. Corrective measures have to be undertaken. They include grafting and the careful use of topical hemostatic agents (Gearhart and Callan, 1986).

Parental Decision. Circumcision is an *elective* surgical procedure and as such is a matter of personal choice. The parents' decision to have their newborn circumcised is usually based on one or more of the following factors: hygiene, religious conviction, tradition, culture, or social norms. Some people do not like to touch their infant's genitals. For these parents, circumcision may be the wisest choice.

Regardless of the reason for the decision, it should be made only after parents have the available facts and sufficient time to review their options. The American Academy of Pediatrics (1975) reaffirmed its position that no medical indications for circumcision of the newborn are valid and that a program of good personal hygiene offers all the advantages of circumcision without the attendant surgical risks. The academy recommended that physicians provide parents with information about the risks of circumcision as well as options regarding this surgical procedure well in advance of delivery.

Parents need to begin learning about circumcision during the prenatal period (NAACOG, 1985a). However, circumcision often is not discussed with the parents before labor. In many instances, it is during admission to the hospital or labor unit that the mother confronts the decision regarding circumcision. The stress of the perinatal period makes this a difficult time for parental decision making. Although consenting to their boy's circumcision is ultimately the parents' personal choice, the fact that there are no medical indications for the procedure is emphasized.

Procedure. In circumcision the prepuce (foreskin) of the glans penis is excised to expose the glans (Fig. 22-12). The operation is performed in the hospital before the infant's discharge. The procedure is no longer done immediately after birth because the amount of cold stress had proved detrimental to the infant. Clotting factors drop somewhat immediately after birth and return to prebirth levels by the end of the first week. Therefore performing the circumcision after the baby is a week old has a firmer physiologic basis. The circumcision of a Jewish male is performed on the eighth day after birth unless the infant is unwell.

For the circumcision procedure the infant is positioned on a plastic restraint form so that his movements are restricted (Fig. 22-13). The penis is cleansed with soap and water. The infant is draped to provide warmth and a sterile field. The sterile equipment is readied for use.

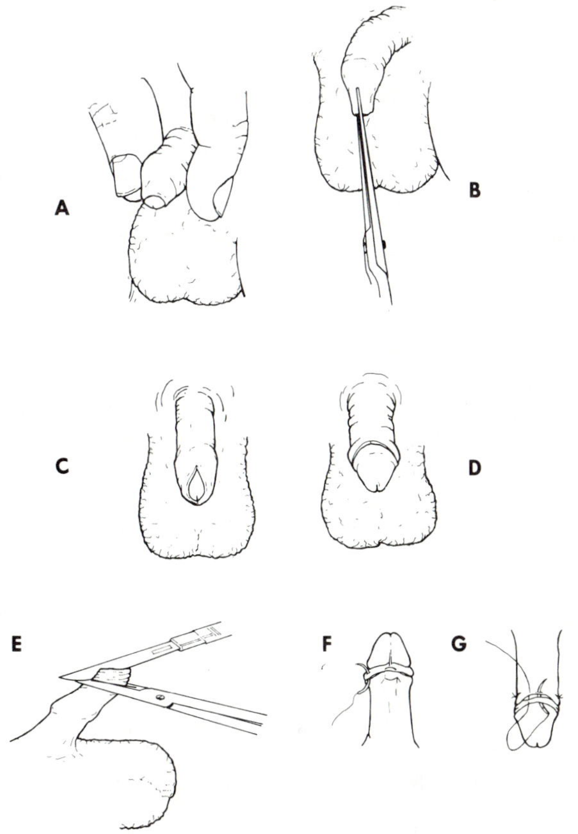

Fig. 22-12 Technique of circumcision. **A** to **D**, Prepuce is stripped and slit to facilitate its retraction behind glans penis. **E**, Prepuce is now-clamped and excessive prepuce cut off. **F** and **G**, Suture material used is plain 00 or 000 catgut in very small needle, but some physicians prefer silk.

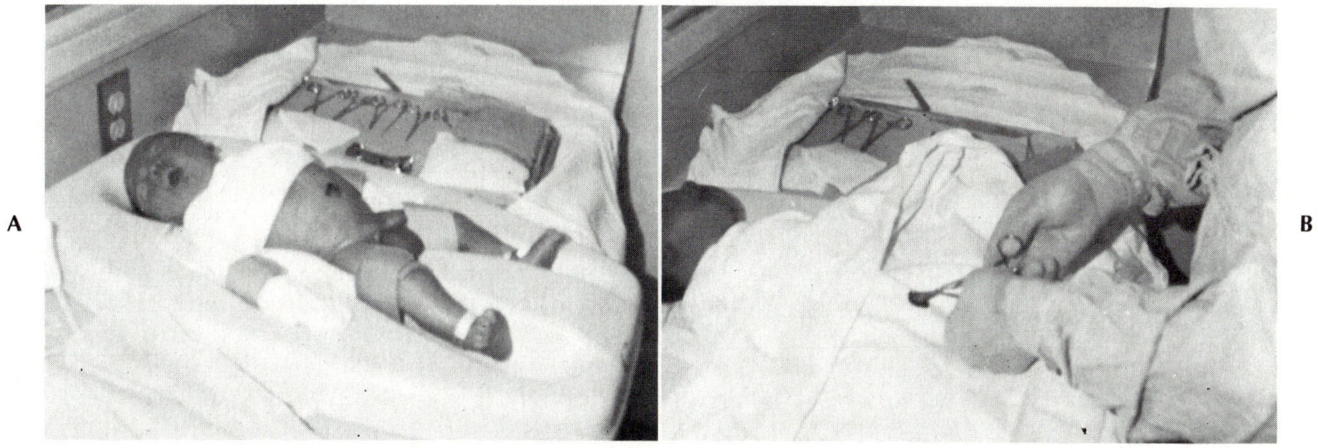

Fig. 22-13 **A**, Proper positioning of infant in Circumstraint. **B**, Physician performing circumcision. Baby is completely covered to prevent cold stress.

Numerous instruments have been designed for circumcision. The Yellen clamp, for instance, may make this an almost bloodless operation. Once the procedure, which takes only a few minutes, is completed, a small petrolatum gauze dressing may be applied for the first day to prevent a cloth diaper from adhering. If a Plastibell is used, the bell applies constant direct pressure to prevent hemorrhage. It also protects against infection, sticking to the diaper, and pain with urination. The bell is fitted over the glans. The suture is tied around the rim of the bell. Excess prepuce is cut away. The plastic rim remains in place for about a week until it falls off, after healing has taken place (Fig. 22-14). Petrolatum gauze is not needed when the bell is used.

Discomfort. If the infant has undergone this surgery without anesthesia, he is comforted until he is quieted. Then he is returned to his crib. These infants usually are fussy for about 2 to 3 hours and may refuse a feeding.

In the Jewish ritual the newborn is given a few drops of wine to relax him in preparation for the surgery. In an article advocating dorsal block for the circumcision, Kirya and Werthmann (1978) wrote:

> Anyone who circumcises a neonate using any of the available techniques senses the pain and stress that the manipulative stages of this procedure generate. During the procedure when the prepuce is clamped with forceps, the infant cries vigorously, trembles, and tries to wiggle out of the restraint. He may eventually become plethoric (flushed), dusky, and mildly cyanotic because of prolonged crying. Occasionally this results in respiratory pauses or regurgitation of feeding.

Pain may not end when the operation is over because the wound requires as long as a week to heal.

Care of the Newly Circumcised Penis. The nurse observes the infant for bleeding. If bleeding is noted from the circumcision, the nurse applies gentle pressure to the site of bleeding with a folded sterile gauze pad, 4 in. × 4 in. If bleeding is not easily controlled, a blood vessel may need to be ligated. One nurse notifies the physician and prepares equipment (circumcision tray and suture) while the other nurse maintains pressure *intermittently* until the physician arrives. The penis is checked hourly for bleeding for 12 hours; if the parents take the baby home before the end of 12 hours, they have to be taught the actions described previously. Before discharge, the nurse checks to see that the parents have the physician's phone number.

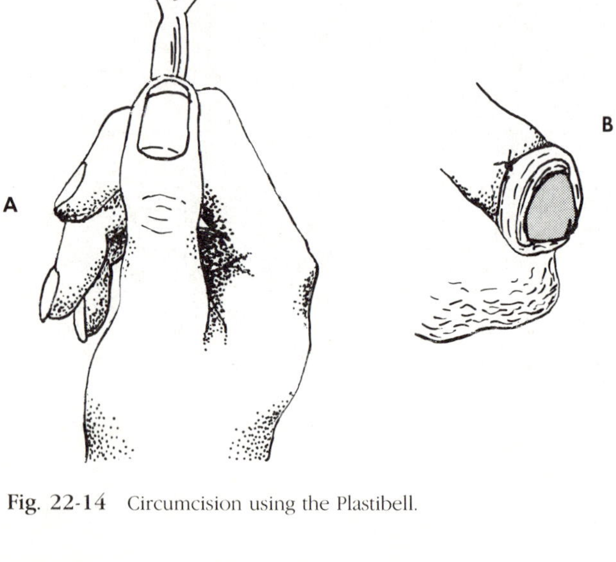

Fig. 22-14 Circumcision using the Plastibell.

Nursing actions are planned and implemented to prevent infection. The nurse washes the penis gently with water to remove urine and feces and reapplies a fresh (sterile) petrolatum gauze around the glans after each diaper change. The glans penis, normally dark red in appearance during healing, becomes covered with a yellow exudate in 24 hours. This is part of the normal healing process, not an infective process. No attempt is made to remove the exudate, which persists for 2 to 3 days.

Cloth diapers are applied loosely for 2 to 3 days because the incised area at the base of the glans penis remains tender and also because blood absorbed by cloth is easier to see than blood absorbed by a disposable diaper. Cloth diapers are used for about a week or until the glans is completely healed.

Teacher/Counselor and Support Person

Caregiving activities for the newborn are shared by the nurse and the mother. The nurse acts as teacher and support person. As soon as the mother feels physically able she is encouraged to participate in her child's care. The mother's need for knowledge and the factors that may impede her learning are determined through questioning and observation. The content taught and teaching aids used should reflect the mother's level of understanding. Films and tapes can be valuable timesavers in teaching. Most hospitals provide written instructions in infant care for parents. The care given the child is supervised, and the parents are encouraged to ask questions.

Positioning and Holding. After feeding, positioning the infant on the right side promotes gastric emptying into the small intestine (Fig. 22-5). Placing the infant in the crib in a side-lying position also permits drainage of mucus from the mouth and applies no pressure to the cord or the sensitive circumcised penis. The infant's position is changed from side to side to help develop even contours of the head and to ease pressure on the other parts of the body.

Anatomically the infant's shape—barrel chest and flat, curveless spine—makes it easy for the child to roll and startle.

A folded or rolled blanket against the spine will prevent rolling to the supine position and will promote a feeling of security. Care must be taken to prevent the infant from rolling off of flat, unguarded surfaces. The parent or nurse who must turn away from the infant even for a moment keeps one hand securely on the infant. If left on the parent's bed, the infant is walled in with pillows.

The infant is held securely with support for the head because newborns are unable to maintain an erect head posture for more than a few moments. Fig. 22-15 illustrates various positions for holding an infant with adequate support. Too much stimulation is avoided after feeding and before a sleep period.

Umbilical Cord Care. The care of the umbilical cord is the same as that for any surgical wound. The goal of care is prevention and early identification of hemorrhage or infection. If bleeding from the blood vessels of the cord is noted, the nurse checks the clamp (or tie) and applies a second clamp next to the first one. If bleeding is not stopped immediately, the nurse calls for physician assistance at once.

Hospital protocol directs the time and technique for routine cord care. The nurse cleanses the cord and skin area around the base of the cord with the prescribed preparation (for example, erythromycin solution, triple blue dye, or alcohol) and checks daily for signs of infection. The cord clamp is removed after 24 hours (Fig. 22-16).

Diaper Rash. Treatment of diaper rash involves exposing the rash to warmth and air. Immediately washing and drying the wet and soiled area and changing the diaper after voiding or defecating prevent and help treat diaper rash. The warmth can be achieved with a 25-watt bulb placed 45 cm (18 in) from the affected area. Parents must be cautioned to prevent the lamp from falling on the baby.

The most severe type of diaper rash occurs when the area becomes infected, indurated (hardened), and tender. Medical advice should be sought and a specifically ordered medication applied.

A rash on the face may result from the infant's scratching (excoriation) or from rubbing the face against the sheets, particularly if regurgitated stomach contents are not washed off promptly.

Clothing. Parents commonly ask how warmly they should dress their infant. A simple rule of thumb for parents is to dress the child as they dress themselves, adding or subtracting clothes and wraps for the child as they do for themselves. A shirt or diaper may be sufficient clothing for the young infant. A bonnet is needed to protect the scalp and minimize heat loss if it is cool or to protect against sunburn and shade the eyes if it is sunny and hot. Wrapping the infant snugly in a blanket maintains body temperature and promotes a feeling of security. Overdress-

A

B

C

D

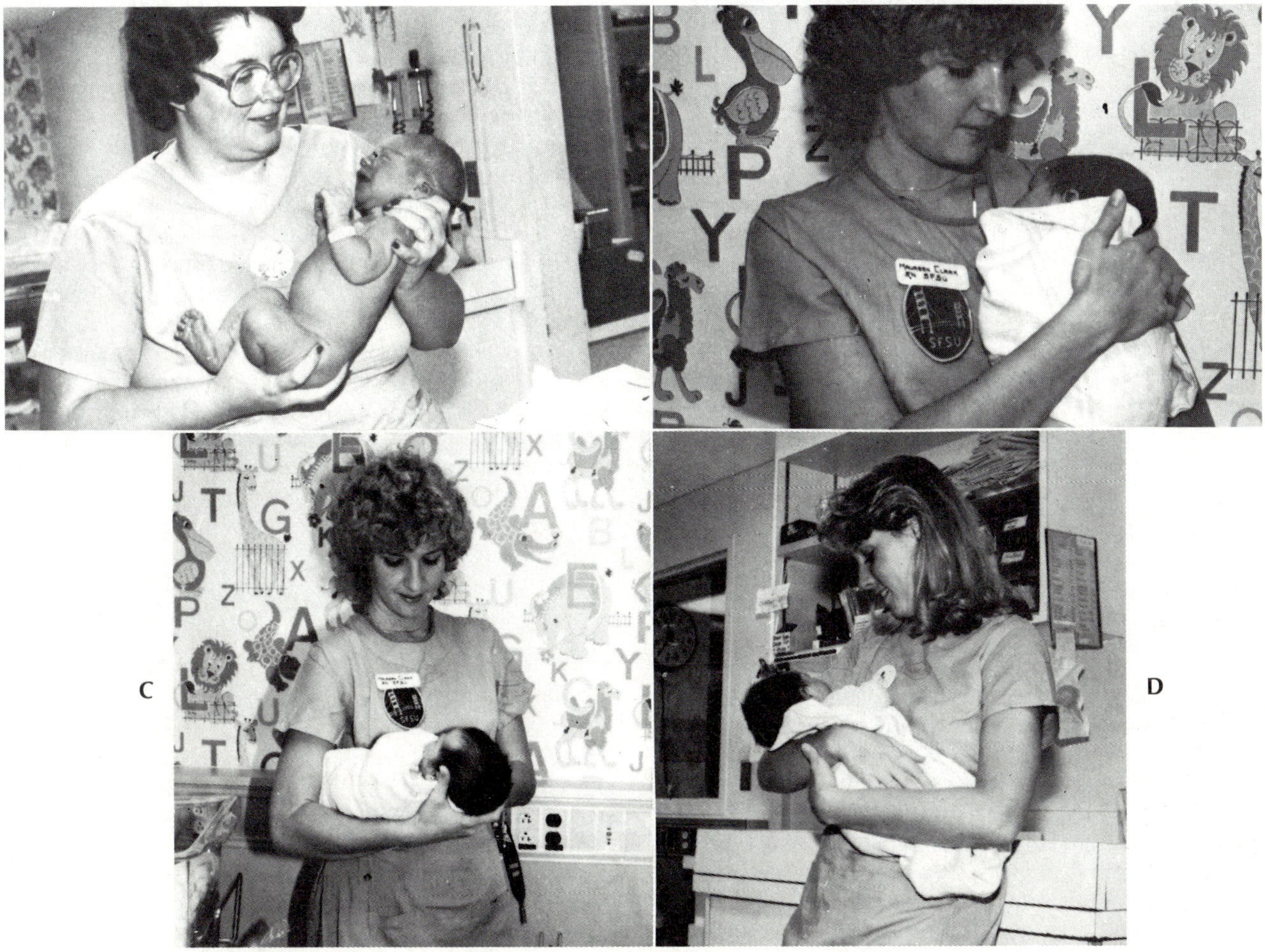

Fig. 22-15 Holding baby securely with support for head. **A,** Holding infant while moving infant from one place to another. Baby is undressed to show posture. **B,** Holding baby upright in "burping" position. **C,** "Football" hold. **D,** Cradling hold.

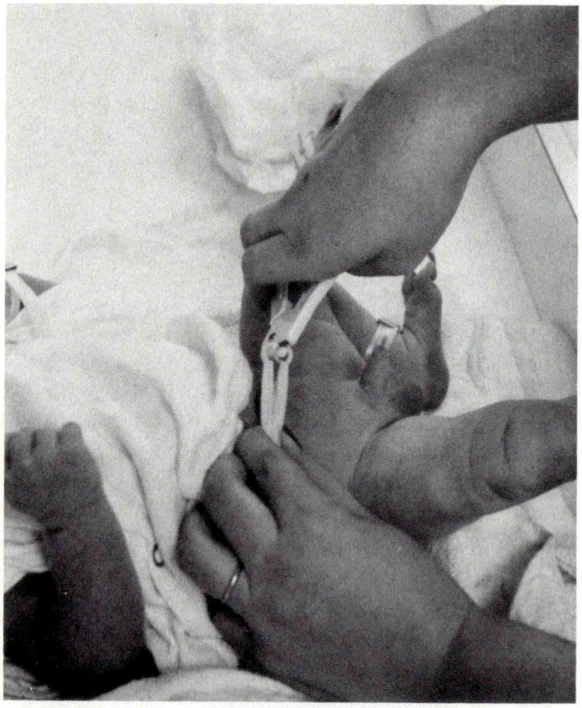

Fig. 22-16 Removal of cord clamp when cord is dry.

ing in warm temperatures can cause discomfort and prickly heat; underdressing in cold weather can also cause discomfort. Cheeks, fingers, and toes can readily become frostbitten. The incident noted below shows the need for teaching a young parent.

> A nurse was called to make a home visit to see an infant because the "baby just sleeps and sleeps and doesn't have any energy." In the apartment the thermostat was set for 33° C (92° F) because the mother "thought that babies need it warm." The mother was wearing a sleeveless dress because she could barely tolerate the extreme heat. The baby was found heavily wrapped in blankets. Lowering the thermostat and dressing the infant to match the temperature resulted in normal newborn behavior.

Care of the Infant's Linens. Care of the infant's clothes and bedding is directed toward minimizing cross infection and removing residues from soap, feces, or urine that may irritate the infant's skin. In the hospital, clothing and bedding are washed separately from other linens and are autoclaved. Some hospitals use disposable shirts and diapers. At home the baby's clothes should be washed separately, with a mild detergent or soap and hot water. A double rinse usually removes traces of the potentially irritating cleansing agent or acid residue from the urine or stool. If possible, dry the clothing and bedding in the sun to neutralize residues. Parents who have to use coin-operated machines to wash and dry clothes may find it expensive or impossible to wash and rinse the baby's clothes well.

Bedding requires frequent changing. The plastic-coated, firm mattress must be washed daily and the crib or bassinet damp dusted. The infant's toilet articles may be kept separate and convenient for use in a box or basket.

Bathing. Bathing serves a number of purposes. It provides opportunities for (1) a complete cleansing of the infant, (2) observing the infant's condition, (3) promoting comfort, and (4) parent-child-family socializing. The initial bath is postponed for 6 hours or until the infant's skin temperature stabilizes at 36.5° C (97.6° F) or core temperature stabilizes at 37° C (98.6° F) for 2 hours. Until the initial bath is completed, personnel must wear gloves when handling the newborn. In some hospitals the infant is given the initial bath, and then cleansing of the genitals as necessary is deemed sufficient for the first 3 to 4 days. Bathing with warm water is sufficient for the first week. Then a mild soap may be used (NAACOG, 1985b). If a documented staphylococcal skin infection outbreak occurs in a nursery, the newborn is bathed with dilute hexachlorophene detergent (pHisoHex) (less than 3%), followed by thorough rinsing of the skin. As pHisoHex is a potential neurotoxin, particularly for infants who weigh less than 2000 g, it is no longer used in many nurseries. Guidelines for client teaching (p. 536), are provided for use with mothers who need instruction in the bathing of their infants. The nurse does not need to wear gloves during the bath demonstration for the parent(s) (Fig. 22-17).

Questions have arisen about some routine practices: use of soap, oils, powder, lotion, and sponging. Nursing research can provide needed answers. One of the most important considerations in skin cleansing is preservation of the skin's "*acid mantle*," which is formed from the uppermost horny layer of the epidermis, sweat, superficial fat, metabolic products, and external substances such as amniotic fluid, microorganisms, and cosmetics (Whaley and Wong, 1987). The infant's skin surface has a pH of about 4.95 soon after birth, and this offers important bacteriostatic effects. Consequently, only plain warm water should be used for the bath (NAACOG, 1985b). Alkaline soaps such as Ivory, oils, powder, and lotions are not used because they alter the acid mantle, thus providing a medium for bacterial growth. The sponging technique is generally used. However, bathing the newborn by immersion has been found to cause less heat loss and less crying (Henningsson et al., 1981).

Infant's Social Needs

The sensitivity of the caregiver to the social responses of the infant is basic to the development of a mutually satisfying parent-child relationship (chapters 21 and 25). Sensitivity increases over time as parents' awareness of their infant's social capabilities becomes more acute.

Parental Awareness. The "Mother's assessment of the behavior of her infant" (MABI) determines how mothers perceive their infants (Field et al., 1978). It was found that mothers perceived their infants in much the same way as the professional examiners did. For example, the mothers noted the postmature infants were not as adaptable or in tune rhythmically with parents. There was one notable exception: mothers were not as aware of the social capabilities of their infants as were the examiners.

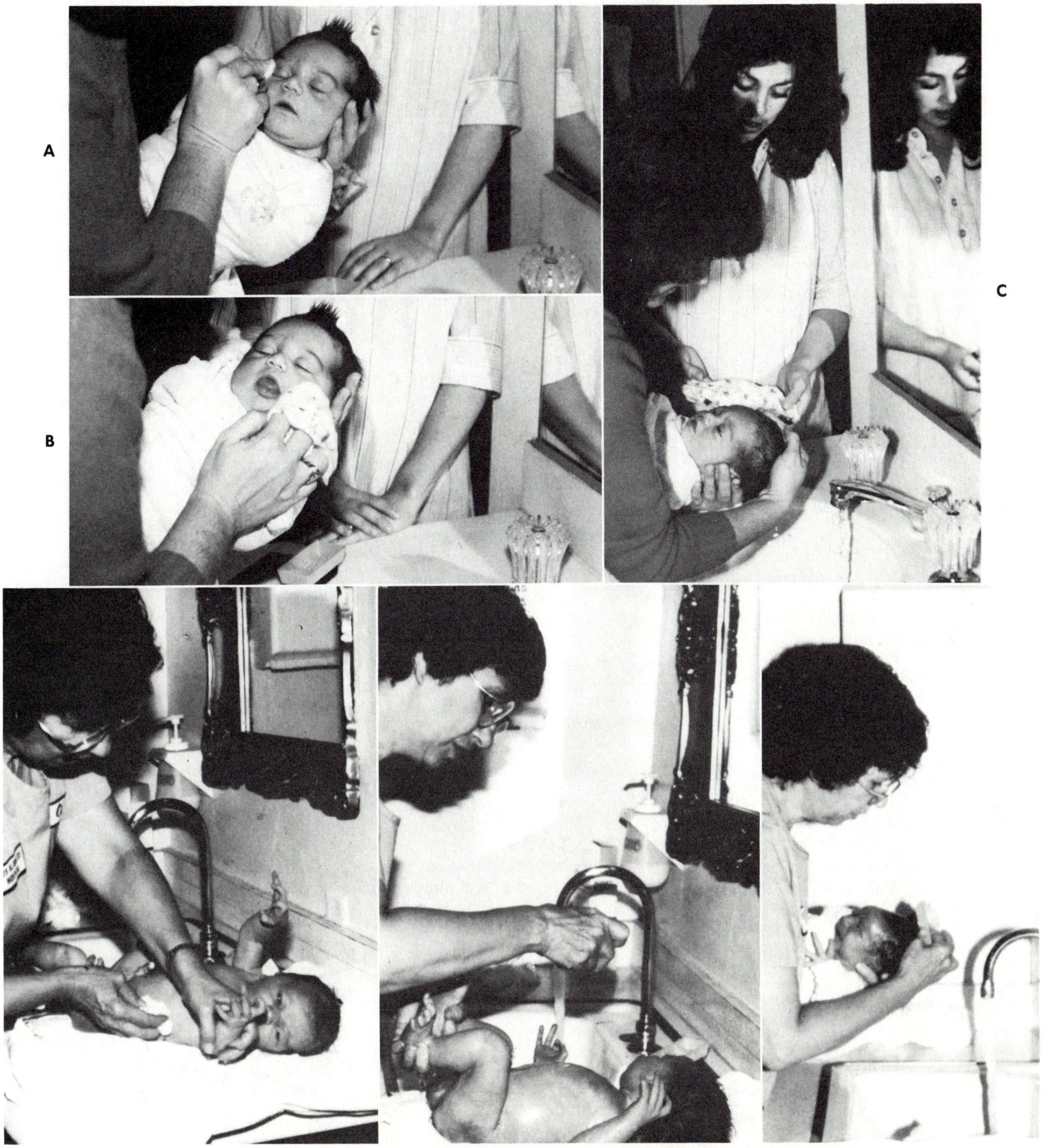

Fig. 22-17 Demonstration baby bath. **A**, Eyes. **B**, Face. **C**, Head and hair. **D**, Sponge-bathing baby. **E**, Rinsing baby. **F**, Brushing hair. Mother in **A**, **B**, and **C** is being supervised. Note in **D** and **E** that nurse keeps one hand on baby at all times. (Gloves are used only until baby has first bath to remove blood and amniotic fluid.)

Courtesy Marjorie Pyle, RNC, Lifecircle, Costa Mesa, Calif.

Guidelines For Client Teaching

BATHING AN INFANT

ASSESSMENT

1. Woman has just delivered her first child, a boy.
2. She has little experience with the care of children.
3. Woman exhibits a readiness to learn by asking many questions.
4. Woman's culture does not have specific prescriptions or proscriptions for this activity.

NURSING DIAGNOSES

Knowledge deficit related to bathing an infant.
Anxiety, mild, related to care of newborn infant.

GOALS

Short-term

To have woman learn infant bathing technique.

Intermediate

To have woman become skilled in bathing and handling infant.

Long-term

To have woman adjust bathing technique to developing child.

REFERENCES AND TEACHING AIDS

Texts; hospital or clinic-prepared instructions; film or video of parent bathing a baby; and parent's class on bathing a baby.

CONTENT/RATIONALE	TEACHING ACTIONS
To review the purposes for bathing: It provides opportunities for (1) a complete cleansing of the infant, (2) observing the infant's condition, (3) promoting comfort, and (4) parent-child-family socialization.	Introduction: Set tone. Have mother seated comfortably (she may need a pillow or doughnut to sit on). Make sure she can see demonstration. Welcome father (or other family member) if present, and include in the process.
To help woman fit baths into her schedule: Initial bath: The initial bath is postponed until the infant's skin temperature stabilizes at 36.5° C (97.6° F) or core temperature stabilizes at 37° C (98.6° F) for 2 hours. Daily bath: a daily bath may be given at any time convenient to the parent but not immediately after a feeding period, since the increased handling may cause regurgitation of the feeding.	Ask mother when father and siblings would be available for infant bath. To prevent cold stress.
To prevent heat loss: The temperature of the room should be 24° C (75° F), and the bathing area should be free of drafts. Heat loss in the infant is greater than in the adult because of the relatively large ratio of skin surface to body mass in the newborn. Heat loss must be controlled during the bath period to conserve the infant's energy. Bathing the infant quickly, exposing only a portion of the body at a time, and thorough drying is therefore part of the bathing technique.	Review material pertinent to care before beginning bath to prevent heat loss. Explain that infants do not shiver to increase body temperature, as adults do. Explain mechanism of burning fat for heat maintenance in the infant and the amount of energy it requires. Show a chart depicting this mechanism simplified.
To prevent skin trauma: The fragile skin can be injured by too vigorous cleansing. Vernix, the white, cheesy-looking material on the skin is not removed, since it is attached to the upper layer of the skin. Too vigorous removal results in removal of the protective skin layer. Vernix may be left on for 48 hours; if it persists beyond that time, it may be washed off gently. If stool or other debris has dried and caked on the skin, soak the area to remove it. Do not attempt to rub it off because abrasion may result. Gentleness, patting dry rather than rubbing, and use of a mild soap without perfumes or coloring are recommended. Chemicals in the coloring and perfume can cause rashes in sensitive skin.	Review material pertinent to skin care before beginning bath to prevent heat loss. Review possible sources of skin damage (for all members of family): dyes, perfumes.

Guidelines For Client Teaching—cont'd

CONTENT/RATIONALE	TEACHING ACTIONS
Supplies and clothing are made ready. Clothing suitable for wearing indoors: diaper, shirt; stretch suit or nightgown optional. Unscented, mild soap. Baby lotion, not powder. Baby powder can be inhaled by the infant.	Arrange work area while explaining process. Comment on equipment and clothing so that mother sees importance of preparing area before child is brought in.
Pins, if needed for diaper, are placed well out of baby's reach	Sticking them in a bar of soap both lubricates them and keeps them away from the infant.
Cotton balls. Towels for drying infant and a clean washcloth. Receiving blanket.	
Bring infant to bathing area when all supplies are ready. The infant is never left alone on bath table or in the bath water, not even for a second. If the mother or nurse has to leave, the infant is taken along or put back in the crib.	Model holding of infant and protecting him with hand (Fig. 22-17). Review major cause of death in small children: drowning.
Test temperature of the water. It should feel pleasantly warm to the inner wrist (about 98 to 99° F).	Demonstrate testing water. Let mother feel.
The infant's head is washed before unwrapping and undressing to prevent heat loss.	Explain that the infant is washed from head to toe starting with the eyes and ending with the genitals. Demonstrate cleansing the eyes and washing the face (Fig. 22-17, *A* and *B*).
Cleanse the eyes from the canthus outward, using a **clean** wash-cloth. For the first 2 to 3 days a discharge may result from the reaction of the conjunctiva to the substance (erythromycin) used as a prophylactic measure against infection. Any discharge should be considered abnormal and reported to the physician. When removing eye discharge avoid contamination of one eye with the discharge from the other by using a separate cotton swab and water source (running water from a tap is best) for each eye.	Teach general hygiene measure to prevent spread of infection.
The **scalp** is washed daily with water and mild soap. It must be rinsed well and dried thoroughly. Scalp desquamation, called **cradle cap**, can often be prevented by removing any scales with a fine-toothed comb or brush after washing. If condition persists, the physician may prescribe an ointment to massage into the skin.	Demonstrate washing and drying head. Use football hold (Fig. 22-17, *C*). Teach mother now (or later) to use football hold.
Creases under the chin and arms and in the groin may need daily cleansing. The crease under the chin may be exposed by elevating the infant's shoulders 5 cm (2 in) and letting the head drop back.	Demonstrate washing creases. Teach potential of warmth, moisture, and unwashed areas for providing an excellent condition for skin break down and infection.
Cleanse the **ears** and **nose** with twists made of moistened cotton.	Demonstrate cleansing of ears and nose. Review reason for the saying, "Do not put anything smaller than your elbow into your ear."
Undress baby and wash body and arms and legs. Pat dry gently. Baby may be tub bathed after the cord drops off.	Demonstrate sponge bath of infant. Rinse well. Pat dry (Fig. 22-17, *C* to *E*).
To teach care of the cord:	Demonstrate care of cord.
Use a cotton swab. Dip swab in solution the physician has ordered and cleanse around base of the cord, where it joins the skin. Notify your physician of any odor, discharge, or skin inflammation around the cord. The clamp is removed when the cord is dry (about 24 to 48 hours) (Fig. 22-16). When you diaper the infant, the diaper should not cover the cord. A wet or soiled diaper will slow or prevent drying of the cord and foster infection. When the cord drops off in a week to 10 days, small drops of blood can be seen when the baby cries. This will heal itself. It is not dangerous.	Ask mother what she would report. Ask mother what she has heard about the cord and cord care.

Continued.

Guidelines For Client Teaching—cont'd

CONTENT/RATIONALE	TEACHING ACTIONS
To teach care of hands and feet: Wash and dry between the fingers and toes daily.	Check between fingers and toes.
Fingernails and toenails are not cut immediately after birth. The nails have to grow out far enough from the skin so that the skin is not cut by mistake. Before the nails can be cut, if the baby scatches himself, you can apply loosely fitted mitts over each hand. Do so as a last resort, however, since it interferes with the baby's ability to console himself. When the nails have grown, the **fingernails** and **toenails** can be cut more readily with manicure scissors (preferably with rounded tips) when the infant is asleep. Nails are kept short.	Show picture of mitts. Review safety measures.
To cleanse genitals: Cleanse the **genitals** of infants daily and after voiding and defecating. For girls, cleansing of the genitals may be done by separating the labia and gently washing from the pubic area to the anus. For uncircumcised boys, gently pull back (retract) the foreskin. Stop when resistance is felt. Wash the tip (glans) with soap and warm water and replace the foreskin. The foreskin must be returned to its original position to prevent constriction and swelling. In the majority of newborns, the inner layer of the foreskin adheres to the glans. By the age of 3 years, in 90% of boys the foreskin can be retracted easily without pain or trauma. For others, the foreskin is not retractable until the teens. As soon as the foreskin is partly retractable, and the child is old enough, he can be taught self-care.	Demonstrate cleansing of genitals. Review foreskin-purposes, cultural factors, anatomy and physiology—as necessary. Demonstrate technique and explain rationale while doing it.
To review dressing the infant: When dressing the child, do not pull shirts roughly over the face or catch fingers in shirt sleeves. Bunch up the shirt in both hands and expand the neck opening before placing the neck opening over the face; then slip the shirt over the rest of the head.	Demonstrate technique and explain rationale while doing it (Fig. 22-18).
Diapering the infant may be done before and after feeding (Fig. 22-19). It is not necessary to wake the infant for changing.	
If cloth diapers are used, absorbency can be increased by bringing the bulk of the diaper in the front for a boy and in the back for a girl. This will help absorb urine so that skin is protected. The diaper between the infant's legs should not be bulky because it can cause outward displacement of the hips. A soaker pad can be placed under the infant as a protection for the blanket. The continued use of plastic or rubber pants may lead to diaper rash.	
Store infant's towels, wash-cloths, and supplies apart from the family for 4 to 4 months to prevent infection.	Clean and tidy area. Reassure mother you will be with her when she gives the bath tomorrow.

EVALUATION Woman gives return demonstration that shows competence.

One way nurses can promote parental sensitivity is to share with the parents the process of the Brazelton assessment. Examples of comments of parents involved in such teaching about their infants include the following (Edelstein, 1975) (Chapter 21):

> "After the examination I seemed to notice the various things that were pointed out. Also, I myself tested the baby once we were home. Through the testing I realize more so now that the baby is quite aware of what goes on around him, and since, I've noticed I talk to the baby more now."
>
> "I was assured that my baby was normal and healthy. Also, it was fascinating to discover all the things he was already aware of. I learned more about him (and babies in general) from participating in the test."

Planning Times for Social Interactions. The activities of daily care during the neonatal period offer the best times for infant and family interaction. While caring for their baby, mother and father can talk to the infant, play baby games, and caress and cuddle the child. In Fig. 22-20, mother, father, and infant engage in arousal, imitation of facial expression, and smiling. Older children's contact with a newborn needs to be supervised for strength of hugs, exploring of eyes and nose, and attempts to feed the baby. Parents often keep baby books that record their infant's progress.

Discharge Planning

For the new parent, child care activities can cause much anxiety. Support from the nursing staff in the mother's beginning efforts can be an important factor in her seeking

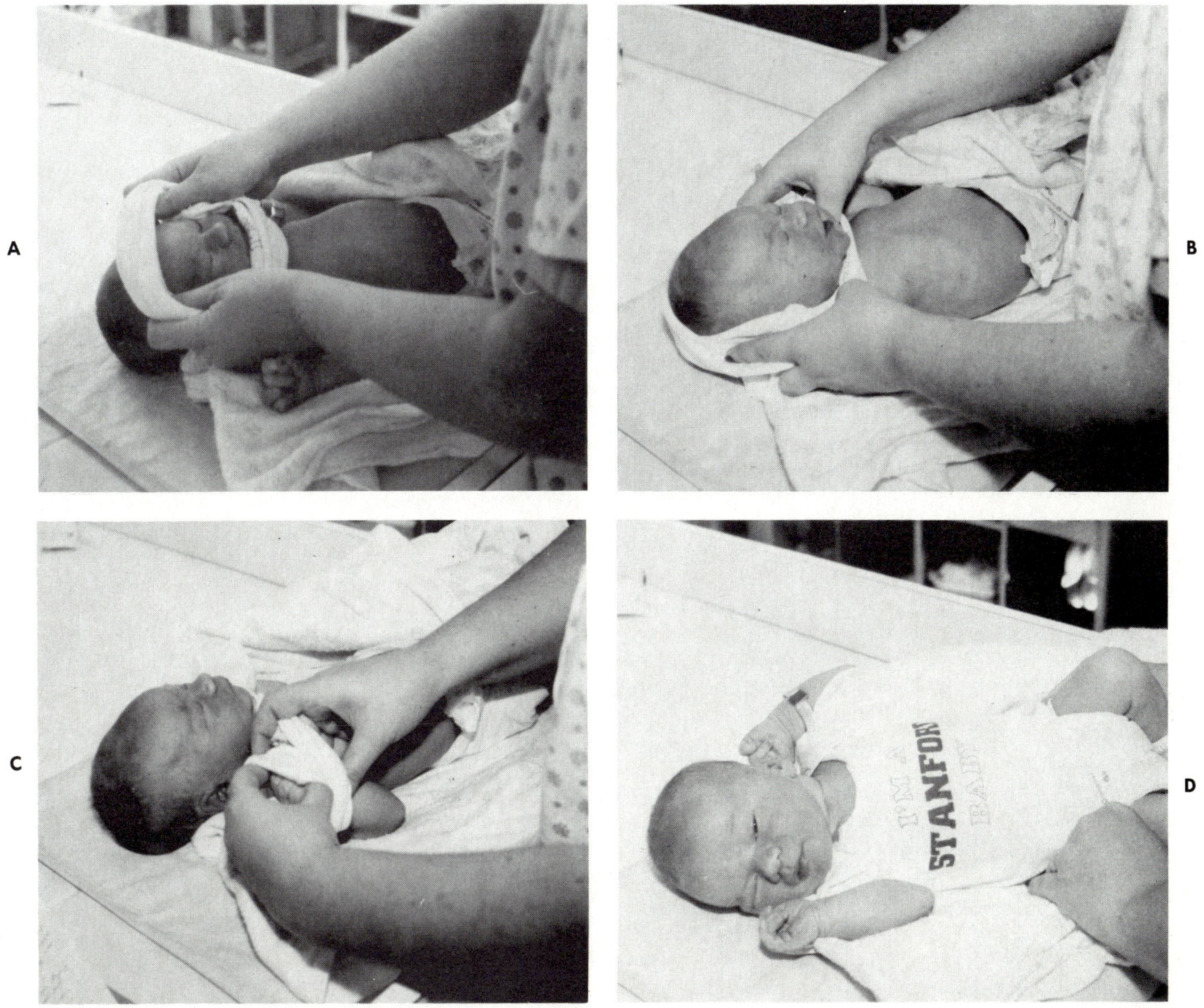

Fig. 22-18 **A**, Placing enlarged neck opening to avoid dragging it across face. **B**, Drawing shirt down over back of head, still avoiding face. **C**, Reaching into shirt sleeve to grasp baby's hand to pull arm through without snagging fingers. **D**, Pulling shirt down to cover trunk.

and accepting help in the future. Whether or not this is the couple's first baby, parents appreciate *anticipatory guidance* in the care of their child. The following topics can be included in discussions with parents. Avoid covering all content at once. The parents can be overwhelmed and become anxious. Follow parental cues to set priorities for teaching. Normal growth and development and the changing needs of the infant (for example, for stimulation, exercise, and social contacts) should be inlcuded in discussions with parents, as well as the following topics.

Temperature. Review the following:

1. The causes of elevation in body temperature (such as exercise, cold stress with resultant vasoconstriction, minimum response to infection) and the body's response to extremes in environmental temperature.
2. Symptoms to be reported, such as high or low temperatures with accompanying fussiness, stuffy nose, lethargy, irritability, poor feeding, and crying.
3. Ways to reduce body temperature, such as giving a cool tub bath, dressing the infant appropriately for the temperature of the air; protecting the infant from long exposure to sunlight, and using warm wraps in cold weather.

Respirations. Review the following:

1. Normal variations in the rate and rhythm.
2. Reflexes, such as sneezing to clear the air passage.
3. The need to protect the infant from the following:
   a. People with upper respiratory tract infections (an efficient mask can be made by wrapping toilet tissue around the head to cover the mouth and nose if the parent or another has a cold).
   b. Pollution from a smoke-filled environment.
   c. Suffocation from loose bedding, drowning (bath water), entrapment under excessive bedding, anything tied around the infant's neck, poorly constructed playpens, bassinets, or cribs. The pediatrician or pediatric nurse can supply printed directions for making the house safe for an infant.
   d. Aspiration pneumonia: A commonly aspirated substance is baby powder, which is usually a mixture of talc (hydrous magnesium silicate) and other silicates (Whaley and Wong, 1987). Although the use of talc has been discouraged, it is a common baby care product and can cause severe and often fatal aspiration pneumonia. One of the factors involved in talc aspiration is the similar appearance of baby

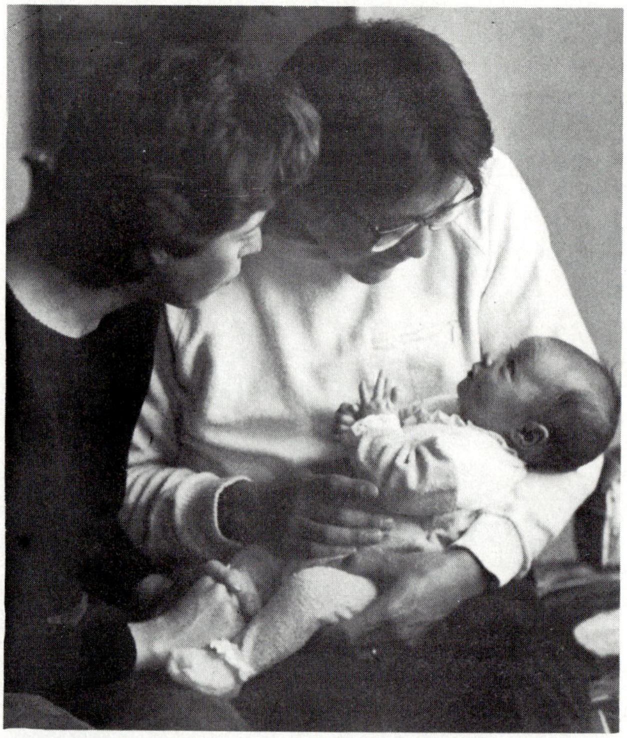

Fig. 22-20 Mother-father-baby interaction.
Courtesy Colleen Stainton.

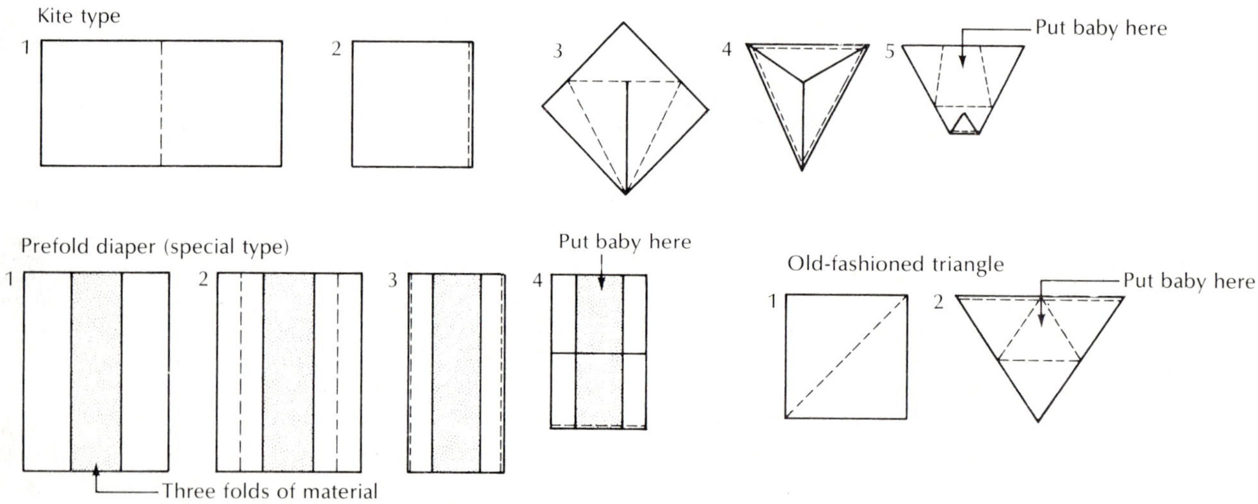

Fig. 22-19 Diapering infant. Dotted lines indicate folds. For kite type, start with large, regular diaper if single thickness is thin.

powder containers and nursing bottles. Talc containers often become favorite playthings and are placed in the mouth (Mofenson et al., 1981). Improper use of powder by sprinkling it directly on the skin creates a cloud of talc dust that is easily inhaled. Parents are advised of the danger of baby powder and discouraged from using it. If they prefer to use a powder, a cornstarch preparation can be substituted. Whenever a powder is used, it should be placed in the hand and then applied to the skin, never shaken directly from the container to the skin. The container is kept closed and immediately stored in a safe place, especially away from curious toddlers who often imitate caregiving activities and may accidentally shake it on the infant.

4. *Symptoms of the common cold:* nasal congestion, coughing, sneezing, difficulty in swallowing (sore throat), low-grade fever. Advise the parents on measures to help the infant: for example, feed smaller amounts but feed more frequently to avoid overtiring the infant; hold the baby in an upright position to feed; offer extra sterile water; for sleeping, raise the infant's head and chest by raising the mattress 30 degrees (do not use pillow); avoid drafts; do not overdress the baby; use only medications prescribed by a physician (do not use nose drops, since aspiration may result in lung involvement); cover the upper lip with a light film of petrolatum to minimize excoriation from nasal secretions.

Elimination. Review the following:

1. Changes to be expected in the color of the stool and the number of bowel evacuations, plus the odor of stools for breast- or bottle-fed infants.
2. The color of normal urine and the number of voidings to expect each day.

Safety. Review the need for the following:

1. Protecting the infant from trauma; for example, keeping objects such as pins and scissors closed and well out of baby's reach. When infant clothes are purchased, the type of closure used should be considered. A front button can easily be pulled off and swallowed. Even though a young infant may not search for buttons or other small objects now, practicing this good habit from the beginning prevents future injuries.
2. Preventing overheating or chilling.
3. Care in transporting infants, particulary in automobiles (Fig. 22-21).
4. Supervising brothers' and sisters' attention to the new baby.

Pacifiers/Thumbsucking. Sucking is the infant's chief pleasure. It may not be satisfied by breast-or formula-feeding (Whaley and Wong, 1987). It is such a strong need that infants who are deprived of sucking, such as those with a cleft lip repair, will suck on their tongue. Some newborns are born with sucking pads on their fingers that developed from in utero sucking activity. Several benefits of nonnutritive sucking have been documented, such as increased weight gain in premature infants and decreased crying (Anderson, 1986).

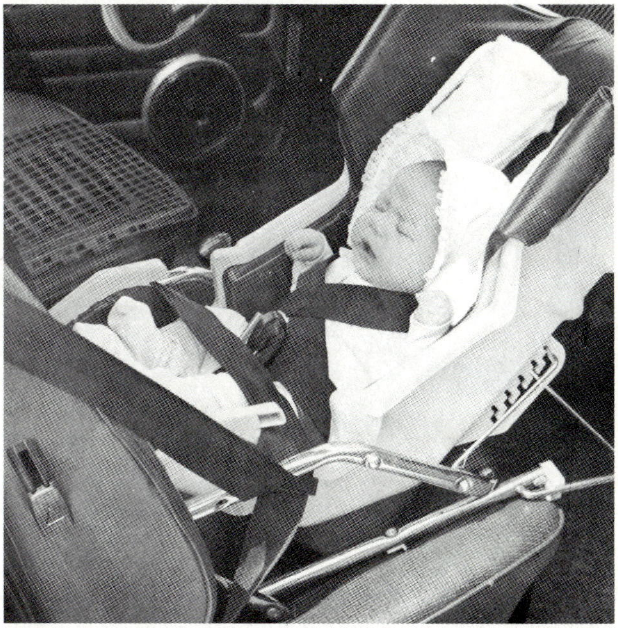

Fig. 22-21 Rearward-facing shell car seat. Infant is placed in car seat when going home from hospital.

From Whaley, LF, and Wong, DL: Nursing care of infants and children, ed 3, St Louis, 1987, The CV Mosby Co.

Problems arise when parents are concerned about sucking of fingers, thumb, or pacifier and attempt to restrain this natural tendency. Before giving advice, nurses investigate the parents' feelings and base guidance on this information. For example, some parents may see no problem with the use of a finger but may find the use of a pacifier repulsive. In general, there is no need to restrain either unless thumb sucking persists past 4 years of age or past the time when the permanent teeth erupt. Parents are advised to work with their pediatrician and pediatric nurse-practitioner about this topic.

To decrease dependence on nonnutritive sucking, sucking pleasure can be increased by prolonging feeding time. A small-holed, firm nipple causes stronger sucking and slower feeding. Also the parent's excessive use of the pacifier to calm the child should be explored. It is not unusual for parents to place a pacifier in the infant's mouth as soon as crying begins, thus reinforcing a pattern of distress-relief (Whaley and Wong, 1987). If the child uses a pacifier, safety considerations in purchasing one must be stressed (Fig. 22-22). A home-made or poorly designed pacifier can be dangerous because the entire object may be aspirated if it is small, or a portion may become detached from the handle and become lodged in the pharynx. Improvised pacifiers, such as those commonly made in hospitals from a padded nipple, also present dangers. The nipple may separate from the plastic collar and be aspirated (Millunchick and McArtor, 1986). In addition, parents may continue to offer this pacifier to the infant at home. Safe pacifiers should be of one-piece construction, have a shield or flange that is large enough to prevent entry into the mouth, and have a handle that can be grasped.

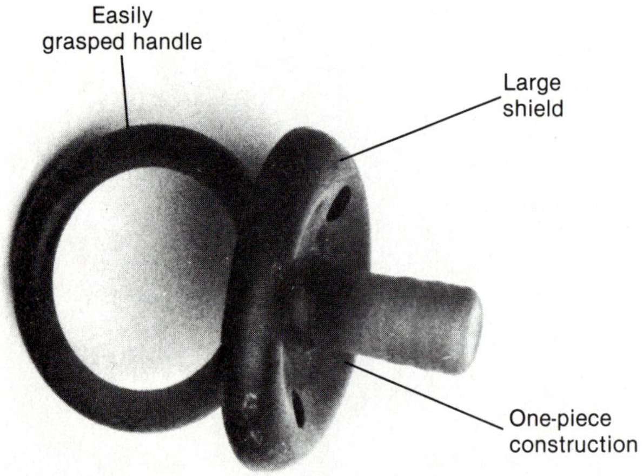

Fig. 22-22 Design of a safe pacifier.
From Whaley, LF, and Wong, DL: Nursing care of infants and children, ed 3, St Louis, 1987, The CV Mosby Co.

Immunizations. Review schedule for immunizations. The *ability* to protect against antigens by formation of antibodies *develops sequentially.* The fetus or infant must be developmentally capable of responding to antigens. This is the reason for planning sequential immunizations in infants. See Appendix J. A form of passive immunity is present in colostrum and breast milk. It is specific for microbial agents present in the mother's own gastrointestinal tract. As the newborn is being freshly colonized, *these antibodies limit bacterial growth in the gastrointestinal tract and protect against overgrowth* (see also Chapter 6). This information helps health care professionals plan for the use of polio vaccine in breast-fed infants. According to Korones (1986):

> Oral polio vaccine depends, for its effectiveness, on multiplication in the intestinal tract. The vaccine fails to immunize babies on breast milk from mothers with high antibody titers to poliovirus because vaccine virus is inactivated in the gut by secretory IgA from breast milk.

Infant Follow-up Care. Plan for infant health follow-up care, that is, at 2 to 4 weeks of age, then every 2 months until 6 to 7 months of age, then every 3 months until 18 months, at 2 years, 3 years, preschool, and every 2 years thereafter.

The newborn's record serves as a documented means of communication among all members of the health-care team. The record contains accurate and complete recordings of the history, physical examination, and laboratory test results, sequential observations, goals, interventions, and the newborn's responses. The record should be readily accessible to the health-care professionals caring for the infant and family. Documentation of the parent's health education, counseling, and responses to information are included. These data provide valuable information for the pediatrician and nurse for the infant's follow-up care and serve as a reservoir for data for future research.

Application of the nursing process when the newborn exhibits symptoms of mucus and molding is demonstrated in the specific nursing care plan that follows.

Specific Nursing Care Plan

NEWBORN WITH MUCUS AND "CONE HEAD"

Carol is a 24-year-old, married woman who gave birth to her first child, a term baby girl weighing 3500 g (7 lb 12 oz). Carol's labor progressed smoothly over 12 hours and she had a spontaneous vaginal delivery without complication. The parents were pleased their daughter could remain in Carol's room. About 4 hours after delivery, Carol called the nurse because the infant was "gagging, spitting up, and was a little blue." After the infant's immediate care was completed, Carol commented about the infant's "poor little cone head."

ASSESSMENT	NURSING DIAGNOSIS (ND)/ PLAN (P)/GOAL (G)	RATIONALE/ IMPLEMENTATION	EVALUATION
Child is gagging and regurgitating mucus.	ND: Ineffective airway clearance (potential) related to excess secretions. P: Facilitate removal of secretions. G: Infant will maintain open airway.	*To ensure maintenance of a clear airway, the nurse will:* Hold infant face downward with head slightly lowered and aspirate mouth and nose with bulb syringe. Position child on side to facilitate drainage from mouth.	

Specific Nursing Care Plan

ASSESSMENT	NURSING DIAGNOSIS (ND)/ PLAN (P)/GOAL (G)	RATIONALE/ IMPLEMENTATION	EVALUATION
		Note efficiency of cough, sneeze, gag, and swallow to maintain clear airway.	Child maintains clear airway.
		Assess breath sounds.	
		Evaluate for signs of respiratory distress.	Child remains free of respiratory distress.
		Comfort infant after a bout of gagging and regurgitation.	
Parents concerned about child's gagging and regurgitation of mucus.	ND: Potential for altered parenting related to lack of understanding of this neonatal characteristic and its management. P: Increase parent's coping through information and demonstration. G: Parents will learn about cause and management of gagging and regurgitation.	*To teach parents about the normal physiologic processes and to learn skill of keeping airway clear the nurse will:* Explain the physiologic processes (second period of reactivity). Reassure parents that gagging, coughing, and sneezing are normal and expected to clear infant's airway. Assist parents in positioning child in ways that promote drainage of secretions. Demonstrate and encourage practice with positioning and use of bulb syringe.	Parents verbalize understanding of instruction. Parents demonstrate skill in helping infant keep a clear airway.
Parents verbalize concern about infant's "cone head".	ND: Knowledge deficit related to the normal molding during the birth process. P: Provide information. G: Parents will learn about normal molding.	*To teach the client about the molding process and evaluate the child's head, the nurse will:* Explain the process of molding and its purpose in a successful vaginal delivery.	Parents verbalize understanding of molding.
		Reassure parents that the child's head will resume its normal shape within a few days.	Child's head will resume rounded shape within a few days.
		Measure, evaluate, and record the child's head circumference within the first hours of life, and again in two days, for baseline growth assessment.	
		Evaluate child's head for soft tissue edema or bruising, and document.	If edema or bruising of the head is present, these areas will resolve within a maximum of six weeks and the child's head circumference will grow within normal limits.

Evaluation

Evaluation is a continuous process. To be effective, it needs to be based on measurable criteria, which reflect the parameters used to measure the goals for care. Parental skill in infant caretaking techniques and their knowledge of their infant's needs and growth patterns form the context in which newborn care is given.

SUMMARY

The care the newborn receives in the first months of life is reflected in the normal growth and development of a healthy infant. The nurse in the various roles as teacher and support person acts as an advocate for the vulnerable infant. The nurse's skills in caring for the newborn and teaching these skills to parents are of paramount importance. Nurses are present during the formative stages of parent-child interactions. From their unique perspective they can do much to help both parents and child.

KEY CONCEPTS

- Assessment of the newborn requires data from the prenatal, intranatal, and postnatal periods.
- Knowledge of the biologic and behavioral characteristics is essential for guiding assessment and interpreting data.
- Providing a protective environment is a key role for the nurse that includes such actions as careful identification procedures, restraining techniques, measures to prevent infection, and support of physiologic functions.
- Maintenance of adequate ventilation includes ensuring an adequate airway and body temperature.
- Each nurse must develop skill in CPR and relieving airway obstruction.
- Parent education is a major role for the nurse and includes involving parents in all phases of the nursing process.
- Circumcision is an elective surgical procedure.
- The newborn has social, as well as physical, needs.
- Whether or not this is the couple's first baby, parents appreciate anticipatory guidance in the care of their child.

STUDY QUESTIONS AND ACTIVITIES

1. Observe or assist in the physical and behavioral assessment of an infant immediately following birth, on admission to the nursery, and during routine assessment.
2. Observe an experienced nurse instruct and explain the behavioral assessment of an infant to the parents.
3. Develop a written plan of care for an infant and her or his parents using a nursing diagnosis as the focus.
4. Practice restraining an infant by several methods.
5. Prepare and teach one class in infant care to parents.
6. Practice the manipulation of various types of equipment found in the newborn nursery.
7. Role-play a nurse caring for and educating a mother during a routine assessment of the infant after discharge from the hospital; include proper attention to one of the following problems:
   a. Skin problems show that the infant is not being bathed properly.
   b. Interactions of siblings with the newborn show that they have not accepted the necessity for correct handling and attitudes toward the newborn.
   c. The mother shows a lack of knowledge concerning the newborn's jaundice.
   d. The mother quotes family members regarding proper care of the umbilicus; the infant is wearing a flannel belly band.
8. Rehearse neonatal CPR and clearing of an airway obstruction in the laboratory setting.

References

American Academy of Pediatrics, Committee on Fetus and Newborn: Report of the Ad Hoc Task Force on Circumcision, Pediatrics 56:610, 1975

Anderson, G: Pacifiers: the positive side, MCN 11(2):122, 1986

Committee on Accidents and Poison Prevention, American Academy Pediatrics: Revised first aid for the choking child, Pediatrics 78:177, 1986

Edelstein, J: The effect of nursing intervention with the Brazelton Neonatal Behavioral Assessment Scale on postpartum adjustment and maternal perception of the infant, unpublished masters thesis, 1975

Field, R, et al: Mother's assessments of the behavior of their infants, Infant Beh Dev 1:156, 1978

Gearhart, J, and Callan, N: Complications of newborn circumcision, Contemp OB/GYN 27:57, Jan 1986

Henningsson, A, et al: Bathing or washing babies after birth, Lancet 2:1401, Dec 1981

Kirya, C, and Werthmann, M: Neonatal circumcision and penile dorsal nerve block: a painless procedure, J Pediatr 92:998, June 1978

Korones, SG: High-risk newborn infants: the basis for intensive care, ed 4, St Louis, 1986, The CV Mosby Co

Millunchick, E, and McArtor, R: Fatal aspiration of a makeshift pacifier, Pediatrics 77(3):369, 1986

Mofenson, HC, et al: Baby powder—a hazard! Pediatrics 68(2):265, 1981

Murray, AD, et al: Effects of epidural anesthesia on newborns and their mothers, Child Dev 52(1):71, 1981

NAACOG: Nurses' role in neonatal circumcision, OGN Nursing Practice Resource 14:3, 1985a

NAACOG: Neonatal skin care, OGN Nursing Practice Resource 12:3, March 1985b

NAACOG: CDC reports caution about AIDS virus, NAACOG Newsletter 13(6): June 1986

Nursing '87 Books: 1987 Nursing photobook annual, Springhouse, Penn, 1987, Springhouse Corp

Pritchard, JA MacDonald, and Gant: Williams obstretics, ed 17, New York, 1985, Appleton-Century-Crofts

Speck, WT: Jaundice and phototherapy: Wonder where the yellow went? Paper presented at "The Fetus and the Newborn," Contemporary Forums, San Diego, 1985

Standards for Cardiopulmonary Resuscitation (CPR) and Emergency Cardiac Care (ECC): Part IV. Pediatric basic life support, JAMA 255(21):2954, 1986

Whaley, LF, and Wong, DL: Nursing care of infants and children, ed 3, St Louis, 1987, The CV Mosby Co

Witchell, M: The circumcision decision and the role of the health provider, ICEA News 24(3):4, 1985

Bibliography

Anderson, CJ: Enhancing reciprocity between mother and neonate, Nurs Res 30(2):89, 1981

Avery, M, et al: An early postpartum hospital discharge program: implementation and evaluation, JOGN Nurs 11:200, 1982

Axnic, K, and Yarborough, M: Infection control: an integrated approach, St Louis, 1984, The CV Mosby Co

Baker, SP, and Fisher, RS: Childhood asphyxiation by choking or suffocation, JAMA 244(12):1343, 1980

Bampton, B, Jones, J, and Mancini, J: Initial mothering patterns of low-income black primiparas, JOGN Nurs 10:174, 1981

Barnard, KE, et al: Early parent-infant relationship, White Plains, NY, 1978, The National Foundation, March of Dimes

Boyer, D: Routine circumcision of the newborn: reasonable precaution or unnecessary risk? J Nurse Midwife 25(6):27, 1980

Bull, M, and Lawrence, D: Mothers' use of knowledge during the first postpartum weeks, JOGN Nurs 14(4):315, 1985

Bullongh, VL, and Bullongh, B: Sexuality from the neonate to the adolescent, Pediatr Basics, Gerber Number 48, p 2, 1987

Consullo, M, et al: An instrument for the measurement of infant-adult synchrony, Nurs Res 36(4):244, 1987

Crawford, J: A theoretical model of support network conflict experienced by new mothers, Nurs Res 34:100, March/April 1985

Cronenwett, LR: Parental network structured and perceived support after birth of first child, Nurs Res 34:347, Nov/Dec 1985b

DelGiudice, GT: The relationship between sibling jealousy and presence at a sibling's birth, Birth 13(4):250, 1986

Dodge, J: When childbirth is a family affair, RN 48(12):20, 1985

Dunn, DM, and White, DG: Interactions of mothers with their newborns in the first half-hour of life, J Adv Nurs 6:271, 1981

Ellison, S, et al: Sucking in the newborn infant during the first hour of life, J Nurse Midwife 24(6):18, 1979

Eoff, M, et al: Temperature measurements in infants, Nurs Res 23:457, 1974

Färdig, J: A comparison of skin-to-skin contact and radiant heaters in promoting neonatal thermoregulation, J Nurse Midwife 25(1):19, 1980

Finholdt, D, et al: The heart is under the lower third of the sternum, Am J Dis Child 140:646, 1986

Fuller, RZ: Upper respiratory obstruction in the neonate: a case of neonatal rhinitis Pediatr Nurs 14(1):30, 1988

Gibbons, MB: Circumcision: the controversy continues, Pediatr Nurs 10(2):103, 1984

Goebel, JB et al: Infant car seat usage: effectiveness of a postpartum education program, JOGN Nurs 13:33, 1984

Goodwin, BA: Pediatric resuscitation, Crit Care Nurs Q 10(4):69, 1988

Harpin, VA, and Rutter, N: Barrier properties of the newborn infant's skin, J Pediatr 102(3):419, 1983

Harvey, K: Mother-baby nursing, Nurs Management 13(7):22, 1982

Herrera, AJ, et al: Parental information and circumcision in highly motivated couples with higher education, Pediatrics 71:233, 1983

Hiser, PL: Concerns of multiparas during the second postpartum week, JOGN Nurs 1(5):195, 1987

Hutton, N, and Schreiner, R: Urine collection in the neonate: effect of different methods on volume, specific gravity, and glucose, JOGN Nurs 9(13):165, 1980

Jaundiced babies bloom with home phototherapy, Clin News 84(7):871, 1984

Judd, JM: Assessing the newborn from head to toe, Nursing '85 15(12):34, 1985

Kesselman, S: Circumcision reconsidered: neither harmless nor healthful, routine circumcision no longer seems justified, Childbirth Educator 1(3):43, 1982

Kowba, MD, and Schwirian, PM: Direct sibling contact and bacterial colonization in newborns. JOGN Nurs 14:412, Sept/Oct 1985

Krozy, RE, et al: Auto safety, pregnancy and the newborn, JOGN Nurs 14:1, Jan/Feb 1985

Kunst-Wilson, W, and Cronewett, LR: Nursery care for the emerging family: promoting paternal behavior, Res Nurs Health 4:201, 1981

Locklin, M: Assessing jaundice in full-term newborns, Pediatr Nurs 13(1):15, 1987

Lowrey, G: Growth and development in children, ed 8, Chicago, 1986, Year Book Medical Publishers, Inc

Maisals, MJ, et al: Circumcision: the effect of information on parental decision, Pediatrics 71:453, 1983

Marecki, M, et al: Early sibling attachment, JOGN Nurs 14:418, Sept/Oct 1985

McFadden, R: Decreasing the infant's respiratory compromise during suctioning, Am J Nurs 81(12):2148, 1981

Mercer, RT: Parent-infant attachment. In Sonstegard, LJ, et al, editors: Women's health, vol 2, Childbearing, New York, 1982, Grune & Stratton, Inc

Merrifield, EB, and Ryberg, JW: What parents should know about pacifiers, Child Nurse 3(4):1, 1985

Orlowski, J: Optimum position for external cardiac compression in infants and young children, Ann Emerg Med 15:667, 1986

Pelosi, MA, and Apuzzio, J: Making circumcision safe and painless, Contemp OB/GYN 24(1):42, 1984

Perry, D: The umbilical cord: transcultural care and custom, J Nurse Midwife 27(4):25, 1982

Perry, SE: Parents' perceptions of their newborn following structured interactions, Nurs Res 32(4):208, 1983

Queenan, JT, moderator: Managing pregnancy in patients over 35, Contemp OB/GYN 29(5):180, 1987

Reid, T: Newborn cyanosis, Am J Nurs 82(8):1230, 1982

Riesch, S, and Munns, S: Promoting awareness: the mother and her baby, Nurs Res 33:271, Sept/Oct 1985

Roberts, FB: Infant behavior and the transition to parenthood, Nurs Res 32(4):213, 1983

Rödholm, M: The behavior of human male adults at their first contact with a newborn. Unpublished doctoral dissertation. Department of Psychology, University of Goteberg, Goteberg, Sweden, 1981

Rutledge, DL, and Pridham, KF: Postpartum mothers' perceptions of competence for infant care, JOGN Nurs 16(3):185, 1987

Saco-Pollitt, C: Birth in the Peruvian Andes: physical and behavioral consequences in the neonate, Child Dev 52(3):839, 1981

Schiffman, RF: Temperature monitoring in the neonate: a comparison of axillary and rectal temperatures, Nurs Res 31(5):274, 1982

Shibley, B: Now newborns can stay home for phototherapy, RN p 69, Feb 1988
Stainton, MC: Parent-infant interaction: putting theory into practice, Calgary, Alberta, Canada, 1981, University of Calgary Faculty of Nursing
Stainton, MC: Maternal newborn attachment origins and processes, III. Interactional synchrony: the prelude to attachment, doctoral thesis, University of California, San Francisco, 1985
Stang, HJ, et al: Local anesthesia for neonatal circumcision: effects on distress and cortisol response, JAMA 259(10):1507, 1988
Strohback, ME, and Kratina, S: Diaper versus bag specimens: a comparison of urine specific gravity values, MCN 7(3):198, 1982
Tedder, JL: Newborn circumcision, JOGN Nurs 16(1):42, 1987
Tobiason, S: Touching is for everyone, Am J Nurs 81(4):728, 1981
Vanderzanden, E: Anticipatory guidance for the first two months of life, J Nurse Midwife 24(5):28, 1979
Wagner, TJ, and Hindi-Alexander, M: Hazards of baby powder? Pediatr Nurs 10(2):124, 1984
Walker, LO, Crain, H, and Thompson, E: Mothering behavior and maternal role attainment during the postpartum period, Nurs Res 35(6):352, 1986
Wallerstein, E: Circumcision: an American health fallacy, New York, 1980, Springer Publishing Co, Inc
Walz, BL: Maternal tasks of taking on a second child in the postpartum period, Maternal Child Nurs J 12(3):185, 1983
Wayland, J, and Higgins, P: Neonatal circumcision: a teaching plan to better inform parents, Nurse Pract 7(6):26, 1982
Winslow, W: First pregnancy after 35: what is the experience? MCN 12(2):92, 1987
Wranesh, B: The effect of sibling visitation on bacterial colonization rate in neonate, JOGN Nurs 11(4):211, 1982
Yu, V: Body position and gastric emptying, Arch Dis Child 50:500, 1975

CHAPTER 23

Newborn Nutrition and Feeding

Learning Objectives

Correctly define the key terms listed.

Evaluate nutrient needs in relation to infant's growth and development during the first few months of life.

Identify factors that affect parent and newborn readiness for feeding.

Compare nutrition supplements recommended for the breast-fed and formula-fed infant.

Review the physiology of lactation in relation to breast development, stages of lactation, and maternal breast-feeding reflexes.

Explore cultural aspects of breast-feeding.

Formulate nursing diagnoses relative to the infant's nutritional status and the parents' needs and preferences.

Examine breast-feeding in relation to advantages, care of breasts, diet and fluids, infant responses, secretion of drugs in milk, maintaining a job, and infant-related and maternal-related concerns.

Discuss formula-feeding.

Develop guidelines for client teaching for breast-feeding, formula-feeding, and formula preparation.

Key Terms

bottle-feeding
breast massage
colostrum
demand feeding
engorgement
extrusion reflex
failure to thrive
feeding reflexes
formula preparation (terminal heating and aseptic methods)
growth
lactation
lactoferrin
lactogenesis
let-down reflex
manual expression of milk
milk ejection
milk secretion
nipple erection reflex
plugged ducts
prolactin reflex
pumping the breasts
readiness for feeding
rooting reflex
sore nipples
sucking reflex
suckling process
supplemental feeding
swallowing reflex
water intoxication
weaning

Skillful health supervision of infants requires knowledge of their nutritional needs. The adage that "as the twig is bent the tree's inclined" is appropriate when considering nutrition experiences in infancy and possible health consequences in later life. This chapter focuses on nutrition needs for normal growth and development from birth to 3 months. Breast-feeding and bottle-feeding are addressed.

INFANT DEVELOPMENT AND NUTRITION NEEDS

Growth and Development

Discussion of the child's growth pattern is often the starting point for effective communication with parents regarding proper nutrition for their child.

Weight, Length, and Head Circumference. The full-term infant will generally double the birth weight by the age of 5 months and triple it in 1 year. The small reduction in birth weight experienced by newborns the first few days after birth is regained by most full-term infants within 10 days. Weight loss of up to 10% is acceptable without concern, with small infants losing proportionately less than larger ones.

Length increases about 50% during the first year. Doubling of birth length does not occur until about 4 years of age. Head circumference also increases rapidly during the first year in conjunction with rapid growth of the brain.

Body Fat. At birth the normal infant has a body composed of about 16% fat (by weight). Between 2 and 6 months of age, the increase in adipose tissue is more than twice as great as the increase in muscle mass; fat deposition occurs at a steady pace until about 9 months of age. Throughout infancy, girls add a greater percentage of weight as fat than boys do; this trend continues throughout the remaining developmental years.

Growth Charts. To assist in the clinical evaluation of physical growth of children in the United States, growth "standards." or "norms," have been developed for height or length, body weight, and head circumference.

Comparison of the measurements for an individual child against the National Center for Health Statistics (NCHS) percentiles indicates where the child ranks relative to all contemporary American children of the same age and sex (Hamill et al., 1979). Measurements outside the extreme percentiles may indicate nutritional problems sufficiently severe to affect growth. On the other hand, measurements within the control or intermediate percentiles indicate that growth is within normal limits by current standards.

Readiness for Feeding

Healthy term neonates are capable of ingesting and digesting selected foods. They also possess the social capabilities necessary to elicit and maintain the mother's interest in feeding them.

Digestive System. All the secretions of the infant's digestive tract contain enzymes especially suited to the digestion of human milk. The ability to handle foods other than milk depends on the physiologic development of the infant. The capacities for salivary, gastric, pancreatic, and intestinal digestion increase with age, indicating what may be a natural pattern for introduction of various solid foods (Table 23-1).

Renal System. Kidney function of the full-term infant is not completely mature. Well-developed glomeruli filter the blood presented to the kidneys satisfactorily. The tubules, which are functionally less mature, are somewhat limited in their ability to resorb water and some solutes. Therefore it is important that the kidneys not be presented with excess solutes (renal solute load) to excrete. For this reason

Table 23-1 *Digestion in Infancy: Birth to 3 Months*

Location	Function	Effect on Feeding
Salivary	Lactose is not produced in salivary secretions; amylase not available in significant quantities.	Salivary enzymes play no role in digestion of milk.
Gastric	Hydrochloric acid (HCl) and pepsin precipitate casein into curds; separate and acidify whey protein.	Protein digestion begins; lactose ($C_{12}H_{22}O_{11}$) digestion partly begins; fat is not digested in stomach.
Pancreatic and intestinal	Pancreatic and intestinal enzymes digest proteins into amino acids, reduce carbohydrate to monosaccharides, and split fatty acids from triglycerides in the small intestine.	Protein from human milk is 95% digested, and a similar percentage of protein is digested from commercial formulas that are heat treated and sufficiently dilute to produce a soft curd.
	Disaccharidases are present in border of the intestinal mucosa.	Lactose in human milk and lactose or other carbohydrates in commercial formulas are digested in intestinal mucosa.
	Pancreatic amylase is present in small quantities.	Complex carbohydrates are poorly used.
	Pancreatic lipase is present in sufficient quantity.	A total of 80% of human milk fat is digested at birth, and almost 95% is digested by 1 month.
	Lipase, naturally found in human milk, is activated by bile salts.	Digestion of fats from commercial formulas equals that of human milk; fat from other sources (butterfat) is poorly digested.

Modified from Willis, NH: Infant nutrition, birth to 3 months: a syllabus, Philadelphia, 1980, JB Lippincott Co.

protein beyond that needed for growth and the extra sodium sometimes added to foods as sodium chloride (NaCl) should be avoided.

The percentage of body water decreases from 75% at birth to 60% at 1 year of age. This reduction is almost entirely in extracellular water. The ability to retain body water through kidney function improves in the early months of life. To the infant this means that risk of dehydration decreases as renal concentrating capacity becomes better.

Neuromuscular System. The development of feeding behavior depends on the maturation of the central nervous system (CNS) (Table 23-2). The rooting, sucking, and swallowing reflexes are present in the term neonate. The infant also has an extrusion reflex that automatically pushes food out of the mouth when it is placed on the tongue. Between 3 and 6 months of age the extrusion reflex becomes less pronounced.

Psychosocial Development. Early emotional, psychologic, and social attachment of the mother to the infant may determine future aspects of the infant's personality. Feeding is the main means by which the newborn establishes a human relationship with the mother (parent). Development of trust is built on the close relationship between mother and infant. If the infant's needs are satisfied through food and love, a sense of trust is developed between the child and the mother. Food becomes the infant's means of bringing her or his mother and her or his world together. The newborn communicates by vigorous and sustained crying to express hunger, thirst, pain, and discomfort.

The mother's feeding practices from birth, whether breast-feeding or formula-feeding, determine the infant's exposure to tactile stimulation. This stimulation is essential to the infant's physical and emotional growth (Table 23-2).

Energy Needs (Calories)

The energy requirements of the infant may be considered in three areas: (1) the basal energy requirement that sustains organ metabolic function, (2) the energy needed for physical activity, and (3) the energy needed for growth. During the first 4 months of life 50% of the infant's energy is expended for basal metabolism, 25% for physical activity and other maintenance functions, and 25% for growth.

During the first year energy allowances range from 120 kcal/kg at birth to 100 kcal/kg at the end of the year (Food and Nutrition Board, 1980). The recommended daily dietary allowance (RDA) for energy is therefore stated as ap-

Table 23-2 *Neuromuscular and Psychosocial Development: Birth to 3 Months*

Neuromuscular	Psychosocial	Implication for Feeding
Month 1		
Sucking and swallowing reflexes are present at birth; stimulus in mouth leads to rhythmic sucking and swallowing pattern; tongue protrusion predominates.	Early emotional, psychologic, and social attachment of mother and infant may determine future aspects of infant's personality. Mother's feeding practices determine exposure to tactile stimulation, which is essential to infant's physical and emotional growth.	Oral reflex is a definite adaptive food-seeking reflex for survival. On reaching satiety, infant withdraws head from breast or bottle and falls asleep. If infant's needs are satisfied through food and love, trust is developed between child and mother. Feedings are main means by which infant establishes human relationship with mother.
Month 2		
Corners of mouth are well approximated but not active in sucking; open gap separates lateral portions of lips. Tonic grasp is disappearing.	Strong emotional bond develops between mother and infant and can be viewed as beginning of social interaction of infant.	Infant is individual who shapes her or his own behavior and feeding schedule. Infant learns to equate mother with food. Infant eats about 5 times each day and may sleep through night.
Month 3		
Lip movement begins to refine; lower lip pulls in; infant may smack lips. Tongue protrusion, still present, but infant may swallow with less protrusion. Infant can hold onto object without focusing on it. By end of third month, control of head and eyes is achieved.	More tactile stimulation exists with breast-fed infant. Basic trust factor (if established) is manifested in infant's responses to mother. Infant ceases to cry with hunger when mother approaches. Infant stares into mother's face while feeding and shows response to human voice.	Infant recognizes bottle or breast as source of food. Milk runs out of sides of mouth when nipple is withdrawn. Infant still does not readily accept cup.

Modified from Owen, AL, et al: Infant feeding guide, Bloomfield, NJ, 1980, Health Learning Systems, Inc.

proximately 115 kcal/kg (52 kcal/lb) for the first 6 months and 105 kcal/kg (47 kcal/lb) for the second half of the year. During the first 4 months about one third of the energy (calories) is used for growth. Both human milk and infant formulas supply approximately 67 kcal/dl (20 kcal/oz); thus 720 ml (24 oz) of human milk formula will supply about 480 kcal.

Fluid Needs

The fluid requirement for normal infants is about 105 ml (3.5 oz)/kg/24 hours. This amount is usually consumed from the breast or in properly prepared formulas. Infants receiving this amount of water have approximately 100 ml/24 hours available for secretion of urine.

Water intoxication resulting in hyponatremia, weakness, restlessness, nausea, vomiting, diarrhea, polyuria or oliguria, and convulsions can result from excessive feeding of water to infants (David et al., 1981). This also may occur when water is fed as a replacement for milk (Partridge et al., 1981). In one reported case, water intoxication resulted from an infant swallowing too much water while swimming in the home pool (Knopp and Schwartz, 1982).

Nutrient Needs

Protein. The protein requirement is greater per unit of body weight in the newborn than at any other time of life. The RDA for protein during the first 6 months is 2.2 g/kg.

The *protein* content of human milk, lower than that of unmodified cow's milk, is sufficient for the infant. Human milk contains far more lactalbumin in relation to casein, which reduces the amount of potential curd formation in the gut of the infant. The *amino acid* composition of human milk is ideally suited to the newborn infant's metabolic capabilities. For example, phenylalanine and methionine levels are low and cystine and taurine levels are high.

Fat. For infants to acquire adequate calories from the limited amount of milk or formula they are able to consume, at least 15% of the calories provided must come from fat. The fat must be easily digestible. Fecal loss of fat and therefore of energy may be excessive if whole or evaporated milk without added carbohydrate is fed to infants.

Fat in human milk is easier to digest and absorb than that in cow's milk. This is caused in part by the arrangement of fatty acids on the glycerol molecule. It also is related to the natural lipase activity present in non-heat-treated human milk.

Carbohydrate. Lactose is the primary carbohydrate of milk and is the most abundant carbohydrate in the diet of infants to 6 months of age. Lactose provides calories in an easily available form. Its slow breakdown and absorption probably benefit calcium absorption. The lactose content in human milk is significantly higher than that in cow's milk.

Minerals and Vitamins. Most of the recommended minerals and vitamins are present in appropriate amounts in human milk and formula-feedings. The mineral content of cow's milk is considerably greater than that of human milk, with the exception of iron and fluoride. Although the amount of iron is low in both types of milk, the iron in human milk is much better absorbed by the infant. Another difference is the amount of calcium and phosphorus, minerals especially needed by the rapidly growing infant. Cow's milk contains more of these minerals but a lower calcium/phosphorus ratio (low calcium and high phosphorus). Because of the infant's immature regulatory mechanisms, calcium is excreted, resulting in tetany in young infants fed with whole unmodified cow's milk (Whaley and Wong, 1987). Human milk contains a smaller but more balanced proportion of these minerals and a higher calcium/phosphorus ratio, which are adequate to meet the infant's needs. Both types of milk contain adequate amounts of zinc, a mineral identified as essential to the human. However, the zinc in human milk is more readily absorbed. Both types of milk are low in fluoride and supplementation is recommended (see p. 568). There has been less concern over inadequate intakes of iodine for infants with the increase of iodine in food. Soy-based formulas for infants are fortified with iodine to counteract the effect of goitrogens (substances that cause the development of goiters, enlargement of the thyroid gland) found in soy products.

Both human and cow's milk provide adequate amounts of vitamins A and B complex. Vitamin C is low in cow's milk but higher in human milk provided the mother's intake is adequate. Vitamin D is low in human milk but adequate depending on the mother's intake and the infant's exposure to sunlight. Cow's milk and its preparations are usually fortified with vitamin D. Human milk contains only one fourth the amount of vitamin K as cow's milk, requiring supplementation at birth (see p. 568). Human milk is higher in vitamin E and will meet the infant's requirement, whereas cow's milk is low and will not meet the RDA.

PHYSIOLOGY OF LACTATION

Lactation is under the control of numerous endocrine glands, particularly the pituitary hormones prolactin and oxytocin. It is influenced by the suckling process and by maternal emotions. The establishment and maintenance of lactation in the human is determined by at least three factors:

1. The anatomic structure of the mammary gland and the development of alveoli, ducts, and nipples
2. The initiation and maintenance of milk secretion
3. The ejection or propulsion of milk from the alveoli to the nipple.

Breast Development

The female human breast, a large exocrine gland, is largely quiescent during most of the woman's life span. It is composed of about 18 segments embedded in fat and connective tissues and lavishly supplied with blood vessels, lymphatic vessels, and nerves. The *size of the breast* is largely related to the amount of fat present and *gives no indication of functional capacity.* The principal feature of mammary growth in pregnancy is a great increase in ducts and alveoli under the influence of many hormones (see

Chapter 10). Fig. 23-1 shows terminal glandular (alveolar) tissue of each lobule leading into the duct system. This eventually enlarges into lactiferous ducts and sinuses (ampullae). Lactiferous sinuses rest beneath the areola and converge at the nipple pore. Late in pregnancy there is maximum development of the lobuloalveolar system and presumably a sensitization of glandular tissue for action by prolactin. Colostrum is secreted in small amounts during the last 3 months of pregnancy.

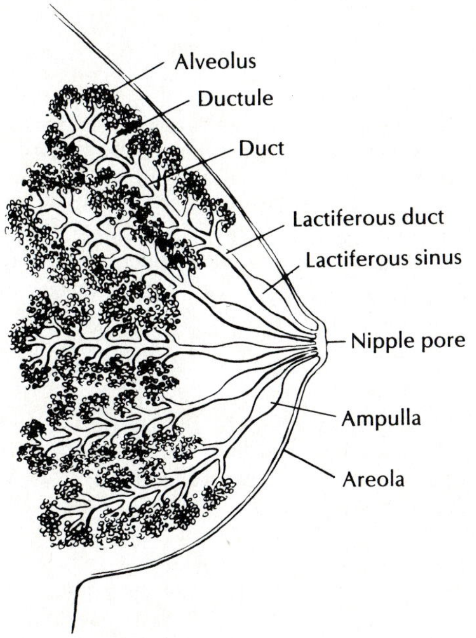

Fig. 23-1 Detailed structural features of human mammary gland.
From Worthington-Roberts, B, Vermeersch, J, and Williams, SR: Nutrition in pregnancy and lactation, ed 2, St Louis, 1981, The CV Mosby Co.

Stages of Lactation

Lactation, or more properly the process of breast-feeding, results from the interplay of (1) hormones and (2) instinctive reflexes and learned behavior of the mother and newborn.

Lactogenesis (milk initiation) commences during the latter part of pregnancy, when secretion of colostrum occurs as a result of stimulation of the mammary alveolar cells by placental lactogen, a prolactin-like substance. It continues after birth as an automatic process.

The continuing secretion of milk is mainly related to (1) sufficient production of the anterior pituitary hormone prolactin and (2) maternal nutrition. Milk secretion occurs by a process of extrusion from the cells.

Movement of milk from alveoli, where it is secreted, to the mouth of the infant is an active process within the breast. This process is brought by the let-down, or milk-ejection, reflex.

The last stage of human lactation is the ingestion of milk by the suckling baby. The full-term, healthy newborn baby possesses three instinctive reflexes needed for successful breast-feeding: the rooting, sucking, and swallowing reflexes (see Chapter 21).

Maternal Breast-feeding Reflexes

Three major maternal reflexes involved in breast-feeding are secretion of prolactin, nipple erection, and the let-down reflex.

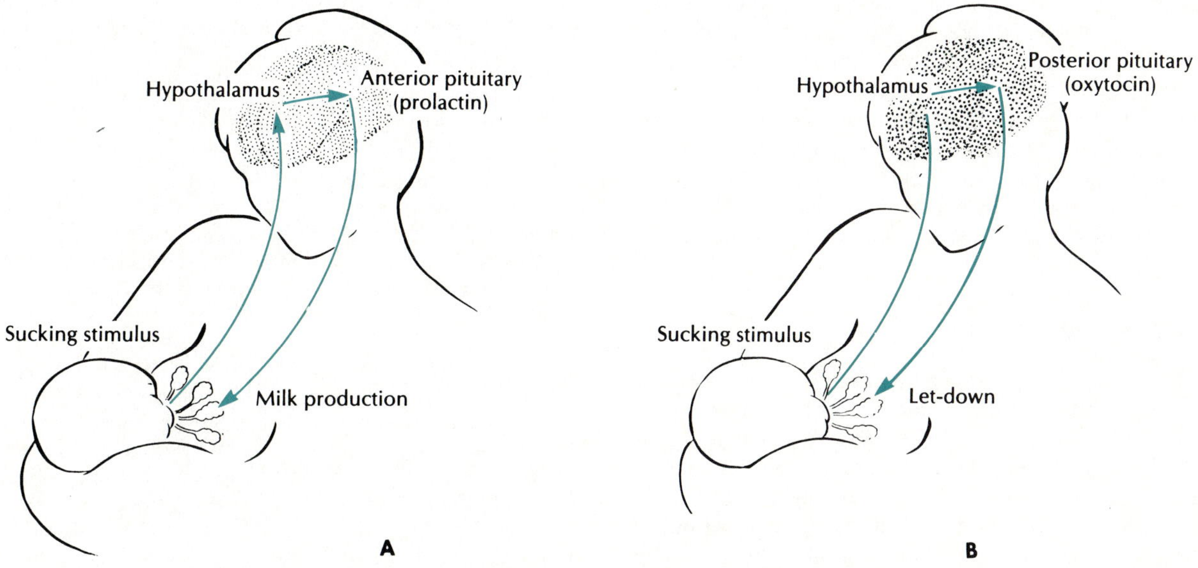

Fig. 23-2 Maternal breast-feeding reflexes. **A**, Milk production. **B**, Let down.
From Worthington-Roberts, B, Vermeesch, J, and Williams, SR: Nutrition in pregnancy and lactation, ed 2, St Louis, 1981, The CV Mosby Co.

Prolactin Reflex. Prolactin can be considered the key lactogenic hormone in initiating and maintaining milk secretion. Its production by the anterior pituitary is mainly the result of the prolactin reflex, resulting from the infant's suckling at the breast. The sucking stimulus provided by the baby sends a message to the hypothalamus. The hypothalamus stimulates the *anterior* pituitary to release **prolactin**, the hormone that promotes milk production by the alveolar cells of the mammary glands (Fig. 23-2, *A*). The amount of prolactin secreted, and hence the milk produced, are related to the amount of sucking stimulus, that is, the frequency, intensity, and duration with which the baby breast-feeds.

Nipple Erection Reflex. Stimulation of the breast nipple by the infant's mouth leads to nipple erection. The stimulation makes the nipple more prominent. This assists in the propulsion of milk through the lactiferous sinuses to the nipple pores.

Let-Down Reflex. The ejection of milk from the alveoli and milk ducts occurs as a result of the let-down, or milk-ejection reflex. The let-down reflex is regulated in part by the CNS. Fig. 23-2, *B,* illustrates the basic features of the let-down reflex. The sucking stimulus arrives at the hypothalamus, which promotes release of **oxytocin** from the *posterior* pituitary. Oxytocin stimulates contraction of the myoepithelial cells around the alveoli in the mammary glands. Contraction of these musclelike cells causes milk to be propelled through the duct system and into the lactiferous sinuses, where it becomes available to the breastfeeding infant.

The let-down reflex appears to be sensitive to small differences in circulating oxytocin levels. Signs of successful let down are easily recognized by the breast-feeding mother. Common and significant occurrences include milk dripping from the breasts before the baby starts to suckle, milk dripping from the breast opposite to the one being used, and uterine cramps during feeding, caused by the action of oxytocin on the uterus. Minor emotional and psychologic disturbances may influence the ease with which breast milk is released to the baby. The attitude of the mother toward breast-feeding (positive, doubtful, or negative) is a powerful factor in achieving successful lactation, influencing milk production, and facilitating the art of breast-feeding. Even minimal breast-feeding can be successful and rewarding for many women (see research highlight).

Cultural Aspects of Lactation

In the Philippines, if the mother's milk does not flow regularly, a meal of chicken and green papaya boiled in coconut "milk" is suggested (Hart, 1965). According to Hart (1965), the Filipino mother is also advised to eat a soup of boiled clams and ginger. Hart stated that Filipinos use hot applications of special medicinal preparations to stimulate lactation. Furthermore, the Filipino mother believes that raising either arm over her head while lying down will decrease, if not actually stop, lactation. Hart also noted the Filipino women's belief that heavy work will make their milk "hot." Korean mothers eat seaweed soup with rice to increase milk production (Chung, 1977). Currier (1978) reported that Spanish Americans believe that exposing mothers to cold diminishes the flow of milk. Yaqui women massage their breasts to drain them (Shutler, 1977).

RESEARCH HIGHLIGHT

Minimal Breast-Feeding

Purpose

To describe minimal breast-feeding patterns where mothers maintain lactation by breast-feeding once or twice a day without expressing between feedings.

Sample

This descriptive study was conducted using a convenient sample of 30 mothers who breastfed their infants once or twice a day without expressing the breasts between feedings.

Methodology

For the purpose of the study, this pattern of feeding was labeled "minimal breast-feeding." Phone interviews, using a semistructured format, were conducted every fourth week until the infant was weaned.

Findings

Three reasons were given for initiating minimal breast-feeding: (1) for convenience (e.g., return to work), (2) for comfort in nursing, and (3) as a method of weaning the infant slowly. Eleven mothers (37%) adopted minimal breast-feeding because they had a desire to involve the infant's father and to make the infant less dependent on themselves. "Comfort-nursing" was used by 8 mothers (27%). The mothers in this group appeared more relaxed and worried less about an adequate milk supply and stated that they continued to breast-feed for psychologic support of the infant rather than to provide nourishment. Mothers who used minimal breast-feeding for weaning reported a sense of completion of the breast-feeding phase rather than regret that may accompany forced weaning.

Mothers were able to manage minimal breast-feeding with little physical discomfort. They reported that their breasts adjusted to breast-feeding once or twice a day once breast-feeding was established. None of the mothers used decreased maternal fluid intake or reported complications such as mastitis, engorgement, or cracked nipples.

Implications

The investigators identified the limitations inherent in the study and made suggestions for additional research.

Working mothers reported satisfaction with "quiet time with baby." Most mothers felt completion of nursing phase at weaning rather than regret that may accompany forced weaning.

Morse, JM, et al: Minimal breastfeeding, JOGN Nurs 15(4):333, 1986.

Table 23-3 *Newborn Readiness for Feeding*

	Rationale
Newborn's age in hours or infant's age in days	During reactivity periods, excessive mucus with gagging may occur. Feeding increases the danger of aspiration. In general, reactivity times occur at birth and at 4 to 6 hours of age.
Condition at birth	Infants with Apgar scores of 6 or less (depressed) or the infant with low birth weight (2500 g or less) may display a delayed reactivity. This may occur after 12 to 18 hours of age.
Possibility of congenital anomalies of gastrointestinal or respiratory tract; incidence of congenital anomalies higher in preterm infants	With choanal atresia, the neonate is unable to breathe and feed simultaneously. With esophageal atresia, the infant will regurgitate and may aspirate. With tracheoesophageal fistula, feeding may enter trachea directly. With lower gastrointestinal tract obstruction (stenosis, atresia), regurgitation, vomiting, or abdominal distension may compromise respirations (Chapter 40).
Gastric capacity	Limited stomach capacity dictates smaller feedings. To provide adequate nutrition, feedings are scheduled more frequently.
CNS maturity	Sucking and swallowing reflexes may not be well developed and synchronized (even in a term baby, the suck and swallow reflex may not be well coordinated during first few hours).
Energy level	Premature infant or infant with respiratory distress may not have sufficient energy to divert to the process of feeding.
Type of feeding; plain sterile water	Until infant's ability to feed is assessed, danger of aspiration exists. Plain sterile water is less irritating to the respiratory tract. Formula may cause aspiration pneumonia. Glucose water may cause inflammatory response in the respiratory tract similar to response to aspirated formula.

Assessment

Feeding an infant involves the infant and the primary caregiving parent, usually the mother. Therefore both need to be assessed.

Infant

The infant is assessed for developmental readiness for feeding, nutritional needs, and success of the feeding program (Owen et al., 1980). Infant factors affecting readiness for feeding (Table 23-3) are assessed shortly after birth for the breast-fed and bottle-fed infant.

As the infant grows and matures, nutrition needs reflect the change. The infant who is obtaining the necessary nutrients and fluid will exhibit a steady increase in weight, good skin and muscle tone, vigorous feeding behavior, and satisfaction. The satisfied newborn sleeps, cries in moderation, and is interested in socializing.

Mother

The mother (couple) is assessed as follows:

1. Physical ability and psychologic readiness for feeding the newborn
2. Knowledge of the advantages of breast- and formula-feeding so an informed choice of method can be made
3. Knowledge of the infant's nutrition needs and capabilities
4. Knowledge and skill in feeding methods
5. Knowledge of an adequate and safe diet during lactation

The techniques used to assess these areas include primarily interviews, discussions, and observation of skill in feeding methods.

Nursing Diagnoses

When dietary data have been collected and analyzed, nursing diagnoses relative to the infant's nutrition status can be made. Examples include the following:

- Knowledge deficit related to
  - Normal growth and development of the infant and her or his nutritional needs
  - Feeding skills
- Situational low self-esteem related to
  - Difficulties encountered in breast-feeding

Planning

Teaching and counseling concerning the feeding of infants are part of the daily care plan for maternity clients. The benefits of both breast-feeding and formula-feeding are presented so that the mother can make an intelligent choice as to how to feed her baby. Counseling should begin in the first or second trimester of pregnancy when the mother is unrushed and has time to consider her choices.

Women are encouraged to express their opinions and feelings so that they can be discussed and any misinformation can be corrected. During the last months of pregnancy, counseling on the process of lactation is made available to women who have decided to breast-feed. Fathers are encouraged to participate in counseling sessions because their encouragement and emotional support contribute to successful lactation. Many mothers have never seen a woman breast-feeding an infant; they therefore find it especially helpful to have a woman who has successfully breast-fed an infant available to answer questions and provide reinforcement.

With the birth of the infant, the parents' choice of feeding method is accepted and supported. Feeding is an emotionally charged area of infant care. Culturally, the size and growth of an infant are equated with excellence and evidence of mothering ability. The infant who is a fussy eater can raise parental anxiety levels. The anxious parent appears to compound the problem, and a vicious cycle can develop. Relatives or friends can take over a feeding period or two. This seems to break the cycle so that the mother can view the feeding session in a more relaxed manner, not as a condemnation of her care. Mothers need positive feedback to develop a feeling of confidence in their own ability. Often just listening and praising is the most effective intervention. Tension tends to lessen milk production. The first few days the mother is home with the new baby are often filled with excitement and anxiety about mothering activities, so entertaining company or undertaking extended family commitments may have to be restricted, as the following incident illustrates.

The mother reported her 6-day-old son (2604 g [5 lb, 13 oz]) had taken 90 ml (3 oz) at 11 PM, 45 ml (1.5 oz) at 3 AM, 30 ml (1 oz) at 6 AM, and now at the 10 AM feeding, "was sleepy and seemed to want only 45 ml (1.5 oz)." The nurse suggested she keep track of the total amount taken over 24 hours. The mother interrupted to say, "I know what is wrong—yesterday all the relatives visited and held him. I think he's tired out." The nurse agreed that this could be so. She also commented on how aware the mother was of her baby's intake.

The next day the mother reported he was eating very well and noted, "I'm glad my instincts were right—it was just too busy a day for him."

Many mothers need considerable assistance with infant feeding. Both group and individual teaching are necessary. Hospitals usually provide excellent teaching aids. A sample care plan appears on p. 570.

Goals. The goals for the *infant* include the following:

1. To provide the levels and types of nutrients to support the infant's body composition, activity, and growth.
2. To minimize the physiologic stress associated with digestion, metabolism, and excretion of nutrients.
3. To supply sufficient water to maintain adequate body water control.

The goals for the *mother* (parent) include the following:

1. To provide knowledge that can be used for sound nutritional selection and feeding practices.
2. To help her become skilled in the feeding method of her choice.
3. To foster mother-child closeness and pleasure.

Implementation

Nurses act as teachers, counselors, and advocates in helping parents learn about feeding their infants. They act as change agents in motivating parents to adopt healthful eating behaviors for themselves and their families. In doing so they help parents clarify goals and make decisions. Parents need assistance in the techniques of breast- and bottle-feeding. They seek counseling for specific concerns and welcome anticipatory guidance.

Early feeding is feeding within 6 to 8 hours after birth. For the term, nonstressed newborn, early oral or parenteral feeding prevents dehydration, spares the available stores of glycogen, maintains blood glucose levels, and lessens initial weight loss. Serum bilirubin levels within normal limits often follow. Protein catabolism that would result in metabolic acidosis, hyperkalemia, or elevated BUN levels is curtailed. Energy is conserved for growth. The sucking response is stimulated.

Breast-feeding

Milk from a healthy mother is the food of choice for a healthy infant. Breast-feeding offers many advantages: nutritional, immunologic, and psychologic (Hughes, 1984). The following are some of these advantages:

1. The infant receives immunoglobulins to protect against some infections.
2. The infant usually experiences less diarrhea or constipation.
3. The type of protein ingested is less likely to cause allergic reactions.
4. The infant has fewer problems with overfeeding; the need to "empty the bottle" is eliminated.
5. Bottle washing, preparation of formula, and refrigeration are unnecessary.
6. Maternal organs return more quickly to their nonpregnant condition (Madgic, 1986).

Women who have had no contact with other mothers who breast-feed and who have had little or no contact with newborns often require considerable assistance to become proficient (Riordan, 1983). The guidelines for client teaching outline a plan for helping an inexperienced mother with the first breast-feeding session with her baby.

Immunologic Benefits. There is evidence that the newborn infant acquires certain important elements of host resistance from breast milk while maturation of her or his own immune system is taking place. Human milk contains high levels of immunoglobin A (IgA) and affords protection against several bacterial and viral diseases, especially those of the respiratory and gastrointestinal systems (Whaley and Wong, 1987).

Guidelines for Client Teaching

BREAST-FEEDING

ASSESSMENT

Primipara planning to breast-feed her infant girl who weighs 3360 g (7 ½ lb).

NURSING DIAGNOSIS

Knowledge deficit related to breast-feeding and lactation.

GOALS

Short-term

To have infant breast-feed successfully.

Intermediate

To establish a feeding pattern satisfactory to infant and mother.

Long-term

Mother able to adjust feedings to needs of newborn daughter by recognizing the infant's cues for hunger and satiety. Mother able to breast-feed successfully while maintaining chosen life-style.

REFERENCES AND TEACHING AIDS

Hospital pamphlets about infant nutrition, films on breast-feeding, posters, booklets, etc.

Text such as:

Pyle, M, RNC: Breast feeding, a family affair, Costa Mesa, Calif, 1985, Life circle.

Riordan, J: St Louis, 1983, The CV Mosby Co.

Pamphlets and books available through the La Leche League.

CONTENT/RATIONALE	TEACHING ACTIONS
To review general content tell mother: Before putting the baby to breast, I want to review some facts with you:	Fill in gaps in knowledge.
You can assume any comfortable position. Let the breast fall forward without tension. Leave one hand free to guide the nipple into the child's mouth.	Have mother experiment with positions. Have her assume the position that feels most comfortable (Fig. 23-3).
I'll review the structure of the breast. The nipple can be made more prominent by gently rolling it between your fingers. The areolar area will be put in the baby's mouth with the nipple. This prevents bruising the nipple.	Have woman expose her breast. Have woman prepare her nipple. Point out areolar tissue.
Colostrum is the yellow fluid you can express from your breasts now. It is good for the baby. It contains some fat and protein and helps baby resist infections.	Demonstrate technique for expressing milk from the breast. Have woman express some colostrum.
Milk may be expected to appear 48 to 96 hours after delivery. Before the milk comes in, the breasts feel soft to the touch. After the milk comes in, the breasts feel full and warmer.	Have woman touch breasts to feel softness.
To teach breast-feeding technique: Have mother hold the baby so that her cheek touches the breasts. The pressure against the outer angle of the lip begins the rooting reflex. The baby will turn toward the nipple. She can smell the colostrum and milk and this will also make her turn toward the nipple.	Demonstrate rooting reflex by touching finger to infant's lips and cheek.
Have woman put the baby to breast by guiding the nipple and areolar tissue into the infant's mouth and over the tongue. Compress breast with thumb above and fingers below areola to permit infant to latch on effectively.	Have the woman practice (Fig. 23-3, *A*). Tell her to avoid holding the breast like a cigarette.
To teach expected infant responses and maternal sensations tell woman: At first the baby sucks in short bursts of three to five sucks followed by single swallows. In 1 to 2 days a sucking pattern evolves. This consists of 10 to 30 sucks followed by swallowing. The infant's lips and jaws exert pressure on the areola and the tongue "cradles" the nipple so that the tip is not eroded. The pressure combined with negative intraoral pressure brings milk into the mouth (Fig. 23-4).	Bring infant to mother. Have her assess her baby's suck by placing her finger in the baby's mouth with the finger pad touching and stroking the palate. She should be able to feel the tongue cushioning the joint of the finger and stroking the finger, while keeping the gum covered. She should not feel an insecure or loose suction on the finger, or a tapping of the gum on the finger alone or combined with the tongue slipping back and forth across the gum (licking).

Continued.

A B C D

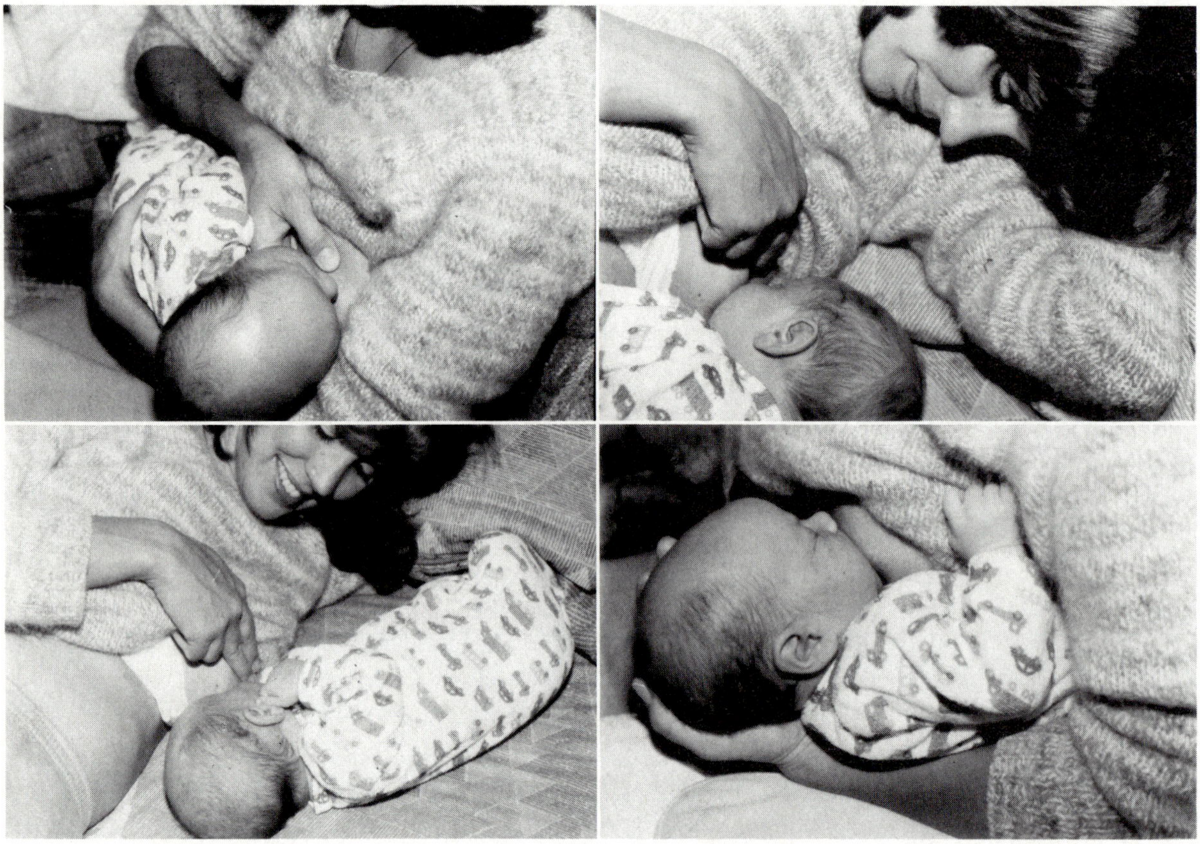

Fig. 23-3 Positioning the baby: series **A**, Cradle hold. One arm and hand supports baby. Other hand supports breast (thumb above and fingers below). Breast is guided into baby's mouth. **B**, Side-lying position. Pillows support mother's head. Baby is turned toward mother. Mother depresses breast to facilitate baby's breathing. **C**, Variation on side-lying position. **D**, Football hold. Baby is held in one arm with hand supporting head.

Courtesy Marjorie Pyle, RNC, Lifecircle, Cost Mesa, Calif.

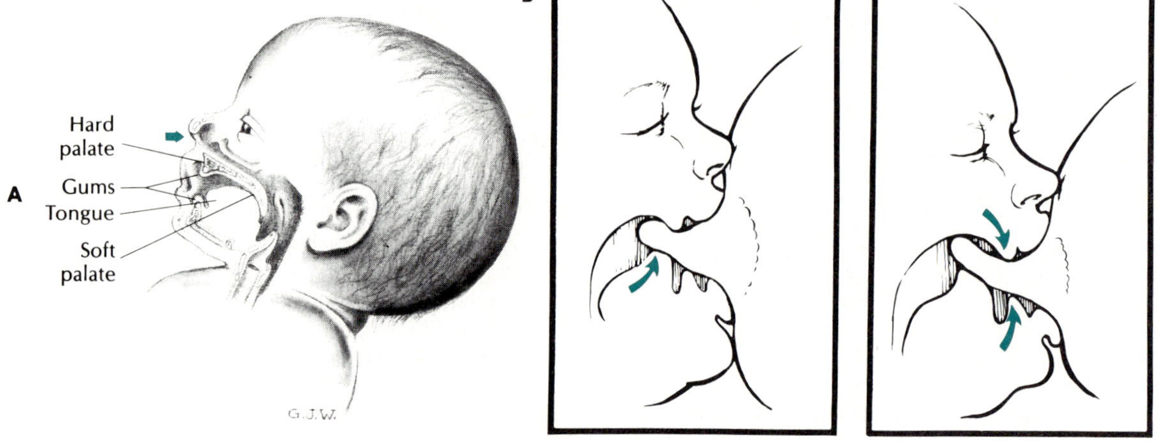

Fig. 23-4 Suckling process: **A**, Infant breathes through nose (arrow). Tongue and palate meet closing esophagus. **B**, Tongue thrusts up and forward to grasp nipple. **C**, Gums compress areola and tongue moves backward creating negative pressure for suction.

B and **C** from Riordan, J: A practical guide to breastfeeding, St Louis, 1987, The CV Mosby Co.

Guidelines for Client Teaching—cont'd

CONTENT/RATIONALE	TEACHING ACTIONS
When the baby is sucking properly, there is no "clicking" noise. This clicking noise means she is sucking on her own tongue in the back of the throat, past the nipple. You should hear the rhythmic suck-swallow breathing pattern that indicates milk is flowing. Some mothers can sense if the infant has drawn the areolar tissue into the mouth along with the nipple.	Have mother suck her own tongue at the back of the throat to hear the clicking sound.
Now let's get the baby ready and put her to breast; first making sure she is awake.	If necessary, waken the baby by stroking her cheek, rubbing her feet, and talking to her.
Now put her to breast by bringing the baby to the breast not the breast to the baby. The baby's face, chest, genitals, and knees should all be facing your body. Touch her upper lip with your nipple: see how she turns toward you and opens her mouth. Pull baby as close to you as you can (Fig. 23-3, *D*).	Help mother position baby so that the head is directly facing the breast and the nipple is not pulled to one side. Guide woman through feeding. Point out and explain sensations she is feeling.
Feel how the baby's jaws fit behind the nipple and the nipple is deep in her mouth?	
If infant needs more breathing space, lift your breast; or make a "dimple" in your breast for breathing space (Fig. 23-3, *B, C*).	Caution woman that making a "dimple" may be done too vigorously and the nipple will be dislodged.
You may need to hold your nipple throughout the entire feeding for a few weeks.	Observe technique, degree of relaxation, offer praise.
I will be back to help you put her to the other breast. It is a good idea to use both breasts at each feeding. Once the milk has come in you can tell which breast to start with next time by feeling the weight. The heaviest one has the most milk, so start with that one. In the meantime, put a safety pin on your bra on the side that you finished, so you will know which side to start out with next time.	Review need to empty both breasts since an empty breast signals woman's body to produce more milk.
To remove the baby from the breast, place a finger in the corner of the baby's mouth until the suction is broken. The breast can then be comfortably removed. I will be back in about 15 minutes or use your call bell if you need help. Leave mother to enjoy her baby.	Return in about 15 minutes to supervise mother removing baby from the breast. Remind her that breast-feeding time is not limited (L'espance and Frantz, 1985; Slaven, 1981).
Before putting the baby to the other breast I will show you how to burp her. Some babies never burp, others do frequently. Gently rub or pat the baby's back.	Demonstrate burping (Fig. 23-5). Supervise mother putting baby to other breast.
After feeding, place the baby on her right side. This allows air in stomach to come up and not bring the milk with it.	Show woman a picture of an infant on right side.

EVALUATION Mother demonstrates competency in breast-feeding.

Immunoglobulins are believed to function directly in the infant's gastrointestinal tract by diminishing antigen contact with intestinal mucosa until the infant's own antibody responses are developed. *Lactoferrin* is secreted in human milk and is believed to play a role in controlling bacterial growth in the gastrointestinal tract. It works by competing with microorganisms that require iron for replication. The presence of these factors is believed to explain the reduced incidence of illness in breast-fed babies that has been reported not only in developing countries but also in the United States.

IgA also probably protects against development of food allergies. In addition, human milk contains numerous other host defense factors, such as macrophages, granulocytes, and T- and B-lymphocytes (Hanson et al., 1985).

Care of Breasts. Daily washing of the breasts with water is sufficient for cleanliness. A lubricant such as liquid petrolatum or lanolin may then be massaged gently into the nipple area. If feasible, the breasts can be exposed to the air for 20 to 30 minutes. The lubricant should not contain alcohol, since the drying effects of the alcohol tend to encourage cracking of the tissue. Some infants object to either

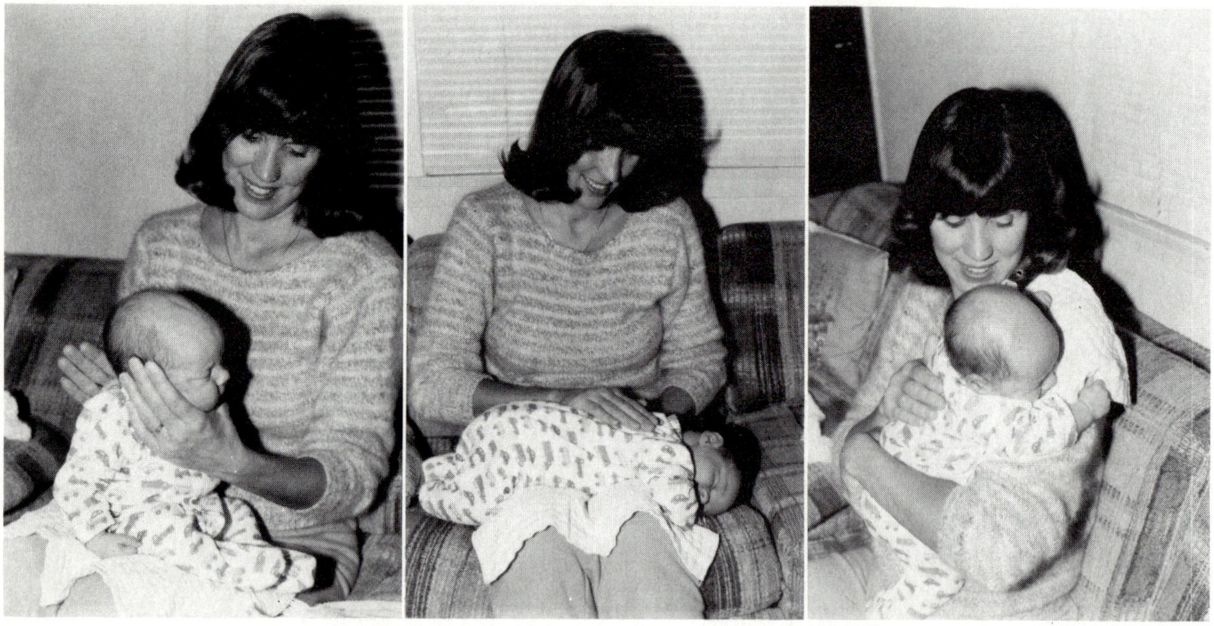

A B C

Fig. 23-5 Positions for burping a baby. **A**, Upright. **B**, Across the lap. **C**, Shoulder position.
Courtesy Marjorie Pyle, RNC, Lifecircle, Costa Mesa, Calif.

the taste or smell of ointments and will refuse to suckle until the breast has been washed.

The brassiere needs to be well-fitted, with broad shoulder straps and the flaps over the breasts large enough to release the breasts without discomfort. Milk leaking from the breasts, particulary just before the next feeding (milk-ejection reflex), can be uncomfortable and embarrassing. The brassiere can be padded with folded squares of soft cotton, a perineal pad cut in two, or commercially designed pads. A tingling sensation in the nipple area precedes leaking of the milk. Pressure with the heel of both hands over the nipple areas will often prevent the milk from forming so that leaking from the breasts is forestalled. Lining the brassiere cup with plastic material is not recommended, since moisture tends to soften the nipple and predispose it to erosion.

Diet and Fluids. During lactation there is increased need for maternal energy, protein, minerals, and vitamins. This increase covers the cost of secreting milk, provides amounts secreted in milk for nourishment of the infant, and protects the mother's stores. A well-balanced diet containing an extra 500 calories per day (per baby) is necessary for both mother and infant. See Chapter 15 for additional information about nutrition. The breast-feeding mother requires *extra fluids,* as much as 3 L per day. These can be taken routinely before each feeding. Glasses of water, fruit juices, decaffeinated tea, or milk can be alternated. The mother can keep a pitcher of water close by when breast-feeding, as she often becomes thirsty. The use of beer or wine to aid lactation is *not* recommended (Blume et al., 1987).

Breast-Feeding Twins. Breast-feeding twins takes planning and patience. If the mother elects the rooming-in regimen, the added care of two infants may prove too taxing to her strength. However, many mothers have stated that the early adjustment made going home easier. It is suggested that these mothers remain longer in the hospital unless there is help at home. It is important to establish a feeding schedule as soon as possible. The mother may use a modified demand schedule. She can feed the first baby who wakes up, then wake up the second baby. She may decide to breast-feed them simultaneously (Fig. 23-6).

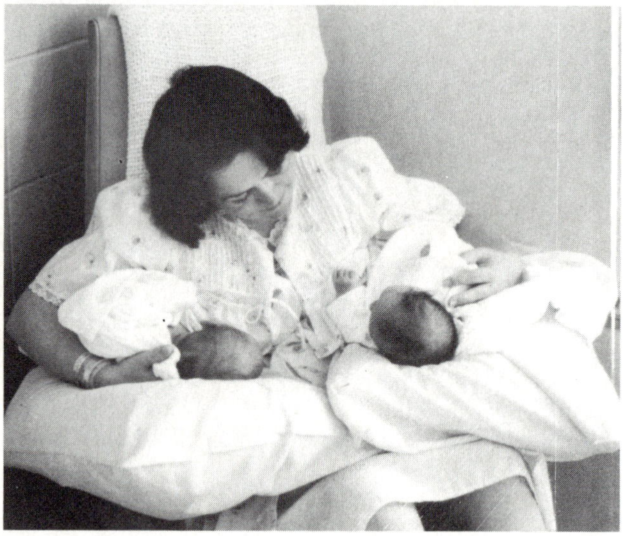

Fig. 23-6 Breast-feeding twins. Note support with pillows. Infants in "football hold" position.
Courtesy Colleen Stainton.

A record of the feeding times, which breast was used by which baby, and which side was used first is essential during the early weeks. If one twin feeds more readily than the other, an effort should be made to have that twin feed on alternate breasts to equalize stimulation. If feeding simultaneously, the mother should experiment with positions. Each baby may be supported on pillows and in the football hold. One may be held in the football hold and the other in the cradle hold. Obviously the mother with twins will need extra assistance from her family, extra nourishment, and extra rest. She will need sufficient energy not only to care for and breast-feed each baby but also to provide the mothering each child needs.

Breast-Feeding in Diabetic Women. Breast-feeding is encouraged in diabetic women not only for its psychologic benefits and its advantages for the infant but also for its antidiabetogenic effect. Breast-feeding decreases the insulin dosage for insulin-dependent women. The insulin dosage must be readjusted at the time of weaning. (See Fig. 32-1, *F* to *G*.)

Infant Responses. Breast-fed babies may wish to feed more often than formula-fed babies. If the baby wants to breast-feed, there is no reason not to do so. Breast-fed babies consume what they need and no more. Breast-feeding whenever the baby is hungry is easy to do because the milk is always ready. Some babies may be hungry as frequently as every hour or two on some days, on other days only every 4 hours. The more often the baby nurses, the more milk the breasts produce. Thus whenever a woman's supply is low (e.g., during or after an illness), she should breast-feed more often. If the woman has too much milk, the baby may need to breast-feed on only one side at a feeding for a while. This will reduce overall stimulation and reduce the milk supply.

Crying does not always mean that the baby is hungry (see Chapter 26). The baby may be physically uncomfortable or just want to be held, burped, or changed. Mother can be reassured that she is producing sufficient milk if the infant has 6 to 10 voidings of pale, straw-colored urine in 24 hours. In warm weather the baby may be thirsty. The mother can give the baby a bottle of water (preboiled in areas with poor sanitation) (1 to 2 oz) or increase the number of breast-feedings.

The *stools* of breast-fed babies are loose. Some infants have a bowel movement at each feeding, whereas others may go up to 5 days without one. Babies who are fed only breast milk do not become constipated, although they may strain considerably in passing the stool. The stool is not irritating to the skin.

Contaminants in Maternal Milk

Nonnutrients enter human milk from the bloodstream of the lactating mother. Such compounds include environmental pollutants, nicotine, methadone, marijuana, caffeine, and alcohol (see Appendix I and Chapter 39). The distribution of a compound across the membrane between plasma and milk is influenced by (1) its solubility in fat, (2) its degree of ionization, (3) its degree of protein binding, and (4) active versus passive transport (Chapter 9).

Comments on advising substance abusers who choose to breast-feed are made in Chapter 34.

Substance abuse poses significant concern for the nursing infant. Regular use of *alcohol* is common in our society. However, during both pregnancy and lactation, even moderate drinking can pose problems for the unborn child or infant. *Smoking* by the lactating woman can cause a decrease in her milk supply. Another reason not to smoke is the second-hand smoke in the baby's atmosphere. This smoke can aggravate or even trigger asthma symptoms, and babies of parents who smoke have a higher incidence of lung disease. *Caffeine* should be taken in moderation by the breast-feeding mother. While only 1% of the mother's ingested caffeine passes through to the milk, the baby's immature system cannot get rid of the caffeine as effectively as an adult can. Some babies are sensitive to even a small amount of caffeine. Caffeine is found in coffee, tea, chocolate, and some soft drinks. It is best to limit these drinks to no more than 24 oz per day total. If *cathartics* are taken, they may cause loose stools in the infant.

Effect of Oral Contraceptives. If *oral contraceptives* are taken sooner than 6 weeks after delivery, the amount of milk a woman produces may be diminished. Experience indicates that most women will not have difficulty producing an adequate amount of milk if they do not use oral contraceptives until after weaning the infant.

Effect of Menstruation. If menstruation occurs, the mother can continue to breast-feed. Although some babies may act fussy, the quality and quantity of the milk are not affected.

Maternal Commitments. On occasions when the mother needs to be away from the infant at feeding time, a bottle of breast milk, expressed earlier, can be substituted. If the mother returns to work, she can continue to breast-feed (MacLaughlin and Strelnick, 1984; Price and Bamford, 1983). (See directions in the boxed material.) The length of time a woman breast feeds her infant will depend on her own feelings and situation. Milk will continue to be produced as long as it is taken from the breast.

Concerns. The inexperienced breast-feeding mother is likely to encounter major or minor problems in the course of adjusting to breast-feeding. Success or failure at the breast-feeding effort may depend largely on the availability of help in the early weeks and the support of a clinician or friend who provides useful tips. Problems relating to the infant are presented in Table 23-4.

Women may encounter problems in relation to breast-feeding (Chapman et al., 1985). Individual counseling by a skilled clinician can greatly simplify the process of learning to cope with the problem. Table 23-5 presents mother-related problems in breast-feeding.

Text continued on p. 564.

HOW TO HAVE A TOTALLY BREAST-FED BABY AND WORK TOO! (GOING BACK TO WORK AT 6 WEEKS POSTPARTUM)

Starting out
- First 3 to 4 weeks breast-feed only to establish your milk supply.
- Nurse your baby every 2 to 3 hours to build up your milk supply.
- RELAX AND ENJOY 6 weeks of nursing totally.

Establishing a home milk supply by pumping your breasts
- Do NOT attempt to pump until the fifth week home from the hospital.
- Weeks 5 and 6 when baby doesn't nurse every 3 hours . . . PUMP. This will mean you are either feeding or pumping every 3 hours.
- In the beginning you will only be able to pump approximately ½ to 1 ounce of breast milk . . . DON'T PANIC . . . after practicing *and* believing, you will be able to pump 1 to 3 ounces or more!

How to pump at home
- RELAX . . . and drink plenty of fluids.
- Take a warm shower or use warm compresses on your breasts.
- Pump 15 minutes on each side . . . or . . . pump while nursing the baby by propping the baby on your lap with pillows on one side and pumping the other side. Baby feeding facilitates milk "let-down" and you will be able to obtain more breast milk while pumping. The baby will be well fed from one-sided nursing.
- Pump at EVERY first morning feeding and you will get a good amount of breast milk for your reserve supply because baby has gone longer between feedings.

Pumping at work
- Pump every 3 to 4 hours to increase your milk supply . . . or . . . more often.
- Pump after 6 to 8 hours away from the baby or when engorgement is felt. This will give you 4 to 12 ounces of milk, enough to feed your baby the next day when added to your supply at home.

Storage
- Freeze IMMEDIATELY after pumping even at work. You can carry home the milk pumped at work in a small ice cooler . . . remember that breast milk is now more precious than gold.
- Freeze in 1 to 2 ounce amounts in plastic baby bottle liners sealed with twist ties. Sit plastic bags in glass to freeze any spillage.
- Date milk and use oldest first.

Equipment
- Breast pads—Evenflo or Sears
- Handpump—Kaneson
- Electric pump—Eggnell (suggested that the equipment be rented). The cost is 80% to 100% covered by insurance if prescribed by your doctor. Have your doctor prescribe the pump in the hospital.
- Plastic baby bottles and nipples . . . always use the same brand.

Preparation of frozen breast milk for feeding baby
- Hold plastic bag under hot running water until thawed and warm.
- Pour into plastic bottle and feed the baby.

Courtesy Fountain Valley Community Hospital, Fountain Valley, Calif, 1983, Childbirth education.

Table 23-4 *Infant-Related Concerns in the Initiation of Breast-feeding*

Concern	Nursing Action
The infant does not open wide enough to grasp the nipple.	Help the mother depress the infant's lower jaw with one finger as she guides the nipple into the mouth.
The infant grasps the nipple and areolar tissue correctly but will not suck.	Help the mother stimulate sucking motions by pressing upward under the baby's chin. Expression of colostrum results, and the infant is stimulated by the taste to begin sucking.
The infant makes frantic rooting, mouthing motions but will not grasp the nipple and eventually begins to cry and stiffen her or his body in apparent frustration.	Help the mother interrupt the feeding, comfort the infant, and take time to relax herself, and then she may begin again.
The infant may suck for a few minutes and then fall asleep.	Help the mother interrupt the feeding and take time to awaken the infant. Stimulation may include loosening the wraps, holding the baby upright, talking to the baby, or gently rubbing her or his back or the soles of the feet. A sleepy infant will not nurse satisfactorily. If it is impossible to wake the baby, it is better to postpone the feeding.
The infant starts by sucking vigorously and, as the milk flows freely, develops a long, slow, rhythmic sucking. The sucking then changes to a short, rapid sucking with frequent rest periods. This behavior indicates a slowing of the flow of milk.	Help the mother massage the breasts toward the nipple. This starts the milk flowing freely again, and the infant will revert to the slow, rhythmic sucking. As soon as sucking resumes, the massage is discontinued so that the infant will not be overwhelmed and choked by the milk flowing too rapidly.

TABLE 23-5 *Mother-Related Problems in Breast-Feeding*

Problem	Nursing Action
Engorged Breasts	
If feeding has been on demand since birth, painful engorgement of the breasts is not likely to occur. However, because of the lag between the production of milk and the efficiency of the ejection reflexes, engorgement of the breasts may occur for up to 48 hours after the milk comes in. The mother often complains that the breast is tender and that the tenderness extends into the axilla. The breasts usually feel firm, tense, and warm as a result of the increased blood supply, and the skin may appear shiny and taut. The unyielding areolae makes it difficult for the infant to grasp the nipple. Breast-feeding can be uncomfortable to the mother and frustrating for both mother and infant.	1. Application of moist heat: apply wet cloths as hot as can be endured to the whole breast and, at the same time, express milk from the nipple. As the wet cloth cools, replace with another one. Shower and direct the hot water to the breasts. 2. Breast massage (Fig. 23-7): **A**, Begin by placing one hand over the other above the breast. **B**, Gently, but firmly, exert pressure evenly with the thumbs across the top and fingers underneath the breast. **C**, Come together with the heel of the hand on each side and release at the areola, being careful not to touch the areola and nipple. **D**, Then gently lift the breast from beneath and drop lightly. Repeat 4 to 5 times with each breast. 3. Manual expression of milk (Fig. 23-8) **A**, Place the thumb and forefinger on opposite sides of the breast just outside the areola, press downward into the rib cage, and then **B**, gently squeeze together and downward; the nipple should not be pulled outward. Repeat the procedure moving the thumb and forefinger around the nipple until as much milk as desired has been expressed. If the milk is to be used later, *it should be expressed into a sterile bottle and frozen.** Milk expression is not easy for some women at first, but persistence usually brings success if the mother takes the time.
Sore Nipples	
The nipples may become sore during the early days of breast-feeding. Soreness may be prevented or limited by using a correct position and avoiding undue breast engorgement. If soreness occurs, it is always temporary until the nipples become accustomed to the baby's sucking (Borovies, 1984).	1. Expose the nipples to air. 2. Use a heat lamp to dry the nipples after the feeding (40-watt bulb in a desk lamp, positioned 45 cm [18 in] from breast). 3. If soreness occurs, limit sucking time to 5 minutes on each breast, the time it takes to empty the breasts of milk. 4. Use a pacifier if the infant's sucking needs have not been met. 5. Use a nipple shield (Fig. 23-9). 6. Discontinue breast-feeding for 48 hours. During this time the milk is expressed manually or with a breast pump, collected in a sterilized glass, and given to the baby by bottle. Precautions for maintaining the milk in a safe condition must be followed. Bottles and nipples must be sterilized by immersing them in water and boiling for 10 minutes; any milk not immediately consumed must be refrigerated or frozen.
Plugged Ducts	
Occasionally a milk duct will become plugged, creating a tender spot on the breast, which may appear lumpy and hot. This might result from inadequate emptying of the milk ducts or from wearing a brassiere that is too tight.	1. Offer the sore breast first so that it will be emptied more completely. 2. Nurse longer and more often; if the breast gets too full, the plugged duct becomes worse and infection may develop. 3. Change positions at every feeding so that the pressure of the feeding will be applied to different places on the breast. 4. Apply warm compresses to the breasts between feedings to reduce the risk of infection by keeping the ducts open.
Increased Lochial Flow	
The breast-feeding mother may note an increase in lochial flow once feeding begins. At times afterpains are intensified to such a degree that the mother becomes uncomfortable, and her tension interferes with feeding the infant.	Offer a mild analgesic for pain 40 minutes before the feeding period. The mother may be reassured that this discomfort is transitory and will be gone in about 2 days.
Sexual Sensations	
For some women the rhythmic uterine contractions occurring while breast-feeding are akin to those experienced during orgasm. These unexpected sexual sensations within the context of child care may be disturbing.	Reassure as to normalcy of such feelings.

*Freeze milk that will not be used within a few hours (see box, p. 560).

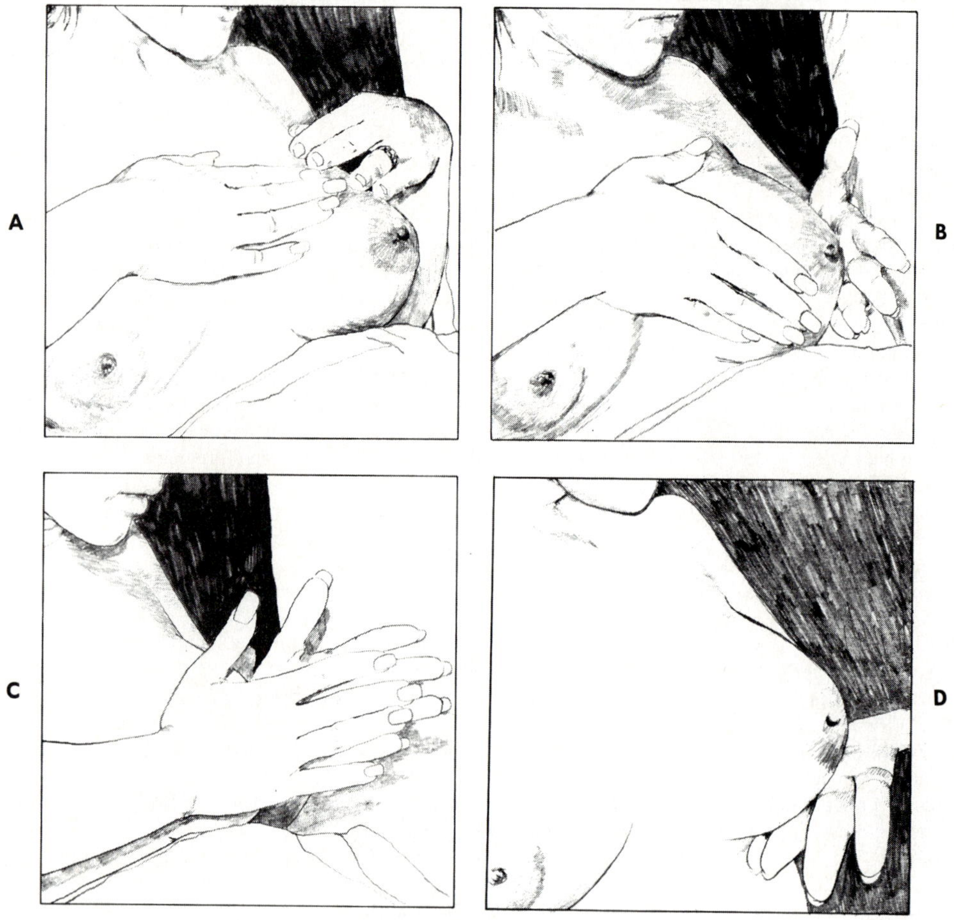

Fig. 23-7 Breast massage.
Courtesy Marjorie Pyle, RNC, Lifecircle, Costa Mesa, Calif.

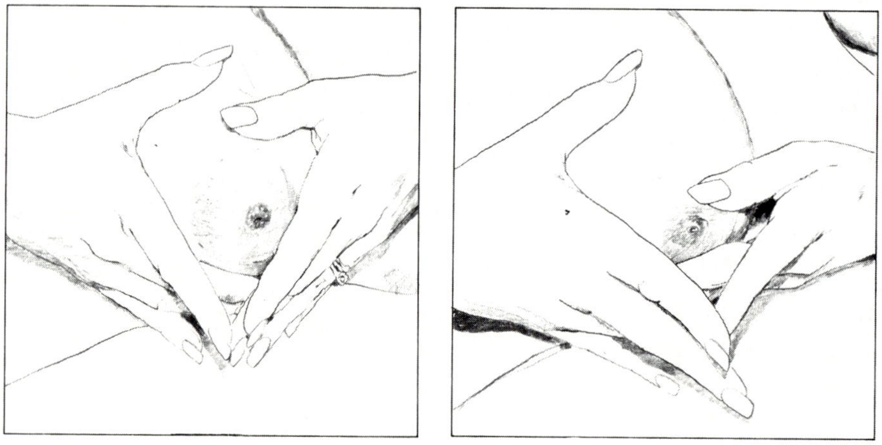

Fig. 23-8 Manual expression of human milk.
Courtesy Marjorie Pyle, RNC, Lifecircle, Costa Mesa, Calif.

TABLE 23-5 *Mother-Related Problems in Breast-Feeding—cont'd*

Problem	Nursing Action
Relactation	
Occasionally a mother starts breast-feeding late or discontinues it but decides at a much later date that she would like to begin again. After adopting an infant, a minority of women decide to attempt lactation even though they have never done so before or, at best, have breast-fed a previous baby of their own. With much sucking stimulus, lactation can be induced but only with great perseverance and in most cases only if a woman has once carried a pregnancy well into the second trimester. Since the mammary glands complete their development for lactation during the first 6 months of pregnancy, a woman who has never been pregnant or never carried a pregnancy beyond the first trimester is a poor candidate for successful induction of lactation.	Instruct the mother to attempt relactation or induced lactation through providing the infant substantial opportunities to suck at the breast. With much sucking stimulus over several days' time many patient and persistent women can initiate the lactation process late or once again. Their volume of milk production may be less than the infant demands, in which case a supplemental feeding following breast-feeding may be necessary. Alternatively, some women find the Lact-Aid Nursing Trainer to complement their own milk production (Fig. 23-10). While the baby sucks at the breast she or he also obtains milk via suction through a small tube leading to a bag of fresh formula that is clipped to the mother's brassiere. While the infant sucks, the mother's milk supply is built up and the infant receives adequate nutrition through the Lact-Aid feeding device.
Breast Pumping	
For a number of reasons, mothers may wish to remove milk from their breasts and save it for a later feeding, take it to their hospitalized newborn, or donate it to a milk bank. Under such circumstances, milk can be expressed by hand and for some women this method is satisfactory. For many women, however, a manual or electric breast pump provides a better stimulus for milk flow and a more efficient mode of milk collection.	Instruct the mother in the use of the breast pump (Fig. 23-11).
Failure of Infant to Thrive	
Insufficient milk supply is rarely a problem for the well-nourished mother. Since sucking stimulates the flow of milk, feeding on demand for adequate duration should supply ample amounts of milk. Occasionally, however, an infant will fail to thrive while seemingly feeding properly.	1. Assist in the explanation of potential problems (Fig. 23-12). 2. Encourage mother to turn to commercial infant formula for at least partial nutrition support of the infant, if the cause of the problem cannot be identified or the defined problem cannot be corrected (Fig. 23-10). 3. Refer the mother to a pediatrician if condition continues, or prn (Fig. 23-12).
Maternal Infection	
If breast tenderness is accompanied by fever and a general flulike feeling, a breast infection is probably present (see Chapter 30).	Instruct the mother to notify her physician immediately.

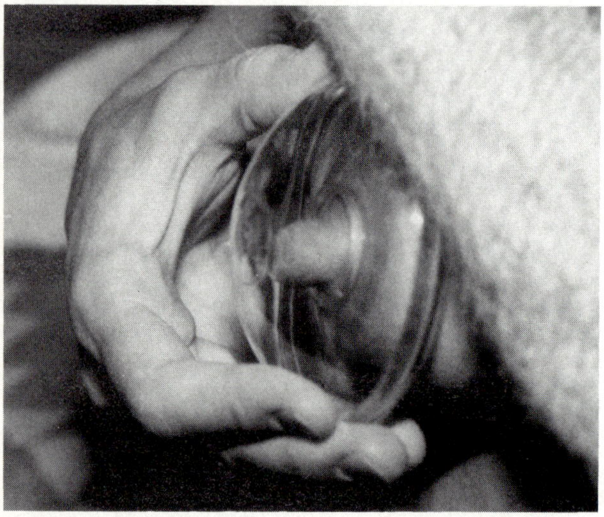

Fig. 23-9 Nipple shield. *Avoid use of breast shields,* since they do not prevent or help sore nipples.
Courtesy Marjorie Pyle, RNC, Lifecircle, Costa Mesa, Calif.

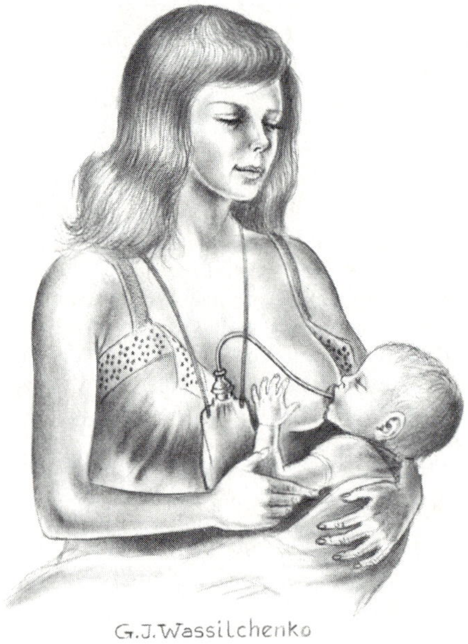

Fig. 23-10 Lact-Aid Nursing Trainer in use.

Formula-feeding

Formula-feeding has proven a successful substitute for breast-feeding in certain instances. These include the following:

1. The family decides against breast-feeding or the mother is unable to breast-feed because of disease or anomalies.
2. The mother's schedule does not permit her to breast-feed.
3. Special formula is required because of infant allergies or special dietary needs.
4. Supplemental feedings are required.
5. The infant is adopted.

Formulas are recommended by physicians based on the infant's nutrition needs, cost, need for refrigeration, convenience, and the mother's ability to prepare the formula accurately and safely. The physician provides written instructions as to the amounts of formula to be fed the infant over 24 hours and when to increase the amounts to ensure meeting the growing infant's nutrition needs.

Hospitals today use commercially prepared formula. It comes prepackaged and can be stored at room temperature. Many parents elect to use similar brands. One consideration in the use of commercially prepared formulas is their cost. It is wise to advise parents to do comparison shopping, since one preparation can be considerably more expensive than another. Also there are a variety of formula-feeding bottles and nipples from which to choose.

Feeding Process. Inexperienced mothers who are formula-feeding their infants need the same teaching, counseling, and support as do the mothers who are breast-feeding. They need assistance with the feeding process and with problems they experience. Some mothers who elect formula-feeding will express concern that the baby will suffer as a result of their decision. They need assurance that knowledge of their infant's nutrition needs and skill in use of formula-feeding can be an acceptable substitute for

A

B

C

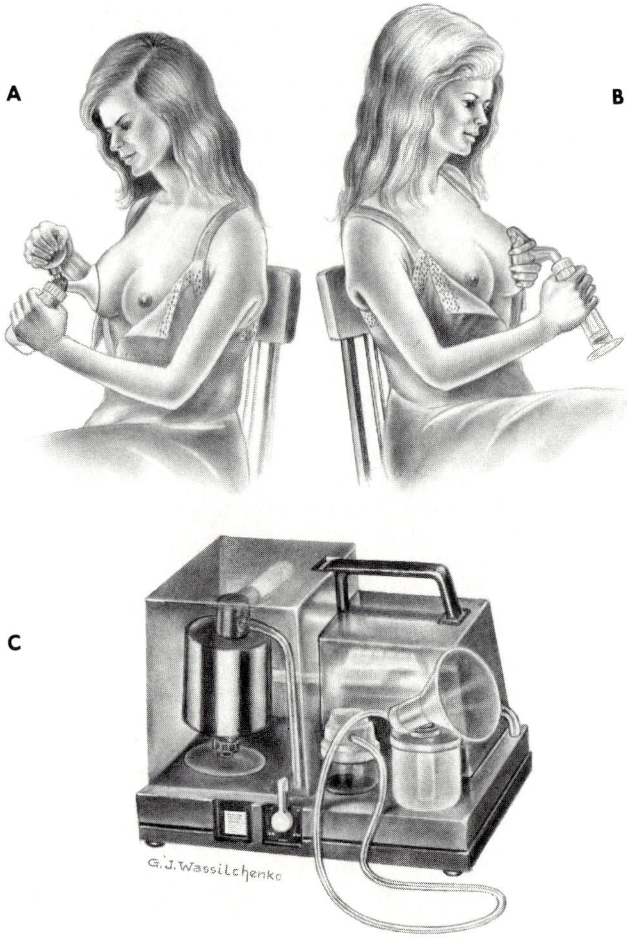

Fig. 23-11 Commonly used breast pumps. **A**, Swedish pump. **B**, Syringe pump. **C**, Electric pump.

breast-feeding. Emphasis on the beneficial use of the feeding time for close contact with their infant can help relieve their tensions. The guidelines for client teaching on formula-feeding, p. 566, can be used to help an inexperienced woman.

Home-Prepared Formulas. Some parents wish to prepare their own formulas. Instruction in the preparation of formula includes methods for sterilizing and storing it. The guidelines for client teaching on formula-feeding can be used as an instruction guide to help the inexperienced mother.

The two traditional ways of preparing formula are the terminal heat method and the aseptic method. In the terminal heat method all the utensils and formula are boiled together for 25 minutes. In the aseptic method the equipment is boiled separately, after which the formula is poured into the bottles. Under improved sanitary conditions, neither of these methods is essential. The clean technique is satisfactory. The nurse must be aware when sanitation in any community warrants the use of a traditional method of formula preparation.

Recent recommendations for labeling commercial infant formulas require that the directions for preparation and use of the formula include pictures and symbols for nonreading individuals. In addition manufacturers are translating the directions into foreign languages, such as Spanish and Vietnamese, to prevent misunderstanding and errors in formula preparation. It is important to impress upon families that the proportions *must not be altered*—neither diluted to extend the amount of formula nor concentrated to provide more calories (Whaley and Wong, 1987).

Evaporated Milk. Although home-prepared evaporated milk formula may be least expensive, it is not generally recommended because of the increased chance of improper measurement and bacterial contamination during preparation of the formula. Often the families who could benefit most by savings are least able to understand the importance of sanitary precautions and accurate measurements in preparing the formula. Special counseling is needed for parents who choose to use evaporated milk formula.

To control growth of bacteria, single feedings should be prepared as needed rather than all feedings for a 24-hour period. A formula may be prepared as follows:

Evaporated milk: 3 oz (90 ml)
Water: 4.5 oz (135 ml)
Corn syrup: 2 tsp

An opened can of evaporated milk should be covered and refrigerated. Evaporated milk is fortified with vitamin D and forms an easily digested curd because of the heat processing it undergoes. Supplements of vitamin C and iron are needed for the infant fed with evaporated milk formulas. Fluoride supplements may be needed also.

Evaporated milk must not be confused with condensed milk, which is a form of evaporated milk with 45% more sugar. Because of its high carbohydrate concentration and disproportionately low fat and protein content, condensed milk is not used for infant feeding.

Powders or Concentrates. Instructions for mixing powdered or concentrated formulas should be followed accurately to prevent overdilution or underdilution. When formulas are underdiluted with water, the renal solute load is increased and may lead to dehydration of the infant. If ov-

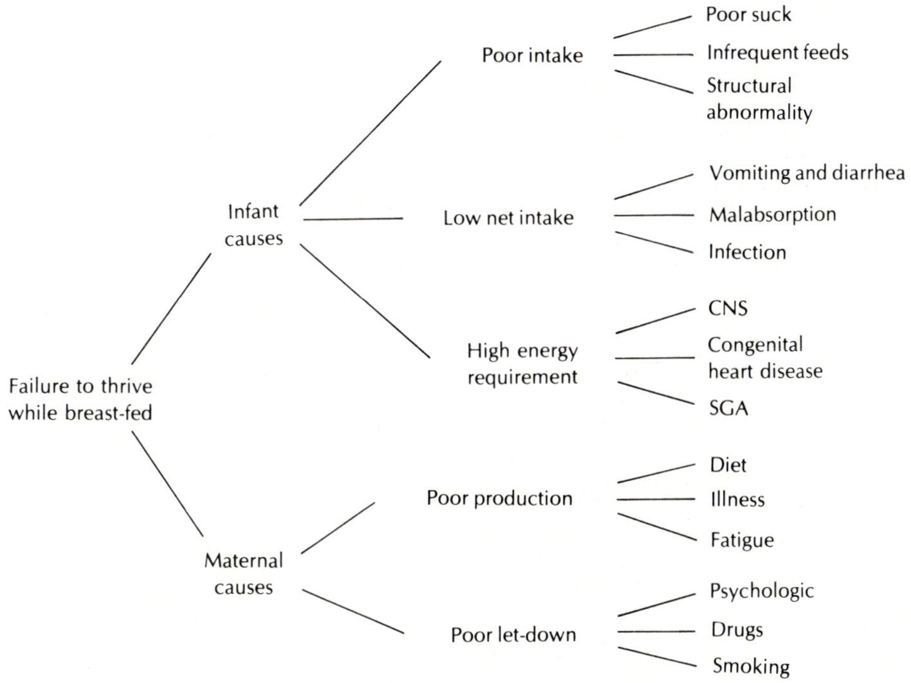

Fig. 23-12 Diagnostic flow chart for failure to thrive.
From Lawrence, R: Breast feeding: a guide for the medical profession, ed 2, St Louis, 1985, The CV Mosby Co.

Guidelines For Client Teaching

FORMULA FEEDING

ASSESSMENT

Sharon, age 17, delivered her daughter 6 hours ago. The infant is a healthy term baby weighing 2912 g (6 1/2 lb). The nurse fed the infant (sterile water) initially at 2 hours of age. Her sucking and swallowing reflexes were normal. The mother is anxious about bottle-feeding her infant. Up to now she has had no contact with babies.

NURSING DIAGNOSES

Knowledge deficit related to bottle-feeding an infant.
Anxiety, mild, related to being a new parent.

GOALS

Short-term

To teach Sharon how to bottle-feed her baby.

Intermediate

To help Sharon assess the amount of feeding her daughter requires.
To teach Sharon how to prepare the formula.

Long-term

To increase Sharon's awareness of her infant's needs.

REFERENCES AND TEACHING AIDS

Posters, films, and hospital and commericial booklets from formula companies related to formula-bottle-feeding an infant. Bottle, nipple; cork and needle.
Cans of formula; ready to feed, and that which has to be mixed with water.

CONTENT/RATIONALE	TEACHING ACTIONS
To review general content tell mother: Before starting to feed the baby I'll go over a few points that will help you feed her.	Give baby to the mother to hold while the discussion goes on.
Baby needs to be wide awake, like the one in the picture.	Show Sharon picture of baby (Fig. 23-13).
These are hospital bottles of formula. They can be stored at room temperature. You may use this brand or the one your pediatrician recommends. They contain 4 oz of formula (120 ml). Your baby will probably drink 2 to 3 oz (60 to 90 ml) at a feeding for a few days and then increase. If you do not use all the formula, throw the remainder away, since it spoils once opened.	Show Sharon a sample bottle of formula.
You can keep track of how many ounces the baby drinks in 1 day by writing it down. When you take the baby for a check-up, your physician or nurse will ask you the amount of intake.	Show Sharon how to note time and amount.
Your baby will probably be hungry every 2 1/2 to 3 hours. If she fusses or cries in between feedings, check her diaper or her need to be picked up and cuddled. As she gets older, she may be thirsty. Check with the pediatrician concerning water supplementation.	
Test the temperature of the formula by letting a few drops fall on the inside of your wrist. If the formula feels comfortably warm to you, it is the correct temperature. If the formula is refrigerated, warm it by placing the bottle in a pan of hot water. Check it often for correct temperature.	Shake a few drops of formula on Sharon's inside writst. Dry her wrist with a facial tissue.
Test the size of the nipple hole by holding the bottle and nipple upside down. The formula should drip from the nipple. If it runs in a stream, the hole is too big. If it has to be shaken for the formula to come out, the hole is too small. To correct this you can try a softer nipple or enlarge the hole in the nipple or both. To enlarge hole, heat a needle stuck into a cork (used as a handle) and insert the hot needle into the nipple. New nipples may be softened by boiling for 5 minutes before using. If nipple collapses, unscrew bottle lid to let air in.	Demonstrate how to check nipple hole. Demonstrate with needle embedded in cork. Heat over match flame and enlarge the hole on the sample nipple.

Guidelines For Client Teaching—cont'd

CONTENT/RATIONALE	TEACHING ACTIONS
Some babies need burping. They tend to swallow air when sucking. Burp the baby before feeding, if she has been crying, then after every ounce of formula. As she gets older and you get more experienced, you will know when to burp her.	Show pictures of mother burping baby (Fig. 23-5). Demonstrate burping technique with Sharon's baby.
To feed the baby, place the nipple in the baby's mouth over her tongue. It should rest against the roof of her mouth. This stimulates sucking reflex.	Show Sharon picture (Fig. 23-13). Have her practice.
Hold the bottle like a pencil. Keep nipple filled with milk so baby doesn't suck air.	Point out on picture (Fig. 23-13). Demonstrate.
Start out with baby away from you until nipple is in her mouth. If she is too close, she will turn toward you and not the nipple, this is the rooting reflex.	Have Sharon hold baby away from herself.
After she starts feeding then you can hold her close.	Help Sharon start feeding.
Some infants take longer to feed than others. Slow, patient feeding, keeping the infant awake and encouraging her to take more may be necessary.	Reassure Sharon that this is a characteristic of infant feeding and not poor mothering.
The stools of a formula-fed baby are soft but formed. They will be yellow with a characteristic odor. She will probably defecate either during the feeding or after. Change the diaper immediately since the composition of the stool is irritating to the skin.	Show picture of type of stool baby will have once meconium has passed.
To review safety measures tell mother: While she is feeding I will review some safety tips.	Use poster to show dangers. Ask Sharon to demonstrate what to do if baby chokes. Place bulb syringe.
Don't prop the bottle, the nipple may fall against the throat and block the air, or the baby could drown in her formula or aspirate any that was regurgitated.	
Infants should never be left alone while feeding until they are old enough to remove bottle from their mouth.	
Bottles taken to bed can lead to early dental problems in young children (baby bottle syndrome).	
Let's practice how to hold baby and use the bulb syringe in case she should choke.	
I will be back in 10 minutes if you have any questions.	Check amount of formula for hospital record.
After baby is finished, place the baby in her crib on her right side so air can come up easily.	Supervise burping the baby. Show picture (see Fig. 22-5).

EVALUATION Sharon demonstrates competence and skill in formula/bottle-feeding her infant and asks appropriate questions.

erdilution occurs, inadequate calories and nutrients are provided, and failure to thrive may result. When the safety of the community or home water supply is in doubt, water sterilized by boiling for 15 minutes is recommended for diluting formulas.

CAUTION: *Honey* is sometimes used as a sweetener for home-prepared infant foods or formula, and occasionally it is recommended for use on pacifiers to promote sucking in hypotonic babies. Use of honey for any of these purposes, however, is discouraged because some sources contain spores of *Clostridium botulinum* (Arnon et al., 1979; Whaley and Wong, 1987). These spores are extremely resistant to heat and therefore are not destroyed in the processing of honey. If ingested by an infant, spores may germinate, and lethal toxin may be released into the lumen of the bowel. Infant botulism may ultimately develop, and in some cases it is known to be fatal.

Commercial Formulas. The Committee on Nutrition of the American Academy of Pediatrics proposed standards for infant formulas in 1976. Recommendations for minimum desirable concentrations of major nutrients were largely based on levels found in mature human milk.

Commercial formulas prepared from nonfat cow's milk are readily available and generally are used for feeding in early infancy. Most commercial formulas provide 20 kcal/oz. Several brands are marketed, with and without added iron. A number of vitamins have been added to each different brand: almost all are fortified with vitamins A and D, ascorbic acid, and vitamin B_6; some also contain vitamin E, folic acid, and vitamin B_{12}; and others contain B-complex

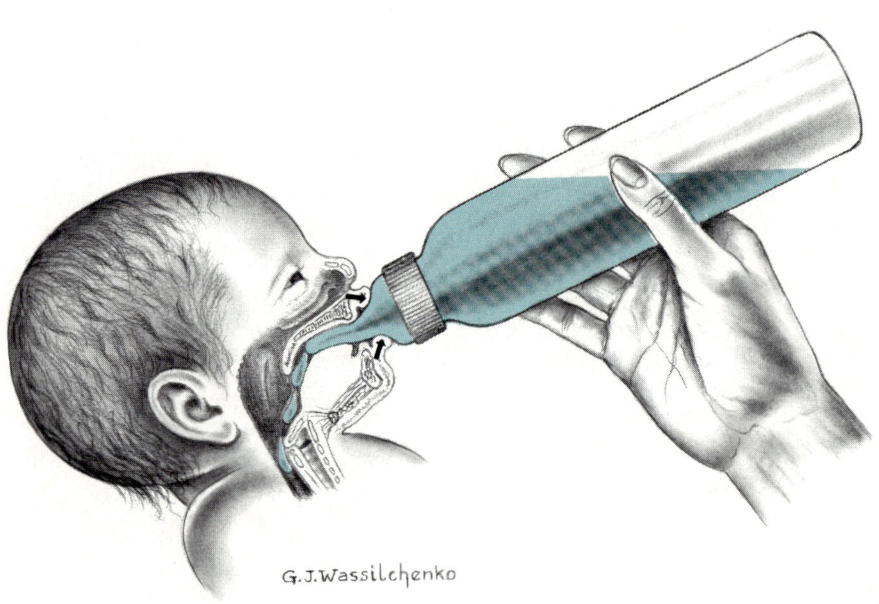

Fig. 23-13 Bottle-feeding. Bottle is held in hand like a pencil. Note milk must cover nipple area so infant will not suck in air.

vitamins. Commercial formulas are also modified in one or more of the following ways:

1. Butterfat is removed and vegetable oils are added to increase the amount of unsaturated fatty acid, particularly linoleic acid, an essential fatty acid. This makes the cow's milk formula more like human milk in essential fatty acid content. Fat in this form is better tolerated by the infant.
2. Protein is treated to produce a softer, more flocculent curd that is more easily digested by the infant.
3. Protein and mineral concentrations are adjusted to more nearly resemble those in human milk. To achieve adequate levels of calories, sugar is added. This is usually in the form of lactose or corn syrup solids.

Most formulas are available in the following forms:

1. Concentrated: requires dilution with water.
2. Ready-to-use (bulk): requires measuring into bottles.
3. Ready-to-use (individual feedings): sold in disposable bottles.
4. Dry powder form: requires mixing with water according to label instructions.

Unmodified Cow's Milk

Regular unmodified cow's milk is not suitable for infants during the early months of life (Williams, 1989). It may cause gastrointestinal bleeding, and its solute load is too heavy for the infant's renal system to handle. However, after the infant is 6 months of age cow's milk may be used, along with a reasonable quantity of solid foods. Since regular milk is low in vitamin C and iron, the diet needs to supply food sources of these nutrients, such as fruit juices and iron-fortified dry cereals. During the first year of life infants should *not* use milks of reduced fat content, such as skim or 2% milk (American Academy of Pediatrics, 1983a, b, 1984), for two reasons: (1) *insufficient energy* to support maintenance requirements, causing the mobilization of body fat to make up the deficit; and (2) *linoleic acid* in the fat portion of milk is an essential fatty acid needed for growth and development of body tissues. A specific form of eczema has been observed in infants deficient in linoleic acid.

Mineral and Vitamin Supplementation

Shortly after birth, vitamin K is administered intramuscularly to prevent hemorrhagic disease of the newborn (Chapter 21). Normally, vitamin K is synthesized by the intestinal flora. However, since the infant's intestine is sterile at birth, and since breast milk contains low levels of vitamin K, the supply is inadequate for at least the first 3 to 4 days.

The normal infant receiving breast milk from a well-nourished mother needs no specific vitamin and mineral supplements, with the exceptions of fluoride in a dose of 0.25 mg daily (regardless of the fluoride content of the local water supply) and iron by 6 months of age (when fetal iron stores are depleted). Supplements of 400 IU of vitamin D daily may be indicated if the mother's vitamin D intake is inadequate or if the infant does not benefit from adequate ultraviolet light because of dark skin color or little exposure to light (American Academy of Pediatrics, 1980a, b).

Like human milk, commercial iron-fortified formula supplies all the nutrients needed by the infant for the first 6 months. The only supplementation required is 0.25 mg of fluoride if the local water supply is not fluoridated or if the infant is given ready-to-feed formula, which eliminates the use of fluoridated tap water (Whaley and Wong, 1987).

If evaporated milk formula is given, supplemental iron, vitamin C, and fluoride (depending on local water supply) are required. Commercially prepared vitamin/iron preparations with or without fluoride are available to meet the specific needs of the infant. The nurse needs to assess the type of formula given and the fluoride content of local water before advising the parent.

Discharge Planning

Anticipatory guidance can be given before the mother leaves the hospital or at the well baby checkups if the mother elects early discharge. Knowledge such as the following is helpful to the parent (Pyle, 1985).

Frequency of Feeding. During the daytime, awaken and feed the infant so that she or he is not sleeping more than 3 hours at a time. At night, let baby sleep and only feed if baby awakens. Make the night feedings businesslike so that baby learns that nights are not play time. At the beginning, most mothers prefer to take the baby to bed to breast- or formula-feed. Mothers also find that baby will sleep better if laid across her upper abdomen, so that baby hears her heartbeat and has the warm body contact.

Ideally for the newborn, feeding schedules are determined by the infant's hunger. Feeding infants when they signal readiness is called *demand feeding. Scheduled feedings* are arranged at predetermined intervals to meet family routines. The newborn will feed every 1½ to 3 hours during the daytime, and usually every 3 to 5 hours at night. Breast-fed infants need to feed *at least every 3 hours* during the daytime. "Good" babies who rarely cry, sleep, and only awaken to nurse every 4 to 6 hours, usually do not have an adequate weight gain, and the mother may not maintain an adequate milk supply. Most babies will average 10 feedings during a 24-hour period. The following provides a guide for formula-fed infants' average intake of formula:

Age	*Quantity per Feeding*	*Number of Feedings per 24 Hours*
Birth to 3 weeks	2 to 3 oz (60-90 ml)	6 to 10
3 weeks to 2 months	5 oz (150 ml)	5 to 8
2 to 3 months	5 to 7 oz (150-210 ml)	5 to 6

Supplemental Feedings for Breast-fed Babies. Supplemental feedings should *not* be offered to breast-fed infants in the nursery because, if satiated, they will not suck vigorously at the breast (Whaley and Wong, 1987). Lactation depends on emptying the breast at each feeding. If milk is allowed to accumulate in the ducts, breast engorgement and ischemia result, suppressing the activity of the acini (milk-secreting cells). Consequently milk production is reduced. In addition, the process of sucking from a bottle is different from breast-nipple compression. The relatively inflexible rubber nipple prevents the tongue from its usual rhythmic action. Infants learn to put the tongue against the nipple holes to slow down the more rapid flow of fluid. When infants use these same tongue movements during breast-feeding, they may push the human nipple out of the mouth and may not grasp the areola properly (Lawrence, 1985).

Usually by 3 to 4 weeks of age, lactation is well established and a feeding schedule has been formed. Formula-fed infants retain about 2 to 3 ounces of formula at each feeding and are fed about 6 times a day. Breast-fed infants may feed as frequently as 10 to 12 times daily. Larger infants are able to retain increased amounts because of greater stomach capacity; as a result they generally sleep through the night sooner than smaller infants. After the milk supply is established, an occasional bottle will not affect lactation and breast-feeding.

Appetite Changes. Mothers will notice appetite spurts between 10 days and 2 weeks; 6 weeks and 9 weeks; and 3 months and 6 months. These appetite spurts correspond to growth spurts. The infant wants to breast-feed more frequently and for longer periods. For the breast-feeding baby, increasing the feedings results in a greater production of milk. The satisfied infant then tapers off her or his demands. For the formula-fed baby, the amount of formula offered can be increased by 2 to 4 oz (60 to 120 ml).

Most 2- to 3-month old babies *may* lengthen the time between feedings to a 3- to 4-hour schedule during the daytime, and longer at night. By 4 to 6 months of age, some infants may sleep through the night without feeding.

Weaning. Weaning may take place because the infant has signified a desire to drink from a cup or because the mother will be absent. Some infants wean themselves, gradually refusing more and more feedings until only the early morning and night feedings are left. Other infants resist attempts to wean them, and mothers have to substitute other social times to compensate them for their loss. Ideally the process is a gradual one extending over several weeks.

Introducing Solid Foods. The infant receives the right balance of nutrients from breast milk or formula during the first 4 to 6 months (Broussard, 1984). It is not true that when solids are given it will help the baby sleep through the night. Introduction of solid foods before the infant is 4 to 6 months of age may result in overfeeding and decreased intake of breast milk or formula (Madgic, 1986). The infant cannot communicate feeling full like an older child can by turning her or his head away. The proper balance of carbohydrate, protein, and fat for an infant to grow properly is in breast milk or formula.

The infant's individual growth pattern should help determine just the right time to start solids. The physician will advise when to introduce solid foods. The schedule for introducing solid foods and the types of foods to serve will be discussed during well-baby supervision visits with the pediatrician and pediatric nurse (American Academy of Pediatrics, 1980 b, 1983 a, b).

Referrals. Referral procedures provide an opportunity for individuals and groups to take advantage of services available from other sources. A properly coordinated health service delivery for infants and children that includes a registered dietitian can contribute to a sense of continuity and to consistency of care and advice. The mother is encouraged to contact the local association that assists with breast-feeding (Appendix K).

A general nursing care plan for newborn nutrition and feeding follows.

General Nursing Care Plan

NEWBORN NUTRITION AND FEEDING

ASSESSMENT	NURSING DIAGNOSIS (ND)/ PLAN (P)/GOAL (G)	RATIONALE/ IMPLEMENTATION	EVALUATION
Prenatal: Prenatal assessment of infant feeding preferences. Cultural, religious, social, and financial considerations influencing feeding choice. Practices of woman's friends and her mother. Personal (and father's) goals and preferences.	ND: Knowledge deficit related to infant feeding. P: Establish a comprehensive data base. G: Client will make an informed decision about breast- or formula-feeding her infant.	*To aid a woman in choosing a method of feeding her infant, the nurse will:* Evaluate woman's (couple's) goals and preferences for feeding. Discuss the pros and cons of both methods of feeding. Encourage questions, concerns, or feelings surrounding newborn nutrition and feeding. Dispel misconceptions surrounding the feeding choice. Encourage the woman to discuss her decision with those members of the family who will be active in child care.	Client chooses a method of infant feeding suitable to her needs and life-style.
First day of life: Assess infant's ability to breast- or formula-feed. 1. Reflexes—suck, swallow, gag. 2. No structural abnormalities (e.g. choanal atresia). Assess infant's readiness for feeding (e.g., rooting reflex, infant's responsiveness). Assess amount and frequency of feeds.	ND: Ineffective airway clearance related to poor suck, swallow, or gag reflexes. ND: Altered nutrition: potential for less than body requirements, related to infant's lack of interest in feeding or regurgitation. P: Perform comprehensive physical assessment. G: Infant will possess readiness to feed and demonstrate intact reflexes.	*To evaluate the infant's ability to feed, the nurse will:* Have infant suck on finger. Remove excess mucus from nose and mouth, burp prn. Feed infant initial feeding of sterile water. Initiate and evaluate mother's preferred choice of feeding as soon as possible.	Reflexes (root, suck, swallow, and gag) are present and sufficiently developed to permit feeding by breast or bottle. Infant accepts, swallows, retains, and assimilates feeding.
Assess woman's ability to feed infant.	ND: Knowledge deficit related to infant feeding. P: Provide information, demonstrate, and observe return demonstration. G: Client will learn how to successfully feed her infant.	*To aid in successful feeding efforts by the mother, the nurse will:* Encourage the use of wakeful periods for feeding infant. Assist the mother with the feeding technique she has chosen. Instruct as to feeding techniques and nutritional needs of the infant.	Client successfully feeds her infant.

General Nursing Care Plan—cont'd

ASSESSMENT	NURSING DIAGNOSIS (ND)/ PLAN (P)/GOAL (G)	RATIONALE/ IMPLEMENTATION	EVALUATION
		Demonstrate and supervise care needed if infant chokes, gags, or spits up. Record amounts of formula or time at breast and note infant's response.	
Assess infant's ability to defecate and urinate.	ND: Constipation related to a structural or mechanical defect. P: Perform a complete physical examination and monitor pattern of elimination daily. G: Infant will demonstrate a normal pattern of elimination	*To evaluate infant elimination, the nurse will:* Record urine amounts and time. Record character of stool and time. Notify physician if no urine within the first 8 hours of life or no stool within the first 24 hours of life. Report and record any structural defects noted (e.g., imperforate anus).	Infant demonstrates normal pattern of elimination.
Parity. First breast-feeding experience? Knowledge about breast-feeding. Support system for breast-feeding experience. Assess breast-feeding problems—mother-related and infant-related.	ND: Knowledge deficit related to breast-feeding and its complications. P: Provide information, demonstrate, and observe return demonstration. G: Client will breast-feed successfully and comfortably and will establish a pattern satisfactory to infant and herself.	*To teach breast-feeding techniques, the nurse will:* See guidelines for client teaching: breastfeeding, p. 555. See Table 23-5, Mother-related concerns in breast-feeding.	Client successfully and comfortably breast-feeds with a pattern that is satisfying to her and her infant.
Parity. Has she bottle-fed previously? Knowledge about bottle-feeding and amounts of formula required. Financial status (WIC Program).	ND: Knowledge deficit related to preparation of formula and bottle-feeding an infant. P: Provide information, demonstrate, and observe return demonstration. G: Client will learn how to prepare formula and bottle-feed her infant and assess the amount of feeding the child requires.	*To teach client to bottle-feed and assess the amount of formula an infant requires, the nurse will:* See guidelines for client teaching: formula feeding, p. 566. See guidelines for client teaching: formula feeding, p. 566.	Client successfully prepares formula and bottle-feeds her infant and demonstrates an awareness of the infant's needs (formula, frequency of feeds, etc.).
Follow-up care: Assess weight gain. Assess growth pattern. Assess hydration status (weight, skin, turgor, sunken eyes or fontanels, moistness of mucous membranes). Assess frequency of feeds, amounts of formula, or breast-feeding time.	ND: Altered health maintenance related to poor nutritional patterns or elimination problems. ND: Altered nutrition: less or more than body requirements related to infant feeding pattern. ND: Knowledge deficit related to growing	*To evaluate infant's nutritional status the nurse will:* Weigh and measure length. Evaluate growth according to age. Note and report poor or excessive growth. Note, report, and seek treatment for dehydration.	Client adjusts feeds according to child's needs. Child receives adequate nutrition to grow within the normal limits for age. Child establishes a regular elimination pattern.

Continued.

General Nursing Care Plan—cont'd

ASSESSMENT	NURSING DIAGNOSIS (ND)/ PLAN (P)/GOAL (G)	RATIONALE/ IMPLEMENTATION	EVALUATION
Assess child's satisfaction between feeds. Assess elimination pattern.	infant's nutritional needs. P: Provide information, demonstrate, and observe return demonstration. G: Client will be adept at adjusting feeding process to meet infant's nutritional needs. G: Infant will grow and gain weight within the normal limits for age. G: Infant will establish a regular elimination pattern.	Discuss feeding pattern and amounts with mother and evaluate child's satisfaction. Encourage client to verbalize feeding problems. Evaluate and report problems with elimination. Teach client infant satisfaction signs.	

Evaluation

The process of evaluation is continuous. As the infant matures, the norms for nutritional intake are adjusted to meet growth needs. The criteria are measurable in terms of the infant's growth, energy levels, and appearance. Parental knowledge is a key factor in infant nutrition and feeding. Parental knowledge and infant well-being and the findings that represent normal response form the basis for selecting appropriate nursing actions and evaluating their effectiveness.

SUMMARY

Providing nutrition services to parents and their infants is a function of the health care team. Physicians, nurses, registered dietitians, social workers, and health educators are major contributors to the care. One of the most important contributors, the nurse, can assist with nutrition assessment and provide education and counseling. Nurses can help interpret dietary prescriptions and make appropriate referrals of more complicated problems to nutritional personnel.

KEY CONCEPTS

- Healthy term babies are developmentally ready for feeding.
- Use of honey in home-prepared formulas can be fatal in some cases; parents should be warned.
- The attitude of the mother (and spouse) toward breast-feeding is a powerful factor in achieving successful lactation.
- The size of the breast gives no indication of its functional capacity.
- The composition and characteristics of commercial formulas are based on those of mature human milk.
- Teaching and counseling concerning the feeding of infants are important aspects of the daily care plan for maternity clients.
- The mother (parent) is presented with the benefits of both breast-feeding and formula-feeding as a basis for decision making.
- Feeding is an emotionally charged area of infant care.
- Most parents benefit from teaching related to chosen method of feeding.
- Limiting of breast-feeding time does not prevent nipple soreness.

STUDY QUESTIONS AND ACTIVITIES

1. Teach a new mothers class on breast-feeding, including:
   a. technique
   b. care of breasts
   c. common problems and treatments
   Use charts or visual aids when appropriate.
2. Prepare a nutritional diary for an infant. Describe factors that may be problem areas and develop a counseling plan to meet the needs of the infant and mother.
3. Conduct a group discussion of feelings and cultural conditioning regarding breast-feeding. At a later meeting, ask a lecturer from the LaLeche League or a similar support group to speak, and follow the presentation with another discussion of how or why your feelings have or have not changed on the subject.
4. Observe new mothers breast-feed and formula-feed their infants. Report on the clients' responses and any

prejudices expressed and observe for the interaction between mother and baby.

5. Research vegetarian diets. Bring findings to a discussion of the influence of such diets on the nutrition of a breast-fed infant.

References

American Academy of Pediatrics, Committee on Nutrition: Commentary on breast-feeding and infant formulas, including proposed standards for formulas, Pediatrics 57:278, 1976

American Academy of Pediatrics, Committee on Nutrition: Vitamin and mineral supplement needs in normal children in the United States, Pediatrics 66(6):1015, 1980a

American Academy of Pediatrics, Committee on Nutrition: On the feeding of supplemental foods to infants, Pediatrics 65(6):1178, 1980b

American Academy of Pediatrics, Committee on Nutrition: The use of whole cow's milk in infancy, Pediatrics 72(2):253, 1983a

American Academy of Pediatrics, Committee on Nutrition: Toward a prudent diet for children, Pediatrics 71(1):78, 1983b

American Academy of Pediatrics, Committee on Nutrition: Imitation and substitute milks, Pediatrics 73(6):876, 1984

Arnon, SS, et al: Honey and other environmental risk factors for infant botulism, J Pediatr 95:331, 1979

Blume, S, et al: Beer and breast-feeding mom, JAMA 258 (15):2126, 1987

Borovies, D: Assessing and managing pain in breast-feeding mothers, MCN 9:272, 1984

Broussard, A: Anticipatory guidance: adding solids to the infant's diet JOGN Nurs 13:239, July/Aug 1984

Chapman, J, et al: Concerns of breast-feeding mothers from birth to 4 months, Nurs Res 34:374, Nov/Dec 1985

Chung, HJ: Understanding the Oriental maternity patient, Nurs Clin North Am 12:67, 1977

Currier, RL: The hot-cold syndrome and symbolic balance in Mexican and Spanish-American folk medicine. In Martinez, RA, editor: Hispanic culture and health care: fact, fiction, folklore, St Louis, 1978, The CV Mosby Co

David, R, et al: Water intoxication in normal infants: role of antidiuretic hormone in pathogenesis, Pediatrics 68:349, 1981

Food and Nutrition Board: Recommended dietary allowances, Washington, DC, 1980, National Academy of Sciences

Hamill, PVV, et al: Physical growth: National center for health statistics percentiles, Am J Clin Nutr 32:607, 1979 (data from the Fels Research Institute, Wright State University School of Medicine, Yellow Springs, Ohio)

Hanson, LA, et al: Protective factors in milk and the development of the immune system, Pediatrics 75(suppl):172, 1985

Hart, DV: From pregnancy through birth in a Bisayan Filipino village. In Hart, DV, Rajadhon, PA, and Coughlin, RJ, editors: Southeast Asian birth customs: three studies in reproduction, New Haven, Conn, 1965, Human Relations Area Files

Hughes, R: Satisfaction with one's body and success in breast feeding, Issues in Comprehensive Pediatric Nursing 7:141, 1984

Knopp, RM, and Schwartz, JF: Water intoxication from swimming, J Pediatr 101:947, 1982

Lawrence, R: Breast-feeding: a guide for the medical profession, ed 2, St Louis, 1985, The CV Mosby Co

L'Esperance, C, and Frantz, K: Time limitation for early breastfeeding. JOGN Nurs 14(2):114, 1985

Madgic, D: Nutrition notes for new mothers, Stanford, Calif, 1986, Department of Dietetics, Stanford University Hospital

MacLauglin, S, and Strelnick, E: Breast feeding and working outside the home, Issues in Comprehensive Pediatric Nursing, 7:67, 1984

Owen, AL, et al: Infant feeding guide, Bloomfield, NJ, 1980, Health Learning System

Parsons, L: Weaning from the breast: for a happy ending to a satisfying experience, JOGN Nurs 7:12, 1978

Partridge, JC, et al: Water intoxication secondary to feeding mismanagement, Am J Dis Child, 135:38, 1981

Price, A, and Bamford, N: The breast feeding guide for the working woman, New York, 1983, Simon and Schuster

Pyle, M: Breast feeding is a family affair, Costa Mesa, Calif, 1985, Lifecircle

Riordan, J: A practical guide to breastfeeding, St Louis, 1983, The CV Mosby Co

Shutler, ME: Disease and curing in a Yaqui community. In Spicer, EH, editor: Ethnic medicine in the Southwest, Tucson, Ariz, 1977, The University of Arizona Press

Slaven S: Unlimited sucking time improves breastfeeding, Lancet 8216:392, 1981

Whaley, LF, and Wong, DL: Nursing care of infants and children, ed 3, St Louis, 1987, The CV Mosby Co

Williams, SR: Nutrition and diet therapy, ed 6, St Louis, 1989, The CV Mosby Co

Bibliography

Aberman, S, et al: Infant feeding practices, mother's decision-making, JOGN Nurs 14:394, Sept/Oct 1985

American Academy of Pediatrics, Committee on Nutrition: Iron supplementation for infants, Pediatrics 58:765, 1976

American Academy of Pediatrics, Committee on Nutrition: Fluoride supplementation: revised dosage schedule, Pediatrics 63:150, 1979

Bachrach, S, et al: An outbreak of vitamin D deficiency rickets in a susceptible population, Pediatrics 64:871, 1979

Balkam, JA: Guidelines for drug therapy during lactation, JOGN Nurs 15(1):65, 1986

Breastfeeding Your Twins, 1984, *Health* Education Associates, 520 School House Lane, Willow Grove, PA 09190

Chapman, JJ, et al: Concerns of breast-feeding mothers from birth to 4 months, Nurs Res 34(6):374, 1985

Chase, HP, et al: Kwashiorkor in the United States, Pediatrics 66:972, 1980

Dallman, RP, et al: Iron deficiency in infancy and childhood, Am J Clin Nutr 33:86, 1980

De Carvalho, M, et al: Effect of frequent breast-feeding on early milk production and infant weight gain, Pediatrics 72(3):307, 1983

Dilts, CL: Nursing management of mastitis due to breastfeeding, JOGN Nurs 14(4):286, 1985

Dwyer, JT, et al: Risk of nutritional rickets among vegetarian children, AM J Dis Child, 133:134, 1979

Ellis, DJ, and Hewat, RJ: Mothers' postpartum perceptions of spousal relationships, JOGN Nurs 14(2):140, 1985

Evans, CJ, Lyons, NB, and Killien, MG: The effect of infant formula samples on breastfeeding practice, JOGN Nurs 15(5):401, 1986

Fomon, SJ, and Ziegler, E: Skim milk in infant feeding, US Department of Health, Education, and Welfare pub no (HSA) 77-5102, Washington, DC, Aug 1977, The Department

Gaull, GE, Wright CE, and Isaacs, CE: Significance of growth modulators in human milk, Pediatrics 75(suppl):142, 1985

Hughes, RB, et al: Outcome of teaching clean vs. terminal methods of formula preparation, Pediatr Nurs 13(4):275, 1987

Jordan, PL: Breastfeeding as a risk factor for fathers, JOGN Nurs 15(2):94, 1986

Kearney, MH: Identifying psychosocial obstacles to breastfeeding success, JOGN Nurs 17(2):98, 1988

Lauwers, J, and Woessner, C: Pain—more than discomfort to breastfeeding women, Int J Childbirth Ed 2(2):30, 1987

McKay, S, and Mahan, C: Ways to upgrade postpartal care, Contemp OB/GYN 27:6:63, Nov 1985

Morse, JM, Harrison, MJ, and Prowse, M: Minimal breastfeeding, JOGN Nurs 15(4):333, 1986

Niebyl, JR: Making the breastfeeding decision, Contemp OB/GYN 28(3):43, 1986

Pipes, P: Nutrition in infancy and childhood, ed 2, St Louis, 1981, The CV Mosby Co

Pittard, WB, III, et al: Bacteriostatic qualities of human milk, J Pediatr 107(2):240, 1985

Reiff, MI, and Essock-Vitale, SM: Hospital influences on early infant-feeding practices, Pediatrics 76(6):872, 1985

Reifsnider, E, and Myers, ST: Employed mothers can breastfeed too! MCN 10(4):256, 1985

Saarinen, UM: Iron absorption in infants: high bioavailability of breast milk iron as indicated by the extrinsic tag method or iron absorption and by the concentration of serum ferritin, J Pediatr 91:36, 1977

Schafer, O: The impact of culture on breastfeeding patterns, J Perinat 6(1):62, 1986

Walker, M: How to evaluate breast pumps, MCN 12(4):270, 1987

Weyl-Feyling, DN: Breast feeding: what do you tell the mother? UCSF antepartum and intrapartum management conference, San Francisco, June, 1987

Williams, SR: Basic nutrition and diet therapy, ed 8, St Louis, 1988, The CV Mosby Co

Willis, NH: Infant nutrition: birth to 6 months: a syllabus, Philadelphia, 1980, JB Lippincott Co

Wolf, DM, and Coachman-Moore, VE: The consulting nutritionist in perinatal health care, J Perinat 6(4):335, 1986

Wong, S, and Stepp-Gilbert, E: Lactation suppression: nonpharmaceutical versus pharmaceutical method, JOGN Nurs 14(4):302, 1985

Worthington-Roberts, B, Vermeersch, J, and Williams SR: Nutrition in pregnancy and lactation, St Louis, 1981, The CV Mosby Co

Zinaman, MJ: Breast pumps: ensuring mothers' success, Contemp OB/GYN, 30:Oct 1987 (special issue)

Zmora, E, et al: Multiple nutritional deficiencies in infants from a strict vegetarian community, Am J Dis Child 133:141, 1979

UNIT

VI

Normal Postpartum Period

The postdelivery period is a time of significant change for the childbearing family. The mother experiences physiologic changes as her body regains its nonpregnant status and psychologic changes as she adjusts to a new phase of motherhood with a separate but dependent infant. The family members have new roles to assume as the newborn becomes established as part of the family unit. Chapter 24 presents content basic to understanding the physiologic adjustments of the woman during the puerperium. Chapter 25 presents family responses to the birth of a child from the perspective of mother, father, sibling(s), and grandparents. It discusses adaptive and maladaptive adjustments of family members. The chapter also includes content related to the impact of the infant's responses and temperament on the parent-child relationship. Chapter 26 draws on content in the previous two chapters in the application of the nursing process to the care of the family during its adjustment in the puerperium.

Nursing research highlights are included. Following are abstracts of examples of relevant nursing research:

Chapter 24: Return of functional ability after childbirth.

Chapter 25: Social support and psychologic outcomes.

Chapter 26: Postpartum anxiety and depression in mothers of term and preterm infants.

CHAPTER

24

Maternal Anatomic and Physiologic Recovery

Learning Objectives

Correctly define the key terms listed.

Describe maternal anatomy and physiology during the postpartum recovery and return to the nonpregnant state.

Review characteristics and measurement of normal uterine involution and lochia.

List expected values for vital signs and blood pressure, deviations from normal findings, and probable causes.

Compare and contrast four types of headaches that may occur during the early puerperium.

Key Terms

adynamic ileus
afterpains
anovulatory
autolysis
bradycardia
catabolism
colostrum
diaphoresis
diastasis recti abdominis
diuresis
engorgement (breast)
exfoliation
fourth trimester
hemorrhoids
human placental lactogen (hPL)
involution
lochia: alba, rubra, serosa
oxytocic medication
physiologic puerperal amenorrhea
prolactin
puerperium (early and late)
splanchnic engorgement
thromboembolism

Many factors influence the mother's responses to her newborn infant, among which are her energy level, her freedom from discomfort, the health of her newborn, and the care and encouragement supplied by professional persons. (See research highlight, below.) To provide care beneficial to the mother, the infant, and the family, the nurse synthesizes knowledge from maternal anatomy and physiology of the recovery period, the newborn's physical and behavioral characteristics, child care activities, and family response to the birth of the child. The nurse, in short, uses a holistic approach to nursing care. This chapter is devoted to the anatomic and physiologic changes in women after delivery.

RESEARCH HIGHLIGHT

Return of Functional Ability After Childbirth

Purpose

Descriptions of recovery from childbirth traditionally focus on healing of reproductive organs and fail to consider women's recovery of full functional ability. Therefore the purpose of this retrospective exploratory study was to compare rates of recovery of full functional ability for women who had cesarean deliveries with those who had vaginal deliveries. Full functional ability was defined as resumption of household, social and community, and occupational activities and assumption of infant care responsibilities.

Sample

The Childbirth Impact Profile, Form MQ (CIP-MQ), an investigator-developed semistructured questionnaire, was administered. The sample included 70 women who had delivered full-term infants within 5 years before data collection. Of these women, 30 had vaginal deliveries and 40 were cesarean delivered.

Methodology

The CIP-MQ contains 45 items about resumption of household, social and community, and occupational activities that had been engaged in before delivery and assumption of infant care. One item, regarding length of time to regain usual level of physical energy, was used as an overall index of functional ability.

Findings

Only 51% of the women reported they had regained their usual level of physical energy by 6 weeks after delivery. Several women reported that although they had resumed certain activities and had even returned to work within a short time after delivery, they had not regained their energy until quite a while later. These women reported they had to resume the activities before being ready because of family obligations, financial constraints, or their own need to appear to be recovered. The latter was true of the cesarean group.

Implications

The findings from this study support implications of previous research that recovery of full functional ability requires more than 6 weeks and that cesarean-delivered women require considerably more time than their vaginally-delivered counterparts. Clinically, more knowledge is needed about the adjustment to parenthood and the impact of the demands following childbirth on recovery.

Tulman, L, and Fawcett, J: Return of functional ability after childbirth, Nurs Res 37(2):77, 1988.

REPRODUCTIVE SYSTEM AND ASSOCIATED STRUCTURES

Uterine Corpus Changes

Uterine Involution. At the end of the third stage of labor the uterus is in the midline, about 2 cm *below* the level of the umbilicus with the fundus resting on the sacral promontory. At this time, uterine size approximates the size at 16 weeks of gestation (about the size of a grapefruit). The uterus is about 14 cm (5½ in) long, 12 cm (4¾ in) wide, and 10 cm (4 in) thick and weighs about 1000 g (2 lb). When relaxed, the uterus is discoid; when contracted, it is globular.

Within 12 hours the fundus may be approximately 1 cm *above* the umbilicus (Fig 24-1). From then on, involution progresses rapidly, and with the "take-up" and improved tone of the uterine supports, the fundus descends about 1 to 2 cm every 24 hours. By the sixth postpartum day the fundus normally will be half the distance from the symphysis pubis to the umbilicus. The uterus should not be palpable abdominally after the ninth postpartum day.

The uterus, which at full term weighs about 11 times its prepregnant weight, rapidly involutes to about 500 g (1 lb) 1 week after delivery and 350 g (11 to 12 oz) 2 weeks after delivery. A week after delivery the uterus lies in the true pelvis once again. At 6 weeks it weighs 50 to 60 g (Figs. 24-1 and 24-2).

Levels of estrogen, which stimulated myometrial growth primarily by increase in cell size, and of progesterone, which was responsible for much of the increased uterine weight and collagen formation during gestation, drop rapidly after delivery. Uterine involution within 4 to 6 weeks occurs principally by a decrease in the size of individual myometrial cells. However, the augmentation of connective tissue and elastin in the myometrium and blood vessels and the increase in the total uterine cell number are permanent. Hence uterine size is increased slightly after each pregnancy.

Uterine Contractions. The intensity of uterine contractions increases significantly immediately after delivery, presumably in response to the greatly diminished intrauterine volume. During the first 1 to 2 postpartum hours, uterine activity decreases smoothly and progressively and stabilizes. Uterine contractions become uncoordinated unless coordination is reestablished with exogenous (injected) oxytocin or endogenous oxytocin (released in response to nipple stimulation from suckling, for example). Uterine myometrial activity (tonus; the "living ligature" [see Fig. 6-11]) contributes to hemostasis by compressing the intramural blood vessels.

Afterpains. In primiparas the tone of the uterus is increased so that the fundus generally remains firm. Periodic relaxation and contraction are the rule for multiparas and may cause uncomfortable **afterpains** that persist throughout the early puerperium. Breast-feeding commonly intensifies these afterpains because oxytocin is released by the posterior pituitary gland in response to stimulation of the nipple.

Placental Site. Immediately after the placenta and membranes are delivered, the placental site is elevated, irregular, and partially obliterated by vascular constriction and thrombosis. According to Williams' classic description (Pritchard, MacDonald, and Gant, 1985), exfoliation (shedding) occurs because the site is undermined by an upward growth of endometrial tissue from the basal layer that remains after the separation of the placenta. Upward growth of the endometrium prevents scar formation that is characteristic of normal wound healing. This unique healing process enables the endometrium to resume its usual cycle of changes and to permit implantation and placentation in future pregnancies. Endometrial regeneration is completed by the end of the third postpartum week except at the pla-

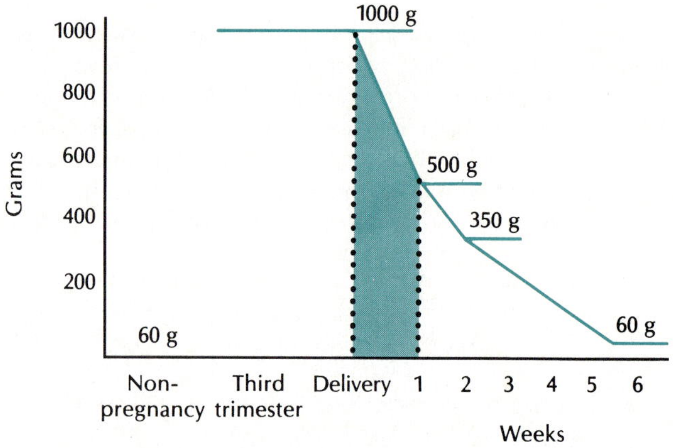

Fig. 24-2 Uterine weight before, during, and after pregnancy. Greatest change is in first week after childbirth.
Redrawn from Wiggins, JD: Childbearing: physiology, experiences, needs, St Louis, 1979, The CV Mosby Co.

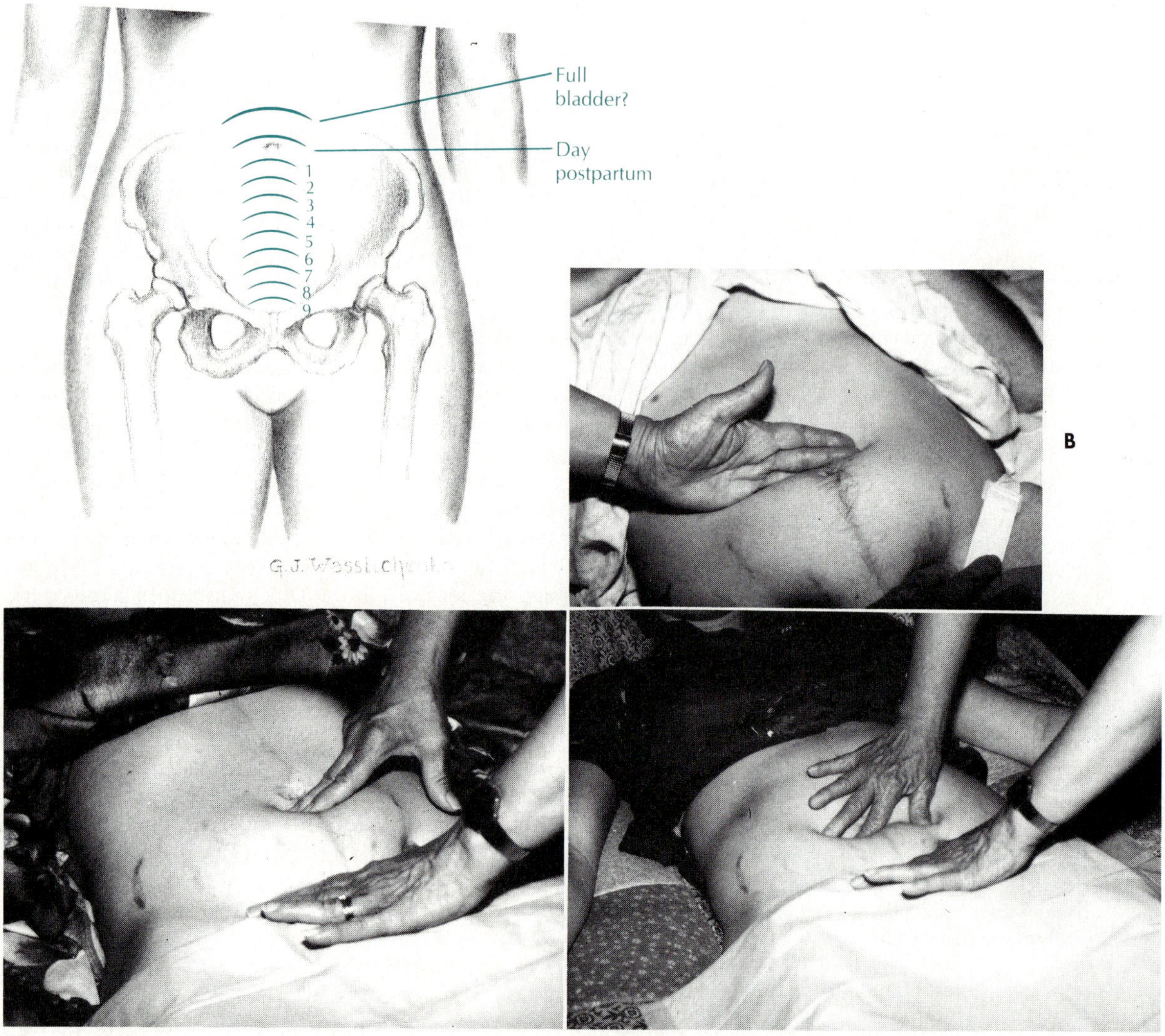

Fig. 24-1 Assessment of involution of uterus after delivery. **A,** Normal progress, days 1 through 9. **B,** Size and position of uterus 2 hours after delivery. **C,** 2 days after delivery. **D,** 4 days after delivery.
B, C, and **D** courtesy Marjorie Pyle, RNC, Lifecircle, Costa Mesa, Calif.

cental site. Regeneration at the placental site usually is not complete until 6 weeks after delivery.

Failure of the placental site to heal completely is called **subinvolution of the placental site.** Women with this condition have persistent lochia and episodes of brisk, painless bleeding. Curettage usually is required.

Lochia. Postdelivery uterine discharge initially is bright red, changing to dark red or reddish brown (lochia rubra). **Lochia rubra** consists mainly of blood, and decidual and trophoblastic debris. The flow pales, becoming pink or brown after 3 to 4 days (lochia serosa). **Lochia serosa** consists of old blood, serum, leukocytes, and tissue debris. About 10 days after delivery, the drainage becomes yellow to white (lochia alba). **Lochia alba** consists of numerous leukocytes, decidua, epithelial cells, mucus, serum, and bacteria. Lochia alba may continue until about 2 to 6 weeks after delivery.

The amount of lochia is described as scant, light, moderate, and heavy (Jacobson, 1985):

scant Blood only on tissue when wiped or less than 2.5 cm (1 in) on a peripad (see Fig. 20.3).
light Less than 10 cm (4 in) stain on a peripad.
moderate Less than 15 cm (6 in) stain on peripad.
heavy Saturated peripad within 1 hour.

Lochia refers only to uterine discharge. The blood seen on the peripad or bed linens may be from a different source (Table 24-1). Regardless of the source of bleeding, if the peripad is soaked through in 15 minutes or less, the flow is considered excessive.

If the woman has received an oxytocic medication, the flow of lochia is usually scant until the effect of the drug has disappeared. If the medication is administered intravenously, the effect persists for 30 minutes after the intravenous medication is discontinued; if the medication is administered intramuscularly, the effect persists for 30 to 60 minutes. If the woman is receiving ergonovine (Ergotrate) maleate, 0.2 mg by mouth 3 to 4 times a day for 2 days, lochia is usually scant.

Persistence of lochia rubra early in the postpartum period suggests continued bleeding as a result of retained fragments of the placenta or membranes. Recurrence of bleeding about 10 days after delivery indicates bleeding from the placental site, which is healing. However, after 3 to 4 weeks bleeding may be caused by infection or subinvolution of the placental site. Continued lochia serosa or lochia alba may indicate endometritis, particularly if fever, pain, or tenderness is associated with the discharge. Lochia should smell like normal menstrual flow; an offensive odor usually indicates infection. Lochia clots, whereas normal menstrual blood does not (Chapter 6).

Table 24-1 *Lochia and Nonlochia Bleeding*

Lochia	Nonlochia Bleeding
Lochia usually trickles from the vaginal opening. The steady flow is greater as the uterus contracts.	If the bloody discharge spurts from the vagina, there may be cervical or vaginal tears in addition to the normal lochia.
A gush of lochia may result as the uterus is massaged. If it is dark in color, it has been pooled in the relaxed vagina, and the amount soon lessens to a trickle of bright red lochia (in the early puerperium).	If the amount of bleeding continues to be excessive and bright red, a tear may be the source.

Cervix. The cervix up to the lower uterine segment remains edematous, thin, and fragile for several days after delivery. The ectocervix (portion of the cervix that protrudes into the vagina) is soft, appears bruised, and has some small lacerations, optimum conditions for the development of infection. It remains easily distensible; two fingers may still be introduced for the first 4 to 6 days after delivery; only the smallest curette may be introduced by the end of 2 weeks. By the eighteenth hour the cervix has shortened, has a firm consistency, and has regained its form. By the end of the first week, recovery is almost complete. The external os, however, does not regain its prepregnant appearance; it is no longer shaped like a circle but appears as a jagged slit often described as "fish mouth" (see Fig. 6-12). Production of cervical and other estrogen-influenced mucus and mucosal characteristics may be delayed in the lactating woman.

Vagina and Perineum. Postpartum estrogen deprivation is responsible for the thinness of the *vaginal mucosa* and the absence of rugae. The greatly distended, smooth-walled vagina gradually returns to its prepregnant size by 6 to 8 weeks after delivery. Rugae reappear by about the fourth week, although they are never as prominent as they are in the nulliparous woman. Most rugae may be permanently flattened. The mucosa remains atrophic in the lactating woman at least until menstruation begins again. Thickening of the vaginal mucosa occurs with the return of ovarian function. Profuse vaginal discharge is usually not present at 4 to 6 weeks after delivery unless there is an associated vaginitis. The hypoestrogenic condition of the vaginal epithelium is responsible for the decreased amount of vaginal mucus production and thinner vaginal mucosa. Local dryness and coital discomfort may persist until ovulation and menstruation resume.

Initially the *introitus* is erythematous and edematous, especially in the area of the episiotomy or laceration repair. Careful repair, prevention or early treatment of hematomas, and good hygiene during the first 2 weeks after delivery usually result in an introitus barely distinguishable from that of a nulliparous woman. The torn hymen heals with the development of fibrosed nodules of mucosa called *hymenal caruncles.*

Most *episiotomies* are visible only if the woman is lying on her side and her buttock is raised. A good light source is essential for visualization of some episiotomies. The healing process of an episiotomy is the same as for any surgical incision. Signs of infection (pain, redness, warmth, swelling, or discharge) or loss of approximation (separation) of the incision edges may occur.

Hemorrhoids (anal varicosities) are commonly seen. The women commonly experience associated symptoms such as itching, discomfort, and bright red bleeding with defecation.

Pelvic Muscular Support. Injury of the supporting structures of the uterus and vagina may occur during childbirth and may become gynecologic problems later in life. The term *relaxation* refers to the lengthening and weakening of the fascial supports of pelvic structures. These include the uterus, upper posterior vaginal wall, urethra, bladder, and rectum. Although relaxations can occur in any woman, most are direct but delayed sequelae to childbirth (Chapter 41).

Abdominal Wall. When the woman stands up during the first days after delivery, abdominal muscles cannot retain abdominal contents. The abdomen protrudes and gives her a still-pregnant appearance (Fig. 24-3). During the first 2 weeks after delivery the abdominal wall is relaxed. About 6 weeks are required before the abdominal wall almost returns to its nonparous state. The skin regains most of its previous elasticity, but some striae persist. The return of muscle tone depends on previous tone, proper exercise, and amount of adipose tissue. On occasion, with or without overdistension because of a large fetus or multiple fetuses, the abdominal wall muscles separate, a condition termed *diastasis recti abdominis* (see Fig. 10-11). Peristence of this defect may be disturbing to the woman, but surgical correction is rarely necessary. With time, the defect becomes less apparent.

Breasts. The concentrations of hormones that stimulated breast development during pregnancy (estrogen, progesterone, human chorionic gonadotropin, prolactin, cortisol, and insulin) decrease promptly after delivery. The time it takes for the return of these hormones to prepregnancy levels is determined in part by whether the mother breastfeeds her infant.

Nonbreast-feeding Mothers. The breasts feel generally nodular (in nonpregnant women they feel granular). The nodularity is bilateral and diffuse.

If the woman chooses not to breast-feed and no antilactogenic medication is taken, prolactin levels drop rapidly. Colostrum secretion and excretion persists for the first few days after delivery. Palpation of the breast on the second or third day, as milk production begins, reveals tissue tenseness. On the third or fourth postpartum day the breasts become **engorged.** They are distended (swollen), firm, tender, and warm to the touch (vasocongestion makes them feel warm). Milk can be expressed from the nipples. Axillary breast tissue (the tail of Spence) and any accessory breast or nipple tissue along the milk line may be involved. Breast distension is primarily caused by temporary congestion of veins and lymphatics rather than from an accumulation of milk. Engorgement resolves spontaneously, and discomfort decreases usually within 24 to 36 hours. If suckling is never begun (or is discontinued), lactation ceases within a few days to a week.

Breast-feeding Mothers. As lactation is established, a mass (lump) may be felt; however, a filled milk sac will shift position from day to day. Before lactation begins, the breasts feel soft and a yellowish fluid, colostrum, can be expressed from the nipples. After lactation begins, the breasts feel warm to the touch and firm. Tenderness persists for about 48 hours. Bluish white milk (skim-milk appearance) can be expressed from the nipples. The nipples are examined for erectility as opposed to inversion and for cracks or fissures.

For a discussion of breast changes associated with lactation, see Chapter 23.

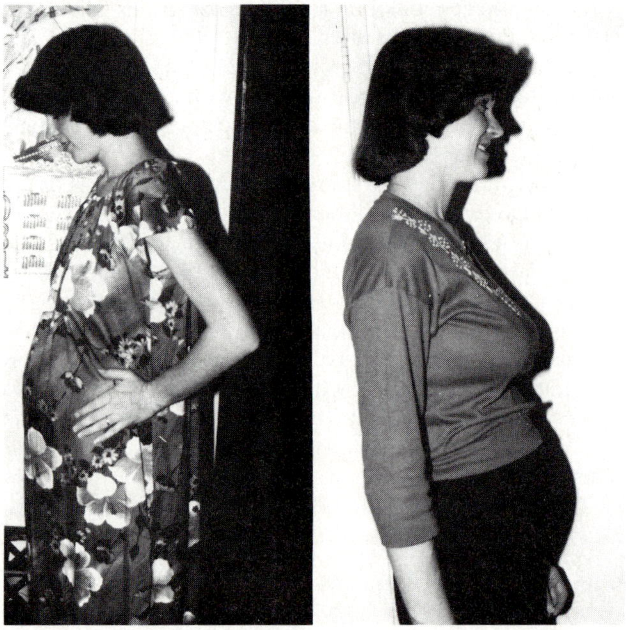

A B

Fig. 24-3 Abdomen after delivery. **A**, Two hours after delivery. **B**, Eight days after delivery.
Courtesy of Marjorie Pyle, RNC, Lifecircle, Costa Mesa, Calif.

ENDOCRINE SYSTEM

Placental Hormones. Plasma levels of placental hormones fall rapidly after delivery. *Human placental lactogen* (hPL) levels reach undetectable levels within 24 hours (see also discussions of growth hormone and carbohydrate metabolism). *Human chorionic gonadotropin* (hCG) declines rapidly, so that standard urinary pregnancy tests are usually negative by the end of the first week.

Estrogen levels in plasma fall to 10% of the prenatal value within 3 hours after delivery; the lowest levels occur about day 7. The significant decline in estrogen is accompanied by the onset of breast engorgement on about postpartum day 3, a coincidence that supports the view that high estrogen levels suppress lactation despite elevated prolactin levels. Plasma levels of estrogen do not increase to follicular levels until 19 to 21 days after delivery. In lactating women, return to normal estrogen levels is somewhat delayed.

Progesterone levels in plasma fall below luteal levels by the third postpartum day and cannot be detected in serum after the first postdelivery week. Progesterone production begins with the first ovulation.

Pituitary Hormones. *Prolactin* levels in blood rise progressively throughout pregnancy. After delivery, in nonlactating women, prolactin levels decline, reaching the prepregnant range within 2 weeks. Initially, suckling and lactation are accompanied by dramatic increases in prolactin concentration. Serum prolactin levels are influenced by the number of times per day breast-feeding occurs. Normal basal values of prolactin are reached by 6 months if breast-feeding occurs only 1 to 3 times per day. High prolactin levels persist for more than a year if suckling occurs more than 6 times per day.

Levels of *follicle-stimulating hormone* (FSH) and *luteinizing hormone* (LH) are low in all women for 10 to 12 days after delivery.

Hypothalamic-pituitary-ovarian Function. Little is known about the physiology of the hypothalamus, the pituitary gland, and the ovaries during the puerperium after term gestation. The exact nature of the changing endocrine milieu is unclear at this time (Danforth and Scott, 1986). However, considerable information is available on the time of appearance of the first ovulation and the reestablishment of menstruation for lactating and nonlactating women. For all women, the first menses *usually* follows an *an*ovulatory cycle or a cycle associated with inadequate corpus luteum function (low LH and progesterone).

Among lactating women, 15% resume menstruation by 6 weeks, and 45% by 12 weeks. Among nonlactating women, 40% menstruate by 6 weeks, 65% by 12 weeks, and 90% by 24 weeks. For lactating women, 80% of first menstrual cycles are anovulatory; for nonlactating women 50% of first cycles are anovulatory (Vorherr, 1979; Danforth and Scott, 1986).

Much of the variability in the reestablishment of menstruation and ovulation observed in lactating women may result from individual differences in the strength of the suckling stimulus. Partial weaning (formula supplementation) and breast-feeding less than 6 times per day also may play a role. This emphasizes the fact that **breast-feeding is not a reliable form of birth control.**

The first menstrual flow is usually heavier than normal. Within 3 to 4 cycles the amount of menstrual flow has returned to the woman's prepregnant volume.

Other Endocrine Changes. *Growth hormone* secretion remains depressed during late pregnancy and the early puerperium. The low level of growth hormone and the rapid decline in the hormones hPL, estrogens, and cortisol and in the placental enzyme, insulinase, *reduce the anti-insulin factors* in the early puerperium. Therefore new mothers have low fasting plasma glucose levels, and insulin requirements for insulin-dependent diabetic women usually fall after delivery (see Chapter 32). Normal hormonal alterations render the early puerperium a transitional period for *carbohydrate metabolism* so that interpretation of glucose tolerance tests is difficult at this time.

Rapid fluctuations in many indices confound evaluation of *thyroid* function during the early puerperium. Postpartum hypothyroidism is suspected if the woman fails to lactate or recovery from childbirth is delayed.

A progressive increase of plasma levels of *corticosteroids* during pregnancy and labor is followed by a decline to nonpregnant values by the end of the first week after delivery. Within 2 hours after delivery, *plasma renin* and *angiotensin II* levels drop to within the normal nonpregnant range. This finding may indicate that the fetoplacental unit is one source of maternal plasma renin.

Basal Metabolic Rate. The basal metabolic rate remains elevated for 7 to 14 days after delivery. Normal nonpregnant values for respiratory system function are given in Appendix E.

Fatigue. Fatigue is customary during the first few days after delivery. Extra rest and sleep are required. The underlying cause is unclear, but may be related to the rapid endocrine changes.

CARDIOVASCULAR SYSTEM

Blood Volume. Changes in blood volume depend on several variable factors, for example, blood loss during delivery, and mobilization and subsequent excretion of extravascular water (physiologic edema). Blood loss results in immediate but limited decrease in total blood volume. Thereafter, normal shifts in body water result in a slow decline in blood volume. By the third to fourth week after delivery the blood volume usually has regressed to nonpregnant values (Fig. 24-4).

Maternal Response to Normal Blood Loss. Pregnancy-induced hypervolemia (increase of at least 40% from 1 to 2 L near term) allows most women to tolerate a considerable blood loss at delivery. Many women lose 300 to 400 ml of blood during vaginal delivery of a single fetus and about twice this amount during cesarean delivery.

Retrogressive changes (readjustments) in the maternal vasculature after delivery are dramatic and rapid. The wom-

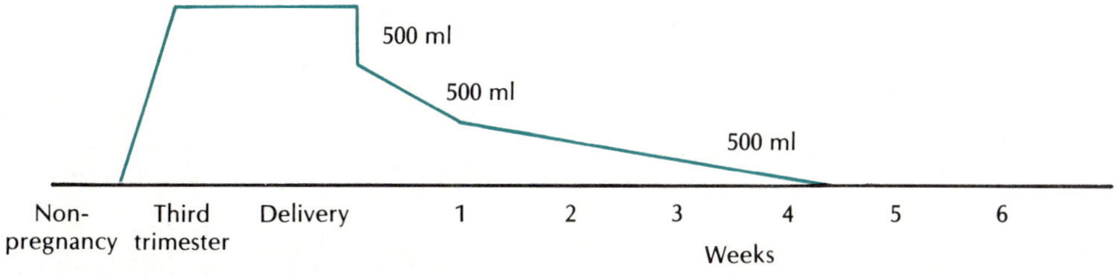

Fig. 24-4 Rate of loss of 1500 ml in blood volume during first postdelivery month. Greatest change at delivery, then in week after childbirth.

From Wiggins, JD: Childbearing: physiology, experiences, needs, St Louis, 1979, The CV Mosby Co.

an's response to blood loss during the early puerperium differs from that in a nonpregnant woman. Three postpartum physiologic changes protect the woman: (1) elimination of uteroplacental circulation reduces the size of the maternal vascular bed by 10% to 15%, (2) loss of placental endocrine function removes the stimulus for vasodilation, and (3) mobilization of extravascular water stored during pregnancy occurs.

Cardiac Output. The cardiac output continues to increase during the first and second stages of labor. The cardiac output peaks during the early puerperium whether the delivery was vaginal or abdominal. A few minutes after delivery, cardiac output has declined to about 50% of prelabor levels; within 2 to 3 weeks, cardiac output is at nonpregnant levels (Fig. 24-5). Although the mean values are slightly lower, the same changes occur if delivery takes place with conduction anesthesia.

Vital Signs and Blood Pressure. Few alterations in vital signs and blood pressure are seen under normal circumstances (Table 24-2). Respiratory function returns to nonpregnant levels by 6 months after delivery. After the uterus is emptied, the diaphragm descends, the normal cardiac axis is restored, and cardiologic features (point of maximal impulse [PMI], ECG) are normalized.

Blood Constituents

Hematocrit. During the first 72 hours after delivery, there is a greater loss in plasma volume than in blood cells. The decrease in plasma volume plus the increase in red blood cell (RBC) mass of pregnancy is associated with a rise in hematocrit by the third to seventh day after delivery. There is no RBC destruction during the puerperium, but any gain will disappear gradually in accordance with the life span of the RBC. In uncomplicated cases the hematocrit will have returned to the normal nonpregnant range by the fourth or fifth postdelivery week.

White Blood Cell Count. Normal leukocytosis of pregnancy averages about 12,000/mm^3. During the first 10 to 12 days after delivery, values between 20,000 to 25,000/mm^3 are common. Neutrophils are the most numerous WBCs with a consequent shift to the left. Leukocytosis coupled with the normal increase in erythrocyte sedimentation rate may confuse the interpretation of acute infections at this time.

Coagulation Factors. An extensive activation of blood-clotting factors occurs after delivery. This activation, together with immobility, trauma, or sepsis, encourages thromboembolism. Factors I, II, VIII, IX, and X decrease within a few days to prepregnant levels. The elevated levels

Table 24-2 *Vital Signs and Blood Pressure After Delivery*

Normal Findings	Deviations from Normal Findings and Probable Causes
Temperature	
During first 24 hours, may rise to 38° C (100.4° F) as a result of dehydrating effects of labor. After 24 hours the woman should be afebrile.	A diagnosis of puerperal sepis is suggested if a rise in maternal temperature to 38° C (100.4° F) is noted after the first 24 hours after delivery and recurs or persists for 2 days. Other possibilities are mastitis, endometritis, urinary tract infections, and other systemic infections.
Pulse	
Bradycardia is a common finding for the first 6 to 8 days after delivery. Bradycardia is a consequence of increased cardiac output and stroke volume. The pulse returns to nonpregnant levels by 3 months after delivery. A pulse rate of between 50 and 70 beats/min may be considered normal.	A rapid pulse rate or one that is increasing may indicate hypovolemia secondary to hemorrhage.
Respirations	
Respirations should fall to within the woman's normal predelivery range.	Hypoventilation and hypotension may follow an unusually high subarachnoid (spinal) block.
Blood Pressure	
Blood pressure is altered *slightly* if at all. Orthostatic hypotension, as indicated by feelings of faintness or dizziness immediately after standing up, can develop in the first 48 hours as a result of the splanchnic engorgement that may occur after delivery.	A low or falling blood pressure may reflect hypovolemia secondary to hemorrhage. However, it is a late sign, and other symptoms of hemorrhage usually alert the staff. An increased reading may result from excessive use of vasopressor drugs or oxytocic drugs. Since pregnancy-induced hypertension (PIH) can persist into or occur first in the postpartum period, routine evaluation of blood pressure is needed. If a woman complains of headache, hypertension must be ruled out as a cause before analgesics are administered. If the blood pressure is elevated, the woman is confined to bed and the physician notified. (See also Chapter 29).

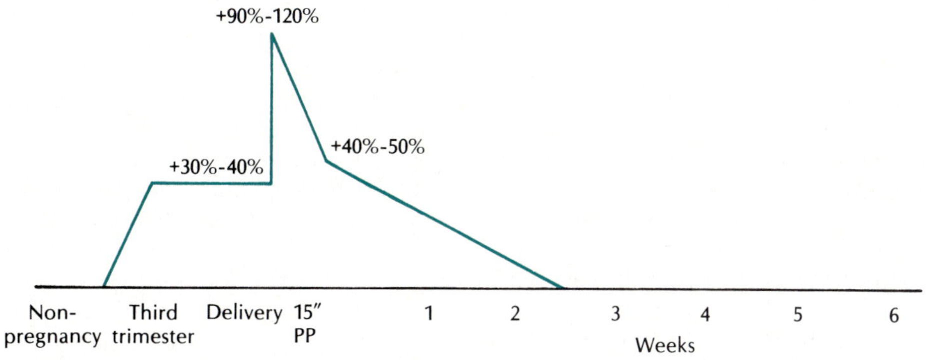

Fig. 24-5 Cardiac output. Work of heart increases during labor and decreases significantly immediately after birth of baby.

From Wiggins, JD: Childbearing: physiology, experiences, needs, St Louis, 1979, The CV Mosby Co.

of fibrin split products are probably the result of their release from the placental site.

Thromboembolism. The woman's legs are examined daily for signs of thrombosis (pain, warmth, and tenderness; swollen reddened vein that feels hard or solid to touch). There may or may not be a positive Homans' sign (dorsiflexion of foot [see Fig. 14-2], which causes calf muscles to compress tibial veins and produce pain if thrombosis is present). It is important to remember that deep venous thrombosis may be silent, that is, not cause pain.

Varicosities. Varicosities of the legs and around the anus (hemorrhoids) are common during pregnancy. Varices, even the less common vulvar varices, regress (empty) rapidly immediately after delivery. Surgical correction of varicosites is not considered during pregnancy. Total or the nearly total regression is anticipated after delivery.

URINARY SYSTEM

Renal Function. The hormonal changes of pregnancy (high steroid levels) contribute to the increase in renal function, and conversely the diminishing steroid levels after delivery may partly explain the reduced renal function during the puerperium. Kidney function returns to normal within a month after delivery. About 6 weeks are required for the pregnancy-induced hypotonia and dilation of the ureters and renal pelves to subside. In a small percentage of women, dilation of the urinary tract may persist for 3 months.

Urine Constituents. The renal glycosuria induced by pregnancy disappears. *Lactosuria* may be expected in lactating women. However, it cannot be detected by use of the Clinitest, since this test is specific for the presence of glucose, not lactose, in urine. The *blood urea nitrogen increases* during the puerperium as autolysis of the involuting uterus is accomplished. As a result of the catalytic processes of involution, *mild proteinuria* (+ 1) is a normal finding for 1 to 2 days after delivery in about 50% of women. *Acetonuria* may even occur in women with an uncomplicated delivery or after a prolonged labor with dehydration.

Reversal of Water Metabolism of Pregnancy. **Profuse diaphoresis**, especially at night (night sweats), is not unusual for 2 to 3 days after delivery. Diaphoresis is a mechanism to reduce the retained fluids of pregnancy and usually is not a symptom of infection.

The renal plasma flow and glomerular filtration rate that increased by 25% to 50% during pregnancy remains elevated for at least the first postpartum week. Normally a **marked diuresis** begins within 12 hours after delivery. The volume of urinary output along with the insensible water loss through perspiration accounts for a large portion of the **weight loss** during the early puerperium. This weight loss is approximately 5.5 kg (12 lb) after delivery of the fetus, placenta, and amniotic fluid and an additional 4 kg (9 lb) during the puerperium because of excretion of fluids and electrolytes accumulated during pregnancy. The mechanism that facilitates elimination of the excess tissue fluid accumulated during pregnancy is often referred to as the *reversal of the water metabolism of pregnancy.*

Urethra and Bladder. Trauma occurs to the urethra and bladder as the infant passes through the pelvis. The bladder wall is hyperemic and edematous, often with small areas of hemorrhage. Clean-catch or catheterized urine specimens after delivery often reveal hematuria from bladder trauma. Later in the puerperium, hematuria may be a sign of urinary tract infection. The urethra and urinary meatus may be edematous. Birth-induced trauma and the effects of analgesia, especially conduction anesthesia, cause relative insensitivity that depresses the urge to void. In addition, pelvic soreness caused by the forces of labor, vaginal lacerations, or the episiotomy reduces or alters the voiding reflex. This alteration, together with postpartum diuresis, may allow rapid filling of the bladder.

Distension of the bladder can readily occur as the water metabolism of pregnancy is reversed and fluids are mobilized in the elimination of end products of protein catabolism. Overdistension can make the bladder more susceptible to infection as well as impede the resumption of normal voiding. If prolonged bladder overdistension occurs, further damage to the bladder wall (atony) may result.

GASTROINTESTINAL SYSTEM

Appetite. The mother is usually hungry shortly after delivery and can tolerate a light diet. After full recovery from analgesia, anesthesia, and fatigue, most new mothers are ravenously hungry. Requests for double portions of food and frequent snacks are not uncommon. For a discussion of diet during lactation, see Chapter 15.

Motility. Typically, decreased muscle tone and motility of the gastrointestinal tract persists for only a short time after delivery. Excess analgesia and anesthesia could delay a return to normal tonicity and motility.

Bowel Evacuation. A spontaneous bowel evacuation may be delayed until 2 to 3 days after delivery. This can be explained by decreased muscle tone (*adynamic ileus*) in the intestines during labor and the immediate puerperium, prelabor diarrhea or a predelivery enema, lack of food, dehydration, or perineal tenderness because of episiotomy, lacerations, or hemorrhoids. Regular bowel habits must be reestablished after delivery once bowel tone returns.

NEUROLOGIC SYSTEM

Neurologic changes during the puerperium are those resulting from a reversal of maternal adaptations to pregnancy and those resulting from trauma during labor and delivery.

Pregnancy-induced neurologic discomforts abate after delivery. Elimination of physiologic edema through the diuresis that follows delivery relieves *carpal tunnel syndrome* by easing the compression of the median nerve. The periodic numbness and tingling of fingers that afflict 5% of gravidas usually disappear after delivery unless lifting and carrying the baby aggravates the condition. For a discussion of nerve injury incurred during childbirth, see Chapter 41. *Headache* requires careful assessment. Four types of headaches are compared in Table 24-3.

MUSCULOSKELETAL SYSTEM

Adaptations in the mother's endocrine system are reversed in the puerperium. The adaptations include those that contribute to relaxation and subsequent hypermobility of the joints and in the change in the mother's center of gravity because of the enlarging uterus. *Stabilization of joints* is complete by 6 to 8 weeks after delivery. However, although all other joints return to their normal prepregnant position before restabilization, those in the parous woman's feet do not; the new mother may notice a permanent increase in shoe size.

Table 24-3 *Comparison of Postpartum Headaches*

	Postsubarachnoid Anesthesia	Stress Headache	Meningeal Irritation	Pregnancy-Induced Hypertension (PIH)
Cause	Leakage of cerebrospinal fluid through puncture in dura into extradural space	Anxiety, muscle tension especially in neck, shoulders; fatigue, hunger	Aseptic chemical meningeal irritation	Etiologic factors of PIH (e.g., vasospasm)
Onset	Days 1-2	Variable		Late in the development of PIH; a frequent forerunner of eclampsia (convulsions)*
Location	Forehead, deep behind eyes; radiates to both temples and to occipital area	Band around head; occipital		Frontal or occipital, or generalized
Intensity	Severe to mild	More or less constant ache		Severe, constant throbbing or "splitting"
Modifiers	Increased intensity in sitting or standing position; eases in supine position	Relieved by physical and psychologic rest, food	Not relieved by lying down	Resistant to relief from analgesics
Duration	1-3 days to several weeks	Variable	1-3 days	Duration of severe PIH
Therapy	Increase oral fluids Supplement oral fluids with at least 1000 ml 5% dextrose in normal saline solution Administer analgesics Assist physician in establishing extradural "blood patch" wtih client's own blood Tight abdominal binder	Implement good communication techniques to help her identify concerns, to ventilate feelings regarding labor/delivery experience; facilitate rest; offer food and fluids; administer medications as necessary; utilize comfort measures (e.g., back rubs, etc).	Administer analgesics, fluids, and other supportive measures	Treatment for PIH (see Chapter 29)

*Pritchard, JA, MacDonald, PC, and Gant, NF: Williams obstetrics, ed 17, Norwalk, Conn, 1985, Appleton-Century-Crofts.

INTEGUMENTARY SYSTEM

Chloasma of pregnancy usually disappears at the termination of pregnancy. *Hyperpigmentation* of the areolae and linea nigra may not regress completely after delivery.

Vascular abnormalities such as spider angiomas (nevi), palmar erythema, and epulis generally regress in response to the rapid decline in estrogens after termination of pregnancy. For some women, spider nevi persist indefinitely.

The abundance of fine *hair* seen during pregnancy usually disappears after delivery; however, any coarse or bristly hair that appears during pregnancy usually remains. *Fingernails* return to their prepregnant characteristics of consistency and strength.

Diaphoresis is the most noticeable change in the integumentary system (see reversal of water metabolism of pregnancy, p. 583).

IMMUNE SYSTEM

The mother's need for *rubella vaccination* or for prevention of Rh isoimmunization is determined.

For discussion of acquired immune deficiency syndrome (AIDS) and other questions concerning immunology, see the section on immunology in Chapter 6.

SUMMARY

The maternity nurse needs a solid understanding of normal physiologic responses during the postpartum period. This will enable the nurse to provide quality nursing care. Knowledge of normal findings will allow the nurse to plan for care and encourage client participation. Women and their families will be better able to anticipate and adjust to postpartum changes if they have been provided with adequate health information. The nurse is in a key role to provide health education to women and their families. The nurse can help ease the transition from pregnancy to motherhood.

KEY CONCEPTS

- The uterus involutes rapidly after delivery, returning to the true pelvis within 1 week.
- The rapid drop in estrogen and progesterone following delivery of the placenta is responsible for many of the anatomic and physiologic changes in the puerperium.
- Assessment of the lochia is vital to monitor normal involution and potential problems.
- Breast-feeding is a *not* a reliable form of birth control.
- Puerperal changes in the blood constituents may be clinically confusing if the clinician is unaware of them.
- The woman's response to blood loss during the early puerperium differs from that in the nonpregnant woman.
- Bradycardia is a common finding for the first 6 to 8 days.
- The early puerperium is marked by a reversal of the water metabolism of pregnancy.

STUDY QUESTIONS AND ACTIVITIES

1. Develop a class for new mothers that will cover all aspects of the postpartum anatomic and physiologic changes and correlate discussion with prenatal adaptations. Research available audiovisual aids.
2. Assess individual multiparous and primiparous women and use findings as the basis of a group discussion of similarities and differences.
3. Observe the return visit of a postpartum client to the clinic and note especially assessment of involution progress, laboratory tests, and physical problems.
4. Prepare an educational session that will explain to the new mother the mechanisms behind physiologic puerperal amenorrhea and correct any misinformation as to the efficacy of breast-feeding as a contraceptive.
5. In a group conference, answer and give rationale for the following questions:
   a. Women who breast-feed often ask whether one can become pregnant while breast-feeding. What should the nurse answer?
   b. Early ambulation of the mother following delivery promotes what normal functions?

References

Danforth, DN, and Scott, JR, editors: Obstetrics and gynecology, ed 5, Philadelphia, 1986, JB Lippincott Co

Jacobson, H: A standard for assessing lochia volume, MCN 10(3):174, 1985

Pritchard, JA, MacDonald, PC, and Gant, NF: Williams obstetrics, ed 17, Norwalk, Conn, 1985, Appleton-Century-Crofts

Vorherr, H, editor: Human lactation, Semin Perinatol 3:191, 1979

Bibliography

Ferguson, H: Planning letter-perfect postpartum care, Nurs '87 17(5):50, 1987

Fischman, SH, et al: Changes in sexual relationships in postpartum couples, JOGN Nurs, 15(1):58, 1986

Gorrie, TM: Postpartal nursing diagnosis, JOGN Nurs, 15(1):52, 1986

Hans, A: Postpartum assessment: the psychological component, JOGN Nurs 15(1):49, 1986

McKay, S, and Mahan, CS: Ways to upgrade postpartal care, Contemp OB/GYN 27:63, 1985

Myles, MF: Textbook for midwives with modern concepts of obstetric and neonatal care, ed 9, New York, 1981, Churchill Livingstone, Inc

Oxorn, H: Oxorn-Foote human labor and birth, ed 5, Norwalk, Conn, 1986, Appleton-Century-Crofts

Quistad, C: How to smooth mom's postpartum path, RN 47:40, April 1984

Willson, JR, and Carrington, ER: Obstetrics and gynecology, ed 8, St. Louis, 1987, The CV Mosby Co

Zuspan, F, and Quilligan, E: Practical manual of obstetric care, St. Louis, 1982, The CV Mosby Co

CHAPTER

25

Family Dynamics After Childbirth

Learning Objectives

Correctly define the key terms listed.

Discuss the parenting process.

List and discuss five preconditions that influence attachment.

Review the sensual responses that strengthen attachment.

Differentiate the three periods in parental role change following childbirth.

List six parental tasks and responsibilities.

Determine infant behaviors that facilitate and inhibit parental attachment.

Identify the three phases of maternal adjustment.

Describe and discuss mothers who need additional supportive counseling.

Explain paternal adjustment.

List three ways to facilitate parent-infant adjustment.

Discuss parenthood after 35.

Review effects of a parent's sensory impairment on the parent-child attachment process.

Assess sibling adjustment to the newborn and the parents.

Examine grandparent adjustment.

Key Terms

attachment
biorhythmicity
claiming process
cognitive-affective skills
cognitive-motor skills
engrossment
entrainment
executive behaviors
fingertip exploration
habituation
infant-parent adjustment
- behavioral repertoires
- responsivity
- rhythm

maternal adjustment
- dependent phase
- dependent-independent phase
- interdependent phase

mothering function
mutuality
parental preconditions
parental roles
paternal responses
- expressive
- instrumental
- observer

positive feedback
sensual responses
signaling behaviors
significant other
taking-in phase

The birth of a child poses a fundamental challenge to the existing interactional structure of a family. The marital relationship between spouses must now accomodate the relationship between parents and child. If there is another child (or children) in the family, parents must adjust their own life space to include another child, and the firstborn children must adjust to another person's claim on parental time and love (Walz and Rich, 1983). This chapter reviews the parenting process and parent, sibling, and grandparent adjustments to childbirth.

PARENTING PROCESS

Biologic parenthood for both parents begins with the union of ovum and sperm. During the prenatal period the mother is the primary agent in providing an environment in which the unborn child may develop and grow. This close symbiotic union of mother and child ends with birth. Others may then assume partial or complete involvement in the infant's care. Whoever—whether biologic or substitute parent, woman or man—assumes the parental role enters into a crucial relationship with a child that will persist throughout the life of each. Men and women, of course, may exist without a child; thus, in essence, parenthood is optional. Parenthood may serve as a maturation factor in the life of a man and woman regardless of whether it is biologically based. For children, parenthood is all important; their continued existence depends on the quality of care they receive.

The tasks, responsibilities, and attitudes that make up parenting care have been designated by Steele and Pollack (1968) as the "mothering function." It is a process in which an adult (a mature, caring, capable, self-sufficient person) assumes the care of an infant (an immature, helpless, dependent person). Either parent may exhibit "motherliness." Motherliness is now recognized to be a non-gender-related ability. The ability to show gentleness, love, and understanding and to place another's welfare above one's own is not limited to women—it is a human characteristic.

Steele and Pollack (1968) describe parenting as one process with two components. The first, being practical or mechanical in nature, involves cognitive and motor skills; the second, emotional in nature, involves cognitive and affective skills. Both components are essential to the infant's well-being and future development.

Cognitive-motor Skills

The first component in the process of parenting includes childcare activities such as "feeding, holding, clothing, and cleaning the infant, protecting it from harm, and providing mobility for it" (Steele and Pollack, 1968). These task-oriented activities do not appear automatically as efficient caretaking behaviors at the birth of one's child. The parents' abilities in these respects have been influenced by cultural and personal experiences. Many parents have to learn how to do these tasks, and this learning process can be difficult. However, almost all parents with the desire to learn and with the support of others become adept in caregiving activities.

Cognitive-affective Skills

The psychologic component in childcare, motherliness or fatherliness, appears to stem from the *parents'* earliest experiences with a loving, accepting mother figure. In this sense parents may be said to "inherit" the ability to show concern and tenderness and to pass on this ability to the next generation by repeating the kind of parent-child relationship they experienced. The cognitive-affective component of parenting includes attitude of tenderness, awareness, and concern for the child's needs and desires. This component influences the environment of the child. It has a profound effect on the manner in which the practical aspects of childcare are performed and on the emotional response of the child to the care. Benedek (1950) describes a positive parent-child relationship as mutually rewarding. This relationship is fundamental to a person's development of confidence in the expectations that others will be willing to help and that the person is worth helping. Erikson's concept (1959, 1964) of "basic trust" is similar. He postulates that such a psychologic entity forms the basis for the adult's eventual relationships with others and ability to trust others. Persons who experienced a positive parent-child relationship tend to be social or outgoing and able to seek and accept assistance from others. In contrast, those deficient in a sense of trust tend to be alienated and isolated. They are most likely to have crises because of their inability to make use of situational supports in times of stress.

PARENTAL ATTACHMENT

Although much research has been directed toward unraveling the process by which a parent comes to love and accept a child and a child comes to love and accept a parent (Fig. 25-1), we still do not know what motivates and commits parent and child to decades of supportive and nurturing care of each other. We do know that it begins as a process of attachment. The attachment process has been described as linear, beginning during pregnancy, intensifying during the early postdelivery period, and being con-

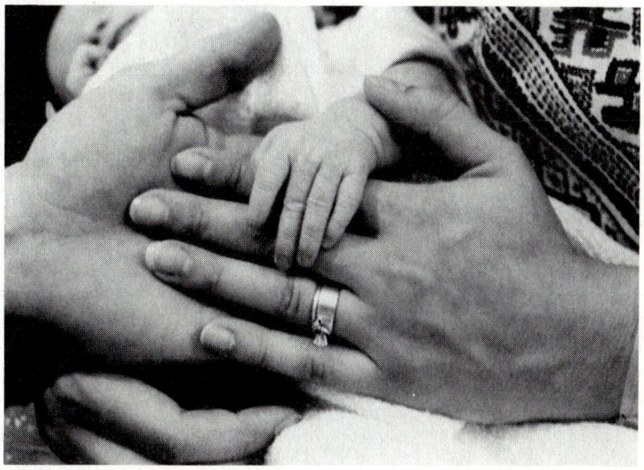

Fig. 25-1 Hands.
Courtesy St. Luke's Hospital, Kansas City, Mo.

stant and consistent once established. It is critical to mental and physical health across the life span (Parkes and Stevenson-Hinde, 1982).

Mercer (1982) lists **five preconditions that influence attachment**:

1. A parent's emotional health (including the ability to trust another person)
2. A social support system encompassing mate, friends, and family
3. A competent level of communication and caregiving skills
4. Parental proximity to the infant
5. Parent-infant fit (including infant state, temperament, and sex)

If any of these preconditions is not present or is distorted, skilled intervention is necessary to ensure the attachment process.

According to Stainton (1983b), attachment is a mutual exchange of feelings predicated by attractiveness, responsiveness, and satisfaction and is subject to changes in intensity as circumstances change over time. Attachment is developed and maintained by proximity and interaction. As with any developmental process, it is characterized by periods of progress and regression, and temporary or permanent withdrawal from attachment figures can occur.

Mercer (1982) notes that attachment is facilitated by **positive feedback.** "Positive feedback includes the social, verbal and nonverbal responses, either real or perceived, that indicate acceptance of one partner by the other." She goes on to say that attachment occurs through "a mutually satisfying experience." The newborn infant grasps a finger or a strand of hair, becoming attached to the parent. A mother commented on her son's grasp reflex, "I put my finger in his hand, and he grabbed right on. It is just a reflex, I know, but it felt good anyway" (Fig. 25-1).

Various theories have attempted to explain the basis for attachment. Freudian psychoanalytic theory emphasizes the development of a bond between child and mother as a result of the mother's satisfying the infant's innate needs. These needs are related to the human need to socialize with another and the physical needs for survival. Social learning theory contributed the principles of reinforcement to the attachment process. As discomfort is reduced or removed by the mother (or other caretaker) and pleasure substituted, the mother becomes associated with the pleasurable feeling of being satisfied. She becomes important to the infant, is loved, and can therefore act as a reinforcing agent or event. The mother becomes a **significant other** in the infant's life.

Bowlby (1958) and others (Ainsworth, 1969, 1970; Ainsworth and Bell, 1970; Brazelton, 1963, 1973) have extended the concept of attachment to include **mutuality**; that is, the infant's behaviors and characteristics call forth a corresponding set of maternal behaviors and characteristics. The infant possesses a repertoire of behaviors that initiate and maintain contact with the mother. **Signaling behaviors** such as crying, smiling, and cooing bring the mother near the child. **Executive behaviors** such as rooting, suckling, grasping, and postural adjustments maintain the contact.

The *infant* influences the caregiver and plays an important role in creating a mutually satisfying experience. The caregiver is attracted to an alert, responsive, cuddly infant and repelled by an irritable, apparently disinterested infant. Attachment occurs more readily with the infant whose temperament, social capabilities, appearance, and gender fit the parent's expectations. If the child does not meet these expectations, resolution of disappointment can delay the attachment process. An important part of attachment is the family **identification of the new baby** (Fig. 25-2). The infant's identity gradually expands, beginning with the **claim-**

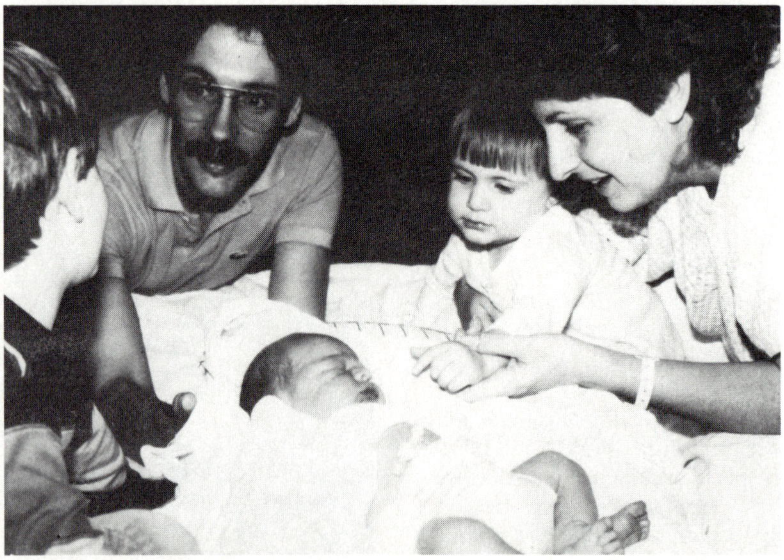

Fig. 25-2 The family examines the new baby. They discuss her appearance and admire her.
Courtesy Marjorie Pyle, RNC, Lifecircle, Costa Mesa, Calif.

ing process; that is, the child is first identified in terms of "likeness" to other family members, then in terms of "differences," and finally in terms of "uniqueness." The unique newcomer is thus *incorporated* into the family. Mothers and fathers scrutinize an infant carefully. They point out characteristics that the child shares with other family members and indicate recognition of a relationship between them. Mothers make comments such as the following that reveal the claiming process: "Russ held him close and said, 'He's the image of his father,' but I found one part like me—his toes are shaped like mine. Look, he's smiling; he likes his mother's jokes."

On the other hand, some mothers react negatively. They "claim" the infant in terms of the discomfort or pain the baby causes the mother. The mother interprets the infant's normal responses as being derogatory to the mother. The mother reacts to her child with dislike or indifference. She does not hold the child close or touch the child to be comforting; for example, "The nurse put the baby into Marie's arms. She promptly laid him across her knees and glanced up at the television. 'Stay still 'til I finish watching—you've been enough trouble already.'"

Parental responses have direct implications for nursing. Nurses can establish an environment that enhances positive parent-child contacts. They can encourage parental awareness of infant responses and ability to communicate, provide support and encouragement as parents attempt to become competent and loving in their role, and enhance the attachment process.

Sensual Responses

Attachment is strengthened through the use of sensual responses or abilities by both partners in the parent-child interaction. The sensual responses and abilities include the following.

Touch. Touch or the tactile sense is used extensively by parents and other caregivers as a means of becoming acquainted with the newborn. The fingertip, one of the most touch sensitive areas of the body, is used to explore the infant's head, face, and body surfaces. The open palms and arms are used to handle the infant (Tulman, 1985). Many mothers reach out for their infants as soon as they are born and the cord is cut. They lift them to their breasts, enfold them in their arms, and cradle them. Research has demonstrated that the newborn does not lose body heat if reasonable precautions are taken (e.g., if the infant is placed on the mother's abdomen after birth and dried thoroughly). Once the child is close to them again they begin the exploration process with their fingertips. For some other mothers and other caregivers (fathers, nursing and medical students) studies have depicted a predictable pattern of touch behavior (Rubin, 1961; Klaus et al., 1982; Tulman, 1985). The caregiver begins with a **fingertip exploration** of the infant's head and extremities. Within a short time the caregiver uses the palm to caress the baby's trunk and eventually enfolds the infant in her or his arms. Gentle stroking motions are used to soothe and quiet the infant. Mothers pat or gently rub their infant's back after feedings. Infants pat the mother's breast as they nurse. Mothers and fathers want to touch, pick up, and hold their infant (Fig. 25-3). They comment on the softness of the baby's skin and are aware of milia and rashes. Infant massage helps relax the baby and promotes attachment (see guidelines for client teaching: infant massage).

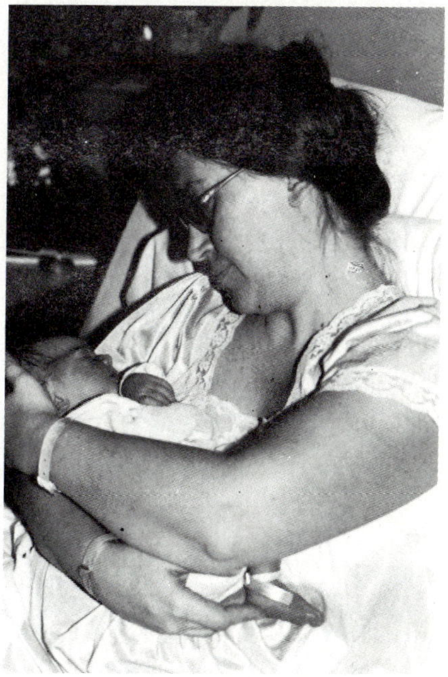

Fig. 25-3 Mother interacts with daughter through touching infant's head and feet.
Courtesy Judy Bamber, San Jose, Calif.

Parents and child seem to enjoy sharing each other's body warmth. Mothers will say, "I love her warm little body against mine."

Parents can be helped to recognize and respond to the similarities of their child's responses before and after birth. *The unborn comes "not as a stranger" but as one known to the parents and alert to the sound of their voices and their soothing actions.* Increasing sensitivity to the infant's like or dislike of types of touch brings parents closer to their babies. Stainton (1983b) reports the following instance:

> The unborn baby was perceived to be distressed at times and communicated this to the parents through excessive movement, especially kicking, indicating a need for, in their words, "calming down." One or both parents typically responded by rubbing the baby's body through the abdominal wall and all reported this resulted in a "settling" or quieting." The majority stated the unborn baby liked to be rubbed. Mothers and fathers were observed rubbing or patting the abdomen.

Eye-to-eye Contact. Interest in having eye contact is demonstrated again and again. Some mothers remark that once their babies have looked at them, they feel much closer to them (Klaus et al., 1982). Others have also noted this response: "I was a mother and looked into his eyes so clear; fell into his eyes, and in love" (Lang, 1972). Parents spend much time getting their babies to open their eyes

Guidelines For Client Teaching

INFANT MASSAGE

ASSESSMENT

1. Parent desires to learn about infant massage.
2. Parent lacks knowledge of infants and their care.
3. Parent needs to learn methods of relaxation.
4. Parent wants to ensure quality time with healthy infant under 6 months of age.

NURSING DIAGNOSIS

Knowledge deficit related to infant characteristics, needs, and care.

Knowledge deficit related to relaxation methods.

GOALS

Short-term

For the mother to continue the connection with the infant similar to that she had with the child before birth.

To meet the knowledge needs regarding infant massage.

To begin practice of massage technique.

Intermediate

To report continued use of technique because of perceived satisfaction of and benefit to parent and child.

Long-term

To expand knowledge and skill base in self-care methods of communication and relaxation.

To expand knowledge base for using therapeutic touch for health.

REFERENCES AND TEACHING AIDS

Booth, CL, Johnson-Crowley, N, and Bernard, KE: Infant massage and exercise: worth the effort? MCN 10(3):184, 1985.

Leboyer, F: Loving hands, New York, 1981, Alfred A. Knopf, Inc.

Schneider, V: Infant massage: handbook for loving parents, New York, 1982, Bantam Books, Inc.

Environment (preferably in the home) in which to demonstrate and practice; doll or baby under 6 months of age.

CONTENT/RATIONALE	TEACHING ACTIONS
To identify benefits: Help parents recognize infant's cues. Soothe baby and reduce effects of stress caused by potentially overwhelming new environment. Provide baby with regular nurturing attention. Deepen attachment between parent and child. Provide fun and feel good.	Set tone of environment. Review benefits. Share quotation from Schneider, p. 47: When from the wearying ware of life/I seek release,/I look into my baby's face/And there find peace./Martha F. Crow Demonstrate communication with doll or infant (probably should teach on doll first).
To have appropriate materials: Assemble 2-3 pillows, 2 towels, a change of diapers and clothes. Purchase cold-pressed vegetable oil: almond, apricot kernel, sunflower, safflower, or coconut oil; powder.	Assemble a variety of materials. Caution against mineral oil (leaches vitamins D, E, and K from skin) and scented oils or use of any product if baby has developed rashes to it.
To provide conducive environment: Choose place that is warm, quiet, dimly lit, out of mainstream of activity. Choose time when parent and baby are in good mood; use relaxation methods first if needed before starting.	Demonstrate. Discuss reasons. Review relaxation techniques.
To avoid injury to baby: Handle infant gently; avoid jerking, pulling. Place infant on lap or sit on floor with infant between legs. Avoid creating cloud of powder near infant's face.	Discuss. Demonstrate. Demonstrate powdering of hands away from baby.
To avoid stressing baby: Watch for infant's cues to end massage: fussing, squirming, turning away. Talk to infant, sing, hum, smile. Limit massage to 20 minutes.	Discuss. Role model.
To perform massage: Read Schneider or LeBoyer reference and follow pictures, since not all of the technique can appear here.	Demonstrate. Watch parent, who performs massage simultaneously. Alert parents to changes in baby's cues and state.

Guidelines For Client Teaching—cont'd

CONTENT/RATIONALE	TEACHING ACTIONS
*To perform techniques:** Greet infant: "Hi" I love you."	Role model this interaction.
Head	
• Do gentle head 'tapping' around base of neck and skull.	Do not use oil on head and face.
• Once eyes are closed, place thumbs together over bridge of nose and move thumbs outward gently over eyes; repeat over bridge of nose and outward over cheeks; repeat over lips and move thumbs outward in a 'smile.'	Caution parents against jabbing or poking. Demonstrate technique using gentle pressure as thumbs are moved outward. Smile at baby while demonstrating.
• With two fingers of each hand starting at forehead, make small circles around face at hairline and under chin.	Demonstrate.
• Gently massage each ear between thumb and forefinger; do one ear at a time.	When using a baby for demonstration, bring parents' attention to baby's responses.
Chest Apply 1 to 2 tablespoons vegetable oil over hands.	
• Do 'open book' over infant's stomach. Starting with both hands flat over chest, make heart-shaped pattern down sides and over groin three or four times.	Use this pattern: 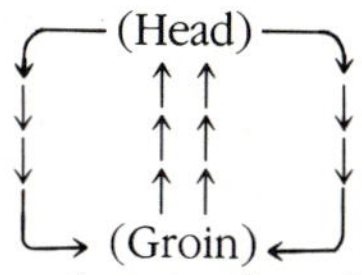 Repeat each technique three or four times.
• Place hands together over abdomen, press in gently, and push outward to sides.	
• Do 'butterfly.' Place one hand on infant's shoulder, pull downward to opposite groin; repeat with other hand.	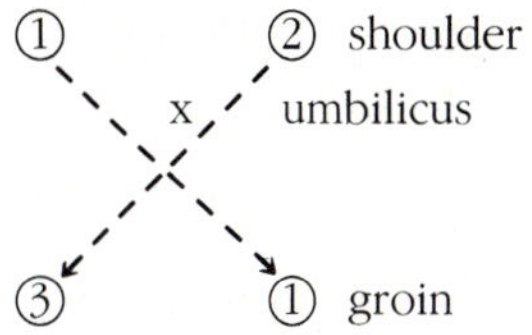
Stomach	
• Do waterwheel: with outside edge of one hand, start at umbilicus and move hand downward to groin; alternate hands like a waterwheel.	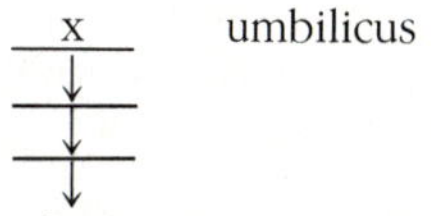 Explain that this technique is good for helping the baby with gas.
• Place thumbs together in center of abdomen, then pull out to sides.	Demonstrate holding baby under buttocks while thumbs are on abdomen.
• Perform 'I love you' using pattern at right.	Role model while talking to baby: 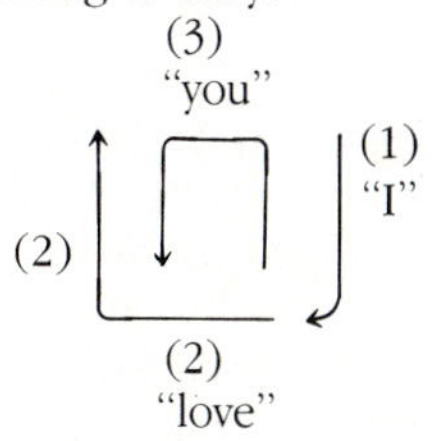
• Perform 'walking': tap with fingers of both hands simultaneously, over infant's abdomen.	Demonstrate.
Arms	
• Perform 'Indian (Swedish) milking': hold one hand at wrist, encircle wrist with other hand and 'milk' downward. Repeat with other arm.	Discuss several possible types: pitstop, Indian (Swedish) milking, squeeze and twist, top of hand, small circles around wrist, rolling.
• Perform rolling: between palms of both hands, roll infant's arm back and forth; repeat with other arm.	Demonstrate and watch parents perform one or two rollings.

* = each bullet starts a new technique

Continued.

Guidelines For Client Teaching—cont'd

CONTENT/RATIONALE	TEACHING ACTIONS
Hands	
• Make little circles in palms of each hand; then gently pull on each finger.	Remind parents to support infant's arm during this technique.
Legs and feet	
• Push on bottom of foot with both thumbs, making small circles; pull on each toe; roll leg between both hands; press on dorsal surface of foot to gently plantar-flex foot.	Draw attention to similarity of these techniques to those used on arms and hands, with addition of pushing on bottoms of feet. Alert parents to any change in infant's state.
Back	
Carefully turn infant back onto abdomen.	Demonstrate care in and bring parents' attention to supporting head during turning.
• Perform 'butterfly' technique making an "X" over baby's back down to the buttocks, starting at the shoulders. Use one hand at a time.	
• Make small circles over baby's back with fingers of both hands simultaneously; start at shoulders and move down to buttocks.	
• Perform 'milking' with one hand, starting at shoulders, moving to feet. Use other hand to support infant.	
Ending	
• 'Comb' infant's back with fingers of both hands simultaneously, starting at shoulders, moving to feet. Gradually lighten pressure so that last 'combing' is barely touching skin.	Demonstrate lessening of pressure and quieting of response to infant.
Variations	
Teach older child who can perform massage on doll with mother.	Teach as one method to cope with sibling rivalry.
Learn technique during prenatal period by practicing on maternal abdomen.	Use technique to enhance parent-fetal relationship to be carried into neonatal period.

EVALUATION The nurse may be reasonably assured that teaching was effective when the mother reports increased knowledge of infant's cues, skill in helping infant relax, and pleasure and satisfaction in learning and using therapeutic touch for health.

and look at them. In our culture eye contact appears to have a cementing effect on the development of a beginning and trusting relationship and is an important factor in human relationships at all ages.

As newborns become functionally able to sustain eye contact, parents and child spend much time gazing at one another (Fig. 25-4). We need to examine medical and nursing practices that thwart this exchange. Instillation of protective eye drops can be withheld until the infant and parents have some time together. Lights can be dimmed so that the child's eyes will open. Newborns can be held close enough to see the parents' faces.

Voice. The shared response of parents and infant to each other's voice is also remarkable. Parents wait tensely for the first cry. Once it has reassured them of the baby's health, they begin comforting behaviors. As the parents talk in high-pitched voices, the infant is alerted and turns toward them.

Odor. Another behavior shared by parents and infant is responsive to each other's odor. Mothers comment on the smell of their babies when first born and have noted that each child has a unique odor. Infants learn rapidly to distinguish the odor of their own mother's breast milk (Stainton, 1985).

Entrainment. Newborns have been found to move in time with the structure of adult speech (Condon and Sander, 1974). They wave their arms, lift their heads, kick their legs, seemingly "dancing in tune" to their parent's voice. This means that the infant has developed *culturally determined rhythms* of speech long before using the spoken language in communicating. A *carryover* (entrainment) occurs once the child begins to talk. This shared rhythm also acts to give the parent positive feedback and to establish a positive setting for effective communication.

Biorhythmicity. The unborn child can be said to be in tune with the mother's natural rhythms, such as heartbeats.

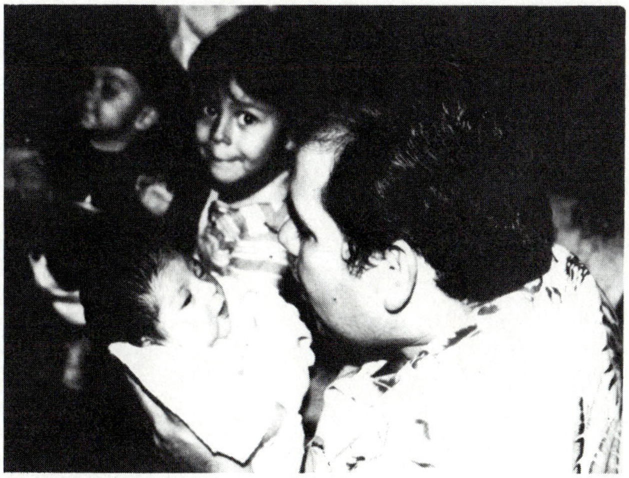

Fig. 25-4 Father and new baby make eye contact.
Courtesy Marjorie Pyle, RNC, Lifecircle, Costa Mesa, Calif.

After birth one of the baby's tasks is to establish a personal rhythm. Parents can help in this process by giving consistent loving care and by using their infant's alert state to develop responsive behavior and thereby increase social interactions and opportunities for learning. The more quickly parents become competent in child-care activities, the more quickly their psychologic energy can be directed toward observing the communication cues the infant gives them.

Early Contact

Research with mammals other than humans indicates that early contact between mother and offspring is important in developing future relationships. *To date, no scientific evidence has demonstrated that immediate contact after birth is essential for the human parent-child relationship.* According to Siegel (1982), findings from carefully controlled replicated investigations appear to document that—

> Early contact, irrespective of its supplementation by extended contact, favorably affects maternal affectional behavior during the first postpartum days. The results are consistent across low and middle socioeconomic status mother-infant pairs as well as in developed and less developed countries.

He also notes that early contact has a positive effect on the duration of breast-feeding. However, long-range effects of early contact have yet to be documented (Lamb, 1982).

A study by Klaus et al. (1982) has emphasized the need to respect the moments and hours after birth as a sensitive time for mother-infant interaction. Their study has been instrumental in facilitating the humanization of birthing practices. The physiologic benefits of early contact between mother and infant have been documented (Klaus and Kennell, 1982). For the mother, levels of oxytocin and prolactin rise; for the infant, sucking reflexes are employed early. The process of developing active immunity begins as the infant inhales flora from the mother's skin.

Early close contact may *facilitate* the attachment process between parent and child. This is not to say a delay will negate this process (humans are too resilient for that), but additional psychologic energy may be needed to accomplish the same effect. For parents unable or unwilling to expend this energy the delay may affect the infant's future well-being.

In one of the first texts on newborn disorders, Budin (1907) notes that "mothers separated from their young soon lost all interest in those whom they were unable to nurse or cherish." Subsequent investigators have brought to light similar behaviors when interactions between parent and child meet interference. Bowlby's work (1958, 1969) emphasizes the attachment process between infant and mother and details the effects of loss of that attachment to the infant. Research in the area of child abuse documents the greater percentage of neglect, abuse, and failure to thrive among infants separated from parents for relatively long periods because of illness or preterm birth (Barnett et al., 1970; Hefler and Kempe, 1965; Klaus and Kennell, 1982; Leifer et al., 1972).

Parents who desire but are unable to have early contact with their newborn infant *can be reassured that such contact is not essential for optimum parent-child interactions.* Otherwise, adopted infants would not form the usual affectional ties with their parents. Nor does the mode of infant-mother contact after delivery (skin-to-skin versus wrapped) appear to have any important effect. The mode of infant-mother contact after delivery is just one of many variables affecting mother-infant attachment (Curry, 1979). Nurses need to counsel mothers to allay fears that their emotional bond to their infant is not necessarily weaker because they missed early contact or because the contact was not skin to skin (Curry, 1979). Women who have experienced a long and difficult labor often are too exhausted to respond other than in a perfunctory way to the newborn. They may welcome the attention of others and be grateful that the infant is healthy, but their primary need centers on recovery from the physical and emotional aspects of pregnancy and childbirth. Infants born at risk as a result of either fetal or maternal disabilities, usually are transferred to the intensive care nursery as quickly as possible. Concerns for their need for intensive medical and nursing care supersede concerns about providing close contact between the infant and the mother or father. Opportunities to be with the infant in the intensive care nursery, to touch or hold her or him if at all possible, and to receive reports of the infant's progress must be part of the nursing plan.

Consumer Demands

The recent upsurge in demand by parents for home rather than hospital delivery is attributable in some measure to the parents' desire to share the birth process and to have immediate and continuous contact with their infant. The development in hospitals of family-centered maternity care units also reflects this demand. In December 1977 the American Medical Association adopted a policy on parent-newborn interaction that gives official medical sanction to efforts of groups identifying hospital practices that may frustrate family-oriented childbirth in the United States.

One widely used method of family-centered care is the provision of rooming-in facilities for the mother and her baby. The infant is transferred to the area from the transitional nursery after evidencing satisfactory postdelivery adjustment. The father is encouraged to visit and to participate in the care of the infant. Some hospitals have established family birth units (Chapter 14). The mother is accompanied by the father during the delivery of the infant, and all three may remain together until discharged. Medical and nursing personnel are available for any care necessary for the mother and child. Other hospitals arrange for the discharge of mother and infant any time from 2 to 24 hours after delivery if the condition of the mother and that of the child warrants it. Follow-up care with nursing personnel from a health agency is part of this plan.

Until recently, in our efforts to physically safeguard mothers and babies, the maternity client and her newborn were restricted in contact with family members. This practice served a useful purpose earlier when infection was a persistent threat to hospitalized women and their newborns. Unfortunately the practice persisted or was used inconsistently long after the need was no longer apparent. It took many years for professional workers to concede that a father could scrub, gown, and maintain good medical asepsis. As a result, much of the ritual of birth that acted as a ceremony to usher in parenthood and its many responsibilities was lost. Every child born depends for survival on the care given by concerned, loving adults. Any methods undertaken to enhance the nurturing quality of this care are worth serious consideration.

PARENTAL ROLE AFTER CHILDBIRTH

For the biologic parent the parental role does not begin at birth but rather enlarges and intensifies. Care and nurturing of the child is not initiated in the postdelivery period. Before birth the mother who carried out the dictates of health (e.g., diet, rest, exercise) for the "good of her baby," the father who supported and sheltered her, and the parents who became aware of and attached to their unborn child were functioning in the parental role.

During the postdelivery period, new tasks and responsibilities arise and old behaviors need to be modified or new ones added (see research highlight). Mothers' and fathers' responses to the parental role change over time and tend to follow a predictable course.

Early Period. During the early period parents have to reorganize their relationship with their child. The child's needs for shelter, nourishment, protection, and socializing continue. What was accomplished through the biologic process of pregnancy now requires an array of caregiving activities. This period is characterized by intense learning and need for nurturing. The family structure and functioning as a system has been forever altered. The duration of this period varies with people but lasts about 4 weeks.

Consolidation Period. The next period represents a time of drawing together and uniting the family unit. This period involves negotiations as to roles (wife-husband, mother-father, parent-child, sibling-sibling). It involves a stabilizing of tasks, a coming to terms with commitments. Parents demonstrate growing competence in child-care activities and become sensitive to the meaning of their infant's behavior. This period lasts approximately 2 months and in conjunction with the early period forms what is now termed the *fourth trimester.*

RESEARCH HIGHLIGHT

Network Structure, Social Support, and Psychological Outcomes of Pregnancy

Purpose

To measure social network characteristics and perceived social support during the third trimester of pregnancy and at 6 weeks postpartum.

Sample

A convenient sample of 50 primigravid couples participated in this study.

Methodology

The Social Network Inventory (SNI) was developed by the investigator to measure emotional, material, information, and comparison support. It was administered in the third trimester and at 4 weeks postpartum. In addition, the Postpartum Self-Evaluation Questionnaire (PSQ) was administered at 4 weeks postdelivery.

Findings

A greater percentage of relatives in the network and more overlap with the spouse's network were important factors associated with positive postpartum outcomes for men, but not for women. Emotional and instrumental support were important variables in explaining 6-week postpartum outcomes. Information and appraisal support were not significant variables during this period. Men scored lower than women on the PSQ scale measuring confidence in ability to cope with the tasks of parenting.

Implications

The findings from this study can influence the delivery of nursing care in the following ways. First, father participation in child care positively influences the mother's perception of the quality of her relationship with her spouse. If both parents can be helped to plan and enact roles that are mutually satisfactory, the quality of the marital relationship will not suffer as much as a result of the birth of the child. Second, in this study primigravid couples contained few members who were in the same stage of family development. Nurses may compensate for this deficit by suggesting opportunities for postpartum appraisal support. Finally, fathers in this study expressed significantly less confidence than did mothers in their ability to cope with the tasks of parenting. Nurses need to recognize fathers' real need for emotional support regarding their parental role.

Cronenwett, LR: Network structure, social support, and psychological outcomes of pregnancy, Nurs Res 34(2):93, 1985.

Growth Period. Parents and children grow in their roles until separated by death. The most outstanding feature of the lifelong process of parent-child interaction is change, consistent evolution over time. The people involved deal not only with the present but also with the future. They need support and care in the here and now and anticipatory guidance for coming changes.

Parental Tasks and Responsibilities

1. *Parents need to reconcile the actual child with the fantasy and dream child.* This means coming to terms with the infant's physical appearance, sex, innate temperament, and physical status. If the real child differs greatly from the fantasy child, parents may delay acceptance for a period. In some instances they may never accept the child. Mothers describe the differences between the real and the imagined child as follows (Stainton, 1983a):

> In the words of one mother, "I was surprised that she seemed to me to be a complete person with a personality of her own. I expected a blank tablet, a piece of clay for me to mold or a sponge for me to fill." Another, "I could not believe how determined and demanding he could be. I was going to control him and get him fitted into our life-style."

Some parents are startled by the appearance of the infant—size, color, molding of the head, or bowed appearance of the legs (Chapter 21). Many parents have never seen or had contact with a newborn infant and find themselves disturbed by their feelings. Mothers and fathers may interpret the physical characteristics that are normal in all newborns as physical or mental deficiencies. Many fathers have commented that they thought the odd shape of the child's head (molding) meant the child would be mentally retarded.

Disappointment over the sex of the infant can take time to resolve. The mother or father may be able to give adequate physical mothering but may find it difficult to be sincerely involved with the infant until these feelings have been resolved. As one mother remarked:

> I really wanted a boy, I know it is silly and irrational, but when they said, "She's a lovely little girl," I was so disappointed and angry—yes, angry—I could hardly look at her. Oh, I looked after her okay, her feedings and baths and things, but I couldn't feel excited. To tell the truth, I felt like a monster not liking my child. Then one day she was lying there and she turned her head and looked right at me. I felt a flooding of love for her come over me, and we looked at each other a long time. It's okay now. I wouldn't change her for all the boys in the world.

Nursing care plans need to include time for explanations about the child's appearance. Nurses need to provide opportunities for parents to discuss their lack of motherly feelings without fear of censure or ridicule. Often the expression of doubts and concerns provides relief and makes it easier for parents to accept help with such feelings.

2. *Parents need to establish the newborn as a person separate from themselves*, that is, as someone having many dependency needs and requiring much nurturing.

3. *Parents need to become adept in the care of the infant.* This includes the following:

a. Caregiving activities
b. Noting the communication cues given by the infant to indicate needs
c. Responding appropriately to the infant's needs

4. *Parents need to establish reasonable evaluative criteria to use in assessing the success or failure of the care given the infant.*

a. Infant responses. Parents are surprisingly sensitive to infant responses. One father told of his first attempt to give his child a kiss. At that moment the child turned her head. The father felt hurt, although he understood that the baby was totally unaware of her own movements. How the infant responds to the parental care and attention is interpreted by the parent as a comment on the quality of the care being given. These responses may include crying, weight gain or loss, or sleeping at a designated time. Continued responses deemed negative by the parent can result in alienation of parent and child to the infant's detriment (Table 25-1).
b. Competence in caregiving activities. Self-esteem grows with competence. Mothers of premature infants have noted that the adept handling of their infants by nurses was recognized as evidence of care yet at the same time was resented. It made *their* efforts to sustain their child appear inadequate. Mothers who have supplied breast milk for their infant comment that this makes them feel they are contributing in a unique way to the welfare of their child.
c. Opinion of significant others. Criticism, real or imagined, of new parents' ability to provide adequate physical care, nutrition, or social stimulation for their infant can prove devastating. These "critics" may need constructive direction. Assistance, including advice by husbands, wives, mothers, mothers-in-law, and professional workers, can be seen as supportive. Conversely, it can be seen as an indication of how inept these persons have judged the new parent to be.

5. *Parents must establish a place for the newborn within the family group.* Whether the infant is the first born or last born, all family members must adjust their roles to accommodate the newcomer. An only child needs support to accept a rival to parental affections. An older child needs support when losing a favored position. The parents are expected to negotiate these changes.

6. *Parents need to establish the primacy of their adult relationships to maintain the family as a group.* Since this includes reorganizing many roles, for example, sexual

Table 25-1 *Infant Behaviors Affecting Parental Attachment*

Facilitating Behaviors	Inhibiting Behaviors
Visually alert; eye-to-eye contact; tracking or following of parent's face	Sleepy; eyes closed most of the time; gaze aversion
Appealing facial appearance; randomness of body movements reflecting helplessness	Resemblance to person parent dislikes; hyperirritability or jerky body movements when touched
Smiles	Bland facial expression; infrequent smiles
Vocalization; crying only when hungry or wet	Crying for hours on end; colicky
Grasp reflex	Exaggerated motor reflex
Anticipatory approach behaviors for feedings; sucks well; feeds easily	Feeds poorly; regurgitates; vomits often
Enjoys being cuddled, held	Resists holding and cuddling by crying, stiffening body
Easily consolable	Inconsolable; unresponsive to parenting, caretaking tasks
Activity and regularity somewhat predictable	Unpredictable feeding and sleeping schedule
Attention span sufficient to focus on parents	Inability to attend to parent's face or offered stimulation
Differential crying, smiling, and vocalizing; recognizes and prefers parents	Shows no preference for parents over others
Approaches through locomotion	Unresponsive to parent's approaches
Clings to parent; puts arms around parent's neck	Seeks attention from any adult in room
Lifts arms to parents in greeting	Ignores parents

From Gerson, E: Infant behavior in the first year of life, New York, 1973; Raven Press, Copyright © 1973. With permission.

roles, child-care roles, career roles, and community roles, time and energy must be provided for this vital task.

Maternal Adjustment

Three phases are discernible as the mother adjusts to her version of the parental role. These phases are characterized by dependent behavior, dependent-independent behavior, and interdependent behavior.

Dependent Phase. During the first 1 to 2 days after delivery the mother's dependency needs predominate. To the extent that these needs are met by others, the mother is able to divert her psychologic energy to her child rather than to herself. She needs "mothering" to "mother." Rubin (1961) has aptly described these few days as the "taking-in phase": a time when nurturing and protective care are required by the new mother.

For a few days following birth, mature and apparently healthy women appear to suspend involvement in everyday responsibilities. They rely on others to respond to their needs for comfort, rest, nourishment, and closeness to their families and newborn.

This phase is a time of great excitement, and most parents are extremely talkative. They need to verbalize their experience of pregnancy and birth. Focusing on, analyzing, and accepting these experiences help the parents move on to the next phase. Some parents are able to use the staff or other mothers as an "audience." Others are unable to do this and need the opportunity to be with family or friends.

Since anxiety and preoccupation with her new role often narrow a mother's perceptual field, information may have to be repeated. The new mother may require reminders to rest, or conversely, to ambulate enough to promote recovery. Ward routine does not necessarily loom large in the new mother's order of priorities; showers are taken when examinations are scheduled, and telephone conversations preclude "being ready" for the baby. Regulations seem cumbersome, and sometimes mothers and their families have difficulty accepting rules that interfere with their needs to share reactions about their child.

Physical discomfort arising from an episotomy, sore nipples, hemorrhoids, afterpains, and occasionally a sprained coccygeal joint can interfere with the mother's need for rest and relaxation. The judicious use of comfort measures and medication depends on the nurse. Many women hesitate to ask for medication, believing that any pain they experience is normal and to be expected; few have a knowledge of the use of heat or cold to relieve local pain.

Dependent-independent Phase. If the mother has received adequate nurturing in the first few days, by the third day her desire for independent action reasserts itself. She alternates between a need for extensive nurturing and acceptance by others and the desire "to take charge" once again. She responds enthusiastically to opportunities to learn and practice the care of the baby or, if she is an accomplished mother, to carry out or direct this care.

The reality of parenthood must be experienced to be understood fully regardless of the desire for the baby and the amount of prenatal preparation undertaken. One young mother expressed it as follows (Lang, 1972):

> But then in my second week, as my strength began to return, my energies began to focus on the overwhelming task of motherhood that stood before me. And I realized then that I faced that task alone. Not that my husband wouldn't stand by me, not that my friends would not share experiences with me, but I stood alone with the realization that only I could be the child's mother.

In the period of 6 to 8 weeks after delivery the mastery of the tasks of parenthood are crucial. Realistic expectations facilitate the subsequent functioning of the family as a unit.

Some women adjust with considerable difficulty to the isolation of themselves with their babies and resent the endless coping with home and child-care responsibilities. The mothers who appear to need additional supportive counseling include:

1. Primiparas inexperienced in child care
2. Women whose careers had provided outside stimulation
3. Women who lack friends or family members with whom to share delights and concerns

Depressive states are not uncommon during this phase. **Feelings of extreme vulnerability** may arise from a number of factors. Psychologically the mother may be overwhelmed by the actuality of parental responsibilities. She may feel deprived of the pregnant state, with its concomitant supportive care of family members and friends. Some mothers regret the loss of the mother-unborn child relationship and mourn its passing. Still others experience a letdown feeling when labor and birth are complete. They had girded themselves for an elemental experience, a walk "through the shadows," and now it is safely over.

Once immediate tasks and adjustments have been undertaken and brought under control, a plateau is reached. At this time the life-long effects of the parents' new responsibilities come into focus. Some parents experience a feeling of being trapped and wonder what life is all about.

Occasionally the mother becomes increasingly fatigued during the last month of pregnancy, when sleep is interrupted by shortness of breath and urinary frequency. Leg cramps, or inability to lie in a comfortable position can disturb sleep. **Fatigue** following delivery is compounded by around-the-clock demands of the new baby and can accentuate the feelings of depression. It has been suggested that a lowered level of circulating glucocorticoids or a condition of subclinical hypothyroidism may exist during the puerperium. This physiologic state could explain some minor degrees of depression.

Depressive reactions are not necessarily expressed verbally. A depressive state signified by typical behaviors (withdrawal, loss of interest in surroundings, and crying) can be manifested.

It is hoped that toward the end of the dependent-independent phase the tasks and adjustments of daily routine will begin to follow a pattern. The baby begins to take an established position in the family. Many of the feeding problems, whether related to breast-feeding or bottle-feeding, have been largely resolved. The mother's physical energy and strength return; the "taking-hold phase" (Rubin, 1961) is ending. By the fifth week the infant has been examined by the physician and the mother also has been examined or has made arrangements for a checkup. It is time to move on to the next phase of adjustment.

Interdependent Phase. In this phase interdependent behavior reasserts itself, and the mother and her family move forward as a system with interacting members. The relationship of husband and wife, although altered by the introduction of a child, resumes many of its former characteristics. A primary need is to establish a life-style that includes but in some respects excludes the child. Husband and wife must share interest and activities that are adult in scope.

Most couples begin intercourse by the third or fourth week after the child is born; some begin earlier, as soon as it can be accomplished without discomfort for the woman. Sexual intimacy increases the man-woman aspect of the family, and the adult pair shares a closeness denied to other family members. Many new fathers speak of the alienation experienced when they observe the intimate mother-child relationship, and some are frank in expressing feelings of jealousy toward the interloper. The resumption of the marital relationship seems to bring the parents' relationship back into focus. See guidelines for client teaching: resumption of sexual intercourse.

The interdependent phase is often one of stress for the parental pair. Career patterns of men from their 20s through their 40s show intense activity centering around advancement in their profession or job. This often necessitates long hours away from the home or moving from one locality to another. Meanwhile the women are engrossed in home activities directed toward the care of the young children. Interests and needs diverge, and there may be a gradual estrangement, which is glossed over for the time being because of the individual needs of each. A special effort must be undertaken to strengthen the adult-adult relationship as a basis for the family unit.

Paternal Adjustment

During the last decade a growing interest in the relationship of the father and the child has become evident. It is now recognized that the mother-child relationship does not exist in a vacuum but within the context of the family system. Parent's attitudes toward and expectations of one another's parental behavior affect the behavior of each dyad. In our culture the newborn has been found to have a powerful impact on the father. Fathers have demonstrated intense involvement with their babies. Greenberg and Morris (1976) named the father's absorption, preoccupation, and interest in the infant *engrossment.* These researchers delineate a number of characteristics of engrossment. Some of the sensual responses relating to touch and eye-to-eye contact are the same as discussed earlier. The father's keen awareness of features both unique and similar to himself is another characteristic related to the father's need to claim the infant. An outstanding response is one of *strong attraction* to the newborn. Much time is spent "communicating" with the infant and taking delight in the infant's response to the father. Fathers feel a sense of increased self-esteem, a sense of being "proud, bigger, more mature, and older" after seeing their baby for the first time. Studies have shown a difference in father-infant relationships. Fathers tend to take the lead in initiating play and other social situations. Mothers tend to take the lead in caregiving activities (Clarke-Stewart, 1978). The subtle and more overt differences in stimulation from two sources, mother and father, provide a wider social experience for the child. In addition the child has improved chances of developing at least one good parenting relationship (Kunst-Wilson and Cronenwett, 1981).

Much has still to be learned about the relationships between fathers and their offspring. The mother's biologic re-

Guidelines For Client Teaching

RESUMPTION OF SEXUAL INTERCOURSE

ASSESSMENT

1. Couple needs information on how and when to resume sexual intercourse postdelivery.
2. Couple states they would like to resume sexual intercourse by third or fourth postdelivery week if bleeding has stopped and the episiotomy is healed.
3. Couple has heard that the first experience with intercourse following delivery may be uncomfortable.
4. Couple has heard that response to sexual stimulation may be altered for a short time after delivery.
5. Couple needs to keep the lines of communication open to remain close and not hurt each other's feelings.

NURSING DIAGNOSES

Knowledge deficit related to resumption of sexual intercourse following delivery:

1. Timing of first intercourse.
2. Need for contraception if pregnancy is not desired.
3. Need for understanding the woman's emotional status at this time.

Anxiety related to knowledge deficit of postdelivery physiology and healing.

Pain related to dryness of vaginal mucosa.

Potential pain related to healing abdominal incision (post cesarean delivery).

Potential pain related to newly healed episiotomy.

Ineffective family coping related to lack of knowledge of:

1. Timing for resumption of sexual intercourse.
2. Measures needed to promote comfort.
3. Precautions to prevent unplanned pregnancy (see guidelines for client teaching: postdelivery contraception, p. 600).

Potential for infection related to lack of understanding of hygienic measures.

GOALS

Short-term (within 3 to 4 weeks)

Woman or couple verbalizes understanding of instructions and content.

Couple discusses subject freely between them and mutually agree to their course of action.

Couple learns to discuss subject with regard to each other's feelings.

Intermediate

Couple resumes sexual intercourse by mutual agreement.

Experience is without discomfort.

No pregnancy results.

Couple continues to communicate effectively with one another.

Long-term

Couple maintains open lines of communication.

Couple mutually agrees on choice of fertility management for present time.

Couple maintains closeness and sexual satisfaction that was part of their lives before the baby arrived.

REFERENCES AND TEACHING AIDS

Printed instructions.

Illustrations.

Texts relevant to subject.

CONTENT/RATIONALE	TEACHING ACTIONS
To provide information about postdelivery physiology and its effects on resumption of sexual intercourse:	Share information with woman and couple.
The couple can safely resume sexual intercourse by the third or fourth postdelivery week if bleeding has stopped and the episiotomy has healed. For the first 6 weeks to 6 months the vagina does not lubricate well because steroid depletion inhibits the vasocongestive response to sexual tension.	Encourage open discussion between couple. Lead discussion by being candid and using open-ended questions. Encourage the couple to ask questions. Encourage couple to problem-solve the situation together.
Physiologic reactions to sexual stimulation for the first 3 postdelivery months are marked by a reduction in both rapidity and intensity of response. Vasocongestion of the labia majora and minora is delayed well into the plateau phase. The walls of the vagina are thin and pink, a condition similar to senile vaginitis. This results from the hormonal starvation of the involutional period. Finally, the size of the orgasmic platform and strength of the orgasmic contractions are reduced.	Suggest slowly building up to the act of intercourse by allowing for caressing, kissing, and shared tenderness.

Guidelines For Client Teaching—cont'd

CONTENT/RATIONALE	TEACHING ACTIONS
A water-soluble gel, cocoa butter, or a contraceptive cream or jelly might be recommended for lubrication. If some vaginal tenderness is present, the partner can be instructed to insert one or more clean, lubricated fingers into the vagina and rotate them within the vagina to help relax it and to identify possible areas of discomfort. A coital position in which the woman has control of the depth of the penile penetration is also useful. The side-by-side or female-superior position is often recommended.	Provide as many alternatives as possible to serve as a basis for discussion and to provide choices. Acknowledge that this may be a difficult area for some people to talk about freely. Provide pictures and explanations of these alternatives.
The presence of the baby influences postdelivery lovemaking. Parents hear every sound made by the baby; conversely they may be concerned that the baby hears every sound they make. In either case any phase of the sexual response cycle may be interrupted by hearing the baby cry or move, leaving one partner or both frustrated and unsatisfied. The amount of psychologic energy expended by the parents in child care activities may lead to fatigue. Newborns require a great deal of attention and time, not to mention what is necessary to take care of twins or triplets, and older children as well.	Validate that although these responses are within normal expectations, it still may be difficult to deal with frustration at times.
Some women have reported sexual stimulation to plateau and orgasmic levels when nursing their babies. Although nursing mothers have a longer delay in ovarian steroid production, they are often interested in returning to sexual activity before nonnursing mothers. Nursing mothers also report higher levels of postdelivery eroticism.	Suggest that the woman take a rest during the day when the baby sleeps.
In the event of fetal or newborn death or the birth of an infant that is small, sick, or deformed, the emotional energy required of the woman and her partner, the mother's depleted physical state, and the stress of burying the dead child or of visiting the hospitalized child strain all relationships. Professional caregivers can only speculate about the effect on sexual relationships during these stressful times as a result of little definitive data.	Help parents cope with grief (see Chapter 28). Provide information on support groups. They can be of tremendous help at a time like this; lending a sympathetic ear and offering advice and comfort to the couple.
The woman should be instructed to follow the Kegel's exercises to strengthen her pubococcygeal muscle. This muscle is the major sphincter of the pelvis. It is associated with bowel and bladder function and with vaginal perception and response during intercourse.	Teach Kegel's exercises (see Chapter 8). Provide written instructions for the woman to take with her.

EVALUATION This is a private subject, the nurse must use tact when speaking to the woman or the couple about the attainment of goals. The nurse's care and teaching was effective if the couple's goals were met: sexual intercourse has been resumed to the satisfaction of the couple and without physical or emotional discomfort; the couple confirm continued effective communication.

lationship with the child can be a basis for predicting behaviors in the mother-child relationship. But the knowledge that a man is the father of a child gives us no clues as to his relationships or behaviors with the child.

There is no evidence as yet as to what effect individual styles have on the father's actual experience with this child. Despite their active involvement in the perinatal period, fathers tend to gravitate toward more traditional roles as they become more involved in job-related activities and less in child-care activities. However, if the father does involve himself in caregiving, he responds much as the mother in talking to the infant (Field, 1978a).

Infant-parent Adjustment

The infant-parent interaction is characterized by a "set of rhythms, behavioral repertoires, and responsivity or response styles" (Field, 1978a). These traits are unique to each partner. Interactions can be facilitated in any of three ways: (1) modulation of rhythm, (2) modification of behav-

Guidelines For Client Teaching

POSTDELIVERY CONTRACEPTION

ASSESSMENT

1. Woman or couple request information regarding contraception after delivery.
2. Woman has idea that she cannot become pregnant while breast-feeding.

NURSING DIAGNOSES

Knowledge deficit related to the many methods of contraception.

Potential for ineffective breast-feeding related to the resumption of hormonal contraception.

Potential for ineffective family coping related to the stress of an unplanned pregnancy.

GOALS

Short-term

Woman or couple verbalizes understanding of content discussed.

Couple discusses postdelivery contraceptive methods available to them.

Intermediate

Couple mutually agrees on and employs simple barrier methods of contraception: (i.e., condoms, contraceptive gels or foams, diaphragm).

Couple discusses any problems they may have with these methods of contraception.

Long-term

Couple discusses and mutually agrees on a choice of fertility management.

Couple maintains open lines of communication.

Couple will reevaluate method of contraception as time goes on, or if there are any adverse effects from the one they are employing.

REFERENCES AND TEACHING AIDS

Inserts from packages of chosen contraceptive.

Hospital/clinic teaching materials.

Flip chart showing anatomy of pelvic structures or total body plastic medical models.

Hospital or clinic audiovisual teaching materials.

Samples of contraceptive device, basal body temperature charts, and thermometer.

Fresh egg white (for teaching about cervical mucus).

Handouts of printed information.

CONTENT/RATIONALE	TEACHING ACTIONS
To provide content about contraception (see Chapter 42).	Discuss and outline a tentative plan on discharge from hospital. Continue discussion of fertility management at the first postpartum visit.
Women *may* not ovulate while they successfully breast-feed their infants because ovarian functions are *usually* suppressed by a high level of serum prolactin.	Share information with woman and couple. Encourage questions. Promote open discussion between couple.
Follicle formation is usually suspended, and ovulation usually does not occur. Women who do not breast-feed frequently or on demand (e.g., every 3 to 4 hours) or *who supplement the infant's feeding* do not maintain an effectively high level of serum prolactin. If these women do not employ contraceptives, they may conceive again, sometimes without having a menstrual period following the previous pregnancy.	Encourage couple to problem-solve the situation together. Provide as many alternatives as possible to provide choices and serve as a basis for discussion. Teach woman (couple) cervical mucus and symptothermal method as one means of determining resumption of ovulatory menstrual cycles.
If the mother is not breast-feeding, she may resume use of oral contraceptives (after delivery) under the physician's direction. If she is breast-feeding, barrier contraception, such as a diaphragm, condom, gel, or foam, should be employed until the first postdelivery examination, at which time the desired method can be instituted (see Chapter 42).	Acknowledge that this may be a difficult area for some people to talk about.

EVALUATION Teaching actions have been effective when the couple's goal of preventing unwanted pregnancy has been achieved. The couple states they discussed and mutually agreed on a choice of fertility management. They consult the clinic or physician when they have questions.

ioral repertoires, and (3) mutual responsivity.

Rhythm. To modulate the rhythm, both parent and infant must be able to interact. Therefore the infant must be in the alert state, one of the most difficult of the sleep-wake states to maintain. The alert state occurs most often during a feeding or in face-to-face play. The parent must work hard to help the infant maintain the alert state long enough and often enough for interactions to take place (Fig. 25-5). Evidently mothers learn how to do this: multiparous mothers show particular sensitivity and responsiveness to their infant's feeding rhythms. The mother who is sensitive to feeding rhythms reserves stimulation for pauses in sucking activity. For example, the mother learns not to talk or smile excessively while the infant is sucking because the infant will stop feeding to interact with her (Field, 1978b). With maturity the infant can sustain longer interactions by modulating activity rhythms, that is, limb movement, sucking, gaze alternation, and habituation (Fig. 25-6). "In the interim, the adult learns to attend to these rhythms, modulate her or his own rhythms, and thereby facilitate a rhythmical turn-taking interaction" (Field, 1978a).

Repertoires. Both contributors to the infant-parent interaction have a repertoire of behaviors they can use to facilitate interactions. Fathers and mothers engage in these behaviors depending on the amount of contact and caregiving of the infant.

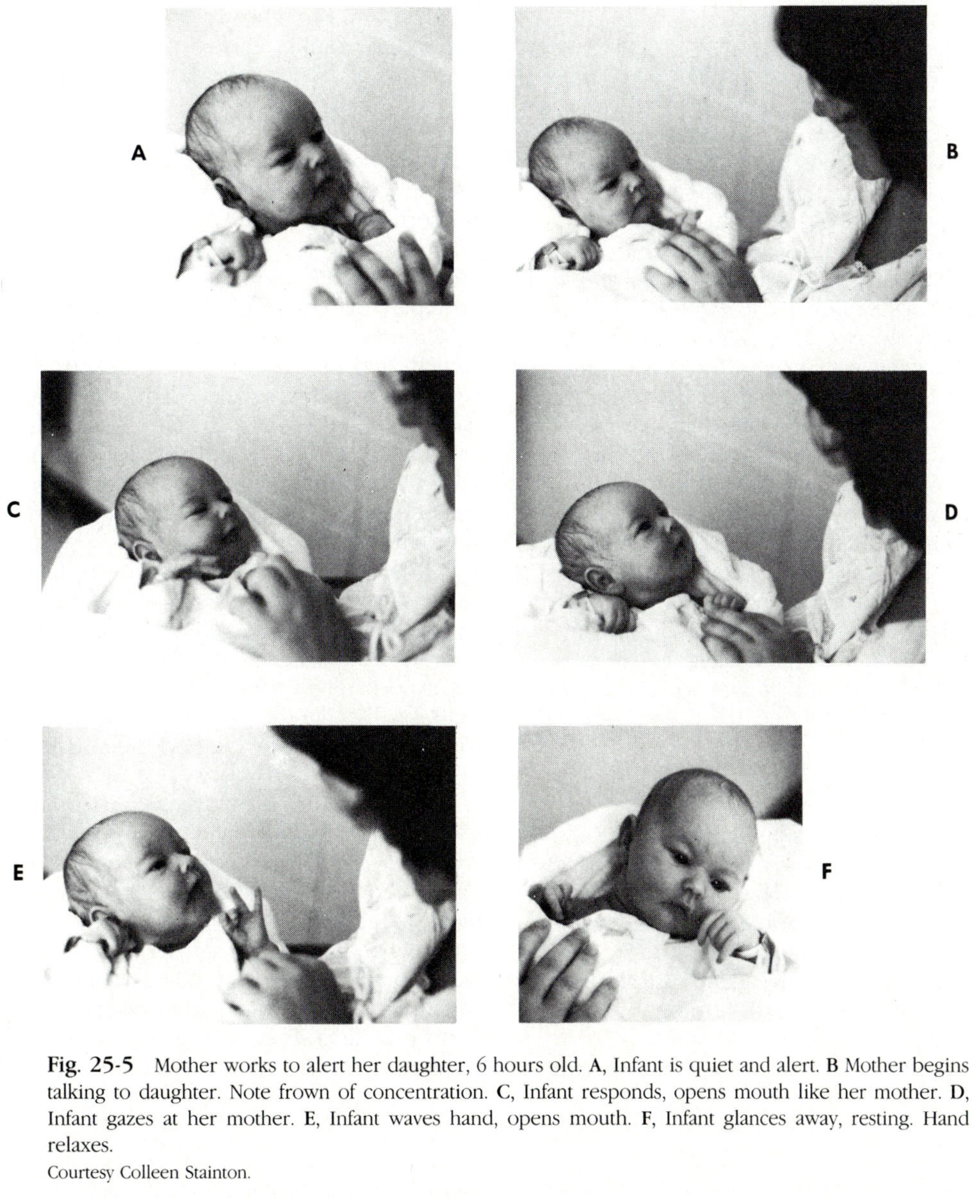

Fig. 25-5 Mother works to alert her daughter, 6 hours old. **A,** Infant is quiet and alert. **B** Mother begins talking to daughter. Note frown of concentration. **C,** Infant responds, opens mouth like her mother. **D,** Infant gazes at her mother. **E,** Infant waves hand, opens mouth. **F,** Infant glances away, resting. Hand relaxes.

Courtesy Colleen Stainton.

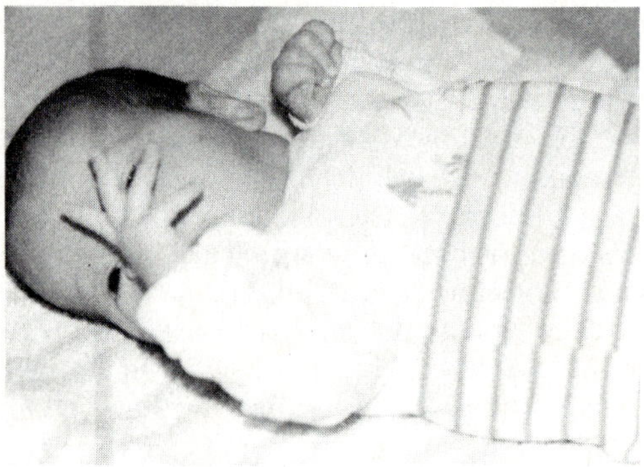

Fig. 25-6 Habituating.
Courtesy Colleen Stainton.

Infant's Repertoire

1. Gaze behaviors. The infant is able to focus and follow the human face from birth. The infant is also able to use gaze alternation. These abilities are under voluntary control. "The infant appears to look away from the mother's face when under- or over-aroused to modulate his or her arousal level and process the stimulation he or she is receiving" (Field, 1978a). Brazelton et al. (1974) suggest that one of the key responses for the parents to learn is *sensitivity to the infant's capacity for attention and inattention.* Developing this sensitivity is especially important in interacting with premature infants (Sammons and Lewis, 1985). Field (1978b) states, "Mothers who are more active or 'overstimulating' and less sensitive or responsive to their infant's pauses or turning away during the conversation are less able to elicit or hold their infants' gaze."
2. Vocalizing and facial expressions. Body gestures form a part of the infant's "early language." Babies greet parents with waving hands or with a reaching out of hands. They can raise an eyebrow or soften their expression to elicit loving attention. They can be stimulated to smile or laugh with game playing. To end an interaction they use pouting or crying, arching of the back, and general squirming.

Parents Repertoire

1. Constant looking at the infant and noting the infant's behavior. New parents often remark they are exhausted from looking at the baby and smiling.
2. Infantilizing speech. Adults slow the tempo, loudness, rhythms, and emphasis to help the infant "listen" to the speech. They also repeat phrases frequently. Infantilizing does not mean "baby talk" with its distortion of sounds.
3. Slowing and exaggerating facial expressions.
4. Game playing with the infant. "Peek-a-boo" is an example.
5. Imitating the infant's behaviors. For instance, if the baby frowns, the adult frowns.

Responsivity. Contingent responses that occur within a specific time and are similar in form to a stimulus behavior. They elicit a feeling in the person originating the behavior of having an influence on the interaction. In other words, they act as positive feedback. Adults view infant behaviors such as smiling, cooing, and sustained eye contact as contingent responses. The adults are encouraged to continue the same game when the infant responds in such a way. These responses act as rewards to the initiator. When the adult imitates the infant, the infant appears to enjoy the responses. The infant in turn imitates behaviors of adults soon after birth. The parent shows progression in presenting behaviors for the baby to imitate; for example, in early interactions the parent will grimace rather than laugh, which is in keeping with the infant's developmental level. Such "turnabout" behaviors sustain interactions and promote harmony in the relationship.

Factors Influencing Parental Responses

Adolescent Parenthood. Adolescent pregnancy and parenthood are significant issues in North America. The special needs of these parents are addressed in Chapter 35.

Parenthood After 35

Fatigue and Recovery. Fatigue and the need for more rest seems to be the major concern of older parents with newborns (Queenan, 1987; Winslow, 1987). Many of these mothers, being less resilient than younger women, need more than 12 hours in the hospital before they go home. Third-party payers should recognize this fact.

Measures designed to assist the mother in regaining strength and muscle tone (e.g., prenatal and postdelivery exercises) are emphasized. Some older mothers may find that the care of the new infant exhausts their physical capabilities. If economic and social conditions are adverse, referral to community agencies may be needed. Many women could benefit from supportive references (Scott, Meredith, and Angwin, 1986).

Multiparas. Multiparas can anticipate the postpartum course more realistically than can nulliparas. Time for rest is expected. Often older siblings assist with the care of the newborn and household responsibilities. The multipara has had experience in adjusting to changes in roles and relationships. Despite the number and quality of her previous experiences, each new mother's nursing care plan must be individualized.

Primiparas. In the early infancy period this group needs careful follow-up and supportive care, including opportunities to discuss alternative parenting approaches. The nurse needs to be aware of community resources developed to meet the needs of this group.*

Response of Family and Friends. The families and friends of the parents and their newborn child form an important dimension of the parent's social network. Social networks provide a support system on which parents can rely for assistance (Cronenwett, 1985a, b; Crawford, 1985). Pos-

*For example, Parenthood after Thirty is a project sponsored by the Foundation for Comprehensive Health Services and funded by grant no. 80-63575 from the Office of Family Planning, State of California Department of Health Services. For further information contact Parenthood after Thirty, 451 Vermont, Berkeley, CA 94704 (415) 524-6635 (Lucy Scott, Ph.D., Project Director).

itive emotional and affectional relationships appear critical to the enhancement of parenting skills and nurturance of children (Gottlieb, 1980; Schronkoff, 1984). Social networks promote the growth potential of children and the prevention of their maltreatment. Mercer (1982) and Crawford (1985) found that social networks provided support but were also a source of conflict. Parents or in-laws who assisted with household responsibilities and who did not intrude into the parents' privacy or critically judge them were most appreciated. Sometimes a large network caused problems in that it generated conflicting advice to the new parents.

Socioeconomic Conditions. Parents whose economic condition is made worse with the birth of each child and who are unable to use an acceptable method of fertility management may find childbirth compounded by concern for their own health and a sense of helplessness. Mothers who are alone, deserted by husband, family, and friends, or who are in an untenable economic state may view the birth of the child with dread. The difficulties in which they find themselves may overcome any desire for mothering the infant (Chapter 34).

Nursing measures designed to help persons in these circumstances involve social and economic community agencies as well as health agencies. Satisfactory outcomes of such problems often require long-term commitments from both the woman or couple and the community. Adequate situational supports need to be instituted in the prenatal period.

Interference with Personal Aspirations. For some women parenthood interferes with or curtails their plans for personal freedom or advancement in their career. Resentment concerning their loss may not have been resolved during the prenatal period. If this resentment is not resolved, it will spill over into caregiving activities and may result in indifference and neglect. Or, conversely, it may result in oversolicitousness and the setting of impossibly high standards by the mother for her behavior or the child's performance (Shainess, 1970).

Nursing intervention includes providing opportunities for parents (1) to vent their feelings freely to an objective listener; (2) to discuss measures to permit personal growth of the parent, for example, by parttime employment, volunteer work, and use of agencies that provide babysitting care or mother substitutes during parents' vacations; and (3) to learn about the care of the child.

PARENTAL SENSORY IMPAIRMENT

In the early dialogue between parent and child, all senses—sight, hearing, touch, taste, and smell—are used by both to initiate and sustain the attachment process. A parent who is deprived of one of the senses needs to develop an enriched use of the remaining sensory sources.

The Blind Parent

Although mothers who are blind need the presence as well as the support of another responsible person, they can become adept in some child-care activities, as the following report indicates:

> We had always planned to have a child. My family and Dick's both wanted us to have the happiness of children and were willing to help us with the baby care. First I bathed and changed a doll; then I practiced caring for my sister's baby. I would feel in all the creases with my finger to see if they were clean and dry. We used disposable diapers that do not need pins. My mother made baby clothes with fastenings of press cloth (Velcro) so I would not have to fiddle with buttons. I feel really confident now. I know I can't do everything for her, but I can do enough to feel like a "mother," and I know she will have all the love she needs.

One of the major difficulties blind mothers experience is the skepticism, overt or covert, of the professional worker. Blind persons sense a reluctance on the part of others to concede that they have a right to be parents. One blind mother-to-be noted that the best approach by the nurse is for the nurse to assess the mother's capabilities (Asrael, 1983). From that basis the nurse can make plans to assist the woman (i.e., the same as for a sighted mother). Another mother talked about the shyness, fear, or reluctance she sensed in nurses that resulted in her being left alone or being involved in awkward conversations:

> I took it upon myself to put the nurses at ease. I was forthright about my condition and asked for specific help and supervision of my baby care efforts. Don't forget, I've had some 25 years' experience in dealing with the sighted public. I have considerable skill now in being blind.

Another mother expressed how sensitive the blind can become to other sensory output. She remarked that she could tell when her infant was facing her because she could feel his breath on her face.

Three mothers who are blind volunteered the following suggestions for providing care for the needs of women such as themselves during childbearing. The first mother noted that "sometimes they [health care providers] act like they're afraid they're going to catch our blindness" (example of avoidance). She offered the following suggestions:

1. Clients who are blind need verbal teaching from health care providers because maternity information is not accessible to blind people.
2. Clients need an orientation to the hospital room that allows the client to move about the room independently. For example, "Go to the left of the bed and trail the wall until you feel the first door. That is the bathroom."
3. Clients need explanations of routines.
4. Clients need opportunities to feel devices (e.g., monitors, pelvic models) and to hear descriptions of the devices.
5. Clients need "a chance to ask questions!"
6. Clients need the opportunity to hold and touch their baby after delivery. "When they put him on my stomach he was warm; I could feel his heart going. That gave me

the moment to see that he was really OK," and "Blind fathers like to cut cords, too."

7. Nurses need to demonstrate baby care by touch and to follow with, "Now let me see you do it."
8. Nurses need to give instructions such as "I'm going to give you the baby. The head is on the left side."

The second mother made the following observations:

> We tend to respond as we're treated, as everyone does. If treated as inadequate, you can tend to overcompensate to try to prove you're adequate, or you can withdraw. People need to be recognized as people. I always tell people I'm not a blind person, I'm a person who happens to be blind. If you could take that one message to people, I know I shared something worthwhile.
>
> I'm not saying blindness doesn't have its problems and adjustments, because it does. But I tend to think we do overemphasize blindness sometimes, especially when it comes to childbirth, pregnancy, and the basic delivery.
>
> I can't think of a time when my hospital care wasn't good. People introduced themselves and said what they were about to do. I was assertive; I got what I wanted. I told the doctor during my prenatal visits about what kind of delivery I wanted. During delivery I put my hands down and felt the head of my child.

Her suggestion to promote attachment was to make certain the mother can "feel the head and face. Comb the hair with your fingers, kiss the cheeks. Breast-feed right away if the baby wants to. Ask the nurse for help with positioning."

The third mother noted that "everyone is so visually oriented they can't see beyond their eyes. They don't think anything can be done without eyes." Her suggestions follow:

1. "Treat us like human beings. That's what we are!"
2. "Relate verbally. Explain! Don't say 'Do it like this' and assume we know what you're doing over there.
3. "Put bells on the baby's shoes to help keep track of them."
4. "Pull a stroller instead of pushing it."

Eye-to-eye contact is considered important in our culture. With a parent who is blind, this critical component in the parent-child attachment process is obviously missing. However, since the mother has no experience in using this strategy to promote relationships, she cannot be said to miss it. The infant will need other sensory input from the blind mother. Perhaps an infant looking into the eyes of a mother who is blind is not conscious that the eyes are unseeing. Other persons in the newborn's environment can participate in active eye-to-eye contact to supply this lack. Another problem may arise if the parent who is blind has an impassive facial expression. One observer noticed an infant making repeated attempts to engage in face play with his mother, who was blind. After repeated failure of his efforts, he abandoned the behavior with his mother and intensified it with his father. This problem might be overcome by the person's learning to accompany talking and cooing to the infant with head nodding and smiling.

The Deaf Parent

The mother who has a hearing impairment faces another set of problems, particularly if the deafness dates from birth or early childhood. About 2 of every 1000 Americans are deaf. An accepted definition for the deaf is persons who cannot hear or understand the spoken word with or without a hearing aid. The mother and her partner are likely to have established an independent household. A number of devices that transform sound into light flashes are now marketed.* The infant's room can be fitted with such a device to permit immediate detection of crying. Even if the parents are not speech trained, their vocalizing can serve as both stimulus and response to the infant's early vocalizing. Parents can provide additional vocal training by use of records and television so that from birth onward the child is aware of the full range of the human voice. Sign language is acquired readily by the young child, and the first sign used as varied as the first word. One mother reported her child first signed "good boy," and another reported "candy" as her child's first effort.

Baranowski (1983) described childbirth education classes for expectant deaf parents: "The students were attentive, asked questions, and readily participated in discussions. Their regular attendance indicated that they were interested in the classes."

Section 504 of the Rehabilitation Act of 1973 requires that hospitals and other institutions receiving funds from the U.S. Department of Health and Human Services use various communication techniques and resources with the deaf, including staff members or a certified interpreter who are proficient in sign language. The nurse who is bilingual has an advantage in providing care for clients. Magilvy et al. (1979) point out that sign language is as complex as any spoken language and that deaf persons are linguistically and cognitively competent.

Much more research in the areas of sensory impairment and the parent-child attachment process needs to be undertaken.†

SIBLING ADJUSTMENT

Introduction of the infant into a family with one or more children may pose problems for the parents. They are faced with the task of caring for a new child while not neglecting the others. Parents need to distribute their attention in a manner that they consider fair.

Older children have to assume new positions within the family hierarchy. The older child's goal is to maintain a leading position. The child who is next in birth order to the infant has to gain a superior position over the newcomer (Kreppner et al., 1982). As the infant develops and begins to assert herself or himself, the older child works toward dominance. "He or she takes away toys and other

*A price list for the Crying Light and other useful visual alarms can be obtained from Applied Communication Corp, PO Box 555, Belmont, CA 94002.

†We welcome information in this area. Address correspondence to IM Bobak, Department of Nursing, San Francisco State University, 1600 Holloway Ave, San Francisco, CA 94132.

objects the younger child is grasping for, thereby demonstrating that he or she has control over the situation. The older child also intervenes more openly when parents are interacting with the younger child" (Kreppner et al., 1982). One 3-year-old child encouraged his mother to put the new baby "out with the garbage because we've seen enough of her."

Regression to an infantile level of behavior may be seen in some children. They may revert to bed-wetting, whining, or refusing to feed themselves. An older child who is still young wavers between thinking "I'm big now" and thinking "I'm still a baby, so look after me." Jealous reactions are to be expected once the initial excitement of having a new baby in the home is over, since the baby absorbs the time and attention of the important persons in the other children's lives.

Parents, especially mothers, spend much time and energy promoting sibling acceptance of a new baby. Other children are involved actively in preparation for the infant, and involvement intensifies after the birth of the child. Mother and father face a number of tasks related to sibling adjustment. The tasks include the following:

1. Making the older child feel loved and wanted.
2. Managing guilt arising from feelings that older children are being deprived of parental time and attention.
3. Developing feelings of confidence in her or his ability to nurture more than one child.
4. Adjusting time and space to accommodate the new baby.
5. Monitoring behavior of older children toward the more vulnerable infant and diverting aggressive behavior.

The new parent can learn many innovative techniques by listening to other parents describe their efforts to ease the older siblings' acceptance of the new child (See guidelines for client teaching: sibling preparation, p. 233). Walz and Rich (1983) have described a number of creative parental interventions.

1. A mother took her firstborn on a tour of her hospital room and pointed out similarities to the first child. "This is the same room I was in with you, and I think the baby is in the same cot that you were in."
2. The newborn was described as a "special gift" for the older child.
3. The children were in the group (grandparents, sister) who were *first* to see the newborn.
4. Time was planned for both children. A mother remarked, "When I get home, I'll arrange my day so that I can have the baby's care done in the morning while Sam (first child) is at school. Maybe the baby will sleep part of the afternoon and I can spend some time with Sam." Another mother said, "When I'm breast-feeding I'll have one arm for the baby and one arm for my daughter (first child)."

Fathers were enlisted as the main support for mothers reallocating time to include older children. "My husband will take care of Becca (first child) and I will have the baby, because he can do things with Becca she will enjoy. I will give the baby things my husband can't." Other husbands were expected to help with the care of the newborn to permit the mother to spend more time with the older child. One mother said, "My husband took his vacation now. This will give me time to spend with my daughter (first child). I'll take her on the new swings we bought her and I'll read to her."

Many parents related difficulties with siblings when they are devoting attention to feeding the infant, either by breast or bottle. The other children seem to sense the closeness of the mother and child in this act and resent it. To counter these reactions some mothers have let the older children drink from a bottle or breast too. The tediousness and effort needed to obtain milk by this method often rapidly discourage them.

Both girls and boys seem to enjoy helping in the care of the baby or a substitute baby (doll). One mother reports that her young son routinely "breast-fed" his doll while she breast-fed the new baby. They had conversations at this time. She believed that sharing this experience seemed to give her son pride in his adult behavior of drinking from a cup. Children 6 years or older pose less of a problem than younger children. They have more significant others to turn to. They often assume "second parent" roles and boast about the new baby to friends and teachers.

Another difficulty arises when well-meaning relatives or friends concentrate on the new baby to the exclusion of the older children. Thoughtful adults often bring gifts to the older children and shower attention on them as well as paying attention to the baby.

Many hospitals permit younger children to visit the mother and newborn (Fig. 25-7). The early visits tend to

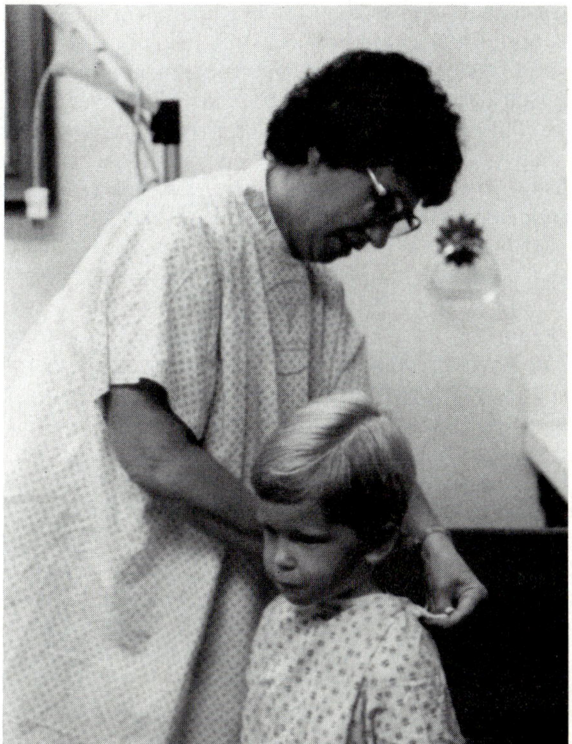

Fig. 25-7 Nurse helps brother don gown before visiting his mother and new baby sister.
Courtesy Marjorie Pyle, RNC, Lifecircle, Costa Mesa, Calif.

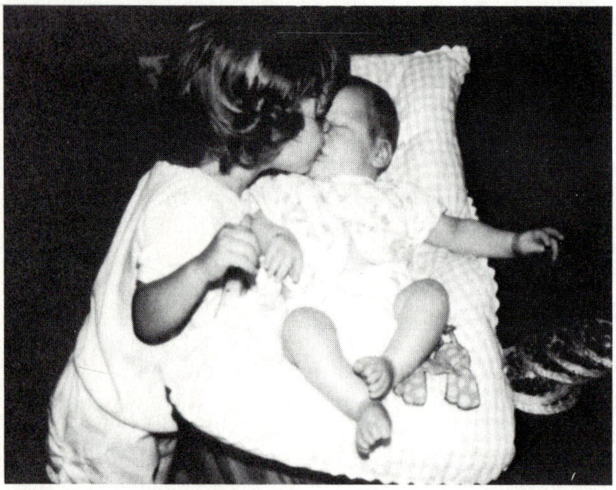

Fig. 25-8 Sister kisses her new brother. Family contacts are important for newborn and siblings.
Courtesy Marjorie Pyle, RNC, Lifecircle, Costa Mesa, Calif.

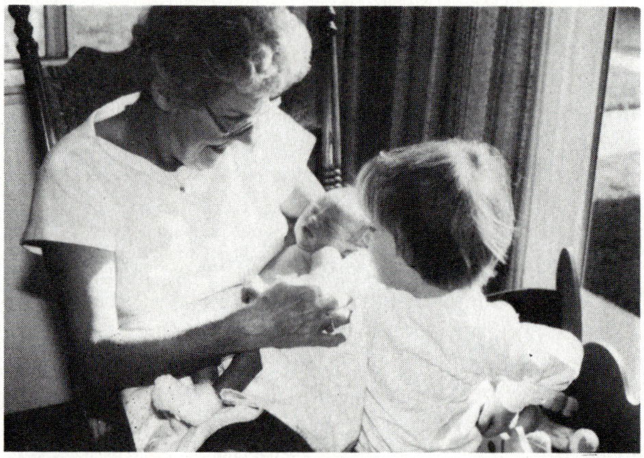

Fig. 25-9 Grandmother holds new baby as older brother looks on.
Courtesy Marjorie Pyle, RNC, Lifecircle, Costa Mesa, Calif.

reduce the older children's feelings of being deserted by the mother and help bring about faster integration of the newborn into the family. Studies (Umphenour, 1980; Kowba et al., 1985; and Wranesh, 1982) have demonstrated that healthy newborns who have direct sibling contact are not at risk for exposure to pathogenic organisms. Therefore separation of neonates and older siblings does not appear to be warranted.

The initial adjustment of older children to a newborn takes time. Parents will be faced with readjustments as the newborn matures and develops ability for more independent social and physical interactions (Kreppner et al., 1982). To expect a young child to accept and love a rival for the parents' affection assumes a too-mature response. Sibling love grows as does other love, that is, by being with another person and sharing experiences (Fig. 25-8).

GRANDPARENT ADJUSTMENT

The amount of involvement of grandparents in the care of the newborn depends on many factors, for example, willingness of the grandparents to become involved, proximity of the grandparents, and ethnic and cultural expectations of the role grandparents play (Grosso et al., 1981).

The woman's mother is an important model for childrearing practices (Rubin, 1975). She acts as a source of knowledge and as a support person (Fig. 25-9). Grandchildren are tangible evidence of continuity, of immortality. Often grandparents comment that the presence of grandchildren helps relieve loneliness and boredom. (See guidelines for client teaching: grandparent preparation, Chapter 14).

Grandparents and the Adult Child. "There are many ways to encourage new parents to include the grandparents, enriching their child's life and benefiting from the extended family themselves" (Olson, 1981). As parents are assisted in working through differing opinions and unresolved conflicts (e.g., dependency, control) between themselves and their parents, they can move toward mastery of the developmental tasks of adulthood. Grandparental support can be a stabilizing influence for families undergoing developmental crises such as childbearing and new parenthood (Newell, 1984). Grandparents can foster the learning of parental skills and preserve tradition. One simple technique to help people span the generation gap is through a printed "letter to new parents," which can be included in prenatal kits distributed in childbirth preparation classes and made available to all family members on the postpartum unit (Olson, 1981). In the letter, feelings and needs of grandparents and parents are verbalized and foster open discussion between the generations.

Grandparents and the Grandchild. "There are certain things that a grandmammy and granddaddy can do for a child that no one else can. It's sort of like stardust—the relationship between grandparents and children" (Haley, 1977). Grandparents who are free to love the grandchild crazily, blindly, lavishly, and without reservation (LeShan, 1975) can have a significant positive influence on the child's life. Praise and encouragement from a significant person fosters the development of a positive self-image and a sense of being worthy. Long-range include future relationships with others and preparation for the developmental tasks of adulthood: "With the removal of grandparents . . . from the world in which the child is reared, the child's experience of the future is shortened by a generation and his links to the past are weakened" (Mead, 1970).

SUMMARY

The childbearing family faces a constant challenge of maintaining balance between the integration of new family members and changing established interaction patterns and problem-solving strategies. The family's ability to meet the challenge is critical for parents and children. Nursing actions designed to strengthen family bonds and facilitate the mother's and father's attainment of parental roles serve an important social purpose.

KEY CONCEPTS

- The birth of a child poses a fundamental challenge to the existing interactional structure of a family.
- Either parent may exhibit "motherliness."
- Attachment is the process by which parent and child come to love and accept each other.
- Attachment is strengthened through the use of sensual responses or abilities by both partners in the parent-child interaction.
- Early contact with the newborn is not essential for optimum parent-child interactions.
- For the biologic parent, the parental role does not begin at birth, but rather enlarges and intensifies.
- Three phases are discernible as the mother adjusts to her version of the parental role.
- Since anxiety and preoccupation with her new role often narrow a mother's perceptual field, information may have to be repeated.
- A primary need of parents is to establish a life-style that includes, but in some respects excludes, the child.
- In Western culture the newborn has been found to have a powerful impact on the father.
- Modulation of rhythm, modification of behavioral repertoires, and mutual responsivity facilitate infant-parent adjustment.
- Many factors influence parental responses (e.g., their age, socioeconomic level, and their expectations of what their child will be like).
- Parents face a number of tasks related to sibling adjustment that require creative parental interventions.
- As parents work through differing opinions and unresolved conflicts between themselves and their parents, they can move toward mastery of the developmental tasks of adulthood.

STUDY QUESTIONS AND ACTIVITIES

1. Compare and contrast parental responses to an infant. Discuss in a group the rationale for such responses. What type of attachment behavior did you observe? Why was the behavior normal or abnormal? Discuss possible reasons for differences in behaviors.
2. Discuss in a group how one's own feelings regarding parenthood may alter one's perception of parenting, and how these experiences might affect their own parenting style.
3. Take turns role-playing a blind or deaf mother interacting both with her newborn and with the nurse who is attempting to provide client education. Follow with a discussion of the responses and frustrations experienced by each party.
4. Develop a client teaching program that explains the reasons for sibling jealousy and provides possible interventions the parents might employ to counteract the problem.
5. Discuss parenthood after 35.
6. In the group setting, discuss own relationships with grandparents and how these experiences compare with the text discussion of the grandparent role.
7. Collect data from personal experience, contact with clients of a culture different from your own, or from selected readings about maternity care in various cultures. Discuss findings in a group setting. Construct a nursing care plan that can be used as a framework for care of the postpartum mother.

References

Ainsworth, MD: Object relations, dependency, and attachment: a theoretical review of the infant-mother relationship, Child Dev 40:969, 1969

Ainsworth, MD: The development of infant-mother attachment. In Caldwell, BM, and Reccurti, HN, editors: Review of child development research, vol 3, New York, 1970, Russell Sage Foundation

Ainsworth, MD, and Bell, SM: Attachment, exploration and separation: illustrated by the behavior of one-year-olds in a strange situation, Child Dev 41:49, 1970

Asrael, W: Disabled women and childbearing: the nurse's role, NAACOG Update series, 1 (lesson 8), 1983

Baranowski, E: Childbirth education classes for expectant deaf parents, MCN 8:143, 1983

Barnett, CR, et al: Neonatal separation: the maternal side of interactional deprivation, Pediatrics 54:197, 1970

Benedek, T: Adaptation to reality in early infancy, Psychoanal Q 7:200, 1950

Bowlby, J: The nature of the child's tie to his mother, Int J Psychoanal 39:350, 1958

Bowlby, J: Attachment and loss, vol 1: Attachment, New York, 1969, Basic Books, Inc, Publishers

Brazelton, TB: The early mother-infant adjustment, Pediatrics 32:931, 1963

Brazelton, TB: Effect of maternal expectations on early infant behavior, Early Child Dev Care 2:259, 1973

Brazelton, TB, et al: The origins of reciprocity: the early mother-infant interaction. In Lewis, M, and Rosenblum, LA, editors: The effect of the infant on its caregiver, New York, 1974, John Wiley & Sons

Budin, P: The nursling, London, 1907, Caxton Publishing Co

Clarke-Stewart, K: And daddy makes three: the father's impact on mother and young child, Child Dev 49:466, 1978

Condon, W, and Sander, L: Neonate movement is synchronized with adult speech: interactional participation and language acquisition, Science 183:99, 1974

Crawford, J: A theoretical model of support network conflict experienced by new mothers, Nurs Res 34:100, March/April 1985

Cronenwett, LR: Network structure, social support, and psychological outcomes of pregnancy, Nurs Res 34:93, March/April 1985a

Cronenwett, LR: Parental network structured and perceived support after birth of first child, Nurs Res 34:347, Nov/Dec 1985b

Curry, MS: Contact during first hour with the wrapped or naked newborn: effect on maternal attachment behaviors at 36 hours and three months, Birth Fam J 6:4, Winter 1979

Erikson, EH: Identity and the life cycle: selected papers. In Psychological issues, vol 1, no 1, New York, 1959, International Universities Press, Inc

Erikson, EH: Childhood and society, New York, 1964, WW Norton & Co, Inc

Field, T: The three Rs of infant-adult interactions: rhythms, repertoires, and responsibility, J Pediatr Psychol 3:131, 1978a

Field, T: Visual and cardiac responses to animate and inanimate faces by young term and preterm infants, Child Dev vol 49, 1978b

Gottlieb, BH: The role of individual and social support in preventing child maltreatment. In Garbarino, J, and Stocking, S, editors: Protecting children from abuse/neglect, San Francisco, 1980, Jossey-Bass, Inc., Publishers

Greenberg, M, and Morris, N: Engrossment: the newborn's impact on the father, Nurs Digest 4:19, Jan/Feb 1976

Grosso, C, et al: The Vietnamese American family . . . and grandma makes three, MCN 6:177, 1981

Haley, A: Haley's Rx: talk, write, reunite (interview), Time 109:72, Feb 14, 1977

Hefler, RE, and Kempe, CH: The battered child, Chicago, 1965, University of Chicago Press

Klaus, MH, and Kennell, JH: Parent-infant bonding, ed 2, St Louis, 1982, The CV Mosby Co

Klaus, MH, and Robertson, M: Birth, interaction and attachment, Pediatric Round Table 6, 1982, Johnson & Johnson Baby Products Co

Klaus, MH, et al: Maternal attachment and mothering disorders, Pediatric Round Table 1, 1982, Johnson & Johnson Baby Products Co

Kowba, MD, et al: Direct sibling contact and bacterial colonization in newborns, JOGN Nurs 14:412, Sept/Oct 1985

Kreppner, K., and others: Infant and family development: from triads to tetrads, Hum. Dev. 25:373, 1982

Kunset-Wilson, W, and Cronenwett, L: Nursing care for the emerging family: promoting paternal behavior, Res Nurs Health 4:201, 1981

Lamb, M: Early contact and maternal-infant bonding: one decade later, Pediatrics 70:325, 1982

Lang, R: Birth book, Ben Lomond, Calif 1972, Genesis Press

Leifer, AD, et al: Effects of mother-infant separation on maternal attachment behavior, Child Dev 43:1203, 1972

LeShan, E: The wonderful crisis of middle age, New York, 1975, Warner Books, Inc

Magilvy, K, et al: Stereotyping, words, and concepts (letter), MCN 4:254, 1979

Mead, M: Culture and commitment: a study of the generation gap, Garden City, New York, 1970, Doubleday & Co

Mercer, RT: Parent-infant attachment. In Sonstegard, LJ, et al: editors: Women's health, vol 2: Childbearing, New York, 1982, Grune & Stratton, Inc

Newell, NJ: Grandparents, the overlooked support system for new parents during the fourth trimester, NAACOG Update Series 1 (lesson 21), 1984

Olson, ML: Fitting grandparents into new families, MCN 6:419, 1981

Parkers, CM, and Stevenson-Hinde, J: The place of attachment in human behavior, New York, 1982, Basic Books, Inc, Publishers

Queenan, JT, moderator: Managing pregnancy in patients over 35, Contemp OB/GYN 29(5):180, 1987

Rubin, R: Maternal behavior, Nurs Outlook 9:682, 1961

Rubin, R: Maternal touch at first contact with the newborn infant, Nurs Outlook 11:828, 1963

Rubin, R: Maternal tasks in pregnancy, Matern Child Nurs J 4:143, Fall 1975

Sammons, WA, and Lewis, JM: Premature babies: a different beginning. St Louis, 1985, The CV Mosby Co

Schornkoff, JP: Social support and the development of vulnerable children, Am J Public Health 74:310

Scott, L, Meredith, A, and Angwin, J: Time out for motherhood: a guide for today's working woman to the financial, emotional and career aspects of having a baby, Los Angelos, 1986, Jeremy P Tarcher, Inc

Shainess, N: Abortion is no man's business, Psychology Today, p. 18, March 1970

Siegel, E: A critical examination of studies of parent-infant bonding. In Klaus, M, and Robertson, M, editors: Birth, interaction and attachment, Evansville, Inc, 1982, Johnson & Johnson Baby Products Co

Stainton, MC: A comparison of prenatal and postnatal perceptions of their babies by parents, paper presented to the First International Congress on Pre- and Para-natal Psychology, Toronto, July 8, 1983a

Stainton, MC: Maternal newborn attachment origins and processes, III. International synchrony: the prelude to attachment, doctoral thesis, University of California, San Francisco, 1983b

Stainton, MC: Origins of attachment: culture and cue sensitivity. Dissertation Abstracts International, *46,* 3786-B. (University Microfilms No. 8600606), 1985

Steele, B, and Pollock, C: A psychiatric study of parents who abuse infants and small children. In Helfer, RE, and Kempe, C, editors: The battered child, Chicago, 1968, University of Chicago Press

Tulman, L: Mothers and unrelated persons' initial handling of newborn infants, Nurs Res 34:205, July/Aug 1985

Umphenour, JH: Bacterial colonization in neonates with sibling visitation, JOGN Nurs 9:73, 1980

Walz, B, and Rich, O: Maternal tasks of taking on a second child in the postpartum period, Matern Child Nurs J 12:3, Fall 1983

Winslow, W: First pregnancy after 35: what is the experience? MCN 12(2):92, 1987

Wranesh, BL: The effect of sibling visitation on bacterial colonization rate in neonates, JOGN Nurs 11:211, 1982

Bibliography

American College of Obstetricians and Gynecologists: The development of family-centered maternity/newborn care in hospitals, Washington, DC, 1978, The College

Avanti, K: Anxiety as a potential factor affecting maternal attachment, JOGN Nurs 10:416, 1981

Bing, E, and Colman, LL: Having a baby after thirty, New York, 1980, Bantam Books

Brandon, HK: The blind mother, Am J Nurs 75:414, 1975

Celotta, B: New motherhood: a time of crisis, Birth Fam J 9(1):21, 1982

Craig, J: Birth of a grandchild brings time of reflection, Menninger Perspect 11:23, Autumn 1980

deVore, N: Parenthood postponed, Am J Nurs 83:1160, 1983

Dunn, J, and Kendrick C: The arrival of a sibling, changes in patterns of interactions between mothers and first-born child, J Child Psychol Psychiatry 21:119, 1980

Dunn, J, Kendrick, C, and McNamee, R: The reaction of first born children to the birth of a sibling: Mothers' reports, J Child Psychol Psychiatry 22(1):1, 1981

Fardig, JA: A comparison of skin-to-skin contact and radiant heaters in promoting neonatal thermoregulation, J Nurse Midwife 25:19, Jan/Feb 1980

Fawcett, J, and York, R: Spouses' physical and psychological symptoms during pregnancy and the postpartum, Nurs Res 35(3):144, 1986

Fawcett, J, Bliss-Holtz, V, Haas, MB, et al: Spouses' body image changes during and after pregnancy: a replication and extension, Nurs Res 36(4):220, 1986

Fischman, SH, et al: Changes in sexual relationships in postpartum couples, JOGN Nurs, 15(1):58, 1986

Fortier, JC: The relationship of vaginal and cesarean births to father-infant attachment, JOGN Nurs 17(2):128, 1988

Gorrie, TM: Postpartal nursing diagnosis, JOGN Nurs 15(1):52, 1986

Hans, H: Postpartum assessment: the psychological component, JOGN Nurs 15(1):49, 1986

Humenick, SS, and Bugen, LA: Parenting roles: expectation versus reality, MCN 12(1):36, 1987

Jones, C: Father to infant attachment: effects of early contact and characteristics of the infant, Res Nurs Health 4:193, 1981

Kendrick, C, and Dunn, J: Caring for a second baby: effects on interactions between mother and first child, Dev Psychol 16(4):303, 1980

Lunch, A: Maternal stress following the birth of a second child. In Klaus, M, and Robertson, M, editors: Birth, interaction and attachment, Evansville, Ind, 1982, Johnson & Johnson Baby Products Co

May, KA: A typology of detachment/involvement styles adopted during pregnancy by first-time expectant fathers, West J Nurs Res 2:445, 1980

McCauley, CS: Pregnancy after thirty-five, New York, 1976, EP Dutton

McCrae, M: Bonding in a sea of silence, MCN 4:29, 1979

McKay, V: The decade of the eighties: significant trends and developments for hearing impaired individuals, Rehabil Lit 42:2, Jan/Feb 1981

Mercer, RT, and Stainton, MC: Perceptions of the birth experience: a cross-cultural comparison, Health Care of Women International 5:29, 1984

Morris, M: Psychological miscarriage: an end to mother love, Transactions, p 11, Jan/Feb 1966

Moss, JR: Concerns of multiparas on the third postpartum day, JOGN Nurs 10:421, 1981

Phillips, CR, and Anzalone, JT: Fathering, participation in labor and birth, ed 2, St Louis, 1982, The CV Mosby Co

Porter, R, et al: The importance of odors in mother-infant interactions, Matern Child Nurs J 12:147, Fall 1983

Price, J: You're not too old to have a baby, New York, 1977, Farrar, Strauss, & Giroux, Inc

Robertson, JF: Grandmotherhood: a study of role conception, J Marriage Fam 39:165, 1977

Rubin, SP: It's not too late for a baby, Englewood Cliffs, NJ, 1980, Prentice-Hall

Schiff, NB: Communication problems in hearing children of deaf parents, J Speech Hear Disord 41:348, 1976

Seitz, S, and Marcus, S: Mother-child interactions: a foundation for language development, Except Child 42:445, 1976

Stein, A: Pregnancy in gravidas over age 35 years, J Nurse Midwife 28(1):17, 1983

Stainton, MC: Parent-infant interaction: putting theory into practice, Calgary, Alta, Canada, 1981, University of Calgary Faculty of Nursing.

Sullivan, D, and Beeman, R: Satisfaction with postpartum care: opportunities for bonding, reconstructing the birth and instruction, Birth Fam J 8:3, Fall 1981

Sussman, AE, and Steward, LG: Counseling with deaf people, New York, 1971, New York Deafness Research and Training Center

Sweeney, A: Genetic counseling in families with hearing impairment, J Rehabil Deaf 12:1, July 1978

Sweet, PT: Prenatal classes especially for children, MCN 4:82, 1979

Tentoni, S, and High, J: Culturally induced postpartum depression: a theoretical position, JOGN Nurs 9:246, 1980

Ventura, J, and Boss, P: The family coping inventory applies to parents of new babies, J Marriage Fam 83:867, 1983

CHAPTER

26

Nursing Care During the Postpartum Period

Learning Objectives

Correctly define the key terms listed.

Review the components of the postpartum interview, physical examination, and laboratory tests.

Outline the progression of puerperal changes and schedule from day 1 through day 3.

Formulate examples of potential nursing diagnoses for physical and emotional care.

Identify goals for postpartum physical and emotional care.

Summarize general care for rest, ambulation and exercise, bed rest, immunizations, and safety.

Compare and contrast parental responses to the birth of a child focusing on adaptive and maladaptive behaviors of the mother, infant, and family.

Explain mother's need to integrate the birth experience.

Examine crisis prevention as a component of postpartum emotional care.

Relate importance of home visits.

Explore the cultural aspects of postpartum care, both physical and emotional.

List physical danger signs during the postpartum period.

Determine the nurse's responsibilities related to discharge

Key Terms

adaptive behaviors
boggy uterus
catheterization
cultural proscriptions
depressive states ("the baby blues")
hemorrhoids
Homans' sign
infant massage
"living ligature"
lochia
maladaptive behaviors
oxytocic medications
parenting difficulties
parenting disorders
perineum
pollution state
$Rh_0(D)$ immune globulin
rubella vaccination
sibling rivalry
sitz bath
state of balance
stimulation of uterine tone
suppression of lactation
"taking-hold"
"taking-in"
thromboembolism
thrombosis

The approach to care of women during the postpartum (puerperal) period has changed from one modeled on the concept of sick care to one that is wellness oriented. Women are concerned about their comfort and recovery, desirous of having contact with their infants, motivated to learn about newborn care, and eager to share their experiences with their families and friends. Their health care is now a collaborative effort on the part of all involved—mother, nurse, physician, and family—to achieve certain goals.

Knowledge of physiologic changes in the mother and emotional changes in the entire family are essential in appropriately evaluating assessment findings. Nursing diagnoses, planning, and implementation consider the need of the mother and family to learn the essentials for self-care. Early discharge, within 24 hours after delivery, is the preference for some. For others, early discharge is a necessity for various reasons (e.g., no insurance coverage, minimum coverage). Evaluation of ongoing learning is important. Effects of learning may not be evident because of the short-term contact with childbearing families after delivery. Long-term effects are yet to be identified through nursing research.

This chapter focuses both on the mother's physiologic needs and on the family's emotional needs. The first portion of the chapter provides the nurse with several procedures for care and guidelines for client teaching. The second portion addresses the emotional needs and care of the family. The nurse makes a significant contribution to providing total care to the woman and her family. Kunst-Wilson and Cronenwett (1981) make the following comment:

> [Nurses'] unique ability to deal with both the physical and psychological spheres, and the interactions of each on the other, especially important in childbearing, makes nursing's potential contribution more comprehensive than that of related disciplines. The nurse has the professional skills to deliver services personally in the office, home, or hospital setting, depending on the family's needs. Thus no major aspect of the normal childbearing experience is beyond the bounds of the nurse's skills.

PHYSICAL CARE

Assessment

The initial assessment includes the report from the nurse in the labor unit. The admitting nurse is given a brief description of all pertinent information (see Table 20-3). The woman's record is reviewed for information from the prenatal and labor records that is necessary for her nursing care plan.

Interview. During the assessment the nurse can determine the mother's emotional status, energy level, degree and location of physical discomfort, hunger, and thirst. To some degree, her knowledge level concerning self-care and infant care can also be determined. If appropriate, ethnic and cultural expectations are assessed regarding postpartum recovery patterns. The nursing care plan must consider individual variations in maternal behaviors and degree of participation in self-care and in infant care.

Physical Examination. Postpartum assessment is based on expected maternal changes. Progression of puerperal changes for the 72 hours after delivery is presented in Table 26-1.

The length of the fourth stage and the time of transfer to the postpartum unit varies. Therefore the schedule for assessment varies. To help the nurse plan assessments, a schedule starting with delivery is displayed in Table 26-2.

Laboratory Tests. After normal childbirth, few laboratory tests are routine. Hemoglobin and hematocrit determinations are required. Clean catch or catheterized urine specimens are sent for culture, sensitivity, and routine analysis for some women. The prenatal record alerts the health care team to the woman's need for rubella vaccination and potential for Rh isoimmunization. Postnatal assessment of fetal cord blood provides information about the woman's need for $Rh_0(D)$ immune globulin.

Nursing Diagnoses

Although women experience similar problems during the postpartum period, certain factors act to make each woman's experience unique. The labor a woman experienced (whether it was long or short), whether she plans to bottle-feed or breast-feed, whether she had an episiotomy, and whether she has other children are some factors to consider. Nursing diagnoses lend direction to types of nursing actions needed to implement a plan of care. Examples of nursing diagnoses follow:

- Knowledge deficit related to
  - Importance of voiding as deterrent to hemorrhage
- Sleep-pattern disturbance related to discomfort of
  - Breast engorgement
  - Episiotomy
  - Afterpains
  - Hemorrhoids
- Bathing/hygiene self-care deficit related to
  - Knowledge deficit of perineal hygiene as promoter of healing during the puerperium
- Potential for infection related to
  - Childbirth trauma to tissues
- Constipation or urinary retention related to
  - Post-childbirth discomfort
- Situational low self-esteem related to
  - Knowledge deficit of expected anatomic and physiologic changes during the puerperium

Planning

The nursing plan is used for the care of women postpartum as it is for other clients. Once the nursing diagnoses are formulated, the nurse decides what nursing measures would be appropriate and which are to be given priority. The organization of care must take the newborn into consideration. The day actually revolves around the baby's feeding and care times.

The mother assumes increasing responsibility for her own self-care. The nurse is responsible for consistent as-

Table 26-1 *Progression of Puerperal Changes: Days 1 Through 3*

Assessment	2-24 Hours (Day 1)	25-48 Hours (Day 2)	49-72 Hours (Day 3)
Temperature	Elevated (38° C [100.4° F])	Within normal range	Within normal range
Pulse	Bradycardia: 50-70 beats/min	Bradycardia may persist or rate may return to within normal range	Bradycardia may persist or rate may return to within normal range
Blood pressure	Within normal range	Within normal range	Within normal range
Energy level	Euphoric, happy, excited, or fatigued; may show need for sleep	Often tired, slow moving	Anxious to go home; level within normal range, but variable
Uterus	At umbilicus or just below	1 cm or more below umbilicus	2 cm or more below umbilicus
Lochia	Rubra; moderate; few clots, if any; fleshy odor of normal menstrual flow	Rubra to serosa; moderate to scant; odor continues to be "fleshy" or absent	Rubra to serosa; scant; odor continues to be "fleshy" or absent
Perineum	Edematous; clean, healing	Edema lessening; clean, healing	Edema lessening or absent; clean, healing
Legs	Pretibial or pedal edema; Homans' sign negative	Edema lessening; Homan's sign negative	Edema minimal or absent; Homans' sign negative
Breasts	Remain soft to palpation Colostrum can be expressed	Begin to feel firmer Occasionally feel lumpy	Increase in vascularity and initiation of swelling Feel firmer and warmer to touch Milk expected within 2-4 days after delivery
Appetite	Excellent; may ask for double helpings, snacks	Usually remains excellent	Varies; appetite may have returned to normal range or may lessen (especially if client is constipated)
Elimination			
Voiding	Up to 3000 ml	Large amounts	Amount/24 hours is lessening
Defecation	None expected	None expected	Usually defecates; may need enema, etc.
Discomfort	Generalized aching; perineal area: episiotomy, hemorrhoids	Muscle aches; perineal area: episiotomy, hemorrhoids	Possible tension headache, perineal area: usually lessening; breasts, nipples

Table 26-2 *Minimum Schedule of Assessments After Delivery*

	Hour															
	1				2		3	4	5	6	7	8	9-24	25-48	49-72
Assessment Factor	15″	15″	15″	15″	30″	30″	60″	60″	60″	60″	60″	60″	Every 4 Hours	Every 8 Hours	Every 8 Hours
Temperature	—	—	—	X	—	—	—	X	—	—	—	X	×4	×3	×3
Pulse, respirations, blood pressure	X	X	X	X	X	X	X	X	—	—	—	X	×6	×3	×3
Fundus, lochia	X	X	X	X	X	X	X	X	—	—	—	X	×4	×3	×3
Bladder	X	X	X	X	X	X	X	X	—	—	—	X	amount (ml)		
Perineum	—	—	—	X	—	—	—	X	—	—	—	X	×4	×3	×3
Breasts, legs	—	—	—	—	—	—	—	—	—	—	—	X	×4	×3	×3
Psychosocial factors	X	X	X	X	—	—	—	X	—	—	—	X	×4	×3	×3
Bowels	—	—	—	—	—	—	—	—	—	—	—	—	Daily	Daily	Daily

sessment of actual or potential problems. In some areas "couple nursing" (mother and baby) has been introduced. The nurse acts as the primary nurse for both mother and infant even if the newborn is kept in the central nursery. This approach is a variation of rooming-in, in which mother and child room together and mother and nurse share the care of the infant.

The nursing care plan will include assessments to detect deviations from normal, comfort measures to relieve discomfort or pain, and safety measures to prevent injury or infection. The nurse also will provide teaching and counseling measures designed to promote a mother's (and father's) feeling of competence in the care of herself and newly born child. The nurse evaluates continuously and is ready to change the plan if indicated. The nurse's ability to adapt the care plan to specific medical and nursing diagnoses results in individualized care for the client.

Standardized care plans are used by almost all facilities and health care providers (Fig. 26-1) and are found in many nursing textbooks. A standard care plan is an aid for students and new graduates in grasping concepts or setting priorities and selecting appropriate actions for real or potential problems (see nursing care plans in this chapter). In addition, it can be used as a checklist for giving general direction for implementing the nursing process with a client. Caution is advised against total reliance on a standardized plan: the uniqueness of the individual may be overlooked.

Goals

1. Prevent hemorrhage, infection, and other biophysical complications
2. Promote involution and physiologic recovery from childbirth
3. Promote physical comfort, rest, activity, and safety
4. Facilitate return of woman's normal pattern of bowel and bladder elimination
5. Meet learning needs for recovery from childbirth, normal involution, and self-care
6. Enhance woman's self-concept by teaching self-care and infant-care skills to increase competence
7. Encourage continued health maintenance through self-care and use of home and community health care delivery systems

Implementation

Maintenance of Infection-free Environment. Facilities (unit kitchens, bathroom, and bed units) and supplies (linens) must be kept scrupulously clean. Frequent changes of draw sheet and a daily change of linen are recommended. Supervision of use of facilities to prevent cross infection among women is necessary (e.g., common sitz bath must be scrubbed after each woman's use, ventilation system is monitored). Personnel must be conscientious about their hand-washing techniques to prevent cross infection. In many institutions nurses are required to wear a face mask when carrying out perineal care. Personnel with colds, coughs, or skin infections (e.g., a cold sore on the lips [herpes simplex virus, type 1]) must follow hospital protocol when in contact with women during the puerperium.

Client Identification. The first step in providing individualized care is to confirm the client's correct identity by checking her arm band. At the same time, the infant's identification number is matched with the corresponding band on the mother's wrist. The nurse demonstrates caring and respect by determining how the mother wishes to be addressed and then notes her preference in her record and on the card index (Kardex).

Orientation to Environment. The woman and her family are oriented to their surroundings. Familiarity with the unit, routines, resources, and personnel reduces one potential source of anxiety—the unknown. The mother is reassured through knowing whom and how she can call for assistance and what she can expect in the way of supplies and services. If the woman's usual daily routine before admission differs from the facility's routine, the nurse works with the woman to develop a mutually acceptable and workable routine.

Ethnic and cultural variations in care of the woman after delivery can be discussed and plans for modifying nursing actions made (see pp. 644 to 647). An example of a cultural variation follows:

A Vietnamese woman who had been in the United States for 4 years requested rooming-in facilities following delivery. Instead of participating in the care of her infant, she refused to do so, remained in bed, wore a woolen cap, and appeared distressed and angry. The staff were nonplussed by her behavior. One nurse decided to put newly learned concepts concerning cross-cultural nursing into effect. She began by praising the woman's ability to speak English and after eliciting a smile, remarked, "Every country has developed good ways to look after mothers and babies. Would you tell me about the care in Vietnam?" There was an immediate response. The woman explained that in her country women remained in bed for 10 days after delivery and the biggest danger to their health was getting a cold. The baby was kept in the room with his mother, but either a grandmother or nurse took complete charge of the care.

Evidently the woman was operating in tune with her cultural expectations, and the nurses were operating within theirs. This rather simple approach to resolving a nursing problem also proved successful in subsequent cases.

Rest. The excitement and exhilaration experienced after the birth of the infant may make rest difficult. The new mother, who is often anxious about her ability to care for her infant or is uncomfortable, may also have difficulty sleeping. Backrubs, other comfort measures, and medication for sleep for the first few nights may be necessary.

Ambulation and Exercise. Early ambulation has proved successful in reducing the incidence of thromboembolism and in women's more rapid recovery of strength. Confinement to bed is not required for women who had general anesthesia, who had *epidural* or *caudal anesthesia,* or who had local anesthesia such as paracervical or pudendal

Name: Room:	Grav: Para: Ab: Stb: Marital status: Occupation: Rh: Type: Rubella antibody titer:	Infant Sex: Wt: Length: Time: Day: Date: Pediatrician: Feeding: Baby's Rh: Type: Coombs: Condition of baby: Date:	Family: Adults: Siblings:
Short-term goal:		Long-term goal:	
Emergency number:	Person:	Relationship:	Address:

Date	Nursing diagnoses	Evaluative criteria	Nursing actions

Client teaching: **Mother**
Breast care
Perineal care; hemorrhoids
Lochia flow norms
Postpartum nutrition and fluid needs
Exercise/rest
Family schedules
Sexual relations
Emotional adjustments
Cesarean delivery
Tubal occlusion

Infant
Characteristics
Bathing
Cord/circumcision
Thermometer use
Bulb syringe
Breast feeding
Storage of milk
Formula feeding
Positioning/handling
Clothing; Diapering
Signs of illness
Safety/poison control
Car seats; CPR
Family planning options
Importance of follow-up care for self and infant

Discharge planning

1. Mother will have follow-up care for self and infant arranged prior to discharge.
2. Mother has received and verbalized understanding of discharge instructions re: care of breasts, perineum, stitches, nutrition, rest/exercise, resumption of sexual activity, danger signs to report to physician.
3. Mother demonstrates comfort and competence in caregiver skills with own infant.

Return visit:

Referrals: ( ) social work
( ) home care

Date/ resolution	Client problem(s)	Expected outcome (short/long-term goals)	Date outcome to be reached	Nursing action	Signature
/	Potential postpartum hemorrhage	Will verbalize lochia flow norms, how to report abnormal signs.		Teach lochia flow norms: color, amount, odor, length of flow, and how to report to nurse/physician.	
/				Assess fundal tone, height, position q15 min first hour postpartum, massage uterus prn.	
/				Assess q½h x 2, then q shift and prn.	
/				Teach mother how to massage fundus.	
/	Potential infection	Will verbalize lochia flow norms, how to report abnormal signs.		Alert woman to report temp. of 100.4° F, foul-smelling lochia, abdominal pain, general feeling of not being well.	
/		Will demonstrate appropriate hygiene and care of perineum, stitches.		Teach use of surgigator, squeeze bottle, sitz bath, avoidance of tampons, intercourse, swimming until postpartum checkup.	
/	Potential anxiety secondary to lack of knowledge/experience in care taking of infant, feeding.	Will demonstrate competence in infant care taking and feeding techniques.		Provide early contact with infant and encourage eye-to-eye, skin-to-skin contact.	
/				Assess readiness for learning, provide frequent opportunity for observing/practicing infant care skills, feedings.	
/				Provide emotional support and positive reinforcement with learned skills.	

Fig. 26-1 Plan of nursing care for woman after normal delivery.
Adapted from Fountain Valley Community Hospital, Fountain Valley Calif.

block. Free movement is permitted once the anesthetic wears off unless an analgesic has been administered. After the first vital rest period is over (usually about 8 hours), the mother is encouraged to ambulate frequently. Postpartum exercises are begun as soon as the woman indicates readiness (see guidelines for client teaching: postpartum exercises). Exercise also promotes rest.

Bed Rest. Parturients who received *intrathecal subarachnoid spinal anesthesia* should remain flat in bed with one flat pillow to align the head with the shoulders for at least 8 hours before they are allowed to ambulate. This position prevents leakage of spinal fluid through the dural membrane at the site of the needle puncture (a potential fistula tract), which causes a severe **"spinal" headache.**

Guidelines for Client Teaching

POSTPARTUM EXERCISES

ASSESSMENT

1. Woman has just completed a full-term pregnancy.

NURSING DIAGNOSES

Knowledge deficit related to postpartum exercises.
Knowledge deficit related to diastasis of rectus abdomini muscle.
Potential body image disturbance related to postpartum body changes.

GOALS

Short-term

Woman verbalizes understanding of exercise program.
Woman begins exercise recommended for the first postpartum day.

Intermediate

Woman follows exercise program without problems or untoward responses (i.e., fatigue, increased pain).

Long-term

Woman continues with a balance between rest and exercise or activity.
Woman verbalizes satisfaction with way she feels and looks.

REFERENCES AND TEACHING AIDS

Handout with illustrations and descriptions of exercise program.
Filmstrip.
Demonstration of exercises by the nurse.

CONTENT/RATIONALE	TEACHING ACTIONS
To inform the woman about exercise and help her define realistic expectations, the nurse presents the following content:	
Rigorous exercise may initiate uterine bleeding, fatigue, or discomfort.	Caution woman against too rigorous and taxing exercises, regardless of the physical fitness of the woman.
Toning of the abdominal muscles takes time. Program progresses slowly from easy to more demanding exercises.	Review exercise program (Fig. 26-2). Encourage woman not to rush.
Girdles or other abdominal supports tend to make the woman "forget" to keep abdominal muscles contracted and therefore delay regaining tone.	Discourage woman from wearing girdles or other abdominal supports.
Fatigue or discomfort drain energy needed for recovery and care of newborn and of self.	Remind woman to stop if exercise makes her too tired.
Kegel's exercises begun soon after delivery, or as soon as anesthesia has worn off, aid in the recovery of the pubococcygeal muscle, which is stretched during vaginal delivery.	Assess woman's knowledge of Kegel's exercises and review as needed.
To counsel the woman who has diastasis (separation) of the rectus abdomini muscle, reinforce the fact that there is no known therapy to prevent or treat the condition.	Encourage discussion of woman's feelings about the facts that the separation usually lessens with time, but if the separation is quite wide, it may not return to pre-pregnant state; and exercise or girdles have not been known to speed the rate of recovery.

EVALUATION Teaching has been effective when the nurse observes that the woman learns how to do the exercises, and, at the follow-up visit to the physician or clinic, she indicates she has followed the exercise program and verbalizes she is pleased with the way she looks.

Since mothers automatically raise their heads to view their infants, the nurse needs to warn the mother to remain flat in bed. The nurse then positions or holds the infant so that the mother can see the child. Bathroom privileges are curtailed, and infant feeding by the mother may be delayed until she can sit up (check hospital protocol).

Prevention of **thrombosis** is part of the nursing care plan. If a woman is confined to bed longer than 8 hours

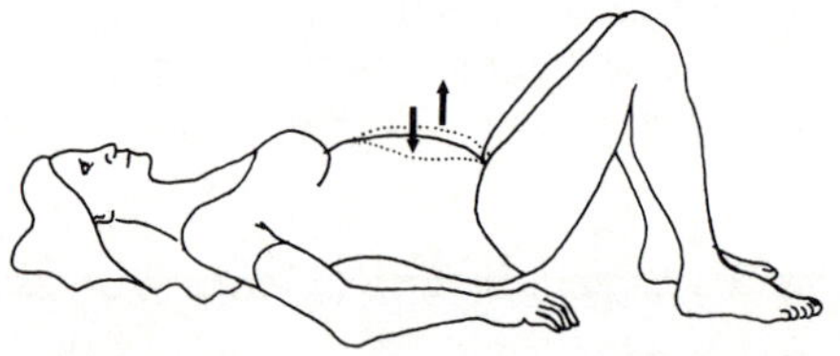

Abdominal Breathing. Lie on back with knees bent. Inhale deeply through nose. Keep ribs stationary and allow abdomen to expand upwards. Exhale slowly but forcefully while contracting the abdominal muscles; hold for 3 to 5 seconds while exhaling. Relax.

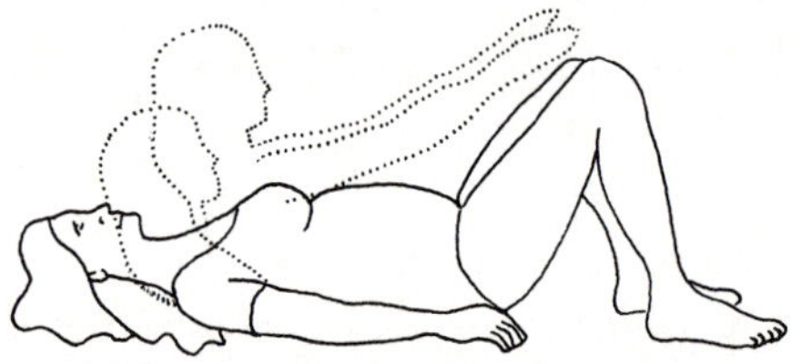

Reach for the Knees. Lie on back with knees bent. While inhaling deeply lower chin onto chest. While exhaling, raise head and shoulders slowly and smoothly and reach for knees with arms outstretched. The body should only rise as far as the back will naturally bend while waist remains on floor or bed (about 6 to 8 inches). Slowly and smoothly lower head and shoulders back to starting position. Relax.

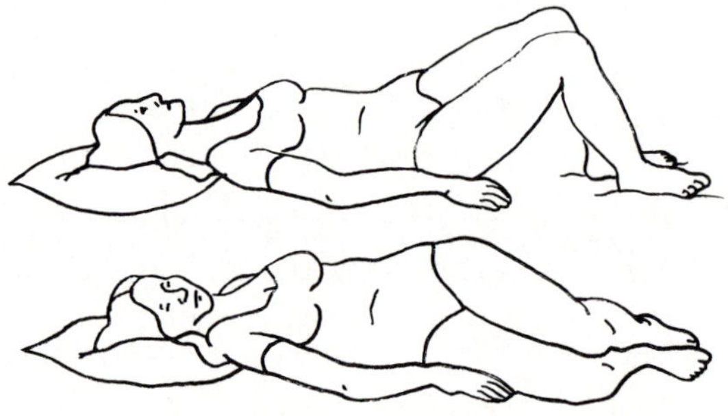

Double Knee Roll. Lie on back with knees bent. Keeping shoulders flat and feet stationary, slowly and smoothly roll knees over to the left to touch floor or bed. Maintaining a smooth motion, roll knees back over to the right until they touch floor or bed. Return to starting position and relax.

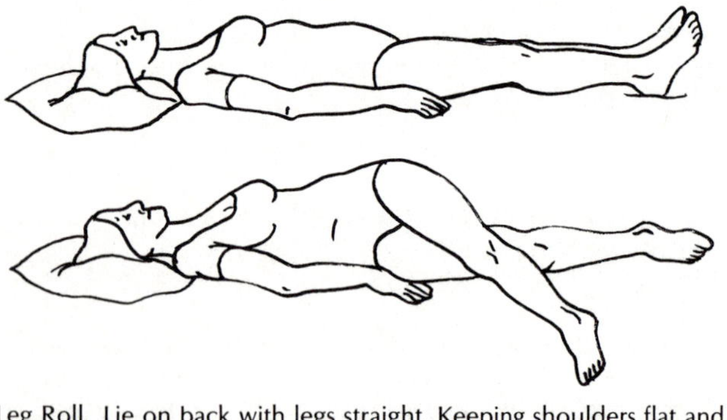

Leg Roll. Lie on back with legs straight. Keeping shoulders flat and legs straight, slowly and smoothly lift left leg and roll it over to touch the right side of floor or bed and return to starting position. Repeat, rolling right leg over to touch left side of floor or bed. Relax.

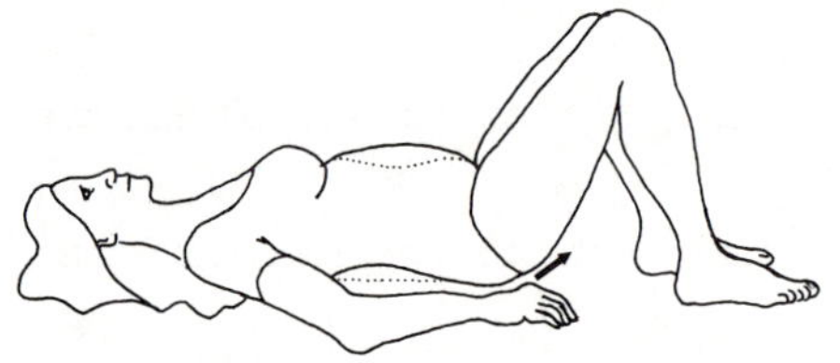

Combined Abdominal Breathing and Supine Pelvic Tilt (Pelvic Rock). Lie on back with knees bent. While inhaling deeply, roll pelvis back by flattening lower back on floor or bed. Exhale slowly but forcefully while contracting abdominal muscles and tightening buttocks. Hold for 3 to 5 seconds while exhaling. Relax.

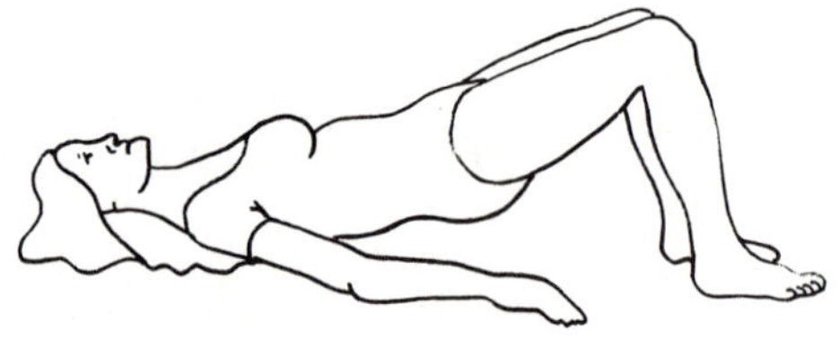

Buttocks Lift. Lie on back with arms at sides, knees bent and feet flat. Slowly raise buttocks and arch back. Return slowly to starting position.

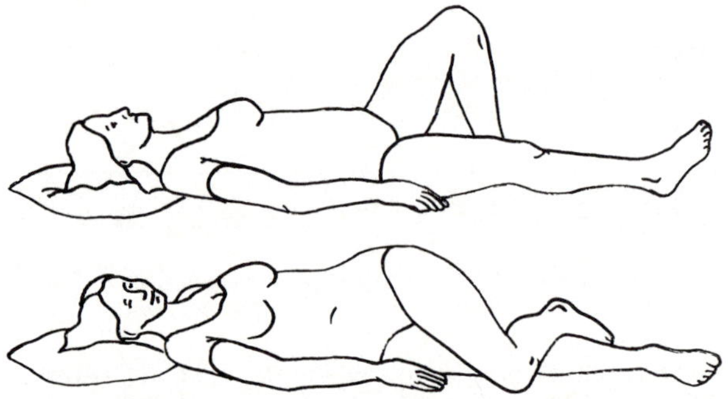

Single Knee Roll. Lie on back with with right leg straight and left leg bent at the knee. Keeping shoulders flat, slowly and smoothly roll left knee over to the right to touch floor or bed and then back to starting position. Reverse position of legs. Roll right knee over to the left to touch floor or bed and return to starting position. Relax.

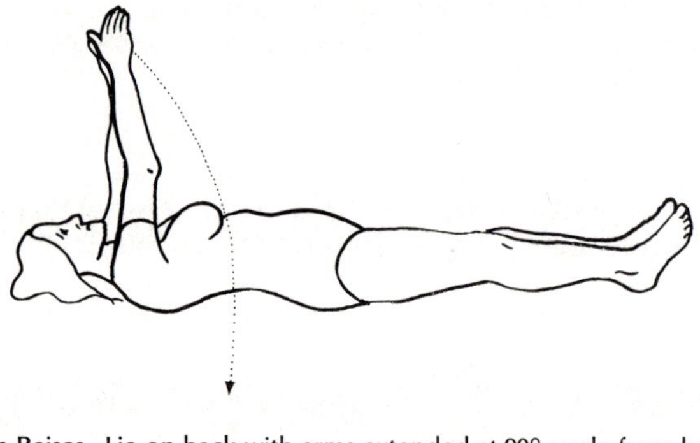

Arm Raises. Lie on back with arms extended at 90° angle from body. Raise arms so they are perpendicular and hands touch. Lower slowly.

Fig. 26-2 Postpartum exercise should begin as soon as possible. The woman should start with simple exercises and gradually progress to more strenuous ones.

(e.g., after spinal anesthesia or cesarean birth), exercise to promote circulation in the legs is indicated:

1. Alternate flexion and extension of feet
2. Rotate feet
3. Alternate flexion and extension of legs
4. Press back of knee to bed surface; relax

If the woman is susceptible to **thromboembolism**, the physician may avoid use of estrogens to inhibit or suppress lactation. Women with varicosities are encouraged to wear support hose. The woman is encouraged to walk about actively for true ambulation and discouraged from sitting immobile in a chair. If a thrombus is suspected, notify the physician immediately; meanwhile the woman should be confined to bed, with the affected limb elevated on pillows.

Immunizations. Rubella vaccination and $Rh_0(D)$ immune globulin are administered during the puerperium as necessary. For a detailed discussion of the Rh factor and isoimmunization, see Chapter 40; for a general discussion of the immune system, see Chapter 6.

During the puerperium the nurse apprises the mother of the recommended schedule of immunizations for the infant (Appendix J).

Rubella Vaccination. For women who have not had rubella (10% to 20% of all women) or women who are serologically negative (i.e., titer of 1:8 or less) rubella virus vaccine is recommended in the immediate postdelivery period to prevent fetal anomalies in future pregnancies. Seroconversion occurs in approximately 90% of women vaccinated after delivery. The live attenuated rubella virus is not communicable; therefore nursing mothers can be vaccinated. However, the live attenuated rubella vaccine is made from duck eggs, so women who have allergies to these eggs may develop a hypersensitivity reaction to the vaccine, for which they will need adrenalin. A transient arthralgia or rash is common in vaccinated women but is benign. Since the vaccine may be teratogenic the client should sign an informed consent and should receive written information about the vaccine, its side effects and risks, and the necessity for practicing contraception for a period of 2 to 3 months after vaccination.

Prevention of Rh Isoimmunization. Injection of $Rh_0(D)$ immune globulin within 72 hours of delivery will prevent sensitization in the Rh-negative woman who has had a fetomaternal transfusion of Rh-positive fetal red blood cells (RBCs). The administration of 300 μg of $Rh_0(D)$ immune globulin is usually sufficient to prevent maternal sensitization. $Rh_0(D)$ immune globulin promotes lysis of fetal Rh-positive RBCs circulating in the maternal bloodstream before the mother forms her own antibodies against them. If a large fetomaternal transfusion is suspected, the dose needed can be assessed by either the Betke-Kleihauer or the D^u test, which detects 20 ml or more of Rh-positive fetal blood in the maternal circulation. The $Rh_0(D)$ immune globulin is administered after all known abortions (gestational age of 8 weeks or more), since the risk of sensitization after abortion is about half the risk after a full-term pregnancy.* **It is administered after delivery to any woman who meets the following three criteria:** (1) the mother must be $Rh_0(D)$ negative with no Rh antibodies (i.e., indirect Coombs' test is negative), (2) the infant must be $Rh_0(D)$-positive or D^u-positive, and (3) results of direct Coombs' test on the cord blood must be negative. If the woman meets these criteria, a 1:1000 dilution of $Rh_0(D)$ immune globulin* is cross-matched to the mother's red cells to ensure compatibility. The same precautions are followed when administering a blood transfusion to ensure that the immune globulin is administered to the correct woman. *If administered to an Rh-positive person, immune globulin will act to promote lysis of the Rh-positive RBCs.* The dose is administered to the mother intramuscularly (*never* intravenously or to the infant).

Comfort. Most women during the early postpartum period need occasional pharmacologic analgesia for general muscle aches, perineal discomfort, incision or episiotomy pain, afterpains, engorgement, or mild tension headaches. Most physicians routinely order a variety of prn analgesics, including both narcotic and nonnarcotic choices, and dosage and time frequency ranges. When administering an analgesic the nurse must make a clinical judgment on the type, dosage, and frequency from the medications ordered. Research has shown that nurses, as well as physicians, underestimate the woman's pain and usually undermedicate. Whereas most research has been with oncology and medical clients, it would seem that this finding may be even more true when caring for postpartum women experiencing mild to moderate pain and in otherwise good health. It has been reported that postpartum women use more analgesia when self-administered medication systems are instituted. This is an area for further nursing research.

The woman's description of the type and severity of her pain is the nurse's best guide in choosing between analgesics. One method used to quantify pain is to have the woman rate her pain on a 10-point scale with 10 being the most severe pain she can imagine. To confirm the location and extent of discomfort the nurse inspects and palpates areas of pain as appropriate for redness, swelling, discharge, and heat and observes for body tension, guarded movements, and facial tension. Blood pressure, pulse, and respiration may be elevated in response to acute pain. Diaphoresis may accompany severe pain. A lack of objective symptoms does not necessarily mean there is no pain.

Nursing actions are chosen so that the pain sensation is eliminated or reduced to a tolerable level that allows the woman to perform self-care activities and begin infant care. Individuals vary in their attitudes about involvement in their own care. Many women may initially have great fatigue and not want to or not be able to participate fully in analgesic decisions. Severe pain also interferes with active participation in choosing pain-relief measures.

If an analgesic is to be given, the nurse informs the client of the prescribed analgesic, their common side effects, and presence in breast milk if she is breast-feeding. A woman may prefer another analgesic or pain control measure if a side effect is felt to be unacceptable. For example, a new mother planning to keep her infant at her bedside may not be comfortable with an analgesic that may

*For prenatal prophylaxis, see Chapters 6 and 40.

*A blood product. Certain religions proscribe use of blood or blood products.

make her drowsy. Pain is a frightening, lonely experience and a woman should feel confident that her needs for pain relief will be attended to. Therefore the nurse evaluates the effectiveness of the analgesic every 15 minutes until acceptable pain relief is achieved.

If there is no improvement in reported pain in 30 minutes, to enhance the analgesic, the nurse institutes appropriate nonpharmacologic pain measures that were not previously instituted, such as ice packs, warm compresses, distraction, imagery, therapeutic touch, and relaxation. Pain relief is enhanced by using more than one method or route.

If acceptable pain relief has not been achieved in 1 hour and there has not been a change in the initial assessment, the nurse may need to contact the physician for additional pain relief orders or directions. Unrelieved pain results in fatigue, anxiety, and worsening perception of pain. Once pain has become severe larger doses or stronger analgesia is required.

When acceptable analgesia has been achieved the nurse evaluates with the woman her pain relief and her expectation and desire to participate in pain control. The nurse identifies any changes the mother desires in her regimen and adds changes to the care plan. A woman's belief regarding what is helpful to achieve pain relief is vital to the success of any pain regimen.

Nursing Care Related to Physiologic Adaptations. All nursing care given during the postpartum period is provided simultaneously with teaching. The rationale for each action can be provided and questions encouraged during each encounter with the new mother. The short span of time allotted the nurse to provide care necessitates that every opportunity for teaching be used. The puerperium period is characterized by heightened interest in learning and readiness to change by the new mother and often by her family as well. The general nursing care plan outlines assessment findings, nursing actions, and evaluation. Evaluation of short-term goals that can be achieved during the hospital stay is readily done. However, it may not be possible to determine to what degree other goals have been met if the nurse has no further contact with the family after the woman returns home.

Decision Trees, Procedures, and Guidelines for Client Teaching. The nurse's instrumental role and the roles as technician, teacher/counselor/advocate are highlighted in this section. Decision trees to assist the nurse caring for clients with boggy uterus and full urinary bladder are provided. To help the nurse meet the physical care needs of the woman after childbirth, procedures for boggy uterus, care of episiotomy or laceration, care of full urinary bladder, and suppression of lactation follow. Table 26-3 includes measures to stimulate uterine tone. Several guidelines for client teaching have been developed to help the nurse fulfill the role of teacher. These include general teaching in the early postpartum period, care of hemorrhoids and postdelivery fertility management (see Chapter 25). Guidelines for client teaching for prevention of urinary tract infection and breast self-examination are in Chapter 8.

Text continued on p. 630.

General Nursing Care Plan

EARLY POSTPARTUM

ASSESSMENT	NURSING DIAGNOSIS (ND)/ PLAN (P)/GOAL (G)	RATIONALE/ IMPLEMENTATION	EVALUATION
Vital signs Temperature Increased pulse Record of blood loss or anemia	ND: Potential for infection related to significant problems that can arise during labor, delivery, and postpartum. ND: Potential knowledge deficit related to signs and symptoms of infection. P: Prevention or timely identification and treatment of infection. P: Meet woman's information needs. G: Woman does not develop signs and symptoms of infection. Woman increases her knowledge about infection and fever.	*To identify infection the nurse will assess for:* Chills or fever of 38° C (100.4° F) or more. Localized redness, heat, pain anywhere on body. Urinary frequency, pain, or burning on urination. Foul-smelling lochia.	Woman reports any symptoms she experiences immediately. Woman is aware of normal ranges of vital signs. Woman does not develop infection; or if she does, identification and resolution are timely.

General Nursing Care Plan—cont'd

ASSESSMENT	NURSING DIAGNOSIS (ND)/ PLAN (P)/GOAL (G)	RATIONALE/ IMPLEMENTATION	EVALUATION
	ND: Potential for hyperthermia related to infection. P: Identify and treat hyperthermia. G: Woman will learn and use temperature reduction techniques and temperature will return to within normal limits.	*To initiate measures to lower temperature the nurse will:* Report fever to physician. Encourage oral fluids or continue IV fluids as ordered. Decrease environmental temperature, remove blankets or heavy clothing. Administer antipyretic medication as ordered.	Woman uses same temperature reduction techniques at home. Woman understands information presented. Woman's temperature returns to within normal range.
Increased blood pressure Decreased blood pressure	ND: Potential for injury maternal, related to hypertension/hypotension. P: Monitor for signs and symptoms of deviations from normal values; monitor per hospital protocol and woman's needs. G: Woman will remain normotensive.	*To promote normotensive state in new mother the nurse will:* Give anticipatory guidance for prevention (i.e., diet, exercise, medication). Teach woman about orthostatic hypotension related to splanchnic engorgement.	Woman aware of normal range. Woman implements preventive measures. Woman takes precautions against fainting during first ambulation; calls for assistance.
Headache	ND: Pain: headache related to stress, increased blood pressure, spinal anesthesia. P: Help woman prevent headache; monitor for headache; implement appropriate therapy. G: Woman will not have headache; or, headache and its cause are identified and treated promptly.	*To prevent or decrease headache the nurse will:* Teach relaxation and stress reduction techniques. Administer medications for increased blood pressure as ordered. Have woman lie down. Keep woman recovering from spinal anesthesia flat for prescribed number of hours. Administer medications as ordered. Increase fluid intake. Prepare for blood patch procedure.	Woman knows and uses relaxation techniques. Woman knows importance of taking antihypertensive medications. Woman understands reason for headache and complies with prevention or treatment.
Uterus Position, size Tone Response to gentle massage Rate of involution Afterpains	ND: Potential for injury related to hemorrhage from an atonic uterus postdelivery. P: Prevent atonic uterus, prevent hemorrhage through teaching and direct care. G: Hemorrhage does not occur. ND: Pain related to uterine involution/afterpains. P: Prevent or minimize discomfort.	*To prevent hemorrhage from atonic uterus the nurse will:* Assess tone and response to gentle massage. Use nonpharmacologic or pharmacologic measures to maintain tone and relieve discomfort of afterpains. Teach woman how to assess fundus. Teach woman how to massage uterus.	Woman understands purpose of firm uterus and follows through with self-massage.

Continued.

General Nursing Care Plan—cont'd

ASSESSMENT	NURSING DIAGNOSIS (ND)/ PLAN (P)/GOAL (G)	RATIONALE/ IMPLEMENTATION	EVALUATION
	G: Woman states that afterpains are tolerable and she is satisfied with measures used.		
Lochia Color and character Amount Size, number of clots Odor ("fleshy")	ND: Potential for infection/hemorrhage related to conditions causing abnormal lochia. P: Detect/prevent underlying causes of deviations from normal. G: Woman's lochia remains within normal limits.	*To prevent possible hemorrhage and infection of endometrium the nurse will:* Monitor amount and character of lochia. If heavy, reassess source of bleeding, uterine tone, and degree of bladder distension. Expelled clots should be charted as to size and amount. Teach expected regression (color and amount) during involution. Teach woman about atony of the uterus and subsequent hemorrhage, and explain that clots prevent the living ligature from working.	Woman verbalizes understanding and reports any unusual symptoms. Lochia is moderate or less with no clots or just a few small clots.
Perineum Healing of episiotomy/laceration Swelling, bruising Hematoma Size, number of hemorrhoids	ND: Impaired skin integrity related to episiotomy/lacerations acquired during delivery. P: Promote healing, prevent further complications. G: Woman's childbirth-related tissue trauma heals without difficulty. ND: Pain, related to episiotomy, laceration, hemorrhoids, swelling, bruising, or hematoma. P: Prevent or minimize discomfort. G: Woman's discomfort is prevented or minimized.	*To ensure proper healing and prevent infection and development of other problems the nurse will:* Monitor perineal healing. Provide comfort measures. Wash hands before and after care of perineum. Teach woman comfort measures—ice packs, sitz baths, heat lamp, anesthetic sprays or creams, witch hazel pads (Tucks). Give woman opportunity to look at perineum and its repair (if interested). Describe to woman what to expect while perineum is healing and hemorrhoids are regressing. Teach woman to avoid contamination of perineum and vulva by—washing hands before and after pericare; wiping from front to back; changing peripads often; changing underwear daily and when soiled.	Perineum heals well. Hemorrhoids regress. Woman employs comfort measures. Comfort is maintained. Woman verbalizes understanding of information presented, uses proper pericare.

General Nursing Care Plan—cont'd

ASSESSMENT	NURSING DIAGNOSIS (ND)/ PLAN (P)/GOAL (G)	RATIONALE/ IMPLEMENTATION	EVALUATION
Urinary tract Symptoms of infection Distension Completeness of emptying Ability to void Total amount in 24 hours	ND: Potential for infection related to bladder trauma during delivery, or retention and stasis of urine. P: Prevent distension and stasis of urine. G: Woman does not experience bladder distention.	*To avoid potential for urinary tract infection the nurse will:* Teach woman to wipe from front to back. Use strict aseptic technique when catheterization is necessary. Help woman void and empty bladder completely. Teach woman symptoms of urinary tract infection: urgency; frequency and burning on urination; and blood in urine.	Woman doesn't develop urinary infection. Woman understands symptoms and reports development of same.
	ND: Urinary retention related to anesthesia and bladder trauma. P: Assist woman to void; catheterize if necessary. G: Woman resumes normal pattern of urine elimination.	*To assist woman in voiding the nurse will:* Encourage oral fluids. Assist to bathroom, if possible. Run water in sink for encouragement. Pour warm water down perineum or immerse in warm sitz bath. Catheterize per physician's order. Teach Crede's method (use of manual pressure on bladder to express urine).	Woman voids and empties bladder completely at least every 4 hours. Bladder distension does not occur. If catheterization is necessary, infection or loss of self-esteem does not occur.
Bowels Bowel sounds Passing flatus Abdominal distension Bowel movement Constipation Diarrhea Hemorrhoids	ND: Constipation related to fear of tearing stitches or pain, medications, decreased peristalsis, hemorrhoids. P: Prevent bowel problems through teaching and direct care. G: Woman does not experience bowel problems.	*To assist woman with first bowel movement the nurse will:* Encourage and assist with early ambulation, fluids, foods with roughage. Encourage immediate response to urge to defecate. Administer stool softeners as prescribed. Employ care of perineum. Counsel woman on: fluids, foods; exercise; bowel habits; hygiene after defecation. Check chart for record of last bowel movement during labor and delivery.	Woman's bowel elimination pattern restored. Woman has minimum discomfort. Woman continues to use preventative and comfort measures learned during hospitalization.
Breasts Soft, filling, firm Engorged Painful Mastitis	ND: Pain of engorged breasts related to lactation or suppression.	*To assist woman with suuppression of lactation the nurse will:*	Lactation is suppressed with minimum discomfort.

Continued.

General Nursing Care Plan—cont'd

ASSESSMENT	NURSING DIAGNOSIS (ND)/ PLAN (P)/GOAL (G)	RATIONALE/ IMPLEMENTATION	EVALUATION
	P: Assist with comfort measures for lactation or suppression; meet information needs. G: Woman's goal of lactation or suppression is met with little if any discomfort.	Teach newborn nutrition and feeding. Tell woman to wear a good supporting bra or provide a binder. Place ice packs to breasts for engorgement as ordered. Give medications as prescribed: bromocriptine, Deladumone (use of this medication requires the woman's signed informed consent).	Lactation initiated successfully with minimal or no discomfort.
		To assist woman with lactation and breast-feeding the nurse will: Teach newborn nutrition and feeding. Teach hygiene: use warm water, no soap; wash breasts first with fresh washcloth. Tell woman to wear good supporting bra (nursing bra, if possible). Teach use of breast pump and manual expression. Teach positioning for breast-feeding. Give information on breast-feeding support groups (i.e., La Leche League).	Woman is satisfied with breast-feeding experience.
Nipples Protruding Inverted Sore or tender Cracked or bleeding	ND: Impaired skin integrity related to learning to breast-feed and take care of nipples. P: Teach feeding techniques and care of nipples. G: Woman learns feeding techniques and care of nipples.	*To teach care of nipples the nurse will:* Assist woman with breast-feeding. Employ preventative and comfort measures: Masse' cream, rotation of newborn's position at breast, correct latching-on, correct removal of baby from breast by breaking suction with finger first.	Woman learns feeding techniques and care of nipples. Nipples are not injured or uncomfortable.
Hemoglobin and hematocrit May be decreased at this time	ND: Altered cardiopulmonary tissue perfusion related to anemia. P: Detect and correct anemia to prevent complications. G: Anemia is detected if present and corrective measures are initiated.	*To monitor hemoglobin and hematocrit:* Order laboratory work as ordered. Retrieve information and place on chart. Alert physician to low levels and implement orders, as necessary.	Values are within normal limits. Woman learns self-care through nutrition. Woman prevents anemia in self and family.

General Nursing Care Plan—cont'd

ASSESSMENT	NURSING DIAGNOSIS (ND)/ PLAN (P)/GOAL (G)	RATIONALE/ IMPLEMENTATION	EVALUATION
	ND: Knowledge deficit related to anemia. P: Increase woman's knowledge about anemia, its cause, treatment, and prevention. G: Woman's anemia is resolved; future occurrence is prevented.	*To meet woman's knowledge needs, the nurse will discuss:* Rationale for tests. Range of normal values and where woman's values fit within that range. Relationship to nutrition.	
Coagulation factors Thrombus formation Intravascular coagulation: local or disseminated (DIC)	ND: Pain from thrombus formation related to alterations in coagulation process. ND: Potential for injury related to development of DIC. P: Monitor to detect and correct problem to prevent further complications. G: Woman develops no problem related to coagulation.	*To protect woman from thrombus formation or other coagulopathies the nurse will:* Monitor for and teach woman symptomatology of thrombus formation (Homans' sign). Monitor for and teach woman problems with ambulation and exercise, redness or swelling of calf or leg. Monitor for symptoms of DIC. Teach woman rationale for assessment, measures to take should symptomatology of thrombus occur.	No coagulation problems occur. Woman recognizes and seeks therapy for symptomatology of thrombus formation.

Procedure 26-1

NURSING ACTIONS FOR UTERINE ATONY (BOGGY UTERUS)

DEFINITION

Loss of uterine muscle tone causing the blood vessels at the site of previous placental attachment to bleed profusely. Also known as "boggy uterus."

PURPOSE

To prevent hemorrhage by maintaining muscle tone.

EQUIPMENT

None required.

NURSING ACTIONS	RATIONALE
Wash hands before and after touching woman or linens and equipment.	To prevent nosocomial infection and to implement universal precautions.
Assess uterine fundus for tone (firmness). Assess lochial bleeding.	No further action must be taken if firm, and lochial discharge is appropriate.
If uterus is not contracted, massage gently.	To stimulate muscle contraction without causing muscle fatigue.
Teach woman to locate and expel clots; reassess in 15 minutes.	To encourage self-care. To empty uterus so that "living ligature" can function. To verify cessation of bleeding.

Continued.

Procedure 26-1—cont'd

NURSING ACTIONS	RATIONALE
Prevent bladder distension:	Distended bladder can cause uterine relaxation:
Encourage spontaneous voiding; give rationale.	Spontaneous voiding helps woman maintain sense of control over her body. Knowing why bladder needs to be emptied completely adds to woman's knowledge base and encourages self-care.
Catheterize as needed; give rationale for need to catheterize vs. inability to void and need for bladder emptying.	Knowing rationale may decrease woman's sense of powerlessness over her body functions.
Put baby to suckle at breast.	To stimulate release of oxytocin from posterior pituitary gland.
If uterus is not maintaining tone, stay with woman and call for assistance.	Continuous manual compression until intravenous infusion is started with pitocin decreases blood loss and is reassuring to woman.
Maintain a calm manner, provide explanations.	
Implement physician's orders to maintain uterine tone.	Uterus may need temporary stimulation from exogenous source of oxytocin to maintain tone.

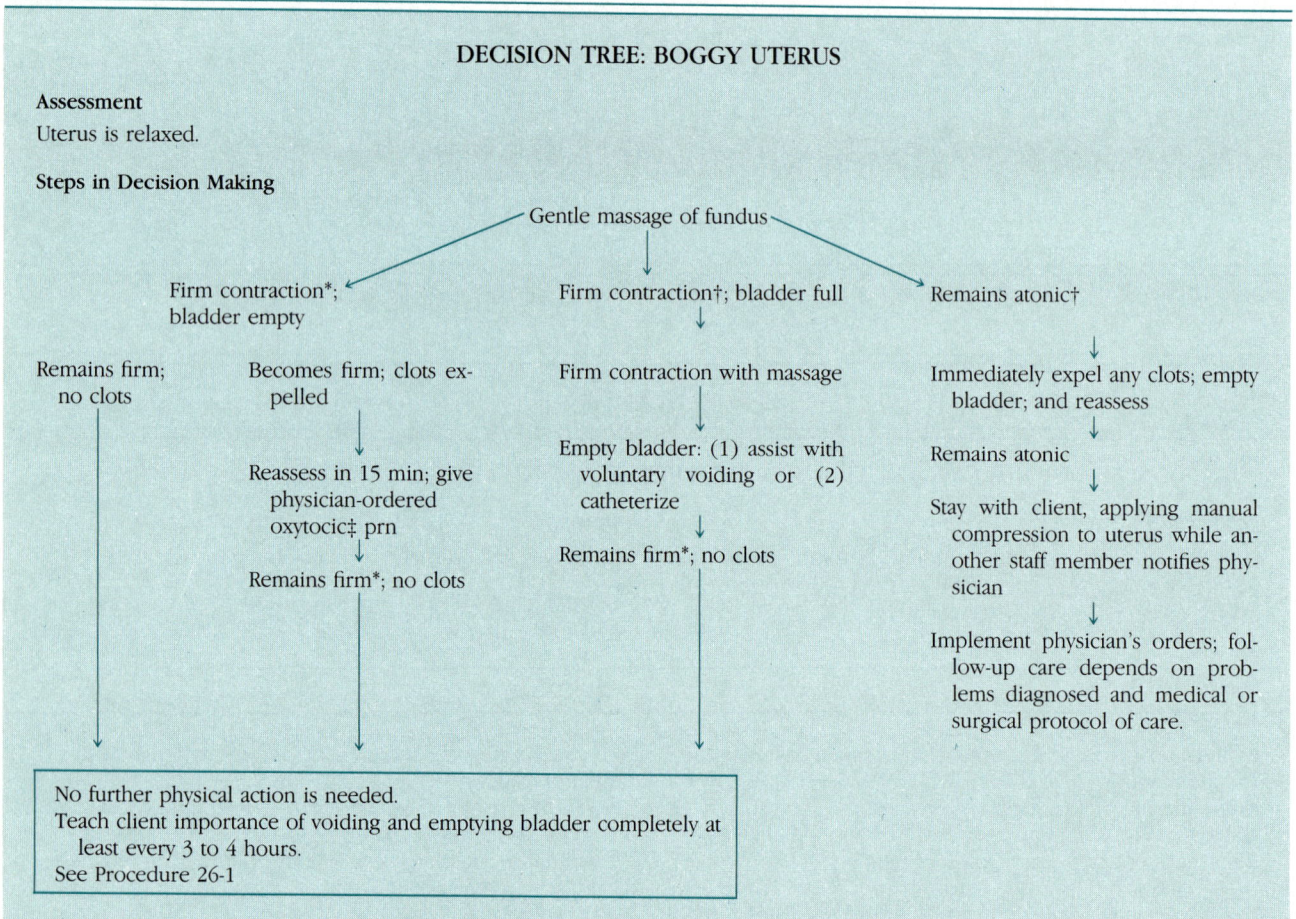

DECISION TREE: BOGGY UTERUS

Assessment

Uterus is relaxed.

Steps in Decision Making

Gentle massage of fundus →

1. Firm contraction*; bladder empty
   - Remains firm; no clots → (see box below)
   - Becomes firm; clots expelled → Reassess in 15 min; give physician-ordered oxytocic‡ prn → Remains firm*; no clots → (see box below)
2. Firm contraction†; bladder full → Firm contraction with massage → Empty bladder: (1) assist with voluntary voiding or (2) catheterize → Remains firm*; no clots → (see box below)
3. Remains atonic† → Immediately expel any clots; empty bladder; and reassess → Remains atonic → Stay with client, applying manual compression to uterus while another staff member notifies physician → Implement physician's orders; follow-up care depends on problems diagnosed and medical or surgical protocol of care.

> No further physical action is needed.
> Teach client importance of voiding and emptying bladder completely at least every 3 to 4 hours.
> See Procedure 26-1

*Fundus is in midline, at level appropriate for time since delivery.

†Fundus is above umbilicus or at level higher than appropriate for time since delivery; uterus may or may not be displaced to right (usually by full bladder or full rectum).

‡See Table 26-3.

Procedure 26-2

CARE AFTER REPAIR OF EPISIOTOMY OR LACERATION

DEFINITION

Treatment of the surgical incision of the perineum, done electively to facilitate delivery of the baby and prevent perineal lacerations (a torn, jagged wound).

PURPOSE

To promote healing, increase comfort, teach mother self-care techniques, and identify and treat complications.

EQUIPMENT

Ice pack with cover; squeeze bottle; sitz bath and thermometer (Fig. 26-3), or surgi-gator (if available) (Fig. 26-4); towels, as necessary; anesthetic cream or spray; witch hazel pads (Tucks).

NURSING ACTIONS	RATIONALE
Wash hands before and after touching woman and equipment. Glove, prn.	To prevent nosocomial infection and to implement universal precautions.
Gather equipment.	To improve efficiency.
Explain procedure to woman.	To decrease anxiety and elicit cooperation.
ICE PACK	
Apply a covered ice pack to perineum.	To decrease chance of "burn" from cold pack.
1. During first 2 hours after delivery.	To decrease edema formation at this time and increase comfort later. To provide anesthetic effect.
2. After the first 2 hours after delivery.	To provide anesthetic effect.
SITZ BATH	
Built-in type (Fig. 26-3):	
Prepare bath by thoroughly scrubbing with cleaning agent and rinsing.	To decrease possibility of infection from another woman; prevents irritation from cleaning agent.
Pad with towel before filling.	To promote comfort and keep woman from slipping (padding before filling keeps towel from floating).
Fill ½ to ⅓ full with water of correct temperature 38° to 40.6° C, or 45° C (100.4° to 105° F, or 113° F)	To provide temperature soothing to some women. The increased blood flow to area is thought by some to facilitate healing; others think that this causes swelling and adds to discomfort.*
Encourage woman to use twice a day or more often once she is ambulating, for 20 minutes.	To provide comfort and aid healing.
Place call bell within easy reach.	To ensure safety since the warm water and other factors (i.e., increased blood supply to perineum, lochial discharge, weakness) may cause woman to feel faint and need assistance.
Teach woman to enter bath by tightening gluteal muscles and keeping them tightened and then relaxing them after she is in the bath.	To decrease perineal discomfort while sitting down. To allow water to reach perineum.
Place dry towels within reach.	To increase comfort and ensure safety.
Ensure privacy.	To show respect for woman.
Check woman in 15 min; assess pulse as needed.	To ensure safety. Increased or irregular pulse may indicate cardiovascular stress; assist woman back to bed.
Apply anesthetic cream or spray.	To decrease perineal discomfort, use sparingly 3 to 4 times per day.
Use witch hazel pads (Tucks) after voiding or defecating; woman pats perineum dry from front to back, then applies witch hazel pads.	To decrease swelling and promote healing
Disposable type:	
Clamp tubing and fill water bag.	To prevent spillage.

*Other authors propose cool sitz bath (Droegemueller, 1980; Ramler and Robers, 1986).

Continued.

Procedure 26-2—cont'd

NURSING ACTIONS	RATIONALE
Raise toilet seat, place bath in bowl with overflow opening directed toward front of toilet.	To allow water to drain into toilet bowl.
Place container above toilet bowl.	To drain water bag by gravity.
Attach tube into groove at front of bath.	To situate tubing below level of water.
Loosen tube clamp to regulate rate of flow; fill bath to about ½ full; continue as above for built-in sitz bath.	See rationale for built-in sitz bath.
SQUEEZE BOTTLE	
Demonstrate for and assist woman; explain rationale.	To cleanse perineum after voiding. To encourage self-care.
Fill bottle with tap water warmed to approximately 38° C (100° F) (comfortably warm on the wrist).	To provide comfortable temperatures.
Instruct woman to position nozzle between her legs so that squirts of water reach perineum as she sits on toilet seat.	To cleanse and soothe perineum.
Explain that it will take several squirts of water over perineum.	To cleanse perineum well.
Remind her to blot dry with toilet paper or clean wipes (provided by the agency).	To avoid tissue trauma and promote comfort.
Remind her to avoid contamination from anal area.	To prevent infection.
SURGI-GATOR	
Assemble Surgi-Gator (Fig. 26-4).	To cleanse and provide comfort to perineum.
Instruct woman regarding use and rationale.	To encourage self-care.
Explain that each woman is issued her own applicator.	To prevent infection.
Follow package directions.	To promote maximum benefit of appliance.
Instruct her to sit on toilet with legs apart and to put nozzle so tip is just past the perineum, adjusting placement as needed.	To provide the jets of water to the perineal area.
Remind her to return her applicator to her bedside stand.	To prevent loss or cross infection.
DRY HEAT	
Inspect lamp for defects.	To prevent fires or burns.
Cover lamp with towels.	To prevent burns if lamp touches skin.
Position lamp 50 cm (20 in) from perineum; use three times a day for 20 min periods.	To provide comfortable warmth. To promote comfort. For some women, keeps area dry and thereby promotes healing.
Teach regarding use of 40-watt bulb at home.	To provide effective "heat" lamp in the home.
Provide privacy by careful draping over woman since knees must be kept up and separated for benefit.	To promote privacy. To demonstrate respect and caring.
If same lamp is being used by several woman, clean it carefully between uses.	To prevent cross infection.
TOPICAL APPLICATIONS	
Teach regarding use of sprays, ointments, or witch hazel pads (Tucks) that are applied directly to sutured area.	To add to woman's knowledge base and encourage self-care.
CLEANSING SHOWER	
Wash perineum with mild soap and warm water at least once daily.	To minimize fear of "breaking the stiches" or pain which deters women from washing perineum.
Cleanse from symphysis pubis to anal area.	To prevent contamination of the vagina and urethra with fecal material.
Apply peripad from front to back, protecting inner surface of pad from contamination.	To prevent infection from contamination.
Wrap soiled pad and place in covered waste container.	
Change pad every time she voids or defecates or at least 4 times per day.	To prevent infection.
Wash hands before and after changing pads.	To prevent infection.
Assess amount and character of lochia with each pad change.	To identify possible complications early.

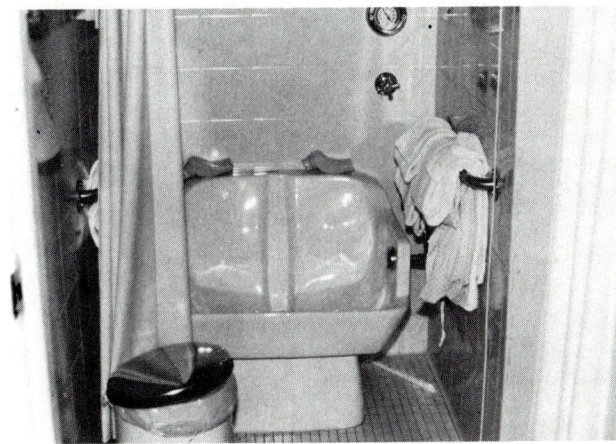

Fig. 26-3 Sitz bath.
Courtesy Marjorie Pyle, RNC, Lifecircle, Costa Mesa, Calif.

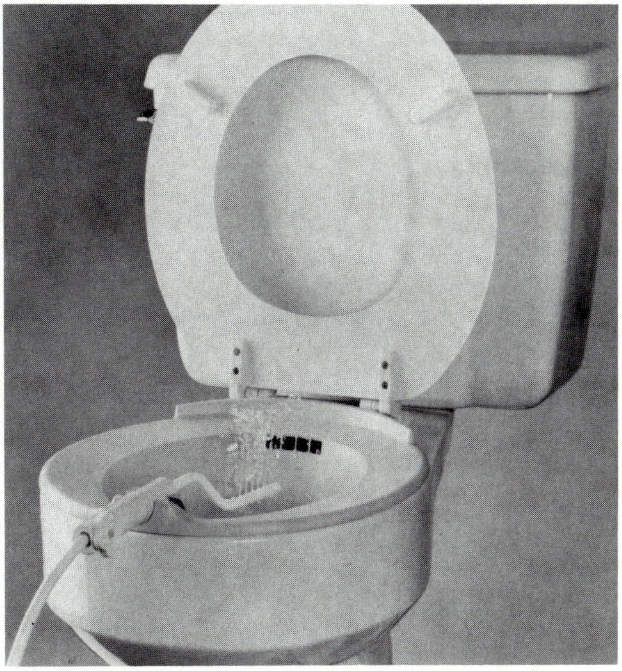

Fig. 26-4 Hygienic sitz bath (Surgi-Gator) for perineal care.
Courtesy Andermac, Inc, Yuba City, Calif.

DECISION TREE: FULL URINARY BLADDER

Assessment

Uterine fundus is well above umbilicus on the right; full bladder is palpated; I&O record indicates intake is considerably greater than output; client states no urge to void or has urge to void but cannot; last voiding, 4 hours ago.

Steps in Decision Making

Inform client that she needs to empty bladder

→ Able to void voluntarily; empties urinary bladder
→ No further physical action is needed.

→ Able to void voluntarily; does not empty bladder completely
→ If perineal discomfort is a factor, employ comfort measures and administer prescribed medications
→ Able to void voluntarily; empties bladder completely
→ No further physical action is needed.

→ Unable to void or does not empty bladder completely
→ If postanalgesia or postanesthesia effect is a factor, try spirits of peppermint; if unsuccessful, catheterize
→ Unable to void voluntarily or cannot empty bladder completely when distended again; insert closed system retention catheter or institute other action per physician's order

No further physical action is needed.
Teach client importance of voiding and emptying bladder completely at least every 3 to 4 hours.
See Procedure 26-3.

Procedure 26-3

NURSING ACTIONS FOR FULL URINARY BLADDER

DEFINITION

Emptying urinary bladder.

PURPOSE

To prevent bladder distension to decrease potential for bladder wall atony, infection, and uterine hemorrhage.

EQUIPMENT

Catheter tray, as needed.

NURSING ACTIONS	RATIONALE
Facilitate spontaneous voiding	
If woman is ambulatory, assist her to bathroom.	To verify woman's ability to walk without difficulty.
Assist her onto bedpan; provide privacy, pour warm water over the vulva, sound of running water, and provide call bell.	To facilitate spontaneous voiding.
Provide ordered medications if discomfort of the perineum is hindering spontaneous voiding.	To minimize discomfort that increases difficulty of spontaneous voiding.
Some women can void spontaneously if they know it is permissible to void in the sitz bath (then follow the bath with a shower) or while squirting water over perineum (see Procedure 26-2).	To relax woman, and dilute the urine, thus increasing woman's comfort.
Teach techniques to facilitate spontaneous voiding (e.g., void immediately when the urge is present; straddle the toilet seat facing the tank or sit on toilet in regular fashion and lean forward; push all the urine out even if it "makes noise").	To assist natural response to physiologic event. To direct the flow of urine away from repair of episiotomy and lacerations. To give woman permission to "make noise" (many learned to "pee quietly" as little girls to be more "ladylike"). Urinating with force is more likely to empty the bladder completely.
Expose the urinary meatus to fumes from peppermint spirits.	To help woman void spontaneously if at all possible to decrease possibility of infection from catheterization and to give her a sense of control over her body functions.
Verify that woman knows rationale for need to empty bladder.	To add to her knowledge base and encourage self-care.
Catheterize, if needed, per physician's order	To overcome the swelling, pain, and residual effects of analgesia/anesthesia that may prevent spontaneous voiding.
If spontaneous voiding has not occurred by 6 hours after delivery, catheterization is usually ordered.	To ensure emptying of the bladder.
Use aseptic technique.	To minimize infection.
If urinary meatus is difficult to visualize because of swelling, with a dry sterile swab, gently brush upward from the vagina to the clitoris.	To cause the meatus to gape so that catheter can be inserted with the least amount of trauma.
Observe for symptomatology of infection: pain or burning on voiding, fever.	
Provide catheter care.	To minimize infection.
Obtain urine specimen to send for culture, sensitivity, and routine urinalysis.	To identify infection or other complication early.
If urinary antibiotic is started, counsel woman to continue to take antibiotic for the full time it is prescribed (usually 1 week).	To prevent infection that may flare up again if antibiotic is stopped too early.
If a drug such as sulfisoxazole (Gantrisin) is ordered, caution woman to avoid drinking cranberry juice.	To ensure safety. Cranberry juice and sulfisoxazole (Gantrisin) combine to form a precipitate that causes considerable discomfort and requires therapy for about a week to clear out of the urinary tract.
After catheterization, assess for adequacy of spontaneous voiding (e.g., record times and amounts).	To ensure bladder functioning and adequacy of emptying.
Report retention with overflow.	
Teach woman symptomatology of urinary tract infection (see guidelines for client teaching, Chapter 8).	To provide identification and therapy to reduce morbidity. To prevent bladder infections that reduce the body's ability to fight other infections.

Procedure 26-4

SUPPRESSION OF LACTATION

DEFINITION

Process of inhibiting the synthesis and secretion of milk from the breasts.

PURPOSE

To discourage lactation by mechanical suppression or pharmacologic suppression, increase comfort, teach mother self-care techniques.

EQUIPMENT

Tight compression "uplift" breast binder or well-fitted supporting brassiere, covered ice packs.

MEDICATIONS

Analgesics, bromocriptine mesylate (Parlodel), other antilactogenics and consent forms.

NURSING ACTIONS	RATIONALE
Wash hands before and after touching woman and equipment. Glove, prn.	To prevent nosocomial infection and to implement universal precautions.
Assess woman and inquire as to whether she wants to breast- or bottle-feed.	Infant feeding is a personal choice.
Mechanical suppression	Treatment of choice.
Apply a tight compression "uplift" binder for about 72 hours; advise woman to use a snug brassiere after 72 hours (some hospitals do not use binders, women are told to wear a snug brassiere from the very beginning).	To give body message that milk production is not needed. Stimulus for lactation and discomfort usually ease after 72 hours.
Avoid any stimulus that could support lactation (e.g., breastfeeding the infant, expression of colostrum, pumping of the breast, using warm water on the breasts).	Nipple stimulation releases prolactin from posterior pituitary. Emptying breast is the primary stimulus for lactation.
Use covered ice packs or analgesics as necessary.	To promote comfort.
Do *not* restrict fluid intake or use diuretics.	These methods do not suppress lactation.
Remind mother that breast firmness, tenderness, and distension (engorgement) are temporary.	Symptoms usually decrease starting about the third day.
Administration of bromocriptine mesylate (Parlodel)	To suppress lactation by preventing the secretion of prolactin.
Confirm physician's explanation of drug to woman.	This nonhormonal, nonestrogenic agent does not act on mammary tissues.
Begin medication after vital signs and blood pressure have stabilized but no sooner than 4 hours after delivery	*One side effect is hypotension in some women.*
Remain with woman when she ambulates for the first time. Assess blood pressure every 4 hours for 72 hours.	Precautionary measure against injury from fainting. Identifies hypotension.
Instruct woman:	To encourage self-care.
Recommended therapeutic dosage is 1 2.5 mg tablet twice daily with meals.	To teach accepted method of taking medication.
Medication is continued for 14 days, or if necessary, for 21 days.	
A rebound of breast secretion, congestion, or engorgement is experienced by a percentage of women.	To prepare woman for possible breast tenderness and need to start mechanical suppression methods.
Breast symptoms are usually only mild to moderate in severity.	To relieve anxiety by knowing that this occurrence is normal.
Use mechanical suppression method to suppress symptomatology.	To encourage self-care. To add to woman's knowledge base.
Administration of other antilactogenics Follow hospital protocol for obtaining an informed consent. Administer medication per physician's directions. Observe woman for thrombus formation as per regular assessment schedule (Table 26-2).	The administration of estrogens or androgens is not used often today and is not recommended to suppress lactation. Research has implicated the use of estrogens or other hormones as lactation-suppressant drugs in the cause of endometrial cancer. The woman must give informed consent to the use of these drugs. Estrogens have also been implicated in the occurrence of thromboembolism after delivery, particularly after cesarean delivery or complicated vaginal delivery.

Evaluation

Evaluation is a continuous process. To be effective, evaluation is based on measurable criteria. The criteria reflect the parameters used to measure attainment of goals. The mother's recovery from childbirth is marked by definitive signs and symptoms. These signs and symptoms form the basis for continued evaluation of the involution process. The nurse's role as support person in providing emotional care to the new mother and family is as vital as the instrumental role and the roles of technician, teacher/advocate/counselor.

EMOTIONAL CARE: THE NURSE AS SUPPORT PERSON

Nurses have a leadership role in efforts to provide holistic client care in the postpartum period. Interventions intended to establish healthy early family relationships can be

Guidelines for Client Teaching

CARE OF HEMORRHOIDS

ASSESSMENT

1. Multipara 12-hours-postpartum. Large painful hemorrhoids protruding from anal opening.

NURSING DIAGNOSES

Pain, related to swollen hemorrhoids.
Knowledge deficit related to the care and treatment of hemorrhoids.
Bathing/hygiene self-care deficit related to hemorrhoid care.

GOALS

Short-term

To reduce hemmorhoidal swelling and promote comfort.

Intermediate

To reduce or eliminate pain and itching.

Long-term

To teach mother self-care techniques.

REFERENCES AND TEACHING AIDS

Charts and pamphlets explaining what hemorrhoids are.
List of instructions for woman to take with her explaining symptoms and treatments.

CONTENT/RATIONALE	TEACHING ACTIONS
To provide content about hemorrhoids: Hemorrhoids are anal varicosities that are precipitated by pregnancy and constipation. The pressure on the pelvic floor by the presenting part and the act of expulsion causes them to protrude and become inflamed.	Show woman picture of chart explaining this.
To provide information for self-care: I will show you what to use to reduce the swelling and decrease the discomfort. First, try a covered ice pack, Leave the pack in place for 20 minutes, repeat every 4 hours. This will reduce the swelling. Cover the ice pack to avoid possibility of a cold "burn."	Show woman the witch hazel pads (Tucks), an ice pack, ointments prescribed by her physician, sitz bath, and rubber glove or finger cots.
Next, apply the cold witch hazel pads, using each one once and discarding after you urinate or defecate. Always wipe from front to back. This stops contamination of episiotomy and open vaginal orifice.	Demonstrate this technique.
A sitz bath will provide an anesthetic effect.	Teach woman the procedure for this (Procedure 26-2).
If the hemorrhoids are still bothersome, put on a glove or a finger cot, lubricate it with water-soluble lubricant and push the hemorrhoid back inside the anus. This may have to be repeated after a bowel movement. Anal reflex will extrude the hemorrhoid again.	Teach woman how to replace the hemorrhoid after putting on a glove and applying lubricant. Once the hemorrhoid is reduced maintain digital pressure for 1 to 2 minutes.
Unless the condition was present before pregnancy, it will correct itself once the increased blood supply and pressure symptoms of pregnancy are diminished and regular bowel habits are reestablished.	Reassure woman and encourage self-care.

EVALUATION Woman establishes self-care and discomfort is diminished.

the unique contribution of nursing. Healthy family relationships promote the growth potential of the newborn and other family members. Caregivers need to be alert to parents who have positive family circumstances, as well as to those who exhibit warning signs during the postdelivery period (Table 26-4). The care described in this part of the chapter is based on careful assessment and formulation of nursing diagnoses. It includes planning for and implementing appropriate nursing actions and evaluating their effectiveness.

Assessment

Woman's Reaction to Birth Experience. Women indicate a need to review the birth experience (Rubin, 1961; Mercer, 1981; Konrad, 1987). The mother's critical self-evaluation of her intrapartum behavior is indicative of one of the important psychologic tasks of the postpartum period. The nurse needs to identify the mother's perception of the fit between her prenatal expectation for her behavior and the intrapartum reality.

Parental Responses. Parental responses to the birth of a child include behaviors that are either adaptive or maladaptive. Both mother and father exhibit these behaviors, although to date most research has centered on the mother. Parents who are faced with the crisis of a severe life stress may not be able to provide supportive parenting for their child. Life stress reduces both psychologic well-being and physical health. These are two important factors in establishing and maintaining relationships with others (Tansig, 1982; Thoits, 1983). Another critical factor is a feeling of

Table 26-3 *Summary of Measures to Stimulate Uterine Tone*

Nonpharmacologic Measures	Rationale
Massage	Causes reflex contraction of muscles. Overstimulation could lead to muscle fatigue and atony.
Remove clots, if present	Keeps uterus empty to allow muscle fibers to contract completely.
Keep bladder empty	Prevents bladder distension, which elevates and displaces uterus, resulting in uterine atony.
Stimulate breasts or nipples (manually or by suckling infant)	Causes release of oxytocin from posterior pituitary.

Pharmacologic Interventions	Action, Uses During Puerperium	Onset of Effect, Duration, Usual Dose	Contraindications, Precautions	Comments
Oxytocin injection, USP (10 U/ml) (Pitocin, Syntocinon, Uteracon), oxytocic, synthetic posterior pituitary hormone	Stimulates phasic uterine muscle contraction, promotes milk-ejection (let-down) reflex, facilitates flow of milk during engorgement.	IV injection, 10 U; onset in 1 min. IV infusion, 10-40 U/1000 ml 5% dextrose or physiologic electrolyte solution. IM injection, 3-10 U; onset in 3-7 min; duration 30-60 min.	Hypersensitivity; return of atony when effect wears off. May cause severe hypertension if client is also receiving ephedrine, methoxamine, or other vasopressors.	**Alert:** Assess for return of atony; store in cool place.
Ergonovine maleate, USP, NF (Ergotrate maleate); oxytocic, ergot alkaloid	Stimulates prolonged, nonphasic uterine contractions.	Oral: 0.2-0.4 mg every 6-12 hr for 48 hr; onset in 6-15 min. IM injection: 0.2 mg (1 ml) if nausea precludes oral preparation, onset "in a few minutes." Initial response: firm, titanic contraction. Subsequent response: alternating minor relaxations and contractions for 1½ hr; then vigorous rhythmic contractions for 3-4 hr after injection.	Severe hypertensive episodes may occur if given to hypertensive clients or those receiving vasoconstrictors; hypersensitivity; nausea, vomiting; sudden change in blood pressure or pulse.	**Alert:** Assess for changes in blood pressure, pulse; store in cool place.
Methylergonovine maleate, NF (Methergine); oxytocic, ergot alkaloid and congener of lysergic acid (LSD)	Stimulates rapid, sustained titanic uterine contractions; used in treatment of subinvolution; has only minimum vasoconstrictive effect.	Oral: 0.2 mg tab, every 6-8 hr for maximum of 1 wk; onset in 5-10 min. IM injection 0.2 mg (1 ml) every 2-4 hr; onset in 2-5 min. IV infusion *(emergency only)*: 0.2 mg (1 ml) *slowly over 60 sec;* onset immediate.	Nausea, vomiting; transient hypertension; dizziness, headache; tinnitus; diaphoresis; palpitations; temporary chest pains.	**Alert:** Do not administer with Percodan—may result in hallucinations; assess blood pressure; store in cold place, away from light.

Table 26-4 *Family Behaviors*

Adaptive Behaviors	Maladaptive Behaviors
Marriage is stable. Father has stable job. Mother's intelligence and health are good. Parents have their own home and stable living conditions. Parents can have fun together and enjoy personal interests or hobbies. Parents had helpful role models when growing up. Parents have a good friend or relative to turn to, a sound "need-meeting" system. Parents exhibit coping abilities, i.e., capacity to plan and understand need for adjustments because of new baby. Baby was planned or wanted. Parents see likable attributes in baby, see baby as separate individual. Father is supportive to mother and involved in care of baby. Baby is healthy and not too disruptive to parents' life-style. Either parent can rescue the child or relieve the other in crisis. Future fertility management is planned.	Husband's or family's reactions to the baby have been negative or nonsupportive. Mother is receiving little or no meaningful support from anyone. There are sibling rivalry problems or a complete lack of understanding of this possibility. Husband is jealous of the baby's drain on mother's time, energy, and affection. Parents have expectations of development far beyond the child's capabilities. Parents remain disappointed over the sex of the child. Negative identification of the child: significance of name, who she or he looks like or acts like. Mother doesn't have fun with the baby. Mother avoids eye contact with the baby and avoids the direct *en face* position.* Verbalizations to the infant are negative, demanding, harsh, etc. Most of mother's verbalizations to others about the child are negative. Mother is bothered by crying; it makes her feel hopeless, helpless, or like crying herself. Mother does not comfort the baby when she or he cries. Feedings: the mother sees the baby as too demanding; she is repulsed by her or his messiness or ignores her or his demands. Changing diapers is seen as a negative, repulsive task. Mother lacks control over the situation. Mother is not involved, nor does she respond to the baby's needs, but relinquishes control to the doctors or nurses. When attention is focused on the child in her presence, mother does not see this as something positive for herself. Mother makes complaints about the baby that cannot be verified.

Reproduced by permission and adapted from Gray, JD, Christy, AC, Dean, GD, and Kempe, CH: Prediction and prevention of child abuse, Semin Perinatol 3:35, Jan 1979.

*Eye contact is an important facet of attachment in Western culture; however, it is not seen as important universally.

personal control. Personal control is a "key element in the attitudes toward self and the world that are characteristic of the competent self" (Turner and Avison, 1985). Those people who do not possess a sense of control seem less able to make the purposive decisions that are necessary to plan for the future of their families (Turner and Avison, 1985).

Many new mothers will experience *parenting difficulties* until their skills become established. Once they feel confidence in their skills, the increase in self-esteem promotes a positive affective response to the child. However, some parents will exhibit *parenting disorders* (a matter of degree) that place the child in jeopardy and at risk. Protocols for the physical screening of high-risk gravidas and fetuses have been developed and confirmed. However, tools predicting high-risk parenting behaviors require more replication over larger population samples before they can be used with the same precision (see box, p. 633).

The quality of motherliness or fatherliness in parent's behavior prompts nurturing and protection as opposed to neglect or abuse of the child. Cues indicating the presence or absence of this quality appear early in the postdelivery period as parents react to the newborn child and continue the process of establishing a relationship (Table 26-5).

Adaptive Behavior. Adaptive behaviors stem from the parent's realistic perception and acceptance of their newborn's needs and her or his limited abilities, immature social responses, and helplessness (Steele and Pollock, 1968). According to Morris (1966):

> Mother-infant unity can be said to be satisfactory when a mother can find pleasure in her infant and in the tasks for and with him; understand his emotional states and comfort him; read his cues for new experience, and sense his fatigue points.

Maladaptive Behavior. Maladaptive behavior is exhibited when parents respond inappropriately to the needs of their infant. They expect responses from the infant far in excess of the infant's ability to perform. They interpret inadequate responses as defiance or as negative judgment of parental capabilities. They obtain no pleasure from physical contact with their child. Such infants tend to be handled roughly. They are held in a manner that allows the head to dangle without support, and are not cuddled. The parents see the child as unattractive. The child caring tasks of bath-

PARENT-BABY INTERACTION

Type of delivery: Vaginal ☐ Cesarean ☐ Time after birth ______ hours Para ☐ ☐ ☐ ☐ Gravida ☐ ☐ ☐ ☐

Marital status ______ Age of mother ______

Father present for delivery of ☐Yes ☐No

Circle "M" and "F" for the best description in each of the five behavioral categories, to achieve a total score for Mother and Father: 8-10 requires *usual* nursing support for bonding; 5-7 requires *extra* nursing support for bonding; 0-4 requires *intensive* nursing support for bonding.

First Contact

Two (2) Points		One (1) Point		Zero (0) Points	
Asks for information about baby, e.g. condition, sex, appearance	M F	Listens to information given about baby without comment	M F	Expresses concern for self only	M F
Reaches out to baby, touching baby if possible	M F	Looks toward baby without reaching out or touching	M F	Does not look toward or touch baby	M F
Spontaneously speaks to baby in affectionate terms or tone	M F	Speaks to baby when prompted to do so	M F	Does not speak to baby (state reason why, if known)	M F
Holds baby in "en face" position and makes eye contact when possible	M F	Holds baby without maintaining *en face* or eye contact	M F	Does not hold baby (state reason why, if known)	M F
Expresses generally positive feelings about the labor and delivery experience	M F	Expresses dissatisfaction or anger at outcome of labor	M F	Even with assistance, expresses no feelings about outcome of labor	M F

Mother's total score ____ Father's total score ____

Other Observations ______

Day 2

Seeks contact with baby	M F	Accepts contact with baby	M F	Avoids contact with baby	M F
With assistance, explores baby's whole skin surface	M F	Explores baby's body, avoiding some areas, e.g., genital area, back	M F	Avoids touching baby's skin	M F
Asks for interpretation of baby's appearance and behavior	M F	Interested when baby's appearance or behavior is interpreted but does not ask questions	M F	Shows little interest in baby's appearance or behavior	M F
Consistently positions baby in *en face* position and seeks eye contact with baby	M F	Positions baby in *en face* position and makes intermittent eye contact	M F	Does not hold baby in *en face* position	M F
Describe feelings about infant and her or his responses	M F	Needs assistance in describing feelings about infant and her or his responses	M F	Does not express feelings about infant or her or his responses	M F

Mother's total score ____ Father's total score ____

Other Observations ______

Day 3

Holds baby close to body when feeding or cuddling, using both hands and arms	M F	Holds baby with a space between own and baby's body	M F	Unable, reluctant, or refusing to hold baby	M F
Spontaneously talks to baby, using name, "son," or endearing terms or tones	M F	Speaks about baby but does not speak directly to baby	M F	Does not speak to baby	M F
Consistently positions baby in *en face* position and maintains eye contact	M F	Positions baby in *en face* position and makes intermittent eye contact	M F	Does not make eye contact with baby	M F
Describes some infant's characteristics to listener (e.g., "He's strong")	M F	Responds with interest when infant's characteristics are pointed out	M F	Does not express any interest in infant characteristics	M F
Seeks opportunities to carry out care giving of baby	M F	Needs prompting with all care-giving of baby	M F	Unable, reluctant, or refusing to care for infant	M F

Mother's total score ____ Father's total score ____

Other observations ______

______
Signature

Table 26-5 *Mothering Behaviors*

Adaptive Behaviors	Maladaptive Behaviors
Feeding	
Offers appropriate amount and type of food to infant	Provides inadequate type or amount of food for infant
Holds infant in comfortable position during feeding	Does not hold infant, or holds in uncomfortable position during feeding
Burps baby during and after feeding	Does not burp infant
Prepares food appropriately	Prepares food inappropriately
Offers food at comfortable pace for infant	Offers food at pace too rapid or slow for infant's comfort
Infant Stimulation	
Provides appropriate verbal stimulation for infant during visit	Provides no, or only aggressive, verbal stimulation for infant during visit
Provides tactile stimulation for infant at times other than during feeding or moving infant away from danger	Does not provide tactile stimulation or only that of aggressive handling of infant
Provides age-appropriate toys	No evidence of age-appropriate toys
Interacts with infant in a way that provides for infant's satisfaction	Frustrates infant during interactions
Infant Rest	
Provides quiet or relaxed environment for infant's rest, including scheduled rest periods	Does not provide quiet environment or consistent schedule for rest periods
Ensures that infant's needs for food, warmth, and dryness are met before sleep	Does not attend to infant's needs for food, warmth, and dryness before sleep
Perception	
Demonstrates realistic perception of infant's condition in accordance with medical and nursing diagnoses	Shows unrealistic perception of infant's condition
Has realistic expectations for infant	Demonstrates unrealistic expectations of infant
Recognizes infant's unfolding skills or behavior	Has no awareness of infant's development
Shows realistic perception of own mothering behavior	Shows unrealistic perception of own mothering
Initiative	
Shows initiative in attempts to manage infant's problems, including actively seeking information about infants	Shows no initiative in attempts to meet infant's needs or to manage problems; does not follow through with plans
Recreation	
Provides positive outlets for own recreation or relaxation	Does not provide positive outlets for own recreation or relaxation
Interaction with Other Children	
Demonstrates positive interaction with other children in home	Demonstrates hostile-aggressive interaction with other children in home
Mothering Role	
Expresses satisfaction with mothering	Expresses dissatisfaction with mothering

Reprinted by permission from Mercer, RT: In Sonstegard, LJ et al, editors: Women's health: childbearing vol 2, New York, 1982, Grune & Stratton, Inc.

ing and changing are viewed with disgust or annoyance. There is a lack of discrimination in responding to the infant's signals relative to hunger, fatigue, need for soothing or stimulating speech, and need for comforting body or eye contact. The parents of these infants often show excessive concern over the health of their child and cannot distinguish between the expected minor illnesses of childhood and serious disabilities. It appears difficult for them to accept their child as healthy and happy.

Interpretation of Infant Behaviors. The parents' response is profoundly affected by their interpretation of the infant's behaviors. Feedback is an important component in any relationship. Mothers and fathers make value judgments about their infant's behavior and respond as though the baby had either "praised" or "criticized" them. Table 26-6 provides a listing of infant behaviors and their evaluation by parents as either adaptive (positive feedback) or maladaptive (negative feedback) (Mercer, 1982).

Parent-baby Interactions. To assess parent and child relationships and competency in child care, the nurse observes parental attitudes toward themselves and their responsibilities. She or he assesses the mother's perceptual acuity and the amount of physical and psychic energy the mother possesses. Cultural or ethnic variations in maternal and paternal roles are also noted. This information provides the context within which the parents will give care to their child. Competency in child care can be determined during feeding periods or when the mother or father is giving general care to the infant (Fig. 26-5).

Stainton (1981) has devised scoring tools for assessing parent-child interaction for use in the postdelivery period (see box, p. 633). The tools reflect the change in the mother's and father's responses as they move from first contact after delivery through the early puerperium. The tools are concise enough for easy application. They can help the nurse assess behaviors that may indicate adaptation or maladaptation to the parental role.

Nursing Diagnoses

After analyzing the data obtained from assessment, the nurse establishes nursing diagnoses that will act as guides to action. The following are examples of diagnoses made for specific clients:

- Altered family processes related to
  - Unexpected birth of twins
- Impaired verbal communication related to
  - Client's deafness
- Altered parenting related to
  - Long, difficult labor
- Knowledge/skill deficit related to
  - Usual infant behaviors
  - Holding, cuddling, interacting with infant
- Anxiety related to
  - Newness of parenting role, sibling rivalry, or grandparental response
- Potential for situational low self-esteem, related to
  - Lack of knowledge of infant characteristics or of caregiving skills
  - Grandparental responses

Planning

The postnatal period is a crucial one for the family. It contains the potential for crisis in family adjustment. Developing a plan of care that recognizes family strengths and provides support for family weaknesses does much to help family members take on new tasks and responsibilities.

Goals. The goals for care include the following:

1. Promotion of self-concept: self-esteem for all family members
2. Promotion of healthy, parent-child relationships
3. Increase in parents' participation in successful care of their newborn, themselves, and other family members

Implementation

Adaptation to the parental role is a complex process. The nurse's application of knowledge in the care of new parents can help them with this role transition. One of the

Table 26-6 ***Infant Behaviors***

Adaptive Behaviors	Maladaptive Behaviors
Sleeping	
Receives adequate sleep for normal growth—at least 17 hours each day without restless sleep patterns or prolonged crying at nap or bedtime after other needs have been met	Receives inadequate sleep for normal growth—less than 16 hours each day; shows restless sleep patterns or prolonged crying at nap or bedtime
Feeding	
Actively seeks food offered	Resists food offered
Actively sucks and swallows food	Does not suck effectively
Demonstrates pleasurable relief after eating	Remains fussy after adequate amount of feeding—no pleasurable relief
Response to Environment	
Demonstrates active response to environment by ignoring or reaching-out behavior	Seems apathetic to environment
Vocalizing	
Demonstrates vocalizations when alert if developmentally ready	Makes infrequent or no vocalizations during visit although developmentally ready
Smiling	
Demonstrates smiling behavior if older than 2 months	Does not demonstrate smiling behavior during visit
Cuddling	
Cuddles when held	Resists being held or stiffens when held

Reprinted by permission from Mercer, RT: In Sonstegard, LJ, et al, editors: Women's health: childbearing, vol 2, New York, 1982 Grune & Stratton, Inc.

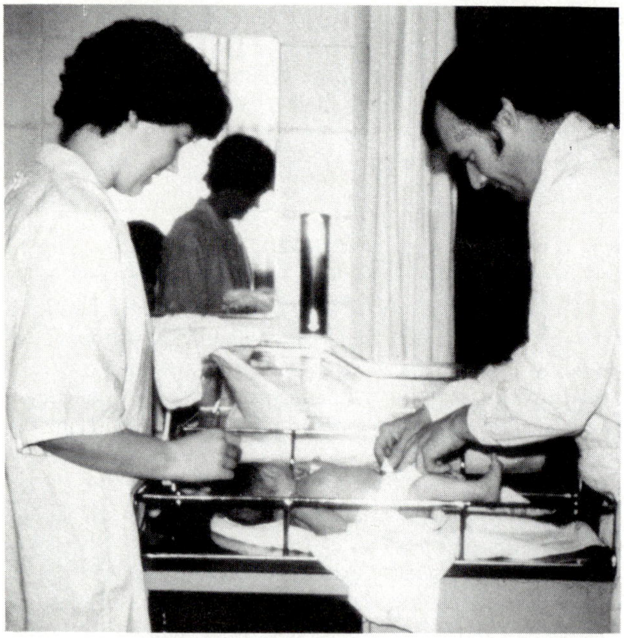

Fig. 26-5 Father bathes his infant with support of nursing student. Courtesy Colleen Stainton.

new mother's first psychologic tasks is to integrate the birth experience.

Integration of the Birth Experience. The nurse who interviews a new mother about her birth experience in a thoughtful, sensitive manner has already intervened therapeutically. Inviting the new mother to review the events and describe how she felt helps her understand what happened and begin the integration process. The new mother usually initiates this portion of the interview with such statements as, "I'm sorry I. . ."; "You should have seen how I screamed. . ." "I just can't remember some things." Feelings of anger and resentment and vocalizing are understandable, temporary responses to an acute, stressful situation. The normalcy of these reactions can be validated by the nurse. However, statements such as "everyone does it" puts all women in the same category and may be perceived as a lack of regard for the individual (Konrad, 1987). Restating or rephrasing are useful communication techniques (Chapter 2). These techniques help the woman fill in the whole picture for herself, reflect on her meaning behind her words, and identify connections between this experience and previous ones. The need for input regarding the birth experience is consistent with Rubin's (1961) "taking-in" phase seen in the early postpartum period. Assisting the new mother with this postpartum psychologic task is a valuable function of the nurse.

Crisis Prevention: Components. Nursing is directed toward increasing the mother's mastery of the "art of motherhood," thereby increasing or sustaining her self-esteem. Nursing care encompasses measures that encourage assertive, self-reliant behaviors in family members. Research by Sullivan and Beeman (1981) indicates that parents express satisfaction with postpartum nursing care if efforts are made to facilitate parent-child relationships by providing instruction in the care of self and infant.

Nursing interventions may be grouped under those pertaining to the crisis intervention theory: perception, situational supports, and coping mechanisms (see Chapter 2).

Perception. One of the main concepts to be stressed repeatedly is that parenthood is a learned role. As with any other learned role, it takes time to master, improves with experience, and evolves gradually and continually as the needs of the parents and child change. Rubin (1961) proposed that for 2 or 3 days after the birth of a child, a mother is receptive to learning about her new role. Rubin termed this the *taking hold phase.*

Caplan (1957) noted that intervention during the early peurperium had a much greater influence on the attitudes of family members than it did at periods of stability of emotional functioning. Care during the early puerperium needs to reflect the mother's and father's psychological readiness for learning new skills. Table 26-7 outlines strategies the nurse can use to help the father adjust to his new role.

Mothers have been found to be receptive to information regarding their infants' interactive capabilities during the early puerperium. During this time mothers' awareness of their own behavioral responses toward their infants can be enhanced. The mother's anxiety level distorts her ability to learn.

Care of the newborn may be limited to feeding during the first few days. When the mother's strength returns, she also may wish to bathe and change the infant. Demonstrations of these techniques and supervision of her efforts are incorporated into the nursing care. Through the loving and attentive manner nurses exhibit while providing physical care to the newborn and to the mother, they act as role models. As one nurse described it:

> I found the mother crying and distraught as she wrapped and unwrapped her baby. She said, "I don't seem to be able to do anything right." I took the baby from her and talked to him. "What are you doing to your mother? You've got her all upset!" The baby alerted to my voice and looked at me. Then I said to the mother, "Now, you talk to him." She said, "You're a big lovely boy, don't cry so much." The baby hearing her voice promptly turned his head from me to look at her. I said, "You see, he knows his mother's voice and prefers it to mine." The mother was surprised and seemed very pleased and excited. We then reviewed how to wrap a baby snugly.

Recognition and praise of her successes increase the mother's feeling of competence and control in her ability to mother. Feelings of self-esteem in the mother are increased through positive feedback. Fig. 26-6 shows a feedback circle in which the left side presents an example of a positive mother-infant interaction based on the sequence outlined on the right side.

Researchers in their studies of mother-infant interac-

Table 26-7 ***Strategies to Support and Promote the Role of the Father, by Stages of Pregnancy***

Antepartum	Intrapartum	Postpartum
Include father in initial antepartum visit and encourage his participation in all subsequent visits. Encourage father's involvement in birthing and parenting classes. Include educational materials that portray "active" father and joint parental involvement in infant care. Raise questions directly related to concerns fathers are likely to experience around childbirth and infant care. Host one session for fathers only. Invite "highly involved" fathers to come and discuss parenting issues. Encourage parents to negotiate parenting "roles" and infant care issues. Offer to serve as a facilitator of those discussions.	Encourage father's presence during labor and delivery. Support his planned role in labor, if appropriate. Allow time for father to hold and fondle newborn. Allow time for father and mother to be alone with newborn after delivery. Encourage father to "room in" with mother during hospitalization, if appropriate. Support father's active involvement with infant during hospitalization (feeding, holding, changing the infant, etc.).	Encourage father to come to follow-up pediatric visits. Conduct postpartum classes for both parents to discuss infant care and related issues. Raise specific questions about difficulties experienced in sharing infant care responsibilities. Offer to help parents renegotiate a plan for sharing infant care, if appropriate. Support formation of father, mother, or joint postpartum lay support groups. Offer to provide consultation to support group or to individuals, as needed.

From Kunst-Wilson, W, and Cronenwett, L: Res Nurs Health 4:201, 1981.

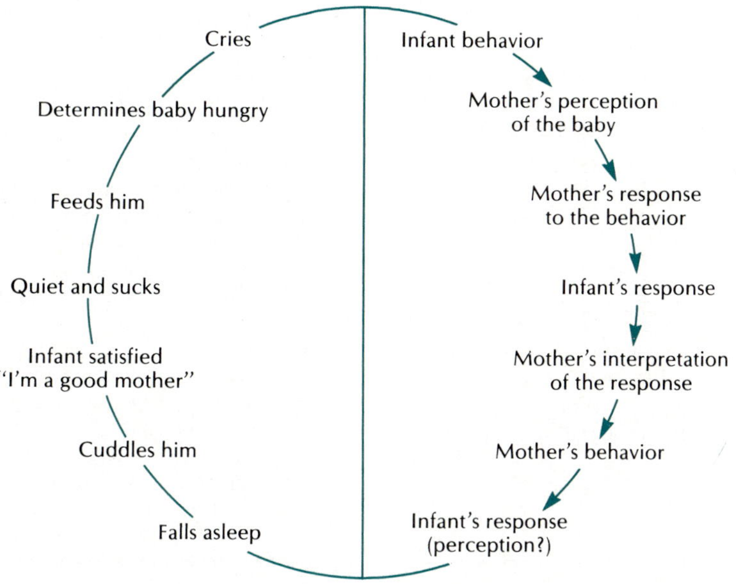

Fig. 26-6 Maternal-infant feedback mechanisms.
From Stainton, MC: Assessment and support of healthy parent-child relationships, Proceedings of POGP: Pediatrics, Obstetrics and Gynecology Workshop for Nurses, Saskatoon, 1977, University of Saskatchewan.

tions have used various techniques to promote the mother's awareness of the behavioral and social capabilities of their newborns. In one of Field's early studies (1977) mothers were asked to imitate their babies rather than attempt to keep their babies' attention. By doing this the mothers decreased their activities and increased responsiveness to infant behavior. By advising mothers to repeat phrases and to be silent during gaze aversion, Field noted mothers were increasingly sensitive to their infants' behavioral cues and responsive to their signals. Anderson (1981) combined providing information to the mother about neonatal behavior with a demonstration of the infant's behavior as a means of enhancing the quality of mother-infant interaction. Riesch and Munns (1985) provided an audiotape with accompanying text for the mothers to listen to privately. They reported the following:

> Mothers who received the intervention to inform them of the neonate's social capabilities and of the maternal behaviors to enhance and support their infants reported significantly more of their own behavior than did mothers who did not receive the treatment. Awareness of one's own behavior undoubtedly was a significant factor in the mother's reporting of her own behavior that her infant noticed. The new mother is concerned about how she will perform her new role; she needs to meet her own expectations and those of others in the performance of her maternal role (Rubin, 1961; Humenick and Bugen, 1987). The mother's expectations may or may not be realistic. Unrealistic expectations may serve as a detriment to a mother's accomplishments. Informing the mother of the responses she can initiate in order to enhance or support her particular infant may relive some of her role uncertainty, thus allowing her to interact freely with her infant (Riesch and Munns, 1985).

Because of the sheltered environment provided after delivery, women may misjudge the actual amount of physical and psychic energy they possess. They may expect to resume tasks too soon and then feel discouraged when they are not able to do so. Their still-pregnant look prompts well-meaning people to ask them when they expect their baby (Fig. 26-7). These remarks can add to the mother's feelings of discouragement. In addition, the baby's behavior does not always meet expectations. Sore nipples, worry about adequate milk supply, or even lack of sensations anticipated with breast-feeding can lead to a mother's disappointment. Some babies cry more than expected or do not seem satisfied with their feedings. Many babies have fussy periods that do not respond to any ministrations:

> But my husband, too, was disconcerted at first, for the intense, unending plaintive cries of our firstborn reached to the very depths of our hearts. And we both had really believed that, somehow, a baby born naturally at home and never separated from his mother would not be so fretful. However, it becomes apparent that all babies cry (Lang, 1972).

Depressive reactions after delivery, often called "the baby blues," are not dismissed lightly. Their prevalence has deprived many women of the support they need (see research highlight regarding postpartum anxiety and depression). Recognition of the state, helping the woman verbalize her feelings, and conveying warmth in touch and tone of voice are helpful actions. Setting up tasks the woman can accomplish easily and successfully are interventions that also can help counteract the feelings of depression.

Mothers also are faced with the need to help siblings adjust to the new sister or brother (see guidelines for client teaching, Chapter 14). **Sibling rivalry** may require parental time and attention to be handled successfully. Even if the children have participated in planning for the new baby, they may be unable to accept the reality of diminished parental attention. Their behavior may reflect their feelings of frustration (see specific nursing care plan).

Forewarning about the possibility of such happenings even in the best regulated homes permits the parents to judge themselves less harshly. They are better prepared to

RESEARCH HIGHLIGHT

Postpartum Anxiety and Depression in Mothers of Term and Preterm Infants

Purpose

There are conflicting reports of anxiety and depression between mothers of term and preterm infants. Therefore the purpose of this study was to compare the levels of anxiety and depression experienced by mothers of term and preterm infants in the immediate postpartum period and over the first 7 postpartum weeks.

Sample

Mothers of 41 preterm infants were matched with 41 mothers of term infants on parity, type of delivery, age, and race. Twelve mothers in both term and preterm groups had cesarean deliveries, and 29 mothers in each group had vaginal deliveries. Criteria for inclusion of preterm infants included: no congenital anomalies, less than 37 weeks gestational age, and weight between 1000 and 2000 g.

Methodology

The 20-item State Scale of the State-Trait Anxiety Inventory was used because it has been found to be a sensitive indicator of changes in transitory anxiety. The second tool used for the study was the Depression Adjective Check List. Data were collected for 7 consecutive weeks.

Findings

A statistically significant difference was found between mothers of term and preterm infants in anxiety and depression in the first postpartum week. There were no differences in maternal anxiety or depression when mothers were grouped according to their infant's risk categories. Neither parity, type of delivery, or the interaction of these two variables has an effect on postpartum anxiety over time. Similar results were found regarding postpartum depression.

Implications

Both groups of mothers experienced a similar response over time and were able to regain psychologic equilibrium within a short time. These findings suggest that even mothers with relatively healthy infants are initially likely to experience heightened anxiety and depression. However, since mothers of premature infants experienced higher anxiety and depression in the first postpartum week than mothers of term infants, they may well benefit from nursing interventions designed to validate the normalcy of their emotional response.

Gennaro, S: Postpartal anxiety and depression in mothers of term and preterm infants, Nurs Res 37(2):82, 1988.

Specific Nursing Care Plan

NURSING CARE DURING POSTPARTUM PERIOD

Laura and Jim had their second child, a girl, 4 days ago. The first child, Scott, is now 3 years old. Laura's HMO insurance promotes early discharge with a home health nurse that visits 24 hours after her return home. When the home health nurse arrives, Laura reports two problems to her:

1. She is having trouble with her first bowel movement. She had had an episiotomy and has hemorrhoids. She is concerned about being hurt and uncomfortable.

2. The 3-year-old son, Scott, is jealous of the new baby. He is whiny and fretful. He has begun to wet his pants again.

Jim's mother is staying with them to help out. She is annoyed with Scott. She says "He is very spoiled. If he were mine, I'd spank his bottom."

The nurse's assessment findings include intact and healing episiotomy and three moderate-sized hemorrhoids. The grandmother has taken Scott with her to the grocery store. The infant is asleep. Laura has been taking fluids well and has eaten well-balanced meals with plenty of fresh fruits and vegetables. She confided that she is "just afraid to be alone" while having the bowel movement.

ASSESSMENT	NURSING DIAGNOSIS (ND)/ PLAN(P)/GOAL(G)	RATIONALE/ IMPLEMENTATION	EVALUATION
Elimination Gave birth 4 days ago. Had a midline episiotomy that is now intact and healing. Has three moderate-sized hemorrhoids that hurt and itch. Last bowel movement was the day of delivery.	ND: Constipation, related to fear of injury and pain at episiotomy site. P: Facilitate return to usual elimination pattern without injury. G: Laura experiences a bowel movement without injury to episiotomy. ND: Pain, related to constipation, episiotomy, and hemorrhoids. P: Facilitate return to usual elimination pattern without discomfort. G: Laura experiences no aggravation of hemorrhoids or discomfort.	*To stimulate bowel elimination and minimize discomfort the nurse will:* Share assessment data. By doctor's order; prepare Laura for and administer a commercially available physiologic enema solution. Stay within shouting distance as enema is expelled. Note results. Reassess perineum and share findings with Laura.	Laura states she feels so much better having a nurse available at this time. Laura states the enema was not as uncomfortable as expected. Laura states she is glad there was a nurse to "explain things."
Laura states she knows little about care of hemorrhoids.	ND: Knowledge deficit related to care of hemorrhoids. P: Teach self-care for hemorrhoids. G: Laura reports confidence in self-care for hemorrhoids.	Review care of hemorrhoids with Laura (guidelines for client teaching: care of hemorrhoids).	Laura states she understands care of hemorrhoids.
Coping—stress tolerance Three-year-old sibling jealous of new baby and has regressed, is now wetting pants again.	ND: Anxiety (Scott) related to fear of losing his mother's attention. P: Minimize anxiety and fear. Reassurance that mother still loves him.	*To relieve Scott's stress Laura will:* Plan time with Scott alone. Plan playing "older level" games with child. Involve father with son.	Scott's anxiety lessens as shown by his returning to his pattern of remaining dry and being away from mother for longer periods.

Continued.

Specific Nursing Care Plan—cont'd

ASSESSMENT	NURSING DIAGNOSIS (ND)/ PLAN(P)/GOAL(G)	RATIONALE/ IMPLEMENTATION	EVALUATION
	G: Scott is less anxious regarding his status in family.		
Grandmother intolerant of Scott's response to new sister.	ND: Ineffective family coping; compromised, related to conflict in method of supporting and disciplining child. P: Facilitate family communication to problem solve situation. P: Provide information regarding discipline (e.g., eliminate use of physical violence as a method of discipline). G: Family will develop a plan that is mutually satisfying; spanking will not be used as a means of discipline.	*To relieve stress-provoking situation: the nurse will develop a plan that may include:* Assigning grandmother to care for newborn during time Scott is usually fretful. Assigning grandmother to take over care of older child (i.e., changing pants, etc.). Praising grandmother for help she is giving the family. Planning outing for father, grandmother, and Scott.	Grandmother becomes more understanding of Scott's acting out. Grandmother verbalizes pleasure with outing and this time to get better acquainted with the men and boys in her life.

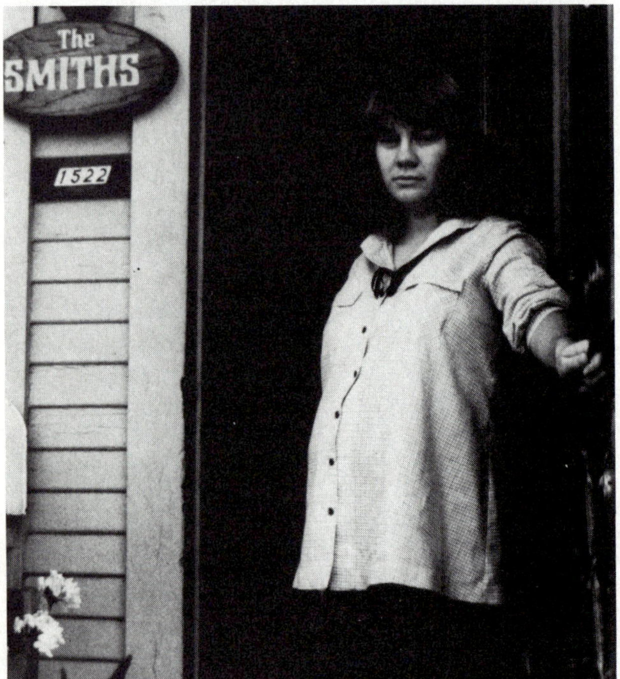

Fig. 26-7 Lack of abdominal muscle tone shortly after delivery gives mother still-pregnant appearance.
Courtesy Marjorie Pyle, RNC, Lifecircle, Costa Mesa, Calif.

seek assistance, change routine, or accept the happening as a passing phase.

Support Systems. The North American culture emphasizes the instinctual components of motherhood. As a result, many parents hesitate to seek help from nurses, physicians, family, and friends. Long-term support by nurses or physicians is a positive factor in the ultimate adjustment of the family. Besides providing emotional support, families and friends can assist with housework, and baby-sitting with older children, and eventually, the new baby. Being able to share experiences verbally with others who are interested and experienced also tends to reassure the new mother. A mother, in discussing visits by the family to see the new baby, commented as follows:

> I want the family to come. You people praise him so and think he is the most wonderful baby. All my friends have their own babies and are too busy trying to get compliments for them to give us any. All babies need aunties and grandmothers!

Being given information about the availability of health facilities and how to get in touch with the nurse or physician relieves new parents of feeling total responsibility for the health of the new baby. A physician reported one aspect of his plan for new mothers as follows:

I make sure they have my phone number and ask them to call me day or night if they are worried. Since I've done this, the frantic calls have decreased to almost nothing. Knowing they can call seems to take the "steam" out of their concern. I feel it has worked both ways, for their benefit and mine.

Home visits by nurses can be used to relieve stress and help parents anticipate and prepare for other possible stresses. Hospital stays are short; the parents leave the hospital in the "honeymoon" phase of transition. The realities of recovery and the parenting role become evident quickly, especially for those without assistance in the home. Parental expectations of each other, even if discussed thoroughly prenatally, usually do not go as expected by either partner (Humenick and Bugen, 1987). Parents need to be encouraged to communicate openly with each other regarding their stresses. Some anticipatory guidance before discharge and during the home visit may enable new parents to negotiate constructively any role dissonance they may experience and to have more realistic expectations of each other and the baby and baby care. Visits may be spaced to take into account potential stress times, such as 2 or 3 days after coming home from the hospital and the third and sixth weeks at home (Fig. 26-8).

The supportive care given at such times includes care for the entire family. Parents are as concerned with the ups and downs of other family members as they are with those of mother and child. The nurse may give supportive care by listening to (1) accounts of successes and failures, (2) individuals' feelings about the new baby, and (3) individuals' comments about what they expect of others (e.g., family members and friends) in their new roles. One prime requisite is set up a climate for the safe expression of doubts and anger, as well as happiness. The family will test the nurse's intent and knowledge, and the nurse must recognize and accept this.

Coping Mechanisms. Family commitments involve having both time and energy for individual family members—mother, father, and children. In addition to new parents learning the techniques for care of themselves and their babies, other suggestions have proved helpful to parents in coping with readjusting their lives. A list of these suggestions can be given to new parents, but discussion of specific ways of handling them is also necessary. Discussion with the parents should include the following suggestions:

1. Set priorities for tasks. Many tasks can be left for a later period or done by others. Be adamant about not taking on extra tasks for family, friends, or community. Try not to schedule a move to a new location soon after giving birth.

2. Do not become overly concerned with appearances—tidiness in the home is not as important as time spent with the family. Taking up the role of "super housekeeper" can be postponed until other adjustments are made.

Sometimes new mothers become overburdened with visits from relatives eager "to take over the baby." The husband can help his wife redirect these wellmeaning people toward helping with housework and cooking. This leaves the parent free to interact with the child.

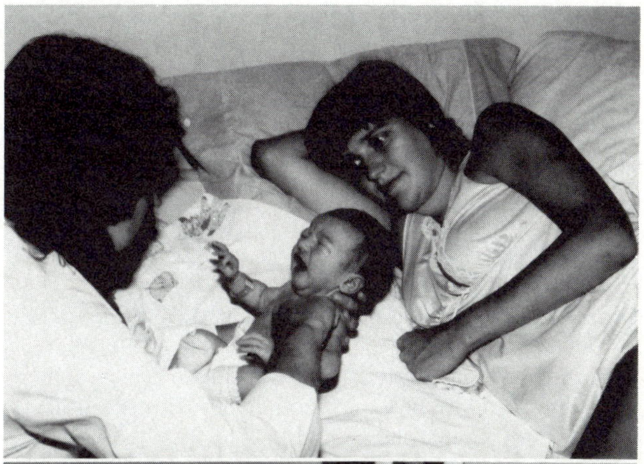

A

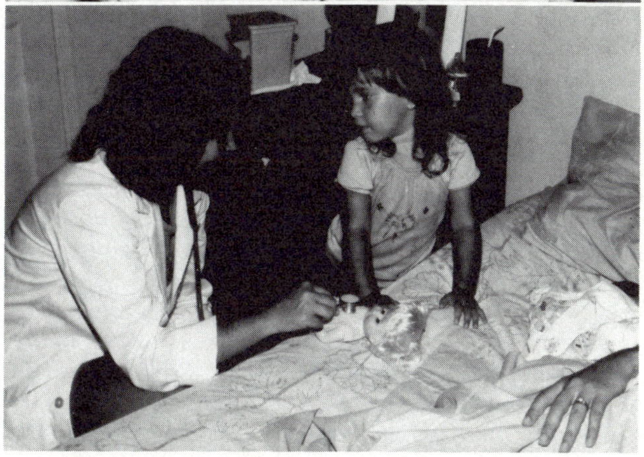

B

Fig. 26-8 **A**, Nurse-midwife assesses newborn with mother watching. **B**, Nurse-midwife reviews assessment of newborn for older sister using sister's doll.
Courtesy Marjorie Pyle, RNC, Lifecircle, Costa Mesa, Calif.

3. Get plenty of rest and sleep; rearrange schedules if necessary. Since naps may not be possible if there are other children in the family, going to bed early is recommended; let friends know when to visit.

4. Do not undertake the care of another incapacitated relative at this point; such responsibilities should be undertaken by other family members.

5. Arrange for some time away from the baby; enlist the help of friends, family, or others for baby-sitting. Relaxation for both husband and wife is necessary. Baby-sitting, if at all possible, must be planned and a regular schedule developed. This includes time off for the mother during the day so that she can get away from the home and its responsibilities. In some localities, churches or other agencies have developed programs attuned to the needs of mothers. The young children are cared for while the mothers take part in activities with other mothers. This helps them establish relationships with others who are also involved in the

care of young children. A mutual sharing of successes and failures in this regard helps the new mother maintain a feeling of equilibrium.

At the very least the mother needs to plan to get out of the house at least once each day. Access to a car and being able to drive are assets. Taking the baby out for a walk or shopping helps break up the daily routine.

6. Make plans regarding fertility management before intercourse is resumed and the possibility of pregnancy arises.

7. Be open in your communication with others. Share incidents of delight or of worry with others. Be open in your requests for support. Discussions with other mothers are helpful. The multiparous mother provides practical advice for the primiparous mother.

8. Learn what health facilities are available, for example, well-baby centers and immunization clinics, and how to get in touch with the physician or nurse. If you have questions, remember that the hospital is open all day and night and you can call the emergency department at any time.

9. Prepare for returning to work. Most women are physically able to return to work by the end of the sixth week. If plans for child care were not made before the birth, adjustments for child care must be made. Ideally a substitute parent would be one who could come to the home and provide love, as well as care, for the child. Some parents are fortunate enough to have grandparents or other relatives willing and able to fill such a role. Others must take the child to another person's home or a day-care center early in the morning and pick the child up at night. The care provided by day-care centers is needed by some children whose mothers must work to help support them or who are the sole support of the child. For families who require this type of service, assistance in locating such help can be obtained from the local health department. Unfortunately there are not enough quality places available for all children requiring day care.

10. Include the father in care-giving activities. Research shows that most fathers participate to the extent that the mother allows (Stainton, 1985). Table 26-7 outlines strategies that the nurse can use to help the father promote growth in his role as parent.

Crisis Prevention: Infant's Crying. Babies cry because they are hungry or wet, too hot or too cold, because they are ill, or simply because they want attention. And, if the baby is crying just to be held, who is to say that this is not a legitimate reason to cry? The way babies cry seems to contain the message they want to convey. Parents soon recognize the difference between cries. When parents want to respond to their baby's cry, they need to be encouraged not to be put off by friends or relatives who say they are spoiling the child. A tiny infant cannot be spoiled. Bell and Ainsworth (1972) found that "Mothers who ignore and delay in responding to the crying of an infant when he is tiny have babies who cry more frequently and persistently later on." A baby's cry requires an investigation to identify the specific need.

Nurses, and often knowledgeable grandparents, have a special role in helping parents and baby synchronize (Darbyshire, 1985). Reciprocal signaling and responding is an important part of parenting (Thoman, 1983; Lamb, 1981). Attachment is greatly enhanced for the mother (parent) who is able to detect and respond to the baby's distress signals and who can comfort and console the baby effectively (Darbyshire, 1985). Conversely, the effect on a mother (parent) faced with a crying, fussing, irritable, and unconsolable baby can be devastating for all concerned (Kirkland, 1985; Mortimer and Kevill, 1985).

Life with a crying baby is a crisis situation. Eventually, parents are "ground down," worrying that something is wrong, facing guilt and loss of self-esteem about their inability to comfort a crying baby. Physical and emotional fatigue compound the crisis.

Parents benefit from concrete suggestions. Knowing that "all parents go through this" is not helpful. If the crying signal is not yet set, several possibilities are explored and tested—hunger, cold, wet diaper. Pain is suspected if there are areas of redness or diaper rash. Loneliness, the need to make contact, may be the sole cause. First the cold, hunger, wet diaper, and pain are treated. Then other comforting techniques are used—**carrying and rocking, sounds, nonnutritive sucking, swaddling, and infant massage.**

People who care for newborns soon become aware that rocking a crying baby vertically and intermittently promotes a "bright-alert" state, whereas continuous horizontal rocking induces the baby to sleep (Byrne and Horowitz, 1981). Studies have also shown that the ideal rate to rock a baby is around 60 to 90 rocks a minute (Pederson, 1975; Ter Vrugt and Pederson, 1973).

The sound of a human voice or soft music can be an effective means to soothe a baby. The old practice of swaddling (wrapping snugly) has been found to pacify some infants. Nonnutritive sucking on a pacifier is another effective method. (See Chapter 22 about the use of safe pacifiers.) Infant massage has benefits for both parent and child (see Chapter 25).

Crisis Prevention: Siblings. Preparation of siblings and of parents for the reactions of siblings begins before childbirth. Preparation of siblings is discussed in guidelines for client teaching: sibling preparation, Chapter 11.

Crisis Prevention: Grandparents. Classes for grandparents-to-be are designed to help the givers and receivers of advice understand one another (Chapter 11) and update them to contemporary thinking. Examples of contemporary child-rearing theories that grandparents may be unfamiliar with are that one cannot spoil a newborn, breast-feeding is superior to formula-feeding, and bright colors are better than pastels for the baby's room since they are more stimulating. Safer infant car seats and disposable diapers are advances that most grandparents readily appreciate.

Few people move gracefully or fearlessly into new identities. Nurses support the grandparents who are the role models and support network for the new parents. Nurses also help new parents bridge the generation gap by keeping communication open. On occasion, the nurse suggests the scripts parents need to work toward to have the kind of loving relationship they would like to have. Many hospitals distribute pamphlets concerning the topic of helping the new parents "without interfering". Several publications on the topic are available at local bookstores.

Nursing Strategies to Meet Changing Family Needs. Nursing care during the postpartum period reflects the changing needs of parents, infants, and family. Parents become more knowledgeable of the infant, proficient in child care, and skillful in negotiating a place for the newborn in the family unit. Table 26-8 reviews nursing strategies specific to the early, consolidation, and growth periods (Chapter 25) of parent-infant-family relationships.

Table 26-8 *Nursing Strategies to Meet Changing Parental Needs*

Early Periods	Consolidation Period	Growth Period
Infant		
The contacts between parents and infant are as follows: 1. Timed to make use of infant's normal patterns of sleeping and waking; at birth, at about 4 to 6 hours, and every 2 to 5 hours thereafter. 2. Provided at important times for parental attachment to take place (preferably at birth or as soon thereafter as the infant's and mother's conditions permit). 3. Long and often enough to permit parents to hold, examine, care for, and enjoy their child. 4. The nurse reviews the normal characteristics of the newborn and gives the parent a report on the infant's initial physical examination. Later the nurse examines the infant in the parents' presence and reviews findings with them. Written instructions as to feeding, medications, and so on are provided. A daily report on the infant's progress and behaviors (e.g., eating, sleeping, voiding, defecating) is given.	The nurse and clients discuss the normal rhythms of the child and the parents' awareness of how the child communicates needs. The parents are advised to take time to study their infant and discover what different types of crying mean and when wakeful periods occur—morning, afternoon, or evening. The nurse identifies problems (e.g., infant crying, sleeping) and assists with solutions. Together, nurse and clients note successes and failures in caregiving activities, and the nurse helps the parents with accumulating successful coping mechanisms and discarding unsuccessful ones.	The infant is examined at the time of the postbirth examination of mother or at 4 weeks of age. The findings are reviewed with the mother and father. The nurse reviews and assesses parental knowledge of the following: 1. The signs and symptoms of illness and measures instituted to effect a cure or obtain medical assistance. 2. The infant's developmental needs: a. Accommodation to physical growth (e.g., introduction of solid foods into diet or weaning). b. Use of longer wakeful periods to increase stimulation of infant and social interaction with siblings and other family members. c. Adaptation to infant's persisting dependency, as well as ability to conform socially or show awareness of others' needs. d. The need for establishing routine pediatric care.
Parents		
The nurse provides a demonstration of infant care and explains hospital routines. When the infant goes from nursing area to mother's bedside, the nurse discusses and demonstrates identification of infant, emergency care of infant if gagging or choking occurs, and protective measures used to minimize the possibility of cross infection. Nursing personnel are available to give infant care or assist with caregiving activities and infant feeding techniques. Parents are encouraged to participate in infant care and, whenever possible, to use techniques developed by themselves.	The nurse and clients discuss the normal responses of parents to the complex role of being a parent. The nurse provides an opportunity for safe revelation of feelings. Nurse and client discuss parental criteria for success in parenting skills (i.e., infant responses, competence in caregiving activities, and opinions of significant others). Success is praised, and parents are encouraged to be open-minded about expectations of their roles and those of others (siblings, grandparents). They are encouraged to make realistic assessment of their infant's needs and abilities. The mother is helped to conserve her energy (e.g., resting when the infant sleeps, lying down while feeding the infant). For some parents whose behavior indicates consistent rejection of the child's infancy	The nurse provides the opportunity for mother and father to discuss problems such as the parents' reactions to the infant and the infant's needs and demands. Discussion of feelings of depression or helplessness and how such feelings affect care the parents can give the child can be helpful. The nurse gives recognition to parental success in nurturing their child. If necessary, the family is helped to obtain further assistance from public health agency personnel or social workers to help them develop more adequate coping mechanisms. Some communities have established around-the-clock telephone centers where parents can obtain help for emotionally based problems with the child.

Continued.

Table 26-8 *Nursing Strategies to Meet Changing Parental Needs—cont'd*

Early Periods	Consolidation Period	Growth Period
	and dependency needs, intensive nursing support is needed as follows: 1. Plan and implement repeated contacts with parents (i.e., contact the mother by telephone on the second day after discharge; provide more frequent office visits; accept phone calls at home; provide regular home visits by public health nurse or nurse visitor). 2. Provide additional attention to the mother, i.e.: use compliments rather than criticism; promote maternal attachment to the newborn; emphasize accident prevention. 3. Enlist the help of other supportive personnel, such as a social worker.	These centers are in addition to emergency medical services. If parenting disorders are noted, the parents are referred to follow-up agencies such as the county public health department.
Family		
Infant is introduced to the family. Young siblings may need reassurance that their mother will not leave them again, and they may respond to their loss by withdrawing from the mother for a short time. Older children are usually excited and pleased and are eager to take on the care of the baby.	The nurse discusses typical reactions of siblings to the newcomer to the family. She encourages parents to share with other parents their successful techniques of helping siblings adjust (Fig. 26-9). She encourages a return of family involvement in their community and going beyond family boundaries for support and encouragement.	The nurse discusses balancing the infant's needs with those of other family members (e.g., jealousy of siblings, husband's or wife's feelings of alienation), the parents' need to modify infant's behavior to meet their expectations (e.g., toilet training, sleeping patterns, stopping crying when admonished), and the infant's relative ability to conform.

Cultural Aspects of Postpartum Care. The greatest conflict between Western and non-Western beliefs and practices in childbearing occurs in the postpartum period (Fig. 26-10). If a woman delivers in the hospital, she and her family are directly confronted with culturally related problems that are not as easily resolved as those encountered in the prenatal and labor and delivery stages. Moreover, the nurses caring for these mothers may view the woman's behavior as totally incomprehensible since it varies so dramatically from Western health care provider's expectations.

Cultural proscriptions during the postdelivery period exist (1) to hasten the recovery of the mother, (2) to assist her physically and emotionally in her assumption of her new maternal role, and (3) to protect and care for the newborn child.

The behavior patterns for many cultures include a period of seclusion for women lasting from 7 to 40 days with a minimum of activity allowed for mothers. These practices are based on two beliefs: that delivery has upset the balance of the mother's body and that the mother, infant, and those caring for them are in a state of pollution.

Maintenance of a State of Balance. Cultures that subscribe to a belief in the necessity of body balance believe that the body has lost a great deal of heat during the labor and delivery process and that the mother is therefore subject to a number of illnesses. Thus certain practices must be followed to restore the balance of heat and cold. Adherents of both humoral and yin and yang theories have prescriptions and proscriptions for restoration of balance of heat and cold (Currier, 1978).

Food. Food is one way in which heat can be restored and cold diminished. The classic Chinese diet (Campbell and Chang, 1975) represents an effort to decrease yin forces, which are cold. Included are an abundance of hot foods. The quality of heat and cold cannot always be measured by actual temperature. The essence of cold might be in a food even if the food is heated. Pillsbury (1978) notes that some foods are considered cold because they are grown in the damp earth or in watery places. Green vegetables, fruits, meats, and fish are commonly considered cold foods. Asians rank rice, eggs, and chicken high on the heat scale and thus believe they should be eaten frequently. Many cultures consider chicken the most desirable hot food. It is obvious that many, if not most, of the foods served on hospital trays, such as meats, vegetables, fruits, and fruit juices, are considerd cold. These will probably not be eaten by many Asian, Southeast Asian, and Spanish-speaking women.

However, if a hot substance is added to boiled water, it may counteract the coldness. For example, the chicken soup is so powerful that the cold quality of the water with which it is made is counteracted. Ginger added to hot wa-

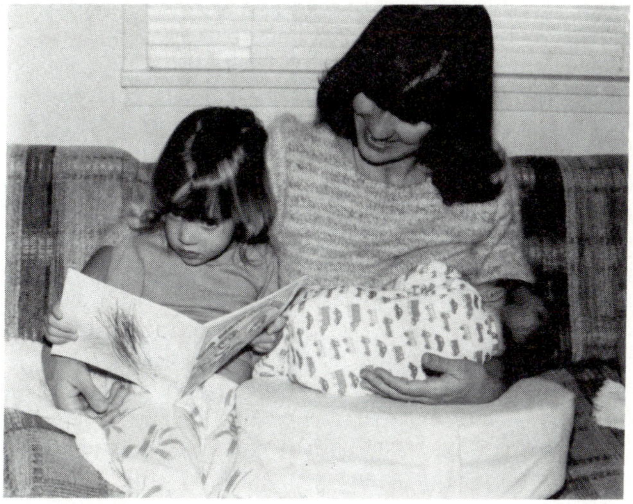

Fig. 26-9 Mother shares feeding time of newborn with older sibling. Baby is supported on an adjustable pad (Keiki Designs). Courtesy Marjorie Pyle, RNC, Lifecircle, Costa Mesa, Calif.

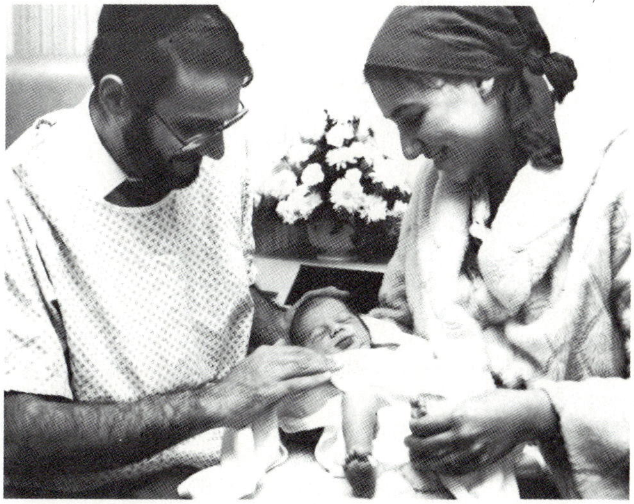

Fig. 26-10 Parents admire their new baby.

ter that has been boiled may cause the same effect. It is obvious then, that ice water, used frequently in hospitals, is forbidden.

Clark (1970) wrote that Mexican-American women are forbidden to eat "cold" foods such as hot chilies, pickles, any food prepared with vinegar, tomatoes, spinach, any pork product, and most fruits. Fruits such as bananas and grapefruit and other citrus fruits must be avoided because of their acidity and because they are believed to cause varicose veins in mothers. Although fruits and vegetables are also prohibited in the pregnant Vietnamese woman's diet, pork legs and knuckles are allowed because pork is believed to improve the secretion of milk (Coughlin, 1965. Hart (1965) reported that to prevent stomachaches, Filipino women avoid "cold" foods such as eels, oysters, squash, and uncooked fruits and vegetables. Filipino women also refrain from eating sour foods because they supposedly cause the mother's milk to curdle. "Tasty" foods with strong, rich flavor, such as peanuts, canned fish, and fatty meats, are avoided because they are believed to cause lactation to stop. The nurse should also understand that Filipino and Chinese women prefer to drink warm water instead of ice water (Campbell and Chang, 1975; Hart, 1965). According to Campbell and Chang, two possible reasons for this preference are (1) the belief that drinking ice water "shocks" the body and (2) the history of poor sanitation in the Philippines and China, which has made it a custom for people in these countries to boil drinking water.

Since, according to Hart (1969), disagreement occurs among Latin Americans and Filipinos about the classifications of basic foods into hot and cold categories, nurses should use clients as their major cultural informants. With flexibility and creativity, the nurse can plan with clients and with other health team members nutritious and culturally acceptable diets (Table 15-7). With little difficulty the nurse can advise the pregnant woman in selecting those foods in the hospital that are healthy, as well as those that the woman considers culturally appropriate. Similarly, the nurse can allow, as much as possible, family members to bring foods to the mother that are not readily available in the hospital but are highly recommended in the woman's culture.

Lactation. In the Philippines, if the mother's milk does not flow regularly, a meal of chicken and green papaya, boiled in coconut "milk" is suggested (Hart, 1965). Chicken soup is also believed important in the production of a nursing mother's milk. According to Hart (1965), the Filipino mother is also advised to eat a soup of boiled clams and ginger. Hart stated that Filipinos use hot applications of special medicinal preparations to stimulate lactation. Furthermore, the Filipino mother believes that raising either arm over her head while lying down will decrease, if not actually stop, lactation. Hart (1965) also noted the Filipino women's belief that heavy work will make their milk "hot." Korean mothers eat seaweed soup with rice to increase milk production (Chung, 1977). Currier (1978) reported that Spanish-Americans believe that exposing mothers to cold diminishes the flow of milk. Yaqui women massage their breasts to drain them (Shutler, 1977).

Activities of Daily Living. In addition to food, contact with air and wind is proscribed by Asians, Filipinos, Mexican-Americans, and southern blacks. Cold must be prevented from entering the body, to counteract further imbalance. Air is considered cold, whatever the temperature, and thus windows and doors must be kept closed. The Chinese belief that a woman's pores are open for 30 days after delivering a baby coincides with the period in which they believe the mother has an excess of cold (Campbell and Chang, 1973; Pillsbury, 1978). Air conditioners are a source of fear for women in the hospital. Fans are to be avoided. New mothers will keep themselves totally covered with blankets despite how hot the temperature of the room may be. The Chinese believe that for these 30 days after birth, cold air can enter the body through the vagina (Campbell and Chang, 1975). This is consistent with the

Chinese belief that during the postdelivery period some balance of the yang, or "hot" air, should be returned by decreasing the yin energy forces, or "cold" air in the body. Similarly, Spanish women believe that during the 40-day postdelivery period they should avoid exposing themselves to any condition that could cause bad air *(malaire)* to enter the vagina (Baca, 1973).

Water is considered cold at all times, even if it is heated. Therefore not bathing for a period of time is a widely held belief. Recognizing these beliefs, the nurse can encourage the mother to take frequent sponge baths and to emphasize perineal care, breast care, and other hygienic and comfort measures. Some mothers will take all kinds of measures to avoid the daily shower but will not directly refuse, complying by going to the shower room, turning on the water, and remaining in such a position that the water will not touch them. Pillsbury (1978) notes that Chinese women who have been westernized in so many ways still adhere to the postpartum practice of avoiding water. They must not wash themselves, their dishes, or their clothes. To the Chinese and other Asians, contact with water, considered cold, causes wind to enter the body and will result in future years in asthma, arthritis, and chronic aches and pains.

In some cultures women use abdominal binders during the pregnancy, as well as during the postdelivery period. Some Mexican-Americans use binders during the first 40 days of the puerperium (Clark, 1970). It is believed by these persons that binders help organs in the stomach return to their normal positions, push the hips together, and firm up the stomach muscles. Binders are used in conjunction with massage to help the woman with the "slipped" uterus (Hart, 1965). According to Hart (1965), in some regions in the Philippines, binders are worn by women both during pregnancy and after delivery to prevent *buhî-buhî. Buhî-buhî* is a syndrome in which ascending gas, starting under the lower left rib, produces symptoms ascribed to postdelivery hemorrhage, such as tachycardia, vertigo, partial blindness, and impaired respiration. The use of the binder is also thought to prevent the postdelivery expansion of the uterus. Another reason this practice is followed by Filipino women is the notion that the "cold" womb should be protected.

Pollution State. In addition to an imbalance of hot and cold, several cultures consider that the mother and infant are in a state of pollution after delivery. A certain time must elapse and certain rituals must be performed before purity is restored. A state of seclusion is commonly compulsory, during which time the mother is encouraged to limit her activities. This is in contrast to the hospital practice of early ambulation following delivery, early infant care responsibilities, and early discharge from the hospital. Mexican-Americans may observe *la cuarentina* for 40 days after birth of babies (Clark, 1970). For the Chinese mother, going out during the first month after birth will offend the gods because dirty birth blood remains throughout the month (Pillsbury, 1978). The Filipino mother (Stern et al., 1980) is commonly misunderstood as lazy and not caring when she refuses to do what is requested in the hospital and at home. Recently, in a personal communication from a group of Cambodian women, concern was expressed about how they will manage after the baby is born because they do not have an extended family to assist during the required time of seclusion and limited activity. The fear of subsequent illness, especially arthritis, in later years is very real to them. Homemaker services are not available to them because according to the Western view, they are able bodied and assistance cannot be justified. Their hope for the future is based on the belief that counteracting the bad effects of not carrying out cultural prescriptions for the postpartum period can be accomplished only by going through a follow-up pregnancy correctly. Their chances of doing future pregnancies "correctly" are remote, however. The cultural quandary for these women is clear.

Snow (1974) described the view of southern blacks that blood is a pollutant that carries contaminants from the body. Southern blacks and others believe that an adequate lochia flow is essential and going outside in the wind or air could thicken and halt the flow of blood, extending the time of pollution. Some Filipino mothers may remain bedfast for 2 weeks, after which time a special bath is taken to further remove the debris of pregnancy believed to be found in perspiration.

"Mother roasting" is a Southeast Asian custom (Hart, 1965). In this practice the mother sits on a cane-bottom (or bamboo-slat) chair draped in a blanket from head to floor, while a bowl of glowing hot coals is placed under her (Nydegger and Nydegger, 1963). There she "roasts" until the coals are cold. This is repeated daily for 11 to 30 days. According to Stern et al. (1980), "roasting" is practiced by Filipinos in the most remote provinces only (Chapter 25). The purpose of this is to hasten the healing process, much like perineal heat lamps used in recent times.

Filipinos believe that this practice (1) stops the blood, (2) fixes the uterus in position, and (3) alleviates birth soreness (Hart, 1965). Vietnamese women practice roasting for the following reasons: (1) the mother's blood must be kept "warm," (2) the mother's uterus will contract properly and consequently prevent unhealthy distortion of the woman's figure, and (3) steam baths will prevent the woman from having a bad body odor during her entire life (Coughlin, 1965). At the end of the 30 to 40 days, the woman usually takes a cleansing bath. Then she resumes her normal activities in the community. Since she has been "cleansed," members of the community need not avoid contacts with a formerly pregnant woman.

An extension of the yin and yang principle is the belief that the mother and the baby should be protected from early exposure to the "unclean" or "defiled" world (Chung, 1977). Chung also stated that in addition to showing a reluctance to go outdoors, zealous believers of this principle cease communications with others to avoid anything evil emanating from the "unclean" outside world.

Horn (1982) supplies a recent example of acculturated behavior. After the birth of her first child, a Greek-American mother followed the ancient proscription of participation in church activities for 40 days. While her husband attended the church wedding of a friend, this woman did her weekly shopping at the local supermarket. In most cultural groups sexual relations are prohibited until after the seclusion period and sometimes throughout lactation.

Some cultural groups have unique practices. For example, the women of Northern Thailand bind their wrists with string. The purpose of wrist binding is to prevent the loss of the soul, which may lead to wind disease, a specific complex of symptoms indicating a state of humoral imbalance characterized by weakness, nausea, and hypersensitivity to odors (Kundstadter, 1978). Northern Thai women giving birth will most likely have their wrists bound and would be extremely frightened and upset if the strings were removed.

The preceding examples indicate that, from the time of delivery to a certain designated time afterward, mothers in many cultures are considered highly susceptible to ensuing illness, either immediately or at an unspecified time in the future. Furthermore, their state of pollution requires that only certain persons contact them during the specified time they remain in seclusion. Most of their activities are carried on by others, usually members of the extended family or friends. The end of the time of seclusion is often marked by a ceremony and includes ritual cleansing of the woman, child, and place of seclusion (Brownlee, 1978). It is important for nurses to understand these factors, assist women in carrying out their beliefs and practices insofar as is possible, and assist them with necessary adjustments when their expectations are not feasible.

Discharge from Hospital

Discharge Planning. Discharge planning begins with the first contact with the client, when the client's physical, emotional, social, and economic profiles start to emerge. The goals listed on p. 618 and p. 639 in the nursing care plans in this chapter serve as guidelines for assessing the client's needs at discharge. In the preparation of a client for discharge, the nurse does the following:

1. Identifies gaps in knowledge and reviews these points, if necessary:
   - (a) Self-care activities and infant-care activities
   - (b) Danger signs (see box, above)
   - (c) Return of ovulation and menstruation
   - (d) Lactation and weaning or suppression of lactation
   - (e) Resumption of sexual intercourse and fertility management
   - (f) Medications that have been prescribed for the client
2. Helps the client develop a support system for help with cooking, cleaning, child care, shopping, and so on
3. Identifies the need for referral to community resources (e.g., homemaker or child care services, food stamps) and offers suggestions, when appropriate
4. Provides the client with a printed instruction sheet that includes phone numbers to call day and night in case of questions or problems

Early Discharge. The duration of hospitalization and the subsequent convalescence at home are still under debate. Most women who do not experience complications return home before the third postdelivery day. Some women who are carefully screened by the nurse, obstetrician, and pediatrician leave much earlier—anywhere from 12 to 24 hours after delivery. Because these clients are in particular need of follow-up care for themselves and their infants, hospitals have established early discharge programs to assist with such care. These programs provide an alternative mode of mother-infant care.

Planning for early discharge begins in the prenatal period and involves the nurse, physician, and other appropriate members of the health care team. The families who participate should meet the following criteria: (1) live within a reasonable distance of the hospital, (2) have taken preparation-for-parenthood classes that include content related to assessment of the mother's recovery, care of the mother during the puerperium, and identification and reporting of possible complications, (3) have someone at home to assist in the care of the infant and mother, and (4) have no major medical problems. If a family is interested in early discharge, they are asked to notify the attending physician and nursing staff at the beginning of prenatal care. Opportunities are provided to meet the nurse who will be making home visits during the puerperium for health assessment and any teaching that is necessary. Women with complications, however, should be asymptomatic for at least 24 hours and capable of personal care before leaving the hospital.

Return Visit. Since biblical times, the puerperium has been considered to last 6 weeks. Hence a return visit and examination have been scheduled traditionally 6 weeks after delivery. This is illogical because many problems, such as leukorrhea, may be identified and successfully treated earlier. Individualization is important, therefore, but a more logical date for return to the physician or clinic would be 3 or 4 weeks after delivery.

Closing the Client's Chart. Just before the time when the client would be leaving the maternity unit, the nurse reviews the client's chart (audits the chart) to see that laboratory reports, medications, signatures, and so on are in order. Some hospitals have a checklist to follow before the client's discharge. The nurse verifies that medications, if ordered, have arrived on the unit, that any valuables kept secured during the client's stay have been returned to her and that she has signed a receipt for them, and that the infant is ready to be discharged.

Escorting the Client from the Hospital. The nurse is

DANGER SIGNS

Postpartum (Physical)

1. Fever, with or without chills
2. Foul-smelling or irritating vaginal discharge
3. Excessive lochia or vaginal discharge
4. Recurrence of bright red vaginal bleeding after the lochia has changed to rust color
5. A swollen area on the leg that is painful, red, or hot to the touch
6. Localized swelling or a painful, hot area on the breast
7. A burning sensation during urination or an inability to urinate
8. Pelvic or perineal pain

careful not to administer any medication that would make the mother sleepy if she is the one who will be holding the baby on the way out of the hospital. In some instances, the woman is seated in a wheelchair and is usually given the baby to hold. Some families leave unescorted and ambulatory, depending on hospital protocol. The woman's possessions are gathered and taken out with her and her family; usually they are placed on some type of cart or carried by family members. Of course, the woman's and the baby's identification bands have been carefully checked. As the client and the baby are assisted into the car, the nurse should make sure that there is a car seat in which to secure the baby. If there is not, the nurse should return both to the unit and arrange with a social worker, if necessary to provide one for the trip home.

CAUTION: Whether or not the woman and her family have chosen early discharge, the nurse and the physician are held responsible if the woman is discharged before her condition has stabilized within normal limits. If complications occur, the medical and nursing staff could be sued for "abandonment."

Recorder

The postpartum client's record serves as a documented means of communication among all members of the health care team. The record contains accurate and complete recordings of the history, physical examination, and laboratory test results. It also contains sequential observations, goals, interventions, and client responses. The record should be readily accessible to the health care professionals caring for the woman and family. Documentation of client health education, counseling, and responses to information are included. The postpartum nurse reassesses and updates the client's care plan, including maternity/gynecologic follow-up and appropriate referrals, to meet client needs. This type of record serves as a reservoir for future research study.

Evaluation

Evaluation is a continuous process. Parental, infant, and family relationships are consistently assessed as indicators of healthy family adjustments after the birth of a child. To be effective, evaluation needs to be based on measurable outcome criteria. The criteria reflect the parameters used to measure the goals for care. The clinical findings that represent normal responses are presented as outcome criteria in the general nursing care plan, the specific nursing care plan, and the summary of nursing actions in this chapter. These criteria are used as a basis for selecting appropriate nursing actions and evaluating their effectiveness.

SUMMARY

The normal postpartum period is a time of rapid change. Change takes place in the physiologic and psychosocial dimensions of the woman, the newborn, and their family. The nurse who makes pertinent assessments, plans and implements client-centered care, and evaluates the effectiveness of the care is enacting an important role in the health of the child-bearing family.

KEY CONCEPTS

- Postpartum care is modeled on the concept of health.
- The nursing care plan includes assessments to detect deviations from normal, comfort measures to relieve discomfort or pain, and safety measures to prevent injury or infection.
- The nurse provides teaching and counseling measures designed to promote a mother's (and father's) feeling of competence and control in the care of herself and newly born child.
- The nurse's clinical expertise is required to implement many therapeutic measures for physical care including care of the boggy uterus, the full urinary bladder, the need for pharmacologic relief of discomfort, care after repair of episiotomy or laceration, care of hemorrhoids, and suppression of lactation.
- Nurses have a leadership role in helping clients establish healthy early family relationships.
- The parents' response is profoundly affected by their interpretation of the infant's response.
- Crisis prevention is an important function of the nurse and includes anticipatory guidance for infant's crying, sibling responses, and interactions with the grandparents.
- Mothers (and fathers) often misjudge the actual amount of physical and emotional energy required for the role transition to parenthood.
- The behaviors of the infant, the spouse, and others may not always meet expectations.
- Family commitments involve having time and energy for individual family members—mother, father, and children— and for the couple, away from the child (or children).
- The greatest conflict between Western and non-Western beliefs and practices in childbearing occurs in the postpartum period.

STUDY QUESTIONS AND ACTIVITIES

1. Assess, plan, implement, and evaluate nursing care of a multipara and a primipara. Formulate the nursing diagnoses to reflect the health-centered philosophy of postpartum care.
2. Research in-depth various cultures' attitudes toward the postpartum woman, including health beliefs and prescribed and proscribed behavior. Present findings in group discussion on how such beliefs and practices can and cannot be integrated with procedures at your hospital.
3. Using the parent-infant interaction assessment tool in this chapter, assess a client during the hospital stay and, if possible, later. Discuss findings with the group.

4. Assess own attitudes and concepts regarding parenting. Use these reports as the basis for group discussion and self-disclosure that works toward a better understanding of lack of parental attachment.
5. In the newborn nursery, select a baby that you "really like" and one that you "can't stand." Identify those characteristics of the newborn that influence your response to the babies; process record a 3 to 5 minute interaction with each one. Reflect on what you would do if *your* baby had the characteristics of the one you "can't stand." Devise strategies for intervention for the mother (or father) whose baby does not meet their expectations.
6. Prepare a client for discharge, including teaching and documentation in the medical record.

References

Anderson, CJ: Enhancing reciprocity between mother and neonate, Nurs Res 30:89, 1981

Baca, J: Some health beliefs of the Spanish-speaking. In Reinhardt, AM, and Quinn, MD, editors: Family-centered community nursing, St Louis, 1973, The CV Mosby Co

Bell, RQ, and Ainsworth MDS: Infant crying and maternal responsiveness, *Child D* 43:1171, 1972

Booth, CL, Johnson-Crowly, and Barnard, KE: Infant massage and exercise: worth the effort? MCN 10(3):184, 1985

Brownlee, AT: Community, culture, and care: a cross-cultural guide for health workers, St Louis, 1978, The CV Mosby Co.

Byrne, JM, and Horowitz, FS: Rocking as a soothing intervention: The influence of direction and type of movement, *Infant Behavior and Development* 4:207, 1981

Campbell, T and Chang, B: Health care of the Chinese in America. In Spradley, BW, editor: Contemporary community Nursing, Boston, 1975, Little, Brown, Co, Inc

Caplan, G: Psychological aspects of maternity care, Am J Public Health 47:25, 1957

Chung, HJ: Understanding the Oriental maternity patient, Nurs Clin North Am 12:67, 1977

Clark, M: Health in the Mexican-American culture: a community study. Berkely, Calif, 1970, University of California Press

Coughlin, R: Pregnancy and birth in Vietnam. In Hart, D, Rajadhon, PA, and Coughlin, RJ, editors: Southeast Asian birth customs: three studies in human reproduction New Haven, Conn, 1965, Human Relations Area Files, pp 205-273

Currier, RL: The hot-cold syndrome and symbolic balance in Mexican and Spanish-American folk medicine. In Martinez, RA, editor: Hispanic culture and health care: fact, fiction, folklore, St Louis, 1978, The CV Mosby Co

Darbyshire, P: Comfort for the crying child, Nurs Times, p 59, Sept 11, 1985

Field, TM: Effects of early separation, interactive deficits, and experimental manipulation on infant-mother face-to-face interaction, Child Dev 48:763, 1977

Gottlieb, BH: The role of individual and social support in preventing child maltreatment. In Garbarino, J, and Stocking, S, editors: Protecting children from abuse/neglect, San Francisco, 1980, Jossey Bass, Inc, Publishers

Hart, DV: From pregnancy through birth in a Bisayan Filipino village. In Hart, DV, Rajadhon, PA, and Coughlin, RJ, editors: Southeast Asian birth customs; three studies in reproduction, New Haven, Conn, 1965, Human Relations Area Files, pp 1-113

Hart, DV: Bisayan Filipino and Malayan humoral pathologies: folk medicine and ethnohistory in Southeast Asia, New York, 1969, Cornell University Southeast Asia Program, pp. 43, 46

Horn, BM: Northwest coast Indians: the Muchleshoot. In Kay, MA, editors: Anthropology of human births, Philadelphia, 1982, FA Davis Co

Humenick, SS, and Bugen, LA: Parenting roles: expectation versus reality, MCN 12(1):36, 1987

Konrad, CJ: Helping mothers integrate the birth experience, MCN 12(4):268, 1987

Lamb, ME: The development of social expectations in the first year of life. In Lamb, M, Sherrod, L, editors: *Infant social cognition,* Hillside, New Jersey, 1981, Erlbaum

Lang, R: Birth book, Ben Lomond, Calif, 1972, Genesis Press

Kirkland, J: *Crying and babies: helping families cope,* Kent, 1985, Croom Helm Ltd

Kundstadter, P: Do cultural differences make any difference? Choice points in medical systems available in Northwestern Thailand. In Kleinman, A, et al, editors: Culture and healing in Asian societies, Cambridge, Mass, 1978, Schenkman Books, Inc

Kunst-Wilson, W, and Cronenwett, LR: Nursery care for the emerging family: promoting paternal behavior, Res Nurs Health 4:201, 1981

Mercer, RT: The nurse and maternal tasks of early postpartum, MCN 6:341, Sept/Oct 1981

Mercer, RT: Parent-infant attachment. In Sonstegard, LJ, et al, editors: Women's health, vol 2, Childbearing, New York, 1982, Grune & Stratton, Inc

Morris, M: Psychological miscarriage: an end to mother love, Transactions, p 11, Jan/Feb 1966

Mortimer, P, and Kevill, F: Infant care: frustration and despair, *Nurs Times, Community Outlook,* p. 19, May 1985

Nydegger, WF, and Nydegger, C: Tarong: an Ilocos barrio in the Philippines. In Whiting, BB, editor: Six cultures: studies of child rearing, New York, 1963, John Wiley & Sons, Inc

Pederson, DR: The soothing effects of rocking as determined by the direction and frequency of movement, *Can J Behav Sci* 7:237, 1975

Pillsbury, BLK: "Doing the month": confinement and convalescence of Chinese women after childbirth, Soc Sci Med 12:11, 1978

Ramler, D, and Roberts, J: A comparison of cold and warm sitz baths for relief of postpartum perineal pain, JOGN Nurs 15(6): 471, 1986

Riesch, S, and Munns, S: Promoting awareness: the mother and her baby, Nurs Res 33:271, Sept/Oct 1985

Rubin, R: Puerperal change, Nurs Outlook 9:753, 1961

Schornkoff, JP: Social support and the development of vulnerable children, Am J Public Health 74:310, 1984

Shutler, ME: Disease and curing in a Yaqui community. In Spicer, EH, editor: Ethnic medicine in the Southwest, Tucson, Ariz, 1977, The University of Arizona Press

Snow, L: Folk medical beliefs and their implications for care of patients, Ann Intern Med 81:82, 1974

Stainton, MC: Parent-infant interaction: putting theory into practice, Calgary, Alberta, Canada, 1981, University of Calgary Faculty of Nursing

Stainton, MC: Maternal newborn attachment origins and processes. III. Interactional synchony: the prelude to attachment, doctoral thesis, University of California, San Francisco, 1985

Steele, B, and Pollock, C: A psychiatric study of parents who abuse infants and small children. In Helfer, RE, and Kempe, C, editors: The battered child, Chicago, 1968, University of Chicago Press

Stern, PN, et al: Culturally induced stress during childbearing: the Filipino-American experience, Issues Health Care Women 2(3-4):67, 1980
Sullivan, D, and Beeman, R: Satisfaction with postpartum care: opportunities for bonding, reconstructing the birth and instruction, Birth Fam J 8:3, Fall 1981
Tansig, M: Measuring life events, J Health Soc Behav 23:52, Jan 1982
Ter Vrugt, D, and Pederson, DR: The effects of vertical rocking frequencies on the arousal level in two-month-old infants, *Child Dev* 44:205, 1973
Thoits, PA: Dimensions of life events that influence psychological distress: an evaluation and synthesis of literature, In Kaplan, HB, editor: Psychosocial stress: trends in theory and research, New York, 1983, Academic Press
Thoman, EB, Acebo, C, and Becker, PT: Infant crying and stability in the mother—infant relationship: a systems analysis, *Child Dev* 54:653, 1983
Turner, RJ, and Avison, WR: Assessing risk factors for problem parenting: the significance of social support, J Mar Fam 47:881, Nov 1985

Bibliography

American Cancer Society, How to examine your breasts, Pamphlet no 2088-LE, June 1978, The Society
Avery, M, et al: An early postpartum hospital discharge program: Implementation and evaluation, JOGN Nurs 11:200, 1982
Bing, E, and Colman, L: Making love during pregnancy, New York, 1977, Bantam Books, Inc
Brooten, DA, et al: A comparison of four treatments to prevent and control breast pain and engorgement in nonnursing mothers, Nurs Res 32:225, 1983
Bull, M, and Lawrence, D: Mother's use of knowledge during the first postpartum weeks, JOGN Nurs 14:315, July/Aug 1985
Carr, KC, and Walton, VE: Early postpartum discharge, JOGN Nurs 11:29, 1982
Censullo, M, et al: An instrument for the measurement of infant-adult synchrony, Nurs Res 36(4):244, 1987
Claypool, JM: Rubella protection for maternal child health care providers, MCN 6:53, 1981
Clinton, JF: Expectant fathers at risk for couvade, Nurs Res 35(5):290, 1986
Clinton, JF: Physical and emotional responses of expectant fathers throughout pregnancy and the early postpartum period, Int J Nurs Stud 24(1):59, 1987
Consullo, M, et al: An instrument for the measurement of infant-adult synchrony, Nurs Res 36(4):244, 1987
Crawford, J: A theoretical model of support network conflict experienced by new mothers, Nurs Res 34:100, March/April 1985
Cronewett, LR: Network structure, social support, and psychological outcomes of pregnancy, Nurs Res 34:93, March/April 1985a
Cronewett, LR: Parental network structured and perceived support after birth of first child, Nurs Res 34:347, Nov/Dec 1985b
Croog, EH, and Zigrossi, ST: Parenting luncheons on the postpartum unit, MCN 8:277, 1983
Danforth, DN, and Scott, JR, editors: Obstetrics and gynecology, ed 5, Philadelphia, 1986, JB Lippincott Co
Devaney, SW, and Lavery, SF: Nursing care for the relinquishing mother, JOGN Nurs 9:375, 1980
Donaldson, NE: The postpartum follow-up nurse clinician, JOGN Nurs 4:249, 1981
Donovan, M, editor: ***Pain Control,*** Nurs Clin North Am, Sept, 1987
Droegemueller, W: Cold sitz bath for relief of postpartum perineal pain, Clin Obstet Gynecol 23:1039, 1980
Edwards M: The crisis of fourth trimester, Birth Fam J 1:19, Winter 1973-1974
Fawcett, J, and York, R: Spouses' physical and psychological symptoms during pregnancy and the postpartum, Nurs Res 35(3):144, 1986
Fischman, SH, et al: Changes in sexual relationships in postpartum couples JOGN Nurs 15:58, Jan/Feb 1986
Goebel, JB, et al: Infant car seat usage: effectiveness of a postpartum education program, JOGN Nurs 13:33, 1984
Goodlin, RC, and Frederick, IB: Postpartum vulvar edema associated with the birthing chair, Am J Obstet Gynecol 146:334, 1983
Gorrie, TM: Postpartal nursing diagnoses, JOGN N 15:52, Jan/Feb 1986
Gosha, J, and Brucker, MC: A self-help group for new mothers: an evaluation, MCN 11:20, Jan/Feb 1986
Haight, K: What you should know about epidural analgesia, Nurs '87, 17(9):58, 1987
Hans, A: Postpartum assessment: the psychological component, JOGN Nurs 15:49, Jan/Feb 1986
Harvey, K: Mother-baby nursing, Nurs Management 13(7):22, 1982
Henderson, JS: Effects of a prenatal teaching program on postpartum regeneration of the pubococcygeal muscle, JOGN Nurs 12:403, 1983
Hensleigh, PA: Preventing rhesus isoimmunization, Am J Obstet Gynecol 146:749, 1983
Hiser, PL: Concerns of multiparas during the second postpartum week, JOGN Nurs 16(5):195, 1987
Horn, M, and Manion, J: Creative grandparenting: bonding the generations, JOGN Nurs 14(3):233, 1985
Jacobson, H: A standard for assessing lochia volume, MCN 10:174, May/June 1985
Jankowski, H, and Wells, S: Self-administered medications for obstetric patients, MCN (12):199, 1987
Jiminez, MH, and Niles, N: Activity and work during pregnancy and the postpartum period: a cross cultural study of 202 societies, Am J Obstet Gynecol 135:198, 1979
Keefe, MR: The impact of infant rooming-in on maternal sleep at night, JOGN Nurs 17(2):122, 1988
Kegel, AH: Progressive resistance exercise in the functional restoration of the perineal muscles, Am J Obstet Gynecol 56:238, 1948
Ketter, DE, and Shelton, BJ: In-hospital exercises for the postpartal woman, MCN 8:120, 1983
Kowba, MD, and Schwirian, PM: Direct sibling contact and bacterial colonization in newborns, JOGN Nurs 14:412, Sept/Oct 1985
Lane, G, Cronin, K, and Peirce, A: Flow charts: clinical decision making in nursing, Philadelphia, 1983, JB Lippincott Co
LaDu, EB: Childbirth care for Hmong families, MCN 10(6):382, 1985
Lee, PA: Health beliefs of pregnant and postpartum Hmong women, Western J Nurs Res 8(1):83, 1986
Leininger, M: Transcultural nursing: an essential knowledge and practice field for today, Can Nurse 80:41, Dec 1984
Mansell, KA: Mother-baby units: the concept works, MCN 9:132, 1984

Marecki, M, et al: Early sibling attachment, JOGN Nurs 14:418, Sept/Oct 1985

McCaffery, M: Nursing management of the patient with pain, Philadelphia, 1979, JB Lippincott Co

McCaffery, M: Patient-controlled analgesia: more than a machine, Nurs '87 17(11):62, 1987

McKay, S, and Mahan, CS: Ways to upgrade postpartal care, Contemp OB/GYN 27:63, Nov 1985

McKenzie, CA, et al: Comprehensive care during the postpartum period, Nurs Clin North Am 17:23, 1982

Mercer, RT: The relationship of developmental variables to maternal behavior, Res Nurs Health, 9:25, 1986

Mercer, RT: Relationship of the birth experience to later mothering behaviors, J Nurs Midwife 30:204, July/Aug 1985

Mercer, RT: The relationship of age and other variables to gratification in mothering, Health Care Women International 6:295, 1985

Mercer, RT, and Stainton, MC: Perceptions of the birth experience: a cross-cultural comparison, Health Care Women 5:29, 1984

Mueller, LS: Pregnancy and sexuality, JOGN Nurs 14(4):289, 1985

Mynick, A: Instituting a postpartum self-medication program, MCN 6:419, 1981

NAACOG: Nurses offer home health-care alternatives, NAACOG Newsletter 15(5): 4, 1988

Newell, NJ: Grandparents: the overlooked support system for new parents during the fourth trimester, NAACOG Update Series, 1(lesson 21), Washington, DC, 1984, The Association

Nurses Association of the American College of Obstetricians and Gynecologists: Standards for obstetric gynecologic and neonatal nursing, ed 3, Washington, DC, 1986, The Association

Olson, ML: Fitting grandparents into new families, MCN 6:419, 1981

Pritchard, JA, MacDonald, PC, and Gant, NE: Williams obstetrics, ed 17, Norwalk, Conn, 1985, Appleton-Century-Crofts

Quistad, C: How to smooth mom's postpartum path, RN 47:40, April 1984

Rödholm, M, and Larsson, K: Father-infant interaction at the first contact after delivery, Early Hum Dev 3:21, 1979

Russell, TR: Managing hemorrhoids during and after pregnancy, Contemp OB/GYN 21:March 1983 (special issue)

Rutledge, DL, and Pridham, KF: Postpartum mothers' perceptions of competence for infant care, JOGN Nurs 16(3):185, 1987

Stolte, K: Postpartum 'missing pieces': sequela of a passing obstetrical era? Birth 13(2):100, 1986

Strang, VR, and Sullivan, PL: Body image attitudes during pregnancy and the postpartum period, JOGN Nurs 14:332, July/Aug 1985

Strelinck, EG: Postpartum care: an opportunity to reinforce breast self-examination, MCN 7(4):249, 1982

Tilkian, SM: Clinical implication of laboratory tests, ed 4, St. Louis, 1987, The CV Mosby Co

Tomlinson, PS: Spousal differences in marital satisfaction during transition to parenthood, Nurs Res 36(4):239, 1987

Tucker, SM, et al: Patient care standards, ed 4, St Louis, 1988, The CV Mosby Co

Vestal, KW: A proposal: primary nursing for the mother-baby dyad, Nurs Clin North Am 17:3, 1982

Wadd, L: Vietnamese postpartum practices: implication for nursing in the hospital setting, JOGN Nurs 12:252, 1983

Walker, LO, Crain, H, and Thompson, E: Mothering behavior and maternal role attainment during the postpartum period, Nurs Res 35(6):352, 1986

Wong, S, and Stepp-Gilbert, E: Lactation suppression: nonpharmaceutical versus pharmaceutical method, JOGN Nurs 14(4):302, July/Aug 1985

Woods, NF: Human sexuality in health and illness, ed 3, St Louis, 1984, The CV Mosby Co

Zalar, MK: Human sexuality: a component of total patient care, Nurs Digest 3:40, 1975

Zalar, MK: Sexual counseling for pregnant couples, MCN 1:176, 1976

UNIT

VII

Complications of Childbearing

Of the approximately 3 million births that occur in the United States each year, 500,000 will be categorized as high risk. The united efforts of all members of the obstetric team and close collaboration with other medical personnel are required to adequately care for the high-risk client. This unit reviews the maternal conditions that predispose or commit the client to an abnormal response to pregnancy.

In Chapter 27 the high-risk client and the factors associated with diagnosis of high risk are identified. Chapter 28 focuses on loss and grief, states experienced by high-risk clients and families. Chapter 29 focuses on hypertensive states during pregnancy that may occur as a pregnancy-induced disease or may predate the pregnancy. Chapter 30 contains content relevant to maternal infections during the antepartum, childbirth, and postdelivery periods. Maternal hemorrhagic conditions are identified in Chapter 31. Endocrine and metabolic disorders receive special attention in Chapter 32. Dystocia, and preterm and postterm labor are discussed in Chapter 33. Chapter 34 contains content about many medical, surgical, and psychosocial conditions. Poverty, emotional complications, and abuse of psychoactive substances are included. Chapter 34 addresses the unique characteristics and needs of adolescent pregnancy and parenthood.

Nursing research highlights are included.

Following are abstracts of examples of relevant nursing research.

Chapter 28: Women's perceptions of first trimester spontaneous abortion.

Chapter 30: Nurses call out for AIDS information.

Chapter 33: Antenatal education for cesarean birth: extension of a field test; and, women's important relationships during pregnancy and the preterm labor event.

Chapter 35: First trimester nausea in pregnant teenagers: incidence, characteristrics, and interventions.

CHAPTER

27

Assessment for Risk Factors

Learning Objectives

Correctly define the key terms listed.

Explore the scope of high-risk pregnancy.

Assess regionalization of health care services.

List risk factors identified through interview, physical examination, and diagnostic techniques.

Understand the various diagnostic techniques and implications of findings.

Explain diagnostic techniques to clients and their families.

Summarize biochemical monitoring.

Summarize biophysical monitoring.

Explain client-teaching for antenatal monitoring.

Key Terms

acoustic stimulation
alpha-fetoprotein (aFP)
amniocentesis
amnioscopy
amniotic fluid assessment
antepartum testing
Apt test
biochemical monitoring
biophysical profile
biparietal diameter (BPD)
chorionic villi sampling (CVS)
contraction stress test (CST)
Coombs' test
daily fetal movement count (DFMC)
Doppler mode
estriol
fetal activity-acceleration determination (FAD)
fetal breathing movements (FBM)
fetoscopy
intrauterine growth retardation (IUGR)
lecithin/sphingomyelin (L/S) ratio
magnetic resonance imaging (MRI)
meconium-stained amniotic fluid
neonatal respiratory distress
nonstress test (NST)
percutaneous umbilical blood sampling (PUBS)
regionalization of health care
shake test
ultrasonography

Of the approximately 3 million births that occur in the United States each year, 500,000 will be categorized as high risk because of maternal or fetal complications. The united efforts of all members of the obstetric team and close collaboration with other medical personnel are required to adequately care for the high-risk client. In this chapter the high-risk client and the factors associated with diagnosis of high risk are identified. Techniques of biophysical monitoring of fetal health are emphasized.

DEFINITION AND SCOPE OF THE PROBLEM

A high-risk pregnancy is one in which the life or health of the mother or offspring is jeopardized by a disorder coincidental with or unique to pregnancy. For the mother the high-risk status extends (arbitrarily) through the puerperium, that is, until 29 days after delivery. Postdelivery maternal complications are usually resolved within a month of birth, but perinatal morbidity may continue for months or years.

A better understanding of human reproduction has greatly reduced maternal morbidity and mortality. Knowledge of the fetus and neonatal disorders has increased dramatically in the last 10 to 15 years. This has led to a gratifying drop in perinatal morbidity and mortality during this period.

Of the 5 to 10 million pregnancies that occur in the United States each year, 2 to 3 million terminate as spontaneous abortions. Many of the abortions are caused by genetic faults or infection. About 1 million early gestations end as elective abortions. Approximately 3.5 million pregnancies reach viability (22 to 24 weeks' gestation), but of these at least 45,000 fetuses fail to survive. About the same number of newborns die during the first month of life. Another 40,000 babies have severe but perhaps correctable congenital anomalies. Pregnancy and delivery complications may be at least partly responsible for mental retardation in approximately 90,000 individuals. In addition, these complications have partially handicapped more than 150,000 persons, who have difficulty coping in our complex society (see statistical picture and definitions, Chapter 2).

Even excluding fetuses who have not reached viability, perinatal mortality exceeds that of all other causes of death combined until 65 years of age. When viewed in this perspective, high-risk pregnancy presents one of the most critical and urgent problems of modern medicine.

A new social emphasis on the quality of life has developed. Family planning has reduced family size and the number of unwanted pregnancies. With these trends the wanted child has become increasingly important. As a consequence, periodic maternal and perinatal assessment is essential to emphasize safe delivery of normal infants who can develop to their maximum potential.

It is well known that pregnancy is a **maturational crisis** in both the physiologic and psychologic sense. The diagnosis of high risk imposes another crisis, a **situational crisis** (e.g., the pregnancy terminates before the anticipated date; the woman develops gestational diabetes mellitus with its potential complications; a neonate is born who does not meet cultural, societal, or familial norms and expectations). Understanding of the high-risk client will allow the nurse to provide individualized therapeutic nursing care.

Maternal Health Problems

Different parts of the world have different leading causes of maternal death attributable to pregnancy. In general three major causes have persisted for the last 35 years: hypertensive disorders, infection, and hemorrhage.

Causes of Mortality	*Percent*
Hypertensive disorders	21
Infection	18
Hemorrhage	14
Other (cardiac, diabetes mellitus, trauma)	46

In the United States, maternal mortality for white women is still less than for all other women, although the gap that existed 30 years ago has been narrowed dramatically. Today the mortality ratio for white women and all others is 2:3. This decline is attributed to changes in social and economic factors and to availability of health care, for instance, to:

1. Advances in medical management
2. Greater knowledge and capability to apply the knowledge
3. Emergence of a philosophy of maternity care that recognizes the advantages of client participation in health care and that focuses on childbirth as a healthy event
4. Public acceptance of prenatal care

Fetal and Neonatal Health Problems

Fetal Death. Fetal death (demise) is defined as the death in utero before complete expulsion of the product of human conception irrespective of the duration of pregnancy. It does not result from therapeutic or elective abortion. It is also called intrauterine death.

Neonatal Death. Neonatal death is the death of a liveborn neonate at 20 weeks' gestation or more. A liveborn neonate is one who shows any evidence of life after birth, even if only momentary (respiration, heartbeat, voluntary muscle movement, or pulsation within the umbilical cord), and who dies at 28 days or less.

Perinatal Death Rate. Perinatal death rate is defined as the sum of fetal and neonatal death rates. This statistic is considered the most sensitive indicator of the effectiveness of perinatal care.

The incidence of each cause of **infant mortality** (Chapter 2) is expressed as the number of deaths per 100,000 live births.

As Table 27-1 demonstrates, the majority of the 10 leading causes of death during infancy continue to occur during the perinatal period; almost 75% of all infant deaths occur within the first 20 days of life. Although a number of perinatal problems have benefited from improved treatment, congenital anomalies continue to be the leading

Table 27-1 *Leading Causes of Death in Infants Under 1 Year of Age, United States, 1984 (Estimated Rates per 100,000 Live Births)*

Rank	Causes of Death	Rate
1	Other conditions originating in the perinatal period	272.7
2	Congenital anomalies	228.1
3	All other causes	170.2
4	Sudden infant death syndrome	131.7
5	Respiratory distress syndrome	103.9
6	Disorders relating to short gestation and unspecified low birth weight	93.3
7	Intrauterine hypoxia and birth asphyxia	26.2
8	Pneumonia and influenza	17.0
9	Birth trauma	8.9
10	Certain gastrointestinal diseases	7.6

From National Center for Health Statistics: Annual summary of births, marriages, divorces, and deaths: United States, 1984. Monthly vital statistics report 33(13):8, DHHS Pub No (PHS) 85-1120, Sept 26, 1985.

cause of infant mortality, accounting for about 22% of those deaths. The incidence of most birth defects has neither substantially decreased nor increased (Whaley and Wong, 1987). Infant mortality includes the neonatal death rate. Problems related to low birth weight and preterm birth are chiefly responsible for deaths during the first 4 weeks of life.

When infant mortality is categorized according to race, a disturbing difference is seen. The infant mortality for whites is considerably lower than for all other races in the United States, with blacks having almost twice the rate for whites. Although the birth rate of both groups has declined, the gap has remained fairly constant (Whaley and Wong, 1987).

These statistics are used to determine health care needs for the general population. Funds and facilities are allocated to those segments of the population within a community or to the geographic location of the United States where the needs are the greatest. In addition, the identified causes of mortality are used in planning for (1) the type and distribution of health care services (e.g., research, location of regional centers) and (2) the development of curricula for educational programs for health care providers.

Regionalization of Health Care Services

There is excellent evidence that mortality decreases when high risk is identified and intensive care applied. In addition, follow-up studies have shown that serious residual handicaps (physical and mental) of surviving infants have been dramatically reduced.

It is neither feasible nor reasonable for each hospital to develop and maintain the full spectrum of medical and nursing specialists, laboratory capabilities, and facilities with equipment. As a consequence, care is being regionalized; that is, all levels of care will be available within a given area, but facilities will be organized to provide different levels of care. A coordinated system within a region first requires the designation of certain hospitals for provisions of levels of care based on their capacity to provide the care required. To provide appropriate services and continuity of care for each client, an effective pattern of communication for consultation and for transport of clients is mandatory. Fundamental to all these activities is a regional program for continuing education of personnel.

Ideally, a regionalized system includes primary care and three levels of facilities within a designated geographic area. Level I facilities have three main functions: (1) the management of normal pregnancy, labor, and delivery, (2) the earliest possible identification of high-risk pregnancy and high-risk neonates, and (3) the provision of component care in the event of unanticipated obstetric or neonatal emergencies.

Level II facilities provide care for a number of maternal and neonatal complications, as well as offer a full range of maternity and neonatal care in uncomplicated cases.

Level II facilities provide care for a number of maternal and neonatal complications, as well as offer a full range of maternity and neonatal care in uncomplicated cases.

Level III facilities, the **regional centers**, have the capacity to manage the most complex disorders, as well as uncomplicated maternity and neonatal cases. In addition, the regional centers provide outreach services; for example, consultation and continuing education for obstetricians, pediatricians, and nurses within the region.

INTERVIEW AND PHYSICAL EXAMINATION

Serious biologic handicaps, health problems, obstetric disorders, and social deprivation may compromise the mother and the infant in subtle or more obvious ways. Early or late fetal damage may occur. The baby may be small for gestational age (SGA), preterm, or postterm. Occasionally the infant may be preterm but of excessive size; that is, large for gestational age (LGA). In other instances the postterm infant is large. Such hazards and their management are unique perinatal problems.

Research and experience have led to the identification of factors that jeopardize the pregnant and postdelivery woman and the fetus-neonate. This knowledge has permitted the development of increasingly effective preventive and therapeutic measures that can minimize the incidence of morbidity, disability, and death of the mother or infant. Commonly it is the alert nurse, conversant and familiar with deviations from normal, who notes and reports potential or real high-risk factors (Tables 27-2 and 27-3 and boxes, p. 660 and p. 661). The interrelationship of risk factors that influence pregnancy outcome are summarized schematically in Fig. 27-1, p. 661.

Text continued on p. 660.

Table 27-2 *Factors that Place the Pregnancy and Fetus-neonate at High Risk by Trimester and During Labor*

Category	Factors that Result in Risk
First Trimester	
Anatomic	Maternal
	Ectopic pregnancy
	Uterine abnormality
	Retroversion of uterus
Physiologic	Fetal
	Gross chromosomal defect
	Hydatidiform mole
	Multiple pregnancy
	Poor trophoblast invasiveness
	Folate deficiency
	Endocrine deficiency
	Hyperemesis gravidarum
	Defective sperm
Psychologic	Psychologic shock
	Drugs
Therapeutic	Elective abortion (aspiration, saline solution, prostaglandin) before this pregnancy
	Drug therapy
	X-ray therapy
Infection	Viral infection
Genetic	Sporadic mutation
	Inherited characteristics
	Sex-linked disease
Environmental	Poverty
	Drugs, tobacco, alcohol
	Inadequate nutrition
Second Trimester	
Anatomic	Maternal
	Uterine abnormality
	Incompetent cervical os
	Fetal
	Gross abnormality
	Acute hydramnios
	Multiple pregnancy
	Poor implantation
Maternal complications	Rh incompatibility
	Cyanotic heart disease
	Hypertension
	Renal disease
	Urinary tract infections
	Accidents
	Anoxia of hypertensive disease or epilepsy
Infections	Polio, syphilis, hepatitis, TORCH,† AIDS
Genetic	Amniocentesis
Environmental	Poverty, drugs, tobacco, alcohol
	Inadequate nutrition
Third Trimester	
Anatomic	Malpresentation
	Cord complications
	Placenta previa*
Maternal complications	Hypertensive disease*
	Rh incompatibilities
	Diabetes
	Thyrotoxicosis
Infections	Viral infection*
	Pneumonia
Nutritional	Protein lack
	Iron deficiencies
	Abruptio placentae*
Therapeutic to mother	Antibacterial drugs
	Tetracycline
	Antithyroid drugs
	Corticosteroids
	Anticonvulsants
	Anticoagulants
Fetal complications	Premature rupture of membranes
	Preterm labor; postmaturity
	Hydramnios or oligohydramnios
	Multiple gestation
Environmental	Poverty
	Drugs, tobacco, alcohol
	Inadequate nutrition
Labor	
Anatomic	Fetal head compression
	Malpresentation
	Umbilical cord prolapse
	Breech presentation
	Placenta previa; abruptio placentae
	Rigid soft tissues
	Multiple gestation
	Placental or umbilical cord compression
	Excessive or inadequate fetal size
Physiologic	Dehydration
	Ketosis
	Fetal acidosis (pH 7.25 or less in the first stage of labor)
	Meconium staining of amniotic fluid
	Fetal bradycardia or tachycardia (longer than 30 minutes)
	Abnormal nonstress test or oxytocin challenge test
	Falling urinary estriol levels
	Immature fetal lungs
	Severe preeclampsia-eclampsia
Maternal complications, iatrogenic	Sedative depression
	Hypotension; anesthesia; supine position
	Oxytocin (Pitocin) augmentation or induction of labor
	Prolonged labor; precipitous labor (less than 3 hours)
	Operative delivery: cesarean, forceps, vacuum extraction
Uterine and placental	Uterine hypotonicity, hypertonicity, inertia
	Placental insufficiency

Modified from Fogel, CI, and Woods, NF: Health care of women: a nursing perspective, St Louis, 1981, The CV Mosby Co.
*Associated with intrauterine growth retardation (IUGR).
†Toxoplasmosis, rubella, cytomegalovirus, and herpes simplex.

Table 27-3 *Psychosocial Perinatal Warning Indicators for Families at High Risk for Abnormal Parenting Practices**

Pregnancy	Labor and Delivery	Postpartum
Parents' Physical and Psychologic Well-Being		
Pregnancy is perceived as very difficult or burdensome Mother feels her health will suffer from childbearing or child rearing Mother intellectually subnormal Mother shows great depression over pregnancy Mother persists in feeling frightened and alone, especially before delivery; careful explanations do not dissipate the fear Excessive visits for health care or expresses multiple psychosomatic complaints Evidence of emotional instability or mental illness History of drug or alcohol abuse Child wanted to fill unmet need in parents' lives Evidence of low self-esteem ("I'm no good"), particularly re parenting ability Mother aged under 20 years Previous pregnancy terminating in spontaneous abortion, fetal or neonatal death, or birth of a damaged child History of previous child's death or removal from home because of abuse or neglect	Mother experiencing excessive discomfort, fatigue, drug effects, or physical complications immediately following delivery Mother or father perceive labor or delivery as traumatic or unsatisfactory Obvious lack of supportive interaction between couple Hostile interaction between couple	Mother does not see attention focused on infant as something positive for herself Mother bothered by infant's crying; makes her feel helpless, hopeless, or unloved Mother relinquishes control to doctors and nurses for meeting needs of infant Evidence of low self-esteem ("I'm no good"), especially re parenting ability Parents express excessive feelings of failure re performance during labor or delivery Parents express resentment or anger toward infant over childbirth experience Express excessive doubt re ability to care for infant
Characteristics of Child	Premature Physically or mentally defective Immature or defective reflex behaviors Unresponsive Condition necessitates separation from parents "Wrong" sex Looks or behavior perceived in negative way by parents	As in column 2 Perceived by parent as being different or "not normal" despite normal findings Sex of infant remains unacceptable to parent Denies or exaggerates handicapped infant's capabilities Difficult feeder Unresponsive, i.e., sleepy baby Irritable or difficult to console Hyperreflexive infant Rigid or noncuddly infant
Parent-child Attachment		
Pregnancy unplanned or unwanted Parents considered abortion or relinquishment Denial of pregnancy, i.e., unwilling to gain weight, refusal to talk about pregnancy	Mother looks distressed, disappointed Does not talk to infant in affectionate terms Makes negative or hostile remarks to infant Expresses disappointment with sex of infant	Does not comfort infant when crying and does not heed physical needs Appears apathetic toward or disinterested in infant Expresses excessive doubt about ability to care for infant Remains disappointed over sex of infant
In advanced pregnancy, mother dresses and acts as though she is not pregnant Absent or disturbed response to quickening Mother perceives fetal movement as abusive or aggressive actions Mother reports an experience she fears will damage baby (i.e., a "scare," accident, etc.) Undue concern re infant's sex or performance Absence of any fantasies about what baby will be like or predominantly negative fantasies Mother attributes negative characteristics to fetus	Mother makes inappropriate verbalizations, glances, or disparaging remarks about or toward infant Avoids eye contact and direct *en face* position Mother does not hold, touch, or examine infant Mother handles infant in rough manner	Frequently voices negative feelings about or toward infant Repelled by messiness and diaper changing Negative identification of infant by name or association with someone disliked No feelings of attachment toward infant after 1 month Mother does not appear to enjoy playing with infant

Modified from Ledger, KE, and Williams, DL: Parents at risk: an instructional program for perinatal assessment and preventive intervention, Victoria, BC, Canada, 1981, Ministry of Health and Queen Alexandra Solarium for Crippled Children Society.

*It must be noted that it is not merely the presence or number of warning indicators that signify a high-risk situation. It is the unique combination of these indicators and their degree of expression in each individual family situation that is of importance. Factors such as culture, educational level, age of parents, receptiveness to change, etc. *must* be taken into consideration.

Table 27-3 *Psychosocial Perinatal Warning Indicators for Families at High Risk for Abnormal Parenting Practices*—cont'd*

Pregnancy	Labor and Delivery	Postpartum
Apparent lack of concern for physical well-being of unborn fetus, as evidenced by refusal to make health and life-style changes (i.e., poor nutrition, excessive use of drugs and alcohol, etc.) Absence of "nesting" behavior in the third trimester (i.e., preparation of clothing, equipment, space for infant)		
Parenting Knowledge, Beliefs, and Expectations		
Perceive own upbringing as abusive or neglectful Experienced harsh physical punishment during childhood Express belief that physical force is necessary in rearing and disciplining children Express a strong desire to parent in manner different from own parents Express inaccurate knowledge of infant care and development Express rigid or unrealistic expectations for infant re physical characteristics, behavior, development, etc.		As in column 1 Unaware of infant's characteristics and ability See infant as demanding or manipulative Inadequate preparation for child rearing Express expectations developmentally far beyond infant's capabilities Express fear of "spoiling" the infant
Support Systems		
No spouse, mate, or significant other Express dissatisfaction with spouse or mate relationship Chronic marital discord, especially if focus of conflict is around childbearing or child rearing Chronic conflict with or alienation from one's own mother or other female relatives History of loss of mother's own mother before her own puberty Mate or family's reaction to pregnancy is negative or nonsupportive Lack or loss of support systems, i.e., no supportive friends or relatives nearby Show evidence of social isolation, i.e., no phone, outside interests, use of community resources	Mother expresses hostility toward father, who "put her through all this" As in column 1	As in column 1
Family Circumstances		
Parent seems unaware or denies impact of new baby on relationship with mate, own time, other siblings Express concern that this child is going to be "one too many" Inadequate housing for family's needs Children too closely spaced Recent death or loss of loved one Have recently moved Financial, health, social, or interpersonal problems in the family Parents describe stresses of chaotic nature (i.e., physical fights, heavy drinking, and arguments among immediate family members, abandonment by mate, etc.) Parents exhibit few skills for dealing with stress Express inability to cope with present life circumstances Dissatisfied with career or career change	As in column 1	As in column 1

CATEGORIES OF HIGH-RISK PREGNANCY

Maternal Age and Parity Factors

1. Age 16 years or under
2. Nullipara 35 years or over
3. Multipara 40 years or over
4. Interval of 8 years or more since last pregnancy
5. High parity (5 or more)
6. Pregnancy occurring 3 months or less after last delivery

Nonmarital Pregnancy

PIH, Hypertension, Kidney Disease

1. Preeclampsia with hospitalization before labor
2. Eclampsia
3. Kidney disease—pyelonephritis, nephritis, nephrosis, etc.
4. Chronic hypertension, severe (160/100 mm Hg or over)
5. Blood pressure 140/90 mm Hg or above on 2 readings 30 minutes apart

Anemia and Hemorrhage

1. Hematocrit 30% or below in pregnancy
2. Hemorrhage (previous pregnancy)—severe, requiring transfusion
3. Hemorrhage (present pregnancy)
4. Anemia (hemoglobin below 10 g) for which treatment other than oral iron preparations is required (hemolytic, macrocytic, etc.)
5. Sickle cell trait or disease
6. History of bleeding or clotting disorder at any time

Fetal Factors

1. Two or more previous premature deliveries (twins = one delivery)
2. Two or more consecutive spontaneous abortions (miscarriages)
3. One or more stillbirths at term
4. One or more gross anomalies
5. Rh incompatibility or ABO immunization problems
6. History of previous birth defects—cerebral palsy, brain damage, mental retardation, metabolic disorders such as phenylketonuria (PKU)
7. History of large infants (over 4032 g [9 lb])

Paternal Age (?) and Other Factors (?)

Dystocia (History of or Anticipated)

1. Contracted pelvis or cephalopelvic disproportion (CPD)
2. Multiple pregnancy in current pregnancy
3. Two or more breech deliveries
4. Previous operative deliveries, e.g., cesarean or midforceps delivery
5. History of prolonged labor (more than 18 hours for nullipara; more than 12 hours for multipara)
6. Previously diagnosed genital tract anomalies (incompetent cervix, cervical or uterine malformation, solitary ovary or tube) or problem (ovarian mass, endometriosis)
7. Short stature (1.5 m [60 in] or less)

History of or Concurrent Conditions

1. Diabetes mellitus; gestational diabetes
2. Hyperemesis gravidarum
3. Thyroid disease (hypothyroidism or hyperthyroidism)
4. Malnutrition or extreme obesity (20% over ideal weight for height; 15% under ideal weight for height)
5. Organic heart disease
6. Syphilis and TORCH infections: toxoplasmosis, rubella in first 10 weeks of *this* pregnancy, cytomegalovirus (CMV), and herpes simplex; AIDS
7. Tuberculosis or other serious pulmonary pathologic condition (e.g., emphysema, asthma)
8. Malignant or premalignant tumors (including hydatidiform mole)
9. Alcoholism, drug addiction
10. Psychiatric disease or epilepsy (documented)
11. Mental retardation

Those with Previous History of

1. Late registration
2. Poor clinic attendance
3. Home situation making clinic attendance and hospitalization difficult
4. Mothers, including minors, without family resources (including desertions, adoptions, injuries, separations, family withdrawals, sole support)

Modified from Fogel, CI, and Woods, NF: Health care of women: a nursing perspective, St Louis, 1981, The CV Mosby Co.

DIAGNOSTIC TECHNIQUES

Ultrasonography

When directional beams of sound strike an object, an echo is returned. The time delay between the emission of the sound and the return of the echo is noted, as well as the direction from which the echo comes. From these data the object's distance and location can be calculated. Sonar (underwater) and radar (air) are familiar uses of very high frequency sound.

First introduced in the 1960s, diagnostic ultrasound has developed rapidly to enjoy a principal position in medical imaging today. Ultrasound is sound having a frequency higher than that of normal human hearing. The range of human hearing extends from 20 Hz to 20 kHz (20,000 Hz). Bats and some insects use ultrasound in the range of about 100 kHz to navigate. Diagnostic ultrasound is beyond audible range but well below that used by sonar and radar. Medical diagnostic ultrasound covers the range from approximately 1 to 10 MHz; 2.25 MHz (2,250,000 Hz) is generally used in obstetric and gynecologic imaging.

The biophysical principles of diagnostic ultrasound are beyond the scope of this text, but several excellent resources are available. See references and bibliography at the end of this chapter.

Operational Modes. Table 27-4 presents a summary of modalities, imaging, and principal uses of diagnostic ultra-

FACTORS THAT PLACE THE POSTPARTUM WOMAN AND NEONATE AT RIGH RISK

Specific factors that place **mother in high-risk** category:

1. Hemorrhage
2. Infection
3. Abnormal vital signs
4. Traumatic labor or delivery
5. Psychosocial factors

Criteria for selection of high-risk infants for admission to neonatal intensive care units:

1. Specific factors that place **infant in high-risk** category:
   a. Infants continuing or developing signs of respiratory distress syndrome (RDS) or other respiratory distress
   b. Asphyxiated infants (Apgar score of less than 6 at 5 minutes); resuscitation required at birth
   c. Preterm infants; dysmature infants
   d. Infants with cyanosis or suspected cardiovascular disease; persistent cyanosis
   e. Infants with major congenital malformations requiring surgery; chromosomal anomalies
   f. Infants with convulsions, sepsis, hemorrhagic diathesis, or shock
   g. Meconium aspiration syndrome
   h. Central nervous system (CNS) depression for longer than 24 hours
   i. Hypoglycemia
   j. Hypocalcemia
   k. Hyperbilirubinemia
2. Factors indicating **moderate-risk**:
   a. Dysmaturity
   b. Prematurity (weight between 2000 and 2500 g)
   c. Apgar score of less than 5 at 1 minute
   d. Feeding problems
   e. Multiple birth
   f. Transient tachypnea
   g. Hypomagnesemia or hypermagnesemia
   h. Hypoparathyroidism
   i. Failure to gain weight
   j. Jitteriness or hyperactivity
   k. Cardiac anomalies not requiring immediate catheterization
   l. Heart murmur
   m. Anemia
   n. Central nervous system depression for less than 24 hours

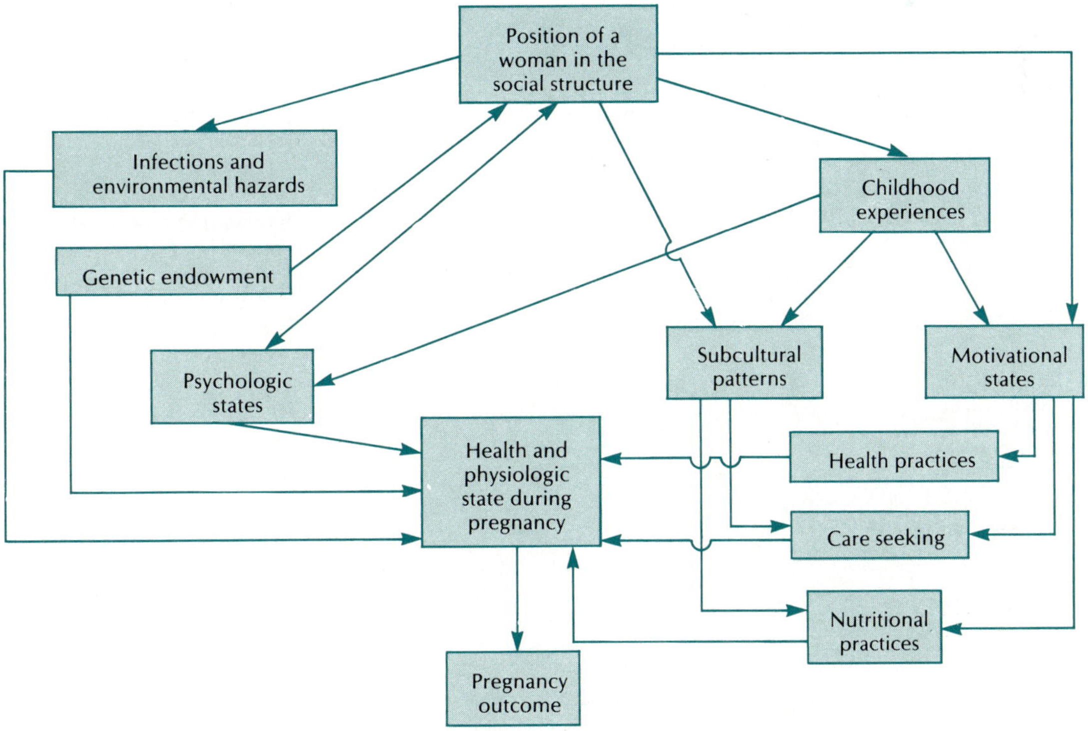

Fig. 27-1 Summary of risk factors that may affect pregnancy outcome.
From Fogel, CI, and Woods, DF: Health care of women, St Louis, 1981, The CV Mosby Co.

Table 27-4 *Diagnostic Ultrasound: Operational Modes†*

Modality	Product	Principal Use
Pulsed wave*	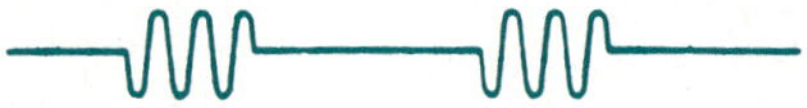	
A mode	Static image	Diagnostic evaluation of brain
B mode (gray scale)†	Static image	Images of abdominal and pelvic structures
M mode	Dynamic imaging	Monitoring of heart and measuring of heart wall displacement
Real time†	Static image and dynamic imaging	Provides dynamic imaging and static images
Continuous wave	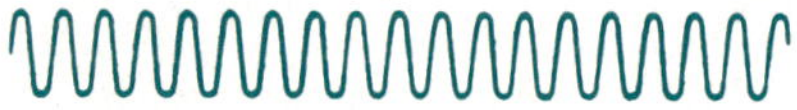	
Doppler mode†	Ranging mode	Fetal heart monitoring

*Pulsed wave—sound emitted at intervals; continuous wave—sound emitted continuously; A mode—one-dimensional image that appears as spikes on a horizontal base; distance between spikes can be measured (e.g., biparietal diameter [BPD]; B mode (gray scale)—rough, two-dimensional image of various tissue densities for visualizing tissue texture and contour; M mode—time-related tracings showing straight lines for motionless structures and wiggly lines for structural motion (e.g., atrial septal defects and patent ductus arteriosus); static—stationary; dynamic—moving; Doppler mode—detection of change in frequency (wavelength) of structures in motion (e.g., blood flow in umbilical cord and placenta, closure of fetal cardiac valves); real time—dynamic imaging (limb and respiratory movements), as well as static images (BPD, placental location).

†Used extensively in obstetrics and gynecology.

Table 27-5 *Major Indications for Obstetric Sonography*

First Trimester	Second Trimester	Third Trimester
Confirm pregnancy Confirm viability Rule out ectopic pregnancy Confirm gestational age* Birth control use Irregular menses No dates Postpartum pregnancy Previous complicated Pregnancy Caesarean delivery Rh incompatibility Diabetes mellitus Fetal growth retardation Clarify dates/sizes discrepancy Large for dates—rule out Leiomyomata Bicornuate uterus Adnexal mass Multiple gestation Poor dates Molar pregnancy Small for dates—rule out Poor dates Missed abortion Blighted ovum	Establish or confirm dates† If no fetal heart tones Clarify dates/size discrepancy Large for dates—rule out Poor estimate of dates Molar pregnancy Multiple gestation Leiomyomata Polyhydramnios Congenital anomalies Small for dates—rule out Poor estimate of dates Fetal growth retardation Congenital anomalies Oligohydramnios If history of bleeding—rule out total placenta previa If Rh incompatibility—rule out fetal hydrops	If no fetal heart tones Clarify dates/size discrepancy Large for dates—rule out Macrosomia (diabetes mellitus) Multiple gestation Polyhydramnios Congenital anomalies Poor estimate of dates‡ Small for dates—rule out Fetal growth retardation Oligohydramnios Congenital anomalies Poor estimate of dates‡ Determine fetal position—rule out Breech Transverse lie If history of bleeding—rule out Placenta previa Abruptio placentae Determine fetal lung maturity Amniocentesis for lecithin/sphingomyelin ratio Placental maturity (grade 0-3) If Rh incompatibility—rule out fetal hydrops

From Athey, PA, and Hadlock, FP: Ultrasound in obstetrics and gynecology, ed 2, St Louis, 1985, The CV Mosby Co.

*Accuracy ± 3 days.

†Accuracy ± 1 to 1½ weeks.

‡Accuracy only ± 3 weeks.

sound. Static image scanners are useful for gynecologic, as well as obstetric diagnosis. Dynamic image scanners provide direct visualization of indicators of fetal viability—fetal cardiac and body movement. The usual examination takes only about 5 minutes. Since the scanner can be moved about, it can be taken directly into labor and delivery rooms for directing amniocentesis or evaluating the source of vaginal bleeding.

Current Applications in Pregnancy. Major indications for obstetric sonography by trimester appear in Table 27-5. During the **first trimester,** ultrasound examination is performed to obtain the following information: (1) number, size, and location of gestational sacs (Fig. 27-2), (2) presence or absence of fetal cardiac and body movement, (3) presence or absence of uterine abnormalities (e.g., bicornuate uterus, fibroids) or adnexal masses (e.g., ovarian cysts, ectopic pregnancy), (4) pregnancy dating (e.g., biparietal diameter [BPD], crown-rump length), and (5) coexistence and location of an intrauterine device (IUD).

During the **second** and **third trimesters** the following information is sought: (1) fetal viability, number, position, gestational age, growth pattern, and anomalies, (2) amniotic fluid volume, (3) placental location and maturity, (4) uterine fibroids and anomalies, and (5) adnexal masses. An example of the application of the findings is presented in Table 27-6. In general, the use of ultrasound has hastened diagnoses so that appropriate therapy can be instituted early in the pregnancy. Early therapy may decrease the severity and duration of morbidity, both physical and emotional of the mother (family). Early diagnosis of fetal anomaly, for instance, makes possible choices such as (1) intrauterine surgery or other therapy for the fetus, (2) discontinuation of the pregnancy, and (3) preparation of the family for the care of a child with a disorder or planning for placement of child after birth.

Findings

Fetal Viability. Fetal heart activity can be demonstrated as early as 6 to 7 weeks by real-time echo scanners and at 10 to 12 weeks by Doppler mode. This information assists in management when the woman experiences vaginal bleeding; incomplete, complete, and missed abortion can be differentiated. By 9 to 10 weeks, molar pregnancy can be diagnosed as a missed abortion (Fig. 27-3).

Gestational Age. Not all women are candidates for the use of ultrasound to determine gestational age. Several indicators have been established for need. Indications for ultrasonographic estimation of fetal age include (1) uncertain dates for the last menstrual period or last normal menstrual period, (2) recent discontinuation of oral hormonal suppression of ovulation (birth control pills), (3) bleeding episode during the first trimester, (4) amenorrhea of at least 3 months' duration, (5) uterine size that does not agree with dates, (6) previous cesarean birth, and (7) other high-risk conditions. Four methods of estimation of fetal age are used: (1) determination of gestational sac dimensions (about 8 weeks), (2) measurement of crown-rump length (between 7 and 14 weeks), (3) measurement of femur length (after 12 weeks), and (4) measurement of the BPD (starting at about 12 weeks).

Fetal BPD at 36 weeks should be approximately 8.7 cm. Term pregnancy and fetal maturity can be diagnosed with some confidence if the biparietal cephalometry by ultrasonography is greater than 9.8 cm (Fig. 27-4 and Table 27-7).

Table 27-6 *Application of Sonography During Pregnancy*

Condition	Sonographic Evidence	Intervention
Impending abortion (before eighth menstrual week)	Poorly formed or "sagging" gestational sac	Eliminate time trying to save pregnancy; possibly decrease blood loss and sequelae of blood loss or of treatment for blood loss
Fetal death (after eighth menstrual week)	No cardiac activity	Empty uterus before development of *retained dead fetus syndrome*
Ectopic pregnancy	Adnexal mass	Early surgical intervention to prevent emergency situation
Molar pregnancy	"Snow storm" appearance within enlarged uterus (Fig. 27-3)	Terminate pregnancy to decrease morbidity from preeclampsia and begin surveillance of hCG* levels
Developmental uterine abnormalities	Resembles coexistent solid neoplasm; variable appearance	Avoid misdiagnosis with inappropriate therapy; provide time to consider type of delivery
IUD (not a rare occurrence)	Locate site Imbedded in myometrial wall apart from gestational sac and placenta	Pregnancy usually goes to term with no IUD-related problem
	Located partially or totally within gestational sac or within placenta	Pregnancy usually ends in spontaneous abortion and may be associated with generalized sepsis

*Human chorionic gonadotropin.

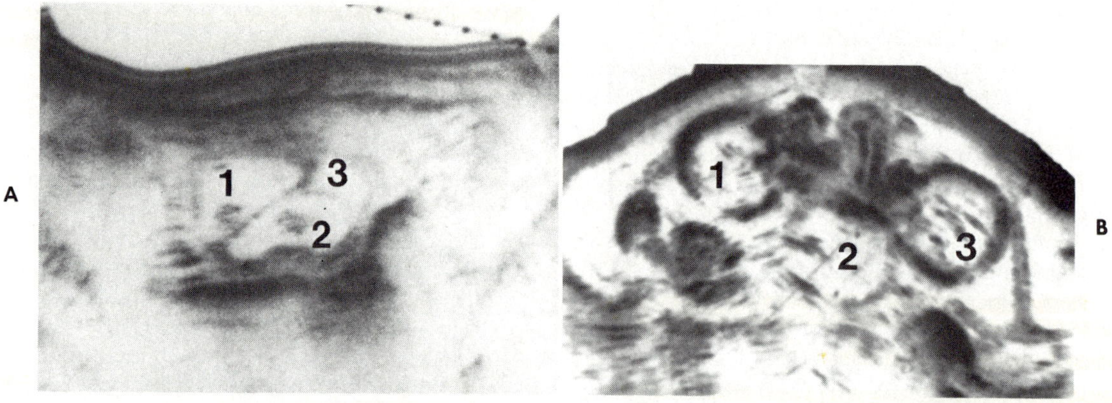

Fig. 27-2 A, Transverse static image scan demonstrates three well-formed gestational sacs. B, Subsequent static image scan demonstrates three well-defined fetal heads in this woman carrying triplets.
From Athey, PA, and Hadlock, FP: Ultrasound in obstetrics and gynecology, ed 2, St Louis, 1985, The CV Mosby Co.

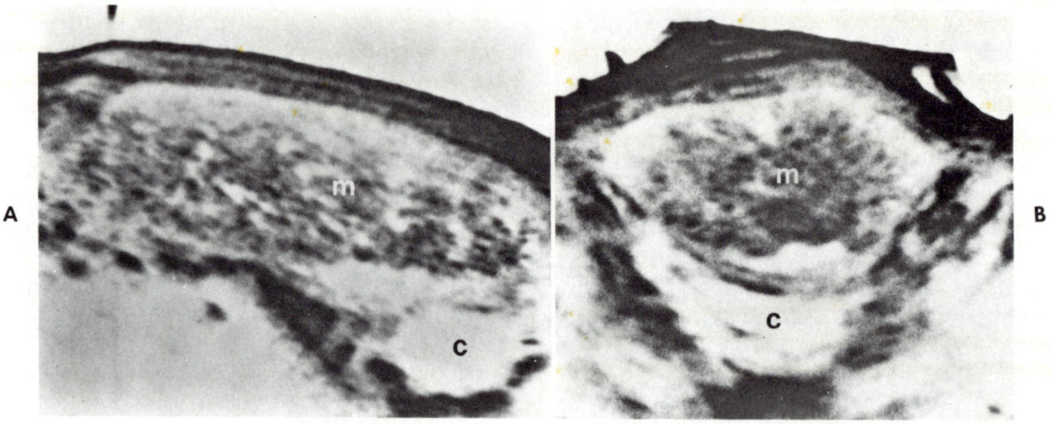

Fig. 27-3 A, Longitudinal and B, transverse scans of molar pregnancy *(m)*. Note typical vesicular (grape-like) pattern. Also demonstrated are multiloculated lutein ovarian cysts *(c)* in cul-de-sac.
From Athey, PA, and Hadlock, FP: Ultrasound in obstetrics and gynecology, ed 2, St Louis, 1985, The CV Mosby Co.

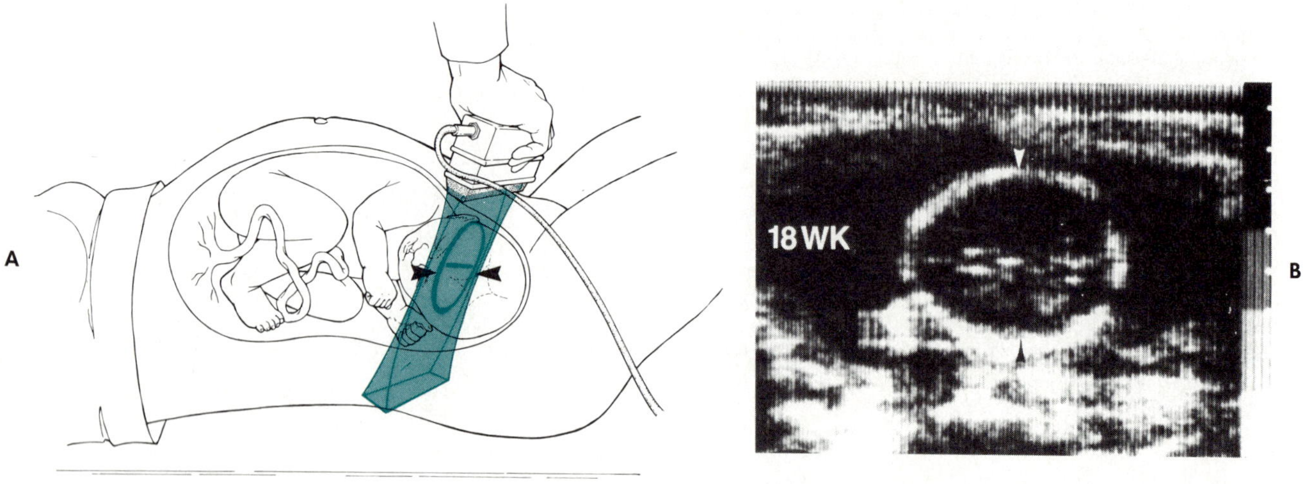

Fig. 27-4 A, Biparietal (arrow) cephalometry by ultrasound. B, Linear-array, real-time image demonstrates fetal BPD *(arrow)* at 18 weeks.
B, From Athey, PA, and Hadlock, FP: Ultrasound in obstetrics and gynecology, ed 2, St Louis, 1985, The CV Mosby Co.

Table 27-7 *Correlation of Fetal Weight and BPD*

BPD (cm)	Estimated Fetal Weight
8.2	2290 g (5 lb, 1 oz)
8.5	2500 g (5 lb, 8 oz)
8.8	2730 g (6 lb, 0 oz)
9.4	3180 g (7 lb, 0 oz)
10.0	3630 g (8 lb, 0 oz)
10.6	4070 g (9 lb, 0 oz)

Fetal Growth. Fetal growth may be jeopordized under certain conditions. Some of the conditions that serve as indicators for ultrasound assessment of fetal growth include the following: poor maternal weight gain or pattern of weight gain; previous **intrauterine growth retardation (IUGR)**; chronic infections (especially urinary tract infections); ingestion of drugs such as anticonvulsants or heroin; maternal diabetes mellitus, pregnancy-induced or other hypertension; multiple pregnancy; and other medical or surgical complications. Serial evaluations of BPD and limb length can differentiate between wrong dates and true IUGR. IUGR may be symmetric (the fetus is small in all parameters) or asymmetric (head and body growth vary). Symmetric IUGR may be caused by low genetic growth potential, intrauterine infection, maternal undernutrition or heavy smoking, or chromosomal aberration. Asymmetric IUGR may reflect placental insufficiency secondary to hypertension, renal disease, or cardiovascular disease. Therapy varies with the probable cause.

The BPD, head circumference, abdominal circumference, and estimated fetal weight for a normal 32-week fetus are illustrated in Fig. 27-5.

Adjunct to Amniocentesis. The safety of amniocentesis is increased when the physician knows the exact position of the fetus, placenta, and pockets of amniotic fluid. Ultrasonography has greatly reduced previous risks associated with amniocentesis.

Fetal Anatomy. Depending on the gestational age, the following structures may be identified: head (including ventricles and blood vessels), neck, spine, heart, stomach, small bowel, liver, kidneys, bladder and limbs. Structural defects may be identified before delivery. Advances in technology may make fetal surgery and genetic engineering a reality for many conditions in the next few years.

Placental Position and Function. The pattern of uterine and placental growth and the fullness of the bladder influence the apparent location of the placenta. During the first trimester, differentiation of the endometrium and the small placenta is difficult and adds to the difficulty of performing an amniocentesis. During the middle of the second trimester the placenta can be clearly defined, but if it is seen to be low lying, its relationship to the internal cervical os can sometimes be altered dramatically by changing the *degree of fullness of the maternal bladder.* In approximately 15% to 20% of all pregnancies in which ultrasound scanning is done in the second trimester, the placenta seems to be overlying the os; at term the incidence of placenta previa is only 0.5%. Three factors may be responsible for the seeming "migration" of the placenta: (1) the maternal bladder can distort the uterine cavity, (2) the lower uterine segment elongates as pregnancy progresses, and (3) poor imaging or misinterpretation of the image can result in an inappropriate diagnosis. The diagnosis of *placenta previa* can seldom be confirmed until the third trimester.

Fetal Well-being. Among the many physiologic measurements that can be accomplished with ultrasound are the following: heart motion, beat-to-beat variability, fetal breathing movements (FBMs), fetal urine production (following serial measurements of bladder volume), fetal limb and head movements, and analysis of vascular waveforms from the fetal circulation (McCallum, 1984). It has been noted that FBMs are decreased with maternal smoking and alcohol ingestion and increased with hyperglycemia. Fetal limb and head movements serve as an index of neurologic development.

Biophysical Profile. Manning, Platt, and Supos (1980) used dynamic ultrasound imaging to evaluate fetal health by observing 5 variables for approximately 30 minutes: FBMs; fetal body movements; fetal tone (shown, for example, when the fetus exhibits extension of any extremity with quick return to the flexed position); amniotic fluid volume; and response to nonstress testing. Findings from the assessment of these variables comprise the fetal biophysical profile (Manning, Platt, and Supos, 1980; Manning et al., 1985; Dauphinee, 1987). A score of 2 is assigned to each variable that is present. A significantly greater perinatal mortality was seen in fetuses and neonates who had scored less than 6 compared with those with higher scores (Manning, Platt, and Supos, 1980; Danforth and Scott, 1986).

Preparation of the Woman. The woman is directed to come for the examination with a full bladder.* The full bladder supports the uterus in position for the imaging. If her bladder is empty, the test may be delayed for about 1 hour until she is able to fill her bladder; it takes only a few moments to empty the bladder if this is needed for the examination. The woman is positioned comfortably with small pillows under her head and knees. The display panel should be positioned so that the woman can observe the images on the screen if she wishes (Fig 27-6). Some women do *not* want to watch.

Safety of the Diagnostic Ultrasound. Biologic effects of extremely high intensities of sound persisting over long periods of time can result in (1) *thermal* changes within the cells, (2) *cavitation,* or formation of tiny gas bubbles that can lead to rupture of cell membranes, and (3) *viscous* stresses. However, no biologic damage has been measured at ultrasonic intensity of less than 100 mW/cm^2, even for extended periods of exposure time. Diagnostic ultrasonic beams all have intensities less than 10 mW/cm^2 and are applied for relatively short periods of time (Athey and Hadlock, 1985).

*Directions for transvaginal ultrasound vary (see Chapter 44); Modica and Timor-Tritsch, 1988.

There is no conclusive evidence that humans have been harmed by diagnostic ultrasound during the 20 years it has been used. No detrimental effects have been observed to date on the fetus or mother either histologically, functionally, or embryologically in experimental work; however, there is a hypothetical risk that cannot be ignored or overlooked. Benefit must be weighed against hypothetical risk. Gravidas should be informed of the clinical indication for ultrasound, specific benefit, potential risk, and alternatives, if any. In addition, a record should be kept of the exposure time, mode, and ultrasound frequency.

Magnetic Resonance Imaging

Magnetic resonance imaging (MRI) is a noninvasive tool that can be used for obstetric and gynecologic diagnosis. In a relatively brief time, MRI has progressed from a primitive imaging modality to one whose image quality and diagnostic abilities rival or surpass all other imaging procedures (Kanal and Wolf, 1986). Like computerized tomography (CT), MRI provides excellent pictures of soft tissue; unlike CT, ionizing radiation is not used. After MRI signals are generated and analyzed, they are displayed on an oscilloscope screen.

In utero imaging during first-, second-, and third-trimester pregnancies in Europe has produced excellent visualization of fetal anatomy. Direct scanning of the placenta with or without paramagnetic contrast agents may further increase the capacity to evaluate placental positioning or fetal maturity. In North America, most MRI has been confined to second- or third-trimester pregnancies because of unproved concerns about the effects of this modality on fetal development. Fetal growth and fetal subcutaneous fat thickness can be directly measured, and studies are being

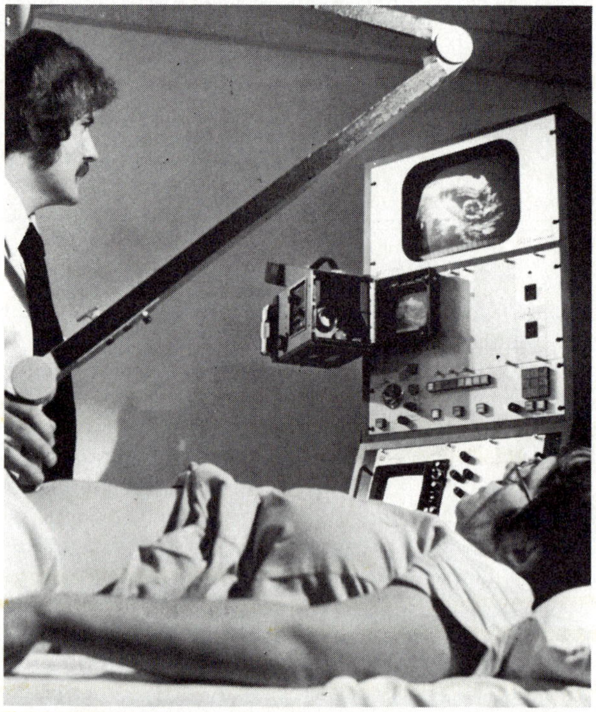

Fig. 27-6 Ultrasonography.
Courtesy March of Dimes.

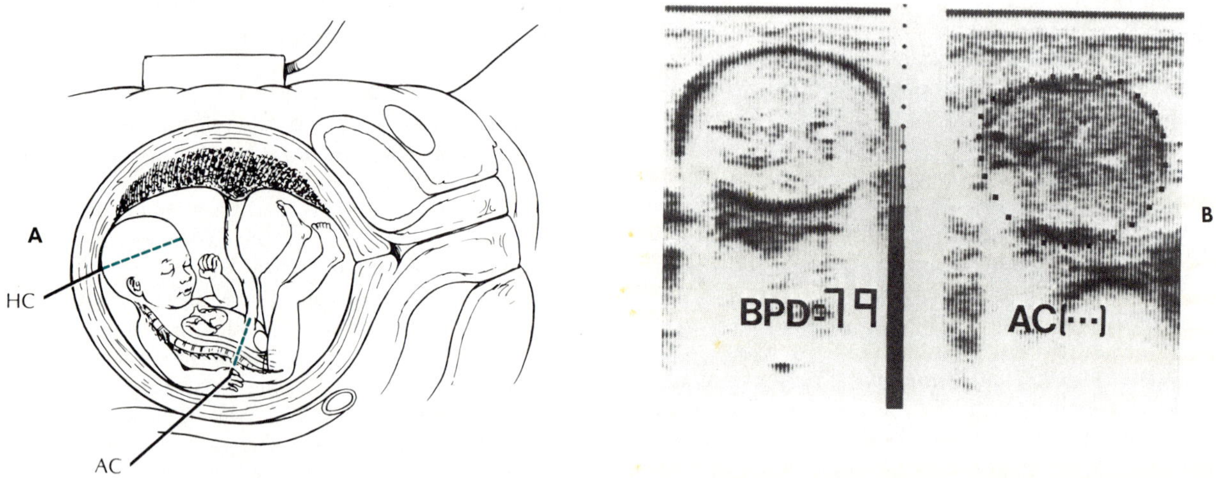

Fig. 27-5 **A**, Schematic presentation of appropriate planes of sections *(dotted lines)* for BPD, head circumference *(HC),* and abdominal circumference *(AC).* **B**, Real-time ultrasound image demonstrates typical head and body images that correspond to planes in **A**. Using these two images, one can determine BPD (7.9 cm), HC (30 cm), AC (28 cm), and estimated fetal weight *(EFW)* (1840 g) in this normal 32-week fetus.
From Athey, PA, and Hadlock, FP: Ultrasound in obstetrics and gynecology, ed 2, St Louis, 1985, The CV Mosby Co.

performed to assess a possible role for MRI in such disorders as intrauterine fetal growth retardation (Kanal and Wolf, 1986).

Fetoscopy

Direct visualization of the fetus is possible with fetoscopy via a tiny telescope-like instrument with the caliber of a large hypodermic needle. The fetoscope is introduced into the uterus through the abdominal wall with the woman under local anesthesia. This method is not used extensively because there is a risk of causing premature labor. The fetoscope is most often used to obtain fetal blood samples for diagnosing serious hereditary blood disorders (e.g., sickle cell anemia). Risks to the fetus from fetoscopy range from 3% to 5% (Goldberg, 1987).

Percutaneous Umbilical Cord Blood Sampling

In percutaneus umbilical cord blood sampling (PUBS), the placenta and cord insertion site are localized with a high-resolution sector ultrasound scanner after 18 weeks' gestation. Mother (and fetus) is anesthetized with intravenous (IV) sedation. A local anesthetic is used at the insertion site. A long (9 cm [3½ in]) spinal needle is used to obtain 1 to 2 ml of heparinized fetal blood for analysis. Indications include the need for chromosomal analysis and indentification of hemoglobinopathies, coagulopathies, and intrauterine infections. Current complications include fetal loss, prematurity, and infection; no statistics are available. Anticipated future use includes assessment of fetal well-being and fetal therapy such as intrauterine transfusion (Goldberg, 1987).

Amnioscopy

Fetal hypoxia is known to result in meconium passage by the mature fetus. Transcervical visualization of greenish amniotic fluid through the intact membranes (amnioscopy) indicates fetal asphyxia. Unfortunately, since the cervix must be more than 1 cm dilated and special equipment (amnioscope with tungsten lamp) is needed, this technique is used rarely.

Roentgenography

A special x-ray technique, termed *amniography* or *fetography,* allows visualization of gross structural abnormalities during the third trimester. There has been little experience with its use in early pregnancy. The procedure involves the instillation of a radiocontrast medium into the amniotic fluid. The medium adheres to fetal skin to produce a clear fetal silhouette on the x-ray film.

The presence of distal femoral ossification centers indicates a fetal age of 36 weeks. If the proximal tibial centers are present, the fetus has reached 40 weeks' gestational age. X-ray visualization of the distal femoral and proximal tibial epiphyseal centers also indicates term pregnancy. This procedure is used with great caution because of the danger of fetal and maternal gonadal damage. In addition, there is growing concern over the use of ionizing radiation because of potential carcinogenic, teratogenic, and mutagenic effects on developing embryonic or fetal tissues. Amniography and fetography (following injection of radiocontrast materials) may be indicated to detect fetal death or anomaly.

Chorionic Villi Sampling

Chorionic villi sampling (CVS) could partially replace amniocentesis for genetic diagnosis. Although there are risks to the fetus, the greatest advantage in this new technique is that genetic diagnosis can be moved ahead from the second to the first trimester—as early as the eighth week—and can produce results rapidly. This increases the potential for improving fetal treatment by allowing earlier intervention (Golbus, 1987). Earlier diagnosis also reduces a couple's waiting period, imposes less social and psychologic stress, permits the couple "privacy" because the pregnancy is not obvious as yet, and allows for an earlier and safer abortion if the couple so chooses.

This procedure is done between weeks 8 and 14 (Fig. 27-7) and involves the removal of a small tissue specimen from the fetal portion of the placenta. Since chorionic villi originate in the zygote, that tissue reflects the genetic makeup of the fetus. The specimen is removed either from the chorion frondosum or the chorion laeve.

Real-time ultrasound is used to guide the procedure. The aspiration cannula and obturator must negotiate the cervical canal, must be placed at a suitable site, and must avoid rupturing the amniotic sac.

Two other techniques used in CVS are direct vision biopsy using a hysteroscope and transabdominal aspiration guided by ultrasound. The magnitude of the risk in CVS is unknown, but the types of complications (e.g., spontaneous abortion, infection, hematoma, intrauterine death, growth retardation, rhesus isoimmunization, and trauma) are predictable. At present, if the risk of a fetal genetic disorder (e.g., hemoglobinopathies) is 25% or more, CVS is one possible diagnostic alternative.

Maternal Urine Assessments

Glucosuria, Acetonuria, and Proteinuria. See index for the pages in which these findings are discussed. See Appendix E for laboratory values.

Infection. Maternal and neonatal infection are discussed in Chapters 30 and 39.

Urinary Estriol Determinations. The steroid precursor produced by the fetal adrenals is synthesized into estriols in the placenta and is excreted by the mother's healthy kidneys. The estriol level in maternal urine (24-hour specimen) is an indicator of the normalcy of the fetoplacental unit. Estriol levels are elevated in multiple pregnancy, but they are extremely low in the presence of a failing pregnancy, anencephaly, or fetal death. Estriol levels fall in dysmaturity, PIH, complicated diabetes mellitus, and partial separation of the placenta. Serial estriol determinations

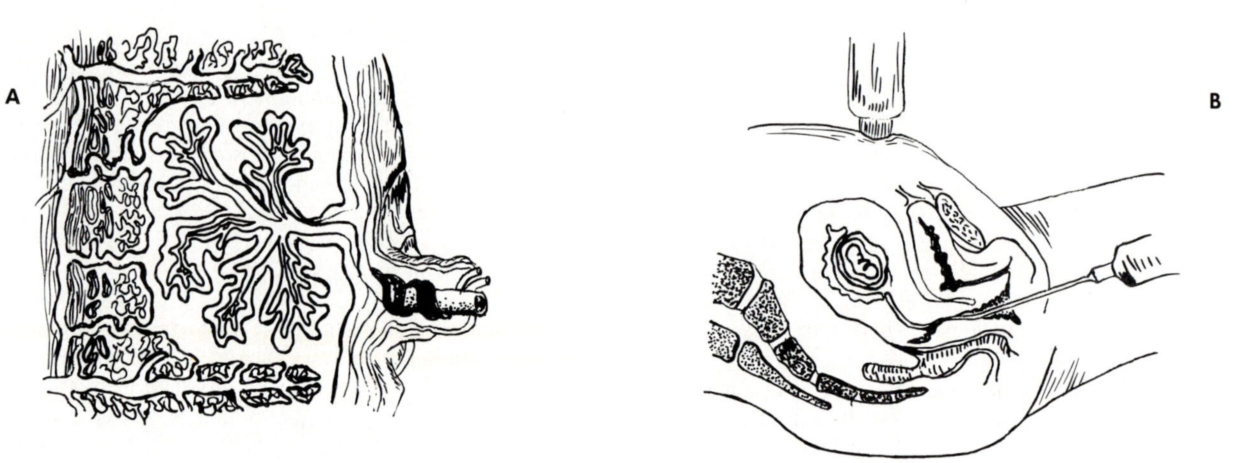

Fig. 27-7 Chorionic villi sampling. **A**, Chorionic villi at time of sampling (between 8 and 14 weeks). **B**, Taking sample by transcervical method.

(never a single estimate) are essential to the establishment of a trend to justify delivery of a fetus.

Correct estimates of the estimated date of delivery (EDD) based on estriol levels in maternal urine are unlikely with obesity, multiple pregnancy, or pelvic tumors, because the EDD will often be an early estimate. Growth retardation of the fetus, oligohydramnios, or fetal death may falsely suggest a later EDD.

The woman is told the purpose of the urine tests; that is, "to assess the health of your developing baby." Printed instructions are given to the woman,* to void and discard the first morning urine; to collect all urine for the next 24 hours, storing it in the refrigerator; and then to bring it to the laboratory. The woman will need the following equipment: two collection bottles, one sieve, and a preservative solution.

Estriol determinations are possible by 20 weeks. A more reliable baseline is possible after 28 weeks. Best results are obtained after 32 weeks. Closely spaced serial evaluations are required to get the slope of increase or decrease. One reading at one point is useless. The same technician should do all the tests for a particular woman to increase reliability of the results. A false reading is likely if the woman is taking any of the following medications: corticosteroids, ampicillin, or methenamine mandelate (e.g., Mandelamine) for urinary tract infection. The methods of specimen collection and preservation are also factors in the accuracy of findings.

High estriol levels with a rising slope are associated with a good prognosis for the fetus (Table 27-8). Low estriol levels *may* be associated with a compromised fetus. NOTE: Factors not strictly related to fetal health may be associated with abnormal values (e.g., a true 24-hour specimen is not collected, gestational age is overestimated, or there is a high level of urinary glucose). If the woman's kidney clearance ability is questioned, the woman has diabetes mellitus, or the woman is unable to give a true 24-hour urinary specimen, plasma estriol may be assayed.

*The client's ability to read, comprehend, and comply with the printed instructions must be assessed as well.

Maternal Blood Assessments

Plasma Estriols. Plasma estriols may be assayed as either unconjugated, or free, estriol (8% to 10% of total estriol) or as total estriol. Plasma assays *do* reflect the fetoplacental production and secretion of estriols, and 24-hour urine specimens do not have to be collected. Plasma estriols are less affected by disorders of the mother's liver or kidneys.

Human Placental Lactogen. Human placental lactogen (hPL), also called human chorionic somatomammotropin (hCS), is produced by the syncytiotrophoblast. However, assay for this hormone is of little value in assessing placental integrity. Other, more accurate and reliable tests, have replaced the routine assessment for hPL levels (Haesslein, 1987).

Coombs' Test. Coombs' test for Rh incompatibility is discussed at length in Chapter 40. If Coombs' titer is greater than 1:8 to 1:16, amniocentesis for delta optical density (ΔOD) is indicated to determine need for intrauterine transfusion.

Amniocentesis

An amniocentesis is performed when there is an indication of problems with the pregnancy or fetus (e.g., to diagnose genetic problems [Chapter 40], to estimate fetal maturity, and to diagnose fetal hemolytic disease). Amniocentesis is possible after the fourteenth week, when the uterus becomes an abdominal organ and when there is sufficient amniotic fluid for this procedure (Table 27-9 and Fig. 27-8).

Preparation. The mother and family are informed of the need for the surgical procedure and appraised of the risks. An informed consent statement and a surgical permit are signed by the woman (Chapter 4). Ultrasonography is performed to locate the placenta. If the pregnancy is less than 20 weeks, a full bladder helps brace the uterus (see

Table 27-8 ***Summary of Biochemical Monitoring Techniques***

Test	Results	Significance of Findings
Maternal Urine Estriols	High and rising levels	General fetal well-being
	Low and falling levels	Possible fetal jeopardy
Maternal Blood		
Human placental lactogen	High levels	Large fetus; multiple gestation
	Low levels	Threatened abortion, IUGR, postmaturity
Unconjugated plasma estriol	High and rising levels	General fetal well-being
	Low and falling levels	Possible fetal jeopardy
Heat-stable alkaline phosphatase	Normally elevated during pregnancy	Poor correlation with fetal outcome
Oxytocinase	200-400 U at term	General fetal well-being
	Low levels	Associated with fetal death, postmaturity, IUGR
Coombs' test	Titer of 1:8 and rising	Significant Rh sensitization
Alpha-fetoprotein	See below	
Amniotic Fluid Analysis		
Color	Meconium	Possible hypoxia or asphyxia
Lung profile		Fetal lung maturity
L/S ratio	>2	
PGL[*]	Present	
Creatinine	>2 mg/dl	Gestational age > 36 weeks
Billirubin (ΔOD[†] 450/nm)	<0.015	Gestational age > 36 weeks, normal pregnancy
	High levels	Fetal hemolytic disease in rhesus isoimmunized pregnancies
Lipid cells	>10%	Gestational age > 35 weeks
Alpha-fetoprotein	High levels after 15-week gestation	Open neural tube or other defect
Osmolality	Decline after 20-week gestation	Advancing nonspecific gestational age
Genetic disorders	Dependent on cultured cells for karyotype and enzymatic activity	
Sex-linked		
Chromosomal		
Metabolic		

From Tucker, SM: Fetal monitoring and fetal assessment in high-risk pregnancy, St Louis, 1978, The CV Mosby Co. In an effort to summarize these studies in tabular form, generalization must be made.

[*]Phosphatidylglycerol.

[†]Delta optical density.

bladder preparation under ultrasonography, p. 665).

Complications. Overall complications are less than 1% for both mother and fetus and include the following:

Maternal: hemorrhage, fetomaternal hemorrhage with possible maternal Rh isoimmunization, infection, labor, abruptio placentae, inadvertent damage to the intestines or bladder, amniotic fluid embolism.

Fetal: death, hemorrhage, infection (amnionitis), direct injury from the needle, abortion or premature labor, leakage of amniotic fluid.

The amniocentesis procedure can be used as a basis for teaching the woman and her family.

Genetic Problems. Cells are cultured for *karyotyping* of chromosomes (see Fig. 9-2). Chromosomal aberrations appear in fetuses of 1% to 2% of women between 35 and 38 years of age, 2% of women between 39 and 40 years of age, and 10% of women over 45 years of age.

Fetal cells are assessed for *sex chromatin.* Sex determination is important if a sex-linked disorder (especially in the male fetus) is suspected. *Biochemical analysis* of enzymes produced from a cell culture is done to detect inborn errors of metabolism (over 60 types can be detected). Alpha-fetoprotein (AFP) levels in supernatant fluid are determined to detect neural tube defects, such as spina bifida and anencephaly. The recurrence risk of neural tube defects after one affected fetus is 2%; after two affected fetuses, 6% to 8% (Anderson, 1987). AFP may also be elevated with severe fetal hemolytic disease, esophageal atresia, congenital nephrosis, omphalocele, fetal hemorrhage into amniotic fluid, and fetal death. Levels may also be elevated in a normal multiple pregnancy. The amount of AFP should decrease to 18.5 μg/ml at 15 weeks and to 0.26 μg/ml at term.

Fetal Maturity. Greater accuracy in estimating fetal maturity is now possible through use of amniotic fluid or its exfoliated cellular content. Term pregnancy and fetal maturity can be demonstrated by the following laboratory studies.

Lecithin/Sphingomyelin Ratio. A *lecithin/sphingomyelin* (L/S) *ratio* greater than 2 indicates adequate lung maturity for extrauterine life (Chapter 9). This is generally achieved by 36 weeks gestational age. A practical means of determining the L/S ratio is the rapid surfactant test, also known as the **shake test** or bubble test. Equal parts of fresh amniotic fluid and normal saline solution are added to two parts 95% ethyl alcohol. The mixture is shaken vigorously for 30 seconds. If bubbles are still present at the meniscus 15 minutes after shaking, the fetal lung is judged to be mature. See Chapters 9 and 37 for discussions of other phospholipids and lung maturity.

Bilirubin. A ΔOD of *bilirubinoid pigments* of 450 nm <0.01 indicates a gestational age of greater than 38 weeks. Bilirubin disappears after 36 weeks.

Creatinine. When the *creatinine* (estimate of renal maturity) value is greater than 1.8 mg/dl, the gestational age is greater than 36 weeks in the absence of maternal renal disease and dehydration or of fetal anomaly.

Lipid cells. After *fetal lipid-containing exfoliated cells* are stained with Nile blue sulfate, a finding of more than 20% orange-staining cells indicates a gestational age of greater than 35 weeks; the fetus probably weighs 2500 g. (For information regarding the use of amniocentesis in estimating fetal health, see Procedure 27-1.)

Fetal Hemolytic Disease. Identification and follow-up of fetal hemolytic disease in isoimmunized pregnancies is another indication for amniocentesis. The first ΔOD analysis for amount of bilirubin in amniotic fluid is postponed until 24 to 25 weeks. Therapy by intrauterine transfusion of packed, Rh-negative, type O red blood cells is not possible before that time (Chapter 40).

Rupture of Membranes

Tests for rupture of membranes and assessment of the color, character, and amount of amniotic fluid are discussed at length in Chapter 18.

Table 27-9 *Typical Amniotic Fluid Increase During Pregnancy*

Weeks' Gestation	Amniotic Fluid Volume (ml)
12	50
14	100
16	175
18	250
20	325

From Queenan, JT: Contemp OB/GYN 15:61, Feb 1980.

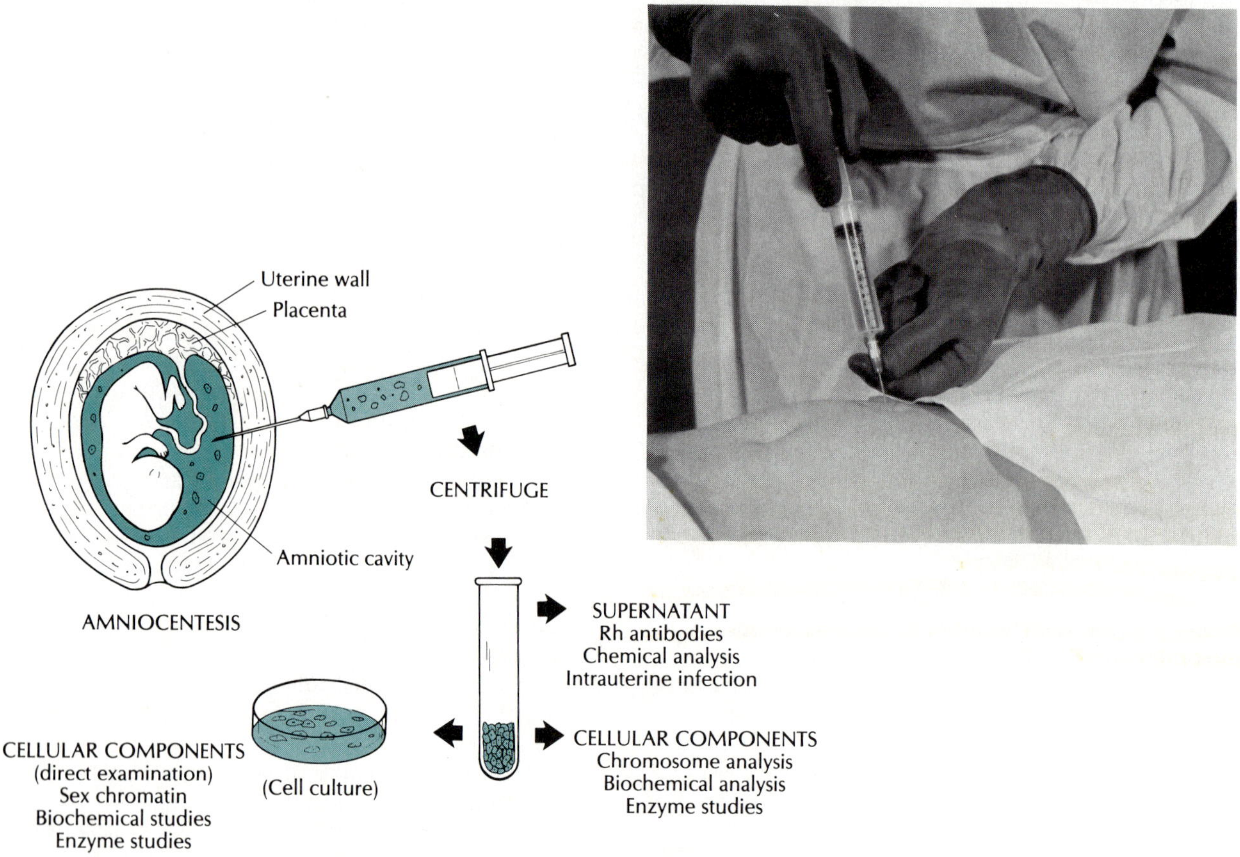

A

B

Fig. 27-8 **A**, Amniocentesis and laboratory utilization of amniotic fluid aspirant. **B**, Transabdominal amniocentesis.

A from Whaley, LF: Understanding inherited disorders, St Louis, 1974, The CV Mosby Co. **B** courtesy March of Dimes.

Procedure 27-1

AMNIOCENTESIS

DEFINITION

The removal of a small amount of amniotic fluid for laboratory analysis and prenatal diagnosis.

PURPOSE

To establish prenatal diagnosis of genetic problems, estimate gestational age, identify and monitor isoimmune disease, accomplish amniography and fetography, perform second-trimester elective abortion (see Chapter 42), estimate fetal lung maturity (L/S ratio).

EQUIPMENT

Amniocentesis tray; electronic fetal monitor; flashlight; amber-colored test tubes (or test tubes wrapped in aluminum foil); razor (to shave abdomen); bandage; antibacterial cleanser; sterile gowns, masks, and gloves; ultrasound machine and conductive gel.

NURSING ACTIONS	RATIONALE
Wash hands before and after touching woman and equipment. Glove, prn.	To prevent nosocomial infection and to implement universal precautions.
Prepare woman for procedure:	Collaborative effort facilitates procedure.
Take baseline vital signs and fetal heart rate (FHR).	To assess subsequent values.
Premedicate (if ordered).	To assist woman in relaxing.
Place woman in supine position with her hands under her head or across her chest.	To position woman in a way that facilitates procedure.
Prepare the abdomen with a shave and a scrub with povidone-iodine (Betadine), if ordered by physician.	To minimize possibility of infection.
Draw blood sample.	To compare with postprocedure blood sample for assessing probable fetomaternal hemorrhage. To assess levels of AFP.
Act as a support person during procedure:	As with any surgical procedure, the woman and family will be tense and anxious as to the outcome.
Explain reason for such a long needle.	The needle passes through layers of fat and muscle before reaching the uterus. Actually only a small portion of the needle enters the uterus. Show woman that the ultrasound guides the doctor in placement of the needle.
Reinforce the physician's explanation for not using local anesthetic.	The physician will not use a local anesthetic for two reasons: (1) It "stings" and (2) it would mean two needles. Once the skin is pierced, there is a sensation of pressure, but not pain.
Assist the physician:	To collaborate in the completion of the procedure accurately and with least potential for injury to maternal-placental-fetal unit.
Label three sterile tubes.	To identify specimen.
If bilirubin determination is needed, darken the room, use a flashlight, and immediately cover the filled amber-colored or aluminum foil-wrapped tube.	To prevent light from altering bilirubin, since a true reading cannot be obtained if the fluid is exposed to light.
After fluid is withdrawn, wash all povidone-iodine off the abdomen and apply a bandage.	To prevent skin burn.
Assist with or draw blood sample.	To assess for the presence of fetomaternal hemorrhage. To assess AFP level.
Continue monitoring the FHR for 30 minutes and assess for uterine contractions.	To identify complications.

Apt Test. The Apt test is used to differentiate maternal and fetal blood when there is vaginal bleeding during pregnancy or labor. It is performed as follows: Add 0.5 ml bloody fluid to 4.5 ml distilled water. Shake. Add 1 ml 0.25N sodium hydroxide. Fetal and cord blood remain pink for 1 or 2 minutes. Maternal blood becomes brown in 30 seconds.

Meconium in Amniotic Fluid

Antenatal Period. Antenatal amniotic fluid meconium may be just physiologic passage without association with poor fetal status or outcome. With the advent of more sophisticated, noninvasive tools to assess fetal health, the clinical significance of amniotic fluid meconium has been reduced (Danforth and Scott, 1986).

Intrapartum Period. Intranatal amniotic fluid meconium is an indication for more careful evaluation. The recent trend is *not* to rely on the presence of meconium as an indication for intervention (Danforth and Scott, 1986); now there is increased reliance on electronic fetal monitoring (EFM) and fetal scalp blood sampling for evaluation of fetal status.

When membranes are ruptured and fetal head can be touched, fetal well-being can be screened. Those fetuses who increased their heart rates with a brisk acceleration in response to *fetal scalp stimulation* uniformly had a scalp blood pH >7.23, suggestive of fetal well-being (Harvey, 1987).

There are three possible reasons for the passage of meconium during the intrapartum period: (1) it is a normal physiologic function that occurs with maturity; (2) it is the result of hypoxia-induced peristalsis and sphincter relaxation, and (3) it may be a sequela to umbilical cord compression–induced vagal stimulation in mature fetuses (meconium passage is infrequent before weeks 32 to 34, with an increased incidence after 38 weeks).

The following new criteria are proposed for evaluating meconium passage during the intranatal period (Danforth and Scott, 1986):

1. Consistency: "old and thin" versus "new and thick." A new and thick consistency is more likely to be the result of fetal stress.
2. Timing: thick, fresh meconium passed for the first time in late labor, associated with nonremediable severe variable or late fetal heart rate (FHR) decelerations, is an omninous sign. However, the presence of meconium alone is not necessarily a sign of fetal distress.
3. Presence of other indicators: meconium passage and nonremediable severe variable or late decelerations (especially with poor baseline variability) with or without acidosis confirmed by scalp-blood sampling are ominous signs.

Table 27-10 presents a listing of conditions that can be diagnosed prenatally by the procedures described. This table is given here for reference only.

Biophysical Monitoring

Evaluation of fetal well-being and maturity is essential in the management of the high-risk pregnancy. The nonstress test (NST), or fetal activity determination (FAD), the contraction stress test (CST), and the biophysical profile have been widely employed for the determination of fetal well-being. In addition, daily fetal movement count (DFMC), as recorded by the expectant mother, has proved to be an additional method of assessing fetal well-being.

The desired goals of antepartum monitoring are to prevent intrauterine fetal death and avoid unnecessary premature intervention.

Indications for both the NST and the CST include:

Maternal diabetes mellitus
Chronic hypertension
Hypertensive disorders in pregnancy
IUGR
Sickle cell disease
Maternal cyanotic heart disease
Suspected postmaturity
History of previous stillbirth
Rhesus sensitization (isoimmunization)
Meconium-stained amniotic fluid (at amniocentesis)
Abnormal estriol excretion pattern
Hyperthyroidism
Collagen diseases
Older gravida
≥40 weeks' gestation
Chronic renal disease

There are no contraindications for the NST. Absolute contraindications for the CST are rupture of membranes and previous classical cesarean delivery. The following are considered relative contraindications for the CST: multiple pregnancy, previous premature labor, placenta previa, hydramnios, and previous low transverse cesarean delivery. As a rule, reactive patterns with the NST or negative results with the CST are associated with favorable outcomes. In general, biophysical assessment is considered reliable, but false negatives and false positives do occur (Danforth and Scott, 1986; Haesslein, 1987).

Nonstress Test (Fetal Activity Determination). The basis for the NST, or FAD, is that the normal fetus will produce characteristic heart rate patterns. Acceleration of FHR in response to fetal movement is the desired outcome of the NST. This then allows most high-risk pregnancies to continue, with the test being repeated twice a week. A **reactive pattern suggests fetal well-being** with an associated good perinatal outcome.

The nurse observes the strip chart for signs of *fetal activity* and a concurrent acceleration of FHR. If evidence of fetal movement is not apparent on the chart paper, the woman is asked to depress a button on a handheld event marker that is connected into the appropriate outlet on the monitor when she feels fetal movement. The "event" of fetal movement is then noted by a spike or arrow printed by the stylus on the uterine activity panel of the strip chart. The test usually takes 20 to 30 minutes but may take longer if the fetus needs to be moved or awakened because of a sleep state (Fig. 27-9).

Table 27-10 *Partial List of Conditions Diagnosed Prenatally*

Disorder	Prenatal Diagnosis
Chromosomal Anomalies	Chromosome analysis of cultured amniotic fluid cells
Congenital Defects	
Cardiac defects	Ultrasound
Central nervous system anomalies	
Anencephaly	AFP in amniotic fluid and maternal serum Ultrasound Fetoscopy Radiography
Hydrocephaly	Ultrasound AFP Radiography
Microcephaly	Ultrasound Radiography
Spina bifida cystica	AFP Fetoscopy Ultrasound
Gastrointestinal defects	
Diaphragmatic hernia	Amniography Ultrasound
Esophageal atresia	Amniography Fetography
Gastroschisis; omphalocele	AFP Ultrasound
Meconium ileus (cystic fibrosis)	Ultrasound Radiography
Skeletal deformities (general)	Ultrasound Radiography
Osteogenesis imperfecta	Elevated amniotic fluid pyrophosphate
Fetal Infections	
Cytomegalovirus	Cytomegalovirus from amniotic fluid
Rubella	Rubella virus from amniotic fluid
Syphilis	Radiography (fetal abnormalities)
Hematologic Disorders	
Erythroblastosis fetalis	Amniotic fluid bilirubin Ultrasound Amniography Fetal blood sample
Sickle cell anemia	Fetal blood sample DNA analysis of amniotic fluid cells
Thalassemia	DNA analysis of amniotic fluid cells Fetal blood sample
Inborn Errors of Metabolism	Amniotic fluid analysis
Argininosuccinicaciduria	C argininosuccinic acid in cultured cells Increased argininosuccinic acid levels
Combined immune deficiency disease	Deficient adenosine deaminase activity in cultured cells
Congenital adrenal hyperplasia	Elevated 17-α-hydroxyprogesterone, Δ^4-androstenedione, and pregnanediol levels in fluid
Congenital erythropoietic porphyria	Massive amounts of porphyrin in fluid
Cystinosis	Elevated cystine in fluid
Fabry's disease	Deficient α-galactosidase activity in cultured cells
Farber disease	Deficient ceramidase activity in cultured cells
Galactosemia	Deficient galactose-1-phosphate uridyl transferase activity in cultured cells
Glutaric acidemia	Gluteric acid in fluid Deficient glutaryl-CoA dehydrogenase in cultured cells

Continued.

Table 27-10 *Partial List of Conditions Diagnosed Prenatally—cont'd*

Disorder	Prenatal Diagnosis
Hyperlipoproteinemid, type II	Absence of LDL cell surface receptors on cultured cells
Hypophosphatasia (congenitally lethal)	Ultrasound Deficient bone and liver alkaline phosphatase isoenzyme activity in cultured cells Deficiency of total alkaline phosphatase activity in cultured cells
Krabbe's disease	Deficient cerebroside β-galactosidase activity in cultured cells
Hunter's syndrome (mucopolysaccharidosis, type II)	Deficient iduronate sulfate activity in fluid Accumulation of S-mucopolysaccharides in cultured cells
Hurler's syndrome (mucopolysaccharidosis, type I)	Decreased α-L-iduronidase activity in fluid Accumulation of S-sulfate mucopolysaccharides in cultured cells
Lesch-Nyhan syndrome	Deficient hypoxanthine-guanine phosphoribosyl transferase activity in cultured cells
Maple syrup urine disease	Deficient branched chain keto-acid decarboxylase in cultured cells
Menke's syndrome (kinky-hair disease)	Increased incorporation of copper into cultured cells
Niemann-Pick disease	Deficient sphingomyelinase activity in cultured cells
Pompe's disease	Deficient α-1, -4-glucosidase in cultured cells
Porphyria (acute, intermittent)	Decreased activity of uroporphyrinogen I synthetase in cultured cells
Sanfilippo's syndrome	Deficient heparin sulfamidase activity in cultured cells Increased heparin sulfate in amniotic fluid
Tay-Sachs disease	Deficient β-N-acetyl-hexasaminidase A and B activity in cultured cells
Wolman's disease	Deficient acid lipase activity in cultured cells
Miscellaneous Conditions	
Cystic fibrosis	Reduced methylumbelliferyl-guauidinobenzoate reactive proteases in amniotic fluid
Duchenne muscular dystrophy	Elevated creatine phosphokinase levels in fetal blood
Fetal sex determination	Ultrasound—fetal outline Chromosome analysis of fluid cells Elevated testosterone levels and decreased follicle-stimulating hormone levels in amniotic fluid (male fetus)
Multiple pregnancy	Ultrasound Radiography
Tumors and cysts	Ultrasound Radiography Amniography
Placental Conditions	
Abruptio placentae	Ultrasound
Blighted ovum	Ultrasound
Ectopic pregnancy	Ultrasound
Placenta previa	Ultrasound

A guide for interpretation of the NST follows:

Result	***Interpretation***
Reactive	Two or more accelerations of FHR of 15 beats per minute (bpm) lasting 15 seconds or more, associated with each fetal movement in a 20-minute period
Nonreactive	Any tracing with either no FHR accelerations or accelerations less than 15 bpm or lasting less than 15 seconds throughout any fetal movement during testing period
Unsatisfactory	Quality of FHR recording not adequate for interpretation

The clinical significance of the interpretation of the NST is as follows:

Reactive NST	As long as twice weekly NSTs remain reactive, most high-risk pregnancies are allowed to continue
Nonreactive NST	Further indirect monitoring may be attempted with abdominal fetal electrocardiography in an effort to clarify FHR pattern and quantitate variability; external monitoring should continue, and a CST should be done
Unsatisfactory	Test is repeated in 24 hours, or a CST is done, depending on the clinical situation

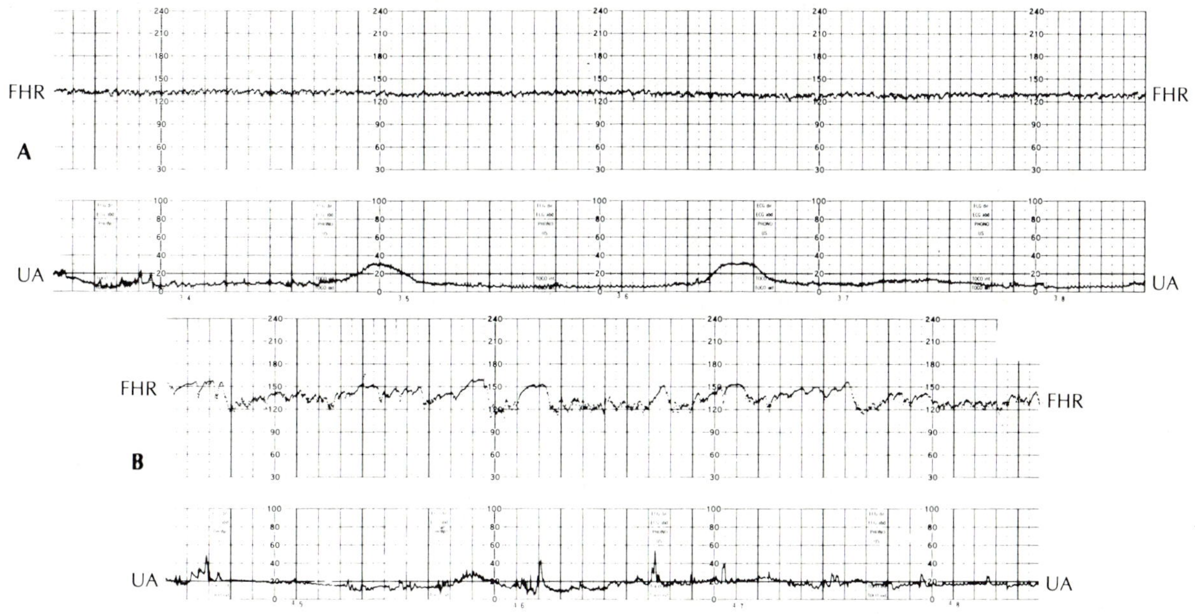

Fig. 27-9 Nonstress test. **A**, Decreased variability caused by fetal sleep cycle. **B**, Reactive nonstress test, indicative of fetal well-being, 15 minutes later.
From Perez, RH: Protocols for perinatal nursing practice, St Louis, 1981, The CV Mosby Co.

The *acoustic stimulation* test is another method of testing antepartum FHR response. The test takes approximately 10 minutes to complete, with the fetus monitored for 5 minutes before fetal acoustic stimulation to obtain a baseline FHR. The sound source is then applied on the maternal abdomen over the fetal head. Monitoring continues for another 5 minutes, and the strip chart is assessed.

A guide for interpretation of the acoustic stimulation test follows:

Reactive acoustic stimulation test	FHR acceleration of at least 15 bpm for at least 120 seconds or two accelerations of at least 15 bpm for at least 15 seconds within 5 minutes of stimulus
Nonreactive acoustic stimulation test	Inability to fulfill either criterion for reactivity as described above within 5 minutes

Contraction Stress Test. The basis for the CST is that a healthy fetus can withstand a decreased oxygen supply during the physiologic stress of an oxytocin-stimulated contraction, whereas a compromised fetus will demonstrate late decelerations that are nonreassuring and indicative of uteroplacental insufficiency. **A negative test suggests fetal well-being.**

Nipple-stimulated Contraction Stress Test. The woman is monitored indirectly, and the nurse observes the strip chart for 10 minutes before initiating nipple-stimulated contractions. If the woman has three or more spontaneous contractions within a 10-minute period, the nipple-stimulated contractions need not be initiated. If less than three spontaneous contractions occur within the period, and if late decelerations do not occur with intermittent spontaneous contractions, nipple stimulation can be initiated. The nurse explains the procedure to the woman and then proceeds by applying warm, moist washcloths to both breasts for several minutes. The woman is instructed to massage or roll the nipple of one breast for 10 minutes. If uterine contractions do not occur, both breasts should be stimulated for 10 minutes. The breasts should be restimulated intermittently as needed to maintain uterine contractions. If nipple stimulation does not produce the desire uterine activity, the nurse should proceed with an oxytocin-stimulated CST.

Oxytocin-stimulated Contraction Stress Test. The physician orders the dosage, which usually starts at 0.5 mU/min.* The oxytocin is always diluted in an IV solution and piggybacked into the tubing of the main IV. The infusion is usually delivered by an infusion pump or controller to ensure accurate dosage. The oxytocin infusion is usually increased by 0.5 mU/min at 15- to 20-minute intervals until three uterine contractions of good quality are observed within a 10-minute period. The FHR pattern is then interpreted. The oxytocin infusion is discontinued and the maintenance IV solution infused until such time as uterine activity has returned to the preoxytocin infusion level. The IV is then removed, and the fetal monitor is discontinued. The woman can be sent home on the physician's orders.

*See Table 33-5 for calculating dosage of oxytocin (Pitocin) and drops per minute.

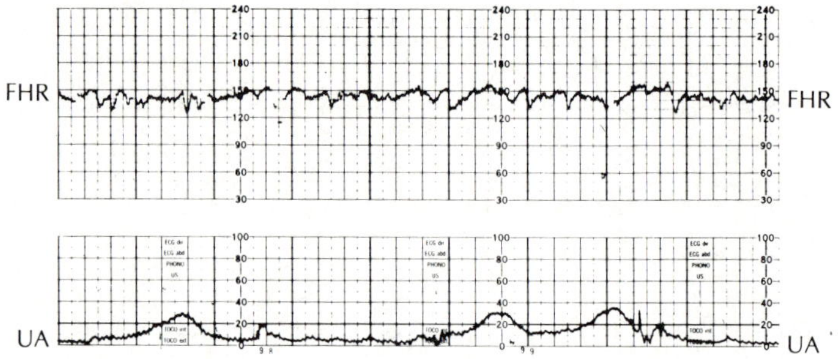

Fig. 27-10 Negative CST: fetal well-being.

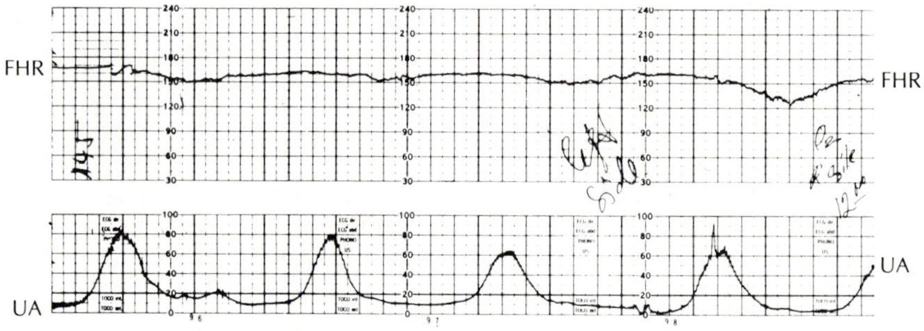

Fig. 27-11 Positive CST: compromised fetus.
From Perez, RH: Protocols for perinatal nursing practice, St Louis, 1981, The CV Mosby Co.

A guide for the interpretation of the CST follows:

Result	*Interpretation*
Negative	No late decelerations with a minimum of three uterine contractions lasting 40 to 60 seconds within a 10-minute period (Fig. 27-10)
Positive	Persistent and consistent late decelerations occurring with more than half the contractions (Fig. 27-11)
Suspicious	Late decelerations occurring with less than half the uterine contractions once an adequate contraction pattern has been established
Hyperstimulation	Late decelerations occurring with excessive uterine activity (contractions more often than every 2 minutes or lasting longer than 90 seconds) or a persistent increase in uterine tone
Unsatisfactory	Inadequate uterine contraction pattern or tracing too poor to interpret

The clinical significance of the CST is as follows:

Result	*Interpretation*
Negative CST	Reassurance that the fetus is likely to survive labor, should it occur within 1 week; more frequent testing may be indicated by the clinical situation
Positive CST	Management lies between use of other tools of fetal assessment and termination of pregnancy; a positive test indicates that the fetus is at increased risk for perinatal morbidity and mortality; the physician may perform an expeditious vaginal delivery following a successful induction or may proceed directly to cesarean delivery
Suspicious, hyperstimulation, or unsatisfactory	NST and CST should be repeated within 24 hours; if interpretable data cannot be achieved, other methods of fetal assessment must be used

Daily Fetal Movement Count (DFMC). Frequent movements of the fetus, as perceived by the mother, have been reassuring signs for centuries. Various investigators have recently reported a marked decrease in fetal movement before an episode of fetal distress or fetal death.

DFMCs, as reported by the mother, have been compared with movements recorded electronically, revealing that almost 90% of all fetal movements can be identified by the mother. This simple, inexpensive, readily applied "test" is continuously available away from the clinical area and relatively easy for the woman to do accurately. Maternal perception of a minimum of 10 movements during the daylight hours is considered reassuring (Haesslein, 1987).

Should a woman complain of decreased fetal movement, she may be asked by the physician to lie down for a period of 1 hour and count all the fetal movements. If she feels three or more during that time, she can be reassured. However, she is cautioned to continue to be aware of fetal movements and report the hourly observations should the problem recur. An immediate NST is usually performed if only one or two movements are felt. If the NST is reactive, no further testing is done unless there are some other risk factors. A nonreactive NST would be followed by a CST, the potential outcomes and significance of which have been previously described.

SUMMARY

Assessment of risk is the focus of this chapter. Assessment through interview, physical examination, and diagnostic techniques is discussed. Risk assessment identifies a population that requires special attention. Early identification of risk facilitates prospective planning and implementation of client and family care management throughout the childbearing cycle.

KEY CONCEPTS

- A high-risk pregnancy is one in which the life or well-being of the mother or offspring is jeopordized by a biophysical or psychosocial disorder coincidental with or unique to pregnancy.
- Factors that place the pregnancy and fetus-neonate at risk include anatomic, physiologic, therapeutic, environmental, and idiopathic events.
- Psychosocial perinatal warning indicators include characteristics of the parents, the child, their support systems, and family circumstances.
- Diagnostic techniques include ultrasonography, MRI, PUBS, CVS, and EFM.
- Biochemical monitoring techniques involve assessment of maternal urine and blood, and of amniotic fluid and its components.
- Maternal and perinatal mortality for whites is considerably lower than for all other races in the United States.
- There is excellent evidence that mortality decreases when high risk is identified early and intensive care applied.
- CVS could partially replace amniocentesis for genetic diagnosis.
- Evaluation of fetal well-being and maturity, essential in the management of the high-risk pregnancy, requires the knowledgeable and willing cooperation of the gravida and her family.
- A *reactive* NST and a *negative* CST suggest fetal well-being.

STUDY QUESTIONS AND ACTIVITIES

1. Observe an ultrasound test being performed. Have the examiner or interpreter explain the results.
2. Assist with an amniocentesis and obtain copies of the results. Have a physician assist you in interpreting the results and their implications.
3. Role-play a nurse attending a woman undergoing amniocentesis for determination of the possibility of genetic defect. Discuss the nurse's responsibilities for client education in this situation.
4. Using Tables 27-2 and 27-3 as guides, review several clients' charts. Identify risk factors and give rationale for each choice.
5. Assist with a CST or NST. Evaluate the fetal monitor strip and determine if it is an example of a reactive nonstress test or a nonreactive nonstress test; a positive oxytocin challenge test or a negative oxytocin challenge test.

References

Athey, PA, and Hadlock, EP: Ultrasound in obstetrics and gynecology, ed 2, St Louis, 1985, The CV Mosby Co

Anderson, RL: Maternal serum alpha-fetoprotein screening, Paper presented at UCSF antepartum and intrapartum management conference, San Francisco, June 1987

Danforth, DN, and Scott, JR, editors: Obstetrics and gynecology, ed 5, Philadelphia, 1986, JB Lippincott Co

Dauphinee, JD: Antepartum testing: a challenge for nursing, J Perinat and Neonat Nurs 1(1):29, 1987

Goldberg, JD: Antepartum fetal blood sampling, Paper presented at UCSF antepartum and intrapartum management conference, San Francisco, June 1987

Golbus, MS: Chorionic villus sampling or amniocentesis? Paper presented at UCSF antepartum and intrapartum management conference, San Francisco, June 1987

Haesslein, HC: Antepartum fetal assessment, Paper presented at USCF antepartum and intrapartum management conference, San Francisco, June 1987

Harvey, CJ: Fetal scalp stimulation: enhancing the interpretation of fetal monitor tracings, J Perinat and Neonat Nurs 1(1):13, 1987

Kanal, E, and Wolf, GL: Magnetic resonance imaging: an overview, Fam Pract recertification 8(9):35, 1986

Manning, FA, Platt, LD, and Supos L: Antepartum fetal evaluation: development of a fetal biophysical profile, Am J Obstet Gynecol 136:787, 1980

Manning, FA, Morrison, I, Lange, IR, et al: Fetal assessment based on fetal biophysical profile scoring: experience in 12,620 referred high risk pregnancies, Am J Obstet Gynecol 151:343, 1985

McCallum, WD: Ultrasound applications in pregnancy, Mid-coastal California Perinatal Outreach Program, Jan 1984

Modica, MM, and Timor-Tritsch, IE: Transvaginal sonography provides a sharper view into the pelvis, JOGN Nurs 17(2):89, 1988

Whaley, LF, and Wong, DL: Nursing care of infants and children, ed 3, St Louis, 1987, The CV Mosby Co

Bibliography

American College of Obstetricians and Gynecologists: *Standards for obstetric and gynecologic services,* ed 6, Washington, DC, 1985

Blank, JJ: Electronic fetal monitoring: Nursing management defined, *J Obstet Gynecol Neonatal Nurs* 14:463, 1985

Bobak, IM, and Jensen, MD: A modular study guide to maternity care, St Louis, 1983, The CV Mosby Co

Bowen, PA: Regional centers. I. A comparison of nursing responsibilities in level II and level III centers, Issues Health Care Women 2(5-6):1, 1980

Bowen, PA: Regional centers. II. The newborn transport system, Issues Health Care Women 2(5-6):5, 1980
Bowen, PA: Regional centers. III. Three regions' educational efforts and infant mortality rates, Issues Health Care Women 2(5-6):19, 1980
Bracero, LA, Schulman, H, and Baxi, LV: Fetal heart rate characteristics that provide confidence in the diagnosis of fetal well-being, Clin Obstet Gynecol, 19:3, March 1986
Brucker, MC, and MacMullen, NJ: CVS: counseling your patient, Nurse Pract 12(8):34, 1987
Carey, J, Seamonds, JA, and Galligan, M: Infant-death rate: rise linked to health-care cuts, US News & World Report, Feb 24, 1986, p 67
Chatterjee, MS: Paternal age and Down's syndrome, Contemp OB/GYN 21(5):171, 1983
Clark, SL: Consultations via facsimile telecopiers, Contemp OB/GYN 30: p 65, Oct 1987 (special issue)
Clark, SL, and Paul, RH: Intrapartum fetal surveillance: The role of fetal scalp blood sampling, *Am J Obstet Gynecol* 153:717, 1985
Dahlberg, NL: A perinatal center based antepartum homecare program, JOGN Nurs 17(1):30, 1988
DiMaio, M, et al: Screening for fetal Down's syndrome in pregnancy by measuring maternal serum alpha-fetoprotein levels, N Engl J Med 317(6):342, 1987
Doctors have doubts on placenta tests (CVS), San Francisco Chronicle, Dec 25, 1987
Douvas, SG, et al: Intrapartum fetal heart rate monitoring as a predictor of fetal distress and immediate neonatal condition in low-birth-weight (under 1,800 grams) infants, Am J Obstet Gynecol 148:300, 1984
Droegemueller, W, et al: Comprehensive gynecology, St Louis, 1987, The CV Mosby Co
Dwyer, JM: Manual of gynecologic nursing, Boston, 1986, Little, Brown & Co, Inc
Fenton, MV: Development of the scale of humanistic nursing behaviors, Nurs Res 36(2):82, 1987
Ferguson, HW: Biophysical profile scoring: the fetal Apgar, Am J Nurs 88(5):662, 1988
Freitas, CA, Helmer, FT, and Cousins, N: The development and management uses of a patient classification system for a high-risk perinatal center, JOGN Nurs 16(5):330, 1987
Gaffney, SE: Intrauterine fetal surgery: the ramifications for nurses, MCN 10:250, July/Aug 1985
Gantes, M, et al: The use of daily fetal movement records in a clinical setting, JOGN Nurs 15(5):390, 1986
Gantes, M, Kirchhoff, K, and Wark, B: Breast massage to obtain contraction stress test, Nurs Res 34(6):338, 1985
Grant, A: Controlled trials of routine ultrasound in pregnancy, Birth, p 16, Dec 1986 (special supplement)
Green, D: Prenatal diagnosis: when reality shatters parents' dreams, Nurs '88, 18(2):61, 1988
Hammer, RM, and Tufts, MA: Chorionic villi sampling for detecting fetal disorders, MCN 11:29, Jan/Feb 1986
Hogge, JS, Hogge, WA, and Golbus, MS: Chorionic villus sampling, JOGN Nurs 15(1):24, 1986
Hogge, WA, Schonberg, SA, and Golbus, MS: Chorionic villus sampling: experience of the first 1000 cases, Am J Obstet Gynecol 154(6):1249, 1986
Holtzman, NA: Prenatal screening for neural tube defects, Pediatrics 71:658, 1983
Horwell, DH, et al: Assessment of transcervical aspiration technique to chorionic villus biopsy in the first trimester of pregnancy, Br J Obstet Gynaecol 90:196, 1983
Jaffe, MS, and Melson, KA: Laboratory and diagnostic cards: clinical implications and teaching, St Louis, 1988, The CV Mosby Co
Jennings, BH: Social support: a way to a climate of caring, Nurs Admin 11(4):63, 1987
Kyba, FN, Ogburn-Russell, L, and Rutledge, JN: Magnetic resonance imaging: the latest in diagnostic technology, RN 17(1):44, 1987
Ledger, KE, and Williams, DL: Parents at risk: an instructional program for perinatal assessment and preventive intervention, Victoria, BC, Canada, 1981, Ministry of Health, Province of British Columbia, and Queen Alexandra Solarium for Crippled Children Society (Queen Alexandra Hospital, 2400 Arbutus Rd, Victoria, BC, Canada V8N IV7)
Lewis, C, and Mocarski, V: Obstetric ultrasound: application in a clinic setting, JOGN Nurs 16(1):56, 1987
Lehmann, D, and Chism, J: Pregnancy outcome in medically complicated and uncomplicated patients aged 40 years or older, Am J Obstet Gynecol 157(3):738, 1987
Marshall, C: The nipple stimulation contraction stress test, JOGN Nurs 15(6):459, 1986
Martin, AO, et al: Chorionic villus sampling in continuing pregnancies, Am J Obstet Gynecol 154(6):1353, 1986
Mashini, IS, et al: Comparison of uterine activity induced by nipple stimulation and oxytocin, Obstet Gynecol 69(1):74, 87
McCluggage, NA: Nursing interventions: nipple stimulation contraction stress test, J Perinatol 5:56, Summer 1985
Moberg, LJ, and Garite, TJ: Latest advances in EFM equipment, Comtemp OB/GYN, p 73, Oct 1987
Moenning, RK, and Hill, WC: A randomized study comparing two methods of performing the breast stimulation stress test, JOGN Nurs 16(4):253, 1987
Mole, R: Possible hazards of imaging and Doppler ultrasound in obstetrics, Birth, p 23, Dec 1986 (special supplement)
Murray, ML, Canfield, S, and Harmon, J: Nipple stimulation-contraction stress test, MCN 11(5):331, 1986
NAACOG-OGN Nursing Resource: Maternal neonatal transport, Washington, DC, 1983, The Association. (The Nurses Association of the American College of Obstetricians and Gynecologists, 409 12th Street SW, Washington, DC, 20024-2191, 202/638-0026)
Neilson, JP: Indications for ultrasonography in obstetrics, Birth p 11, Dec 1986 (special supplement)
Neldam, S: Fetal movements as an indicator of fetal well being, Lancet 1:1222, 1980
Nurses' Association of the American College of Obstetricians and Gynecologists: Electronic fetal monitoring: nursing practice competencies and educational guidelines, Washington, DC, 1986, NAACOG
Nurses' Association of the American College of Obstetricians and Gynecologists: Standard for obstetric, gynceologic and neonatal nursing, ed 3, Washington, DC, 1986, Nurses Association of the American College of Obstetricians and Gynecologists
Nurses' Association of the American College of Obstetricians and Gynecologists and American College of Obstetricians and Gynecologists: Electronic fetal monitoring: joint ACOG-NAACOG statement, Washington, DC, NAACOG, ACOG, 1986
Oakley, A: The history of ultrasonography in obstetrics, Birth p 5, Dec 1986 (special supplement)
Oki, E: A protocol for the nipple-stimulation CST, Contemp Obstet Gynecol 22(4):157, 1983
Parer, JT: Handbook of fetal heart rate monitoring, Philadelphia, 1983, WB Saunders
Petrie, RH: Intrapartum fetal monitoring, Clin Obstet Gynecol 19:1, March 1986

Platt, LD: Transvaginal ultrasound, Contemp OB/GYN, 30:99, Oct 1987 (special issue)
Poland, M, Ager, J, and Olson, J: Barriers to receiving adequate prenatal care, Am J Obstet Gynecol 157(2):299, 1987
Queenan, JT: OB ultrasound in the office, Contemp OB/GYN 22:134, 1984 (technology sumposium)
Queenan, JT: Old questions about a new procedure (chorionic villi sampling) (editorial), Contemp OB/GYN 22:3, 1984 (technology symposium)
Quirk, JG, and Miller, FC: FHR tracing characteristics that jeopardize the diagnosis of fetal well-being, Clin Obstet Gynecol 19:12, March 1986
Richardson, BS: Fetal activity: measure of well-being, Contemp OB/GYN 22(3):211, 1983
Richart, RM, and Pringle, P: A state-of-the-art guide to colposcopes, Contemp OB/GYN, 30:107, Oct 1987, (special issue)
Sadovsky, E: Fetal movements and fetal health, Semin Perinatol 5:131, 1981
Schifrin, BS, Weissman, BA, and Wiley, J: Electronic fetal monitoring and obstetrical malpractice, Law Med Health Care 13:100, 1985
Serafini, P, et al: Antepartum fetal heart rate response to sound stimulation: the acoustic stimulation test, Am J Obstet Gynecol 148:41, 1984
Simpson, JL: Advances in prenatal genetics: past, present, and future, Contemp OB/GYN 21(1):193, 1983
Stewart, N: Women's views of ultrasonography in obstetrics, Birth p 34, Dec 1986 (special supplement)
Stringer, MR: Chorionic villi sampling: a nursing perspective, JOGN Nurs 17(1):19, 1988
Thacker, SB: Research strategies for the use of imaging ultrasound as an obstetric screening tool, Birth, Dec 1986, (special supplement)
US National Center for Health Statistics: Vital Statistics of the United States, 1980, Washington, DC, 1982, US Government Printing Office
Ward, RH: Chorionic villi sampling: its promise and its problems, Contemp OB/GYN 22:31, 1984 (technology symposium)

CHAPTER

28

Loss and Grief

Learning Objectives

Correctly define the key terms listed.

Compare the three stages of grieving according to Lindemann and the five stages described by Kübler-Ross.

Identify ways in which the loss reaction is influenced by growth and development, cultural and spiritual beliefs, sex roles, relationships with significant others, and socioeconomic status.

Describe behavioral patterns useful as assessment criteria for the grieving client.

Identify the nurse's role in assisting clients with problems related to loss, death, and grief.

Formulate at least five examples of nursing diagnoses related to grief.

Review interventions for grieving clients to provide therapeutic communication, maintain self-esteem, and promote a return to normal activities.

Describe how the nurse helps meet the special needs of the woman and her family experiencing spontaneous abortion, fetal or neonatal death, maternal death, premature labor, and birth of a neonate with a disorder.

Develop criteria to evaluate nursing care for grieving clients.

Evaluate possible reactions of the nurse when caring for clients experiencing loss and grief.

Key Terms

acceptance
acute mourning
anticipatory grief
bargaining
denial
developing awareness
family's response
grandparents' response
grieving process
maternal death
nurse's response
pathologic mourning
resolution
role-playing
shock and belief
siblings' response

How often one hears that the "maternity ward is the happiest place in the whole hospital." This type of comment is most often expressed by those with no experience on a maternity service. However, experienced maternity nurses recognize the need to be prepared to meet the grief and grieving needs of women and their families.

Pregnancy and birth constitute an identity crisis situation in which everything is expected to proceed normally. During this natural transition in the woman's life cycle, she examines and actively relates to her femininity, sexuality, and capacity for motherhood. An unnatural or unexpected interruption in the process poses a potential threat to a woman's self-esteem and femininity. Possible threats to maternal health include abortion (spontaneous, elective, or therapeutic), non-marital pregnancy, premature or postmature delivery, birth trauma, placing the baby for adoption, stillbirth, neonatal death, or the birth of a child with a defect.

The death of a mother during the perinatal period is an unexpected tragedy. Even if the mother had been designated as "high risk," maternal death sends ripples of shock throughout the maternity unit. "Death of the mother completely disrupts the family structure and often leaves the father with the care of a baby at a time when his emotional reserves are lowest" (Johnson, 1986). For the family the sense of loss and grief is enormous.

When expectations of birth and joy are replaced by loss, the nurse's role is critical. The nurse must be able to cope constructively with her own response to loss and grief to meet the woman's needs. As in any crisis situation, the nurse's problems may be reactivated by those presented by the woman and her family. The nurse also becomes vulnerable as these internal conflicts emerge while she helps with the woman's problems. An understanding of loss and the normal grieving process is fundamental to the implementation of the nursing process.

THE GRIEVING PROCESS

When an individual experiences a loss, the person's reactions usually follow a predictable pattern. Effects of maternal analgesia or general anesthesia may affect the mother's grieving process. Phases of mourning have been described by Lindemann (1944) and Kübler-Ross (1969) and may be compared as follows:

Lindemann (Three Phases)	*Kübler-Ross (Five Stages)*
1. Shock and disbelief	1. Denial and isolation: "No, not me!"
	2. Anger: "Why me?"
	3. Bargaining: "If I . . ."
2. Developing awareness and acute mourning	4. Depression and acute grief: "How can I . . ."
3. Resolution or acceptance	5. Acceptance: "I can, I must."

The phases of mourning according to Lindemann are explained further.

Shock and Disbelief. During the period immediately after the loss the person struggles with the reality of the event and may even deny its existence. Mental symptoms may include restlessness, confusion, and apathy. The following somatic manifestations are common: dizziness, lightheadedness or syncope, pallor, perspiration, tachycardia, palpitations, nausea, and other gastrointestinal tract symptoms.

Developing Awareness and Acute Mourning. Reality of the loss begins to penetrate awareness; interest in daily affairs and activity diminishes. Feelings of sadness, self-depreciation, depression, guilt, helplessness, and hopelessness surface. Intense feelings of loneliness or emptiness, a strong urge to cry, and preoccupation with the loss are common. Blame may be internalized or projected onto others. Anger is a common characteristic in this phase. Exhaustion and shortness of breath may occur occasionally.

Resolution or Acceptance. Recovering from grief may take a year or longer, although the acute period lasts approximately 6 weeks. With resolution of the mourning process, the person gradually resumes daily activities, reestablishes precrisis relationships in light of the crisis event, forms new relationships, and becomes less preoccupied with the loss.

Pathologic Mourning. The following signs *may* signal pathologic mourning:

1. Cheerfulness
2. Avoidance of the topic
3. Marked or persistent hostility toward the staff, her husband, or the maternal or paternal family
4. Marked or persistent guilt feelings regarding the event
5. Viewing the sick or premature infant or the infant with a disorder as normal or deceased

NURSING CARE

The critical period for intervention is in the immediate crisis period. The goal of crisis intervention is to help the woman and her family begin *now* to mourn appropriately.

The nurse must be aware of possible individual differences and cultural prescriptions for mourning and the expression of grief when assessing the appropriateness of the grief response.

Assessment

Nursing assessment of the grieving client explores the meaning of the loss for the client, considers variables affecting the client's reaction, and assesses the client's progression through the grieving process. Many *factors* influence the client's individual reaction.

The client's level of growth and development affects the person's concept of loss, experience with past losses, and perception of loss in personal and social contexts. Cultural and spiritual beliefs may hinder or promote the expression and resolution of grief. Societal expectations about sex role behavior influence the expression of grief, with women generally more open in expression than men. The nature of the relationship one has with a signficant other affects how one grieves if the other dies or has a loss. Assessment of socioeconomic factors is important because of the individual's or family's resources for coping with loss.

The mother and family members are assessed for behaviors common to the stages of grieving. Verbal and nonverbal responses to loss are assessed. The nurse also assesses the woman's and family's external support system—who they are, their availability, their effect on the woman and her family (i.e., does she seem comforted by them?). The nurse notes that woman's and family's desire for spiritual support (e.g., baptism of the conceptus or newborn).

Nursing Diagnoses

Nursing diagnoses may include physiologic and psychosocial problems related to grieving or problems occurring in the grieving process itself. Examples of nursing diagnoses include the following:

- Anxiety or situational low self-esteem related to
  - Lack of understanding of the grieving process
- Ineffective individual (or family) coping related to
  - Perinatal death of fetus or newborn or mother
- Altered family processes related to
  - Loss of a family member or birth of a child with a disorder
- Knowledge deficit related to
  - Loss and the grieving process
- Altered parenting related to
  - Loss of a family member, maternal morbidity, or birth of a child with a disorder
- Powerlessness related to
  - Loss and grief
- Sleep pattern disturbance related to
  - Grieving process
- Spiritual distress (distress of the human spirit) related to
  - Loss and grieving process

Planning

During this important step, goals are set in client-centered terms. The goals are prioritized. Nursing actions are selected to meet the goals.

Goals

1. The woman retains a positive sense of self-esteem and self-worth as a woman, mother, and sexual being.
2. The woman and family appraise the situation realistically (e.g., ambivalent or negative feelings toward the pregnancy did not cause the loss).
3. The woman and family receive anticipatory guidance regarding components of the grieving process and possible reactions of family and friends.
4. The woman and her family can verbalize their feelings and an understanding of the grieving process.

Implementation

Implementation of nursing actions are individualized. General actions to assist the nurse who is helping families cope with loss related to childbearing are presented in the tables and nursing care plans that follow. Following are the most commonly encountered situations:

1. Spontaneous abortion
2. Fetal death (before admission to hospital for delivery)
3. Intranatal death (stillbirth) or neonatal death
4. Premature labor
5. Birth of a newborn with a defect or disorder

Maternal death is rarely encountered. Suggestions for nursing actions with her family are discussed in some detail.

Regardless of the specific loss experienced, some nursing actions are appropriate to all. Therapeutic communication techniques help the mother and family understand the meaning of the loss, share feelings, and move less stressfully through the grieving process. Intervention to maintain the client's self-esteem involve listening, responding positively to requests, maintaining confidentiality, providing comfort and support, and meeting spiritual needs.

Interventions to promote a return to activities of daily living include encouraging clients to participate in decisions, as well as specific adaptations. Nursing care of a client's body after death requires respect and dignity for the body and meeting of the family's needs. The baby is usually removed to a work area, and all instruments are removed from the baby. The cord is occluded with a tie or plastic clamp. The baby is baptized if so requested by parents or if not explicitly denied by parents. The baby is measured and weighed. The baby is identified with one baby band; the other band is placed on mother's wrist. The completed stillborn certificate is attached to the baby. The baby is wrapped in a shroud. The second copy of the stillborn certificate is pinned to the shroud and the baby and placenta are taken to the designated area in the hospital.

If the mother or family does not want to see the fetus or newborn, a photograph is stored with the chart. Often the family requests to see the photograph at a later date.

Baptism. The rite of baptism is particularly significant to Roman Catholic, some Episcopalian, and Greek Orthodox religious groups. If death appears inevitable, the clergy should be notified according to the family's wishes. If death is imminent, any adult, preferably of the same faith, may baptize the infant. Water is poured down the head or other skin surface and the following words spoken: "I baptize you, in the name of the Father, of the Son, and of the Holy Spirit." If an abortion or fetal death occurs, the expelled products of conception are baptized. The parents and the priest or minister should be notified of the baptism and a notation made on the record.

Filing Certificate of Death. Requirements may vary among states within the United States. California requires that each death shall be registered with the local registrar of birth and death registration in the district in which the death was officially pronounced or the body was found, within 5 days after death and before any disposition of the human remains.

The medical and health section data and the time of death shall be completed and attested to by the physician last in attendance, provided such physician is legally authorized to certify and attest to these facts or by the coroner

General Nursing Care Plan

PERINATAL LOSS

ASSESSMENT	NURSING DIAGNOSIS (ND)/ PLAN (P)/GOAL (G)	RATIONALE/ IMPLEMENTATION	EVALUATION
Assess maternal emotional response: A. Quiet, composed. B. Denial: "I just don't believe it." Euphoric, animated. C. Overtly upset, crying. D. Angry toward staff, others, "Why do I have to feel anything? Give me something now." "If the doctor had only . . ." "If I had only . . .", sad, tearful. Review her obstetric history: A. Was there difficulty conceiving? B. Any previous abortions? C. Was there anything done to initiate abortion? Note mother's age—adolescent's needs are different from those of a middle-aged woman.	ND: Ineffective individual (or family) coping related to perinatal death of fetus, newborn, or mother. ND: Powerlessness related to loss and grief. P: Provide information and listen actively to assist woman (family) with grieving. G: The woman retains a positive sense of self-esteem and self-worth as a woman, mother, and sexual being.	*Verbal repetition of experience helps one cope with a situation, therefore the nurse will:* Be available and indicate willingness to sit and listen to woman and family. Encourage and assist verbalization: A. Feelings of loss. B. Woman's fear of "having something wrong with her." C. Any feelings, actions, or lack of action that woman or family may believe caused the loss. D. Reflections on previous pregnancies, labors, or any grieving experience. Provide physical care and meet dependency needs in thoughtful and unhurried manner. Be cognizant of own nonverbal messages. Do not minimize event with comments such as "You are still young," or "You'll have others."	Evaluation of the effectiveness of nursing actions is difficult when working with perinatal loss. The grieving response takes a considerable amount of time and the nurses contact with the family may be limited. Therefore the nurse must rely on the knowledge that supportive and understanding care is significant to the family's successful resolution of their loss.
Assess woman's external support system: A. Presence of relatives. B. Behavior of relatives (does she seem reassured by their presence and actions?) C. Family's interest and ability to stay with her, to provide comfort measures, etc. Are there definite cultural (or religious) influences that help mother define death and direct her grieving process?	ND: Knowledge deficit related to the loss. ND: Spiritual distress (distress of the human spirit) related to loss and grief. P: Provide information and act as sounding board. G: The woman and family appraise the situation realistically (e.g., ambivalent or negative feelings toward the pregnancy did not cause the loss).	*People experiencing loss may need to ask some questions repeatedly from same or other people, therefore the nurse will:* Act as advocate to physician in regard to woman's questions concerning cause and her biologic functioning capacity. Fill in gaps in information and clarify misconceptions. Make appropriate referrals: spiritual leader, family planning, psychiatric social worker, genetic counselor. Maternal loss: child care, homemaker service, home health care.	Woman is able to identify and ask questions. Woman indicates she understands information. Woman is able to utilize community and family resources for support.

Continued.

General Nursing Care Plan—cont'd

ASSESSMENT	NURSING DIAGNOSIS (ND)/ PLAN (P)/GOAL (G)	RATIONALE/ IMPLEMENTATION	EVALUATION
If the person experienced a previous loss, what coping mechanisms were effective and what actions aided toward acceptance. Assess the support systems in the different areas of the family's life (e.g., work, children, school). If possible, assess the older child's (children's) reactions. Assess the parents' reactions as they face the need to tell the older child, children, other family members, and friends.	ND: Anxiety, or situational low self-esteem related to lack of understanding the grieving process. ND: Knowledge deficit related to loss and grieving process. ND: Altered parenting related to the loss of a family member, maternal morbidity, or birth of a child with a disorder. ND: Altered family process related to loss of a family member, or birth of a child with a disorder. P: Provide information and assist with problem-solving for coping. G: The woman and family will receive anticipatory guidance regarding components of the grieving process and possible reactions of family and friends.	*Individuals experiencing a loss need to understand grief reactions to help dispel fear of the unknown and know that their feelings are "normal," therefore the nurse will:* Alert family to characteristics of grieving process: A. Personal responses. B. Variations in responses to be expected at different developmental levels. C. Duration for child versus adult. Encourage mother (couple) to verbalize concerns perhaps to role play different approaches regarding ways to inform siblings, other family members and friends. Encourage family to discuss event openly with adolescent.	Mother (family) is able to verbalize understanding of grieving process. Mother (family) openly communicate their concerns and reactions. Mother (family) rehearse (role-play) approaches to communicate loss and grieving response to family and friends. Children attend community group that provides support for coping with loss.
Assess the family's need or desire to see or hold the lost fetus/infant. Assess the family's need to have the nurse, clergy, physician present during the viewing. Assess for desire to have fetus/infant baptized.	ND: Anxiety related to initiating the grieving process. ND: Ineffective individual or family coping related to initiating the grieving process. P: Provide tangible proof of loss and opportunity to say good-bye. G: The family will identify and validate the loss, which will permit the grieving process to begin.	*Some people experiencing a loss need to see or hold the fetus/infant to identify and validate the loss.* If mother, spouse, or relatives wish to see or hold infant: A. Prepare family for sight of infant and tell them you will stay with them as long as they desire. B. Prepare infant: bathe and bundle. C. Provide private space; physician, member of clergy, nurse or other should stay close by for support. D. Give permission to cry by your actions, (giving tissues) by saying, ("It's worth crying over.") Assemble keepsakes such as name bracelet, picture, footprints for parents to take with them or acquire at a future time. Arrange for baptism and record event in progress notes.	Mother (family) hold or see the fetus/infant. Mother (family) verbalize satisfaction with the experience. Parent's religious beliefs are respected.

Specific Nursing Care Plan

PARENTS EXPERIENCING FETAL DEATH

Ann, age 27, gestational week 20, was admitted to the labor floor after complaining of severe abdominal cramping and leaking small amounts of pink vaginal discharge. Ann and her husband are placed in a private examining room. As the nurse enters the room she hears Ann state, "I don't want to lose this baby—I feel so close to it now that I have felt it move—I'm scared." After several unsuccessful trials of drug therapy to cease labor, and cessation of a FHR; Ann is being prepared for her imminent delivery. The physician is currently reviewing the assessment with Ann and her husband and explaining choices of anesthesia for delivery.

ASSESSMENT	NURSING DIAGNOSIS (ND)/ PLAN (P)/GOAL (G)	RATIONALE/ IMPLEMENTATION	EVALUATION
Ann's response is one of being scared and upset. Spouse is at bedside listening to Ann's feelings. Ask if Ann wishes anyone else at the hospital as a support person and make effort to contact individual.	ND: Powerlessness related to loss and grief. ND: Potential ineffective individual (or family) coping related to death of a fetus. P: Establish data base to meet support needs. G: Ann will verbalize her needs and discuss her concerns and feelings.	*Focus to remain on Ann and husband.* Do not listen for FHR or apply contraction monitor to Ann. *Be available and open for communication.* Introduce yourself and immediately indicate your awareness of the situation. ("This is a very difficult and sad time for you.") Encourage and assist verbalization of feelings. Be cognizant of own nonverbal messages. Provide physical care and meet dependency needs in thoughtful and unhurried manner.	Ann verbalizes her immediate needs to the nurse or through her husband. Spouse is able to remain at bedside as a support to Ann.
Persistent preterm labor despite drug therapy. Pink serous vaginal discharge. 20 week gestation fetus (nonviable). No FHR noted. Parents informed by physician of imminent delivery of a stillborn fetus. Assess parents' understanding of cause of fetal loss and choices regarding anesthesia and the birth process.	ND: Knowledge deficit related to fetal loss. ND: Knowledge deficit related to the birth process. P: Be available to parents to answer questions. G: Ann will ask questions about the cause of fetal death. G: Ann will make an informed decision regarding choice of anesthesia for delivery	*To keep Ann informed of past and upcoming events, the nurse will:* Act as advocate to physician in regard to woman's questions concerning cause of death and events she will experience during delivery. Fill in gaps in information and clarify misconceptions. Respect Ann's choice of anesthesia. If she wishes to be awake or if couple wishes father to be present at birth; prepare them for the following: (a) Silence and tension at delivery. (b) Sight of still, pale, or reddish infant; infant's peeling skin and markedly molded head.	Ann asks questions about the cause of fetal loss. Ann chooses a method of anesthesia for delivery. Ann and husband express satisfaction with care received.

Continued.

Specific Nursing Care Plan—cont'd

ASSESSMENT	NURSING DIAGNOSIS (ND)/ PLAN (P)/GOAL (G)	RATIONALE/ IMPLEMENTATION	EVALUATION
Assess the couple's desire to hold or see the fetus. Assess for desire to have the fetus baptized.	ND: Potential anxiety related to initiating the grieving process. ND: Potential ineffective individual or family coping related to initiating the grieving process. ND: Potential spiritual distress (distress of the human spirit) related to loss and grief. P: Facilitate couple's grieving. G: The couple will identify and validate the loss that will permit the grieving process to begin.	*Some people experiencing a loss need to see or hold the fetus to identify and validate the loss.* If mother, spouse, or relatives wish to see or hold infant: (a) Prepare family for sight of fetus, and identify individuals for viewing. (b) Bathe and wrap the infant. (c) Provide privacy for viewing and stay close by for support. (d) Give permission to cry, (giving tissues) by saying, ("It's a sad time, and it's OK to cry.") Arrange for baptism if desired and record event in progress notes.	Ann and her husband initiate the grieving process. Ann and her husband identify their support system. Family expresses satisfaction in viewing and holding infant. Baptism or other religious rite is performed.
Assess any previous loss the couple might have had and identify effective coping mechanisms and support systems utilized.	ND: Knowledge deficit related to grief and grieving. P: Provide needed information. G: The couple will receive anticipatory guidance regarding components of the grief process.	*To aid the couple in understanding the grief process, the nurse will:* Explain characteristic patterns of the grief response. Identify and examine any previous effective coping mechanisms. Identify couple's support system.	The couple verbalizes understanding of the grief process.

in those cases in which he is required to complete the medical and health section data and certify and attest to these facts.

The medical and health section data and the physician's or coroner's certification shall be completed by the attending physician within 15 hours after the death. It should also be completed by the coroner within 3 days after examination of the body.

Evaluation

Evaluation of the effectiveness of nursing actions is somewhat more difficult when working with loss and grief. The grieving response takes a considerable period of time. The nurse's contact with the family may be limited. The nurse must rely on the knowledge that supportive and understanding care is significant to the family's successful resolution of their loss.

LOSS OF THE FETUS OR NEWBORN

Conception affirms the woman's ability to initiate her biologic role. Any event that interferes with her ability to carry a normal fetus to term causes her to question her biologic intactness. The event may be perceived as an assault to the woman's self-concept and feelings of self-worth. She may feel cheated. Many women experience ambivalent feelings toward the idea of pregnancy; many harbor thoughts of self-abortion. Coincident loss of the pregnancy may precipitate a guilt reaction for real or imagined negative thoughts or actions.

Spontaneous Abortion and Ectopic Pregnancy

For the woman who has a history of difficulty in conceiving and carrying a pregnancy to viability (about 24 weeks), negative feelings about herself as a complete woman may be expected. Nursing care of such a woman

Table 28-1 *Psychosocial Role of Nurse in Care of Parents Experiencing Spontaneous Abortion or Ectopic Pregnancy*

Assessment	Plan/Implementation	Rationale
Assess woman's behavior: Euphoric, talkative Quiet, nonverbal Denial or acknowledgment Review her obstetric history: Was there difficulty conceiving?* Any previous abortions?† Was anything done to initiate abortion? Assess family's response.	Be available and indicate willingness to sit and listen to woman and family. Encourage and assist verbalization of: Feelings of loss, of being cheated Woman's fear of not being able to ever carry to term, of having something wrong with her Any feelings, actions, or lack of action that woman or family may believe caused this Reflections on previous pregnancies, labors, etc. Act as advocate to physician in regard to woman's questions concerning cause and her biologic functioning capacity. Make appropriate referrals: family planning, psychiatric social worker, genetic counselor, etc.	Verbal repetition of experience helps one cope with a situation and integrate experience into one's perception of self in nonthreatening manner. People experiencing loss may need to ask same questions repeatedly from same or other people. Answers may need to be given frequently, with patience and understanding. People experiencing grief feel alienated from others, lonely, and helpless; they may exhibit anger in presence of or toward accepting, understanding, and caring other, such as nurse.

*For a discussion of the grief response and infertility, see Chapter 42.
†For a discussion of the nurse's response and the woman's response to elective abortion, see Chapter 42.

and her family should focus on helping them verbalize their feelings openly and honestly. Sympathetic, active listening by the nurse may help the woman in retaining or regaining her self-esteem and feelings of self-worth (Table 28-1; research highlight).

One woman who suffered spontaneous abortion submitted these "thoughts on being a habitual aborter" (Zlomke, 1986):

> The term "habitual aborter" is an insidious one, and one which I believe no woman should ever hear. It is a phrase which implies that she could have control over her life if she would only exert herself, as though she were a smoker or a nail biter. The truth is that she has lost all control over her life. With the death of each baby a little more of her future dies until she finally can bear it no longer and gives up. The pain is so great that even after having had a healthy baby since my last miscarriage, I notice that I wrote this whole paragraph in the third person.

Definition of Fetal Death

Fetal death is defined as death before the complete expulsion or extraction from its mother of a product of conception (irrespective of the duration of pregnancy); the death is indicated by the fact that after such separation the fetus does not breathe or show any other evidence of life, such as beating of the heart, pulsation of the umbilical cord, or definite movement of voluntary muscles. Fetal death is required to be registered if the twentieth week of gestation has been reached.

Fetal Death

Fetal movements may cease before the onset of labor, that is, between 20 weeks and term. The mother may deny a lack of fetal activity: "Maybe he's just asleep . . . he's quiet sometimes." She may call the physician for reassurance that everything is all right. Subsequently she may be admitted to the hospital for tests of fetal status. Even in light of evidence from the tests and clinical symptoms, some women cling tenaciously to the hope that the infant will be born alive and well.

Other women acknowledge fetal death by a change in their behavior. One woman arrived on a maternity unit in active labor. A review of her chart showed that she had kept all her clinic appointments until 4 weeks before labor. She stated she was feeling well and described her labor so far. She said nothing as the nurse checked for the fetal heart rate (FHR). When none were heard, the nurse inquired about fetal activity. Quietly and unemotionally, the mother replied, "They stopped a month ago."

Occasionally it is the nurse who responds with denial. The nurse may rationalize the absence of FHR and funic and uterine souffles as "positional," "too much noise in the room," "defective fetoscope," and the like. The nurse may choose to avoid the woman or to avoid open communication on the subject. The nurse has several therapeutic alternatives available, however (see the general nursing care plan for loss of the fetus or newborn, p. 683).

Intranatal Fetal or Newborn Death

FHR may be lost late in the first stage of labor or during the second stage. The atmosphere in the labor unit becomes tense and subdued. There is a sudden change from joyful anticipation to dread. Silence accompanies the birth. Resuscitative measures are attempted. All persons present focus on the newborn. Shock and disbelief are experienced by parents and staff alike.

RESEARCH HIGHLIGHT

Women's Perceptions of First Trimester Spontaneous Abortion

Purpose

To explore women's response to spontaneous abortion. Pregnancy represents a significant event in a woman's life; 15 to 20% of all pregnancies end in spontaneous abortion.

Sample/Methodology

A convenient sample of nine women were asked to complete a questionnaire relating their experiences surrounding their miscarriages.

Findings

Sadness, preoccupation, thinking and dreaming about the baby, irritability, disbelief, and anger were present at some level of concern. Eating and sleeping were not identified as problems. However, seven women experienced episodes of crying, five prayed for the lost infant, eight experienced depression, and six experienced disbelief.

Although most of the women were satisfied with the care they received from health care professionals, one woman reported that, "When I went into the hospital I was asked if I had done this myself."

Implications

Findings from this study show the importance of recognizing the special difficulties and needs of women who abort spontaneously in the first trimester. Knowledge of the emotional impact that accompanies a loss of pregnancy is especially important for enhancing therapeutic communication and intervention between health care professionals and the women who miscarry.

Wall-Haas, CL: Women's perceptions of first trimester spontaneous abortion, JOGN Nurs 14(1):50, 1985.

The supportive role of the nurse in the care of parents who experience the death of their infant during labor and delivery is presented in the specific nursing care plan for the family following the death of a fetus on p. 685.

Nurse and Parent Reactions and Interactions

The nurse may undergo a period of self-recrimination relevant to her own behavior surrounding the incident, for example: Could the physician have been called earlier? Were the fetal heart tones really there and was the rate normal when they were last checked? Was it judicious to give that last medication at the time it was given? Were there any clues earlier? Did the nursing care (ability to assess labor and the maternal-fetal condition during labor, ability to resuscitate) cause the fetal or neonatal death? The nurse's self-examination can undermine self-confidence as a nurse. In their search for answers and to vent angry feelings, the mother and family may also probe. The nurse may perceive the questioning as challenges to her capabilities as a nurse. At times like this even the most competent and self-assured nurse may need peer or other support to identify feelings and verbalize them and to regain perspective.

The nurse may be unaware of personal struggles with reactions to grief. The nurse may resort to reassuring and comforting the grieving individual or individuals in a manner that does not foster a healthy grieving response. Some commonly heard responses given by physicians, nurses, and well-meaning friends *should be avoided:*

- "There was a reason why God wanted this baby. Have faith."
- "It's God's will. We have to have faith that it was for the best."
- "It's probably better this way. This often happens when the baby has something wrong with it."
- "You are so young. There's time for more."
- "Be thankful you have those other lovely children at home. They'll be a solace and comfort to you."

This baby is important *now.* The mother needs to talk about *this* baby. She does not want or need to focus on her other children or any suggestions for substitutes for her loss.

Certain behaviors give the message that to face grief is "bad" for a person and to avoid facing it is better for all concerned. An example might be avoiding talking about the infant, quelling tears, and forbidding the mother to see and hold the infant.

Somehow it is thought that to avoid an issue is the healthiest and easiest way. It does prevent "scenes." Out of sight is out of mind. But out of sight is not out of the mother's mind. The mother has felt life. She has developed a relationship with the infant through shared internal physical sensation and fantasy. If the child lives for a few hours or days after birth, the mother's relationship with the child has progressed even further. Even after delivery the hormones that sustain an attachment between mother and child are still present. The physical signs and discomforts that occur during the normal postpartum period also exist. At home are the baby clothes and furniture, family, and friends, awaiting the hoped-for new arrival. Resolution of grief is important *now* and can be a healthy growth-inducing process.

Mothers and families look to the hospital staff to meet their needs. Having had an unfortunate maternity experience, these mothers may suffer a severe blow to their sense of worth associated with the ability to give life. Their role concept, self-esteem, and femininity may be diminished. Nursing interventions that assist the grieving family in coping with this ego-threatening experience may foster a healthy mourning process and can be incorporated easily within the busiest nursing assignment.

Death is often equated with powerlessness, an end, and failure. However, the nurse need not be professionally and personally helpless. Preventive mental health measures are well within the scope of the nurse. Some therapeutic nursing interventions are as follows:

1. Parents need an objective listener, one who is genuinely interested and willing to face true feelings and who will not try to "talk them out of it." The nurse acts as a role model for open communication in facing grief and for feeling safe and comfortable in dealing with an unpleasant situation.

2. Parents need to feel that those around them know that it is natural for them to feel sad, weepy, and easily distracted.

3. Nurses should convey to parents that grieving takes time and that they may never really "get over it," although the pain does ease with time; good memories then tend to persist.

4. Nurses should be prepared for the anger and self-blame parents may feel and help the parents identify these feelings: "You may be wondering if you did or did not do something to cause this." Parents may not be able to work through their anger before discharge; some parents return or write many months later to apologize for their behavior and to thank those who were able to see beyond their anger and help them with their needs.

5. Coping with grief and recovering from childbirth exact a heavy toll on the mother's resources. Although the grieving process often makes sleep difficult and appetite nonexistent, adequate rest and diet must be assured to replenish the mother's vitality. Thoughtful nursing actions (e.g., back rubs, just sitting quietly with her) can meet very real, critical needs. Sleeping pills may delay the grieving process.

6. The nurse should prepare the parents for returning home, for example, what to expect of themselves emotionally and physically and what they can expect from the other children. Siblings may feel that the parent or parents lied to them about the coming of a new baby. The older child may feel that it is her or his fault that the baby died because she or he may not have wanted a new sibling now, or wanted a boy but got a girl, so that the girl then died. Older siblings may act out their feelings in other ways. Older children may need verbal explanations as well as assistance in voicing feelings and thoughts. Discussion about the fetal or newborn death as well as death in general should be an open subject in the family. The cause of the death should be openly presented so that the child may cope with any existing feelings of guilt. A small child who cannot understand verbal explanations needs demonstrations of love and affection to provide reassurance and security. He may be unable to express frightening thoughts that he is experiencing. Occasionally the small child may resort to misbehavior to draw attention or may cling excessively to his parents. Euphemisms such as, "The baby went away (or to sleep)" or "God took him" are usually meant to help the child, but more often they can be threatening. Regardless of the way parents handle the reaction to death, some children may manifest their inner disturbance in nightmares, bed-wetting, school problems, or other ways.

Physical symptoms that parents may experience include sleep problems with fatigue, anorexia, muscle aches and "knots," gastrointestinal symptoms, and palpitations.

Psychologic or emotional symptoms that parents may experience include an inability to concentrate for long on any one activity (i.e., their minds may wander or they may feel everything is whirling around in their heads) and pressure in the head. People commonly express the fear of "going crazy" when they experience reactions that they do not expect or understand. The mother may hold her abdomen and state she feels "empty" and that her arms "ache to hold a baby." Parents may fear being alone, wish to go away somewhere, or become overconcerned about or disinterested in their older children. Irritability with or disinterest in the other children may compound guilt feelings.

LOSS OF THE MOTHER

Childbirth is viewed as a normal physiologic event. When the mother dies, the survivors may respond in a wide variety of ways. The newborn infant may be targeted as the cause of the mother's death. Family members who feel that the newborn is somehow responsible may find it difficult to develop a positive, caring relationship with the child. The loss leaves the father emotionally drained at this time when the newborn and older children need him most. In the back of his mind, he may experience guilt for his role in family planning. He may wonder how the family can manage financially regardless of whether the wife had contributed to the family income.

Families have a need to know why the event occurred. Consent for autopsy is usually given. The physician may gain more information with which to discuss the maternal death with the family.

Grandparents feel the loss intensely as well. Parents expect that their children will survive them in the "natural order" of things. The death of their daughter is a break in the continuity. Furthermore the maternal grandparents may be faced with the possibility that the husband will remarry and thus create a distance between them and their grandchild.

Denial is the prominent defense mechanism used intermittently by children of all ages. Denial is used even though intellectually death is comprehended. The pain of coming to grips with the loss extends over a long period of time. For varying lengths of time there is hope and expectation that the loved one will return.

The time to offer counseling is at the time when a death occurs, before conflicts and anxieties have resulted in behavior difficulties or symptom formation. Important areas involve helping the bereaved around burial services. This includes clarifying with the parent the importance of discussing the nature of the illness so that the child can achieve his own differentiation and supporting the bereaved in their grief so that they in turn can allow the expression of grief in their children (Sahler, 1978).

Working with the family who suffers this type of loss is challenging but also potentially rewarding (Table 28-2).

Children Under 5 Years of Age. There is a special necessity for preventive work with children under 5 when a parent dies. Children under 5 form the most vulnerable age group (Sahler, 1978). Such children depend solely on parental support for their ego development and mastery of the instinctual drives. Their reality testing is limited. They are easily overwhelmed with anxiety. Their capacity to verbalize affects is not fully developed. They need adult help in identifying feelings. Symptoms of anxiety and inner stress are prone to take the form of physical activity (e.g., regression behaviors, over or under activity, or psychosomatic symptoms).

Table 28-2 *Psychosocial Role of Nurse in Care of Family After Maternal Death*

Assessment	Plan/Implementation	Rationale
1. Assess husband's and family's emotional response: a. Quiet, composed. b. Denial: "I just don't believe it"; euphoric, animated. c. Overtly upset, crying. d. Angry toward staff, others; "If only the doctor had . . ."; "If I had only . . ."; said, tearful. e. Responses toward newborn and older children. 2. Assess external support system. a. Presence of relatives. b. Behavior of relatives. Do husband and children seem reassured by their presence and actions? c. Family's interest and ability to stay with husband or siblings. d. Ask if they wish to contact clergy or members of their church. 3. Young children (under 5 years): a. Concept of death. b. Behavioral responses. 4. Children of any age: a. Use of denial. b. Concept of death. 5. Adolescent: a. Level of maturity. b. Prominant developmental tasks: identity, including sexual identity; moving toward independence. c. Assess for suicidal ideation.	1. Be available and indicate willingness to sit and listen. 2. Encourage and assist verbalization of: a. Feelings of loss, of being cheated. b. Any feelings, actions, or lack of action that family may believe caused this. 3. Act as advocate of family with physician regarding questions concerning cause. 4. Fill in gaps in information and clarify misconceptions. Help family formulate questions for physician; help them understand what physician tells them. 5. Alert family to characteristics of grieving process: a. Personal responses. b. Variations in responses to be expected at different developmental levels. c. Duration for child versus adult. 6. Assist family with concerns such as, "Are you wondering how to tell the other children, the grandparents, etc.?" 7. Make appropriate referrals: home health care, child care, psychiatric social worker, homemaker service.	1. Verbal repetition of experience helps one cope with a situation and integrate experience into one's perception of self in nonthreatening manner. 2. People experiencing loss may need to ask same questions repeatedly from same or other people. Answers may need to be given frequently, with patience and understanding. 3. People experiencing grief may feel alienated from others, lonely, and helpless; they may exhibit anger in presence or toward accepting, understanding, and caring other, such as nurse. 4. Response to loss and grief is influenced by a number of factors, some of which are: a. Age, developmental level of survivor. b. Events leading up to her death. c. Circumstances related to social aspects of this pregnancy. 5. When medical and nursing staff are able to communicate comfortably and openly about death and grief reactions and feelings, the family may be better able to face and cope with situation. Knowledge about any situation helps dispel fear of unknown, misconceptions, fantasy. Knowledge supports ego strength. Open communication and being available physically and psychologically helps in following ways: a. It fosters open communication between husband and significant others and between family and staff. Energy does not have to be diverted to keeping up a front. b. It gives permission to grieve, validates appropriateness of grieving here and now in a manner acceptable to them, and gives permission to speak of death.

Adolescent Reactions. Because of greater ego maturity the normal adolescent is better able to cope with the finality of death. The predominant task of adolescence is to move toward independence, to free oneself from close dependence on parents. Adolescents need repeated attempts to break away, to try various activities outside the family. Although critical of and hostile to parents at times, adolescents have an option to return and be cared for. When one parent is no longer available to meet this need for comfort and care, the struggle toward independence may be disrupted. Guilt is common. The child wonders if the parent might have lived if he had done something different (e.g., been nicer, not rebelled so much).

The relationship between the adolescent and the surviving parent needs consideration. The living parent may be preoccupied with his own grief. Thus the adolescent is doubly deprived. Attempts to console the father may be met with anger and irritation. The adolescent may turn away with a sense of being a failure. The potential for suicide often arises in the adolescent group. Many develop a renewed interest in immortality. Deutsch (1967) has made the point that as the adolescent struggles with intense anxieties, she or he is confronted with one of life's sharpest paradoxes—namely, that on the threshold of a new life, she or he feels the threat of death.

Adolescents are struggling with their sexual identity as well. The death of their mother during childbirth can have a negative effect on both the female and male adolescent. Open communication is essential in helping the adolescent identify these feelings and differentiate herself or himself from the deceased (Sahler, 1978).

Adults often mourn at a faster pace than children. When the two generations are out of phase in their grieving, a sensitive nurse is aware that children may be confused, especially if the father remarries. The nurse can play a supportive role by alerting the family to expect this reaction. The adolescent needs much emotional support and opportunities to verbalize her or his concerns so that misconceptions about death can be clarified.

BIRTH OF A COMPROMISED NEWBORN

The birth of a premature child (see Chapters 33 and 34) or a child with an obvious defect is a shattering experience for parents and a disturbing experience for those who attended the birth. Parents feel devastated and inadequate; anticipated joy ends in despair and confusion. A flurry of activity often follows such a birth. The child may then be examined by specialists, often at a facility far from the mother's hospital. Physicians and others (e.g., clergy) may talk with the parents. The natural order of postdelivery phychologic tasks is disrupted, and the new parents are in crisis. The nurse is in a unique and critical position. Of all the members of the health team, the nurse alone can be available 24 hours a day. A nurse can help plan for discharge and postdischarge care. Although clinical intervention will vary with each situation, in every case the nurse must establish herself as a caring, knowledgeable, resourceful person.

Whether the child is premature, ill, or has a defect, the parental responses and needs are similar in many respects. In general, the couple's needs can be summarized to include (1) mourning the loss of the fantasized perfect baby, (2) immediate diagnosis and management of the newborn, (3) clinical evaluation and diagnosis of the causes of the infant's disorder, (4) when appropriate, preparation and planning for the continued care of the affected newborn, (5) redefinition of the parental role in their social network (i.e., reentrance into their society), and (6) family planning and genetic counseling. Nursing management is planned to help parents meet these needs.

Mourning Loss of Perfect Child. Grieving is the first difficult task of the new parents of a premature child or a child with a malformation or disorder. Psychologic shock, commonly coupled with the necessity of physical separation from the infant, makes this period trying. The parents are vulnerable. Resolution of grief for the lost, assumed-perfect child precedes the development of acceptance or attachment to the real imperfect child or any decisions regarding her or his placement. The period of acute grief is usually about 6 weeks; however, in the continued presence of a child with a defect, grief may become chronic and persist for a lifetime.

The parents are profoundly affected by the manner and attitudes of those around them, especially the medical and nursing personnel. Parents are sensitive to and respond quickly to nonverbal cues from others that may connote nonacceptance, revulsion, or blame. Voice inflections, facial expressions, or the posture of the nurse who witnesses parental grief reactions or views the infant is quickly noted and internalized. Nurses also are representatives of society and may reflect society's reactions to them as parents of a child who is less than perfect.

Early Parent-child Relationship. The very small premature infant, the sick infant, or a child with a serious congenital disorder may have to be taken to another institution immediately after birth. This event can cause the mother to feel psychologically estranged from her infant.

Continuing Parent-child Relationship. The skilled medical and nursing care required by the infant in this period, which the parents cannot provide, may be overwhelming. In fact, they may focus on the gadgetry—the machines, tubes, and bottles—associated with the infant's care rather than on the infant.

Parents need to "keep in touch" with the infant somehow. This may be accomplished by viewing the infant frequently and at close range and hearing frequent progress reports and answers to their questions. At other times, parents may be permitted to touch, fondle, and stroke the infant when it is still not practical to involve them in actual feeding and bathing. During these initial contacts, and until parents gain self-confidence, the nurse should remain nearby, offering support as needed.

If the infant's hospitalization is prolonged, the nursing staff should keep the parents informed of the infant's progress. This can be accomplished with telephone calls and notes "from the baby."

The parents and nurse may feel frustrated, uncomfortable, and even helpless when faced with the birth of a child with a defect. However, the parents and nurse can grow from a mutually shared experience. Touching and sharing another's experience of loss can be threatening but also rewarding.

Grandparents Reactions. Grandparents are also touched by the birth of an infant at risk. Grandparents can be supportive to the young family, having the natural response to protect their offspring. For others, birth of a grandchild who is less than perfect seems to lower their self-esteem. They may resort to blaming the young parents or their child's spouse for acts of omission or commission in precipitating the problem with remarks such as, "We've never had this happen in *our* family before—ever." Other comments commonly heard include, "The women in *our* family have never had problems having babies" and "I told him [her] that nothing good would come of this marriage [relationship]." Comments such as these from members of the parents families may mask hidden feelings. Such feelings might include inadequacy about themselves, feelings of helplessness in the situation, or concern that there may be no grandchild and therefore no "immortality" for them. Many other emotional reactions are possible.

The nurse must avoid the pitfall of taking sides. The nurse provides patience, tact, and warm sympathy. This is coupled with efforts to help family members identify and explore feelings, clarify misconceptions, and provide simple, cogent explanations that may contribute to the comfort, strength, and unity of the entire family.

A nursing care plan is incomplete without an assessment and plan for action regarding grandparental responses.

Siblings' Reactions. As discussed earlier, preparation of parents of a high-risk infant begins long before the infant is discharged from the hospital. Preparation of the older children also needs to be undertaken before the infant goes home. The young child can easily "forget" the existence of a brother or sister in the hospital. If possible, visits to see the new baby should be encouraged. For the older child the idea of an imperfect baby can be clarified by seeing him and having a chance to discuss fears and misconceptions. One 8-year-old boy was given the job of "explaining" all about his premature sister to the visiting grandparents. He discussed the care of the baby and use of supportive equipment surprisingly well.

Immediate Diagnosis and Management of Child. Diagnosing the disorder and initiating appropriate therapy is the physician's responsibility; however, the nurse must be conversant with diagnostic techniques and rationale for therapy to reinforce and clarify the physician's explanations. If possible, the nurse should sit in with the parents and physician during their sessions to know what is being said. Open lines of communication between physician and nurse, always essential, are vital now. One nursing function is to help parents identify and verbalize their questions as well as their misgivings and fears. The nurse must deal with those questions and concerns within her realm of expertise and channel others to appropriate health care team members.

The history taking and diagnostic procedures necessary to uncover the etiology are exacting. One is asked to look for disorders in ancestors, to explore prenatal acts of omission and commission (e.g., nutrition, drugs), and to seek out other environmental factors.

Parents may express feelings of shame and embarrassment lest they be carrying a "bad" gene or be responsible for exposure to a devastating environmental agent. Others are anxious to fix the blame somewhere. Many women remember transient (or persistent) negative feelings about the pregnancy or baby and interpret these feelings as punishment for their real or imagined transgressions.

The nurse's role must be supportive. This includes preparing parents for what to expect and allowing for anticipatory worry, listening actively, and assisting with the formulation of questions and the ventilation of feelings.

Long-term Management of Child. Long-term management of a child with a disorder necessitates multidisciplinary planning and cooperation. A coordinated program of continual guidance and counseling of the parents is essential. The emotional, physical, and financial status of the parents, available community resources, and the child's condition must be evaluated.

The nurse's role varies with the situation: Is the defect obvious? Is it curable? Is it treatable? How do parents perceive the disorder? Skillfully executed, the nurse's supportive function aids parents in decision making and in self-acceptance regarding their decisions (e.g., surgical procedures, institutionalization).

If the child requires medications, diet, or physical manipulation, the nurse should assist in teaching how, when, and why. Parents will benefit from supervised practice before discharge and frequent positive reinforcement of their ability to perform necessary tasks.

Community resources should be tapped to assist with the financial burden, equipment, drugs, and psychologic support (see Appendix K). For example, in the San Francisco Bay area, there is a group of parents of children with cleft lip and palate who meet to share feelings, problems, techniques, and new developments. A social worker may have the prime responsibility in this area of management, but the nurse should be cognizant of resources also. Visiting nurse associations may be involved in the follow-up care in the home.

Continued guidance and counseling are essential in helping the family and its members live in harmony with each other, increasing their comfort and strengthening their unity. The child with a defect needs love, affection, and social and physical stimulation as much as or more than any other child. At the same time, the child's special needs and reactions must be considered. Other family members also need love, a sense of fulfillment, and recognition as worthwhile persons. Meeting all these needs requires much energy from each family member. The nurse can help family members understand the special dynamics of their situation and cope with the inevitable tensions and resentments that arise.

Redefinition of Parental Role and Social Network. A society expects adults to produce healthy children to perpetuate that society. A social stigma is attached to bearing a defective child, a reality with which the parents must learn to cope.

After parents grieve and come to terms with their failure to produce a healthy offspring, they still face several hurdles. One is to make a decision regarding the disposition of the child—institution or home. If the child comes home, they must learn to meet her or his special needs and introduce the child to society.

Another hurdle is facing others—the other children, family, friends, and strangers. Even during the hospital stay, parents experience society's adverse reaction. Subtle or blatant expressions of social isolation are evident. The cards, flowers, and other gifts of congratulation are sparse. Commonly the cheery forms of congratulations come only from those unaware of the "situation." Telephone conversations are guarded. Even medical personnel, unhappily, may shun these parents. Families may be insinuating blame on each other. At home, callers do not ask to see the baby. If they do, verbal response may be stilted, although nonverbal response is poignant.

The entire health team and community resourses such as clergy must accept the task of helping parents reenter the outside world. Several of the techniques already discussed are helpful, but others also may prove helpful.

One simple technique is **role playing.** The anticipated

meetings with the other children, family, and friends are acted out. Another approach is to discuss how parents will handle the curiosity of friends, acquaintances, and strangers. These techniques help in several ways. First, by anticipating the words and reactions of others, they verbalize their own. Second, the practice augments their store of coping strategies. Both techniques may uncover feelings that can be dealt with here and now, although resolution of these feelings may not come until much later. Each encounter may serve to strengthen coping mechanisms and bring the resolution of feelings a step closer.

SUMMARY

Stuart and Sundeen (1987) summarize the nurse's role in loss and grief as follows. Although death is the most certain aspect of life, fear of it is universal. Because of this and because of their proximity to the situation of dying, death is a necessary concern for nurses. Attitudes toward death are culturally learned. Personal reactions have their basis in the psychologic maturity and personality characteristics of the individual. The individual's own values, beliefs, and experiences influence the cognitive aspects of dying.

The nurse needs to have a cognitive grasp of the developmental aspects of the concept of death, the stages and processes associated with grief, and resources available to the individual and family. It is important to assess one's own viewpoints and attitudes toward death, since these often transfer over into the caregiving situation.

Understanding of the dying process is closely linked to the level of maturity and cognitive abilities of the child and adults involved. Helping children and adults learn to express their fears about death can help diminish some of the emotional strain of grief work. Adaptation to changes within the existing family structure and interactions are invariably necessary. Change is difficult. The family may require support from community resources. The death of a newborn or the mother is a shattering experience.

Nurses are expected to provide physical care, comfort, understanding, and emotional support to the individual and family. However, nurses must recognize that there are limitations and immense emotional strains that pervade the caregiving situation. Nurses caring for the bereaved need a professional support system of their own.

KEY CONCEPTS

- An unnatural or unexpected interruption in pregnancy and birth poses a potential threat to a woman's self-esteem and femininity.
- Death of the mother completely disrupts the family structure and often leaves the father with the care of a baby at a time when his emotional reserves are lowest.
- When expectations of birth and joy are replaced by loss, the nurse's role is critical.
- An understanding of loss and the normal grieving process is fundamental to the implementation of the nursing process.
- Many factors influence the client's response to loss—level of growth and development, cultural and spiritual beliefs, societal expectations, nature of the relationship among family members, socioeconomic status.
- The nurse is also vulnerable when caring for clients experiencing loss and grief.

STUDY QUESTIONS AND ACTIVITIES

1. Interview labor-delivery nurses who in their work have experienced the delivery of an imperfect child or an unexpected fetal death. What were their feelings? What were the behaviors of staff persons? Who assisted the parents?
2. Discover what community resources and support groups exist to assist parents who have experienced:
   a. a premature birth
   b. birth of an imperfect child
   c. a fetal death
3. After viewing a film on death and grieving, discuss the kinds of behavior the group observed of the grieving person.

Inexperienced students may be quite uncomfortable in situations of grief and loss. Exercises should focus on developing self-awareness of feelings regarding loss and how these feelings can transfer to parents. Activities that are beneficial are:

4. Develop a role-playing situation wherein a student acts as a nurse assisting parents of an imperfect child. Anticipate meetings with older children, families, and friends.
5. Invite a speaker from a local support group to describe her or his work with parents and families.
6. Compare and contrast the grieving process as it might affect the family experiencing the fetal death of a perfect child and the family whose child is born defective.

References

Deutsch, H: Selected problems of adolescence, Monogr Ser Psychoanal Study Child no 3, 1967, International Universities Press, Inc

Johnson, SH: Nursing assessment and strategies for the family at risk: high-risk parenting, ed 2, Philadelphia, 1986, JB Lippincott Co

Kübler-Ross, E: On death and dying, New York, 1969, Macmillan Publishing Co

Lindemann, E: Symptomatology and management of acute grief, Am J Psychol 101:141, 1944

Sahler, OJ, editor: The child and death, St Louis, 1978, The CV Mosby Co

Stuart, GW, and Sundeen, SJ: Principles and practice of psychiatric nursing, ed 2, St Louis, 1987, The CV Mosby Co

Zlomke, E: Personal correspondence, Spring, 1986

Bibliography

Arms, S: To love and let go, New York, 1983, Alfred A Knopf, Inc

Barnes, J: Reactions to the death of a mother, Psychoanal Study Child 19:334, 1964

Beckey, RD, et al: Development of a perinatal grief checklist, JOGN Nurs 14:194, May/June, 1985

Bethea, SW: Primary nursing in the infant special care unit, JOGN Nurs 13:202, May/June 1985
Blackburn, S, and Lowen, L: Impact of an infant's premature birth on the grandparents and parents, JOGN Nurs 15:173, March/April 1986
Carr, D, and Knupp, SF: Grief and perinatal loss: a community hospital approach to support, JOGN Nurs 14(2):130, 1985
Cefalo, RC: Managing missed abortion and antepartum fetal death, Contemp OB/GYN 22(3):17, 1983
Consolvo, CA: Relieving parental anxiety in the care-by-parent unit, JOGN Nurs 15(2):154, 1986
Cordell, A, Apolito, R: Family support in infant death, JOGN Nurs 10(4):281, 1981
Dahlberg, NLF: A perinatal center based antepartum homecare program, JOGN Nurs 17(1):30 1988
Drane, JF: The defective child: ethical guidelines for painful dilemmas, JOGN Nurs 13(1):42, 1984
Eager, M, and Exoo, R: Parents visiting parents for unequaled support, MCN 5:35, 1980
Ehrenkranz, RA: Neonatal death: caring for parents, Contemp OB/GYN 22(3):24, 1983
Elsea, SF: Ethics in maternal-child nursing, MCN 10:303, Sept/Oct 1985
Estok, P, and Lehman, A: Perinatal death: grief support for families, Birth 10(1):17, 1983
Furlong, RM, and Hobbins, JC: Grief in the perinatal period, Obstet Gynecol 61:497, 1983
Furman, E: A child's parent dies; studies in childhood bereavement, New Haven, 1974, Yale University Press
Gennaro, S: Anxiety and problem-solving ability in mothers of premature infants, JOGN Nurs 15(2):160, 1986
Gilbert, ES, and Harmon, JS: High-risk pregnancy and delivery: nursing perspectives, St Louis, 1986, The CV Mosby Co
Grabauskas, P, et al: Helping the parents after a baby's death, RN, p 31, Aug 1987
Green, D: Prenatal diagnosis: when reality shatters parents' dreams, Nurs '88, 18(2):61, 1988
Gulanick, M, et al, editors: Nursing care plans: nursing diagnosis and intervention, Michael Reese Hospital and Medical Center, St Louis, 1986, The CV Mosby Co
Hawkins-Walsh, E: Diminishing anxiety in parents of sick newborns, MCN 5:20, 1980
Helping patients and doctors cope with perinatal death (symposium), Contemp OB/GYN 20(2):98, 1981
Jenkins, RL, and Tock, MK: Helping parents bond to their premature infant, MCN 11(1):32, 1986
Jenkins, RL, and Westhus, NK: The nurse role in parent-infant bonding: overview, assessment, intervention, JOGN Nurs 10:114, March/April 1981
Kaplan, DM, and Mason, EA: Maternal reactions to premature birth viewed as an acute emotional disorder, Am J Orthopsychiatry 30:118, July 1960
Laufer, M: Object loss and mourning during adolescence, Psychoanal Study Child 21:269, 1966
Ledger, KE, and Williams, DL: Parents at risk: an instructional program for perinatal assessment and preventive intervention, Funded by Ministry of Health, Province of British Columbia and Queen Alexandra Solarium for Crippled Children Society, Canada (Queen Alexandra Hospital, 2040 Arbutus Road, Victoria, BC, Canada, V8N 1V7)
Malcolm, N, and Wooten, B: It's hard to say Goodbye, Can Nurse 83(4):27, 1987
Merenstein, GB, and Gardner, SL: Handbook of neonatal intensive care, St Louis, 1986, The CV Mosby Co
Mina, CF: A program for helping grieving parents, MCN 10:118, March/April 1985
Monsen, R: Phases in the caring relationship: from adversary to ally to coordinator, MCN 11(5):316, 1986
Ney, PG: Helping patients cope with pregnancy loss, Contemp OB/GYN 29(6):117, 1987
Quimette, J: Perinatal nursing: care of the high-risk mother and infant, Boston, 1986, Jones and Bartlett Publishers
Raff, BS: Nursing care of high-risk infants and their families: introduction, JOGN Nurs 15:141, March/April 1986
Raff, BS: The use of homemaker-home health aids' perinatal care of high-risk infants, JOGN Nurs 15:142, March/April 1986
Rothenberg, LS: Down's syndrome babies: decisions not to feed and the letter from Washington, J Calif Perinatal Assoc 2(1):78, 1982
Sadler, ME: When your patient's baby dies before birth, RN, p 28, Aug 1987
Schwab, F, et al: Sibling visiting in a neonatal intensive care unit, Pediatrics 71:835, 1983
Steele, K: Caring for parents of critically ill neonates during hospitalization: Strategies for health care professionals, MCN 16(1):13, 1986
Stewart, D: Spiritual care of the neonate, Periscope (published by the California Perinatal Association), pp. 1-2, June 1980
Thornton, J, Berry, J, and DalSanto, J: Neonatal intensive care: the nurse's role in supporting the family, Nurs Clin North Am 19(1):125, 1984
Veach, SA: Down's syndrome: helping the parents of a special infant, Nurs '83, 13(9):42, 1983
Wessel, M: Death of an adult—and its impact upon the child, Clin Pediatr 2:28, 1973
Wessel, M: The adolescent and death of a parent. In Galagher, R, Heald, F, and Garrelagher, D, editors: Medical care of the adolescent, New York, 1976, Appleton-Century-Crofts
Whaley, LF: Genetic counseling in maternity nursing. In McNall, LK, and Galeener, JT, editors: Current practice in obstetric and gynecologic nursing, vol I, St Louis, 1976, The CV Mosby Co
Whaley, LF and Wong, DL: Nursing care of infants and children, ed 3, St Louis, 1987, The CV Mosby Co
Whitaker, CM: Death before birth, Am J Nurs 86:156, Feb 1986

CHAPTER

29

Hypertensive States in Pregnancy

Learning Objectives

Correctly define the key terms listed.

Differentiate between pregnancy-induced hypertension (PIH) and chronic hypertension.

Review etiologic theories of PIH.

Describe pathophysiology of PIH.

Evaluate maternal, fetal, and newborn morbidity and mortality attributable to PIH.

Describe the HELLP syndrome.

List assessment techniques for PIH.

Formulate nursing diagnoses for mild and severe PIH.

Summarize the management of mild and severe PIH.

Assess the use of the anticonvulsant magnesium sulfate.

Review management of convulsions.

Key Terms

affect
antihypertensives
arteriolar spasm
calcium gluconate
chronic hypertension
clonus
convulsion care
deep tendon reflex (DTR)
eclampsia
gestational hypertension
HELLP syndrome
hyperreflexia
magnesium sulfate
mean arterial pressure (MAP)
oliguria
pitting edema
preeclampsia
pregnancy-induced hypertension (PIH)
proteinuria
roll-over test
seizure precautions
toxemia

Pregnancy-induced hypertension complicates approximately 5% to 7% of pregnancies in otherwise normal primigravid women, and as many as 20% to 40% of pregnancies in women with chronic renal disease or vascular disorders such as essential hypertension, diabetes mellitus, and lupus erythematosus (Danforth and Scott, 1986). In many regions of North America and in many parts of the world, hypertension complicating pregnancy is the leading cause of maternal and infant morbidity and mortality. Diminished placental perfusion secondary to arteriolar vasospasm places the fetus at risk. Eclampsia (seizures) from profound cerebral effects is the major maternal hazard. Early recognition and timely intervention are vital to arrest the progression of the disorder when possible, to prevent eclampsia, and to effect a safe delivery of the infant. The joint efforts of physicians and nurses can do much to prevent and treat the condition and thereby promote satisfactory outcomes for mother and baby.

CLASSIFICATION

Confusion over classification terminology continues. Recently the Committee on Terminology of the American College of Obstetricians and Gynecologists prepared a new classification to distinguish the various hypertensive states of pregnancy. The classification differentiates pregnancy-induced hypertension (PIH) from concurrent hypertension and pregnancy (CHP). PIH encompasses those hypertensive disorders that begin during pregnancy and subside completely following delivery. The causes of CHP states are unrelated to pregnancy. This classification of PIH and CHP is described in Table 29-1 (Gilbert and Harmon, 1986). PIH, especially preeclampsia–eclampsia, is the primary focus of this chapter.

Gestational Hypertension. Gestational hypertension is defined as an elevation of systolic and diastolic pressure equal to or exceeding 140/90 mm Hg. An alternative definition that is more sensitive to individual variations is a rise in systolic pressure of 30 mm Hg or a rise in diastolic pressure of 15 mm Hg above the woman's baseline values. The latter definition is useful because blood pressure varies with age, race, physiologic state, dietary habits, and heredity. Gestational hypertension is not accompanied by other evidence of preeclampsia or hypertensive vascular disease; it disappears within 10 days following parturition.

The blood pressure elevation must be present on 2 occasions 6 hours apart. Techniques of measurement must be standardized, for instance, always taken with the woman sitting *or* supine *or* in a lateral position. The technique used must be noted in the client's record to provide data to guide interpretation of previous, present, and future readings.

The appearance of de novo third-trimester hypertension in a nullipara, regardless of whether other signs are present, is sufficient reason to proceed with hospitalization and treatment as if she had preeclampsia. Third-trimester hypertension is defined as a diastolic blood pressure of 85 mm Hg or more or a mean arterial pressure (MAP) exceeding 95 mm Hg (Lindheimer and Katz, 1985).

Preeclampsia. The presence of **proteinuria** distinguishes preeclampsia from gestational hypertension. Preeclampsia may be accompanied by **edema,** which is a generalized accumulation of interstitial fluid (face, hands, abdomen, sacrum, tibia, ankles) after 12 hours of bed rest or a *weight gain* of more than 2 kg (4 to 4½ lb) per week. The presence of edema is less significant than the rapidity of weight gain.

Eclampsia. Eclampsia includes the symptoms of severe preeclampsia and one or more of the following: (1) tonic and clonic **convulsions or coma,** with the coma possibly following an unobserved seizure related to other seizure disorders, (2) **hypertensive crisis,** or (3) **shock.**

Chronic Hypertensive Disease. Hypertension may predate the pregnancy and be a manifestation of primary or

Table 29-1 *Classification of the Hypertensive States of Pregnancy*

Type	Description
Pregnancy-induced Hypertension (PIH)	
Gestational hypertension	The development of hypertension after 20 weeks of gestation in a previously normotensive woman without proteinuria; the blood pressure returns to normal within 10 postpartum days
Preeclampsia	The development of hypertension and proteinuria with or without edema in a previously normotensive woman after 20 weeks of gestation or early postpartum; in the presence of trophoblastic disease it can develop before 20 weeks of gestation
Eclampsia	The development of convulsions or coma in a preeclamptic woman
Superimposed preeclampsia or eclampsia	The development of preeclampsia or eclampsia in a woman with concurrent hypertension
Concurrent Hypertension and Pregnancy (CHP)	
Chronic hypertension	Hypertension that develops before pregnancy or before week 20 of gestation that is not pregnancy associated

Modified from Gilbert, ES, and Harmon, JS: High-risk pregnancy and delivery: nursing perspectives, St Louis, 1986, The CV Mosby Co.

Table 29-2 *Differential Diagnosis of Essential Hypertension and Preeclampsia (PIH)*

Features	Essential Hypertension	Preeclampsia (PIH)
Onset of hypertension	Before pregnancy; during first 20 weeks of pregnancy	After 20 weeks of pregnancy (exception: trophoblastic tumors*)
Duration of hypertension	Permanent; hypertension beyond 3 months postdelivery	Hypertension absent 10 days postdelivery
Family history	Often positive	Usually negative, may be positive
Past history	Recurrent "toxemia"	Psychosexual problems common
Age	Usually older	Generally teenaged or in early 20s
Parity	Usually multigravida	Usually primigravida
Habitus	May be thin	Usually eumorphic
Retinal findings	Often arteriovenous nicking, tortuous arterioles, cotton-wool exudates, hemorrhages	Vascular spasm, retinal edema; rarely, protein extravasations
Proteinuria	Often none	Usually present; absent at 6 weeks postdelivery

Reproduced with permission, from Benson, RC, editor: Current obstetric and gynecologic diagnosis and treatment, ed 5. Copyright 1984 by Lange Medical Publications, Los Altos, Calif.

*Hydatidiform mole (molar pregnancy).

secondary chronic hypertensive disease (Table 29-2). Primary (essential) hypertensive disease, in which no cause can be determined, is the diagnosis in about 85% of nonpregnant, premenopausal hypertensive women. The remaining 15% of women with hypertension have secondary hypertensive vascular disease, caused by disorders such as chronic pyelonephritis or glomerulonephritis, renal artery stenosis, or coarctation of the aorta. Occasionally, when the hypertensive woman is seen initially late in pregnancy, studies after the puerperium may be required before the cause of hypertension can be determined. Often the etiologic factors are obscure, and the tentative impression may be one of "essential hypertension" (see Table 29-2).

With chronic hypertensive disease, the physician treats the symptomatology during pregnancy. The pregnancy is usually permitted to continue if the woman responds to therapy. Frequent estriol determinations after the thirty-second week will be ordered in an attempt to allow the woman to carry the fetus to 34 to 36 weeks (Chapter 27). Protracted or maternal central nervous system (CNS), cardiac, or renal complications may develop. If the woman's blood pressure reaches 200/110, immediate medical attention is necessary. The physician will usually order antihypertensive drugs such as hydralazine (see Table 29-4) and assess the need for a prompt delivery.

The nursing care of women with chronic hypertensive disease is the same as that of women with preeclampsia. Preeclampsia superimposed on chronic hypertension is more difficult to manage than preeclampsia alone and carries a grave prognosis for mother and fetus. If and when cardiac involvement is diagnosed, the nursing care of the woman with cardiac disease is superimposed on the original plan (see Chapter 34). The woman and her family must be aware of the possibility of premature delivery and of the need for careful and continuous supervision during the prenatal, intranatal, and postdelivery periods.

The *prognosis* for the pregnant woman with chronic hypertension depends on the cause, the degree of hypertension, the woman's symptoms, and her response to treatment. Whatever the cause, the fetus may be severely affected by hypertension and its sequelae. Early delivery may be lifesaving for the mother and fetus.

ETIOLOGY

The cause of PIH has been the subject of extensive research and much speculation for decades. No known theory as yet accounts for all symptoms. Evidently PIH is somehow related to the physiologic changes of pregnancy because it disappears after the termination of pregnancy. Therefore the gravid uterus, placenta, or fetus could be the central factor in the condition. Pritchard, MacDonald, and Gant (1985), note that pregnancy-induced or aggravated chronic hypertension is much more likely to develop in the woman who is exposed to *chorionic villi* for the first time, or is exposed to a superabundance of chorionic villi, as with twins or hydatidiform mole (one form of trophoblastic disease discussed in Chapter 44). Common theories implicate nutritional deficiency, immunologic dysfuntion, genetic predisposition, and uterine ischemia.

Nutritional deficiency, especially in protein and calories, compromises hepatic sufficiency. Hepatic conjunction of estrogen and progesterone is impaired. The resultant accumulation of these placental steroid hormones may trigger the disorder (Brewer, 1966). A deficiency in calcium, iron, and vitamins may also be etiologic factors (Belizan and Villar, 1980). Nutritional deficiencies may interfere with the synthesis of prostaglandin and thus increase sensitivity to angiotensin. However, Zlatnick and Burmeister (1983) presented convincing evidence that in their study population, the incidence of PIH was *not* directly related to the level of dietary protein.

An *immunologic response* may be an etiologic factor. The presence of the foreign protein, the placenta, and fetus may trigger an overwhelming immune response.

In most cases, an immunoprotective response (Chapter

6) prevents the development of effector lymphocytes and antibodies against the expanding invasive trophoblast (Chapter 9). If effector lymphocytes and antibodies are produced against trophoblastic tissue, lipid accumulates, fibrin is deposited, and occlusion of some placental vessels can occur (Alanen and Lassila, 1982; Gilbert and Harmon, 1986), resulting in cellular damage. Thromboplastic and fibrin–fibrinogen products are released. The release of these products has several consequences, including coagulopathy; specifically a decrease in platelet count. Deposition of these products in the liver and renal glomerulus may excite generalized vasospasm, a type of immune system response that may explain in part the increase in risk experienced by primigravidas or by multigravidas when having a child by a new father.

A *genetic* predisposition may be an etiologic factor of PIH (Cooper and Liston, 1979). The higher incidence of PIH in daughters of mothers who experienced the disorder supports the theory of hereditary tendency.

Uterine ischemia, insufficient blood flow through the uterus, may initiate a vasospastic response (Dennis, McFarland, and Hester, 1982). Ischemia may explain the increased incidence in primigravidas and in gravidas with multiple gestation (e.g., twins) when uterine growth and development do not keep pace with increased demands for blood flow.

PHYSIOLOGY

Knowledge of normal maternal physiology (Chapter 6) is necessary to understand the pathophysiology of PIH. Increases in total blood volume, cardiac output, and glomerular filtration rate (GFR) characterize maternal changes (Chapter 10). Increased estrogen levels raise levels of renin, angiotensin II, and aldosterone. While aldosterone exerts a sodium and water retention effect on the kidneys, progesterone blocks that effect; the normal net effect is sodium depletion. Angiotensin II stimulates a rise in blood pressure, except during normal pregnancy. During normal pregnancy, resistance to the pressor effect may be related to increased levels of such vasodilator prostaglandins as PGE_2 (Valenzuela, Hayashi, and Johns, 1983). Despite the increased blood volume, this decreased peripheral resistance is credited with the slight drop in maternal blood pressure during the second trimester. A return to nonpregnant blood pressure readings is expected in the third trimester.

In dependent limbs, fluid moves from the intravascular compartment to the extravascular space. "Physiologic anemia" (normal hemodilution), results in decreased plasma colloid osmotic pressure. Mechanic pressure from the weight of the gravid uterus increases venous capillary hydrostatic pressure. The net effect is physiologic edema of dependent limbs during the third trimester (Gilbert and Harmon, 1986). Physiologic edema is expected to disappear after 8 to 12 hours of bed rest.

Pathophysiology

In some pregnant women vascular sensitivity to angiotensin II increases. This increased vascular sensitivity occurs before the onset of *hypertension* (see roll-over test, p. 700). Vasospasm results. Vasospasm decreases the diameters of blood vessels, impeding blood flow, and raising blood pressure. Blood flow to all body organs is decreased. Function in organs such as the placenta, kidneys, liver, and brain is depressed by 40% to 60%. Many pathophysiologic sequelae are seen.

Impaired placental perfusion leads to early *degenerative aging of the placenta and possible intrauterine growth retardation* (IUGR) of the fetus. The theory that impaired prostaglandin synthesis (p. 697) may be a factor in PIH is important to recall. Uterine activity and sensitivity to oxytocin is increased. Therefore increased sensitivity to the effects of oxytocin must be taken into account when the drug is used for induction or augmentation of labor.

Reduced kidney perfusion decreases the GFR and leads to degenerative glomerular changes. *Protein, primarily albumin, is lost in the urine.* Uric acid clearance is decreased. Sodium and water are retained. Plasma colloid osmotic pressure decreases as serum albumin levels fall. Fluid moves out of the intravascular compartment, resulting in *hemoconcentration,* increased blood viscosity, and tissue *edema.* The hematocrit increases as fluid leaves the intravascular space (Pritchard, MacDonald, and Gant, 1985). Therefore a rising hematocrit is seen as the condition worsens; a falling hematocrit (to normal levels) accompanies improvement of the condition. In severe preeclampsia, blood volume may fall to or below nonpregnant levels, severe edema develops, and *rapid weight gain* is seen (Danforth and Scott, 1986).

Decreased perfusion of the liver leads to impaired function. Hepatic edema and subcapsular hemorrhage, experienced by the gravida as *epigastric or right upper quadrant pain,* is one sign of impending eclampsia (convulsion). Rupture of the liver is a rare but catastrophic complication of PIH (Pritchard, MacDonald, and Gant, 1985). Liver enzyme levels (e.g., SGOT) rise in the wake of liver damage.

Arteriolar vasospasms and decreased blood flow to the retina lead to *visual symptoms* such as scotoma (blind spots) and blurring. The same pathology leads to cerebral edema and hemorrhages, and increased *CNS irritability.* CNS irritability is expressed as headache, hyperreflexia, positive ankle clonus, and occasionally convulsions (p. 703). Affectual changes are often seen.

Debate continues whether PIH contributes to or is the result of disseminated intravascular coagulation (DIC) or whether DIC occurs with PIH. Pritchard, MacDonald, and Gant (1985) contend that DIC is a characteristic feature of PIH and plays a dominant role in the pathogenesis of the syndrome. Danforth and Scott (1986) state that DIC is rarely seen with PIH and that there is no evidence that the coagulopathy causes the hypertensive syndrome. Danforth and Scott (1986) and Gibson et al. (1982) report a **selective reduction in platelet count** (thrombocytopenia) without a significant alteration in other coagulation factors. Bern et al. (1981) report that microangiopathic thrombocytopenia is the consequence of interaction between platelets and vascular endothelium. This interaction could be produced by defective prostaglandin production. Thrombocytopenia is being increasingly recognized as a sign of severe PIH, regardless of the degree of hypertension (Danforth and

Scott, 1986). See also the discussion of the HELLP syndrome (p. 700).

If the hypertension is difficult to bring under control, cardiac and pulmonary complications can occur. Heart failure, a common cause of maternal death attributed to PIH, is rare in young, otherwise healthy women (Danforth and Scott, 1986). Sudden circulatory collapse and shock may occur in the older women with a history of repeated hypertensive pregnancies. A rapid fall in systolic blood pressure by 70 mm Hg or more is most often seen *a few hours after delivery* although it may occur before or during labor.

Typically, pulmonary edema caused by PIH is associated with severe generalized edema but electrocardiographic tracings are normal. Intravenous (IV) fluid infusion is an iatrogenic cause of fluid overload. Pulmonary edema and congestive heart failure are virtually the only accepted indications for diuretic therapy during pregnancy (Danforth and Scott, 1986).

See Fig. 29-1 for a summary of pathophysiologic changes associated with PIH.

MORBIDITY AND MORTALITY

Placental abruption with or without hypofibrinogenemia or DIC (Chapter 31) may occur with eclampsia. During a convulsion the woman may bite her tongue or lips; ribs or vertebrae may be fractured; and retinal detachments may occur. Eclampsia occurs in 0.05% to 0.2% of all pregnancies and in 1.5% of twin gestations (Anderson, 1987). About 8% of women with eclampsia die of the disease or its complications. The most common causes of death are intracranial hemorrhage and congestive heart failure.

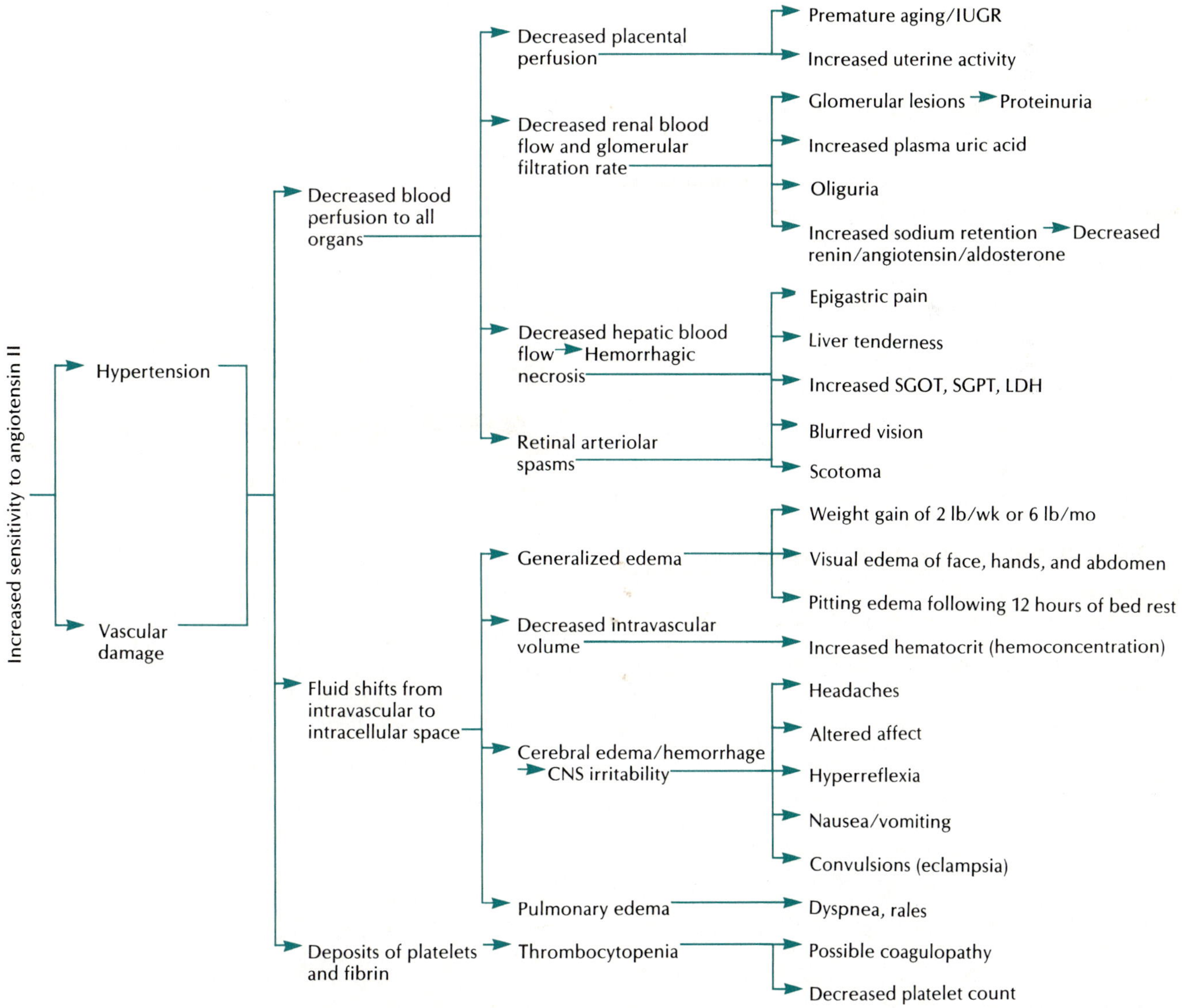

Fig. 29-1 Pathophysiology of PIH.
Modified from Gilbert, ES, and Harmon, JS: High-risk pregnancy and delivery: nursing perspectives, St Louis, 1986, The CV Mosby Co.

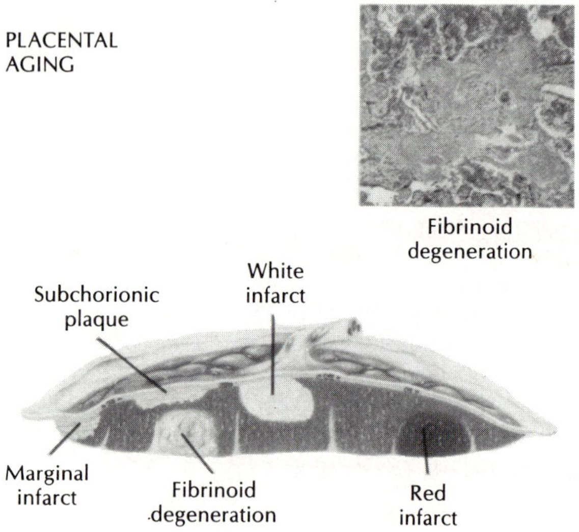

Fig. 29-2 Effects of severe PIH on placenta with resultant placental insufficiency.

Perinatal morbidity is high, because most women with PIH deliver before the thirty-seventh week of gestation. The fetal outcome of maternal hypertension is questionable because of placental insufficiency (Fig. 29-2). Generally the fetus is small for gestational age (SGA). However, these infants generally do better than other preterm infants of the same weight and gestational age born of nonhypertensive mothers. This is probably because of intrauterine stress that increases the rapidity of fetal lung maturation.

In many parts of North America the *perinatal mortality* is at least 20% with eclampsia. This is mainly because of the effects of hypoxia, prematurity, or acidosis during maternal convulsions. A single maternal convulsion increases the prospect of perinatal death at least fivefold.

The HELLP Syndrome

The HELLP syndrome (H: hemolysis, EL: elevated liver enzymes, and LP: low platelet count) represents an extension of the pathology of severe preeclampsia–eclampsia (Danforth and Scott, 1986). The initial symptoms of the HELLP syndrome usually appear early in the third trimester. A circulating immunologic component may be the underlying cause.

For a woman to be diagnosed as having the HELLP syndrome, her platelet count must be <100,000/mm^3, her liver enzyme levels must be elevated (SGOT/SGPT), and some evidence for intravascular hemolysis must be present (schistocytes or burr cells on peripheral smear). The hemolysis that occurs accounts for the large drop in hematocrit out of proportion to blood loss that is found in the majority of new mothers with HELLP syndrome during the postpartum period (Weinstein, 1986). A unique form of coagulopathy (not DIC) occurs with the HELLP syndrome.

Recognition of the clinical and laboratory findings of the HELLP syndrome is important if early, aggressive therapy is to be initiated to prevent maternal and neonatal mortality (Weinstein, 1986; Anderson, 1987).

The unfavorable cervix and the aggressive nature of this disorder support cesarean delivery. Prolonged induction could increase maternal morbidity. Fresh-frozen plasma may be needed if bleeding persists. The major laboratory manifestations of the disease, however, may not appear until the early postpartum period (48 to 72 hours). Delayed transfusion of packed cells is often necessary because of the continued hemolysis. It is important to attempt to lower the blood pressure if the diastolic is consistently greater than 110 mm Hg. **Hypoglycemia** may be present in the women with the HELLP syndrome and, when the blood sugar is <40 mg/dl, is associated with a high maternal mortality (Egley, Gutliph, and Bowes, 1985).

It is possible that some immunologic component crossing the placenta is responsible for the leukopenia seen in some neonates (Weinstein, 1986). Similar findings of the thrombocytopenia and leukopenia of the newborn from the mother with the HELLP syndrome have been reported by Brazie, Gumm, and Little (1982).

Assessment

Interview and Physical Examination

PIH can occur without warning or with the gradual development of symptoms. Therefore each woman is assessed for etiologic factors during the first visit. During each subsequent visit the woman is assessed for symptomatology that suggests the onset or presence of PIH.

In addition to the determination of the systolic and diastolic pressures, the *blood pressure* may be evaluated by two other methods: by the MAP and by the roll-over test. A blood pressure of 140/90 represents an *MAP* of 107 mm Hg. (MAP is calculated by adding the diastolic pressure to one third of the pulse pressure, p. 266.)

The *roll-over test* may be of some predictive value to detect women at risk for PIH. To perform this test, measure the blood pressure with the woman in the lateral recumbent position until the pressure is stable. Roll the woman to the supine position and measure the blood pressure immediately; repeat blood pressure measurement in 5 minutes. A *positive test* is defined as an increase of 20 mm Hg or more in diastolic pressure at the 5-minute reading. A *negative test* is defined as less than a 20 mm Hg rise in the diastolic pressure at the 5-minute reading (Knuppel and Drukker, 1986). The mechanism by which the supine position effects a rise in blood pressure is not clear, but it is another manifestation of intrinsic vascular hypersensitivity in women destined to develop PIH (Pritchard, MacDonald, and Gant, 1985; Reiss, 1987).

Although it is not a simple test to perform and not absolutely accurate, the roll-over test may indicate most women who are in danger of developing preeclampsia. Israel (1985) studied the predictive value of the roll-over test in women with mild preeclampsia.

One intent of the assessment of the blood pressure, weight, and urine in pregnant women is the prompt identification of complications such as PIH. Observation of edema plus assessment findings warrant additional investigation. *Edema* is assessed for distribution, degree, and pitting. If periorbital or facial edema is not obvious, the grav-

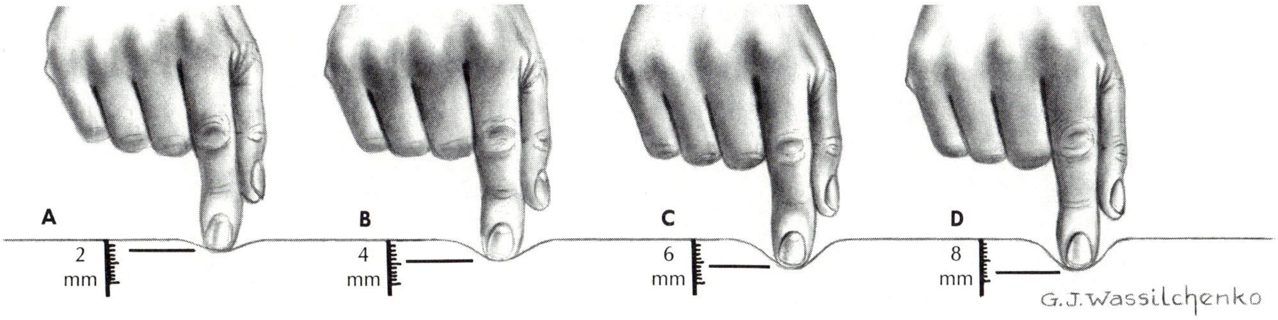

Fig. 29-3 Assessment of pitting edema: **A**, +1; **B**, +2; **C**, +3; **D**, +4.

ida is asked if it was present when she awoke. As the day progresses, gravity is responsible for movement of fluid to dependent body parts. In more severe preeclampsia, facial edema is obvious. Edema may be described as dependent, pitting, or nonpitting (Kozier and Erb, 1987).

Dependent Edema. Dependent edema is edema of the lowest or most dependent parts of the body, where hydrostatic pressure is greatest. If a person is ambulatory, this edema may first be evident in the feet and ankles. If the person is confined to bed, the edema is more likely to occur in the sacral region.

Pitting Edema. Pitting edema is edema that leaves a small depression or pit after finger pressure is applied to the swollen area. The pit is caused by movement of fluid to adjacent tissue, away from the point of pressure. Within 10 to 30 seconds the pit normally disappears. Pitting may be slight (+1) as in Fig. 29-3, *A*, or increase up to +4 as in Fig. 29-3, *D*.

Although the amount of edema is difficult to quantitate, the following method may be used to record relative degrees of edema formation:

+1 Minimum edema of the pedal and pretibial areas
+2 Marked edema of the lower extremities
+3 Edema of the face and hands, lower abdominal walls, and sacrum
+4 Anasarca (generalized massive edema) with ascites

Nonpitting Edema. Nonpitting edema is edema in which the fluid in edematous tissues cannot be moved to adjacent spaces by finger pressure. Nonpitting edema is not a sign of extracellular fluid excess. It often accompanies infections and traumas that cause fluid to collect and coagulate in tissue spaces. The coagulation prevents displacement of fluid to other areas by pressure.

Symptomatology reflecting CNS and visual system involvement usually accompanies facial edema. Although it is not a routine assessment during the prenatal period, evaluation of the fundus of the eye yields valuable data. An initial baseline finding of normal *eyegrounds* assists in differentiating preexisting from new disease process (Fig. 29-4). The woman may be unable to relate other symptoms such as epigastric pain or oliguria. Respirations are assessed for rales.

Deep tendon reflexes (DTRs) are evaluated if preeclampsia is suspected. The biceps and patellar reflexes and clonus are assessed and the findings recorded (Fig. 29-5; see also Table 29-6). To elicit the **biceps reflex** a downward blow is struck over the thumb, which is situated over the biceps tendon. *Normal response is flexion of the arm at the elbow.* Elicit the **patellar reflex** with the woman's legs hanging freely over the end of the examining table, or with the woman in the supine position. A blow with a percussion hammer is dealt directly to the patellar tendon, inferior to the patella. *Normal response is the extension or kicking out of the leg.* To assess for hyperactive reflexes **(clonus)** at the ankle joint, support the leg with the knee flexed. With one hand, sharply dorsiflex the foot and maintain dorsiflexed position for a moment, then release the foot. *Normal (negative clonus) response* is elicited when, while the foot is held in dorsiflexion, no rhythmic oscillations (jerking) are felt. When the foot is released, no oscillations are seen as foot drops to plantar flexed position. Abnormal (positive clonus) response is recognized by rhythmic oscillations felt when the foot is in dorsiflexion and seen as foot drops to the plantar flexed position.

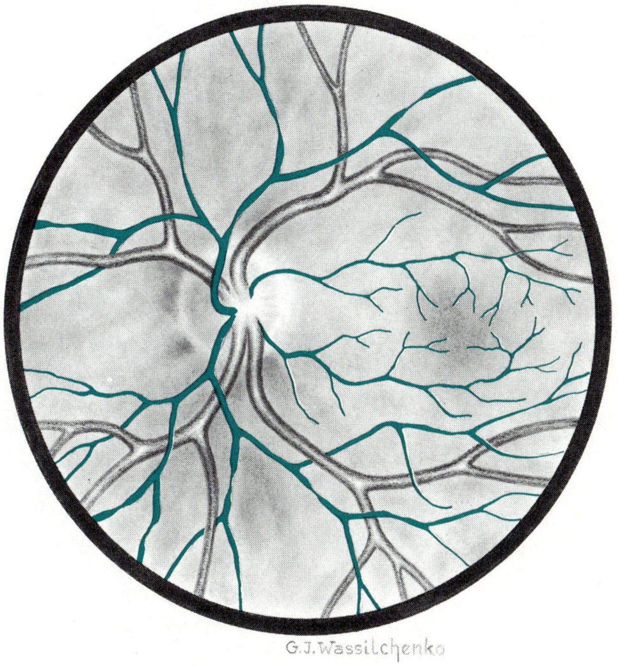

Fig. 29-4 Funduscopic evidence of severe PIH: arteriospasm, edema, hemorrhages, arteriovenous nicking, and exudates.

The fetal heart rate (FHR) and rhythm are assessed. Fetal movement and growth are determined by Leopold's ma-

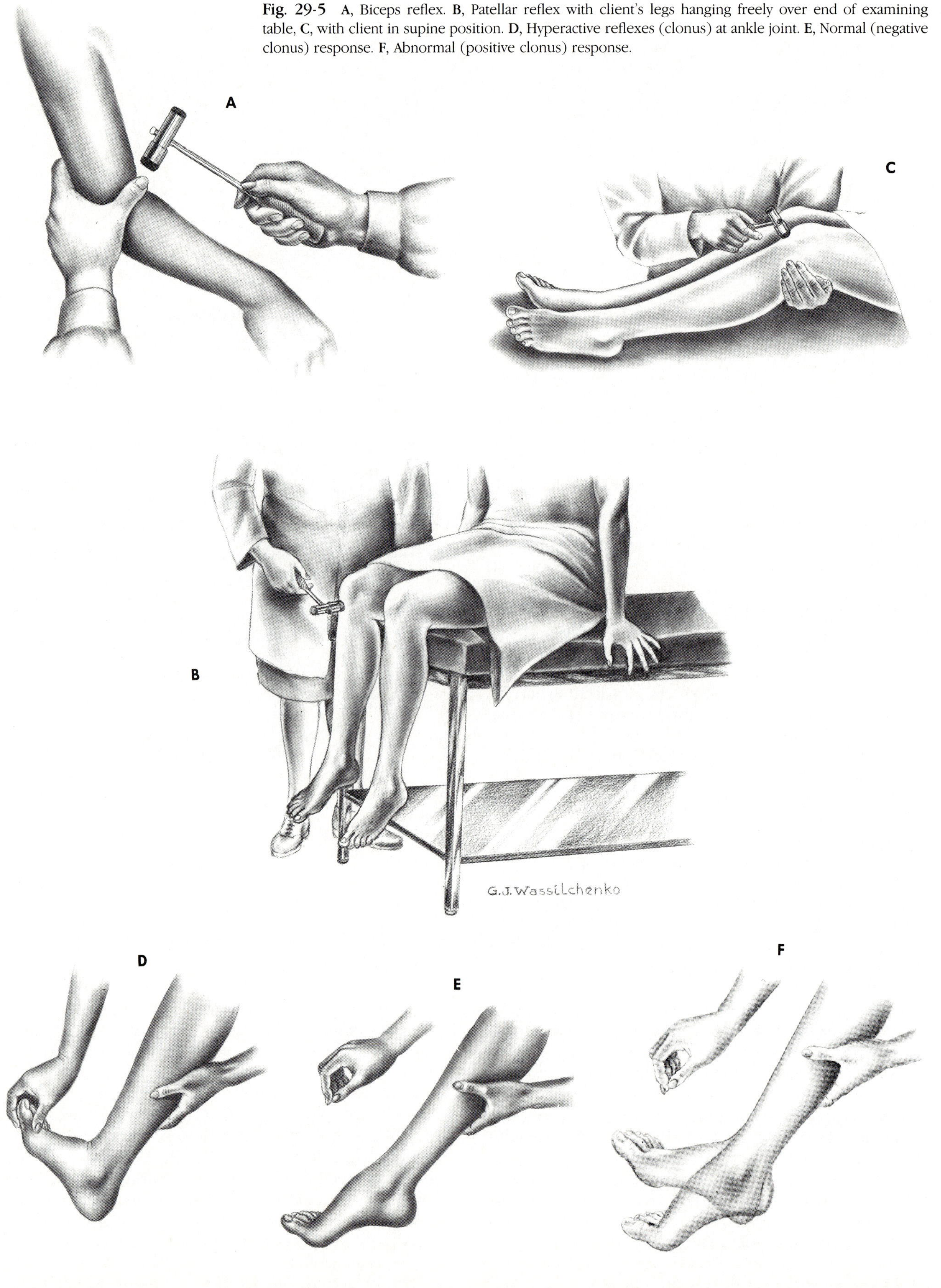

Fig. 29-5 A, Biceps reflex. B, Patellar reflex with client's legs hanging freely over end of examining table, C, with client in supine position. D, Hyperactive reflexes (clonus) at ankle joint. E, Normal (negative clonus) response. F, Abnormal (positive clonus) response.

neuvers (Chapter 16). Fundal height is measured. Biophysical or biochemical monitoring for fetal well-being may be ordered (Chapter 27).

Uterine tonicity is evaluated for signs of labor and abruptio placentae (Chapter 31). If labor is suspected, a vaginal examination for cervical changes is indicated.

During the physical examination, the gravida is scrutinized for signs of decreased platelets (Chapter 31). Ecchymotic areas, history of bruising with mild trauma, and bleeding from gums may manifest coagulopathy.

Danger signs of preeclampsia are summarized in the box at right.

Eclampsia is usually preceded by various premonitory symptoms and signs, including headache, severe epigastric pain, hyperreflexia, and hemoconcentration, but convulsions can appear suddenly and without warning in a seemingly stable woman with only minimum blood-pressure elevations (Lindheimer and Katz, 1985; Pritchard, MacDonald, and Gant, 1985).

The convulsions that occur in eclampsia are an awesome, frightening sequence to observe. Increased hypertension precedes the tonic-clonic convulsions; hypotension and collapse follow. Stertorous breathing and coma are the aftermath of a seizure. Nystagmus and muscular twitching persist for a time. Disorientation and amnesia cloud the immediate recovery. Oliguria and anuria are notable. A more detailed description of tonic-clonic convulsions is given in the box below.

TONIC-CLONIC CONVULSIONS

Stage of invasion: 2 to 3 seconds; eyes fixed; twitching of facial muscles.

Stage of contraction: 15 to 20 seconds; eyes protrude and are bloodshot; all body muscles in tonic contraction (e.g., arms flexed, hands clenched, legs inverted).

Stage of convulsion: Muscles relax and contract alternatively. Respirations are halted and then begin again with long, deep stertorous inhalation. Coma ensues (2 to 3 minutes to hours).

Occurrence: During prenatal, intranatal, or postdelivery period.

Recurrence: Within minutes of first convulsion or never.

Laboratory Tests

Plasma creatinine and urea levels are determined. Urine is monitored for amount per hour and for protein. Proteinuria is defined as protein present in amounts greater than 300 mg/L (+1) in a 24-hour specimen or greater than 1 g/L (+2) in a random daytime urine sample on 2 or more occasions at least 6 hours apart (Table 29-3). The urine must be a midstream clean-catch or catheter-derived specimen if there is the possibility of contamination by vaginal discharge. The woman is assessed for the HELLP syndrome—hemolysis (microangiopathic), elevated liver enzymes (AST or SGOT, ALT or SGPT), and low platelet count (p. 700). The hematocrit is monitored.

DANGER SIGNS

Pregnancy Induced Hypertension

1. Rapid rise in blood pressure
2. Rapid gain in weight
3. Generalized edema
4. Quantitative increase in proteinuria
5. Epigastric pain
6. Marked hyperreflexia; especially transient or sustained ankle clonus
7. Severe headache
8. Visual disturbances
9. Oliguria with urinary output of less than 100 ml in 4 hours
10. Drowsiness, listlessness (dulled sensorium)
11. Nausea and vomiting, severe

Table 29-3 *Protein Readings*

Code	Milligrams per Deciliter
0	
Trace	
+1	30 mg/dl (equivalent to 300 mg/L)
+2	100 mg/dl
+3	300 mg/dl
+4	Over 1000 mg (1 g)/dl

The findings are carefully analyzed to identify preeclampsia. Differentiation of mild and severe preeclampsia precedes planning for care (Table 29-4). Danforth and Scott (1986) have emphasized two principles to guide the care of women with PIH:

1. The importance of even a "mild" degree of hypertension complicating pregnancy must be appreciated
2. No one can accurately predict which women with PIH will develop eclampsia

Nursing Diagnoses

Medical management of preeclampsia requires the coordinated efforts of the entire health care team. Nursing actions will be derived from medical management, physician's directives, and nursing diagnoses. Examples of relevant nursing diagnoses include the following:

"Mild" Preeclampsia

- Knowledge deficit related to
  - PIH and its effects on mother and baby
  - How to obtain assistance
  - How to assess blood pressure
  - How to assess for edema

 - Diet required in PIH (protein intake, sodium intake, and roughage and fluids)
 - Meaning of bed rest and its significance to woman and her infant's condition
- Ineffective individual coping related to
 - Activity restriction
- Impaired home maintenance management related to
 - Activity restriction
- Ineffective family coping related to
 - Mother's restricted activity and concern over a complicated pregnancy

Moderate and Severe Preeclampsia

- Pain, related to
 - Symptomatology
- Sensory-perceptual alteration related to
 - PIH
- Potential for injury related to
 - Therapy or eclampsia
- Altered tissue perfusion (cardiopulmonary) related to
 - PIH or its complications (DIC)
- Ineffective breathing pattern related to
 - Edema
- Altered patterns of urinary elimination related to
 - PIH
- Ineffective individual and family coping related to
 - Stress of experiencing a major complication of pregnancy

Table 29-4 *Differentiation of Mild and Severe Preeclampsia*

	Mild Preeclampsia*	Severe Preeclampsia
Maternal Effects		
Blood pressure	Rise in systolic blood pressure of 30 mm Hg or more. A rise in diastolic blood pressure of 15 mm Hg or more or a reading of 140/90 mm Hg × 2, 6 hours apart.	Rise to 160/110 mm Hg or more on two separate occasions 6 hours apart with pregnant woman on bed rest.
MAP	140/90 = 107.	160/110 = 127.
Weight gain	Weight gain or more than 1.4 kg (3 lb)/month during the second trimester, more than 0.5 kg (1 lb)/week during the third trimester, or a sudden weight gain of 2 kg (4-4½ lb)/week at any time.	Same.
Proteinuria Qualitative dipstick Quantitative 24-hour analysis	Proteinuria of 300 mg/L in a 24-hour specimen or greater than 1 g/L in a random daytime specimen on 2 or more occasions 6 hours apart as protein loss is variable. With dipstick varies from trace to 1+.	Proteinuria of 5-10 g/L in 24 hours or 2+ or more protein on dipstick.
Edema	Dependent edema, some puffiness of eyes, face, fingers; pulmonary rales absent.	Generalized edema, noticeable puffiness of eyes, face, fingers. Pulmonary edema → rales.
Reflexes	Hyperreflexia 3+. No ankle clonus.	Hyperreflexia 3+ or more. Ankle clonus.
Oliguria	Output matches intake.	Oliguria: less than 100 ml/4 hr output.
Headache	Transient.	Severe.
Visual problems	Absent.	Blurred, photophobia, blind spots on funduscopy. Retinal arterial spasm (Fig. 29-3).
Irritability	Transient.	Severe.
Serum creatinine	Normal.	Elevated.
Thrombocytopenia	Absent.	Present.
SGOT elevation	Minimal.	Marked.
Fetal Effects		
Placental perfusion	Reduced.	Decreased perfusion expressed as IUGR in fetus FHR: late decelerations.
Premature placental aging	Not apparent.	At birth placenta appears smaller than normal for the duration of the pregnancy. Premature aging is apparent with numerous areas of broken syncytia. Ischemic necroses (white infarcts) are numerous, and intervillous fibrin deposition (red infarcts) may be recorded.

*No preeclampsia should be considered "mild" (Danforth and Scott, 1986; Knuppel and Drukker, 1986; Lindheimer and Katz, 1985).

Planning

Planning care follows medical diagnosis, choice of home or hospital management, and the woman's and family's resources. A plan is developed mutually with the client, if possible. While the information in this chapter is general in nature, the care plan should be individualized and related specifically to the needs of the client and her family. This chapter includes general nursing care plans for home management of mild preeclampsia and hospital management of severe preeclampsia. Specific care plans for protein, for magnesium sulfate therapy and eclampsia, and client teaching are also in this chapter.

Goals. The overall goals for care during the maternity cycle are as follows:

1. Provision of early adequate prenatal care, including adequate nutrition, specific to the needs of each woman to protect against PIH
2. Prompt intensive therapy for preeclampsia to drastically reduce the incidence of eclampsia and the severity of its complications
3. Prompt initiation of corrective therapy for eclamptic convulsions to reduce maternal and perinatal morbidity and mortality

Implementation

Nurses assume many caregiving roles in the management of gravidas experiencing preeclampsia. The nurse-clinician's roles can be categorized as supportive, teacher/counselor/advocate, instrumental, and recorder. In these roles, the clinician is a consumer of nursing research and is alert to potential research problems.

Supportive Activities. The development of preeclampsia causes anxiety in the woman and her family. There is a threat to the well-being of the mother and her unborn child, and the family's expectations about pregnancy and delivery must be altered. Such disruption in a family constitutes a crisis. The physical nature of the crisis requires the beneficial use of modern technology. The woman and her family's perception of the disease process, the reasons for it and the care received will affect their compliance with and participation in therapy. The family will need to use coping mechanisms and support systems to help them through the experience. A plan of care for the woman suffering for severe preeclampsia is superimposed on the nursing care all women need during labor and delivery.

NOTE: A special relationship develops between the seriously ill gravida and the alert nurse providing long-term hospital care. The woman is under the stress of the disease, anxious about the outcome, and dependent on the nurse. The nurse invests emotional energy in the woman. After delivery, especially if the newborn is healthy, the woman redirects her energies to her family. Nurses may feel "let down" with this shift in the relationship.

Teacher/Counselor/Advocate. The most effective therapy is **prevention.** Sachs, et al. (1987) "observed an association between the receipt of little or no antenatal care and higher maternal (morbidity and) mortality rates. Measures should be taken to improve public education and access to antenatal care."

Nutrition counseling, referral to community resources, mobilization of support systems, and information about normal adaptations to pregnancy are essential components of care.

Encouragement of **early identification** and reporting of symptomatology of physical danger signs during pregnancy (Chapter 12, p. 249) is an essential component of client teaching during pregnancy. The nurse's skills in health assessment for etiologic factors and symptomatology of preeclampsia cannot be overestimated.

Home Management. The most effective therapy for preeclampsia is preventing progression of the condition. Management at home can be satisfactory if the preeclampsia is mild and fetal growth retardation is not a problem. Home therapy includes twice-weekly medical and nursing assessment, encouraging the client to participate in the care, dietary modifications, and bed rest. Application of the nursing process to at-home care of a woman with mild preeclampsia is presented in the general nursing care plan and guidelines for client teaching that follow. This care is given in addition to the general care needed in pregnancy.

Text continued on p. 709.

Guidelines for Client Teaching

HOME CARE OF PREECLAMPSIA

ASSESSMENT

1. Woman with two children pregnant with twins.
2. Thirty-third week of gestation.
3. Mild hypertension.
4. Generalized edema.
5. Proteinuria, +2

NURSING DIAGNOSES

Potential for injury: fetus and mother, related to edema, proteinuria, and hypertension.
Knowledge deficit related to PIH and its effects on mother and baby.
Knowledge deficit related to diet required to PIH.
Knowledge deficit related to assessment of blood pressure and edema.
Fluid volume deficit related to generalized edema.
Altered health maintenance related to activity intolerance.
Potential noncompliance related to two preschoolers at home and woman's need for bed rest.
Activity intolerance: decreased, related to minimizing effects of PIH.
Ineffective individual coping related to activity restriction.
Impaired home maintenance management related to activity restriction.
Ineffective family coping related to mother's restricted activity and concern over a complicated pregnancy.
Potential altered parenting related to family and personal stress.
Constipation, related to decreased activity, decreased gastric motility, pregnancy.

GOALS

Short-term

To increase woman's understanding of PIH and encourage her and her family's participation in her care.
To teach woman (couple) how to monitor severity of PIH.
To teach woman about diet prescribed for her by the physician.
To aid woman in maintaining adequate rest by arranging support systems.

Intermediate

To continue monitoring effects of PIH on woman and fetus.
To have woman comply with decreased activity and diet.

Long-term

To prepare for potential complications such as an early birth.
To decrease anxiety.
To keep PIH under control until delivery of the twins.

REFERENCES AND TEACHING AIDS

Pamphlets and booklets from hospital, clinic, or physician's office explaining PIH and its problems and treatments.
Diagrams or charts to be used in explanation of PIH.
Printed list of potential complications for woman to take home.
List of phone numbers to call for emergency assistance to be placed by the woman's phone.
List of community or social services that may be of assistance to the family while the woman is on bedrest.

CONTENT/RATIONALE	TEACHING ACTION
To increase woman's (couple's) knowledge of PIH, share the following:	Show diagrams and charts while explaining how the condition develops, who's at risk, and what signs to look for.
How the condition can effect woman's fetuses and her.	Show chart to help explain organ system changes.
There is no definite cause for PIH but there are many theories that support the symptoms that occur, which are a result of changes in the functioning of body organs.	Use simple terms and do not scare woman. It is important that she understand what could happen if treatment regimen is not taken seriously, however, it is not necessary to increase her fear and anxiety.
To implement assessment and self-management of PIH: Review assessment and management	
Pitting edema.	Show woman (couple) how to assess extent of edema (Fig. 29-3).
Protein in urine.	Demonstrate chemstrip for protein in urine.
Fetal activity.	Instruct woman how to monitor fetal activity within a certain amount of time.
Daily weight.	Instruct woman to weigh herself daily and record weight.
Intake and output.	Give woman a list of common household measures and instruct her on how to keep a record of her intake and output.
Danger signs.	Give woman a list of the danger signs of PIH that should be reported to the physician immediately (p. 703).

Guidelines for Client Teaching

CONTENT/RATIONALE	TEACHING ACTION
Diet, as it pertains to sodium and protein intake. Rationale for diet: Helps reduce edema and blood pressure. Helps baby grow.	Discuss the diet that was prescribed for her by her physician. Instruct woman as to food groups that are equivalent to 70 to 80 g of protein. Provide a printed list for her to take home with her. Instruct woman as to amounts of salt to use in preparing or serving foods. Advise her to refrain from eating salty convenience or snack foods (i.e., potato chips).
Roughage and fluids.	Advise woman about including ample roughage and fluids, restricted exercise can aggravate constipation.
Bedrest.	Instruct woman (couple) on what is meant by bedrest. Emphasize need to spend most of the day in bed, preferably lying on her left side; ambulation for meals and to go to the bathroom are usually permitted. Discourage going up and down stairs. Restrict outings to visits to the physician's office.
Activity and the need for diversion within woman's restrictions.	Encourage the family to take part in her care and take over care of the house, younger children, cooking, etc.
To assist family in mobilizing support and coping: Social worker or support systems in the community may be needed if there are no family support systems.	Refer to community agencies as necessary.
Open discussion of problems is beneficial in implementing care. Mutual problem-solving facilitates tension reduction, supporting or improving coping skills. Assistance and reassurance facilitate compliance to medical regimen.	To avert potential for impaired family processes, encourage open discussion and problem-solving problems with the pregnancy, younger children, and taking care of the house.

EVALUATION The nurse can be reasonably assured that teaching is effective if woman adheres to medical regimen with family support, woman has a healthy baby, and all goals are met.

General Nursing Care Plan

HOME MANAGEMENT OF PIH

ASSESSMENT	NURSING DIAGNOSIS (ND)/ PLAN(P)/GOAL(G)	RATIONALE/ IMPLEMENTATION	EVALUATION
Populations at risk: Primigravida (<15 to >35) Multiple gestation Diabetes Rh incompatability Renal disease Hypertension Over 20 weeks gestation	ND: Knowledge deficit related to PIH and those women at risk. P: Educate those women at risk to prevent or minimize PIH. G: Woman does not develop PIH.	*To teach woman about PIH the nurse will:* Assess risk factors at each prenatal visit. Take a complete nursing history including family and social history. Discuss problems with woman. Discuss rationale for treatment. Include support person or family in discussions.	Woman verbalizes understanding of information presented. Woman states she will come to all prenatal visits as scheduled.

Continued.

General Nursing Care Plan—cont'd

ASSESSMENT	NURSING DIAGNOSIS (ND)/ PLAN(P)/GOAL(G)	RATIONALE/ IMPLEMENTATION	EVALUATION
Symptomatology of PIH: Sudden weight gain Generalized edema Increase in blood pressure *over baseline:* Systolic: 15 mm Hg Diastolic: 30 mm Hg Proteinuria	ND: Potential for injury: fetus and mother related to hypertension, vasospasm, decreased glomerular filtration rate, and edema. P: Detect and control PIH. G: Woman's PIH remains in control.	*To teach woman how to assess for PIH the nurse will teach her to:* Assess weight every day—watch for an increase of 2 or more pounds per week. Monitor fluid intake and urine output. Observe for pitting edema of lower extremities, tight rings, shoes, facial puffiness. Teach how to use dipstick for assessment of proteinuria.	Woman reports weight, urine output, results of urine dipstick, and edema to nurse every day.
Knowledge of symptomatology Readiness to learn Ability to learn content (as influenced by effects of illness of medications, language barrier, age, or experience, or innate intelligence)	ND: Knowledge deficit related to severity of PIH and effects on mother and fetus. P: Teach woman (family) danger signs and symptoms to look for with increasing severity of disease. G: Woman knows signs and symptoms and has a printed list readily available to her and her family members; promptly reports symptomalogy to health care provider.	*CNS symptomatology:* Blurred vision. Headaches. Nausea and vomiting. Hyperreflexia. Convulsions. *Hepatic symptoms:* Epigastric pain (RUQ). *Urinary output:* Proteinuria >2+. Oliguria. *Fetal distress:* Decreased fetal activity. Changes in fetal activity. *Placentae abruptio:* Vaginal bleeding or spotting. Uterine tenderness. Change in fetal activity. Abdominal pain.	Woman (family) demonstrates understanding of information presented. Woman (family) tests urine several times per day. Woman experience diuresis. Woman reports fetal activity and keeps scheduled appointments. Woman verbalizes understanding of information presented. Woman reports any problems.
Woman overweight or undernourished Excessive sodium intake Inadequate protein and caloric intake Financial status Cultural/religious influences Pitting edema	ND: Altered nutrition: less than or more than body requirements. ND: Knowledge deficit related to diet required in PIH. P: Provide nutrition counseling. G: Woman accepts and learns to follow diet prescribed by physician. ND: Potential intravascular fluid volume deficit related to protein loss and fluid shifts to the extravascular space. P: Provide adequate protein intake. G: Woman consumes adequate diet.	*To help woman with her nutritional status the nurse will:* Provide nutrition counseling (Chapter 15) re: intake of sodium chloride ("salt"), protein, calories; re: physician's orders; re: personal and family preferences, budget, and storage and preparation facilities.	Woman keeps a diet history. Woman verbalizes understanding of limiting salty foods and lowering sodium intake. Woman follows prescribed diet

General Nursing Care Plan—cont'd

ASSESSMENT	NURSING DIAGNOSIS (ND)/ PLAN(P)/GOAL(G)	RATIONALE/ IMPLEMENTATION	EVALUATION
Home situation: resources that would permit woman to be on bed rest and to restrict activity Woman needs help around house Knowledge of stress reduction techniques	ND: Activity intolerance related to the disease process. P: Help woman (family) arrange for home management of PIH. G: Woman (family) implements home care as prescribed.	*To assist woman to comply with bed rest the nurse can:* Teach woman importance of remaining in bed. Teach relaxation (see guidelines for client teaching, Chapter 13). Act as a client advocate and put family in touch with community support systems. Assess family and internal support systems.	Woman remains on bed rest, left side as much as possible. Woman uses relaxation techniques with success. Arrangements are made for help with house and any other children in family.

Instrumental Activities

Manual skills are of particular importance in the care of women with a serious complication of pregnancy. If the woman's condition becomes increasingly severe, hospitalization is recommended.

Severe preeclampsia is diagnosed when one or more of the following are present (Weinstein, 1986): (1) blood pressure of at least 160 mm Hg systolic or 110 mm Hg (MAP 127 or more) diastolic on 2 readings 6 hours apart; (2) proteinuria of ≥5 g/24 hours; (3) oliguria (<400 ml in 24 hours); (4) cerebral or visual disturbances; and (5) pulmonary edema or cyanosis.

The woman may also be hospitalized for lesser degrees of hypertension but with any of the following: (1) proteinuria of 1+ or more; (2) increasing edema, (3) persistent or severe headache; (4) nausea and vomiting; and (5) epigastric pain.

Severe preeclampsia represents an obstetric emergency. Immediate and continuous care by the obstetric team is mandatory to prevent maternal and fetal morbidity or mortality.

Hospital Care for Severe Preeclampsia. The woman is admitted to either the delivery suite or to a private room on the antepartum or postpartum unit. The room must be close to staff and emergency drugs, supplies, and equipment (see box at right). Noise and external stimuli must be minimized.

The extensiveness of health assessment on admission is governed by the severity of the woman's condition. An assessment guide appears in the box on p. 710. Weight is taken on admittance and at least every 2 days thereafter. An indwelling urinary catheter facilitates monitoring of renal function and effectiveness of therapy. If appropriate, vaginal examination reveals the state of the cervix. Abdominal palpation establishes uterine tonicity and fetal size, activity, and position. Electronic monitoring of the mother and fetus may be ordered. The nurse's skill in implementing the

DRUGS AND EQUIPMENT FOR PREVENTIVE TREATMENT OF CONVULSIONS OF ECLAMPSIA

DRUGS	EQUIPMENT
Magnesium sulfate: 2 ampules, 10 ml/ampule (5 g 50%); 500 mg (4 mEq)/ml	Emergency delivery pack
Sodium bicarbonate: 50 ml (7.5%) (44.6 mEq)	Ophthalmoscope
Hydralazine: 5 ampules, 20 mg/ampule	Reflex hammer
Heparin sodium: 10 ml, 5000 USP units/ml	Fetal monitor
Diazepam: 2 ml, 5 mg/ml	Padded tongue blade
Chlordiazepoxide: 5 ml, 20 mg/ml	Plastic airway
Epinephrine: 2:1000, 1 mg/ml	Oxygen and suction
Atropisol, 1% (mydriatic)	Tourniquets
Atropine sulfate: 0.4 mg/0.5 ml	Syringes: 2, 10, and 50 ml
Sterile water ampules	Cutdown tray
Sterile normal saline ampules	IV administration supplies
Calcium gluconate: 10%, 1g/10 ml; 97 mg (4.8 mEq)/10 ml Ca ++	Sphygmomanometer with an appropriate-sized cuff
Phenytoin: 2 ml, 50 mg/ml	Rectal thermometer
Propranolol: tablets 40 mg	Means for obtaining weight
Intravenous barbiturates	Indwelling urinary catheter tray with collection bag
	Urinary dipsticks

techniques described can be reassuring to the woman and her family.

Commonly bed rest is ordered. The nurse's ingenuity may be called on to help the woman cope physically and psychologically with the side effects of immobility. Thromboembolic events, which are a risk factor during normal pregnancy, pose an even greater risk with preeclampsia.

Prevention of Eclampsia and Use of Magnesium Sulfate

One of the important goals of care for the woman with severe preeclampsia is preventing or controlling convulsions. The nurse maintains a matter-of-fact, calm attitude and briefly explains the rationale of treatment (Table 29-5).

To prevent convulsions, various drugs may be used in

CLINICAL ASSESSMENT GUIDE: PREECLAMPSIA

Assessment of Client's Environment

CRITERIA	PRESENT	ABSENT	COMMENTS
Environment			
Quiet			
Nonstimulating			
Lighting subdued			
Seizure precautions			
Oral airway (or padded tongue blade) near head of bed			
Padded side rails			
Suction equipment tested and ready to use			
Oxygen administration equipment tested and ready to use			
Call button within easy reach			
Emergency medication tray immediately accessible			
Magnesium sulfate in or adjacent to woman's room			
Calcium gluconate immediately available in a well-labeled syringe			
Emergency delivery pack accessible			

Assessment of Client

Subjective
- Write what the woman says when you ask her to describe how she feels

Objective
- Record what you see
- Describe facies
- Describe affect
- Observe and note location of edema
- Record temperature, blood pressure, weight
- Auscultate FHR; assess rhythm and quality
- Assess fetal activity
- Check urine amount and protein level
- Auscultate chest; listen for moist respirations or cough
- Test and record deep tendon reflexes
- Assess onset of labor
- Record amount of fluid intake and urinary output in past 24 hours
- Record drug, dosage, and time of medication during the past 24 hours

Table 29-5 *Pharmacologic Control of Hypertension and Its Sequelae in Pregnancy and Labor*

Medication	Target Tissue	Effects of Medication		Nursing Actions
		Maternal	Fetal/Neonatal	
Anticonvulsants				
Magnesium sulfate IV or IM Dosage varies	Myoneural junction: decreases acetylcholine, thereby depressing neuromuscular transmission Thyroid: decreases parathormone secretion, resulting in increased urinary excretion of calcium Placental perfusion dynamics not altered	Minimum hypotensive effect Minimum if any direct effect on CNS because of blood-brain barrier to magnesium Hypocalcemia CAUTION: Do not give excessive dosages that tend to decrease urinary output to depress deep tendon reflexes (DTRs) DANGER: Muscular paralysis (cardiopulmonary) **Antidotes: calcium gluconate**, neostigmine, pentylenetetrazol (Metrazol) Increases duration of labor; amount of oxytocin needed to stimulate labor is higher	Mild depression in small number (6%) Neonatal hypermagnesemia easily treated: calcium; exchange transfusion with citrated blood No effect on FHR variability in healthy term fetus; neonatal toxic effects rare (Sibai, 1987)	Notify perinatal staff Decrease CNS irritability Arrange environment to promote rest Provide continuous nursing care Encourage kidney perfusion with left side-lying position and insert indwelling urinary catheter; monitor urinary output every hour Under 25 ml/hr—do not repeat dose Diuresis—good prognostic sign Repeat dose per order if: DTRs present (Fig. 29-5) Respirations of 12/min or more Urinary output over 1 dl/4 hr Assess maternal condition Hydration Affect Other signs or symptoms of preeclampsia Keep 10 ml of 10% calcium gluconate at bedside; with linen/equipment for delivery, eclamptic tray, oxygen, and suction equipment
Diazepam (Valium)	Thalamus and hypothalamus: direct depressant effect	Effective in initial management of eclamptic convulsions Rapid IV administration may lead to apnea or cardiac arrest	Flattens FHR base line (loss of beat-to-beat variability), an important criterion in assessing fetal oxygenation High levels in newborn: Depressed sucking ability Hypotonia Temperature instability (decrease) Decreased respiratory rate	Notify perinatal staff Assess DTRs, respirations, signs of labor Monitor labor; see Normal labor
Barbiturates (rapid-acting) Phenobarbital sodium: 0.2-0.3 mg IV Amobarbital sodium: 0.25-0.5 g IV	CNS: depressant effect	Controls seizures	Depressant effect on fetus May minimize hyperbilirubinemia	See Diazepam

Continued.

Table 29-5 *Pharmacologic Control of Hypertension and Its Sequelae in Pregnancy and Labor—cont'd*

Medication	Target Tissue	Effects of Medication: Maternal	Effects of Medication: Fetal/Neonatal	Nursing Actions
Antihypertensive*				
Hydralazine (Apresoline, Neopresol) (arteriolar vasodilators) 50 to 200 mg (0) per day	Peripheral arterioles: decreases muscle tone, thereby decreasing peripheral resistance Hypothalamus and medullary vasomotor center; minor decrease in sympathetic tone	Headache Flushing Palpitation Tachycardia Some decrease in uteroplacental blood flow	Minimum effects; some decrease in Po_2	Assess for effects of medications Alert mother (family) to expected effects of medications Assess blood pressure (precipitous drop can lead to shock and perhaps to abruptio placentae) and urinary output Maintain bed rest with side rails for safety
Methyldopa (Aldomet) (used if maintenance therapy is needed): 250-500 mg orally every 8 hr (α_2-receptor agonist)	Postganglionic nerve endings: interferes with chemical neurotransmission to reduce peripheral vascular resistance CNS: sedation	Sleepiness Postural hypotension Constipation Rare: drug-induced fever in 1% of women and positive Coombs' test in 20%	After 4 months of maternal therapy, positive Coombs' test in infant	See Hydralazine
Diuretics†				
Thiazides	Arteriolar smooth muscles: reduces responsiveness to catecholamines	Ineffective in preventing preeclampsia Further reduces already-present decreased plasma volume of preeclampsia Complications Fluid and electrolyte imbalance Pancreatitis Decrease in carbohydrate tolerance Hyperuricemia	Hyponatremia Thrombocytopenia	Arrange to have blood drawn to measure levels of Na, Cl, H_2O, K, and H+ to prevent hyponatremia, hypokalemia, hypochloremia, metabolic acidosis
Furosemide (Lasix): 40 mg IV	Loop of Henle	Relieves pulmonary edema Excessive use results in hypokalemia and hyponatremia	No abnormalities noted	See Thiazides
Ethacrynic acid (Edecrin)	Similar to furosemide	Similar to furosemide	Deafness	See Thiazides
Mannitol (for impending renal failure, oliguria, DIC): 12.5-25 mg IV	Osmotic diuretic: pulls fluid into vascular bed (therefore not recommended for persons with congestive heart failure)	Increases renal plasma flow and urinary output Flushes out kidneys Reduces swelling in ischemic cells in kidney and myocardium	No known effect	See Thiazides
Blood volume expanders				
Salt-poor, serum albumin‡	Intravascular volume	Increases blood volume		

*By midpregnancy, diastolic and systolic blood pressure normally falls by 10 to 15 mm Hg. If diastolic blood pressure is 75 mm Hg or more in second trimester and 85 mm Hg or more in third trimester, statistical increase in fetal mortality occurs.

NOTE: For obese woman, use thigh cuff or ultrasound to obtain accurate readings.

†For control of chronic hypertension, pulmonary edema, renal oliguria, acute renal failure, chronic nephrotic syndrome. If used, physician must be ready to justify action.

‡May not be appropriate for woman with severe preeclampsia–eclampsia.

conjunction with medical and nursing care. The one most commonly used is magnesium sulfate, an anticonvulsant and smooth muscle relaxant.

Administration. Magnesium sulfate may be given intravenously or intramuscularly. Various dosage schedules are used. For example, an initial dose of 4 g of magnesium sulfate in 250 ml of 5% dextrose in water may be given intravenously (infused *slowly* at a rate of 5 ml/30 sec). Then, 4 to 5 grams may be given intramuscularly in each buttock (1% procaine may be ordered added to the solution to reduce the pain of injection). When magnesium sulfate is given *intramuscularly,* levels are adequate during the first 1 to 2 hours of administration, but inadequate for the next 3 to 4 hours (Sibai, 1987). The intramuscular dose can be followed at 4-hour intervals with intramuscular doses of 4 to 5 g.

When magnesium sulfate is given intravenously, the effect is immediate. A therapeutic serum level (4 to 8 mg/dl) is usually maintained by a constant infusion of 2 g/hr (Sibai, 1987; Anderson, 1987).

Monitoring for Toxicity. Early symptomatology of toxicity includes nausea, feeling of warmth, flushing, muscle weakness, and slurred speech.

Blood Pressure. Magnesium sulfate interferes with neuromuscular impulse transmission, resulting in muscle relaxation. It reduces blood pressure by splanchnic vasodilation; therefore severe hypotension can occur. The woman's blood pressure should be monitored continuously while the drug is being administered intravenously and every 15 minutes at other times.

Urinary Output. Urinary output must be closely monitored because magnesium sulfate both increases sodium retention and is excreted by the kidneys.

Hourly urinary output must be measured when magnesium sulfate is administered intravenously. The woman's urinary output must total at least 100 ml every 4 hours. If output is less, assess renal function and notify the physician. Toxic drug levels can occur if magnesium sulfate dose is not decreased when decreased output occurs. If adequate output is not maintained the dose should not be repeated.

A retention catheter is inserted if accurate hourly determination of urinary output is warranted. Hourly measurement is necessary when the woman is receiving a medication such as magnesium sulfate or when decreasing urinary output is suspected or actual.

Diuresis within 24 to 48 hours is an excellent prognostic sign. It is considered evidence that perfusion of the kidney is improved secondary to relaxation of arteriolar spasm. With improved perfusion, fluid moves from interstitial spaces to the intravascular bed, and edema is reduced. Diuresis results in weight loss. In the presence of a large urinary output, the dosage of magnesium sulfate may need to be increased to 3 g/hr IV. If the volume of urine is under 100 ml/4 hr, the dosage of magnesium sulfate is reduced. The physician is notified. The woman is assessed for renal function.

Respirations. Adverse effects of magnesium sulfate also include respiratory paralysis. *Maternal toxicity has been reached when respirations are fewer than 12/min.* The drug is withheld if respirations are fewer than 12/min. The woman receiving magnesium sulfate therapy **should never be left unattended** because $MgSO_4$ toxicity with respiratory arrest may occur.

Reflex Activity. *Maternal toxicity has been reached when reflex activity is absent.* It is imperative that the reflexes be checked before and after each injection of magnesium sulfate (Table 29-6 and Fig. 29-5, on p. 702). If the mother is receiving a continuous IV infusion of magnesium sulfate, patellar reflexes are assessed every hour (Sibai, 1987; Anderson, 1987).

Serum Levels. A response to rise in serum levels of magnesium occurs:

4-8 mg/dl: Convulsions are prevented (therapeutic level)
10-12 mg/dl: Reflexes disappear
15-17 mg/dl: Respirations slow (below 12) or respiratory arrest
30-35 mg/dl: Cardiac arrest is possible; total paralysis

When the anticonvulsant is administered intravenously, serum levels are determined by *volume of distribution*—weight, height, extracellular and intracellular volume—and *renal excretion.* Serum levels are obtained every 4 to 6 hours and as needed.

Table 29-6 *Assessing Deep Tendon Reflexes (DTRs)*

Degree	Grading	Clinical Significance and Nursing Actions
Brisk with sustained clonus	5+	Woman not responding to medications as desired; may be accompanied by apprehension, restlessness, excitability; notify physician
Hyperactive response (brisk with transient clonus)	4+	Woman not responding to medications as desired; may be accompanied by apprehension, restlessness, excitability; notify physician
More than normal (brisk)	3+	Woman responding; however, important to assess frequently
Normal, active	2+	Safe dosage level, therapeutic effect
Low response (sluggish or dull)	1+	Notify physician for medical directives
No response	0	Turn off magnesium sulfate drip; change to "keep open" solution; notify physician for immediate care; prepare antidote (20 ml vial of 10% calcium gluconate) for injection

Fetus. Toxic levels in the fetus cause marked slowing of respirations and hyporeflexia after birth. Sibai (1987) reports that neonatal toxic effects are rare in the healthy term newborn whose weight is within normal range for gestational age. The danger signs for both fetus and mother that are associated with magnesium sulfate toxicity are summarized in the box below.

DANGER SIGNS

$MgSo_4$ Toxicity

1. Sudden hypotension
2. Urinary output less than 25 ml/hr
3. Respiration less than 12/min
4. Hyperreflexia, hyporeflexia, absence of reflexes
5. Serum levels of 10 to 12 mg/dl: reflexes absent*
6. Serum levels of 15 to 17 mg/dl: respiratory arrest
7. Serum levels of 30 to 35 mg/dl: total paralysis and cardaic arrest
8. Sudden decrease in FHR

*Clear sign of toxicity. Discontinue STAT (Sibai, 1987).

Antidote. The antidote for magnesium sulfate toxicity is a calcium salt such as calcium gluconate. A 10 ml vial of a 10% aqueous solution of calcium gluconate should be kept at the bedside. If needed, it is administered over 3 minutes intravenously and repeated every hour until the respiratory, urinary, and neurologic depression has been alleviated. *The maximum number of injections of a calcium salt is 8 injections in a 24-hour period.*

If improvement occurs therapy is continued until labor begins spontaneously. If the fetal age is greater than 38 weeks with a lecithin/sphingomyelin (L/S) ratio of 2:1 and other indications of fetal maturity, labor may be induced (Chapter 27 and 33). If improvement does not occur or the fetus shows signs of stress, the care for severe preeclampsia–eclampsia is initiated.

Immediate Care of Eclampsia

The immediate care during a convulsion is to ensure a patent airway. Once this has been attained, adequate oxygenation must be provided.

Immediate Care of Convulsions

1. If convulsions occur, turn woman onto left side to prevent aspiration of vomitus and supine hypotension syndrome.
2. Insert folded towel, plastic airway, or padded tongue blade into *side* of mouth to prevent biting of lips or tongue and to maintain airway. Do not put fingers into woman's mouth; she may bite them involuntarily.
3. Suction food and fluid from glottis or trachea.
4. Give $MgSO_4$ (and amobarbital sodium for recurrent convulsions) as ordered (Anderson, 1987).
5. Administer oxygen by means of face mask or tent after convulsion ceases (masks and nasal catheters cause excessive stimulation). Oxygen rate may be up to 10 L/min (as opposed to 3 L/min advocated for continuous 0_2 in chronic conditions).
6. Record time and duration of convulsions; include description.
7. Note any urinary or fecal incontinence.

Transfusion. Have the woman's blood typed and matched. Keep the blood available for emergency transfusion; women with eclampsia often develop premature separation of the placenta, hemorrhage, and shock.

Fluids. Give fluids as directed; record the time, the amount and the woman's response. Central venous pressure (CVP) or pulmonary arterial wedge pressure (PAWP) may be required for accurate fluid monitoring in the presence of pulmonary edema or acute renal failure. Hospital protocols vary.

1. Permit nothing by mouth (NPO) if woman is convulsing.
2. Insert indwelling catheter for accurate measurement of urinary output if one is not in place.
3. Assist physician with IV infusion of 200 to 300 ml of 20% glucose solution, 2 to 3 times a day during critical period to support liver function, aid nutrition, and replace fluid; 50% glucose is rarely used, since it often scleroses veins.
4. To correct hypovolemia, crystalloids (0.9% saline or Ringer's lactated solution) are infused intravenously. To maintain a urine output of 30 ml/h, 50 to 125 ml/h is infused.
5. If woman is oliguric or if serum protein level is low, physician may order salt-poor ablumin (25 to 50 ml) or 250 to 500 ml of plasma or serum to be administered intravenously.
6. Note and record maternal response.

Medications. Give medications as directed; monitor and record the woman's response. Record drugs, dosages, and times given.

1. Diuretics are *no longer* advocated (see Table 29-5).
2. Sedatives such as phenobarbital, 0.05 g, may be given orally or intramuscularly on admission to the hospital and repeated to maintain moderate sedation until the woman's condition improves. Monitor for start of labor, since woman may be unaware of sensation.
3. Sodium bicarbonate is given if arterial blood gases (ABGs) reveal a pH $\leq$ 7.10. Maternal acidemia ($\downarrow Po_2$) occurs after aspiration (Anderson, 1987).
4. Magnesium sulfate (IV or intramuscular [IM]) may be ordered as necessary. Before administering magnesium sulfate, the following findings must be present:
    1. DTRs of at least +1
    2. Respirations at least 12/min
    3. Urinary output at least 100 ml/4 hr
5. Multiple medications should be avoided (e.g., phenytoin [Dilantin] and diazepam [Valium] are not given with magnesium sulfate) (Anderson, 1987).
6. Hydralazine (Apresoline) is given for a diastolic pressure $\geq$ 110 mm Hg. The goal is to maintain a diastolic pressure between 90 to 100 mm Hg.

Laboratory Tests. Laboratory tests are ordered to assess for the HELLP syndrome, to have blood typed and crossmatched for packed cells, and to assess for DIC (Chapter 31).

Hygiene. Maintain body hygiene. The vulvar area may be washed with warm, soapy water.

Psychologic Support. The physician or nurse explains procedures briefly and quietly. The woman is never left alone if the condition is severe or if she is receiving magnesium sulfate therapy. The family is also kept informed of management, rationale, and the woman's progress.

Delivery. Preeclampsia–eclampsia and severe hypertensive or renal disease are intensified by the continuation of pregnancy. Termination of gestation is the only practical treatment. The fetus may therefore be premature or otherwise compromised.

1. Eclampsia is controlled before induction of labor is attempted; then labor is induced (Chapter 33). Analgesia with meperidine (Demerol), 25 to 50 mg, is suggested (Anderson, 1987).
2. Vaginal delivery with local infiltration, pudendal block, or balanced general anesthesia is preferred. However, if labor cannot be induced readily, if the woman is bleeding, or if there is fetal distress, cesarean delivery should be effected. Abruptio placentae is associated in 20% of women with preeclampsia (Chapter 31).
3. Pediatrician and pediatric (intensive care nursery) nurse are present to provide immediate care for the newborn.

A general nursing care plan for the woman experiencing severe preeclampsia and two specific nursing care plans follow.

Evaluation

Evaluation is a continuous process. To be effective, it needs to be based on measurable criteria, which reflect the parameters used to measure the goals for care. That is, the woman's condition improves; CNS irritability is reduced; convulsions (if any) are terminated; hypertension is reduced (normal values usually return by 10 days after delivery); water imbalance, acid-base imbalance, and other electrolyte imbalances are corrected; proteinuria is reduced, and serum protein level is increased; fetal well-being continues; and placental complications are absent or controlled, and delivery proceeds as previously planned whether vaginal, induced, or cesarean.

If the gravida's condition does not improve, the nurse assists in care for elective delivery, that is, induction of labor or cesarean birth, the woman and family are aware of need for care, cause of symptoms, and prognosis. Informed consent forms are completed. If the outcome for the mother or baby is unfavorable, the family is assisted to cope with loss and grief.

General Nursing Care Plan

HOSPITAL MANAGEMENT OF SEVERE PREECLAMPSIA

ASSESSMENT	NURSING DIAGNOSIS (ND)/ PLAN(P)/GOAL(G)	RATIONALE/ IMPLEMENTATION	EVALUATION
Blood pressure, 160/110 or more. Proteinuria, 3+, 4+. Urinary output, scant, dark color. Weight gain, 2 kg (4 lb) in less than a week. Hematocrit increases (hemoconcentration). Generalized edema.	ND: Potential for injury: maternal and fetal, related to edema, proteinuria, hypertension. P: Decrease severity of disease to ensure a healthy mother and baby. G: Mother and fetus suffer no adverse sequelae to PIH. ND: Decreased cardiac output related to arteriolar constriction and increased peripheral resistance. ND: Altered cardiopulmonary tissue perfusion related to edema and expansion of extravascular fluid. P: Reduce edema and increase tissue perfusion. G: Normalization of intravascular volume and tissue profusion	*To monitor and minimize severity of disease and effects of edema, proteinuria, and hypertension the nurse will:* Keep woman on absolute bedrest with side rails up. Start IV and maintain rate to keep line open. Insert indwelling catheter. Have woman select people she wishes to stay with her. Limit other visitors. Maintain calm unhurried approach to care. Give rationale for care. Report on woman's progress. Assure woman that her family will be kept informed.	Woman's symptomatology of PIH regresses. Woman remains quiet. Woman's (family's) stress and anxiety kept to a minimum. Family members are kept informed.

Continued.

General Nursing Care Plan—cont'd

ASSESSMENT	NURSING DIAGNOSIS (ND)/ PLAN(P)/GOAL(G)	RATIONALE/ IMPLEMENTATION	EVALUATION
Platelets decrease.	ND: Potential for injury: maternal and fetal, related to undetected hemoconcentration and clotting disturbances. P: Monitor for coagulopathy. G: Woman does not develop coagulopathy.	*To minimize problems with cardiac output and tissue perfusion the nurse will:* Continue surveillance of blood pressure every 1 hour or more, check for generalized edema, weight, and urinary output, hematocrit, platelets, and SGOT daily or as ordered. Report deviations immediately. Implement physician-ordered therapies.	Symptoms improve. Woman does not develop complications.
Epigastric or right upper quadrant pain. Nausea and vomiting. Headaches. Blurred vision. Hyperreflexia. Changes in level of consciousness (LOC). Seizures. Retinal detachment. Blindness.	ND: Pain related to stretching of the hepatic capsule or cerebral edema. ND: Potential for injury, maternal and fetal, related to possible seizure activity or aspiration of stomach contents. ND: Sensory-perceptual alterations related to edema, proteinuria, hypertension. P: Prevent progression of PIH; or, identify symptomatology of increasing severity, and institute appropriate therapy. G: Woman and fetus suffer no adverse sequelae to PIH.	*To prevent adverse sequelae to severe PIH, the nurse will:* Control amount of external stimuli. Monitor symptoms. Assess LOC. Assess reflexes. Record findings of funduscopic examination. Report any changes. Implement physician-ordered therapy.	Seizures are prevented. Woman rests comfortably. Symptoms improve. Woman remains lucid. Eyegrounds do not change.
Presence of rales. Pulmonary edema.	ND: Impaired gas exchange related to pulmonary edema. P: Continue surveillance. G: Respiratory function remains within normal limits.	*To monitor gas exchange; the nurse will:* Listen periodically to lung sounds. Check for pulmonary edema and rales.	Breath sounds remain within normal limits.
Fetal growth retardation. Fetal distress. Late decelerations of fetal heart rate (FHR).	ND: Potential for injury: fetus, related to inadequate placental perfusion. P: Facilitate placental perfusion. G: FHR remains stable; fetus born healthy.	*To increase placental perfusion; the nurse will:* Prevent supine hypotensive syndrome: place woman on left side; when on back, raise headrest and place a wedge under right hip.	Woman remains on side. FHR remains stable.
Levels of creatinine and urea increase. Oliguria (<100 ml/4 hr). Increased proteinuria.	ND: Altered patterns of urinary elimination related to decreased renal perfusion and GFR.	*To check urinary eliminations; the nurse will:* Check urinary output every hour.	Urinary elimination remains within normal limits. Diuresis occurs. Proteinuria decreases.

General Nursing Care Plan—cont'd

ASSESSMENT	NURSING DIAGNOSIS (ND)/ PLAN(P)/GOAL(G)	RATIONALE/ IMPLEMENTATION	EVALUATION
Generalized edema. Sudden weight gain.	P: Continue surveillance. G: Urinary elimination remains within normal limits. Diuresis occurs. Proteinuria decreases/stops.	Report output of <100 ml/4 hr. Keep accurate intake and output records. Check urine for protein every 4 hours. Send blood specimen to laboratory for measurement of creatinine; check results against previous tests.	Creatinine remains within normal limits.
Administration of $MgSO_4$	ND: Potential for injury: maternal and fetal, related to $MgSO_4$ side effects/toxicity. P: Minimize or prevent side effects/toxicity. G: Side effects/toxicity do not occur.	*To administer $MgSO_4$, the nurse will:* Follow hospital protocol (see also specific nursing care plan): Check hospital's procedure manual. Check blood levels of $MgSO_4$ periodically. Observe for toxicity. Assess reflexes and LOC periodically. Keep calcium gluconate on hand.	Further complications from $MgSO_4$ administration do not occur.
Woman (couple) anxious. Fearful of injury to fetus.	ND: Anxiety related to sudden change in condition. P: Relieve anxiety. G: Woman's (family's) anxiety is minimized. ND: Ineffective individual and family coping related to stress of disease process. P: Give support and information. G: Woman (family) develop increased coping skills.	*To monitor coping mechanisms; the nurse will:* Assess affect, restlessness, anxiety. Assess response to support person. Observe for adverse behavior. Keep woman (couple) informed of progress.	Woman feels free to express concerns. Support person does not make woman more anxious.
Preterm labor.	ND: Potential for injury: fetus, related to preterm birth. P: Monitor for labor; if labor occurs, minimize injury. G: Woman's pregnancy and labor result in a healthy mother and baby.	*To monitor for labor; the nurse will:* Observe woman for progress of labor. Assess for complications of labor. Prepare for delivery. Prepare woman (couple) for delivery by answering questions, supplying information and reinforcing information given to her by the physician.	Preterm labor does not occur; or, labor progresses normally. Healthy mother and baby result.

Specific Nursing Care Plan

PROTEIN INTAKE AND PSYCHOSOCIAL PROBLEMS

Sheila J., age 36, is pregnant for the third time. Both Sheila and her husband, Bob are pleased about the pregnancy. The pregnancy had been uneventful up to the thirty-third week, when Sheila was diagnosed with mild PIH and told to go home and maintain bed rest. The physician also prescribed a 70 g protein, low sodium diet. This has been a problem for Sheila and her family. Bob was laid off from his job 5 weeks ago. Sheila had been doing typing and other secretarial services from her home to bring in some extra money while not having to pay a babysitter for the 2 other children who are ages 7 and 5. To economize, they have been eating mostly pasta, tuna, hamburger meat, breadstuffs, eggs, and milk. Very little fruits and vegetables were used because of their high price. They have no family support and Bob is too proud to accept food stamps.

ASSESSMENT	NURSING DIAGNOSIS (ND)/ PLAN(P)/GOAL(G)	RATIONALE/ IMPLEMENTATION	EVALUATION
Blood pressure 140/90. Generalized edema: puffy eyes, swollen fingers. Proteinuria +2.	ND: Potential for injury: maternal and fetal, related to edema, proteinuria and hypertension. P: Minimize present signs and symptoms of PIH. G: Sheila's symptomatology of PIH abates.	*To monitor severity of maternal response to PIH, assess twice a week to note any change in following:* Vital signs and blood pressure. Edema. Weight gain. Proteinuria.	Sheila's symptomatology of complications subside and parameters remain within normal limits.
Sheila does not understand diet as prescribed.	ND: Knowledge deficit related to diet required in PIH. P: Meet Sheila's knowledge needs. G: Sheila follows diet as ordered by physician.	*To maintain an adequate protein intake:* Provide rationale for diet: Helps lower blood pressure. Helps decrease edema. Helps baby grow. Instruct Sheila on dietary food groups that are equivalent to 70 g protein.	Sheila verbalizes understanding of information presented. Sheila demonstrates knowledge of food groups.
Family's budget is limited. Sheil i does not understand "salt"—sources, amount needed.	ND: Situational low self-esteem related to financial status. P: Arrange for financial support (for nutrition needs) that is acceptable to family. G: Sheila's and family's nutrition needs are met without a loss of self-esteem.	Introduce Sheila to federal programs that supply necessary protein foods to pregnant woman and their children (i.e., MIC, WIC). *To maintain adequate but not excessive sodium intake:* Instruct Sheila on amounts of salt to use in food preparation. Advise her to refrain from salty or high sodium foods: potato chips, peanuts, certain cheeses.	Sheila contacts agencies and takes advantage of their programs. Sheila complies with diet and demonstrates knowledge by reporting on foods eating.
Sheila does not understand self-care for constipation.	ND: Constipation related to diet and pregnancy. P: Teach self-care for constipation. G: Sheila's constipation is relieved through her use of new knowledge.	*To minimize constipation:* See specific nursing care plan, Chapter 15. Advise about including ample amounts of roughage and fluids in the diet. Instruct on the fruits and vegetables that provide fiber and roughage.	Constipation minimized or prevented. Sheila expresses pleasure with learning self-care for constipation.

Specific Nursing Care Plan—cont'd

ASSESSMENT	NURSING DIAGNOSIS (ND)/ PLAN(P)/GOAL(G)	RATIONALE/ IMPLEMENTATION	EVALUATION
Sheila does not understand what is meant by bedrest and its significance to her care.	ND: Knowledge deficit related to meaning of bedrest and its significance to her condition and that of her fetus. P: Teach content related to bedrest and mutually develop a plan for its implementation. G: Sheila remains on bedrest as much as possible.	*To help Sheila maintain adequate rest the nurse will:* Instruct Sheila and her family on what is meant by bedrest: avoid stairs, limit outings to visits to health care provider, spend most of the day in bed, preferrably lying on her left side, and ambulate for meals and to use bathroom. Act as a client advocate by putting Sheila in touch with a social service worker to network for outside help and support while on bedrest (i.e., church group volunteers, senior citizen volunteers).	Sheila remains on bedrest as ordered.
Limited financial resources. Stress between husband and wife. Family stress.	ND: Ineffective individual and family coping related to stress of monetary problems and Sheila's illness. P: Help family develop positive coping strategies. G: Family will develop positive coping strategies.	*To help Sheila (family) reduce tension:* Encourage open discussion of problems. Help family seek solutions to problems (i.e., community resources, support of neighbors and friends). Friends neighbors or community resources provide homemaker services (e.g., laundry, shopping, child care, food preparation with instructions).	Sheila and family accept temporary disability and accept assistance.
Husband and Sheila upset with situation—spend very little time with 5 and 7 year old.	ND: Potential altered parenting related to stress of family situation. P: Help Sheila and her husband develop a plan. G: Positive family processes are implemented.	*To maintain family unity;* Have family spend time together at mother's bedside. Have parents read stories to children. Suggest that husband take children to park or playground in afternoon. Have family watch television together. Suggest family have picnic meals at mother's bedside. Instruct children on little things they can do around the house "for mommy," for example, dust furniture, put clothes away, answer door or phone, bring things to her. Children of this age want to help; it makes them feel like a useful part of the family unit.	Family unit remains intact and positive.

Specific Nursing Care Plan

PREVENT $MgSO_4$ TOXICITY; CARE OF WOMAN DURING CONVULSION

Tiara Stewart, a 15-year-old primigravida was diagnosed as having moderate to severe PIH. She was admitted to the hospital 2 days ago through the emergency room when she started to convulse at home. Her mother states she has not been complying with the prescribed diet and has continued to be out of bed, especially when her friends come over to visit her. Tiara's mother works all day and has no one to sit with Tiara.

In the emergency room, an IV was started and a loading dose of $MgSO_4$ was administered. Maintenence dose of $MgSO_4$ will be continued afterwards. Assessment of the fetus and the pregnancy is ongoing and prevention of further seizures is extremely important.

ASSESSMENT	NURSING DIAGNOSIS (ND)/ PLAN(P)/GOAL(G)	RATIONALE/ IMPLEMENTATION	EVALUATION
15-year-old primigravida, 32 weeks gestation. PIH with CNS involvement.	ND: Potential for injury, maternal and fetal, related to PIH and siezures of eclampsia. P: Prevent further seizures. G: Tiara has no further seizures. ND: Altered cardiopulmonary tissue perfusion related to vasoconstriction and vasospasms. P: Treat PIH and increase tissue perfusion. G: Tissue perfusion is maintained. ND: Sensory-perceptual alterations (visual, kinesthetic) related to loss of consciousness and seizures. P: Check level of consciousness periodically, prevent further deterioration of CNS. G: Tiara suffers no adverse CNS sequelae.	*To prevent further seizures the nurse will:* Assess CNS status periodically: Headache. Visual disturbances. Level of consciousness. Irritability. Fundoscopic changes. Assess for impending seizures: Deep tendon reflexes—hyperactive. Ankle clonus. Epigastric pain. Oliguria. Decrease environmental stimuli: Dimly lit room. Limit noise. Limit visitors. Cluster procedures. Promote rest.	Tiara remains quiet and further seizures are prevented.
$MgSO_4$ maintenance	ND: Activity intolerance related to maintaining an IV with $MgSO_4$. P: Keep Tiara quiet but occupied. G: Tiara follows treatment regimen.	*To increase tissue perfusion the nurse will:* Keep Tiara on bed rest, lying on left side. Administer oxygen as ordered. Administer medications as ordered.	Tissue perfusion increased.
	ND: Sensory-perceptual alterations (kinesthetic) related to effects of $MgSO_4$. P: Prevent further problems. G: Tiara experiences no adverse effects of $MgSO_4$ therapy. ND: Potential for injury, maternal and fetal, related to hypermagnesia and	*To prevent $MgSO_4$ toxicity the nurse will:* Monitor vital signs, blood pressure, and reflexes. Monitor serum magnesium levels. Keep calcium gluconate available. Observe level of consciousness and urinary output.	$MgSO_4$ toxicity prevented.

Specific Nursing Care Plan—cont'd

ASSESSMENT	NURSING DIAGNOSIS (ND)/ PLAN(P)/GOAL(G)	RATIONALE/ IMPLEMENTATION	EVALUATION
	toxic reactions of $MgSO_4$. P: Prevent $MgSO_4$ toxicity. G: Tiara does not experience $MgSO_4$ toxicity.		
Seizure	ND: Potential for injury related to seizure. P: Prevent or minimize injury. G: Tiara is not injured and labor nor DIC occur.	*To prevent injury during a seizure the nurse will:* Turn Tiara on side to prevent aspiration of stomach contents. Administer oxygen. Suction nose and mouth as needed. Not restrict Tiara's movements, but prevent her from injuring herself. Loosen tight clothing. Document seizure in nurse's notes. Monitor for signs of labor. Observe for other problems (i.e., DIC).	Tiara is protected during seizure. Labor does not occur; or, if labor occurs, Tiara and her baby suffer no adverse sequelae.

POSTDELIVERY NURSING CARE

The nursing care of the woman who experiences hypertensive disease differs from that required in a normal postpartum period in a number of respects. The following content emphasizes the specific nursing strategies needed by these women.

Assessment

Blood pressure is measured every 4 hours for 48 hours or more frequently as the woman's condition warrants. Even if no convulsions occurred before delivery, they may occur within this period.

The woman is asked to report headaches, blurred vision, etc. The nurse assesses affect, alertness, or dullness. Blood pressure is reassessed before giving analgesic for headache.

NOTE: No ergot products are given because they increase blood pressure.

The woman's and family's responses to labor are monitored. Regular postpartum assessment is performed.

Nursing Diagnoses

Examples might include the following:

- Situational low self-esteem related to
  - Inability to accept high-risk nature of delivery experience
- Potential anxiety of mother related to
  - Initial occurrence of hypertension during puerperium
- Potential altered family processes related to
  - Stress during high-risk prenatal, intranatal, and postdelivery periods

Plan/Implementation

Postpartum care for the woman with hypertensive disease includes care related to normal involution. In addition the woman and her family need opportunities to discuss their emotional response to complications. The nurse also provides information concerning the prognosis. Preeclampsia–eclampsia does not necessarily recur in subsequent pregnancies, but careful prenatal care is essential.

The nurse reaffirms the physician's advice that evaluation must be thorough during the postdelivery examination to rule out chronic hypertension. The woman needs family planning information (the next pregnancy should be delayed for 2 years; the woman is not a candidate for oral contraceptive use) (Chapter 42).

Evaluation

The nurse uses the following criteria to evaluate the plan of care:

1. Recovery from PIH is complete *or* woman begins therapy for chronic hypertension not related to pregnancy.
2. Woman's self-concept is not impaired.
3. Infant is healthy *or* has minimum impairment.

Recorder. The woman's record serves as a documented means of communication among all members of the health care team. The record contains accurate and complete recordings of the history, physical examination, and laboratory test results, sequential observations, goals, interventions, and the woman's responses. The record should be readily accessible to the health care professionals caring for the woman and her family. Documentation of the parent's health education, counseling, and responses to information are included. These data provide valuable information for the obstetrician and nurse for the woman's follow-up care and serve as a reservoir for data for future research.

SUMMARY

Hypertensive states during pregnancy constitute a physiologic risk for the woman and her fetus-newborn. This complication also imposes a psychologic risk for the woman and her family. Client teaching is central to the prevention of PIH and home care of "mild" preeclampsia. Technical skill is important in the care of women with severe preeclampsia. Knowledge of the use of magnesium sulfate as an anticonvulsant is essential. The seriousness and the unique problems posed by the HELLP syndrome challenge the nurse's assessment and care skills. Appropriate management depends on accurate differentiation of the various hypertensive states in pregnancy.

KEY CONCEPTS

- PIH is characterized by hypertension and proteinuria often accompanied by edema occurring after the twentieth week of pregnancy or during the early postpartum.
- The cause of PIH is unknown.
- PIH involves every organ in the body.
- Severe PIH is an obstetric emergency where the central goal for care is the prevention of eclampsia.
- The anticonvulsive drug of choice, magnesium sulfate, requires careful monitoring.
- Diuresis following therapy for PIH is an excellent prognostic sign.
- Since it is not possible to predict accurately which women will develop eclampsia, the importance of even a mild degree of hypertension complicating pregnancy must not be underestimated.
- Management of an eclamptic convulsion directs the caregivers to act to prevent self-injury, to ensure adequate oxygenation, to reduce risk of aspiration, to establish control with magnesium sulfate and to correct maternal acidemia.
- The presence of chorionic villi (trophoblastic tissue) in certain women incites vasospasm and hypertension that is cured only by their complete removal (e.g., evacuation of the gravid uterus).
- Magnesium sulfate toxicity is evident by such signs as absence of patellar reflex, respirations less than 12/min, and a urinary output of less than 100 ml/4 hr.
- The HELLP syndrome, a serious finding in some women with severe preeclampsia, usually becomes apparent during the early third trimester.

STUDY QUESTIONS AND ACTIVITIES

1. Visit a high-risk prenatal center. Interview a nurse and a nutritionist on the latest trends in treating PIH.
2. Develop a plan of care, utilizing nursing diagnoses, for a client with PIH. Be certain to include potential problems.
3. Arrange for a nurse and a nutritionist to speak to the group on the latest trends in treating PIH.
4. Role-play a nurse attempting to provide client teaching for a woman with PIH who resists the need for complete bed rest. Have the group suggest additional strategies.

References

Alanen, A, and Lassila, O: Deficient natural killer cell function in preeclampsia. Obstet Gynecol **60**:631, 1982

Anderson, GD: A systematic approach to eclamptic convulsion, Contemp OB/GYN 29(3):65, 1987

Belizan JM, and Villar, J: The relationship between calcium intake and edema, proteinuria and hypertension gestosis: a hypothesis, Am J Clin Nutr **33**:2202, 1980

Brazie, JE, Gumm, JK, and Little, VA: Neonatal manifestations of severe maternal hypertension occurring before the thirty-sixth week of pregnancy. J Pediatr 100:265, 1982

Brewer, T: Metabolic toxemia of late pregnancy, Springfield, Ill 1966, Charles C Thomas, Publisher

Cooper, D, and Liston, W: Genetic control of severe preeclampsia, J Med Genet **16**:409, 1979

Danforth, DN, and Scott, JR, editors: Obstetrics and gynecology, ed 5, Philadelphia, 1986, JB Lippincott Co

Dennis, E, McFarland, K, and Hester, L: The preeclampsia-eclampsia syndrome. In Danforth, D, editor: Obstetrics and gynecology, ed 4, Hagerstown, Md, 1982, Harper & Row, Publishers, Inc

Egley, CC, Gutliph, J, and Bowes, WA: Severe hypoglycemia associated with HELLP syndrome, Am J Obstet Gynecol 152:576, 1985

Gibson, B, Hunter, D, Neame, PB, and Kelton JG: Thrombocytopenia in preeclampsia and eclampsia, Thromb Haemost 8:234, 1982

Gilbert, ES, and Harmon, JS: High-risk pregnancy and delivery: nursing perspectives, St Louis, 1986, The CV Mosby Co

Israel, R: Predictive value of roll-over test in women with mild preeclampsia, Am J Obstet Gynecol 153(1):77, 1985

Knuppel, RA, and Drukker, JE: High-risk pregnancy: a team approach, Philadelphia, 1986, WB Saunders Co

Kozier, B, and Erb, G: Fundamentals of nursing, ed 2, Menlo Park, Calif, 1987, Addison-Wesley Publishing Co, Inc

Lindheimer, MD, and Katz, AI: Current concepts: hypertension in pregnancy, N Engl J Med 313(11):675, 1985

Pritchard, JA: Management of preeclampsia and eclampsia, Kidney Int. 18:259, Aug 1980

Pritchard, JA, MacDonald, PC, and Gant, NF: Williams obstetrics, ed 17, New York, 1985, Appleton-Century-Crofts

Reiss, RE, et al: The blood pressure source in primiparous pregnancy: a prospective study of 383 women, J Reprod Med 32:523, 1987

Sachs, BP, et al: Maternal mortality in Massachusetts: trends and prevention, N Engl J Med 316(11):667, 1987

Sibai, BM: Seeking the best use for magnesium sulfate in preeclampsia–eclampsia, Contemp OB/GYN 29(1):155, 1987

Valenzuela, G, Hayashi, R, and Johns, A: Effects of magnesium sulfate upon uterine contractility in humans, Magnesium 2:120, 1983

Weinstein, L: The HELLP syndrome: a severe consequence of hypertension in pregnancy, J Perinat 6(4):316, 1986

Zlatnik, FJ, and Burmeister, LF: Dietary protein and preeclampsia Am J Obstet Gynecol 147:345, 1983

Bibliography

Bern, MM, Driscoll, SG, and Levitt, T: Thrombocytopenia complicating preeclampsia, Obstet Gynecol 57:289, 1981

Brengman, SL, and Burns, MK: Hypertensive crisis in L & D, Am J Nurs 88(3):325, 1988

Campbell, WA, and Vintzileos, AV: Are α-blockers safe for hypertension during pregnancy? Contemp OB/GYN 31(1):178, 1988

Droegemueller, W, et al: Comprehensive gynecology, St Louis, 1987, The CV Mosby Co

Hill, MN: Hypertension: what can go wrong when you measure blood pressure, Am J Nurs 80:942, 1980

Hoffmaster, J: Detecting and treating pregnancy-induced hypertension, MCN 8:398, 1983

Kasser, NS, et al: Roll over test, Obstet Gynecol 54:411, 1980

Kelley, M: Maternal position and blood pressure during pregnancy and delivery, Am J Nurs 82:809, 1982

Kelley, M, and Mongiello, P: Hypertension in pregnancy, labor, delivery and postpartum, Am J Nurs 82:813, 1982

Knor, ER: Decision making in obstetrical nursing, 1987, BC Decker, Inc (Distributed by The CV Mosby Co, St Louis)

Kotchen, JM, et al: Blood pressure of young mothers and their children after hypertension in adolescent pregnancy: six-to-nine year follow-up, Am J Epidemiol 115:861, 1982

Martin, RW, and Morrison, JC: Oral magnesium for tocolysis Contemp OB/GYN 39(4):111, 1987

McCubbin, JH, et al: Cardiopulmonary arrest due to acute maternal hypermagnesemia, Lancet 9:105, 1981

McKay, DG: Chronic intravascular coagulation in normal pregnancy and preeclampsia, Contrib Nephrol 25:108, 1981

Moore, LG, et al: The incidence of pregnancy induced hypertension is increased among Colorado residents at high altitude, Am J Obstet Gynecol 144(14):423, 1982

Queenan, JT, and Hobbin, JC, editors: Protocols for high-risk pregnancies, Oradell, NJ, 1982, Medical Economics Books

Rayburn, W, Zuspan, F, and Piehl, E: Self-monitoring of blood pressure during pregnancy, Am J Obstet Gynecol 148:159, 1984

Repke, JT: Approaches to chronic hypertension during pregnancy, Contemp OB/GYN 29(6):69, 1987

Rose, B, Spencer, R, and Hensleigh, P: Resolution of oliguria in a pre-eclamptic after treatment with magnesium sulfate, J Perinat 7(3): 215, 1987

Ruge, CA: Catheter-related UTIs: what's the best way to prevent them? Nurs '87 17(12):50, 1987

Ruiz, AR, and Sibai, BM: Glucocorticoids for lung maturation in preeclampsia, Contemp OB/GYN 29(4):147, 1987

Shannnon, DM: HELLP syndrome: a severe consequence of pregnancy-induced hypertension, JOGN Nurs 16(6):395, 1987

Sibai, BM, et al: Maternal-perinatal outcome associated with the syndrome of hemolysis, elevated liver enzymes and low platelets in severe preeclampsia, AM J Obstet Gynecol 155:501, 1986

Sibai, BM: Pregnancy-induced hypertension, Contemp OB/GYN 31(5):51, 1988

Tcheng, D: When pregnancy threatens mother and child (preeclampsia), RN p 46, Dec, 1986

Weinstein, L: Preeclampsia/eclampsia with hemolysis, elevated liver enzymes, and thrombocytopenia, Obstet Gynecol 66:657, 1985

Zuspan, FP: Treatment of severe preeclampsia and eclampsia, Clin Obstet Gynecol 9:954, 1986

CHAPTER

30

Maternal Infections

Learning Objectives

Correctly define the key terms listed.

Summarize care of clients with sexually transmitted diseases.

Summarize care of clients with TORCH infections.

Summarize care of clients with urinary tract infections.

Summarize care of clients with puerperal infections.

Summarize care of clients with toxic shock syndrome.

Summarize care of clients with vaginal infections.

Summarize care of clients with bacteremic shock.

Summarize care of clients with acquired immune deficiency syndrome (AIDS).

Review infection control to minimize nosocomial infections and occupational risk for infection.

Key Terms

acquired immune deficiency syndrome (AIDS)
bacteremic shock
condylomata acuminata
disseminated intravascular coagulation (DIC)
endogenous
fomite
human papillomavirus (HPV)
human immunodeficiency virus (HIV)
infestations
leukorrhea
mean arterial pressure (MAP)
nosocomial
puerperal infection
sexually transmitted disease (STD)
TORCH infections
toxic shock syndrome (TSS)
universal precautions
urinary tract infections (UTI)
vaginitis

Sexually transmitted diseases and other infections are responsible for significant morbidity. Financial costs are substantial. However, the personal costs of suffering imposed by the disease process and its sequelae cannot be measured. Some consequences persist for a lifetime, such as congenital infection that compromises a child's quality of life, and infertility and sterility. The latter problems are discussed in Chapters 40 and 42.

The focus of this chapter is to present conditions associated with gynecologic infections and related medical and nursing care. Maternal and fetal and neonatal effects of the disease processes and therapeutic measures are emphasized.

Pregnancy confers no immunity against infection and both mother and fetus must be considered when the pregnant woman carries an infection. In some disorders, such as tuberculosis, the fetus is almost always spared, even though the mother may be dying. In other diseases, such as rubella, the fetus may be critically compromised, whereas the mother may be only slightly ill.

Preventive medicine is particularly important in obstetrics. Many tragedies can be averted by informed anticipation. For example, vaccination against rubella before pregnancy currently is the only means to control this disorder. No cure is available for rubella. Women are becoming more knowledgeable about factors such as infections, which can jeopardize fetal development. The large number of infections, the varying responses of the fetus or newborn, and the range of nursing and medical actions necessitate a readily available resource. The box at right and Tables 30-1 to 30-3 provide this information.

SEXUALLY TRANSMITTED DISEASE

Venereal diseases (named after Venus, the goddess of love), now termed *sexually transmitted diseases* (STDs), often share common characteristics. They have a predilection for genital and perigenital sites, perhaps because of genital pH, temperature, moisture, and hormonal influences. The causative organisms are relatively unstable when removed from their natural habitat. They are either completely or predominantly transferred from one person to another sexually (see box below).

SEXUALLY TRANSMITTED DISEASE (STD)

Historically Defined Venereal Diseases

Syphilis: acquired, congenital (annual worldwide incidence is estimated at 50 million people, with 40,000 in the United States)
Gonorrhea (annual worldwide incidence is estimated at 250 million people, with 3 million in the United States)
Chancroid
Lymphogranuloma venereum (*Chlamydia trachomatis,* L-1, L-2, L-3)
Granuloma inguinale

Newly Defined STDs

Hepatitis B (serum hepatitis)
Herpes genitalis
Balanoposthitis; balanitis
Proctitis
Human papillomavirus: condylomata acuminata
Genital candidiasis
Gardnerella vaginalis
Chlamydial infection (serovars D through K)
Acquired immune deficiency syndrome (AIDS)

Enteric Diseases That May Be Sexually Transmitted

Salmonellosis
Amebiasis
Typhoid
Giardiasis
Shigellosis

Diseases Spread by Body Contact But Not Necessarily by Coitus

Pediculosis
Molluscum contagiosum
Scabies

Chlamydia Trachomatis

Chlamydial infections are epidemic in the United States. These infections are 3 times more prevalent than gonorrhea and 30 times more prevalent than syphilis. *Chlamydia trachomatis* is the most common sexually transmitted bacterial pathogen in the United States. This pathogen is responsible for substantial morbidity, personal suffering, and heavy economic burden. Estimated cost exceeds $1.4 billion per year (Loucks, 1986; Washington et al., 1987a,b).

Maternal effects are usually mild. Infection of the cervix may be asymptomatic or be evident by appearance of congestion, edema, mucopurulent discharge, dyspareunia, and bleeding. Lymphogranuloma venereum, urethritis, dysuria, acute salpingitis with symptoms of pelvic inflammatory disease (PID), sterility, or infertility may occur. Other conditions include conjunctivitis, sore throat, and perihepatitis.

Fetal or neonatal effects are common. Stillbirth and neonatal death are 10 times more common than in noninfected women. Preterm birth may result. The newborn may acquire the infection by direct contact with an infected birth canal. Newborn infection may be asymptomatic. **Inclusion conjunctivitis** occurs in one third of exposed newborns. Conjunctivitis appears after 3 to 4 days. Chronic follicular conjunctivitis with conjunctival scarring and corneal neovascularization contributes to vision sequelae. About 25% of newborns with *Chlamydia* **pneumonia** can exhibit symptoms of serious tachypnea, dyspnea, or apnea that require hospitalization (Schachter et al., 1986).

Counseling. *Trachomatis* is an obligatory parasitic bacterium. That is, the organisms can exist only within living cells. Therefore transmission occurs directly from one person to another (Larson, 1984). There are 15 known serovars. Serovars D through K are responsible for neonatal infections (Chapter 39) and for adult ocular and genital infections. Serovars L-1, L-2, and L-3 are responsible for lymphogranuloma venereum, a sexually transmitted disease rare in North America (Marvin and Slevin, 1987; Loucks,

1986; Bourcier and Seidler, 1987). There are 3 to 4 million adults infected each year; 800,000 of these are males with urethritis. Yearly, the number of cases of newborn conjunctivitis (73,800) and of pneumonia (37,100) are equally impressive (Perlman, 1986). This infection is implicated in cervical dysplasia on Papanicolaou smear, in ectopic pregnancy, and in sterility in the female; as well as in genital inflammation and damage to the prostate and sperm in the male.

Populations at risk have been identified (Loucks, 1986; Washington et al, 1987a,b; Perlman, 1986; Marvin and Slevin, 1987; Corbett and Meyer, 1987). The sexually active female under 20 years of age is 2 to 3 times more likely to become infected than women between 20 and 29. Women over 30 have the lowest rate. Women and men with multiple sexual partners are at highest risk. People who *do not* use barrier methods of birth control (condom, spermicide, diaphragm) have a higher incidence. Lower socioeconomic status may be a risk factor. Sexually active males under 20 are at high risk for urethritis. In men, the infection is linked to nongonococcal urethritis (NGU). The infection rate among homosexual males is one-third that of heterosexual males. However, 4% to 8% of infected homosexual males have rectal chlamydial infection (Loucks, 1986).

In 1985, the Centers for Disease Control (CDC) guidelines specified screening the populations at risk, treating all those who are presumably infected, and educating the medical profession and public (Marvin and Slevin, 1987). Combination antibiotic therapy is recommended for heterosexual men and women with gonorrhea since 20% to 50% harbor *C. trachomatis.* Homosexual men with gonorrhea have a low incidence of concurrent chlamydia infection. Of people infected with chlamydia, 15% of males and 26% of females also have gonorrhea.

Ceftriaxone (or amoxicillin with probenecid) initially and tetracycline subsequently is the treatment of choice. Erythromycin is substituted if the woman is sensitive to penicillin or if she is pregnant.

Laboratory diagnosis is possible (Bennett, 1987). Tissue culture provides a definitive test. However, it is expensive, requires skill to perform, and requires 4 to 7 days for results. There are two antigen detection methods: (1) a direct immunofluorescent test (e.g., MicroTrak) that requires a fluorescent microscope and takes 30 minutes; and (2) an enzyme-linked immunosorbent assay (ELISA) test (e.g., Chlamydiazyme) that gives a color signal in 4 hours. The 30-minute test is more appropriate for screening low-risk populations; the ELISA test, for high-risk populations.

Human Papillomavirus

Condylomata acuminata are sexually transmitted lesions caused by human papillomavirus (HPV). There are over 46 HPVs that infect skin and mucosal surfaces. HPV-6 and HPV-11 are among the 15 HPVs known to infect the genital tract (Howett and Rapp, 1986; Jenson et al., 1986; Kreider, 1987; Byrne et al., 1987; Bourcier and Seidler, 1987; Ferenczy, 1987; Corbett and Meyer, 1987).

The incidence of reported cases in the United States has increased dramatically:

1966	169,000
1981	>1,000,000
1987	>40,000,000

Disease occurs at the site of entry of the virus after an incubation period of 1 to 6 months. *HPV is not disseminated through the bloodstream.* HPV is clinically significant because various types are associated with congenitally derived respiratory papillomatosis in children (Chapter 39) and cervical carcinoma in adult women (Chapter 44).

Condylomata acuminata are dry, wartlike growths on the vulva, vagina, cervix, or rectum. They may be small or large, single or multiple, or have a cauliflower appearance. Chronic vaginal discharge, pruritus, or dyspareunia can occur. Diagnosis is by colposcopy and direct visualization of the growths, biopsy, or presence of koilocytes (nuclear abnormalities in squamous cervical epithelium) seen in Papanicolaou smears.

In the immunocompetent person, condylomata acuminata may regress spontaneously. The condition is difficult to treat in many people, however. Available therapy is primarily cytotoxic or destructive. *Cytotoxic* agents are podophyllin (podophyllum resin) and 5-gluorouracil (5-FU). Podophyllin, 20% to 30% in tincture of benzoin, is used for lesions 2 cm or less in diameter, but not in the vagina or on the cervix. Petrolatum is used to protect surrounding skin because podophyllin is caustic and cytotoxic. The woman must wash the medication off after 4 hours or sooner if burning occurs. She is treated weekly for 6 weeks. Therapy may not produce a cure. The recurrence rate is 70%. **Podophyllin is not to be used during pregnancy.** The use of podophyllin during pregnancy is associated with fetal death and preterm labor (see also Chapter 30). The more effective cytotoxic agent is 5-FU in 5% cream. This highly toxic agent is used for resistant condylomata. The cure rate approaches 90%. There are no systemic effects when it is administered intravenously since only 5% to 6% is absorbed. Local pain and epithelial erosions are side effects of local application. Treatment with 5-FU is most effective when used in conjunction with laser therapy.

The most effective *destructive* method is a carbon dioxide laser used with local anesthesia. It is precise and sterile, and is accompanied by minimum bleeding and trauma. The treated area does not regain its normal pigmentation for several years. Post-laser-therapy instruction follows:

1. Keep area clean by irrigating with warm water twice a day
2. Dry with electric hair dryer
3. Apply antibacterial cream twice a day
4. Use gauze dressing to prevent rubbing against clothing
5. Use lidocaine ointment 5% for discomfort
6. Return to clinic as instructed
7. Use latex condoms until disease is cured in the woman. Today condoms are dense enough to prevent passage of viruses (500 A° = size of HPV).

Trichloroacetic acid, 50% solution, is a destructive therapy that is somewhat safer to use than podophyllin. It can be self-applied with a cotton swab and does not need to be washed off.

Therapy during pregnancy is determined on an individual basis. About 30% of pregnant women harbor HPV in the genital tract (Ferenczy, 1987). Large, outward-growing lesions on the vulva that may interfere with delivery or episiotomy are usually treated. Carbon dioxide laser treatment has been used to treat genital warts between 30 and 32 weeks gestation. Treatment is usually followed by vaginal delivery with no complications (Ferenczy, 1984, 1987). Flat lesions do not pose mechanical problems for vaginal delivery. However, they too may be associated with transmission of the virus to the newborn (Chapter 39). The woman is advised of the risk that if she delivers vaginally, her child may be one of the 300 children per year who are diagnosed with recurrent juvenile respiratory papillomatosis (Ferenczy, 1987; Huffman and Blanco, 1987). The woman can make an informed decision concerning vaginal or abdominal birth.

Gardnerella Vaginalis

Gardnerella vaginalis is the type of bacteria implicated in bacterial vaginosis (Bennett, 1987). It affects vaginal pH, thus altering the flora of the vagina. Incidence varies with the population. *Gardnerella vaginalis* is formed in 15% of female university students, 15% to 20% of pregnant women, and 30% of women who attend clinics for treatment of sexually transmitted diseases. Diagnosis is based on clinical signs. The vaginal fluid pH is elevated, usually ≥4.5. The homogeneous vaginal discharge has an amine (fishy) odor when mixed with 10% potassium hydroxide. "Clue cells" are seen on microscopic examination of vaginal discharge.

The *maternal effect* of infection with this bacteria is usually a mild illness. The bacterial vaginosis is expressed by a milklike discharge. Itching, burning, and pain may be present in the vagina and around the introitus. Obstetric complications can occur, especially in untreated cases. Amniotic fluid infection, premature rupture of membranes (PROM), preterm labor and delivery, and postpartum endometritis have been linked to this infection. *Fetal and neonatal effects* include septicemia and death.

Counseling. *G. vaginalis* is transmitted through sexual contact, especially when estrogen levels are high. It is often seen with other infections of the vagina. Because therapy is often a sulfa-based medication (suppository, cream), each woman is assessed for sensitivity to sulfonamides before medication is prescribed.

An 85% to 95% cure rate is achieved with oral metronidazole 500 mg 2 times per day for 7 days. Best results are obtained if the woman and her partner(s) are treated at the same time. The sexual partner is usually only treated, though, if the woman exhibits symptoms of recurrent infection. Adjunctive topical medication may include metronidazole, sulfonamides, povidone-iodine, or chlorhexidine.

Gonorrhea

Gonorrhea ("clap," "drip") is caused by *Neisseria gonorrhoeae,* a type of diplococci bacteria. Although gonorrhea is an STD, it is also spread by direct contact with infected lesions and fomites. Self-inoculation with contaminated hands is common. Secretions on fomites such as washcloths, towels, bed linens, and clothing are often implicated. Thus this bean-shaped gram-negative organism is responsible for genitourinary, anorectal, oropharyngeal, and systemic infections.

Gonorrhea often is only mildly symptomatic in women, or the diplococci may persist unsuspected in the lower genital tract. Symptomatology of lower urogenital tract infection includes dysuria and frequency, heavy green-yellow purulent discharge at the cervical os, cervical tenderness, vulvovaginitis, bartholinitis, dyspareunia, and postcoital bleeding. Swollen and painful Bartholin's glands and tenderness in the lymph nodes in the groin usually accompany infection. In 10% to 15% of cases, the upper urogenital tract is affected in the later stage of infection. Lower abdominal pain, cervical tenderness, fever, nausea, and vomiting are accompanying symptoms. Adnexal abscess and pelvic tenderness indicate PID. PID is implicated in ectopic pregnancy or sterility. Chronic pelvic pain and low backache may be seen. Anorectal infection is diagnosed by local inflammation, burning, and pruritus. Oropharyngeal infection may be asymptomatic or result in inflammation and sore throat. Systemic infection results in gonococcemia, skin rashes, arthritis, pericarditis, and meningitis. Gonococcal perihepatitis (Fitz-Hugh and Curtis syndrome) is discussed in Chapter 35.

Maternal effects are seen. After the third month of pregnancy, gonorrheal salpingitis rarely occurs, perhaps because with progressive pregnancy, the chorion laeve fuses with the decidua parietalis, thus obliterating the endometrial cavity. Postdelivery maternal complications of untreated gonorrhea include gonococcal endometritis, acute salpingitis, dermatitis, and arthritis.

Neonatal effects include **ophthalmic neonatorum** and pneumonia. Ophthalmitis with partial or total blindness can occur. Neonatal sepsis is characterized by temperature instability, hypotonia, poor feeding, and jaundice.

Counseling. Prevention is achieved by limiting the number of sexual partners; using barrier contraception, including nonoxynol-9 spermicide; and avoiding oral-genital sexual activity. The incubation period is 2 to 5 days. In the woman, the early stage may be asymptomatic. In addition, 5% of women with gonorrhea also have syphilis.

The woman and her sexual partner(s) must be treated simultaneously to prevent reinfection (the ping-pong effect). Gravid women allergic to penicillin can be given erythromycin or spectinomycin; nongravid women can be given cephalosporins and kanamycin. Erythromycin is contraindicated in women with liver disease.

After therapy the woman is advised to abstain from sexual intercourse or to have her partner(s) use condoms until cultures are negative at two consecutive follow-up visits. Oral-genital sex especially should be avoided.

Syphilis

Syphilis ("lues") is caused by the spirochete, *Treponema pallidum,* after an incubation period of several weeks. The spirochete is responsible for chancre, condylomata lata, cardiovascular disease, neurologic disease, and congenital syphilis.

Several methods of assessment of syphilis are available:

1. Dark-field microscopic examination or direct fluorescent antibody staining of material from lesions or umbilical cord
2. Assessment of clinical signs
3. Roentgenographic evidence of characteristic bone involvement
4. Serologic testing for antibodies known as reagins

Any test for antibodies may be negative in the presence of active infection because it takes time for the body's immune system to develop antibodies to any antigen.

Nonspecific serologic tests for nontreponemal antigens used for screening purposes are of two types: complement fixation (Kolmer, Wasserman) and flocculation (Kahn, RPR [rapid plasma reagin], VDRL [Venereal Disease Research Laboratories]). The VDRL test will not be positive until 10 to 90 days after infection; that is, 50% are positive in 3 weeks, 90% in 6 weeks, and 100% in 13 weeks. Therefore infection may exist in the presence of a negative result from the VDRL test. If the antibodies have been acquired from the mother, titers should drop to zero by 3 months. False-positive results may occur if the newborn has an acute infection of any kind or a collagen disease. Even in the presence of a syphilitic infection a false-negative result may occur, for example, if the mother became infected late in pregnancy. A false-positive result may occur in the presence of heroin dependence.

Specific tests for treponemal antigen are more expensive, used for differential diagnosis. These tests include TPI (*T. pallidum* immobilization), FTA-ABS (fluorescent treponemae antibody absorption), and FTA-ABS IgM (fluorescent treponemal antibody absorption, immunoglobulin M). The FTA-ABS IgM is most specific for neonatal syphilis; a positive result is especially valuable in diagnosis of the condition in the asymptomatic child. Results of the FTA-ABS IgM test may be negative, however, in the presence of active disease if infection occurred late in pregnancy and the fetus or newborn had insufficient time for an IgM response. In questionable cases the test is repeated.

NOTE: Yaws, a nonvenereal contagious disease, is caused by the spirochete *Treponema pertenue.* This spirochete is closely related to the causative organism of syphilis. Yaws is spread by contact with secretions or sores from an infected person. Both syphilis and yaws give a positive result in the serologic test for syphilis (STS). Yaws is a common disease in equatorial Africa, Hawaii, South America, and the East and West Indies. It is effectively treated with antibiotics, especially penicillin.

Early syphilis infection may be asymptomatic. During the *primary stage,* a chancre forms at the portal of entry of this STD. The chancre has a red base with firm, rolled edges and is painless. The local lymphadenopathy clears without treatment in 4 to 6 weeks.

The *secondary stage* begins about 6 weeks after healing of the primary lesion. A symmetric, nontender rash may appear anywhere over the body, including palms of hands and soles of feet. If the rash develops on the scalp, loss of hair is seen. Condylomata appear on any moist skin surface. Systemic infection causes malaise, fever, and headache. This secondary stage also clears without treatment in 2 to 6 weeks.

Latent stages appear at varying times. An early latent stage may appear up to 4 years after the primary infection. At this time, lesions reappear. For 50% to 70% of people, the latent stage lasts a lifetime, during which time there is no outward evidence of disease.

The *tertiary stage* brings clinical evidence of disease throughout the body. Obliterative endarteritis leads to cell damage and death and to the formation of gumma nodules of dead tissue. The acronym PARESIS summarizes possible sequelae seen in changes in the following: *P*ersonality, *A*ffect, *R*eflexes, *E*ye function, *S*ensorium, *I*ntellect, and *S*peech.

Fetal and neonatal effects are seen. Syphilis probably continues to be a major cause of late abortion throughout the world, despite widespread success of diagnosis and treatment of this disease. Primary and secondary stages of untreated syphilis lead to stillbirth. Latent and tertiary stages of untreated syphilis lead to secondary syphilis (congenital syphilis) in the newborn.

Congenital syphilis occurs when the spirochetes cross the placenta after the sixteenth to eighteenth week of gestation. The following sequelae are seen: snuffles (rhinitis), rhagades (cracks, fissures around the mouth), hydrocephaly, and corneal opacity. Later, saddle nose, saber shin, Hutchinson's teeth (notched, tapered canines), and diabetes develop in untreated children. There are no residual effects if the mother is treated adequately before the fifth month. Destruction of tissue that occurs before treatment cannot be reversed, but additional tissue destruction is prevented by adequate treatment.

Therapy for syphilis includes the following possible regimens (Corbett and Meyers, 1987; Tramont, 1987): penicillin G benzathine, tetracycline if allergic to penicillin, or erythromycin if unable to take penicillin or tetracycline. However, there is a steady flow of treatment failures. One possible reason may be developing organism resistance (Guinan, 1987). A second reason may be an alteration in the immune status of the infected person (Tramont, 1987; Johns, Tierney, and Felsenstein, 1987; Berry et al., 1987). Neurologic complications of syphilis have developed in persons infected with AIDS.

TORCH INFECTIONS

Toxoplasmosis, **o**ther infections (e.g., hepatitis), **r**ubella virus, **c**ytomegalovirus, and **h**erpes simplex viruses, known collectively as TORCH infections, comprise a group of organisms capable of crossing the placenta and adversely affecting the development of the fetus. TORCH infections, their maternal, fetal, and newborn effects, are outlined in Table 30-1.

Table 30-1 *Maternal Infection: TORCH*

Infection	Maternal Effects	Fetal or Neonatal Effects	Counseling: Prevention, Identification, and Management
Toxoplasmosis (protozoa)	Acute infection: similar to influenza; lymphadenopathy	With maternal acute infection: parasitemia Less likely to occur with maternal chronic infection Abortion likely with acute infection early in pregnancy (See Table 39-1)	Avoid eating raw meat and exposure to litter used by infected cats; if cats in house, have toxoplasma titer checked If titer is rising during early pregnancy, abortion may be given to the mother as an option
Other:			
Hepatitis A (infectious hepatitis) (virus)	Abortion—cause of liver failure during pregnancy Fever, malaise, nausea, and abdominal discomfort	Exposure during first trimester; fetal anomalies; fetal or neonatal hepatitis; premature birth; intrauterine fetal death	Usually spread by droplet or hand contact especially by culinary workers; γ-globulin can be given as prophylaxis for hepatitis A
Hepatitis B (serum hepatitis) (virus)	May be transmitted sexually Symptomatology variable: fever, rash, arthralgia, depressed appetite, dyspepsia, abdominal pain, generalized aching, malaise, weakness, jaundice, tender and enlarged liver	Infection occurs during birth See Table 39-1 Maternal vaccination during pregnancy should present no risk for fetus; however, data are not available. See Chapter 39 for information about vaccination of children at risk for hepatitis B	Generally passed by contaminated needles, syringes, or blood transfusions; can also be transmitted orally or by coitus, however, but incubation period is longer; hepatitis B immune globulin can be given prophylactically after exposure Hepatitis B vaccine recommended for populations at risk; vaccine consists of series of 3 IM doses Populations at risk: women from Asia, Pacific islands, Haiti, sub-Africa, Alaska (women of Eskimo descent) Other women at risk include health care providers
Rubella (3-day German measles, virus)	Rash, fever, mild symptoms; suboccipital lymph nodes may be swollen; some photophobia Occasionally arthritis or encephalitis Abortion	Incidence of congenital anomalies; first month, 50%; second month, 25%, third month, 10%, fourth month, 4% Exposure during first 2 months: malformations of heart, eyes, ears, or brain, abnormal dermatoglyphics Exposure after fourth month: systemic infection, hepatosplenomegaly, intrauterine growth retardation, rash At 15-20 years of age, may experience deterioration of intellect and development or develop epilepsy	Vaccination of pregnant women contraindicated, **pregnancy should be prevented for 2 months after vaccination**; hemagglutinin-inhibition-antigen-negative parturients can be safely vaccinated after delivery
Cytomegalovirus (CMV) (a herpes virus)	Respiratory or sexually transmitted asymptomatic illness or mononucleosis-like syndrome; may have cervical discharge	Fetal or neonatal death or severe, generalized disease—hemolytic anemia and jaundice; hydrocephaly or microcephaly; pneumonitis; hepatosplenomegaly	Virus may be reactivated and cause disease in utero or during delivery in subsequent pregnancies; fetal infection may occur during passage through infected birth canal; disease is commonly progressive through infancy and childhood
Herpes genitalis (herpex simplex virus; HSV II)	See discussion that follows		

Herpes Simplex Virus

Herpes simplex virus type 1 (HSV-1) infections predominate during childhood. The virus is transmitted primarily by contact with *oral* secretions and causes cold sores and fever blisters. HSV-2 infections usually occur after puberty as sexual activity increases. HSV-2 is transmitted primarily by contact with *genital* secretions. Although it has been shown that HSV can survive for many hours on objects like doorknobs, faucets, and toilets, scientists do not believe that people are likely to be infected by contact with such objects (March of Dimes, 1984; Nerurkar et al., 1983). Public health experts believe that within the United States from 10 million to 40 million people carry the HSV-2. Many genital infections show a mixture of HSV-1 and HSV-2.

HSV interacts with epithelial or neuroepithelial cells and neurons. The incubation period is between 2 and 4 weeks. During the initial infection, HSV migrates to one or more sensory nerve ganglia, where it remains latent and dormant indefinitely (Fig. 30-1, *A*). An intact immune system cures the infection at the portal (place of entry). The *primary* infection involves mucocutaneous cells; recurrent infection involves stratified epithelial cells. Stressor stimuli trigger recurrent infection (Fig. 30-1, *B*). Fever, another infection, emotions, menstruation, and ultraviolet light are some common stressors (Blankenship, 1987). Infections seem to be more severe in the woman during pregnancy.

HSV is diagnosed by cytologic testing and microscopic examination. A Papanicolaou smear of the lesion is positive for multinucleated giant cells with ground glass nuclear appearance and cervical dysplasia. A wet-mount preparation of lesion secretions is positive for polymorphonuclear leukocytes (Corbett and Meyer, 1987).

HSV infections may involve external genitals, the vagina, and cervix. Symptomatology is more pronounced with first infections of HSV. Painful blisters form, rupture, and then drain, leaving shallow ulcers that crust over and disappear after 2 to 6 weeks. A vaginal discharge is seen if the cervix or vaginal mucosa is involved. The woman may experience fever, malaise, anorexia, painful inguinal lymphadenopathy, dysuria, and dyspareunia.

Recurrences are sometimes preceded by itching, a burning sensation in the genital area, tingling in the legs, or a slight increase in vaginal discharge. Repeated recurrence may result in keratitis, encephalitis, and possibly cervical carcinoma (Chapter 44). Symptomatic therapy is available (see guidelines for client teaching: genital herpes). No specific cure has been identified.

Maternal effects include preterm labor and the possibility of cesarean delivery. The Committee on Fetus, Newborn and Infectious Diseases of the American Academy of Pediatrics proposed guidelines for delivery of women with HSV (Table 30-2) (Blankenship, 1987). For asymptomatic women, vaginal samples can be taken at birth (Petit, 1987). Test results are available in a few days. If results are positive, staff and parents can be vigilent for signs of neonatal illness. Early intervention in the disease greatly boosts chances of survival (Prober, 1987).

Fetal and neonatal effects are serious. Abortion and pre-

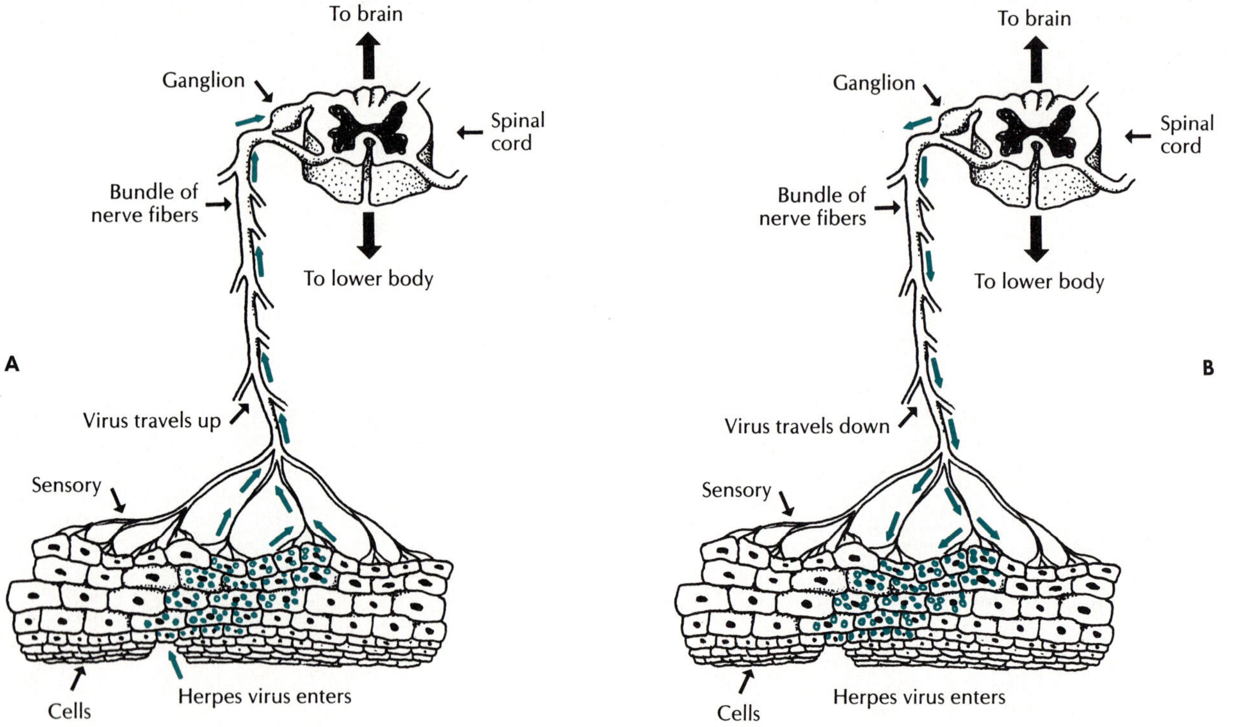

Fig. 30-1 **A**, Initial herpes infection takes place when virus (colored dots) enters cells of mucous membranes, eyes, or skin. They reproduce and travel up (colored arrows) the sensory nerves until they reach a ganglion (cluster of nerve cell bodies). There they are protected by the body's immune system, which overcomes the infection at the place of entry. **B**, Though the entry wound soon heals, when conditions allow, the virus may later travel back down the nerve pathway to reinfect skin cells again.

Guidelines for Client Teaching

GENITAL HERPES

ASSESSMENT

1. Woman has genital herpes (Herpes Simplex Virus Type II).
2. Woman is 9 months pregnant.

NURSING DIAGNOSES

Pain, related to active genital herpes.
Knowledge deficit related to symptomatic therapy for and prevention of neonate contracting genital herpes.
Impaired skin integrity related to active herpes lesions.
Potential for injury: fetus, related to active herpes virus.

GOALS:

Short-term

Relief from discomfort. Teach woman about the disease.

Intermediate

Woman learns possible newborn problems if infant born vaginally while disease is active.
Woman reports rupture of membranes or any other signs of impending labor to the clinic or physician.

Long-range

Infant does not contract herpes infection.
Woman's herpes goes into remission.
Recurrence of genital herpes kept to a minimum.

REFERENCES AND TEACHING AIDS

Pamphlets from clinic, hospital, or March of Dimes describing genital herpes disease.
Pictures and diagrams.
Films or videos.
Printed instructions for woman to take home for reference.

CONTENT/RATIONALE	TEACHING ACTION
To describe genital herpes: Genital herpes is caused by virus that is spread by sexual contact. The incubation period is approximately 3 to 14 days for primary infection and secondary infection may occur after 7 to 10 days.	Provide printed material for her to follow along. Ask woman if she has had subsequent outbreaks.
She may have had flu-like symptoms followed by the outbreak of painful vesicals in her genital area that rupture and may become secondarily infected from other organisms. An itching or tingling sensation may precede the pain when the vesicles are first forming. Lymph nodes in the inguinal area may be swollen.	Show woman pictures of active herpes lesions. Describe the symptoms and ask woman if she has had them before. Show a diagram or chart depicting the placement of the inguinal lymph nodes.
To provide information regarding prevention of spread to fetus/newborn: Fetus can be infected with the disease as it comes down the birth canal, since the lesions are in the genital tract. It is important for the physician or clinic to know if your disease is active before you deliver; neonatal herpes is serious and can cause eye or nerve damage to the baby, or even death.	Show picture of fetus coming down the birth canal.
When your disease is active, that is, open vesicles in your genital area, a cesarean delivery is favored, because it bypasses the birth canal.	Show picture of vesicles. Show diagram of cesarean delivery.
The physician will schedule your appointments weekly during your last month of pregnancy. The reasons for this are: (1) to check on you and your fetus for signs of impending labor, (2) keep an eye on the herpes infection, and (3) schedule a cesarean delivery before you go into labor. There is no effecive treatment at present for genital herpes, however, symptomatic treatment may help your discomfort while the lesions are active.	Give her a printed schedule of appointments for the last month of her pregnancy.
To teach self-care: The printed information I am giving you will outline these symptomatic treatments.	Provide printed instructions for her to follow at home. Encourage discussions of feelings regarding infection and its therapy.

Continued.

Guidelines For Client Teaching—cont'd

CONTENT/RATIONALE	TEACHING ACTIONS
Take warm sitz bath for 15 minutes at a time with a drying agent such as Domeboro (two packets or tablets to a shallow tub of warm water) three to five times daily. Keep the genital area dry and clean. Drying the genital area with a blow dryer after showering is useful.	Describe purpose of each measure that: Provides comfort.
Wash hands after using the toilet, and do not touch face after genital contact. Urinating through an empty toilet paper tube is helpful in preventing pain during urination.	Prevents inoculation of self and others.
Pour warm water over urethra and vulva while urinating.	
Cold milk baths or soaks with aluminum acetate (Burrow's solution 1:20).	
Avoid any sexual contact during the entire time that lesions are present. Using condoms and spermicides 6 weeks after the lesions disappear will help prevent the spread of herpes (p. 746).	
Avoid strong deodorant soaps, creams, and ointments.	Prevents recurrence and irritation of skin in the genital area.
Wear 100% cotton underwear.	
Avoid tight-fitting jeans, pants, and pantyhose with nylon inserts.	
Taking care of your physical and mental health is important. Being run-down makes you more vulnerable to infection.	
Yearly Papanicolaou smears are advisable since herpes type II may have a causal role in the development of cervical carcinoma.	Screens for tissue dysplasia (Table 30-2).
When you are pregnant, you should inform the physician that you have herpes.	Alerts physician to develop plan of care according to your condition.
Topical medications that may be ordered by your physician include: acyclovir ointment 5%, miconazole nitrate vaginal cream 2%, povidone-iodine, chlohexidine, or triple sulfonamides.	Some not tested or approved for pregnant or lactating women, but you may use at a later time.

EVALUATION Woman verbalizes understanding of instructions and follows them accordingly. Woman experiences less discomfort. Newborn shows no sign of infection

Table 30-2 ***Guidelines for Delivery of Women with Herpes genitalis***

Maternal Condition	Risk of Transmission	Mode of Delivery	Postpartum Placement: Mother	Postpartum Placement: Newborn
Virologic or cytologic studies are negative 1 week before delivery	Low	Vaginal	Private room	Nursery permissible
Cervical lesion present *or* culture is positive *and* membranes intact or ruptured less than 4 hours before	Low	Abdominal (cesarean)	Private room	Room-in with mother
Cervical lesion present or culture is positive and membranes ruptured more than 4 hours before	High (regardless of mode of delivery)	Vaginal	Private room	Room-in with mother

term birth occur. Transplacental infection is rare but the consequences are serious. Microcephaly, mental retardation, retinal dysplasia, patent ductus arteriosus, and intracranial calcification are sequelae. Following intranatal infection, signs appear in 4 to 7 days. The signs include lethargy, poor feeding, jaundice, bleeding, pneumonia, convulsions, opisthotonus, bulging fontanels, and skin and mouth lesions. Neonatal infection with disseminated disease results in 82% mortality. Survivors suffer central nervous system (CNS) or ocular sequelae and face recurrence in the first 5 years of life. According to the CDC (1986) substantial numbers of intrauterine or postpartum infections occur and cannot be prevented by cesarean delivery.

Counseling. If cervical lesions are acquired, the infection initiates a chain of events that leads to invasive carcinoma in middle age. The cervical cells are more vulnerable just after puberty when they change from columnar to squamous epithelium. This vulnerability lasts until about the age of 17 years. Frequent intercourse with numerous different male partners, without using a diaphragm or condom, exposes the cervix to multiple sperm specimens and infections with HSV or HPV. The combination of these events is thought to be carcinogenic.

Drug therapy is limited. Acyclovir (Zovirax) is the first drug approved by the Food and Drug Administration (FDA). It is most effective for primary lesions. Researchers are seeking a herpes vaccine. For symptomatic therapy, see guidelines for client teaching: genital herpes.

Infection control measures start with good handwashing by the nurse and family. Gloves should be worn when touching lesions or their secretions. Hospital and home areas occupied by the mother need routine cleaning. A family member with an oral lesion is cautioned against kissing the newborn; masks may be appropriate. The family is reassured that strict personnel policies are used. Anyone with an oral HSV lesion or skin lesion (herpetic whitlow) should not give care to a mother or infant until the lesion is dried and crusted (Blankenship, 1987).

Other infections of the vulva and vagina may appear independently or co-exist with STDs or TORCH infections (Table 30-3).

GENERAL INFECTIONS

Many infections place the woman at risk during the childbearing cycle. Following are some maternal infections the nurse may encounter.

Coxsackievirus B. This virus may cause mild illness in the *mother*. It is responsible for death, cardiovascular anomalies, myocarditis, and meningoencephalitis in the *fetus*.

Chickenpox (Varicella, a Herpes Virus Infection). *Maternal effects* vary. The infection may appear as herpes zoster (shingles). The severe disseminated epidemic type of varicella during pregnancy may be fatal for the mother (and fetus) because of necrotizing angitis (inflammation of blood and lymph vessels).

Fetal and neonatal effects are also seen. Abortion or fetal death may occur. Infected newborns may exhibit defects of skin, bone, and muscle; chorioretinitis; or hydrocephalus.

Table 30-3 *Other Infections of the Vulva and Vagina*

Clinical Situation	Clinical Symptoms and Gross Findings	Nursing Actions and Management
Vulvar dermatitis	Pain; pruritus; formication*; ulceration exudation	
Eczema	Moist dermatitis	Remove antigen or irritant
Psoriasis	Red, slightly elevated flat lesions (in body folds)	Dermatologist; topical steroid
Viral infections		
Herpes genitalis	See p. 730	See guidelines for client teaching: genital herpes
Herpes zoster (shingles)	Burning, pain along sensory nerves	Analgesic, bed rest, compresses (Burow's solution of aluminum acetate)
Warts (verruca vulgaris or plana)	On skin or mucosa	May not respond to treatment, surgery, cryotherapy
Condylomata acuminata	See p. 726	
Other infections		
Impetigo—hemolytic *Staphylococcus aureus* or streptococcus	Pruritus, formication, vesicles and bullae	Isolate; topical antibiotic
Furunculosis—staphylococcus	Perifollicular abscesses, pain	Incision and drainage (I and D); isolate; systemic antibiotics
Erysipelas—β-hemolytic streptococcus	Red, raised, confluent induration; pain, fever, burning, aching, chronic exudative sores	Isolate; systemic antibiotics; hot, wet compresses (Burow's solution of aluminum acetate)
Tuberculosis—*Mycobacterium tuberculosis*	See p. 734	Systemic antituberculosis chemotherapy with vitamin B_6 replacement

*Abnormal skin sensation

Zoster immunoglobulin (IG) may be given prophylactically to exposed gravidas.

Group B β-hemolytic Streptococcus. Group B β-hemolytic streptococcus is a type of bacteria that can cause *maternal effects* of septicemia, cellulitis (erysipelas), fever, puerperal infection, impetigo, scarlet fever, and abortion. *Fetal and neonatal effects* are also serious, including death within 2 to 12 hours of birth, blindness, deafness, spinal meningitis, mental retardation, and learning or behavior problems in survivors. Penicillin is the drug of choice.

Influenza. Influenza is caused by a virus. *Maternal effects* can be serious if complicated by pneumonia. Abortion and premature labor may result. *Fetal and neonatal effects* include death, preterm birth, and occasionally, anencephaly or meningomyelocele. If the woman is not pregnant, she may be given polyvalent influenza virus (attenuated live virus) vaccine.

Listeriosis. Listeriosis is caused by gram-positive bacterium, *Listeria monocytogenes.* This organism is harbored in the vagina or cervix by 4% of pregnant women. Listeriosis may exhibit influenza-like symptoms. It occurs most commonly in summer or fall. Other symptoms include vaginitis, urinary tract infection (UTI), and enteritis. *Fetal and neonatal effects* are serious. This infection may result in abortion. Amnionitis or placentitis is evidenced by dirty brown amniotic fluid. With neonatal infection, generalized skin rash and meningitis is seen. Pneumonia carries a 50% mortality. Meningitis, which appears most often in term males, may appear later in the neonatal period. Treatment with penicillin or erythromycin is usually successful. Unfortunately the diagnosis of listeriosis is often obscure or delayed; hence the prognosis for the fetus or newborn generally is poor.

Malaria. Malaria is caused by the protozoan, *Plasmodium falciparum. Maternal effects* include chills and fever, abortion, and premature labor. Labor may be prolonged, hazardous, fatiguing, and end in cesarean birth. There is often a recurrence during the puerperium. *Fetal and neonatal effects* occur. There is extensive involvement of the placenta. The newborn is small for gestational age (SGA) or stillborn if the maternal infection does not cause abortion. Infection occurs in 10% of newborns of infectious women. Quinine (chloroquine phosphate [Aralen]) given to the mother may be fetotoxic. In severe cases of malaria, however, use of appropriate medications may be an acceptable calculated risk.

Mumps. Parotitis (mumps) occurs rarely in gravidas. In the *mother,* this virus may cause abortion or preterm labor. *Fetal* death may result. Congenital malformation such as endocardial fibroelastosis may be associated with this viral infection in survivors. Prophylaxis for epidemic parotitis is possible with administration of hyperimmune mumps γ-globulin.

Poliomyelitis. *Maternal effects* of poliomyelitis (polio) include an increased susceptibility to the polio virus during pregnancy. If the woman suffers paralysis, labor progresses normally. There is a higher incidence of mortality however. *Fetal and neonatal effects* occur. Occurrence during the first trimester may result in abortion, possible anomalies, and intrauterine growth retardation (IUGR). Neonatal infection during the passage through the birth canal may be diagnosed after the appearance of flaccid paralysis.

Prophylaxis for polio has almost eradicated this disorder in some countries. However, it is still prevalent and potentially devastating in parts of Asia and Africa. Prophylaxis for pregnant women is possible with Salk vaccine (killed virus) but *not* with Sabin vaccine (attenuated live virus). The Salk vaccine confers an immunity of about 2 years; Sabin vaccination is followed by permanent immunization (after pregnancy).

Rubeola. Rubeola, also known as 2-week measles, is caused by a virus. Rubeola during pregnancy is uncommon because most women have had the disease and are immune to it. Should the woman acquire rubeola during pregnancy, there are *fetal and neonatal effects.* Abortion or preterm labor may occur. The newborn may be born with a rash but generally survives, usually without developmental anomalies. Prophylactic γ-globulin may prevent the disease; measles vaccination of susceptible women before (but not during) pregnancy is recommended.

Tuberculosis. Tuberculosis is caused by a gram-negative, acid-fast bacillus. Pulmonary tuberculosis does not jeopardize pregnancy, although urinary and CNS tuberculosis may. Pregnancy does not affect pulmonary tuberculosis adversely. Genital infection is rare. It may be sexually transmitted or be secondary to primary lesions in the lungs. Spontaneous abortion is experienced by 20% of infected women. Many pregnancies are ectopic, or the woman suffers impaired infertility with genital tuberculosis.

The outcome of *fetal* and *neonatal involvement* depends on the stage of tuberculosis infection of the mother. Congenital tuberculosis is rare. Maternal therapy with streptomycin may result in congenital nerve deafness.

Contraception is advocated for women with active tuberculosis; pregnancy is contraindicated until the woman has been free of the disease for 1½ to 2 years. All pregnant women should be evaluated for tuberculosis (tine test or purified protein derivative [PPD]) early in pregnancy and again later if suspicion of the disease exists. Once the infant has been born, she or he should have no intimate contact with mother or others who may have the disease until contagion is no longer a problem. Therapeutic abortion rarely is indicated; cesarean delivery is warranted only for obstetric indications.

URINARY TRACT INFECTIONS

Lower Urinary Tract Infections: Cystitis, Urethritis

Urinary tract infection (UTI) affects about 10% of pregnant women, most of these in the prenatal period. Those who have had UTIs previously are especially prone to develop them again during pregnancy. Cervicitis, vaginitis, obstruction of the flaccid ureters (particularly on the right because of pressure by the pregnant uterus against the slightly dilated flaccid ureters), vesicoureteral reflux, and the trauma of delivery predispose the pregnant women to UTI, generally from *Escherichia coli.* Asymptomatic bacteriuria occurs in about 5% to 15% of all pregnant women. If untreated, pyelonephritis during gestation will develop in approximately 30% of these women. Premature labor and delivery may be more common also.

Urine culture and sensitivity tests should be obtained

early in pregnancy, preferably at the first visit, from a clean-catch urine specimen (Chapter 8). Catheterization should be avoided if possible. If infection is diagnosed, treatment with an appropriate antibiotic drug for 2 to 3 weeks, together with forced fluids and urinary tract antispasmodic medication (e.g., belladonna derivatives) is recommended. Infections caused by the colon aerogenic organisms generally respond well to sulfisoxazole (Gantrisin) or nitrofurantoin. Treatment should be continued for 2 to 3 weeks until 2 negative cultures are obtained, and the infant should be observed for hyperbilirubinemia (Chapter 40). Retreatment of the mother may be necessary if there is a recurrence. Acute pyelonephritis may be confused with appendicitis, cholecystitis, or premature labor.

If infection persists or recurs, urologic investigation is necessary to identify contributory causes such as urinary tract obstruction, stones *(nephroureterolithiasis),* diverticulum, tuberculosis, or poor personal hygiene. Pregnancy causes dilation of the renal hilum and calyces so that small stones often are lodged, and most of these pass painfully. Whether urinary stones form more readily during pregnancy because of urinary stasis, hypercholesterolemia, or increased calciuria and vitamin D is still debated. See general nursing care plan: maternal infection and specific nursing care plan, p. 747.

General Nursing Care Plan

MATERNAL INFECTION

ASSESSMENT	NURSING DIAGNOSIS (ND)/ PLAN (P)/GOAL (G)	RATIONALE/ IMPLEMENTATION	EVALUATION
Prenatal: Assess for general malaise, fever, rashes, gland engorgement, etc. History of UTIs, vaginal infections. Assess whether the woman has any specific risk factors for infection (population, geographical). Physical assessment: 1. Fever. 2. General affect. 3. Signs and symptoms of infection. Laboratory tests: 1. Urinalysis. 2. Blood tests (Hgb, Hct, antibody titers, syphillis, AIDS, diabetes). 3. Cultures: gonorrhea, etc.	ND: Potential for injury related to infection (maternal and fetal). ND: Altered patterns of urinary elimination related to UTI. P: Monitor closely; intervene per physician's orders; provide information; and be available for discussion of concerns and questions. G: Woman will obtain prompt treatment for signs and symptoms of infection. G: Woman will follow treatment regime.	*To identify, treat, and prevent potential spread of infection, the nurse will:* Note and evaluate any complaints suggestive of infection. Note woman's infection and treatment history. Implement universal precautions to protect self and others from spread of infection. Obtain necessary lab work. Assist physician and support woman and family during tests and when test results are explained. Explain necessity of taking all antibiotic tablets as ordered. Viral infections are treated symptomatically. Suggest comfort measures which will help to relieve discomfort. All OTC preparations must be approved by a physician.	Infection is prevented or treated promptly with no or minimum sequelae to mother or infant.
Assess woman's knowledge about infection, its signs and symptoms, treatment and potential sequelae.	ND: Knowledge deficit related to infection, its treatment, and possible sequelae. ND: Altered family processes related to interruption of sexual relations. ND: Body image disturbance, situational low self-esteem, altered role performance, and per-	*To teach woman about infection, its treatment, potential sequelae, and necessary isolation precautions, the nurse will:* Review the signs and symptoms of infection. Explain general care issues: 1. Adequate hydration. 2. Rest.	Woman learns the signs and symptoms of infection. Woman learns how to treat and manage her infection. Woman learns how to prevent spread of infection to others. Woman verbalizes understanding of necessary isolation precautions taken by the health care team.

Continued.

General Nursing Care Plan—cont'd

ASSESSMENT	NURSING DIAGNOSIS (ND)/ PLAN (P)/GOAL (G)	RATIONALE/ IMPLEMENTATION	EVALUATION
	sonal identity disturbance related to contagious infection. ND: Anxiety related to spread of infection. ND: Fear related to possible fetal sequelae. P: Provide information and encourage discussion of concerns. G: Woman will learn the signs and symptoms of infection. G: Woman will learn about her infection, its treatment, and possible sequelae. G: Woman will learn how to prevent spread of infection to others. G: Woman will verbalize understanding of necessary isolation precautions taken by the health care team during care.	2. Adherence to medication regime. 4. Control temperature with fluids, cool bath, and acetaminophen (Tylenol). 5. Well balanced diet. Reinforce physician's explanation of woman's infection, its treatment, and possible sequelae (maternal and fetal). Clarify misconceptions. Help woman formulate questions for physician. Assist woman in preparation to inform partner of infection and any necessary treatment he might need to seek. Teach woman how to prevent spread of infection. Explain any isolation precautions necessary by the health care team to prevent spread of infection to others. Encourage verbalization of concerns and fears. Assist with counseling before proposed therapeutic abortion.	
Postnatal: Assess all prenatal and intrapartal data. Physical assessment: 1. Newborn—assess for symptomatology of infection (Chapter 39). 2. Mother—vital signs, general affect, malaise, rash, gland enlargement; redness, tenderness, warmth, pain over a specific area. Laboratory tests: Culture of any exudate. Blood tests for infection, Urinalysis.	ND: Potential for injury related to infection. ND: Altered patterns of urinary elimination related to UTI. P: Follow prescribed management. G: Woman and infant will receive prompt treatment for infection and will experience no or minimum sequelae.	*To treat an infected mother and newborn, the nurse will:* Obtain specimens ordered for laboratory testing. Administer medications as ordered (medications for symptomatic relief or antibiotics). Ensure adequate rest and nutrition. Provide high risk care to infant (Chapter 39).	Infection is treated promptly with no or minimum sequelae for mother and infant.
Assess knowledge regarding infection: prevention, identification, treatment.	ND: Knowledge deficit related to infection. P: Provide information as needed; provide written instructions. G: Woman will learn how her infection is identified and managed.	*To teach about infection, its treatment, and possible sequelae, the nurse will:* Review possible sequelae from infection that she or her infant might experience. Counsel regarding breastfeeding (some infections are transmitted in breast milk).	Woman learns about prevention, identification and management of infection.

General Nursing Care Plan—cont'd

ASSESSMENT	NURSING DIAGNOSIS (ND)/ PLAN (P)/GOAL (G)	RATIONALE/ IMPLEMENTATION	EVALUATION
		Encourage questions and clarify misconceptions. Teach woman the importance to adhere to the treatment regime and the need for follow-up. Assist woman and family with grieving if indicated (Chapter 28).	
Assess need for isolation precautions for mother and infant.	ND: Potential for injury related to possible spread of infection to others. ND: Alteration in parenting related to fear of spreading infection to newborn. P: Provide information, demonstrate, and observe return demonstration. G: Woman will remain in isolation to prevent potential spread of infection.	*To prevent the spread of infection, the nurse will:* Isolate mother and infant if necessary (explain isolation to the mother). Teach mother how to prevent the spread of infection to her newborn. Encourage mother-infant interaction while reinforcing isolation guidelines.	Spread of infection is prevented. Mother interacts with child while maintaining isolation protocol.

Pyelonephritis

Pyelonephritis is caused by a bacterium. Some maternal infections are asymptomatic. Acute pyelonephritis is distinguished by urinary frequency, urgency, pyuria, dysuria, chills, fever, and backache. Costovertebral angle tenderness and tenderness over the affected kidney are experienced. *Fetal and neonatal effects* are serious. Acute pyelonephritis commonly is associated with preterm labor (Danforth and Scott, 1986). The newborn is then exposed to the hazards of prematurity. Treatment with penicillin or cephalosporin and adequate hydration are warranted. Therapy with sulfonamides may cause icterus, hemolytic anemia, and kernicterus. The newborn may also be at risk as a result of IUGR. Nitrofurantoin therapy for the mother during pregnancy may lead to megaloblastic anemia or G6PD deficiency in the newborn. Acidifying the urine with high doses of ascorbic acid during pregnancy should be avoided. The fetus can become conditioned to a high vitamin C environment and develop scurvy in the neonatal period (Danforth and Scott, 1986). The women who are most vulnerable to UTI are primigravidas, women with difficult labors, and women with diabetes or sickle cell disease.

Glomerulonephritis

Acute glomerulonephritis, is a rare complication of pregnancy. It is characterized by proteinuria, hematuria, edema, and hypertension. Treatment requires antibiotic therapy, bed rest (in side-lying or semi-to high-Fowler's position to facilitate renal perfusion), and fluid-electrolyte and dietary control. Pregnancy does not seriously affect acute early glomerulonephritis.

Women with mild, inactive glomerulonephritis generally can go through pregnancy safely. Women with progressive, chronic glomerulonephritis, that is, severe renal damage associated with proteinuria, hypertension, and an elevated blood urea nitrogen (BUN) level, do not tolerate pregnancy well. If pregnancy is not interrupted, spontaneous abortion is likely; preeclampsia–eclampsia often supervenes, and fetal death may result. Cardiac or renal failure generally is the cause of maternal death.

Postpartum UTIs

Postdelivery UTIs are usually caused by coliform bacteria. UTIs are common because of trauma to the base of the bladder and urethra and catheterization during or after labor.

Suprapubic or costovertebral angle pain, fever, urinary retention, hematuria, dysuria, or urinary frequency often signifies UTI. This symptomatology indicates the need for urinalysis, urine culture, bacterial sensitivity tests, and probable wide-spectrum antibiotic therapy. Substitution of a specific antibacterial drug must await an assessment of the woman's history, response to initial therapy, and the sensitivity report.

Prompt treatment of definite UTIs is indicated. However, prophylactic therapy rarely is warranted. More cases yield to treatment within a week. Urologic consultation is indicated if symptoms persist. Prevention of recurrence of UTI is an important part of therapy. See Chapter 8 for information on teaching UTI prevention.

PUERPERAL INFECTION

Infection of the placenta and membranes may predispose the woman to puerperal infection. *Placentitis,* or infection of the placenta, may be bacterial, viral, rickettsial, or protozoal in origin. The most common agents are bacteria, which also cause the greatest changes in the placenta. Bacterial infections may result in fatal fetal and even maternal septicemia.

Chorioamnionitis may be the cause or the result of PROM. Chorioamnionitis may be followed by placentitis and fetal congenital pneumonia, omphalitis, or septicemia. These conditions often are caused by enteric streptococci, an aerogenic type of colon bacteria. Placentitis and chorioamnionitis may be followed by endometritis and parametritis. The result is serious puerperal sepsis.

Puerperal infection (Puerperal sepsis or "childbed fever") is any clinical infection of the genital canal that occurs within 28 days after abortion or delivery. Infections may result from bacteria commonly found within the vagina *(endogenous)* or from the introduction of pathogens from outside the vagina *(exogenous).* An episiotomy or lacerations of the vagina or cervix may open avenues for sepsis. Even more formidable, however, may be the large placental site. Here the denuded endometrium (decidua basalis) and residual blood after parturition make the uterus an ideal site for a wound infection. The virulence of infecting organisms, the woman's resistance to them, and the rapidity and specificity of therapy determine the efficacy of treatment. Puerperal sepsis occurs after about 6% of deliveries in the United States. Fortunately body defenses generally limit the disease in most instances. Puerperal infection probably is the major cause of maternal morbidity and mortality throughout the world.

The most common infecting organisms are the numerous streptococcal and anaerobic organisms. Fulminating epidemic puerperal sepsis classically is caused by the hemolytic streptococcus. The less virulent anaerobic streptococci may be responsible for other puerperal infections, however, *S. aureus,* gonococci, coliform bacteria, and clostridia are less common but serious pathogenic organisms causing puerperal infection.

Commonly the infection is complicated by medical disorders such as anemia, malnutrition, or diabetes mellitus. Obstetric problems, including PROM, a long, exhausting labor, instrument delivery, hemorrhage, and retention of the products of conception, increase the likelihood and severity of puerperal sepsis.

An *endometritis,* usually at the placental site, permits infection to begin. Localized infection may be followed by salpingitis, peritonitis, and pelvic abscess formation. (Tubal occlusion after salpingitis is a common cause of infertility.) Septicemia may develop. Secondary abscesses may arise in distant sites such as the lungs or liver. Pulmonary embolism or septic shock, often with disseminated intravascular coagulation (DIC), from any serious genital infection may prove fatal. Postdelivery femoral thrombophlebitis ("milk leg") may result in a swollen, painful leg.

Clinical Findings. The symptomatology of puerperal infection may be mild or fulminating. Any fever, that is, **a temperature of 38° C (100.4° F) or more on 2 successive days, not counting the first 24 hours after delivery,** must be considered caused by puerperal infection in the absence of convincing proof of another cause.

General malaise, anorexia, chills, or fever may begin as early as the second postdelivery day. Perineal discomfort or lower abdominal distress, nausea, and vomiting may soon develop. Foul or profuse lochia, hectic fever, tachycardia, ileus, pelvic pain, and tenderness characterize critical puerperal sepsis. Without improvement, bacteremic shock or death may ensue.

Laboratory Findings. Considerable **leukocytosis, a shift to the left** of the differential white blood cell (WBC) count and a markedly increased red blood cell (RBC) sedimentation rate are typical of puerperal infections. Anemia, often an accompaniment, is evidenced by reduced RBC, hemoglobin, and hematocrit values. Intracervical or intrauterine bacterial cultures (aerobic and anerobic) should reveal the offending pathogens within 36 to 48 hours.

The physician must distinguish nongenital from genital sepsis. Mastitis, respiratory and urinary tract infections, and enteritis are considered in that order of probability.

Management. The most effective and cheapest treatment of puerperal infection is prevention. Preventive measures might include good prenatal nutrition to control anemia and intranatal control of hemorrhage. Good maternal hygiene is essential. Strict adherence by all medical personnel to the best aseptic techniques during the entire hospital and delivery period is mandatory. Coitus after rupture of membranes is contraindicated. Dystocia or prolonged labor should be avoided, especially after leaking of amniotic fluid. Traumatic vaginal delivery must be avoided, blood loss replaced, and fluid-electrolyte balance maintained.

Infection measures for cure and comfort are instituted. Fluid and electrolyte balance is vital. Broad-spectrum antibiotics are administered intravenously until the infecting organism is identified. Then organism-specific antibiotic therapy is begun. The mother and infant are separated during the febrile period. Other members of the family are encouraged to nurture the newborn. The mother is positioned in high-Fowler's to facilitate gravity drainage of discharge from the uterus and vagina. Isolation protocol of the agency is warranted.

Surgical measures may be required. These incude surgical procedures such as dilation and curettage (D & C) to remove the retained products of conception, hysterectomy (if the uterus is ruptured), colpotomy to drain a pelvic abscess or ligation or clipping of the vena cava and ovarian veins to prevent septic embolism.

The virulence of the organisms, the resistance of the woman, and her likely response to treatment are the intangibles of prognosis. Prevention, supportive therapy, and prompt massive antibiotic administration have reduced the maternal mortality in the United States to less than 0.4%. Regrettably, in developing countries the death rate may be more than 10 to 20 times this figure.

TOXIC SHOCK SYNDROME

Toxic shock syndrome (TSS) is a potentially life-threatening systemic disorder that has three principal clinical manifestations: **fever of sudden onset, hypotension, and rash** (see box below). The erythematous macular desquamating rash is most prominent on palms and soles. The acute phase to TSS lasts about 4 to 5 days; the convalescent phase, about 1 to 2 weeks.

The CDC (1982) has established diagnostic criteria for TSS that include the above signs plus the following manifestations.

1. Involvement of three or more other organ systems:

System/Area	*Manifestations*
Gastrointestinal	Nausea; vomiting; diarrhea
Renal	Decreased urinary output; pyuria
Hepatic	Jaundice; abnormal values (increased transaminase)
CNS	Altered sensorium (decreased level of consciousness [LOC]); headache
Respiratory	Adult respiratory distress syndrome (ARDS)
Mucous membranes	Inflammation of vaginal oropharyngeal, and conjunctival membranes
Muscular	Myalgia; weakness
Hematologic	Thrombocytopenia; DIC
Cardiac	Ischemic changes on ECG; decreased left ventricular contractility

2. Serologic laboratory tests for Rocky Mountain spotted fever, leptospirosis, and measles are negative. Cultures positive for *S. aureus* can be obtained from blood, urine, or stool. If primary site of infection is tampon related, positive cultures are obtained from the vagina and cervix.

A toxin (pyrogenic exotoxin C [PEC] or enterotoxin F) secreted by strains of *S. aureus* is the causative factor in TSS. About 9% of women harbor the organism normally in their vaginas; about 1% to 5% of sexually active males have urethral cultures that are positive for *S. aureus* without having the disease. Poor perineal hygiene and lack of handwashing before touching the perineal area may increase risk. Commonly associated conditions that may predispose the person to TSS by providing a portal of entry into systemic circulation include the following:

1. Menstruation
2. Chronic vaginal infection (e.g., herpes)
3. Puerperal endometritis
4. Incisional or soft tissue abscess
5. Skin infection following a bee sting
6. Intravenous (IV) injection of heroin
7. Use of high-absorbency tampons or barrier contraceptives (e.g., sponge, diaphragm) (Berkley et al., 1987; Wolf et al., 1987)
8. Neonatal infection concurrent with maternal infection.

The population at greatest risk is women between the ages of 15 and 24 who use tampons during menstruation. Recently influenza B virus has been associated with TSS, an association that provides a basis for a non-tampon-related epidemic of TSS (MacDonald et al., 1987).

Pathophysiology. The toxins may suppress synthesis of IgM antibodies. Toxin-induced injury to capillary endothelium alters capillary permeability. Fluid leaks out, and the volume of venous blood returning to the heart is diminished. Impaired tissue perfusion results in tissue hypoxia and renal and CNS abnormalities. Other problems arise from the toxin's direct damage to target organs. Tissue damage releases thromboplastin, which initiates the coagulation cascade. Thrombocytopenia and coagulopathy (e.g., DIC) are potential hazardous sequelae. In some people, impaired tissue perfusion, with its sequelae, has resulted in loss of toes and fingers following gangrene.

Prognosis. Mortality is associated with TSS. In order of incidence the three causes of mortality are (1) ARDS (see Chapter 34), (2) uncontrollable hypotension, and (3) DIC.

Although most affected women have an uneventful recovery with no recurrence, some suffer adverse sequelae. Infection that does recur does so most often with the next menstrual cycle. Recurrence is most likely if the woman had not been treated with β-lactamase–resistant antibiotics. Some women have persistent abnormalities in intellectual function. Persistent problems include impaired memory, concentration, and calculation ability, abnormal electrocardiogram (ECG), and impaired cerebellar function (hyperreflexia). For a few women sequelae are more serious. Impaired renal function, neuromuscular function (vocal cord paralysis), and peripheral perfusion, especially of the hands and feet may persist after the infection is cured.

Management. Early identification of TSS is essential so that appropriate therapy can be initiated. Nurses must be on the alert for this syndrome because of the increased likelihood of its occurrence in obstetric and gynecologic settings. Nursing care for TSS is summarized in the emergency procedure on p. 740.

DANGER SIGNS

Toxic Shock Syndrome (TSS)

1. **Fever of sudden onset**—over 38.9° C (102° F)
2. **Hypotension**—systolic pressure <90 mm Hg; orthostatic dizziness; disorientation
3. **Rash**—diffuse, macular erythrodema

MASTITIS

Mastitis, or breast infection, affects about 1% of recently delivered women, most of whom are primiparas who are breast-feeding. Mastitis is almost always unilateral and develops well after the flow of milk has been established. The infecting organism generally is the hemolytic *S. aureus*. An

EMERGENCY PROCEDURE

NURSING CARE FOR TOXIC SHOCK SYNDROME (TSS)

DEFINITION

A severe, acute disease, caused by infection with strains of *Staphylococcus aureus,* that produces a unique toxin. It is seen most often in menstruating women.

PURPOSE

Early identification and prompt treatment.
Prevention of complications of TSS. Education for self-care.

EQUIPMENT

Equipment and solutions for initiating and monitoring parenteral therapy; medications, as ordered (e.g., naloxone, dopamine); materials for good oral hygiene; oxygen equipment and external oxygen source; retraints, as necessary; antishock garments, as necessary (MAST trousers).

NURSING ACTIONS	RATIONALE
Identify client and check physician's orders.	To provide the right therapy for the right person.
Wash hands before and after touching woman and equipment. Glove, prn.	To prevent nosocomial infection and to implement universal precautions.
Woman is acutely ill and will probably be accompanied to the hospital by a family member.	To reassure family members, as well as the woman.
Explain all procedures to the woman, as well as the support person. Reinforce information given to them by the physician.	
Combat hypotension and maintain blood pressure:	
A. First priority: fluid resuscitation.	A. To combat hypotension.
1. Assist with the use of central venous pressure (CVP) or pulmonary arterial wedge pressure (PAWP) balloon flotation catheter monitoring devices; assess mean arterial pressure (MAP), pulse, jugular vein pulse, and urinary output.	1. Monitor intravenous fluid infusion. PAWP gives the MAP.
2. Insert intravenous infusion line with a large bore needle; be prepared to administer fluids that may include packed red blood cells or coagulation factors, isotonic crystalloids (normal saline, lactated Ringer's solution), or colloids (plasmanate, salt-poor albumin).	2. In the event that blood or blood products must be used to treat coagulopathy: To combat hypotension. To maintain osmotic pressure.
3. Assess for signs of **fluid overload**: flushed skin, headache, increased pulse, venous distension, coughing (sign of pulmonary edema), and shortness of breath; if symptoms appear, change infusion rate to "keep open" and place the client in high Fowler's position immediately.	3. To correct the condition, **fluid overload requires immediate therapy**
4. Assess for signs of fluid deficit: thready pulse, clammy skin, increased capillary refilling time following pressure on nail beds; increase infusion rate.	4. To combat hypotension.
5. Insert a urinary retention catheter to monitor output: oliguria, equal to input, greater than input.	5. To ensure accurate assessment of output; output <20 ml/hr may indicate impending kidney shutdown.
6. If nausea and vomiting complicate therapy, a nasogastric tube and prochlorperazine (Compazine) may be ordered.	6. To prevent further disturbance of fluid and electrolyte balance.
a. Provide good mouth care.	a. To prevent stomatitis that often accompanies TSS and the irritation that occurs from the nasogastric tube.
b. Apply lidocaine (Xylocaine) or anesthetic spray.	b. To relieve oropharyngeal pain from dryness and nasogastric irritation.
c. Provide hydrogen peroxide, sips of cold water, or ice chips, or apply petrolatum salve or glycerine to lips.	c. To add to comfort by relieving dry mucosa and lip dryness.
d. Apply nystatin (Mycostatin or Nilstat) to affected mucosa; the infection may occur on any mucosa—oropharyngeal, vaginal, or conjunctival.	d. To prevent further debilitation; TSS and antibiotic therapy put the woman at great risk for fungal infections.

EMERGENCY PROCEDURE—cont'd

NURSING ACTIONS	RATIONALE
B. Use antishock garments, per hospital protocol.	B. Used by some hospitals to help raise blood pressure. Known in some institutions as MAST trousers, also used for mass hemorrage.
C. Institute vasopressor therapy, as ordered.	C. To maintain blood pressure.
1. Administer dopamine (IV) in low doses, per order.	1. Dopamine has a weak β-mimetic effect that increases myocardial contractility and heart rate without a disproportionate rise in myocardial oxygen consumption; dopamine also exerts a vasoconstrictive action on skeletal muscle.
2. Administer naloxone (Narcan), per order.	2. Naloxone is used to counter the effect of stress-induced elevated levels of endorphins that depress the cardiovascular system and lower blood pressure.
Cure infection	*To cure infection:*
A. Per order, administer β-lactamase-resistant antibiotics.	A. Effective against the staphylococcal organism only; there is no effect on the toxins already in the blood stream; most *S aureus* strains are penicillin-resistant.
B. Assist with surgical intervention (drainage of an abscess, removal of fetus in a septic pregnancy [septic abortion]).	B. To remove causative factor.
Prevent ARDS, one cause of mortality.	
A. Administer oxygen with mechanical ventilation as necessary and monitor by arterial blood gases (ABGs).	A. To meet oxygenation needs.
B. Prevent fluid overload and shock lung.	B. To decrease possibility of ARDS.
Ensure safety	*To ensure safety:*
A. Provide appropriate restraints or constant bedside observation.	A. May be necessary to prevent injury from falls, pulling out IV lines, etc.; confusion, combativeness, and restlessness characterize the acute phase of the disorder.
B. Reposition the woman frequently and encourage to cough and deep breathe as often as possible.	B. To prevent problems of immobility—thrombus, pneumonia, embolism.
Plan for discharge	*To prevent recurrence through:*
A. If woman had experienced menstruation-related TSS:	A. Avoidance of predisposing conditions.
1. Instruct on good hygiene practices (i.e., washing hands before inserting tampons and changing tampons frequently).	B. Using good hygiene.
2. Caution against the use of tampons for at least 3 months or until cultures for *S. aureus* are negative.	
3. Advise regarding the use of tampons:	
a. Use tampons only during periods of heavy flow, change at least every 1 to 4 hours.	
b. During time of moderate flow, use tampons during day, and pads at night, change every 4 to 8 hours.	
c. During period of light flow, use pads only.	
B. If the woman has never had TSS:	
1. Counsel to use tampons during the period of heavy and moderate flow and to change them according to the above schedule.	
2. During light flow, use tampons or pads during the day, pads at night.	
3. Caution all women against using high-absorbency tampons at any time.	High-absorbency tampons and the diaphragm are thought to provide a portal of entry by causing microulcerations in the vaginal mucosa. Super absorbent tampons contain more oxygen and are retained for a longer time than less absorbant tampons.

infected nipple fissure usually is the initial lesion, but the ductal system is involved next. Inflammatory edema and engorgement of the breasts soon obstruct the flow of milk in a lobe; regional, then generalized mastitis follows. If prompt resolution of the septic process does not occur, a breast abscess is virtually inevitable.

Chills, fever, malaise, and local breast tenderness are noted first. Eventual localization of sepsis and axillary adenopathy are delayed developments.

Intensive antibiotic therapy (such as cephalosporins and vancomycin, which are particularly useful in staphylococcal infections), support of breasts, local heat (or cold), and analgesics are required. Lactation is maintained (if desired) by emptying the breasts every 4 hours by manual expression or breast pump. If an abscess develops, wide incision and drainage must be effected. Most women respond to treatment, and an abscess can be prevented.

Almost all instances of acute mastitis can be avoided by proper breast-feeding technique (see Chapter 23) to prevent cracked nipples. Missed feedings, waiting too long between feedings, and abrupt weaning may lead to clogged nipples and mastitis. Cleanliness practiced by all who have contact with the newborn and new mother also reduces the incidence of mastitis.

MANAGEMENT OF VAGINAL INFECTIONS

Any irritating vaginal discharge should be evaluated promptly and appropriate treatment initiated immediately. Management of vaginal infections becomes more complicated if multiple organisms or agents are involved. Pediculosis pubis, threadworm, varicosities, and allergic response to perineal deodorants may obstruct the differential diagnosis and management. The discomfort imposed by these conditions challenge the woman's emotional, as well as her physical well-being.

Infections must be distinguished from the normal vaginal discharge, leukorrhea. **Leukorrhea** is a whitish discharge. It consists of mucus and exfoliated vaginal epithelial cells secondary to hyperplasia of the vaginal mucosa such as occurs during pregnancy, at the time of ovulation, and just before menstruation. If it is copious, it can cause discomfort from maceration.

Vaginal infections may be sexually transmitted. Trichomonal vaginitis and monilial vaginitis are considered to be sexually transmitted in most, but not all cases. Simple vaginitis may be attributed to faulty hygiene, tight clothing, or emotional stress.

Simple Vaginitis. Infectious organisms such as *E. coli*, staphylococci, and streptococci change the normal acidity of the vagina. A pH of 3.5 to 4.5 is needed to support Döderlein's bacilli, the vagina's main line of defense. The proximity of the urethra to the vagina predisposes the woman with vaginitis to a concurrent urethritis.

Burning, pruritis (itching), redness, and edema of surrounding tissues are characteristic of simple vaginitis. These symptoms are particularly discomforting during voiding and defecating.

Objectives of management of simple vaginitis are to relieve discomfort, to foster growth of Döderlein's bacilli, to eradicate offending organisms, and to prevent recurrence. Interventions may include the following:

1. Maintain scrupulous cleanliness, especially after elimination
2. Douche with a weakly acid solution such as 15 ml (1 tbsp) white vinegar to 1000 ml (1 qt) water (see client teaching: vaginal douching, Chapter 44)
3. Insert a β-lactose suppository (to enhance growth of Döderlein's bacilli)
4. Observe chemotherapy regimen specific for organisms by inserting suppository into the vagina with an applicator or applying cream locally to the area as directed

Atrophic Vaginitis. Low estrogen levels, such as those that occur during preadolescence and lactation and after menopause, result in a thin vaginal lining. Infection may occur from the normal vaginal flora. Antibiotics and hormone replacement therapy comprise this therapy.

Cervicitis. Abnormal discharge may be due to an infection of the cervix and not to vaginitis. Spotting of blood between periods or after intercourse, and cramping during intercourse are characteristic. Sexually transmitted gonorrhea, chlamydia, trichomoniasis, or herpetic infections are the usual infection implicated. Therapy is specific to the causative microbe.

Monilial Vaginitis. *Candida albicans,* a fungus (yeast) normally found in the intestinal tract, contaminates and infects the vagina. Infection with *C. albicans* is also known as moniliasis, thrush, or candidiasis. This infection is seen commonly in women with poorly controlled diabetes mellitus, since the organism thrives in a carbohydrate-rich milieu. Antibiotic or steroid therapy will reduce the number of Döderlein's bacilli and thus can cause monilial vaginitis. Döderlein's bacilli help maintain an acidic pH.

The thick vaginal discharge is irritating and pruritic. Commonly dysuria and dyspareunia are complaints. Speculum examination reveals thick, white, tenacious cheeselike patches adhering to the pale, dry, and sometimes cyanotic vaginal mucosa.

Objectives of treatment are the same as for simple vaginitis with one exception: women with recurrent infection should be checked for diabetes mellitus, and control of diabetes should be instituted if required (see Chapter 32). Guidelines for client teaching are presented below.

C. albicans also causes thrush in the newborn. Infection may occur by direct contact with an infected birth canal or from the contaminated hands of those who take care of the infant. Guidelines for client teaching are presented on p. 743.

Trichomonas Vaginitis. *Trichomonas vaginalis* (trichomoniasis) is a hearty protozoan that thrives in an alkaline milieu. In symptom-free individuals the infection may be identified during a routine examination or with a Papanicolaou smear.

The profuse, bubbly (foamy), white leukorrhea characteristic of this infection causes irritation, hyperemia, edema of the vulva, and dyspareunia (painful intercourse). Urinary frequency and dysuria may occur. In the male partner the protozoan may be harbored in the urogenital tract (without symptoms) and remain a source of reinfection for his mate.

Guidelines for client teaching are presented on p. 744.

Guidelines for Client Teaching

MONILIAL INFECTION

ASSESSMENT

1. Woman diagnosed as having monilial vaginal infection.
2. Woman in third trimester of pregnancy.

NURSING DIAGNOSIS

Knowledge deficit related to care and prevention of monilial vaginal infection.

GOALS

Short-term

Woman verbalizes understanding of measures to care for and prevent monilial vaginal infections.

Intermediate

Woman implements measures to care for present monilial infection.

Infection is cured.

Long-term

Woman does not have a recurrence of monilial vaginal infection.

REFERENCES AND TEACHING AIDS

Printed material such as pamphlets and booklets that are provided by hospitals, clinics, or drug companies.

CONTENT/RATIONALE	TEACHING ACTION
To provide content about infection: Causative agent: *Candida albicans.* Discuss predisposing and aggravating conditions: Pregnancy and oral contraceptives with increased estrogens cause higher levels of glycogen in the vaginal tissue, this supports the growth of the fungus. Diabetic women have higher tissue glucose. Systemic antibiotic use suppresses the normal flora in the vagina and changes the pH of the secretions.	Determine woman's knowledge of the infection and its causes; fill in gaps.
Discuss symptoms of the infection: moderate to severe itching; whitish, thick discharge; red and swollen vulva and perineum; painful intercourse.	Provide printed material that reinforces this information.
To discuss prescribed therapy and self-care: Maintain scrupulous cleanliness, especially after elimination. Use the prescribed medication given to you by the physician. Miconazole nitrate 2% vaginal cream is preferred during pregnancy (Pritchard, MacDonald, and Gano, 1985).	Discuss feelings about having the infection. Identify emotional stressors that may predispose her to the infection. Review physician's instructions.
Cotton underwear or pantyhose with a cotton crotch should be used. Nylon fabric retains too much heat and stops air from circulating, this supports growth of the fungus.	Discuss types of underwear and review reasons.
Abstain from intercourse or use a condom until the infection is cured.	Determine woman's knowledge of need to include sexual partner; discuss partner's willingness to comply.
To provide information about neonatal infection: Discuss how the infant can contract this infection as it comes through the birth canal during delivery. It is called **thrush** in the infant.	Point out in pamphlet.

EVALUATION Woman verbalizes understanding of the instructions given and implements plans to clear up the infection. Infection is cured and recurrence is avoided.

Guidelines for Client Teaching

TRICHOMONAL INFECTION

ASSESSMENT

1. Woman diagnosed as having trichomonal vaginal infection.
2. Woman in third trimester of pregnancy.

NURSING DIAGNOSIS

Knowledge deficit related to care and prevention of trichomonal vaginal infections.

GOALS

Short-term

Woman verbalizes understanding of measures to care for and prevent trichomonal vaginal infections.

Intermediate

Woman implements measures to care for present trichomonal vaginal infection.
Infection is cured.

Long-term

Woman does not have a recurrence of trichomonal vaginal infection.

REFERENCES AND TEACHING AIDS

Printed material such as pamphlets and booklets that are provided by hospitals, clinics, and drug companies.

CONTENT/RATIONALE	TEACHING ACTION
To provide information about the infection:	
Causative agent: *Trichomonas vaginalis.*	
Discuss the disease process:	Determine the woman's knowledge of the disease.
Trichomonal vaginal infection is caused by a protozoan flagellate. It is transmitted sexually most of the time.	Discuss feelings about having the disease.
The symptoms you will have with this infection are:	Inquire whether she has any of these symptoms and discuss them.
Yellow-green frothy or bubbly discharge that is present in copious amounts.	Provide printed material that reinforces this information.
Discharge has a strong, foul odor.	
Vagina and cervix are inflammed, edematous and reddened.	
Moderate to severe itching.	
Dysuria or dyspareunia.	
To discuss prescribed therapy and self-care:	
Metronidazole (Flagyl) is the drug of choice and can be administered orally or vaginally.	Review physician's instructions.
Maintain scrupulous cleanliness, especially after elimination. Cotton underwear or pantyhose with a cotton crotch is best.	Review hygiene and type of underwear to use.
To prevent reinfection by her partner, he should be treated at the same time. Intercourse should be avoided until infection is cured.	Determine her knowledge of need to include sexual partner; discuss partner's willingness to comply.
Relief should be noted in 1 to 2 weeks. Rarely is second course of treatment necessary.	

EVALUATION Woman verbalizes understanding of the instructions given and all goals for care are met. Infection is cured and does not recur. Newborn does not contract the infection.

BACTEREMIC SHOCK

Critical infections, particularly by bacteria that liberate endotoxin, such as enteric gram-negative bacilli, may cause bacteremic (septic) shock. Pregnant women, especially those with diabetes mellitus, or women who are receiving immunosuppressive drugs are at increased risk of having this disorder.

High spiking fever and chills are evidence of serious sepsis. Anxiety is followed by apathy. Concomitantly the temperature often falls to slightly subnormal levels. The skin then becomes pale, cool, and moist. The pulse will be rapid and thready. Marked hypotension and peripheral cyanosis develop. Oliguria occurs.

Laboratory studies reveal marked evidence of infection (blood culture may reveal bacteremia later). Hemoconcentration, acidosis, and DIC may develop. Central venous pressure (CVP) generally is low. ECG may reveal changes indicative of myocardial insufficiency. Evidence of cardiac, pulmonary, and renal failure will be notable. Hypoxia is the major problem, however. Hypoxia is especially noxious to the CNS, myocardium, and lungs.

The physician will initiate antishock theapy. Massive doses of antibiotics and corticosteroids are given intravenously if possible. The woman may be given digitalis. Heart function and urinary output are monitored closely. The infected area is drained or the focus of infection is removed (for example, by hysterectomy or abortion) if the woman's condition will permit.

Prompt diagnosis and intensive treatment afford a fairly good prognosis. Encouraging signs include increasing alertness and the establishment of good urinary flow.

ACQUIRED IMMUNE DEFICIENCY SYNDROME (AIDS)*

Transmission of human immunodeficiency virus (HIV), a retrovirus, occurs primarily through the exchange of body fluids (e.g., blood, semen, perinatal events) (Landesman et al., 1987; Hecht, 1987; Friedland and Klein, 1987). Severe depression of the cellular immune system characterizes acquired immune deficiency syndrome (AIDS) (Chapter 6). Although the populations at high risk have been well-documented, *all* women should be assessed for the possibility of having been exposed to HIV. AIDS in women is commonly reported at a later stage in the disease and they usually enter the hospital for initiation of treatment when the illness is more severe. The delay may be due in part because women may have symptoms different from those of men (Shaw, 1986). Chronic vaginitis is a common presenting problem.

Delay in diagnosis must be avoided when the woman is pregnant. Exposure to the virus has a significant impact on the woman's pregnancy and newborn feeding method and on the newborn's health status (Klug, 1986). The HIV from infected women is transmitted in three ways (Landesman et al, 1987; Friedland and Klein, 1987):

1. To the fetus as early as the first trimester through maternal circulation
2. To the infant during labor and delivery by inoculation or ingestion of maternal blood and other infected fluids
3. To the infant through breast milk

Regardless of whether AIDS is diagnosed, the nursing process is implemented in a culturally sensitive and humane manner. "HIV infection is a biologic event, not a moral comment. It is vital to remember, to model, and to teach that [personal] reactions to particular life-styles, practices, or behaviors must not influence [the nurse's] ability to provide objective, compassionate, and effective health care to all" (Keeling, 1987).

To provide a high level of care, nurses have identified a need for additional information about AIDS. Flaskerud (1987) conducted a national survey to identify these information needs (see research highlight).

Prenatal Period. The incidence of AIDS in pregnant women is expected to increase (Minkoff, 1987a). The health history, physical examination, and laboratory testing must reflect this expectation if women and their newborns are to receive appropriate care. Women who fall into the high-risk category for AIDS should be retested for HIV antibodies late in the third trimester (Minkoff, 1987a). Prenatal testing for conditions associated with AIDS may help identify the woman with AIDS (Kaplan et al, 1987; Minkoff, 1987a; Rhoads et al, 1987; Foster, 1987): gonorrhea, syphilis, prolonged and persistent episodes of herpes, *C. Trachomatis,* hepatitis B, *M. tuberculosis,* candidiasis (oropharyngeal or chronic vaginal infection), cytomegalovirus

RESEARCH HIGHLIGHT

Nurses Call Out For AIDS Information

Purpose

To determine nurses' needs for AIDS information.

Sample

A random sample of 832 nurses was obtained from the membership in community health nursing, medical-surgical nursing, and psychiatric-mental health nursing lists of the National Association of School Nurses. The responding nurses represented 48 states and the District of Columbia.

Methodology

From August 1986 through March 1987 a national survey of these 832 nurses was conducted.

Findings

Of the respondents, 51% considered it likely that they would see a person with AIDS in their work settings during the next 6 months. In addition 75% or more of the respondents indicated needing information in 56% of the categories identified in the survey instrument. The most frequent areas cited were: AIDS symptoms assessment, transmission in the workplace, precautions for health care workers, psychosocial care, and legal and ethical issues. Respondents' informational needs were significantly related to whether they thought they would see a person with AIDS in the next 6 months. The nurses who were surveyed indicated that they were providing education, counseling, and referral help to their fellow workers, as well as to persons with whom they came in contact with their employment settings. The groups who were receiving the least information were prostitutes and their families, police officers, and firefighters.

Implications

Findings from this survey suggest that if nurses are to have an impact in stemming the AIDS epidemic, they will have to focus much of their practice on prevention. The nurses in this survey expressed a need for more knowledge and practice in sexual history taking and counseling and in drug-abuse history taking and counseling.

Flaskerund, JH: Nurses call out for AIDS information, Nurs Health Care 8(10):557, 1987.

*The term "AIDS" is obsolete. "HIV infection" more correctly defines the problem.

(CMV), and toxoplasmosis. About half of AIDS sufferers have elevated CMV titers. Because CMV inclusion disease poses a serious hazard to the fetus (Table 30-3), pregnant women are advised to avoid direct contact with AIDS sufferers.

History of vaccinations and immune status is documented. The titers for chickenpox and rubella are determined, and tuberculosis skin testing (PPD) is done. Previous vaccination with Recombivas HB vaccine (Merck) is noted. (This vaccine is now free of association with human blood or blood products.)

The woman may be a candidate for receiving *$Rh_O D$ immune globulin.* Transmission of HIV has not been traced to the Rh vaccine. The preparation process involves ethyl alcohol, which inactivates the virus. The vaccine is made from blood drawn from an identified group of regular donors. New blood tests that can detect evidence of HIV are used on blood used to produce the vaccine (MMWR, 1987; Francis and Chin, 1987).

Some prenatal discomforts (e.g., fatigue, anorexia, and weight loss) mimic signs and symptoms of HIV infection. Differential diagnosis of *all* "pregnancy-induced" complaints and symptomatology of infections is warranted.

To support any pregnant woman's immune system, appropriate counseling is provided for optimum nutrition; sleep, rest, exercise; and stress reduction. If AIDS is diagnosed, the woman is advised of the possible consequences for her infant. The woman is supported in her decision. Should she choose to continue the pregnancy, she is counseled regarding "safe sex" techniques. Use of condoms and nonoxynol 9 spermicide is encouraged to minimize further exposure to HIV if her partner(s) is the source. Orogenital sex is discouraged. As necessary, the woman is referred for drug rehabilitation to discontinue substance abuse. Abuse of alcohol, amphetamines (speed, crank), marijuana, nitrites (poppers, amyl), or other drugs compromises the body's immune system and increases the risk for AIDS and associated conditions:

1. HIV may require the presence of an already damaged immune system before it can cause disease
2. Alcohol and drugs interfere with many medical and alternative therapies for AIDS
3. Alcohol and drugs affect the judgment of the user, who may become more prone to engage in activities that put people at high risk for AIDS or increase exposure to HIV
4. Alcohol and drug abuse causes stress, including sleep problems, which harms immune system functioning

If the woman wishes to have additional information, she can be referred to any one of many booklets and pamphlets, such as *What Everyone Should Know About AIDS,* Channing L. Bete Co., Inc., South Deerfield, MA 01373. Hotline numbers are available in many communities. Where necessary, universal precautions are taken when working with any client.

Intrapartum Period. Care of the parturient is not substantially altered by asymptomatic infection with HIV (Minkoff, 1987a). The mode of delivery is based on obstetric considerations. The mode of delivery is not an issue because the virus crosses the placenta early in pregnancy.

The primary focus is the prevention of nosocomial spread of HIV and the protection of care providers. The risk of transmission of HIV is considered to be low during vaginal delivery despite the exposure to the infected woman's blood, amniotic fluid, and vaginal secretions. (See precautions for invasive procedures, p. 749.)

External electronic fetal monitoring (EFM) is preferred if EFM is needed. There is a possibility of inoculation of the virus into the newborn if fetal scalp blood sampling is done or if a fetal scalp electrode is applied. In addition, the one who performs either of these procedures, is put at risk by accidental sticks to the finger.

Postpartum Period. Little is known of the clinical course of the postpartum period for the woman infected with HIV. While the immediate postpartum period has not been noted to be remarkable (Update, 1986), longer follow-up has revealed a high frequency of clinical illness in mothers whose children develop disease (Minkoff et al., 1987b,c; Scott, 1985).

The newborn can be with the mother, but breast-feeding is contraindicated (see Chapter 39). Universal precautions are implemented for mother and newborn, as they are with all clients. The woman and her infant are referred to physicians who are experienced in the treatment of AIDS and associated conditions. See specific nursing care plan, p. 747.

INFECTION CONTROL

Infection control measures are essential to protect care providers and prevent nosocomial infection of clients, regardless of the infectious agent. The risk of occupational transmission varies with the disease. Even if that risk is low, as it is with HIV, that any risk exists is significant to warrant *reasonable* precautions.

Precautions against airborne disease transmission are available in all health care agencies. *Universal precautions* from the CDC follow.

Universal Precautions

Since medical history and examination cannot reliably identify all people infected with HIV or other blood-borne pathogens, blood and body-fluid precautions should be consistently used for **all** people. This approach, previously recommended by CDC and referred to as "universal blood and body-fluid precautions" or "universal precautions," should be used in the care of **all** people, especially including those in emergency-care settings in which the risk of blood exposure is increased and the infection status of the person is usually unknown.

1. All health care workers should routinely use appropriate **barrier precautions** to prevent skin and mucous-membrane exposure when contact with blood or other body fluids of any person is anticipated. *Gloves* should be worn for touching blood and body fluids, mucous membranes, or non-intact skin of all persons, for handling items or surfaces soiled with blood or body fluids, and for performing venipuncture and other vascular access procedures. *Gloves should be changed after contact with each patient. Masks and protective eyewear or face shields*

Specific Nursing Care Plan

POSTPARTUM WOMAN WITH HEPATITIS B, POSSIBLY AIDS, AND A UTI

Ann is a 26-year-old, single female who is admitted to the postpartum unit after delivering a 2464 g (5½ lb) boy with Apgar scores of 7^1, 8^5 via an uncomplicated spontaneous vaginal delivery. Ann admits to a history of IV drug abuse and was hospitalized at 20 weeks gestation for Hepatitis B. On that admission, Ann stated that she had been using dirty needles for her drug habit. Ann denies the use of any drugs since her last hospitalization and is currently active in a drug rehabilitation program.

During Ann's initial interview to the labor floor, she complained of having recent night sweats, as well as frequency and urgency of urination. HIV—pending; Urine culture—pending; Urinalysis—specific gravity 1.015; pH 8.0; glucose—negative; protein—negative; blood—large; ketone—negative; WBC—many; bacteria—many.

ASSESSMENT	NURSING DIAGNOSIS (ND)/ PLAN (P)/GOAL (G)	RATIONALE/ IMPLEMENTATION	EVALUATION
Former IV drug abuser (or present?) Hepatitis B at 20 weeks gestation. Night sweats. Assess knowledge of isolation precautions.	ND: Potential for injury related to spread of infection. ND: Knowledge deficit related to isolation guidelines. ND: Situational low self-esteem related to isolation precautions and infection. P: Provide information and be available for discussion of concerns. P: Implement universal precautions and precautions for invasive procedures. G: Ann will be treated without spread of infection to others. G: Ann will verbalize understanding of isolation precautions.	*To isolate for potential spread of Hepatitis B or possible AIDS, the nurse will:* Use gown and gloves when in contact with body/blood fluid. Bathe woman immediately unless unstable. Stress hand washing. Prevent needle/sharps injury. For blood spills, use sodium hydrochloride solution (household bleach). Mother may visit child in special care nursery. Mother may not breast-feed at this time as a result of suspected AIDS. Explain the isolation precautions implemented and answer any questions or concerns the woman might have. Blood and specimens should be double bagged or sealed in an impervious container labeled "blood/body fluids precautions." Equipment and linens soiled with body fluid should be discarded or double bagged and labeled before being sent for decontamination. Immunologically-compromised staff should not care for Ann. Provide education and support for family and staff.	Spread of infection is prevented. Ann verbalizes understanding of isolation procedures and their purpose. Ann demonstrates understanding and acceptance of isolation. Ann learns appropriate methods for feeding and caring for her infant. Ann demonstrates no loss of self-esteem or self-worth. Family supports Ann.

Continued.

Specific Nursing Care Plan—cont'd

ASSESSMENT	NURSING DIAGNOSIS (ND)/ PLAN (P)/GOAL (G)	RATIONALE/ IMPLEMENTATION	EVALUATION
Complains of frequency and urgency during urination. Urine culture pending. Urinalysis: alkaline and concentrated, hematuria, WBC—many; bacteria—many. Access knowledge about identification and treatment of a UTI. Assess knowledge about prevention of UTI.	ND: Potential for injury related to UTI. ND: Altered patterns of urinary elimination related to UTI. ND: Knowledge deficit related to identification and treatment of a UTI. P: Provide information and be available to discuss concerns. G: Ann's urinary tract infection will be treated promptly. G: Ann will adhere to treatment regime.	*To treat Ann's UTI, the nurse will:* Encourage fluids (especially cranberry juice), if she is not being treated with sulfa-based medications. Administer medications as ordered and evaluate results. Evaluate for systemic symptoms (malaise, fever, etc.). Note and report flank pain to physician. Explain importance of taking all prescribed medications. Encourage Ann to seek follow-up care if frequency and urgency persist of reoccur post discharge. Teach preventive measures (see guidelines for client teaching, Chapter 8).	Ann's UTI is treated promptly and she does not experience any potential sequelae. Ann resumes normal pattern of urinary elimination. Ann verbalizes understanding of importance on following treatment regime for a UTI. Ann does not experience recurrence of UTI.
History of acute Hepatitis B 5 months ago. Night sweats. History of IV drug abuse. Assess Ann's knowledge of Hepatitis B and AIDS	ND: Potential for injury related to infection. ND: Knowledge deficit related to infection. ND: Potential anxiety or fear related to infection. P: Provide information and be available to discuss concerns. P: Collaborate with other caregivers to develop a support system to foster her sense of self-esteem. G: Ann will not experience any signs or symptoms of acute hepatitis. G: Ann will be tested for HIV-antibodies and evaluated for other clinical signs. G: Ann will be followed up for her infections.	*To monitor for acute Hepatitis B, and AIDS, the nurse will:* Monitor Ann for signs and symptoms of acute hepatitis. Monitor Ann for other signs and symptoms of AIDS besides night sweats. Note history of recurrent infections. Obtain specimens for lab tests as ordered. Note any wounds that do not seem to heal.	Ann does not experience an acute episode of Hepatitis B. Ann receives report on HIV antibody test and is referred for follow-up care, if positive. Ann learns about her infections, treatment, or possible sequelae.
Assess Ann's understanding and acceptance of her infections and needed therapy.	ND: Spiritual distress related to infections. P: Allow time for discussion.	*To support Ann in her acceptance and understanding of her infections, the nurse will:* Teach Ann about her infections, their course, identification, treatment or possible sequelae.	Ann retains or develops a sense of self-esteem and self-worth.

Specific Nursing Care Plan—cont'd

ASSESSMENT	NURSING DIAGNOSIS (ND)/ PLAN (P)/GOALS (G)	RATIONALE/ IMPLEMENTATION	EVALUATION
	P: Refer to community resources, e.g., clergy, support groups. G: Ann will come to terms with her condition.	Evaluate lab data and support Ann during physicians' report of findings. Answer questions Ann has regarding her diagnosis, condition of her infant, or any concerns or feelings she wishes to express. Refer to follow-up care agency if seropositive for HIV.	At subsequent visits in clinic or home Ann continues to demonstrate: Use of appropriate precautions for control of and prevention of spread of infection. Self-esteem and self-worth.

should be worn during procedures that are likely to generate droplets of blood or other body fluids to prevent exposure of mucous membranes of the mouth, nose, and eyes. *Gowns or aprons* should be worn during procedures that are likely to generate splashes of blood or other body fluids.

2. Hands and other skin surfaces should be **washed** immediately and thoroughly if contaminated with blood or other body fluids. Hands should be washed immediately after gloves are removed.

3. All health care workers should take precautions to **prevent injuries** caused by needles, scalpels, and other sharp instruments or devices during procedures; when cleaning used instruments; during disposal of used needles; and when handling sharp instruments after procedures. *To prevent needlestick injuries,* needles should not be recapped, purposely bent or broken by hand, removed from disposable syringes, or otherwise manipulated by hand. After they are used, disposable syringes and needles, scalpel blades, and other sharp items should be placed in puncture-resistant containers for disposal; the puncture-resistent containers should be located as close as practical to the use area. Large-bore reusable needles should be placed in a puncture-resistant container for transport to the reprocessing area.

4. Although saliva has not been implicated in HIV transmission, to minimize the need for **emergency mouth-to-mouth resuscitation**, mouthpieces, resuscitation bags, or other ventilation devices should be available for use in areas in which the need for resuscitation is predictable.

5. **Health care workers** who have exudative lesions or weeping dermatitis should refrain from all direct client care and from handling client care equipment until the condition resolves.

6. **Pregnant health care workers** are not known to be at greater risk of contracting HIV infection than health care workers who are not pregnant; however, if a health care worker develops HIV infection during pregnancy, the infant is at risk of infection resulting from perinatal transmission. Because of this risk, pregnant health care workers should be especially familiar with and strictly adhere to precautions to minimize the risk of HIV transmission.

Precautions for Invasive Procedures. An invasive procedure is defined as surgical entry into tissues, cavities, or organs or repair of major traumatic injuries (1) in an operating or delivery room, emergency department, or out-of-hospital setting; including both physicians' and dentists' offices; and (2) a vaginal or cesarean delivery or other invasive obstetric procedure during which bleeding may occur. The universal blood and body-fluid precautions listed above, combined with the precautions listed below, should be the minimum precautions for **all** such invasive procedures.

1. All health care workers who participate in invasive procedures must routinely use appropriate barrier precautions to prevent skin and mucous-membrane contact with blood and other body fluids of all clients. Gloves and surgical masks must be worn for all invasive procedures. Protective eyewear or face shields should be worn for procedures that commonly result in the generation of droplets, splashing of blood or other body fluids, or the generation of bone chips. Gowns or aprons made of materials that provide an effective barrier should be worn during invasive procedures that are likely to result in the splashing of blood or other body fluids. *All health care workers who perform or assist in vaginal or cesarean deliveries should wear gloves and gowns when handling the placenta or the infant until blood and amniotic fluid have been removed from the infant's skin and should wear gloves during post-delivery care of the umbilical cord.*

2. If a glove is torn or a needlestick or other injury occurs, the glove should be removed and a new glove used as promptly as client safety permits; the needle or instrument involved in the incident should also be removed from the sterile field.

According to staff members in the AIDS unit at San Francisco General Hospital (Am Nurse, 1986), treatment precautions by health care providers are the same as those for the care of people with hepatitis B (Table 30-2). These precautions for health care providers and the nonpregnant people who come in contact with AIDS sufferers support those described above. In addition the following is appropriate: wash washable surfaces and used equipment with a solution of sodium hypochlorite (household bleach) and water—1 cup of household bleach to 9 cups of water. Remove blood or other fluids before disinfection to avoid neutralizing the bleach solution.

SUMMARY

Infections are potentially hazardous to the woman any time, to the mother and fetus during pregnancy, and to the health care provider. The knowledgeable nurse can help the woman prevent or treat infections successfully. Overall therapeutic measures include educating the general public regarding immunization for nonimmune people. Many states are introducing or passing laws requiring screening for rubella and chickenpox titers. Tests for exposure to syphilis are routine; populations at risk require assessment for chlamydial infection or for AIDS antibodies. Easily accessible and person-oriented (nonjudgmental) clinics should be available to all, so that people are encouraged to use them for diagnosis and treatment.

Health care providers must assume all clients are infectious. The same procedures that protect against exposure to HIV also protect against transmission of other infectious organisms, including hepatitis B.

KEY CONCEPTS

- Pregnancy confers no immunity against infection and both mother and fetus must be considered when the pregnant woman contracts an infection.
- HIV is transmitted through blood, semen, and perinatal events.
- HSV interacts with epithelial or neuroepithelial cells and neurons; after an infection, the HSV migrates to one or more ganglia where it remains latent and dormant until reactivated by one or more stressors.
- *C. trachomatis* is the most common sexually transmitted bacterial pathogen in the United States and is reponsible for substantial morbidity, personal suffering, and heavy economic burden.
- Young sexually active females and males who have multiple sex partners and do not practice safe sex are at greatest risk for STDs.
- TSS is a potentially life-threatening systemic disorder that has three principal clinical manifestations: fever of sudden onset, hypotension, and rash; the first priority of therapy is fluid resuscitation.
- Abuse of alcohol and drugs compromises the body's immune system and increases the risk for AIDS and associated conditions.
- During the intrapartum period, a primary focus of care is the prevention of nosocomial spread of infection and the protection of care providers.
- Since medical history and examination cannot reliably identify all people with HIV or other blood-borne pathogens, blood and body-fluid precautions should be consistently used for all people.
- STDs and genital and perigenital infections are biologic events, for which people have a right to expect objective, compassionate, and effective health care.

STUDY QUESTIONS AND ACTIVITIES

1. Review infection control measures at community agencies used for clinical experience. Observe personnel application of those measures. Compare and contrast observed behaviors with infection control measures.
2. Discuss personal reactions to working with clients who have infections. Role play an interaction with a pregnant woman whose HIV antibody test is positive (seropositive).
3. Divide a group of students into four groups. Each group take one STD or TORCH infection, develop a complete nursing care plan for a 22-year-old who is 10 weeks pregnant. (Woman is married.) When finished, compare and contrast the nursing care plans, noting the similarities and differences.
4. Discuss a general nursing care plan for a young mother who has been diagnosed with AIDS. She is being discharged home with her baby. You are to make a home visit and teach her and the family members about her care and infection control.
5. While reading the text, jot down questions that need further research in the area of nursing care when the client has an infection.

References

Bennett, EC: Sexually transmitted diseases: current approaches, NAACOG Newsletter 14(8):1, 1987

Berkley, SF, et al: The relationship of tampon characteristics to menstrual toxic shock syndrome, JAMA 258(7):908, 1987

Berry, CD, et al: Neurologic relapse after benzathine penicillin therapy for secondary syphilis in a patient with HIV infection, N Engl J Med 316:1587, 1987

Blankenship, R: Herpes in pregnancy, Periscope Newsletter of Calif Perinat Assn p4, Summer 1987

Bourcier, KM, and Seidler, AJ: Chlamydia and condylomata acuminata: an update for the nurse practitioner, JOGN Nurs 16(1):17, 1987

Byrne, JC, et al: Human papillomavirus-11 DNA in a patient with chronic laryngotracheobronchial papillomatosis and metastasis squamous-cell carcinoma of the lung, N Engl J Med 317(14):873, 1987

Centers for Disease Control: Toxic shock syndrome, Center for Prevention Services, CDC, Atlanta, Ga, 1982

Centers for Disease Control; *Chlamydia trachomatis* infections, policy guidelines for prevention and control, Washington, DC, 1985, US Government Printing Office

Centers for Disease Control: Hepatitis B virus and vaccine, Hepatitis Branch, Center for Prevention Services, CDC, Atlanta, Ga, 1986

Centers for Disease Control: Recommendations for prevention of HIV transmission in health-care settings, MMWR Suppl 36(2S): Aug 21, 1987

Corbett, M, and Meyer, JH: The adolescent and pregnancy, Boston, 1987, Blackwell Scientific Publications, Inc

Danforth, DN, and Scott, JR, editors: Obstetrics and gynecology, ed 5, Philadelphia, 1986, JB Lippincott Co
Ferenczy, A: Treating genital condyloma during pregnancy with the carbon dioxide laser, Am J Obstet Gynecol 148:9, 1984
Ferenczy, A, moderator: Symposium: treating condylomata, Contemp OB/GYN 30(3):158, 1987
Flaskerud, JH: Nurses call out for AIDS information, Nurs Health Care, 8(10):557, 1987
Foster, SD: Education, the best defense against AIDS: MCN focus on patient teaching, MCN 12(5):311, 1987
Francis, DP, and Chin J: The prevention of acquired immunodeficiency syndrome in the United States, JAMA 257(10):1357, 1987
Friedland, GH, and Klein, RS: Transmission of the human immunodeficiency virus, 317(18):1125, 1987
Guinan, ME: Treatment of primary and secondary syphilis: defining failure of three- and six- month follow-up, JAMA 257:359, 1987
Hecht, F: Counseling the HIV-positive woman regarding pregnancy, JAMA 257(24):3361, 1987
Howett, MK, and Rapp, F: Basic biology of papillomaviruses, Contemp OB/GYN 28(5):110, 1986
Huffman, DG, and Blanco, JD: Multiple genital papillomatosis: an indication for cesarean section? JAMA 258(22):3309, 1987
Jenson, AB, et al: Papillomaviruses: HPV immunology appears promising, Contemp OB/GYN 28(6):59, 1986
Johns, DR, Tierney, M, and Felsenstein, D: Alteration in the natural history of neurosyphilis by concurrent infection with the human immunodeficiency virus, N Engl J Med 316:1569, 1987
Kaplan, LD, et al: Treatment of patients with acquired immunodeficiency syndrome and associated manifestations, JAMA 257(10):1367, 1987
Keeling, RP: AIDS education: a mandate for schools of nursing, Dean's Notes, 9(2):1, 1987
Klug, RM: AIDS beyond the hospital: children with AIDS, Am J Nurs 86(10):1126, 1986
Kreider, JW: Papillomaviruses: what experimental models of viral infection tell us, Contemp OB/GYN 29(1):105, 1987
Landesman, S, et al: Serosurvey of human immunodeficiency virus infection in parturients, JAMA 258(19):2701, 1987
Larson, E: Intransigent genital infection? suspect chlamydiae, RN 47:42, 1984
Loucks, A: Chlamydia: an unheralded epidemic, Am J Nurs 86(7):920, 1986
MacDonald, KL, et al: Toxic shock syndrome: a newly recognized complication of influenza and influenza like illness, JAMA 257(8):1053, 1987
March of Dimes: Public health education information sheet: herpes simplex, Oct 1987
Marvin, C, and Slevin, A: Chlamydia—cause, prevention, and cure, MCN 12(5):318, 1987
Minkoff, HL: Pregnant women with HIV, JAMA 258(19):2714, 1987a
Minkoff, HL, et al: Pregnancies resulting in infants with acquired immunodeficiency syndrome: description of the antepartum, intrapartum, and postpartum course, Obstet Gynecol 69:285, 1987b
Minkoff, HL, et al: Follow-up of mothers of children with AIDS, Obstet Gynecol 87:288, 1987c
MMWR: Penicillinase-producing *Neisseria gonorrhoeae*—United States, 1986, JAMA 257(12):1579, 1987
Nerurkar, L, et al: Survival of herpes simplex virus in water specimens collected from hot tubs in spa facilities and on plastic surfaces, JAMA 250:3081, 1983
Perlman, D: Antibiotic found to protect unborn from a common VD, San Francisco Chronicle, Feb. 1, 1986.
Petit, C: Stanford researchers find flaw in herpes test, San Francisco Chronicle, p 24, Jan 29, 1987
Rhoads, JL, et al: Chronic vaginal candidiasis in women with human immunodeficiency virus infection, JAMA 257(22):3105, 1987
Schachter, J, et al: Erythromycin in the routine treatment of chlamydial infections in pregnancy, N Engl J Med 314:276, Jan 30, 1986
Scott, GB, et al: Mothers of infants with the acquired immunodeficiency syndrome: evidence for both symptomatic and asymptomatic carriers, JAMA 253:363, 1985
Shaw, NS: Serving your patients in the age of AIDS, Contemp OB/GYN 28(4):141, 1986
Tramont, EC: Syphilis in the AIDS era, N Engl J Med 316(25):1600, 1987
Update: human immunodeficiency virus infection in health care workers exposed to blood of infected patients, MMWR 36:285, 1987
Washington, AE, Browner, WS, and Korenbrot, CC: Cost-effectiveness of combined treatment for endocervical gonorrhea considering co-infection with *Chlamydia trachomatis,* JAMA 257(15):2056, 1987a
Washington, MD, Johnson, RE, and Sanders, LL: *Chlamydia trachomatis* infections in the United States, JAMA 257(15):2070, 1987b
Wolf, PH, et al: Toxic shock syndrome, JAMA 258(7):908, 1987

Bibliography

Abrams, DI: AIDS: clinical update, part 1, Calif Nurs Rev 53:4, Oct 1986
Abrams, DI: AIDS: battling a retroviral enemy, Calif Nurs Rev 8(6):10, 1986
Abrams, D: AIDS: in search of hope, Calif Nurs Rev 9(1):4, 1987
AIDS virus can invade cells directly, report says, San Francisco Chronicle, p A26, Feb 5, 1988
The American National Red Cross: The American Red Cross AIDS prevention program for youth, Washington DC, 1987, The Association
Anderson, D: AIDS: an update on what we know now, RN p 49, March 1986
Baker, J, et al: Unsuspected human immunodeficiency virus in critically ill emergency patients, JAMA 257(19):2609, 1987
Becker, L, and Lagomarsino, W: Isolation guidelines for perinatal patients: creating a new protocol, MCN 12(6):400, 1987
Bennett, J: Aids: what precautions do you take in the hospital? Am J Nurs 86(8):952, 1986
Bennett, J: Nurses talk about the challenge of AIDS, Am J Nurs 87(9):1150, 1987
Berman, SM, et al: Low birth weight, prematurity, and postpartum endometritis: association with prenatal cervical *Mycoplasma hominis* and *Chlamydia trachomatis* infections, JAMA 257(9):1189, 1987
Birdsall, C, and Ruggio, J: Clinical savvy: mouth-to-mouth resuscitation—is there a safe, effective alternative? Am J Nurs 87(8):1019, 1987
Boucher, M, et al: Adult respiratory distress syndrome: a rare manifestation of *Listeria monocytogenes* infection in pregnancy, Am J Obstet Gynecol 149(6):686, 1984
Brown, ZA: Effects on infants of a first episode of genital herpes during pregnancy, N Engl J Med 317(20):1246, 1987

Burnhill, MS: Treating persistent and recurrent vulvovaginitis, Contemp OB/GYN 31(3):71, 1988
Buying guide: tampons, University of California Berkeley Wellness Letter 3(1):3, 1986
California Nurses Association (CNA): Infection control precautions, Correspondence, Sept 1987, The Association
Centers for Disease Control: Safety of therapeutic immune globulin preparations with respect to transmission of human T-lymphotropic (sic) virus type III/lymphadenopathy-associated virus infection, MMWR 35:231, 1986
Centers for Disease Control: CDC reports caution obstetric personnel, patients about AIDS virus, NAACOG Newsletter 13(6):1, 1986
Cleary, PD, et al: Compulsory premarital screening for the human immunodeficiency virus, JAMA 258(13):1757, 1987
Coleman, DA: How to care for an AIDS patient, RN p 16, July 1986
Conti, MT, and Eutropius, L: Preventing UTIs: what works? Am J Nurs 87(3):307, 1987
DeBrow, ME: Safer sex, NSNA/IMPRINT ISSUES, p 33, Feb/Mar, 1988
Dhundale, K, and Hubbard, PM: Home care for the AIDS patient: safety first, Nurs '86, 16(9):34, 1986
Douching: Am Fam Physician 35:376, March 1987
Douglas, RG: Infectious disease, JAMA 258(16):2252, 1987
Droegemueller, W, et al: Comprehensive gynecology, St Louis, 1987, The CV Mosby Co
Editorial: Toxic shock syndrome: back to the future, JAMA 257(8):1094, 1987
Editorial: Control of sexually transmitted Chlamydial infections, JAMA 257(15):2073, 1987
Editorial: Human immunodeficiency virus infection in women, JAMA 257(15):2074, 1987
Editorial: Syphilis in the AIDS era, N Engl J Med 316(25):1600, 1987
Emmons, J, and Courter, P: Toward control of chlamydial infections, Nurs Pract 10:15, Nov 1985
Ferenczy, A, Silverstain, S, and Crum, CP: Papillomaviruses: importance of latency in HPV infections, Contemp OB/GYN 30(5):71, 1987
Fischl, MA, et al: Evaluation of heterosexual partners, children, and household contacts of adults with AIDS, JAMA 257(5):640, 1987
Fogel, CI, et al: Gonorrhea in women: a serious health problem, *Health Care Women Int* 8(1):75, 1987
Forster, GE, et al: Papanicolaou smears in diagnosis of endocervical chlamydial infection, Am J Obstet Gynecol 156(1):257, 1987
Friedman-Kien, AE, et al: Natural interferon alfa for treatment of condylomata acuminata, JAMA 259(4):533, 1988
Friedrick, EG: Vaginis: Candida, Gardnerella, Trichomonas, Am J Obstet Gynecol 152(3):247, 1985
Gerberding, JL, et al: Risk of transmitting the human immunodeficiency virus, cytomegalovirus, and hepatitis B virus to health care workers exposed to patients with AIDS and AIDS-related conditions, J Infect Dis 156:1, 1987
Gershon, A: Chickenpox: how dangerous is it? Contemp OB/GYN 31(3):41, 1988
Gillespie, L: When cystitis is suspected, what's the next step? NAACOG Newsletter 14(10):1, 1987
Gilstrap, LC, and Cox, SM: An aggressive approach to UTI, Contemp OB/GYN 30(5):23, 1987
Goldsmith, MF: Some advice on using condoms against STDs: what every man (and woman) should know, JAMA 257(17):2266, 1987
Gravett, MG, et al: Independent associations of bacterial vaginosis and *Chlamydia trachomatis* with adverse pregnancy outcome, JAMA 256:1899, 1986
Greene, WH, and Gerberding, JL: Infection-control policies and AIDS, N Engl J Med, 316(23):1479, 1987
Gross, TP, and Rosenberg, ML: Shelters for battered women and their children: an underrecognized source of communicable disease transmission, Am J Public Health 77(9):1198, 1987
Guidelines for control of perinatally transmitted Human T-Lymphotropic Virus-Type III/Lymphadenopathy-Associated virus infection and care of infected mothers, infants, and children, San Francisco Epidemiologic Bulletin (Suppl) 2(1): April 1986
Guinan, ME, and Hardy, A: Epidemiology of AIDS in women in the United States: 1981 through 1986, JAMA 257:2039, 1987
Haggerty, L: TORCH: a literature review and implications for practice, JOGN Nurs 14:124, Mar/Apr 1985
Hodges, LC, and Poteet, GW: The tragedy of AIDS: a new trial for nursing education, Nurs Health Care 8(10):656, 1987
Hoff, R, et al: Seroprevalence of human immunodeficiency virus among childbearing women: estimation by testing samples of blood from newborn, Engl J Med 318(9):526, 1988
Horowitz, BJ, Edelstein, SW, and Lippman, L: Sexual transmission of candida, Obstet Gynecol 69(6):883, 1987
Jackson MM, et al: Clinical savvy: Why not treat all body substances as infectious? Am J Nurs 87(9):1137, 1987
Johnson, JR: Heterosexual transmission of acquired immunodeficiency syndrome, JAMA 257(17):2288, 1987
Karnes, N: Don't let ARDS catch you off guard, Nurs '87, 17(5):34, 1987
Kaunitz, AM, et al: Prenatal care and HIV screening, JAMA 258(19):2693, 1987
Kennedy, M: AIDS: coping with the fear, Nurs '87, 17(4):44, 1987
King, J: Vaginitis, JOGN Nurs 13:41s, 1984
Koff, RS: Hepatitis in pregnancy (editorial), N Engl J Med 314(24):1581, 1986
Koop, CE: Physician leadership in preventing AIDS, JAMA 258(15):2111, 1987
Krieger, LM: Battling AIDS: a report from the front lines, San Francisco Examiner Image, p 12, May 31, 1987
Larson, E: Chlamydia: the most prevalent cause of sexually transmitted disease, *Health Care Women Int* 8(1):19, 1987
Leads from the MMWR. Progress toward achieving the national 1990 objectives for sexually transmitted diseases. *JAMA* 257(April 24):2141, 1987
Leishman, K: Heterosexuals and AIDS: the second stage of the epidemic, The Atlantic Monthly p 39, Feb 1987
Lewis, HE: Acquired immunodeficiency syndrome: state legislative activity, JAMA 258(17):2410, 1987
Lewis, HR, and Lewis, ME: What you and your patients need to know about safer sex, RN 53, Sept 1987
Lobel, HO: Use of prophylaxis for malaria by American travelers to Africa and Haiti, JAMA 257(19):2626, 1987
Loveman, A, Colburn V, and Dobin, A: AIDS in pregnancy, JOGN Nurs 15(2):91, 1986
Marion, RW, et al: Human T cell lymphotrophic virus type III (HTLV-III) embryopathy: a new dysmorphia syndrome, Am J Dis Child 140:638, 1986
Markowitz, L, et al: Toxic shock syndrome, JAMA 278(1):75, 1987
Martin, PW, et al: Importance of confirmation tests after strongly positive HTLV-III screening tests, N Engl J Med 314(24):1577, 1986

Matthews, GW, and Neslund, VS: The initial impact of AIDS on Public Health Law in the United States—1986, JAMA 257(3):344, 1987

Medical news and perspectives: sex in the age of AIDS calls for common sense and 'condom sense,' JAMA 257(17):2261, 1987

Mendez, H, et al: Human immunodeficiency virus (HIV) infection in pregnant women and their offspring (abstract) Pediatr Res 21:1466A, 1987

Miles, PA: Sexually transmitted diseases, JOGN Nurs 13:102s, 1984

Mitchell, C, and Smith, L: Dilemmas in practice: if it's AIDS, please don't tell, Am J Nurs 87(7):911, 1987

Morbidity and Mortality Weekly Report (MMWR): Lack of transmission of human immunodeficiency virus through Rh_o (D) immune globulin (human), MMWR 36(44): 1987 (reported in JAMA 258[22]:3225, 1987)

NEA Higher Education Advocate: The facts about AIDS: a special NEA Higher Education Advocate report, 4(13):Aug 1987

Nelson, W: Clinical management of AIDS patients, CNA Calif Nurse 82(4):10, 1986 (special issue)

Nurses Association of the American College of Obstetricians and Gynecologists: Toxoplasmosis during pregnancy threatens fetal health, NAACOG Newsletter 11:1, 1984

Nze, R: Supporting the mother and infant at risk for A.I.D.S., Nurs '87 17(11):44, 1987

Osborne, NG, and Pratson L: Sexually transmitted diseases and pregnancy, JOGN Nurs 13:9, 1984

Ouimette, J: Perinatal nursing: care of the high-risk mother and infant, Boston, 1986, Jones & Barlett Publishers, Inc

Papillomavirus raises risk of cervical Ca, Contemp OB/GYN 27(6):168, 1986

Pass, RF, et al: Young children as a probable source of maternal and congenital cytomegalovirus infection, N Engl J Med 316(22):1366, 1987

Petit, C: Most common VD: chlamydia fight gets new hope, San Francisco Chronicle, Sept 7, 1987

Plantemoli, LV: When the patient has a Foley, RN 47(3):42, 1984

Population Reports: AIDS—a public health crisis, Issues in World Health Series L(6):L-193, July/Aug 1986

Potter, PA, and Perry, AG: Fundamentals of nursing, ed 2, St Louis, 1989, The CV Mosby Co

Prevention of human immune deficiency virus infection and acquired immune deficiency syndrome, Washington, DC, 1987, American College of Obstetricians and Gynecologists

Prober, CG: Low risk of herpes simplex virus infections in neonates exposed to the virus at the time of vaginal delivery to mothers with recurrent genital herpes simplex virus infections, N Engl J Med 316:240, 1987

Pyun, KH, et al: Perinatal infection with human immunodeficiency virus: specific antibody responses by the neonate, N Engl J Med 317(10):611, 1987

Quilan, MW: UTI: helping your patients control it once and for all, RN 47(3):39. 1984

Quinn, TC, et al: Serologic and immunlogic studies in patients with AIDS in North America and Africa: the potential role of infectious agents as cofactors in human immunodeficiency, virus infection, JAMA 257(19):2617, 1987

Raymond, CA: Evidence mounts that other infections may trigger AIDS virus replication, JAMA 257(21):2875, 1987

Reckling, JB, and Neuberger, GB: Understanding immune system dysfunction. Nurs '87 17(9):34, 1987

Reid, R, et al: Sexually transmitted papillomaviral infections, Am J Obstet Gynecol 156(1):204, 1987

Remis, RS: When may a couple stop using condoms? JAMA 257(17):2289, 1987

Ritter, SE, and Vermund, SH: Congenital toxoplasmosis. JOGN Nurs 14:435, Nov/Dec 1985

Romanowski, B, and Harris, JR: Sexually transmitted diseases, Clinical Symposa 36:1, 1984

Ruge, CA: Catheter-related UTIs: what's the best way to prevent them? Nurs '87, 17(12):50, 1987

Schmid, GP, et al: Chancroid in the United States: reestablishment of an old disease, JAMA 258(22):3265, 1987

Schwalb, RB, and Stiles, B: Preventing infection during pregnancy—and after (UTI), RN 47(3):44, 1984

Shah, KV, et al: HPV infection: understanding respiratory papillomas, Contemp OB/GYN 29(4):65, 1987

Shaw, FE, and Maynard, JE: Hepatitis B: still a concern for you and your patients, Contemp OB/GYN 27:27, March 1986 (special issue)

Sommers, GM, and Kao, MS: Pharmacology: chemotherapeutic agents used during pregnancy, Contemp OB/GYN 30(3):45, 1987

Soper, DE, Kemmer, CT, and Conover WB: Abbreviated antibiotic therapy for the treatment of postpartum endometritis, Obstet Gynecol 69(1):127, 1987

Stango, S, and Whitley, RJ: Current concepts: herpesvirus infections of pregnancy. II Herpes simplex virus and varicella-zoster virus infections, N Engl J Med 313:1327, Nov 21, 1985

Sumner, SM: Action stat! Septic shock, Nurs '87, 17(2):33, 1987

Sweet, RL: International symposium on vulvovaginal mycoses: importance of differential diagnosis in acute vaginitis, Am J Obstet Gynecol 152(7):921, 1985

Sweet, R, et al: Chlamydia trachomatis infection and pregnancy outcome, Am J Obstet Gynecol 156(4):824, 1987

Symposium: Establishing bacterial vaginosis, Contemp OB/GYN 27:186, Feb 1986

Taketa, M: Fear of AIDS sweeping Asia—new laws aimed at foreigners, San Francisco Chronicle, p 42, April 7, 1987

Tierney, JD, and Felsenstein, D: Alteration in the natural history of neurosyphilis by concurrent infection with the human immunodeficiency virus, N Engl J Med 316:1569, June 1987

Torrington, J: Pelvic inflammatory disease, JOGN Nurs 14:21s, Nov/Dec 1985

Ungvarski, P: Demystifying AIDS: educating nurses for care, Nursing and Health Care 8(10):571, 1987

USPHS AIDS information hotline: 800/342-AIDS

Wells, MA, et al: Inactivation and partition of human T-cell lymphotrophic virus, type III, during ethanol fractionation of plasma, Transfusion 26:210, 1986

Wetzel, AM, and Kirz, DS: Routine hepatitis screening in adolescent pregnancies: is it cost effective? Am J Obstet Gynecol 156(1):166, 1987

Whettam, J: Update on toxic shock: how to spot it and treat it, RN 47(2):55, 1984

Winkler, B: Controlling chlamydial infections, Contemp OB/GYN 30(5):30, 1987

Witter, FR: Pharmocology: TB regimens during pregnancy, Contemp OB/GYN 23:101, 1984

Wolsy, C: Human immunodeficiency virus infection in women, JAMA 257(15):2074, 1987

Yarchoan, R, and Broder, S: Development of antiretroviral therapy for the acquired immunodeficiency syndrome and related disorders, Special Report 316(9):557, 1987

Zuck, TF, et al: More on partitioning and inactivation of AIDS virus in immune globulin preparations, N Engl J Med 314(22):1454, 1986

CHAPTER

31

Maternal Hemorrhagic Disorders

Charlotte Kain

Learning Objectives

Correctly define the key terms listed.

Review causes, signs and symptoms, possible complications, management and care for hemorrhagic disorders during pregnancy.

Formulate nursing diagnoses for hemorrhagic disorders during pregnancy, identify data bases and develop a nursing care plan.

Compare and contrast abruptio placentae and placenta previa.

Discuss clotting disorders in pregnancy with emphasis on disseminated intravascular dissemination (DIC).

Review postdelivery hemorrhage causes, signs and symptoms, possible complications, and management and care.

Describe hemorrhagic shock and its management; discuss hazards of therapy for each disorder.

Summarize the role of the nurse in the health care team approach to the treatment of bleeding disorders.

Key Terms

abortion
abruptio placentae
central venous pressure (CVP)
cerclage
Couvelaire uterus
Cullen's sign
dehiscence
disseminated intravascular coagulation (DIC)
double set-up
ectopic pregnancy
embolism
fluid overload
hematoma
hemorrhagic shock
hydatidiform mole
idiopathic thrombocytopenic purpura (ITP)
incompetent cervix
inversion of uterus
level of consciousness (LOC)
oxygen toxicity
placenta accreta
placenta previa
retained placenta
Sheehan's syndrome
shock lung
subinvolution
trophoblastic disease
uterine atony
velamentous cord insertion
von Willebrand's disease

Hemorrhagic disorders in pregnancy are medical emergencies. They require expert teamwork on the part of physician and nurse to minimize the deleterious effects.

The nurse must be alert to the symptoms of hemorrhage and shock and be prepared to obtain necessary blood replacement and complete laboratory orders. The pregnant woman and her family need much supportive care during this time of stress. Support includes prompt attention to needs, competent technical care, and information regarding the rationale for care and the progress of treatment. The woman's inability to carry a pregnancy to term or to maintain a normal sequence of development to delivery often causes her to question her femininity and capabilities as a woman.

Early in pregnancy, abortion or ectopic pregnancy is the most common cause of excessive bleeding. Later, premature separation of the normally implanted placenta or placenta previa may be the cause of hemorrhage.

Postdelivery hemorrhage is a possibility during any childbirth experience. Specific problems that result in hemorrhage are uterine atony, lacerations of the birth canal, hematomas, episiotomy dehiscence, retained placenta, inversion of the uterus, and subinvolution of the uterus. Postdelivery anterior pituitary necrosis (Sheehan's syndrome) secondary to hypovolemic shock is also discussed.

A general nursing care plan for hemorrhagic disorders of pregnancy is included in this chapter, p. 777; as is a specific nursing care plan, p. 771.

EARLY PREGNANCY

Spontaneous Abortion

Abortion is the termination of pregnancy before viability of the fetus. The abortion may be spontaneous, resulting from natural causes, or the pregnancy may be interrupted deliberately for medical reasons (therapeutic abortion) or for social reasons (elective abortion) (see Chapter 42).

Viability is reached at about 24 weeks' gestation, when the fetus weighs 600 g (1lb 5oz) or more. With today's technology for newborn care, such an infant has at least a chance to survive. An **early spontaneous abortion**, or miscarriage, is one that occurs before 16 weeks' gestation; a **late abortion** is one occurring between 16 and 24 weeks' gestation. About three fourths of these abortions occur before the sixteenth week of pregnancy, and the majority of these take place before the eighth week. More than half of all spontaneous abortions are caused by fetoplacental developmental defects. Most of the other spontaneous abortions result from maternal causes; the reasons for the remainder are speculative. Many early pregnancies are lost for unknown reasons before the diagnosis of pregnancy is even made. The diagnosis of the type of abortion a woman is experiencing is based on the signs and symptoms present (Table 31-1 and Fig. 31-1).

Recurrent (habitual) spontaneous **abortion** is the loss of three or more previable pregnancies.

The causes of repeated early abortion may include (1) endocrine imbalance (e.g., hypothyroidism, diabetes mellitus, deficient endogenous progesterone), (2) infections (e.g., syphilis, bacteriuria, and *Chlamydia trachomatis*), (3) systemic disorders (e.g., lupus erythematosus), (4) psychologic factors (but proof is lacking), (5) genetic factors (about 60% of early abortions display an abnormal chromosomal makeup), and (6) cocaine use, which recently has been linked to spontaneous abortion and premature labor (Cocaine, 1987). An increase in maternal blood pressure and a reduction in uterine blood flow may be etiologic factors (Woods, Plessinger, and Clark, 1987; Cole, 1987). (See chapter 42 for management of infertility.)

Anomalies of the reproductive tract cause second- or third-trimester pregnancy loss. Little can be done to avoid

Table 31-1 *Assessing Abortion*

Type of Abortion	Amount of Bleeding	Uterine Cramping	Passage of Tissue	Tissue in Vagina	Internal Cervical Os	Size of Uterus
Threatened	Slight	Mild	No	No	Closed	Agrees with length of pregnancy
Inevitable	Moderate	Moderate	No	No	Open	Agrees with length of pregnancy
Incomplete	Heavy	Severe	Yes	Possible	Open with tissue in cervix	Smaller than expected for length of pregnancy
Complete	Slight	Mild	Yes	Possible	Closed	Smaller than expected for length of pregnancy
Septic	Varies; usually malodorous; fever present	Varies; fever present	Varies; fever present	Varies; fever present	Usually open; fever present	Any of the above with tenderness
Missed	Slight	No	No	No	Closed	Smaller than expected for length of pregnancy

From Gordon, RT: Emergencies in obstetrics and gynecology. In Warner, CG, editor: Emergency care: assessment and intervention, ed 3, St Louis, 1983, The CV Mosby Co.

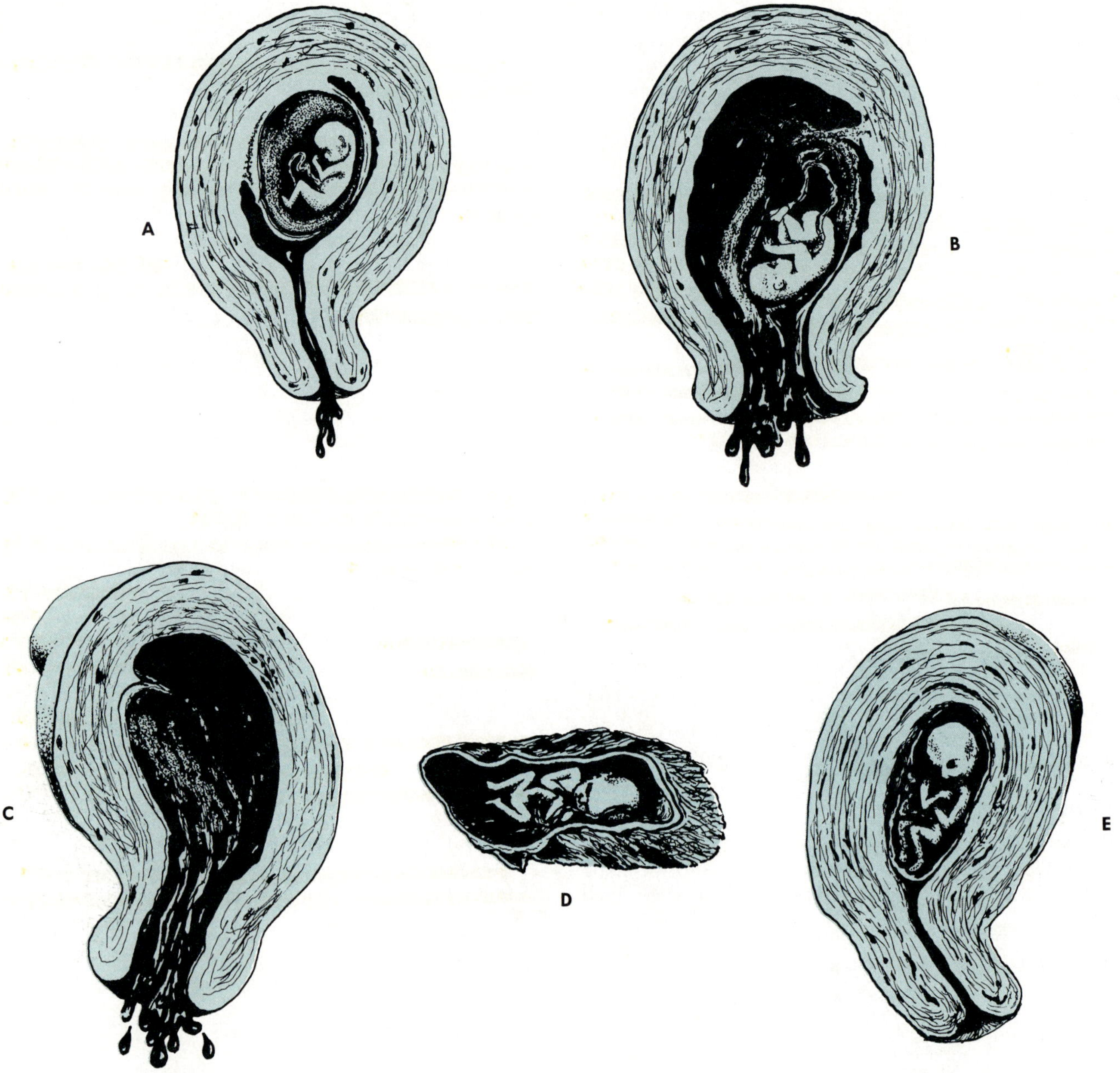

Fig. 31-1 Spontaneous abortion. **A**, Threatened. **B**, Inevitable. **C**, Incomplete. **D**, Complete. **E**, Missed.

genetic causes of pregnancy loss, but prepregnancy correction of maternal disorders, immunization against infectious diseases, proper early prenatal care, and treatment of pregnancy complications will do much to prevent abortion.

Complications of abortion include the following:

1. *Uterine lithopedion, or "womb stone."* A missed abortion is retained for months or years, during which time the products of conception have calcified (see Fig. 31-1).

2. *Hemorrhage or sepsis.* Hemorrhage and sepsis (e.g., salpingitis, peritonitis) occur especially in induced abortion under septic conditions and in instances of neglected care. Death may follow instrumentation and perforation of the soft, slightly enlarged uterus, or septicemia or septic emboli may follow spontaneous incomplete abortion. Even mild infection may be followed by tubal occlusion and infertility.

Signs and symptoms depend on the characteristic of the implantation site, which in turn depends on the duration of pregnancy. Three stages of the development of the implantation site are recognized.

1. *Early, or decidual, stage.* Until the sixth week of pregnancy the conceptus, which is virtually surrounded by decidua, is poorly attached to the uterus. The symptoms are not severe, and bleeding and cramping are minimal.

Table 31-2 *Types of Spontaneous Abortion and Usual Management*

Type of Abortion	Management
Threatened	Bed rest, sedation, and avoidance of stress and orgasm are recommended. Further treatment will depend on client's course.
Inevitable and incomplete	Prompt termination of pregnancy is accomplished usually by dilation and curettage (D & C).*
Complete	No further intervention may be needed if uterine contractions are adequate to prevent hemorrhage and if there is no infection.
Septic	Immediate termination of pregnancy by method appropriate to duration of pregnancy (see Table 42-14). Cervical cultures and sensitivity (C & S) studies are done and broad-spectrum antibiotic therapy (e.g., ampicillin) is started. Treatment for septic shock is initiated if necessary.
Missed	If spontaneous evacuation of the uterus does not occur within 1 month, however, pregnancy is terminated by method appropriate to duration of pregnancy (see Table 42-14). Blood clotting factors are monitored until uterus is empty. Disseminated intravascular coagulation (DIC) and incoagulability of blood with uncontrolled hemorrhage may develop in cases of fetal death after twelfth week if products of conception are retained for longer than 5 weeks (see pp. 766 to 769 for discussion of DIC).

*For a discussion of dilation and curettage, see Chapter 42.

2. *Intermediate, or attachment, stage.* From the sixth to twelfth week of pregnancy the anchor villi in the chorion frondosum (area of the basal plate) become moderately well attached to the myometrium. Moderate discomfort and blood loss are expected because of the larger conceptus and adherence of portions of the placenta.

3. *Late, or placental, stage.* The placenta is fully formed after the twelfth week and is firmly attached to the uterus. Abortion is typified by severe pain, similar to that of labor, because the fetus must be expelled. Bleeding is less than that of women with an intermediate-stage abortion because the placenta does not separate completely until after the fetus has been delivered. At this point uterine contractions generally are strong, checking any brisk bleeding.

Commonly the pregnancy will have been terminated for about a week before signs or symptoms of abortion become definite. For this reason it may be difficult to date the actual termination of pregnancy.

The following **laboratory findings** are characteristic of abortion. A negative or weakly positive *urine* pregnancy test is characteristic of abortion. With considerable or persistent blood loss, *anemia* is likely (hemoglobin level less than 10.5 g/dl). *Sepsis* may develop with incomplete or missed abortion. Temperature is greater than 38° C (100.4° F), and *white blood cell count* (WBC) is greater than 12,000/μl. An increased sedimentation rate is the rule with pregnancy, anemia, or infection. Therefore sedimentation rate is not helpful for differential diagnostic purposes. *Endocrine studies* show that human chorionic gonadotropin (HCG), estrogen, and progesterone titers are minimal or absent in established abortions.

Differential diagnosis may be difficult. Abortion may be an obvious conclusion in pregnant women who are bleeding and in pain. In complicated cases or in those without accurate menstrual background information, however, the diagnosis may be obscure.

Ectopic pregnancy classically involves amenorrhea or menstrual changes, unilateral pelvic pain, uterine bleeding, and a sensitive adnexal mass. Decidua but no placental villi may be found on curettage.

In *membranous dysmenorrhea* the woman suffers pain, uterine bleeding, and the passage of tissue, but none of the usual symptoms of pregnancy can be identified. Moreover, the uterine scraping will contain secretory endometrium but no pregnancy decidua or chorionic villi.

Management (Table 31-2) depends on the classification of spontaneous abortion (see Fig. 31-1). Therefore an early accurate diagnosis of spontaneous abortion is vital.

General preoperative and postoperative care is appropriate for the woman requiring surgical intervention for spontaneous abortion. Before the procedure a full history and a general and pelvic examination should be performed. Laboratory tests include a complete blood count (CBC), blood typing for group and Rh factor and cross matching, and urinalysis. Chest x-ray films and electrocardiogram evaluation are obtained if necessary. Blood, fluid, and electrolyte imbalances are corrected as soon as possible.

Analgesics, or anesthesia appropriate to the procedure, or both are used. Intravenous (IV) administration of oxytocin, 1 ml (10 U) in 500 ml of infusate may be needed to induce abortion. After evacuation of the uterus, 10 to 20 U in 1000 ml of infusate may be given to prevent hemorrhage.

Ergot products such as ergonovine, which contract the uterus and cervix, are contraindicated until the uterus is emptied to avoid retention of fragments of tissue. Retained fragments of fetal or placental tissue predispose to uterine relaxation and puerperal infection. Three or four doses of ergonovine, 0.2 mg orally or intramuscularly every 4 hours, should be given if the woman is normotensive. Antibiotics are given as necessary. Transfusion may be required for shock or anemia. If the woman is Rh negative and has not developed isoimmunization, she is given an intramuscular injection of $Rh_o(D)$ immune globulin within 72 hours of the abortion.

Incompetent Cervix*

Cervical incompetence is a condition characterized by painless dilation of the cervical os without labor or contractions of the uterus. Miscarriage or premature delivery may result. Etiologic factors include a prior traumatic delivery or forceful dilation and curettage (D and C) of the cervix. Other instances may result from a congenitally short cervix or anomalous uterus.

Correction of the weakened cervix is possible by wedge trachelorrhaphy (removal of a wedge from the anterior segment of the cervix with closure) in the nonpregnant woman. During gestation, a cerclage, band of homologous fascia, or nonabsorbable ribbon (Mersilene) may be placed around the cervix beneath the mucosa to constrict the internal os of the cervix (Fig. 31-2). Successful continuation of the pregnancy to viability or beyond occurs in the great majority of women, provided the membranes remain intact and that the cervix is not more than 3 cm dilated or more than 50% effaced at the time of correction.

A general nursing care plan for the woman and family experiencing hemorrhagic disorders of pregnancy is on p. 777.

Ectopic Pregnancy

Ectopic pregnancy is one in which the fetus is implanted outside the uterine cavity (Fig. 31-3). Fully 90% of ectopic pregnancies occur in the fallopian tube, most of these on the right side, for undetermined reasons. Approximately 1 of every 200 pregnancies are ectopic, and at least three fourths of these become symptomatic and are diagnosed during the first trimester. Ectopic pregnancy is a significant cause of maternal morbidity and mortality even in developed countries.

Most extrauterine pregnancies result from abnormalities that impede or prevent the transit of the fertilized ovum through the fallopian tube (e.g., peritubal adhesions following pelvic inflammatory disease). On occasion, an ovum is fertilized within the ovary or soon after ovulation.

Ectopic pregnancy is classified according to the site of implantation (e.g., tubal, ovarian). The uterus is the only organ capable of containing and sustaining a term pregnancy. However, the rare abdominal pregnancy, with delivery by laparotomy, may result in a living infant.

There are no **signs or symptoms** diagnostic of early ectopic pregnancy. A missed period, adnexal fullness, and tenderness may suggest an unruptured tubal pregnancy. In contrast, the following triad is associated with *early* ruptured extrauterine pregnancy in almost 50% of cases:

1. Amenorrhea or an abnormal menstrual period followed by slight uterine bleeding
2. Adnexal or cul-de-sac mass
3. Unilateral pelvic pain over the mass

Additional findings of *acute* rupture may include shock, referred shoulder pain, or evidence of acute blood loss in chronic ruptured tubal pregnancy.

Hysterosalpingography is contraindicated in suspected tubal pregnancy because it may initiate tubal rupture or hemorrhage. In possible advanced abdominal pregnancy, a sonogram showing a fetus high out of the pelvis, often in abnormal presentation, may be diagnostic.

In *chronic* ruptured tubal pregnancy, which represents slightly more than half the total of ectopic pregnancies, internal bleeding usually has been slow and the symptoms atypical or inconclusive. In addition to slight, dark vaginal bleeding, a sense of pelvic pressure or fullness, lower abdominal tenderness, flatulence, and a tense, sensitive, semicystic, perhaps crepitant, cul-de-sac mass may be felt. Slight fever, leukocytosis, and a falling hematocrit or hemoglobin level may be noted. An ecchymotic blueness of the umbilicus (Cullen's sign), which is indicative of hematoperitoneum, may develop in a neglected ruptured intraabdominal ectopic pregnancy.

The following procedures are useful in the **diagnosis** of ectopic pregnancy: a careful *history* with identification of a late last menstrual period (LMP) or an actual missed period followed by slight vaginal bleeding may be indicative; a

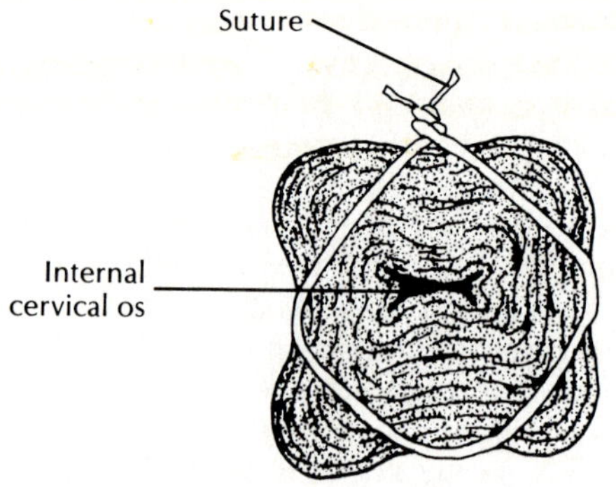

Fig. 31-2 Correction of incompetent cervical os: McDonald operation. Cross-section view of closed internal os.

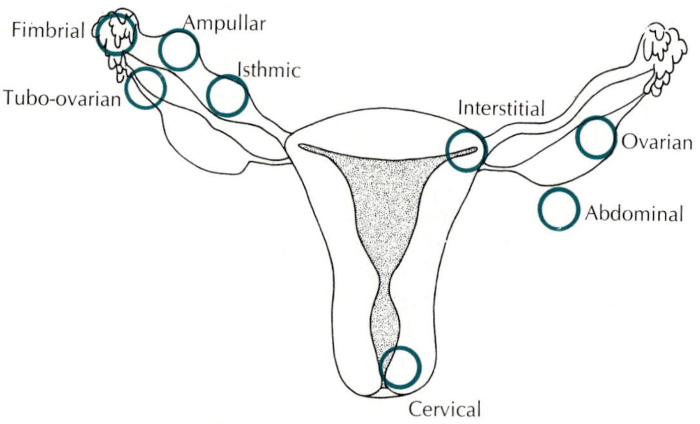

Fig. 31-3 Sites of implantation of ectopic pregnancies. Order of frequency of occurrence is ampulla, isthmus, interstitium, fimbria, tubo-ovarian ligament, ovary, abdominal cavity, and cervix (external os).

*The word "incompetent" is unfortunate. It connotes that the person with an "incompetent" os is deficient, and this can lead to a loss in self-esteem. A better designation may be "premature dilation of the cervix."

thorough *pelvic examination,* under anesthesia if necessary, reveals an adnexal or cul-de-sac mass; *culdocentesis* may yield free blood that will not clot or is already clotted; *culdotomy* may release gross clotted blood, perhaps including the aborted products of an extrauterine pregnancy; *laparoscopy* may disclose an extrauterine pregnancy; *D and C* will produce pregnancy endometrium, without chorionic villi in ectopic pregnancy (however, a uterine pregnancy or perhaps a threatened or incomplete abortion may be encountered); *laparotomy* will reveal the correct diagnosis and provide the best opportunity for treatment. The addition of *ultrasound* as an aid in the management of a woman with an ectopic pregnancy has allowed improved accuracy in the preoperative diagnosis and has reduced the number of unnecessary laparoscopies being performed. An appropriately timed ultrasound examination for the at-risk woman allows earlier diagnosis and a resultant reduction in the mortality and morbidity resulting from this condition (de Crespigny, 1987).

The **differential diagnosis** of ectopic pregnancy involves a consideration of numerous disorders that share many, perhaps all, of the same signs and symptoms. The physician must consider uterine abortion, ruptured corpus luteum cyst, appendicitis, salpingitis, ovarian cysts, torsion of the ovary, and urinary tract infection (Table 31-3).

Prevention of ectopic pregnancy per se is impossible. Early vigorous treatment of gonorrhea should prevent salpingitis or limit tubal disease. Prolonged bleeding or fever after supposedly complete abortion should be treated by D and C and antibiotic therapy to reduce the likelihood of postabortal salpingitis.

The major **management** problem in ectopic pregnancy

Table 31-3 *Differential Diagnosis of Ectopic Pregnancy*

	Ectopic Pregnancy	Appendicitis	Salpingitis	Ruptured Corpus Luteum Cyst	Uterine Abortion
Pain	Unilateral cramps and tenderness before rupture	Epigastric, periumbilical, then right lower quadrant pain; tenderness localizing at McBurney's point; rebound tenderness	Usually in both lower quadrants with or without rebound	Unilateral, becoming general with progressive bleeding	Midline cramps
Nausea and vomiting	Occasionally before, frequently after rupture	Usual; precedes shift of pain to right lower quadrant	Infrequent	Rare	Almost never
Menstruation	Some aberration; missed period, spotting	Unrelated to menses	Hypermenorrhea or metrorrhagia or both	Period delayed, then bleeding, often with pain	Amenorrhea, then spotting, then brisk bleeding
Temperature and pulse	37.2°-37.8° C (99°-100° F); pulse variable; normal before, rapid after rupture	37.2°-37.8° C (99°-100° F); pulse rapid: 99-100	37.2°-40° C (99°-104° F); pulse elevated in proportion to fever	Not over 37.2° C (99° F); pulse normal unless blood loss marked, then rapid	To 37.2° C (99° F) if spontaneous; to 40° C (104° F) if induced (infected)
Pelvic examination	Unilateral tenderness, especially on movement of cervix; crepitant mass on one side or in cul-de-sac	No masses; rectal tenderness high on right side	Bilateral tenderness on movement of cervix; masses only when pyosalpinx or hydrosalpinx present	Tenderness over affected ovary; no masses	Cervix slightly patulous; uterus slightly enlarged, irregularly softened; tender with infection
Laboratory findings	WBC to 15,000/μl; RBC strikingly low if blood loss large; sedimentation rate slightly elevated	WBC: 10,000-18,000/μl (rarely normal); RBC normal; sedimentation rate slightly elevated	WBC: 15,000-30,000/μl; RBC normal; sedimentation rate markedly elevated	WBC normal to 10,000/μl; RBC normal; sedimentation rate normal	WBC: 15,000/μl if spontaneous; to 30,000/μl if induced (infection); RBC normal; sedimentation rate slightly to moderately elevated

Reproduced, with permission, from Benson, RC, editor: Current obstetric and gynecologic diagnosis and treatment, ed 5, copyright 1984 by Lange Medical Publications, Los Altos, Calif.

is hemorrhage; bleeding must be quickly and effectively controlled. The physician must consider blood loss and impending shock. Blood transfusions must be available. Laparotomy may be done immediately after the diagnosis of ectopic pregnancy is made. Blood and clots are evacuated, and bleeding vessels are controlled. Excision of the cornua and fallopian tube is recommended if the tube is grossly involved. The ovary is conserved if possible. Hysterectomy usually is necessary for ruptured cornual or interstitial pregnancy.

Microsurgical techniques permit linear incision of the tube. Salpingostomy and evacuation of a small tubal pregnancy may be feasible in rare instances (Diamond and DeCherney, 1987).

Ovarian pregnancy always requires loss of the ovary, and of the tube if the latter is densely adherent. Concurrent prophylactic appendectomy or other elective procedures are permissible only if the woman's general condition is good, the procedure is not difficult, and the woman has given informed consent.

Advanced **ectopic abdominal pregnancy** requires laparotomy as soon as the woman is fit for surgery (Fig. 31-4). If the placenta of a second- or third-trimester abdominal pregnancy is attached to a vital organ, such as the liver, no attempt at separation and removal should be made. The cord should be cut flush with the placenta and the afterbirth left in situ. Degeneration and absorption of the placenta usually occur without complications.

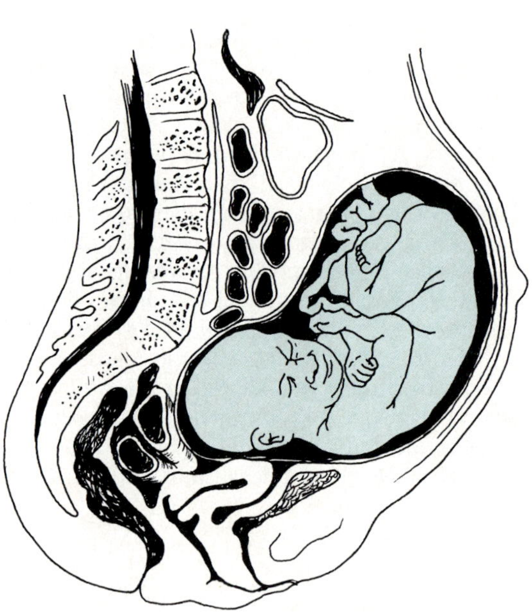

Fig. 31-4 Ectopic pregnancy, abdominal.

Prognosis varies. Maternal death from ectopic pregnancy is about 1 in 800 in North America. Maternal morbidity and secondary surgery are high, however, principally because of inaccurate or delayed diagnosis of ectopic pregnancy. The perinatal mortality in ectopic pregnancy is virtually 100%. Ectopic pregnancy recurs in approximately 10% of women, but more than 50% of women who have had an ectopic pregnancy achieve at least one normal pregnancy thereafter.

A general nursing care plan for women experiencing hemorrhagic disorders of pregnancy is on p. 777.

Hydatidiform Mole

Gestational trophoblastic neoplasms are divided into three groups: hydatidiform mole (H. mole), invasive mole (chorioadenoma destruens), and choriocarcinoma. The latter two are discussed in Chapter 44. There are two distinct types of H. moles: **complete mole**, or classic mole, and **partial mole**, which may or may not be part of the accepted continuum of trophoblastic disease (DePetrillo, 1987; Szulman, 1984).

The complete mole results from fertilization of an egg whose nucleus has been lost or inactivated (Fig. 31-5, *A*). The nucleus of a sperm (23X) duplicates, resulting in the diploid number, 46XX. The mole resembles a bunch of white grapes (Fig. 31-5, *B*). The hydropic (fluid-filled) vesicles grow rapidly, causing the uterus to be larger than expected for duration of pregnancy. Usually, the mole contains no fetus, no placenta, and no amniotic membranes or fluid. Maternal blood has no placenta to receive it. Therefore hemorrhage into the uterine cavity results, and vaginal bleeding is seen. In about 90% of the 46XX diploid H. moles, a progression toward choriocarcinoma occurs.

The *incidence* of complete H. mole in the United States is 1 in 1500 pregnancies. The risk of developing a second mole is 4 to 5 times higher than the risk of the first. There is marked geographic variation; the incidence in the Orient is 5 to 15 times higher than it is in the Western world.

The karyotype of the partial mole is normal diploid, trisomic, or triploid (Fig. 31-6). Maternal genes do exist. The triploid mole is usually the result of two paternal sets and one maternal set of chromosomes (diandry), but could result from one paternal set and two maternal sets (digyny). Triploid karyotype is either 69XXX or 69XXY. There is evidence of an embryo or fetus. Embryonic membranes are present. The potential for malignant transformation is much less than that associated with the complete H. mole (Danforth and Scott, 1986).

Approximately 80% of partial H. moles regress spontaneously; 15% continue as nonmetastatic gestational trophoblastic disease, and 5% become metastatic gestational trophoblastic disease. Of women with metastatic trophoblastic disease, 50% develop the neoplasms as sequelae of a molar pregnancy (Danforth and Scott, 1986). The incidence of partial H. mole is difficult to estimate.

In the early stages the *signs and symptoms* of H. mole cannot be distinguished from normal pregnancy. Later, vaginal bleeding occurs in almost every case. The vaginal discharge may be dark brown (resembling prune juice) or bright red, scant or profuse. It may continue for only a few days or intermittently for weeks. Early in pregnancy about half the women have a uterus significantly larger than expected from the menstrual dates. The percentage of women with an excessively enlarged uterus increases as the length of time from the LMP increases. Approximately 25% of women will have a uterus smaller than would be expected from the menstrual dates.

Anemia from blood loss, excessive nausea and vomiting (hyperemesis gravidarum), and abdominal cramps caused

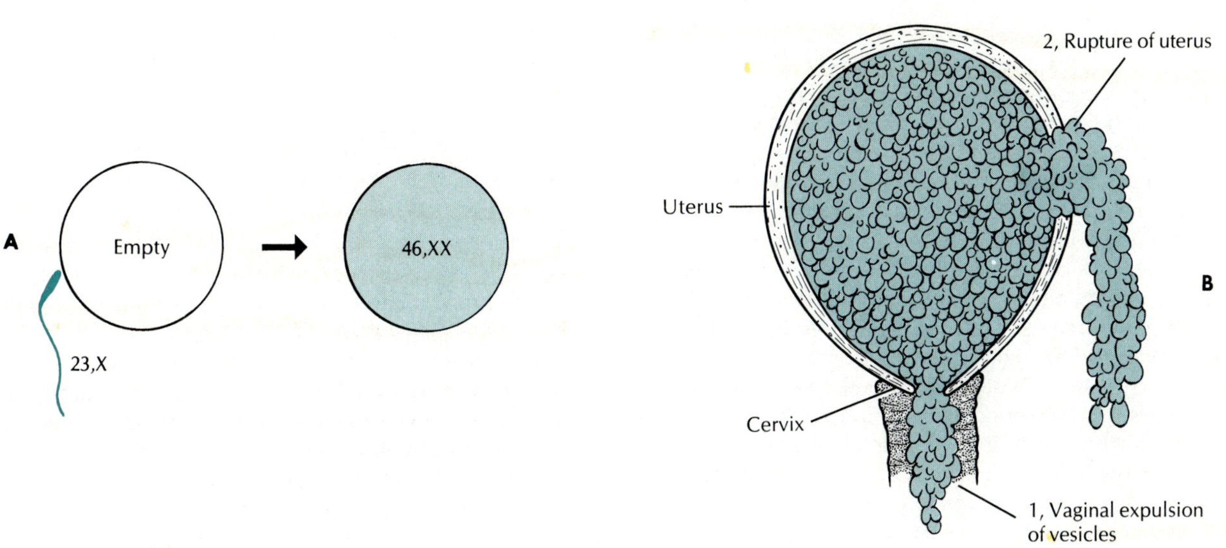

Fig. 31-5 A, Chromosomal origin of a complete mole. A single sperm (green) fertilizes an "empty" ovum. Reduplication of the sperm's 23,X set gives a completely homozygous diploid 46,XX. A similar process follows fertilization of an empty ovum by two sperms with two independently drawn sets of 23,X or 23,Y; therefore, both karyotypes of 46,XX and 46,XY can result. B, Uterine rupture with hydatidiform mole. *1,* Evacuation of mole through cervix. *2,* Rupture of uterus and spillage of mole into peritoneal cavity (rare).

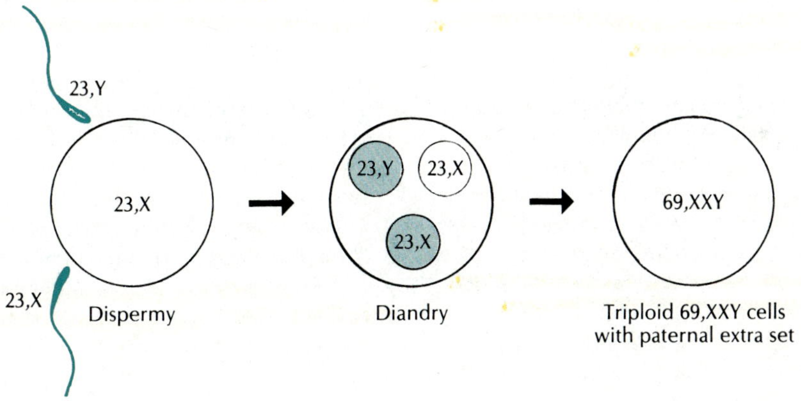

Fig. 31-6 Chromosomal origin of the triploid, partial mole. A normal ovum with a 23,X haploid set is fertilized by two sperms (green) to give a total of 69 chromosomes. A sex configuration of XXY, XXX, or XYY, is possible.

by uterine distension are relatively common findings. Anemia results from intrauterine bleeding. Preeclampsia occurs in about 15% of cases, usually between 9 and 12 gestational weeks. In addition, symptoms of true preeclampsia-eclampsia may occur even though it is well before the twentieth week of pregnancy (Chapter 29). Hyperthyroidism and pulmonary embolization of trophoblastic elements occur less commonly but are serious complications of H. mole. Ovarian enlargement is noted in approximately 10% of women at the time of uterine evacuation; in 20% of cases, ovarian enlargement is detected 1 to 4 weeks after a mole has been evacuated.

Many moles abort spontaneously. When hydropic vesicles are passed vaginally and the woman saves the specimen, the **diagnosis** can be established with certainty. No clinical sign or symptom permits a diagnosis before tissue is passed. The sonographic pattern of a molar pregnancy is characterized by a diffuse "snowstorm" pattern (Athey and Hadlock, 1981). Any uncertainty in diagnosis is usually clarified by an accurate clinical history, an accurate hCG titer, and, if necessary, a repeat sonogram in 2 weeks. A baseline serum hCG level is required before evacuation of the uterus. This is not considered diagnostic, since the required information is usually provided by the history, physical examination, and ultrasound study. hCG concentrations significantly higher than those of normal early pregnancy can be suggestive but are not diagnostic.

According to Danforth and Scott (1986) **immediate man-**

agement of this condition has changed. D and C had been recommended if the uterus was 12 weeks' gestational size or less, and abdominal hysterotomy was recommended if the size of the uterus was larger than 12 weeks' gestational size. More recently, suction curettage has been found to be safe and effective for most H. moles, regardless of size. Although suction curettage is usually appropriate, hysterectomy may be considered for women of high parity, those 40 years of age or older, and those who have completed their desired families. Hemorrhage and its sequelae are identified and treated. The malignancy rate in women over age 40 reaches 35%, and in those of high parity it approximates 15%. After evacuation of the H. mole, if the serum hCG levels regress spontaneously and return to nonpregnant levels within 8 to 12 weeks, the cyclic menses resume.

The following protocol should be adhered to in the **follow-up management** of women with complete H. mole. *Weekly hCG levels* are assayed until complete remission (weekly normal hCG titers for 3 consecutive weeks); after which, β-hCG should be measured by radioimmunoassay every month for 6 months and then every 2 months for the next 6 months. Since hCG levels are essential for monitoring this condition, it is essential that the woman (couple) *avoid pregnancy* for 1 year after evacuation of an H. mole. If there are no contrary indications, oral contraception may be prescribed. *Physical and pelvic examination* at 2-week intervals is necessary until complete remission has occurred, the uterus and ovaries have returned to normal size, and uterine bleeding has ceased. A *chest x-ray film* to detect metastases is obtained at the time of evacuation of the mole. Further chest films are not needed if hCG levels continue to fall spontaneously and complete remission follows. If hCG levels remain within normal limits for a year, the physician may assure the woman or couple that normal pregnancy can be anticipated, with a low probability of recurrence of H. mole if the woman is 40 years of age or younger. A *cure* is defined as complete absence of all clinical and hormonal evidence of disease for 5 years. Persistent trophoblastic disease is discussed in Chapter 44.

A general nursing care plan for a woman with a hemorrhagic disorder of pregnancy is on p. 777.

LATE PREGNANCY

Premature Separation of Placenta

Premature separation of the placenta, also termed **abruptio placentae**, is the separation of part or all of the placenta from its implantation site (Fig. 31-7). Separation occurs in the area of the decidua basalis after the twentieth week of pregnancy, before the birth of the baby.

Premature separation of the placenta is a serious disorder and accounts for about 15% of all perinatal deaths. Approximately one third of infants of women with premature separation of the placenta die. More than 50% of these die as a result of preterm delivery, and many others die of intrauterine hypoxia. Queenan and Hobbin (1982) state that rapid correction of resultant problems of abruptio placentae can decrease perinatal mortality from a high between 35% and 60% to a low of 3.6%

Premature separation of the placenta occurs in about 1 in 86 to 1 in 200 late pregnancies. Certain individuals seem predisposed to premature separation of the placenta. This problem is much more common in women with hypertension of any cause; 40% of women with diastolic pressures of 90 or more experience some degree of abruptio placentae. The incidence is three times greater in women with a gravidity of more than five than in primigravidas. Women with a history of reproductive loss (abortion, premature labor, prenatal hemorrhage, stillbirth, or neonatal death) experience premature separation of the placenta more than twice as often as the average population at risk. Between 15% to 20% of women who have had a previous premature separation of the placenta will have a recurrence. If the woman has had two prior premature separations, the chance in the next pregnancy is at least 25%.

The cause of premature separation of the placenta is unknown in most cases, but a sudden decrease in uterine size (as can occur with rupture of the membranes) may be re-

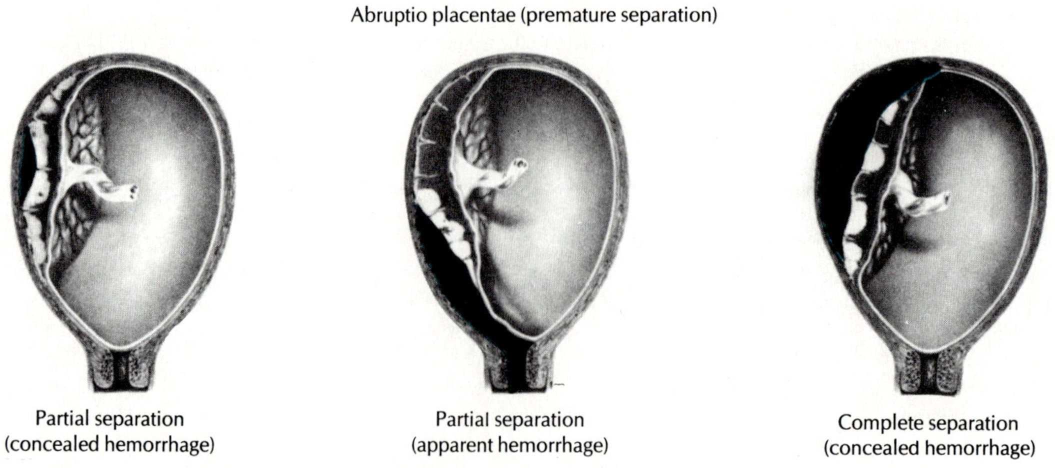

Fig. 31-7 Abruptio placentae. Premature separation of normally implanted placenta.
Courtesy Ross Laboratories, Columbus, Ohio.

sponsible. Precipitating factors include vascular engorgement during compression of the ascending vena cava, followed by sudden uteroplacental vasodilation. Abdominal trauma is a factor in less than 5% of cases, and short cord is identified in less than 1%. *Cocaine use* has been linked to abruptio placenta (Bingol, 1987; Woods, Plessinger, and Clark, 1987; Acker et al., 1983) (see p. 869).

Clinical Manifestations and Differential Diagnosis. The separation may be partial or complete, or only the margin of the placenta may be involved. Bleeding from the placental site may dissect (separate) the membranes from the decidua basalis and flow out through the vagina; it may remain concealed (retroplacental hemorrhage); or it may do both (Fig. 31-7). Clinical symptoms vary with the degree of separation (Table 31-4).

Symptoms include *uterine bleeding* with small to moderate amount of dark-red vaginal bleeding in 80% to 85% of cases. Bleeding may result in hypovolemia (shock; oliguria, anuria) and coagulopthy. *Uterine hypertonicity* (mild to severe) and pain are present. *Pain* is mild to severe, localized over one region of the uterus, or diffuse over the uterus with a boardlike abdomen. Couvelaire uterus (see at right and p. 764) may occur.

Laboratory findings include a positive Apt test (see Chapter 27) of amniotic fluid (indicates presence of maternal blood); a fall in hemoglobin and hematocrit (may appear later); and a fall in coagulation factors. From 10% to 30% of clients will develop consumptive coagulopathies (e.g., DIC) (the majority within 8 hours of hospital admission) and increased clot retraction.

Sonography reveals that the implantation site of the placenta is normal. Initially, retroplacental blood clot may not be visible, but the enlarging clot may be seen when the sonogram is repeated. The fetal position is within the usual distribution (e.g., generally in vertical lie with head presenting). The fetal station is within the usual distribution (e.g., from high [−5 cm] to engaged [0 station] or deeper in the birth canal).

Most of the following **complications** accompany moderate to severe abruptio placentae:

1. Hypovolemic shock, resulting in
   a. Pituitary necrosis (Sheehan's syndrome)
   b. Renal failure
2. Fetal hypoxia, or anoxia with possible fetal death
3. Coagulopathy; disseminated intravascular coagulation (DIC)
4. **Couvelaire uterus** (bleeding into the myometrium resulting in boardlike rigidity of the uterus)
5. Hepatitis as a sequel to
   a. Blood transfusion
   b. Fibrinogen replacement

Hypovolemic shock may result from loss of blood from

Table 31-4 *Summary of Findings: Abruptio Placentae and Placenta Previa*

	Abruptio Placentae			
	Marginal Separation	Moderate Separation	Severe Separation* (More Than 66%)	Placenta Previa
Bleeding: external, vaginal	Minimal	Absent to moderate	Absent to moderate	Minimal to severe and life threatening
Color of blood	Dark red	Dark red	Dark red	Bright red
Shock	Absent	Common	Very common; often sudden	Occasional
Coagulopathy	Rare	Occasional	Common	Rare
Uterine tonicity	Normal	Increased—may be localized to one region or diffuse over uterus; uterus fails to relax between contractions	Tetanic, persistent uterine contraction; board-like uterus	Normal
Tenderness (pain)	Usually absent; if present, is localized	Increased—usually diffuse over uterus	Agonizing, unremitting uterine pain	Absent
Ultrasonographic findings				
Location of placenta	Normal—upper uterine segment	Normal—upper uterine segment	Normal—upper uterine segment	Abnormal—lower uterine segment
Station of presenting part	Variable to engaged	Variable to engaged	Variable to engaged	High—not engaged
Fetal position	Usual distribution†	Usual distribution	Usual distribution	Commonly transverse, breech, or oblique
Concurrent hypertensive state	Usual distribution	Commonly present	Commonly present	Usual distribution

*Onset is usually abrupt; fetus usually dies.
†Usual distribution refers to the usual variations or incidence seen when there is no concurrent problem.

the maternal circulation. Prolonged hypovolemia results in ischemia (and hypoxia). Ischemia of the pituitary gland causes pituitary necrosis (Sheehan's syndrome) (see p. 774). Ischemia of the kidneys leads to renal failure: acute tubular necrosis that may be reversible or acute cortical necrosis that is not reversible.

Continued bleeding that cannot exit easily may rupture through the fetal membranes or spread between the muscle fibers of the myometrium. Pressure from the confined expanding volume of blood may rupture the amniotic sac; the blood imparts a port-wine color to the amniotic fluid.

Extravasation of blood into the myometrium (Couvelaire uterus) has several sequelae:

1. Myometrial tissue is damaged, necrosis results, and thromboplastin is released, thus initiating the clotting mechanism (see p. 767). Fibrinogen and platelet levels fall as these clotting factors are used to form the retroplacental clot, and coagulopathy results.

2. Small amounts of blood in the myometrium cause ecchymosis and a localized increase in tonicity. The woman may or may not experience uterine tenderness.

3. Increasing amounts of blood in the myometrium increase uterine tonicity, irritability, and tenderness that spread over the entire uterus; the ability of the uterus to relax between contractions diminishes or is lost. Electronic fetal monitoring reflects the increasing fetal distress that may finally end in fetal death.

4. After delivery the uterus may feel firm because of the blood between the muscle fibers in the myometrium. Uterine contractile efficiency and therefore its ability to close off bleeding sinuses may be greatly impaired (Danforth and Scott, 1986). The problem may be compounded by a clotting defect (p. 768). However, uterine contractility is seldom affected sufficiently to produce serious postpartum hemorrhage (Pritchard, MacDonald, and Gant, 1985).

Management. The nurse assists the physician in implementing the therapeutic measures. Side-lying position on a wedge placed under the supine woman's right hip facilitates adequate uterine-placental perfusion. Blood lost is restored. If shock is present or appears imminent *and* clotting mechanism is intact, central venous pressure (CVP) or pulmonary artery wedge pressure (PAWP) monitoring is started to monitor blood and fluid replacement accurately. A retention catheter is placed to monitor urinary output accurately for volume and proteinuria. Oliguria and proteinuria are ominous signs. Coagulopathy is anticipated and corrected. The fetus is monitored and delivered when indicated. Hysterectomy may be necessary to control bleeding or if Couvelaire uterus occurs. The woman and her family need emotional support.

Prognosis. Maternal mortality approaches 1% in premature separation of the placenta; this condition remains a leading cause of maternal death. The mother's prognosis depends on the extent of the placental detachment, overall blood loss, degree of DIC, and time between the placental "accident" and delivery. Fortunately, 80% to 90% of all premature separations of the placenta only involve two or three cotyledons, and therefore the prognosis is generally not grave.

Fetal prognosis is poor. At least one third of babies of mothers with premature placental separation die before, during, or soon after birth. Of those who survive, there is an increase in the absolute numbers of neurologically damaged infants. Fetal depression occurs with at least twice the normal frequency. If the Apgar score at 5 minutes is less than 3, the infant may have sustained neurologic damage. If the 5-minute Apgar score is 7 or greater, there is about a 90% chance of normal growth and development. Infants involved in premature separation of the placenta who weigh more than 2500 g (5lb 8oz) and who have good Apgar scores usually develop normally. About 60% of infants involved in premature separation of the placenta who weigh less than 2500 g at birth develop normally.

A general nursing care plan for the woman with a hemorrhagic disorder of pregnancy is on p. 777.

Placenta Previa

In placenta previa the placenta is implanted in the lower uterine segment. The degree to which the internal cervical os is covered by the placenta determines how placenta previa is classified. Placenta previa (Fig. 31-8) often is described as **complete, total, or central** if the internal os is entirely covered by the placenta, when the cervix is fully dilated. **Partial placenta previa** implies incomplete coverage. **Marginal placenta previa** indicates that only an edge of the placenta approaches the internal os. The term **low-lying (low) implantation** is used when the placenta is situated in the lower uterine segment but away from the os. Gestational age and cervical dilation and effacement affect the extent of coverage of the internal os. A better classification of placenta previa is the estimation of percentage coverage of the internal os *at full dilation,* the diameter required for delivery of a mature fetus through the cervix (Fig. 31-9).

In the second trimester approximately 45% of all placentas are implanted in the lower uterine segment. As the lower uterine segment elongates, the placenta seems to move upward. By term only 1 placenta in 150 is still a previa. Those placentas most likely to remain unchanged are the ones classified as central (complete).

The cause of placenta previa is uncertain. Reduced vascularity of the upper segment subsequent to scarring from uterine surgery (abortion, cesarean delivery), molar pregnancy, or tumor necessitating lower implantation of the placenta is a plausible theory. Multiple gestation that requires a larger surface area for placental implantation may be a factor. Vessels of the endometrium involved in previous sites of implantation undergo changes that may reduce the blood supply to those regions, thus predisposing to low implantation in subsequent pregnancies.

The site of implantation and size of the placenta are related. Specifically, because the circulation of the lower uterine segment is less favorable than that of the fundus, placenta previa may need to cover a larger area for adequate efficiency. In placenta previa the surface area may be at least 30% greater than the average placenta implanted in the fundus.

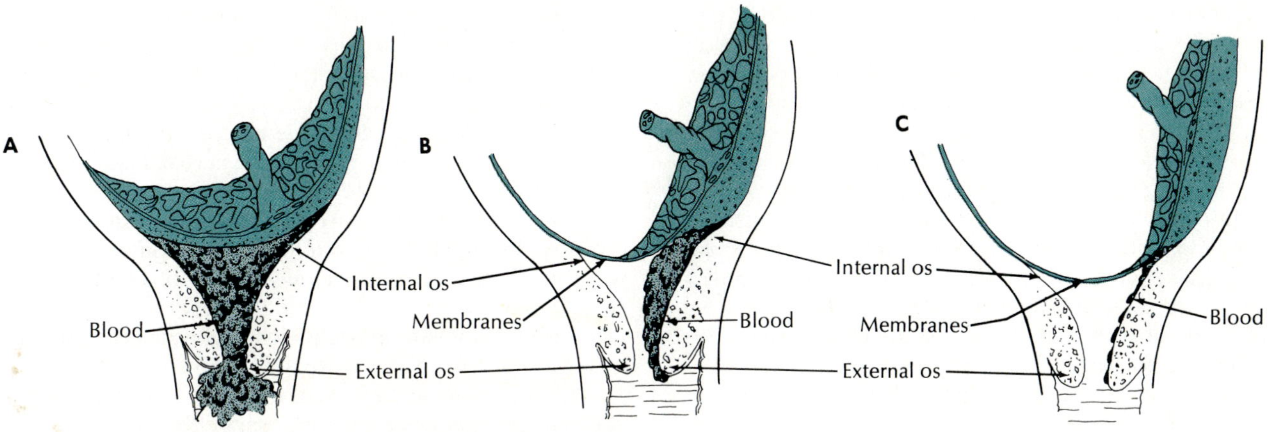

Fig. 31-8 Types of placenta previa after onset of labor. **A**, Complete, or total. **B**, Incomplete or partial. **C**, Marginal, or low lying.

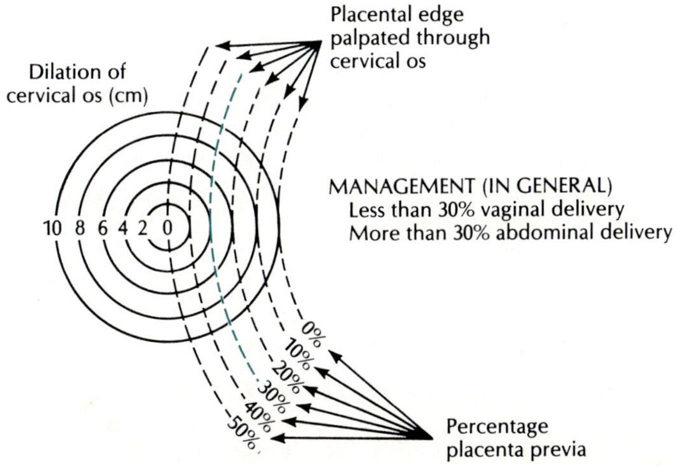

Fig. 31-9 Classification of placenta previa.
Modified from Tatum, HJ, and Mule, JG: Am J Obstet Gynecol 93:768, 1965.

Clinical Manifestations and Differential Diagnosis

Symptoms. *Painless uterine bleeding,* especially during the third trimester, characterizes placenta previa (Table 31-4). Rarely is the first episode life-threatening or a cause of hypovolemic shock. Approximately 7% of placenta previas are without symptoms and are an incidental finding on ultrasonic scans. A few are manifest for the first time at term, when the lower uterine segment stretches and thins; at that time tearing and bleeding occur at the lower implantation site. About 3% of all cases of placenta previa are accompanied by placenta accreta, increta, or percreta (p. 773).

The *bright-red bleeding* may be intermittent, occur in gushes, or, more rarely, may be continuous. It may start while the woman is resting or in the midst of any activity. Fortunately, exsanguination almost never occurs unless vaginal or rectal examination initiates violent bleeding before or during early labor.

The detachment of placenta previa is painless. However, if the first bleeding coincides with the onset of labor, the woman may experience discomfort because of uterine contractions.

Abdominal examination usually reveals a *soft (relaxed), nontender uterus* of normal tone. If the fetus is in a longitudinal lie, the fundal height is usually greater than expected for gestational age because the low placenta hinders descent of the presenting fetal part. Leopold's maneuvers may reveal a fetus in an oblique or breech position or transverse lie because of the abnormal site of placental implantation.

As a rule, fetal distress or fetal death occurs only if a significant portion of the placenta previa becomes detached from the decidua basalis or if the mother suffers hypovolemic shock.

Ultrasonography. Obstetric ultrasound, with either real-time (linear or sector) or static imaging, is the diagnostic method of choice. If ultrasound reveals a normally implanted placenta, a speculum examination is performed to rule out local causes of bleeding (e.g., cervicitis, polyps, or carcinoma of the cervix), and a coagulation profile is obtained to rule out other causes of bleeding.

Amniocentesis. If 35 to 36 weeks' gestation is reached, ultrasound-guided amniocentesis for assessing fetal lung maturity (lecithin/sphingomyelin [LS] ratio or presence of phosphatidyglycerol) is warranted. Immediate delivery by cesarean surgery is recommended to forestall hemorrhage if fetal lungs are mature. (A major problem related to placenta previa is preterm delivery.)

Vaginal Examination. If possible, sterile vaginal speculum examination by the physician for diagnosing placenta previa should be postponed until viability has been reached (preferably after the thirty-fourth week), and after the ultrasound report is available. The vaginal examination, known as the **double-setup procedure**, is a serious undertaking; it is attempted only if the physician is prepared for delivery.

In a double setup a sterile vaginal examination is performed in an operating room with staff and equipment ready to effect an immediate vaginal or cesarean delivery. Since manipulation of the lower uterine segment or cervix may result in profound hemorrhage, preparation for immediate delivery is essential. Readiness implies an IV line in place with a needle large enough to accommodate blood transfusion, two units of matched blood for the mother, sterile tables set up and open, anesthetists present, at least one physician and one nurse scrubbed, and a pediatrician present. Amniotomy for anticipated vaginal delivery (if placenta is low lying, cervix is favorable, and presenting part is low) or cesarean delivery (if placenta encroaches on or covers cervical os or fetus is in oblique or transverse lie) should be performed.

Management. When fetal maturity is near, conservative management (e.g., bed rest in the hospital to extend the period of gestation) is usually possible because initial spontaneous critical bleeding almost never occurs in placenta previa. When fetal lung maturity (L/S ratio of at least 2:1) is achieved and survival is likely, then elective termination of pregnancy can be carried out.

After the diagnosis of placenta previa has been made, the woman should remain in the hospital under close supervision. At least two units of blood, typed and crossmatched, must be available for emergency use. A hematocrit of at least 35% is maintained (Silver, et al, 1984). The duration of pregnancy should be confirmed and, except in an emergency, delivery postponed until after the thirty-sixth week.

If the woman has greater than a 30% placenta previa or if bleeding is excessive, cesarean delivery is indicated, preferably with the woman under light general inhalation anesthesia.

If hemorrhage is in progress and *vaginal delivery* is planned, the membranes are ruptured, if this can be done easily. Rupturing the membranes permits the presenting part to tamponade the edge of an incomplete placenta previa, thus checking brisk bleeding. A semi-Fowler's position with head of bed elevated 20 to 30 degrees encourages the fetal body to act as tamponade. If there is less than a 30% placenta previa, cautious stimulation of labor by continuous IV oxytocin drip is permissible unless bleeding is aggravated. The woman is kept NPO since operative delivery is a possibility. If labor does not ensue within 6 hours and if progress is not rapid, cesarean delivery is indicated. The fetus may have bled through small tears in the placenta; hence the cord is clamped early at cesarean delivery.

Bipolar (Braxton Hicks, internal podalic) version should not be employed because of the serious risk of rupture of the lower uterine segment, cervical laceration, or hemorrhage.

Blood loss may not cease with the delivery of the infant. The large vascular channels in the lower uterine segment may continue to bleed because of the diminished muscle content of the lower uterine segment. The natural mechanism to control bleeding—the interlacing muscle bundles (the "living ligature") contracting around open vessels—so characteristic of the upper part of the uterus is absent in the lower part of the uterus. *Therefore postpartum hemorrhage may occur even if the fundus is contracted firmly.*

The location of the placental site close to the cervical os renders it more accessible to ascending infection from the vagina. Hemorrhage and anemia increase the predisposition to antenatal infection (placentitis) and postpartum (puerperal) infection.

If uterine bleeding cannot be controlled with oxytocic drugs, ligation of the hypogastric (internal iliac) arteries (Fig. 6-14, A) or even hysterectomy may be necessary.

Hypovolemia must be treated without overtransfusion or overinfusion. Precise control of blood and fluid replacement necessitates continuous monitoring of CVP or PAWP (see p. 775).

Prognosis. Maternal morbidity may occur from the placenta previa itself, the management, or the birth. Antenatal hemorrhage may be fatal or nearly fatal. Prolonged hypovolemia and hypotension, more commonly associated with abruptio placentae, lead to cerebral or renal damage.

Complications associated with the management of placenta previa include sepsis, surgery-related trauma to structures adjacent to the uterus, anesthesia complications, blood transfusion reactions, or overinfusion of fluids.

Maternal mortality in placenta previa has dropped almost 50%, to about 0.6%, during the past decade in larger centers in North America because of conservative therapy. The perinatal mortality (resulting primarily from prematurity) still approaches 20% in most hospitals. This figure undoubtedly can be reduced by half with better management. Currently, placenta previa increases the likelihood of death of the newborn by about 10 times.

A general nursing care plan for the woman with a hemorrhagic disorder of pregnancy appears on p. 777.

Cord Insertion and Placental Variations

A **velamentous insertion of the cord** is a rare placental anomaly in which the cord vessels begin to branch at the membranes and then course onto the placenta (Fig. 31-10, *A*). Rupture of the membranes or traction on the cord may tear one or more of the fetal vessels. As a result the fetus may quickly exsanguinate (bleed to death). Battledore (marginal) (Fig. 31-10, *B*) insertion of the cord increases the risk of fetal hemorrhage, especially following marginal separation of the placenta.

Rarely, the placenta may be divided into two or more separate lobes, resulting in **succenturiate placenta** (Fig. 31-10, *C*). Each lobe has a distinct circulation; the vessels collect at the periphery, and the main trunks unite eventually to form the vessels of the cord. Blood vessels joining the lobes may be supported only by the fetal membranes and are therefore in danger of tearing during labor or during the birth of the baby or of the placenta. During delivery of the placenta, one or more of the separate lobes may remain attached to the decidua basalis, preventing uterine contraction.

CLOTTING DISORDERS IN PREGNANCY

Normal Clotting

Normally there is a delicate balance (homeostasis) maintained between two opposing systems, the *hemostatic* system and the fibrinolytic system. The hemostatic system is

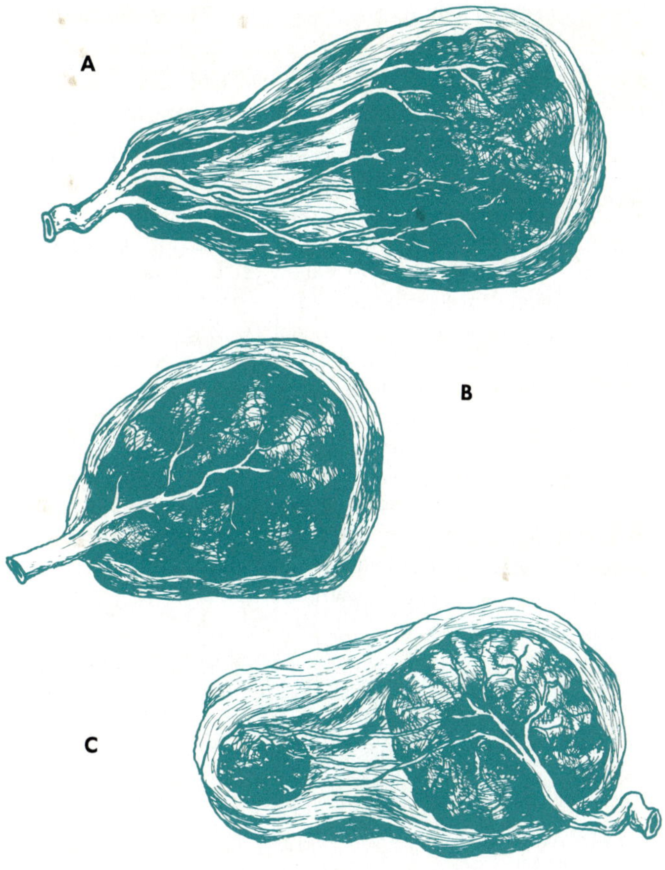

Fig. 31-10 Cord insertion and placental variations. **A**, Velamentous insertion of cord. **B**, Battledore placenta. **C**, Placenta succenturiate.

involved in the life-saving process; this system stops the flow of blood from injured vessels, in part through the formation of insoluble fibrin that acts as a hemostatic platelet plug.* The phases of the coagulation process involve an interaction of the coagulation factors (see Table 31-5) in which each factor sequentially activates the factor next in line in the so-called cascade effect sequence.

The *fibrinolytic* system refers to the process by which the fibrin is split into fibrinolytic degradation products products (FDP) and circulation is restored.

Clotting Problems

A history of abnormal bleeding, inheritance of unusual bleeding tendencies, and a report of significant aberrations of laboratory findings indicate a bleeding or clotting problem (Table 31-6). The comprehension of useful tests of hemostasis is based on the usual mechanisms for the control of bleeding, that is, the function of platelets and the necessary clotting factors.

Disseminated Intravascular Coagulation. Disseminated intravascular coagulation (DIC, defibrination syndrome, defibrination coagulopathy), a pathologic form of clotting, (1) is diffuse rather than localized, (2) injures rather than protects the necessary site of coagulation, and (3) consumes clotting factors, such as platelets and fibrinogen, so avidly that widespread external and internal bleeding follows. Multiple factors are involved, including platelet and coagulation dysfunction. DIC in pregnancy may occur insidiously or with dramatic suddenness. Constant vigilance on the part of the obstetric team is necessary. Unless DIC is treated immediately and effectively, death often results.

*Aspirin inhibits platelet aggregation.

Table 31-5 *Blood Clotting Factors*

Factor	Synonyms
I	Fibrinogen
II	Prothrombin
III	Platelet factor 3, thromboplastin
IV	Calcium
V	Labile factor, proaccelerin, AC globulin (ACG)
VI	Synonymous terms no longer used
VII	Serum prothrombin conversion accelerator (SPCA), proconvertin, autoprothrombin
VIII	Antihemotrophic factor (AHF), antihemophilic globulin
IX	Plasma thromboplastin component (PTC), Christmas factor, autoprothrombin II
X	Stuart-Prower factor, Stuart factor, Prower factor
XI	Plasma thromboplastin antecedent (PTA)
XII	Hagemen factor
XIII	Fibrin (protein) stabilizing factor

Unanticipated, profuse, locally uncontrollable uterine hemorrhage, bleeding from the episiotomy, lacerations or needle puncture sites, or shock often initiates the DIC syndrome in the woman (ecchymosis or bleeding from mucous membranes or gastrointestinal tract may be apparent in the infant).

Spontaneous bleeding from the woman's gums or nose may be noted. Excessive bleeding may occur from the site of a slight trauma (e.g., venipuncture sites, intramuscular [IM] or subcutaneous injection sites, nicks from shaving of perineum or abdomen, injury from insertion of urinary catheter). Laboratory tests reveal reduced platelets, fibrinogen, proaccelerin, antihemophilic factor, and prothrombin (the factors consumed during coagulation). Other factors should be normal. Fibrinolysis is first increased but later is severely depressed. Degradation of fibrin leads to the accumulation of fibrin split-products in the blood. Fibrin split-products have anticoagulant properties and thus prolong the prothrombin time. Bleeding time is normal; coagulation time shows no clot; clot retraction time shows no clot; and partial thromboplastin time (PTT) is increased. DIC must be distinguished from other clotting disorders before initiating therapy.

The primary **management** of all cases of DIC involves correction of the underlying cause, for example, delivery of the dead fetus; treatment of existing infection or preeclampsia–eclampsia; or removal of abrupted placenta (following delivery of fetus by cesarean birth). Packed red blood cells may be transfused to correct anemia. Deficiencies secondary to DIC primarily involve platelets, factors V and VIII, fibrinogen, and prothrombin. Administration of *fresh-frozen plasma* in combination with *platelet concentrates* is effective in all these conditions when replacement therapy is warranted (Danforth and Scott, 1986). The frozen plasma is thawed in the laboratory and should be administered within 15 to 20 minutes, since the factors disintegrate as the plasma warms. Adequate fibrinogen levels can be obtained by infusion of *cryoprecipitate* with significantly less risk of hepatitis transmission (Table 31-7). Each bag of cryoprecipitate contains an average of 250 mg fibrinogen; 16 to 20 bags are required for replacement therapy. The use of blood type-specific cryoprecipitate reduces the risk of blood transfusion reactions (Danforth and Scott, 1986). Disadvantages of cryoprecipitate are variability in plasma fibrinogen response and the large volume that must be infused. CVP monitoring is begun to attempt to maintain CVP within normal limits: 6 to 12 cm H_2O (Fig. 31-11). Supportive measures include keeping the woman's right hip elevated to prevent hypotensive syndrome. Oxygen is administered by a tight-fitting mask at 10 to 12 L/min. The emotional needs of the family are recognized and supported.

Heparin therapy has been recommended to inhibit coagulation activated by thromboplastin release. However, heparin anticoagulation is not recommended for the obstetric client with DIC. DIC secondary to retained dead fetus may be an exception to this generalization. Prognosis depends on the degree and extent of the underlying disorder as well as the response of the woman to prompt and proper treatment. If DIC worsens or does not improve within several hours, retained products of conception, sepsis, and liver disease must be considered.

A general nursing care plan for a woman with hemorrhagic disorders of pregnancy and DIC appears on p. 777.

Autoimmune Thrombocytopenic Purpura. Autoimmune thrombocytopenic purpura (ATP) is an autoimmune disorder in which antiplatelet antibodies decrease the life span of the platelets. The following results of tests are diagnostic: (1) thrombocytopenia, (2) capillary fragility, (3) increased

Table 31-6 *Coagulation Tests*

Test	Comments
Activated partial thromboplastin time (PTT; measures intrinsic system): 25-36 sec	Screening test of choice: very sensitive, relatively easy to perform, inexpensive. All coagulation factors except proconvertin are measured.
One-stage prothrombin time (PT; Quick test; measures extrinsic system); 9.5-11.3 sec	Test for proconvertin (VII), proaccelerin (V), Stuart-Prower factor (X), prothrombin (II), and fibrinogen deficiencies. Unfortunately, it does not measure factors necessary for earlier stages of coagulation.
Thrombin time (plasma): 10-15 sec	Test measures conversion of fibrinogen to fibrin and depends on concentration of fibrinogen or inhibitors such as fibrin split-products, antithrombins, and heparin.
Platelet count: 130,000-370,000/mm³	**Most reliable index for DIC.**
Specific factor assays (e.g., plasma fibrinogen): 195-365 mg/dl	Each of coagulation factors can be assessed by indirect clotting method using natural or synthetic factor-deficient substrates and compared with activity of normal plasma (100%). However, fibrinogen is only factor that can be measured directly by chemical method.
Bleeding time Template: 2-8 min Ivy: 1-7 min Duke: 1-3 min	Finger or earlobe puncture 5 mm deep and 2 mm wide (Bard-Parker blade no. 11) is made after antiseptic preparation of skin. Note time of puncture; touch bleeding point gently with sterile filter paper to absorb blood every 30 sec until bleeding stops.

Table 31-7 *Replacement Clotting Factors*

Infusate and Factors	Need	Risk	Expected Outcome
Fresh-frozen plasma; clotting factors	Depleted clotting factors	Hepatitis B	Increase fibrinogen to 10 mg/dl per unit infused
Cryoprecipitate; I,V,VII,XIII	Fibrinogen concentration below 50 mg/dl; a level of 50,000/mm³ should be sought	Hepatitis	Increase fibrinogen 2 to 5 mg/dl, to 10 mg/dl per unit infused
Platelet concentrate; platelets	<20,000/mm³	Rhesus isoimmunization in Rh negative women	Increase platelet count 7500/μl per unit infused

bleeding time, and (4) a bone marrow smear showing a normal or increased megakaryocyte count with many young forms (Danforth and Scott, 1986).

ATP may result in severe hemorrhage following cesarean delivery or from cervical or vaginal lacerations. The incidence of postdelivery uterine bleeding or vaginal hematomas is also increased in ATP. Neonatal thrombocytopenia occurs in about 50% of the cases and is associated with a high mortality. Platelet transfusions are given to maintain the platelet count at 100,000/cu mm. Corticosteroids are given if the diagnosis is made before or during pregnancy. (Splenectomy is deferred until after the puerperium.) The history taken during the initial prenatal visit should include reference to bleeding in the woman.

Hemophilia. At least nine types of congenital disorders of the clotting mechanism have been identified, including hemophilia A, hemophilia A and C, and von Willebrand's disease. About 75% of hemophiliacs have the A variety, and about 15% have the B variety. These two types represent about 90% of all congenital hemorrhagic diseases caused by defective formation of a fibrin clot.

Classic hemophilia (A) is a bleeding disorder typified by a deficiency of factor VIII antihemophilic factor (AHF), an antihemophilic globulin that is essential in thromboplastin formation in phase 1 of blood coagulation. The source of factor VIII in the body is unknown. All degrees of severity of the disease have been reported. Bleeding occurs most often from the nasal or oral mucosa or from contusions or lacerations. Bleeding into the skin, muscles, or joints may also ensue. Hemophilia B, or Christmas disease, is caused by a genetically determined deficiency of factor IX and is clinically indistinguishable from hemophilia A.

Both hemophilia A and hemophilia B are transmitted as sex-linked recessive traits by the mother. Because they are expressed predominantly in the son and only rarely in the daughter (only in homozygous females), the major problem arising with pregnancy is the birth of an affected infant. Hematomas after injections and bleeding from circumcision are common. However, most affected newborns exhibit no clinical abnormalities. Recording and reporting of such incidences, if they occur, will aid in diagnosis at a later date.

The affected woman requires treatment with cryoprecipitate or fresh frozen plasma to replace factor VIII or factor IX to prevent hemorrhage during and after childbirth.

von Willebrand's Disease. One type of hemophilia is von Willebrand's disease. It is probably the most common of all hereditary bleeding disorders (Rigby, 1987). It results from a factor VIII deficiency and platelet dysfunction. It is transmitted as an incomplete autosomal-dominant trait to

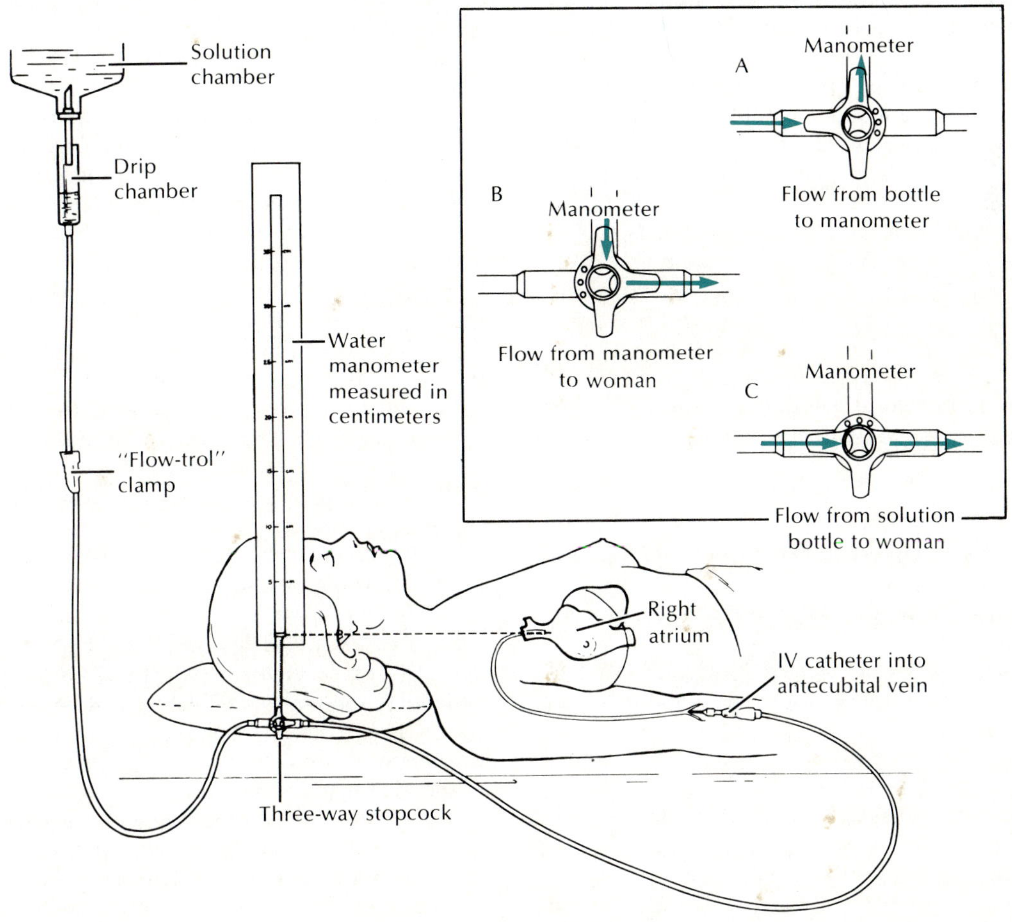

Fig. 31-11 Measurement of CVP with manometer.

both sexes. Although von Willebrand's disease is rare, it is one of the most common congenital clotting defects in American women of childbearing age. The symptoms include a familial bleeding tendency, previous bleeding episodes, prolonged bleeding time (most important test), factor VIII deficiency (mild to moderate), and bleeding from mucous membranes. Since factor VIII increases during pregnancy, this increase may be sufficient to offset danger from hemorrhage during childbirth. However, the woman should be observed for at least 1 week postpartum.

Treatment of von Willebrand's disease consists of replacement of factor VIII, if it is less than 30%, through administration of cryoprecipitate or fresh frozen plasma.

POSTDELIVERY HEMORRHAGE

Hemorrhage is a leading cause of maternal death worldwide. Postdelivery hemorrhage, traditionally the loss of 500 ml of blood or more after delivery, is the most common and most serious type of excessive obstetric blood loss. At least 5% of women suffer postdelivery hemorrhage.

A small woman is less able to withstand the loss of blood than a larger one. It has been noted that the average maternal blood loss can be as much as 10% of the woman's blood volume without immediate critical consequence. Therefore a more meaningful definition of postdelivery hemorrhage is the loss of 1% or more of body weight, a figure easily referable to blood volume because 1 ml of blood weighs 1 g.

Postdelivery hemorrhage may be sudden and even exsanguinating. Moderate but persistent bleeding may continue for days or weeks. Postdelivery hemorrhage may be early, within the first 24 hours after delivery, or late, from 24 hours after delivery until the twenty-eighth day.

Control of bleeding from the placental site is accomplished by prolonged contraction and retraction of interlacing strands of myometrium, the **living ligature**. A firm or contracted uterus does not normally bleed after delivery unless placenta previa had existed. Therefore careful assessment of uterine tone and the maintenance of uterine contractions through manual massage or oxytocic stimulation are important parts of postdelivery care.

Etiology

The causes of postdelivery hemorrhage, in approximate order of frequency, are as follows:

1. Mismanagement of the third stage of labor (e.g., incomplete placental separation)
2. Uterine atony caused by excessive analgesia or anesthesia, prolonged labor, overdistension of the uterus or urinary bladder
3. Lacerations of the birth canal
4. Hematologic disorders (e.g., DIC)
5. Complications of pregnancy (e.g., inversion of the uterus, placenta accreta)
6. Tumors of the cervix or uterus
7. Medical complications of pregnancy (e.g., hyperthyroidism, vitamin K deficiency)
8. Infections of the genital tract (e.g., endometritis)

Early postdelivery hemorrhage almost invariably is caused by uterine atony, lacerations of the birth canal, or DIC. **Late postdelivery hemorrhage** most commonly is the result of subinvolution of the placental site, retained placental tissue, or infection (see specific nursing care plan, p. 777).

Clinical Findings and Differential Diagnosis

It is helpful to consider the problem of excessive bleeding with reference to the stages of labor. From delivery of the fetus until separation of the placenta the character and quantity of blood passed may suggest excessive bleeding. For example, *dark blood* is probably of venous origin, perhaps from varices or superficial lacerations of the birth canal. *Bright blood* is arterial and indicates, for example, deep lacerations of the cervix. *Spurts of blood* with clots may indicate partial placental separation. *Failure of blood to clot* or remain clotted is indicative of coagulopathy.

The period from the separation of the placenta to its delivery may be when excessive bleeding occurs. Commonly this is the result of incomplete placental separation, often caused by poor management of the third stage of labor (e.g., undue manipulation of the fundus). After the placenta has been recovered, persistent or excessive blood loss usually is the result of atony of the uterus (i.e., its failure to contract well or maintain its contraction) or prolapse of the uterus into the pelvis. Late hemorrhage may be the result of partial involution of the uterus and unrecognized lacerations of the birth canal.

Complications of postdelivery hemorrhage are either immediate or delayed. Hemorrhagic (hypovolemic) shock (p. 775) and death may occur from sudden, exsanguinating hemorrhage. Delayed complications provoked by postdelivery hemorrhage include anemia, puerperal infection, and thromboembolism.

Uterine Atony. Uterine atony is marked hypotonia of the uterus. Uterine atony occurs in at least 5% of deliveries, particularly when the woman is a grand multipara; with hydramnios; when the fetus is large; or after the delivery of twins or triplets. In such conditions, the uterus is "overstretched" and contracts poorly. Uterine atony is the principal cause of postdelivery hemorrhage.

Placental separation and expulsion are facilitated by contraction of the uterus, which also prevents hemorrhage from the placental site. The corpus is, in essence, a basketwork of strong, interdigitating, smooth muscle bundles through which pass many large maternal blood vessels. If the uterus is flaccid after detachment of all or part of the afterbirth, brisk venous bleeding will occur and normal coagulation of the open vasculature will be impaired. In contrast, a firm, contracted uterus will not bleed because the myometrium will compress the vasculature, and resolution of the placental site can occur.

Numerous preventable problems may be responsible for uterine atony. For example, undesirable side effects may follow the administration of ill-chosen drugs, of very potent analgesic agents (e.g., morphine) late in the first stage of labor, and of certain anesthetics (e.g., ethyl ether) that are especially efficient smooth muscle-relaxing drugs.

Specific Nursing Care Plan

MATERNAL HEMORRHAGE AND INFECTION

Mindy, age 26, had a normal, healthy, full term pregnancy. Two days ago she gave birth to a 3360 gram (7½ lb) girl after an 8-hour labor. Her only medication for pain was a local anesthetic for repair of the episiotomy. During delivery delayed placental separation resulted in an estimated blood loss of 750 ml of blood. Mindy states she does not understand why she has an infection when her pregnancy was so normal.

ASSESSMENT	NURSING DIAGNOSIS (ND)/ PLAN (P)/GOAL (G)	RATIONALE/ IMPLEMENTATION	EVALUATION
Hematocrit (Hct) 27%. Temperature 38.4° C for last 6 hours. Fundus firm after massage at 1 cm below umbilicus, slightly tender. Persistance of lochia rubra.	ND: Potential for infection secondary to anemia. ND: Knowledge deficit related to prevention and treatment for infection. P: Provide information, implement prescribed treatment and be available for discussion of concerns and questions. G: Mindy will learn signs of infection, its treatment and prevention.	*To treat low Hct, the nurse will:* Administer therapy per orders: blood transfusion, iron preparation. Advise regarding nutrition. *To treat puerperal infection, the nurse will:* Administer IV fluids and antibiotics per physician order. Advise regarding nutrition. Evaluate and notify physician of lab results when complete. *To prevent spread of infection, the nurse will:* Teach methods of good hygiene. Teach methods of preventing spread to newborn.	Hct increases to normal level. Temperature returns to normal range. Uterine involution progresses normally. Newborn does not acquire infection from Mindy. Mindy verbalizes understanding of good nutrition, good hygiene, and preventing spread of infection.
Mindy states she does not understand why she has an infection when her pregnancy was so normal.	ND: Knowledge deficit related to connection between anemia and infection. P: Provide information and be available for discussion. G: Mindy understands association between anemia and infection.	*To increase knowledge about infection, the nurse will:* Teach signs and symptoms of infection. Teach how anemia can increase the potential for infection.	Mindy verbalizes relationship between prevention of anemia (nutrition) and susceptibility to infection.

Mismanagement of the third stage of labor, allowing only partial separation of the placenta or retention of placental fragments, may be associated with uterine atony. Moreover, the poorly contracting uterus may have slipped deep into the true pelvis to cause chronic passive congestion of the organ, an added cause of abnormal bleeding.

The first step in the treatment of uterine bleeding is to elevate and hold the uterus out of the pelvis and to massage the corpus to initiate and maintain a firmly contracted organ (Fig. 20-2). The physician orders oxytocin, 10 U administered intravenously (well diluted), or its equivalent. Moreover, continuous IV administration of oxytocin solution (5 U/500 ml of 5% dextrose in water) should run for 3 or 4 hours. Blood transfusion for the treatment of shock and blood replacement may be urgently needed.

The accoucheur should hasten to palpate the interior of the uterus so that retained products of conception can be removed and possible rupture of the uterus diagnosed. If the blood being lost fails to clot, a coagulopathy (e.g., DIC) may have developed, and prompt appropriate treatment may be lifesaving.

If the procedures outlined are ineffectual and normal clotting of blood is ensured, bilateral ligation of the internal iliac arteries will usually stop the bleeding. Thus the uterus will be preserved for future childbearing. If this is not a serious consideration, if rupture of the uterus is confirmed, or if hemorrhage from uterine atony persists, hysterectomy may be required.

Lacerations of the Birth Canal. Lacerations of the birth canal are second only to uterine atony as a major cause of postdelivery hemorrhage. Therefore prevention, recognition, and prompt, effective treatment of birth canal lacerations are vitally important.

Continued bleeding despite efficient postdelivery uterine contractions demands inspection or reinspection of the birth passage. Continuous bleeding from so-called minor sources may be just as dangerous as a sudden loss of a large amount of blood, although often it is ignored until shock develops. Birth canal lacerations may include injuries to the labia, perineum, vagina, and cervix.

Factors that influence the causes and incidence of obstetric lacerations of the lower genital tract encompass several conditions:

1. Operative delivery
2. Aseptic or unattended spontaneous delivery
3. Congenital abnormalities of the maternal soft parts
4. Contracted pelvis
5. Size, presentation, and position of the fetus
6. Relative size of the presenting part and the birth canal
7. Prior scarring from infection, injury, or surgery
8. Vulvar perineal and vaginal varices
9. Abnormalities of uterine action, for example, precipitate delivery (Chapter 33)

Other associated problems may be abnormal tissue elasticity or friability, the presence of tumors, the general condition of the mother (e.g., exhaustion, dehydration), and the presence of complicating diseases. All these factors may exist alone or in combination.

The diagnosis of birth canal lacerations requires (1) an inherent awareness of their possible occurrence and (2) an immediate routine, meticulous inspection of the entire lower birth canal after each delivery. Prerequisites for an adequate appraisal include aseptic technique (the woman for whom labor and birth has been precipitate must be prepared and draped), standard instruments for surgical repair, an assistant to provide exposure by retraction, and appropriate lighting.

Upward displacement of the cervix after its inspection by means of a "tailed" or "tagged" vaginal pack will greatly facilitate the inspection of the entire vaginal tract. Hence lacerations may be seen and repaired, and hematomas may be identified and treated before they reach serious proportions. A vaginal pack also serves to elevate the uterus, enhancing its contractility and limiting blood loss during repair.

Proper anatomic reapproximation of all tissues is performed immediately after delivery for the following reasons:

1. To ensure hemostasis and to prevent hematomas
2. To eliminate open sources of puerperal infection
3. To correct problems (e.g., a poorly repaired old laceration of the rectal sphincter may be revised when increased vascularity and physiologic hypertrophy of pregnancy may favorably influence healing)

Blood replacement and the administration of appropriate antibiotic agents, when indicated, are important. A retention urinary catheter may be required in specific cases.

Labial Lacerations. Extreme vascularity in the labial and periclitoral areas often results in profuse bleeding. Immediate repair, by means of fine (e.g., 4-0) catgut on an atraumatic needle, is required. Counterpressure with a gauze pad and a T binder may be required.

Perineal Lacerations. Lacerations of the perineum are the most common of all injuries in the lower genital tract. These are classified as first, second, third, and fourth degree (see Chapter 19).

An episiotomy may extend to become either a third- or fourth-degree laceration.

The care of the woman who has suffered lacerations of the perineum is similar to that advocated for episiotomies, that is, analgesia as needed for pain, and heat or cold applications as necessary. To avoid injury to the suture line, a woman with third- or fourth-degree lacerations is not given routine postdelivery rectal suppositories or enemas. Attention to diet and intake of fluids is emphasized, as well as oral stool softeners to assist her in reestablishing bowel habits.

Vaginal Lacerations and Hematomas. Prolonged pressure of the fetal head on the vaginal mucosa ultimately will interfere with the circulation and may produce ischemic or pressure necrosis. The state of the tissues, therefore, together with the type of delivery, may result in deep vaginal lacerations and may predispose to vaginal hematomas.

Vaginal hematomas occur more commonly in association with forceps rotation of a fetus in an occipitoposterior (OP) position. They are often found on the same side as the occiput, perhaps because of long-continued pressure of the fetal head in one posterior quadrant of the vagina.

A vaginal hematoma should be diagnosed at the incipient, or early stage. Most hematomas can usually be detected by routine inspection after delivery. Many vaginal hematomas occur beneath the mucosa opposite the ischial spines in the plane of the midpelvis. Therefore the physician will palpate the vaginal walls to detect a full, crepitant, or fluctuant area that may not have become visible. The large masses will be purple, in contrast to the dark red of the remainder of the vaginal mucosa.

Many small hematomas undoubtedly go undetected and may even be self-limiting. Because all hematomas have a small start, the underlying principle of treatment is the prevention of a large hematoma. The sequelae may include tissue devitalization, serious blood loss, shock, and infection.

During the postdelivery period, if the woman complains of persistent perineal pain or a feeling of fullness in the vagina, a careful inspection of the vulva is made. The woman assumes a side-lying position, the upper buttock is raised, and she is asked to bear down. A large purplish mass may be seen at the introitus.

Once the hematoma is diagnosed, treatment is initiated. The woman is returned to the delivery unit, where (after a suitable anesthetic has been administered) the hematoma is incised and evacuated and deep sutures are placed for control of the bleeding.

If the hematoma is larger than 5 cm in diameter, a catheter is placed in the urinary bladder and a moderately tight vaginal pack inserted. A vaginal pack must be inserted carefully to avoid traumatizing the tissues. To facilitate insertion of the pack, an antibiotic ointment may be spread on the pack or applied within the vagina. The catheter and pack may be removed in 6 to 8 hours. Antimicrobial agents for systemic action are not routinely required.

Episiotomy Dehiscence. An episiotomy dehiscence or hematoma in the absence of infection suggests coagulopathy. Abnormal coagulation factors can cause either poor wound healing or bleeding into the tissues. Any surgical procedure should be delayed until routinely available coagulation tests have been performed and results are within normal limits.

Retained Placenta: Nonadherent. The obstetrician must recognize the normal completion of the third stage of labor, or complications may result. If the operator is hasty, for example, the placenta may not have an adequate opportunity to separate. If one waits too long, needless loss of blood may occur.

After birth of the baby but before recovery of the placenta, some women may have only slight bleeding, but others may have considerable blood loss. If no significant bleeding occurs and with proper management, the normally implanted placenta separates with the first or second strong uterine contraction after delivery of the infant. Placental separation occurs within 15 minutes in about 90% of women. Within 30 minutes after birth, an additional 5% of women will have a separated placenta. If one waits 45 minutes after delivery, only another 1% or 2% will achieve placental separation. Hence there is little to be gained by an extended wait-and-see attitude. If the placenta has not been recovered within 30 minutes of delivery, manual removal should be attempted. Administration of oxytocin intravenously (slowly) or intramuscularly immediately after delivery and elevation of the uterus without manual stimulation should aid separation of the placenta and reduce blood loss. If excessive bleeding develops, manual separation and removal of the placenta are carried out immediately.

Some obstetricians practice elective manual separation and extraction of the placenta to expedite the delivery sequence or to avoid abnormal bleeding, for example, after twin delivery. No supplementary anesthesia will be needed for parturients who have had block anesthesia for delivery. For other women, administration of light nitrous oxide and oxygen inhalation anesthesia or IV thiopental (Pentothal) will suffice for intrauterine exploration, placental separation, and recovery of the placenta.

If delivery occurs early (fifth or sixth month), either spontaneously or by induced abortion, placental retention is the rule because of poor separation of the afterbirth (p. 757). This may be caused by an immature zone of separation, weak uterine contractions, or a relatively large placenta.

Retained placenta may be the result of one of the following:

1. Partial separation of a normal placenta.
2. Entrapment of the partially or completely separated placenta by an hourglass constriction ring of the uterus.
3. Mismanagement of the third stage of labor, for example, massage of the uterus (Credé's method) before separation of the placenta or ill-timed administration of ergot products.
4. Abnormal adherence of the entire placenta or a portion of the placenta to the uterine wall.

In all instances postdelivery hemorrhage or infection may be a critical complicating factor.

Because of the possible complications, ergot preparations should be given only *after* recovery of the placenta. They should always be given intramuscularly or orally, never intravenously.

Retained Placenta: Adherent. Abnormal adherence of the placenta occurs for reasons unknown, but it is thought to be the result of zygote implantation in a zone of defective endometrium. Abnormal adherence of the placenta is diagnosed in only about 1 of every 12,000 deliveries. Approximately 90% of the mothers are multiparous, and many of them have also had abortions. The mother with an abnormally attached placenta is jeopardized mainly by postdelivery hemorrhage leading to hypovolemic shock. Firm placental attachment is associated with increased maternal morbidity and mortality. There are no sure signs of an abnormally adherent placenta during pregnancy.

Factors that predispose to abnormally firm placental attachment are (1) scarring of the uterus such as occurs after cesarean delivery, myomectomy, or vigorous curettage; (2) endometritis, associated with tuberculosis; (3) abnormal site of implantation, such as the cervix or lower uterine segment; or (4) malformation of the placenta.

Unusual placental adherence may be partial or complete, and the following degrees of attachment are recognized.

- **Placenta accreta** (vera): slight penetration of myometrium by placental trophoblast (unusual)
- **Placenta increta**: deep penetration by placenta (rare)
- **Placenta percreta** (destruans): perforation of uterus by placenta (exceptional)

More cases of partial than complete placenta accreta occur. At least 15% of cases of abnormally adherent placenta (all types) are associated with placenta previa.

In all types of abnormal adherence, placentation occurs in an area of deficient, sparse, or absent decidua. Thus the placenta develops on a surface partially or completely devoid of decidua (basalis). The uterine muscle is exposed, and invasion of the trophoblast and chorionic villi of the myometrium soon occurs. A dense fibrous area develops, together with hyalinization of neighboring uterine muscle. **There is no zone of separation:** no cleavage plane can be developed between the placenta and the uterine wall. Attempts to remove the placenta in the usual manner are therefore unsuccessful, and laceration or perforation of the uterine wall may result.

Bleeding with complete or total placenta accreta does not occur unless separation of the placenta is attempted. Partial placenta accreta invariably is associated with excessive intranatal or postdelivery bleeding. The reason is that vessels adjacent to the adherent placenta remain open, and free bleeding prevents clotting.

When manual removal of a placenta accreta is attempted, damage to placental tissue and decidua, both rich in thromboplastin, occurs. When this substance is released in quantity into the circulation, DIC may develop.

At vaginal delivery the diagnosis of an abnormally adherent placenta generally is made when manual separation of a retained placenta is attempted. If the placenta will not separate readily (even a portion), immediate abdominal hysterectomy may be indicated. Persistent attempts at placental removal rarely will be successful, and fatal hemorrhage may result.

Placenta accreta or increta usually is diagnosed at cesarean delivery when an abnormally adherent placenta is discovered. In such cases, especially when surgery was indicated because of placenta previa, total hysterectomy may be the best treatment. If the woman wants to have another child and is in good condition, and if hemorrhage can be controlled, the risk of not removing the uterus may be justifiable. Small retained portions of the placenta may separate or be absorbed, but infection often is an added late complication. A second operation may be necessary because of later hemorrhage. After a subsequent viable pregnancy, elective repeat cesarean delivery will be mandatory because another placenta accreta or increta is likely. Delivery should be followed immediately by total abdominal hysterectomy.

Inversion of the Uterus. Inversion of the uterus (turning inside out) after delivery is a critical obstetric complication. The inversion may be complete or partial. Fundal pressure and traction applied to the fundus, especially when the uterus is flaccid, may result in inversion. More specifically, the causes include straining (Valsalva's maneuver); traction on the cord before the placenta has separated; Credé's method, that is, kneading the uterine fundus in an attempt to separate an adherent placenta; and placental extraction under deep relaxing anesthesia. Occasionally a large uterine tumor may be responsible for inversion.

Profound shock follows complete inversion; postdelivery hemorrhage accompanies partial uterine inversion. Prompt assistance is imperative because maternal mortality may reach 30% without immediate corrective therapy.

Prevention—always the easiest, cheapest, and most effective therapy—is especially appropriate in the avoidance of puerperal uterine inversion. **One must not pull on the umbilical cord unless the placenta has definitely separated.** The fundus should never be used as a piston to "push the placenta out." Credé's method is not used; it is harmful and not useful. Regional anesthesia is employed when feasible. An experienced attendant remains with the woman until the uterus is firm and rounded.

Complete inversion of the uterus is obvious; a large, red, rounded mass (perhaps with the placenta attached) protrudes 20 to 30 cm outside the introitus. Incomplete inversion cannot be seen but must be felt; a smooth mass will be palpated through the dilated cervix, reducing the size of the uterine cavity by at least half.

Management of this condition involves all of the following interventions.

1. Combat shock, which invariably is out of proportion to the blood loss. Give oxytocin intravenously to contract the uterus. (Ergot products are strictly contraindicated because the cervix, as well as the uterus, will contract, and replacement of the uterine inversion may be difficult unless the cervix is severed.)

2. Replace the uterus, after the woman is under deep ether or halothane anesthesia, by inserting and "working" first the lower uterine segment and then, finally, the fundus upward while applying traction to the cervix. Leave the placenta attached if it has not yet separated, and then manually free the placenta. Give the oxytocic as ordered. As the uterus and cervix contract, withdraw the placenta with the hand. Pack the uterus if inversion seems about to recur.

3. Abdominal or vaginal surgery may be necessary to reposition the uterus if successful manual replacement fails.

4. Give the woman a transfusion; initiate broad-spectrum antibiotic therapy; and insert a nasogastric tube to decompress the stomach and to minimize adynamic (paralytic) ileus, a frequent sequela.

Successful, prompt vaginal replacement is likely in about 75% of women. Uterine inversion may occasionally recur in a subsequent delivery.

Subinvolution of Uterus. Late postdelivery bleeding may occur as a result of subinvolution of the uterus. Subinvolution is defined as the delayed return of the enlarged puerperal corpus to normal size and function (Pritchard, MacDonald, and Gant, 1985). The causes of subinvolution include reduced circulation because of malposition, myomas, retained products of conception, and infection.

Subinvolution may complicate the puerperium because of such symptoms as pelvic discomfort or backache. There may be signs of abnormality such as leukorrhea or bleeding from an enlarged, boggy, perhaps tender uterus.

In the absence of frank bleeding, treatment is with ergonovine, 0.2 mg/4 hr for 2 or 3 days, antibiotic therapy, and warm acetic douches. With hemorrhage, D and C to remove stained placental secundines and to freshen the placental site for adequate healing generally is required, together with oxytocics and antibiotics.

The woman needs to be instructed to report symptoms to the physician. Although many women experience a short bleeding episode of up to 3 weeks after delivery, prolonged bleeding must be reported. After 3 to 4 weeks, bleeding may be caused by infection or subinvolution of the placental site.

Postdelivery Anterior Pituitary Necrosis

Postdelivery anterior pituitary necrosis (Sheehan's syndrome) follows ischemia as a result of hypovolemic shock and DIC in about 15% of survivors of severe postdelivery hemorrhage. Infarction of much or all of the anterior hypophysis causes partial or total loss of thyroid, adrenocortical, and gonadal functions. The degree of hormonal deficiency depends on the extent of gland destruction.

Women with Sheehan's syndrome fail to lactate and have a decrease in breast size. Loss of axillary and pubic hair, genital atrophy, and amenorrhea are the rule. Such women are apathetic and easily suffer fatigue (Pritchard, MacDonald, and Gant, 1985).

The prognosis of Sheehan's syndrome depends on the degree of residual anterior pituitary function and the supplementary therapy required. Minimum treatment requires

Table 31-8 *Symptoms of Shock*

	Mild	Moderate	Severe	Irreversible
Respirations	Rapid, deep	Rapid, becoming shallow	Rapid, shallow, may be irregular	Irregular, or barely perceptible
Pulse	Rapid, tone normal	Rapid, tone may be normal but is becoming weaker	Very rapid, easily collapsible, may be irregular	Irregular apical pulse
Blood pressure	Normal or hypertensive	60-90 mm Hg systolic	Below 60 mm Hg systolic	None palpable
Skin	Cool and pale	Cool, pale, moist, knees cyanotic	Cold, clammy, cyanosis of lips and fingernails	Cold, clammy, cyanotic
Urinary output	No change	Decreasing to 10-22 ml/hr (adult)	Oliguric (less than 10 ml) to anuric	Anuric
Level of consciousness (LOC)	Alert, oriented, diffuse anxiety	Oriented, mental cloudiness or increasing restlessness	Lethargic, reacts to noxious stimuli, comatose	Does not respond to noxious stimuli
CVP	May be normal (6-12 cm H_2O)	3 cm H_2O	0-3 cm H_2O	

Modified from Royce, JA: Nurs Clin North Am **8**:377, 1973; and Wagner, MM, Clinical Nursing Specialist, University of Iowa Hospitals and Clinics.

thyroid hormone, cortisone, and estrogen replacement. Infertility, reduced resistance to infection, proneness to shock, and premature aging are problems of women with pituitary cachexia.

HEMORRHAGIC SHOCK

Hemorrhage* is a major threat to the mother during the childbearing cycle. Shock may result. Shock is an emergency situation in which the perfusion of body organs may become severely compromised and death may ensue. Vigorous treatment is necessary to prevent adverse sequelae (e.g., cellular death, fluid overload, shock lung, and oxygen toxicity). A brief explanation of the physiologic mechanisms is provided to assist the nurse in implementing appropriate actions.

Physiologic Mechanisms

Physiologic compensatory mechanisms are activated in response to hemorrhage (or other trauma such as cardiac arrest). The adrenals release catecholamines, causing arterioles and venules in the skin, lungs, gastrointestinal tract, liver, and kidney to constrict. The available blood flow is diverted to the brain and heart and away from other organs, including the uterus. If shock is prolonged, the continued reduction in cellular oxygenation results in an accumulation of lactic acid and acidosis (from anaerobic glucose metabolism). Acidosis (lowered serum pH) causes arteriole vasodilation; venule vasoconstriction persists. A circular pattern is established: decreased perfusion, increased tissue anoxia and acidosis, edema formation, and pooling of blood further decrease the perfusion. Cellular death occurs. Table 31-8 is an assessment guide to assist the nurse in the observation and evaluation of the degree of shock.

*For a discussion of bacteremia (septic shock), see Chapter 30.

Management

Nursing Interventions The following nursing interventions for the client in shock should be considered (Royce, 1973):

1. Stay with the woman. Send others to alert the physician and to obtain needed equipment. An emergency cart should be well supplied and available at all times. It should include equipment to start IV fluid, to give oxygen, and to suction, a retention catheter with urinometer, and blood pressure and CVP or PAWP apparatus.
   Nurses should have standing orders to start IV fluids and know the type of infusion fluid to use and laboratory tests to order.
2. While waiting for the physician, the nurse should perform the following procedures:
   a. Insert an airway to facilitate oxygen administration and suction.
   b. Start IV administration of 5% dextrose in water with 0.45% or 0.2% normal saline solution to maintain peripheral vascular circulation.
   c. Elevate the right hip (if woman cannot be in left side-lying position) to avoid supine hypotensive syndrome. *Trendelenburg's position* (with head down and feet elevated) *is not advised.* This position may interfere with cardiac function. Use this position on physician request only.
3. Assist physician in instituting and monitoring measures to increase tissue perfusion. Monitor IV fluids. Too slow a rate (caused by slowing of drip rate or kinking or occlusion of tubing) may be inadequate to dilute blood viscosity or to maintain peripheral circulation. Too rapid

a rate may result in fluid overload and pulmonary edema.

Fluids to increase blood volume include whole fresh blood, plasma, and albumin. Fluids to dilute hemoconcentration (viscosity) are dextrose in water and Ringer's lactated solution.

4. Monitor, assess, and record respirations, pulse, blood pressure, skin condition, urinary output, level of consciousness (LOC), and CVP (Fig. 31-11) to evaluate effectiveness of management:
   a. **Respirations.** The body rids itself of excess acids by increasing the respiratory rate. Ventilatory assistance with oxygen or respirator or both may be needed.
   b. **Pulse.** The pulse rate increases and becomes irregular as shock progresses in severity.
   c. **Blood pressure.** In later stages of shock the systolic pressure decreases.
   d. **Skin.** Perfusion of the skin is sacrificed in the body's attempt to maintain blood flow to the heart and brain. Therefore the condition of the skin is a valuable index to the severity of shock. The nurse assesses the degree of ischemia or cyanosis of the nail beds, eyelids, and skin inside the mouth (buccal mucosa, gums, tongue). The nurse notes the degree of coolness and clamminess.
   e. **Urinary output.** Measure hourly output. Oliguria (50 ml/hr) may indicate worsening of shock or inadequate fluid therapy; an increased output indicates improvement in the woman's condition.
   f. **Level of consciousness.** The adequacy of cerebral perfusion may be estimated by an evaluation of the woman's LOC. In early stages of decreased blood flow the woman may complain of "seeing stars," feeling dizzy, or feeling nauseous. She may become restless and orthopneic. As cerebral hypoxia increases, the woman may become confused and react slowly or not at all to stimuli. An improved sensorium is an indicator of improvement.
   g. **Heart function.***
      (1) CVP: CVP readings measure the function (e.g., blood pressure) of the right side of the heart. Normal values range between 6 and 12 cm H_2O. A low or falling value indicates inadequate blood volume or hypovolemia. A high or rising value indicates impaired contractility of the heart.
      (2) PA catheter: A multiple-lumen pulmonary artery (PA) catheter is used to measure both right- and left-side heart functions.
      (3) PAWP: A PA catheter, when properly placed and when its flexible latex balloon is inflated, is used to measure the pulmonary artery wedge pressure (PAWP), an indicator of left-side heart function.

Anxiety is contagious. The nurse's calm, confident manner, coupled with brief, simple explanations, is an important adjunct to the interventions just discussed.

*Techniques for measuring hemodynamic pressure are beyond the scope of this text. Excellent references are Daily, E: Techniques in bedside hemodynamic monitoring, ed 3 St Louis, 1984, The CV Mosby Co; 1987 Nursing Photobook Annual, Nursing '87 Books, Springhouse Corp, Springhouse, Penn.

HAZARDS OF SHOCK THERAPY

HAZARD	NURSING ACTION
Fluid overload: moist respirations, stridor, or dyspnea	Alert physician, decrease the drip rate
Shock lung: Tachypnea, dyspnea, anxiety, a rise in blood pressure, cyanosis, and harsh loud breaths	Alert physician, maintain ventilator between 50 and 70 mm Hg
Oxygen toxicity: muscular twitching about the face, followed by convulsions resembling grand mal seizures.	Alert physician; take convulsion precautions

Blood Replacement. Common clinical symptomatology of inadequate intravascular volume (hypovolemia) that necessitates *blood replacement* includes the following:

1. Evidence of hemorrhage: loss of a large amount of blood externally or internally in a short period of time
2. Evidence of hypovolemic shock: signs and symptoms of hypotension, weak and rapid pulse, cool clammy skin, rapid breathing, restlessness, reduced urine output
3. Decrease in hemoglobin (Hgb) and hematocrit (Hct) below acceptable level for trimester of pregnancy or the nonpregnant state:

	Hgb	*Hct*
First trimester	≤11 g/dl	≤37%
Second trimester	≤10.5 g/dl	≤35%
Third trimester	≤10 g/dl	≤33%
Non pregnant	≤12 g/dl	≤37%

Hazards of Therapy. The 24 hours after the shock period are critical. Observe for fluid overload, shock lung, and oxygen toxicity (see box above). *Fluid overload* results in pulmonary and peripheral edema. *Shock lung* may develop after the woman receives mechanical ventilatory assistance, especially if the ventilator is not maintained between 50 and 70 mm Hg. Symptomatology follows alveolar capillary damage. *High concentrations of oxygen* are toxic to the adult as well as the newborn. Irritation of mucous membranes of the upper respiratory tract, substernal pain, and cough may occur. Later neurologic symptoms include tinnitus, euphoria, confusion, and respiratory arrest.

Transfusion reactions may follow administration of blood or blood components. Complications include hemolytic reactions, febrile reactions, allergic reactions, circulatory overloading, and air embolism. Rapid transfusion with ice-cold blood can chill the heart and cause arrhythmia or arrest. Disease transmission may occur with transfusion of some blood components. Careful screening has reduced this risk.

A general nursing care plan for hemorrhagic disorders of pregnancy follows.

General Nursing Care Plan

HEMORRHAGIC DISORDERS OF PREGNANCY

ASSESSMENT	NURSING DIAGNOSIS (ND)/ PLAN (P)/GOAL (G)	RATIONALE/ IMPLEMENTATION	EVALUATION
Vital signs and blood pressure. Affect/LOC (agitated, anxious, uncomfortable, dull). Tenderness (uterine, abdominal, cervical, perineal). Integument (color, warmth, moisture, turgor). Time in child-bearing cycle: Prenatal: duration since LMP. Postnatal: duration since delivery. Events preceding symptoms (falls, vaginal examination, coitus, childbirth). Previous obstetric history: past, current. Amount of bleeding, presence and size of clots. Associated discomfort: amount and location (uterine, referred pain, bladder). Passage of tissue. Blood: Rh and blood group, type and crossmatch as necessary; Hgb, Hct; CBC: WBC, platelets. Urine: Pregnancy test if woman suspected of being in early pregnancy; UTI; chest x-ray study if extrapelvic infection is suspected or if surgery is anticipated.	ND: Decreased cardiac output related to hemorrhage. ND: Fluid volume deficit related to hemorrhage. ND: Impaired gas exchange related to hemorrhage or its therapy. ND: Altered cardiopulmonary tissue perfusion related to hemorrhage. ND: Fluid volume excess related to blood or fluid replacement. ND: Potential for injury related to infection or excessive volume loss. ND: Pain. P: Monitor closely, or provide information, and be available to discuss concerns. G: The client will remain physiologically safe as indicated by: a. Vital signs stabilized within normal limits b. Hemodynamic stability c. Absence of infection d. Absence of pain	*To identify hemorrhage and treat appropriately, the nurse will:* Report and record findings promptly. Monitor vital signs, blood pressure, LOC, CVP, integument. Save all peripads, linens soaked with blood, clots, and tissue. Start IV infusion using large bore catheter in the event blood transfusion is needed. Hang appropriate blood product. Administer medications as ordered, (analgesics, oxytocics, antibiotics). Obtain specimen collection, (blood, urine, culture). Insert retention urine catheter. Provide preoperative and postoperative care as needed, including medications, oxygen; keep woman and family informed. Give Rh_o (D) immune globulin, if indicated (Chapter 40).	Woman's blood loss is minimized. Vitals signs are stablized within normal limits. Complications of blood, fluid, and electrolyte replacement are averted. Fluid and electrolyte balance is maintained. Woman's reproductive capability is maintained. Surgical intervention is successful with no adverse sequelae. Comfort is maximized. Client remains free from infection. Fetus/newborn suffers no sequelae related to maternal condition.
Assess woman's learning needs in regard to hemorrhage, its management, and complications.	ND: Knowledge deficit related to identification of and care during a hemorrhagic disorder. P: Provide information and be available to discuss concerns and questions. G: Woman will be instructed about her condition and its management. G: Woman will learn the danger signals of hemorrhage.	*To teach the woman about hemorrhage, its management and complications, the nurse will:* Carefully explain known causes, management, and expected outcomes. Assist in identifying questions for the physician. Teach woman about danger signs and symptoms (bleeding, fever, cramping, pain) and whom to call should they occur. Counsel regarding antibiotic	Woman and family verbalize understanding of the condition and its management. Woman identifies danger signals and whom to notify.

Continued.

General Nursing Care Plan—cont'd

ASSESSMENT	NURSING DIAGNOSIS (ND)/ PLAN (P)/GOAL (G)	RATIONALE/ IMPLEMENTATION	EVALUATION
	G: Woman will learn the signs and symptoms of infection.	therapy. Counsel regarding nutrition to prevent anemia. Provide information regarding contraceptives as appropriate. Refer to social services (home health care, home service, etc.).	
Assess for previous experience with loss and positive coping mechanisms utilized. Assess support system. Assess current emotional status of woman. Identify spiritual needs for clergy to be present as support or to baptize fetus or newborn.	ND: Anxiety related to actual or potential loss. ND: Body image disturbance, personal identity disturbance, situational low self-esteem, altered role performance. ND: Ineffective individual or family coping related to loss and grief. ND: Powerlessness related to loss or grief. ND: Spiritual distress related to loss or guilt. P: Provide information and be available to discuss concerns and questions. G: Woman and family will accept a loss in a positive manner (Chapter 28). G: Guilt or blame will be averted. G: Self-concept will not be disturbed. G: Spiritual distress will be averted. G: Sense of power will be retained (participates in own care).	*To help woman and family with the experience of loss and initiate the grieving process, the nurse will:* Explain procedures, sensations, expected outcomes; answer questions. Involve family in planning and care. Encourage verbalization of concerns and feelings. Assist woman and family with emotional reactions. Implement care of woman and family experiencing perinatal loss (Chapter 28.) Explain the grief process. Give couples the opportunity to see fetus or inform them of sex. Baptize products of conception or newborn, or summon clergy if requested.	Woman verbalizes understanding of condition and its management. Woman identifies support system. Woman initiates grief process.
Disseminated intravascular coagulation (DIC) Predisposing factors: Retained dead fetus. Infection. PIH. Abruptio placenta. Amniotic fluid embolism. Signs: Spontaneous bleeding (e.g., from gums, nose). Excessive bleeding from site of slight trauma. Reduced laboratory values for platelets, fibrinogen, proaccelerin, antihemophilic factor, and prothrombin.	ND: Anxiety, fear, pain, ineffective individual coping related to signs and symptoms of DIC. ND: Knowledge deficit related to DIC, its causes and management. ND: Fluid volume deficit or excess related to DIC or its management. ND: Altered (cardiopulmonary) tissue perfusion and injury related to DIC. P: Continuous assessment for risk factors and symptomatology and rapid identification and initiation of therapy.	*To implement therapy the nurse will:* Assist physician with treatment or removal of predisposing factors: a. Deliver dead fetus. b. Treat existing infection or PIH. c. Deliver fetus and abrupted placenta. Establish management of hemorrhagic shock or bacteremic shock (Chapter 30). Replace clotting factors (Table 31-7). Assist with treatment of sequelae.	The woman survives the disease with minimum or no damage to body organs or systems. The woman's blood-clotting mechanism returns to normal. The woman and her family understand the disease process and its management. The newborn survives with no adverse sequelae.

General Nursing Care Plan—cont'd

ASSESSMENT	NURSING DIAGNOSIS (ND)/ PLAN (P)/GOAL (G)	RATIONALE/ IMPLEMENTATION	EVALUATION
Ecchymoses (sudden tachycardia, diaphoresis, or restlessness with anxiety). Occurrence of sequelae: Acute renal failure. Pituitary insufficiency (Sheehan's syndrome).	G: For the mother: prompt identification and appropriate therapy to prevent serious sequelae to hemorrhage or its therapy. G: For the fetus or newborn: prevention of hypoxia. G: For the family: a healthy mother and newborn.		

SUMMARY

Bleeding disorders of mother are medical emergencies that demand expert teamwork on the part of the health-care team if negative outcomes are to be avoided. The nurse must be able to assist the physician in minimizing blood loss, analyzing assessment findings to arrive at a correct diagnosis, and implement appropriate actions to maintain the pregnancy where possible, and provide the emergency care needed for both mother and baby. Additionally, the reactions of the woman and her family need to be considered. Anxiety, grief, and altered self-concept can result from fetal or maternal loss.

KEY CONCEPTS

- Blood loss during pregnancy should always be regarded as a danger sign until ruled out by the woman's physician.
- Many spontaneous abortions occur for unknown reasons, but fetoplacental maldevelopment and maternal factors can account for others.
- The type of spontaneous abortion directs the management.
- Ectopic pregnancy is a significant cause of maternal morbidity and mortality even in developed countries.
- There are two distinctive types of H. mole: complete and partial.
- Premature separation of the placenta and placenta previa are differentiated by type of bleeding, uterine tonicity, and presence or absence of pain.
- Clotting disorders are associated with many obstetric complications.
- External fundal pressure and traction on the umbilical cord before placental separation can result in inversion of the uterus.
- Postdelivery hemorrhage is the most common and most serious type of excessive obstetric blood loss.
- Hemorrhagic (hypovolemic) shock is an emergency situation in which the perfusion of body organs may become severely compromised and death may ensue.
- The potential hazards of therapeutic interventions may further compromise the woman experiencing hemorrhagic disorders.

STUDY QUESTIONS AND ACTIVITIES

1. View and discuss a film on obstetric hemorrhage or interview women who have recovered from hemorrhagic disorders. In group discussion, examine reactions to these disorders and the implications for effective nursing care.
2. In small groups, role-play the interaction between the nurse and a client being treated for a molar pregnancy. Present these interactions before other students or videotape the role-play for critiquing.
3. Work with a nurse caring for a client being treated for a severe hemorrhagic disorder. Prepare a care plan based on the nursing diagnoses and discuss the client's needs in group discussion.
4. Role-play a nurse caring for each of the following clients:
   a. A 22-year-old unmarried woman threatened with the loss of her first pregnancy at 14 weeks.
   b. A 35-year-old mother of twins who lost 1500 ml of blood at the time of delivery.
   c. A 28-year-old woman whose second pregnancy is complicated by a suspected placenta previa.
   d. A 42-year-old primigravida admitted at 34 weeks with possible abruptio placentae. She has a history of cocaine use.

References

Acker, D, et al: Abruptio placentae associated with cocaine use, Am J Obstet Gynecol 146:220, 1983

Athey, PA, and Hadlock, FP: Ultrasound in obstetrics and gynecology, St Louis, 1981, The CV Mosby Co

Bingol, N: Teratogenicity of cocaine in humans, J Pediatr 110:93, 1987 (In JAMA 257(13):1806, 1987)

Cocaine use linked to infant defects, San Francisco Chronicle, Jan 19, 1987

Cole, HM, editor: Cardiovascular effects of cocaine, JAMA 257(7):979, 1987
Danforth, DN, and Scott, JR, editors: Obstetric and gynecology, ed 5, Philadelphia, 1986, JB Lippincott Co
de Crespigny, LC: The value of ultrasound in ectopic pregnancy, Clin Obstet Gynecol 30(1):136, 1987
DePetrillo, AD, et al: Symposium: gestational trophoblastic disease: an update, Contemp OB/GYN 29(1):199, 1987
Diamond, MP, and DeCherney, AH: Surgical techniques in the management of ectopic pregnancy, Clin Obstet Gynecol 30(1):200, 1987
Pritchard, JA, MacDonald, PC, and Gant, NF: Williams obstetrics, ed 17, Norwalk, Conn, 1985, Appleton-Century-Crofts
Queenan, JT, and Hobbin, JC, editors: Protocols for high-risk pregnancies, Oradell, NJ, 1982, Medical Economics Books
Rigby, PG: Bleeding: symposium on bleeding disorders in pregnancy, Am J Obstet Gynecol 156(6):1422, 1987
Royce, JA: Shock emergency nursing implications, Nurs Clin North Am 8:377, 1973
Silver, R, et al: Placenta previa: aggressive expectant management, Am J Obstet Gynecol 150:15, 1984
Szulman, AE: Syndromes of hydatidiform moles, J Reprod Med 29:788, 1984
Woods, JR, Plessinger, MA, and Clark, KE: Effect of cocaine on uterine blood flow and fetal oxygenation, JAMA 257(7):957, 1987

Bibliography

Andrinopoulos, GC, and Mendenhall, HW: Prostaglandin $F_2\alpha$ in the management of delayed post-partum hemorrhage, Am J Obstet Gynecol 146:217, 1983
Appelman, Z, and Golbus, MS: Screening for hemoglobinopathies before delivery, Contemp OB/GYN 27:129, April 1986
Brabeck, MC: Ambulatory management of thromboembolic disease during pregnancy with continuous infusion of heparin, JAMA 257(13):1790, 1987
Benson, RC, editor: Current obstetric and gynecologic diagnosis and treatment, ed 3, Los Altos, Calif, 1980, Lange Medical Books
Berkowitz, RS, and Goldstein, DP: Complications of molar pregnancy, Contemp OB/GYN 24:57, 1984
Celeste, SM, and Smith, MD: Gestational trophoblastic neoplasms, JOGN Nurs 15:11, Jan/Feb 1986
Clark, SL, and Phelan, JP: Surgical control of obstetrical hemorrhage, Contemp OB/GYN 24:70, 1984
Crombleholme, WR: Cerclage in managing fetal wastage, USCF Antepartum and intrapartum management conference, p 174, June 1987
Cyganski, JM, Donahue, JM, and Heaton, JS: The case for the heparin flush, Am J Nurs 87(6):796, 1987
DeVore, N, and Baldwin, K: Ectopic pregnancy on the rise, Am J Nurs 86(6):674, 1986
Dimarchi, JM, Kobara, TY, and Kosasa, TS: A new problem: persistent ectopic pregnancy, Contemp OB/GYN 29(1):37, 1987
Douching: Am Fam Physician 35:376, March 1987
Dreyfus, TM, et al: Management of immune thrombocytopenia in pregnancy: response to infusions of immunoglobins, Am J Obstet Gynecol 148:225, 1984
Droegemueller, W, et al: Comprehensive gynecology, St Louis, 1987, The CV Mosby Co
Duff, P: Defusing the dangers of amniotic fluid embolism, Contemp OB/GYN 24:127, 1984
Dunn, DL, and Lenihan, SF: The case for the saline flush, Am J Nurs 87(6):798, 1987
Few, BJ: Prostaglandin F_2 for treating severe postpartum hemorrhage, MCN 12(3):169, 1987
Flint, C: Postpartum haemorrhage at home, Nurs Times, 84(3):47, 1988
Gardeyi, N: Cardiovascular effects of cocaine, JAMA 257(7): 979, 1987
Gordon, RT: Emergencies in obstetrics and gynecology. In Warner, CG, editor: Emergency care: assessment and intervention, ed 3, St Louis, 1983, The CV Mosby Co
Gunning, JE: For controlling intractable hemorrhage: the gravity suit, Contemp OB/GYN 22:22, July, 1983
Hayashi, RH: Heading off disaster in postpartum hemorrhage, Contemp OB/GYN 20:90, 1982
Higgins, SD: Essentials of fluid resuscitation and blood transfusion, Contemp OB/GYN 24:102, 1984
Huff, RW: How to handle third-trimester bleeding, Contemp OB/GYN 20:39, 1982
Jennings, BM: Improving your management of DIC, Nurs '79 9(5):60, 1979
Kuczynski, JJ: Support for the women with an ectopic pregnancy, JOGN Nurs 15(4):306, 1986
Marchbanks, PA, et al: Risk factors for ectopic pregnancy: a population-based study, JAMA, 259(12):1823, 1988
Miller, D: Tips on drawing blood through a heparin lock, RN, p 22, July 1986
Mims, BC: The risks of oxygen therapy, RN, p 20, July 1987
Ney, PG: Helping patients cope with pregnancy loss, Contemp OB/GYN 29(6):117, 1987
Nursing '87 Books: 1987 nursing photobook annual, Springhouse, Penn, 1987, Springhouse Corp
Osguthorpe, NC: Ectopic pregnancy, JOGN Nurs 16(1):36, 1987
Peck, NL: Action stat! Blood transfusion reaction, Nurs '87 17(1):33, 1987
Pelosi, MA, and Apuzzio, J: Surgical management of abdominal pregnancy, Contemp OB/GYN 31(1):144, 1988
Problem-patient conference: habitual aborters, Contemp OB/GYN 27:147, Feb 1986
Purcell, JA: Shock drugs: standardized guidelines, Am J Nurs 82:965, 1982
Querin, JJ, and Stahl, LD: Twelve simple, sensible steps for successful blood transfusions, Nurs '83 13(11):34, 1983
Siskind, J: Handling hemorrhage wisely, Nurs '84 14(1):34, 1984
Strickland, DM, et al: Hypofibrinogenemia as a cause of delayed post-partum hemorrhage, Am J Obstet Gynecol 143:230, 1982
Wall-Haas, CL: Women's perceptions of first trimester spontaneous abortion, JOGN Nurs 14:50, Jan/Feb 1985
Weckstein, LN, Masserman, JS, and Garite, TJ: Placenta accreta: a problem of increasing clinical significance, Obstet Gynecol 69(3):480, 1984
Woods, JR, Plessinger, MA, and Clark, KE: Effect of cocaine on uterine blood flow and fetal oxygenation, JAMA 257(7): 957, 1987

CHAPTER 32

Endocrine and Metabolic Disorders

Learning Objectives

Correctly define the key terms listed.

Differentiate diabetes mellitus types I, II, III, and IV and their respective risk factors in pregnancy.

Summarize the effects of pregnancy on insulin requirements.

Review assessment as it relates to: history and interview, physical examination, fetal surveillance, and laboratory tests.

Formulate nursing diagnoses relevant to assessment data common to many gravidas whose pregnancies are complicated by diabetes mellitus.

Discuss planning and setting goals when the pregnancy is complicated by diabetes mellitus.

Explain nursing interventions implemented when diabetes complicates pregnancy.

Discuss evaluation of nursing care when the pregnancy is complicated by diabetes mellitus.

Assess the significance of hyperemesis gravidarum.

Explain effects of disorders of the thyroid and adrenal glands on pregnancy.

List the effects of maternal phenylketonuria (PKU) on pregnancy.

Key Terms

Addison's disease
diabetes mellitus
hydramnios
hyperadrenocorticism
hyperemesis gravidarum
hyperthyroidism
hypothyroidism
gestational diabetes mellitus
glucose tolerance test
glycemia
euglycemia
hyperglycemia
hypoglycemia
glycohemoglobin (HbA_{1c})
insulin
large for gestational age (LGA)
macrosomia
maternal phenylketonuria (PKU)

DIABETES MELLITUS

Preexisting diabetes mellitus as a complication of pregnancy was a rare occurrence before the discovery of insulin. Before insulin therapy was available, most diabetic girls died before or during puberty; many were amenorrheic and therefore infertile or sterile. When pregnancy did occur, the maternal mortality was 25%; fetal-neonatal loss was 50%. Today, techniques such as home glucose monitoring, multiple doses or constant infusion of insulin, and dietary counseling (American Diabetes Association, 1987) are being used to create a normal intrauterine environment for fetal growth and maturation. These therapeutic modalities most often result in the delivery of an infant who is structurally and physiologically normal (Gabbe, 1985). Such measures have also proved a significant benefit to the mother, providing her with techniques that enable her to be an active participant in her care and remain outside the hospital. If she continues to follow this regimen after she has delivered her child, she may reduce long-term morbidity from diabetes mellitus.

Classification. Following is the 1979 classification of diabetes mellitus issued by the National Diabetes Data Group.

type I diabetes mellitus Formerly called juvenile-onset diabetes or insulin-dependent diabetes; onset in people 40 years or *younger;* etiology: genetic, immunologic, viral. Prone to ketosis.

type II diabetes mellitus Formerly called maturity-onset diabetes or non-insulin-dependent diabetes; occurs in all ages, but more usual in the older, overweight person; etiology: primarily genetic. Resistant to ketosis. In pregnancy, insulin is required to control maternal plasma glucose levels (Hollingsworth, 1985).

type III diabetes mellitus Formerly called gestational diabetes; intolerance to glucose with onset during pregnancy with return to normal glucose tolerance after delivery.

type IV diabetes mellitus Formerly called secondary diabetes; refers to abnormalities in glucose tolerance following pancreatic disease, endocrine disorders (Cushing's syndrome), drug ingestion (oral contraceptives), cirrhosis, and the like.

hyperglycemia Blood levels of glucose that exceed normal values.

White's classification of pregnant diabetic women (1978) considers age at onset, duration, and vascular or renal changes, if any (Table 32-1). Although even mild forms of diabetes pose a threat to mother and infant, the incidence of perinatal death increases with the presence and degree of vascular or renal pathologic changes (classes, D, E, and F).

Incidence. Diabetes mellitus is a complication in about 1% to 2% of pregnant women. It has been found that one in four families has a history of diabetes. The incidence of diabetes mellitus increases with age. About 3.8 in every 100 women will become diabetic. Many of these cases will be diagnosed during pregnancy. As many as 35% to 50% of women who exhibit gestational diabetes will show further deterioration of carbohydrate metabolism during the next 15 years of life (Danforth and Scott, 1986).

Pathogenesis. Diabetes mellitus (types I, II and III) is regarded primarily as a genetically determined syndrome. It is usually inherited as a recessive trait but occurs as a dominant trait in some families. If the β-cells of the islets of Langerhans (pancreas) are deficient either in number or in function, the production of endogenous insulin falls short of the need. As a result, glucose is poorly used, and abnormalities of carbohydrate, protein, and fat metabolism appear. The italicized words in the following paragraph are the four cardinal signs and symptoms of diabetes mellitus.

Insulin lowers blood glucose levels by enabling glucose to enter muscle and adipose cells where it is used for energy. When glucose is poorly used it accumulates in the blood **(hyperglycemia)**. This results in a hyperosmolarity of the blood. The body compensates by attempting to dilute the heavy concentration of carbohydrate by transferring fluids from the cellular and interstitial compartments into the vascular compartment. Thus the person becomes **dehydrated** at the cellular and tissue level while having an excess volume in the vascular compartment. The kidneys then function to excrete large volumes of urine *(polyuria)* in an attempt to regulate the excess vascular volume and to excrete the unusable glucose. Hypertonic glucose serves as a diuretic and results in even more body dehydration with excessive thirst *(polydipsia)*.

The body compensates for its inability to convert carbohydrate into energy by burning proteins (muscle) and fats. Unfortunately the end products of this metabolism are ketones and fatty acids, which in excess quantity produce **acidosis** and **acetonuria**. *Weight loss* occurs in the presence of excessive hunger *(polyphagia)*.

Inheritance of the genetic trait (genotype) for diabetes mellitus does not necessarily mean that the individual will demonstrate diabetic glucose intolerance (phenotype). Many people with the genotype do not show any evidence of diabetes until they experience one or more of a variety of **precipitating factors**. Examples of such stressors include an increase in age, normal developmental periods of rapid hormonal change (menarche, pregnancy, and menopause), obesity, infection, surgery, emotional factors, and tumor or infection of the pancreas (may damage the β-cells so that diabetes occurs secondary to the trauma).

Effects of Pregnancy on Insulin Requirements

First Trimester. During the first trimester the developing embryo-fetus siphons (moves by active transport) glucose across the placenta from the mother. This gestational period is characterized by nausea, vomiting, and often, decreased food intake by the mother while glucose use by the embryo-fetus increases. As maternal glucose is used by the fetus, the maternal glucose level drops, thereby decreasing the need for insulin (Fig. 32-1, *A* to *B*). **Maternal insulin does not cross the placenta.** By the eighth week of gestation the conceptus secretes her or his own insulin at levels adequate to use the glucose obtained from the mother.

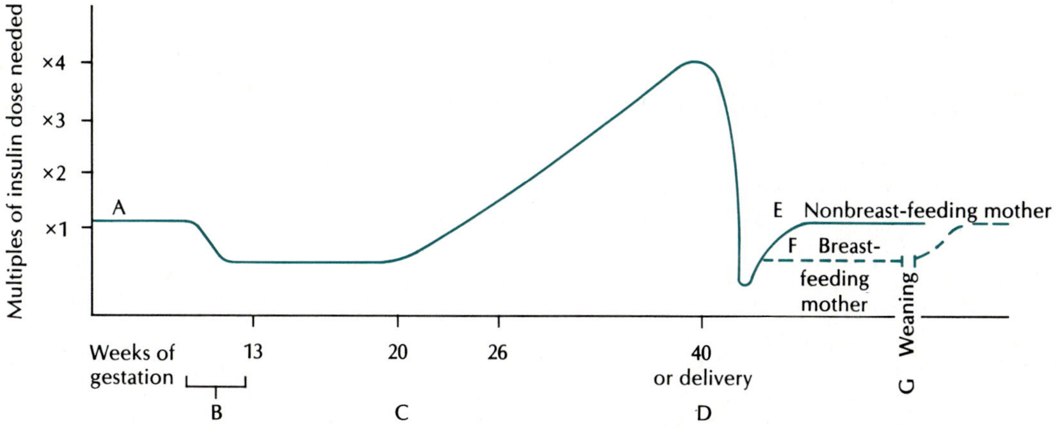

Fig. 32-1 Changing insulin needs during pregnancy caused by properties of placental hormones and enzyme (insulinase) and cortisol.

Second and Third Trimesters. The development of maternal resistance to insulin keeps pace with the increasing levels of placental hormones (especially hPL), insulinase, and cortisol. Insulin resistance is a glucose-sparing mechanism that assures an abundant supply of glucose to the fetus. The mother's need for insulin increases beginning in the second trimester. Insulin requirements may double or quadruple by term gestation (Fig. 32-1, *C* to *D*).

Puerperium. Delivery of the placenta brings about an abrupt drop in levels of circulating placental hormones, insulinase, and cortisol. Maternal tissues quickly regain their prepregnancy sensitivity to insulin. For the nonbreast-feeding mother, prepregnancy insulin-carbohydrate balance usually returns in about 7 to 10 days (Fig. 32-1, *E*). Lactation utilizes maternal glucose, so that the breast-feeding mother's insulin requirements will remain low for up to 6 to 9 months (Fig. 32-1, *F*). Upon completion of weaning, prepregnancy insulin requirement is reestablished (Fig. 32-1, *G*).

Effects of Pregnancy on Diabetes Mellitus

Diabetic control is affected by the pregnancy-induced changes in insulin requirements. Nausea, vomiting, and cravings result in dietary fluctuations. Diabetes-related macrovascular and microvascular disease may progress. Whether pregnancy worsens long-term renal function in women with diabetic nephropathy is a matter of controversy (Nesler et al., 1985). There is little information concerning the effects of pregnancy and the prognosis in women with diabetic cardiomyopathy (Nesler et al., 1985). Whether pregnancy effects retinopathy in the diabetic patient or intensifies the progression of established retinopathy is also a matter of controversy (Kitzmiller, Aiello, Kaldany, and Younger, 1981; Klein et al., 1984; Sinclair, Nesler, and Schwartz, 1985). Maintaining euglycemia, adequate bed rest, and control of hypertension is essential (Jovanovic and Jovanovic, 1984).

Programs instituting care *before* pregnancy, as well as supervision throughout pregnancy, are associated with the best outcomes for the woman and the fetus (Mennuti, 1985).

Effects of Diabetes Mellitus on Pregnancy

Conditions associated with diabetes increase maternal morbidity and mortality. Associated conditions vary slightly with the class of diabetes. In the presence of mild diabetes (classes A to C and glucose intolerance of pregnancy), in which there *is no* associated vascular disease, there is a greater incidence of intensification of preexisting diabetic condition, pregnancy-induced hypertension (PIH; preeclampsia), hydramnios, intranatal fetal death, macrosomia (large for gestational age [LGA]), and large placenta.

In the presence of more advanced diabetes (classes E to F), in which there *is associated vascular disease,* there is a greater incidence of spontaneous abortions, intrauterine growth retardation (IUGR) (small for gestational age [SGA]), and intrauterine fetal deaths and neonatal deaths. Complications associated with mild diabetes (above) occur less commonly.

Insulin dosage per day does not reflect the severity of diabetes. The age of onset and the duration of diabetes are more important to pregnancy outcome.

Infections. Infections are much more common and serious in diabetic women who are pregnant (e.g., pyelonephritis, monilial vaginitis). Disorders in carbohydrate metabolism alter the body's normal resistance to infection. The inflammatory response, leukocyte function, and vaginal pH are all affected. Pregnancy changes predispose any woman to urinary tract infection (UTI). Infection results in increased insulin resistance and ketoacidosis. Unless recognized and treated promptly, ketoacidosis adversely affects the fetus. Ketoacidosis is poorly tolerated by the fetus. Fetal death may occur.

Vascular Damage. The severity of preeclampsia (occurring in 10% to 20% of pregnant diabetic women) is associated directly with the degree of renal vascular involve-

Table 32-1 *Classification of Diabetes During Pregnancy (Priscilla White)*

Class	Characteristics	Implications
Glucose intolerance of pregnancy	Erroneously known as gestational diabetes. Abnormal glucose tolerance during pregnancy; postprandial hyperglycemia during pregnancy.	Diagnosis before 30 weeks' gestation important to prevent macrosomia. Treat with diet adequate in calories to prevent maternal weight loss. Goal is postprandial blood glucose <130 mg/dl at 1 hour, or <105 mg/dl at 2 hours. If insulin is necessary, manage as in classes B, C, and D.
A	Chemical diabetes diagnosed before pregnancy; managed by diet alone: any age at onset.	Management as for glucose intolerance of pregnancy.
B	Insulin treatment used before pregnancy; onset at age 20 or older; duration < 10 years.	Some endogenous insulin secretion may persist. Fetal and neonatal risks same as in classes C and D, as is management.
C	Onset at age 10-20, or duration 10-20 years.	Insulin-deficient diabetes of juvenile onset.
D	Onset before age 10, or duration > 20 years, or chronic hypertension (not preeclampsia), or background retinopathy (tiny hemorrhages).	Fetal macrosomia or intrauterine growth retardation possible. Retinal microaneurysms; dot hemorrhages, and exudates may progress during pregnancy, then regress after delivery.
F	Diabetic nephropathy with proteinuria.	Anemia and hypertension common; proteinuria increases in third trimester, declines after delivery. Fetal intrauterine growth retardation common; perinatal survival about 85% under optimum conditions; bed rest necessary.
H	Coronary artery disease.	Serious maternal risk.
R	Proliferative retinopathy.	Neovascularization, with risk of vitreous hemorrhage or retinal detachment; laser photocoagulation useful; abortion usually not necessary. With active process of neovascularization, prevent bearing-down efforts.

From Benson, RC, editor: Current obstetric and gynecologic diagnosis and treatment, ed 5, Los Altos, Calif, 1984, Lange Medical Publications.

ment. Severe vascular involvement results in deterioration of the placenta and IUGR or death, the need to deliver the baby prematurely because of the risk to the mother in continuing the pregnancy, and possible abruptio placentae (premature separation of the normally implanted placenta, Chapter 31).

Effects of Diabetes Mellitus on Labor and Delivery: Dystocia

Hydramnios. Hydramnios (polyhydramnios) occurs about 10 times as often in pregnancies of diabetic women as in pregnancies of nondiabetic women. Hydramnios (amniotic fluid in excess of 2000 ml) increases the possibility of compression of abdominal blood vessels (vena cava and aorta), causing supine hypotension. Hydramnios also causes maternal dyspnea because of upward pressure on the diaphragm. Hydramnios is associated with premature labor, perhaps because of overstretching of the uterus, and with dystocia (difficult labor and delivery).

Macrosomia. There is a greater likelihood of large fetuses (macrosomia). Large fetuses are associated with dystocia (Chapter 33), often resulting in operative vaginal delivery (episiotomy and forceps), trauma to the mother's soft tissues or to the baby, and cesarean delivery.

Prognosis

The outcome for both the mother and her child from the embryo stage through birth is determined in large measure by the degree to which diabetes is controlled. If there are no complications of pregnancy, and diabetes is well controlled, mortality for the woman with diabetes is about the same as that for any other woman. The infant from a pregnancy complicated by diabetes mellitus is discussed in Chapter 38.

Perinatal mortality increases threefold to fourfold for the diabetic woman who experiences any of the following conditions: pyelonephritis, severe acidosis, PIH, and poor diabetic control (sometimes because of poor compliance by the woman). Perinatal mortality of 50% follows an acute onset of hydramnios or a rapid drop in insulin requirements.

In the woman who experiences glucose intolerance of

pregnancy the glucose tolerance test (GTT) results typically return to within normal range 3 to 5 weeks after delivery.

Assessment

History and Interview. Early identification of glucose intolerance in a woman is essential so that prompt appropriate therapy can be initiated. Factors in a woman's ***history*** that are associated with the risk of glucose intolerance of pregnancy include:

1. Family history of diabetes (first-degree relatives only [i.e., parents, siblings])
2. Poor obstetric history (e.g., spontaneous abortion, unexplained stillbirth, hydramnois, unexplained prematurity or low birth weight)
3. Previous birth of a newborn weighing 4000 g (8 lb 13½ oz) or more
4. Previous birth of a newborn with major congenital anomalies
5. High parity (5 or more) (Hollingsworth, 1985)

These historical risk factors would be unlikely to reveal the likelihood of glucose intolerance during a first pregnancy. Over one third of cases of glucose intolerance of pregnancy in one population were missed when historical risk factors were used in choosing gravidas for laboratory testing. Since emotional stress is a precipitating factor, family and socioeconomic events are reviewed.

Accurate estimation of gestational age is essential (Chapter 12). Fetal growth is evaluated against normal expectations per dates.

Physical Examination. Findings in the current pregnancy that alert the health care team to the possibility of diabetes (in the absence of a previous diagnosis of the condition) include maternal age of 25 years or older, obesity (weight of 90.7 kg [200 lb] or more), recurrent monilial (*Candida albicans* or "yeast") vaginitis that is not responding to therapy, and glycosuria.

Hydramnios and a large fetus palpated during Leopold's maneuvers warrant further assessment. Women with PIH (Chapter 29) should be assessed for diabetes mellitus. A retinal examination should be done routinely for all gravidas for retinopathy of diabetes and also for changes that may occur with PIH.

If the gravida is an insulin-dependent diabetic, her skin is examined for damage at injection sites. Capillary filling time is assessed, especially in the lower extremities.

Fetal Surveillance. Diagnostic techniques for fetal surveillance (Chapter 27) are often ordered for the woman whose pregnancy is complicated by diabetes mellitus. Ultrasonography reveals progress of growth and presence of congenital malformations (e.g., caudal regression syndrome). Maternal blood and urine estriol measurement by radioimmunoassay (RIA) reflects the combined function of the placenta and fetus, as well as the clearance of estriol conjugates by the maternal system. The advent of RIA technology specific for unconjugated estriol in maternal plasma, which is about 10% of the total circulating compound, provides a measure of fetoplacental function independent of maternal renal or hepatic function (Golde and Platt, 1985). Difficulties with this test plus other technologic developments in diagnosis and management have led many physicians to abandon estriol monitoring.

Biochemical analysis of amniotic fluid is done to ascertain fetal lung maturity and congenital malformations (Chapter 27). Since the frequency of neural tube defects in infants of diabetic mothers is more than 10 times that of the general population (Milunsky, Alpert, Kitzmiller, et al., 1982), all gravidas with overt diabetes should be offered serum α-fetoprotein (AFP) testing (Mennuti, 1985). Another diabetes-associated anomaly, renal agenesis, may result in elevated maternal serum AFP.

The diagnosis of imperforate anus accompanying the caudal regression syndrome or as an isolated defect may be confirmed by measurement of intestinal enzymes, such as alkaline phosphatase in the amniotic fluid before 24 weeks' gestation (Mullivor, Mennuti, and Harris, 1979).

Biophysical monitoring is also employed (Chapter 27). Nonstress test (NST), contraction stress test (CST), daily fetal movement count, and biophysical profile are used to expand the data base for assessment. Cardiac anomalies may be reasonably assessed by routine fetal echocardiography (Kleinman, 1982).

Data from all these tests discern some fetuses in jeopardy in pregnancies complicated by diabetes. The specific value of any one test is more difficult to discern. Evidence supports *glucose normalization* as the key to improved perinatal survival (Golde and Platt, 1985).

Determination of Delivery Date for Diabetic Mother. The best time for delivery of the infant is when the intrauterine environment is not yet overwhelmingly hazardous and the fetus has developed sufficiently to exist outside of the uterus. The delivery date (by cesarean delivery or by induction) for the fetus in jeopardy is commonly chosen on the basis of statistics of perinatal mortality: at 32 to 34 weeks there is a 19% mortality, primarily related to hazards of prematurity; **at 36 weeks the mortality is the lowest**, at 11%; and at 37 to 40 weeks, the mortality is the highest, at 26%, primarily because of intrauterine death from acidosis or placental insufficiency. It is unclear whether the placenta is inadequate to meet the nurturing needs of the oversized infant or whether diabetes-induced vascular changes contribute to placental dysfunction.

Improved methods for maintaining glucose levels within the normal range have improved fetal prognosis. Risk management has allowed more women to enter spontaneous labor at term, thereby reducing the need for antepartum assessment of fetal maturity (Golde and Platt, 1985).

Laboratory Tests. Glycosuria can be diagnosed with Tes-Tape or Clinistix. Both of these depend on enzyme reactions *specific for glucose,* not to be confused with fructosuria and lactosuria.

Laboratory tests are required to establish the diagnosis of diabetes mellitus. Two types of laboratory tests are available: tests to identify levels of glucose in blood or plasma (Table 32-2) and a test to determine the percent of normal adult hemoglobin (HbA) that is glycosylated (HbA_{1c}). Some physicians suggest that *all* pregnant women should be screened for plasma glucose using the 50 g, *1-hour glucose screen* during the first prenatal visit. Coustan and Carpenter (1985) believe the most efficient time to perform this test is at 24 to 26 weeks' gestation. Most clinical laboratories

Table 32-2 *Blood Tests for Diabetes Mellitus in Pregnancy*

Test	Instructions	Technique	Findings	Precautions
Fasting blood sugar (FBS): measures amount of glucose in blood when woman is fasting	No food for 12 hr before test, e.g., 8 PM to 8 AM; water is only fluid allowed	Blood drawn by venipuncture and sent to laboratory	Normal: 80-120 mg/dl serum Abnormal: ≥140 mg/dl on 2 occasions, diagnostic of diabetes mellitus	None
Postprandial blood sugar: measures blood sugar following meal	None	Woman eats meal containing 100 g of carbohydrate; blood drawn by venipuncture 2 hr after meal and sent to laboratory	Normal: 80-120 mg/dl serum	None
Oral glucose tolerance test (GTT): measures woman's response to measured dose of glucose	No food for 12 hr before test or during test, but may have water; no smoking, tea, coffee, during test (alter body's response to carbohydrate); minimize activity (alters glucose metabolism); minimize stress (epinephrine and cortisone raise glucose levels by promoting gluconeogenesis)	Weigh woman, obtain fasting blood and urine specimens; administer 100 g of glucose orally in lemon juice; collect blood samples at 1, 2, and 3 hr; mark each specimen with time obtained and send to laboratory	See values, p. 785 Abnormal fasting: elevated or two other values lie outside normal range (below)	Caution woman she may experience dizziness, sweating, weakness, nausea, vomiting, or diarrhea during second and third hour Diuretics and glucocorticoids, may distort findings; do not use if fasting blood sugar (FBS) over 200 mg/dl
Intravenous (IV) glucose tolerance test: preferred test in pregnancy since absorption of glucose from intestinal tract is variable and may result in distorted findings in oral GTT	Same as oral GTT	Weigh woman; obtain fasting blood and urine specimen: administer 50 ml of 50% glucose in distilled water IV over a 4 min period and serial blood specimens obtained until 2 hr is reached, labeled as to time obtained, and sent to laboratory	Plasma glucose level Normal fasting: <100 mg/dl 2 hr: level not higher than fasting level	Caution woman she may experience facial flushing and dizziness as glucose is being administered Other precautions: same as for GTT
Tolbutamide response test not used since tolbutamide may have teratogenic effect on fetus				

are now measuring glucose in plasma by more specific glucose oxidase techniques. The 1-hour glucose screening test can be accomplished in a clinic or office setting on a woman who is not fasting. It is unfortunate that the test is not accurate before the seventh week of gestation when malformation from any preexisting abnormalities of the carbohydrate metabolic state occurs (Hay and Sparks, 1985). If the glucose level is ≥ 135 mg/dl, the 3-hour glucose tolerance test (GTT) is performed (Coustan and Carpenter, 1985).

After a 100 g glucose load the 3-hour GTT is abnormal if 2 or more of the following values are found:

	Plasma (mg/dl)	*Venous Whole Blood (mg/dl)*	*Plasma (Glucose Oxidase) (mg/dl)*
Fasting	≥ 105	≥ 90	≥ 95
1 hour	≥ 190	≥ 165	≥ 180
2 hours	≥ 165	≥ 145	≥ 155
3 hours	≥ 145	≥ 125	≥ 140

The above criteria are the same regardless of age, duration of pregnancy, or obesity.

With prolonged hyperglycemia, some of the hemoglobin remains saturated with glucose for the life of the red cell. Therefore a test for HbA_{1c} is a reflection of serum glucose over a period of weeks (Corbett, 1987). HbA_{1c} is useful for assessing overall control in type I (insulin-dependent) diabetes. It has not proved useful in screening for glucose intolerance of pregnancy. Glycosylated hemoglobin measures three components of HbA: A_{1a}, A_{1b}, and A_{1c}. Values are as follows (Corbett, 1987):

$\leq$ 7.5%	Good diabetic control
7.6% to 8.9%	Fair diabetic control
$\geq$ 9%	Poor diabetic control

Values for the measurement of HbA_{1c} *only* are as follows (Corbett, 1987):

2.2% to 4.8%	Nondiabetic adult
2.5% to 5.9%	Good diabetic control
6.0% to 8.0%	Fair diabetic control
$\geq$ 8.0%	Poor diabetic control

A decreased incidence of congenital anomalies is associated with HbA_{1c} values that are within normal limits. No preparation is needed for this test. A 5 ml specimen of venous blood is collected in an ethylenediamine tetraacetic acid (EDTA) (lavender-top) tube. It is put on ice and sent to the laboratory promptly (Corbett, 1987).

Nursing Diagnoses

Each woman's experience with the serious diagnosis of diabetes mellitus is unique to her and her family. Nursing diagnoses must be carefully formulated to reflect the actual or potential altered health-related responses that can be influenced, improved, or alleviated by nursing interventions. Examples of possible nursing diagnoses follow:

- Anxiety (or fear) related to
  - The diagnosis
- Knowledge deficit related to
  - The disorder, its management, and prognosis for self and baby
- Potential for injury to self and fetus related to
  - Poor control of diabetes
- Noncompliance related to
  - Insufficient funds or lack of transportation to grocery store
- Altered nutrition: less than body requirements
- Altered nutrition: more than body requirements
- Powerlessness related to
  - Unexpected diagnosis that disrupts expectations of "normal" pregnancy
- Body image disturbance
- Personal identity disturbance
- Altered role performance
- Situational low self-esteem
- Spiritual distress

Planning

Planning care for women and their families is given direction from identified nursing diagnoses and the medical management of this complication. The plan is individualized, relating specifically to needs identified by the caregivers and to those mutually identified by the woman and caregivers. The information in this chapter is general in nature; not all women experience all problems discussed nor require all facets of care described. See the nursing care plans and client teaching in this chapter.

Goals. The goals of management are several:

1. Minimize the risk to the mother
2. Minimize the need for antepartum hospitalization to maintain or restore diabetic control
3. Educate the woman and her family about diabetes mellitus and its control
4. Prevent perinatal morbidity and mortality
5. Help the mother maintain her self-esteem
6. Foster mutuality and support among family members

Implementation

Nurses assume many caregiving roles with women whose pregnancies are complicated by diabetes mellitus. The nurse's roles may be described as supportive, teacher/counselor/advocate, instrumental, and recorder.

Supportive Activities

Assisting the woman with stress reduction is central to the care needed by these women. Stress reduction and relaxation, discussed in Chapter 13, are taught as needed.

Space, privacy, and time are provided for the woman and her family to voice their feelings and questions, as well as to problem-solve among themselves. It takes time to adjust to any change in self-concept and expectations. In addition to the support needed in light of this complication, nursing interventions to meet the care needs of any gravida and her family are provided.

Fetal surveillance techniques may identify a congenital malformation incompatible with survival. Parents need supportive care as they consider the option of early pregnancy termination. The early detection of serious fetal malformations allows for exploration of various options in planning delivery and immediate care of the newborn. The parents may also benefit from the time to prepare for the birth of a child with a congenital abnormality. Even though the testing methods are noninvasive, the investigation of a pregnancy for fetal malformations should be conducted under conditions that are both voluntary and informed (Chapter 4). The risks, accuracy, and limitations of the tests should be discussed. The benefits of diagnosis and the options available when a positive diagnosis is obtained should be discussed in advance (Mennuti, 1985).

Teacher/Counselor/Advocate

Engaging the woman as an active participant in the health care team maintains or enhances her self-esteem and develops her self-confidence that she will be able to care for herself and her baby. The responsive, reliable, self-assured woman, who has learned to assess her own blood glucose and maintain euglycemia and who communicates openly and frequently with the physician and nurse, often can be seen at the clinic or the office on the same schedule as the nondiabetic gravida. Open communication is encouraged to facilitate client participation in self-care. The need for hospitalization during pregnancy to control diabetes and the need for early delivery are minimized. With this approach to care the nurse-clinician or nurse-practitioner is the primary educator for the woman and her family.

Pregnancy

Diet. Dietary or insulin management must be based on blood glucose (not urinary glucose) values. The diet is individualized to allow for increased maternal and fetal metabolic requirements: calories, 35 to 40 kcal/kg ideal body weight*; protein, 1 g/kg ideal body weight; complex carbohydrate, 50% of total kcal; fat should comprise less than 30% (Franz, 1988). Distribution should be two sevenths for each of three meals and one seventh for an evening snack. Women with brittle diabetes may require six small meals a day. The obese woman may need more food to prevent ketoacidosis. Sodium is not restricted; however, excesses are discouraged. An average weight gain of (12.5 kg) 27.5 lb is associated with the lowest incidence of preeclampsia and perinatal mortality.

Exercise. Exercise must be regular. The woman must be capable of making necessary adjustments to diet and insulin intake if the exercise pattern alters.

Insulin Requirements. *Prenatal insulin requirements begin to increase after the eighteenth to twentieth week.* Before that time hypoglycemic episodes may occur because of fetal drain and the low level of hormone antagonists to insulin. Insulin reactions are therefore common.

Monitoring Blood Glucose. The diabetic woman requires instruction as to the relevance of testing urine for glucose levels in pregnancy. By midpregnancy, trace to 1+ glucose is acceptable. Blood glucose levels are monitored by fasting blood sugar (FBS) and 2-hour postprandial tests (Table 32-2).

A recently developed technique using a color graph machine (glucose reflectance meter) reduces or eliminates the necessity of obtaining venous blood samples and thereby "saves" accessible veins. The woman can perform the test at home (Fig. 32-2). Using the Autolet (a disposable lancet on a springboard arm that facilitates finger sticks), the woman obtains a blood sample from the side of a finger (all the fingers are used in rotation). The drop of blood is placed on a glucose reagent strip. After a predetermined number of seconds, the blood is wiped or blotted from the strip and placed in the machine, the color graph is read. The results are recorded and reported to the physician. If blood glucose levels measure less than 100 mg/dl, as a rule the infant is normosomic and has few hypoglycemic problems after delivery.

The advent of home glucose monitoring has been credited with increasing the woman's feeling of control over self, and with decreasing or eliminating hospitalizations and therefore separation from family. It presents the most accurate method to document the degree of control in an out-of-hospital setting. It enables the woman to adjust her insulin dosage on a 24-hour basis. Early detection of hypoglycemia is possible even during sleep (Landon and Gabbe, 1985). If used before conception and early in pregnancy, home glucose monitoring may safeguard the conceptus during organogenesis.

*The actual number of kilocalories the individual woman should receive varies. The woman needs sufficient kilocalories to achieve optimum weight gain and to prevent acidosis.

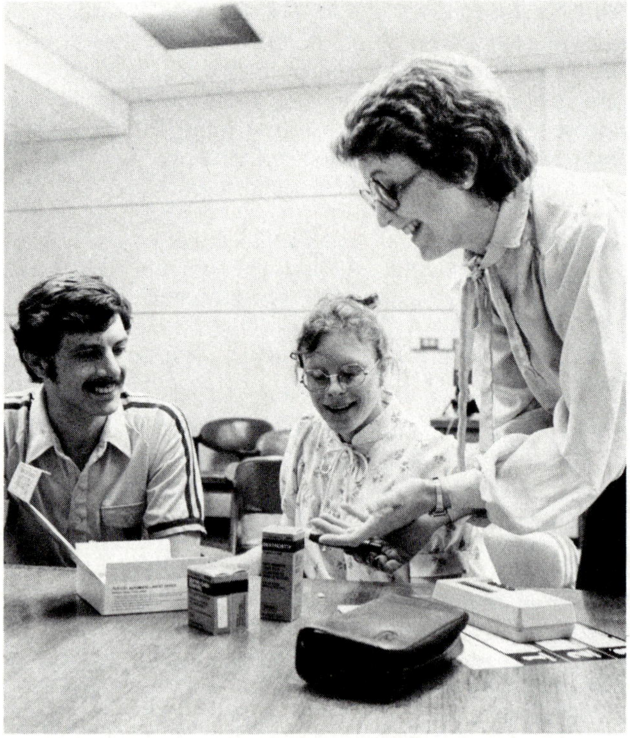

Fig. 32-2 Nurse is teaching family home monitoring for blood glucose. After return demonstration, nurse reviewed with woman how to balance insulin doses with findings.
Courtesy Stanford University Medical Center, Stanford, California.

Continuous Insulin Infusion. Continuous insulin infusion systems (Fig. 32-3) simplify insulin administration for women who need multiple injections per day (Nursing 87). The system infuses insulin at a set basal rate with a bolus dose to cover meals. The infusion tubing from this portable, battery-operated pump can be left in place for several weeks without local complications. Several biochemicals in addition to glucose are also maintained within normal limits, thus decreasing the risk of developing diabetes-related complications.

Supervision. If there is a question about the woman's ability to maintain euglycemia, visits are scheduled a minimum of every 2 weeks for the first 32 weeks and then weekly until delivery. A urine sample is checked at each visit throughout pregnancy for blood, glucose, ketones, protein, bilirubin, and pH. Microscopic examination may reveal asymptomatic UTIs, which are frequent and can cause fetal demise. Women having poor control need to be carefully assessed for infection; for example, asymptomatic UTIs may significantly change a woman's insulin requirements. Mycotic vaginitis in the diabetic pregnant woman is more common and difficult to control.

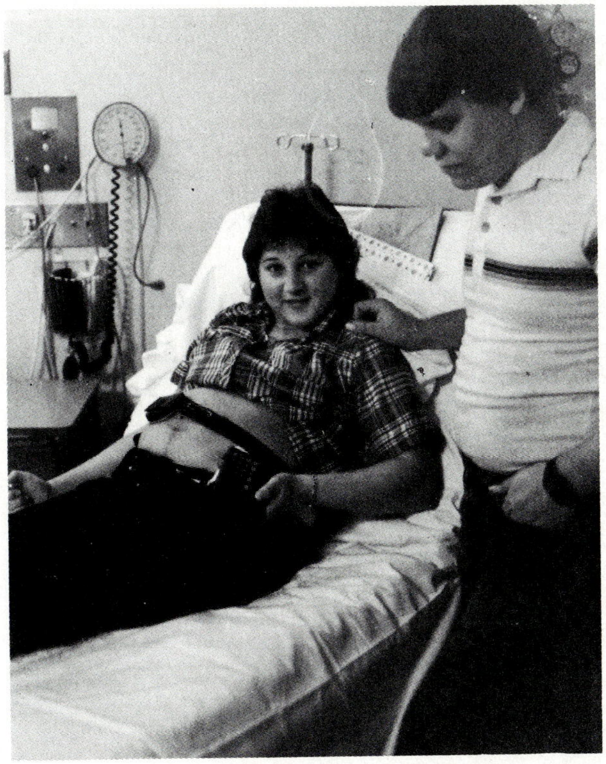

Fig. 32-3 Continuous insulin infusion regulated closely with home monitoring of glucose makes tighter control of diabetes mellitus possible.

Fetal well-being is monitored closely (Chapters 17 and 27). The stress of frequent monitoring can be relieved somewhat by meeting the woman's knowledge needs, by referring the woman to social service agencies for assistance with child care and transportation, and by providing a private time and space to discuss concerns.

Hospitalization. Despite the advances in home glucose monitoring some women may require hospitalization for regulation of insulin. Before pregnancy a woman may have been taking tolbutamide, but during pregnancy she may have to change to regular insulin. She may have poor control ("brittle diabetes") so that daily evaluation is necessary. If she develops an infection, IV antibiotic therapy may be indicated. Close monitoring of fetal health may be required as a basis for early termination of the pregnancy.

Complications. The diabetic pregnant woman is provided with written instructions as to the need for prompt reporting of **nausea, vomiting,** and **infections,** (see guidelines for client teaching, p. 791, and general nursing care plan, p. 793).

Labor and Delivery

Insulin Therapy. Most women utilize large amounts of energy (calories) to accomplish the work and manage the stress of labor and delivery. However, each woman expends different amounts of calories. Blood sugar levels must be controlled carefully during labor. To accomplish this, an IV line is inserted for infusion of glucose and insulin. Hourly determinations of blood glucose are made. Insulin and glucose are titrated to maintain blood glucose levels of 70 to 100 mg/dl (Robertson, 1987).

Intranatal insulin requirements involve a prescribed dose of insulin added to 100 ml of 10% dextrose in water for IV solution. NOTE: insulin, a protein, is attracted chemically to the plastic in the IV tubing. It leaves the solution and adheres to the lining of the tubing. Adherence to the tubing can be prevented by flushing the line first with 100 ml of normal saline and 10 units of insulin, which will completely coat the lining. Then the prescribed solution of insulin is begun and will remain stable. (A protein [albumin] may be added to the solution instead; however, it is more expensive.)

General Care. The mother should assume a side-lying position during bed rest in labor to prevent supine hypotension because of a large fetus or polyhydramnios. If strong labor and good progress do not ensue within 6 to 8 hours, cesarean delivery may be considered. Poorly controlled diabetes or obstetric indications such as fetopelvic disproportion, positive oxytocin challenge test (OCT), change in estriol levels, or preeclampsia–eclampsia are also indications for a cesarean delivery. The woman is observed and treated for diabetic complications such as hyperglycemia, ketosis, ketoacidosis, and glycosuria (Table 32-3). A pediatrician should be present at delivery to initiate proper neonatal care.

Puerperium

Insulin Requirements. The woman must be closely monitored. She may require only one half to two thirds of her prenatal dosage on the first postpartum day if she is eating a full diet. It takes several days after delivery to reestablish carbohydrate homeostasis (Fig. 32-1). The insulin-dependent woman must realize that *she must eat on time.* This is true even if the baby needs feeding or other pressing demands exist.

Complications. Possible complications include preeclampsia–eclampsia, hemorrhage, and infection. *Preeclampsia* occurs in one fourth of all diabetic new mothers and in one third of all diabetic new mothers, class C or D. *Hemorrhage* is a possibility if the mother's uterus had been overdistended (hydramnios, macrosomic fetus) or overstimulated (oxytocin induction). Monilial *infection* of the vagina or nipples or other infections are more likely to occur in a woman suffering from diabetes.

Breast-feeding. Breast-feeding is encouraged. Besides the advantages of maternal satisfaction and pleasure, breast-feeding also has an antidiabetogenic effect. Breast-feeding decreases the dosage for insulin-dependent women. The insulin dosage must be readjusted at the time of weaning (Fig 32-1, *F* to *G*).

Fertility Management. The new mother needs information for *family planning* and *contraception.* To assist in their decision making, couples need to be informed that if the mother has type I diabetes, the offspring have a 22% chance of developing diabetes; if she has type II diabetes, the offspring have a 4% chance. Nearly 100% of offspring of parents who both have noninsulin-dependent diabetes develop that type of diabetes. Only 45% to 60% of the offspring of both parents who have insulin-dependent diabe-

Table 32-3 *Differentiation of Hypoglycemia, Ketoacidosis, and Hyperglycemic Hyperosmolar Nonketotic Coma (HHNK)*

	Hypoglycemia (Insulin Reaction)	Ketoacidosis (Diabetic Coma)	HHNK
Causes	Too much insulin Not enough food (delayed or missed meals) Excessive exercise or work Indigestion, diarrhea, vomiting	Too little insulin Too much or wrong kind of food Infection, injuries, illness Insufficient exercise	Abnormally high glucose levels without ketoacidosis in mild or suspected diabetic—pancreatic disorders that lower production of insulin Complication of extensive burns, excess steroids (i.e., with steroid therapy), acute stress, TPN,† hemodialysis, peritoneal dialysis
Onset	Sudden (regular insulin) Gradual (modified insulin or oral agents)	Slow (days)	Rapid if woman dehydrated
Symptomatology	Hunger Sweating Nervousness Weakness Fatigue Blurred or double vision Dizziness Headache (especially with NPH insulin* or PZI) Pallor, clammy skin Shallow respirations Normal pulse Laboratory values Urine: negative for sugar and acetone Blood glucose: 60 mg/dl or less	Thirst Nausea or vomiting Abdominal pain Constipation Drowsiness Dim vision Increased urination Headache Flushed, dry skin Rapid breathing Weak, rapid pulse Acetone (fruity) breath odor Laboratory values Urine: positive for sugar and acetone Blood glucose: 250 mg/dl	Polyuria Thirst (intracellular dehydration) Hypovolemia Blood serum levels FBS: 600-3000 mg/dl Acetone level: normal or slightly elevated Dry skin Coma, death
Nursing actions	Notify physician Give low-fat milk If orange juice is given for a fast supply of sugar, follow it later with milk Obtain blood and urine specimens for laboratory testing	Notify physician Keep woman flat in bed and warm Record intake and output Check and record vital signs	Administer insulin in line with blood glucose levels Monitor IV therapy (sodium and water deficits corrected without extreme shift of fluid into intracellular compartment with no reduction of hyperosmolarity of blood) Monitor woman for dehydration; record intake and output Check and record vital signs Notify physician of changes in symptomatology

Modified from form used at Santa Clara Valley Medical Center, San Jose, Calif.
*NPH: neutral protamine Hagedorn; PZI: protamine zinc insulin
†TPN (total parenteral nutrition) replaces the term *hyperalimentation.*

tes will develop the syndrome.* The risk of diabetes doubles with every 20% of excess weight, and this figure applies to the young, as well as to the older diabetic person. Diabetes is now the sixth leading cause of death by disease in adults and the first leading cause of new cases of blindness between the ages of 20 and 75. If contraception is chosen, the woman may be advised to use the *diaphragm with spermicide.* The use of oral hormonal contraceptives is questioned because of their effect on carbohydrate metabolism. However, much more serious is the possibility of increased risk of ischemic heart disease and cerebrovascular accidents (Steele, 1985) (Chapter 42). The use of triphasic pills may carry less risk.

Intrauterine devices (IUDs) are associated with an increased risk of infection. In the presence of severe renal disease and proliferative retinopathy, sterilization may be advised (Steele, 1985).

Instrumental Role

Technical skills are required to implement nursing care. The nurse obtains and assesses urine specimens and mon-

*Prediction of risk varies from author to author (Steele, 1985).

itors blood glucose. Insulin injections, heparin locks, and IV therapy are often needed. In addition, the woman and her family are taught to obtain and test urine and blood specimens and to administer insulin subcutaneously.

Recorder. Accurate documentation is necessary for comprehensive care and facilitates communication among the health care team. Future plans for management are based on client responses to present care. A complete record meets legal requirements and serves as a reservoir of data that could prove helpful in nursing research.

Evaluation

Evaluation is a continuous process. The woman's responses to the disorder are assessed constantly. Adjustments in the care plan are made in regard to measureable outcome criteria. Clinical findings that represent expected responses are presented as outcome criteria in the nursing care plans.

Text continued on p. 799.

Guidelines for Client Teaching

DIABETES

ASSESSMENT

1. Pregnant woman of >25 years old.
2. Obese prepregnant and pregnant weight.
3. Glycosuria.
4. One hour blood sugar >190 mg/dl.
5. Large fetus.
6. Hydramnios.

NURSING DIAGNOSES

Knowledge deficit related to gestational diabetes.
Altered nutrition: more than body requirements related to obesity.
Altered nutrition: less than body requirements related to dysfunctional carbohydrate metabolism.
Potential for injury: mother and fetus, related to dysfunctional carbohydrate metabolism.
Potential self-care deficit related to procedures necessary to maintain euglycemia.
Fluid volume excess related to fluid retention and vascular changes.

GOALS

Short-term

Woman will learn about gestational diabetes.
Woman (couple) will learn how to test blood sugar with fingerstick.
Woman (couple) will learn how to assess glycosuria with chemstrip.
Woman (couple) will learn basics of diet management.
Woman (couple) will learn insulin administration.

Intermediate

Woman will learn to maintain euglycemia.
Woman will maintain proper nutrition and exercise.

Long-term

Woman will have a healthy baby with minimal or no problems postpartum.

REFERENCES AND TEACHING AIDS

Pamphlets from insulin manufacturers (i.e., Lilly, SKF).
Pamphlets from chemstrip and blood sugar testing apparatus manufacturers.
A-V materials on diabetes.
Chemstrips for urine.
Insulin needle, sterile water, alcohol sponges, orange or grapefruit.
Chart showing injection sites.

CONTENT/RATIONALE	TEACHING ACTIONS
To inform woman (couple) about diabetes:	
Discuss pathophysiology of diabetes with woman and support person.	Using a chart or A-V materials, show couple (woman) where insulin is manufactured in the body. Discuss what insulin does in carbohydrate metabolism. Show how diabetes changes this regulatory mechanism and how it effects the mother and the fetus.
Explain how the glucose gets into the urine from the bloodstream.	Demonstrate how to test a sample of woman's urine with a chemstrip. Ask for a return demonstration and observe the accuracy with which she interprets the results. Show woman how to record the results.

Continued.

Guidelines For Client Teaching—cont'd

CONTENT/RATIONALE	TEACHING ACTIONS
To discuss self-assessment: Discuss how to do the fingerstick and test it for glucose. Allow for woman to be ready to learn (demonstrate understanding and caring).	Demonstrate how to test blood for glucose level. If woman is shy about sticking her own finger, ask the support person to do a return demonstration on the woman. Show how to read the results and where to record it. If the woman is on a sliding scale of insulin, show woman (couple) how to read the scale and interpret how much insulin she should have at that time.
To teach self-administration of insulin: Explain the use of the equipment for the procedure by using the exact equipment the woman will use at home. This avoids confusion and gives the woman (couple) hands-on experience. Stress importance of accuracy. Stress importance of using correct syringe with correct insulin. Teach and stress importance of rotating sites. Current bottle of insulin can be used at room temperature, unused bottle to be kept refrigerated.	Show woman (couple) the procedure for drawing up the insulin, reading the syringe, and administering the insulin. For practice injections, use the fruit. When it comes time for the real injection, ask the woman (couple) to give a return demonstration to you while you supervise. The first injection is usually the most difficult. Nurse may have to help the woman (support person) pierce the skin.
To avoid complications through self care: Review signs and symptoms of ketoacidosis. Point out that illness, especially infection, vomiting, diarrhea may precipitate ketoacidosis.	Review adverse effects of ketoacidosis.
Stress importance of continuing urine and blood testing during sick days and staying in constant contact with the physician.	Review relationship between available glucose and insulin needs.
Explain causes and dangers of hypoglycemia to woman (couple).	Review causes and dangers of hypoglycemia to woman (couple).
Describe care and treatment and prevention of hypoglycemia. List foods to take during an insulin reaction, discuss amount to take. Discuss what to do in case of insulin coma. Support person must understand what to do (Glucagon injection).	Stress importance of carrying fast-acting sugar and consuming extra carbohydrate before exercise. Stress importance of bedtime snack. Stress relationship between diet and exercise. Give Medic-Alert information.
Explain importance of carrying identification pointing out woman is a diabetic. Discuss diet management. Have registered dietition (RD) see woman/couple. Reinforce information given by him/her.	Teach role diet plays in disease management. Provide printed material for woman to take home for future reference.
Discuss increased susceptibility to infection, eye problems, neurologic changes.	Discuss with woman importance of good skin and foot care. Stress importance of wearing proper fitting shoes, discourage extremes of temperature.
Explain role of exercise in helping to balance insulin and blood glucose. Discuss exercise ad activities that have been prescribed for her by the physician.	Stress that exercise enhances use of glucose and decreases need for insulin. Talk about the exercises and activities that she is to do regularly.
Explain the importance of contacting her physician before any long-term travel. Review dangers of not being prepared for complications.	Stress the importance of not doing any unnecessary long-term travel. Stress importance of carrying insulin, syringes, fast-acting sugar. Wear ID bracelet and carry an exchange list for dietary needs.
Stress the need for follow-up care during this time.	Give woman (couple) appointment for next time. Write down numbers of importance for the woman (couple) and give them to her to take with her. Allow time for questions.

EVALUATION Woman (couple) is receptive to information presented. Competence is evident in return demonstrations and questions. Woman and fetus complete pregnancy with no adverse sequelae to diabetes mellitus.

General Nursing Care Plan

DIABETES MELLITUS

ASSESSMENT	NURSING DIAGNOSIS (ND)/ PLAN (P)/GOAL (G)	RATIONALE/ IMPLEMENTATION	EVALUATION
How long has woman had diabetes mellitus? Has woman administered insulin? Knowledge about diabetes. Knowledge about care needed during pregnancy to prevent sequelae for the mother and fetus. Assess feelings about diabetes.	ND: Knowledge deficit related to diabetes mellitus, its management, and potential effects on the pregnant woman and fetus. ND: Ineffective individual coping related to woman's responsibility in managing her diabetes mellitus during pregnancy. P: Provide information, be available for discussion, demonstrate, and observe return demonstration. G: Woman will learn about diabetes mellitus, its management, and potential sequelae during pregnancy. G: Woman will demonstrate technique of home monitoring tests and verbalize understanding of the results she should report. G: Woman will verbalize her concerns and feelings about her disease and its possible sequelae.	*To teach woman about diabetes mellitus, its management, and effects on pregnancy, the nurse will:* Review pathophysiology of the disease. Encourage verbalization of concerns and feelings. Assist woman in formulating questions for the physician. Clarify misconceptions. Teach home monitoring tests, demonstrate techniques, interpretation, and recording of results. (Urine test should be controlled at +1 sugar to avoid hypoglycemia, which is extremely dangerous to the fetus). Review the effects of diabetes on the pregnant woman and fetus (especially the uncontrolled diabetes sequelae). Teach (written and oral) the danger signs of diabetes and whom to notify. Stress importance of weekly prenatal visits during second half of pregnancy. Refer woman to community diabetic support group.	Woman verbalizes understanding of instruction. Woman accurately demonstrates how to perform home monitoring tests. Woman verbalizes her concerns and feelings about her disease and its possible sequelae, without undue anxiety. Woman keeps all scheduled appointments. Woman notifies caregiver if danger signs appear. Woman joins and participates in community diabetic support group.
Assess verbal and nonverbal actions regarding diabetes and pregnancy. Assess woman's support system. Note previous successful coping mechanisms.	ND: Anxiety, fear, ineffective individual coping, dysfunctional grieving, powerlessness, body image disturbance, self-esteem disturbance, altered role performance, personal identity disturbance, spiritual distress, altered family processes related to diabetes and its potential sequelae on the pregnant woman and fetus. P: Establish a therapeutic relationship, provide information, be available for discussion, and assist with problem solving.	*To assist woman in verbalizing concerns and adjusting to the strict management of her disease, the nurse will:* Provide private area for conversation. Discuss issues in an unhurried manner. Provide consistency in caregivers. Encourage verbalization of concerns and feelings. Answer questions honestly. Assist woman in formulating questions for physician. Clarify misconceptions. Offer woman choices when possible.	Woman verbalizes her concerns and feelings. Woman participates in her plan of care. Woman identifies her support system. Woman identifies previous successful coping mechanisms.

Continued.

General Nursing Care Plan—cont'd

ASSESSMENT	NURSING DIAGNOSIS (ND)/ PLAN (P)/GOAL (G)	RATIONALE/ IMPLEMENTATION	EVALUATION
	G: Woman will verbalize concerns and feelings regarding diabetes and its potential sequelae on the pregnant woman and fetus. G: Woman will identify her support system. G: Woman will identify previous successful coping mechanisms.	Compliment woman on successful learning, problem solving, and coping. Identify previous successful learning, problem solving, and coping. Identify with woman her support system. Involve significant others in plan of care. Refer to community diabetes support group. Refer to psychologist, clergy, social worker, etc.	
Assess knowledge regarding insulin and its administration.	ND: Knowledge deficit related to insulin effects and its administration. ND: Potential for injury related to improper insulin administration. P: Provide information and time for discussion, demonstration, and observation of return demonstration. G: Woman will learn the purpose and effects of insulin in the body. G: Woman will administer insulin to herself correctly.	*To teach woman about insulin, its effects on the body, and proper administration, the nurse will:* Explain insulin's effect in the body. Review peak action of insulin and signs of hypoglycemia. Stress importance of administration of correct dose with correct syringe. Demonstrate correct withdrawal and administration of insulin. Explain importance of site rotation and identify the sites that can be used. Teach proper techniques of insulin storage. Monitor woman's self-administration of insulin until techniques are learned and understood. Explain why insulin needs will be higher during the third trimester.	Woman learns the purpose and effect of insulin. Woman administers her own insulin properly. Woman understands changing insulin needs during pregnancy.
Assess knowledge of hyperglycemia.	ND: Knowledge deficit related to hyper- or hypoglycemia. ND: Potential for injury related to hyper- or hypoglycemia to the pregnant woman and fetus. P: Provide information to woman conducive to discussion for woman and other family members. G: Woman will verbalize the signs and symptoms of hyper- or hypoglycemia.	*To teach woman about hyperglycemia, the nurse will:* Explain that illness, infection, vomiting, and diarrhea can precipitate ketoacidosis. Encourage woman to call physician when illness occurs and continue to administer insulin. Teach danger signs of ketoacidosis.	Woman learns the signs and symptoms of hyperglycemia. Woman verbalizes danger signs and whom to notify if they occur. Woman notifies caregiver promptly if danger signs appear. Woman experiences no episodes of hyperglycemia.

General Nursing Care Plan—cont'd

ASSESSMENT	NURSING DIAGNOSIS (ND)/ PLAN (P)/GOAL (G)	RATIONALE/ IMPLEMENTATION	EVALUATION
	G: Woman will seek medical attention when danger signs and symptoms occur. G: Woman will use preventive measures to avoid hyper- and hypoglycemia.		
Assess knowledge of hypoglycemia, its signs and symptoms, and its treatment. Assess knowledge of preventive measures for hypoglycemia.		*To teach woman about hypoglycemia, the nurse will:* Teach signs and symptoms of hypoglycemia. Review causes and dangers of insulin reaction. Stress importance of carrying fast-acting sugar when traveling and of having milk on hand at home. Review relationship of exercise and diet. Explain importance of seeking medical attention for hypoglycemia because of its dangerous effects on self and fetus. Give Medic-Alert information and encourage woman to wear bracelet or necklace. Review the signs of hypo- and hyperglycemia with significant others and who to notify when danger signs occur.	Woman verbalizes signs and symptoms of hypoglycemia. Woman carries supply of fast-acting sugar and verbalizes having milk on hand at home. Woman wears Medic-Alert bracelet at all times. Woman experiences no episodes of hypoglycemia. Family verbalizes knowledge of signs of hypoglycemia and its treatment.
Review knowledge of diabetic diet. Assess cultural and financial influences on food served. Who prepares the meals? Who buys the food? Woman's likes/dislikes.	ND: Knowledge deficit related to the diabetic diet and its importance to a woman with diabetes during pregnancy. ND: Altered nutrition: less or more than body requirements, related to diabetes and pregnancy. P: Provide information and climate conducive to discussion. G: Woman will learn about the diabetic diet and verbalize the importance of adhering to its protocol during pregnancy.	*To teach the woman about diabetes diet management during pregnancy, the nurse will:* Consider cultural and financial implications when planning teaching. Ascertain type of diet woman is to follow at home. Refer to registered dietitician (RD). Explain importance of a balanced diet. Encourage woman to design sample menus. Stress importance to maintain or achieve appropriate weight and pattern of weight gain during pregnancy.	Woman verbalizes understanding of instruction. Woman gains weight according to protocol for the pregnant woman with diabetes. Woman implements diet prescribed by and developed with caregiver.

Continued.

General Nursing Care Plan—cont'd

ASSESSMENT	NURSING DIAGNOSIS (ND)/ PLAN (P)/GOAL (G)	RATIONALE/ IMPLEMENTATION	EVALUATION
Intranatal: Perform assessments for normal laboring woman. Assess for signs of hypoglycemia. Assess for signs of preeclampsia. Assess fetal monitor strip. Assess anxiety level. Assess for excessive uterine size associated with hydramnios and fetal macrosomia. Assess for dyspnea and supine hypotension related to excessive uterine size.	ND: Potential for injury related to hypoglycemia. ND: Potential for injury related to preeclampsia. ND: Anxiety related to labor. ND: Altered (cardiopulmonary) tissue perfusion related to supine hypotension. P: Monitor maternal-fetal well-being, prevent supine hypotension, and identify and treat complications promptly. G: Woman will be monitored closely and treated for signs of hypoglycemia, preeclampsia and supine hypotension. G: Fetus will be monitored closely for signs of distress.	*To monitor woman and fetus for signs of labor complications the nurse will:* Monitor vital signs, especially blood pressure, frequently. Monitor and report signs and symptoms of preeclampsia and hypoglycemia. Evaluate and record labor pattern. Continuously monitor fetal heart rate (FHR) and report fetal distress. Monitor IV fluids of 10% dextrose in water and insulin as ordered; titrate infusion to frequent blood glucose determinations to maintain euglycemia. Monitor the administration of oxytocin for induction as ordered. Provide supportive labor nursing which is especially important to prevent hypoglycemia secondary to anxiety. Prepare for induction or cesarean delivery (fetal distress, fetopelvic disproportion, lack of labor progression). Alert pediatrician and nursery personnel.	Woman is monitored and treated promptly for preeclampsia and hypoglycemia. Supine hypotension is avoided. Euglycemia is maintained. Woman remains free of anxiety. Woman experiences no adverse sequelae to fluid therapy and oxytocin induction or augmentation of labor. Fetus remains free from distress as indicated by FHR.
Postnatal: Perform normal postpartum assessment. Note frequent blood and urine glucose levels. Note signs and symptoms of hypo- or hyperglycemia. Assess signs and symptoms of hemorrhage and infection.	ND: Potential for injury related to fluctuating blood glucose levels after delivery. ND: Potential for injury related to complications of involution (hemorrhage, infection), or postpartum appearance of preeclampsia. P: Monitor woman's progress, provide information, and be available for discussion. G: Woman's blood glucose level will be monitored closely for initial 24-48 hours postdelivery and remain within normal limits.	*To monitor and treat womans' fluctuating glucose levels, the nurse will:* Perform frequent fractional urine tests. Obtain blood for glucose level as ordered. Monitor foods and fluids taken. Evaluate for signs and symptoms of hypo- or hyperglycemia. Adjust insulin intake according to protocol ordered. Explain the need to triple caloric intake and decrease insulin by one-half to successfully produce breast milk. If mother develops acetonu-	Woman's blood glucose stabilizes within normal limits; woman minimum experiences or no sequelae from hypo- or hyperglycemia. Woman remains free of hemorrhage, infection, or preeclampsia. Woman verbalizes understanding of instruction.

General Nursing Care Plan—cont'd

ASSESSMENT	NURSING DIAGNOSIS (ND)/ PLAN (P)/GOAL (G)	RATIONALE/ IMPLEMENTATION	EVALUATION
	G: Woman will progress through normal involution without complication.	ria discard her breast milk until resolved. Explain that hypoglycemia decreases milk production. Counsel woman to eat every meal on time even if it means others must wait. *To monitor involution, the nurse will:* See postpartum general care plan, (Chapter 26).	Woman progresses through involution without complication.

Specific Nursing Care Plan

GESTATIONAL DIABETES

Susan Burke is a married, 27-year old newspaper editor. Susan is now in her 30th week of pregnancy and has received regular prenatal care. At 20 weeks gestation, she was diagnosed with gestational diabetes and was insulin-dependent by 23 weeks. Susan quickly learned her diabetic regime and verbalized understanding of her condition and its possible sequelae.

Susan notified her obstetrician complaining of severe fatigue and nausea effecting her work schedule. For the past 24 hours, her blood glucose has ranged from 200-400 ml/dL and urine has tested +4 for glucose but negative for acetone.

ASSESSMENT	NURSING DIAGNOSIS (ND)/ PLAN (P)/GOAL (G)	RATIONALE/ IMPLEMENTATION	EVALUATION
Stressful active job, insulin-dependent, fatigue, nausea, blood glucose 200-400, urine +4 sugar, urine negative acetone. Assess recent diet/exercise/rest/illness. Assess for signs and symptoms of ketoacidosis.	ND: Potential for injury related to hyperglycemia. P: Identify cause so that appropriate plan can be developed and implemented. G: Susan's hyperglycemia will be controlled promptly and she and her fetus will suffer minimum or no sequelae.	*To monitor and treat Susan's hyperglycemia, the nurse will:* Monitor frequent blood glucose levels. Monitor fractional urines. Adjust insulin doses as ordered. Review signs of hypoglycemia with Susan. Note and report signs of ketoacidosis or hypoglycemia. Teach Susan about ketoacidosis, its signs, and possible sequelae for her and the fetus. Review need for proper diet, exercise, and rest, even if it means her job and others must wait. Monitor fetal heart rate (FHR).	Susan achieves a euglycemic state. Susan and her fetus suffer minimum or no sequelae from the hyperglycemic episode. Susan and caregiver identify cause and develop a plan to avoid recurrence.

Continued.

Specific Nursing Care Plan—cont'd

ASSESSMENT	NURSING DIAGNOSIS (ND)/ PLAN (P)/GOAL (G)	RATIONALE/ IMPLEMENTATION	EVALUATION
		Perform NST as ordered.	
Sudden hyperglycemic episode. Note frequency or urgency of urination. Send urine specimen to identify asymptomatic UTI. Note vaginal itching or increased vaginal discharge. Note other signs and symptoms of infection.	ND: Potential for injury related to infection. ND: Knowledge deficit related to recognition of signs and symptoms of infection. P: Identify infection and implement appropriate care (Chapter 30). G: Susan's infection will be identified and treated promptly. G: Susan will learn and report signs of infection.	*To identify and treat infection, the nurse will:* Obtain specimens for culture (urine, vaginal smear). Identify systemic or local signs of infection. Administer prophylactic antibiotics as ordered. Teach Susan the signs and symptoms of infection. Explain that infection increases insulin resistance and ketoacidosis, thus signs of infection should be reported immediately.	Susan remains free from infection. Susan's infection is identified and treated promptly. Susan learns the signs of infection and whom to notify if they occur.
Stressful career, "fatigue and nausea affecting work schedule." Hyperglycemic episode.	ND: Ineffectual individual coping related to a stressful career as manifested by a poor diet, little exercise, and insufficient rest. P: Identify cause and develop plan with Susan to avoid recurrence. G: Susan will acquire proper diet, adequate exercise, and sufficient rest. G: Susan will achieve a euglycemic state.	*To teach the importance of strict adherence to the diabetic regime, the nurse will:* Explain the possible sequelae to the fetus and Susan as the result of glucose shifts. Review diet/exercise/rest protocol. Emphasize the importance that for the next 10 weeks, Susan and her regime must come before work or family. Encourage Susan to consider time off from work or to work a lighter schedule. Explain that gestational diabetes is a temporary condition but can have long-lasting effects if not controlled. Answer questions, listen to concerns and feelings. Involve significant others in encouraging Susan to adhere to her regime.	Susan acquires proper diet, exercise, and rest. Susan achieves a euglycemic state.

HYPEREMESIS GRAVIDARUM

Hyperemesis gravidarum is defined as excessive or pernicious vomiting during pregnancy, leading to dehydration and starvation. Many pregnant women suffer nausea and vomiting at some time during early gestation. The indisposition is mild in most cases, but in about 1 of every 1000 pregnant women, severe intractable emesis will require hospitalization and perhaps even therapeutic abortion.

The cause of hyperemesis during pregnancy is still debated. Psychologically unstable women whose established reaction patterns to stress involve gastrointestinal disturbances often are affected. In some women, however, psychologic causes cannot be elicited. Other causes could be multiple pregnancy, hormonal abnormalities (elevated thyroxine [T_4]), or trophoblastic disease (hydatidiform mole).

In extreme cases **dehydration** leads to fluid-electrolyte complications, particularly acidosis. Rarely does vomitus contain only gastric acid fluids. Most vomiting involves loss of contents (alkali) from deeper within the gastrointestinal tract. This leads to the development of **metabolic acidosis. Starvation** causes hypoproteinemia and hypovitaminosis. Degenerative changes produce characteristic symptomatology. Jaundice and hemorrhage secondary to vitamin C and B-complex deficiency and hypothrombinemia lead to bleeding from mucosal surfaces. The embryo or fetus may die, and the mother may die from irreversible metabolic alterations. In most cases hyperemesis gravidarum will respond to therapy; hence the prognosis is good. The woman is discharged home when fluid and electrolyte balance is restored and weight gain begins. A general nursing care plan for hyperemesis gravidarum follows.

General Nursing Care Plan

HYPEREMIS GRAVIDARUM

ASSESSMENT	NURSING DIAGNOSIS (ND)/ PLAN (P)/GOAL (G)	RATIONALE/ IMPLEMENTATION	EVALUATION
Assess for signs and symptoms: Excessive vomiting. Dehydration: rapid weight loss, poor skin turgor. Metabolic acidosis: headache, mental dullness, hyperpneic leading to disorientation, stupor, coma, and death. Starvation: hypoproteinemia and hypovitaminosis.	ND: Potential fluid volume deficit and impaired gas exchange related to vomiting and metabolic acidosis. ND: Altered nutrition: less than body requirements related to nausea and vomiting. P: Maintain constant vigilence for excessive vomiting. G: Woman's vomiting episodes are eliminated, fluid and electrolyte balance returns, and adequate nutrition is assured.	*To support women's physiologic processes, the nurse will:* Assist physician or initiate intravenous fluid therapy per physician's order. Give antiemetics as ordered. Maintain woman NPO as ordered. Support woman's nutritional needs through TPN, addition of nutrients (vitamins, etc) into peripheral or central lines. Keep room clean and fresh with adequate ventilation. When oral foods/fluids are allowed, provide small amounts of attractively served foods to fit her preferences.	Hyperemesis gravidarum abates and does not recur. Fluid/electrolyte balance is restored. Adequate nutrition is reestablished.
Assess woman's affect, emotional state, and support system.	ND: Potential ineffective family or individual coping related to age, lifestyle, pregnancy, hyperemesis, or other disturbance.	*To support woman's emotional/psychologic processes, the nurse will:* Provide safe, confidential, private space for identifying and discussing	Woman is able to identify and discuss her concerns and begin to problem-solve solutions. Support system is mobilized, it is determined

General Nursing Care Plan—cont'd

ASSESSMENT	NURSING DIAGNOSIS (ND)/ PLAN (P)/GOAL (G)	RATIONALE/ IMPLEMENTATION	EVALUATION
	P: Assist with identification of etiologic factor(s) and with therapeutic management to meet her emotional/psychologic needs. G: Etiologic factor(s) is (are) identified and appropriate therapy initiated.	concerns. Mobilize support group/ person of her choice. Maintain 'no visitor' policy or monitor her visitors, prn. Keep woman and family informed of maternal and fetal status.	whether etiologic factors had an emotional or psychologic basis. Woman states she felt comfortable with and part of the team.
Assess for etiologic factors.	ND: Potential fluid volume deficit and impaired gas exchange related to persistence of etiologic factors. P: Assess collaboratively with appropriate team members (e.g. endocrinologist). G: Etiologic factor(s) is (are) identified and managed so that hyperemesis does not recur.	*To assist with assessment the nurse will:* Follow-through with collection of specimens and prescribed therapies. Carefully document woman's responses.	Etiologic factor(s) is (are) identified, appropriate therapy is instituted, and hyperemesis does not recur.
Assess knowledge and understanding of the disorder.	NP: Knowledge deficit related to condition, its cause, and management. P: Meet woman's knowledge needs. G: Woman states she understands condition.	*To meet woman's knowledge needs, the nurse will:* Provide content in amount and manner to meet individual woman's needs. Provide sufficient time for discussion, repetition, etc.	Woman states content accurately, and, after discharge reports early signs/symptoms of recurrence immediately.
Assess for severe (rare) complications of jaundice, hemorrhage, fetal distress.	ND: Potential for injury related to severe complications. P: Maintain careful surveillance; report signs, symptoms immediately. G: Woman and fetus suffer no adverse sequelae.	*To prevent progression of severe complications, the nurse will:* Remain vigilent for complications. Report findings immediately and initiate therapy as ordered.	Woman and fetus suffer no adverse sequelae related to hyperemesis gravidarum or its management.

DISORDERS OF THE THYROID GLAND

Hyperthyroidism

Hyperthyroidism, which affects about 1 of every 1500 pregnant women, may seriously complicate gestation or endanger the fetus. Hyperthyroidism may be responsible for anovulation and amenorrhea, but the disease is not a cause of abortion or fetal anomaly. Hyperthyroidism is associated with an increased incidence of premature labor and delivery. Symptoms include weakness, sweating, weight loss (or poor gain), nervousness, loose stools, and heat intolerance. Warm, soft, moist skin, tachycardia, exophthalmos, tremor, and goiter (enlarged gland) with a bruit are characteristic. Enlargement of the thyroid gland is symmetric. Laboratory findings, particularly the basal metabolic rate and the free T_4 index, will be elevated.

Radioactive iodine must not be used in testing or in therapy because it may destroy or compromise the fetal thyroid. Other antithyroid drugs such as iodine or the thiouracils may be employed to control the overactive maternal thyroid, provided the free T_4 index remains normal and that leukopenia does not develop.

Partial thyroidectomy, also an acceptable treatment for toxic goiter, requires preoperative preparation by antithyroid medication, usually Lugol's iodine solution. Hypothyroidism, which occurs in at least 20% of hyperthyroid women postoperatively, must be treated promptly to spare the fetus. A free T_4 index determination on the cord blood at birth should be run to aid in determining the status of the infant.

Any maternal therapy for thyroid dysfunction may induce fetal thyroid insult. Determination of free T_4 index in cord blood of such an infant is necessary.

Hypothyroidism

Hypothyroidism may be responsible for anovulation in the woman with impaired fertility. Moreover, thyroid deficiency may cause spontaneous abortion, fetal maldevelopment, or fetal goiter. Mild degrees of hypothyroidism in women may go unrecognized or may suggest a disease process of another system, for example, menorrhagia. In the latter instance diagnosis depends largely on laboratory tests. Simple goiter generally is caused by iodine lack, and the woman is only slightly thyroid deficient.

Early hypothyroidism is characterized by easy fatigability, cold intolerance, lethargy, constipation, dry skin, or headache. Thin brittle nails, dry skin, alopecia, poor skin turgor, and delayed deep tendon reflexes are typical. During pregnancy laboratory findings may reveal normal or reduced protein-bound iodine (PBI), reduced thyroxine (T_4) (column or D), reduced triiodothyronine (T_3) (resin), and a reduced T_4 index (normal range is 0.75 to 2.5 units if T_4 by column is used; 1.3 to 5 units if T_4[D] is used with resin T_3 uptake).

Malignant Disease. Surgical treatment rather than use of radioisotopes is preferred when malignant thyroid disease complicates pregnancy. It is permissible to follow with well-shielded radiation therapy. Hill and associates (1966) found that pregnancy subsequent to the diagnosis of thyroid malignancy seems to have no effect on the outcome of this disease.

DISORDERS OF THE ADRENAL GLAND

Hyperadrenocorticism

Hyperfunction of the adrenal cortex occurs in Cushing's syndrome, Cushing's disease, adrenogenital syndrome, hyperaldosteronism, and pheochromocytoma. The individual's principal problem in all these disorders is abnormal loss of salt, as well as hypertension and its related complications. Such women do not easily become pregnant because of amenorrhea and anovulation. A tumor (e.g., pituitary, adrenal) should be identified if present and removed if feasible. Adrenocortical hyperplasia and hyperfunction may be controlled with one of the cortisones. Preeclampsia–eclampsia, infection, osteoporosis, and shock may be associated problems. The frequency of fetal anomaly is not increased in hyperadrenocorticism, but there is a risk of premature delivery.

Hypoadrenocorticism (Addison's Disease)

Hypoadrenocorticism, idiopathic in more than 50% of cases and caused by tuberculosis in most of the rest, is an uncommon complication of pregnancy. These women, whose fluid-electrolyte balance may be precarious, especially after pernicious nausea and vomiting of pregnancy, are susceptible to infection and especially to shock. A low plasma sodium chloride level, reduced 17-ketosteroid and 17-hydroxycorticoid levels, a low or absent plasma cortisol level, together with eosinophilia and lymphocytosis, are diagnostic laboratory findings in Addison's disease. With cortisone replacement therapy, electrolyte supplementation, and the avoidance of hemorrhage, the woman usually can go through pregnancy successfully. Therapeutic abortion rarely is indicated; vaginal delivery is desirable. Whether cortisone is teratogenic in humans is still debated.

People with Addison's disease display easy fatigability, anorexia, and frequent episodes of nausea, vomiting, and diarrhea. They also have sparse axillary hair and increased skin pigmentation and suffer hypotension.

MATERNAL PHENYLKETONURIA

Phenylketonuria (PKU) is an inborn error of metabolism caused by an autosomal recessive trait that creates a deficiency in the enzyme phenylalanine hydroxylase. Absence of this enzyme results in the inability to metabolize phenylalanine to tyrosine. Prompt diagnosis of this disorder in the newborn and subsequent dietary intervention has made it possible for individuals to live a productive life with the exception of reproduction. Homozygosity for this disorder in a woman whose fetus is heterozygous produces disastrous fetal results.

Elevated maternal blood phenylalanine levels during pregnancy result in fetal hyperphenylalaninemia. Maternal risk in this disorder is not a factor; however, for the fetus, intrauterine and postnatal growth retardation, including mental retardation, is almost universal. About one-fourth of fetuses are malformed. Apparently, a maternal diet low in phenylalanine has questionable preventive value unless followed *before conception* (Hayes et al., 1987). A simple urine test (Phenostix) is available and is applied routinely to every woman in early pregnancy.

• • •

Other endocrine disorders, for example, hypoparathyroidism and hyperparathyroidism, are rarely encountered during pregnancy. The nurse is referred to medical texts and the references at the end of this chapter.

SUMMARY

Maternal endocrine and metabolic disorders have immediate and long-term consequences for the mother and her fetus or newborn. The woman who becomes an active participant in her care has the most potential for preventing or minimizing the adverse effects of the disorder and improving the prognosis for herself and her offspring. The tremendous strides in the management of diabetes are of value only if the woman is willing to utilize the care available. Public education that leads to prepregnancy care that continues throughout the childbearing experience leads to the best results for women whose pregnancies are complicated by diabetes mellitus, hyperemesis gravidarum, disorders of the thyroid or adrenal gland, or PKU.

KEY CONCEPTS

- Alteration in the maternal metabolic milieu characteristic of diabetic mellitus may be responsible for congenital malformations that occur sometime before the fourth to the seventh week of gestation.
- Maternal hyperglycemia results in elevated fetal glucose concentrations.
- Maternal insulin does not cross the placenta.
- Fetal insulin secretion (begun at 10 weeks' gestation) is directly related to fetal glucose concentration.
- After the tenth week of gestation, fetal hyperinsulinism results from maternal hyperglycemia (fetal hyperinsulinism is responsible for fetal disorders, discussed in Chapter 38).
- A decrease in insulin requirements in later weeks of pregnancy is a grave prognostic sign for the fetus; the decreasing need reflects decreasing placental function.
- Home monitoring for glucose, multiple doses or constant infusion of insulin, and dietary counseling are being used to create a normal intrauterine environment for fetal growth and maturation.
- Poor control of diabetes mellitus during pregnancy is responsible for dystotic labor from hydramnios and macrosomia, infections, vascular damage, and an increased risk for PIH.
- The woman who is being treated for hyperemesis gravidarum is discharged home when fluid and electrolyte balance is restored and weight gain begins.
- Elevated maternal blood phenylalanine levels during pregnancy result in fetal hyperphenylalaninemia responsible for intrauterine and postnatal growth retardation and mental retardation.

STUDY QUESTIONS AND ACTIVITIES

1. Develop a teaching plan for the pregnant diabetic woman, using audiovisual aids where feasible. If possible, present a class for diabetic women at a prenatal clinic.
2. Interview several diabetic mothers in the postpartum period and determine their feelings during pregnancy, the amount of hospitalization required before delivery, tests undergone, and medication costs. In group discussion, present this information and discuss and compare the mothers' perceptions of their experiences.
3. Develop plans of care for a woman with hyperemesis gravidarum, including psychologic considerations.
4. Develop a care plan for a woman who does not follow her prescribed treatment. Role play one part of the care plan in front of a group. Explore the feelings, beliefs, and values that emerge in the group discussion that follows.

References

American Diabetes Association: Position statement: Nutritional recommendations and principles for individuals with diabetes mellitus: 1986, *Diabetes Care* 10:126–32, 1987

Corbett, JV: Laboratory tests and diagnostic procedures with nursing diagnoses, ed 2, Norwalk, Conn, 1987, Appleton & Lange

Coustan, DR, and Carpenter, MW: Detection and treatment of gestational diabetes, Clin Obstet Gynecol 28(23):507, 1985

Franz, MJ: Nutrition recommendations for the eighties, Practical Diabetology 7(4):1, 1988

Gabbe, SG: Diabetes in pregnancy, Clin Obstet Gynecol 28(3):455, 1985

Golde, S, and Platt, L: Antepartum testing in diabetes, Clin Obstet Gynecol 28(3):516, 1985

Hay, WW, and Sparks, JW: Placental, fetal, and neonatal carbohydrate metabolism, Clin Obstet Gynecol 28(3):473, 1985

Hayes, JS, et al: Managing PKU: an update, MCN 12(2):119, 1987

Hill, CS, Jr, et al: Effect of pregnancy after thyroid carcinoma, Surg Gynecol Obstet 122:1219, 1966

Hollingsworth, DR: Maternal metabolism in normal pregnancy and pregnancy complicated by diabetes mellitus, Clin Obstet Gynecol 28(3):457, 1985

Jovanovic, R, and Jovanovic, L: Obstetric management when normoglycemia is maintained in diabetic pregnant women with vascular compromise, Am J Obstet Gynecol 149:617, 1984

Kitzmiller, JL, Aiello, LM, Kaldany, A, and Younger, MD: Diabetic vascular disease complicating pregnancy, Clin Obstet Gynecol 24:107, 1981

Klein, BEK, Davis, MD, Segal, P, et al: Diabetic retinopathy: assessment of severity and progression, Ophthalmology 91:10, 1984

Kleinman, CS: Fetal echocardiography, Sanders R, editor: Ultrasound annual, New York, 1982, Raven Press

Landon, MG, and Gabbe, SG: Glucose monitoring and insulin administration in the pregnant diabetic patient, Clin Obstet Gynecol 28(3):496, 1985

Mennuti, MT: Teratology and genetic counseling in the diabetic pregnancy complicated by diabetes mellitus, Clin Obstet Gynecol 28(3):486, 1985

Milunsky, A, Alpert, E, Kitzmiller, JL, et al: Prenatal diagnosis of neural tube defects. VIII. The importance of serum alphafetoprotein screening in diabetic pregnant women, Am J Obstet Gynecol 142:1030, 1982

Mullivor, RA, Mennuti, MT, and Harris, H: Origin of the alkaline phosphatases in amniotic fluid, Am J Obstet Gynecol 135:77, 1979

National Diabetes Data Group: Classification and diagnosis of diabetes mellitus and other categories of glucose intolerance, Diabetes 28:1039, 1979

Nesler, CL, et al: Diabetic nephropathy in pregnancy, Clin Obstet Gynecol 28(3):528, 1985

Nursing 87 Books: 1987 Nursing photobook annual, Springhouse, Penn, 1987, Springhouse Corp

Robertson, C: When your pregnant patient has diabetes, RN, p 18, Nov 1987

Sinclair, SH, Nesler, CL, and Schwartz, SS: Retinopathy in the pregnant diabetic, Clin Obstet Gynecol 28(3):536, 1985

Steele, JM: Prepregnancy counseling and contraception in the insulin-dependent diabetic patient, Clin Obstet Gynecol 28(3):553, 1985

White, P: Classification of obstetric diabetes, Am J Obstet Gynecol 130:228, 1978

Bibliography

American Diabetes Association: Position statement: use of noncaloric sweeteners, *Diabetes Care* 10:546, 1987

American Diabetes Association and The American Dietetic Association: *A guide for professionals: diabetes nutrition and meal planning,* Alexandria, Vir, 1988, American Diabetes Association

Barnico, LM, and Cullinane, MM: Maternal phenylketonuria: an unexpected challenge MCN 10:108, March/April 1985

Bates, S, and Ahern, JA: Tight control: what does it mean? Am J Nurs 86(11):1256, 1986

Byrnes, CA: What's new in the diabetic diet, Nurs' 87 17(8):58, 1987

Caro, I: Cutaneous manifestations of diabetes mellitus, Practical Diabetology 7(2):20, 1988

Christman, C: Diabetes: new names, new test, new diet, Nurs' 87 17(1):34, 1987

Coustan, DR, and Carpenter, MW: Detection and treatment of gestational diabetes, Clin Obstet Gynecol 28:507, Sept 1985

Coustan, DR: Home glucose monitoring becomes more sophisticated, Contemp OB/GYN 20:7, Oct 1982 (Special issue, Technology 1983)

Coustan, DR: Is insulin necessary for gestational diabetes, Contemp OB/GYN 29(6):35, 1987

Dibble, CM, Kochenour, NK, Worley, RJ, et al: Effect of pregnancy on diabetic retinopathy, Obstet Gynecol 59:699, 1982

Droegemueller, W, et al: Comprehensive gynecology, St Louis, 1987, The CV Mosby Co

Duhamel, B: From the mermaid to anal imperforation: the syndrome of caudal regression, Arch Dis Child 36:152, 1961

Flavin, K, and Haire-Joshu, D: The pharmacologic repertoire, Am J Nurs 86(11):1244, 1986

Fredholm, NZ: The insulin pump: new method of insulin delivery, Am J Nurs 81(11):2024, 1981

Gabbe, SG: Diabetes in pregnancy, Clin Obstet Gynecol 28:455, Sept 1985

Haire-Joshu, D, Flavin, K, and Clutter, W: Contrasting type I and type II diabetes, Am J Nurs 86(11):1239, 1986

Haire-Joshu, D, Flavin, K, and Santiago, JV: Intensive conventional insulin therapy, Am J Nurs 86(11):1251, 1986

Hollander, P: Gestational diabetes: the diabetes of pregnancy, Practical Diabetology 7(2):14, 1988

Hughes, B: Diabetes management: the time is right for tight glucose control, Nurs '87 17(5):63, 1987

Jovanovic, L: Insulin on the go, Practical Diabetology 7(2):10 1988

Kalhan, S, Schwartz, R, and Adam, P: Placental barrier to human insulin in insulin-dependent diabetic mothers, J Clin Endocrinol Metab 40:139, 1975

Kitzmiller, JL: Recent progress in the management of diabetes mellitus, UCSF antepartum and intrapartum conference, San Francisco, Calif, June, 1987

Lenke, RR, and Levy, HL: Maternal phenylketonuria and hyperphenylalaninemia: an international survey of the outcome of untreated and treated pregnancies, N Engl J Med 303:1202, 1980

Lipman, AG: Drugs that interfere with urine glucose tests, Mod Med, Aug 15-Sept 15, p 195, 1978

McAdams, RC, and Birmingham, D: When diabetes races out of control, RN, p 46, May 1986

Messner, RL, and Gorse, GJ: Nursing management of peripheral intravenous sites, FOCUS on critical care 14(2):25, 1987

Miller, E, Hare, JW, and Cloherty, JP: Elevated maternal hemoglobin A_{1c} in early pregnancy and major congenital anomalies in infants of diabetic mothers, N Engl J Med 304:1331, 1981

Mills, JL, Baker, L, and Goldman, AS: Malformations in infants of diabetic mothers occur before the seventh gestational week: implications for treatment, Diabetes 28:292, 1979

National Diabetes Data Group, Classification and diagnosis of diabetes mellitus and other categories of glucose intolerance, Diabetes 28:1039, 1979

Ney, DM: Nutritional management of diabetes during pregnancy, Practical Diabetology, 7(2):1 1988

Pederson, JF, Pedersen, LM, and Mortensen, HB: Fetal growth delay and maternal hemoglobin A_{1c} in early diabetic pregnancy, Obstet Gynecol 64:351, 1984

Queenan, JT: Managing polyhydramnios, Contemp OB/GYN 22:17, Aug 1983

Robertson, C: When an insulin-dependent diabetic must be NPO, Nurs '86 16(6):30, 1986

Robertson, C: Interpreting blood glucose studies, Nurs '86 16(8):64, 1986

Robertson, C: When the patient is also a diabetic, RN, p 33, July 1987

Robertson, C: When your pregnant patient has diabetes, RN, p 18, Nov 1987

Warram, HJ, Krolewski, AS, Gottlieb, MS, and Kahn, CR: Differences in risk of insulin-dependent diabetes in offspring of diabetic mothers and diabetic fathers, N Engl J Med 311:149, 1984

Zigrossi, ST, and Riga-Ziegler, M: The stress of medical management on pregnant diabetics, MCN 11(5):320, 1986

CHAPTER 33

Labor and Delivery at Risk

Learning Objectives

Correctly define the key terms listed.

Discuss assessment for each type of labor and delivery at risk.

Formulate nursing diagnoses based on assessment.

Compare and contrast interventions for different types of dystocia.

Evaluate needed alterations in the nursing process for clients experiencing operative obstetrics.

Examine alterations in nursing process for clients experiencing multiple pregnancy.

Explain management of preterm labor at home and in the hospital setting.

Review management of postterm labor.

Discuss evaluation criteria for nursing process for labor and delivery at risk.

Key Terms

amniotomy
Bishop's scale
breech presentations
cesarean delivery
dysfunctional labor
dystocia
eutocia
external cephalic version
Ferguson's reflex
fetal lung maturity
fetopelvic disproportion
forceps delivery
iatrogenic
induction of labor
magnesium sulfate
oxytocin
pelvic dystocia
postterm birth
precipitate labor
preterm labor
prolonged labor
prostaglandin
ritodrine hydrochloride
soft tissue dystocia
tocolysis
trial of labor
vacuum extraction
vaginal birth after cesarean delivery (VBAC)

Complications during the birth period can cause death or injury to both mother and infant. Prevention and detection of complications and consequent institution of remedial measures require the concerted efforts of the obstetric team. Many of the complications can be diagnosed before the beginning of labor, and preparation can limit their effects. Others arise suddenly, thus only the critical judgment of those present safeguards the mother or infant. The care afforded the expectant mother through normal labor must be adjusted to meet additional needs (Fig. 33-1). Equipment necessary for high-risk pregnancy, includes labor bed with side rails, oxygen flowmeter, call bell, blood pressure apparatus on wall behind bed, fetal monitoring equipment to left of bed, intravenous (IV) stand and drip meter to right of bed, and stethoscopes on overhead table. Clients and support persons need careful explanation of use of this equipment to reduce anxiety when seeing it for first time.

DYSTOCIA

Dystocia is defined as difficult birth as opposed to easy (normal) birth, or eutocia. Dystocia results from differences in the normal relationships between any of the five essential factors of labor (see Chapter 16). The five factors are as follows:

1. Passageway
   a. Configuration and diameters of the maternal pelvis (pelvic dystocia)
   b. Distensibility of the lower uterine segment, cervical dilation, and capacity for distension of the vaginal canal and introitus (soft tissue dystocia)
2. Powers (dysfunctional labor)
   a. Primary powers: intensity, duration, and frequency of uterine contractions
   b. Secondary powers: bearing-down efforts
3. Passenger
   a. Fetus: gestational age, size, attitude, presentation, and position of the fetus; number of fetuses (dystocia of fetal origin)
   b. Placenta: type, sufficiency of, and site of implantation; cord insertion (Chapter 31)
4. Position of the mother: standing, walking, sidelying, squatting, hands and knees, sitting
5. Psychologic response: previous experiences, emotional readiness, preparation, cultural-ethnic heritage, support systems, and environment

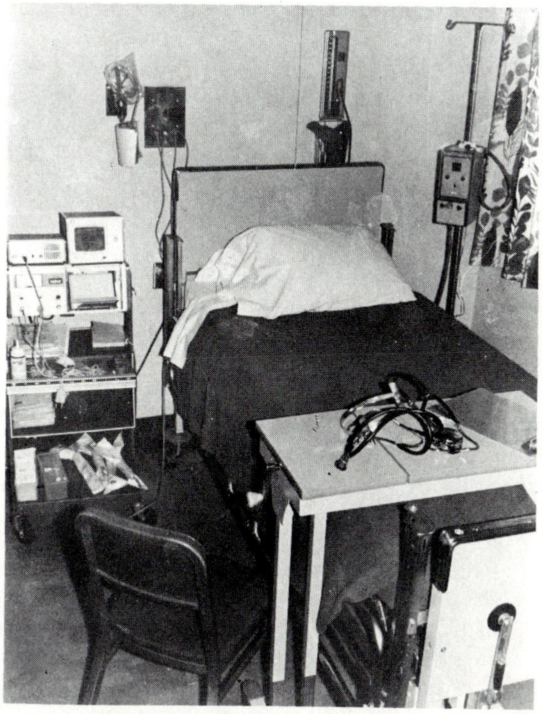

Fig. 33-1 Labor room for high-risk pregnancy.

The differences between dystocia and eutocia relate to **changes in the pattern of progress in labor**. Abnormal labor patterns are reflected in the following aspects:

1. Alterations in the characteristics of uterine contractions
2. Lack of progress in effacement or dilation of the cervix
3. Lack of progress in descent and expulsion of the fetus

Dystocia is classified according to the area or tissue of the birth canal that is involved. The condition may occur singly or in combination with another. Tables 33-1 to 33-3 present descriptions of the various types of conditions that cause dystocia. They include a description of the condition of dystocia, changes in the pattern of labor, potential maternal and fetal effects, and the medical management. The nursing care of the woman with any type of dystocia is similar to that associated with prolonged labor (p. 810).

Passageway

Pelvic Dystocia. Pelvic dystocia may occur with significant shortening of one or more of the internal diameters of the bony pelvis. Such diminution in capacity is termed *pelvic contracture.* The *mechanism* of labor depends on the configuration of the interior of the pelvis (see Chapter 16). However, the *outcome of labor* is affected more by the size of the pelvis than by pelvic configuration. Table 33-1 presents an overview of the various types of pelvic contracture.

Pelvic deformities may be secondary to automobile accidents or childhood poliomyelitis. Unilateral lameness from polio distributes the body weight unevenly. This causes the "good" side of the pelvis to move upward, inward, and backward (Compton, 1987).

Soft Tissue Dystocia. Soft tissue dystocia results from obstruction of the birth passage by an anatomic abnormality other than that of the bony pelvis. The obstruction may result from placenta previa (low-lying placenta), that partially or completely obstructs the internal os of the cervix. Care relative to placenta previa is discussed in Chapter 31.

The most common pelvic mass associated with pregnancy is a *uterine myoma* (Bezjian, 1980). The incidence of myomata in pregnancy is approximately 1%. The most common complications of myomas in pregnancy are abortion, premature labor, malpresentations, obstructed labor, and postpartum hemorrhage (Myerscough, 1982; Compton, 1987). Myomas may affect the progress of labor either by causing a fetal malpresentation, such as a face or a brow,

Table 33-1 *Pelvic Dystocia*

Factor	Inlet Contracture	Midpelvic Contracture	Outlet Contracture
Description	Diagonal conjugate less than 11.5 cm (see Fig. 16-9)	Sum of interischial spinous and posterior sagittal diameters of midpelvis 13.5 cm or less (see Fig. 16-10) Interischial spinous diameter less than 9 cm (see Fig. 16-10)	Interischial spinous diameter 8 cm or less Outlet contraction alone, without midplane contraction, rare
Change in pattern of labor	**Rupture of membranes, early, spontaneous** **Dilation of cervix slows or ceases** **Descent does not occur**	**Descent arrested (transverse arrest of the fetal head); fetal head cannot undergo internal rotation and descend** **Contractions decrease in frequency and intensity** **Dilation of cervix slows**	**Descent arrested**
Potential maternal effects	Intrauterine infection Rupture of abnormally thinned lower segment of uterus (see Fig. 16-14, *E*) Pathologic retraction ring develops Formation of fistulas Psychologic trauma from difficult delivery	Rupture of uterus Exhaustion Psychologic trauma from difficult delivery	Extensive perineal lacerations Exhaustion
Potential fetal effects	Fetal asphyxia Fetal and neonatal death Excessive molding of fetal head Prolapse of cord	Fetal asphyxia Fetal death Excessive molding of head	Fetal asphyxia Fetal death
Medical management	Cesarean delivery if safe vaginal delivery not possible	Cesarean delivery if fetal head cannot pass obstruction Forceps delivery if fetal head passes obstruction (head descends, perineum bulges, vertex is visible) Vacuum extractor when cervix fully dilated	Extensive mediolateral episiotomy

or by actually causing an obstruction in the birth canal. Generally, myomas in the upper part of the uterus do not cause these problems, in spite of many of them being extremely large at the time of delivery. However, myomas located in the lower segment, if of sufficient size, can cause dystocia during labor (Compton, 1987).

Bandl's ring, a pathologic retraction ring (Fig. 16-14, *E*) may cause second-stage dystocia. Uncommonly, a *vaginal* longitudinal *septum* divides the vagina partly or completely into two compartments. The physician may opt to incise them early in labor before they tear or obstruct delivery of the fetal head (Compton, 1987).

All types of *ovarian tumors* may be associated with pregnancy, but the most common are cystic. If the cyst is particularly large, it can fill the whole true pelvis and cause dystocia (Compton, 1987).

A **distended bladder** may on occasion act as an obstruction to labor, especially during the second stage of labor. Straight catheterization of the bladder during the second stage of labor may be all that is needed to correct what had previously appeared to have been a second stage arrest (Compton, 1987). A **full rectum** may have the same effect.

Pelvic ectopic kidneys are a rare finding in pregnancy. Women who become pregnant after a renal transplantation are becoming much more common. The transplanted kidney is placed in the pelvis. A borderline pelvis theoretically could cause an obstruction (Compton, 1987).

In obese women weighing more than 136.4 kg (300 lb), the amount of adipose tissue found in the pelvis can be impressive (Compton, 1987). Often the bony pelvis, both on clinical examination and on x-ray pelvimetry, appears to be adequate. However, in spite of excellent uterine contractions and an average size infant, dystocia may develop in the later stages of labor. In the absence of significant molding, dystocia probably occurs because of decreases in the pelvic diameters secondary to *pelvic adipose tissue.* Occasionally, **cervical edema** occurs in labor when the cervix is caught between the presenting part and the symphysis. Cervical edema prevents complete dilation of the cervix.

Powers: Dysfunctional Labor

Hypotonic Uterine Dysfunction. When uterine contractions are too weak, too short, irregular, or infrequent (Figs. 33-2 and 33-3), progressive cervical dilation and effacement and descent of the presenting part do not occur.

Uterine dysfunction complicates almost 5% of all labors at term, and approximately 90% of the women are nulliparas. It is classified as follows:

1. *Primary uterine inertia:* inefficient contractions persist from the onset of labor
2. *Secondary uterine inertia:* well-established, efficient contractions become weak and inefficient or stop altogether

Table 33-2 presents a summary of dysfunctional labor.

Hypertonic Uterine Dysfunction. Hypertonic uterine contractions may result in "precipitate" labor. Precipitate labor is defined as a rapid labor that lasts less than 3 hours. It is characterized by tetanic-type contractions. If the birth canal is in a relaxed state, effects on the mother can be minimal. However, if the birth canal is not readily distensible, uterine rupture or lacerations of the birth canal can occur. Pritchard, McDonald, and Gant (1985) note "**The uterus that contracts with unusual vigor before delivery is likely to be hypotonic after delivery with hemorrhage from the placental implantation site as the consequence.**" The fetus may suffer from hypoxia as a result of diminished placental perfusion secondary to tetanic-type contraction.

Inadequate Voluntary Expulsive Forces. Bearing down efforts are compromised by large amounts of analgesic. Anesthesia may block the bearing down reflex and alter the effectiveness of voluntary efforts. Exhaustion from lack of sleep or long labor and fatigue from inadequate hydration and food affect the woman's voluntary efforts. Maternal position can work against the forces of gravity, as well as decrease the contraction's strength and efficiency. Gravity adds 10 to 35 mmHg to the pressure exerted by the presenting part (Fenwick and Simkin, 1987).

Passenger: Dystocia of Fetal Origin

Fetal dystocia is the result of an unfortunate relationship between fetal anatomy and maternal pelvic capacity (Per-

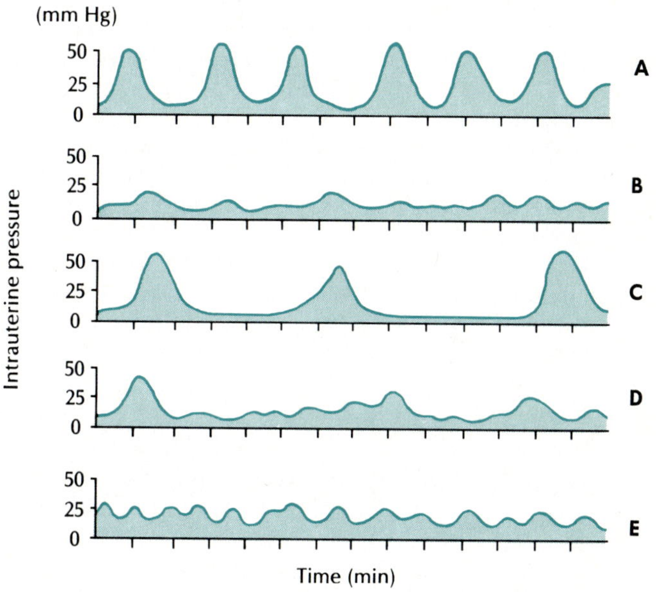

Fig. 33-2 Uterine contractility patterns in labor. **A,** Typical normal labor. **B,** Subnormal intensity, with frequency greater than needed for optimum performance. **C,** Normal contractions, but too infrequent for efficient labor. **D,** Incoordinate activity. **E,** Hypercontractility.

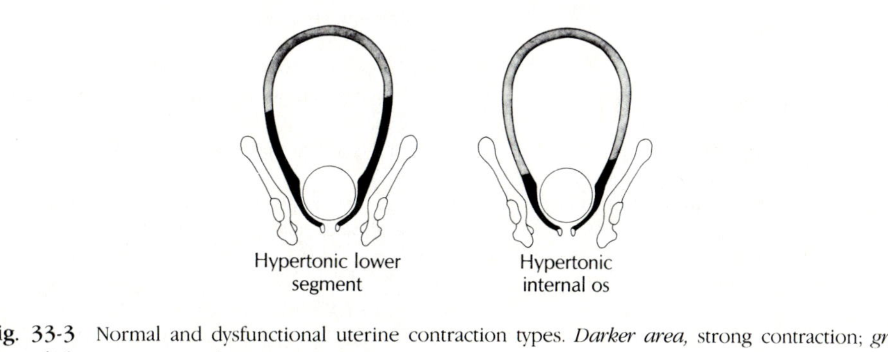

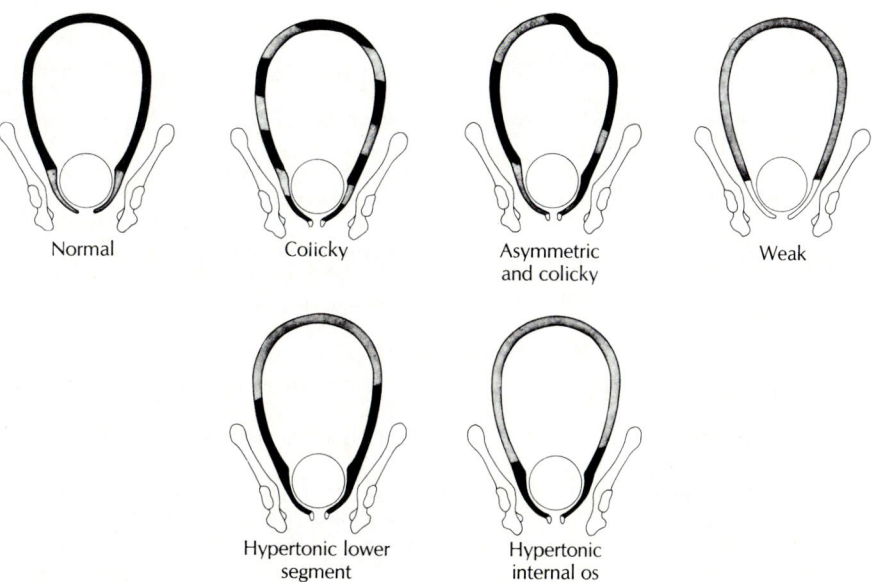

Fig. 33-3 Normal and dysfunctional uterine contraction types. *Darker area,* strong contraction; *grey area,* slight contraction, *white area,* atonic areas.

kins, 1987). It may be caused by fetal anomalies such as gross ascites or abdominal tumor, myelomeningocele, and hydrocephalus, excessive size, or malpresentation or malposition of the fetus (Table 33-3). Although these conditions are uncommon, they constitute obstetric emergencies.

Fetal dystocia may be classified according to the cause of the abnormality as follows:

Fetopelvic Disproportion. Excessive *fetal size* is arbitrarily 4000 g (8 lb. 13½ oz) or more in North America. Shoulder dystocia can be anticipated in large fetuses (Lee, 1987). Such large fetuses represent about 5% of term births. Commonly excessive size is a result of diabetes mellitus, obesity, maternal multiparity, or the large size of one or both parents.

Fetal Malposition. The most common fetal malposition is *persistent occiput posterior (OP) position.* Other fetal malpositions are encountered rarely, for example, *transverse lie* (see Fig. 16-5, *D*).

Fetal Malpresentation. *Breech presentation* is the most common example of malpresentation. Concern surrounding vaginal delivery in breech presentation arises from the vulnerability of the fetal brain stem, cerebellar fossa, and vertebral artery from subluxation of the occipital bone (Perkins, 1987).

Multiple Pregnancy. Multiple pregnancy is the gestation of twins, triplets, quadruplets, or more infants (Chapter 9). Infants of multiple pregnancies account for 2% to 3% of all viable births. Of twins, more than 15% weigh less than 2500 g. Most of these are preterm. Twins occur in about 1 in 99 conceptions; triplets and quadruplets occur much less frequently (Fig. 9-11). Multiple pregnancy is most common in blacks, least common in Orientals, and of intermediate occurrence in whites. Almost 30% of twins are monozygotic (Fig. 9-9); nearly 70% are dizygotic (Fig. 9-10). Fewer males than females are born in multiple pregnancies. Maternal morbidity and mortality are greatly increased in multiple pregnancy because of medical and obstetric complications. The prenatal diagnosis of multiple pregnancy is made in only about 75% of cases and often late in gestation. This is regrettable, since much can be done for the mother and her infants if treatment is instituted early.

In twin pregnancy, both fetuses will present by the vertex in about one half of cases; one will present by the vertex and one by the breech in approximately one third of

Table 33-2 *Dysfunctional Labor: Primary and Secondary Powers*

Factor	Hypotonic Uterine Dysfunction	Hypertonic Uterine Dysfunction	Inadequate Voluntary Expulsive Forces
Description	Cause may be contracture and fetal malposition, overextension of uterus (twins), or unknown (primary powers) (Figs. 33-2 and 33-3)	Usually occurs before 4 cm dilation; cause not yet known, may be related to fear and tension (primary powers) (Figs. 33-2 and 33-3)	Involves abdominal and levator ani muscles Occurs in second stage of labor; cause may be related to conduction anesthesia, heavy analgesia, paralysis or intense pain with contractions (secondary powers)
Change in pattern of progress	**Contractions decrease in frequency and intensity** **Uterus easily indentable even at peak of contraction** **Uterus relaxed between contractions (normal)**	**Pain out of proportion to intensity of contraction** **Pain out of proportion to effectiveness of contraction in effacing and dilating the cervix** **Contractions increase in frequency** **Contractions uncoordinated** **Uterus is contracted between contraction (basal hypertonus), cannot be indented.**	**No voluntary urge to push or bear down**
Potential maternal effects	Infection Exhaustion Psychologic trauma	Loss of control related to intensity of pain and lack of progress Exhaustion	Spontaneous vaginal delivery prevented
Potential fetal effects	Fetal infection Fetal and neonatal death	Fetal asphyxia with meconium aspiration	Fetal asphyxia
Medical management	Oxytocic stimulation of labor (p. 814) Prostaglandin stimulation of labor (p. 814)	Analgesic (morphine, meperidine) if membranes not ruptured or fetopelvic disproportion not present Relief of pain permits mother to rest; when she awakens, normal uterine activity may begin	Coach mother in bearing down with contractions Analgesia to counteract pain Cesarean delivery only if fetal distress

Table 33-3 *Dystocia of Fetal Origin*

Factor	Fetopelvic Disproportion	Malposition	Malpresentation: Breech
Description	Fetal macrosomia with normal or small pelvis Fetal anomaly	Persistent occiput posterior position (OP) Leopold's manuevers reveal small parts against abdominal wall Abdominal contours differ (Fig. 33-4) Vaginal examination: the cervix may need to be fully dilated before examiner can feel direction of suture lines in relation to fontanels	Related to prematurity; most infants assume a longitudinal lie with vertex presenting at term Related to multiple fetuses, hydramnios, oligohydramnios, fetal or maternal anomalies Breech presentations revealed by abdominal and vaginal examinations, x-ray films, and sonography Breech presentation occurs in four types (Fig. 33-5)
Change in pattern of progress	**Engagement does not occur** **Descent does not occur** **Uterus unusual size or contour** **Membranes rupture early** **Cervical dilation slows** **Contractions decrease in frequency and intensity**	**Contractions are diminished in frequency and intensity** **Backache is accentuated** **Cervical dilation slows** **Descent is delayed** **Second stage of labor may be prolonged**	**Heart sounds loudest slightly above the umbilicus (Fig. 18-5)** **Labor not unduly prolonged** **Spontaneous complete expulsion seldom successfully accomplished** **Aftercoming head does not have time to mold during descent and therefore expulsion may be prevented**
Potential maternal effects	Infection Development of pathologic ring Rupture of uterus Vaginal fistulas	Exhaustion Increased sensitivity to pain Extension of episiotomy Psychologic trauma from prolonged labor	Morbidity and mortality increased as result of operative delivery including cesarean delivery
Potential fetal effects	Infection Prolapse of cord Excessive molding of the head; may result in intracranial hemorrhage	Fetal asphyxia	Prematurity Congenital anomalies Birth trauma, asphyxia from cord compression or placental separation during birth Fetal death Infant has little molding of the head
Medical management	Cesarean delivery if vaginal delivery poses a potential threat to mother or fetus	Conservative approach followed as most of fetuses (70%) in OP position: • Rotate spontaneously to an anterior position and deliver spontaneously • May deliver in the face-to-pubes position if posterior position persists Mediolateral episiotomy done to permit manual or forceps rotation Low forceps delivery of vertex may be needed Cesarean delivery if head does not engage, rotation cannot be accomplished or face-to-pubes delivery not possible	External version may be attempted after 34 weeks gestation (Fig. 33-6) Extra sterile towels and **Piper forceps** (Fig. 33-9) are added to delivery table for mechanism of labor shown in Fig. 33-7 Cesarean delivery is commonly used in nulliparas and in multiparas with fetuses estimated to be larger than 3360 g (7¼ lb) if labor is ineffective or when hazardous complications arise

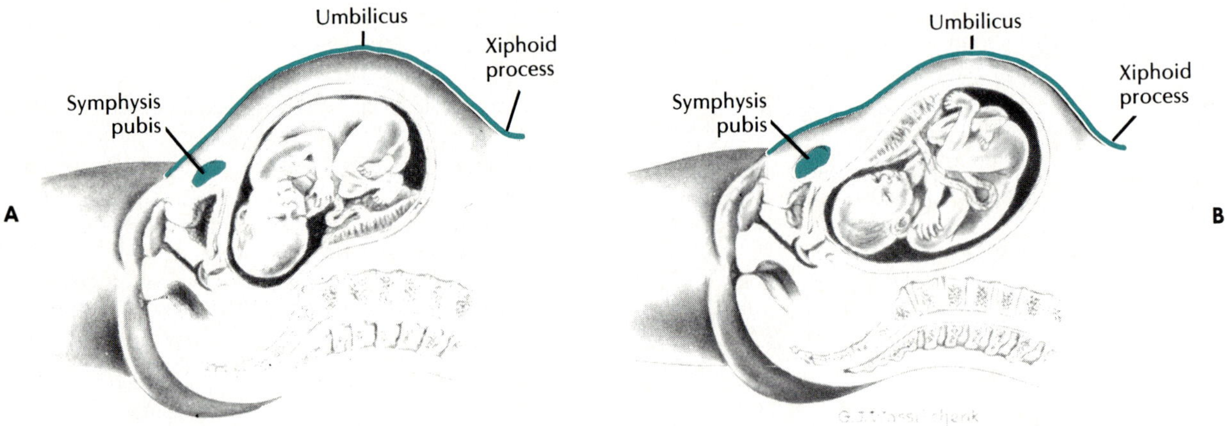

Fig. 33-4 Comparison of abdominal contours with fetus in occiput anterior (OA) position (colored), **A**, and occiput posterior (OP) position. **B**, The indentation between fetal chin and small parts forms a concavity above the level of the symphysis (may be obscured by a full bladder).

the total births. Other combinations are uncommon. Conjoined twins (1:50,000 pregnancies) result in dystocia as a result of fetopelvic disproportion (Perkins, 1987).

Position of the Mother

The functional relationships between the uterine contractions, the fetus, and the mother's pelvis are altered by maternal positioning. In addition, positioning can provide either a mechanical advantage or disadvantage to the mechanisms of labor by altering the effects of gravity and the relationships among body parts that are significant to labor progress (Fenwick and Simkin, 1987). Discouraging maternal movement or restricting labor to the recumbant or lithotomy position may compromise labor. The positions commonly chosen by laboring women for comfort may also reduce the length of labor, thus reducing the possibility of dystocia (Fenwick and Simkin, 1987). Freedom of movement (e.g., walking, squatting, sitting) offers a greater variety of angles to the presenting part, increasing the chances of a better fit between fetus and pelvis (Chapters 16, 17, and 19).

Psychologic Response

Hormones released in response to stress can cause dystocia. Sources of stress vary for each individual, but pain and the absence of a support person are two accepted factors. Maternal position can decrease the efficiency of labor and increase pain (Caldeyro-Barcia, 1979). Confinement to bed and restriction of maternal movement add a potential psychologic stress to compound the physiologic stress of immobility in the unmedicated parturient. Women who are upright in the second stage of labor produce lower levels of stress-related hormones (β-endorphin, adrenocorticotropic hormone [ACTH], cortisol, and epinephrine) than women who are supine. These women report less tension and anxiety when sitting upright. The labor-inhibiting effects of excessive levels of these hormones are well documented (Simkin, 1986) and may be associated with dystotic labor patterns (Fenwick and Simkin, 1987).

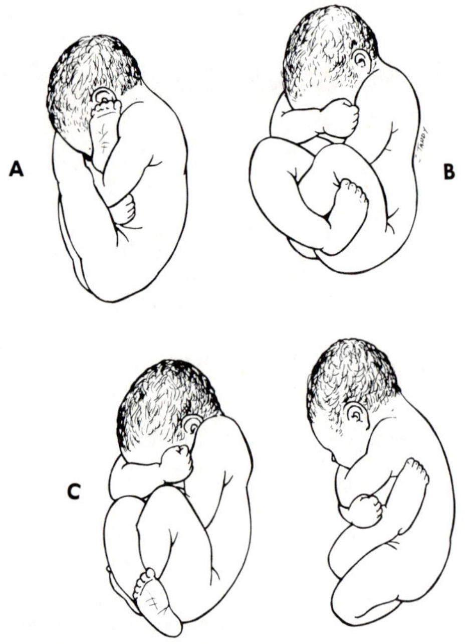

Fig. 33-5 Types of breech presentation. **A**, Frank breech: thighs are flexed on hips; knees are extended. **B**, Complete breech: thighs and knees are flexed. **C**, Incomplete breech: foot extends below buttocks. **D**, Incomplete breech: knee extends below buttocks.

Prolonged Labor

Determination of when labor begins may be the source of considerable perplexity and produce errors of variable magnitude (Sheen and Hayashi, 1987). The onset of the active phase is apparent on the graphs, because the rate of cervical dilation begins to change acutely and the labor curve becomes more steeply inclined (Figs. 18-7 and 18-8).

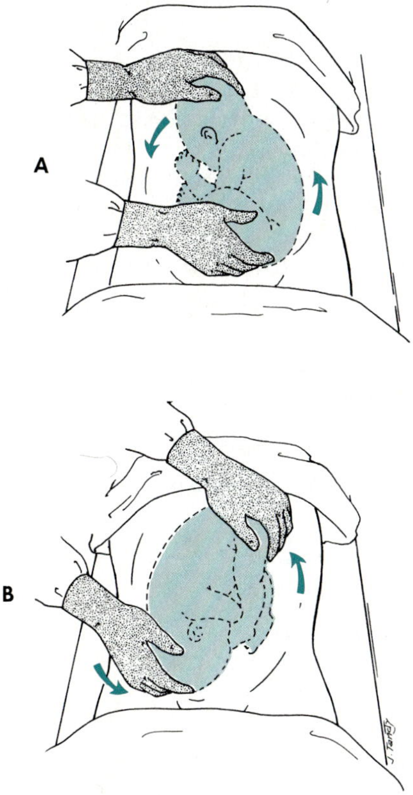

Fig. 33-6 External version of fetus from breech to vertex presentation. This must be achieved without force. **A**, Breech is pushed up out of pelvic inlet while head is pulled toward inlet. **B**, Head is pushed toward inlet while breech is pulled upward.

The Terminology Committee of the American College of Obstetricians and Gynecologists suggests that *prolonged labor* is active labor that continues more than 20 hours. Most obstetricians are satisfied that 18 hours is the upper limit for normal labor. (Danforth and Scott, 1986).

Prolonged labor may result from varying causes. Pelvic contractures, fetopelvic disproportion, or inadequate uterine contractions can occur singly or in combination. The cervix may be *unfavorable,* that is, not relaxed and partially dilated in preparation for labor. Progress in either the first or second stage is delayed or protracted. Fig. 33-8 compares and contrasts the partogram of a normal labor with major types of deviation from normal progress of labor.

The partogram in Fig. 33-8, *A,* is a graphic appraisal of the time factor in normal labor for a primigravida. The *latent phase* includes that portion of the first stage between the onset of labor contractions and the acceleration in rate of cervical dilation. The upswing in the curve denotes the onset of the *active phase* of the first stage of labor, which includes the *acceleration phase,* the *phase of maximal slope,* and the *deceleration phase.* Compare this with Fig. 33-8, *B,* which show major types of deviation from normal progress of labor. These can be detected by noting the dilation of the cervix at various intervals after labor begins. If a woman exhibits an abnormal labor pattern as depicted by the broken lines, the physician should be notified immediately! (Sheen and Hayashi, 1987.)

1. Cervical dilation patterns: report to physician
   a. Prolonged latent phase: 20 hours or longer in the nullipara and 14 hours or longer in the parous woman
   b. Protracted active phase: cervical dilation of less than

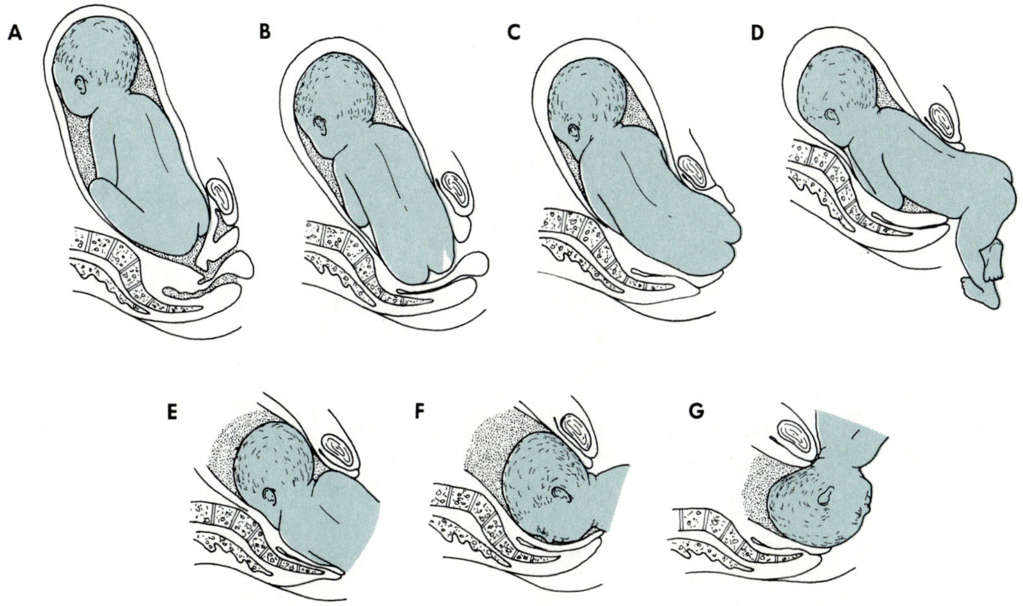

Fig. 33-7 Mechanism of labor in breech position. **A**, Breech before onset of labor. **B**, Engagement and internal rotation. **C**, Lateral flexion. **D**, External rotation or restitution. **E**, Internal rotation of shoulders and head. **F**, Face rotates to sacrum when occiput is anterior. **G**, Head is delivered by gradual flexion during elevation of fetal body.

1.2 cm/hr in the nullipara and less than 1.5 cm/hr in the parous woman
   c. Arrest of the active phase: no progress in the active phase for more than 2 to 4 hours
   d. Precipitate labor: labor of less than 3 hours
2. Descent patterns: report to physician
   a. Protracted descent pattern in the active phase: rate of descent less than 1 cm/hr in the nullipara and less than 2 cm/hr in the parous woman
   b. Arrest of descent in the active phase: no progress for 1 hour or more in the nullipara and 30 minutes in the parous woman
   c. Failure of descent during deceleration and second stage

The labor patterns in normal and prolonged labor are given in the box on p. 813.

Fetal mortality increases sharply after 15 hours of the active first stage of labor. Maternal morbidity and mortality may occur as a result of uterine rupture, infection, serious dehydration, and postpartum hemorrhage. A long difficult

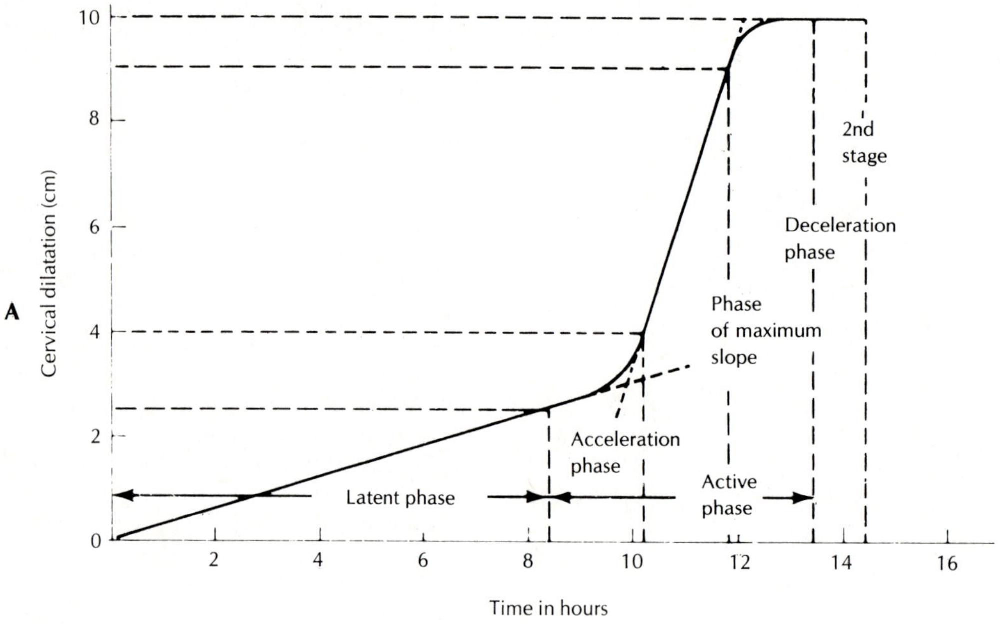

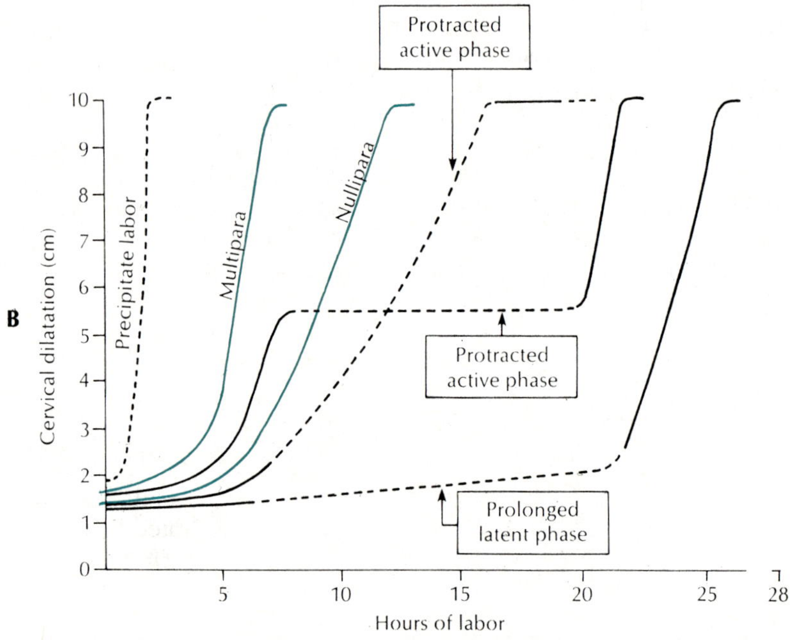

Fig. 33-8 **A**, Partogram of a normal labor. **B**, Arrest of descent in the active phase: no progress for 1 hour or more in the nullipara and 30 minutes in the parous woman.

labor can have an adverse psychologic effect on the mother, father, and family.

Assessment

Risk assessment is a continuous process. Findings from the history and interview, physical examinations, biochemical and biophysical monitoring, and laboratory tests are analyzed (Chapter 27). The progress of labor is monitored for signs of dystocia and maternal and fetal compromise.

Nursing Diagnoses

Nursing diagnoses will vary with the type of dystocia and the individual problems of the woman and her family. Several nursing diagnoses can be anticipated in light of the characteristics of dystocia:

- Pain
- Potential for injury: fetal compromise
- Potential for injury: maternal
- Powerlessness related to
  - Loss of control
- Ineffective individual coping related to
  - Disappointment, pain, fear, or exhaustion
- Knowledge deficit
- Situational low self-esteem related to
  - Inability to labor and give birth to baby as expected

Planning

Nursing diagnoses provide direction for care. During this important step, goals are set in client-centered terms, and the goals are prioritized. Nursing actions are selected with the client, as appropriate, to meet the goals.

Goals. Goals for the woman who is experiencing dystocia include the prevention of hemorrhage, infection, and embolytic complications; control of pain; and promotion of feelings of self-esteem. Goals for the infant include maintenance of a healthy intrauterine environment and healthy adjustment to extrauterine life. The promotion of positive mother-family-infant relationships is a vital goal for the family.

Implementation

Nurses assume many caregiving roles when labor is complicated. The nurse's roles are both supportive and teacher/counselor/advocate. Knowledge of medical management for each condition is essential to implementation of the nursing process. This knowledge enables the nurse to work collaboratively with the physician and to meet the client's knowledge and emotional needs. The nurse should also be a consumer of nursing research and alert to potential areas for future nursing research.

LABOR PATTERNS IN NORMAL AND PROLONGED LABOR

Normal Labor

1. Dilation: continues
   a. Latent phase: <4 cm and low slope
   b. Active phase: >5 cm or high slope
   c. Deceleration phase: ≥ 9 cm
2. Descent: active at ≥ 9 cm dilation
3. Normal labor progresses rapidly; multiparas faster than nulliparas

Prolonged Labor Patterns	Nulliparas	Multiparas
1. Prolonged latent phase	>20 hr	>14 hr
2. Protracted active-phase dilation	<1.2 cm/hr	<1.5 cm/hr
3. Secondary arrest: no change for	≥2 hr	≥2 hr
4. Prolonged deceleration phase	>3 hr	>1 hr
5. Protracted descent	<1 cm/hr	<2 cm/hr
6. Arrest of descent	≥1 hr	≥½ hr

Trial of Labor

A trial of labor is a reasonable period (4 to 6 hours) of active labor allowed for assessment of the possibility of a safe vaginal delivery for mother and infant. Examples of when it is done are previous cesarean section, a "questionable" pelvis, and fetal malpresentation (i.e., breech presentation). In the presence of such conditions, if x-ray pelvimetry and fetal sonography demonstrate no fetopelvic disproportion, and the cervix is soft and dilatable, a trial of labor is reasonable. Active labor includes adequate contractions, engagement and descent of the presenting part, and progressive effacement and dilation of the cervix. Trial of labor is seldom induced artificially.

Assessment of the response of the woman and fetus during this time provides the data for the physician's choice of delivery. Should evidence of maternal or fetal compromise arise, the nurse initiates appropriate action and notifies the physician.

Induction of Labor.

Induction of labor is the deliberate initiation of uterine contractions before their spontaneous onset. The need for initiating labor may arise from maternal or fetal sources, for instance, severe pregnancy-induced hypertension (PIH) or postterm pregnancy. Such conditions may harm the mother or infant if birth does not occur. Elective induction also may be indicated for the woman who has a history of precipitous labors (less than 3 hours). Labor is induced under controlled conditions to avoid an unexpected out-of-hospital birth.

There are a number of medically approved methods to induce labor. They include chemical inductions of labor, with prostaglandins (PGE) and oxytocins, and mechanical methods, such as rupture of membranes (amniotomy).

Prostaglandin. A prostaglandin gel for local application to the cervix has been formulated. The gel is used to soften or prime the cervix and induce labor (Schulman and Farmakides, 1987). The cervix is assessed using the Bishop's scale (Table 33-4). For those women whose cervix is unfavorable, induction using prostaglandins is more effective than using oxytocin.

The woman is admitted to the labor suite, and routine assessments are completed. The dilation and effacement of the cervix are determined. A Bishop's scale score of 5 or more is required. A 30-minute electronic monitoring of the fetal heart rate (FHR) and uterine contractions is done to establish baseline data. The physician instills 0.5 mg of PGE gel intracervically at the level of the internal os, using a flexible catheter (Glazer and Hulme, 1987). The catheter is then removed. The woman remains in bed for 1 hour; then she may ambulate.

The FHR, blood pressure, and pulse are monitored at least every 30 minutes. Ideally the monitoring is done electronically. Contractions usually begin a half-hour after administration of the gel. The time of the beginning of contractions is recorded. An amniotomy is performed at 4 cm cervical dilation, and internal fetal monitoring is applied. Progress of labor is then recorded as it is for all clients.

The local application of prostaglandins appears to minimize side effects. Any hypertonic contractions of the uterus are reported immediately. If the woman does not deliver within 24 hours, the cervix is reassessed using the Bishop's scale, and an induction using oxytocin is done if indicated. Use of PGE to prepare the cervix may permit a lower concentration of oxytocin during induction (Schulman and Farmakides, 1987).

During induction by this method the nurse observes for and intervenes appropriately for side effects (Glazer and Hulme, 1987). Possible side effects include uterine hypertonus, fetal distress, and diarrhea. Left lateral recumbant position, oxygen, and IV fluid support fetal perfusion. Analgesics and tocolytics may be ordered. Cesarean delivery is a possibility. Continued reassurance and support help the woman and her family cope with the situation.

Oxytocin. Oxytocic stimulation of labor may be used either to induce the labor process or to augment a labor that is progressing slowly because of inadequate uterine contractions. It can also be used to assess fetal response to the stress of labor contractions (oxytocin challenge test [OCT]); see Chapter 27.

The *indications* for oxytocin induction of labor include the following:

1. Slowing of progress of labor
2. Management of abortion, to stimulate the uterus to pass the conceptus
3. Prolonged rupture of the membranes
4. Prolonged pregnancy (42 to 43 weeks)
5. Preterm delivery in diabetic mother or infant with severe isoimmunization
6. Severe preeclampsia, abruptio placentae, or fetal death necessitating termination of the pregnancy artificially

Table 33-4 *Bishop's Scale*

	Score*			
	0	1	2	3
Dilation (cm)	0	1-2	3-4	5-6
Effacement (%)	0-30	40-50	60-70	80
Station (cm)	−3	−2	−1	+1
Cervical consistency	Firm	Medium	Soft	
Fetal position	Posterior	Midline	Anterior	

*Parous woman can be induced at score of 5; nulliparous woman, at score of 7.

7. Multigravidas with a history of precipitate labor who live a long distance from the hospital

The management of stimulation of labor is the same regardless of indication. Because of the potential dangers associated with the use of injectable oxytocin in the prenatal and natal periods, the Food and Drug Administration has issued restrictions on its use.

Contraindications to oxytocic stimulation of labor include the following:

1. Fetopelvic disproportion
2. Fetal distress
3. Previous uterine surgery (e.g., cesarean birth)
4. Overdistended uterus (hydramnios, multiple birth)
5. Grand multiparity (over four)

Hazards of oxytocin stimulation to both mother and infant include the following:

1. Maternal
   a. Tumultuous labor and tetanic contractions, which may cause premature separation of the placenta, rupture of the uterus, laceration of the cervix, or postdelivery hemorrhage
   b. Sequelae to above complications: infection, disseminated intravascular coagulation (DIC), amniotic fluid embolism
   c. Fear or anxiety: may be compounded if the procedure is not successful (the woman must be aware of this possibility and of what other techniques can be used)
2. Fetal
   a. Fetal asphyxia and neonatal hypoxia from too frequent and prolonged uterine contractions
   b. Physical injury
   c. Prematurity, if the estimated date of delivery (EDD) has been estimated inaccurately

The responsibility for initiating oxytocin stimulation of labor belongs to the physician, although the procedure is often administered by the nurse (see Procedure 33-1). The physician must determine the correct amount of oxytocin to be added to the infusion bottle, together with the number of drops per minute that will deliver a specific oxytocin dose in milliunits per minute. The number of milliunits of oxytocin *per milliliter* of parenteral solution depends on

Procedure 33-1

INDUCTION OF LABOR

DEFINITION

An obstetric procedure in which labor is started or augmented artificially by means of amniotomy or administration of oxytocics.

PURPOSE

To initiate or augment the uterine contractions of labor.

EQUIPMENT

Oxytocin (Pitocin) or synthetic oxytocin (Syntocinon); container of 1000 ml 5% dextrose in water or normal sterile saline for oxytocin solution; container of 1000 ml 5% dextrose in water or normal sterile saline for piggyback set-up (maintenance IV); infusion pump (IVAC) or standard pump (Harvard); amnihook or Allis clamp (for AROM); bedpan or fracture pan.

NURSING ACTIONS	RATIONALE
Wash hands before and after touching woman and equipment. Glove.	To prevent nosocomial infection and to implement universal precautions.
Apply fetal and maternal electronic monitor before beginning induction.	To obtain constant, accurate recording of FHR and contractions. To obtain baseline information.
Explain technique, rationale, and reactions to expect: IV fluid route and rate: what "piggyback" is for. Reasons for use: induce labor, improve labor.	To promote cooperation of woman and family. To lessen anxiety over technique. To assure woman and family of careful monitoring. To prepare woman and family for chances of success.
Discuss: Reactions to expect—nature of contractions: Intensity of contraction increases more rapidly, holds the peak longer, and ends more quickly. The contractions will begin to come regularly and more often.	To prepare woman for sensations. Preparation dispels fear of the unknown.
Monitoring to expect: Maternal: blood pressure, pulse, uterine contractions, uterine tone. Fetal: heart rate, activity	To reassure woman of continued care.
Success to expect: reaffirm physician's explanation that if inertia is not overcome in 8 hours or less (using 5 U of oxytocin), the chance of success is minimal.	To help woman orient herself in time; to know an end point.
Position woman in left lateral position.	To maximize placental perfusion and oxygenation of fetus.
Prepare solutions and administer according to prescribed orders with pump delivery system: Set up infusion pump and solution. Flag solution containing oxytocin (Pitocin) with a red label. Connect piggyback solution to IV line.	To promote safety, a piggyback setup is used; this permits the induction solution to be stopped while the vein remains open with the second solution.
Begin induction with 1 mU/min (Table 33-5).*	To ensure that the least amount of medication necessary is used for a favorable outcome.
Increase dose arithmetically by 2 mU increments (e.g., 1,3, and 5 mU/min at 15 min intervals) (Table 33-5).	To determine minimum amount of medication necessary for success.
Maintain dose when: Intensity of contraction results in intrauterine pressures of 50 to 75 mm Hg (by internal monitor). Duration of contraction is 40 to 60 seconds. Frequency of contraction is 2 ½ to 4-minute intervals.	To maintain needed stimulation and avoid overstimulation.
Discontinue use of oxytocin per hospital protocol: keep line open with nonmedicated solution.	Woman is in active labor, further stimulation is not required.
Keep woman and family informed of progress.	To reduce anxiety.

*If the pregnancy is complicated by diabetes mellitus, higher doses of oxytocin are usually needed.

Procedure 33-1—cont'd

NURSING ACTIONS	RATIONALE
Discontinue infusion of oxytocin and keep vein open with plain solution if these **danger signs** occur:	To prevent further complications.
Contractions: excessive intrauterine pressure above 75 mm Hg, duration over 60 seconds, and frequency more often than every 2 to 3 minutes.	Overstimulation of the uterine muscle can cause tetany and rupture of the uterus.
Fetal stress: fetal bradycardia, tachycardia, or heart irregularity (oxytocin is stopped and 5% dextrose in water is infused).	Fetoplacental unit may not be strong enough or able to withstand the stress of labor.
For amniotomy:	
Position woman on bedpan or fracture pan.	To catch amniotic fluid when amniotic sac is torn.
Person performing procedure puts on gloves and inserts first two fingers of one hand into cervix until membranes are identified.	To maintain clean environment. To serve as a guide for the amnihook or Allis clamp.
Amnihook or Allis clamp is inserted alongside fingers and membranes are hooked and torn by the instrument.	To allow for release of amniotic fluid.
Assess color, odor, and consistency of fluid.	Discoloration or foul odor signals meconium passage by fetus or infection.
Assess fetal heart rate.	To check for compression or prolapse of umbilical cord.

the amount of oxytocin in units added to the infusion and the time factor over which the solution is to be infused. See Table 33-5 for oxytocin administration using a volumetric infusion pump.

Artificial Rupture of Membranes. Transcervical amniotomy or artificial rupture of the membranes (AROM) can be used to stimulate labor. The cervix should be soft, partially effaced, and slightly dilated, preferably with the presenting part engaged or engaging. Simple rupture of the membranes using a hook or other sharp instrument passed over a finger into the cervix will allow the drainage of amniotic fluid. The mother can be assured that neither she nor the infant will feel any pain from the amniotomy. Within 6 to 8 hours, labor may be under way. Some obstetricians prefer to first stimulate the uterus with IV oxytocin and, as soon as good contractions are evident, rupture the membranes. Others prefer merely to rupture the membranes, knowing that oxytocin stimulation often is unnecessary.

Methods Not Recommended for Stimulation of Labor. Several methods are not recommended for stimulation of labor. Intramuscular or intranasal oxytocin and "stripping of the membranes" are potentially dangerous to the fetus. Occasionally nurses will need to care for women exposed to these actions. The nurse must monitor these women for hyperstimulation of the uterus and prolapse of cord, bleeding, or sepsis.

Forceps Delivery

Obstetric forceps are made from two double-curved, spoonlike articulated blades. They are used to assist in the expulsion of the fetal head. This instrument, regarded by many as one of the greatest inventions of all time, was devised by Peter Chamberlen about 1625. The commonly employed forceps have a cephalic curve shaped similarly to that of the fetal head. A pelvic curve of the blades conforms to the pelvic axis (Fig. 33-9). The blades are joined by a pin, screw, or groove arrangement. These locks prevent the forceps from compressing the fetal skull. Indications for the use of forceps include the following:

1. Maternal: to shorten the second stage in dystocia (difficult labor), or when the mother's expulsive efforts are deficient (e.g., she is tired or she has been given spinal anesthesia), or when the woman is endangered (e.g., cardiac decompensation).
2. Fetal: to rescue a jeopardized fetus (e.g., premature labor or fetal distress close to delivery).

Prerequisites for Forceps Operations. The following conditions must apply for successful forceps delivery:

1. *Fully dilated cervix.* Severe lacerations and hemorrhage may ensue if a rim of cervical tissue remains.
2. *Head engaged.* The extraction of a mature fetus with a "high" (unengaged) head usually is disastrous.
3. *Vertex presentation or face presentation* (mentum anterior). Other presentations require wider-than-average pelvic diameters.
4. *Membranes ruptured* to ensure a firm grasp of the forceps on the fetal head.
5. *No cephalopelvic disproportion.* If there is engagement, there must be no outlet contracture or gross sacral deformity.
6. *Empty bladder and bowel* to avoid visceral laceration and fistula formation.

Level of Forceps Application. The station of the head determines the level of forceps application and, generally, the relative difficulty to be expected in forceps operations.

High Forceps. The biparietal diameter of the vertex is

Table 33-5 ***Oxytocin Administration Using a Volumetric Infusion Pump***

	Dilution of Oxytocin in IV Fluid (mU min)		
Milliliters per Hour (ml/hr)	5 U Oxytocin in 1000 ml Fluid	10 U Oxytocin in 1000 ml Fluid	20 U Oxytocin in 1000 ml Fluid
1.5	0.125	0.25	0.5
3	0.25	0.5	1
6	0.5	1.0	2
9	0.75	1.5	3
12	1.0	2.0	4
15	1.25	2.5	5
18	1.5	3.0	6
21	1.75	3.5	7
24	2.0	4.0	8
27	2.25	4.5	9
30	2.50	5.0	10
33	2.75	5.5	11
36	3.0	6.0	12
39	3.25	6.5	13
42	3.5	7.0	14
45	3.75	7.5	15
48	4.0	8.0	16
51	4.25	8.5	17
54	4.5	9.0	18
57	4.75	9.5	19
60	5.0	10.0	20
63	5.25	10.5	21
66	5.5	11.0	22
69	5.75	11.5	23
72	6.0	12.0	24
75	6.25	12.5	25
78	6.5	13.0	
81	6.75	13.5	
84	7.0	14.0	
87	7.25	14.5	
90	7.5	15.0	
93	7.75	15.5	
96	8.0	16.0	
99	8.25	16.5	
102	8.5	17.0	
105	8.75	17.5	
108	9.0	18.0	
112	9.25	18.5	
115	9.50	19.0	
118	9.75	19.5	
119	10.0	20.0	

above the ischial spines (not engaged) when the forceps are applied. Most hospitals have policies against the high-forceps application because of the high potential for fetal and maternal compromise.

Midforceps. The vertex is at the ischial spines, almost to the ischial tuberosities on application of the forceps. The delivery often is difficult, depending on the size of the vertex, its position, and the pelvic architecture and diameters. The use of midforceps remains controversial (Friedman, 1987; Hayashi, 1987).

Outlet (Low) Forceps: The vertex is distending the introitus with outlet forceps. This should be an "easy" forceps delivery. The blades are applied principally to provide control and guidance of the head.

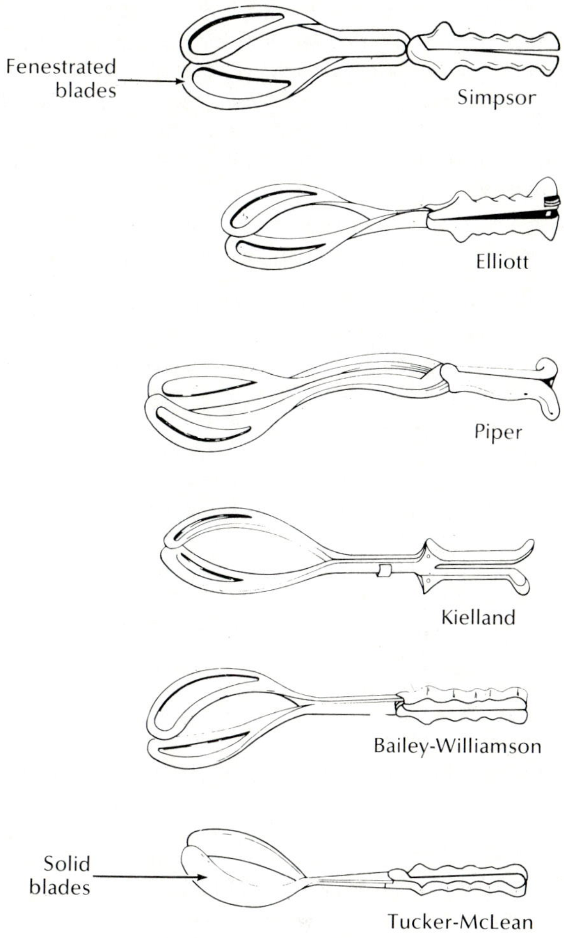

Fig. 33-9 Types of forceps.

Nursing Care. The nurse obtains forceps designated by physician (Fig. 33-9) The FHR is checked, reported and recorded *before* forceps are *applied.* The mother is informed that the forceps blades fit like two tablespoons around an egg. The blades come over the baby's ears. The FHR is rechecked, reported, and recorded *before traction* is applied after application of forceps. Compression of the cord between the fetal head and the forceps would cause a drop in FHR. The physician would then remove and reapply the forceps.

Vacuum Extraction

Vacuum extraction is delivery of a fetus in *vertex* presentation with the use of a cup-suction device that is applied to the fetal scalp for traction. Indications for use of the vacuum extractor (ventouse) are similar to those for simple outlet forceps delivery. This instrument, widely used in Europe, often speeds labor and delivery, obviating difficult forceps procedures or even cesarean delivery. The vacuum extractor adds traction to the involuntary and voluntary efforts and is more physiologic than forceps extraction. Fetal scalp ecchymoses must be expected; even cephalhematomas occur with the ventouse. When there is a prolonged application of the vacuum extractor (30 minutes), there may be severe damage to the scalp, or subgaleal hematomas may develop.

External Cephalic Version

If the Leopold's maneuvers disclose a breech presentation the question of external version arises. External cephalic version is an old technique that is being reconsidered as a possible treatment for unfavorable presentations, especially breech presentations. It consists of converting a breech presentation to a vertex presentation by an external maneuver. It is done after the 37th week and before labor to avoid the need for a cesarean delivery. Some frank breech presentations cannot be turned because of the fetal configuration or the situation of the placenta. Others, after being converted to a vertex presentation, often revert. However, some breeches spontaneously turn to vertex during the last trimester.

Complications such a abruptio placentae or cord compression made this procedure unsafe in the past. Now with the use of (1) ultrasound to visualize the placenta site to avoid any force against it and to evaluate the adequacy of amniotic fluid volume, (2) a tocolytic agent such as terbutaline or ritodrine to relax the uterus and facilitate manipulation, and (3) an electronic fetal monitor to detect any fetal distress immediately the technique is being reevaluated as to its safety and usefulness (Gilbert and Harmon, 1986).

The procedure is usually done between 37 and 40 weeks of gestation in a controlled environment where a cesarean delivery could be performed immediately if indicated. The presenting part should be unengaged, the membranes should be intact, and a nonstress test should be reactive before version is attempted.

Immediately an ultrasound examination is carried out, blood is drawn for a complete blood count and blood type, an IV infusion is started with an 18-gauge intracatheter, and a 15 to 30 minute fetal monitor strip is obtained to determine the baseline FHR. The tocolytic agent is prepared in the same manner and concentration as that used for tocolysis in preterm labor. It is piggybacked into the main IV line. The usual rate is 5 μg/min of terbutaline or 100 μg/min of ritodrine.

The nurse places the woman in slight Trendelenburg's position to "float" the presenting part. With one hand over each pole, the physician gently displaces the breech laterally out of the pelvis while guiding the head in the opposite direction (Fig. 33-6). Commonly, the fetus will "somersault" or roll into the vertex presentation. Manipulations are stopped during a uterine contraction. If turning is not possible one way, an attempt is made to turn the fetus in the opposite direction. The vertex is held in the new presentation for a time to permit the head to "settle-in." The nurse checks FHR frequently. External version is discontinued if fetal or maternal distress develops or turning is difficult. On completion of the procedure, the IV tocolytic drug is discontinued. The external fetal monitor reapplied to assess the FHR pattern and to assess for the development of uterine contractions. If the version is successful, greater than 90% of the fetuses will present in labor in a vertex presentation. The procedure is repeated in a week if necessary.

The occurrence of fetal and maternal hemorrhage during this procedure has been reported; therefore, Rh immune globulin should be given to all Rh-negative women with Rh-positive partners.

Contraindications to external version include marked oligohydramnios, placenta previa, rupture of the membranes, previous third-trimester bleeding, and previous myomectomy or metroplasty. It appears that external cephalic version in selected cases is a safe alternative for management of the fetus in the breech presentation near term.

Cesarean Delivery

Cesarean delivery is the delivery of a fetus through a transabdominal incision of the uterus. Although the myth persists that Julius Caesar was delivered in this manner, the derivation of the term is more likely from the Latin word *caedo* meaning "to cut." Whether cesarean delivery is planned (elective) or unplanned (emergency), the loss of the experience of delivering a child in the traditional manner may have a negative effect on a woman's self-concept. In an effort to maintain the focus on the *birth* of a child rather than the operative procedure, the term *cesarean delivery* or *cesarean birth* has come into common usage. The mother experiences abdominal rather than vaginal birth.

The basic purpose or use of cesarean delivery is to preserve the life or health of the mother and her fetus. The use of cesarean delivery is based on evidence of maternal or fetal stress. Maternal and fetal morbidity and mortality have decreased since the advent of modern surgical methods and care. However, cesarean delivery still poses threats to the health of both mother and infant. The technique of cesarean surgery has changed. Today incisions into the lower uterine segment rather than into the muscular body of the uterus permit a more effective healing. These findings are presented in the box on p. 819.

Cesarean Delivery Rates. The rate for cesarean delivery has increased dramatically. From the mid-1960s to the early 1980s the cesarean delivery rate has increased from less than 5% to more than 15% (Morrison and others, 1982). Concern about the rising cesarean delivery rates in the United States prompted the National Institute of Health to convene a Consensus Development Conference in 1980 (Petitti, 1985). Recommendations included the following:

1. "Women with low transverse incision be permitted a trial of labor in properly equipped hospitals and in the absence of other indications for a repeat cesarean" (Petitti, 1985).
2. The category "dystocia" as an indication for cesarean delivery be investigated further.
3. Vaginal delivery of the *term breech* be considered an acceptable alternative in carefully selected cases.

In spite of these recommendations and support from the

INDICATIONS FOR CESAREAN DELIVERY AND MATERNAL AND FETAL EFFECTS

INDICATIONS FOR CESAREAN DELIVERY	EFFECTS OF CESAREAN DELIVERY	TYPE OF UTERINE INCISIONS
Maternal 1. Fetopelvic disproportion 2. Previous cesarean delivery 3. Breech presentation 4. Medical complications (e.g., PIH) 5. Placental abnormalities (i.e., placenta previa, premature separation of the placenta) 6. Infections (e.g., herpes virus, type 2) 7. Trauma to the pelvis	**Maternal** 1. Mortality (1:1000) from a. Anesthesia b. Severe sepsis c. Thromboembolic episodes 2. Morbidity higher than with vaginal delivery because of: a. Infection b. Injury to the urinary tract	**Classic Cesarean Incision** Incision is vertical through skin and vertical through contractile portion of uterus (Fig. 33-10, *A*). It is used when rapid delivery is necessary, in shoulder presentation, and in placenta previa when the placenta is implanted on the anterior wall. Classic cesarean delivery is useful when general anesthesia is unavailable, since this operation can be carried out with local infiltration anesthesia. The potential for rupture of the scar (1% to 2%) with a subsequent pregnancy and the frequent occurrence of small bowel adhesions to the anterior suture line have limited the use of this type of cesarean delivery.
Fetal 1. Fetal hypoxia 2. Prolapse of cord 3. Breech presentations 4. Malpresentations (e.g., shoulder) 5. Fetal anomalies (e.g., hydrocephalus)	**Fetal** 1. Mortality has declined where cesarean delivery is used in conjunction with improved perinatal care 2. Morbidity a. Birth trauma is reduced b. Reduced morbidity in breech deliveries, transverse lie of the fetus, and placenta previa	**Lower Segment Cesarean Incision** Lower segment cesarean delivery is possible by means of a vertical incision (Fig. 33-10, *B*) or a transverse incision (Fig. 33-10, *C*). The transverse incision is the preferred method. It "(1) results in less blood loss, (2) is easier to repair, (3) is located at a site least likely to rupture with extrusion of the fetus into the abdominal cavity during a subsequent pregnancy, and (4) does not promote adherence of bowel or omentum to the incisional line" (Pritchard, McDonald, and Gant, 1985).

American College of Obstetricians and Gynecologists, rates have not declined (Gleichner, 1984).

There is considerable disagreement as to whether the decrease in prenatal mortality is a direct result of the use of cesarean delivery. Some researchers contend that recent advances in perinatal care have an equal or greater effect (O'Driscoll and Foley, 1983). Pritchard, McDonald and Gant (1985) note that "final answers with respect to the frequency, indications, results in terms of safety to the mother and fetus, and the legal, ethical, and economic consequences of cesarean section are unlikely to become apparent for several years."

Elective Cesarean Delivery. These women have time for psychologic preparation. The psychic response of women in these groups may differ. Those women scheduled for *repeat surgery* may have disturbing memories of the conditions preceding the initial surgical delivery and their experiences in the postoperative recovery period. The added burden of care of an infant while recovering from a surgical operation may be faced with great concern. Some women elect the repeat cesarean birth because they can exert more *control* over events. Women who face elective cesarean delivery for the *first time* share with other surgical clients the same apprehensive concerning surgery. These anxieties are coupled with the uncertainty of being able to cope with child care after a major operation.

Emergency Cesarean Delivery. Women in this group share with their families abrupt changes in their expectations for birth, postdelivery care, and the care of the new baby at home. This may be an extremely traumatic experience. The woman approaches surgery usually tired and discouraged after a fruitless labor. She is worried and fretful about her own and the child's condition. She may be dehydrated, with low glycogen reserves. All preoperative procedures must be done quickly and competently. The time for explanation of procedures and of operation is short. Since maternal and family anxiety levels are high, much of what is said is forgotten or perhaps misconstrued. Postoperatively, time must be spent reviewing the events preceding the operation and the operation itself to ensure that the woman understands what has happened. Fatigue is often noticeable in these women. They need much supportive care.

Many women who experience a cesarean birth speak of the feelings that interfere with their maintaining an adequate self-concept. These feelings include fear, disappointment, frustration at losing control, anger (the "why me" syndrome), and loss of self-esteem as their body image is not sustained. Success in mothering activities and in the recovery process can do much to restore these women's self-esteem. Some women see the scar as mutilating, and worries concerning sexual attractiveness may surface. Some men are fearful of resuming intercourse because of the fear of hurting their mates.

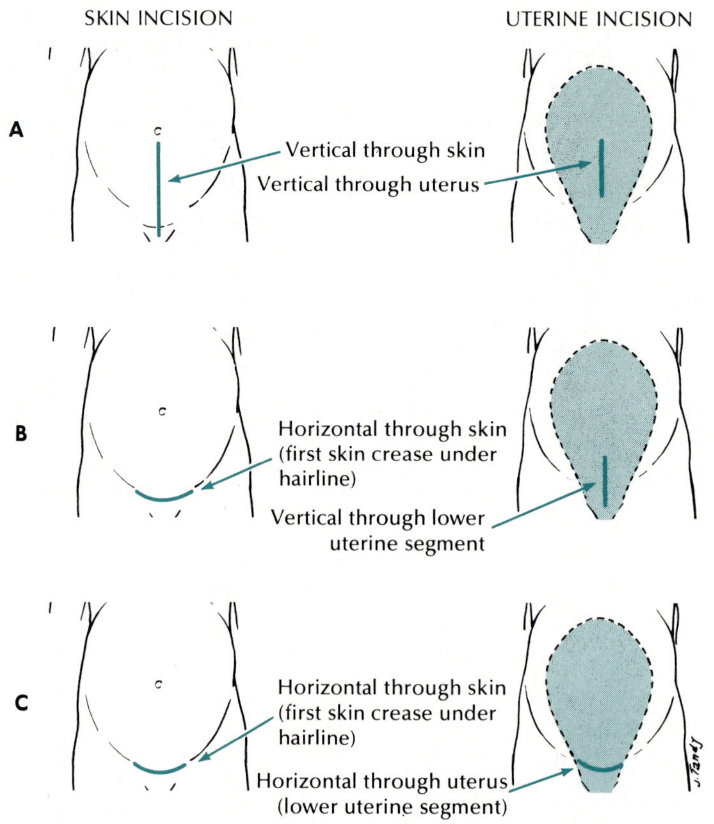

Fig. 33-10 Cesarean delivery: skin and uterine incisions. **A,** Classic: vertical incisions of skin and uterus. **B,** Low cervical: horizontal incision of skin; vertical incision of uterus. **C,** Low cervical: horizontal incisions of skin and uterus.

The separation of mother and child may prove detrimental to the establishment of parent-child bonds, particularly if other negative factors are present. They need to view their mothering ability positively. One mother expressed her feelings about the impact of an unexpected cesarean delivery regarding her self-concept as follows:

> At first I was despondent over not being able to deliver vaginally, but then I comforted myself with the thought, you were a good mother for 9 months, no 12-hour period (delivery) can alter that. My baby and I have our whole lives to be mother and daughter.

Professional staff can expect some anger directed toward them. Parents will wonder if it was absolutely necessary for them to have a cesarean delivery. Such feelings may surface even years later.

Prenatal Preparation for Cesarean Birth. Concerned professional and lay groups in the community have established councils for cesarean birth in an attempt to meet the needs of these women and their families. Such groups advocate including preparation for cesarean birth in all parenthood preparation classes (see research highlight). No woman can be guaranteed a vaginal delivery, even if she is in good health and there is no indication of danger to the fetus before the onset of labor. Every woman needs to be aware of and prepared for this eventuality. The unknown and unexpected are ego weakening. Each woman or couple needs accurate data to build new coping abilities or to strengthen old ones. "Walking through," role playing, or worry work before a crisis situation increases one's sense of control in that situation and minimizes the sense of loss experienced.

Childbirth educators stress the importance of emphasizing the similarities as well as differences between cesarean and vaginal birth. Also, in support of the philosophy of family-centered birth, many hospitals have changed policies to permit fathers to share in these births as they have in vaginal ones. Women undergoing cesarean birth agree that the continued presence and support of their partners have helped them experience a positive response to the whole process:

> Knowing that he would be there and that he would be among the first to hold and nurture our baby made a tremendous difference to me. Even though "I" as the woman couldn't participate as directly as I had anticipated, "we" as the family could. I felt a sense of control, not a sense of being a passive . . . well . . . organ.

RESEARCH HIGHLIGHT

Antenatal Education for Cesarean Birth

Purpose

Unanticipated cesarean births occur often enough to warrant inclusion of cesarean birth information in Lamaze childbirth preparation classes.

Sample/Methodology

After field testing a 20-page cesarean childbirth education pamphlet, the investigators incorporated the pamphlet into Lamaze classes. Focused discussion about cesarean birth was included in the classes when this topic related to other content on labor and delivery. The pamphlet was distributed at the third class when feelings about cesarean delivery was discussed.

A 3-question open-ended evaluation questionnaire was mailed to 58 women and 57 male partners approximately 1 week after the birth of their child. Questionnaires were returned by 75% of the sample.

Findings

Using content analysis, 160 reactions to the pamphlet were classified as either positive or negative. The number of positive reactions was greater than the number of negative reactions to the pamphlet.

Implications

The findings from this study of predominately upper-middle class to upper class parents indicated that the educational program prepared them for unanticipated cesarean births.

Fawcett, J, and Henkein, JC: Antenatal education for cesarean birth: extension of a field test, JOGN Nurs 16(1): 61, 1987.

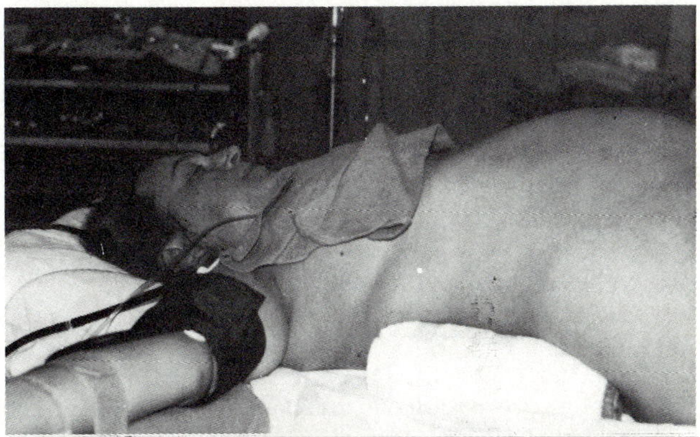

A

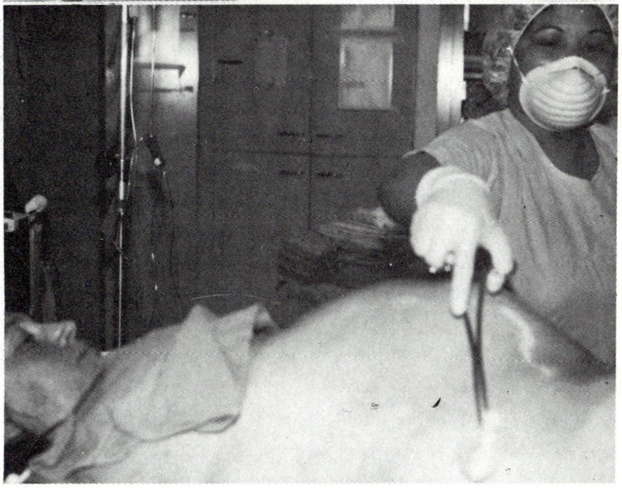

B

Fig. 33-11 **A**, Preparation for cesarean birth. Pad under hip tilts abdomen and prevents supine hypotension. **B**, Scrub nurse prepares abdomen for surgery.
Courtesy Judy Bamber, San Jose, Calif.

Client teaching to prepare the expectant woman and her family is on p. 822.

Care During Cesarean Delivery. The goal for the woman and her family is family-centered care for a cesarean delivery. Facing cesarean delivery relates to (1) the option for father to be present at the birth, (2) availability of regional as well as general anesthesia, and (3) receiving support from the health care staff. The box on p. 823 reviews the options that can be made available to couples.

The *preparation* of the woman for cesarean birth is the same for either elective or emergency surgery. The obstetrician discusses the need for the cesarean delivery and the prognosis for mother and infant with the woman and her family. The anesthesiologist assesses the woman's cardiopulmonary system and presents the options for anesthesia. Informed consent is obtained for the procedures. Procedure 33-2 contains the nursing care necessary in preparation for surgery.

Once the woman has been taken to surgery her care becomes the responsibility of the obstetric team, surgeon, anesthesiologist, pediatrician, and nursing staff (Figs. 33-11, above, and 33-12, p. 824). If possible, the father, gowned appropriately, accompanies the mother to the surgical unit and remains close to her.

Care of the infant is delegated to a pediatrician and a nurse because these infants are considered to be at risk until there is evidence of physiologic stability after delivery (Fig. 33-13, p. 826). A crib with resuscitative equipment is readied before surgery. Those responsible for care are expert in resuscitative techniques, as well as in observational skills for detecting normal infant responses. After birth, if the infant's condition permits, she or he is given to the father to hold and to show to the mother (Fig. 33-14, p. 826). The attachment process can continue uninterrupted. Some mothers are able to breast-feed the infant in the recovery room area. However, many are not ready for this direct participation. They need to be reassured that the parent-child attachment process will not be impaired.

If compromised, the infant is transported immediately to the infant intensive care unit. Personnel keep the family informed of the infant's progress. Father-child contacts are initiated as soon as possible.

If the family-oriented approach is not feasible, the family

Guidelines for Client Teaching

PREPARATION FOR CESAREAN DELIVERY

ASSESSMENT

1. Woman in third trimester of pregnancy.
2. Woman to be prepared for possible cesarean delivery.
3. Woman to have repeat cesarean delivery.

NURSING DIAGNOSES

Knowledge deficit related to cesarean delivery.

Knowledge deficit related to testing for fetal well-being and fetal lung maturity.

Anxiety and fear related to possible or actual cesarean delivery.

Self-esteem disturbance related to unsatisfied planned birth experience.

Potential altered parenting.

Personal identity disturbance related to loss of control over decisions and powerlessness.

GOALS

Short-term

Woman (couple) will learn that a cesarean delivery can be a positive birth experience.

Woman (couple) will learn the reasons for the cesarean delivery.

Intermediate

Woman (couple) will learn the rationale for prenatal testing and how the results determine cesarean delivery.

Woman (couple) will learn rationale for testing for fetal lung maturity.

Woman (couple) will learn about medications and forms of anesthesia given for cesarean deliveries.

Long-term

Woman (couple) will take a tour of the operating room/delivery room.

Woman (couple) verbalizes feelings about cesarean delivery.

Woman (couple) will learn immediate preoperative preparation for cesarean delivery.

Woman (couple) understands breast-feeding is still an option.

Woman understands that pain relief will be provided.

REFERENCES AND TEACHING AIDS

Books and pamphlets describing cesarean delivery in a positive way.

Discussion and lecture, use of slides, charts, illustrations.

Films or videos depicting a cesarean birth.

Tour of the hospital's labor and delivery suite, including the operative area and recovery area.

Discussions with parents who have experienced cesarean delivery.

CONTENT/RATIONALE	TEACHING ACTIONS
To meet information needs regarding cesarean delivery and rationale:	
Explain the anatomy and physiology pertaining to cesarean delivery and how it differs from a vaginal delivery.	Use charts, diagrams, audio-visual aids to show difference between a vaginal and cesarean delivery.
Discuss prenatal testing and how it illustrates fetal well-being.	Use diagrams or audio-visual aids if possible; discuss parents' questions and concerns.
Nonstress test (NST); used as a screening test, looking for accelerations of FHR in conjunction with fetal movement. Reactive test shows at least 2 FHR accelerations >15 beats per minute above the baseline and lasting 15 seconds or more in conjunction with fetal movements in a 10-minute period. Nonreactive test does not fulfill the above criteria and is an indication for further evaluation.	Discuss rationale behind each test. Explain where these tests are done and by whom. Discuss questions and concerns.
Contraction Stress Test (aka oxytocin stress test, stress test). This test evaluates fetal response to labor contractions (i.e., can the fetus withstand the stress of normal labor?)	
Negative test shows no late decelerations of FHR during 3 contractions over a 10-minute period.	
Positive test—late decelerations are observed during this time; shows fetoplacental unit cannot withstand the stress of normal labor. There are terms of classification in between. For this test, intravenous oxytocin may be administered or the woman may be asked to provide nipple stimulation to produce natural oxytocin in the body.	Indicate that interpretations of this test will be explained by the physician at the time the test is taken.

Guidelines For Client Teaching—cont'd

CONTENT/RATIONALE	TEACHING ACTIONS
Ultrasonography, either done alone or in cojunction with an amniocentesis, provides information on approximate gestational age and maturity of the fetus.	Explain what ultrasound testing is and what information it provides the physician. Show a picture of the machine, a diagram of how it works, and a picture of a fetus from an ultrasound done previously.
Biophysical profile, a combination of ultrasonography, NST, fetal movement, and placental grading; tells the physician how the maternal-fetal-placental unit is working.	Explain the parameters of this test and what the significance of the test shows.
Amniocentesis (Procedure 27-1) may be done to provide information on fetal lung maturity by way of L/S ratio, phosphatidylglycerol (P/G) ratio, or Foam Stabilizing Index (FSI).	Explain what information this test provides.
Discuss the types of medications the woman may be given to mature the fetal lungs if a cesarean delivery is necessary	Review what the physician's instructions were at this point. Clarify any questions.
To provide anticipatory guidance for pre- and postoperative care:	
Discuss types of anesthesia that are used for cesarean delivery.	Show a diagram or picture of a woman receiving an epidural or spinal.
Explain the difference between epidural and spinal anesthesia. If continuous morphine or fentanyl is used in your institution, explain what this is.	
Explain preoperative preparation and postoperative assessment that will be implemented.	Explain shaving the abdomen, insertion of an indwelling urinary catheter, starting intravenous infusion. Discuss what will be done in the recovery area after the operation. Reassure woman, if she is up to it, and her newborn is well, she may hold the baby at this time.
Discuss alternate positions for breast-feeding so that the incision is not interfered with.	Reassure her that she may still breast-feed.
Arrange for a tour of the labor and delivery area, include the operating and recovery areas.	Take woman (couple) on a tour. Point out important sights, sounds, and smells at that time. Leave time for questions.

EVALUATION Couple verbalizes understanding of information presented, they ask appropriate questions. Woman (couple) sees cesarean delivery as a positive, alternate method of childbirth, and it is a satisfying experience for them.

OPTIONS TO FACILITATE FAMILY-CENTERED CESAREAN BIRTHS*

1. Admission to the hospital on the morning of the birth for elective cesareans so that parents can spend the previous night together (provided they have had previous orientation).
2. Father to remain with the mother during the physical preparation, e.g., shave, catheterization.
3. The choice of regional anesthesia where possible, and explanation of the differences between regional and general anesthesia.
4. Father in the delivery room when either regional or general anesthesia is the choice.
5. Mirror and/or ongoing commentary from a staff member for mother and/or father.
6. Photographs or video taken in the delivery room-if even one parent is unable to witness the birth.
7. Mother's hand freed from restraint for contact with husband and baby.
8. Opportunity for both parents to interact with the baby in the delivery room and/or postanesthetic recovery room.
9. Opportunity for breast-feeding in the delivery room or postanesthetic recovery room.
10. Modified Leboyer practices, e.g., father to submerge baby in warm water until relaxed and alert in the delivery room or in the nursery, if available for vaginal delivery.
11. Delayed antimicrobials in baby's eyes.

From Leach, L, and Sproule, V: Meeting the challenge of cesarean birth, JOGN Nurs 13:193, May/June 1984.
*In an effort to make the cesarean delivery more family-centered, the following options should be available where safety permits.

Continued.

OPTIONS TO FACILITATE FAMILY-CENTERED CESAREAN BIRTHS—cont'd

12. If father not in the delivery room:
    a. A support person should replace him at the mother's side;
    b. Father to be given baby to hold en route to nursery;
    c. Father to have the birth experience relayed to him by a staff member.
13. Father to accompany baby to the nursery and remain with infant until both are reunited with the mother.
14. Family reunited in postanesthetic recovery room if possible.
15. Father to be in postanesthetic recovery room to tell his wife about the birth if she has had a general anesthetic.
16. If it is difficult to reunite the family in postanesthetic recovery room, the mother's condition should be judged individually to allow the family to be reunited as soon as possible.
17. Baby's condition to be judged individually so that time alone in an incubator in the nursery can be avoided if possible.
18. Provision of time alone for the family in those first critical hours.
19. Rooming-in as soon as possible, i.e., if mother feels well enough she may be able to manage rooming-in on the first day.
20. Father to be included in the teaching of caregiving skills.
21. Siblings to be included where possible.

A

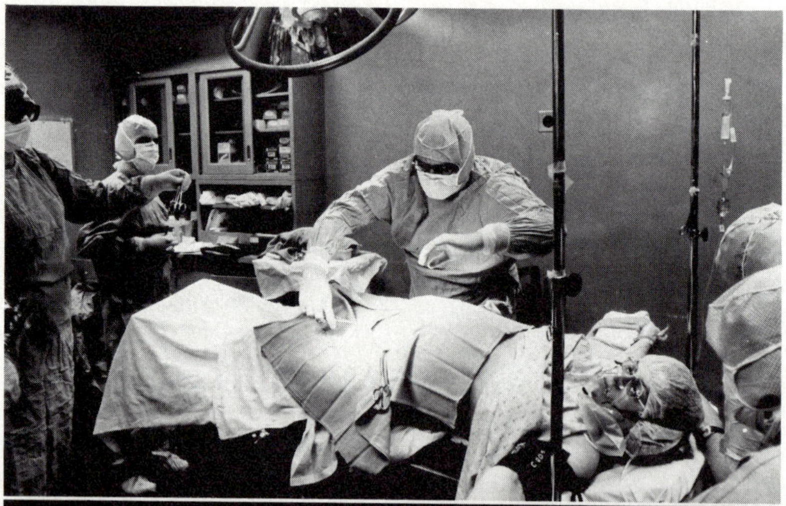

B

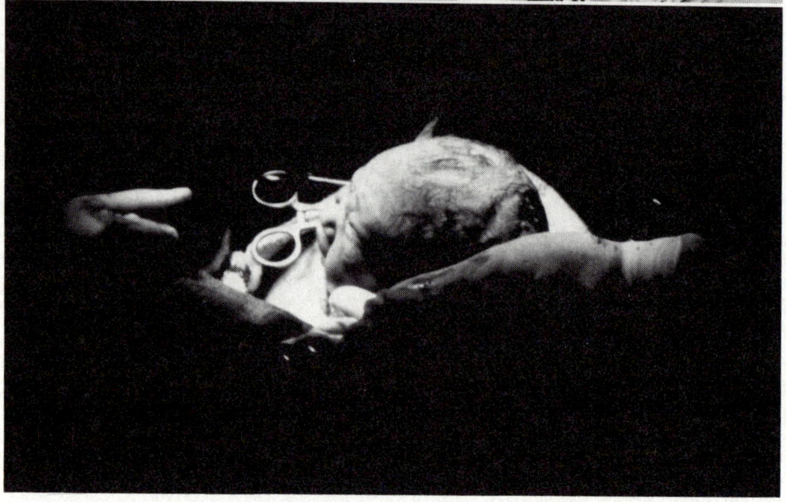

Fig. 33-12 **A**, Surgical team preparing woman for surgery. **B**, Birth of infant.

A courtesy Jose Mercado. From News and Publication Service, Stanford University, Stanford, California. **B**, courtesy Marjorie Pyle, RNC Lifecircle, Costa Mesa, Calif.

Procedure 33-2

CESAREAN DELIVERY: PREPARATION

DEFINITION

Delivery of the fetus by an abdominal and uterine incision.

PURPOSE

To complete the preparation for surgery as competently and quickly as possible.

To provide emotional support through a caring attitude, calm manner, and technical competence.

To decrease client anxiety by reassurance.

EQUIPMENT

Skin preparation kit (for shaving); retention (Foley) catheter kit; IV infusions (as ordered); medications (as ordered).

NURSING ACTIONS	RATIONALE
Wash hands before and after touching woman and equipment. Glove, prn.	To prevent nosocomial infection and to implement universal precautions.
Explain procedures to be carried out.	To keep the family informed, decrease anxiety, and elicit cooperation.
Complete preoperative preparation of abdomen. The abdomen is shaved beginning at the level of the xiphoid process and extending to the flank on both sides and down to the pubic area.	To minimize potential for infection.
Insert a retention catheter (Foley). It is attached to a continuous drainage system. Care must be taken that catheter is placed properly within the bladder and is draining adequately.	To ensure the bladder remains empty during the operation.
Administer preoperative medications as ordered:	
Analgesia.	To promote relaxation before surgery.
Atropine.	To minimize amount of secretions in bronchial tree.
Antacid.	To prevent irritative pneumonia if aspiration of gastric juice from stomach occurs.
If spinal or epidural anesthesia is used, an antacid may be the only medication administered.	
Begin IV infusion. 1000 ml Ringer's lactate solution, or 5% dextrose in water or saline.	To maintain hydration. To have a line open for administration of blood, medications, etc. if needed.
Send specimens to laboratory for analysis.	To replace blood loss during surgery or postpartum if excessive.
Send blood for typing and cross-matching. Two units of matched blood are kept in reserve for 48 hours after surgery.	
Send urine for routine analysis.	To establish baseline data.
Send blood for CBC and chemistry.	To establish baseline data.
Take and record vital signs, blood pressure, FHR.	To establish baseline data.
Complete preoperative care including removal of dentures, contact lenses, rings, and fingernail polish. Valuables are given to support person or put into safekeeping.	To protect client.
Ready the woman's chart for use in surgery and to see whether permission forms for care of the mother and infant are signed. If the woman has received an analgesic or anesthetic, the responsible adult accompanying the woman signs the necessary forms.	To provide data base for future comparison. To provide data base for implementation of the next steps in the nursing process. To promote collaboration with other members of the health care team.
Provide as much information as possible to the woman and her family while carrying out the necessary care.	To relieve apprehension and promote understanding

A

B

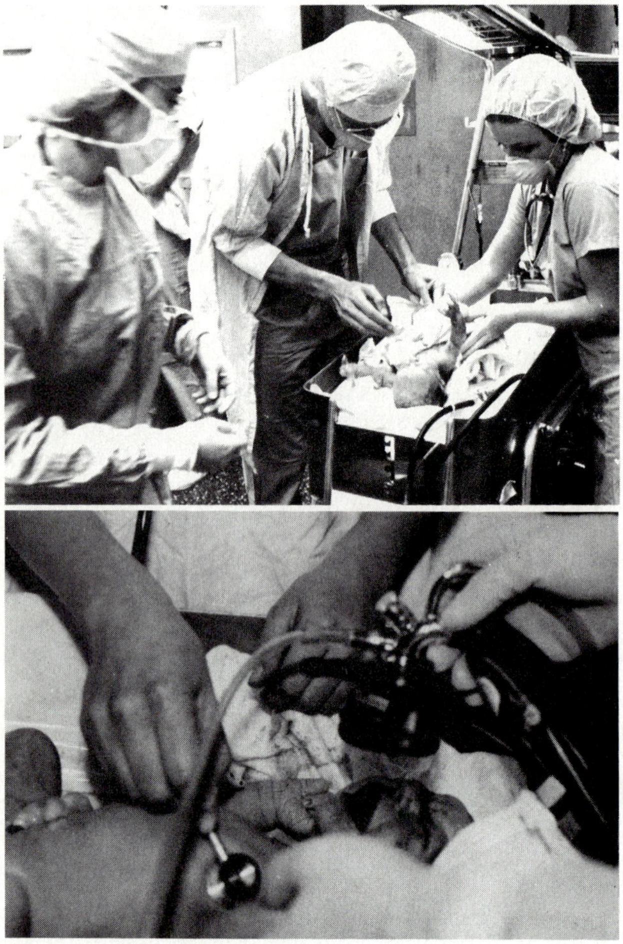

Fig. 33-13 Pediatrician administers oxygen. Note mask is held above infant's face; oxygen is heavier than air and will sink to face level. Nurse is assessing fetal heart rate. Infant is crying; note muscle tone now. Arms and legs are flexed and not resting on bed.
Courtesy Judy Bamber, San Jose, Calif.

is directed to the surgical waiting room. The physician reviews with the family members the condition of the mother and child after the birth is completed. Family members may accompany the infant as she or he is transferred to the nursery. This gives the family opportunity to see and admire the infant.

Postpartum Period. The care of the woman after cesarean delivery combines surgical and obstetric nursing. Once surgery is completed, the mother is transferred to the recovery room for intensive care until her condition stabilizes. Then she is moved to the postdelivery unit. See nursing care plan: after delivery by cesarean on p. 827.

Vaginal Birth After Cesarean (VBAC)

Data are gradually accumulating concerning the safety of vaginal delivery after cesarean delivery (Meier and Parreco, 1982; Gellman et al., 1983). In the past, when the incision was directed through the uterine fundus, once a woman had a cesarean delivery, all future deliveries were elective cesarean deliveries. The risk of rupture through a lower

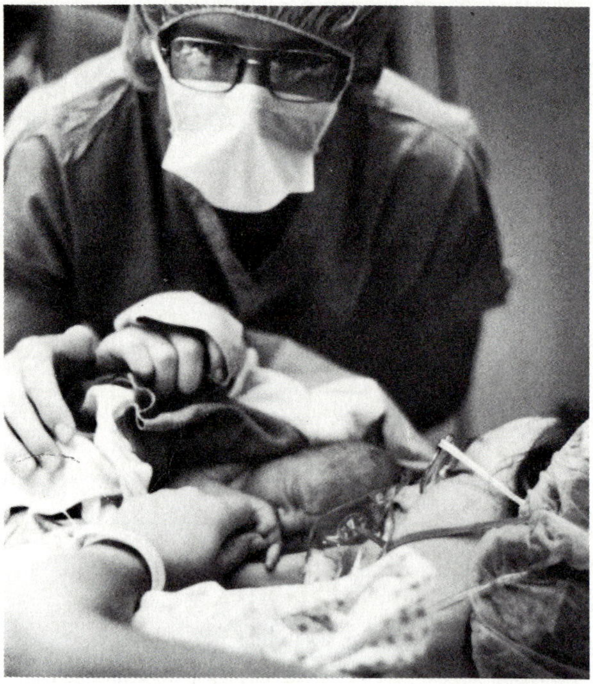

Fig. 33-14 Parents and their newborn.
Courtesy Jose Mercado. From News and Publications Service, Stanford, Calif.

uterine segment scar is only 0.5% (Knuppel and Drukker, 1986). In the past, the woman was often counseled to limit the number of pregnancies to three. Today the type of subsequent delivery is a decision to be made by the woman after full consultation with her physician. Danforth (1982) states that in general, suitable candidates for future vaginal deliveries are (1) those women whose operation was of the low cervical (not classic) type, (2) those women who begin labor before EDD, and (3) those women who enter the labor suite with the fetal head well-engaged and the cervix soft, anterior, effaced, and dilated at least 3 cm.

If the original indication for the cesarean delivery is still present in a subsequent pregnancy, for example, a grossly contracted pelvis, repeat cesarean delivery is indicated. Moreover, a cesarean delivery is recommended for women who had a classic cesarean incision or any cesarean delivery marred by a septic course wherein questionable healing of the scar may result in rupture during labor. The expectant woman and her family need positive reinforcement that whatever decision they make is acceptable. Contact with mothers who have experienced vaginal birth after cesarean can provide role models for these women.

When the *original complication* for which a cesarean delivery was initially done *has not recurred* a trial of labor is recommended. A trial of labor and vaginal delivery are considered to be too great a risk for mother and fetus, however, unless the woman is in a center where facilities are available for emergency surgery, anesthesia, continuous electronic monitoring for FHR and uterine activity, and blood transfusion.

Trial labor occurs under close observation with equipment for immediate cesarean delivery or hysterectomy

Specific Nursing Care Plan

CARE AFTER CESAREAN DELIVERY

Jessie R., a primipara, has an unplanned cesarean delivery for cephalopelvic disproportion (CPD) and moderate fetal distress. Jessie and her husband had attended childbirth education classes and were looking forward to an uncomplicated vaginal delivery.

ASSESSMENT	NURSING DIAGNOSIS (ND)/ PLAN (P)/GOAL (G)	RATIONALE/ IMPLEMENTATION	EVALUATION
Primigravida with failure to progress.	ND: Knowledge deficit related to unplanned cesarean birth. P: Provide time to discuss birth at earliest possible time. G: Jessie and husband understand rationale for cesarean delivery.	*To help Jessie and husband understand need for cesarean birth the nurse will:* Review and reinforce information given to them by physician. Answer any questions. Remain with Jessie and provide reassurance and emotional support.	Jessie and husband verbalize understanding of information presented.
Fetal distress. Cephalopelvic disproportion.	ND: Potential for injury: fetus, related to CPD and fetal distress. P: Monitor closely; report fetal distress; intervene appropriately (Chapter 17). G: Injury is minimized or prevented.	*To assure birth of a health baby the nurse will:* Assess Jessie's vital signs, blood pressure, and FHR. Monitor fetal well-being. Assess for abnormal or unusual FHR patterns on monitor strip. Alert physician to any changes in condition of mother or fetus.	Jessie verbalizes understanding of procedures being performed. If fetal distress occurs, it is relieved with appropriate intervention.
Cesarean delivery is scheduled.	ND: Potential for injury: mother, related to emergency cesarean birth. P: Perform preoperative preparation. G: Injury and complications are minimized or prevented.	*To assist Jessie through delivery with little or no complications the nurse will:* Assess Jessie's physical and emotional status. Affirm that consent form is signed. Obtain relevant baseline information: laboratory tests, vital signs, blood pressure. Perform necessary preoperative procedures with as little trauma as possible. Inquire as to last food taken—prevent aspiration of stomach contents by administering antacid as ordered and observing postoperatively for vomiting.	Jessie verbalizes understanding of information presented and procedures being done. Jessie does not vomit or aspirate stomach contents.
Jessie and husband give verbal and nonverbal cues that they are anxious.	ND: Anxiety: moderate to severe, related to dystocia and emergency cesarean birth. P: Help couple minimize and cope with anxiety.	*To decrease Jessie's anxiety the nurse will:* Provide information. Reassure husband and Jessie. Help Jessie and husband	Jessie shows trust in health care providers by discussing feelings openly.

Continued.

Specific Nursing Care Plan—cont'd

ASSESSMENT	NURSING DIAGNOSIS (ND)/ PLAN (P)/GOAL (G)	RATIONALE/ IMPLEMENTATION	EVALUATION
	G: Jessie and husband appear less anxious and verbalize less anxiety.	cope with possible disappointment and feelings of failure.	
Postcesarean delivery. Jessie is experiencing postoperative pain.	ND: Pain resulting from cesarean delivery. P: Utilize assessment data to monitor need for and response to medication. G: Jessie will verbalize comfort and rest/sleep.	*To help ease discomfort, the nurse will:* Assess vital signs, blood pressure. Assess fundus, lochia, incision, and bladder distension. Provide comfort measures. Administer pain medication as ordered.	Jessie verbalizes a decrease in pain. Assessment data stabilize within normal limits.
Disappointment with change from birth plans.	ND: Potential altered parenting related to dystocia and need for emergency cesarean delivery. P: Help couple integrate experience (see Chapter 20). G: Couple verbalizes acceptance of selves and method of delivery and begins attachment to infant.	*To assist Jessie (couple) in accepting situation and begin attachment to their infant, the nurse will:* Assess emotional status of couple. Provide information to assist with integration of experience. Provide reassurance. Provide quiet time for interaction with infant, if possible.	Couple accepts cesarean delivery as necessary and successfully integrates the experience (guidelines for client teaching: emotional factors during the fourth stage of labor, Chapter 20).
Surgical incision (see Fig. 33-15).	ND: Potential for infection related to surgical procedure. P: Implement postsurgical care (Chapter 34) and universal precautions (Chapter 30) to prevent nosocomial infection and maintain asepsis. G: Jessie/neonate/staff do not develop infection.	*To avert post-partum or incisional infection, the nurse will:* Assess vital signs, incision healing, odor of lochia. Provide good preoperative skin prep (shave) and postoperative incision care Provide good perineal care periodically. Maintain nutrition and hydration. Administer postdelivery antibiotics as ordered.	Jessie reports any unusual findings to nurse. Jessie, neonate, and staff do not develop infection.
Potential for postsurgical complications secondary to immobility.	ND: Potential for injury related to sequelae of immobility. P: Avoid sequelae of immobility. G: Jessie experiences no adverse sequelae to immobility.	*To avert postoperative sequelae to immobility the nurse will:* Perform health assessments as scheduled with particular attention to breath sounds, respiratory rate; signs and symptoms of thromboembolic processes; intake and output; bowel sounds and function; affect and emotional responses. Teach and coach coughing and deep breathing and use of incentive spirometer.	Jessie experiences no respiratory, gastrointestinal, neuromuscular, emotional, or cardiovascular problems secondary to immobility.

Specific Nursing Care Plan—cont'd

ASSESSMENT	NURSING DIAGNOSIS (ND)/ PLAN (P)/GOAL (G)	RATIONALE/ IMPLEMENTATION	EVALUATION
		Encourage and assist with ambulation, range of motion, self-care. Provide nutrition, maintain hydration, and ensure good hygiene. Medicate and provide comfort measures to promote mobility	
Powerlessness.	ND: Situational low self-esteem related to loss of control and emergency cesarean delivery. P: Foster open communication, encourage verbalization of feelings, and provide information as necessary. G: Jessie (couple) discusses feelings openly and participates in decision-making process when appropriate.	*To assist Jessie in resolving negative feelings the nurse will:* Assess Jessie's (couple's) verbal/nonverbal communication. Encourage open discussion. Provide information. Provide couple time for beginning attachment to infant. Provide options for care when appropriate. Prepare couple for return home: mother's fatigue and recovery after childbirth and abdominal surgery; parenting needs of neonate and family; and responses of each family member to the new baby and their changing roles in the family (see Unit 3 and Chapter 25).	Couple verbalizes understanding of information given. Couple indicates satisfaction with participation in discussion and in decision-making. During postdischarge follow-up, parents express satisfaction with assistance they received to be able to meet demands of early weeks following birth.

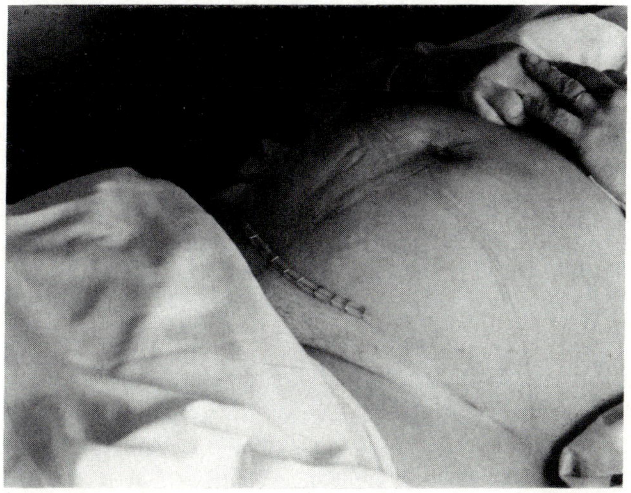

Fig. 33-15 Typical incision for cesarean birth. Note "skin clips" used to suture incision.

available in an emergency. The woman is admitted following onset of spontaneous labor whenever possible. The woman is not left unattended. Unless an intrauterine catheter for uterine contractility is used, a nurse-client ratio of 1:1 is instituted. Without the intrauterine catheter, the nurse keeps one hand on the parturient's abdomen for continuous assessment of uterine contractility. Maternal and fetal vital signs and responses, and the progress of labor are monitored closely.

Symptomatology of *ruptured classical cesarean scar* includes the following (O'Sullivan et al., 1981; Knuppel and Drukker, 1986): a continuous, tearing pain, then relief; cessation of contractions; distension and tenderness of abdomen; and fetal distress or death. The fetus may be extruded into the abdomen. The woman may exhibit signs of shock, such as tachycardia, restlessness, and collapse.

Symptomatology of *ruptured low segment cesarean scar* includes the following: pain; suprapubic tenderness; continued contractions; an irregularity or suprapubic swelling that may be palpated. Fetal distress occurs occasionally but fetal death is rare. The woman may have an increased pulse, but restlessness and collapse are rare. Cervical dilation may continue. Vaginal bleeding may occur late in the first stage or postpartum. Hematuria may be seen.

In the absence of rupture, spontaneous or low forceps-assistance delivery occurs; after which the physician explores the uterine cavity to rule out uterine rupture, which requires immediate treatment (Danforth and Scott, 1986).

During the early postpartum period the woman must be assessed for concealed bleeding into the abdominal cavity or broad ligaments. Concealed bleeding may be suspected if the woman develops tachycardia, restlessness, hypotension, thirst, tachypnea, air hunger, or abdominal pain. A broad ligament hematoma must be ruled out if the fundus rises and is pushed to one side in the presence of an empty bladder. On vaginal examination, fullness anteriorly (after bladder emptying) or in either parametrial region also suggests bleeding and warrants further evaluation. Any abnormal bleeding, either associated with a defect or not easily explained or controlled, warrants laparotomy (Knuppen and Drukker, 1986).

Evaluation

Evaluation of a woman with dystotic labor requires moment-to-moment assessment to adjust the care plan to the woman's needs. Care can be considered effective if the mother completes labor with the least amount of fatigue, remains relatively comfortable, and suffers no adverse sequelae such as hemorrhage. Optimum physical and emotional well-being of the mother and healthy adaptation to extrauterine life of the child are excellent indicators that evaluative criteria have been met. When the family members state that they are satisfied with the management of the labor, the nurse can feel relatively reassured that emotional and physical supportive care goals were met.

MULTIPLE PREGNANCY

A pregnancy with more than one fetus places the mother and fetuses at risk. Maternal blood volume is increased in multiple gestations resulting in an increased strain on the maternal cardiovascular system. Anemia often develops because of a greater demand for iron by the fetuses. Marked uterine distension and increased pressure on the adjacent viscera and pelvic vasculature occur in multiple pregnancies. Diastasis of the two recti abdominis muscles (in the midline) may occur. Placenta previa develops more frequently in multiple pregnancies because of the large size or placement of the placentas (see Fig. 9-9, *A,* note placement of placentas). Premature separation of the placenta may occur before the second and subsequent fetuses are born.

Weight of each twin and her or his placenta usually are less than an infant and placenta of a singleton pregnancy after the thirtieth week. However, the aggregate weight is almost twice that of a singleton near term. The mean weight of twins in the United States is more than 2270 g (5 lb). Congenital malformations are twice as frequent in monozygotic twins as in singletons. There is no increase in the incidence of congenital anomalies in dizygotic twins. Two-vessel cords, that is, cords with a single umbilical artery, occur more often in twins than in singletons, and this abnormality is most common in monozygotic twins. The most serious problem for the fetus is the local shunting of blood between placentas (twin-to-twin transfusion) (Fig. 9-9*B, C,*). The *recipient* twin is larger. However, this twin may develop congenital heart failure during the first 24 hours after birth. The *donor* twin will be small, pallid, dehydrated, malnourished, and hypovolemic. Prematurity is a serious problem for the newborns.

Clinical diagnosis of multiple pregnancy is accurate in only about three fourths of cases. A correct diagnosis of twins may be possible in most instances by the twenty-fourth to twenty-sixth week based on the following:

1. History of dizygous twins in the female lineage
2. Abnormally large maternal weight gain (inconsistent with diet or edema)
3. Hydramnios
4. Palpation of excessive number of small or large parts
5. Asynchronous fetal heart beats or more than one fetal electrocardiographic (EEG) tracing
6. Radiographic or ultrasonographic (B-scan) evidence of more than one fetus (Chapter 27)

Prenatal Care

Prenatal care will include changes in the pattern of care and modifications in other aspects such as weight gain and diet. Prenatal visits by the mother with multiple pregnancy are scheduled at least every 2 weeks in the second trimester and weekly thereafter.

Diet and weight control are supervised to allow weight gain of about 50% or more than the average woman with a singleton pregnancy (as much as 18 kg [40 lb] above the woman's ideal nonpregnant weight). Iron and vitamin supplementation is desirable. Attempts are made to prevent preeclampsia–eclampsia and vaginitis; if they do develop, they are treated early and properly.

Support from a well-fitted maternity girdle may be welcomed. The considerable uterine distension can cause increase in backache. Elastic stockings or tights may control leg varices.

Abstinence from coitus or masturbation to the point of orgasm during the last trimester is recommended. This may help prevent preterm labor.

Enforced rest periods, begun as soon as pregnancy is diagnosed, may help to avoid untimely early labor. The mother needs to assume the left lateral position.

Untimely early labor should be avoided. Delivery after the third-sixth week increases the likelihood of survival of the newborns.

Labor and Delivery

Delivery in a maternity center where specialty care is always available is advisable when there is a multiple pregnancy. The woman is admitted to the hospital at the first sign of labor.

First stage. The woman is placed on bed rest in a left

lateral position. Her blood is typed and cross-matched, and several units of bank blood are kept available in the delivery room for emergency transfusion. Parenteral infusion of 5% dextrose in water (or other infusate) is started through a no. 16 or 18 needle (that can accommodate blood if needed) in the first stage of labor and is continued until the fourth stage is completed. Blood or drugs, if indicated, are administered intravenously at a slow rate. Analgesia must be limited drastically since the infants often are premature. If no complications occur, management of the first stage in multiple pregnancy does not differ from the single pregnancy with the same presentation.

Cesarean delivery is performed only for accepted obstetric reason. Multiple pregnancy itself is not an indication. However, feto-disproportion (e.g., conjoined twins), fetal distress, or monoamniotic twins (diagnosed by amniography) warrant cesarean delivery.

Second Stage. A physician and nurse team for each newborn is scrubbed, gowned, and gloved for the multiple birth delivery. After the first twin is born the cord is clamped promptly to prevent the second twin of a monozygotic pregnancy from partially exsanguinating through the first cord. The time of birth is noted, and the infant is labeled as Baby A.

The optimum time for delivery of the second child is 5 to 20 minutes after delivery of the first child. The physician's objective is to deliver the second child without difficult operative procedures. Some physicians prefer to deliver this fetus by cesarean birth. The second child is labeled Baby B and so on.

Third Stage. The third stage of labor must be managed with care. Excessive blood loss is common with multiple pregnancy. Oxytocin (Pitocin), 1 ml (10 units) intravenously, is administered immediately after delivery of the last child. The IV 5% dextrose in water infusion is continued. The fundus is elevated. It is not massaged until after the uterus contracts and expels the separated placenta. An ergot preparation such as ergonovine (Ergotrate), 0.1 mg intravenously, is then given if the woman is not hypertensive. Gentle massage and elevation of the fundus are continued for 15 to 30 minutes. The physician manually separates and extracts the placenta if separation of the placenta is delayed or bleeding is brisk.

Postpartum Care

The mother with multiple pregnancy requires the same physical care as any other parturient. She is more prone to develop postdelivery hemorrhage because of excessive uterine distension. Therefore she must be carefully assessed.

Psychologically, however, even the most willing of mothers can find their coping mechanisms overwhelmed by both the idea and reality of caring for two or more infants. Mother-child attachment takes longer because the mother attaches first to one newborn and then to the other. Parents must organize simplified and flexible plans of care. The almost constant attention required until the infants' schedule of care can be synchronized may prove exhausting. If possible, help is obtained, particularly to guarantee sufficient rest for the mother. The added expense can also be burdensome to a young family. One mother expressed anger at the surprise birth of twins. The explanation of such errors did not placate her. She needed time to vent these feelings before she could be helped with changing her anticipated plan for care.

Most parents are anxious to know if their children are identical or fraternal. Gross examination of the placenta at birth cannot prove whether twins are identical. Therefore it is best to tell parents differentiation in the type of twinning cannot be made at this time.

If the infants are born prematurely or are small for gestational age, their prolonged hospital stay can cause parental separation anxiety. If this is the case, the mother may be encouraged to visit or care for the infants in the hospital. She can use this waiting time to recover as much physical strength as possible. It provides time for the family to prepare for the infants' homecoming. Introduction of multiple siblings into a family also can result in intense rivalry. All children compete for the mother's attention. Substitute mothering by interested relatives can do much to ease the strain.

PRETERM LABOR AND BIRTH

Preterm birth is traumatic for both child and parent. The infant is faced with adjustment to extrauterine existence before final readiness for the event. Parents are faced with an unexpected emotional crisis as a result of the natural process of pregnancy and birth being altered. Parents and child often are separated. The separation extends over a period of time. Death or disability of the infant is a possibility that must be faced. The elements that foster parent-child attachment, that is, closeness, positive perception of the self and the child, and infant responsiveness, are radically changed. Child and parents experiencing the crisis of premature labor and birth need the concerted support of all members of the health care team.

Preterm birth is that which occurs after the twentieth but before the end of the thirty-seventh week of gestation. It results in the birth of a premature infant usually weighing less than 2400 g (5 lb 5 oz). The overall incidence of premature birth in the United States is 6% to 7%; in blacks the incidence is 10% to 11%. The *diagnosis* of preterm labor contractions may be difficult to distinguish from painful Braxton Hicks contractions or false labor. True labor is progressive and associated with cervical dilation, effacement, or both.

Infant Mortality and Morbidity

Premature birth is responsible for almost two-thirds of infant deaths. The infant born prematurely does not possess the growth and development necessary for uncomplicated adjustment to extrauterine life. Her or his prospects for survival or good health may be severely compromised. Infants weighing more than 2500 g (5½ lb) and delivered after 37 weeks of pregnancy have the best prospects of survival. There is a dramatic reduction in mortality in infants, regardless of weight, who are delivered after the thirty-sixth week of gestation. The prognosis for low-birth-weight infants weighing more than 1800 g (4 lb) is more favorable than for those weighing 1500 to 1800 g (3 to 4 lb). The mortality is less than 5% if the pregnancy has progressed to 35 weeks and the fetus weighs more than 2000 g (4½ lb). With these guidelines it is illogical to try to stop labor if the duration of pregnancy is 37 weeks or longer. The hazardous zone is 34 to 37 weeks, and the fetus should weigh more than 1800 g.

Etiology

Maternal and Fetal Factors. Debilitating maternal disorders, trauma, abdominal surgery, maternal injury, preeclampsia–eclampsia, uterine anomalies or tumors, cervical incompetence, and sepsis often are preludes to premature labor. Smoking, heavy work, single parenthood and other psychosocial factors are implicated.

Gross placental abnormalities such as placental separation or extrachorial placenta are associated with premature labor. Transplacental infections such as rubella, toxoplasmosis, or syphilis may be responsible for preterm labor. Multiple pregnancy, hydramnios, and premature rupture of the membranes are also notable. Congenital adrenal hyperplasia is usually associated with premature labor.

Iatrogenic Factors. Premature labor can result from elective delivery because of misjudgment of fetal maturity or miscalculation of the EDD. Iatrogenic prematurity accounts for slightly less than 10% of preterm babies.

Unknown Factors. In approximately two-thirds of preterm deliveries, no definite cause can be identified. Thirty to fifty percent of preterm labors occur after premature rupture of the membranes (PROM). It is important for nurses to convey this information to parents experiencing preterm labor.

Management of Preterm Birth

Obstetric management of prematurity involves (1) early detection of preterm labor, (2) suppressing uterine activity, and (3) improving intrapartum care of the fetus destined to be born early.

Over the past 25 years, little if any progress has been made in preventing preterm birth, and the incidence of low-birth-weight babies has remained unchanged. At present the United States ranks sixteenth among industrialized nations in perinatal mortality, mainly because of the high incidence of preterm birth. Consequently it is unlikely that this ranking will improve substantially unless this high incidence is lowered.

Client Education Program. Many women are unaware of the danger of preterm delivery and need to be informed of how they might reduce the risk. Client education programs have been established by concerned professional groups for the purpose of early detection of preterm labor. If preterm labor can be detected, early preventive therapy can be initiated. Research indicates treatment needs to be started in the early latent phase of labor to be successful (Spisso, Harbert, and Thiagarajah, 1982; Pritchard, McDonald, and Gant, 1985). One such program was developed by the nursing staff in a perinatal nursing program (Herron and Dulock, 1982).

All pregnant women are screened according to risk factors associated with preterm labor at their initial prenatal visit. They are assessed at 22 to 26 weeks of gestation. Women who are considered at high risk for preterm labor are followed in the preterm labor clinic.

Women in the high-risk group for preterm labor are seen weekly. They receive education in the symptoms of preterm labor (guidelines in Chapter 14—Preterm Labor Recognition), and instruction in palpation and timing and reporting of uterine contactions. Recently an ambulatory tocodynomometer device (Fig. 33-16) was developed to detect excessive uterine contractions before they can be perceived by the woman herself. The data is transmitted twice per day, via the telephone, to the hospital for analysis. Ambulatory home monitoring may represent a new and effective means for accurate and early diagnosis of preterm labor. Data from the tocodynomometer or from frequent assessment of the cervix are analyzed and appropriate therapy instituted if labor is suspected.

Therapy for Prevention of Preterm Birth. Attempts to arrest labor are justified if the following conditions are present.

1. Labor is diagnosed. There are three or more contractions of moderate intensity and duration per 20 minutes; the cervix is dilated no more than 4 cm or effaced no more than 50%; but the membranes must be intact with no bulging.
2. The fetus must be live and viable (some hospitals specify 20 to 36 weeks; others, 27 to 37 weeks' inclusive gestation). Estimation of gestational age by ultrasonography is the preferred technique.
3. There are no signs of fetal distress or disease.
4. There must be no medical or obstetric disorder or clinically significant abnormalities in laboratory findings that are a contraindication to the continuation of pregnancy.
5. The woman is both willing and capable of giving an informed consent. She should be able to comply with the prescribed regimen of medication (on an out-of-hospital basis) and weekly visits until delivery and to return for the 6-week postdelivery examination.

Home Management. Preterm labor may be treated by bed rest in the home. See guidelines for client teaching, p. 833.

In-hospital Suppression. Various drugs have been used to suppress labor. They are known as tocolytic drugs. *Toko-* or *toco-* are Greek roots referring to obstetrics; *-lytic* means "to break down or stop."

Ritodrine hydrochloride (Yutopar) (Ueland, 1981; Pritchard, McDonald, and Gant, 1985) is the first β-sympathomimetic drug approved in the United States for use in preterm labor. The administration of ritodrine must be closely supervised by persons having knowledge of the pharmacology of the drug. They must be qualified to identify and manage complications of drug administration or pregnancy.

Drug action. Ritodrine hydrochloride stimulates type II β-adrenergic receptors. These cause uterine muscle relaxation, vasodilation, bronchodilation, and muscle glycogen-

A B

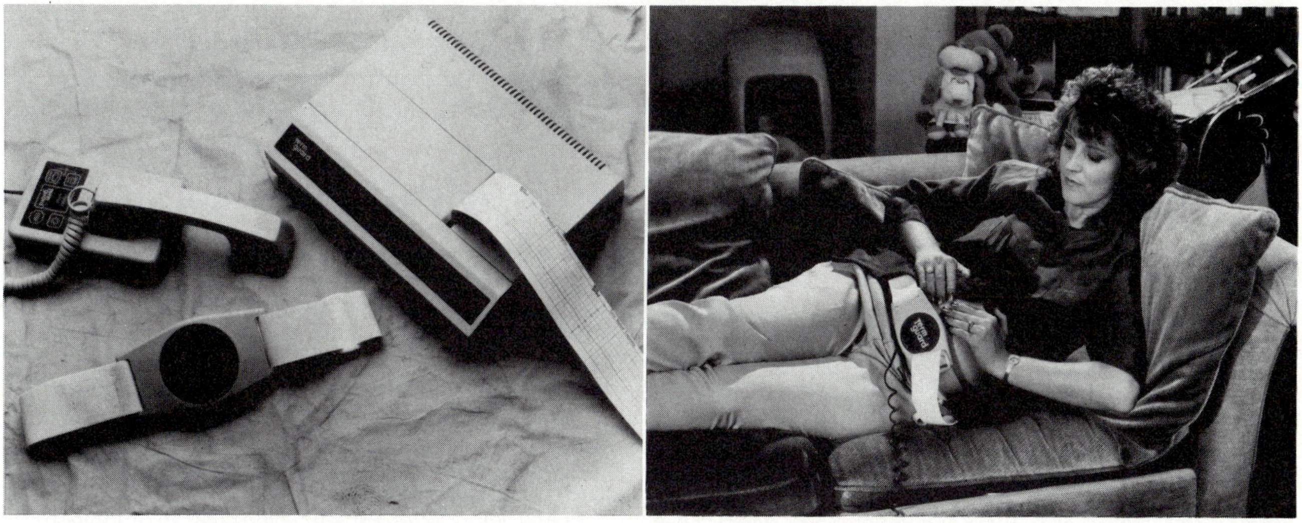

Fig. 33-16 Home uterine activity monitoring. **A**, Lightweight ambulatory tocodynamometer and recording unit used to transmit data over the phone. **B**, Tocodynamometer in place at center of abdomen below umbilicus.

Guidelines for Client Teaching

PRETERM LABOR: HOME MANAGEMENT

ASSESSMENT

Gravida 2 carrying twins, 30 weeks gestation.
First baby born at 34 weeks gestation.
Preterm labor has been diagnosed and treated; woman is now ready for discharge with medication; or,
Preterm labor is to be treated at home.

NURSING DIAGNOSES

Knowledge deficit related to management of preterm labor.
Potential for injury: maternal and fetal, related to recurrence of preterm labor and delivery.
Anxiety, mild to moderate, related to possible recurrence of preterm labor and delivery.

GOALS

Short-term

Gravida learns home management after preterm labor episode.

Intermediate

Gravida implements home management.

Long-term

Gravida carries pregnancy to or near term and gives birth to healthy mature twins.

REFERENCES AND TEACHING AIDS

Printed materials available through drug companies, hospitals, and clinics.

CONTENT/RATIONALE	TEACHING ACTIONS
To understand preterm labor, its causes, signs, and symptoms:	
Review guidelines for client teaching: preterm labor recognition, Chapter 14.	Implement teaching actions as required from guidelines, Chapter 14.
To foster understanding and self care:	
Bed rest	
Bed rest is intended to keep the pressure of the fetus off the cervix and to enhance uterine perfusion. Kneeling or sitting in bed does not keep the fetus from pressing on the cervix. Physical rest is facilitated by peace of mind. Someone other than the mother must assume care of older children, cooking, and cleaning. Many women are allowed out of bed only for use of the bathroom.	Develop care plan mutually with woman/couple/family. Mobilize assistance for home management. Advise woman to lie on her left side with her head flat or raised on a small pillow.

Continued.

Guidelines For Client Teaching—cont'd

CONTENT/RATIONALE	TEACHING ACTIONS
Medications	
If the woman is being maintained at home on an *oral* dose of tocolytic medication (ritodrine hydrochloride or terbutaline), woman must know rationale, side effects, and danger signs (boxes, p. 835).	Medications are reviewed and the woman is given written instructions regarding care. Inform woman about the action and side effects of the drug. Instruct her how to take her pulse and report any rate greater than 120 beats per min to her physician, how to report symptoms, including palpitations, tremors, agitation, and nervousness.
Some over-the-counter drugs may cause deleterious effects. Oral administration may be better tolerated when taken with food.	Caution her not to use ritodrine with any over-the-counter drugs unless her physician approves.
Sedation is often ordered to facilitate relaxation and rest.	Advise and give written instructions (for herself and her family) regarding the medication. This includes the prescription for sedation, dosage, times for administration, and side effects.
Avoidance of activities that could stimulate labor:	
Sexual stimulation is contraindicated because (1) prostaglandins in semen can stimulate labor in a susceptible woman and (2) touching the cervix or pressure against the posterior wall of the vagina may stimulate Ferguson's reflex (the increase in myometrial contractility that follows mechanical stretching or touching of the cervix). Nipple stimulation may induce oxytocin production that can cause recurrence of uterine activity.	Encourage discussion of this sensitive topic.
To identify hazards and intervene in a timely manner:	
Review danger signs, boxes, p. 835. Review danger of infection if membranes are not intact.	Review verbally and provide written instructions regarding: a. What to do and whom to notify in case of onset of labor or rupture of membranes. b. Maintaining personal hygiene if membranes have ruptured earlier. c. Assessing for signs of infection (e.g., odor of vaginal discharge, increase in body temperature).
To assist with home maintenance:	
Social service consultation may be helpful if the woman has to be transported into a center from an outlying area. Living arrangements, meals, transportation, and financial assistance may be needed for some families.	Refer to appropriate agency after discussion and mutual planning with family.

EVALUATION The nurse can be reasonably assured that teaching was effective if the goals for care are achieved. The woman and her family are able to implement self-care so that preterm labor is stopped, there are no adverse sequelae to medication, and positive family processes are maintained. The woman delivers healthy infants at or near term.

olysis. Decrease in serum potassium levels may cause arrhythmias.

Contraindications for use. Not all fetuses can benefit from prolonging intrauterine life. An adverse uterine environment may be more detrimental than premature birth. Contraindications to inhibition of labor include the following conditions (NAACOG, 1984):

a. Fetal death confirmed by ultrasound
b. Antepartum hemorrhage; requires immediate delivery
c. PIH (degree to be evaluated individually)
d. Dilation more than 3 to 4 cm (tertiary consultation should be attained if dilation greater than 4 cm)
e. Maternal cardiac pathology (β-mimetics contraindicated)
f. Insulin-dependent diabetes
g. Maternal hyperthyroidism
h. Gestational age less than 20 weeks, confirmed by ultrasound
i. Ruptured fetal membranes (PROM), afebrile mother (controversy; some physicians delay delivery to mature fetal lungs)
j. Chorioamnionitis
k. Mother already taking β-mimetics for a previously existing medical condition; should not be receiving additional β-mimetic therapy

Beneficial effects. A delay of premature delivery is potentially beneficial to the fetus. In addition the tocolytic agents currently available are usually able to delay delivery long enough for the use of glucocorticoids to effect fetal pulmonary maturation.

Toxic effects. Cardiopulmonary complications are possible. Therefore careful assessment and monitoring are essential. Because of the possible cardiopulmonary effects an electrocardiogram may be ordered before the treatment. A cardiac monitor for the mother may be indicated to maintain continuous assessment for *tachycardia* and *arrhythmia.* See Procedure 33-3 for a summary of the hazardous complications and the care required for a client receiving ritodrine hydrochloride. See box below for danger signs for ritodrine and terbutaline toxicity. The danger box for terbutaline is included because this drug is used by some physicians.

DANGER SIGNS

Ritodrine Toxicity

1. Central nervous system: severe nervousness or anxiety, tremulousness, headache, restlessness.
2. Respirations: dyspnea, hyperventilation.
3. Cardiovascular system: severe palpitations or cardiac irregularities, chest pain; pulmonary edema.
4. Gastrointestinal: severe nausea or vomiting, epigastric distress, diarrhea.

Terbutaline Toxicity

1. Central nervous system: severe dizziness, drowsiness, headache, nervousness, restlessness; clouded sensorium.
2. Blood pressure: severe hypertension.
3. Heart rate: continuous palpitations.
4. Musculoskeletal: severe muscle cramps and weakness.
5. Gastrointestinal: continuous nausea and vomiting.

Administration and dosage. The drug may be administered either intravenously or orally. IV administration precedes the oral administration. The dosage is determined by the physician. **Magnesium sulfate** in sufficiently high concentrations can suppress uterine contractions (Spisso, Harbert, and Thiagarajh, 1982; Niebyl, 1986). The *precautions* taken during administration of magnesium sulfate are *the same* regardless of whether the rationale for therapy is the suppression of labor or the prevention of eclampsia (see Chapter 29).

Pharmacologic Stimulation of Fetal Lung Maturity. Respiratory distress syndrome (RDS) was formerly known as hyaline membrane disease of the newborn (HMD). It is common in small premature twins who have fetal lung immaturity. The incidence and severity of RDS has been found to be reduced if glucocorticoids are administered to the mother at least 24 to 38 hours before the delivery. The fetus must be less than 34 weeks gestation. The administration must be made at least 24 hours before delivery and no longer than 7 days before delivery (Liggins and Howie, 1974; Brown et al., 1979). Children who have been exposed to the stated levels of glucocorticoids in utero appear to grow and develop normally during the early years of life (Liggins, 1976, 1982). Hence some authorities consider that the chance of benefit to the fetus far outweighs the chance of harm. Pritchard, McDonald, and Gant (1985) note that controversy still exists over the efficacy of glucocorticoid prophylaxis. The following are recognized as contraindications for glucocorticoid therapy:

1. Multiple pregnancy
2. Maternal infection, such as tuberculosis
3. Complications of pregnancy, such as PIH
4. Imminent delivery

Care During Irreversible or Acceptable Preterm Birth. The labor is conducted according to the principles that apply to a low-birth-weight (easily compromised) fetus. If vaginal delivery is chosen, the analgesia is limited, and continuous FHR monitoring is applied. AROM is delayed until the cervix is more than 6 cm dilated, and there is sufficient descent of the presenting part to avoid prolapse of the cord.

If the augmentation of labor is advisable, a low concentration of oxytocin is infused continuously. Pudendal block anesthesia is desirable. An episiotomy is done to limit the length of the second stage and excessive pressure on the fragile fetal head. Outlet (low) forceps are used for delivery unless easy spontaneous birth is likely. A pediatrician and a nurse from the infant intensive care unit are present at the birth so that resuscitative and supportive care for the infant can be initiated immediately if necessary (see Unit VIII). The newborn is permitted several breaths before clamping the cord; if resuscitation is required, however, the cord is clamped and cut immediately.

Parental concern for the well-being of the infant is apparent during labor. Parents need to be aware of the interest and support of the staff. However, false assurance of fetal health must be avoided. For some parents the reality of the situation is not appreciated until they see their daughter or son in the intensive care unit. For others who experience fetal or neonatal death, the loss intensifies once the stress of labor and delivery is over (see Chapter 28).

During the postpartum period physical care of the mother is similar to that required for any vaginal delivery. However, the family will be very anxious concerning the health and prognosis of their infant (Sammons and Lewis, 1985). Nursing care of the preterm infant involves not only medical and nursing personnel but also the participation of the parents (see Chapter 37). The nurse must be aware of the impact that preterm birth may have on family dynamics (see research highlight, p. 837).

Procedure 33-3

NURSING CARE OF A WOMAN RECEIVING RITODRINE HYDROCHLORIDE

DEFINITION

The use of a β-sympathomimetic agent to stop the uterus from contracting, thereby stopping preterm labor.

PURPOSE

Suppression of preterm labor.

EQUIPMENT

Intravenous infusion equipment, sphygmomanometer, stethoscope, equipment for cardiopulmonary arrest, fetal monitoring equipment.

HAZARDOUS SYMPTOMS

See danger signs: ritodrine hydrochloride, p. 835.

NURSING ACTIONS	RATIONALE
Identify client and check physician's orders.	To provide the right therapy for the right person.
Wash hands before and after touching client or equipment. Glove, prn.	To prevent nosocomial infection and to implement universal precautions.
Assess maternal vital signs and FHR.	To obtain baseline data.
Monitor vital signs and blood pressure every 15 minutes until stable and then follow hospital protocol. *Maternal pulse should not exceed 140 beats per minute for more than 10 minutes.* Note regularity and quality.	To detect complications: cardiac arrhythmias are adverse effects of β-adrenergic therapy, pulmonary edema, and fluid overload.
Prepare mother for use of cardiac monitor.	
Note breath sounds when counting respiratory rate.	
Monitor FHR: *should not exceed 180 beats per minute.* Intermittent evaluation should continue during oral therapy also.	
Observe for any untoward symptoms.	
Ask woman to report symptoms.	To elicit subjective symptoms.
Send blood samples to laboratory for analysis of levels of glucose, potassium, and hematocrit.	To assess for hypokalemia and acidosis. As glucose moves into cells, potassium shifts from the extracellular space.
Maintain absolute bed rest during intravenous infusion.	To minimize stress and reduce pressure on cervix.
Prevent hypotension; keep woman in left-lateral position or place wedge under right hip if in supine position.	To maintain placental perfusion.
Apply antiembolism stockings.	To prevent pooling of blood in lower extremities.
Do not use under knees. Encourage passive leg exercises.	
Maintain adequate hydration, 2000 to 3000 ml daily.	To maintain cardiac output.
Prevent overhydration:	
Measure intake and output.	To detect overhydration.
Weigh daily.	
Prevent undue stress:	To promote relaxation through anticipatory guidance.
Prepare woman for potential side effects (i.e., agitation, palpitations, nervousness, tremors, tachycardia).	
Instruct woman to report symptoms.	To elicit subjective symptoms.
Treat for complications:	
Hold medication. If intravenous, keep line open with plain solution.	To minimize effects of medication.
Notify physician and prepare antidote as ordered.	To initiate immediate therapy.
Maintain woman in high Fowler's position.	To minimize effects of possible pulmonary edema.
Administer oxygen.	To maintain sufficient oxygenation.
Initiate CPR for arrest if necessary.	To maintain oxygenation and body functions.

RESEARCH HIGHLIGHT

Women's Important Relationships During Pregnancy and the Preterm Labor Event

Purpose

There is a lack of information concerning factors antecedent to the onset of premature labor. This study sought to determine (1) important relationships identified by the pregnant woman, and (2) an evaluation of the relationships as either satisfactory or unsatisfactory.

Sample

A convenient sample of 45 women participated in the study.

Methodology

This study compared the descriptions and evaluations of important relationships identified by woman who experienced premature labor with those of woman experiencing essentially normal pregnancies. Premature labor was experienced by 30 women, and 15 women experienced essentially normal pregnancies. Women in the premature labor group were interviewed in their hospital rooms (21 to 35 weeks gestation). The normal pregnancy subjects were interviewed at a maternity outpatient clinic at approximately the 32nd week of pregnancy.

The three relationship categories were: 1) husband (or baby's father), 2) parental figures, and 3) peers. Relationships were described as either satisfactory or unsatisfactory (worrisome).

Findings/Implications

Findings indicated that premature-labor subjects reported more unsatisfactory relationships with husbands and parental figures. Although not statistically significant, premature labor subjects reported more problems with peers than did normal-pregnancy subjects. In this study premature-labor subjects described having more problems with and receiving less help and affection from the people upon whom they depend.

Richardson, P: Women's important relationships during pregnancy and the preterm labor event, W J Nurs Res 9(2):203, 1987.

POSTTERM BIRTH

The postterm pregnancy persists beyond the end of the forty-second week, 2 weeks beyond the EDD figured from Naegele's rule. The infant whose gestational age is beyond 42 weeks is referred to as "postterm" if healthy and "dysmature" if adversely affected by the delayed birth (see Chapter 37).

Maternal risks are related to the delivery of an excessively sized infant. Fetal risks appear to be twofold. The first is related to the possibility of birth trauma and asphyxia through fetopelvic disproportion. The second risk is felt to result from the compromising effects on the fetus of an "aging" placenta. Danforth and Scott (1986) note "the normal life span of the placenta is about 40 weeks; after this time, its capacity and reserve are progressively reduced in the face of increasing demands by the growing fetus." Oligohydramnios and consequent cord compression are also suspected to affect fetal well-being (Leveno et al., 1984). There is still considerable controversy over the predominant cause of postterm fetal effects (Shearer and Estes, 1985).

The decision whether to initiate labor is difficult. Pritchard, McDonald, and Gant (1985) report five problems that can affect the decision:

1. Gestational age is not always precisely known. Thus the fetus may actually be less mature than thought.
2. Precise identification of those fetuses who are likely to die or develop serious morbidity if left in utero is difficult.
3. Most fetuses fare rather well.
4. Induction of labor is not always successful.
5. Cesarean delivery appreciably increases the risk of serious maternal morbidity not only in this pregnancy but also to a degree in subsequent ones.

SUMMARY

Complications during birth have both physical and emotional sequelae. The mother faces hazards to her life. Prolonged and difficult labor can be physically debilitating. The consequent fatigue may interfere with the initial interactions with her newborn. Memories of a difficult birth can resurface years later as a stress factor in subsequent births. The family will be faced with long-term grief reaction if the infant suffers disability. If death of either mother or infant occurs, the family, as it was, no longer exists. Parents, during this time of crisis, need the best possible medical and nursing care that our technically and psychologically knowledgeable society can offer.

KEY CONCEPTS

- Dystocia results from differences in the normal relationships between any of the five essential factors of labor.
- The differences between dystocia and eutocia relate to changes in the pattern of progress in labor.
- The functional relationships between the uterine contractions, the fetus, and the mother's pelvis are altered by maternal positioning.
- Uterine contractility is increased by oxytocin and PGE and is decreased by tocolytics.
- All expectant parents benefit from learning about operative obstetrics (e.g., use of forceps, cesarean delivery) and preterm labor during the prenatal period.
- The basic purpose of cesarean delivery is to preserve the life or health of the mother and her fetus.
- Under certain conditions, vaginal birth is possible after previous cesarean birth.
- The gravida and her family can be taught to treat preterm labor at home with bedrest, tocolytics, and avoidance of activities that stimulate the uterus.
- In-hospital treatment for preterm labor involves the use of tocolytics and pharmacologic stimulation of lung maturity.
- Postterm birth poses a risk to both the mother and the fetus.

STUDY QUESTIONS AND ACTIVITIES

1. Develop a plan for client education for the client concerning:
   a. Self-assessment, to identify preterm labor with and without use of an ambulatory tocodynomometer.
   b. Home management intended to prevent preterm birth.
   c. In-hospital tocolysis and pharmacologic stimulation of fetal lung maturity
2. Using several examples of partograms that indicate various types of dystocia, identify the type of dystocia, and discuss its management.
3. Role-play a nurse providing care to the woman experiencing:
   a. Prolonged labor
   b. Postterm labor
4. In small groups, develop nursing care plans for the following types of labors; in the total group, compare and contrast the care plans. Select from the following, or from actual cases on your unit:
   a. Woman experiencing preterm labor; previous labor was also preterm and the infant died at 3 days of age.
   b. Woman is having a cesarean delivery scheduled during the prenatal period because of a known obstetric problem.
   c. Woman is having an emergency cesarean delivery.
   d. Woman is having prolonged labor; she is in optimum condition and fetal monitor tracings indicate her twins are responding well to labor.
5. Follow a woman through the perioperative period of a cesarean delivery. What preparation was provided to her? What needs are expressed in the postpartum period that are different from postpartum needs of women who have had a vaginal delivery?

References

Bezjian, AA: Pelvic masses in pregnancy. In Sabbagha RE, editor: Diagnostic ultrasound applied to obstetrics and gynecology, 1980, Harper & Row Publishers, Inc 1980:229

Brown, ER, et al: Reversible induction of surfactant production in fetal lambs treated with glucocorticoids, Pediatr Res 13:491, 1979

Caldeyro-Barcia, R: The influence of maternal position on time of spontaneous rupture of the membranes, progress of labor, and fetal head compression, Birth Fam J 6:7, 1979

Compton, AA: Soft tissue and pelvic dystocia, Clin Obstet Gynecol 30(1):69, 1987

Danforth, D, and Scott, J, editors: Obstetrics and Gynecology, ed 5, Philadelphia, 1986, JB Lippincott Co

Fenwick, L, and Simkin, P: Maternal positioning to prevent or alleviate dystocia in labor, Clin Obstet Gynecol 30(1):83, 1987

Friedman, EA: Midforceps delivery: no? Clin Obstet Gynecol 30(1):93, 1987

Gellman, E, et al: Vaginal delivery after cesarean section, JAMA 249:2935, 1983

Gilbert, ES, and Harmon, JS: High-risk pregnancy and delivery: nursing perspectives, St Louis, 1986, The CV Mosby Co

Gleichner, N: Cesarean section rates in the United States: the short-term failure of the National Consensus Development Conference in 1980, JAMA 252:3273, 1984

Glazer, G, and Hulme, MA: Prostaglandin gel for cervical ripening, MCN 12(1):28, 1987

Hayashi, RH: Midforceps delivery: yes? Clin Obstet Gynecol 30(1):90, 1985

Herron, MA, and Dulock, HL: Preterm labor: a staff development program in perinatal nursing care, 1982, March of Dimes Birth Defects Foundation

Knuppel, RA, and Drukker, JE: High-risk pregnancy: a team approach, Philadelphia, 1986, WB Saunders Co

Lee, CY: Shoulder dystocia, Clin Obstet Gynecol 30(1):77, 1987

Leveno, KJ, et al: Prolonged pregnancy. I. Observations concerning the causes of fetal distress, Am J Obstet Gynecol 150:465, 1984

Liggins, GC: The prevention of RDS by maternal beta-methasone administration. In Lung maturation and the prevention of hyaline membrane disease. Report of the Seventieth Ross Conference on Pediatric Research, Columbus, Ohio, 1976, Ross Laboratories

Liggins, GC: Report on children exposed to steroids in utero, Contemp OB/GYN 19:205,1982

Liggins, GC, and Howie, RN: The prevention of RDS by maternal steroid therapy. In Gluck L, editor: Modern perinatal medicine, Chicago, 1974, Year Book Medical Publishers Inc

Meier, PR, and Parreco, RP: Trial of labor following cesarean section: a two-year experience, Am J Obstet Gynecol 144:671, 1982

Morrison, et al: Cesarean section: what's behind the dramatic rise? Perinatal Neonatal, 6:87, 1982

Myerscough, PR: Munro Kerr's operative obstetrics, ed 10, London, 1982, Bailliere Tindall

NAACOG: Preterm labor and tocolytics, Nurs Pract Res 10:1, Sept 1984

Niebyl, J, et al: Tocolytics: when and how to use them, Contemp OB/GYN 27(6):146, 1986

O'Driscoll, K, and Foley, M: Correlation of decrease in perinatal mortality and increase in cesarean section rates, Obstet Gynecol 61:1, 1983

O'Sullivan, MJ, Fumia, F, Holsinger, KK, et al: Vaginal delivery after cesarean section, Clin Perinatol 8:131, 1981

Perkins, RP: Fetal dystocia, Clin Obstet Gynecol 30(1):56, 1987

Petitti, E: Recent trends in cesarean delivery rates in California, Birth 12:25, Spring 1985

Pritchard, J, McDonald, P, and Gant, N: Williams obstetrics, ed 17, New York, 1985, Appleton-Century Croft

Sammons, WA, and Lewis, JM: Premature babies: a different beginning, St. Louis, 1985, The CV Mosby Co

Schulman, H, and Farmakides, G: Role of the unfavorable cervix in the induction of labor, Clin Obstet Gynecol 30(1):50, 1987

Shearer, M, and Estes, M: A critical review of the recent literature on postterm pregnancy and a look at women's experience, Birth 12:95, Summer 1985

Sheen, PW, and Hayashi, RH: Graphic management of labor: alert/action line, Clin Obstet Gynecol 30(1):33, 1987

Simkin, P: Stress, pain and catecholamines in labor, Part 1: a review, Birth 13:8, 1986

Spisso, KR, Harbert, GM, Jr, and Thiagarajah, S: The use of magnesium sulfate as the primary tocolytic agent to prevent premature delivery. Am J Obstet Gynecol 142:840, 1982

Ueland, K: Ritodrine hydrochloride (Yutopar) for treatment of preterm labor, Periscope, p 4, April 1981

Bibliography

Adamsons, K, and Wallach, RC: Treating preterm labor with diazoxide, Contemp OB/GYN 31(1):161, 1988

Alley, A: Pre-operative teaching for cesarean birth, AORN 34:846, 1981

Andrews, CM: Changing fetal position through maternal posturing. In: Raff, BS, editor: Perinatal parental behavior: nursing research and implications for newborn health, White Plains, NY, 1981, March of Dimes Foundation

Atwood, RJ: Parturitional posture and related birth behavior, Acta Obstet Gynecol Scand (suppl 57):5, 1976

Banta, D, and Thacker, S: The risks and benefits of episiotomy: review, Birth 9:25, 1982

Baxi, LV, and Petrie, RH: Pharmacologic effects on labor: effects of drugs on dystocia, labor, and uterine activity, Clin Obstet Gynecol 30(1):19, 1987

Bell, R: The prediction of preterm labour by recording spontaneous uterine activity, Br J Obstet Gynaecol 90:884, 1983

Buchan, PC, and Nicholls, JAJ: Pain after episiotomy—a comparison of two methods of repair, JR Coll Gen Pract 30:297, 1980

Carlson, JM, Diehl, JA, Sachtelben-Murray, M, et al: Maternal positioning during parturition in normal labor, Obstet Gynecol 68:443, 1986

Cetrulo, CL, and Cetrulo, LG: Medicolegal dystocia, Clin Obstet Gynecol 30(1):106, 1987

Cranley, M, et al: Women's perceptions of vaginal and cesarean deliveries, Nurs Res 32:11, 1983

Creasy, RK, and Katz, M: Basic research and clinical experience with beta adrenergic tocolytics in the United States. In: Fuchs, F, and Stubblefield PG, editors: Preterm birth: causes, prevention and management, New York, MacMillan Publishing Co

Cox, B, and Smith, E: The mother's self-esteem after a cesarean delivery, MCN 7:309, 1982

Droegemueller, W, et al: Comprehensive gynecology, St Louis, 1987, The CV Mosby Co

Engelmann, GJ: Labor among primitive peoples, Reprint of 1882 edition, New York, 1977, AMS Press, Inc

Fawcett, J, and Henklein, JC: Antenatal education for cesarean birth: extension of a field test, JOGN Nurs 16(1):61, 1987

Filly, RA: Twins: sonographic aids to management, UCSF Antepartum and intrapartum management, San Francisco, Calif, June 1987

Finley, BE, et al: Emergent cesarean delivery in patients undergoing a trial of labor with a transverse lower-segment scar, Am J Obstet Gynecol 155:936, 1986

Flanagan, T, et al: Management of term breech presentation, Am J Obstet Gynecol 156(6):1492, 1987

Galvan, BJ, and Broekhuizen, FF: Obstetric vacuum extraction, JOGN Nurs 16(4):242, 1987

Garfield, RE: Cellular and molecular bases for dystocia, Clin Obstet Gynecol 30(1):3, 1987

Gill, PJ, and Katz, M: Early detection of preterm labor: ambulatory home monitoring of uterine activity, JOGN Nurs 15(6):439, 1986

Grundy, HW: Tocolysis: who to treat? When to start? UCSF Antepartum and intrapartum management conference, San Francisco, Calif, June 1987

Herron, MA: Preterm labor. I. Preventing preterm births, NAACOG update series, lesson 2, 1983

Integration of the cesarean birth experience—the various adjustment cycles, Perinatal Press 4:136, 1980

International Medical News Service, Standing, sitting during delivery not dangerous. Report of a presentation by H. Nagai at the 11th World Congress of Gynecology and Obstetrics in Berlin, Obstet Gynecol News 20:10, 1985

Jacobs, MM: Role of prostaglandins in cervical ripening—should you be using it? UCSF Antepartum and intrapartum management, San Francisco, Calif, June 1987

Katz, MM: The role of home tocodynamometry in clinical practice, UCSF Antepartum and intrapartum management conference, San Francisco, Calif, June 1987

Katz, M, and Gill, PJ: Comprehensive preterm birth prevention program, Clin Res 32(2):296A, 1984

Katz, M, and Gill, PJ: Initial evaluation of an ambulatory system for home monitoring and transmission of uterine activity data, Obstet Gynecol 66(2):273, 1985

Knor, ER: Decision making in obstetrical nursing, 1987, BC Decker, Inc

Kopelman, JN: Computed tomographic pelvimetry in the evaluation of breech presentation, Obstet Gynecol 68:455, 1986

Lam, F: Tocolytic infusion at home, UCSF Antepartum and intrapartum management conference, San Francisco, Calif, June 1987

Laros, RK: Twins: current obstetrical management, UCSF Antepartum and intrapartum management, San Francisco, Calif, June 1987

Leach, L, and Sproule, V: Meeting the challenge of cesarean birth, JOGN Nurs 13:19, May/June, 1984

Levine, MG, Holroyde, J, and Woods, JR, et al: Birth trauma: incidence and predisposing factors, Obstet Gynecol 63:792, 1984

Lipson, J: Repeat cesarean birth, social and psychological issues, JOGN Nurs 13:157, May/June 1984

Lupe, PJ, and Gross, TL: Maternal upright posture and mobility in labor: a review, Obstet Gynecol 67:727, 1986

Main, D, Gabbe, S, Richardson, D, and Strong, S: Can preterm deliveries be prevented? Am J Obstet Gynecol 151:892, 1985

Mondanlou, HD, Dorchester, WL, Thorosian, A, and Freeman, RK: Macrosomia: maternal, fetal and neonatal implications, Obstet Gynecol 55:420, 1980

NAACOG: The nurse's role in the induction/augmentation of labor, OGN Nursing Practice Resource, Jan 1988 (PO Box 71437, Washington, DC 20024-1437)

Nager, CW, Key, TC, and Moore, TR: Cervical ripening and labor outcome with preinduction intracervical prostaglandin E_2 (Prepidil) gel J Perinatal 7(3):189, 1987

NICHD: Consensus Report by the Task Force on Cesarean Childbirth, Bethesda, Md, NICHD, 1980

Notzon, FC, et al: Comparisons of national cesarean-section rates, N Engl J Med 316(7):386, 1987

Odent, M: Birth reborn, New York, 1984, Random House, Inc

Ogburn, MD: The mystery of preterm labor, Childbirth Educator p 20, Summer 1986

Richardson, P: Women's important relationships during pregnancy and the preterm labor event, W J Nurs Res 9(2):203, 1987

Seitchik, J: The management of functional dystocia in the first stage of labor, Clin Obstet Gynecol 30(1):42, 1987

Speer, DP, and Peltier, LF: Pelvic fractures and pregnancy, J Trauma 12:474, 1972

Stewart, DB: The pelvis as a passageway. I. Evolution and adaptions, Br J Obstet Gynecol 91:611, 1984

Struyk, APHB, and Treffers, PE: Ovarian tumors in pregnancy, Acta Obstet Gynecol Scand 63:421, 1984

Stubblefield, PG, and Heyl, PS: Treatment of preterm labor with subcutaneous terbutaline, Obstet Gynecol 59(4):457, 1982

Stubblefield, PG: Causes and prevention of preterm birth: an overview. In: Fuchs, F, and Stubblefield PG, editors: Preterm birth: causes, prevention and management, New York, 1984, MacMillan Publishing Co

Tucker, SM, et al: Patient care standards: nursing process, diagnosis, and outcome, ed 4, St Louis, 1988, The CV Mosby Co

Symposium: Alternatives to cesarean section, Contemp OB/GYN 31(1):191, 1988

Weiss, JD: Management of dystocia, UCSF Antepartum and intrapartum management, San Francisco, Calif, June 1987

Young, J, and Poppe, C: Breast pump stimulation to promote labor, MCN 12(2):124, 1987

CHAPTER

34

Medical, Surgical, and Psychosocial Conditions Complicating Pregnancy

Learning Objectives

Correctly define the key terms listed.

Review the management of women with cardiovascular disorders.

Discuss anemia during pregnancy.

Discuss pulmonary disorders with emphasis on adult respiratory distress syndrome.

Summarize disorders of the gastrointestinal, integumentary, and neurologic systems that complicate some pregnancies.

Relate the care of women whose pregnancies are complicated with autoimmune disorders.

Explain the nursing process for women experiencing abdominal surgery or trauma during pregnancy.

Review the care of women experiencing emotional complications during the childbearing cycle.

Explain the care of women who use, abuse, or are dependent on drugs such as alcohol, opioids, and cocaine.

Assess the effects of poverty on the childbearing cycle.

Key Terms

adult respiratory distress syndrome (ARDS)
affective disorders
aortic dissection
autoimmune diseases
cardiac decompensation
chorea gravidarum
depressive reactions
intoxication
manic reactions
McBurney's point
mitral valve prolapse
peripartum cardiomyopathy
physiologic anemia of pregnancy
postpartum psychosis
primary pulmonary hypertension
psychoactive drugs
reflex bradycardia
schizophrenia
sickle cell hemoglobinopathy
systemic lupus erythematosus
trauma care
withdrawal (drug)

The effects on pregnancy of selected preexisting medical disorders and the nursing care that can lead to their effective management are presented in this chapter. These conditions are sometimes first diagnosed during pregnancy.

Some surgical procedures and injuries and the related nursing roles are also discussed. Surgical interruption of pregnancy and surgical termination of fertility are discussed in Chapter 42.

Three psychosocial conditions that have implications for the health of the mother and child that can interfere with family integration and restrict bonding with the infant, are dealth with: emotional disorders, psychoactive substance abuse and dependence, and poverty.

CARDIOVASCULAR DISORDERS

Every pregnancy taxes the cardiovascular system (Chapter 10). The strain is present during pregnancy and is maintained for a few weeks after delivery. An increase in blood volume begins by the tenth or twelfth week of gestation, reaches a maximum increase of 30% to 50% at 20 to 26 weeks, and levels off after the thirtieth week. Blood volume returns to nonpregnant levels within the first 2 to 3 weeks after delivery. The increase in blood volume is correlated with total birth weight and thus tends to be greater in multigravidas and women with multiple pregnancies. The relaxation of the great veins causes a decrease in systemic vascular resistance, a decrease in blood pressure (p. 205) and pulse pressure, and an increase in cardiac output. The cardiac output and stroke volume at rest reflect the increase in the blood volume but return to normal by 6 weeks after delivery. The heart rate is accelerated by a maximum of 15 to 20 beats per minute in the last trimester. The point of maximal intensity (PMI) is laterally displaced (see Fig. 10-8). A split develops in the first heart sound because of increased venous return to the heart. As many as 90% of women may develop a systolic ejection murmur. With delivery of the placenta and closure of the placental vascular shunt, venous hypertension occurs during the first 24 hours after childbirth.

The normal heart can compensate for these and associated burdens so that pregnancy and delivery are generally well tolerated. If myocardial or valvular disease develops, or if a congenital heart defect is large, cardiac decompensation is likely.

Incidence and Characteristics. Heart disease is the leading cause of *non*obstetric maternal mortality. A maternal mortality of 1% to 3% is likely with severe heart disease. It ranks fourth overall as a cause of maternal death. A perinatal mortality of up to 50% must be expected with persistent cardiac decompensation. Some degree of cardiac impairment affects 0.5 % to 2% of pregnant women (Roberts and Chestnut, 1987). Cocaine use is associated with various cardiac complications (p. 868) and vascular phenomena (e.g., abruptio placentae).

Effects of Pregnancy on Heart Disease. The effects of pregnancy on heart disease result from the maternal adaptations during pregnancy. The stress these place on a heart whose function is already taxed can cause cardiac decompensation. Cardiac failure can develop during the last few weeks of pregnancy, during labor, and during the postdelivery period (Pritchard, MacDonald, and Gant, 1985).

Effects of Heart Disease on Pregnancy. The woman who has rheumatic heart disease secondary to rheumatic fever may experience **chorea gravidarum** (Sydenham's chorea). This condition is characterized by involuntary purposeless contractions of the muscles of the trunk and extremities, anxiety, and impairment of memory. Recovery occurs within 6 to 10 weeks of delivery. Treatment consists of rest for the body and mind.

Spontaneous abortion is increased, and premature labor and delivery are more prevalent in the pregnant woman with cardiac problems. Probably because of the low Po_2 level, fetal growth retardation commonly occurs.

The differential diagnosis of heart disease involves ruling out respiratory problems, primarily arrhythmias. The diagnosis of heart disease depends on the history, physical examination, x-ray films, and ultrasonograms when required.

Classification. The degree of dysfunction (disability) of the woman with cardiac disease often is more important in the treatment and prognosis of cardiac disease complicating pregnancy than the diagnosis of the valvular lesion per se. The New York Heart Association's functional classification of organic heart disease, a widely accepted standard, is as follows:

Class I: asymptomatic at normal levels of activity
Class II: symptomatic with increased activity
Class III: symptomatic with ordinary activity
Class IV: symptomatic at rest

No classification of heart disease can be considered rigid or absolute, but this one offers a basic practical guide for treatment, assuming frequent prenatal visits, good client cooperation, and proper obstetric care. Medical therapy is conducted as a team approach with a cardiologist. The functional class of the disease is determined at 3 months and again at 7 or 8 months.

Assessment

During the *prenatal period* the woman is assessed at weekly intervals at home or on a continuous basis if hospitalized. The nurse assesses for factors that would increase stress on the heart, such as anemia, infection, or a home situation that includes responsibility for the house, other children, or extended family members. The client is observed for signs of **cardiac decompensation**, that is, **progressive generalized edema, rales at the base of the lungs, or pulse irregularity** (see box, p. 842). Symptoms of cardiac decompensation may appear abruptly or gradually. Medical intervention must be instituted immediately to correct cardiac status. Unfortunately dyspnea, chest pain, palpitations, and syncope occur commonly in pregnant women and can mask the symptoms of a developing or worsening cardiovascular disorder.

The routine assessment continues for the prenatal period, including monitoring weight gain and pattern of weight gain, edema, vital signs, discomforts of pregnancy,

DANGER SIGNS

Cardiac Decompensation

Gravida: Subjective Symptoms

1. Increasing fatigue or difficulty breathing or both with her usual activities
2. Feeling of smothering
3. Need to cough frequently
4. Rapid pulse; feeling that her heart is "racing"
5. Swelling of feet, legs, fingers (rings do not fit anymore), or face

Nurse: Objective Signs

1. Irregular rapid pulse (≥100 beats per minute)
2. Progressive, generalized edema
3. Rales at base of lungs
4. Orthopnea; increasing dyspnea
5. Rapid respirations (≥25 per minute)
6. Frequent cough
7. Increasing fatigue

urinalysis, and blood work. The nurse keeps careful check of the side effects and interactions of all medications—including supplemental iron—that the woman is taking and reports them to the physician. Their use also is documented on the client's record.

During the *intrapartum period* assessment includes the routine assessments for all laboring women as well as assessments for cardiac decompensation. The latter include taking vital signs at least every 10 to 30 minutes. **The physician is alerted if the pulse rate is 100 beats per minute or greater or if respirations are 25 per minute or greater.** Respiratory status is checked constantly for developing dyspnea, coughing, or rales at the base of the lungs. The color and temperature of the skin are noted. Pallor, cooling, and sweating may indicate cardiac shock. The woman is carefully watched for symptoms of emotional stress.

The *immediate postdelivery period* is hazardous for a woman with a compromised heart. Cardiac output increases rapidly as extravascular fluid is remobilized into the vascular compartment. At the moment of delivery, intraabdominal pressure is reduced drastically; pressure on veins is removed, the splanchnic vessels engorge, and blood flow to the heart is increased. When blood flow increases to the heart, a **reflex bradycardia** may result. Fluid begins to move from the extravascular spaces into the bloodstream. Some physicians favor the application of the abdominal binder or alternating tourniquets on the extremities to minimize the effects of this rapid change in intraabdominal pressure.

Cardiac monitoring for decompensation continues through the first weeks after delivery because it has been known to occur as late as the sixth postpartum day. Routine assessment as for any newly delivered woman is instituted, for example, vital signs, bleeding, uterine contractility, urinary output, pain, rest, diet, and daily weight. Laboratory (e.g., hemoglobin, hematocrit, and urinalysis) results are noted and reported if indicated to the physician. It is important to assess the woman's support systems, since activity will be curtailed until the cardiac system is recovered. The family response to the birth and infant needs to be observed because the mother may not be directly involved in the infant's care for a period of time (e.g., prematurity of infant, health of mother).

Nursing Diagnoses

Following are examples of nursing diagnoses that may be formulated. As always, individualization of diagnoses is vital.

Prenatal

- Fear related to
  - Increased peripartum risk
- Potential altered tissue perfusion related to
  - Hypotensive syndrome
- Impaired home maintenance management related to
  - Mother's confinement to bed

Intrapartum

- Anxiety related to
  - Fear for infant's safety
- Fear of dying related to
  - Perceived physiologic inability to cope with the stress of labor

Postpartum

- Self-care deficit related to
  - Need for bed rest
- Situational low self-esteem related to
  - Restriction placed on involvement in care of infant

Planning

The nursing diagnoses derived from analyses of clinical findings act as guides to develop a plan of care. (See general nursing care plan p. 845). This plan addresses the specific needs of the client. The mother who has cardiovascular problems faces curtailment of her activities. The restrictions can have physical and emotional implications. The community health nurse, social worker, and pediatrician are some of the resource people whose services may need to be incorporated into the plan of care. Goals such as the following might be appropriate.

Goals. General goals for care include the following:

1. Woman and family understand the disorder, management, and probable outcome.
2. Woman and family understand their role in management, including when and how to take medication, diet, and preparation for and participation in treatment.
3. Woman and family cope with emotional reactions to pregnancy and infant at risk.

Implementation

General Care

Therapy is focused on minimizing stress on the heart. Factors that increase the risk of cardiac decompensation are treated. The work load on the cardiovascular system is reduced by appropriate treatment of any coexisting emotional stress, hypertension, anemia, hyperthyroidism, or obesity. Infections are treated promptly since respiratory, urinary, or gastrointestinal tract infections can complicate the condition by accelerating heart rate and by direct spread of organisms (e.g., *Streptococcus*) to the heart structure. Sodium intake is restricted and accompanied by careful monitoring for hyponatremia. The sodium ion, with its ability to attract and hold fluid, affects the quality and the amount of the circulating volume. The woman's intake of potassium is monitored to prevent hypokalemia. Hypokalemia is associated with heart and other muscular weakness and dysfunction. Anticoagulant therapy, if used, is monitored. Tests for fetal maturity and well-being, and placental sufficiency may be necessary. Other therapy is directly related to the functional classification of heart disease.

Class I. The pregnant woman with class I heart disease should limit stress to protect against cardiac decompensation. Additional rest at night and after meals, frequent evaluations, and the early and effective treatment of respiratory and other infections should be stressed. Therapeutic abortion is never medically warranted. If there are no obstetric problems, vaginal delivery is recommended. This is accomplished using pudendal block anesthesia with forceps for shortening of the second stage of labor.

Class II. A program similar to that for class I should be followed for the pregnant woman with class II heart disease. However, the woman should be admitted to the hospital near term (if signs of cardiac overload or arrhythmia develop) for evaluation and treatment.

Penicillin prophylaxis of nonsensitized pregnant women against bacterial endocarditis in labor and during the early puerperium may be ordered. Mask oxygen and pudendal block anesthesia are important. Ergot products should not be used because of increases in blood pressure. Dilute intravenous oxytocin immediately after delivery may be employed to prevent postdelivery hemorrhage. Tubal sterilization may be performed, but surgery is delayed several days at least to ensure homeostasis. If sterilization is not achieved, effective contraception must be provided.

Class III. Bed rest for much of each day is necessary for pregnant women with class III cardiac disease. About 30% of these women experience cardiac decompensation during pregnancy. With this possibility the woman may be hospitalized for the remainder of pregnancy and the early puerperium. Early therapeutic abortion may be suggested, particularly a previous episode of cardiac failure. Breastfeeding is contraindicated. Sterilization should be postponed until a later date, but explicit contraceptive advice must be given.

Class IV. Because persons with class IV cardiac disease have decompensation even at rest, a major initial effort must be made to improve the cardiac status of pregnant women in this category. Early therapeutic abortion, although not innocuous, may be feasible with regional anesthesia in some cases. Prophylactic antibiotic therapy may be ordered with the procedure. Vaginal delivery of women with class IV lesions is the safest approach if abortion is not done. Maternal mortality approaches 50% in class IV heart disease; the perinatal mortality is even higher.

Operative Care. Operations for the correction of congenital or acquired heart disease should be done before pregnancy if possible. Closed cardiac surgery such as release of a stenotic mitral orifice can be accomplished with little risk to mother or fetus. However, open heart surgery requires extracorporeal circulation, and under these circumstances, hypoxia may develop. As a consequence the risk of fetal damage or loss rises to almost 30%. If anticoagulant therapy is required during pregnancy, **heparin** should be used because this large-molecule drug does not cross the placenta. Even though heparin is the anticoagulant of choice during pregnancy, it is not without risk. Heparin use can result in maternal hemorrhage, preterm birth, and stillbirth. Oral anticoagulants, such as warfarin (Coumadin) compounds, cross to the fetus and may cause anomalies or hemorrhage in the infant. However, valvuloplasty clients should receive penicillin or other antibiotic prophylaxis against bacterial endocarditis during gestation.

Prenatal Period

Signs and symptoms of cardiac decompensation are reviewed during the prenatal period. The woman requires *adequate rest.* She should sleep 8 to 10 hours every day and 30 minutes after meals. Her activities are restricted; for example, if the woman is at home, she needs to limit housework, shopping, and laundry to the amount allowed for her functional classification of heart disease. *Nutrition* counseling is necessary for her in the presence of her family. Adequate nutrition may be difficult to achieve especially when someone else shops and cooks for her. The woman needs a diet high in iron and protein and adequate enough in kilocalories to gain 10.8 kg (24 lb) during pregnancy. To prevent pyrosis (heartburn) the woman is advised to assume a semi- or low-Fowler's position after eating.

The woman may need to learn to self-administer *heparin.* She is cautioned to avoid foods high in vitamin K, such as raw, deep green, leafy vegetables, which counteract the effects of the heparin. Therefore she will require a substitute source of folic acid in her diet.

Infection adds considerable stress on cardiac function. The woman should notify her physician at the first sign of infection or when she is exposed to infection. Hospitalization may be required until the infection is cured.

The nurse may need to reinforce the physician's explanation for the need for close medical supervision. Information about management of the woman's labor and her early postdelivery period is reviewed. The woman and her family will need time to plan for the necessary extra care the mother will require.

Intrapartum Period

Nursing care during the intrapartum period focuses on the promotion of cardiac function. *Anxiety is alleviated* through maintaining a calm atmosphere and keeping the woman and her family informed. *Uterine perfusion* is facilitated by placing the woman in a side-lying position. *Cardiac function* is supported by keeping her head and shoulders elevated and body parts resting on pillows. *Discomfort* is relieved with medication and supportive care. For delivery the nurse will assist in the administration of pharmacologic relief of discomfort.

The woman may require other types of medication (e.g., anticoagulants, prophylactic antibiotics). If evidence of cardiac decompensation appears, the physician may order *deslanoside* (Cedilanid-D) for rapid digitalization, *furosemide* (Lasix) for rapid diuresis, and *oxygen* by intermittent positive pressure to decrease the development of pulmonary edema.

Delivery is accomplished with the woman in the left side-lying position, or if placed in the supine position, a pad is positioned under the right hip to minimize the danger of supine hypotension. The knees are flexed, and the feet are flat on the bed. Stirrups are not used to prevent compression of popliteal veins and an increase in blood volume in the chest and trunk as a result of the effects of gravity. An episiotomy and the use of outlet forceps also decrease the work of the heart.

Postpartum Period

Care in the postpartum period is tailored to the woman's functional capacity. Positioning in bed is the same as that for the labor; that is, the head of the bed is elevated and the woman is encouraged to lie on her side. Bed rest may be ordered with or without bathroom privileges. The nurse may need to help the woman meet her grooming and hygiene needs and even help her with turning in bed, eating, and other activities. Boredom and respiratory and circulatory sequelae to immobility must be addressed. Progressive ambulation may be permitted as tolerated. The nurse assesses the woman's pulse, skin, and affect before and after walking.

Bowel and bladder elimination requires special attention. Bowel movements without stress or strain are promoted with stool softeners, diet, and fluids, plus mild analgesia and local anesthetic spray. Overdistension of the bladder is prevented. A distended bladder can result in an atonic uterus and hemorrhage. Anemia may result. Anemia adds additional stress to cardiac function. Rapid emptying of the bladder is avoided however. Rapid decompression of the bladder results in a precipitous drop in intraabdominal pressure, leading to **splanchnic engorgement** and generalized hypotension. The woman must be protected from infection. A private room is one method to restrict traffic into her room.

Mother-child interactions receive special planning. The interactions should not stress the mother. The mother may direct care of the infant by a designated family member. The mother can breast-feed if her condition warrants. That is, women in classes I and II may breast-feed; those whose functional capacity is classified as class III or IV are advised against breast-feeding.

The fed baby can be brought regularly to the mother, held at her eye level and by her lips, and brought to her fingers so that she can establish an emotional bond with her baby with a low expenditure of her energy. At the same time, involving the mother passively in her infant's care helps the mother feel vitally important—as she is—to the infant's well-being (e.g., "You can do something no one else can: provide your baby with your sounds, touch, and rhythms that are so comforting"). Perhaps the mother can be encouraged to make a tape recording of her talking, singing, or whispering, to be played for the baby in the nursery, to help the infant feel her presence and be in contact with her voice.

Before discharge the nurse assesses the home support for the woman and infant. Preparation for discharge is carefully planned with the woman and family. Provision of help in the home for the mother by relatives, friends, and others must be addressed. If necessary, the nurse refers the family to community resources (e.g., for homemaking services). Rest and sleep periods, activity, and diet must be planned. The couple will want information about reestablishing sexual relations, contraception, sterilization of the man or the woman (especially if the woman is classified as classes II, III, or IV), and medical supervision.

A general nursing care plan for a childbearing woman with heart disease follows.

Evaluation

The nurse uses the following criteria as *overall indications* for the success of therapy:

1. The woman is able to tolerate the stresses imposed by pregnancy. These include increase in cardiac output by more than one third, increase in pulse rate by 10 beats per minute, expansion of blood volume by 25%, and psychologic stress common to pregnancy and related to the heart condition.
2. Congestive heart failure, the primary cause of maternal mortality in women with cardiac disease, is prevented.
3. The home situation is controlled, with assistance provided as necessary.
4. The mother and family accept the limitations imposed on the woman by the presence of heart disease.
5. The parent and child relationship is fostered by the family.

Miscellaneous Cardiovascular Conditions

Primary pulmonary hypertension (PPH) is a rare disorder. It is associated with a mortality approximately of 50% during pregnancy (Danforth and Scott, 1986). Pulmonary artery pressure is high with progressive right ventricular hypertrophy. There is no pulmonary edema. Death is usually caused by right ventricular failure or ventricular arrhythmia. The last months of pregnancy and the early puer-

Text continued on p. 848.

General Nursing Care Plan

HEART DISEASE AND CHILDBEARING

ASSESSMENT	NURSING DIAGNOSIS (ND)/ PLAN (P)/GOAL (G)	RATIONALE/ IMPLEMENTATION	EVALUATION
Prenatal care: Assess for factors that increase stress on the heart (anemia, infection, household activities). Assess for signs of cardiac decompensation: generalized edema, rales at the base of lungs, pulse irregularity. Patterns of weight gain. Vital signs. Edema. Discomforts of pregnancy. Urinalysis (protein, blood acetone, glucose). Blood work (Hgb, Hct, WBC, platelets). Check for side effects and interactions of medications. Assess dietary patterns.	ND: Altered tissue perfusion related to hypotensive syndrome. ND: Increased cardiac output related to pregnancy. ND: Impaired home maintenance management related to mother's restricted household activities or confinement to bed. P: Provide information, be available for discussion, and continuing ongoing surveillance for maternal well-being. Home visit may be considered. Explore community resources for home assistance. G: Woman will maintain adequate perfusion as exhibited by stable blood pressure, clear lung fields, no edema, and regular pulse. G: Woman will attend scheduled appointments. G: Woman will avoid restricted activities and achieve adequate rest. G: Woman will self-administer heparin as ordered.	*To closely monitor a woman with heart disease for decompensation, the nurse will:* Reinforce physician's explanation for need of close medical supervision. Schedule weekly appointments and evaluate problems pertaining to missed appointments. Review symptoms of cardiac decompensation. Monitor weight and dietary patterns. Monitor vital sign patterns. Note and report edema ("Are your shoes getting tight?") Obtain urine and blood specimens, and evaluate and report results. Monitor for side effects and interactions of medications. Encourage adequate rest. Restrict activities such as housework and shopping and refer to child care and home health agencies. Teach woman how to self-administer heparin as ordered.	Woman remains free from cardiac decompensation. Woman attends weekly health care appointments. Woman obtains adequate rest and avoids restricted activities. The home situation is controlled with assistance provided as necessary. Woman self-administers heparin as ordered by a physician.
Assess client's baseline knowledge of her heart disease. Assess client's knowledge of how pregnancy will affect her heart disease.	ND: Knowledge deficit related to care required by a woman with heart disease during pregnancy. ND: Fear related to increased peripartum risk. P: Provide information, be available for discussion, and mobilize resources and support. G: Woman and family will learn how to monitor and care for her heart disease during pregnancy. G: Woman and family will learn the risks of preg-	*To teach the heart disease client how to care for herself during pregnancy, the nurse will:* Review effects pregnancy will have on her health. Help woman formulate questions for the physician. Evaluate woman's desire to continue with the pregnancy given all the peripartum risks and review her option for termination of the pregnancy. Teach symptoms of cardiac decompensation (verbal and written). Review restricted activities	Woman and family verbalizes an understanding of the risks of pregnancy on woman's health. Woman learns how to care for herself during pregnancy and knows whom to contact should danger signs present. Woman and famility utilize community resources and support. Woman and family follow prescribed diet and treatment regimen.

Continued.

General Nursing Care Plan—cont'd

ASSESSMENT	NURSING DIAGNOSIS (ND)/ PLAN (P)/GOAL (G)	RATIONALE/ IMPLEMENTATION	EVALUATION
	nancy on her heart disease.	and need for rest. Teach nutrition and the need for a high iron, high protein, and adequate caloric diet to gain about (10.8 kg) 24 lb during pregnancy. Tell woman to avoid foods high in Vitamin K if she is receiving heparin therapy. Teach woman regarding danger of infection, its signs, and symptoms. Review information pertaining to management of labor and the early postdelivery period.	
Intrapartum care: Routine assessments for a laboring woman. Vital signs every 10 to 30 minutes. Alert physician to heart rate > 100 or > 25 respirations per minute. Assess respiratory status frequently for dyspnea, coughing, or rales at base of lungs. Note and record color and skin temperature. Assess for signs of cardiac shock. Assess for suspicious FHR deceleration patterns (Chapter 17).	ND: Increased cardiac output related to the stress of labor and delivery. ND: Altered (cardiopulmonary) tissue perfusion related to hypotension (maternal or fetal). P: Promote cardiac function, provide emotional support, and remain alert for potential complications. G: Woman will maintain adequate perfusion, exhibited by stable blood pressure, regular pulse, warm pink extremities, and clear lung field. G: Woman will maintain adequate perfusion to the placenta as exhibited by a stable FHR during labor.	*To increase perfusion by alleviating cardiac stress, the nurse will:* Promote cardiac function by: A. Alleviating anxiety. B. Placing woman in side-lying position. C. Medicating or sedating for discomfort. D. Preventing, recognizing, reporting, and treating hypotension, which may follow anesthesia. For delivery, place on left side or supine with left hip elevated. Administer medications and report signs of cardiac decompensation. Monitor contractions and FHR response.	Woman maintains adequate perfusion during labor and delivery. Fetus will remain adequately perfused in utero as demonstrated by acceptable FHR patterns.
Watch for symptoms of emotional stress.	ND: Anxiety related to fear for infant's safety. ND: Fear of dying related to perceived inability to control stress of labor. P: Minimize or eliminate emotional stress. G: Woman will be comforted and anxiety relieved by stress reduction techniques.	*To control the client's level of stress, the nurse will:* Answer any questions of concern the client might have about labor and delivery. Help client formulate questions for the physician. Correct misconceptions. Explain upcoming procedures, feelings, or sensations she might experience. Encourage support person to provide comfort techniques (back rub, pressure to lumbar spine, etc.). Encourage support person to remain at bed side	Woman reports comfort or demonstrates reduced anxiety by measures instituted.

General Nursing Care Plan—cont'd

ASSESSMENT	NURSING DIAGNOSIS (ND)/ PLAN (P)/GOAL (G)	RATIONALE/ IMPLEMENTATION	EVALUATION
		with the woman as a comfort measure. Administer medications for discomfort or sedation as ordered.	
Postdelivery care: Close assessment for cardiac decompensation. Routine postpartum assessments. Assess for signs and symptoms of infection and hemorrhage. Monitor intake/output closely.	ND: Decreased cardiac output related to fluid shifts after delivery. ND: Altered (cardiopulmonary) tissue perfusion related to rapid fluid shifts on a compromised cardiovascular system. ND: Potential for injury related to hemorrhage or infection. ND: Knowledge deficit regarding methods to reduce stress on cardiac system. P: Promote cardiac function and involution, provide emotional support, and remain alert for potential complications. G: Woman will not demonstrate signs of cardiac decompensation after delivery.	*To monitor for, and prevent cardiac decompensation, the nurse will:* Evaluate for cardiac decompensation up to 7 days after delivery. Perform all routine postpartum care and teaching. Apply abdominal binder or tourniquets as ordered by a physician after delivery. Administer medications as ordered (oxygen, digitalization therapy, etc.) Elevate head of bed and encourage side-lying. Teach regarding stool softeners, fluids and diet to reduce strain of bowel movements. Prevent overdistended bladder after delivery. Isolate from sources of infection. Prevent or promptly treat hemorrhage or infection. Facilitate mother-infant interactions that do not stress the mother.	Woman remains free from signs and symptoms of cardiac decompensation. Woman remains free from hemorrhage and infection. Woman verbalizes understanding of instructions. Woman experiences normal involution.
Assess woman's support system. Assess family's response to the birth and infant. Assess the need for outside resources (home care, child care).	ND: Ineffective family coping: compromised, related to added child care and household tasks. ND: Altered family processes related to assuming woman's responsibilities after delivery. ND: Self-care deficit related to need for bed rest. ND: Situational low self-esteem related to restriction placed on involvement in care of infant. P: Facilitate parent-child relationship and mutually develop a plan for care utilizing outside resources as necessary. G: Woman will rest and recuperate after delivery. G: Woman will not be stressed by child care or household activities after delivery	*To assure that the woman has the needed rest to recuperate, the nurse will:* Identify with the client her support systems. Observe the family's response to the infant and child care activities. Examine the family's time and resources to assist the client with child care and household tasks. Notify outside resources to assist with the care of the woman, house, and child (homemaker, child care, home health care). Encourage woman to spend "quiet moments" with her child but to allow family to provide most of the child care activities. Remind woman that she can assume all child care activities once she allows her body to recuperate from childbirth.	Woman achieves the needed rest to recuperate. The mother and family accept the limitations imposed on the woman by the presence of heart disease. Woman's family or outside services assumes responsibility of children and household tasks until client recuperates. The parent-child relationship is fostered by the family.

perium are especailly dangerous. Increased blood volume and cardiac output may be responsible. Management includes bed rest from 20 weeks' gestation, digitalis, and diuretics.

Mitral valve prolapse (MVP) is a common condition occurring in 6% to 10% women of reproductive age (Danforth and Scott, 1986). The mitral valve leaflets prolapse into the left atrium during ventricular systole, allowing some backflow of blood. Midsystolic *click* and late systolic *murmur* are hallmarks of this syndrome. Most women are asymptomatic. A few women have a peculiar chest pain or palpitations, which usually respond to β-blockers such as propranolol (Inderal). Pregnancy is usually well tolerated.

Marfan's syndrome is an autosomal dominant disorder. About 90% of individuals with this symptom have mitral valve prolapse, and 25% have aortic insufficiency. There is an increased risk of *aortic dissection* and rupture during pregnancy, and maternal mortality is reported at 25% to 50% (Danforth and Scott, 1986). Management during pregnancy is by restricted activity and propranolol (Inderal) therapy.

Cardiovascular accidents (CVAs) can occur. Uncontrolled hypertension can result in cerebral hemorrhage (Chapter 29) (Pritchard, MacDonald, and Gant, 1985). CVAs have been reported with cocaine (Cregler and Mark, 1986).

Some women who are asymptomatic **after cardiac surgery** undergo frightening deterioration during pregnancy. This is especially experienced by women with prosthetic heart valves (Metcalfe, McAnulty, and Ueland, 1986). The hemodynamic demands of pregnancy compromise their cardiac status. Should such a woman become pregnant, abortion before the hemodynamic demands are fully manifest is the most therapeutic course if it is acceptable to the woman and her family. Most women opt for careful contraception to avoid pregnancy rather than for therapeutic interruption.

PERIPARTUM CARDIOMYOPATHIES

Peripartum cardiomyopathies comprise a syndrome of cardiac failure (1) occurring during the peripartum period, (2) with no previous history of heart disease, and (3) with no specific etiologic factors (Demakis and Rahimtoola, 1971). When not associated with pregnancy, cardiomyopathy is known by an array of names: hypertrophic cardiomyopathy (HCM), idiopathic hypertrophic subaortic stenosis, and asymmetric septal hypertrophy. It is a commonly diagnosed disease of the heart muscle. Its exact cause is unknown, although it may be genetically transmitted.

Most clients are asymptomatic until late adolescence or early adulthood (childbearing years) or more rarely middle age. Symptoms include angina pectoris, exertional dyspnea, supraventricular and ventricular arrhythmias, dizziness, and syncope. Most deaths associated with HCM are sudden, unexpected, and unrelated to functional status. HCM may be precipitated by physical or emotional stress, and the myocardial ischemia resulting from stress may promote ventricular fibrillation.

The incidence of peripartum cardiomyopathies has been reported as 1 in 3000 to 4000 pregnancies. It occurs more often in the multiparous woman. The maternal mortality has been estimated in the range of 30% to 60%, the infant mortality approximately 10%.

Clinical findings are those of congestive heart failure (left ventricular failure). Findings include breathlessness, tachyarrhythmias, and edema (Fig. 34-1) with radiologic findings of cardiomegaly.

The *prognosis* is good if cardiomegaly is not persistent after 6 months. The prognosis for women whose hearts remain enlarged is not as favorable.

Future pregnancies usually result in some cardiac failure (50% to 88%). Mortality has been estimated as high as 60%.

Medical Management. Bed rest is advocated up to 7 months, with some women requiring 20 to 22 months. The rationale for instituting bed rest is to decrease the heart rate, stroke volume, and arterial pressure.

Low sodium intake (1.5 to 2 g per day) is ordered for women with severe congestive failure. The use of diuretics, digitalis, and anticoagulants require close medical supervision to detect toxicity. Suppression of lactation is often recommended with no particular rationale other than to minimize stress. (All women experience some rise in blood pressure at the onset of lactation.)

Nursing Care. The nursing care of clients with peripartum cardiomyopathies is essentially the same as for those with other types of cardiac problems. The use of Trendelenburg's position for relief of syncope has been demonstrated. The necessity for prolonged bed rest can pose social and economic hardships for a family; therefore referral to community resources for assistance may be necessary. Because sudden death is a feature of this condition, the family needs to be trained in cardiopulmonary resuscitation. Clients need to have ready access to emergency care. (Some hospitals provide special numbers to dial for immediate dispatch of a medically staffed ambulance.)

ANEMIA

Anemia, the most common medical disorder of pregnancy, affects at least 20% of pregnant women. These women have a higher incidence of puerperal complications such as infection than do pregnant women with normal hematologic values.

Anemia results in reduction of the oxygen-carrying capacity of the blood. An indirect index of the oxygen-carrying capacity is the packed red blood cell volume (PCV), or hematocrit level. The normal hematocrit range in nonpregnant women is 38% to 45%. However, normal values for pregnant women with adequate iron stores may be as low as 34%. This has been explained by hydremia (dilution of blood), or the **physiologic anemia of pregnancy.**

About 90% of cases of anemia in pregnancy are of the iron-deficiency type. The remaining 10% of cases embrace a considerable variety of acquired and hereditary anemias, including folic acid deficiency and hemoglobinopathies.

Normal Values During Pregnancy. Normal and abnormal changes confuse the hematologic profile during pregnancy. The blood values of pregnant women differ significantly from those of nonpregnant women. All the

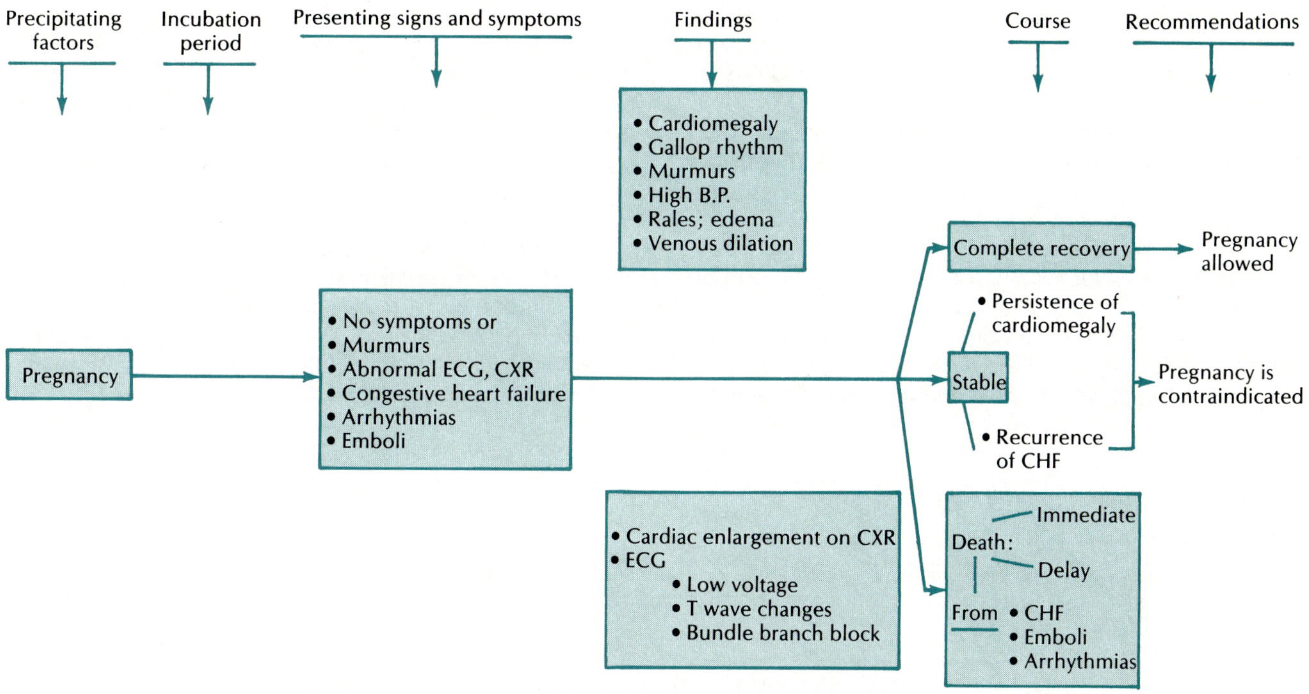

Fig. 34-1 Summary of course of peripartum cardiomyopathy.
From Veille, JC: Am J Obstet Gynecol 148:805, 1984.

constituents of blood normally increase during pregnancy: plasma volume, by 30% to 35%; red cell volume, by 20% to 30%; and hemoglobin mass, by 12% to 15%. The dilution of red blood cells and hemoglobin resulting from the relatively greater increase in plasma volume does not significantly change cell indices such as the mean corpuscular volume (MCV). However, this dilution does affect red blood cell count (RBC), hemoglobin, and hematocrit values. Laboratory values drop progressively to a low between the thirtieth and thirty-fourth weeks of pregnancy.

Definition of Anemia During Pregnancy. At or near sea level, during the *first* trimester, the pregnant woman is anemic when her hemoglobin level is less than 11 g/dl or her hematocrit level falls below 37%. She is anemic in the *second* trimester when the hemoglobin level is less than 10.5 g/dl or the hematocrit level falls below 35%; and she is anemic in the *third* trimester when the hemoglobin level is less than 10 g/dl or the hematocrit level is less than 33%. Much higher values are indicative of anemia in areas of high altitude; for example, at 1500 m (5000 ft) above sea level, a hemoglobin level less than 14 g/dl indicates anemia.

Iron Deficiency Anemia

Without iron therapy even pregnant women who enjoy excellent nutrition will conclude pregnancy with an iron deficit. Diet alone cannot replace gestational iron losses. Inadequate nutrition without therapy will certainly mean iron deficiency anemia during late pregnancy and the puerperium.

Successful iron therapy during pregnancy can be carried out in the vast majority of cases with oral iron supplements (e.g., ferrous sulfate, 0.3 g 3 times a day). Some pregnant women cannot tolerate or fail to take the prescribed oral iron. In such cases the woman should receive parenteral iron such as the iron-dextran complex (Imferon).

Folic Acid Deficiency Anemia

Folic acid deficiency anemia occurs in at least 2% of pregnant women in North America, an incidence much higher than that suspected even 5 years ago. Anemia compromises the women's defenses, making her more vulnerable to urinary tract infections and hemorrhage.

Poor diet, cooking with large volumes of water, or canning of food may lead to folate defficiency. Also, malabsorption or increased folate use may play a part in the development of anemia caused by a lack of folic acid.

During pregnancy the recommended daily intake is 150 μg of folic acid. In folate deficiency a dosage of about 5 mg per day orally for several weeks should ensure a remission. A generous maintenance dose each day should prevent a relapse. Because iron deficiency anemia may also accompany folate deficiency, augmented iron intake should also be provided.

Sickle Cell Hemoglobinopathy

Sickle cell trait (SA hemoglobin pattern) is sickling of the red blood cells but with a normal RBC life span. Pregnant women with sickle cell trait are susceptible to urinary tract infection. Hematuria is common.

Sickle cell anemia (sickle cell disease) is a recessive, hereditary, familial hemolytic anemia peculiar to those of black or Mediterranean ancestry. These individuals usually have abnormal hemoglobin types (SS or SC). Persons with sickle cell anemia have recurrent attacks (crises) of fever and pain in the abdomen or extremities beginning in childhood. These attacks are attributed to vascular occlusion (from abnormal cells), tissue hypoxia, edema, and red blood cell destruction. Crises are associated with normochromic anemia, jaundice, reticulocytosis, positive sickle cell test, and the demonstration of abnormal hemoglobin (usually SS or SC).

Almost 10% of blacks in North America have the sickle cell trait, but less than 1% have sickle cell anemia. The anemia is often complicated by iron and folic acid deficiency.

Pregnant women with sickle cell anemia are prone to pyelonephritis, leg ulcers, bone infarction, and cardiopathy. (Oral contraceptives are contraindicated.) An aplastic crisis may follow serious infection. Medical therapy, including transfusions to maintain the hematocrit level at least 30% is essential. Cesarean delivery is warranted only on obstetric indications.

Pregnancy may impose critical complications in sickle cell disease. Maternal mortality often ranges between 5% and 10%. The perinatal mortality may reach 30%. Therapeutic abortion is not medically indicated.

Table 34-1 identifies some potential problems faced by the woman with sickle cell disease and some preventive and maintenance interventions.

Table 34-1 ***Sickle Cell Disease: Potential Problems, Prevention, and Maintenance***

Potential Problem	Prevention and Maintenance
1. Inadequate oxygen to meet needs of labor and prevent sickling	1. a. Monitor hemoglobin level and hematocrit to maintain hemoglobin at 7 g or more and hematocrit at 20% or more b. Assist with transfusions c. Administer oxygen d. Coach for relaxation and to lessen anxiety (Chapter 13)
2. Infection resulting from anemia: urinary tract infection, pyelonephritis, pneumonia	2. a. Continue actions as under no. 1 b. Maintain adequate hydration c. Administer antibiotics, as ordered d. Maintain strict asepsis e. Encourage frequent voiding to keep bladder empty
3. Sequestration crisis caused by need for and destruction of RBCs	3. Administer folic acid supplement (15-30 mg) to decrease erythropoietic demands and reduce probability of capillary stasis
4. Crisis caused by hypoxia, hypotension, acidosis, dehydration, exertion, sudden cooling, low-grade fever	4. a. Continue actions as under no. 1 b. Avoid supine hypotension c. Maintain adequate hydration d. Maintain comfortable room temperature; use warm blankets or cool cloths as needed e. Assist with analgesia and anesthesia
5. Pseudotoxemia (hypertension, and proteinuria; *no* large weight gain); often accompanies bone pain crisis	5. a. If true PIH occurs, care is the same as for PIH (Chapter 29) b. Monitor blood pressure and urine c. Administer heparin, as ordered
6. Thrombophlebitis (from increased blood viscosity)	6. a. Monitor for positive Homans' sign b. Initiate bed rest if Homans' sign is positive or if reddened, warm areas, or a lump are found c. Maintain adequate hydration d. Administer heparin, as ordered e. Apply warm compresses f. Apply antiembolism stockings
7. Congestive heart failure	7. a. Assess pulse, respiratory rate every 15 minutes b. Auscultate for rales frequently c. Place in semirecumbent position d. Administer oxygen and medications (e.g., digitalis, antibiotics, diuretics, analgesics) e. Prevent bearing down; reassure woman about low forceps delivery under anesthesia (local or regional)
8. Pulmonary infarction (hemoptysis, cough, temperature to 38.9° C [102° F], friction rub)	8. Assess for this possible complication to facilitate early diagnosis
9. Postpartum hemorrhage (resulting from heparin therapy)	9. Administer ordered oxytocic medication

Thalassemia

Thalassemia (Mediterranean or Cooley's anemia) is a relatively common anemia in which an insufficient amount of hemoglobin is produced to fill the red blood cells. Thalassemia is a hereditary disorder that involves the abnormal synthesis of the α- or β-chains of hemoglobin. β-Thalassemia is the more common variety in the United States and is often diagnosed in individuals of Italian, Greek, or southern Chinese descent. The unbalanced synthesis of hemoglobin leads to premature red blood cell death resulting in severe anemia. Thalassemia major is the homozygous form of the disorder; thalassemia minor is the heterozygous form.

Thalassemia major may complicate pregnancy. Preeclampsia is more common in women with thalassemia major. Thalassemia major may be associated with low-birth-weight infants and increased fetal wastage. Placental weight often is increased, perhaps secondary to maternal anemia. The frequency of fetal distress from hypoxia is greater than in control women. Therefore pregnant women with thalassemia major should be monitored more closely than normal pregnant women.

Regular transfusion may be necessary. Folic acid should be given to avoid folate deficiency. Partial exchange transfusion may be warranted in severe thalassemia. Splenectomy may be necessary if enlargement and pain occur. Women with thalassemia major may die of chronic infection or progressive hepatic or cardiac failure, the result of excessive iron deposition.

Persons with *thalassemia minor* have a mild persistent anemia, but the RBC may be normal or even elevated. However, no systemic problems are caused by the anemia that is a part of the minor form of the disease. Thalassemia minor must be distinguished principally from iron deficiency anemia.

Pregnancy will neither worsen thalassemia minor nor will it be compromised by the disease. The anemia will not respond to iron therapy. Prolonged parenteral iron can lead to harmful, excessive iron storage. Infants born to parents with thalassemia will inherit the disorder. Persons with thalassemia minor should have a normal life span despite a moderately reduced hemoglobin level.

PULMONARY DISORDERS

Bronchial Asthma

Bronchial asthma is an acute dramatic respiratory illness caused by allergens, marked change in ambient temperature, or emotional tension. In many cases the actual cause may be unknown. A family history of allergy is likely in about 50% of all persons with asthma. Almost 2% of individuals in the United States have bronchial asthma, but less than 1% of pregnant women suffer from this disorder. The effect of pregnancy on asthma is unpredictable. Psychologic alterations induced by pregnancy do not make the pregnant women more prone to asthmatic attacks. Asthma increases the incidence of abortion and premature labor, but the fetus per se is unaffected. In severe cases, asthma may be life threatening for the gravida. The prognosis for both mother and fetus will be good in most cases.

Therapy for bronchial asthma has two objectives: (1) relief of the acute attack and (2) prevention or limitation of later attacks. In all asthmatics, known allergens should be eliminated and a comfortable home temperature maintained. Tranquilizers (but not sedatives) should be given to relieve apprehension. Respiratory infections should be treated and mist or steam inhalation employed to aid expectoration of mucus. Bronchial asthma therapy is initiated. Acute episodes may require steroids, aminophylline, oxygen, and correction of fluid-electrolyte imbalance. Mild or moderate bronchial asthma responds well to epinephrine (1:1000) or isoproterenol inhalation (1:200 aqueous solution) by nebulizer for one or two inhalations. See medical-surgical texts for general care. Precautions specific for obstetrics include the following:

- Do not use morphine in labor, since it may cause bronchospasm. Meperidine (Demerol) usually will relieve bronchospasm.
- Avoid or limit ephedrine and corticotropins (pressor drugs) in preeclampsia–eclampsia.
- Opt for vaginal delivery using local or regional anesthesia, whenever possible.

Adult Respiratory Distress Syndrome

Adult respiratory distress syndrome (ARDS, shock lung) occurs when the lungs are unable to maintain levels of oxygen and carbon dioxide within normal limits. Marked tachycardia, dyspnea, and cyanosis that does not respond to nasal oxygen or intermittent positive pressure breathing are the most noted signs. ARDS is not a condition specific to pregnancy; it can also result from chest trauma, drug ingestion, or pneumonia. When ARDS is associated with pregnancy, pulmonary embolism, disseminated intravascular coagulation (DIC) (see Chapter 31), and aspiration pneumonia are the precipitators.

The postpartum incidence of ARDS is not affected by the means of delivery, but by the amount of trauma experienced during pregnancy and delivery. It also may occur after spontaneous or medically induced abortion.

It has been noted that during pregnancy there is an increase in some of the coagulation factors. This increase in coagulation results in shortening of the partial thromboplastin time (PTT). This state predisposes the woman to an increase in rapidity of blood clotting and an increased tendency to form blood clots (hypercoagulability).

Laboratory reports are important in identifying the origin of acute pulmonary problems. The important observations for the nurse to note are vital signs, signs of thrombophlebitis, and hemorrhage.

Vital Signs. Temperature elevation may indicate the development of thrombophlebitis. The pulse rate increases to compensate for respiratory insufficiency of any origin. The severity of the pulmonary problem increases as the pulse rate rises. An initial rise in blood pressure occurs as cardiac output increases to try to supply the bloody tissue with oxygen. When lung damage is severe, the blood pressure drops. Respiratory changes are the most important indicators of ARDS. The rate, depth, respiratory pattern, symmetry of chest movement, and use of accessory muscles should be noted; therefore observation of respiratory characteristics after activity is important. If there is any indication of abnormality, count respirations for a full minute; an error of plus or minus four may be highly significant. During the postdelivery period, apprehension, distended neck veins, cyanosis, diaphoresis, or pallor may be clues to watch for. Also mental confusion or disorientation may be noted.

On auscultation of the lungs, rales, rhonchi, wheezes, or a pleural friction rub need to be reported, especially when they have occurred since an earlier normal assessment. The pregnant woman should be positioned for breathing comfort. Oxygen and emergency equipment should be available while the physician is notified. Reassure the woman so that her anxiety is lessened.

Thrombophlebitis. The lower extremities need to be checked for swelling, pain, inflammation, venous distension, and Homans' sign. If thrombophlebitis is suspected, the woman should be kept on bed rest until the physician can be notified. Sudden movement or straining can dislodge a clot and lead to pulmonary embolism.

Postdelivery Hemorrhage. Petechiae, ecchymosis, hematuria, and epistaxis are important indications of DIC. Replacement of clotting factors and heparin therapy may be required for DIC. Sources of trauma should be identified and eliminated so that outside causes of hemorrhage are avoided.

Pulmonary Embolus. Pregnancy also brings about changes in the vascular system. Alterations in vein distensibility have been noted, possibly because of softening of collagen induced by humoral influences. The combination of vein distensibility and obstruction of venous blood return from the lower extremities (caused by fetal pressure on veins, especially in the last trimester) predisposes a woman to pooling of blood. In addition, hypercoagulation and pooling may lead to thrombophlebitis. Thrombophlebitis can result in ARDS (emboli from thromboembolism cause obstruction in the pulmonary circulation).

Aspiration Pneumonia. Aspiration pneumonia can be caused by changes in the gastrointestinal system during pregnancy. Progesterone has been known to relax smooth muscles. When the resting tone is lowered, the cardiac sphincter becomes weak and reflux of the stomach contents can easily occur. Increased intraabdominal pressure (because of fetal growth) further predisposes the mother to gastric reflux. Food eaten as long as 24 to 48 hours before labor can be vomited and then aspirated. Aspiration of solid foods and liquids may cause bronchial obstruction leading to bronchoconstriction, which in turn can result in ARDS. Large particles can be removed by coughing, suctioning, or bronchoscopy, but liquids are harder to remove. The hydrochloric acid in the aspirated stomach contents may cause an asthmatic-like syndrome with necrotizing bronchitis. For this reason an antacid is given preoperatively as a prophylactic measure.

GASTROINTESTINAL DISORDERS

Compromise of gastrointestinal function during pregnancy is apparent to all concerned. There are psychogenic overtones generally admitted in nausea and vomiting of pregnancy. However, a capricious food choice is observed in many women during pregnancy. In addition, obvious physiologic alterations, such as the greatly enlarged uterus, and less apparent changes, such as hypochlorhydria, require understanding for proper diagnosis and treatment.

Peptic Ulcer

Peptic ulcer is less common in women than in men, and this problem is even more uncommon during pregnancy. Moreover, women with a diagnosed peptic ulcer generally improve during gestation. Therefore hemorrhage and perforation are unlikely. Fortunately emergency surgery for peptic ulcer complications rarely jeopardizes the pregnancy. Postdelivery reactivation of the ulcer may occur. Medical therapy is similar to that recommended for nonpregnant individuals.

Cholelithiasis and Cholecystitis

Women are more likely to have cholelithiasis (gallstones) than are men, and pregnancy seems to play a part in its development. It is known that gallstones are more commonly diagnosed in women of advanced parity than in nulliparas of the same age and background. Increased biliary cholesterol and biliary stasis are probable causes. Cholecystitis does not commonly occur during pregnancy.

Generally, gallbladder surgery should be postponed until the puerperium. Impaction of a stone in the cystic or common duct during pregnancy may require cholelithotomy or cholecystectomy. Meperidine (Demerol) or atropine alleviates ductal spasm and pain. Morphine may be given also.

Ulcerative Colitis

The cause of ulcerative colitis is unknown. Its effect on pregnancy is minimal unless there is marked debilitation, whereupon spontaneous abortion, fetal death, or premature delivery may occur. In general, when pregnancy coincides with active ulcerative colitis, the great majority of women will experience a severe exacerbation of the disease. When pregnancy occurs during a period of inactivity of the disorder, a flare-up is unlikely. There is no specific therapy for ulcerative colitis, but adrenocorticosteroids and antibiotics may be beneficial.

INTEGUMENTARY DISORDERS

Dermatologic disorders induced by pregnancy (see Table 13-2) include melasma (chloasma), herpes gestationis, noninflammatory pruritus of pregnancy, vascular spiders, palmar erythema, and pregnancy granulomas (including epulides). Skin problems generally aggravated by pregnancy are acne vulgaris (in the first trimester), erythema multiforme, herpetiform dermatitis, granuloma inguinale, condylomata acuminata, neurofibromatosis, and pemphigus. Dermatologic disorders usually improved by pregnancy include acne vulgaris (in the third trimester), seborrhea dermatitis, and psoriasis. An unpredictable course during pregnancy may be expected in atopic dermatitis, lupus erythematosus, and herpes simplex.

Therapeutic abortion or early delivery may be justified for some dermatologic conditions. These conditions include herpes gestationis, disseminated lupus erythematosus, and neurofibromatosis (von Recklinghausen's disease).

Explanation, reassurance, and common sense measures should suffice for normal skin changes (see Table 13-2). In contrast, disease processes during and soon after pregnancy may be extremely difficult to diagnose and treat.

NEUROLOGIC DISORDERS

Epilepsy

Epilepsy may result from developmental abnormalities or injury. Epilepsy seriously complicates about 1 of every 1000 gestations. Convulsive seizures may be more frequent or severe during complications of pregnancy, such as edema, alkylosis, fluid-electrolyte imbalance, cerebral hypoxia, hypoglycemia, and hypocalcemia. On the other hand, the effects of pregnancy on epilepsy are unpredictable.

The differential diagnosis of epilepsy versus eclampsia may pose a problem. Epilepsy and eclampsia can coexist. However, a past history of seizures, the absence of hypertension, generalized edema, or proteinuria, and a normal plasma uric acid level point to epilepsy. Electroencephalography (EEG) rarely is diagnostic.

Grand mal seizures can be controlled by intravenous sodium amobarbital or magnesium sulfate. Phenytoin (Dilantin) and its analogues may be fetotoxic (Chapter 40). Diazepam (Valium) or chlordiazepoxide (Librium) are safe analeptic drugs. Epilepsy is not an indication for therapeutic abortion or cesarean delivery. Diazepam and chlordiazepoxide affect the newly delivered infant.

Multiple Sclerosis

Multiple sclerosis, a patchy demyelinization of the spinal cord and central nervous system (CNS), may be a viral disorder. Multiple sclerosis commonly develops initially after a pregnancy and is more common during the childbearing years. Multiple sclerosis may occasionally complicate pregnancy, but exacerbations and remissions are unrelated to the pregnant state. For this reason medically indicated therapeutic abortion is illogical. The burden of pregnancy and subsequent care of the child may warrant early interruption of pregnancy and sterilization in extreme cases. Women with multiple sclerosis occasionally may have an almost painless labor. The character of uterine contractions is unaffected by the disease, however.

Myasthenia Gravis

Myasthenia gravis, an autoimmune motor (muscle) end plate disorder that involves acetylcholine use, affects the motor function at the myoneural junction. Muscle weakness, particularly of the eyes, face, tongue, neck, limbs, and respiratory muscles results. The peak prevalence of myasthenia gravis is about 25 years of age. Pregnancy may complicate the disorder, although some women experience a remission during gestation. Pregnancies in women with this disease can be carried to safe delivery if certain precautions are taken. Moreover, congenital myasthenia gravis is rare. Therefore the disorder is not an indication for therapeutic abortion.

The nurse and physician should be alert to symptomatology, which includes easy fatigue, intermittent double vision, upper eyelid drooping, and facial muscle weakness. In more serious cases, upper arm weakness and breathing difficulty are seen. Infections may precipitate the onset or relapse and must be treated aggressively during pregnancy.

Parturients with myasthenia gravis usually tolerate labor well, because they already have some degree of muscle relaxation. Meperidine is the obstetric analgesic of choice. Local anesthesia is preferred. If a general anesthetic is required, a combination of nitrous oxide, oxygen, and cyclopropane generally is best. Oxytocin may be given, but scopolamine and muscle relaxants are contraindicated. After delivery, women must be carefully supervised, because relapses often occur during the puerperium.

Occasionally an infant born to a mother with severe myasthenia gravis also shows myasthenic signs sufficient to require neostigmine treatment for 1 to 2 months. Complete recovery of the infant is the rule. However, infants born with the disorder do not have as good a prognosis as do infants born without the disorder.

Bell's Palsy

An association between idiopathic facial paralysis and pregnancy was first cited by Bell in 1830, but it was not until 1975 that Hilsinger and colleagues proved this association. Not all neurologists agree with this association, however (Aminoff, 1978). There does not seem to be any causative relationship between the appearance of Bell's palsy and any of the complications of pregnancy.

No effects of maternal Bell's palsy have been observed in infants. Maternal outcome is generally good. Electromyography and nerve conduction velocity studies are useful in predicting the outcome. Evidence of a complete block in conduction carries a worse prognosis. Loss of taste also carries a less favorable prognosis. Steroids are sometimes prescribed for the condition. In most affected women, 90% or more return of facial function can be expected.

Adaptation to Pregnancy by Spinal Cord Injured Women

Debra I. Craig

In 1982 it was estimated that approximately 10,000 people would suffer spinal cord injuries. Of these 10,000, approximately 1000 of the injuries would occur in women aged 15 to 25. It was also predicted that this number would increase each year (Axel, 1982). Role function is influenced by one's self-expectation and the expectations held by others (Sarbin and Allen, 1968). It is an accepted role function of women to bear children, and one's feminine identity may be tied to the ability to give birth. As spinal cord injured (SCI) women enter the childbearing process, it is essential that nurses be prepared to assist these women in the development of a positive experience throughout the perinatal period. Axel (1982) states that there is a correlation between a positive self-image and role definition and the ability to achieve pregnancy in SCI women.

There is no physiologic reason for SCI women to believe that they cannot achieve a normal pregnancy. Fertility is not impaired by their injury and there is no greater incidence of spontaneous abortion or fetal abnormalities among this population (Goller and Paeslack, 1971, 1972; Ohry, et al., 1978; Young, Kutz, and Klein, 1983). However, the SCI woman must deal with her own expectations regarding parenting, the expectations of her significant others, and the perceived expectations of both the medical profession and society. Women with spinal cord injuries experience reactions similar to other women when their pregnancies are confirmed. That is shock, elation, disbelief, relief, and joy. The reactions of significant others range from shock and joy to concern regarding the effect of the pregnancy on the woman. SCI women receive a variety of responses to their impending or confirmed pregnancy from the medical profession. Some have been counseled to seek psychologic help, others to avoid becoming pregnant because it may be too dangerous, or to consider abortion. SCI women have had to search for physicians willing to take them as patients, although some have found supportive physicians from the onset of their pregnancies.

These women encounter a variety of responses within the hospital environment. They perceive the staff to be ill-at-ease in caring for them. "Perhaps the nurses were unsure about our needs and what to expect from us during labor," was a comment made by one paraplegic mother. Another quadriplegic woman stated she felt like she had been "raped" by the system because no one seemed to listen to her requests and desires. Spinal cord injured women tend to be more in touch with their bodies and its responses because of their injuries and are more directive in their care. They find that hospitals are not designed to accommodate people who spend their lives in wheelchairs. Most of the rooms are too small, as are the showers and bathrooms. The quadriplegic woman may need a specialized call light to obtain help. Commonly, these lights are not readily available to them.

The SCI woman also needs additional help in providing care to her newborn. Her concerns regarding her ability to care for the newborn are often verbalized during pregnancy, but not readily considered by hospital staff. SCI mothers express appreciation for those nurses who take extra time to help problem-solve infant care needs. SCI women have been very imaginative in developing adaptive equipment for the safety and care of their children. Some of the adaptations include redesigning the crib so that the side can be raised and the baby moved directly onto the mother's lap. Mothers have also designed special equipment to pick a baby up from a play pen or the floor. In addition to worrying about the physical care of their children, the mothers worry about how the child will adapt to her disability. The children of SCI parents are usually accepting of their parents disability and commonly educate their classmates regarding the functional ability of their parents.

Physiologically the SCI woman encounters many of the same problems that pregnant women in general experience. All woman suffer from urinary frequency during their pregnancy. This is more of a problem for the SCI women because of their alteration in voiding methods. Some SCI women use an indwelling catheter, some catheterize themselves at specific intervals, and others crede themselves to empty their bladder. Generally the increased urine production of pregnancy forces the women to increase the number of times they void daily, which increases the number of times they must transfer and undress themselves. Pressure on the bladder by the enlarging uterus increases the incidence of incontinence. Most SCI women find that a padding system is needed, especially during the third trimester. The most common materials used for padding are disposable diapers, either infant or adult size, and sanitary napkins. Many SCI women are unable to return to their prepregnant level of bladder functioning and must continue to wear padding after the birth of the baby.

The alteration in bladder functioning increases the SCI woman's susceptibility to bladder and kidney infections. Urinary tract infections (UTIs) affect about 10% of the pregnant nonspinal cord injured population and the majority of pregnant SCI women. SCI women generally experience an increase in the number and frequency of UTIs beginning in the second trimester and continuing through delivery. The SCI woman must work closely with her urologist and obstetrician to treat the infection without hurting the fetus.

Constipation is another problem that plagues the pregnant woman. The SCI woman has developed a bowel program as part of her routine of daily living. This usually includes either stool softeners or bulk-producing medication. During pregnancy the bowel program must be altered to accommodate both the hormonal effect, slowing the gastrointestinal tract, and pressure from the enlarging uterus on the intestinal tract. Adaptations used during pregnancy to combat constipation include increasing the frequency and amount of stool softeners or bulk producers, increasing the frequency of bowel movements, adding more roughage to the diet, and maintaining a high fluid intake.

Having to use the bathroom more frequently is just one of the mobility problems that the SCI woman encounters. SCI women use the prone position to sleep to relieve pressure on the ischial spines and gluteal muscle and to straighten joints. As a pregnancy progresses it becomes impossible for the SCI woman to lie prone. This necessitates more frequent repositioning during the night and often involves the significant other more dramatically in the caregiving. Transfers to and from the wheelchair, bathroom, bed, and car become more difficult as the pregnancy progresses. This difficulty in transfering threatens to hinder the woman's independence. Mobility is also a question that must be faced when the SCI woman visits the obstetrician. Is there room for her to undress? How does she get on and off of the examining table? Does the office staff know how to assist her with her needs?

A decrease in mobility correlates with the increased risk of developing pressure areas. Young, Kutz, and Klein (1983) list the development of decubiti as a major complication of SCI women. A recent unpublished study indicates that only a small proportion of SCI women develop decubiti (Craig, 1985). SCI women are aware of the possibility of developing pressure areas and take proactive measures to prevent their development.

It has been assumed that since SCI women have impaired sensation they will not be able to tell when they are in labor. This has not proven to be true. They may not experience labor in the same manner as other women, but because they are in tune with their bodies they know that something is happening. Some sense their abdomen tightening, others suffer increased spasms, others have a rhythmic need to void or defecate, and still others who had sparing (incomplete cord damage with occasional areas of remaining sensation) experience menstrual-like cramps or actual labor. Women who are injured at the level of T5 or above may correlate increasing symptoms of autonomic dysreflexia with labor.

Autonomic dysreflexia results from hyperstimulation of the splanchic nerves and loss of central control over sympathetic spinal reflexes. Hyperstimulation may result from distension of pelvic viscera, uterine contractions, muscle spasms, bladder or bowel distension, or chest pressure. Autonomic dysreflexia may be manifested by sweating, facial flushing, a pounding headache, pilomotor erection, and severe hypertension (Tabsh, Brinkman, and Reff, 1982). The symptoms of dysreflexia are more prevalent during the end of the first stage of labor and all of the second stage as perineal pressure and distension occur. These symptoms, a pounding headache and an increased blood pressure, must not be confused with pregnancy induced hypertension. The most common treatment for dysreflexia is epidural anesthesia and/or the delivery of the baby.

Delivery of the infant is usually accomplished vaginally. The SCI woman experiences no higher incidence of cesarean birth than a noninjured woman. There is no reduction in the power of the uterine contractions and spontaneous labor. Adequate contractions can and do occur even when the cord transection is above the motor nerve supply of the uterus. The SCI woman has no difficulty with a vaginal delivery even though she has no ability to push. Uterine contractions plus a relaxed perineum facilitate a vaginal delivery. The indications for a cesarean delivery are the same for a SCI woman as for any other woman.

After the delivery of the baby the SCI woman is confronted with the problem of maintaining the integrity of the episiotomy. Ohry et al. (1978) state that the use of nonabsorbable sutures to repair episiotomies reduces infections, abcesses, and the probability of dehiscence in the SCI woman. The woman must be assisted in checking their episiotomies at least twice a day for healing, especially since they experience decreased or absent perineal sensation. Sitz baths cannot be used because of the woman's inability to transfer into or onto one. Heat lamps must be used with extreme caution since the SCI woman has little or no sensation and might suffer a burn. The long sanitary napkins used in maternity are ideal for the SCI woman since they decrease the possibility of the pad causing a pressure area. Pressure areas may also result from the use of sanitary belts, and the women should be cautioned against their use.

During pregnancy both the SCI and the noninjured woman must adapt to physiologic and psychologic changes. The SCI woman has already made major adaptations in her life-style. With pregnancy she must make additional adaptations, but she has a background in successful problem solving to assist her. Through education and timely interventions, nurses can assist with these adaptations and facilitate a positive perinatal experience.

AUTOIMMUNE DISORDERS

Autoimmune disorders have a predilection for women in their reproductive years; therefore associations with pregnancy are not uncommon (Danforth and Scott, 1986). Pregnancy may affect the disease process. Some disorders adversely affect the course of pregnancy or are detrimental to the fetus. Autoimmune disorders include rheumatoid arthritis, systemic lupus erythematosus, hyperthyroidism, myasthenia gravis (p. 853), and immunologic thrombocytopenic purpura (Chapter 31). Autoantibodies from rheumatoid arthritis do *not* cross the placenta; those of the other disorders do. The woman with immunologic thrombocytopenic purpura may deliver a child who demonstrates thrombocytopenia. Petechiae and bleeding into the gastrointestinal and genitourinary tracts and into the brain may be evident. If the mother has myasthenia gravis, the newborn may exhibit a weak cry, sucking mechanism, and facial muscles and may have respiratory problems. Thyrotoxicosis is probable in the newborn of the mother with hyperthyroidism.

Rheumatoid Arthritis

Approximately three of every four women with rheumatoid arthritis (RA) find that the severity of symptoms decreases during pregnancy (Cecere and Persellin, 1981). For this reason many affected women attempt to become pregnant as often as possible; however, many are subfertile because of the RA. During normal pregnancy an increase in α_2-glycoprotein surpasses 40 mg/dl in about 75% of women (Cecere and Persellin, 1981). In addition, total plasma and free cortisol (especially estrogens and progesterones) show an increase (Nolten and Reuckert, 1981). This combination apparently leads to depressed cellular immunity (Persellin, 1981). Women in whom the rheumatoid factor (autoantibodies found in the synovial fluid) decreases during pregnancy report improvement in their symptoms. Researchers are now investigating the possibility of a positive effect on RA associated with the use of oral contraceptives (see also Table 6-10).

The woman with RA needs to be informed of the positive and negative aspects that accompany pregnancy. She must be cautioned that although symptoms may subside during pregnancy, she should anticipate a return of her symptoms after delivery. Exacerbations often recur about a month after delivery. "In short, she will be trading off a 75% chance that she will feel better against the strong possibility that she could 'crash' when the infant is about a month old" (Baum, 1984).

Management of rheumatoid arthritis during pregnancy

includes an appropriate balance of rest and exercise, heat and physical therapy, and salicylates, 3 to 6 g per day as tolerated (Danforth and Scott, 1986). Aspirin probably remains the safest and most useful antiinflammatory drug in these women. Mild hemostatic changes in the infant and an increase in the average length of gestation are attributed to maternal ingestion of large doses of aspirin, however. Systemic corticosteroids can reduce the inflammatory response, but because of the complications associated with chronic use, their place in rheumatoid arthritis is limited to acute situations in which other methods are ineffective.

Although proof that the breast-fed infant can be harmed is lacking, nonsteroidal antiinflammatory medications are not recommended for mothers who breast-feed. These drugs have been demonstrated in breast milk.

Systemic Lupus Erythematosus

One of the most common serious disorders of childbearing age, systemic lupus erythematosus (SLE), is a chronic multisystem inflammatory disease. The condition is not rare; more than 250,000 persons are known to have SLE, with an estimated 50,000 new cases per year. Although the antibody may be formed in response to a virus, a familial tendency seems to be involved (see also Table 6-10).

The vague early symptoms, such as fatigue, may be overlooked. Eventually all organs become involved. The condition is characterized by a series of exacerbations and remissions. A subcommittee of the American Rheumatism Association has proposed an extensive set of criteria to standardize the diagnosis.

If the diagnosis has been established and the woman desires a child, she is advised to wait for 2 years. At that time, if the disease has been controlled well on low doses of corticosteroids, pregnancy may be reasonably considered (Danforth and Scott, 1986). Oral contraceptives are contraindicated; diaphragms and condoms, are the preferred methods of fertility management if pregnancy is desired in the future, but sterilization is suggested if no more children are desired. The outlook for persons with SLE has improved markedly in the past few years. The survival rate is now more than 90% for 5 years and more than 80% for those who survive for 10 years after diagnosis.

Although the effect of pregnancy on SLE seems inconsistent, most maternal deaths occur during the puerperium or after abortion (Danforth and Scott, 1986). The rate of spontaneous abortion is high. Maternal complications correlate with the degree of cardiac or renal involvement. Renal failure, hypertension, and death are associated with diffuse proliferative lupus glomerulonephritis. When the kidneys are involved, gravidas are subject to superimposed preeclampsia, stillbirths, preterm delivery, and small-for-gestational age infants. However, if the disease is stable during pregnancy, the risk that the disease will worsen with gestation is only slight.

Obstetric management includes surveillance of the woman's renal and cardiovascular status and determination of fetal status. Corticosteroid (prednisone) therapy is maintained throughout pregnancy; hydrocortisone is administered intravenously during labor and delivery. Corticosteroid therapy is continued for about 2 months after delivery.

The relationship with immunosuppressive drugs (such as corticosteroids) and infection must be appreciated. Infection is now a leading cause of death among people with SLE. Nursing care is presented in the specific nursing care plan on p. 857.

Although the antibodies cross the placenta, their amount varies so that the effect on the fetus also varies. The most severely affected newborns suffer from discoid lupus, anemia, neutropenia, thrombocytopenia, and congenital complete heart block. Great strides in diagnosis, drug therapy, and knowledge about the immune system provide hope for the future.

SURGERY DURING PREGNANCY

The need for immediate abdominal surgery occurs as frequently among pregnant women as among nonpregnant women of comparable age. Diagnosis is more difficult in the pregnant woman, however. An enlarged uterus and displaced internal organs may prevent adequate palpation and alter the position of the surgical procedure.

Differential diagnosis includes consideration of obstetric complications (e.g., ectopic pregnancy and premature separation of the placenta) and the onset of labor. Mild leukocytosis and increased serum values of alkaline phosphatase and amylase are characteristic of pregnancy, as well as surgical intraperitoneal processes. Rising or abnormally high laboratory values are suspect, however. X-ray evaluation, a valuable adjunct to diagnosis, is contraindicated, particularly in the first trimester, except in extreme cases. The surgeon is confronted with both a surgical and an obstetric problem.

Laparotomy or laparoscopy may be required. Hazards of these procedures include abortion and premature labor. But surgical or anesthetic intervention does not affect the incidence of congenital malformations.

Assessment

Fetal vital signs and activity and uterine contractility (labor may have begun) are monitored, and constant vigilance for symptoms of impending obstetric complications is maintained. The woman and her family may have heightened concerns regarding effects of the procedure and medication on fetal well-being and the course of pregnancy.

Assessment of the mother is directed by the type of problem that requires surgery. The general guidelines for health assessment discussed in Chapter 8 are appropriate. The extent of presurgery assessment is determined by the immediacy of surgical intervention.

Nursing Diagnoses

Nursing diagnoses also vary with the surgical condition and the immediacy of surgical intervention. Nursing diagnoses may include the following:

- Knowledge deficit related to
  - The surgical condition
  - The surgical procedure

Specific Nursing Care Plan

POSTPARTUM CARE OF WOMAN WITH LUPUS ERYTHEMATOSUS

Dora S. was diagnosed as having systemic lupus erythematosus (SLE) 3 years ago after her first baby was born with complete heart block. Dora is a black female, 33 years old. Her SLE, discoid rash, and nondeforming arthritis were controlled with prednisone before and during this pregnancy. Dora is recovering from a spontaneous vaginal delivery 16 hours ago. Preliminary assessments show her daughter to be a normal newborn. Dora is very tired and has a poor appetite. The physician has ordered laboratory tests for the evaluation of her SLE. He has also ordered medication for her musculoskeletal pain. The rheumatologist has suggested she not breast-feed since the medications are expressed in the breast milk. This disappoints her, since she could not breast-feed her other child either because he was so ill.

ASSESSMENT	NURSING DIAGNOSIS (ND)/ PLAN (P)/GOAL (G)	RATIONALE/ IMPLEMENTATION	EVALUATION
Dora has SLE. Dora 16 hours postpartum and very tired. Dora experiencing musculoskeletal and joint pain.	ND: Pain, related to nondeforming arthritis and episiotomy. P: Minimize discomfort. G: Dora will be free from pain.	*To minimize or prevent pain the nurse will:* Assess sources of pain. Provide comfort measures such as: Warmth. Proper body alignment. Range of motion to maintain joint mobility. Teach proper body mechanics. Administer medication as ordered. Teach perineal care for episiotomy. Arrange for sitz baths as ordered.	Dora verbalizes a decrease in pain. Dora retains joint mobility. Dora performs self-care.
Activity intolerance.	ND: Activity intolerance: decreased, related to labor and delivery and decrease in stamina related to SLE. P: Ensure appropriate rest and exercise. G: Dora has enough energy for self-care and to take care of her newborn.	*To conserve energy and increase activity tolerance the nurse will:* Cluster treatments and tests. Provide quiet time for rest periods. Keep visitors to a minimum with Dora's authorization. Assist with activities of daily living (ADL) and newborn care.	Dora accepts more responsibility for ADL and newborn care.
Poor appetite.	ND: Altered nutrition: less than body requirements related to poor appetite and fatigue. P: Maintain adequate caloric oral intake. G: Dora's appetite improves and she consumes a diet that is adequate in calories and well-balanced.	*To maintain adequate nutrition the nurse will:* Collaborate with Dora and dietition to plan small, frequent meals with snack before bedtime. Make meals colorful and appetizing. Compile a list of Dora's favorite foods. Request family members to bring favorite cultural foods from home. Make mealtime unhurried and atmosphere pleasing.	Dora's appetite improves. Dora indicates that she is satisfied with her diet that is well-balanced and adequate in calories. Intravenous fluids are not necessary.

Continued.

Specific Nursing Care Plan—cont'd

ASSESSMENT	NURSING DIAGNOSIS (ND)/ PLAN (P)/GOAL (G)	RATIONALE/ IMPLEMENTATION	EVALUATION
Discoid rash. Episiotomy. Dora requests information about care of rash.	ND: Impaired skin integrity related to skin lesions of SLE and episiotomy. ND: Potential for infection related to impairment of skin integrity. P: Prevent infection, promote healing. G: Dora's skin lesions heal well.	*To prevent infection and promote healing of skin lesions and episiotomy, the nurse will:* Skin lesions: Implement specified medical regimen as ordered by physician. Discuss proper cleansing and medication techniques. Advise Dora to wear loose, nonirritating clothing, to use non-irritating make-up, if lesions on face, and to keep hands clean and nails short and clean. Episiotomy: Teach perineal care: cleansing, proper wiping, frequent change of pads; cleansing perineum after each void or stool. Provide sitz bath and instruction on how to use it.	Skin lesions remain dry—no inflammation or infection develops. During her follow-up visit, Dora states she is implementing care for her rash and that she is more comfortable. Episiotomy heals without infection or inflammation.
Dora upset about not being able to breast-feed.	ND: Potential altered parenting related to unfulfilled goal to breast-feed. ND: Situational low self-esteem related to formula-feeding her infant. P: Facilitate acceptance of formula-feeding and attachment and foster self-esteem. G: Dora states she feels "OK" about formula-feeding.	*To help Dora develop effective parenting skills and faster attachment, the nurse will:* Provide time to discuss feelings of disappointment. Explain positive aspects of formula-feeding. Provide time to mother and infant during feeding for cuddling and closeness. Observe feeding behaviors and assist if necessary.	Dora begins to develop close bond with infant and demonstrates proper feeding techniques.

  - Recovery
  - Potential sequelae for self and infant
- Potential for injury related to
  - Effects of postoperative immobility
- Spiritual distress related to
  - High-risk status

Planning

The preoperative and postoperative plans for care incorporate consideration for the family's and woman's concern for the infant, as well as for the woman.

Goals. Goals for care vary with each individual client. However, general goals apply in all situations. These general goals include:

1. Spiritual care* needs of woman and family are met.
2. Woman and family understand the condition, rationale for surgical intervention, expected outcome, and postoperative course and management.
3. Well-being of maternal-fetal-placental unit is maintained.
4. Mother and fetus-neonate suffer no adverse sequelae.

*Spiritual care is "care of the incorporeal part of [people] that includes religious, intellectual, cultural, ethical, and moral beliefs" (Tucker et al., 1988).

Table 34-2 *Preoperative Management*

	Collect Data	Psychologic Preparation	Physical Preparation	Legal Status
Physician	Aid in medical diagnosis Determine need, type, and extent of surgery Identify potential complications requiring medical intervention Obtain baseline data for future comparison	Explain need, type, and extent of surgery to woman and significant others Explain effect on fetus and pregnancy	Prescribe and carry out tests Prescribe diet, drugs Prescribe actions to ensure safety and comfort during surgery	Obtain informed, signed consent for procedure Complete physician's preoperative orders
Nurse	Identify psychologic readiness for surgery Identify knowledge of events that will occur Identify potential complications requiring nursing intervention Obtain baseline data for future comparison	Verify woman's understanding and clarify as indicated Give explanations about tests Give opportunities to express feelings and concerns Support significant others	Assist woman and physician in carrying out tests Help woman meet basic needs in preparation for surgery Assist woman in carrying out physician's orders	Ensure that identification bands are on and correct Complete preoperative checklist

Modified from Phipps, WJ, Long, BC, and Woods, NF: Medical-surgical nursing: concepts and clinical practice, ed. 3, St Louis, 1987, The CV Mosby Co.

5. Mother complies with scheduled postoperative follow-up care.

Implementation

Preoperative Period. Preoperative care for a pregnant woman differs from that for a nonpregnant woman in one significant aspect: the presence of at least one other person, the fetus. Procedures such as preparation of the operative site and the time of insertion of intravenous lines and urinary retention catheters vary with the physician and the facility. However, in every instance there is a total restriction of solid foods and liquids or a clear specification of the type, amount, and time at which clear liquids may be taken before surgery. Food by mouth is restricted for several hours before a scheduled procedure. Even if she has had nothing by mouth, but, more important, if surgery is unexpected, the woman is in danger of vomiting and aspirating, and special precautions are taken before anesthesia is administered (Chapter 17).

General preoperative observations and ongoing care are the same as for any surgery, with the addition of fetal surveillance. Preoperative management by the physician and nurse is summarized in Table 34-2. Following are the data suggested by Phipps, Long and Woods (1987) that should accompany the gravida to surgery:

Name	Hearing
Age	Vision
Height and weight	Respiratory status
Consciousness level	Allergies
Language and speech	Special problems*

*Fetal age and status; uterine activity.

In addition, a notation of FHR and fetal status is important.

Postoperative Period. Most recovery rooms have special forms used as checklists for assessing the client's postoperative status and progress. General observations and ongoing care pertinent to postoperative recovery are initiated. This general care includes maintaining fluid and electrolyte balance by diligent attention to intake and output. The nurse promotes physical and emotional rest through the appropriate use of nurse-ordered comfort measures and physician-ordered medications and procedures. If intrauterine pregnancy continues, fetal monitoring and monitoring of uterine activity are continued (Chapter 17).

Some causes of vital sign changes early in the postoperative phase are listed in Table 34-3.

Client safety remains an important component of care. The family is called on to assist in maintaining client safety through orientation of the woman (and her family and friends) to the need to use side rails, to call for assistance when getting out of bed, to protect the intravenous infusion and incision sites, and to cleanse the perineum.

Discharge Planning. Planning for discharge begins when the gravida first enters the health care delivery system. The extent to which the goals of care can be met before surgery is reviewed, and adjustments are made accordingly. For example, if the surgery was an emergency such as for appendicitis, there is little time for preoperative preparation. After the woman has recovered from the effects of the surgery, the nurse needs to take time to encourage her to voice her fears, concerns and questions. She may have questions regarding the effect of the surgery and anesthesia on the fetus. If she is unable to express these concerns to the physician, the nurse acts as client-advocate and informs the physician.

Table 34-3 *Some Causes of Vital Sign Changes in Early Postoperative Phase*

Increase	Decrease
Temperature	
Stress reaction (low-grade fever)	Cold operating room and recovery room
Pulse rate	
Jarring during transfer	Digitalis overdose
Shock, hemorrhage	Cardiac arrhythmias
Hypoventilation	
Acute gastric dilation	
Pain	
Anxiety	
Cardiac arrhythmias	
Respiratory Rate	
Hypoventilation: poor positioning, right chest or upper abdominal dressing, obesity, gastric dilation	Drugs: anesthetics, narcotics, sedatives
Blood Pressure	
Anxiety (↑ systolic)	Jarring during transfer
Pain	Severe pain
	Cardiac arrhythmias
	Shock: fluid loss, hemorrhage, acute gastric dilation

From Phipps, WJ, Long, BC, and Woods, NF: Medical-surgical nursing: concepts and clinical practice, ed 3, St. Louis, 1987, The CV Mosby Co.

The participation of the woman and her family in discharge planning is necessary to individualize the care to fit with the available family support systems, the home situation, and the facilities. If the woman is to perform some type of treatment or exercises at home, the family member or friend who will be caring for her is included when she is taught these activities, and her mastery is evaluated. The woman may be demonstrating symptoms of grief and loss, and her participation in discharge planning may be minimal. She may need assistance coping with these feelings (Chapter 28).

The woman may need referral service to various community agencies for evaluation of the home situation, child care, home health care, and financial or other assistance. All arrangements for her return home and for convalescent care should be completed as early as possible before the expected date of discharge. Topics covered vary but may include the following:

1. Care of incision site.
2. Return of gastrointestinal function: diet, elimination.
3. Signs and symptoms of developing complications: wound infection, thrombophlebitis, pneumonia. These should be given to the woman in printed form as well.
4. If the woman is expected to assess her temperature, she will need a thermometer and must know how to use it.
5. Resumption of activities of daily living. For example, the woman should not lift heavy objects and usually should not resume driving for 2 to 4 weeks or longer.
6. Treatments and medications ordered.
7. List of resource people and phone numbers that can be used for different services.
8. Schedule of follow-up visit.

The follow-up examination at the physician's office is scheduled usually 1 to 2 weeks after discharge. The nurse plays a vital role in helping clients understand the importance of follow-up care.

Evaluation

The nurse can be reasonably assured that care has been effective if the goals of care have been achieved.

Appendicitis

Acute suppurative appendicitis complicates about 1 in every 1000 pregnancies. This disorder poses the following special problems during gestation:

1. Appendicitis is more difficult to diagnose during pregnancy. The appendix is carried high and to the right, away from McBurney's point, by the enlarged uterus (Fig. 34-2).
2. Appendiceal rupture and peritonitis occur 2 to 3 times more often in pregnant women than in nonpregnant women.
3. Maternal and perinatal morbidity and mortality are greatly increased when appendicitis occurs during pregnancy.

Most cases of acute appendicitis occur during the first 6 months of gestation, with decreasing frequency through the third trimester, labor and puerperium. The differential diagnosis of appendicitis during pregnancy is also difficult because of gastrointestinal or genitourinary problems that may be confused with appendicitis. A high level of suspicion is important in the diagnosis of appendicitis.

Management. Appendectomy before rupture is extremely important. Antibiotic therapy before rupture is of questionable value; after rupture it may be lifesaving. Therapeutic abortion is never indicated in appendicitis. Cesarean delivery at or near term may be justified in association with appendectomy.

Prognosis. Maternal mortality increases to about 10% in the third trimester and is about 15% when appendicitis develops during labor. Perinatal mortality is approximately 10% with unruptured appendicitis but is at least 35% with peritonitis.

Intestinal Obstruction

Although intestinal obstruction (dynamic ileus) is not common during pregnancy, any woman with a laparotomy scar is more likely to suffer intestinal obstruction during gestation. Adhesions, an enlarging uterus, and displacement of the intestines are etiologic factors.

Persistent abdominal, cramplike pain, vomiting, auscul-

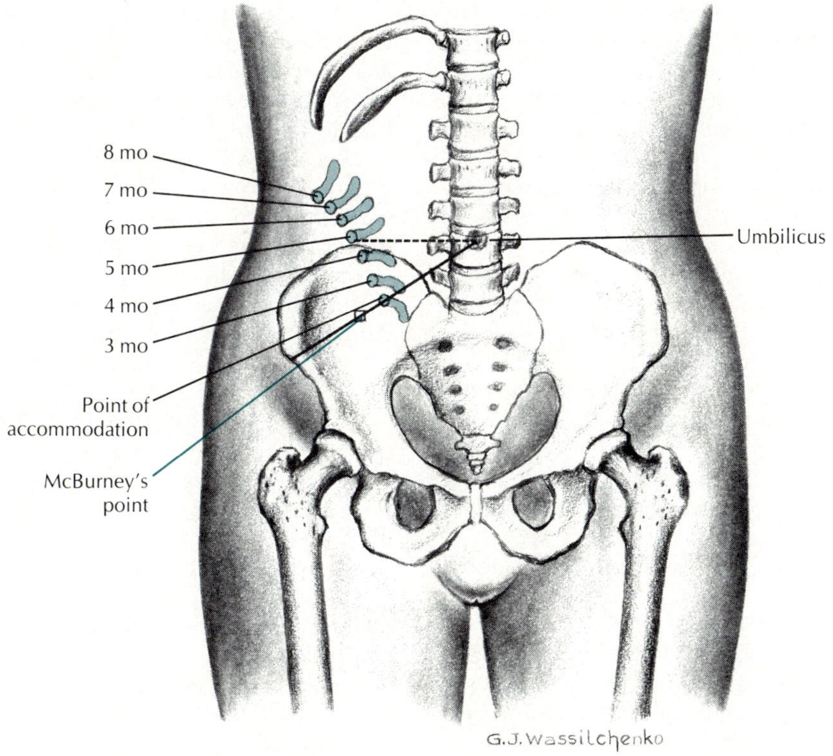

Fig. 34-2 Change in position of appendix during pregnancy.

tatory rushes within the abdomen, and "laddering" of the intestinal shadows on x-ray films aid in the diagnosis of intestinal obstruction. Immediate surgical intervention is required for release of the obstruction. Pregnancy is rarely affected by the surgery, assuming the absence of complications such as peritonitis. Cesarean delivery is not indicated in intestinal obstruction.

Abdominal Hernias

The incidence of abdominal hernias and related incarceration of the bowel is reduced during pregnancy despite permanent enlargement of umbilical or incisional hernial rings. Displacement of a nonadherent bowel by the enlarging uterus and its shielding of so-called weak areas of the abdominal wall are responsible. In fact, temporary spontaneous reduction of some abdominal wall hernias occurs during gestation. In contrast, however, the uncommon irreducible or adherent hernias may become incarcerated as pregnancy progresses.

Straining or bearing down during the second stage of labor may be contraindicated for women with hernias. Therefore low forceps delivery may be planned. Abdominal hernia is not an indication for cesarean delivery; herniorrhaphy should be done as an interval procedure (i.e., between pregnancies).

Gynecologic Problems

Ovarian cysts and twisting of ovarian cysts or adnexal tissues may occur. Pregnancy predisposes a woman to ovarian problems, especially during the first trimester. Conditions include retained or enlarged cystic corpus luteum of pregnancy, ovarian cyst, and bacterial invasion of reproductive or other intraperitoneal organs.

Laparotomy or laparoscopy is required to discriminate between ovarian problems and early ectopic pregnancy, appendicitis, or other infectious processes. See Chapter 30 for a discussion on common vaginitis.

INJURIES DURING PREGNANCY

Minor injury during pregnancy is a common occurrence; most trauma (more than 50%) occurs during the third trimester. Maternal adaptations to pregnancy are responsible for syncope, loss of balance, and general clumsiness. Discomfort such as a contracting uterus or vigorous fetal movement may be distracting while the woman is driving or working; an estimated 7% of pregnant women sustain accidental injury (Smith and Payne, 1984). The leading cause of death in women of reproductive age is accidents and not neoplasms or obstetric complications (Higgins, 1983).

Assessment

The woman's condition is the initial concern. The injury sustained determines the type and extent of assessment conducted. Attention is focused first on the basic ABCs: airway, breathing, and circulation. The woman's abdomen is assessed for ruptured uterus and uterine activity. As indicated, health assessment techniques described in Chapter 8 are performed. When available, the woman's prenatal record is reviewed.

Physical examination. Findings from the injury must not be confused with the normal physiologic changes during pregnancy:

1. Usual signs of organ rupture (i.e., guarding, rebound tenderness, and rigidity) may only be responses to stretching of the abdominal wall.
2. Examination of the woman in a supine position results in hypotension and a systolic value as low as 80; changing her position to left lateral or simply moving the fetus raises the systolic value to more than 100.
3. A "silent" abdomen, a sign of bowel trauma, may be a normal finding because of the decreased motility found during pregnancy.
4. Delayed emptying time of the stomach during pregnancy poses a threat of vomiting and possible aspiration if the woman has eaten within the last several hours.
5. During pregnancy, the woman may sustain a significant blood loss (about 30% reduction in circulating blood volume) without the usual signs and symptoms of hypovolemia. Pelvic blood vessels (retroperitoneal and parametrial arteries) enlarge greatly during pregnancy so that they are damaged and perhaps rupture more easily as a result.
6. The large uterus can compartmentalize and hide hemorrhage originating in the liver and spleen.
7. A rapid pulse may reflect only the usual increase of 10 to 15 beats per minute, or it may be a sign of hypovolemia.

Laboratory Tests. The type of test is determined by the type of injury. Appropriate blood studies include tests for serum amylase and blood gases; baseline bleeding profile; and complete blood count, typing and cross-matching. In normal pregnancies a white blood count of 18,000/mm^3 in the last trimester and 25,000/mm^3 during labor is usual; these same values are also indicative of intraabdominal hemorrhage. DIC can complicate severe trauma, abruption, and sepsis.

An indwelling urinary bladder catheter for drainage facilitates management of fluid therapy and aids diagnosis; for example, difficulty in passing the catheter suggests urethral disruption and hematuria suggests a ruptured bladder. The catheter also provides access for retrograde cystogram X-ray examination.

Intraperitoneal hemorrhage must be detected. The physician places a peritoneal lavage catheter for detecting intraperitoneal hemorrhage. The procedure is performed under local anesthesia through a small incision into the peritoneum. The test is positive for bleeding if the aspirate exceeds 10 ml of nonclotting blood or if, after instillation of 1 liter of lactated Ringer's solution, bloody fluid is recovered. Radiographic studies may be necessary to guide management.

Posttraumtic Uterine and Fetal Surveillance. When the mother has been stabilized, attention is turned toward monitoring the fetus and monitoring for premature labor and placental abruption. Usually, if these complications occur, they happen within 24 to 48 hours after the accident.

In the case of minor trauma, the woman is hospitalized and evaluated for the following: vaginal bleeding, uterine irritability, abdominal tenderness, abdominal pain or cramps, evidence of hypovolemia, a change in or absence of fetal heart tones, and leakage of amniotic fluid (Rothenberger, 1978).

After injury, if **placental abruption** (abruptio placentae) is to occur, it usually manifests itself within 48 hours. **Uterine rupture** can occur at the traditional site of a previous scar or over the site of implantation, which is weakened by increased vascularity at the site. Expulsion of the uterine contents into the abdominal cavity may occur and is usually followed by massive hemorrhage.

Nursing Diagnoses

The nursing diagnoses are formulated from assessment findings. Examples of possible nursing diagnoses include the following:

- Anxiety, fear related to
  - Uncertainty of outcome for the gravida and fetus
- Knowledge deficit related to
  - Inadequate pretreatment preparation time
- Potential for injury related to
  - Recent food intake before need for anesthesia

Planning

Planning with the gravida may not be possible in all situations. The gravida and family are included in planning at the earliest possible time. Goals are derived from the injury, its management and course, and based on the gravida's and family's individual needs.

Goals

1. Injuries resulting from accidents are diagnosed and treated accurately and rapidly.
2. Woman and fetus sustain no permanent adverse sequelae.
3. Woman and family grieve appropriately.
4. Injuries are prevented through prenatal education on safety in view of normal maternal adaptations to pregnancy (e.g., balance).

Implementation

Prevention. Intervention begins with prevention. The woman is counseled to discontinue activities requiring balance and coordination, to use seat belts appropriately, to recognize early symptoms, and to seek therapy immediately. If the woman is hospitalized only for observation, she is involved in assessment for signs and symptoms of complications.

Immediate Care. Immediate trauma care consists of attention to the ABCs. While hypoxia and hypovolemia are being corrected, the woman should be transferred to a trauma center with obstetric and neonatal backup, if possible. During transfer, attendants must remember the aortocaval syndrome and position the woman on her side or

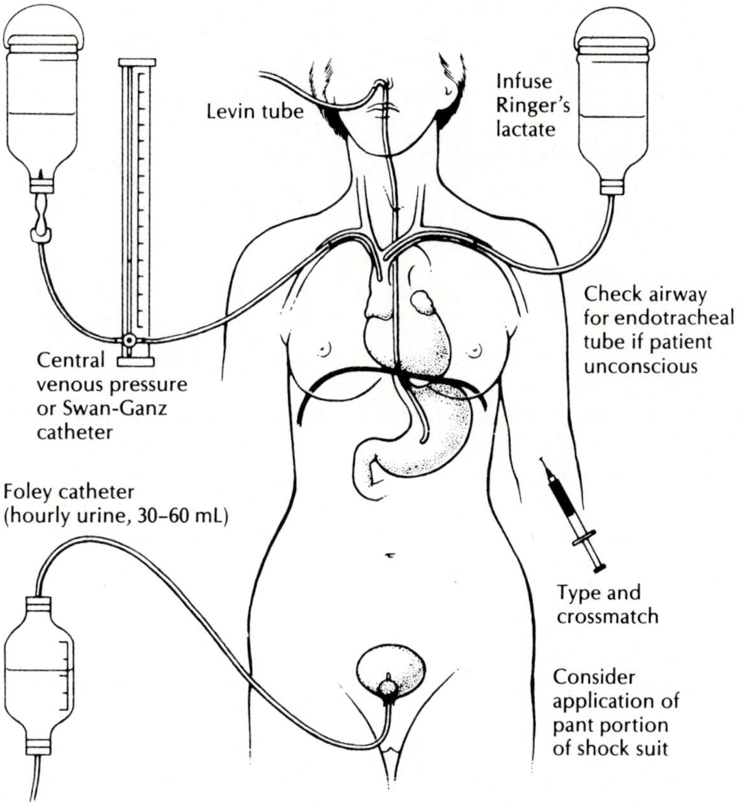

Fig. 34-3 Summary of technique used for resuscitation. Trauma care should begin in field where injury occurred, always with attention to basic ABCs: airway, breathing, and circulation.
From Higgins, SD: Contemp Obstet Gynecol **21**(3):32, 1983.

displace the uterus laterally by a uterine displacer or by a pillow placed under her right hip to prevent compromise of cardiac output followed by a decrease of blood to the fetus.

Subsequent Care. A nasogastric tube is inserted, if indicated, because delayed gastric emptying time and increased intestinal transit time increase the risk of vomiting and aspiration (Fig. 34-3). Mouth care and reassurance is used to counter the annoyance the woman may feel because of the presence of the tube.

Fluid and electrolyte replacement (Chapter 31) is instituted and monitored. Oxygen need is met. Properative care is provided if surgery is indicated.

Laparotomy. Penetrating abdominal wounds, internal hemorrhage, and ruptured uterus are all indications for immediate surgical intervention. Wounds high in the abdomen have most likely penetrated a vital structure because organs such as the bowel, liver, and spleen have been displaced upward by the enlarging uterus.

Cesarean Delivery. Indications for immediate cesarean delivery (Chapter 33) include fetal distress and maternal infection, ruptured diaphragm, unstable spinal fractures, and complicated pelvic fractures. The enlarged uterus can hamper control of hemorrhage and repair of vital structures. A ruptured diaphragm must be repaired immediately, but the family must be informed that even in nonpregnant persons, the morbidity and mortality are high. During pregnancy, increased intraabdominal pressure generated by the uterus and bearing-down efforts during labor increase the risk. Unstable spinal fractures cannot be tolerated by the pregnant woman because of inability to remain in the supine position and of the stress of vaginal delivery. A pelvis distorted by extensive fracture in itself is incompatible with vaginal delivery, but vaginal delivery may also cause extensive damage to the urethra and bladder that does not have the protection of an intact and well-formed pelvis.

Postmortem Cesarean Delivery. Fetal outcome of the uninjured fetus is likely to be good if the interval is less than 10 but no more than 20 minutes since the mother's death. The family will need supportive care to deal with the grief of losing a loved one (Chapter 28).

Evaluation

The nurse can be assured that care has been effective if the goals of care have been achieved.

EMOTIONAL COMPLICATIONS

Mental health problems can complicate pregnancy, childbirth, and the puerperium. Medical diagnoses of psychiatric health problems are broadly differentiated as *neurotic* or *psychotic.* The problems are further classified by the American Psychiatric Association (1980) in the *Diagnos-*

tic and Statistical Manual of Mental Disorders (DSM-III). In 1985 a revision of DSM-III (DSM-III-R) was drafted (American Psychiatric Association, 1985).

DSM-III-R uses a five-axis system that gives attention to certain types of disorders, aspects of the environment, and areas of functioning that might be overlooked if one focused exclusively on the single presenting problem. Axes I and II comprise the entire classification of mental disorders. Axis III allows the clinician to identify any current physical disorder or condition that is potentially relevant to the understanding or treatment of the individual. Axis IV documents the severity of the psychosocial stressors on a scale of one to seven, with pregnancy seen as a moderate stressor, receiving a score of four; and the birth of a child, seen as a severe stressor, receiving a score of five. Axis V allows the clinician to rate an individual's psychologic, social and occupational functioning on a continuum of mental health-illness. Ratings are made on a nine-point global assessment of functioning with the score of nine representing good functioning, and one representing the poorest functioning.

Psychiatric nurses will utilize all five axes of the DSM-III-R with the related nursing diagnoses in planning and implementing nursing care. The maternity nurse will need to document observations carefully and collaborate with psychiatric nurses to provide care to women suffering from mental health problems during pregnancy, childbirth, and the puerperium.

Etiology and Characteristics

Developmental and personality disorders generally have an onset in childhood or adolescence. They usually persist in a stable form into adulthood (Stuart and Sundeen, 1987). Mental retardation, autism, and disruptive behavior disorders are examples.

Mental health disorders generally predate pregnancy. Sleep and arousal disorders, schizophrenic disorders, delusional (paranoid) disorders, and anxiety disorders are a few behavioral categories.

Pregnancy per se is not a cause of psychiatric illness. The psychologic and physical stresses relating to pregnancy or to the formidable new obligations of motherhood may, however, precipitate an emotional crisis (Affonso, 1984). The principal emotional disturbances complicating gestation are mood (affective) disorders and schizophrenia. Organic mental syndromes and disorders (non-substance-induced) may also be seen. The mood disturbances include depression or depression with manic episodes (bipolar disorders). Paranoia or other disorganizational problems may characterize schizophrenic disorders. Toxic delirium associated with substance abuse, excessive analgesia, or serious metabolic disorders is not common. Rarely, psychosis secondary to alcoholism or syphilis may complicate both prenatal and postdelivery progress. Psychoactive substance–induced organic mental disorders are discussed in the section that follows.

No one single factor has been isolated as responsible for precipitating an episode of postpartum mental illness. Predisposing factors have been categorized by Herzog and Detre (1976) as follows: (1) genetic-constitutional, (2) social environmental, and (3) physiologic-endocrine.

Emotional illnesses arising during the puerperium are diagnosed by their initial features: affective, schizophrenic or organic. Those illnesses that do not meet the criteria for any of these disorders are designated "postpartum psychoses" (American Psychiatric Association, 1980).

Mood (Affective) Disorders

Although the cause of affective depressive disorders is unknown, the family history may record one or more adults who have had this problem. Moreover, women who have psychiatric complications during the course of pregnancy often have had similar crises previously.

Over 50% of pregnancy-related mental illnesses are affective reactions. Of these, about 10% are predelivery manic or depressive states; the remainder disturb the postdelivery period. Younger women seem more prone to manic reactions, but depression is the more common problem for most women.

Rejection of the infant, often caused by abnormal jealousy, is a prominent feature of affective disorders. The mother may be obsessed by the notion that the offspring may supplant her in her husband's affections. In other instances, guilt regarding aversion to pregnancy, attempted abortion, or other personal conflicts may be the basic problem.

Depressive reactions, far more common than manic reactions, may begin as a mild feeling of discouragement (the "baby blues") during the first week after delivery. However, anxiety, anorexia, and exaggerated fatigue soon color the despondency. The woman seems helpless; she is self-accusatory and often expresses strange or inappropriate thoughts or feelings. Occasionally a disconsolate mother may kill her infant and herself.

Depression may continue for weeks or months. Amphetamines are not helpful and may add to agitation. However, a tranquilizer with a prominent stimulatory effect, such as trifluoperazine (Stelazine), may be beneficial. Psychotherapy must be intensive and often prolonged. Meanwhile, separation of mother and infant will be necessary. If the depression lifts within several weeks, the prognosis is good. However, women who have been depresssed previously, especially those who have had even longer depressions, have a poor prognosis.

Manic reactions often occur during the first or second week of the puerperium, perhaps after a brief depression. Agitation, excitement, and volubility, often with rhyming or punning, develop. The woman becomes disinterested in personal care and food. Because dehydration or exhaustion may ensue, prompt and effective supportive treatment is essential.

Psychiatric therapy may include a tranquilizer with a prominent sedative effect, for example, promethazine hydrochloride (Phenergan). Lithium carbonate may be given later for more prolonged control. Psychotherapy is essential. The usual duration of the manic state is 1 to 3 weeks.

The prognosis for mother and infant is good after initial separation and gradual reunion.

Schizophrenia

Schizophrenic reactions, now suspected of being a disorder of cerebral metabolism, affect adolescents and younger adults rather than older persons. Abnormal personality features are common. Unusually shy, retiring, hypersensitive, or overly suspicious women are prone to schizophrenic break. A sudden onset of delusions or hallucinations may alter a seemingly well-accepted normal pregnancy. The symptoms indicate the woman's inability to adjust to and cope with her new obligations as a mother.

The husband and infant are totally rejected. Hostility toward the spouse and the medical staff is obvious. Often the excited, confused woman believes hers to have been an immaculate conception, or she may believe that she is being influenced by the Deity. The woman abandons reality and retreats completely into her own world of unreality. The mother totally neglects her infant. Suicide is unlikely. A phenothiazine type of tranquilizer, for example, chlorpromazine (Thorazine), will be useful. Transfer of the woman to a psychiatric hospital usually is necessary. Electroshock therapy and psychotherapy usually are effective.

A good prognosis is likely with the first psychotic episode, especially if it occurs unexpectedly during the puerperium. The child probably will never suffer from schizophrenia, despite speculation regarding hereditary tendencies.

Assessment

The nursing care plan must reflect the expected behavioral responses of the particular disorder. Characteristics of the woman and her specific circumstances are utilized to individualize the plan.

Nursing Diagnoses

Nursing diagnoses relevant to any emotional illness or developmental disorder such as mental retardation may include, but are not restricted to, the following:

- Potential for injury to fetus related to
  - Psychotropic medication
  - Maternal suicide
- Potential for injury to newborn related to
  - Unmet needs (e.g., hygiene, nutrition) and safety precautions
  - Mother's poor impulse control
- Ineffective family coping: compromised, related to
  - Increased care needs of mother-fetus-newborn
- Impaired home maintenance management related to
  - Increased care needs of mother-fetus-newborn
- Potential altered parenting related to
  - Lack of supervised opportunities for attachment to infant
- Potential altered growth and development (infant) related to
  - Lack of intellectual stimulation

Planning

Planning focuses on the mother's dependency needs, attachment to the infant, family integration, parenting skills and care of the infant, and home maintenance management. Supervision of the mother and family in the home is a prime concern.

Goals. Goals of care may include the following:

1. Maintaining the physical well-being of the mother and infant.
2. Establishing effective individual and family coping.
3. Continuing healthy growth and development in each family member.

Implementation

Community resources such as the community health nurse, homemaker service, or foster care are utilized as necessary. Discharge planning carefully developed with the family in collaboration with a hospital-community health care team is vital.

Evaluation

Evaluation of interventions occurs over a varying period of time. "Postpartum psychoses" may resolve in a period of weeks. Other disorders, including mental retardation, extend indefinitely.

• • •

Discussions follow of inhospital management of the psychotic pregnant woman and of the woman experiencing a postpartum emotional complication.

Prenatal Hospitalization

Inhospital psychiatric treatment is often required to treat psychotic pregnant women. Maternal physiologic adaptations and fetal movement often result in intensification of delusional ideas in the schizophrenic woman. Women with bipolar mood (affective) disorders may respond well during pregnancy and childbirth. After delivery, however, these women are prone to worsening of psychotic symptoms and depression (Spielvogel and Wile, 1986). Hospitalized women present treatment challenges in three areas: psychotropic medication, legal sanctions, and management in an acute hospital setting. A brief overview of these difficulties is given here. Psychiatric texts must be consulted for specifics.

Psychotropic Medications. All psychotropic medications pass through the placenta to the fetus and through breast milk to the infant. The risks of medication are weighed against the risks of maternal agitation and potentially self-destructive behavior. Children exposed to psychotropics between 8 and 10 weeks' gestation show a higher rate of congenital anomalies (5.4%) than the population with no such exposure (3.2%) (Edlund and Craig, 1984). A higher perinatal death rate (Edlund and Craig, 1984) and an increased incidence of an extrapyramidal syndrome consisting of "tremors, hypertonia, weakness, and poor sucking and other reflexes" complicate the neonatal period (Hauser, 1985). Medication dosage is balanced between the mother's needs and fetal response determined by nonstress tests. Some medications may be behavioral teratogens with short- and long-term effects (Vorhees, Brunner, and Butcher, 1979).

Bipolar affective disorders are often treated with **lithium.** A high incidence of fetal cardiovascular abnormalities is linked to lithium taken during the first trimester. Maternal shifts in fluid balance may require doubling the lithium dose to achieve a therapeutic level (Spielvogel and Wile, 1986). At delivery, renal clearance is reduced. Therefore toxicity can result if the lithium dose is not decreased by at least 50% 1 week before birth—if the delivery date can be correctly anticipated. Regardless of dose, the neonate may show signs of toxicity: cyanosis, lethargy, low Apgar scores, absent Moro's reflex.

Legal Sanctions. Women with mental health problems who can care for themselves may be unable to do so for themselves and the fetus. Hospital care may be mandated during pregnancy. Delusions about the pregnancy and its medical monitoring may necessitate legal intervention. Other legal issues arise closer to delivery. These issues surround the care of the mother and her infant and fertility management (Spielvogel and Wile, 1986).

Inhospital Management. Schizophrenic pregnant women often experience an intensification of their disorder. These women usually remain ambivalent toward the fetus and resist examination and procedures. Since they seem unaware of signs of labor, the staff must be keenly alert to behavioral and physical indicators of labor. Even though disorganization often improves, specific delusions may persist. The new mother may not be able to be close to her baby or to recognize or meet the baby's needs.

Pregnant women with bipolar effective disorders usually respond well to pregnancy, the fetus, and delivery. The new mother's responses may not be consistent or appropriate to the baby, however. After delivery, psychotic symptoms or depression worsen. Mothers need to be supervised carefully when visiting with their babies to safeguard their safety.

Postpartum Mental Illness

Postpartum mental illness may be acute or chronic and appears cross-culturally. It ranges from a transitory depression to severe postpartum emotional disturbances. The transitory depression, "maternity blues" or "baby blues," may occur in 30% to 80% of all childbirths (Ketai, 1979).

Transitory depression begins the second or third day after birth. The symptoms include anxiety, poor concentration, tearfulness, and despondency. The symptoms usually subside within the first week. No hospitalization is required. However, approximately 40% of women with mild depression have symptoms that persist as long as 1 year (Gelder, 1978; Tentoni and High, 1980). Illnesses of intermediate severity occur in 11% of all childbirths (Hayworth, 1980).

Severe postpartum emotional disturbance is noted in only 1% to 2% of all normal childbirths. However, 2% to 9% of women admitted to mental hospitals are admitted for conditions related to childbearing (Ketai, 1979; Weiner, 1982).

The onset of postpartum psychosis is usually abrupt and occurs within days of delivery. The symptoms center around the mother's relationship with the baby. The mother's response may be of an overprotective or of a rejecting nature (Hurt, 1985). The mother may be convinced that someone is trying to take her baby from her and will clutch it protectively. Or she may believe that the baby is dead or defective or that God is caring for it and so the baby does not need care.

The presenting symptoms form the basis for management (American Psychiatric Association, 1980; Hurt, 1985). Schizophrenia-like symptoms are treated with psychotropic medications. Lithium may be prescribed with or without psychotropic medications for bipolar affective disorders. Depression may be treated with electroconvulsive therapy (ECT) if suicidal or infanticidal thoughts are identified. Women may need assistance for alterations in patterns of sleep-rest, self-care (basic hygiene), nutrition and fluid balance, elimination, self-esteem, and family coping and processes. Discharge planning focuses on preparation for meeting the demands of an infant while the mother is still integrating her experience with psychosis, supporting the husband, and exploring the effects of the illness on their family (Hurt, 1985).

Hurt (1985) describes one psychiatric unit's protocol for acquaintance and maternal attachment and for the family system. The mother's depression or psychosis prevents her from engaging in the mutual interaction with the baby that is needed for acquaintance and subsequent attachment (bonding). Within the hospital setting the reintroduction of the mother and baby can occur at the mother's own pace. During these interactions the mother's readiness to care for the baby after discharge is evaluated. The interactions are carefully supervised and guided. A schedule is set for increasing hours over 3-to-4 days, culminating in the infant's admission to the unit for an overnight stay. The over-night stay allows the mother to experience the infant's being there and giving up sleep for the baby, a situation difficult for new mothers under ideal conditions. During this time the nurses observe her for "bonding behaviors." Bonding behaviors are defined as eye-to-eye contact (*en face* position), physical contact of holding, touching, cuddling, talking to the baby and calling the baby by name, and initiating care for the baby when appropriate. A staff member is assigned to keep the baby within sight at all times. Indirect teaching, praise, and encouragement are designed to bolster the mother's self-esteem and self-confidence. Staff work with the father is provided concurrently. Administrative and clinical support in this psychiatric unit has facilitated comprehensive care to women who develop a psychosis in the puerperium and to their families.

PSYCHOACTIVE SUBSTANCE USE

The use of mind-altering substances is pandemic. In this discussion, substance abuse is defined as the use of any mind-altering agent to such an extent that it interferes with the individual's biologic, psychologic, or sociocultural integrity (Stuart and Sundeen, 1987). Interference with biologic integrity might be exemplified (during pregnancy) in poor nutrition leading to poor weight gain, anemia, and a predisposition to infection and PIH. Some drugs (morphine, heroin, diazepam, and others) induce platelet disorders that predispose the woman to hemorrhage (Danforth and Scott, 1986). Psychologic consequences may include acute psychosis in a pregnant teenager who has been taking PCP or the inability of a new mother to "bond" with her infant (see discussion of emotional disturbances). Expectant and new mothers using mind-altering substances receive negative feedback from society, as well as from health care providers who condemn them for endangering the unborn and the infant and who may withhold support.

This discussion focuses on the use and abuse of alcohol, opioids, and cocaine. Many other substances are abused. The care needed by the individual varies with the particular circumstances of that individual and the substance abused. However, the nursing process is similar for all.

It has been estimated that 75% of pregnant women who are drug dependent do not seek prenatal care until labor begins (Finnegan and Macnew, 1974). They will take the drug just before seeking admission; therefore withdrawal symptoms can be delayed until 6 to 12 hours after delivery. The care of the substance-dependent pregnant woman is based on historical data, symptoms, physical findings, and laboratory results. As a result of the woman's defensiveness and frequent denial, history taking has to be done in a sensitive and competent manner (Bodendorfer et al., 1979).

The woman dependent on a drug tends to exhibit a passive response to life and its responsibilities. She may show a high degree of depression. Drug use has meant a way for her to relieve psychologic distress, to encourage social interaction, and to blunt the feelings of loneliness and emptiness that are part of depression. Pregnancy is not planned. It occurs as an "accidental" phenomenon. It may serve as a positive event, confirming her worth as a woman.

After birth, however, the woman is faced with the parental tasks of caring for and nurturing a completely dependent infant and of forming a warm, close, intimate relationship with the child. Care of the woman addicted to a drug offers a tremendous challenge to nursing.

Realization of the difficulty of the nursing challenge becomes apparent. The demands of motherhood are being made of a person who is herself dependent and arrested at the stage of taking and receiving rather than giving. Most substance-dependent people are unable to establish positive intimate relationships and lack a meaningful support system. The mother's ability to care for her infant after discharge from the hospital should be assessed by frequent observations, including some in the home setting.

The *goals* for her care would include the following:

1. Provide the woman with optimum and comprehensive antenatal care.
2. Prevent preterm delivery, perinatal loss, and neonatal drug dependence.
3. Involve the woman in long-term medical, social, psychiatric, and vocational rehabilitation.

Alcohol

Assessment

Identification of the woman with an alcohol problem may be difficult. Denial of the problem or its consequences is seen commonly. A concerned, nonjudgmental, matter-of-fact approach is used in the hope that the woman admits a problem if it exists. Inability to form positive relationships is often secondary to manipulative behavior. A low tolerance for frustration or anxiety and expressions of guilt related to alcoholic behavior patterns may be evident. Physical signs and symptoms may also be present (Table 34-4). During withdrawal, CNS agitation is expressed as fatigue, insomnia, agitation, restlessness, and belligerence. Bruises, rashes, and other injuries may be found on observation. Poor physical hygiene and malnutrition are potential problems, especially in the chronic alcoholic. Assessment for maternal and fetal well-being follows the protocols discussed for other clients.

Nursing Diagnoses

The following are examples of nursing diagnoses formulated from the assessment data:

- Ineffective individual coping related to
  - Low self-esteem
  - Poor parenting in own childhood
  - Lack of healthy mechanisms for recognition and release of anger
- Noncompliance related to
  - Manipulative behaviors with staff
- Chronic low self-esteem related to
  - Feelings about alcoholism
- Potential altered health maintenance management related to
  - Poor personal hygiene
- Potential fluid volume deficit and altered nutrition related to
  - Effects of excessive alcohol consumption
- Potential for injury to self, fetus, or newborn related to
  - Sensory effects of alcohol consumption
- Knowledge deficit related to
  - Effects of alcohol on developing fetus

Planning

Planning for care must be accomplished with recognition of the woman's life-style and habits. The ideal long-

Table 34-4 *Psychoactive Substance Effects*

Drug	Psychologic Signs	Physiologic Signs
Alcohol		
Intoxication	Mood lability or change Impaired attention or memory Irritability Talkativeness	Slurred speech Flushed face Incoordination, unsteady gait Nystagmus
Withdrawal	Anxiety Depressed mood or irritability Maladaptive behavior	Nausea and vomiting Malaise or weakness Autonomic hyperactivity Coarse tremor of hands, tongue, eyelids Orthostatic hypotension
Opioid*		
Intoxication	Euphoria, dysphoria Psychomotor retardation Apathy Maladaptive behavior Impaired attention or memory	Pupillary constriction Drowsiness Slurred speech
Withdrawal	Insomnia	Lacrimation, rhinorrhea Pupillary dilation Piloerection; sweating Diarrhea Yawning Mild hypertension Tachycardia Fever
Cocaine		
Intoxication	Psychomotor agitation Elation Grandiosity; talkativeness Hypervigilance Maladaptive behaviors	Tachycardia Pupillary dilation Hypertension Perspiration; chills Nausea; vomiting
Withdrawal	Depressed mood Disturbed sleep Increased dreaming	Fatigue
Phencyclidine (PCP)	Euphoria Psychomotor agitation Increased anxiety Emotional lability Grandiosity Sensation of slowed time Synesthesias Maladaptive behaviors	Vertical or horizontal nystagmus Hypertension Increased heart rate Numbness Decreased response to pain Ataxia; dysarthria

*Most commonly abused narcotics: heroin (the most potent), codeine, morphine.

term goal would be total abstinence. However, the woman may be unable to face that level of commitment at this time. The thought of relinquishing the substance forever is anxiety provoking. It is rare for a substance-dependent person to stop use of that substance suddenly. Short-term goals are necessary. The woman must participate in the decision-making process in formulating the goals. It is particularly important that the goals be phrased so that it is clear that the woman has responsibility for her behavior. The goals are written into a contract signed by the woman and the nurse (or physician). One copy is kept by the woman.

Short-term Goals

1. Stabilize woman's physiologic status
2. Initiate a withdrawal program
3. Instill importance of keeping appointments for prenatal (or postpartum) care
4. Minimize adverse effects on fetus; or ensure care and safety of newborn

Implementation

Most busy obstetric or maternity services cannot provide the comprehensive care needed by an alcoholic pregnant woman or new mother. Referral to social services or to Alcoholics Anonymous (AA) or a similar group may be warranted. Planning for participation in a support group is the joint effort of the woman and maternity and mental health staff. The woman may need to attend group support meetings more than once per week. These support services focus on the woman's (and family's) behavioral defenses, emotional stability, and socioeconomic problems.

The woman may be hospitalized for CNS agitation, acute intoxication, or for alcohol use–related injuries or physical problems. Stabilization of vital signs, rehydration, and nourishment take priority. Hospitalization may be in a psychiatric unit.

The primary focus of care is the woman. Usually she is already acutely aware of the dangers to the fetus resulting from her behavior. Emphasis on the fetus's well-being instead of on her own may add to her guilt, frustration, and low self-esteem.

Evaluation

Attendance and participation in group meetings is one desired outcome. Increased interest in prenatal or postnatal care, improved nutrition and personal hygiene, and abstinence from alcohol are hoped-for outcomes.

Cocaine

The cocaine abuser often has a constellation of cocaine-related problems: family problems, employment difficulties, various health issues, psychologic stress, guilt, and anger (Landry and Smith, 1987). Coexisting psychiatric disorders cloud differential diagnosis. Decreased amounts of **norepinephrine** and **serotonin**, have been implicated in people with biologically based depression. Dysfunction of **serotonin** metabolism is seen in disorders such as violence, rage, and maladaptive behavior. Cocaine raises norepinephrine and serotonin levels rapidly and then depletes them precipitously. Schizophrenics display excessive dopamine levels in some areas of the brain. The biochemical systems of norepinephrine, serotonin, and dopamine play a vital role in mood regulation and mental health; all three systems are affected by cocaine. Diagnostic protocol to distinguish between drug use and drug addiction requires considerable knowledge and is beyond the scope of this text. An appropriate plan of care is designed depending on the diagnosis (i.e., substance use problems or addiction disease) (Landry and Smith, 1987). The focus of this section is the identification of the pregnant cocaine-user and the effects of cocaine on the pregnancy. The care of the cocaine-affected neonate is addressed in Chapter 39.

Assessment

The nurse or physician takes a history of the drug abuse (95% are also addicted to heroin or methadone), type of drug and mode of administration, and participation (if any) in drug programs; assesses the woman's feelings and plans for this pregnancy (infant); and determines the expected date of delivery (EDD).

The social worker or psychiatric social worker is brought in to evaluate the woman's social, economic, home, and ethnic problems; welfare requirements; and educational or vocational status and needs.

Medical Complications. Pregnancy is compromised by cocaine-related medical complications that are encountered by the infrequent, as well as frequent, high-dose user. A variety of less serious medical problems is seen, including lack of energy, insomnia, nasal sinus problems, nosebleeds, sore throat, and decreased libido. More serious problems develop as general health deteriorates. The nasal septum perforates. Cardiovascular stress increases, tachycardia, systemic hypertension, ventricular arrhythmias, sudden coronary artery spasm, and myocardial infarction develop. Cocaine-associated complications also include liver damage, intestinal ischemia, seizures, hemorrhagic bronchitis, headache, and death. Needle-borne diseases such as hepatitis B and AIDS are common. "Tracks," septic phlebitis cellulitis and superficial abscesses are seen in intravenous drug users. Many addicts are poorly nourished and commonly have sexually transmitted diseases. Pulmonary disease with acute pulmonary edema is a commonly encountered complication. A toxicology (urine) screen or other laboratory tests for liver damage and anemia may be ordered when drug use is suspected. An assessment of the woman's support system adds valuable data for developing a plan of care. The presence of any of the medical complications, results of laboratory tests, or signs and symptoms of intoxication or withdrawal (Table 34-4) assist in the identification of substance use problems and addictive disease.

Pregnancy. Cocaine users typically mediate the side effects of cocaine by a CNS depressant such as alcohol (Landry and Smith, 1987). Thus the woman and her fetus are exposed to the risks of cocaine and alcohol. In some areas of the United States it is estimated that 10% of pregnant women use cocaine (Chasnoff, et al., 1986).

Cocaine produces tachycardia and a rise in blood pressure by increasing the levels of catecholamines (Woods, Plessinger, and Clark, 1987). During pregnancy, uterine blood vessels are maximally dilated, but they vasoconstrict readily in the presence of catecholamines. Separation of the placenta (abruption) or acute onset of labor following intravenous cocaine administration is probably secondary to acute spasm of uterine blood vessels (Woods, Plessinger, and Clark, 1987). Use of the drug during pregnancy can lead to small-for-gestational-age neonates and fetal death (Woods, et al, 1987). Neonate addiction is discussed in Chapter 39.

Nursing diagnoses

The following are examples of nursing diagnoses formulated from the assessment data:

- Potential for infection related to
  - Life-style
  - Dehydration and malnutrition
- Nutrition, less than body requirements related to
  - Drug use
- Injury related to
  - Method of administration of drug or effects of drug
- Ineffective individual coping related to
  - Lack of support system
- Self-care deficit, bathing/hygiene related to
  - Effects of drug
- Potential for violence related to
  - Maintenance of drug habit

Planning

A multidisciplinary approach is needed to plan for the care of the expectant mother. In increasing numbers, pregnant cocaine users are seen on maternity units. Their presence and needs present special challenges to nurses. A "standardized" nursing care plan may be best developed by the total team of nurses on the maternity unit. A starting point in the development of a care plan may need to be a values clarification experience (Chapter 2). It is not uncommon for nurses to harbor negative feelings for psychoactive drug users' behaviors. Collaboration with psychiatric nurses may be necessary to augment the maternity nurse's therapeutic potential with these clients. Comprehensive care involves many organizations, child protective services, human resource agencies, and the community health department (Mondanaro, 1987).

Goals

1. Stabilize woman's physiologic status
2. Initiate a maintenance (e.g., methadone) or withdrawal program
3. Instill importance of keeping appointments for prenatal (or postpartum) care for herself and her infant if she is keeping the child
4. Minimize adverse effects on fetus; or ensure care and safety of child

Implementation

The need for **biologic support** may be related to overdose, withdrawal, allergy, or toxicity. Physical deterioration results from the deleterious effects of drugs, including conditions such as malnutrition, dehydration, and various infections. The acute physical condition takes priority over the woman's other health needs.

Interactive interventions are initiated as soon as they are appropriate. The type of interactive intervention is directed toward alleviating the stressors that apply to each individual and identified in the nursing diagnoses. Examples of interactive intervention include group support, client education, or individual counseling. Psychiatric nurses are skilled in intervening in denial, dependency, manipulation, and anger. Other required skills include establishing behavioral contracts and increasing self-esteem.

Social support systems are mobilized. Family counseling, self-help groups, transitional living programs, and community treatment programs are involved. Employee assistance programs are now available in many industries, including hospitals (Clemmer, 1987).

Labor room nurses also need to work out a "standardized" plan for care. Typically the woman displays poor control over her behavior and a low threshold for pain, which is especially noticeable when she is in labor. Increased dependency needs are apparent. Intoxication or withdrawal signs and symptoms (Table 34-4) may challenge the staff. Evidence of poor hygiene, nutrition, and fluid balance are usually present.

The management of cocaine detoxification and treatment of addictive disease are beyond the scope of this text.

Evaluation

Evaluation is difficult because the long-range effects cannot be projected. On the short-term basis, noting that the care given to the woman and baby is the best that was possible may be the only gratification the nurse will have.

Opioid: Heroin

Assessment

Assessment of opioid use is similar to that for alcohol and cocaine use. Interview and open discussion may disclose the problem and its extent (e.g., length of addiction, amount needed in cost per day). Physical examination reveals intravenous tracks, cellulitis, and surface abscesses at the administration sites. Further assessment of the peripheral vascular system may reveal burning paresthesia or decreased or absent peripheral pulses (or both) in the extremity used for self-injection. Signs of sexually transmitted diseases (STDs) and urinary tract infections (UTIs) are often present.

Laboratory tests are ordered for toxicology, STDs, hepatitis B, and AIDS antibody. BUN, serum creatinine, total protein levels, albumin-to-globulin ratio, total iron-binding capacity, hemoglobin, and hematocrit values are obtained. Chest x-ray study may be ordered for pulmonary disease. Hilar lymphadenopathy in 95% of addicts, pulmonary edema, bacterial pneumonia, and foreign body emboli (from the substances used to "cut" street drugs) may be revealed.

Initial and serial ultrasound studies are used to determine gestational age because amenorrhea, common among drug users, precludes dating by history of last menstrual period (LMP). However, nonstress and stress testing are not too helpful in assessing fetal well-bing. The addicted fetus is nonreactive. Estriol measurements are inaccurate. The opioid-addicted woman is more likely to experience premature rupture of membranes (PROM) and preterm labor.

Nursing Diagnoses

The following are examples of nursing diagnoses formulated from the assessment data:

- Chronic low self-esteem related to
  - Life-style
- Altered nutrition, less than body requirements, related to
  - Depressed appetite
- Potential for infection related to
  - Intravenous drug use and associated conditions (e.g., poor hygiene, poor nutrition)
- Impaired social interaction related to
  - Dependency needs
- Potential altered parenting related to
  - Lack of social support system

Planning

Planning for care is similar to that which is utilized for women who abuse alcohol and cocaine.

Goals

1. Stabilize woman's physiologic status
2. Instill importance of keeping appointments for prenatal (or postpartum) care
3. Minimize adverse effects on fetus, or ensure care and safety of infant

Implementation

Biologic support to stabilize the physiologic status takes priority. Treatment for intoxication or withdrawal signs (Table 34-4) is provided as necessary. Malnutrition, dehydration, infections, and injuries require immediate attention.

Interactive interventions are directed toward strengthening egos and instilling self-confidence. Dependence needs to be converted to positive supportive mechanisms. Treatment of heroin (or methadone) addiction requires trained professional support. During the prenatal and postpartum periods, initiation of or maintenance in a methadone program is appropriate. In general, the fetus cannot tolerate withdrawal by maternal detoxification and abstinence. The mother will require considerable supervision and assistance with the care of herself and newborn (see care described under psychosocial condition, p. 864).

Social support systems must be mobilized. Methadone maintenance programs provide some of this support. Other community resources must be involved.

Care during labor is critical. Fetal tachycardia and increased fetal activity are indicators of the onset of fetal withdrawal. Fetal withdrawal must be prevented by administering heroin or methadone as required. Any form of anesthesia can be used for delivery. Staffing should be sufficient to ensure strict surveillance of visitors to prevent unsupervised drug administration.

Advice regarding **breast-feeding** is individualized. Small amounts of methadone appear in breast milk and the baby's eating and safety needs must of course be considered. Breast-feeding necessitates a closeness between the mother and child, and the baby may be more irritable and difficult to console. These women, who are already in a fragile state with depleted energy reserves and coping capability, commonly experience severe emotional decompensation. This can be aggravated by breast-feeding and care of the infant, which are exhausting under ideal circumstances. For some women the need to breast-feed and care for the infant provides the impetus to break the habit. Community health agencies may be mobilized for home supervision or guidance in antepartum and infant care or for putting the infant up for adoption. Day-night-center care programs or halfway houses may be indicated.

Discharge planning should begin with the first contact with the woman. If she is to be discharged to the care of her parents, several nursing actions may be employed. The client is involved in decision making whenever possible. The mother is involved with the care of her infant when she is willing. Mother-child attachment is promoted. Angry, argumentative encounters between the mother and nurse are avoided; the nurse needs to respond with patience, sympathy, consistency, and at times, with firmness. The mother's positive maternal responses and feelings are supported even if she is relinquishing her infant for adoption.

Evaluation

Short-term positive achievements are indicators of success (e.g., if the mother keeps her appointments or learns to diaper the baby). It is not reasonable to expect to see evidence of significant strides, such as complete abstinence from drugs and assumption of adult maturity behaviors within a short period of time.

POVERTY

The very poor, the social class of people who consistently live at or below the poverty level, are in a perpetual state of despair. Their limited skills give them no bargaining power in the job market. Education needed to improve their status is beyond them. The poor desire a better life for their children but are trapped in a circular pattern that perpetuates their condition. Their powerlessness to control their fate or condition is a source of fatalism and resignation that is characteristic of the group in general. This fatalistic attitude is a significant impediment to occupational and educational aspirations and to seeking health care (Whaley and Wong, 1987).

The term **poverty** implies both visible and invisible impoverishment. *Visible poverty* refers to lack of money or material resources, which includes insufficient clothing, poor sanitation, and deteriorating housing. *Invisible poverty* refers to social and cultural deprivation such as limited employment opportunities, inferior educational opportunities, lack of or inferior medical services and health-care facilities, and an absence of public services (Spector, 1979).

Factors Related to Poverty

One factor that notably affects women is **employment and wage discrimination.** Poverty and undue stress occur in response to the discrimination and exploitation that women experience in paid employment. Most seriously affected are the swelling numbers of single-parent families headed by women (Griffith-Kenney, 1986).

Throughout the United States are groups of people, geographically segregated, who constitute what is known as "pockets of poverty." These are seen in the dense urban areas, such as the ghettos, and many rural areas, especially those that are geographically isolated from needed facilities and services. The nonurbanized regions identified as poverty areas in the United States are Appalachia, the deep South, the lower Southwest, and northern New England (Spector, 1979).

Certain **ethnic or racial groups** are overrepresented in the impoverished population. The most obvious of these are the blacks, Hispanics, and Native Americans.

Migrant Families

One of the most disadvantaged groups is migrant farm workers and their families. The low position of these families on the economic scale and their rootless, mobile existence subject them to inadequate sanitation, substandard housing, social isolation, and lack of educational opportunities and medical services. This is especially deleterious to the mothers and children. Health care is generally inadequate. Families are apt to live in a number of localities in the course of a year with no continuity in what health care is available. Pesticides and herbicides have been identified as mutagenic and teratogenic. Since both parents work in the fields, both are exposed to potential mutagens; the women may be exposed to teratogens during pregnancy. Accident rates are high and meals may be erratic.

Some migrants have a home base to which they return at the end of a growing season; others travel continuously, migrating north in summer and south in winter. With most there is little if any integration into the dominant culture; therefore migrant groups suffer social isolation. Groups who travel together, especially those with the same ethnic background, develop a cohesiveness and form their own set of values and customs. Sometimes a migrant family will leave the migration stream and become a part of a permanent community. However, this involves adaptation to a new environment and life-style that can be stress provoking to these families (Whaley and Wong, 1987).

Preventive Health Care

The vulnerability of economically and socially deprived persons in our society to health problems is apparent across the spectrum of health care from prevention to rehabilitation. Preventive health is more than the prevention of disease states. It involves those factors in an individual's life that protect the individual and allow for growth and development of potential. Adequate clothing and shelter, proper nutrition, education, a safe environment, all taken for granted by the economically advantaged, are noticeably lacking in the health experience of many low-income groups.

The concept of preventive health is often missing. The development of a concept of preventive health begins in childhood as the child is directed and encouraged to "eat your dinner and grow up to be a strong boy," "clean your teeth," "go to the doctor for a checkup," and "get enough sleep." These repeated admonitions eventually result in a concept of health care that includes prevention as well as cure. For women who have experienced this indoctrination, acceptance of the necessity for prenatal care comes more readily. For those women who have only gone to a physician when they were very ill, the relative health of the pregnant state precludes full use of care available. For some low-income women a choice between prenatal care (preparation for birth) and providing their families with necessities results in their foregoing prenatal care.

In some communities clinics have been established specifically for high-risk mothers and their infants. Adolescent mothers and premature infants make up a large part of the client population at these clinics. Although prevention of the problem is probably the best approach, follow-up care is of great importance. For migrant workers, continuity in care is not likely. Helping mothers develop parenting skills will do much to promote the optimum growth and development of these disadvantaged children. Nursing and nurse-researchers are in the forefront of efforts to provide care for childbearing families.

Pregnancy Outcomes

The differences in pregnancy outcomes related to socioeconomic class have been well documented for over half a century. Studies have consistently demonstrated a relationship between economic class and maternal and infant morbidity and mortality. These discrepancies have been of major concern to nursing groups as they have attempted to improve the health and well-being of all individuals in society. Researchers have repeatedly identified two recurrent factors that predispose low-income women to poor pregnancy outcomes (Osofsky and Kendall, 1973). The first relates to reproductive experience of the women and the second to the specific obstetric and neonatal complications involved.

Reproductive Experience

Low-income individuals tend to begin reproducing at an earlier age and to end at a later age than other women. In addition, they have many pregnancies, and these are adversely affected by the close spacing of the gestations. Birch and Gussons (1970) describes this phenomenon as "too young, too old, and too often." Maternal age and parity are implicated in perinatal mortality. There is increased risk to the fetus, infant, and mother when the mother is at either extreme of age or parity. Prematurity and its complications remain the chief causes in perinatal mortality. Low-income mothers are more likely to give birth to premature infants than are mothers in the population at large.

Complications

Low-income mothers are more predisposed to intercurrent illness and obstetric complications during pregnancy. Obstetric complications such as placenta previa, abruptio placentae, and placental insufficiency often result in preterm births or small-for-gestational-age babies and subsequent infant difficulties. Many obstetric complications have life-threatening consequences for the mother as well as for the infant. Examples of complications include hemorrhage, cardiac disease, or uncontrolled infection.

The problems faced by low-income mothers have direct implication for nursing service. At present much of our current knowledge could be used to ameliorate or prevent the occurrence of the problems. One of the prerequisites to providing assistance to the low-income mother is to bring her into the health care system.

SUMMARY

Pathophysiology, medical treatment, and nursing care of several disorders are presented in this chapter. The chapter dicusses the knowledge base for understanding various disorders to assist the nurse in implementing the nursing process with problems that occur during pregnancy. A general knowledge of medical-surgical and mental health nursing is invaluable to the maternity nurse. As always, sensitivity to the woman and her family during the childbearing experience that is complicated by a physical or psychosocial disorder is as important as expert technologic assistance.

KEY CONCEPTS

- The stress of normal maternal adaptations to pregnancy on a heart whose function is already taxed may cause cardiac decompensation.
- Anemia, the most common medical disorder of pregnancy, affects at least 20% of pregnant women.
- The chance of developing adult respiratory distress syndrome (ARDS) increases with the amount of trauma experienced during pregnancy or delivery.
- Autoimmune disorders (e.g., systemic lupus erythematosus, myasthenia gravis) have a predilection for women in their reproductive years, therefore associations with pregnancy are not uncommon.
- In the gravida, an enlarged uterus, displaced internal organs, and altered laboratory values may confound differential diagnosis when the need for immediate abdominal surgery occurs.
- Preoperative care for a pregnant woman differs from

that for a nonpregnant woman in one significant aspect: the presence of at least one other person, the fetus.

- Psychosocial conditions that may complicate childbearing can interfere with family integration and restrict bonding with the infant.
- Developing a nursing care plan for women who are dependent on psychoactive substances may be most therapeutic if it is a collaborative effort of the total health delivery team following a values clarification experience.
- Low-income mothers are more predisposed to intercurrent illness and obstetric complications during the childbearing cycle.

STUDY QUESTIONS AND ACTIVITIES

1. Visit a high-risk or free prenatal clinic. Assess the risk factors for the clients. What nursing actions may alleviate potential complications for the low-income client? What is the reproductive history of the low-income client?
2. Discover resources in your community that offer financial, counseling, or educational services to pregnant clients with heart disease. What criteria must the client meet to be eligible for service? Interview a staff member and report your findings back to your group.
3. It is difficult to remain objective with substance abuse clients, especially when fetal damage occurs. Activities to raise the awareness might include inviting a speaker from a community agency or half-way house, attending a self-help group meeting, or role-playing two situations:
   a. A nurse caring for a drug-dependent mother who has given birth to an addicted infant.
   b. The same nurse expressing her feelings to a peer. Have the group discuss the implications for effective nursing care.
4. Follow a pregnant client through the perioperative phase. Discuss what considerations were given to the client's obstetric needs and what measures were taken to protect the fetus.
5. Through research and interviews, determine what percentage of the women delivering at your clinical facility have had no prenatal care.

References

Cardiovascular Disorders

Cregler, LL, and Mark, H: Cardiovascular dangers of cocaine abuse, Am J Cardio 57:1185, May, 1986

Danforth, DN, and Scott, JR, editors: Obstetrics and Gynecology, ed 5, Philadelphia, 1986, JB Lippincott Co

Demakis, JG, and Rahimtoola, SH: Peripartum cardiomyopathy, Circulation 44:964, 1971

Metcalf, J, McAnulty, JH, and Ueland, K: Burwell and Metcalfe's Heart disease and pregnancy: physiology and management ed 2, Boston, 1986, Little, Brown & Co, Inc

Pritchard, J, MacDonald, P, and Gant, N: Williams Obstetrics, ed 17, New York, 1985, Appleton-Century-Crofts

Roberts, SL, and Chestnut, DH: Anesthesia for the obstetric patient with cardiac disease, Clin Obstet Gynecol 30(3):601, 1987

Neurologic Disorders

Aminoff, MJ: Neurological disorders and pregnancy, Am J Obstet Gynecol 132:325, 1978

Axel, SJ: Spinal cord injured women's concerns: menstruation and pregnancy, Rehab Nurs 7(5):10, 1982

Craig, DI: Adaptation to pregnancy by spinal cord injured women. Unpublished research for MSN degree requirement, University of San Diego, 1985

Goller, H, and Paeslack, V: our experiences about pregnancy and delivery of the paraplegic woman, Paraplegia, 8:161, 1971

Goller, H, and Paeslack, V: Pregnancy damage and birth complications of paraplegic women, Paraplegia, 10:213, 1972

Hilsinger, RL, et al: Idiopathic facial paralysis, pregnancy, and the menstrual cycle, Ann Otol Rhinol Laryngol 84:433, 1975

Ohry, A, Peleg, D, Goldman, J, et al: Sexual function, pregnancy and delivery in spinal cord injured women, Gyn Obstet Invest 9(6):281, 1978

Sarbin, TR, and Allen VL: Role theory. In Lindzey G, and Aronson, E, editors: The handbook of social psychology, Vol 1, ed 2, Reading, Mass, 1968, Addison-Wesley Publishing Co, Inc

Tabsh, KMA, Brinkman, CR, III, and Reff, RA: Autonomic dysreflexia in pregnancy, Obstet Gynecol 60(1):119, 1982

Young, BK, Kutz, M, and Klein, SA: Pregnancy after spinal cord injury: altered maternal and fetal responses to labor, Obstet Gynecol 62(1):59, 1983

Autoimmune Diseases

Baum, J: Arthritis and pregnancy, Contemp OB/GYN 23(3):97, 1984

Cecere, FA, and Persellin, RH: The interaction of pregnancy and the rheumatic diseases, Clin Rheum Dis 7:747, 1981

Danforth, DN, and Scott, JR, editors: Obstetrics and gynecology, ed 5, Philadelphia, 1986, JB Lippincott Co

Nolten, WE, and Rueckert, PA: Elevated free cortisol index in pregnancy: possible regulatory mechanism, Am J Obstet Gynecol 139:492, 1981

Persellin, RH: Inhibitors of inflammatory and immune responses in pregnancy serum, Clin Rheum Dis 7:769, 1981

Surgery During Pregnancy

Phipps, WJ, Long, BC, and Woods, NF: Medical-surgical nursing: concepts and clinical practice ed 3, St Louis, 1987, The CV Mosby Co.

Tucker, SM, et al, editors: Patient care standards, ed 4, St Louis, 1988, The CV Mosby Co

Injuries

Higgins, SD: Caring for the injured pregnant patient, Contemp Obstet Gynecol 21(3):32, 1983 (special issue)

Rothenberger, D: Blunt maternal trauma: a review of 103 cases, J Trauma 18:173, 1978

Smith, LG, and Payne, T: Pregnant trauma victims, Am J Nurs 84:14, 1984

Emotional Disturbance

Affonso, D: Postpartum depression, In Fields, P, editor: Recent advances in perinatal nursing, New York, 1984, Churchill Livingstone

American Psychiatric Association: Diagnostic and statistical manual of mental disorders, ed 3, Washington, DC, 1980, The Association

American Psychiatric Association: Draft of the DSM-III-R in Development (subject to change), as proposed by the Work Group to Revise DSM-III. American Psychiatric Association, October 1985

Edlund, MJ, and Craig, TJ: Antipsychotic drug use and birth defects: an epidemiologic reassessment, *Compr Psychiatry* 25:32, 1984

Gelder, M: Hormones and postpartum depression. In Sandler, M, editor: Mental illness in pregnancy and the puerperium, New York, 1978, Oxford University Press

Hauser, LA: Pregnancy and psychiatric drugs. *Hosp Community Psychiatry* 36:817, 1985

Hayworth, J, Little, BC, Bonham Carter, S, et al: A predictive study of postpartum depression: some predisposing characteristics *Br J Medical Psychology* 1980; 53:161-167

Herzog, A, and Detre, T: Psychotic reactions associated with childbirth, Dis Nerv Sys 37:229, 1976

Hurt, LD, and Ray, CP: Postpartum disorders: mother-infant bonding on a psychiatric unit, J Psychosocial Nurs 23(2):15, 1985

Ketai, RM, and Marvin, AB: Childbirth-related psychosis and familial symbiotic conflict, *Am J Psychiatry* 136:190, 1979

Spielvogel, A, and Wile, J: Treatment of the psychotic pregnant patient, Psychosomtics 27(7):487, 1986

Stuart, GW, and Sundeen, SJ: Principles and practice of psychiatric nursing, ed 3, St Louis, 1987, The CV Mosby Co

Tentoni, S, and High, K: Culturally induced postpartum depression, JOGN Nurs 9:246, July/Aug 1980

Vorhees, CV, Brunner, RL, and Butcher, RE: Psychotropic drugs as behavioral teratogens, *Science* 205:1220, 1979

Weiner, A: Childbirth related psychiatric illness, Compr Psychiatry 25:143, 1982

Psychoactive Substance Use

Bodendorfer, TW, et al: Obtaining drug exposure histories during pregnancy, Am J Obstet Gynecol 135:490, 1979

Chasnoff, I, et al: Cocaine use in pregnancy, N Engl J of Med 313(11):666, 1985

Clemmer, J: When an addicted nurse comes back to work, RN, p 62, Oct 1987

Danforth, DN, and Scott, JR, editors: Obstetrics and gynecology, ed 5, Philadelphia, 1986, JB Lippincott Co

Finnegan, LP, and Macnew, BA: Nursing care of the addicted infant, Am J Nurs 74:685, 1974

Landry, M, and Smith, DE: Crack: anatomy of an addiction, part 2. Calif Nurs Rev 9(3):28, 1987

Mondanaro, J: Strategies for AIDS prevention: motivating health behavior in drug dependent women, J Psychoactive Drugs 19(2):143, 1987

Stuart, GW, and Sundeen, SJ: Principles and practice of psychiatric nursing, ed 3, St Louis, 1987, The CV Mosby Co

Woods, JR, Plessinger, MA, and Clark, KE: Effect of cocaine on uterine blood flow and fetal oxygenation, JAMA 257:957, 1987

Poverty

Birch, HG, and Gussons, JD: Disadvantaged children: health, nutrition, and failure, New York, 1970, Harcourt Brace & World

Griffith-Kenny, J: Contemporary women's health: a nursing advocacy approach, Menlo Park, Calif, 1986, Addison-Wesley Publishing Co

Osofsky, HJ, and Kendall, N: Poverty as a criterion of risk, Clin Obstet Gynecol 16:103, 1973

Spector, RE: Cultural diversity in health and illness, New York, 1979, Appleton-Century-Crofts

Whaley, LF, and Wong, DL: Nursing of infants and children, ed 3, St Louis, 1987, The CV Mosby Co

Bibliography

Cardiovascular Disorders

Charache, S, et al: Management of sickle cell disease in pregnant patients, Obstet Gynecol 55:407, 1980

Clark, SL: Actions of cardiac drugs during pregnancy, Contemp OB/GYN 30(2):65, 1987

Devees, CB: Hematologic disorders in pregancy, Nurs Clin North Am 17(1):57, 1982

Eikayam, U, et al: Interface: treating arrhythmias of pregnancy, Contemp OB/GYN 23(6):55, 1984

Eilen, B, et al: Aortic valve replacement in the third trimester of pregnancy: case report and reviews of the literature, Obstet Gynecol 57:119, 1981

Fahey, VA: An in-depth look at deep vein thrombosis, Nurs '84 14(3):34, 1984

Gardezi, N: Cardiovascular effects of cocaine, JAMA 257(7):979, 1987

Hankins, GD: Invasive cardiovascular monitoring: an update, Contemp OB/GYN 27:114, Nov 1985

Lavery, JP: When coagulopathy threatens the pregnant patient, Contemp OB/GYN 20(1):190, 1982

Lehmann, D, and Chism, J: Pregnancy outcome in medically complicated and uncomplicated patients aged 40 years or older, Am J Obstet Gynecol 157(3):738, 1987

Masoorli, ST, and Piercy, S: A step-by-step guide to troublefree transfusions, RN 47(5):34, 1984

Morrison, JC, et al: Prophylactic transfusions in pregnant patients with sickle hemoglobinopathies: benefit versus risk, Obstet Gynecol 56:274, 1980

Morrison, JC, et al: Therapy for the pregnant patient with sickle hemoglobinopathies: a national focus, Am J Obstet Gynecol 144:268, 1982

Nagey, DA, et al: Isovolumetric partial exchange transfusion in the management of sickle cell disease in pregnancy. II. Simplified ambulatory technique, Am J Obstet Gynecol 147:693, 1983

Odio, A: Resurgence of acute rheumatic fever, N Eng J Med 317(8):507 1987

Richardson, EA, and Milne, LS: Sickle-cell disease and the childbearing family: an update, MCN 8:417, 1983

Shime, J, et al: Congenital heart disease in pregnancy: Short- and long-term implications, Am J Obstet Gynecol 156(2):313, 1987

Ship-Horowitz, T: Nursing care of the sickle cell anemic patient in labor, JOGN Nurs 12(6):381, 1983

Sullivan, JM, and Ramanathan, KB: Management of medical problems in pregnancy—severe cardiac disease, N Eng J Med 313(5):304, 1985

Woods, JR, Plessinger, MA, and Clark, KE: Effect of cocaine on uterine blood flow and fetal oxygenation, JAMA 257(7):957, 1987

Pulmonary Disorders

Boucher, M, et al: Adult respiratory distress syndrome: a rare manifestation of *Listeria monocytogenes* infection in pregnancy, Am J Obstet Gynecol 149(6):686, 1984

Holbreich, M: Care of the asthmatic during pregnancy, Contemp OB/GYN 21(4):155, 1983

Wotring, KE: Adult respiratory distress syndrome as a complication of pregnancy, MCN 4:314, 1979

Gastrointestinal Disorders

Braverman, DZ, et al: Effects of pregnancy and contraceptive steroids on gallbladder function, N Engl J Med 302:362, 1980

Everson, GT, et al: A critical evaluation of real-time ultrasonography for the study of gallbladder volume and contraction, Gastroenterology 79:40, 1980
Johnston, WG, and Baskett, TG: Obstetric cholestasis: a 14 year review, Am J Obstet/Gynecol 133:299, 1979
Problem-patient conference: when liver disease complicates pregnancy, Contemp OB/GYN 22(3):59, 1983
Raptopoulos, U, et al: Comparison of real-time and grey-scale static ultrasonic cholecystography, Radiology 140:153, 1981
Simeone, JF, and Ferrucci, JT: New trends in gallbladder imaging, JAMA 246:380, 1981
Stauffer, RA, et al: Gallbladder disease in pregnancy, Am J Obstet/Gynecol 144:661, 1982

Integumentary Disorders

Wade, TR, et al: Skin changes and diseases associated with pregnancy, Obstet/Gynecol 52:233, 1978

Neurologic Disorders

Aminoff, MJ: Neurological disorders and pregnancy, Am J Obstet/Gynecol 132:325, 1978
Birk, K, and Rudick, R: Pregnancy and multiple sclerosis, Arch Neurol 43:719, July 1986
Burns, A, Burks, JS, and Franklin, GM: The effects of pregnancy in multiple sclerosis: a retrospective study, Neurology 36(8):1097, 1986
Conley, NJ, and Olshanski, E: Current controversies in pregnancy and epilepsy: a unique challenge to nursing, JOGN Nurs 16(5):321, 1987
Dansky, LV, et al: Anticonvulsants, folate levels, and pregnancy outcome: a prospective study, Ann Neurol 21(2):176, 1987
Donaldson, JO: Neurology of pregnancy, Major Probl Neurol 7:(whole issue), 1978
Drachman, DB: Present and future treatment of myasthenia gravis, N Engl J Med 316(12):743, 1987
Gibbs, CE: Sudden sensorium derangement during pregnancy, Contemp OB/GYN 20(1):452, 1982
Greenland, VC, and Young, BK: The mother who has a spinal cord injury, Contemp OB/GYN 24(2):201, 1984
Greenspoon, JS, and Paul, RH: Paraplegia and quadriplegia: special considerations during pregnancy and labor and delivery, Am J Obstet Gynecol 155(4):738, 1986
Hilsinger, RL, et al: Idiopathic facial paralysis, pregnancy, and the menstrual cycle, Ann Otol Rhinol Laryngol 84:433, 1975
Levine, SE, and Keesey, MC: Successful plasmapheresis for fulminant myasthenia gravis during pregnancy, Arch Neurol 43:197, Feb 1986
McGregor, JA, and Meeuwsen, J: Autonomic hyperreflexia: a mortal danger for spinal cord-damaged women in labor, Am J Obstet Gynecol 151:330, 1985
Nazir, M: When myotonic dystrophy complicates pregnancy, Med Aspects Human Sexuality 21(8):72, 1978
Plum, F, editor: Benign encephalopathy of pregnancy, Neurology Alert 5(3):9, 1986
Weisz, RR: Facial paralysis in a pregnant woman, Clini-Pearls 7(1):5, 1984

Autoimmune Disorders

Baum, J: Arthritis and pregnancy, Contemp OB/GYN 23(3):97, 1984
Cecere, FA, and Persellin, RH: The interaction of pregnancy and the rheumatic diseases, Clin Rheum Dis 7:747, 1981
Chez, RA, and Rizzuto, RS: When your patient develops rheumatoid arthritis, Contemp OB/GYN 23(3):77, 1984
Karacic, B: Antepartal nursing management of Grave's disease, JOGN Nurs 15(3):214, 1986
Linos, A, et al: Case-control study of rheumatoid arthritis and prior use of oral contraceptives, Lancet 1:1299, 1983
Nass, T: Helping the patient who has lupus, RN, 69, Oct, 1987
Nolten, WE, and Rueckert, PA: Elevated free cortisol index in pregnancy: possible regulatory mechanism, Am J Obstet Gynecol 139:492, 1981
Persellin, RH: Inhibitors of inflammatory and immune responses in pregnancy serum, Clin Rheum Dis 7:769, 1981
Petri, M: Outcomes encouraging in mothers with lupus, Contemp OB/GYN 31(3):103, 1988
Unger, A, et al: Disease activity and pregnancy associated alpha-2-glycoprotein in rheumatoid arthritis during pregnancy, Br Med J 286:750, 1983

Surgical Conditions

Bremer, C, and Cassata, L: Trauma in pregnancy, Nurs Clin North Am 21(4):705, 1986
Buchsbaum, HJ: Accidental injury in pregnancy, Contemp OB/GYN 20(1):26, 1982
Cameron, S: OB staff alert, Can Nurse 75:30, Nov, 1979
Clinical News: Pregnant trauma victims, Am J Nurs 84(1):14, 1984
DeVore, GR: Finding causes of nonobstetric abdominal pain in pregnancy, Contemp OB/GYN 24(2):19, 1984
Droegemueller, W, et al: Comprehensive gynecology, St Louis, 1987, The CV Mosby Co
Foster, CA: The pregnant trauma patient, RN 14(11):58, 1984
Fraulini, KE, and Murphy, P: REACT—a new system for measuring postanesthesia recovery, Nurs '84 14(4):101, 1984
Golan, A: Trauma in late pregnancy: a report of 15 cases, South African Med J 57:161, Feb 1980
Lee, TC, and Mariner, DR: When you have to remove the appendix, Contemp OB/GYN 21:42, March 1983 (special issue)
Nursing '87 Books: 1987 Nursing photobook annual, Springhouse, Penn, 1987, Springhouse Corp
Weeks, DD, et al: When leukemia complicates pregnancy, MCN 13(1):28, 1988

Emotional Complications

Beelman, MS: Husband fights postpartum conviction: trying to educate lawmakers about wife's 'baby blues' that led to killing, San Francisco Examiner, Sunday, May 10, 1987
Carmack, BJ, and Corwin, TA: Nursing care of the schizophrenic maternity patient during labor, MCN 5:107, 1980
Dal Pozzo, EE, and Marsh, FH: Psychosis and pregnancy: some new ethical and legal dilemmas for the physician, Am J Obstet Gynecol 156(2):425, 1987
Fisher, LY: Nursing management of the pregnant psychotic patient during labor and delivery JOGN Nurs 17(1):25, 1988
Fisher, LY: Care of the pregnant psychotic patient, Calif Nurs 82(3):4, 1986
Focusing on today's issues in perinatal care: postpartum depression (commentary by Niles Newton), ICEA Rev 4:2, 1980
Hans, A: Postpartum assessment: the psychological component JOGN Nurs 15(1):49, 1986
Koplan, CR: The use of psychotropic drugs during pregnancy and nursing in Bassuk E, Schoonover, S, Gelenberg A, et al, editors: The practitioner's guide to psychoactive drugs, New York, 1983, Plenum Publishing Corp
Lagerlof, JM: Maternal fetal "conflict": balancing our values, Calif Nurs Rev p 34, Jan/Feb, 1988

Linden, S, and Rich, CL: The use of lithium during pregnancy and lactation, J Clin Psychiatry 44:358, 1983
Malasanos, L, et al: Assessment of mental status. In Health assessment, ed 3, St Louis, 1987, The CV Mosby Co
McNeil, TF, Jaij, L, and Malmquist-Larsson, A: Women with non-organic psychosis: mental disturbance during pregnancy, Acta Psychiatr Scand 70: 127, 1984
Nurnberg, HG: Treatment of mania in the last six months of pregnancy, Hosp Comm Psychiatry 31:122, 1980
Petrick, J: Postpartum depression: identification of high-risk mothers JOGN Nurs 13(1):37, 1984
Slayton, RI, and Soloff, PH: Psychotic denial of third-trimester pregnancy, J Clin Psychiatry 42:471, 1981
True-Soderstrom, B, et al: Postpartum depression, Matern Child Nurs J 3:109, 1983
Weinberg, PC, and Turnbull, JM: When to refer psychiatric emergencies, Contemp OB/GYN 22(5):246, 1983
Zajicek, E: Psychiatric problems during pregnancy. In Wolkind, S, and Zajicek, E, editors: Pregnancy, A Psychological and Social Study London, 1981, Academic Press

Psychoactive Substance Use

Alexander, LL: The pregnant smoker: nursing implications, JOGN Nurs 16(3):167, 1987
Amaro, H, Beckman, L, and Mays, V: A comparison of black and white women entering alcoholism treatment, J Studies of Alcohol 48(3):220, 1987
Bingue, N, Fuch, M, Diaz, V, et al: Teratogenicity of cocaine in humans, J Pediatr 110:93, 1987
Chasnoff, IJ, Burns, WJ, and Schnoll, SH: Cocaine use in pregnancy, N Engl J Med 313:666, 1985
Chasnoff, IJ: Cocaine use in pregnancy: perinatal morbidity and mortality, Neurobehav Toxicol Teratol, 1987 (in press)
Chasnoff, IJ, Bussey, ME, Savich, R, et al: Perinatal cerebral infarction and maternal cocaine use, J Pediatr 108:456, 1986
Damjanov, I: Metronidazole and alcohol in pregnancy, JAMA 256(4):472, 1986
Dixon, SD, Coen, RW, and Crutchfield, S: Visual dysfunction in cocaine-exposed infants (abstract), Pediatr Res 21:359, 1987
Estep, R: The influence of the family on the use of alcohol and prescription depressants by women J Psychoactive Drugs 19(2):171, 1987
Fox, N, Habel, R, and Sexton, MJ: Alcohol consumption among pregnant smokers: effects of a smoking cessation intervention program, Am J Public Health 77(2):211, 1987
Hingson, R, et al: Maternal marijuana use and neonatal outcome: uncertainty posed by self-reports, Am J Public Health 76(6):667 1986
Jessup, M, and Green, JR: Treatment of the pregnant alcohol-dependent woman, J Psychoactive Drugs 19(2):193, 1987
Liporati, NC, and Chychula, LH: How you can really help the drug-abusing patient, Nurs '82 12:46, June 1982
Madden JD, Payne TF, and Miller, S: Maternal cocaine abuse and effect on the newborn, Pediatrics 77:209, 1986
Mittleman, HS, Mittleman, RE, and Elser, B: Cocaine, Am J Nurs 84:1092, Sept 1984
Morningstar, PJ, and Chitwood, DA: How women and men get cocaine: sex-role stereotypes and acquisition patterns, J Psychoactive Drugs 19(2):135, 1987
NAACOG: Pregnancy and alcohol: a hazardous mix, NAACOG Newsletter 15(3):1, 1988
Niven, RG: Adolescent drug abuse, Hosp Community Psychiatry 37:596, June 1986
Oro, AS, and Dixon, SD: Perinatal cocaine and methamphetamine exposure: maternal and noenatal correlates, J Pediatr 111(4):571, 1987
Reed, BG: Developing women-sensitive drug dependence treatment services: why so difficult? J Psychoactive Drugs 19(2):151, 1987
Ronkin, S, et al: Protecting mother and fetus from narcotic abuse, Contemp OB/GYN 31(3):178, 1988
Rosenbaum, M, and Murphy, S: Not the picture of health: women on methadone, J Psychoactive Drugs 19(2):217, 1987
Ryan, L, and Erlichs, FL: Outcome of infants born to cocaine using drug dependent women, Pediatr Res 20:338, 1986
Silver, H, et al: Addiction in pregnancy: high risk intrapartum management and outcome, J Perinatol 793):178, 1987
Sward, S: The 'next hit' came before baby: cocaine overwhelms the maternal instinct in addicted women, San Francisco Chronicle, PB3, March 18, 1988, p. B3.
The health consequences of smoking for women: a report of the Surgeon General, Pub No 410-889/1284, Washington, DC, 1983, Department of Health and Human Services
Woods, JR, Plessinger, MA, and Clark, KE: Effects of cocaine in uterine blood flow and fetal oxygenation, JAMA 257:957, 1987
Zacharias, J: A rational approach to drug use in pregnancy, JOGN Nurs 12(3):183, 1983
Zuspan, FP: When drugs and alcohol complicate pregnancy, Contemp OB/GYN 24(1):35, 1984

Poverty

Carter, ER: Quality maternity care for the medically indigent, MCN 11(2):85, 1986
Curry, MA: Nurses study effects of cuts on access to prenatal care, Am Nurs 15:1, 1983
Fogel, CT, and Woods, NF: Health care of women, St Louis, 1983, The CV Mosby Co
Johnson, SH: Nursing assessment and strategies for the family at risk: high-risk parenting, ed 2, Philadelphia, 1986, JB Lippincott Co
Kotelchuck, M: WIC participation and pregnancy outcomes: Massachusettes Statewide Evaluation Project, Am J Pub Health 74:10, Oct 1984
Moleti, CA: Caring for socially high-risk pregnant women, MCN 13(1):24, 1988
Thompson, P: Health promotion with immigrant women: a model for success, Can Nurse, p 20, Dec 1987

CHAPTER 35

Adolescent Sexuality, Pregnancy, and Parenthood

Learning Objectives

Correctly define the key terms listed.

Discuss dynamics of adolescent sexual development.

Explain the decision tree for adolescent sexual decision making.

Examine the incidence and cost of adolescent pregnancy and parenthood.

Compare and contrast the developmental tasks of adolescence and of pregnancy.

Compare and contrast the nutritional needs of the nonpregnant, pregnant, and lactating adolescent.

Describe assessment.

Formulate nursing diagnoses, plan of care, and goals.

Review implementation and evaluation of nursing care.

Discuss nursing care of the adolescent father.

Key Terms

risk-taking behavior
denial
developmental tasks
sexual decision-making tree
physiologic consequences
personal costs
public costs
readiness for childbearing
parenting abilities
infant responsiveness

Adolescents view their world in far different terms than do adults. Much of adolescent behavior consists of experimenting with a variety of activities, many potentially perilous, including sex, substance abuse, and violence (Greydanus, 1987; Goleman, 1987). The combination of thrill-seeking, inability to perceive risks in a situation, and the need to impress peers is a deadly combination (Goleman, 1987). In the United States the adolescent population is the only one that has not experienced improvement in health status (Blum, 1987); it is the only age group with an increasing mortality (Greydanus, 1987).

Violence has replaced communicable diseases as the primary cause of adolescent mortality. Over 77% of deaths in this age group are the result of accidents, suicide, and homicide (Blum, 1987; Litt, 1987). Increasing poverty (Burke, 1986; Rosenbaum and Starfield, 1986), life-style, and risk-taking behaviors are implicated in adolescent morbidity, with associated sequelae of trauma, adolescent pregnancy, substance abuse, and other major health problems (Blum, 1987). Participation in **risk-taking behaviors** is difficult to understand. Indulgence in these behaviors must be considered within the dynamics of adolescent development and today's culture in the United States.

Robinson et al. (1987) suggest that to reduce self-destructive behavior a "social influence resistance model" is needed. Adolescents are bombarded by media in which the social roles portrayed are subordinated to the scriptwriter's values, beliefs, and morals (Litt, 1987). The employment of peer pressure to reduce risk-taking behaviors may be the answer (see also p. 891) (Robinson et al., 1987; Marks and Kreuter, 1987).

DYNAMICS OF ADOLESCENT SEXUAL DEVELOPMENT

Many factors contribute to the increase in teenage sexual activity: peer pressure, sex-oriented media, minimum or no parental supervision, mobility, and a transient society that discourages neighbors from knowing one another (Corbett and Meyer, 1987; Hamburg, Nightingale, and Takanishi, 1987). This young, inexperienced population is thus enticed to sexual activity without adequate preparation (Holder, 1987). For many there is no turning back.

Risk taking and the need to explore new roles and new experiences occur at a time when cognitive development has not yet reached the point where teenagers can make judgments that will keep them out of trouble (Goleman, 1987). Belief in their own invulnerability persuades teenagers that they can take risks safely. In one study (Goleman, 1987), adolescents were found to anticipate that the risk of pregnancy from unprotected intercourse *decreases* with each subsequent occurrence. Further, perception of risks may fade in face of peer pressure (e.g., use of condoms is rejected regardless of risk of pregnancy if peers' view of their use is negative). Worries about long-term consequences are nonexistent; only the immediate experience matters (Goleman, 1987; Sachs, 1986). Adolescent sexuality, masturbation, homosexuality, sexual activity, and myths shared with adults are discussed in Chapter 7.

ADOLESCENT CHOICES

A major task of the adolescent is to develop cognitive ability, the ability to think through alternatives and to make abstractions (Yoos, 1987). The level of cognitive development influences sexual decision making. Recognition of cognitive immaturity aids in understanding adolescent sexual activity and the adolescent's failure to use contraception. Cognitive and behavioral skills are still inadequate to use relevant information effectively. Experience and social interaction are required for movement from one stage of development to another. Decision-making skills can be developed through stage-appropriate learning experiences. The underlying cognitive level may account for the "apparent irrationality" of adolescent decision making in sexual behavior (Yoos, 1987). The adolescent may fail to translate knowledge into behavior because of the manner in which the information is given, a manner ill suited to the adolescent's stage of cognitive development (Yoos, 1987).

Adolescents are faced with making decisions about sexuality in the early teens and regardless of their decision-making ability, will need factual information relative to sexuality, intercourse and parenthood on which to base decisions (Offer, 1987). Fig. 35-1 represents a process of sexual decision making. Unfortunately young teenagers use "denial" as a coping mechanism. They can *deny* the significance of what they hear.

Sexual Activity

Peer group pressure to initiate sexual activity is strong in present-day teen culture. It can supersede the influence of parents or older friends. Often teenagers feel that once virginity has been lost, they have nothing more to lose. Abstinence needs positive reinforcement, but if abstinence is not to be, the next decision for the teenager is whether to use contraception.

Contraception

Although the percentage of adolescents becoming sexually active has leveled off in the past 5 years, there are still significant numbers of adolescents, especially those over the age of 16 years, who would benefit from information on contraception (Emans and Grimes, 1987). Unprotected intercourse is practiced by most sexually active adolescents during a period of a few months to 4 years (Corbett and Meyer, 1987). In a study conducted at a Planned Parenthood clinic it was found that the average 14-year-old engaged in sexual activity for 4.8 months before taking contraceptive precautions, while the 17-year-old risked 10.4 months of unprotected intercourse (Kornfield, 1985). Fear of parental discovery of contraception is a major reason why adolescents will delay seeking contraceptive services for a year or more after initiating sexual intercourse (Zabin and Clark, 1981; Zelnik, 1983).

Fear of pregnancy and a decision to continue to be sexually active is the primary reason why adolescents seek contraceptive services. Oral contraceptives (OCs) are usually the contraceptive of choice because "the pill" is not as

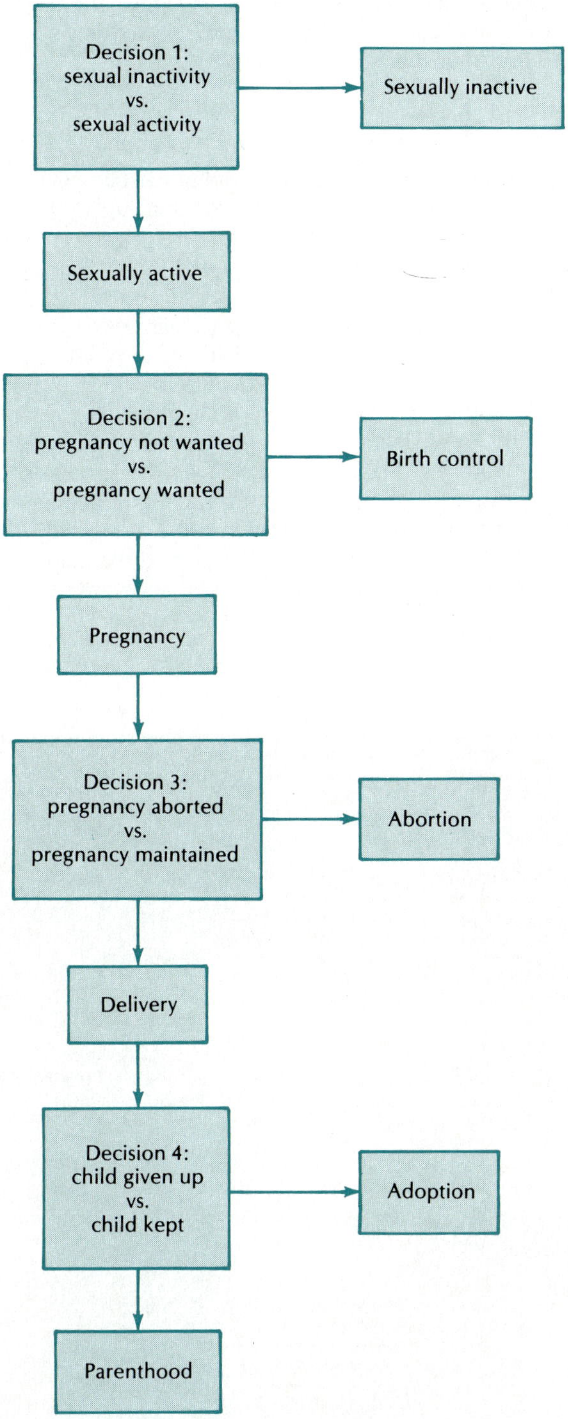

Fig. 35-1 Decision tree for adolescent sexual decision making.
From Kreipe, RE. In McAnarney, E, editor: Premature adolescent pregnancy and parenthood, New York, 1983, Grune & Stratton, Inc. Reprinted by permission.

directly associated with sexual intercourse as barrier methods (Chapter 42). Barrier methods are described by adolescents as messy and disturbing pleasure. However, current public education regarding the significant protection against sexually transmitted diseases afforded by condoms and foam may change the adolescent's use of them.

The female adolescent is the decision-maker concerning sexual relationships, pregnancy risks, and contraception. The coital behavior of the average adolescent female is seldom promiscuous. Few adolescents have more than two or three partners before marriage. Most have a single partner in a monogamous relationship (Corbett and Meyer, 1987).

Factors that influence adolescent contraceptive use are as follows:

1. *Patterns of sexual activity.* Frequency of intercourse, number of partners, and cooperation between the adolescent partners.
2. *Contraceptive services.* Access, staff attitudes, flexibility of appointment schedules, and costs.

Examples of factors contributing to non-use of contraceptives include:

1. Erroneous beliefs regarding conception and a feeling of immunity to pregnancy risk.
2. Fear of exposure and peer disapproval or punishment by parents.
3. Belief that contraceptives are dangerous and harmful—exaggerated fears of side effects.
4. Partners who are unsupportive, uncommitted, or who have a negative attitude toward contraception.

Effective contraceptive methods will not be used when the adolescent has little understanding of the consequences of sexual behavior. Responsible sexuality requires decision-making skills that lead to consistent and correct use of a contraceptive method (Emans and Grimes, 1987). Through personalized contraceptive services and values-clarification, adolescents can learn to utilize effective and safe contraceptive methods consistently from the onset of their sexual activity (Sachs, 1986).

Abortion

Once pregnancy occurs, the adolescent is faced with the choice of abortion or carrying the pregnancy to term. Denial of the pregnancy or a lack of decision-making skills results in delay in informing parents. The teenager who vacillates regarding abortion often makes a decision to have her baby in a roundabout way. Options need to be presented in a nonjudgmental manner to ensure the young person's freedom of choice (Chapter 42). Fewer teenagers are electing abortion today than in the 1970s.

The adolescent may not choose to involve her family in her decision to elect abortion (Holder, 1987). In some states a judge is appointed to determine if the teenager is mature enough to make the decision for herself. In other states, adolescents are considered "mature minors" and may consent to abortion as they may to any other procedures. Where there is doubt of the young adolescent's capacity to understand and give consent to an abortion, parental notification may be considered. However, in cases where the physician or social worker suspects that the pregnant adolescent is the victim of incest or sexual abuse within the household or extended family, parental notification may place her at additional risk. It is generally believed that a great many (perhaps most) pregnant 12 to 14-year-olds are such victims and are not participants in sexual relationships with age-appropriate boyfriends (Holder, 1987; Zdanuk, Harris, and Wisian, 1987). In such cases, child abuse agencies may need to become involved.

Adoption

If the adolescent mother opts to have her child, she can either keep the baby or place it for adoption. The majority of teenagers are electing to keep their infants. If, however, adoption is contemplated, discussion of the adoption process begins in the prenatal period (see specific nursing care plan, p. 899). The adolescent is encouraged to talk freely of her feelings, both for and against the process. If possible, the girl's family and father of the baby are part of the group that help her with her decision. The adolescent needs to be assured that what she is doing is positive and that feelings of sadness and of frustration are bound to occur.

After the baby is born, the young mother may or may not wish to see the baby or to know its sex. It is generally agreed that releasing a child is facilitated if one grieves for an *actual loss* rather than a *fantasy* one; however, the mother has the right to make her own choice. She can be given the information about the infant's health (e.g., "your baby is healthy and strong"), since it may affect her response to her own feelings of self-worth.

Placing an infant for adoption may be accepted by some young parents with varying emotional responses. For some, it may be another episode in a "bad" experience. On the other hand, giving a baby up for adoption may be attended by all the symptoms of grief one would expect at the death of a newborn: "She is only 15 years old, but she loves the baby. Her parents won't take it, so she has to give it up. Her grief was heartbreaking. On the day she went home she came into the nursery to hold her baby for one last time."

It is essential to help the young woman cultivate a positive attitude toward potential future pregnancies. "Subconsciously she may compensate for the loss of this infant by producing another as soon as possible, by drifting into new relationships while seeking support during her grief, by making unreasonable demands on subsequent children, or by becoming overly protective of subsequent offspring" (Sorosky et al., 1978; Polit and Kahn, 1986).

Today the teenager and her parent need to be informed of the possibility that the infant given for adoption may, as an adult, seek to identify her or his biologic parents. It is now a recognized practice to provide adoptive parents with all pertinent biologic knowledge that may affect the infant. It is also helpful for the child to know of psychosocial "successes" in her or his biologic family—musical ability, sports prowess, scientific success—all of which can be part of the adopted baby's history and a source of pride.

The grief of the young parent at her loss has to be balanced with the need of her infant for continued care and nurturing. The experience of relinquishing her child "for the child's good" may be the young woman's first major autonomous decision in her life and as such is an important step toward maturity (Arms, 1983).

Parenthood

Carrying the pregnancy and keeping the baby is also an option in adolescent sexual decision making (Fig. 35-2). When this choice is made, the health care giver, community resources, and the family must be mobilized to assist the adolescent parent. Research findings suggest that children born to adolescent mothers are at greater risk for behavioral, social, intellectual, and perhaps even physical retardation than are children born to older mothers (Baldwin and Cain, 1981; Hardy et al., 1978; Stockard, 1986; White-Traut and Pabst, 1987). In 1979, McAnarney et al. reported that the younger the adolescent mother, the less likely she was to display maternal behaviors such as touching, synchrony with the baby, vocalization, or closeness. In later research, McAnarney et al. (1986) reported that adolescent mothers are less likely to be accepting, cooperative, accessible, and sensitive to their children's needs.

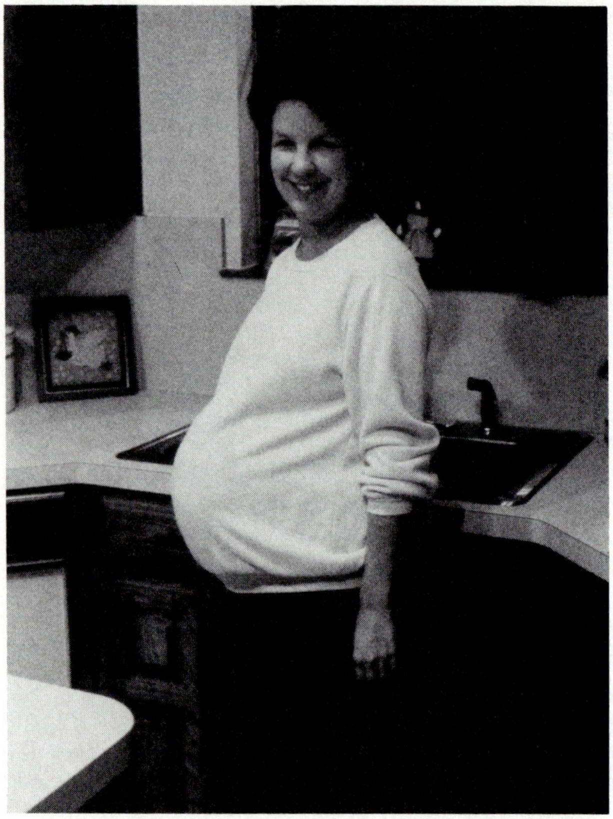

Fig. 35-2 Late adolescent carrying pregnancy to term.

ADOLESCENT PREGNANCY AND PARENTHOOD

Incidence and Costs

Many adults have difficulty understanding the high incidence of adolescent pregnancy when contraception and elective abortion are available. Ignorance about conception and contraception or fear of discovery if contraception is sought and used may be operative. Or perhaps, for their own reasons, some deliberately select pregnancy and motherhood.

Each day more than 3000 teenagers in the United States become pregnant (Stockard, 1986). Each year 1 of 11 adolescent females becomes pregnant; about one third of these are by adolescent males. Every year slightly more than 1 million pregnancies occur to females between the ages of 15 and 19 years. Teenage pregnancy and fertility rates (1987) vary widely among the states, but the average is 11.2 per 1000 aged 15 to 19 (see box at right). Of these pregnancies, 38.7% ended in abortion, 13.4% were estimated to have ended by miscarriage, and the remainder (47.9%) were carried to the birth of a preterm or term infant. Among the developed nations the United States has the highest fertility and abortion rates for adolescent females (Blum, 1987; Rosenfield, 1981; Westoff, Calot, and Foster, 1983).

Physiologic Consequences. The **physiologic consequences** of early adolescent pregnancy seem to be less than previously proposed (Hayes and Crovitz, 1979; Hollingsworth and Kreutner, 1980). However, for the early adolescent, anemia, preeclampsia, cephalopelvic disproportion (CPD), and placental abruption persist as pregnancy sequelae (Blum, 1987; Wallis, 1985; Zuckerman et al., 1987). The maternal mortality from pregnancy complications among females who give birth under age 15 years is much higher (approximately 2.5 times higher) than that for mothers aged 20 to 24 (Stockard, 1986). There is a question of whether age or the adolescent's psychosocial development is the major determinant of the most frequent sequelae for the infant: low birth weight, birth trauma, and preterm birth (Elster, 1984; Lawrence, 1983; Zuckerman, 1983). While high-quality comprehensive prenatal care can limit the physiologic complications experienced by adolescent mothers and their children, such health services are often unavailable. Even if these services are accessible, they often are not used by the adolescent until relatively late in pregnancy (Blum, 1987; Stockard, 1986).

Personal Costs. **Personal costs** of adolescent childbearing are well known. Although most adolescents have the strengths needed to cope successfully with the developmental crises of adolescence, usually they have not yet developed the strengths and skills required of a woman during pregnancy. Social and environmental resources may be limited as well. The adolescent is often without social acceptance of her pregnancy and parenthood, a supportive husband, a stable home, and some financial security. Following delivery, adolescent parents face many obstacles to economic and social success (Blum, 1987; Spivak and Weitzman, 1987). Married or not, the adolescent mother may be ill prepared for the responsibilities she is about to assume.

Data from the National Longitudinal Survey of Work Experience of Youth indicate that among young women who become pregnant, drop out of school, and subsequently

TEENAGE PREGNANCY RATES, PER 1000 GIRLS AGED 15 TO 19, BY STATE

1	Nevada	144
2	California	140
3	Texas	137
4	Florida	131
5	Georgia	130
6	Wyoming	127
7	New Mexico	126
8	Mississippi	125
9	Alaska	124
10	Arizona	123
11	Maryland	122.5
12	Washington	122
13	Oklahoma	119.5
14	Oregon	119
15	Louisiana	118
16	Alabama	117.3
17	Arkansas	117.2
18	Colorado	113.7
18	South Carolina	113.7
20	Tennessee	113
21	Kentucky	111
22	North Carolina	110
23	Virginia	107
24	Missouri	106
25	Delaware	105.6
25	Hawaii	105.6
27	West Virginia	104
28	Michigan	102
29	Indiana	101.9
30	Ohio	101.3
31	Kansas	101
32	New York	100.7
33	Illinois	100.6
34	Idaho	.96
35	New Jersey	95.8
36	Vermont	.95
37	Utah	94.6
38	Montana	.93
39	Pennsylvania	.90
40	Maine	.87
41	South Dakota	.86
42	Massachusetts	85.7
43	Wisconsin	.85
44	Rhode Island	.83
45	Connecticut	80.7
45	Nebraska	80.7
45	New Hampshire	80.7
48	Iowa	.79
49	Minnesota	.77
50	North Dakota	74.8

are delivered of an infant, only 53% have completed their high school requirements by the age of 26 years (Blum, 1987). This compares with a high school completion rate of 95% for women 20 to 26 years of age who bore no children (Mott and Marsiglio, 1985). Adolescent pregnancy seems to be the primary reason for females to terminate their education prematurely. However, those who do become pregnant before completion of a high school education are, on the average, 2 years behind grade level at the time of conception (Blum, 1987; Stockard, 1986). Therefore school failure may be a contributing factor to adolescent motherhood (Blum, 1987). Poverty and leaving school early are closely linked. Lack of a high school diploma makes unemployment far more likely. However, if the adolescent comes from a stable family environment and has emotional and financial support from her family, the return to school rate is high (Corbett and Meyer, 1987). Without this support the school drop-out rate and incidence of subsequent pregnancy is high. If the adolescent misses a full year in school, dropping a grade behind her peers, she has little incentive to return. A lifetime of lost advantages may result if she lacks the educational criteria to enter the labor force. The adolescent who moves away from home and family may suffer increased loneliness, isolation, and poor self-image. The adolescent mother who marries because she is pregnant is predisposed to divorce (i.e., one out of two such marriages ends in divorce) (Corbett and Meyer, 1987).

Public Costs. The **public cost** of teenage pregnancy is staggering (Blum, 1987; Stockard, 1986). Stickle (1981) reported a 26.4% incidence of low birth weight (LBW) infants among mothers under 18 who lacked proper prenatal care. Mothers under 15 are twice as likely to have preterm or LBW infants. Infants at risk secondary to LBW preterm birth or intrauterine growth retardation (IUGR) impose a tremendous cost on society. Initial care in intensive care units is expensive. Sequelae to LBW and IUGR, such as mental retardation, cerebral palsy, and epilepsy, add to society's cost.

During 1986 the United States spent $17.93 billion on all families that had been started when the mother was an adolescent, which calculates to an average exceeding $18,000 per year per child born to an adolescent for each of the first 18 years of life (Blum, 1987; Haffner, 1987). This amount represents outlays for Aid to Families with Dependent Children (AFDC), Medicaid, Women and Infant Care (WIC), and food stamps. Estimates are that costs will reach $5.5 billion during the next 20 years (in 1986 dollars) for care of families started by adolescents in 1986 in the United States. If all 1986 births had been delayed until the mother was in her 20s, the U.S. taxpayers would have saved an estimated $2.2 billion.

Motivation

On a personal level the reasons adolescents give for becoming pregnant vary widely. They include the effect of family relationships, use of coping mechanisms, love and commitment to one another, and the enhancement of self-concept.

Family Relationships. Some adolescents may have faulty relationships within the family. It may be that in mother-daughter conflicts the daughter uses pregnancy to act out her rebellion or as a statement of her growing sexuality as opposed to her mother's declining sexuality. For others there may be a search for nurturance from a mother or father who failed to provide it.

Some adolescents living in certain ethnic and multigenerational families know that their offspring will become family members. In a few instances the pattern for early adolescent pregnancy out of wedlock is a familiar and accepted one. There appears to be a warm, supportive relationship that, once the initial shock to the family system is resolved, results in supportive and nurturing care for the adolescent and her infant.

Coping Mechanisms. If human behavior is purposeful (even if the purpose is obscure), cues to the young girl's behavior may sometimes be gained by having her assess where she is now and where she was before pregnancy. Pregnancy may function as a coping mechanism. For young girls living in poverty, having babies is one form of economic survival. The allotments of money, food stamps, medical and dental care, and special schooling provided by the government establish their economic as well as personal independence. In reality, however, the adolescent's concept of wealth is usually distorted, and a cycle of poverty can be established or perpetuated.

Sometimes an unwanted partner is removed or tested: "Somehow I sensed that if I got pregnant, he wouldn't stand by me. Was I ever right! He abandoned me in a foreign country—just took off. I'm glad I found out his true colors."

Some adolescents view the child to be born as an ally for themselves, someone who will love them in spite of adversity and who will act as a supportive person. The infant's need to be dependent, to be nurtured, and to be viewed as a person apart is not recognized. The young mother's disappointment and bewilderment over her infant's normal behavior can lead to bitterness and eventual neglect.

Love and Commitment. Researchers have found a significant love relationship in some teenage couples (Elster and Panzarine, 1981). They report that a crisis during the pregnancy often arose in the relationship between the father of the baby and the girl's parents. Of those adolescents who keep their children, a substantial number eventually marry; the premarital sexual relationship was part of a longer commitment to one another.

Self-concept. Pregnancy can serve as a rite of passage into adulthood and irrefutable evidence of sexual identity and attractiveness. Some adolescents become pregnant as a result of experimentation with genital sex or sexual intercourse. The teenager assumes this is a normal part of peer activity. One student who worked with school-age mothers remarked:

> I was appalled by their passivity. They seemed to feel that another person had every right to do things to their bodies. I feel what is needed most is for them to value themselves, to see the beauty of their own bodies, and not to allow themselves to be destroyed.

Cultural Beliefs

A country such as the United States represents a mosaic of social, ethnic, and racial groups. Evidence does not support culture as a causative factor in early pregnancy. No culture in the United States promotes premarital pregnancy and childbirth, especially among adolescents. Each group rears its young to accept and act on beliefs considered important to the particular group. Beliefs consist of knowledge, opinions, and faith that dispose persons toward a certain kind of behavior (Horn, 1983). As a result, individuals' beliefs vary considerably, as do the resulting actions. Health care providers need to view the client's situation from the client's perspective. Sensitivity to differences must be reflected to health care plans to increase the likelihood that the needs of all clients are met.

Horn investigated the differences in the beliefs of three groups of young women in the United States (native-born Indian women, black women, and white women) concerning (1) prevention of pregnancy and contraception, (2) the significance of being a mother at an early age, and (3) the kinds of support systems available within their social network. These beliefs were found to be influential in their becoming pregnant, as well as during their pregnancies. Horn found that although all the women were knowledgeable about contraception, beliefs dictated its use: "not until after the first baby is born," "use of birth control pills and IUD not acceptable because menstrual cycle is altered," or "religious belief prevented or encouraged use." The significance of becoming a mother at an early age also differed: "there is a value in early pregnancy—it validates one's feminine role"; "it [pregnancy] is not highly desired but accepted"; and "early motherhood is not valued; it is seen as a failure." With reference to expectations that support would be available, the first two groups believed that it would be, but the third group did not expect assistance (and did not receive it).

Speraw (1987) reported on a cross-cultural perspective of adolescents' perceptions of pregnancy. The results of her study suggest that there are distinct, measurable differences in the ways adolescents from differing backgrounds perceive their pregnancies and the effects of pregnancy on their lives. Adolescents who participated identified themselves as white, black, Hispanic, or Pacific Asian. Response themes within groups had many similarities, but in only a few areas was total or near total agreement found. In no group were answers so alike that they could be classified as characteristic of any one group. Perception of pregnancy was individual and dependent on many variables, only one of which was culture.

Findings showed that within the black community, high value was placed on children and motherhood, and strong family support was usually given. Most negative reactions centered on changes experienced within their bodies. High regard was also felt by Hispanic subjects. However, perceived family support was nonexistent or mixed. Responses of white subjects indicated reluctance to accept their pregnancies and reflected feelings of guilt and regret. Pacific Asian subjects offered no clear initial response to pregnancy, made statements related to the idea of fate, and were least likely to list "family" as the source of support. Many subjects from this group were sent away from home in disgrace; there was an expressed need to maintain the family's good name in the community that overrode the need of the adolescent to feel loved or accepted.

In Speraw's study (1987) adolescents described life changes that were pregnancy related. Necessary clothing changes, social isolation from peers (all groups) and from family (Pacific Asian adolescents, especially), modified recreational activities (no motor bike rides), and altered relationships were concerns. The best part of pregnancy and motherhood was given as "just to have something." The anticipated "worst" part of motherhood was "mothering," concern about child abuse, worry, long hours, loss of freedom, and "being disappointed by your child like you disappointed your parents."

Psychosocial Developmental Tasks

The psychosocial developmental tasks of adolescents are interrupted by pregnancy. As with other developmental sequences, there are critical periods when interference can have traumatic effects. The younger the adolescent when she becomes pregnant, the greater will be the trauma. For the 12- to 14-year-old girl, pregnancy can be a fearful experience. Because of the extreme youth of these younger adolescents, society tends to respond in a more protective way, and there seems to be a generalized effort to minimize the trauma. The 15- to 17-year-old girl, with her mixture of childlike and adult behavior and her more overt conflicts with parents, seems to arouse more societal anger and resentment, perhaps because both family and society must respond in a responsible way to behavior they are at a loss to control. The 18- to 20-year-old girl is viewed somewhat as an adult who, with a modicum of support, can fend more adequately and who can assume that major responsibility for her offspring.

The following developmental tasks may be interrupted by pregnancy in adolescence:

1. *Achievement of new and more mature relations with age mates of both sexes*

The pregnant adolescent may find herself isolated from her peer group. Within some social groups, parents will try to prevent contact between their teenagers and one who has become pregnant—an attempt to proclaim societal condemnation of adolescent behavior. In some areas regular school attendance must be discontinued, which effectively limits meetings with peers. The pregnant adolescent has contact largely with other pregnant teenagers, her boyfriend if he remains available to her, and relatives. Thus the practice time for developing social relationships is curtailed.

2. *Achievement of a feminine social role*

In one sense pregnancy confers overt adult sexuality on the teenager, but in another sense it limits the feminine role to one of procreation. Opportunities for social development of feminine potential are either abandoned or are set aside until early or middle adulthood.

3. *Acceptance of her physique and effective use of the body*

Adolescents are experiencing a period of rapid change in physical growth and become acutely conscious of their bodies and body sensations. The symptoms of pregnancy can cause the teenager much dismay. Elimination, for example, is not necessarily talked about openly, and the need for care related to this area is equated with being infantile or elderly. The frequent urination of early and late pregnancy may be "treated" by restricting fluid intake. This restriction increases the likelihood of severe constipation or bladder infections.

The increase in melanin causes deepening of color in the areolar tissue of the breasts, the formation of the mask of pregnancy, and the appearance of the linea nigra. These changes may be viewed by the adolescent as stigmas. The increased mucoid vaginal secretions may be thought to be caused by infection, and if the adolescent resists care, they may increase her anxiety and fear. Increased sensitivity of the breasts can be a source of discomfort and anxiety. The fatigue of early pregnancy, compounding the fatigue experienced by many adolescents, can cause the adolescent to assume that she is ill.

Until late adolescence, body image is still formative. By midpregnancy the enlarging abdomen and the increasing size of breasts and buttocks may prompt the teenager to try to control her appearance by dieting, with adverse consequences to fetal health and her own growth needs. The shift in the center of gravity as body posture changes to accommodate the protuberant abdomen causes back strain and lack of balance. These are aggravated by the disparity between the rate of growth of the skeleton and the muscles supporting it; the muscles are not strong enough (even in the nonpregnant state) to maintain correct posture. The effects may be severe if the teenager feels compelled to compete in strenuous activities (including dancing) or to wear nonsupportive shoes because of her need to belong to her peer group. Symptoms of abnormalities, vaginal bleeding, and dizziness are sometimes concealed until serious conditions develop.

It is one thing for a woman who is knowledgeable and secure to accept and cope with the symptoms of pregnancy. She may feel compensated by the feeling that the child she is creating will be wanted and loved. For the adolescent whose pregnancy does not have full social approval and whose baby may not be welcomed, the discomforts of pregnancy can assume major proportions. Unfortunately to some they are seen as punishment for their illicit or "sinful" behavior.

4. *Achievement of independence from parents and other adults*

A teenager's move toward independence comes to an end when she becomes pregnant, and she is compelled to turn to her family for nurturance just as she did as a young child. Even with the support provided by social agencies, the school-age mother-to-be finds it almost impossible to separate herself from her family. With that support comes a reestablishment of family dominance and dependency.

For example, a 15-year-old-girl cannot make a decision relative to the continuing care of her infant without family concurrence. She is not able to provide such care for her child unless some adult is willing to provide shelter and assistance for them both. If this support is not forthcoming, the younger teenager must examine other options (e.g., foster care or giving the child up for adoption). The pregnancy may, however, serve as a catalyst to force the family to examine its relationships. In many instances the pregnancy has been a means of resolving parent-child conflicts in a more growth-responsive way.

Although certain areas of independence are curtailed, others may be substituted. The teenager who assumes responsibility may emerge from this life experience as one who can function in an interdependent manner with adults. These responsibilities include attendance at prenatal care classes, following an adequate dietary regimen, and participating in parent-craft groups.

For some adolescents the forced contact with a caring health professional during pregnancy may have a dramatic effect and provide a role model. As one 16-year-old girl expressed it:

> The only thing that was okay with it all was that I met F ________(nursing counselor). She likes me—well, I know she does. Even when I got rough, she'd be there. I never knew grown people were like that, that they cared about me. I would like to be like her, not a nurse, but like someone who loves people.

5. *Establishment of a life-style that is personally and socially satisfying*

A prerequisite of a satisfying life-style is the opportunity to make thoughtful and informed choices in the areas of career, sexual relationships, marriage, family interdependence, and parenthood.

Because of interruptions in schooling, many teenagers who might realistically have had other career goals are relegated to occupations that are not commensurate with their capabilities and temperament. Some never overcome this disadvantage; others must postpone any formal preparations until much later in life.

Precipitate marriage by the older adolescent does not have a good success rate. This results because the adolescent is unprepared for the give-and-take of such a close relationship, beset by economic problems, and living in inadequate housing (often with inlaws). Often the adolescent has no time for the "fun" of growing up. Thus participants in early marriage tend to experience desertion or divorce, intensifying their sense of alienation and defeat. For the early adolescent, pregnancy and parenthood seem not to be recognized as possible consequences of sexual behavior. Pregnancy comes as a surprise. Parenthood is something that happens to parents, from whom the younger teenager is seeking to establish independence, not a state in which giving of oneself to another will be required.

The older adolescent, being less egocentric and more capable of problem solving, often is able to face the reality of pregnancy and parenthood in an adult manner. She can seek assistance from social agencies in her own right. She may find, however, that the care of a child without the emotional and economic support of another caring adult means altering career plans.

6. *Acquisition of a set of values (an ethical system) that will serve as a guide to socially responsible behavior*

Becoming pregnant and producing a child who will not receive mature, concerned parenting cannot be said to be socially responsible behavior. However, by assuming adult responsibilities associated with pregnancy and parenthood, some adolescents emerge as stronger, other-centered individuals. For those who are unable to be helped or who are not helped to use this experience as a time of maturation, pregnancy may become a coping mechanism, albeit an inadequate one, to solve the problems of the moment. For this group recidivism is more prevalent, and the adolescent who sought to become independent through sexual activity remains a dependent person.

Developmental Tasks of Pregnancy

In common with older pregnant women, the adolescent faces certain developmental tasks directly related to becoming a parent. Her response to the implications and challenges of these tasks reflects her cognitive level (Chapter 7). Adolescents are in the period of transition between the inductive reasoning of late childhood (concrete operations) and the deductive reasoning of the older individual (formal operations). For an adolescent whose thoughts are circumscribed by the "here and now" and "seeing is believing," movement toward the "there and then" and predictions of the future may be limited. The old saying that "you cannot put an old head on young shoulders" holds true.

1. *Accepting the biologic reality of pregnancy*

The usual response of the adolescent is denial. Anxiety about the response of her family or boyfriend will often delay the seeking of outside support. Adolescents have reported that sharing their suspicions of pregnancy with their parents was the most difficult part of their pregnancy and assumed crisis proportions. Many parents also have reported how emotionally distraught their daughter became. Evidently the idea of being pregnant comes with a sense of surprise and disbelief: "I can't believe it is happening to me," "I didn't think I could get pregnant; I'm too young," "I keep thinking it is some awful dream and I will wake up." The sense of **denial** is so profound that the girl experiences genuine shock at the consequences of her sexual behavior. Denial is also one means to create time to reevaluate her situation. Recognition that she can no longer control the size and appearance of her body heightens her sense of vulnerability and increases the feelings of alienation imposed by the pregnancy.

Suspicions of pregnancy may first be discussed with a girlfriend, and fantasies about what will happen when the mother is told will be reviewed. Some adolescents leave clues that they hope will be noticed by their mothers. Containers of pills are left in accessible places, diaries previously locked and secreted are left open, or letters to girlfriends are placed so they can easily be read. The parent is expected to note the repetitive nausea and vomiting in early pregnancy and the changing body shape of mid-pregnancy. It is hoped the parent will bring up the subject of possible pregnancy. The girl expects anger, recriminations, and, perhaps physical abuse. She is surprised by the support and nurturing that are often forthcoming.

The end result of the denial of the reality of pregnancy is the postponement of medical care, to the detriment of both the adolescent and her fetus. Abortion as an option may have to be ruled out because of the advanced stage of pregnancy. Infection, drug ingestion, and inadequate nutrition may have already traumatized the fetus. Those who have contact with school-age adolescents need to be particularly alert to changes in their behavior patterns. Often the teacher, school counselor, or school nurse is the first to note symptoms suggestive of pregnancy and to broach the possibility of pregnancy with the girl. In many instances the professional acts as the girl's support in telling her parents of her condition and initiating medical and social care. The older adolescent will often seek professional confirmation of pregnancy before seeking parental or societal help. Once the pregnancy is confirmed and care has been initiated, the adolescent, whatever her age, needs help in assuming the responsibility for continuing the care.

2. *Accepting the reality of the unborn child*

The second task relating to acceptance of the reality of the unborn child develops in the same manner with the adolescent as with the older woman. The idea of a happy, cuddly baby who will love and obey the parent seems a common fantasy. The young adolescent can be enthusiastic about how she will dress her baby, take her baby out for walks, and bathe and play with the baby. In fantasy the infant acquires a doll-like form, but the care of the baby cannot be set aside as can the care of a doll. The all-consuming nature of child care—the problems with alleviating crying, feeding the infant, and washing clothes—can prove frustrating and may result in nonnurturing behavior toward the child. The concept of the infant's growth and development into first a toddler, then a preschooler, next a school-age child, and an adolescent does not occur to them. They tend to be centered in the present.

3. *Accepting the reality of parenthood*

Being a parent implies being loving, concerned, and capable of providing the nurturing care an infant needs. It is the most difficult task for adolescents, as it is for many adult pregnant women. The desire for knowledge about child-care activities, nutritional needs of infants, and infant growth and development is evidenced in this group as in any other. One is impressed by the *desire* of the adolescent to be a good mother. The young adolescent is limited in her ability to fulfill the commitment to her child. This results from her meager life experiences, her own need to grow and develop, and her inability to cope with abstractions and to solve problems on the basis of inference and projection (Yoos, 1987).

The older adolescent, able to project herself into the future, can see herself and her infant more readily as separate entities with differing needs. She is more able to fantasize about her child as a preschooler or even a teenager. However, in spite of her greater ability to propose solutions to problems and follow through on suggestions, the family she will create will remain one of the most vulnerable in our society.

Developmental Tasks of Parenthood

The developmental tasks of parenthood include reconciling the imagined with the actual child, becoming adept in caregiving activities, being aware of the infant's needs, and establishing oneself and one's infant as a family. These tasks will be as important to the new adolescent parent's schema as to the adult's (see also Chapters 25 and 26).

Nutrition. Within the United States the age group with the poorest and most unsatisfactory nutrition status is the adolescent between the ages of 10 and 16 (Corbett and Meyer, 1987). Nutrition requirements are at their highest during this period of rapid weight gain and linear growth. The diet of many adolescents is high in fats, sugar, and salt. These diets ("fast foods") are particularly low in vitamins C and A, folic acid, and fiber. Other deficiencies include riboflavin, thiamin, calcium, iron, and zinc. Although these nutritional imbalances are related to other diseases in later life, this discussion focuses on immediate reproductive consequences. These diets are responsible for such common nutritional concerns as overnutrition and undernutrition and iron deficiency anemia.

The adolescent's appetite is responsive to many competing influences. Desire for slimness, prevention of acne, wearing of braces, fast foods, food fads, and use of drugs affect nutrition. Nicotine and alcohol consumption alter the appetite by displacing food in the diet. These drugs can lead to nutritional deficiency by changing the transport, metabolism, and storage of nutrients.

Calcium is needed for the development and mineralization of skeletal mass; iron is needed for the expansion of blood volume and muscle mass; and zinc is needed for sexual maturity. Vegetarian diets may lead to deficiency in zinc. Iron deficiency anemia is seen in 5% to 15% of adolescents, with increased incidence in the black population.

Thiamin, riboflavin, and niacin are necessary for energy metabolism. Folacin is important for DNA metabolism. Vitain B_{12}, vital to the rapid growth of cells during adolescence, is important for fat, protein, and carbohydrate metabolism.

Acne. Many adolescents develop some degree of acne between the ages of 16 and 20. Acne is not believed to be caused or worsened by eating specific foods; therefore food restrictions have little effect (Corbett and Meyer, 1987). The best advice is probably good hygiene. Vitamin A or zinc sulfate may be recommended in some cases.

Oral Contraception. Many adolescents begin to use OCs during the growth spurt. OCs alter the metabolism of proteins, carbohydrates, lipids, and some vitamins and minerals (Chapter 15) regardless of the adequacy of the dietary intake. No clinical manifestations result and routine supplementation is not indicated. However, should vitamin B_6 deficiency be associated with mental depression, supplementation (1.5 mg B_6 per day) or discontinuation of OCs may be considered. Fluid retention increases body weight, a side effect to which many adolescents object.

The use of OCs should be discouraged in the young adolescent who smokes or has a family history of atherosclerotic disease. The health care provider may need to consider monitoring lipid levels for those with such risk factors.

Pregnancy. Nutrition requirements include those of a normal adolescent as well as the growth and development of maternal and fetal tissues. Nutrition inadequacies are to be expected. Early detection and timely intervention of undernourishment may prevent or minimize negative effects of inadequate nutrition on the fetus. Poor nutrition and poverty have been implicated in complications of preeclampsia, anemia, CPD, and low-birthweight infants.

Adolescent diets restricted out of concern for appearance or by denial of pregnancy can be hazardous to both adolescent and fetal growth and development. Smoking interferes with metabolic processes and often results in below average birth weights. Fetal alcohol syndrome (FAS) is a consequence of alcohol ingestion. For optimum fetal growth the adolescent needs to reach a critial body weight. This point is reached when the woman achieves a weight in *excess of 10% above ideal body weight* by term gestation. This approximates the requirement for adult women: 25 to 30 pounds if the woman is at ideal body weight for height and age at the time of conception. Deficiency in weight must be corrected (see also Chapter 15). Then the 25 to 30 pounds should follow. However, most adolescents, regardless of weight at time of conception, gain less than 25 pounds.

There is a direct correlation between *inadequate weight gain* and LBW infants. Inadequate preconception weight, gestation length, and gynecologic age ($\leq$2 years) also influence birth weight. *Gynecologic age* equals the age of the female at conception minus her age at menarche; that is, if the adolescent's present age is 14 and her menarche occurred at age 12, her gynecologic age is 2. For problems associated with LBW, see Chapter 37.

The outcome for the fetus may not be reflected in lowered birth weight alone. Research indicates that brain growth takes place in an orderly sequence, as does growth of other organs. The first-phase hyperplasia (growth by increase in the number of cells) takes place prenatally. The second-phase hypertrophy (growth by increase in cell size), in combination with hyperplasia, is the growth pattern noted in the first 6 months of life. Maternal malnutrition may therefore contribute to a reduced complement of brain cells in the fetus, and the mother's lack of knowledge of the nutrition requirements of her newborn compounds the problem.

Table 35-1 *Recommended Daily Dietary Allowances for Calories (Kilocalories)**

Growth Percentile	Nonpregnant (by Age in Years) 11-14	15-18	19-22	23-50	Added Pregnancy Allowance
50	2200	2100	2100	1000	300
10	1500	1200	1700	1600	300
90	3000	3000	2500	2400	300

From Frank, D, et al: J Calif Perinatal Assoc 3(1):21, 1981; based on National Center for Health Statistics weight-for-length data and recommendations of the Committee on Maternal Nutrition.

*The allowance for energy is established at the lowest value corresponding to good health. No extra allowance is included.

KILOCALORIE REQUIREMENTS AND SAMPLE MENUS FOR PREGNANT ADOLESCENTS

Calculating Kilocalorie Requirements*	Kilocalories
1. Allow kilocalories for maximum daily growth needs:	123
2. Add RDA† of kilocalories for pregnancy:	300
3. Add average RDA† of kilocalories for age and growth percentile for nonpregnant female.	2100
	2523 total daily
4. *Underweight:* Add 500 additional kilocalories per day, 16% of which should be protein (20 g):	3023 total daily
5. *Overweight:* Use lower range of "normal" suggested values or 38 kcal/kg or 17 kcal/lb pregnancy weight.	

Sample Menus

	DAY 1	DAY 2
Breakfast	Egg and ham on English muffin (fast food) 1 cup milk 1 glass orange juice (6 oz; 180 ml)	1 cup cornflakes with 1 cup milk 2 Tbsp raisins 1 glass orange juice (6 oz; 180 ml)
Snack	1 pkg peanut butter crackers 1 can apple juice (6 oz; 180 ml)	1 pkg nuts 1 carton chocolate milk (8 oz; 240 ml)
Lunch	Cheeseburger on bun with lettuce and tomato 1 carton chocolate milk (8 oz; 240 ml) 1 slice watermelon	"Sub"—1 slice each ham, salami, and cheese with lettuce, tomato, onion, green pepper, 1 Tbsp dressing 1 can apple juice (6 oz; 180 ml)
Snack	Ice cream cone	1 cup buttered popcorn
Dinner	Baked chicken leg and thigh ½ cup rice ½ cup string beans 1 cup milk ½ cup fruit cocktail	2 cups spaghetti and meatballs 1 slice Italian bread Tossed salad—lettuce, tomato, onion 1 Tbsp dressing 1 tsp margarine
Snack	1 slice pizza	Milkshake, vanilla

KILOCALORIES	PROTEIN (G)	FAT (G)	CHOLESTEROL (G)	KILOCALORIES	PROTEIN (G)	FAT (G)	CHOLESTEROL (G)
2604	119	132	286	2857	115	147	248
Underweight: replace cheeseburger with extra-large hamburger deluxe; add 1 cup orange juice to evening snack				*Underweight:* add 1 carton chocolate milk to afternoon snack, extra cheese or cold cuts to lunch, 2 Tbsp dressing for salad			
3149	133	155	334	3353	137	172	278
Overweight: replace ice cream cone with 1 can apple juice (6 oz; 180 ml)				*Overweight:* replace milkshake with 1 cup skim milk			
2354	111	114	270	2400	112	131	196

From Frank, D, et al: J Calif Perinatal Assoc 3(1):21, 1981.

*These calculations are based on the maximum kilocalorie allowance for growth. The best indication of whether a pregnant female is getting sufficient kilocalories is to monitor her growth. If inadequate or excess weight gain occurs, consultation with a nutritionist is recommended.

†Recommended daily dietary allowance.

During the adolescent's growth spurt the recommended daily allowances (RDAs) for pregnancy may be insufficient to meet maternal and fetal needs. Factors such as the adolescent's stage of growth, activity level, and physical and mental health may add to or subtract from her nutritional needs (Table 35-1 and Box, above). Pregnancy increases the needs for certain nutrients that are already deficient in nonpregnant adolescents: kilocalories, protein, iron, folic acid, vitamin C, and other vitamins and minerals. Controversy regarding the need to increase and supplement dietary calcium continues. Most sources support this increase to facilitate mineralization of the fetal skeleton, meet the adolescent's growth needs, and support lactation. A dietary intake of 1200 mg per day is needed.

Breast-feeding. Initially many adolescents respond negatively to the idea of breast-feeding. Fear of permanent alteration in the breasts, a view of breast-feeding as "dirty," other misconceptions, or a lack of role models may inhibit any woman. Peer reactions or negative responses from the spouse or boyfriend are other factors.

Formula-feeding is often the method chosen. The child's nutrition and freedom from infection will depend on the mother's good hygiene in preparation and storage of the formula and in feeding practices.

NURSING CARE

Many interacting biologic and social factors affect the quality of human reproduction, and these in turn are influenced by the preconceptional, maternity, and neonatal care that is made available. The adolescent and her offspring are particulary vulnerable to the risks inherent in pregnancy and parenthood. This is a result of circumstances characteristic of her age group, such as psychologic immaturity, economic dependency, or delayed medical care, and political ineffectiveness. Parental education, age, and parity have been associated with injuries of children. The adolescent's neuromuscular immaturity, impulsivity, use of chemical substances, and lack of safety precautions (i.e., risk-taking behaviors) affect her parenting behaviors (Blum, 1987). For these reasons the care of the adolescent parent requires the concerted effort of physicians, nurses, nutritionists, and social workers. The team approach has proved to be effective in the care of young teenage mothers (Osofsky, 1985; Ouimette, 1986; Siegel, 1987). The nursing process—assessment, formulation of nursing diagnoses, plan, implementation, and evaluation—reflects the particular needs of the adolescent client.

Assessment

An accurate assessment occurs within an atmosphere of trust, understanding, and confidentiality (Fullar, 1986). The nurse must maintain objectivity. A nonjudgmental approach and skillful communication techniques (Chapter 2) are needed to put the adolescent at ease in expressing her feelings and concerns.

Several areas must be assessed. These include the adolescent mother's health status, developmental level, knowledge base and perceived needs, support systems, and parenting characteristics and abilities (Ouimette, 1986). Careful assessment is needed to identify learning and care needs.

Health Status

A thorough health history with a review of systems is needed (Chapter 8). Physical examination and laboratory tests add to the data base. During puberty the vaginal epithelium is thin. Therefore it is more vulnerable to irritation and infection. The adolescent who begins sexual activity at an early age and has an increased number of sexual partners is at greater risk for sexually transmitted diseases (STDs) and associated conditions. Contact vaginitis can result from perfumed soap, powders, and sprays; colored, perfumed toilet paper; and tight jeans or other garments.

Nutrition assessment is essential (Chapter 15). Nutrition problems stemming from the current "in" diet for teenagers can compromise both the mother and fetus (Osofsky, 1985). The life-style of many pregnant teenagers includes abuse of alcohol, smoking, and substance abuse and dependence. These behaviors compromise general health and affect nutrition (Chapters 15 and 34). Adolescent females are at greater risk for scoliosis, which is related to adolescent growth patterns, nutrition, and psychosocial factors (Whaley and Wong, 1987).

Immunization status is assessed. Immunizations such as those against diphtheria, tetanus, polio, measles, mumps, and rubella need to be renewed every 10 years. Tuberculosis is increasing in females, especially within 2 years of menarche. Vision and dental screening must also be considered.

The cardiorespiratory systems must be assessed. If the adolescent smokes, she is asked about a productive chronic cough and shortness of breath, which are indicative of small airway disease. If a positive family history is found for coronary heart disease or stroke, laboratory assessment for blood lipids and cholesterol is warranted. In the presence of severe pleuritic pain with right-upper-quadrant tenderness under the rib cage the young sexually active female is assessed for Fitz-Hugh and Curtis syndrome. This syndrome accompanies perihepatitis that is secondary to gonococcal or nongonococcal pelvic inflammatory disease (PID). Cervical cytology is required to rule out severe dysplasia or even carcinoma in situ (Corbett and Meyer, 1987).

Psychosocial screening includes assessment for reactions to pregnancy, depression, or suicide. For many adolescents the pregnancy results in a private grief that is not publically displayed. The primary language spoken, the school grade completed, and the literacy of the adolescent are also important factors to assess. If possible, it should be determined if the expectant mother is the victim of sexual abuse or incest, which has been found to be the most common cause of pregnancy in those under 15 years of age (Corbett and Meyer, 1987; Holder, 1987; Zdanuk, Harris, and Wisian, 1987).

Careful determination of baseline blood pressure is necessary since teenagers have lower systolic and diastolic pressures than older women. A teenager could be in serious jeopardy for eclampsia with a blood pressure reading of 140/90. Chronic hypertension is found in 1% to 2% of adolescents.

During labor and delivery the young teenager (11 to 14 years) suffers from dystocia more commonly than the older teenager or woman. Therefore the incidence of cesarean delivery is higher. Prematurity, small-for-gestational age (SGA), and fetal perinatal mortality are also increased. The risk of maternal mortality is higher for pregnant teenagers under age 15 than for women in their early twenties (Carey, McCann-Sanford, and Davidson, 1983).

Psychosocial Development

Effective interaction with the adolescent requires an understanding of the level of psychosocial development and tasks of this age group (Chapter 7). The psychosocial development of the teenager reflects the three stages (early, middle, and late) of adolescence. These stages roughly approximate chronologic age but more precisely are characterized by predominant drives, moods, and abilities (Fullar, 1986; Sahler, 1983). Hatcher (1976) described five aspects of personality development that have proved to be good indicators of the adolescent's overall developmental level. The five aspects are as follows:

1. The identity of the parent most related to conflicts (see Table 35-2)

Table 35-2 *Adolescent Development and Readiness for Childbearing*

	Early Adolescence (11-14)	Middle Adolescence (15-17)	Late Adolescence (18-20)
Parent most related to conflicts	Beginning to loosen ties with her mother. Vacillates between wanting to be closer (i.e., a mother herself) and wanting to be babied (i.e., cannot conceive of herself as a mother).	Struggling to break from both parents and become autonomous.	Personal identity stronger; some emotional independence from parents; ready for outside love interest.
Quality and style of relationships with others	Strong relationships with other girls. Experiences crushes on safe (i.e., unattainable) adults.	Relationships with peers intense; parents replaced with peers; difficulty with authority figures, cannot either accept or compromise. Friends are heterosexual but self-identity needs (who am I), not intimacy needs, are uppermost. Sexual experimentation and risk taking.	Conflict with parents lessens, nurturant feelings for others emerge, wants to share love and commitment.
View of herself	Self-concept inconsistent and fluctuating; parallels rapid physical changes and capability changes. Vague sense of self as female.	Self-involvement a critical need. Ambivalence and uncertainty predominate. Senses her femininity and has a beginning awareness of responsibility for actions. Definitive commitments not yet necessary. Unresolved dependency needs preclude her wanting to accept dependency of others.	More realistic about who and what she is. Behaviors and responses more predictable. Capable of personal reflections, more in touch with her own feelings. Accepts adult body.
Defense mechanisms	Primary defense is denial, manifested by unwillingness to hear pertinent information (e.g., almost never protected by contraception during sexual experimentation).	Magical thinking and feelings of greater power pervade fantasy, mood swings experienced, any nonsuccess is a tragedy. Exaggeration of response prevents an accurate assessment of real tragedy.	Uses reality-based strategies to cope with stress. Can think through problems, uses rational thought.
Goals and interests	Is "now" oriented. The immediacy of her needs requires instant gratification. Operates by fixed rules and authority, little ability to "give and take," therefore rigid and punitive. Denial is major defense.	Goals and interest reflect growing ability to problem solve. Dependency-independency needs make her inconsistent in approach. Intensely narcissistic (self-centered). Generally unempathetic and unable to tolerate others' demands that detract from her self-focus. Impulsive, unpredictable behavior.	Goals and interests reflect longer-range view. More ready to accept responsibility for self and others. Recognizes need to develop educational or vocational skills. Approximates the adult in being able to provide warm, nurturing care for a child.

Modified from Sahler, OJ: In McAnarney, ER, editor: Premature adolescent pregnancy and parenthood, New York, 1983, Grune & Stratton, Inc. Reprinted by permission.

2. The quality and style of her relationships with others
3. Her view of herself
4. Her major defense mechanisms
5. Her goals and interests

Sahler (1983) applied these findings to readiness for the task of childbearing.

Knowledge Base and Perceived Needs

Significant factors to consider include the adolescent's cognitive status and time orientation, egocentricity, body image, dependency, and peer and spouse relationships. The adolescent is assessed for her knowledge of reproduction, sexual functioning, and her own sexuality. Basic knowledge of these factors is important to help the pregnant adolescent understand more readily the additional changes during pregnancy.

Support Systems

There appears to be a direct relationship between the amount of social support and prenatal course and evidence of appropriate maternal behavior (Fullar, 1986; Mercer, 1985). Emotional support is seen by the young mothers as being the most important type of support, especially if provided by the mother's family of origin (Colletta and Gregg, 1981).

The pregnant adolescent and mother is particularly sensitive to the attitudes and actions of persons in her support system (Mercer, 1985). These people include parents, boyfriends, or husbands, and health personnel. Pregnant adolescents become introverted. Often they become distanced from their sexual partners, who may not understand this as a normal stage in accepting the pregnancy. Mercer (1985) notes that assessment of the following can provide a basis for supportive care:

1. How the mother perceives her role
2. Who is helpful to her
3. How she views her infant

Parenting Abilities

Studies to date have not produced conclusive evidence to show there are major attitudinal differences between adolescent and adult mothers. However, some differences in parenting behaviors are beginning to be documented. For example, adolescents, although providing warm and attentive physical care, appear to use less verbal interaction than do older parents.

Infants' development of cognitive ability appears to be related to the amount of exposure they have to verbal communication—the more verbal exchanges, the greater the development of cognitive ability. Jones et al. (1980) and Mercer (1983) found that adult mothers were significantly more responsive to their newborn infants than were younger mothers, regardless of race or of socioeconomic or martial status. Other researchers have confirmed clinical observations that some adolescents use aggressive, inappropriate behaviors, for example, poking and pinching their infants. These behaviors are rarely seen in adult mothers (Lawrence et al., 1981). The negative attitudes may reflect the adolescent's self-centeredness and level of cognitive development. Excessive child abuse by adolescent mothers has not been substantiated by research. It may be that neglect, secondary to lack of knowledge, is a more pronounced feature of parenting disorders in the adolescent.

Parenting ability is based on a parent's sensitivity to the infant's needs. Many factors can affect sensitivity, including stress, level of cognitive development, knowledge, infant responses, and support systems.

Stress. The adolescent's ability to function in a mothering role is affected by the level of stress she is experiencing. Adolescents are exposed to many stresses as they undertake the tasks and responsibilities of parenthood, a role that in our culture is traditionally reserved for adults who are financially and educationally secure. Stress can affect the quality of a person's functioning, making her insensitive to other needs. Adolescents' reactions to perceived stress depend on the quality of their support systems, their self-esteem, and their ability to solve problems directly.

Responsiveness to Infant. The responses of teenage mothers to their infant's responses parallel those of the adult mother (Chapter 25). Adolescents certainly respond to positive feedback from their infants. They are pleased when their infants recognize them and prefer them over others. However, studies do indicate that adolescents perceive their infants as more temperamentally difficult than do adult mothers (Field et al., 1980).

The adolescent's knowledge of child development is usually limited. This lack may directly affect parental sensitivity by influencing the mother's perception, interpretation, and responsiveness to infant cues (Elster et al., 1983).

Teenage parents have been found to expect too much of their children too soon. A study of adolescent couples revealed that they consistently overestimated the age at which their child could accomplish certain behaviors, for example, sitting alone at 12 weeks (mothers) or at 6 weeks (fathers) (DeLissovoy, 1973). Jarrett (1982) found a similar lack of knowledge (Table 35-3). In addition, teenage parents were found to possess inaccurate knowledge of their offspring's cognitive, social, and language development.

Nursing Diagnoses

The information gathered during physical examinations, interviews, and laboratory analysis of specimens is analyzed, and nursing diagnoses are formulated. Nursing diagnoses relevant to the adolescent parent might include the following:

- Potential for fetal injury related to
  - Inadequate placental perfusion secondary to preeclampsia
- Knowledge deficit related to
  - Nutritional needs of the mother and baby during pregnancy
- Potential altered health maintenance related to
  - Substance abuse
- Potential infant care deficit related to
  - Ignorance of infant's growth and development needs
- Situational low self-esteem related to
  - Inability to relate to own mother

Table 35-3 *Ages at Which Teenage Mothers Expect Children to Accomplish Specific Behaviors*

Behavior	Norm for Mastery (months)	Mother's Expectations (%) <12 Months	12-18 Months	18-24 Months	>36 Months
Bladder control	18-24	43	43	14	0
Bowel control	14-36	26	30	30	14
Obedience training	>24	80	14	6	0
Recognition of right from wrong	30-36	78	20	2	0

From Jarret, E: MCN 7(2):119, 1982.

Planning

The plan of care reflects the adolescent mother's need for increased surveillance, complying with health care measures, and feelings of positive self-worth. The care begins as early as possible in the prenatal period and extends through the formative period of the new family.

Goals. The goals for care of pregnant adolescents parallel those for care of all pregnant women: to assist them in experiencing a physically safe and emotionally satisfying pregnancy and to promote optimum health in their offspring. Care of teenage mothers also includes the following goals:

1. Early and continued prenatal care
2. Comprehensive obstetric, psychosocial, parenting, and outreach services in one setting
3. Creative forms of health care delivery to maximize services to all pregnant adolescents and their families

Implementation

It is important that persons who work with pregnant adolescents have come to terms with their own sexuality to be able to maintain a nonjudgmental approach. They must be genuinely interested in the adolescent, as well as being enthusiastic, warm, caring individuals able to view adolescents as young persons involved in an exciting growth period. They need to accept the adolescent as someone willing to respond to a concerned adult and who basically wants to be accepted and successful. Nurses need to be able to listen and to respond with honest answers, to be available when needed, and to be capable of accepting repeated "testing" by the adolescent. They need to be able to create a safe and stable environment that engenders trust. Such an environment will enable the professional to determine the adolescent's real problems and to set realistic goals. Accepting some behavior as typically adolescent and not as acting-out or hostile reactions to pregnancy will enable the caregiver to maintain concern for the population served and to remain committed on an individual basis.

Nurses who work with pregnant adolescents need to be knowledgeable concerning (1) the physical attributes of the adolescent and her developmental needs, (2) the adolescent's maturational level relative to personality and cognitive development, (3) maternal responses to pregnancy and the adolescent's interpretation of them, and (4) the cues that indicate stress in the adolescent and difficulties in parenting.

Nurses need to be adept in using a variety of teaching strategies (Fullar, 1986). Group discussions are effective because adolescents have a strong need for peer contact and acceptance. However, because of the immaturity of the participants the nurse will often need to act as leader. Question boxes and anonymous pretests are devices that reveal gaps in knowledge or belief in myths. Demonstrations by the nurse, with group members exhibiting the same skill, are an effective means of assessing the teenager's abilities. Creative approaches, including peer education and computer games, actively involve teenagers in self-care with good results (Siegel, 1987).

As counselors and advocates, nurses are concerned with the adolescent's ability to make decisions, to explore the risks and consequences of her actions, and to assume responsibility for her behavior. Some of the techniques used to encourage growth in these areas include having the adolescent set up a discussion group, decorate a child care space, select a menu, plan a day for herself and her infant, and talk over solutions to problems. Independent function is encouraged; the nurse acts as a catalyst in solving problems, but the problem solving belongs to the adolescent.

Another area in which the adolescent requires assistance is in helping her separate herself from her baby so that she can see the child's unique needs. Information relative to child development and to infant caretaking is basic to this goal.

Nurses can act as role models for adolescent parents in the care of themselves and their infants. Areas particularly important to emphasize to the mother are healthy lifestyles, cleanliness, and good eating habits. The nurse can help the young mother become skillful in taking care of the daily needs of her infant. The nurse's physical assessment skills can be taught to the parent so that she becomes more knowledgeable about her child's needs.

Community Support

Before 1960 the care of pregnant adolescents was centered in maternity residences for unmarried mothers, operated in many cases by either the Salvation Army or the

Florence Crittendon organizations (Appendix K). In the 1960s and 1970s the age of the mother, rather than the legitimacy aspects of the parenthood, became the focus of attention. As a result, community programs with a triad of services—medical, social, and educational—were established. In 1978 Congress passed Public Law 95-625 to improve coordination and linkage between community agencies working with pregnant or parenting adolescents. In 1982 the Act was incorporated into the Maternal and Child Services Block Grant. The 1982 Act placed more emphasis on families, adoption alternatives, research, and evaluation. Federal funding for the various projects is currently being curtailed. Budget cuts may also reduce public health nursing services from health departments, social workers in hospitals and clinics, and Medicaid for prenatal care during a first pregnancy. Child care programs are also vulnerable to budget cuts.

Adolescent Clinics. Because of the circumstances of adolescent pregnancy, programs specifically addressing the problems of the adolescent are being developed across the country (Appendix K). Clinics for adolescents are better equipped to provide health care services responsive to the teenager's unique needs. They also provide for supportive associations with the father of the child and with the girl's parents or other authority figures. They utilize a multidisciplinary team of nurse-midwives, physicians, nurses, nutritionists, and social workers. The outcomes of lower recidivism and increased birth weights are two indicators of their effectiveness (Chanis et al., 1979; Doyle and Widhalm, 1979; Peoples and Barrett, 1799; Neeson et al., 1983; Osofsky, 1985).

Pregnancy

The adolescent is considered to be at risk during her pregnancy. There is an increase in scheduled prenatal visits. Effort is expended to encourage prompt attendance at the clinic; lapses in attendance are followed up by telephone calls or personal contacts.

Prenatal Classes. The content of prenatal classes is chosen with the adolescent's needs in mind. Content relating to maternal adaptations during pregnancy should be presented in terms of how the adolescent can adjust to changes (Fig. 35-3). For example, exercises to promote posture, the care of skin, hair, and nails, and hygiene for increased perspiration and vaginal secretions are discussed. Concrete examples of "what to do" and "what not to do" are needed. Orientation in the present makes it difficult for the adolescent to anticipate the baby's needs.

Teaching requires flexibility, good humor, ingenuity, and at times, ego strength. Standard approaches are not likely to appeal to adolescents. Probaby they will not have anyone with whom to attend the classes. Films that depict a loving couple experiencing classes and birth may cause the unpartnered adolescent to "tune out." The teacher needs to be friendly and welcoming and may need to sit near the adolescent. Teaching must consider the early adolescent's short attention span; the teaching pace is brisk and interesting. Role-playing allows the expectant mother to become a partner in her own care. Audiovisual methods allow her to "be there" without actually being there, giving her an option to pace the input.

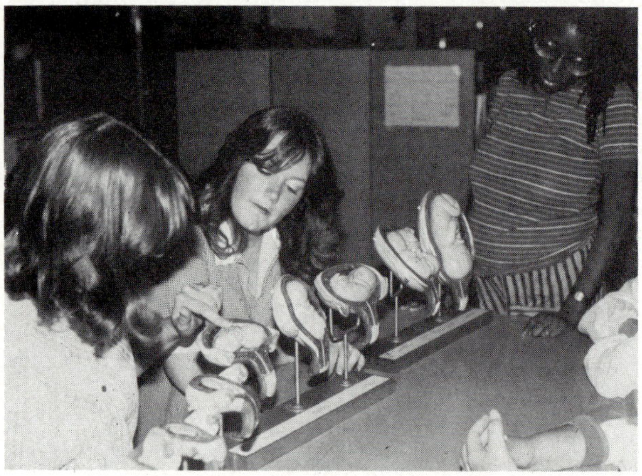

Fig. 35-3 Teenage expectant mothers learn about maternal adaptations to pregnancy.
Courtesy Marjorie Pyle, RNC, Lifecircle, Costa Mesa, Calif.

Information about what happens during labor and delivery and how pain is controlled requires considerable emphasis. Opportunities to discuss feelings and fears with other adolescents who have experienced birth are welcome. Basic information about sex and reproduction is needed to ensure accuracy of the adolescent's knowledge in this area. Birth control information should be included in prenatal classes and presented realistically and nonjudgmentally. Adolescents welcome information about infant care but need help to see the usefulness of information given about child growth and development.

Nutrition Counseling. Adolescence is a period of developing independence. Symbols of home—milk, fresh fruits and vegetables, and a "square meal"—if these were present, are associated with dependency and as such may be threatening (e.g., "peanut butter is for children"). Often there is the desire to "be free" to choose "forbidden" foods. Peers congregate at the hamburger stand; soda, hamburgers, and french fries may be supplemented with candy bars. Nausea and vomiting in pregnancy often compromise an adequate dietary intake (see research highlight).

The young married adolescent may have just learned how to cook. This achievement, as well as her desire to please her husband and meet his preferences, must be considered in nutrition counseling. Supporting her inner desire to assert independence during nutrition counseling sessions lends support to the overall developmental task of this period: movement from the role of child to that of adult. Listen and allow her to talk. Build on what she and her family already know and practice. Reinforce sound dietary patterns and acknowledge adaptations that are willingly made. In planning a teaching strategy to meet the objectives of nutrition counseling, the nurse must first set realistic goals such as the following:

1. To support the pregnant adolescent's psychosocial move toward independence
2. To increase her knowledge of nutrients and daily allowances

RESEARCH HIGHLIGHT

First Trimester Nausea in Pregnant Teenagers: Incidence, Characteristics, Intervention

Purpose

To determine the incidence and characteristics of nausea and vomiting in teenagers during pregnancy, and effective interventions.

Sample

The sample included 78 pregnant teenagers, 75% of whom were black, and 70% of whom were unmarried.

Methodology

A questionnaire was developed to determine which measures were used by teens to control nausea and vomiting and which measures were most effective. The instrument consisted of 14 forced-choice items and 1 open-ended question. Content validity was established using a panel of judges who were practicing nurses. A reading specialist helped establish a sixth-grade reading level. The instrument was pilot tested by a group of nurses and pregnant teenagers.

Findings

Nausea and vomiting during pregnancy (NVP) was experienced by 56% of the subjects. NVP was experienced by 95% of white teens as opposed to only 42% of black teens. The incidence of NVP was correlated with the desire to become pregnant. Girls who wanted the pregnancy were more likely to have experienced NVP than those who did not want to be pregnant.

Implications

The nonpharmacologic measure that was reported by 46% of the teens to be most effective in controlling NVP was to lie down during the episode. This method has not been reported in the literature as a nonpharmacologic treatment of NVP. It has been suggested that NVP may be a result of orthostatic hypotension, since NVP tends to occur upon getting out of bed in the morning. This investigator suggests that controlled studies are needed to determine if a relationship exists between orthostatic hypotension and NVP.

DiIorio, C: First trimester nausea in pregnant teenagers: incidence, characteristics, intervention, Nurs Res 34(6):372, 1985.

3. To teach her how to plan diets for herself and her family
4. To teach her how to select foods to meet nutrition needs, personal preferences, budget requirements, and seasonal availability.
5. To teach her how to prepare foods to ensure optimum nutritive value

Of necessity these goals go beyond the immediate objectives of a healthy pregnancy, an uneventful labor, and a full-term, healthy infant whose weight and maturity are appropriate for gestational age. Subsequently the infant grows and develops normally. Recent animal research has disclosed that two generations are required to counteract the mental and physical retardation resulting from protein deficiency during pregnancy. The young mother who improves her own and her family's dietary patterns is building the foundation for a healthier beginning for generations to follow (see general nursing care plan: teenage pregnancy, p. 895).

The relationship between sound nutrition and physical appearance can be used to gain the attention of adolescents (and perhaps older women as well) for nutrition education. Commonly the condition and appearance of the skin, hair, and nails are uppermost in the minds of adolescents. Body contours in both the male and female adolescent and muscular development in the male teenager are selling points for good nutrition.

Labor and Delivery

The adolescent in labor should have the support of a knowledgeable coach, whether husband, boyfriend, parent, or nurse. Many teenagers come to labor lacking preparation; they are fearful and often alone. If they are admitted early in the first stage, teaching about relaxation with contractions, ambulation, side-lying positions, and comfort measures can be accomplished (Unit IV). According to Mercer (1979) the teenager's rights to grant informed consent and to refuse treatments must be continually acknowledged (Holder, 1987; Morrissey, Hofmann, and Thrope, 1986). This is also true of her right to be informed of her progress and of both her own and her infant's health status. Recognizing the rights of youthful parents fosters their self-esteem and personal development.

Today most adolescents keep their infants and are responsive to the staff's sharing in their delight and joy (Fig. 35-4). For these young parents, efforts to promote parent-child attachment are particularly important.

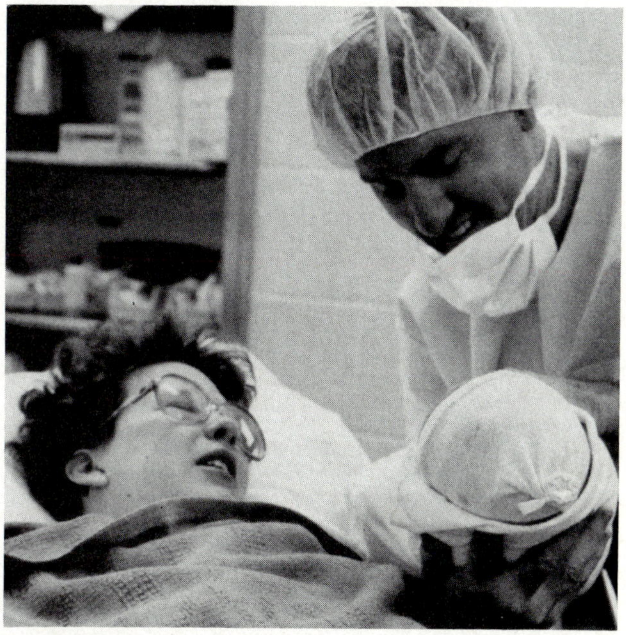

Fig. 35-4 Nurse acquainting young mother with newborn son after cesarean delivery.

The Puerperium

Physically the adolescent mother will require the same care as any woman who had delivered an infant. Increased emphasis on teaching self-care and breast examination is warranted. Explicit directions as to follow-up care for herself and her infant are required. The need for continued assessment of her parenting abilities during the postdelivery period is essential if needed support is to be forthcoming. Although the nurse may be responsive to cues of parenting ability evidenced in the prenatal period, these findings are not as predictive as the cues noted during the reality phase of parenthood.

If possible the young mother and her child are placed in a rooming-in accommodation so that the process of mothering the child can be started as early as possible. This support needs to be sustained after the mother and child return home. The process of continued care should include home visit and group sessions for discussion of infant care or parenting problems. Research indicates that outreach programs concerned with parent-child interactions, child injuries, and instances of failure to thrive and that provide prompt and effective community intervention do prevent more serious subsequent problems (Gray, et al., 1979).

Parenting education needs must be met for the increased number of adolescents who are bearing and rais-

SAMPLE INTERVIEW QUESTIONS

Often girls your age, when they become mothers, find their lives to be different from what they had planned for themselves. They sometimes must drop out of school, and it may be hard for them to find a job they like. Plans they once had for themselves may just seem like unreachable dreams. Let's talk about how you feel regarding these things.

1. Are you going to school now? What do you feel about that?
   If necessary: Are you glad that you are? or Do you wish that you were?
2. Do you have any kind of job right now? What do you feel about it?
   If necessary: Do you like your job? Does it seem adequate to meet your needs? or Do you wish you were working?
3. What would you most like to be doing with your life right now if you could do anything that you wished?
4. What would you most like to do in the future if you had the choice of doing anything that you wanted to do? Is this a possible goal for you? What do you feel about that?

Young mothers often find their lives totally filled with school, job, and caring for their babies. Often they do not have time to do the things they like to do, such as visit with their friends, make new friends, or be with their husband or boyfriend. Sometimes their own mothers seem to use the baby as a means of controlling what their daughters do and do not do. This can sometimes be very frustrating.

5. Do you seem to be able to find time to be by yourself? What do you feel about that? What do you usually do when you have free time for yourself? What would you most like to do during this time?
6. Do you find time to be with your friends? Are you able to see them as often as you would like? What do you feel about that? Have you made any new friends since you had the baby?
   If unmarried: Have you been able to be with your boyfriend or meet and date new guys since you had the baby? What do you feel about that?
7. Do you feel that your mother puts a lot of pressure on you to do things that you should do? What do you feel about that?

Husbands or boyfriends sometimes get involved with the baby, and sometimes they do not. Young mothers often feel isolated and alone and resent the fact that the father is not helping much with the baby. Sometimes mothers feel that they do not get along with the husband or boyfriend as well as they did before the baby came.

8. Does your baby's father seem to enjoy the baby? What type of things does he do with him (her)? Change diapers? Bathe? Feed? Play? Other? Do you get enough help from him? What do you feel about that? Do you seem to be closer, less close, or about the same as you were before the baby was born? What do you feel about that?

It is important what some people think about us, but with other people we do not really care what they think. I'm going to give you a list of people and I want you to tell me whether or not they would agree with the way you take care of your baby and how you feel about whether they agree or not.

9. Mother, Father, Baby's father, Baby's father's parents, Teacher, Employer, Friends, Nutritionist, Social worker, Nurse, Doctor, Church members, Minister or priest, Neighbors, Relatives

Some things about caring for the baby are fun, but others may be very irritating to a mother. I'm going to ask you about different things you do in caring for your baby and about what your baby does. Tell me what you feel about them.

10. First, feeding your baby. What do you feel about this? How much time does it usually take? Does it seem to take a lot out of you?
11. Now let's consider changing your baby's diaper. What do you feel about that?
12. How about bathing your baby?
13. How about playing with your baby? What do you feel about that? Do you find time to play with your baby often? Do you feel that it is important for you to play with her (or him)?
14. Does your baby try to annoy you sometimes? What does the baby do that really annoys you? What do you feel about that? What do you usually do about it? Do you ever find that you need to punish your baby? What types of things does your baby do that need punishment? How do you usually punish your baby when this is necessary?

Reprinted with permission of the publisher of Pediatric Nursing. From Poole, CJ: Pediatr Nurs 2:7, March/April, 1976.

ing children. Inexperience and a lack of knowledge about caring for children (i.e., limited knowledge of growth and development, use of physical punishment for controlling child behavior, and suboptimum social stimulation), are probable causes of problems demonstrated by infants of adolescent mothers.

To enhance learning, motivation to learn must be strengthened, and the content taught must be relevant. The learner must recognize a need for information or learning will not occur (Chapter 2). Howard and Sater (1985) reported on self-perceived health education needs of 66 adolescent mothers. White, Hispanic, and black females were almost equally represented in this group of 14- to 18-year-old participants. Their educational level varied from 7 to 12 years. The care of the infant was rated the area of primary concern. Ways to make the baby feel loved (90.9%), to protect the baby from accidents (89.4%), and to take care of a sick baby (86.4%) topped the list of perceived learning needs.

The adolescent who has an infant who was born prematurely or who is SGA may find it extremely difficult to reconcile this tiny, scrawny infant with her fantasized baby. Her feelings of helplessness when she contemplates the care of a healthy term infant are compounded when she is introduced to her child in the intensive care unit. It may be impossible for her to perceive herself as mothering such an infant. The additional care needed by the infant can overwhelm the coping mechanisms she had built up so trustingly in the prenatal period. The consequent alienation of mother and infant may never be overcome. Intensive teaching and continuous support programs are essential if both the young mother and her vulnerable infant are not to be overwhelmed.

As noted earlier the young adolescent is not able to establish a family unit for herself or her child. The interdependence possible in such a unit is denied her. If the young mother and her child are incorporated into the older family unit, the process in which she was moving from dependent to interdependent behavior must be adjusted to accommodate an essentially dependent individual. Persons who provide counseling that involves the parents of the young mother seek to set realistic goals for developing the independence of the adolescent. Topics for open discussions among all persons concerned should include infant care responsibilities, the teenager's need to continue her education, and her need to work toward maturity. The adolescent's parents will need support as well, since they face a new set of responsibilities and tasks. They, too, in a sense, must adjust a fantasy to an actual child.

When assistance is given to a young mother, efforts are made to determine her feelings toward her infant, the quality of the interaction between mother and infant, her knowledge of an attitude toward infant care activities, and her understanding of her infant's growth and developmental needs. Many young mothers pattern their practice on what they themselves experienced. It is vital, therefore, to determine the kind of support that those close to these young mothers are able or prepared to give and the kinds of community aid that can supplement this support. The sample interview questions developed by Poole (1976) help the nurse obtain information (box, p. 894). The use of the questionnaire reassures the adolescent that there are concerns common to herself and others. This tool is useful in assisting the adolescent in problem identification and problem solving. These skills are essential for the adolescent to accomplish the developmental tasks she faces.

A general nursing care plan and a specific nursing care plan for teenage pregnancy follow.

Text continued on p. 901.

General Nursing Care Plan

TEENAGE PREGNANCY

ASSESSMENT	NURSING DIAGNOSIS (ND)/ PLAN (P)/GOAL (G)	RATIONALE/ IMPLEMENTATION	EVALUATION
Note previous obstetric history. Assess knowledge regarding: pregnancy, childbirth, parenthood. Cultural beliefs. Financial status. View of pregnancy. Does client want to continue with the pregnancy? Does client want to be a parent or put the child up for adoption?	ND: Knowledge deficit related to choices regarding pregnancy, childbirth experience, and parenthood. P: Supply information about choices and community resources and support. G: Client will learn about pregnancy, childbirth, and parenthood. G: Client will learn about	*To teach client about pregnancy, childbirth, and parenthood, the nurse will:* Examine own views regarding sexuality to be able to maintain nonjudgmental approach. Listen and give honest answers. Accept and expect repeated testing from the adolescent.	Client learns about her pregnancy choices, childbirth experience; and parenthood. Client makes a choice with which she is comfortable. Client is able to effectively utilize community resources or support from family or friends.

Continued.

General Nursing Care Plan—cont'd

ASSESSMENT	NURSING DIAGNOSIS (ND)/ PLAN (P)/GOAL (G)	RATIONALE/ IMPLEMENTATION	EVALUATION
Assess teen's support systems: boyfriend, peers, family, outreach service, in community.	her choice to maintain or abort the pregnancy, keep the child, or place the child for adoption.	Create a safe and stable environment that engenders trust. Evaluate which of the three stages of development the adolescent is experiencing. Teach the adolescent about pregnancy choices, childbirth, and parenthood. Utilize group teaching as a means for learning and establishing teen support. Encourage questions and verbalization of fears or concerns. Compliment teen on well-thought-out questions and reference to learned issues. Encourage support person to attend and participate in prenatal care. Refer to childbirth and parenthood class.	
Note teen's current obligations (school, work, home). Accessibility to health care.	ND: Ineffective individual coping, related to situational crises of teen pregnancy. P: Establish a trusting relationship and ensure confidentiality. G: Client will learn the importance of early and continuous prenatal care. G: Client will keep her appointments and participate in her care.	*To encourage client to attend prenatal care, the nurse will:* Provide consistency of caregivers. Explain the need to closely monitor her pregnancy. Create safe, stable environment. Evaluate transportation needs to health care center. Schedule appointments around school or work activities. Use creative forms of health care delivery to maximize services. Note maternal responses to pregnancy and the adolescent's interpretation of them. Provide obstetric, psychosocial, and outreach services in one setting, if possible. Offer teen as many choices as possible and encourage her to take an active role in her plan of care.	Client attends prenatal care. Client participates in her plan of care.
How do you feel about yourself? How do you feel about	ND: Body image disturbance, situational low self-esteem, altered role	*To assist the client in maintaining her self-concept, the nurse will:*	Client verbalizes her concerns and feelings about pregnancy.

General Nursing Care Plan—cont'd

ASSESSMENT	NURSING DIAGNOSIS (ND)/ PLAN (P)/GOAL (G)	RATIONALE/ IMPLEMENTATION	EVALUATION
pregnancy? How do you feel about becoming a mother? What are your goals for the future? Support system.	performance, related to pregnancy. ND: Potential for altered growth and development related to concurrent adolescence and pregnancy. ND: Potential for social isolation from family or peers related to pregnancy. P: Help client increase problem-solving skills to plan for a future, and to communicate caring and support. G: Client will discuss concerns and feelings about pregnancy. G: Client will identify her support system. G: Client will continue to develop in her stage of adolescence during her pregnancy.	Show interest in client, her thoughts and feelings. Provide private place to talk and discuss matters in an unhurried manner. Encourage verbalization. Identify support system with teen. Evaluate teen's adolescent stage to counsel and support her in achieving her developmental tasks. Compliment teen on her appearance, verbalization of feelings, and learning. Refer to outside resources, guidance counselor, tutor.	Client identifies her support system. Client develops in her own stage of maturity.
Assess for teen's use of: alcoholic beverages, smoking, street drugs. Ask if teen's close friends use alcohol, drugs, or tobacco products (see substance abuse, Chapter 34).	ND: Altered health maintenance related to substance abuse. ND: Potential for injury (maternal and fetal) related to substance abuse. ND: Potential for infection related to intravenous drug abuse. P: Provide information and be available for discussion of concerns and questions. G: Client will learn how substance abuse will effect herself and her baby during pregnancy. G: Client will avoid nonprescribed drugs, smoking, and alcoholic beverages during pregnancy.	*To promote a pregnancy free from substance abuse, the nurse will:* Examine teen's substance abuse habit: 1. Duration of abuse. 2. Time and circumstances when substances are used. Explain the dangers of substance abuse on the pregnant woman and fetus. Utilize group teaching to promote peer support against substance abuse. Examine with teen her current peer group and their influence with the use of drugs, smoking, and alcohol. Involve support person in plan to reduce, then eliminate substance abuse. Refer teen to social services and a "quit smoking" or addiction program.	Client learns about the effects of substance abuse on pregnancy. Client avoids nonprescribed drugs, smoking, and alcoholic beverages during pregnancy.
How many meals are eaten daily? Who prepares the meals? Cultural and religious influences on food. Knowledge of the four basic food groups. Client's food likes/dislikes.	ND: Knowledge deficit related to nutritional needs of the mother and fetus during pregnancy. ND: Altered nutrition: less than body requirements, related to in-	*To increase the client's knowledge about nutrition during pregnancy, the nurse will:* Review the four basic food groups. Instruct on the importance of adequate nutrition dur-	Client verbalizes understanding of instruction. Client prepares sample menus that meet the daily nutrition requirements during pregnancy.

Continued.

General Nursing Care Plan—cont'd

ASSESSMENT	NURSING DIAGNOSIS (ND)/ PLAN (P)/GOAL (G)	RATIONALE/ IMPLEMENTATION	EVALUATION
Does she take vitamins? Financial status. (See assessment, Chapter 14).	creased nutrient requirements during pregnancy and adolescence. P: Increase client's knowledge about nutrition and involve her in "taking charge" of what happens to her by mutual planning. G: Client will learn about the nutritional needs of pregnancy. G: Client will design sample meals that are balanced with the basic food groups.	ing pregnancy. Examine cultural and financial considerations when planning nutrition instructions. Refer to financial support agencies for low income cases (welfare, WIC). Mutually select foods to meet nutrition needs, personal preferences, budget requirements, and seasonal availability. Assist client in designing sample menus. Teach client how to prepare foods to ensure optimum nutritive value.	
Note baseline blood pressure and monitor at every prenatal visit. Note edema (are your shoes fitting tight?) Note proteinuria. Note fetal heart rate after 8 to 12 weeks. Note fetal activity after 16 weeks.	ND: Altered tissue perfusion related to inadequate placental perfusion secondary to PIH. ND: Potential for injury: maternal and fetal related to PIH. P: Monitor for potential complications. G: Client will be monitored closely for signs and symptoms of pregnancy-induced hypertension (PIH). G: Client will be treated promptly if she demonstrates PIH.	*Adolescents at great risk for PIH. See PIH general care plan, Chapter 29, pp. 707, 716.*	Client remains free from PIH or condition is identified and treated promptly so mother and fetus demonstrate no or minimum sequelae. Client experiences no complications.
Has adolescent cared for a child before? Who will be assisting in child care? Support system. Knowledge of infant needs.	ND: Knowledge deficit related to infant care activities, growth patterns, and developmental needs. P: Provide information and encouragement, demonstrate, and observe reverse demonstration. G: Client will learn infant care activities, growth pattern, and developmental needs. G: Client will identify her support system for child care.	*To teach adolescent about infant care activities, growth patterns, and developmental needs, the nurse will:* Identify baseline knowledge. Begin infant care activities instruction during prenatal period. Involve support person in teaching sessions. Focus teaching toward adolescent's maturity and cognitive level. Refer client to parenthood classes. Refer to and make initial contact with social services for a future resource person if problems arise in child care.	Client learns infant care activities, growth patterns, and developmental needs. Client identifies her support system. Client's self-esteem increases with increase in skill.

Specific Nursing Care Plan

TEENAGE PREGNANCY

Jane Brady is a 16-year-old girl who is 28-weeks pregnant. She initially sought prenatal care at 16 weeks gestation but has missed several appointments since. Jane expresses concern for her baby and seems to enjoy the teen pregnancy and childbirth class presented by the teen clinic before her prenatal visits. Despite encouragement to bring a support person to the clinic with her, she always comes alone. Upon questioning, the nurse discovers that Jane has several close friends, but feels embarrassed and different around her peers at school with her "big belly."

Jane's parents are divorced and she lives with her mother and older sister who both work full-time. Jane's mother and sister have expressed interest in assisting with child care but Jane verbalizes ambivalence about keeping the baby.

ASSESSMENT	NURSING DIAGNOSIS (ND)/ PLAN (P)/GOAL (G)	RATIONALE/ IMPLEMENTATION	EVALUATION
Missed prenatal appointments. Enjoys prenatal classes. Mother and sister work full-time. Note transportation to clinic.	ND: Potential for injury (maternal and fetal) related to several missed prenatal appointments. P: Identify reason for missed appointments and mutually develop a plan for prenatal care. G: Jane will attend scheduled prenatal care.	*To examine the problems surrounding missed appointments, the nurse will:* Identify transportation problems to the clinic and suggest solutions. Schedule appointments around school activities. Examine feelings or concerns about the prenatal visits. Create safe stable environment. Provide consistent caregiver. Explain the need to closely monitor her pregnancy.	Jane attends her scheduled prenatal visits. Jane identifies her feelings. Jane verbalizes understanding of need for prenatal care.
Jane comes to prenatal visits alone. Jane is in high school. Jane has several close friends. Jane feels embarrassed and different around her peers at school. Parents divorced. Jane is unfamiliar with outside resources.	ND: Situational low self-esteem. ND: Body image disturbance. ND: Altered role performance related to pregnancy and middle stage adolescence. P: Develop a trusting relationship (Chapter 2), provide time and space, and mutually develop a plan of care. G: Jane will discuss concerns and feelings about "fitting in" with her peers at school. G: Jane will participate in problem solving. G: Jane will continue to achieve her education during and after pregnancy. G: Jane will bring a support person to her prenatal visits.	*To encourage participation in problem solving and achievement of teen's educational and support needs, the nurse will:* Take unhurried time discussing Jane's concerns and feelings. Encourage Jane to discuss her thoughts with her close friends. Identify Jane's goals in life and suggest ways to meet those goals (Who am I?) Encourage participation in known problem solving. Compliment Jane on her general appearance, verbalization of fears, and participation in care. Identify with Jane her support system including outside resources (welfare, WIC, home health care, child care, psychologists, guidance counselors, tutors).	Jane discusses concerns and feelings. Jane participates in problem-solving. Jane continues her education during pregnancy. Jane brings a support person to prenatal visits. Jane appears clean and well-groomed. Jane utilizes community resources as needed.

Continued.

Specific Nursing Care Plan—cont'd

ASSESSMENT	NURSING DIAGNOSIS (ND)/ PLAN (P)/GOAL (G)	RATIONALE/ IMPLEMENTATION	EVALUATION
		Refer to guidance counselor if Jane needs tutoring to achieve educational needs. Encourage Jane to choose one person who will attend prenatal care, assist in childbirth, and participate in child care activities with her.	
Expressing ambivalence about keeping child or placing child for adoption. Assess knowledge about adoption. Assess family's feelings about adoption.	ND: Potential ineffective individual coping related to making an informed permanent decision. ND: Knowledge deficit related to parenthood and adoption issues. P: Provide information and be available for discussion of questions and concerns. G: Jane will make an informed decision about keeping her infant or placing the child for adoption.	*To assist Jane in formulating an informed decision about parenthood or adoption, the nurse will:* Evaluate own feelings regarding parenthood and adoption as to not send verbal or nonverbal messages that will influence Jane. Discuss the pros and cons of parenthood and adoption with Jane. Encourage questions and answer honestly. Clarify misconceptions. Suggest solutions to problems such as financial support or educational needs that may be of concern to Jane when evaluating parenthood. Refer Jane to a licensed adoption agency for specific questions surrounding the adoption process. Encourage Jane to discuss the decision with her family but stress that *only she alone* can make the decision. Evaluate Jane's feelings regarding seeing her child after birth or knowing its sex if adoption is chosen. Until adoption papers are signed, Jane should know that she can change her decision.	Jane makes an informed decision regarding parenthood or adoption. Jane's problem-solving skills increase.

Evaluation

The maternity nurse needs to evaluate the care she provides to the adolescent client to see how effective her nursing actions have been. As with all pregnant women, the plan of care will have to be redesigned to meet the unique needs of the individual adolescent client. The maternity nurse has the responsibility of becoming involved in the increasing health needs of the teenage mother.

The descriptions below of three 17-year-old girls illustrate the differences in attitude, acceptance of the pregnancy, readiness of parenthood, and amount and kind of outside support available.

It is obvious that to each of these teenagers, pregnancy had a different meaning; their perceptions of themselves varied, as did their needs. A stereotyped approach to the young pregnant woman is no more successful than a similar approach to the older one.

ADOLESCENT FATHER

The effect of pregnancy and parenthood on adolescent fathers has recently become an area of nursing concern. Three major factors have prompted interest in the problems of these young parents.

1. The critical role of the father in the development of a child has been shown (Lamb, 1981; Parke et al., 1980).

2. Health programs have been developed that consider the needs of both the adolescent mother and the adolescent father (Berland, 1987).

3. The role of the father in the birth process has changed. Fathers are now encouraged to be participants in birth. Responsibilities and rights of fathers are more accepted. For example, the federal government expects the unwed mother to attempt to gain child support from the father of the child before it will grant financial assistance (Moore, 1981). A father has the legal right to petition for custody of his child if the mother wishes to place the baby for adoption (Panner and Evans, 1975). Regardless of the length or even the existence of marriage between teen parents, significant numbers of young men remain involved with their children (Stengel, 1985).

Berland (1987) attempted to establish a young fathers' support group. He assumed that he could entice the fathers to attend by persuading the mothers. He found that the mothers often are powerless in their relationships with the father of the baby. For various reasons, other mothers did not wish to have the fathers involved. When the fathers were reached, Berland found that among his subjects, their children's welfare was not as important as their own personal development. Relating to female friends was as far as they could manage. They appeared unready for parenthood.

Case 1. Sharon, 17 years old and with an attractive, outgoing personality, was married 3 months before the birth of her baby. She was enthusiastic about attending parentcraft classes, and her husband, Bob, came to those relating to support in labor. He was to finish high school in June, 2 months before the baby was born, and would go to work immediately in a local gas station. Their parents were going to help them for 6 months by paying the rent on a small apartment, but they were expected to provide for other necessities. Bob made a cradle for the baby, and she made most of the baby clothes. Both families were excited about the baby and nonjudgmental in their attitudes toward Sharon and her husband.

Sharon had a normal pregnancy and delivery. She was pleased and happy with her baby and found caring for the child rewarding. Bob did well in his job and accepted his new responsibilities.

Case 2. Mary Lou, 17 years old, was a small, fragile-looking young woman. Mary Lou was the youngest of four sisters, all of whom were married and away from home. She had numerous relatives—aunts, uncles, and cousins—in the vicinity. Both her mother and father worked.

Mary Lou never divulged the name of the father of her child. She had no intention of giving the baby up for adoption; she intended to stay home and care for it herself. She refused to attend group classes but was eager and willing for the nurse to teach her individually. When she was taken on the tour of the hospital facilities, she clung to the nurse and needed much reassurance and mothering. The birth was normal, and Mary Lou had a boy. This was an occasion for great family rejoicing, since there had not been a boy for three generations, and her sisters had had girls. Mary Lou came to the hospital with a suitcase containing pretty clothes for herself and lovely baby clothes. The extended family accompanied her to the hospital and were there to greet the new baby. On the first visit to the home, the nurse was extremely aware of the overwhelming presence of the family, particularly Mary Lou's father. Mary Lou was feeding the baby his bottle in a correct but perfunctory manner. Subsequent visits found her increasingly trying to isolate herself. The nurse encouraged Mary Lou to seek additional counseling because she was concerned with Mary Lou's lack of affective response. Mary Lou refused, and within a week ran away from home, leaving the baby behind.

Case 3. Betty, 17 years old, was an overweight young woman. She refused to wear maternity clothes and bought herself an overlarge dress in a dark-brown material with small red flowers. She took no other interest in her appearance. She talked repeatedly about how the father of the child had taken advantage of her, that she was a good girl, and that "he was bad." The baby was to be put up for adoption. She refused to discuss her relationships with her parents, who lived in another city.

Betty had a long, difficult labor. At one time she struck the nurse who was caring for her and screamed for the nurse to "get this monster out of me." She refused to see the baby or to talk about the child. She appeared to deny the whole experience. When the time came for her to return to her home, the nurse accompanied her to the bus. She boarded the bus, and the bus pulled away; the nurse waved, but Betty did not look back.

Nursing Care

The adolescent father, as well as the adolescent mother, is faced with immediate developmental crises, that is, completing the developmental tasks of adolescence and making a transition to parenthood. If the young couple marry, a third stress is added—transition to marriage. The long-range effects of premature parenthood are related to delayed educational and vocational attainment and to lack of stability in marriage.

If at all possible, the father is approached through his pregnant partner. Some clinics make clear that the pregnant adolescent will bring her partner to the clinic and that he will take an active interest in the birth process. At other times the father needs to be contacted directly. Data needed for inclusion of the young father in all aspects of the care are based on the assessment of four areas, (1) the future of the couple together, (2) the adequacy of coping, (3) educational and vocational goals, and (4) the adequacy of health education knowledge (Elster, 1982; Elster and Lamb, 1982).

Adolescent fathers (as all fathers) need support to discuss their emotional responses to the pregnancy. These may include pleasure, ambivalence, or anger. The fathers' feelings of guilt, powerlessness, or bravado deserve recognition, as these may have negative consequences for both parents and children (Berland, 1987). Caparulo and London (1981) characterize them as "adolescents first, fathers second." Counseling needs to be reality oriented. Topics such as child care and expense, parenting skills, and the father's role in the birth experience need to be explored. Teenage fathers also need knowledge of reproductive physiology and birth control options.

The adolescent mother's boyfriend, as well as her family, have an impact on how she will deal with her pregnancy, labor and delivery, and subsequent parenthood. The adolescent partner may continue to be involved in an ongoing relationship with the young mother. In many instances he plays an important role in the decisions she faces in pregnancy. He may influence her decision to continue the pregnancy or have an abortion and to keep the child or place the child for adoption.

The nurse supports the young father by helping him develop realistic perceptions of his role as "father to a child." The nurse encourages his use of coping mechanisms that are not detrimental to his, his partner's, and his child's well-being. The nurse enlists support systems, parents, and professional agencies on his behalf. Promoting mutual responsibility for birth control is a constant necessity.

SUMMARY

Much has still to be done before the problems of adolescent pregnancy and its sequelae for infant, mother, family, and society in general are solved.

There is a definite societal acceptance toward allowing adolescents more freedom to make decisions, and to exercise autonomy and self-determination in their relationships with health care providers and with others in the social system.

Cooperative effort on personal, local, and national levels is mandatory. In spite of the development of many successful programs, adolescent pregnancy remains the most pressing problem in maternity and gynecologic nursing care today.

KEY CONCEPTS

- Adolescents see their world in far different terms than do adults: their major task is the development of cognitive ability.
- Cognitive development influences sexual decision making.
- Increasingly, poverty, life-style, and risk-taking behaviors are implicated in adolescent morbidity, with associated sequelae of pregnancy and other major health problems.
- Physiologic consequences and personal and public costs of adolescent pregnancy and parenthood are staggering.
- The adolescent's perception of pregnancy and parenthood is individual and dependent on many variables.
- The developmental tasks of adolescents are interrupted by pregnancy.
- Poor nutrition and poverty have been implicated in physiologic consequences to the adolescent mother and her fetus and newborn.
- Adolescents' reactions to perceived stress depend on the quality of their support systems, their self-esteem, and their skill in problem identification and problem solving.
- The adolescent's knowledge of child development is usually limited.
- Standard approaches to prenatal and postpartum teaching are not appropriate or appealing for most adolescents.

STUDY QUESTIONS AND ACTIVITIES

1. In a group setting discuss feelings about adolescent pregnancy. Start with a discussion of girls, known to group members, who became pregnant in high school. Discuss the attitudes of their peers and the outcomes of their pregnancies.
2. As a group project discover financial, health, and educational resources in the area that provide services needed by adolescent parents. Each student should visit at least one agency and learn about the attitudes of staff and the services it provides. Compile a directory of resources for the adolescent and a list of services that are lacking in the community.
3. Ask a family counselor or other support person to talk to the group about the problems faced by the adolescent father.
4. Design teaching techniques to meet adolescent cognitive level and learning needs. Construct a class around nutrition, prenatal, or postpartum content.

References

Arms, S: To love and let go, New York, 1983, Alfred A Knopf, Inc

Baldwin, W, and Cain, V: The children of teenage parents. In Furstenberg, F, Lincoln, R, and Menken, J editors: Teenage sexuality, pregnancy and childbearing, Philadelphia, 1981, University of Pennsylvania Press

Berland, A: Young fathers' support group, Pediatr Nurs 13(4):255, 1987

Blum, R: Contemporary threat to adolescent health in the United States, JAMA 257(24):3390, 1987

Burke, V: Poor children: a study of trends and policy, 1968-1984, Subcommittee on Public Assistance and Unemployment Compensation, Committee on Ways and Means, House of Representatives, Washington DC, 1986, Congressional Research Service

Caparulo, F, and London, K: Adolescent fathers: adolescents first, fathers second, Issues in Health Care of Women 3:23, 1981

Carey, W, McCann-Sanford, T, and Davidson, E, Jr: Adolescent age and obstetric risk. In McAnarney, E, editor: Premature adolescent pregnancy and parenthood, New York, 1983, Grune & Stratton, Inc

Chanis, M, et al: Adolescent pregnancy, J Nurse Midwife, 24:18, May/June 1979

Colletta, ND, and Gregg, CH: Adolescent mothers' vulnerability to stress, J Nerv Ment Dis 169:50, 1981

Corbett, M, and Meyer, JH: The adolescent and pregnancy, Boston, 1987, Blackwell Scientific Publications, Inc

DeLissovoy, V: Child care by adolescent parents, Child Today 2:23, 1973

Doyle, MB, and Widhalm, MV: Midwifing the adolescent at Lincoln's Hospital's teenage clinics, J Nurse Midwife 24:27, July/Aug 1979

Elster, AB: Effects of pregnancy and parenthood on adolescent fathers and implications for clinical intervention, J Calif Perinatal Assoc 2(2):44, 1982

Elster, AB: The effect of maternal age, parity, and prenatal care on perinatal outcome in adolescent mothers, Am J Obstet Gynecol 149(8):845, 1984

Elster, AB, and Lamb, ME: Adolescent fathers: a group potentially at risk for parenting failure, Infant Ment Health J 3:148, 1982

Elster, AB, and Panzarine, S: Teenage fathers: a trajectory of stress over time. Presented at the Society for Adolescent Medicine, New Orleans, Oct 29, 1983

Elster, AB, et al: Parental behavior of adolescent mothers, Pediatrics 71:494, 1983

Emans, SJ, and Grimes, DA: Contraceptive choice for teenagers, JAMA 257(24):3419, 1987

Field, TM, et al: Teenage, lower-class black mothers and their preterm infants: an intervention of developmental follow-up, Child Dev 51:426, 1980

Fullar, SA: Care of postpartum adolescents, MCN 11(6):398, 1986

Goleman, D: Why teenagers are reckless, *San Francisco Chronicle* Dec 2, 1987

Gray, JD, et al: Prediction and prevention of child abuse, Semin Perinatol 3(1):85, 1979

Greydanus, DE: Risk-taking behaviors in adolescence, JAMA 258(15):2110, 1987

Haffner, DW: Adolescent pregnancy: incidence and cost, JAMA, 258(14):1890, 1987

Hamburg, DA, Nightingale, EO, and Takanishi, R: Facilitating the transitions of adolescence: council on adolescent development, JAMA 257:3405, June/July 1987

Hardy, JB, et al: Long-range outcome of adolescent pregnancy, Clin Obstet Gynecol 21:1215, 1978

Hatcher, SL: Understanding adolescent pregnancy and abortion, Primary Care 3:407, 1976

Hayes, L, and Crovitz, E: Adolescent pregnancy, South Med J 31:869, 1979

Holder, AR: Minors' rights to consent to medical care, JAMA 257(24):3400, 1987

Hollingsworth, DR, and Kreutner, AKK: Teenage pregnancy: solutions are evolving, N Engl J Med 303:516, 1980

Horn, B: Cultural beliefs and teenage pregnancy, Nurs Pract 8:35, Sept 1983

Howard, JS, and Sater, J: Adolescent mothers: self-perceived health education needs, JOGN Nurs 14(5):399, 1985

Jarrett, GE: Childrearing patterns of young mothers: expectations, knowledge, and practices, MCN 7(2):119, 1982

Jones, FA, et al: Maternal responsiveness of primiparous mothers during the postpartum period: age differences, Pediatrics 65:579, 1980

Kornfield, R: Who's to blame: adolescent sexual activity, J Adolesc 8(1):17, 1985

Lawrence, RA, et al: Aggressive behaviors in young mothers: markers of future morbidity? Pediatr Res 15:443, 1981

Lawrence, R: Early mothering by adolescents. In McAnarney, E, editor: Premature adolescent pregnancy and parenthood, New York, 1983, Grune & Stratton, Inc

Litt, IF: Adolescent medicine, JAMA 258(16):2230, 1987

McAnarney, ER, et al: Premature parenthood: a preliminary report of adolescent mother-infant interaction, Pediatr Res 13:328, 1979

McAnarney, E, et al: Interaction of adolescent mothers and their 1-year-old children, Pediatrics 78:585, 1986

Marks, JS, and Kreuter, MW: Youth pregnancy: a community solution, JAMA 257(24):3410, 1987

Mercer, RT: The adolescent experience in labor, delivery, and early postpartum. In Mercer, RT, editors: Perspectives on adolescent health care, New York, 1979, JB Lippincott Co

Mercer, RT: Assessing and counseling teenage mothers during the perinatal period, Nurs Clin North Am 18(2):293, 1983

Mercer, R: Relationship of birth experience to later mothering behaviors, J Nurse Midwife 30:204, July/Aug 1985

Moore, KA: Government policies related to teenage family formation and functioning: an inventory. In Ooms, T, editor: Teenage pregnancy in a family context: implications for policy, Philadelphia, 1981, Temple University Press

Morrissey, JM, Hofmann, SD, and Thrope, JC: Consent and confidentiality in the health care of children and adolescents: a legal guide, New York, 1986, Free Press

Mott, F, and Marsiglio, W: Early childbearing and the completion of high school, Fam Plann Perspect 17:234, 1985

Neeson, JD, et al: Pregnancy outcome for adolescents receiving prenatal care by nurse practitioners in extended roles, J Adolesc Health 4:94, June 1983

Offer, D: In defense of adolescents, JAMA 257(24):3407, 1987

Osofsky, H: Mitigating the adverse effects of early parenthood, Contemp OB/GYN 25:57, Jan 1985

Ouimette, J: Perinatal nursing care of the high-risk mother and infant, Boston, 1986, Jones & Barlett Publishers, Inc

Panner, R, and Evans, BW: The unmarried father revisited, J School Health 45(5):271, 1975

Parke, RD, et al: The adolescent father's impact on the mother and child, J Soc Issues 36:88, 1980
Peoples, MD, and Barrett, AE: A model for the delivery of health care to pregnant adolescents, JOGN Nurs 8(6):339, 1979
Polit, D, and Kahn, J: Early subsequent pregnancy among economically disadvantaged teenage mothers, Am J Pub Health 76(2):167, 1986
Poole, C: Adolescent mothers: can they be helped? Pediatr Nurs 2:7, 1976
Robinson, TN, et al: Perspectives on adolescent substance use: a defined population study, JAMA 258(15):2072, 1987
Rosenbaum, S, and Starfield, B: Unpublished data, April 1986
Rosenfield, A: The adolescent and contraception: issues and controversies, Int J Obstet Gynecol 19:57, 1981
Sachs, B: Reproductive decisions in adolescence, IMAGE: J Nurs Scholarship 18(2):69, 1986
Sahler, OJ: Adolescent mothers: how nurturant is their parenting? In McAnarney, ER, editor: Premature adolescent pregnancy and parenthood, New York, 1983, Grune & Stratton, Inc
Siegel, DM: Adolescents and chronic illness, JAMA 257(24):3396, 1987
Sorosky, AD, et al: The adoption triangle: the effects of sealed records on adoptees, birth parents and adoptive parents, New York, 1978, Anchor Press.
Speraw, S: Adolescents' perceptions of pregnancy: a cross-cultural perspective, West J Nurs Res 9(2):180, 1987
Spivak, H, and Weitzman, M: Social barriers faced by adolescent parents and their children, JAMA 258(11):1500, 1987
Stengel, R: The missing father myth, Time, p 88, Dec 9, 1985
Stickle, G: Overview of incidence, risks and consequences of adolescent pregnancy and childbearing, Birth Defects 17(3):5, 1981
Stockard, R: Facing the facts on adolescent pregnancy, NAACOG Newsletter, 13(9):1, 1986
Teenage pregnancy and fertility in the United States, 1970, 1974, and 1980, MMWR 36(suppl 1SS):1SS-10SS, 1987
Wallis, C: Children having children, Time, p 78, Dec 9, 1985
Westoff, C, Calot, G, and Foster, A: Teenage fertility in developed nations, Fam Plann Perspect 15:105, 1983
Whaley, LF, and Wong, DL: Nursing of infants and children, ed 3, St Louis, 1987, The CV Mosby Co
White-Traut, RC, and Pabst, MK: Parenting of hospitalized infants by adolescent mothers, Pediatr Nurs 13(20:97, 1987
Yoos, L: Adolescent cognitive and contraceptive behaviors, Pediatr Nurs 13(4):247, 1987
Zabin, LA, and Clark, SD: Why they delay: a study of teenage family planning clinic patients, Fam Plann Perspect 13(5):205, 1981
Zdanuk, JM, Harris, CC, and Wisian, NL: Adolescent pregnancy and incest: the nurse's role as counselor, JOGN Nurs 16(2):99, 1987
Zelnick, M: Sexual activity among adolescents: perspectives of a decade. In McAnarney, ER, editor: Premature adolescent pregnancy and parenthood, New York, 1983, Grune & Stratton, Inc
Zuckerman, B, et al: Neonatal outcome: is adolescent pregnancy a risk factor? Pediatrics 71:489, 1983

Bibliography

Bader, M, Blum, RW, and Haffner, DW: Adolescent pregnancy: incidence and cost, JAMA 258(14):1890, 1987
Bearinger, L, and Gephart, J: Priorities for adolescent health: recommendations of a national conference, MCN 12(3):161, 1987
Benkenstein, S, et al: Pregnant adolescent group for education and support, MMWR 36(33):549, 1987
Brown, MA: How fathers and mothers perceive prenatal support, MCN 12(6):414, 1987
Brown, A: Adolescents and abortion: a theoretical framework for decision-making, JOGN Nurs 12(4):241, 1983
Christensen, ML, et al: An interdisciplinary approach to preventing child abuse, MCN 9:108, 1984
Danforth, DN, and Scott, JR, editors: Obstetrics and gynecology, ed 5, Philadelphia, 1986, JB Lippincott Co
Droegemueller, W, et al: Comprehensive gynecology, St Louis, 1987, The CV Mosby Co
Drug abuse in adolescents, Child Care Newsletter 6(2):1, 1987 (An educational service of Johnson & Johnson, Dept. CCN, Box 836, Somerville, NJ 08876)
Daniels, M, and Manning, D: A clinic for pregnant teens, Am J Nurs 83:68, 1983
Elster, A, et al: The medical and psychosocial impact of comprehensive care on adolescent pregnancy and parenthood, JAMA 258(9):1187, 1987
Emans, SJ, et al: Adolescents' compliance with the use of oral contraceptives, JAMA 257(24):3377, 1987
Foster, SD: Are commercial patient education materials right for you? MCN 12(4):287, 1987
Hepworth, JT, et al: Gynecologic age: prediction in adolescent female research, Nurs Research 36(6):392, 1987
Hollingsworth, D, et al: Impact of gynecologic age on outcome of adolescent pregnancy. In McAnarney, ER, editor: Premature adolescent pregnancy and parenthood, New York, 1983, Grune & Stratton, Inc
Humenick, SS, and Bugen, LA: Parenting roles: expectation versus reality, MCN 12(1):36, 1987
Jay, S, et al: Effect of peer counselors on adolescent compliance with use of oral contraceptives, Pediatrics 73:126, 1984
Kreipe, RE: Prevention of adolescent pregnancy. In McAnarney, E, editor: Premature adolescent pregnancy and parenthood, New York, 1983, Grune & Stratton, Inc
Lane, C, and Kemp, J: Family planning needs of adolescents, JOGN Nurs 13(2):61s, 1984
Lewis, HR, and Lewis, ME: What you and your patients need to know about safer sex, RN, p 53, Sept 1987
MacDonnell, S: Vulnerable mothers, vulnerable children: a follow-up study of unmarried mothers who kept their children, Halifax, Nova Scotia, 1981, Policy Planning and Research Division, Nova Scotia Department of Social Services
Maciak, BJ, et al: Pregnancy and birth rates among sexually experienced US teenagers—1974, 1980, and 1983, JAMA 258(15):2069, 1987
McAnarney, E, and Thiede, H: Adolescent pregnancy and childbearing: what we learned in the 1970s and what remains to be learned in premature adolescent pregnancy and parenthood. In McAnarney, E, editor: Premature adolescent pregnancy and parenthood, New York, 1983, Grune & Stratton
McAnarney, E, et al: Adolescent mothers and their infants, Pediatrics 73:358, 1984
McAnarney, E: Children having babies, Am J Dis Child 141:1053, 1987
McAnarney, E: Children having babies, JAMA 258(14):1863, 1987

Mercer, RT: First-time motherhood: experiences from teens to forties, New York, 1986, Springer Publishing Co, Inc

Mercer, RT: Adolescent motherhood: comparison of outcome with older mothers, J Adolesc Health Care 5:7, Jan 1984

Miller, SH: Childbearing and childrearing, Child Today p 26, May June 1984

Morgan, BS, and Barden, ME: Unwed and pregnant: nurses' attitudes toward unmarried mothers, MCN 10(2):114, 1985

Muscari, ME: Adolescent suicide attempts by acetaminophen ingestion, MCN 12(1):32, 1987

Panel on adolescent pregnancy and childbearing, National Research Council: Risking the future: adolescent sexuality, pregnancy and childbearing, Washington, DC, 1987, National Academy Press

Parrains, J: L'adolescent et ses pairs: élaboration d'un programme d'assistance, L'infirmiere Canadienne, 26:40, Aug 1984

Phillips, DP, and Carstensen LL: Clustering of teenage suicides after television news stories about suicide, N Engl J Med 315:685, 1986

Porter, LS: Parenting enhancement among high-risk adolescents: testing a holistic patient-centered nursing practice model, Nurs Clin North Am 19(1):89, 1984

Ruff, CC: How well do adolescents mother? MCN 12(4):249, 1987

Seidel, HM, et al: Mosby's guide to physical examination, St Louis, 1987, The CV Mosby Co

Spitz, A, et al: Teenage pregnancy and fertility in the United States, 1970, 1974, 1980, MMWR 36(1SS):1-10SS, 1987

Strickland, OL: The occurrence of symptoms in expectant fathers, Nurs Res 36(3):184, 1987

Thompson, ME, and Kramer, M: Methodologic standards for controlled clinical trials of early contact and maternal infant behavior, Pediatrics 73:294, March 1984

Vanzyl York, P: Nutritional needs of women, The Melpomene Report: A Journal for Women's Health Research 6(2):10, 1987

Velasquez, J, et al: Intensive services help prevent chld abuse, MCN 9(2):113, 1984

Vernon, MEL, et al: Teenage pregnancy: a prospective study of self-esteem and other sociodemographic factors, Pediatrics 72:632, 1983

Wallach, EE, moderator: Symposium: caring for younger pregnant teenagers, Contemp OB/GYN 30(5):154, 1987

Yoos, L: Perspectives on adolescent parenting: effect of adolescent egocentrism on the maternal-child interaction, J Pediatr Nurs 2(3):193, 1987

UNIT

VIII

Complications of the Newborn

Identification of risk and general care of the compromised newborn are presented in Chapter 36. Techniques inherent in the nursing care of infants, for example, maintenance of respirations, oxygen therapy, and feeding measures, are included. Chapter 37 describes complications associated with gestational age and birthweight. Chapter 38 focuses on birth trauma and the newborn of a diabetic pregnancy. Chapter 39 offers extensive content about infection and drug dependence. Chapter 40 presents complications of hyperbilirubinemia and congenital anomalies.

As in the other units, content is presented in a manner that facilitates the nursing process in the care of the newborn and their families. Nursing research highlights are included, as well as abstracts of examples of nursing research:

Chapter 36: Gavage tube insertion in the premature infant.

Chapter 37: A randomized clinical trial of early hospital discharge and home follow-up of very-low-birth-weight infants.

Chapter 38: Maternal prenatal attachment in normal and high-risk pregnancies.

CHAPTER

36

Nursing Care of the Compromised Newborn

Sharon Eaton

Learning Objectives

Correctly define the key terms listed.

Outline the assessment of an infant at risk.

Develop a nursing care plan for an infant with respiratory distress.

Explain the importance of temperature support and regulation.

Discuss nursing care related to nutrition, feeding, and elimination.

Describe procedures for meeting the nutrient and fluid needs of infants at risk.

Explore the emotional aspects of care of the high-risk infant and the family.

Compare and contrast the "kangaroo method," and technologic incubator.

Develop a discharge plan for the infant at risk.

Key Terms

cold stress
continuous positive airway pressure (CPAP)
cues of overstimulation
extracorporeal membrane oxygenation (ECMO)
gavage feeding
high-risk neonate
high-risk parenting
infant stimulation
"kangaroo method"
moderate risk neonate
oxygen therapy
parenteral fluid therapy
readiness for interaction
respiratory distress
total parenteral nutrition (TPN)
transcutaneous oxygen tension monitoring ($tcPO_2$)

The high-risk infant is a sick baby whose intact survival is in jeopardy. Health care must support the high-risk newborn's basic functioning while compensating for inadequacies and weaknesses. "Normal" values and parameters vary with the infant's level of maturity and developmental problems. Assessment and therefore supportive care are complicated further by the infant's inability to speak and by nonspecific, generalized responses to dysfunctional problems. Assessment rests heavily on historical data provided by the mother and obstetric team and on current levels of knowledge related to gestational age and disorders of the neonate. Plan and implementation of the nursing process with the high-risk infant focus on the physiologic maintenance of warmth, respiration, and nutrition.

The care of the infant at risk has become highly specialized and beyond the scope of this text.* The following discussion presents general content relevant to the care of the high-risk infant. Care of infants with selected risk factors is discussed in greater detail in the following chapters. *The nurse's actions can influence the health care team to keep the family's childbearing experience in focus rather than concentrate solely on the risk factors.*

TRANSPORT TO A REGIONAL CENTER

Hospitals that are not staffed or equipped to care for the mother and fetus or newborn at high risk arrange for their immediate transfer to a specialized perinatal or tertiary care center (Chapter 27) (Fanaroff and Martin, 1987) (see box, p. 910). If a compromised infant is expected to be born, a maternal transport is arranged, if possible; that is, the anticipated compromised newborn is transported in utero. In utero transport has two distinct advantages: (1) the mother and newborn are not separated so that attachment is facilitated, and (2) neonatal morbidity and mortality are decreased. It is not always possible to transport the mother before delivery for a variety of reasons (e.g., imminent delivery, lack of prior diagnosis). Therefore it is necessary for physicians and nurses to have the necessary skills and equipment for accurate diagnosis and emergency intervention to stabilize the client's physical condition and to maintain it until transport can be effected. (For surgical emergencies of the newborn, see Chapter 40; for specific maternal conditions, see Index.)

Parents of infants who have been transported to regional centers need support, since bonding is interrupted. Parents who are physically separated from their infants feel a loss of control after the transport team gives them a quick glimpse of the baby and they see wires, equipment, and tubes attached to the infant (Merenstein and Gardner, 1985). Before they are transported to regional centers, high-risk infants must be stabilized. Attention is given to six basic physiologic areas:

- Temperature regulation and support
- Oxygen needs and ventilation
- Acid-base balance
- Fluid needs
- Glucose needs
- Vital signs

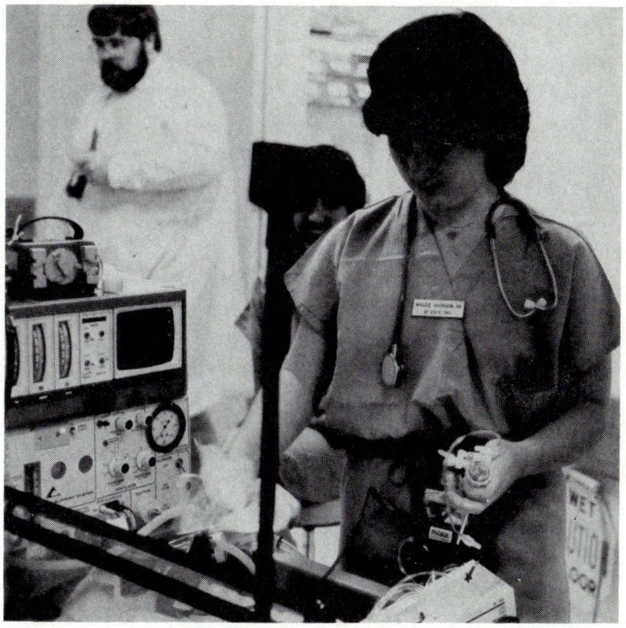

Fig. 36-1 Preparing a total life support system used for transport of compromised newborns to this regional center for postpartum care.

During transport to a regional perinatal center, the following general categories of supplies, equipment, and medications are needed*:

Needed by both mother and fetus/newborn:

Oxygen and equipment for maintaining a clear airway and adequate gas exchange

Intravenous equipment and solutions for meeting hydration needs, for administering medications, for transfusion of blood or blood products, and for obtaining blood samples

Equipment for monitoring of vital signs and blood pressure

Blood-drawing supplies

Supplemental source of electricity

Additional supplies for the mother:

Stretcher with approved restraints or safety belts: linen

Eclamptic tray: supplies, medications, and equipment

Delivery pack

Emesis basin

FHR monitor

Additional supplies for the newborn:

Transport unit with total life support and monitoring capacity (Fig. 36-1)

Thoracotomy tray and thoracentesis set

*See References and Bibliography. Most facilities have developed modular study guides and manuals for procedures and for laboratory values and their management.

*Carefully outlined and specific guidelines are provided in NAACOG-OGN Nursing Practice Resource, Maternal-Neonatal Transport, No 8, June 1983. (The Nurses Association of the American College of Obstetricians and Gynecologists, 409 Twelfth Street, SW, Washington, DC, 20024-2191, 202/638-0026.)

FACTORS THAT PLACE THE NEWBORN AT RISK

Criteria for selection of high-risk infants for transport or admission to neonatal intensive care units:

Specific factors that place **infant in high-risk** category:
- Infants continuing or developing signs of respiratory distress syndrome (RDS) or other respiratory distress
- Asphyxiated infants (Apgar score of less than 6 at 5 minutes); resuscitation required at birth
- Preterm infants; dysmature infants
- Infants with cyanosis or suspected cardiovascular disease; persistent cyanosis
- Infants with major congenital malformations requiring surgery; chromosomal anomalies
- Infants with convulsions, sepsis, hemorrhagic diathesis, or shock
- Meconium aspiration syndrome
- Central nervous system (CNS) depression for longer than 24 hours
- Hypoglycemia
- Hypocalcemia
- Hyperbilirubinemia

Factors indicating **moderate-risk:**
- Dysmaturity
- Prematurity (weight between 2000 and 2500 g)
- Apgar score of less than 5 at 1 minute
- Feeding problems
- Multiple birth
- Transient tachypnea
- Hypomagnesemia or hypermagnesemia
- Hypoparathyroidism
- Failure to gain weight
- Jitteriness or hyperactivity
- Cardiac anomalies not requiring immediate catheterization
- Heart murmur
- Anemia
- CNS depression for less than 24 hours

The transport vehicle should have the capacity for safety precautions:

1. Ground transport: money (change) for telephone call; restraints
2. Air transport: in-flight turbulence precautions (restraints, intravenous fluids in plastic bags) and precautions against changes in atmospheric pressure

NURSING CARE OF THE NEWBORN WITH RESPIRATORY DISTRESS

Any newborn with respiratory difficulty is in jeopardy.* The infant's response to prompt, appropriate treatment bears a direct relationship to the cause, degree of maturity, and other medical problems.

Breathing is a new experience for the infant. In priority of care, it ranks second only to the control of massive hemorrhage. Because of its high priority and its challenging nursing aspects, considerable space in the delivery room is devoted to the initiation and maintenance of respirations.

The alert nurse often is the pivotal point between functional and dysfunctional survival for the infant in respiratory distress. The nurse's alertness and informed observations place the nurse in a preventive, curative, and rehabilitative role.

Assessment

The infant in distress at birth is immediately identifiable. In addition, some infants who at birth appear pink and vigorous, with good muscle tone and respiratory rates and rhythms within normal range, become distressed soon afterward. Respiratory difficulty, with cyanosis and retractions such as occur after aspiration or tension pneumothorax, may appear suddenly. More commonly, respiratory difficulty follows a progressive sequential pattern: The **respiratory rate** initially may increase without a change in rhythm. Flaring of the nares and expiratory grunt are also early signs of respiratory distress. The **apical pulse** increases in rate. **Retractions**, depending on the cause, may begin as subcostal and xiphoid and then progress upward to intercostal, suprasternal, and clavicular retractions (Fig. 36-2). The **color** changes from pink to circumoral pallor, to cir-

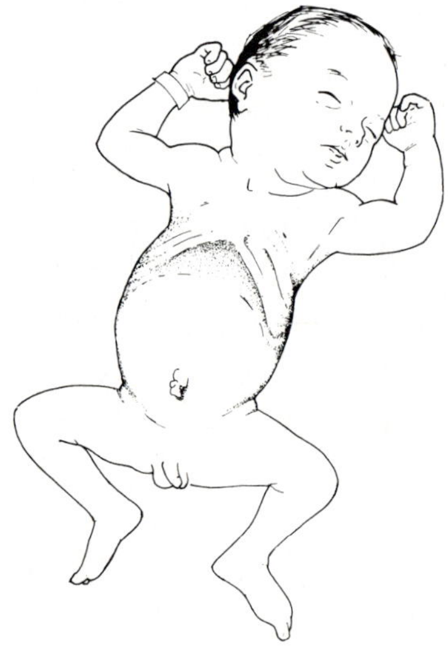

Fig. 36-2 Retraction: substernal, subcostal, and intercostal retractions are evident.
Courtesy Ross Laboratories, Columbus, Ohio.

*See discussion on techniques for suctioning the newborn, oxygen therapy, and resuscitation in Chapter 22.

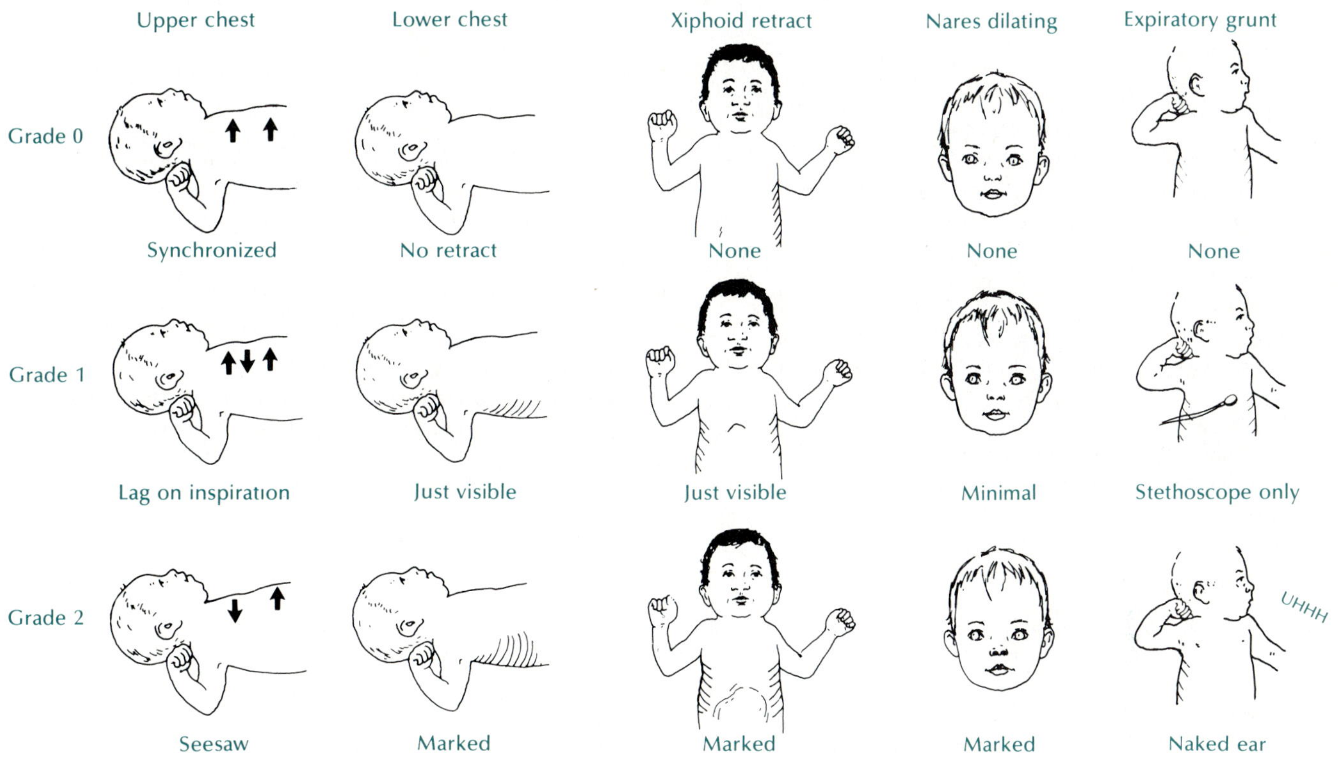

Fig. 36-3 Observation of retractions. Silverman-Anderson index of respiratory distress is determined by grading each of five arbitrary criteria: *grade 0* indicates no difficulty; *grade 1,* moderate difficulty; and *grade 2,* maximum respiratory difficulty. Retraction score is sum of these values; total score of 0 indicates no dyspnea, whereas total score of 10 denotes maximum respiratory distress.
Modified from Silverman, W, and Anderson, D: Pediatrics 17:1, 1956.

cumoral cyanosis, and then to generalized cyanosis; acrocyanosis deepens. **Respiratory effort** and deepening distress are indicated by the following (Fig. 36-3):

1. Chin tug (chin is pulled down [and mouth opens wider] as auxiliary muscles of respiration are activated).
2. Abdominal seesaw breathing patterns (Figs. 21-4 and 36-3).
3. Increased number of apneic episodes.

If the newborn is hypoxic, the **temperature** may begin to drop. (Avoid rapid warming of the newborn; it may evoke apneic episodes.) An accurate and timely **blood pressure** reading can assist in the early diagnosis of cardiorespiratory disease and in the monitoring of fluid therapy. Blood pressure readings are obtained by the Doppler method or electronic monitor. A blood pressure cuff of appropriate size must be used. A too wide cuff results in a false low reading; an overly narrow cuff will give a false elevated reading. For the newborn a cuff of about 2.5 to 3 cm (1 in) wide and 7.5 cm (3 in) long is usually adequate (Fig. 36-4).

The stethoscope should have a pediatric-sized diaphragm for maximum skin contact and localization of sounds. The stethoscope is applied with firm pressure but not so much pressure that transmission of sound and vibrations is compromised.

The Doppler instrument and electronic monitoring device (on a biometric console) are more accurate methods for determining blood pressure. However, this type of equipment is not available in all hospitals or community health settings.

The monitor displays the systolic and diastolic value, the mean systolic/diastolic pressure (the reading is midway between the diastolic and systolic pressures), and the newborn's heart rate. The existing standard normal range for

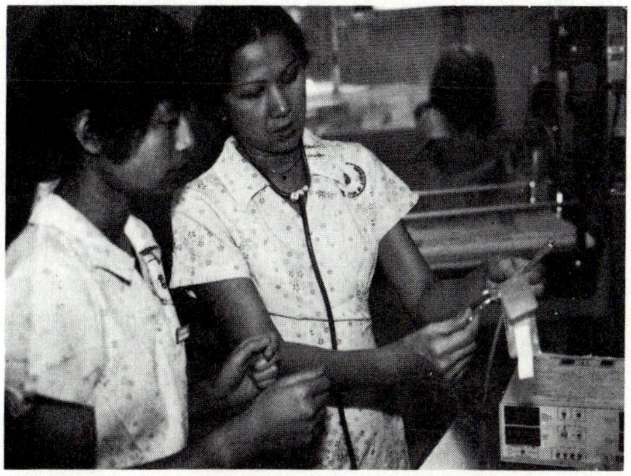

Fig. 36-4 Preparing to assess a newborn's blood pressure electronically.

the mean pressure for infants weighting 2500 g (5½ lb) or more is 30 to 60 mm Hg.

Nursing Diagnoses

Examples of nursing diagnoses for the newborn with respiratory distress include the following:

- Ineffective breathing pattern related to
  - Immaturity
  - Cold stress
- Ineffective airway clearance related to
  - Newborn anatomy, immobility, and increased secretions
  - Meconium aspiration
  - Immaturity or congenital disorder
  - Respiratory depression secondary to narcosis or acidosis
- Impaired gas exchange related to
  - Immaturity (e.g., insufficient surfactant)

Planning

During the important planning step, goals are set to meet the unique needs of the high-risk newborn. The goals are prioritized. Nursing actions are selected to meet the goals. Before nursing care is implemented, the nurse plans carefully to assure that the care provided is goal directed.

Goals

1. Respirations are maintained
2. Bronchopulmonary dysplasia and retinopathy of prematurity (retrolental fibroplasia) do not develop
3. Metabolism meets needs of repair, maintenance, and growth
4. Respiratory needs of all tissues are met, (e.g., blood gases and acid-base balance are maintained within normal limits)
5. Congenital dysfunctions or anomalies are recognized early, and appropriate treatment is initiated
6. Parents are supported in coping constructively with the situation and relating to the infant as a person

Implementation

Supportive Measures. The newborn's respiratory efforts must be supported by careful positioning. When the infant is supine, the arms will be at the sides, flexed, and slightly abducted. Diapers, if used, must be pinned loosely. The prone position recently has been shown to improve respiratory effort, increase PaO_2, and diminish the work of respiration.

Suctioning assists the infant in maintaining a patent airway. An unobstructed airway usually decreases the newborn's labored breathing by improving ventilation. (See discussion of suctioning procedures in Chapter 22.)

A thermoneutral environment is essential for metabolic homeostasis. Cold stress is detrimental to the well-being of any infant, especially the infant at risk. For a discussion of thermogenesis and the prevention of cold stress, see Chapter 22.

Nutrition and feeding of the infant in respiratory distress are as much a challenge for the nurse as for the infant. The extra work of breathing taxes the infant's energy reserves and demands greater caloric input. Breast-feeding and bottle-feeding are not appropriate for the newborn in distress. The newborn in severe distress may require gavage feeding exclusively. Parenteral fluids or total parenteral nutrition (TPN) may be required for the newborn who cannot tolerate gavage feedings (see p. 917).

For the convalescent infant in no respiratory distress who can bottle-feed, a softer nipple with an adequate opening is used (e.g., when the bottle is inverted, fluid should drip at 1 drop per second). Some infants can breast-feed when both mother and child receive supportive guidance (Chapter 23). The airway must be cleared before and during feeding as necessary. Moreover, the infant is "bubbled" before feedings.

If the convalescent infant is feeding at the breast, the nurse remains at the bedside with a bulb syringe at hand. This provides reassurance for the mother and avoids a buildup of tension, which might be transferred from mother to infant. Should the infant gag or choke, the nurse can show the mother how to manage such a situation.

Oxygen Therapy. Oxygen therapy may be lifesaving, but its administration must be carefully monitored, as with any medication. The administration of oxygen to newborns requires clinical judgment supported by laboratory determinations (Fanaroff and Martin, 1987). Indiscriminate use of oxygen may be hazardous, resulting in retinopathy of prematurity (retrolental fibroplasia) and bronchopulmonary dysplasia. See the discussion on oxygen therapy (Chapter 22), retinopathy of prematurity (retrolental fibroplasia), and bronchopulmonary dysplasia (Chapter 37).

When an infant requires supplemental oxygen, despite its potential hazards, the delivery of oxygen is carefully controlled and monitored. Small increases in ambient oxygen can be delivered directly into the incubator. A head box within the incubator is used when oxygen concentrations exceed 30%. The head box more accurately provides the correct concentration while simultaneously limiting significant fluctuations in oxygen, especially when the incubator portholes are opened. Some incubators have an automatic cut-off mechanism when ambient oxygen reaches a preset level. These controls cannot be relied on independently. The ambient oxygen concentration is checked at regular intervals by a paramagnetic oxygen analyzer or continuously monitored by means of an oxygen electrode. To prevent cold stress and drying of respiratory mucosa, oxygen delivered to an infant is warmed and humidified. Periodic measurement of PaO_2, hemoglobin, and pH, in addition to close clinical observation, is the most reasonable and accurate approach to minimizing the risk of both hyperoxic and hypoxic insults to a sick infant (Fanaroff and Martin, 1987).

Continuous Positive Airway Pressure. Continuous positive airway pressure (CPAP) is most commonly administered through nasal prongs or an endotracheal tube (oral or nasal). The purpose of this technique is to reduce the work of breathing. CPAP increases alveolar volume. It employs the same principle as the expiratory grunt (a physiologic adaptation to trap air within the lungs, keeping alveoli open to prevent atelectasis on expiration). CPAP also increases functional residual capacity, improves oxygenation, and decreases pulmonary shunting.

Transcutaneous Oxygen Tension Monitoring. Older methods of monitoring arterial oxygenation in the sick newborn involved such invasive techniques as umbilical artery catheterization and radial and temporal artery puncture or catheterization. Oxygen electrodes placed intravascularly to achieve continuous monitoring of arterial oxygenation have not met with success in recent years.

Today accurate noninvasive transcutaneous (tc) oxygen tension ($tcPo_2$) monitoring is feasible on a continuous basis. The $tcPo_2$ electrode is applied according to the manufacturer's instructions. However, all electrodes are applied to a hairless and greaseless site, and an airtight contact with the skin is secured. The electrode application site is changed every 4 hours to avoid burns. The distinct advantage of this method is that the data are available on a moment-to-moment basis; for example, complications can be identified early, and the efficiency of respiratory therapy can be evaluated readily. Weaning from oxygen therapy is facilitated by $tcPo_2$ monitoring (Procedure 36-1) (Merenstein and Gardner, 1985; Fanaroff and Martin, 1987).

Extracorporeal Membrane Oxygenation. Extracorporeal membrane oxygenation (ECMO) is an innovative technique that offers promise as a means of supporting life during intractable respiratory failure in selected infants (Fanaroff and Martin, 1987). Perfusion and gas exchange are accomplished by means of a cardiopulmonary bypass through a membrane lung (Bartlett, et al., 1985). This allows the infant's heart and lungs to recover at low ventilator settings and inspired oxygen concentrations. This experimental approach may decrease acute and chronic lung disease. Despite the technical challenge and staff time expenditure involved in its delivery, ECMO is considered a useful option for respiratory failure in several major neonatal centers (Fanaroff and Martin, 1987).

Procedure 36-1

WEANING FROM OXYGEN THERAPY

DEFINITION

Withdrawing an infant from ventilator and extraneous oxygen dependency.

PURPOSE

To prepare infant to breathe room air. To stop ventilator use.

EQUIPMENT

Equipment already in use by infant being weaned; pulse oximeter (if available); regular bassinet, blankets, linens as needed after infant is weaned.

NURSING ACTIONS	RATIONALE
Identify client and check physician's orders.	To provide the right therapy for the right person.
Wash hands before and after touching client or equipment. Glove, prn.	To prevent nosocomial infection and to implement universal precautions.
Proceed with weaning process gradually.	To minimize the possibility of complications. The hazards of sudden cyanosis and respiratory collapse become greater with increased time that infant has received oxygen therapy.
Decrease oxygen by 10% every 30 to 60 minutes (or 2 to 4 hours) as child improves.	To minimize the possibility of reopening right-to-left shunts: foramen ovale, ductus arteriosus.
Attach infant to pulse oximeter during weaning.	To provide information on oxygen saturation of the tissues.
Monitor laboratory values simultaneously: blood pH, PaO_2,* partial pressure of carbon dioxide in arterial blood ($PaCO_2$), arterial hemoglobin concentration.	To provide data for modifying rate of weaning process.
Observe infant closely for the following: Pulse. Respiratory effort. Skin color.	To prevent adverse reactions to weaning: Pulse elevation. Respiratory distress. Cyanosis.
If symptoms occur, increase oxygen and proceed with slower weaning process.	

*Blood gas values given in Appendix H. Hospital intensive care units have protocols for care based on blood gas values.

Evaluation

Small improvements such as the slight downward adjustment in the administration of oxygen can represent major milestones in the status of the compromised infant. Successful weaning from ventilatory support systems and development of parental attachment to the infant are signs that goals are being achieved. The nurse can be reasonably assured that goals have been achieved when assessment years later shows no evidence of adverse sequelae (e.g., respiratory, visual, or neurobehavior impairment in the child) and no dysfunctional family processes directly attributable to the child's early illness.

TEMPERATURE SUPPORT AND REGULATION

Assessment

In the non-cold-stressed neonate, measuring *axillary temperature* is the safest, most practical means of monitoring deep body temperature. However, in the cold-stressed neonate, metabolism of brown fat in the axillary area may result in misleadingly high readings.

A *thermistor probe* or transducer taped to the skin is designed to provide accurate temperature readings for the newborn under an overhead radiant heat source or in a Servo-Control incubator. When only a single skin temperature is to be sensed, the thermistor probe is attached to the skin over the liver or between the umbilicus and the pubis. Least favored attachment sites are over bony prominences (one of the least vasoreactive body regions) or extremities (one of the most vasoreactive regions). False temperature measures will occur if the probe is attached near heat-producing transcutaneous gas-monitoring transducers or over areas of bruised or burned skin (Fanaroff and Martin, 1987).

Skin temperature usually decreases first in the cold-stressed infant. Therefore the infant's body and extremities are touched to assess for coolness or warmth. The infant is also assessed for physiologic **signs of cold stress**. The stronger, more mature infant responds by increased physical activity and crying. In other infants, respiratory rate often increases. Color changes may be noted in any infant. These include deepening acrocyanosis, appearance of generalized cyanosis, and mottling of the skin (cutis marmorata). In a male with descended testes, the cremasteric reflex is activated; that is, on exposure to cold, the testes are pulled up into the inguinal canal.

The sigmoid colon bends at a right angle to itself at a depth of 3 cm. Inserting a **rectal thermometer** to a depth of less than 5 cm (2 in) may not accurately reflect core temperature (Fanaroff and Martin, 1987). Insertion of the thermometer to 5 cm to obtain an accurate reading risks perforation of the rectum. Rectal perforation carries a mortality of approximately 70% in reported cases (Merenstein and Gardner, 1985). Therefore routine use of a glass rectal thermometer or an electronic probe is contraindicated for the neonate, even after rectal patency has been demonstrated.

Nursing Diagnoses

Examples of nursing diagnoses related to temperature support and regulation include the following:

- Ineffective thermoregulation, related to
  - Immaturity
  - Congenital disorder
- Potential altered body temperature related to
  - Environmental factors leading to hypothermia or hyperthermia
  - Disease processes such as infection
  - Fluid deficit secondary to hypovolemia
  - Physiologic immaturity of newborn

Planning

During the important planning step, goals are set in client-centered terms. Whenever possible, parents are included in the planning. The goals are prioritized. Nursing actions are selected to meet the goals.

Goals

1. Skin temperature is maintained between 36.1° and 36.7° C (97° to 98° F)*
2. No apneic spells occur
3. Adequate weight is gained
4. Sequelae of cold stress (i.e., sclerema, oxygen deprivation to tissues, metabolic acidosis, hypoglycemia, abnormal blood gases, and dysfunction of CNS) do not develop

Implementation

Nursing care should be planned and implemented to prevent or minimize cold stress. Nursing actions to support thermoregulation include quickly drying the newborn in a warm, absorbent blanket, taking particular care to dry and cover the head (one fourth of body length). (If infant is of good weight and in good condition, she or he may be given to mother to hold.) The nurse prevents cold air from blowing over face because receptors in facial skin are extremely sensitive to cold. The wrapped infant is placed in warm incubator, Kreisselmann, or other heated carrier. Infant may be placed unwrapped under radiant heat source or under plastic wrap to reduce drafts (Fig 36-5). All procedures and observations when infant is unwrapped are done in incubator, under radiant heat, on warm surface, etc. All surfaces and materials touching infant are kept warm. The nurse's hands should be warm when handling neonate. Oxygen or air is warmed before it is administered to infant.

The equipment needs to be maintained in excellent operative condition. The nurse needs to know procedures

*See discussions on techniques for regulating warmth and humidity in infant's environment and for maintaining thermoneutral environment in Chapter 22.

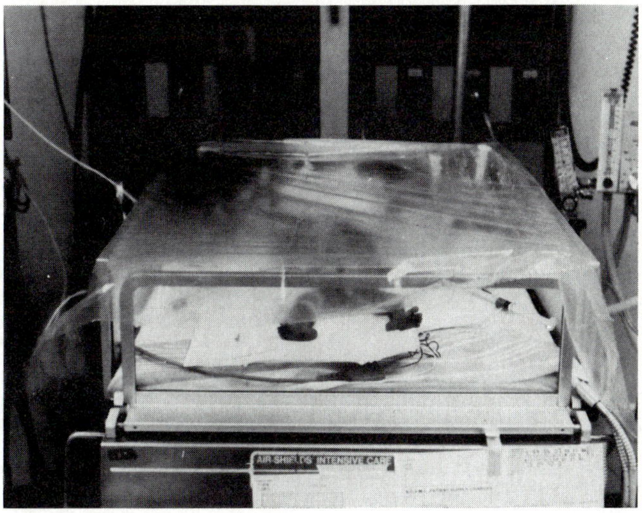

Fig. 36-5 Infant under plastic wrap to ensure a draft-free environment.
Photography by Anne Kunke, San Jose, Calif. From Whaley, LF, and Wong, DL: Nursing care of infants and children, ed 3, St Louis, 1987, The CV Mosby Co.

and rationale for procedures. Equipment is plugged in and operative. The thermostat is set on the control panel. The probe is placed in contact with the skin, and the portholes and lid are closed. The incubator is placed away from windows, fans, and air-conditioning units. Bassinets are placed away from drafts or sources of heat or cold. The infant's temperature is measured periodically to check the accuracy of the equipment.

Abdominal skin temperatures are maintained at 36.1° to 36.7° C (97° to 98° F), and axillary temperature is maintained at 36.5° C (97.7° F). Any rise in temperature over 37.3° C (99° F) or drop of 0.6° to 1° C (1° to 2° F) is reported. If the infant's temperature is too low or too high, the environment is altered to return the infant to the desired body temperature. The nurse checks and readjusts the thermostat setting as necessary and checks to see that the equipment is plugged into an electrical outlet.

The thermistor probe is reapplied if it is wet or detached. Incubator portholes are closed. On incubator portholes with plastic sleeve covers, the sleeve is kept on its track. The infant's clothing and blankets are adjusted as necessary. The placement of the incubator or bassinet is changed as needed to prevent temperature changes from elements such as drafts and sunlight.

Warming the Hypothermic Infant. Rapid warming or cooling may produce apneic spells and acidosis in an infant. Therefore the warming process is increased slowly over a period of 2 to 4 hours.*

The nurse places the infant in a Servo-Control incubator and sets the incubator temperature on the control panel at 1.2° C (2° F) above skin temperature, even if the skin temperature is lower than normal. The thermistor probe is taped to the skin of the anterior abdominal wall. When the skin temperature reaches the predetermined temperature, the incubator temperature is reset. The process is repeated until an abdominal skin temperature of 36.5° C (97.7° F) is achieved.

Weaning the Infant from the Servo-Control Incubator. The incubator weaning process is accomplished slowly over a period of hours or days. The nurse assists the infant through the following measures. The infant is dressed in a diaper and shirt. The incubator temperature is lowered and the temperature readings of both the infant and incubator are recorded. The baby's response is assessed. This procedure is repeated until the incubator temperature equals the room temperature, and the infant's abdominal skin temperature is 36.5° C (97.7° F). The infant is then wrapped in a blanket, the incubator portholes are opened, and the infant's response is reassessed. The baby may be removed to an open crib if the axillary temperature is adequate.

Evaluation

The nurse can be assured that care was effective if the infant's temperature stabilizes within normal limits, apneic episodes do not occur, and sequelae of cold stress do not develop. The plan of care evolves to meet the changing needs of the high-risk infant.

NUTRITION AND ELIMINATION

Low-birth-weight newborns make up the largest number of high-risk infants. Of these, about one third are small for gestational age (SGA) regardless of maturity. About two thirds are preterm and appropriate for gestational age (AGA). SGA newborns may also be preterm.

The feeding and nutrition of the high-risk infant warrant careful consideration. The extent to which nutrition needs are met is directly related to the infant's immediate and long-range well-being. For example, if the low-birth-weight infant with low glycogen stores is not fed promptly, the resultant symptomatic or asymptomatic hypoglycemia may seriously damage carbohydrate-dependent brain cells (see Chapter 37).

Caloric, nutrient, and fluid requirements of the infant at risk may be greater for many reasons. Preterm or dysmature (malnourished) newborns usually have limited stores. Depletion of stores occurs in the newborn who is stressed by one or a combination of factors, including such conditions as birth asphyxia, increased respirations or respiratory effort, insensible fluid loss by evaporation when the infant is under radiant heat or during phototherapy, and a hypothermic environment. The immaturity of the body system affects nutrient requirements. Gastrointestinal tract losses occur through vomiting, diarrhea, and dysfunctional absorption. Renal system losses are caused by inability to concentrate urine and maintain an adequate rate of urea excretion, as well as by an inadequate response to antidiuretic hormone (ADH). Growth demands also affect nutrient requirements. The preterm newborn's growth rate approximates the fetal growth rate during the last trimester, which is 2 or more times that of a term infant after delivery.

*Rapid warming is elected by some authors: Kaplan and Eidelman (1984).

Assessment

General Observations. Weight is measured and plotted daily on a growth grid. Weight loss or rate of weight gain is calculated. Oral feedings are provided when possible. The type of formula, the number of calories per 30 ml (1 oz), and the volume are carefully noted. The infant is monitored closely during feeding. Observations include noting the infant's attempts at sucking, presence or absence of abdominal distension (Fig. 36-6), vomiting or regurgitation, cyanosis, and amount of mucus. The time required for feeding is noted. If feeding is done by gavage, the size of the feeding tube and the route (nasogastric or orogastric) is recorded.

If abdominal distension occurs, the time, degree, and effect on respirations are reported and described. Vomiting and regurgitation are potential problems. When they occur, the color, amount, time in relation to feeding, and character (forcefulness or associated with a burp) are important observations.

Regardless of birth weight, the neurologic or physical status of the infant may prohibit oral feedings. Many infants at risk are nourished by parenteral fluids or TPN. When parenteral fluids are given, the type of fluids, rate per minute, and infusion site are assessed. TPN is assessed per hospital protocol. The care used in starting the infusion, the subsequent nursing care, and the contents of the infusate are factors in determining how long each infusion site will be used (Fanaroff and Martin, 1987).

Elimination patterns are assessed. Frequency of urination, color, and specific gravity are monitored. The amount, frequency, and character of stools are also noted. The stool is assessed for obstipation or constipation (or both), diarrhea, loss of fats (steatorrhea), guaiac, and pH.

Weight and Fluid Loss and Gain. As much as 80% to 85% of the preterm (28 to 34 weeks) newborn's body weight consists of water as compared with 70% in the term infant. Most of this water occupies the extracellular fluid compartment. Even with the early fluid and nutrition intake, the preterm infant's weight and fluid losses seem exaggerated. Several factors predispose to weight and fluid losses. Inadequate fluid intake (e.g., from delayed administration or insufficient volume) predisposes the infant to weight loss.

Insensible water loss (IWL) represents evaporative losses that occur largely through the skin. Approximately 30% of this IWL is from the respiratory tract and most of this is prevented by humidified oxygen—enriched gases that are used for respiratory support in sick infants. Total IWL ranges anywhere from 1.75 to 3.6 ml/kg/hour. The quantity is influenced by gestational age, postpartum age, weight, and use of radiant warmer or incubator and other factors.

Greater fluid demands to meet increased cellular metabolic processes (e.g., from stress, repair, or growth) predispose the newborn to weight and fluid losses.

The limits of acceptable weight loss are as follows: During the newborn's first 3 days of extrauterine life, the preterm infant can lose 12% or less of birth weight. For the term infant of normal weight for gestational age, a weight loss of 10% or less is acceptable. Weight loss of 15% or less is acceptable for infants weighing 4500 g (9 lb 14 oz) or more. For dysmature SGA infants, a loss of 5% or less of birth weight is acceptable.

After the first 3 days, a preterm newborn's loss or gain during each 24-hour period should not exceed 2% of the previous day's weight.

The following examples illustrate how to calculate weight loss and gain, suggesting causes and nursing actions for each case.

EXAMPLE 1

Day 4 1750 g
Day 5 1730 g
20 g loss

$$\frac{20}{1750} = \frac{x\%}{100\%}$$
$$1750x = 2000$$
$$1750\overline{)2000.00} = 1.1$$
$$x = 1.1\% \text{ weight loss}$$

Probable causes: Stool passage
Inadequate fluid: amount and type

Nursing actions: Record and report
Observe infant
Perform blood glucose test

EXAMPLE 2

Day 4 1750 g
Day 5 1790 g
40 g gain

$$\frac{40}{1750} = \frac{x\%}{100\%}$$
$$1750x = 4000$$
$$1750\overline{)4000.0} = 2.3$$
$$x = 2.3\% \text{ weight gain}$$

Probable causes: Overfeeding
Fluid retention

Nursing actions: Record and report
Observe newborn for other symptoms
Collect urine in bag: check amount, specific gravity
Perform blood glucose test

EXAMPLE 3

Day 4 1750 g
Day 5 1715 g
35 g loss

$$\frac{35}{1750} = \frac{x\%}{100\%}$$
$$1750x = 3500$$
$$1750\overline{)3500.0} = 2.0$$
$$x = 2\% \text{ weight loss}$$

Probable causes: Excessive stooling, voiding
Excessive evaporative losses
Inadequate amount and type of fluid
Malabsorption problem

Nursing actions: Record and report
Check incubator and infant for temperature; check incubator for humidity
Observe newborn for other symptoms
Collect urine in bag: check urine for amount and specific gravity; use Clinistix
Perform blood glucose test

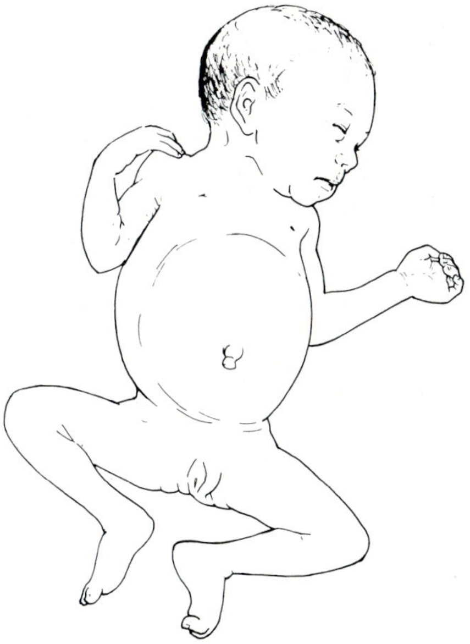

Fig. 36-6 Sudden abdominal distension.
Courtesy Ross Laboratories, Columbus, Ohio.

Nursing Diagnoses

Examples of nursing diagnoses related to nutrition and elimination include the following:

- Altered nutrition, less than body requirements, related to
  - Problems of immaturity
- Fluid volume deficit or overload related to
  - Immaturity or neonatal disorder
- Ineffective breathing pattern related to
  - Sudden abdominal distension

Planning

During the important planning step, goals are set in client-centered terms. Parents are encouraged to be involved to the extent they feel ready. The goals are prioritized. Nursing actions are selected to meet the goals.

Goals

1. Feeding and nutrition of the high-risk newborn are accomplished with the following results:
   a. Minimum respiratory distress; no aspiration or aspiration pneumonia
   b. Minimum expenditure of energy
   c. No hypoglycemic reactions
   d. Acceptable fluid-electrolyte balance
   e. No abdominal distension
   f. No trauma to tissues of the gastrointestinal tract
   g. No diarrhea
2. Sucking satisfaction is maximized
3. Nutrition is sufficient to accomplish the following:
   a. Meet resting metabolic requirements
   b. Provide sufficient energy to perform physical activity
   c. Counter losses through gastrointestinal and urinary tracts
   d. Supply constituents for growth (the infant establishes a steady pattern of appropriate weight gain)
4. Parent-child relationship is fostered in the following ways:
   a. Parent begins to participate in the feeding process in light of the infant's physical capabilities and the parent's desired degree of involvement
   b. Infant begins to associate feeding and eating with pleasure as she or he develops a sense of trust
   c. At discharge parents are comfortable with the feeding method needed by the infant, whether feeding is by breast, bottle, gavage, or gastrostomy

Early Feeding. Early feeding is avoided if the newborn had low Apgar scores at birth. Early feeding of asphyxiated newborns may be an important cause of necrotizing enterocolitis (NEC) (see Chapter 37).

Nourishment Types and Schedules. The formula and feeding schedule of the infant at risk are based on several criteria. The infant's birth weight, pattern of weight gain or loss, and estimated gestational age are factors. The infant's physical condition is also important. Pharyngeal coordination (sucking, swallowing reflexes are present and coordinated), fatigability, malformations, and amount of urine excreted per hour must be taken into account. Laboratory values such as nitrogen balance, electrolyte imbalance, glucose level, serum bilirubin level, and other results also influence the type and schedule of feeding. Variants that influence the feeding of the infant at risk include fluid volume given, caloric requirements, mode of feeding, and formula (breast milk, predigested formula, and calories per ounce).

Parenteral Fluids and Total Parenteral Nutrition. The very small newborn or the newborn who is unable to suck because of developmental or respiratory problems (especially the infant on assisted ventilation) is sustained by parenteral infusions. The electrolytes and nutrients per milliliter, as well as the milliliters of fluid per kilogram of body weight per hour, are carefully calculated by the physician. The nurse monitors the functioning of infusion equipment (tubing, infusion pump), ensures asepsis, secures and protects the needle (catheter) at the insertion site, and assesses and records the newborn's responses. As the infant's condition improves, the infant may be offered fluids by nipple. As the amount of feeding given orally is increased and tolerated, the amount given by infusion is decreased.

Oral Preparations. The nurse assists in assessing the newborn's tolerance for oral feeding by noting:

- Pharyngeal coordination (suck and swallow reflexes present and synchronized)
- Presence and degree of respiratory distress or apneic episodes, if any
- Presence of bowel sounds and absence of abdominal distension
- Residual gastric aspirate of 2 ml or less before feeding

Various milk formulas are available. These vary in calories, protein, and mineral content (see Chapter 23). Breast milk or formula may be fed by continuous flow with a pump and feeding tube inserted into the stomach or jejunum or by intermittent gavage or nipple. During the transition to nipple it may be necessary to use both nipple and gavage to ensure the prescribed intake. Each newborn must be evaluated for ability to handle solute and fluid load.

Oral feedings begin with sterile water. Feedings are advanced by increasing the amount of fluid *or* the number of calories per 30 ml (1 oz) at any one feeding. The maximum number of calories per ounce is 24. During the feeding the newborn's tolerance is observed. For infants weighing less than approximately 1800 g (4 lb) caution and judgment is exercised continuously in advancing the feedings. Too rapid advancement may lead to vomiting, diarrhea, abdominal distension, and apneic episodes. Residual gastric aspirate of 2 ml or more may be present at the time of the next feeding. Retention of fluid with cardiopulmonary embarrassment or marked diuresis with loss of sodium ($Na+$), leading to hyponatremia, may occur. Regurgitation can occur and predispose the infant to aspiration pneumonia.

Procedures. The nurse readjusts the feedings (or infusion) to achieve acceptable weight gain. Observations are recorded accurately. Deviations from the normal range in weight losses or gains guide future diagnostic evaluations.

The nursing care plan is readjusted regarding continuation of gavage feedings or attempting oral feedings based on the infant's responses. Simultaneous sucking satisfaction is offered as soon as possible before the tenth day of life; gavage through nipple if necessary (Bernbaum, 1983). The type and amount of formula and the frequency of feedings are planned in accordance with ongoing assessment (evaluation) and nursing diagnoses. If the infant is taking oral

Procedure 36-2

FEEDING NEWBORN WITH CLEFT LIP AND PALATE

DEFINITION

Congenital defects characterized by a fissure(s) in the palate and upper lip, resulting from the failure to fuse during embryonic development.

PURPOSE

To facilitate feeding when infant has difficulty creating a vacuum and sucking.
To prevent aspiration of feeding.
To prevent discomfort from increased amount of swallowed air.

EQUIPMENT (Fig. 36-7)

Lamb's nipple; Duckey nipple with flange to fit over defect; Brecht feeder; Rubber-tipped Asepto syringe.

NURSING ACTIONS	RATIONALE
Identify client and check physician's orders.	To provide the right therapy for the right person.
Wash hands before and after touching client or equipment. Glove, prn.	To prevent nosocomial infection and to implement universal precautions.
Prepare thickened formula as ordered, usually with dried rice cereal.	To increase gravity flow of fluid into stomach, and prevent aspiration.
Choose appropriate nipple and enlarge hole in nipple as needed.	To assist infant in creating a vacuum during sucking and to encourage development of normal sucking pattern. To permit passage of thickened formula.
Check infant for clear airway.	To minimize possibility of aspiration.
During feeding check infant for the following signs: aspiration—choking and cyanosis; swallowed air—abdominal distention.	To prevent abdominal distension and aspiration that can compromise respirations.
Hold infant in upright position.	To minimize possibility of aspiration and return of fluid through nose and to aid swallowing.
Interact with infant: talk and make eye contact with her or him.	To stimulate psychosocial development. If mother sees nurse doing this, it may facilitate her acceptance of the child.
Burp or bubble infant frequently.	To minimize amount of air that is swallowed when there is unnatural passage between nose and mouth. Technique increases infant's comfort and minimizes regurgitation and aspiration.
When feeding with a rubber-tipped Asepto syringe, place rubber tip on top of and to side of infant's tongue.	To facilitate feeding. To prevent tip of syringe from entering cleft in palate.
Offer feeding slowly.	To allow infant time to swallow.
NOTE: The child with a cleft lip only may be able to feed well with a regular or "preemie" nipple.	

feeding, the type of nipple ("preemie," regular, breast) depends on the infant's ability to master the specific type of nipple and the energy available to spend on the process.

Overfeeding is avoided. Assessment for overfeeding is done by checking the amount of residual gastric aspirate before subsequent feeding. If there is residue, refeed residue and subtract this amount from the feeding. The amount of subsequent feedings is decreased, and perhaps the infant is fed more frequently. The infant is burped or "bubbled" as necessary.

The nurse involves the parents in the actual feeding or teaches them how to give gavage feedings if the child will require such feedings after going home.

Implementation

Feeding the Newborn with Cleft Lip and Palate. The baby born with a cleft lip and palate may be normal in every other way. Surgical repair on the lip is usually done soon after birth if possible to assist parents in the attachment process with their newborn. The palate is usually repaired some months later. The nurse may be called to feed the newborn during the early neonatal period or to teach the parent to do so. Procedure 36-2 and Fig. 36-7 are presented to assist the nurse in feeding the newborn and to serve as a guide for teaching the parent(s).

Gavage Feeding. Gavage feedings are supplied by an indwelling nasogastric tube with continuous flow of formula administered by an infusion pump. Feeding by gavage is the method for choice for the infant who is (1) compromised by respiratory distress, (2) immature or has a weak suck or uncoordinated sucking-swallowing behavior, or (3) easily fatigued even when using a "preemie" nipple. Procedure 36-3 and Fig. 36-8 describe gavage feedings using oral insertion and nasal insertion. Insertion of the gavage feeding tube has been studied (research highlight).

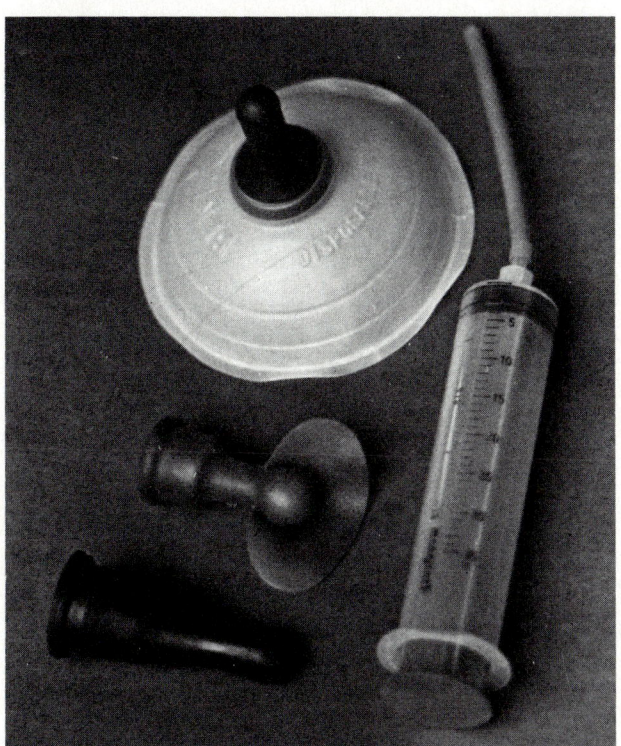

Fig. 36-7 Some devices used to feed infant with cleft palate. *Clockwise,* lamb's nipple, flanged nipple, special nurser, and syringe with rubber tubing (Breck feeder).

From Whaley, LF, and Wong, DL: Nursing care of infants and children, ed 3, St Louis, 1987, The CV Mosby Co.

Parenteral Fluid Administration. Administration of parenteral fluids may be the method of choice for meeting the infant's fluid and caloric needs. Procedure 36-4 and Fig. 36-9 describe monitoring of parenteral fluid therapy.

Total Parenteral Nutrition (TPN). Total parenteral nutrition is the method of choice for the infant who (1) requires several surgeries for repair of gastrointestinal anomalies or obstruction, (2) suffers from chronic diarrhea, or (3) has malabsorption syndrome. This method of meeting the infant's nutrition needs is described in Procedure 36-5.

Text continued on p. 926.

RESEARCH HIGHLIGHT

Gavage Tube Insertion in the Premature Infant

Purpose

This study was done to determine which, if either, of the two conventional gavage tube measurement methods resulted in the most accurate placement in the stomach of 30 premature infants.

Sample

The infants studied had a gestational age at birth of 28 to 36 weeks and required gavage tubes for feeding or gastric decompression. In addition, each infant enrolled in the study was receiving chest or abdominal x-ray studies and had no congenital malformations that might affect feeding tube placement.

Methodology/Findings

A routine review of 85 x-ray films of gavage-fed infants at a regional center revealed that 38% of the nasogastric gavage tubes had been placed incorrectly in relation to the distal tip.

On different days, the two conventional placement methods were used to insert gavage tubes in each infant. Placements were scheduled to coincide with the x-ray studies. The films were examined by the investigators and two physicians to determine proper placement criteria.

Measures to control tube slippage and technique were used in this study. However findings yielded incorrect placement rates of 55.6% and 39.3%, respectively.

Implications

Although these findings are considered preliminary and should be interpreted with caution, the problem must obviously be investigated more fully. These investigators are therefore in the process of studying two modified techniques in an attempt to find a more accurate procedure for inserting nasogastric tubes in premature infants.

Weibley, TT, Adamson, M, Clinkscales, N, et al: Gavage tube insertion in the premature infant, MCN, 12:24, Jan/Feb, 1987.

Procedure 36-3

GAVAGE FEEDING

DEFINITION

A procedure in which a tube is passed through the nose or mouth into the stomach to feed an infant with weak sucking, uncoordinated sucking, and swallow or respiratory distress.

PURPOSE

To meet the nutrition and fluid needs of the infant who cannot suck.

EQUIPMENT

Sterile feeding tube: rubber or plastic, rounded tips, sizes 5 to 10, infant lengths; clearly calibrated syringe for feeding; stethoscope and sterile medication syringe without needle; sterile water for lubrication; feeding formula; medications.

NURSING ACTIONS	RATIONALE
Identify client and check physician's orders.	To provide the right therapy for the right person.
Wash hands before and after touching client or equipment. Glove, prn.	To prevent nosocomial infection and to implement universal precautions.
The infant's anatomy makes it difficult to enter the trachea. One or more of the following tests are done to determine correct stomach placement:	*To assure paper placement of the nasal or oral tube for gavage feedings.*
Use sterile syringe to inject 0.5 ml of air through catheter into stomach, Simultaneously, listen for sound of air bubbling or "growling" in stomach with stethoscope over epigastric region.	Sound of air bubbling confirms tube placement in stomach.
The most complete procedure involves listening with stethoscope first over the epigastrium and then on each side of the anterior chest.	The sound of rushing air heard over the anterior chest should be considerably diminished intensity compared with that heard over the epigastrium.
Aspirate small amount of stomach contents.	Aspiration of stomach contents confirms proper placement of tube.
Fill tube with stomach contents, and pinch off tube; add syringe containing feeding.	This avoids allowing air into stomach with feeding.
Oral insertion: intermittent or indwelling catheter:	*To accomplish oral insertion:*
Position infant: head of mattress up one notch, folded towel under shoulders to slightly extend neck.	Opens oropharynx. Extends and straightens esophagus.
Select size 8 French feeding tube.	Is adequate size for feeding. Less apt to fold over or curl up.
Measure distance between bridge of nose, to earlobe, and then to lower end of xiphoid process. Mark distance with 5 cm (2 in) thin strip of paper tape. Fold tape over tube, leaving two long ends with which to secure tube when it is in place.	Determines length necessary to reach into stomach without folding back on itself. Facilitates anchoring tubing, if it is to be indwelling. Paper tape is usually less irritating to skin.
Lubricate tube in sterile water.	Prevents trauma and infection.
Pass tube along base of tongue, advancing it into esophagus as infant swallows.	Offers less risk of vagal stimulation or of accidental entry into trachea. Stimulates esophageal peristalsis and opens cardiac sphincter.
Test placement of tube.	Avoids introduction of formula, vitamins, and medicines into trachea or esophagus.
Aspirate and measure any residual feeding in stomach. If 1 ml or less, subtract same amount from this feeding. If more than 1 ml, physician may wish to have this feeding skipped.	Avoids overfeeding. Excessive fluid in stomach suggests intestinal obstruction.
Slowly pour warmed formula into syringe barrel and allow it to flow by gravity into stomach. Hold reservoir 15 to 20 cm (6 to 8 in) above infant's head. If gravity flow is too rapid, lower syringe, or insert plunger into syringe, and inject *slowly*. Feeding time should approximate that of nipple feedings (20 minutes or about 1 ml/min.)	Rapid entry of formula into stomach causes rapid rebound response with regurgitation, thus increasing danger of aspiration or abdominal distension, which compromises respiratory effort.
Do not allow level of formula to go below neck of syringe.	Prevents entry of air into stomach to minimize risks of regurgitation and distension.
Observe infant's response.	Prevents respiratory distress. Assists gastrointestinal functioning.

Procedure 36-3—cont'd

NURSING ACTIONS	RATIONALE
Follow formula with specified amount of sterile water.	Gets all formula into stomach and clears tubing of formula.
Pinch tubing (or clamp it off) and withdraw it rapidly.	Prevents entry of air into stomach. Creates vacuum to hold fluid in tubing to prevent dripping it into trachea on withdrawal.
Burp or bubble infant. With left hand, support infant's head and shoulders. Raise to a sitting position and lean infant onto right hand. Right hand supports infant's chest with palm and infant's jaw with thumb and forefinger. Gently rub back with left hand.	Increases comfort. Prevents regurgitation.
Position on right side with small rolled drape or towel.	Facilitates stomach emptying.
Record the following: Amount of residual gastric aspirate Type and amount of feeding, medicine Time of feeding Infant response: fatigue, peaceful sleep, abdominal distension, respiratory distress, type and amount of vomiting or regurgitation; heart and respiratory rate	Provides basis for evaluation and readjustment of feeding regimen. Facilitates communication among personnel.

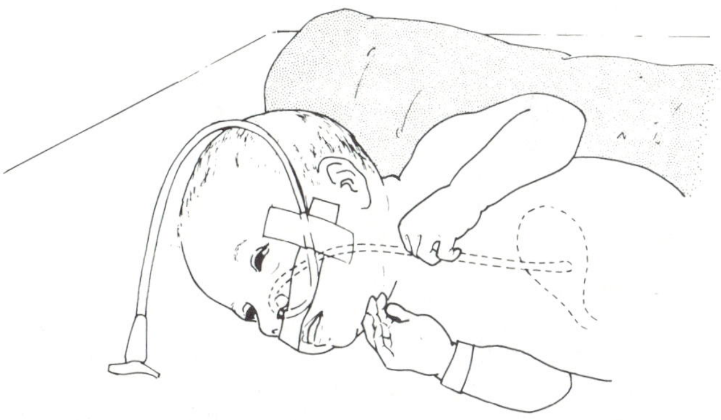

Fig. 36-8 Indwelling gavage tube: nasal route. Infant is propped on right side to facilitate emptying of stomach into small intestine. Note rolled towel for support. (See also Fig. 22-6.)

NURSING ACTIONS	RATIONALE
Nasal route: intermittent or indwelling catheter:	*To accomplish nasal insertion:*
Position as for oral route.	Opens oropharynx. Extends and straightens esophagus.
Select size 3½ to 5 French feeding tube.	Is adequate size for feeding and small enough to allow breathing space around it, since neonates are obligate nose breathers.
If indwelling, change every 2 or 3 days (48 to 72 hours) or more frequently if otitis is present, alternating sides of nares.	Prevents infection, irritation; excess mucus, ulceration, bleeding
Observe infant for respiratory distress.	If tube causes distress, remove it. Infants are obligate nose breathers. Use oral route.
May be preferred route for indwelling tube for continuous drip feeding.	Very small preterm infant often tolerates feeding better by continuous drip, stomach is not overloaded.
Measure distance from bridge of nose to earlobe, and then to xiphoid process (just beyond tip of sternum). Mark spot with 5 cm (2 in) thin strip of paper tape, and overlap tube, leaving ends free	Provides adequate length to reach stomach without curling. Facilitates anchoring of tubing. Decreases risk of skin irritation from tape.
Lubricate with sterile water.	Prevents tissue trauma.
Insert tube, holding it horizontally until it reaches back of nares; then lift tubing slightly and continue to advance. Allow infant to swallow tube while it is being advanced.	Accommodates to bend in back of nares and minimizes direct tissue damage. Stimulates peristalsis and opens cardiac sphincter.
Continue as for oral route.	Same as for oral route.
Nursing care after feedings:	*To provide supportive care after feedings:*
Burp infant gently after feedings.	Promotes comfort and prevents vomiting.
Turn infant's head or position the infant on right side after feeding and burping (Fig. 36-8).	Protects against aspiration of stomach contents if vomiting occurs. Allows release of air from baby's stomach (Fig. 36-8; see also Fig. 22-6).
Postpone postural drainage and percussion for a minimum of 1 hour after feeding.	Promotes retention of feeding.
Avoid feeding the infant within an hour before a laboratory test for blood glucose.	Promotes accurate reading in laboratory tests.

Procedure 36-4

MONITORING PARENTERAL FLUID ADMINISTRATION

DEFINITION

Administration of fluids and nutrients to an infant by a route other than the alimentary canal, usually by intravenous route, either peripheral vein or umbilical artery.

PURPOSE

To meet the newborn infant's fluid needs.

EQUIPMENT

1. Supplies to start or maintain intravenous therapy by way of a peripheral vein, venous cutdown, or umbilical catheter.
2. Supplies to prevent accidental overhydration:
   a. Bottles containing 250 ml of infusion fluid.
   b. Administration sets with enclosed reservoirs and minidropper.
   c. Infusion pump with automatic alarm to signal an empty fluid chamber.
   d. Medicine cup (paper) or other appliance to protect insertion site if using scalp vein (Fig. 36-9).

NURSING ACTIONS	RATIONALE
Identify client and check physician's orders.	To provide the right therapy for the right person.
Wash hands before and after touching client and/or equipment. Glove, prn.	To prevent nosocomial infection and to implement universal precautions.
Prepare equipment.	To avoid searching for missing articles after procedure has begun.
Restrain infant.	To provide for infant's safety and increased ease of starting parenteral fluids.
Provide pacifier to infant if appropriate.	To provide comfort for the infant who can handle a pacifier.
Continue care of intravenous infusion. Regulate rate of flow.	*To provide for adequate infusion.*
Infusion pump: check setting; double-check by counting drops per minute every hour, and note amount infused every 4 hours.	Assures a more accurate and constant flow rate. Double-checks for equipment malfunction.
Reposition extremity or infant's head.	Assures proper body alignment and prevents breakdown of skin. Protects infusion site.
Do not make up deficiency or excess by changing rate of flow without consulting physician.	Fluid may *overload* infant's system. An infant who has received more than prescribed amount for period must be assessed for overhydration and cardiac decompensation.
Check infusion site every hour.	*To prevent trauma to tissues. Assures adequate hydration. Possible complications:* Infection; Thrombophlebitis; Tissue and vein trauma (Fig. 36-10).
Check for tissue infiltration (swelling). Check for tissue trauma: color, temperature. If needle is in extremity, compare and contrast with other extremity.	
If needle is in scalp vein, check head and face for symmetry of contour and movement.	Needle out of vein with injection of fluid into surrounding tissues and possible tissue breakdown.
Evaluate infant's hydration every hour.	*To determine adequate rate of flow.*
Urinary output: collect or weigh diapers.	Assesses amount of urine excreted.
Specific gravity of urine (see Appendix H and Procedure 22-5 for use of urine collectors).	Assists in assessing appropriate solute or fluid infant needs and kidney function.
Weight: infant may be weighed every 8, 12, or 24 hours (same scale, naked, before feeding).	Weight gain or loss greater than 2% of body weight within a 24-hour period is cause for concern.
Urine: check for glucose every 8 to 24 hours.	Presence of excess glucose in the urine would indicate an excessive glucose load in the intravenous fluid.
Other: tissue turgor; fever; sunken fontanels; soft, sunken eyeballs; or behavior changes may be present.	Assesses state of hydration.

Procedure 36-4—cont'd

NURSING ACTIONS	RATIONALE
Record the following:	*To provide complete data.*
Type of fluid being used.	Evaluates treatment.
Amount of fluid absorbed every hour and amount scheduled to have been absorbed.	Meets infant's changing needs.
Amount of fluid in bottle or fluid chamber.	Identifies possible cause of any existing or new problem.
Flow rate.	Provides base line for continuation at present rate or change in rate.
Infant's condition.	Indicates infant's response to this regimen and readiness for progression.
Change intravenous tubing and bottle every 24 hours.	To decrease possibility of infection.
Irrigate intravenously.	*To maintain patency of system.*
Three-way stopcock may be used to connect tubing to needle.	Facilitates flushing needle while decreasing chance of contamination and loss of blood during procedure.
Without three-way stopcock, clamp intravenous tubing and disconnect at junction with needle. Keep tubing end sterile. Attach syringe containing 1 to 3 ml of normal saline solution or heparinized saline solution to needle.	Clears out small occluding clots; prevents formation of clots.
Slowly inject fluid into vein. Disconnect syringe and reconnect to intravenous tubing. Unclamp intravenous tubing and regulate flow of infusion.	Prevent trauma to vein or dislodging the needle.
Never flush a clogged needle.	To avoid pushing blood clot through infant's circulation.
After intravenous fluid is discontinued:	*To ensure adequate nutrition and hydration.*
Observe infant for hypoglycemia for 24 hours.	Hypoglycemia often is seen after discontinuation of parenteral therapy.
Observe infant for adequacy of nutrition and hydration.	Assesses infant's ability to take and utilize nutrients and fluids by mouth or gavage.
Continue to assess infant for thrombophlebitis at previous insertion site and sloughing.	Begins definitive treatment and prevents tissue damage.

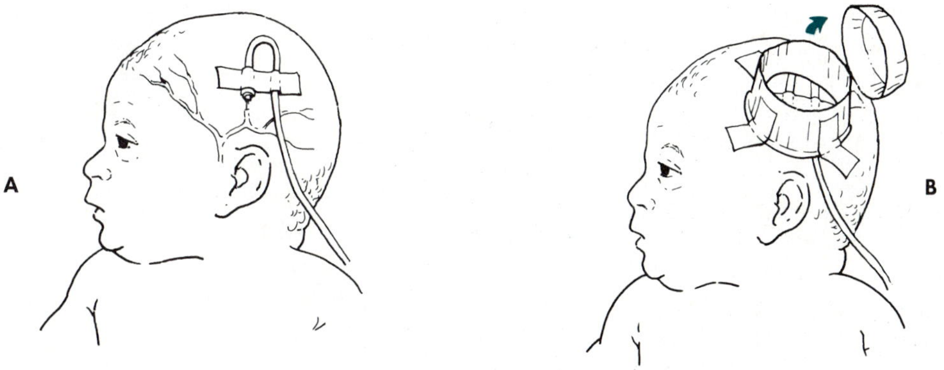

Fig. 36-9 **A**, Venipuncture of scalp vein. **B**, Paper cup protecting venipuncture site.

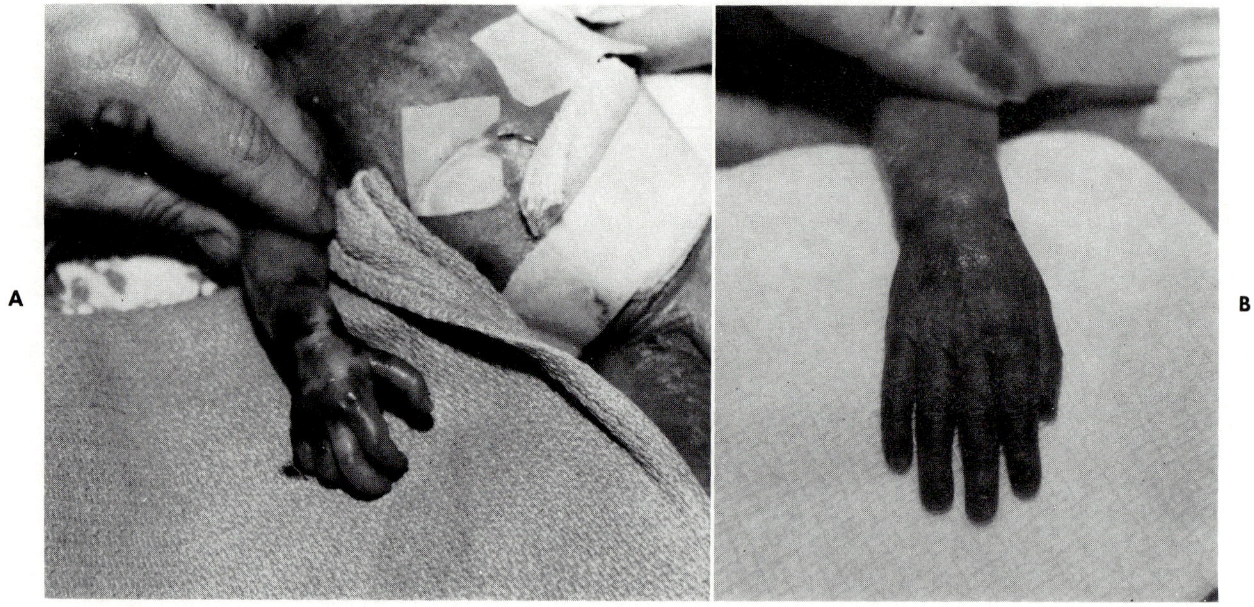

Fig. 36-10 **A**, Intravenous infiltration in small infant can cause severe ischemia. **B**, Fortunately, preterm infant has remarkable regenerative abilities (same hand 1 week later).
Courtesy Mount Zion Hospital and Medical Center, San Francisco.

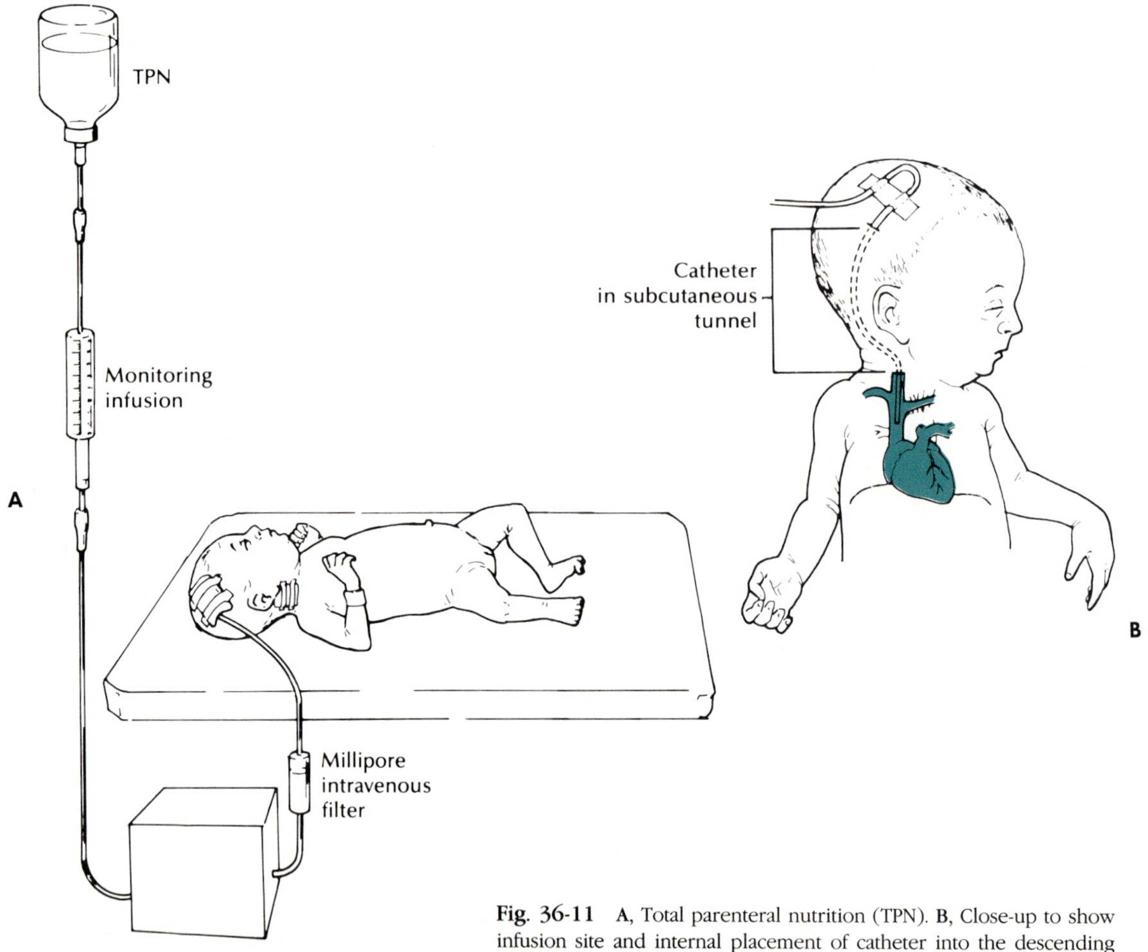

Fig. 36-11 **A**, Total parenteral nutrition (TPN). **B**, Close-up to show infusion site and internal placement of catheter into the descending vena cava. Parenteral nutrition is often used in conjunction with other forms of feeding, particularly when weaning to oral feedings.

Procedure 36-5

TOTAL PARENTERAL NUTRITION (TPN)

DEFINITION

The administration of a nutritionally adequate hypertonic solution consisting of glucose, protein hydrolysates, minerals, and vitamins through an indwelling catheter in the superior vena cava or umbilical artery (Fig. 36-11).

PURPOSE

To provide continuous nutrition at a prescribed rate for extended periods of time.

EQUIPMENT

Equipment for starting intravenous infusion or cut-down; silastic catheter of appropriate size; millipore intravenous filter; constant infusion pump; TPN solution (infusion fluid); pacifier and mobiles; restraints as necessary.

NURSING ACTIONS	RATIONALE
Identify client and check physician's orders.	To provide the right therapy for the right person.
Wash hands before and after touching client or equipment. Glove, prn.	To prevent nosocomial infection and to implement universal precautions.
Gather equipment as necessary.	To be efficient and save time.
Procedure may be done in operating room. Nursing actions are the same as those for care of an infant receiving intravenous therapy, except for the following notable additions:	To maintain strict aseptic technique.
Avoid using the catheter for purposes other than the infusion solution (e.g., not to be used for blood or medications).	To maintain patency; avoid mixing incompatible fluids.
Avoid making up excess or deficit by altering the drip rate without consulting the physician.	To avoid fluid overload or deficit.
Order prescribed mixture from pharmacy. Do not tamper with mixed solution. Do not add to mixture.	To ensure accuracy of amounts and prevent microbial contamination and admixture problems.
Check on rate of flow.	To avoid overfeeding or underfeeding.
Check pump setting.	To avoid using malfunctioning equipment.
Check amount given from calibrated, enclosed reservoir every 2 to 4 hours.	
Change bottle, tubing and Millipore filter every 24 hours.	To decrease risk of microbial contamination.
Change dressing around catheter.	To prevent infection, and allow observation of needle insertion site.
Monitor infant's weight daily, at same time, on same scale, before feeding.	To provide index of response to this form of therapy.
Provide pacifier, mobiles, infant stimulation pictures.	To provide sucking satisfaction and visual stimulation.
Observe infant for complications associated with TPN.	To facilitate prompt identification and treatment of problems:
Catheter and its insertion: local skin infection septicemia, blood vessel thrombosis, obstruction or dislodgment of catheter, cardiac symptoms such as dysarrhythmia. *Candida* septicemia is common.	Sepsis.
Infusion solution—type and amount: glucosuria, dehydration, acidosis, amino acid imbalance.	Metabolic complications.

Evaluation

Nursing care is evaluated to determine if the nursing goals have been met. Success can be measured by small steady increments in weight gain, fluid and electrolyte balance, and absence of gastrointestinal distress. Initiation and maintenance of oral feedings are reassuring to parents and nurses. Parental success and satisfaction with the feeding process and the infant's response to it are indicators that goals are being met.

EMOTIONAL ASPECTS OF CARE

Newborn's Emotional Needs. Premature and sick infants who are not in acute distress or who are convalescing have at least the same emotional and developmental needs that the normal term infant has. It may be difficult to meet the needs of the infant at risk. The sick infant who needs intravenous therapy, nasogastric feedings, heel-stick samples, oxygen by plastic hood, or CPAP cannot be cuddled, fondled, or played with as can the term infant. Instead she or he must experience many painful stimuli, including numerous intrusive procedures, such as having electronic leads taped to and removed from the chest wall. The view through the plastic walls of the incubator is blurred, a cacophony of sounds (e.g., motors, hiss of oxygen) penetrates the infant's closed-in world, and overhead bright lights deny diurnal and nocturnal rhythms.

Without adequate attention to emotional and developmental needs, the premature and sick infant may begin to show signs of great anxiety and tension, including the following:

Failure to thrive (slow or absent recovery, growth, weight gain)

Looking away from or to the side of the people who are caring for her or him

Absent, weak, or infrequent crying (as if to say, "What's the use?")

These are a result of being exposed to life-support measures while being separated from the constant presence of one mothering and comforting person.

Communication Patterns. Babies communicate with the world around them in various ways (Cole, no date). Developing skill in reading these cues is essential for the nurse to individualize a plan of care that maximizes the neonate's potential for healing and growth. Most full-term babies thrive on stimulation. However, the compromised neonate may be overwhelmed by too much stimulation. **Cues of a baby who is ready for interaction** include an overall appearance of relaxation. The neonate looks at the caregiver's face and appears to listen.

Cues of a baby who is overstimulated and needs time-out from interaction include color changes (e.g., pale or flushed). The infant may hiccough, gag, or spit up. The breathing pattern changes. Muscle tone changes. Frequent startles and tremors may be seen. The baby uses several methods to cope with overstimulation. Nurses and parents alike benefit from being on the alert for these cues. The coping strategies include ways to decrease the intensity of incoming cues (avoiding eye contact), to take time away from interaction (yawning, becoming drowsy, and sneezing), and to provide self-gratification (thumb sucking). These strategies allow the child to avoid overload and loss of energy (Cole, no date).

Several methods are available to the nurse to *reduce* the neonate's *incoming stimuli.* Swaddling the infant (when possible), propping the newborn with rolled diapers, covering the crib with a blanket, and organizing care to allow for long stretches of rest in between treatments are a few. Do Not Disturb signs on the crib remind people to give the infant time to rest.

Infant Stimulation. The infant's sense of trust develops when she or he learns the feel, sound, and smell of the

A B

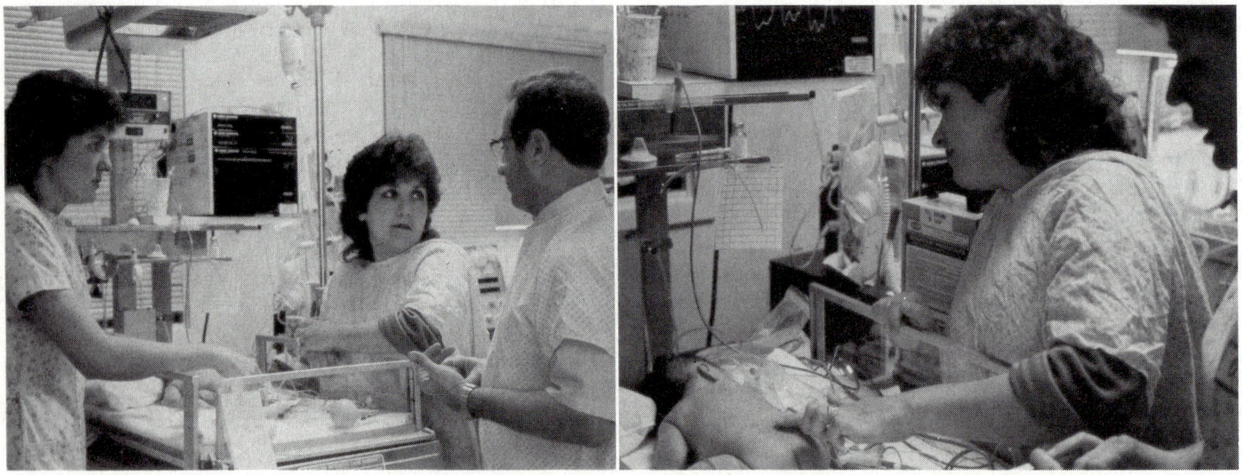

Fig. 36-12 Mother in special care nursery. **A,** Mother listens intently as physician keeps her informed of her baby's condition and progress. Nurse stands by for support. **B,** Note mother's tentative, tender fingertip touch as she begins to explore her baby.

Courtesy Nanci Newell, Fountain Valley Community Hospital, Fountain Valley, Calif.

same mothering person who comforts her or him and who removes uncomfortable stimuli (e.g., hunger, wet or soiled clothing). The infant even learns to anticipate these happenings and soon learns that cries bring this mothering person. These conditions cannot be duplicated in the nursery, but some modifications often can be made in the nursing care plan. In the technologic environment of a premature or sick baby nursery (Fig. 36-12), nursing's focus must be on people, not on equipment. The possibilities are limited only by the parameters of human creativity.

When the baby is ready for stimulation, the nurse has many options.

Time from treatments can be scheduled to stroke the infant's skin. The parents may be encouraged to touch the infant through portholes.

Mobiles and decals that can be changed frequently may be placed inside the incubator.

The nurse can respond to the infant's efforts to cry by reassuring her or him and offering a pacifier while stroking the skin and talking to the infant.

When the infant can tolerate being out of the incubator, even for short periods of time, the nurse can remove, cuddle and rock, and sing to the infant. This activity is beneficial, especially during feedings—even when feeding by gavage or gastrostomy. If possible, the infant may be taken out of the incubator and held to raise bubbles of air from the stomach. If the mother or father is able to visit frequently, both parent and infant will benefit immeasurably from this activity.

If the infant must have feedings by gavage or gastrostomy, the nurse can offer a pacifier during the feeding process (in the absence of respiratory distress). This will provide sucking satisfaction, and the infant will begin to associate this pleasant, self-gratifying, and self-initiated activity with the comforting feeling of a filling stomach.

The nurse can talk, sing, and hum to the infant whenever possible. However loud talking and excessive discordant noise should be avoided (Fanaroff and Martin, 1987). Some nurseries permit the placement of wind-up musical toys in the incubator or crib.

The newborn can be held so that she or he can see the caregiver's face. Eye contact can be established as the nurse talks or sings to the infant.

Even if the infant is undergoing phototherapy, there can be some periods when the baby is not under the lamp. The protective eye patches can be removed so that the infant can see the nurse's or the parent's face during periodic, short comforting sessions.

Technologic versus Human Incubator: "Kangaroo Method"

Vivian Wahlberg

In Western countries and cultures, preterm infants are usually cared for in a technically advanced environment—an incubator—to conserve warmth and energy for repair, maintenance, and growth. Thus these infants are separated from their mothers. They are faced with many technologic treatments and procedures, such as gavage feedings and biometric monitoring. However, in Colombia, South America, it has been possible for recently born healthy preterm infants to be cared for by their mothers. The babies are tucked inside their mother's blouses in a head-up position and are breast-fed as soon as their condition is stable (Ress, 1984; Anderson, Marks, and Wahlberg, 1986). Here, in the "human incubator," the infants have all they need in a natural way: skin-to-skin contact, humidity, nourishment, warmth, and love. Because of its marsupial nature, this initial care of the preterm infant by the mother has become known around the world as the "kangaroo method" (Fig. 36-13). It originated in 1979 in Bogota, Colombia. This method is in sharp contrast to the care of preterm infants in North America and Europe.

The Instituto Materno Infantil at San Juan de Dios Hospital in Bogota is a large maternity hospital with an average of 12,000 deliveries a year. It serves the low-income population of the city and has a large number of high-risk pregnancies. The lack of resources motivated Dr. Rey and Dr. Martinez, two pediatricians working at the hospital, to devise the alternative approach.

The Programma Ambulatorio de Prematuros arose out of severe economic restraints and problems with nosocomial and cross-infections, but is based on a deep respect for natural processes. Premature infants in satisfactory clinical condition, no matter how small, are not kept in intensive care units. Instead they go directly to their mothers as early as 2 to 3 hours after birth and are mostly discharged within 12 to 24 hours after birth. Mother and infant remain together 24 hours a day.

Mothers are requested to breast-feed their infants in self-regulatory fashion. The babies are to feed on demand to satiety. The mothers carry the babies skin-to-skin to maintain their warmth. Reports in 1983 by the founders of the program showed dramatic decreases in mortality, morbidity, and parental abandonment.

The "kangaroo method" (K-method), in a modified form, has now also been introduced in many European neonatal units: Hammersmiths Hospital in London (Whitelow and Sleath, 1985) and Karolinska Hospital in Stockholm. Low-birth-weight (LBW) or preterm infants who are AGA and who no longer require oxygen or intensive care can be nursed by their mothers in the "kangaroo position" with skin-to-skin contact without untoward results.

It has been observed in Columbia, Sweden, and England that the continuity of closeness and mutual stimulation between the mother and preterm infant has reciprocal effects. Mothers reported feelings of emotional harmony and a psychological sense of oneness with their infants. Because the infant's head is in an upright position, the risk of a "pathologic flat" head (seen in many preterm infants) is not observed. In this upright position the risk of regurgitation and aspiration is minimized.

The K-method of caring for the compromised newborn promotes early emotional attachment between mother and infant. Normal growth of the cranium is facilitated. Natural methods of meeting the infant's needs replace technologic means. For infants who are in a stable physical condition, the K-method may also shorten the length of care in the incubator and the hospital and thus decrease cost for care. The experience increases the mothers' sense of comfort

A 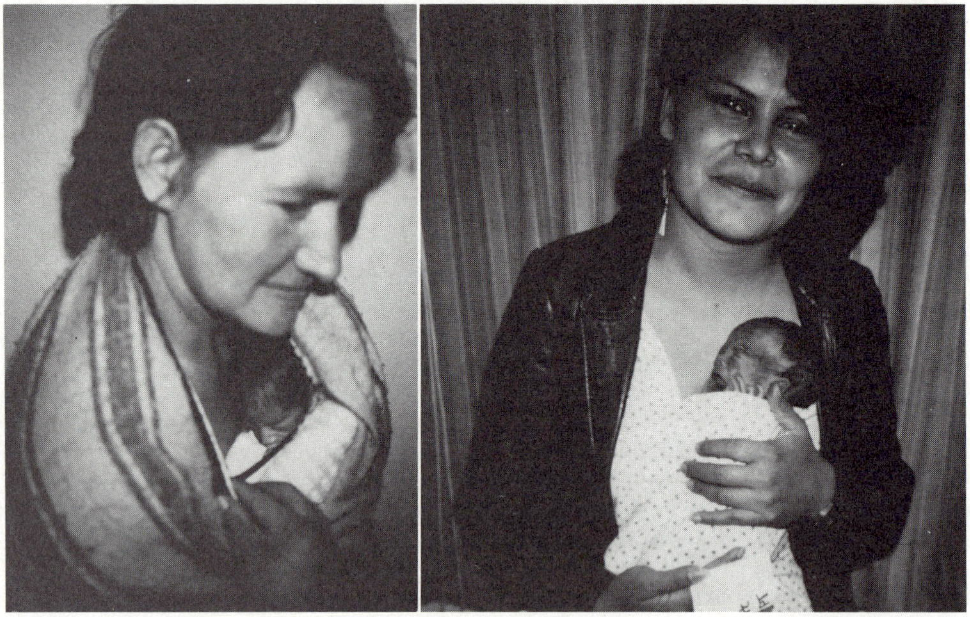 B

Fig. 36-13 The kangaroo method. **A**, Infant snuggled inside wrap. **B**, Infant inside mother's blouse in skin-to-skin contact. (Bogota, Columbia, S.A.).
Courtesy Vivian Wahlberg, R.N., C.M., Dr. Med. Sc., Karolinska, Stockholm.

and confidence in providing care for their premature infants.

Discharge Planning. Adequate discharge planning for the high-risk infant and follow-up arrangements should include general pediatric care, visiting nurse service, parenting classes and training in cardiopulmonary resuscitation (Chapter 22). This is especially true for young or psychosocially high-risk parents (Merenstein and Gardner, 1985). Referrals to county social service departments should be made for single mothers who are eligible for Aid to Families of Dependent Children and Medicaid. For infants with special problems (spina bifida, cerebral palsy, or Down's syndrome), referrals should be made for special programs. These programs provide services for the infants and support groups for parents. Parents whose infants have special medical needs (gavage feedings, tracheostomy or colostomy care, or oxygen) should be evaluated by the medical and nursing personnel. This evaluation will help determine community resources (equipment, supplies, or emergency care) and make appropriate referrals. Home nursing care and homemaker services are sometimes covered by medical insurance. Home visits may be necessary to provide actual nursing activities and to relieve parents from the emotional burden inherent in caring for an infant with medical problems. For infants who are developmentally disabled, infant stimulation programs and follow-up programs provided by many hospitals that have neonatal intensive care units are extremely valuable. Locating babysitters who will care for a child with special problems can be an overwhelming task for parents. Cultivating a resource list for parents and suggesting that parents exchange services with each other can be helpful. Graduate parents and neonatal nurses can provide a useful service to parents in this situation. Lastly, parents should be referred to appropriate funding agencies (Handicapped or Crippled Children's Program, Medicaid, or Social Security Disability) that provide financial assistance.

SUMMARY

The woman, her family, and the compromised neonate are highly vulnerable. Protection of the newborn by maintenance of a warm environment, adequate oxygen, and safety is an important part of the nurse's care. The newborn's nutrition, fluid, and elimination needs must be monitored and met carefully. The family of the woman experiencing a high-risk pregnancy, labor, and delivery and the sick neonate require skilled nursing care. The manner in which parents are counseled and supported initially and subsequently influences parental adjustment and parent-child interactions. The nurse needs to examine her or his own feelings about high-risk pregnancy, compromised neonates, and neonatal death. Coming to terms with these feelings increases the nurse's ability to assist grieving families and parents. The result can be a rewarding and fulfilling experience for the nurse.

KEY CONCEPTS

- Identification of risk situations affecting mother and infant is vital to plan adequate care.
- High risk infants have special problems caused by immaturity, alterations in functioning of systems, and metabolic balances.
- Parents need help to accept, care for, and take home infants who require care for risk conditions.

- The aim of transporting high-risk infants to regional centers is to provide access to the required level of care.
- The alert nurse often is the pivotal point between functional and dysfunctional survival for the infant in respiratory distress.
- A thermoneutral environment is essential for metabolic homeostasis.
- For the child receiving supplemental oxygen, periodic laboratory measurements and close clinical observation are essential to make appropriate adjustments in care to minimize the risk of both hyperoxic and hypoxic insults.
- The extent to which nutrition needs are met is directly related to the infant's immediate and long-range well-being.

STUDY QUESTIONS AND ACTIVITIES

1. For students with no previous experience with intensive care units: in groups of two, walk into an intensive care nursery (ICN) as if you were new parents of a baby who was just admitted. Bring a notebook with you. Limit your visit to 30 minutes, but stay the *full* 30 minutes. Individually, jot down your observations, keeping the following in mind: describe your "gut reactions"; what do you notice first?; using all of your senses, make one observation for each item you observed; stand beside one neonate and focus in on everything you see within 15 cm (6 in) of the baby; spend 15 minutes comparing notes with your partner.
2. Develop a general nursing care plan for the parents starting with the birth of a child at moderate risk until the mother (who is reasonally healthy) is discharged from the hospital.
3. Have students "buddy up" with an ICN nurse for 1 clinical day. The clinical observation day should follow an orientation to the ICN so that the student can focus in on the experience to be described. Choose any of the following:
   a. Observe a complete physical assessment. Compare with the routine physical assessments in the well-baby nursery.
   b. Describe the infant's willingness to interact with caregivers and to engage in eye-to-eye contact. Note your reactions to the neonate. Discuss implications for nursing care of the neonate and family, based on your findings.
   c. Calculate the percentage of weight gain and loss for three high-risk neonates. Identify probable causes and describe nursing actions.
   d. Observe nursing care related to maintenance of respirations, temperature, and nutrition and elimination.
4. Choose an infant at high risk. Identify ethical issues involved. Discuss the identified issues (using content regarding ethical issue decision making in Chapter 4) from the following perspectives:
   a. As the professional nurse working with the baby and family.
   b. As the parent.
   c. As the taxpayer/legislator who must decide how best to allocate funds among a variety of community needs.
5. In the clinical setting or in the laboratory, demonstrate techniques such as oxygen administration and application of thermistor probes, and monitoring of parenteral fluid administration.

References

Anderson, GC, Marks, EA, and Wahlberg, V: Kangaroo care for premature infants, Am J Nurs 86(7):807, 1986

Bartlett, RH, et al: Extracorporeal circulation in neonatal respiratory failure: a prospective randomized study, Pediatrics 76:479, 1985

Bernbaum, JC, et al: Non-nutritive sucking during gavage feeding enhances growth and maturation in premature infants, Pediatrics 71:41, 1983

Cole, JG: The competent preemie: a guide for parents, Project WELCOME, Children's Hospital, Wheelock College, 200 the Riverway, Boston, MA 02215 (no date given)

Fanaroff, AA, and Martin, RJ, editors: Neonatal-perinatal medicine: diseases of the fetus and infant, ed 4. St Louis, 1987, The CV Mosby Co

Kaplan, M, and Eidelman, AT: Improved prognosis in severely hypothermic newborn infants treated by rapid rewarming, J Pediatr 105:468, 1984

Merenstein, GB, and Gardner, SL: Handbook of neonatal intensive care, St Louis, 1985, The CV Mosby Co

Ress, PE: Saving underweight babies in Bogota, Secretariat News 39(13):7, 1984 (United Nations Headquarters, New York)

Whitelaw, A, and Sleath, K: Myth of the marsupial mother: home care of very low birth weight babies in Bogota, Colomia, Lancet 1(8439):1206-1208, 1985

Bibliography

Aberman, S, and Kirchoff, KT: Infant-feeding practices: mothers' decision making, JOGN Nurs 14:394, Sept/Oct 1985

Anand, KJ, and Hickey, PR: Pain and its effects in the human neonate and fetus, N Engl J Med 317(21):1321, 1987

Avery, P, and Olson, IM: Expanding the scope of childbirth education to meet the needs of hospitalized, high-risk clients, JOGN Nurs 16(6):418, 1987

Blackburn, S, and Lowen, L: Impact of an infant's premature birth on the grandparents and parents, JOGN Nurs 15(2):173, 1986

Bobak, IM, and Jensen, MD: A modular study guide to maternity care, St Louis, 1983, The CV Mosby Co

Bowen, PA: Regional centers. I. A comparison of nursing responsibilities in level II and level III centers, Issues Health Care Women 2(5-6):1, 1980

Bowen, PA: Regional centers. II. The newborn transport system, Issues Health Care Women 2(5-6):5, 1980

Bowen, PA: Regional centers. III. Three regions' educational efforts and infant mortality rates, Issues Health Care Women 2(5-6):19, 1980

Boynton, BR, and Boynton, CA: Discharge planning for high-risk infants, J Perinatol 5:44, Fall 1985

Bracero, LA, Schulman, H, and Baxi, LV: Fetal heart rate characteristics that provide confidence in the diagnosis of fetal well-being, Clin Obstet Gynecol, 19:3, March 1986

Brooten, D: RN follow-up plan helps high-risk infants, Am Nurse Feb, 1988

Budreau, G, and Kleiber, C: Nursing management of the infant with an intraoral appliance, JOGN Nurs 16(1):23, 1987
Carey, J, Seamonds, JA, and Galligan, M: Infant-death rate: rise linked to health-care cuts, US News & World Report, Feb 24, p 67, 1986
Censullo, M: Home care of the high-risk newborn, JOGN Nurs 15:146, March/April 1986
Consolvo, CA: Relieving parental anxiety in the care-by-parent unit, JOGN Nurs 15:154, March/April 1986
Douvas, SG, et al: Intrapartum fetal heart rate monitoring as a predictor of fetal distress and immediate neonatal condition in low-birth-weight (under 1,800 grams) infants, Am J Obstet Gynecol 148:300, 1984
Elliot, JP, et al: helicopter transportation of patients with obstetric emergencies in an urban area, Am J Obstet Gynecol 143(2):157, 1982
Elsea, SF: Ethics in maternal-child nursing, MCN 10:303, Sept/Oct 1985
Franck, LS: A national survey of the assessment and treatment of pain and agitation in the neonatal intensive care unit, JOGN Nurs 16(6):384, 1987
Freitas, CA, Helmer, FT, and Cousins, N: The development and management uses of a patient classification system for a high-risk perinatal center, JOGN Nurs 16(5):330, 1987
Gennaro, S: Anxiety and problem-solving ability in mothers of premature infants, JOGN Nurs 15:160, March/April 1986
Glass, SM, and Giacoia, GP: Intravenous drug therapy in premature infants: practical aspects, JOGN Nurs 16(5):310, 1987
Grabauskas, P, et al: Helping the parents after a baby's death, RN, p 31, Aug, 1987
Gunzenhauser, N, editor: Infant stimulation: for whom, what kind, when, and how much? Pediatric Round Table #13. Johnson & Johnson, Baby Products Co, PO Box 836, Somerville, NJ 08876
Harrison, LL, and Twardosz, S: Teaching mothers about their preterm infants, JOGN Nurs 15:165, March/April 1986
Have ecmo, will travel: Am J Nurs 86:117, 1986
Jenkins, RL, and Tock, MK: Helping parents bond to their premature infant, MCN 11:32, Jan/Feb 1986
Johnson, SH: Nursing assessment and strategies for the family at risk: high-risk parenting, ed 2, Philadelphia, 1986, JB Lippincott Co
Kaplow, R, and Fromme, LR: Nursing care plan for the patient receiving high-frequency jet ventilation, Crit Care Nurs 5:25, 1985
Karp, TB, et al: High frequency jet ventilation: a neonatal nursing perspective, Neonatal Network, p 42, April 1986
Keating, SB, and Kelman, GB: Home health care nursing: concepts and practice, Philadelphia, 1988, JB Lippincott Co
Kemp, V, and Page, C: Maternal prenatal attachment in normal and high-risk pregnancies, JOGN Nurs 16(3):179, 1987
Kirkpatrick, BV, et al: Use of extracorporeal membrane oxygenation for respiratory failure in term infants, Pediatrics 72:872, 1983
Korones, SB: High-risk newborn infants: the basis for intensive nursing care, ed 4, St Louis, 1986, The CV Mosby Co
Kunnel, MT, et al: Comparisons of rectal, femoral, axillary, and skin-to-mattress temperature in stable neonates, Nurs Research 37(3):162, 1988
Lagerlof, JM: Nurses and ethics, Calif Nurs Rev 9(5):12, 1987
Long, S, and Henretig, F: Assessment of fever in the neonate, Pediatr Consult 6(1):2, 1987
Lucey, JF, and Dangman, B: A reexamination of the role of oxygen in retrolental fibroplasia, Pediatrics 73:82, 1984
Mammel, MD, et al: Comparison of high-frequency jet ventilation and conventional mechanical ventilation in a meconium aspiration model, J Pediatr 103:630, 1983
Meis, P, Ernest, JM, and Morre, M: Causes of low birth weight in public and private patients, Am J Obstet Gynecol 156(5):1165, 1987
Mina, CF: A program for helping grieving parents, MCN 10(2):118, 1985
Moen, JE, et al: Axillary versus rectal temperatures in preterm infants under radiant warmers, JOGN Nurs 16(5):348, 1987
NAACOG: Ethical decision making in OGN nursing practice, OGN Nurs Pract Res, R26, Oct 1987 The Association. (The Nurses Association of the American College of Obstetricians and Gynecologists, 409 Twelfth Street, SW, Washington, DC, 20024-2191, 202/638-0026)
NAACOG—OGN Nursing Resource: maternal neonatal transport, Washington, DC, 1983, The Association. (The Nurses Association of the American College of Obstetricians and Gynecologists, 409 Twelfth Street, SW, Washington, DC, 20024-2191 202/638-0026)
Pernoll, ML, et al: Diagnosis and management of the fetus and neonate at risk: a guide for team care, ed 5, St Louis, 1986, The CV Mosby Co
Philip, A: Neonatology: a practical guide, ed 3, Philadelphia, 1987, WB Saunders Co
Pridham, K, Chang, A, and Hansen, M: Mothers' problem-solving skill and use of help with infant-related issues: the role of importance and need for action, Res Nurs Health 10(4):263, 1987
Quimette, J: Perinatal nursing: care of the high-risk mother and infant, Boston, 1986, Jones & Bartlett Publishers, Inc
Raff, BS: Nursing care of high-risk infants and their families: introduction, JOGN Nurs 15:141. March/April 1986
Raff, BS: The use of homemaker-home health aides' perinatal care of high-risk infants, JOGN Nurs 15:142, March/April 1986
Ream, S, et al: Infant nutrition and supplements, JOGN Nurs 14:371, Sept/Oct 1985
Sadler, ME: When your patient's baby dies before birth, RN, p 28, Aug, 1987
Sahler, OJ, editor: The child and death. St Louis, 1978, The CV Mosby Co
Sims-Jones, N: Back to the theories: another way to view mothers of prematures, MCN 11(6):394, 1986
Stevenson, DK, Frankel, LR, and Benitz, WE: Immediate management of the asphyxiated infant: facilitating the cardiorespiratory transition from fetus to newborn, J Perinatol 7(3):221, 1987
Styer, GW, and Freeh, K: Feeding infants with cleft lip and/or palate, JOGN Nurs 10:329, 1981
The teflon intravenous catheter: incidence of phlebitis and duration of catheter life in the neonatal patient, JOGN Nurs 17(1):35 1988
Weibley, TT, Adamson, M, and Clinkscales, N: Gavage tube insertion in the premature infant, MCN 12(1):24, 1987
Whaley, LF, and Wong, DL: Nursing care of infants and children, ed 3, St Louis, 1987, The CV Mosby Co
Young, LY, Creighton, DE, and Suave, RS: The needs of families of infants discharged home with continuous oxygen therapy, JOGN Nurs 17(3):187, 1988

CHAPTER

37

Gestational Age and Birthweight

Sharon Eaton

Learning Objectives

Correctly define the key terms listed.

Describe preterm, term, postterm, and postmature newborn infants.

Assess newborn infants according to gestational age and weight.

Rate newborn infants according to the physical maturity scale and the neuromuscular maturity scale.

Explain respiratory distress syndrome (RDS) and treatment measures.

Review prematurity and oxygen therapy.

Discuss retinopathy of prematurity (ROP), bronchopulmonary dysplasia (BPD), and predisposition of premature newborns to these problems.

List the signs and symptoms of perinatal asphyxia.

Describe meconium aspiration syndrome.

Examine nursing care of parents of infants at risk because of gestational age and birth weight.

Key Terms

appropriate for gestational age (AGA)
bronchopulmonary dysplasia (BPD)
corrected age
hypoglycemia
infant stimulation
large for gestational age (LGA)
meconium aspiration syndrome
necrotizing enterocolitis (NEC)
neuromuscular maturity
newborn maturity rating and classification
nonnutritive sucking
perinatal asphyxia
physical maturity
prolonged pregnancy
postmature
postterm
premature
preterm
respiratory distress syndrome (RDS)
retinopathy of prematurity (ROP)
small for gestational age (SGA)
term

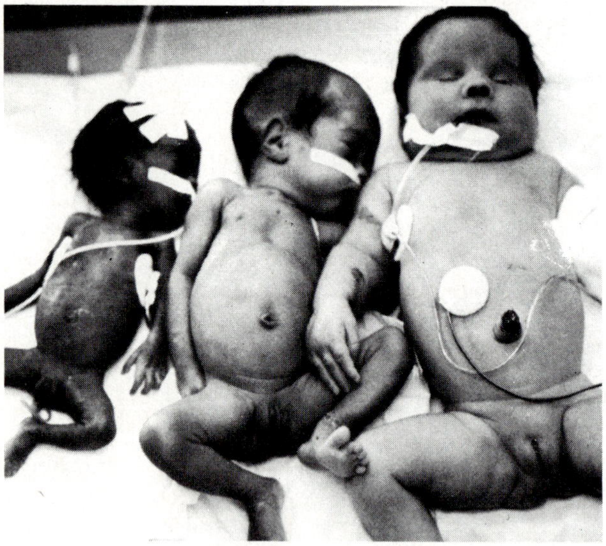

Fig. 37-1 Three babies of same gestational age, with weights of 600, 1400, and 2750 g, respectively, from left to right. Their weights are plotted in Fig. 37-2 at points *A, B,* and *C.*

From Korones, SB: High-risk newborn infants; the basis for intensive nursing care, ed 4, St Louis, 1986, The CV Mosby Co.

Infants born at risk for gestational age and weight problems exhibit physiologic and pathologic states related to the degree of maturity. Modern technology has contributed to the improved survival rate and overall health of preterm infants, but problems remain. These relate to the appearance of "new" diseases such as necrotizing enterocolitis (NEC) and the survival of infants born so small that their expectancy of a "quality life" is questionable. The plan of care for the infant born prematurely must include an understanding of infant behavior. Nursing care emphasizes the need for parental support to give the infant her or his best chance for a healthy, happy life.

Classification of infants according to **gestational age** is as follows:

1. Preterm or premature: infants born before completion of 37 weeks' gestation regardless of birth weight.
2. Term: infants born between the beginning of the thirty-eighth week and the end of the forty-second week of gestation.
3. Postterm: infants born after completion of the forty-second week of gestation.
4. Postmature: infants born after completion of the forty-second week of gestation and who have experienced progressive placental insufficiency.

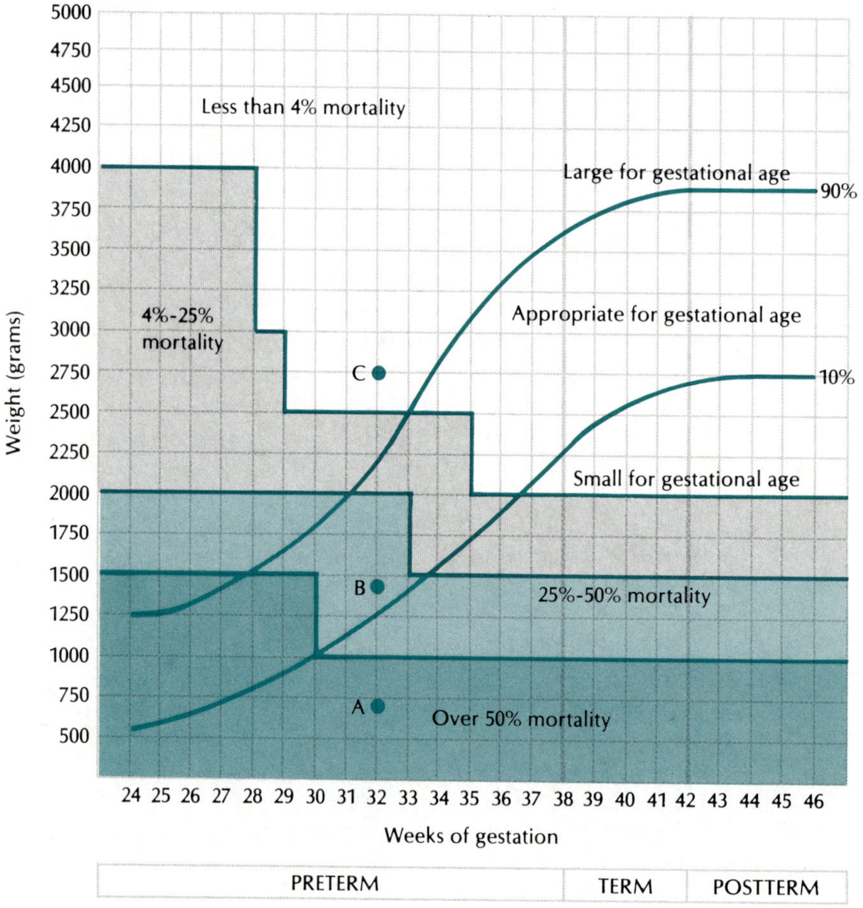

Fig. 37-2 Intrauterine growth status for gestational age and according to appropriateness of growth. Weights of infants shown in Fig. 37-1 are plotted at points *A, B,* and *C.*

Courtesy Mead Johnson & Co, Evansville, Indiana. Modified from Battaglia, FC, and Lubchenco, LO: J Pediatr 71:59, 1967.

The weight of the infant has a normal range for each gestational week (Figs. 37-1 and 37-2). Variations in weight may occur in the preterm, term, postterm or postmature infant. **Classification** of infants by **weight** is as follows:

1. Large for gestational age (LGA): the infant is said to be *large for gestational age* or *large for dates* if at any week the weight is above the 90th percentile (or two or more standard deviations above the norm).
2. Appropriate for gestational age (AGA). The infant is termed *appropriate for gestational age* if the weight falls between the 10th and 90th percentile for her or his age.
3. Small for gestational age (SGA). A baby is *small for gestational age* if the weight is below the 10th percentile (or two or more standard deviations below the norm).

Common causes of LGA newborns include glucose intolerance of pregnancy, true maternal diabetes mellitus, maternal overnutrition, and heredity. SGA newborns may be the result of maternal smoking, hypertensive states, undernutrition, anemia, or nephritis. In addition, the birth of an SGA newborn may be associated with multiple gestation, a discordant twin pregnancy, or congenital anomalies. High altitude, rubella, or intrauterine infection may predispose a woman to the birth of an SGA infant. Fetal malnutrition, intrauterine growth retardation (IUGR), and chronic fetal distress are other processes that may result in the birth of babies who are SGA.

INFANT MORTALITY AND MORBIDITY

Premature birth is responsible for almost two-thirds of infant deaths. The infant born prematurely does not possess the growth and development necessary for uncomplicated adjustment to extrauterine life, and prospects for survival or good health may be severely compromised. Infants weighing more than 2500 g (5½ lb) and delivered after 37 weeks of pregnancy have the best prospects of survival. There is a dramatic reduction in mortality in infants, regardless of weight, who are delivered after the thirty-sixth week of gestation. The prognosis for low-birth-weight infants weighing more than 1800 g (4 lb) is more favorable than for those weighing 1500 to 1800 g (3 to 4 lb). The mortality is less than 5% if the pregnancy has progressed to 35 weeks and the fetus weighs more than 2000 g (4½ lb).

PRETERM INFANT

The preterm infant is at risk because of immaturity of organ systems and lack of reserves. The morbidity and mortality occurring with preterm infants are higher by three to four times than those of older infants of comparable weight (Figs. 37-3 and 37-4). The potential problems and care needs of the preterm infant of 2000 g differ from those of the term, postterm, or postmature infant of equal weight (Philip, 1987).

Preterm infants are at a distinct disadvantage when they face the transition from intrauterine to extrauterine life. *The degree of disadvantage depends primarily on their level of maturity.* Physiologic disorders and anomalous malformations affect their response to treatment as well. In general, the closer they are to the normal term infant in gestational age and weight, the easier will be their adjustment to the external environment.

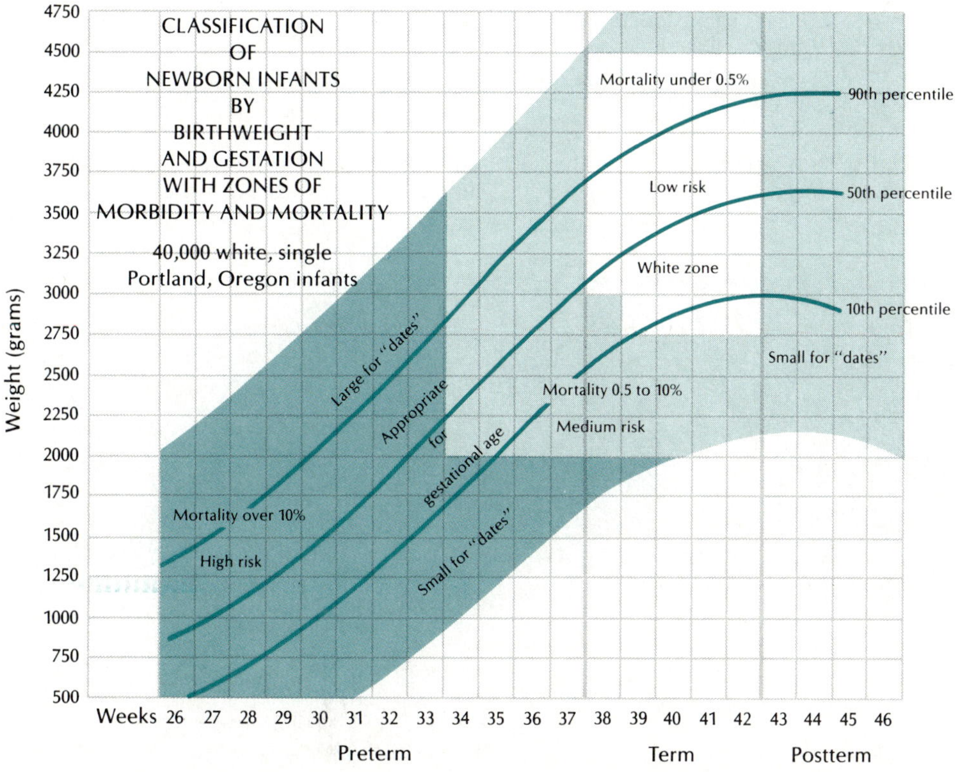

Fig. 37-3 Zones of mortality and morbidity in relation to both weight and gestation.
Modified from Behrman, RE, and Babson, SG: Am J Dis Child 121:486, 1971. Copyright 1971, American Medical Association.

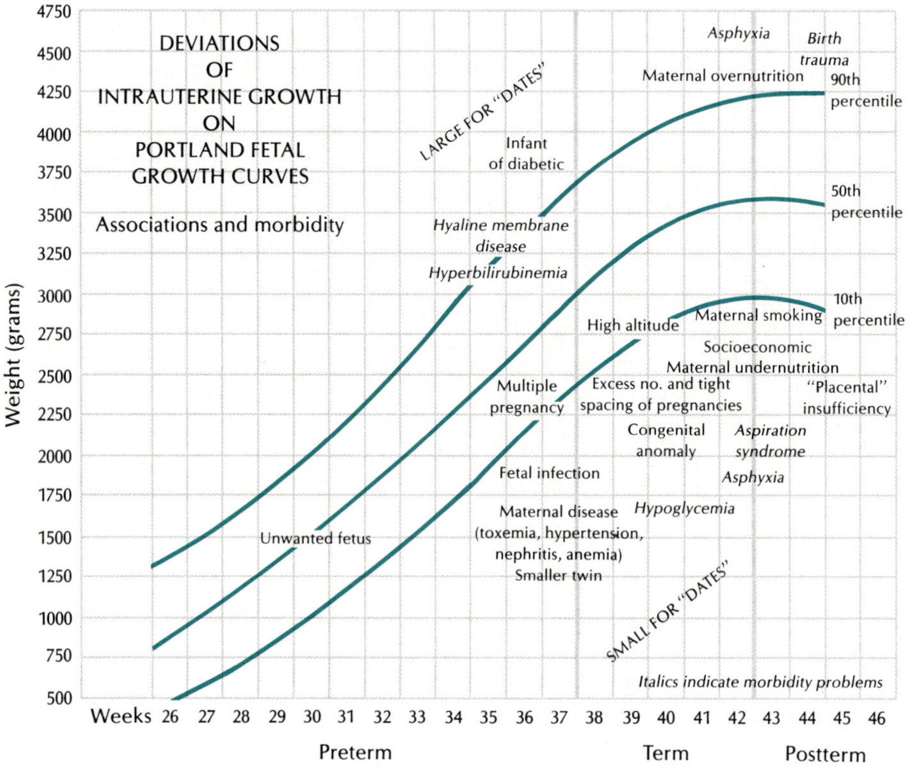

Fig. 37-4 Important associations and morbidity factors of accelerated or reduced fetal growth above 90th percentile and below 10th percentile for gestational age using Portland curves. Fetal growth data obtained from 40,000 single, white, middle-class infants born at sea level.

Modified from Babson, SG, et al: Diagnosis and management of the fetus and neonate at risk, ed 4, St Louis, 1980, The CV Mosby Co.

Assessment

Gestational Age

Physical examination procedures to determine gestational age are based on the procedure devised by Dubowitz and associates (1970). Ideally the tests are performed between 2 and 8 hours of age. For the first hour the infant is recovering from the stress of birth, and this is reflected in muscle movements; for example, the arm recoil is slower in a fatigued infant. After 48 hours some responses change significantly. The plantar creases on the soles of the feet appear to increase in number and become visible as the skin loses fluid and dries. See Figs. 37-5 to 37-9 and Tables 37-1 and 37-2 for the clinical estimation of gestational age. Fig. 37-10 is an example of the recording of the gestational age estimation.

Potential Problems of Preterm Newborn

An accurate assessment of gestational age is a good indicator of the problems a premature newborn is likely to experience (Philip, 1987). The clinical problems occurring

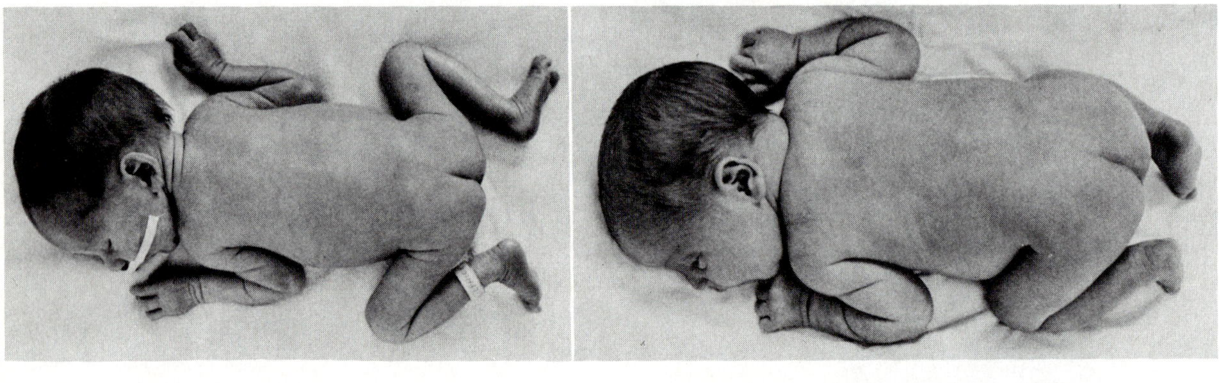

Fig. 37-5 **A**, In prone position, premature infant lies with pelvis flat and legs splayed like a frog's. **B**, Normal full-term infant lies with his limbs flexed, pelvis raised, and knees usually drawn under abdomen.

Courtesy Mead Johnson & Co, Evansville, Indiana.

A

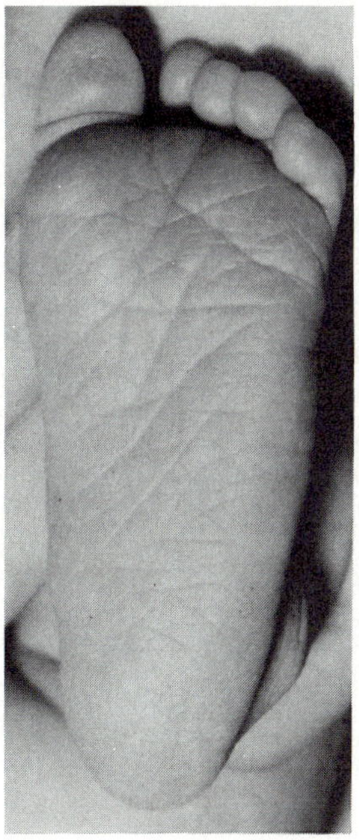

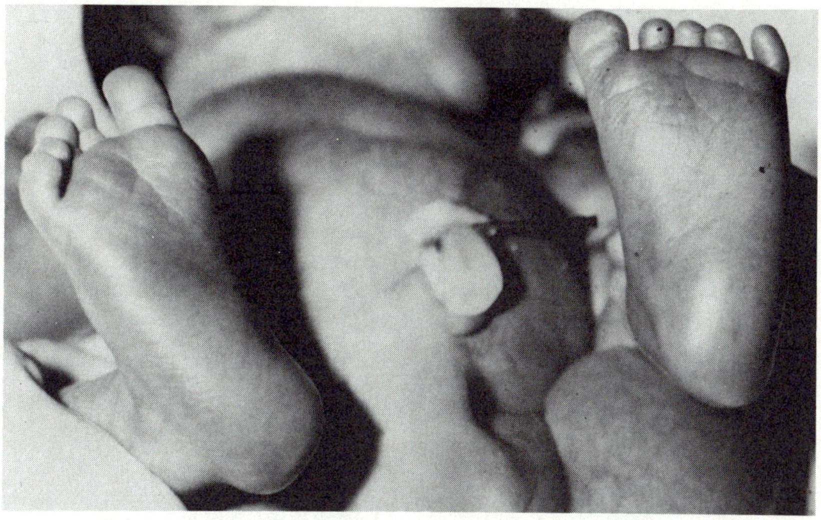

B

Fig. 37-6 A, Normal sole creases of full-term newborn. B, Sole of foot of premature infant. As infant loses interstitial fluid after birth, creases become apparent even in preterm infants. Therefore assessment needs to be done in first 2 hours after birth.

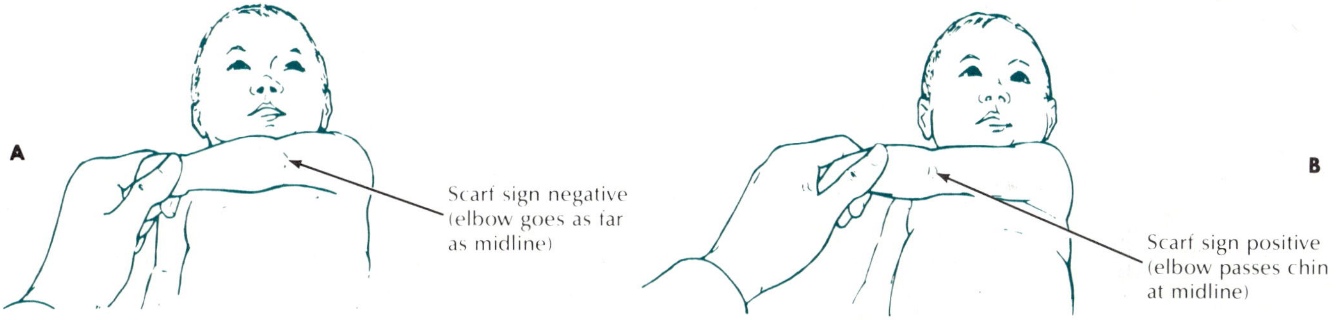

Fig. 37-7 Assessment of gestational age in term newborn, A, and preterm newborn, B.

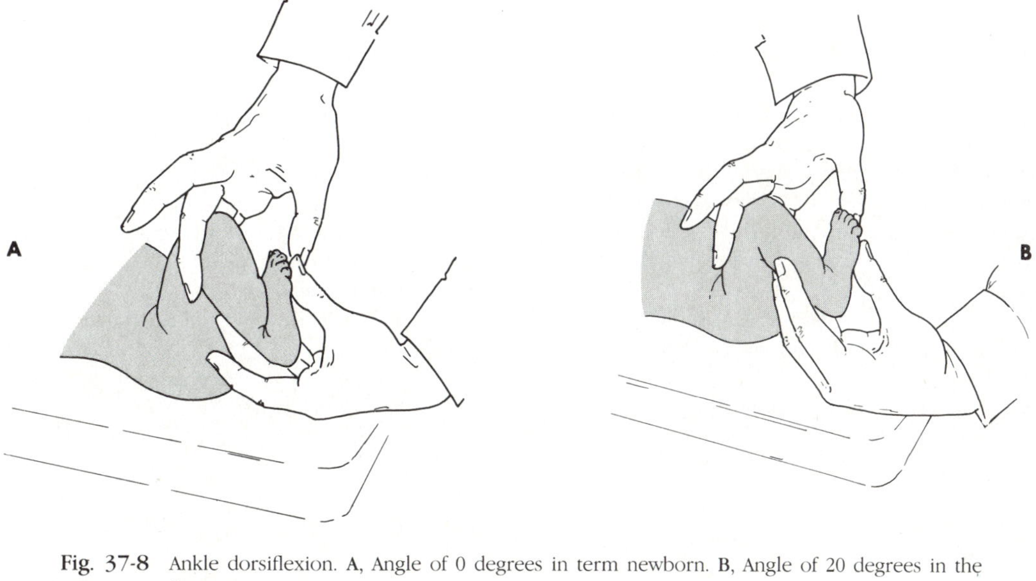

Fig. 37-8 Ankle dorsiflexion. A, Angle of 0 degrees in term newborn. B, Angle of 20 degrees in the preterm newborn.

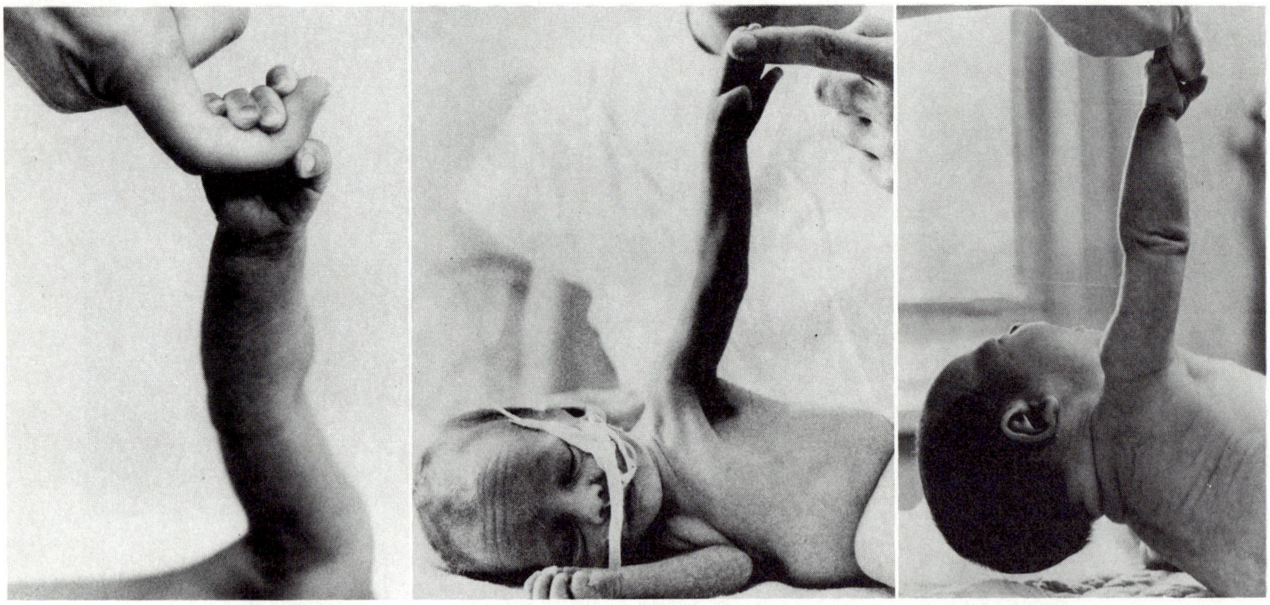

Fig. 37-9 **A**, Primitive grasp reflex present in all normal newborns usually weakens and disappears after 3 months. When palm is stimulated by finger, infant will grasp it. Full-term infant reinforces grip as finger is drawn upward. Dorsum of hand should not be touched, since this excites opposite reflex, and hand opens. **B**, Grasp reflex present in premature infant is distinct from that noted in term infant. Grip can be obtained and arm drawn upward, but when traction is applied, grip opens and there is much less muscle tension. **C**, Once grasp is obtained in term infant, grip is reinforced when the arm is drawn upward. There is progressive tensing of muscles until baby hangs momentarily.
B and **C** Courtesy Mead Johnson & Co, Evansville, Indiana.

in the preterm infant and their physiologic bases are summarized in Table 37-3.

Growth and Development Potential

Although it is impossible to predict with complete accuracy the growth and development potential of each premature newborn, some findings support an anticipated favorable outcome (Bennett, Robinson, and Sells, 1983). The growth and development landmarks are corrected for gestational age.

The age of a preterm newborn is corrected by adding the gestational age and the postdelivery age. For example, if an infant was born at 32 weeks' gestation 4 weeks ago, the infant would be considered 36 weeks of age. The child's **corrected age** 6 months after the birth date, is 4 months. Responses are evaluated against the norm expected for a 4-month-old infant.

Favorable findings that support the prediction of a growth and development pattern within the norm include the following:

1. At discharge from the hospital, which usually occurs between 37 and 40 weeks after the woman's last menstrual period (LMP), the infant exhibits the following characteristics:
   a. Is able to raise the head when prone and is able to hold the head parallel with the body when tested for head lag response. (When the infant is pulled up by the hands, the infant's head lags, but then the head and chest will be in line as the upright position is reached. This alignment will be held momentarily before the head falls forward [pull-to-sit or traction reflex]).
   b. Cries with vigor when hungry.
   c. Shows appropriate weight gain and pattern of weight gain according to growth grid.
   d. Has neurologic responses appropriate for corrected age. The retinas appear normal.
2. At 39 to 40 weeks the infant is able to focus on the examiner's or parent's face and is able to follow with her or his eyes.

At the corrected ages of 6 and 12 months the infant is assessed again for age-appropriate responses. The infant may have continued problems if she or he displays any of the following behaviors:

a. Was and continues to be a poor eater
b. Is irritable
c. Displays sensory, perceptual, intellectual, or motor deviations in development
d. Displays or develops hypertonia or hypotonia

These behaviors must be interpreted with caution and the infant reevaluated by an interdisciplinary team at frequent intervals. Parents will need continued support and attention should these signs appear. Minor behavioral de-

Text continued on p. 942.

Table 37-1 *Elaboration of Physical Maturity Scales*

Criterion	Findings and Assigned Scores					Infant Score*
	0	1	2	3	4	
Skin						____
Edema	Edema evident over hands and feet; pitting seen over tibia	Pitting edema over tibia	No edema obvious	—	—	
Texture and opacity	Gelatinous, transparent; veins seen especially over abdomen	Visible, veins; thin, smooth	Few larger veins seen, especially over abdomen; medium-thick smooth skin	Veins rarely seen; some thickening superficial cracking	No vessels; parchmentlike, thick, cracking; if leathery, very cracked, and wrinkled, give score of 5	
Color	Dark red (infant is quiet for evaluation)	Pink	Pale pink	Pale; pink mainly over palms, soles, lips, and ears		
Lanugo	None	Abundant over body; long; thick	Thinning, especially over lumbosacral area	Bald areas; thinning over other areas	Mostly bald of lanugo; at least half of back bald	____
Plantar creases	No creases seen	Faint red marks on upper half of sole	Red marks obvious over more than upper half; deeper lines over less than one third	Indentations noticeable over more than one third; lines seen over two thirds	Creases cover entire sole (Fig. 37-6)	____
Breast	Nipple barely perceptible; no palpable breast tissue	Flat, smooth areola present around well-defined nipple; some breast tissue	Stippled areola but edge flat; 1-2 mm breast bud	Stippled areola with edges raised; 3-4 mm breast bud	Full areola; 5–10 mm breast bud; may have breast milk	____
Ear Form Cartilage	Pinna flat, soft, easily folded	Slight incurving of pinna; soft, easily folded; slow recoil	Well-incurved pinna; soft; ready recoil	Upper pinna well curved; formed and firm to edge; instant recoil	Thick cartilage; ear stiff	____
Genitals						____
Male	No testes in scrotum and no rugae over scrotum	—	Testes descending; few rugations	Testes within scrotum good rugae	Scrotum pendulous with rugae covering scrotum	
Female	Prominent clitoris and labia minora; labia majora do not cover labia minora	—	Labia majora and labia minora equally prominent	Labia majora appear large; labia minora, small	Labia majora completely cover clitoris and labia minora	
					TOTAL	____

*Highest score possible = 25

Table 37-2 *Elaboration of Neuromuscular Maturity Scales**

Criterion	Method of Assessment	0
Posture (Fig. 37-5)	Position: supine Activity: quiet Assessment: extension and flexion of arms, hips, legs	Complete extension 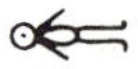
Square swindow (wrist)†	Position: supine Method: with thumb supporting back of arm below wrist, apply gentle pressure with index and third fingers on dorsum of hand; do not rotate infant's wrist Assessment: angle formed between hypothenar eminence and forearm	Very prematue (<30 weeks) 90° 
Arm recoil‡	Position; supine Method; flex forearms on upper arms for 5 sec; pull on hands to full extension and release Assessment: degree of flexion	No recoil; arms remain extended  180°
Popliteal angle	Position: supine; pelvis on flat, firm surface Method: flex leg on thigh; then flex thigh on abdomen; holding knee with thumb and index finger, extend leg with index finger of other hand behind ankle Assessment: degree of angle behind knee	Complete extension; very premature  180°
Scarf sign (Fig. 37-7)	Position: supine Method: support head in midline with one hand; pull hand to opposite shoulder Assessment: position of elbow in relation to midline	Elbow to opposite arm like scarf around neck 
Heel to ear	Position: supine, pelvis is kept flat on surface Method: pull foot up toward ear on same side; do not hold knee Assessment: distance of foot from ear and degree of extension of knee	Toes touch ear; leg completely extended (180°) 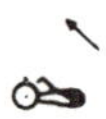

*Compare combined scores for physical and neuromuscular maturity to the "maturity rating" scores and read estimated weeks of gestational age. Estimate of gestational age obtained is accurate only to plus or minus 2 weeks. After gestational age is estimated, infant's length, weight, and head circumference are entered on appropriate graphs. All three measurements should fall within same approximate range, for example, all within SGA, LGA, or AGA. If one measurement is excessively large (falling into LGA range) and other two fall into SGA range, growth deviation should be assessed. **X**, First examination; **O**, second examination.

†Counterpart: ankle dorsiflexion (see Fig. 37-8).

‡Counterpart: leg recoil.

Table 37-2 *Elaboration of Neuromuscular Maturity Scales—cont'd*

Finding and Assigned Scores					Infant Score	
1	2	3	4	5	X	0
Extension of arms; slight flexion of hips, legs 	Extension of arms 	Slight flexion of arms; full flexion of legs 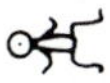	Complete flexion 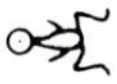	—	________	________
Premature (30-35 weeks) 60° 	Premature (30-35 weeks) 45° 	Maturing (35-38 weeks) 30° 	Term: hand lies flat on ventral surface of forearm 0°	—	________	________
—	Some recoil; sluggish response 100°-180° 	Maturing (35-38 weeks) 90°-100° 	Brisk recoil to complete flexion >90° 	—	________	________
Prematue (30-35 weeks) 160° 	Premature (30-35 weeks) 130° 	Maturing (35-38 weeks) 110° 	Maturing (35-38 weeks) 90° 	Extension is resisted >90° 	________	________
Elbow beyond midline of thorax 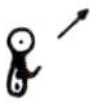	Elbow just beyond midline 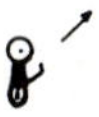	Elbow at midline 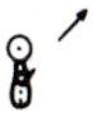	Elbow does not reach midline 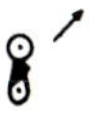	—	________	________
Toes almost reach face (130°) 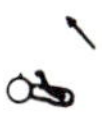	Knees flexed (110°) 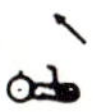	Knees flexed (90°) 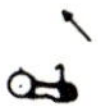	Knees flexed politeal angle is less than 90° 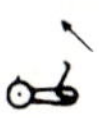	—	________	________
				NEUROMUSCULAR MATURITY TOTALS	________	________
				PHYSICAL MATURITY TOTALS (see Table 37-1)	________	________
				COMBINED SCORE	________	________

See Fig. 37-10 for Maturity Rating.

NEWBORN MATURITY RATING and CLASSIFICATION

ESTIMATION OF GESTATIONAL AGE BY MATURITY RATING

Symbols: X - 1st Exam O - 2nd Exam

NEUROMUSCULAR MATURITY

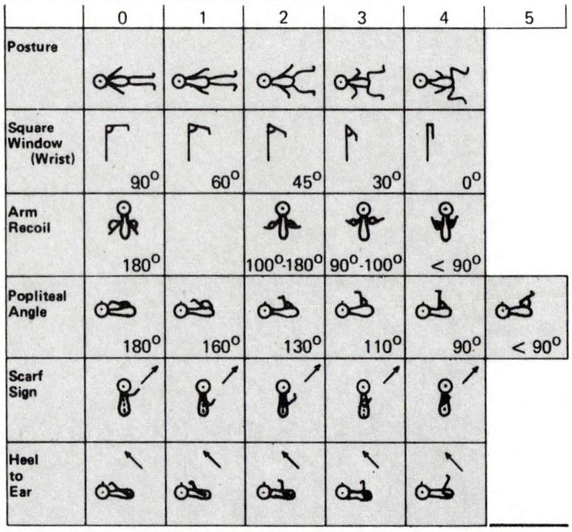

	0	1	2	3	4	5
Posture						
Square Window (Wrist)	90°	60°	45°	30°	0°	
Arm Recoil	180°		100°-180°	90°-100°	< 90°	
Popliteal Angle	180°	160°	130°	110°	90°	< 90°
Scarf Sign						
Heel to Ear						

PHYSICAL MATURITY

	0	1	2	3	4	5
SKIN	gelatinous red, trans-parent	smooth pink, visible veins	superficial peeling &/or rash, few veins	cracking pale area, rare veins	parchment, deep cracking, no vessels	leathery, cracked, wrinkled
LANUGO	none	abundant	thinning	bald areas	mostly bald	
PLANTAR CREASES	no crease	faint red marks	anterior transverse crease only	creases ant. 2/3	creases cover entire sole	
BREAST	barely percept.	flat areola, no bud	stippled areola, 1–2 mm bud	raised areola, 3–4 mm bud	full areola, 5–10 mm bud	
EAR	pinna flat, stays folded	sl. curved pinna, soft with slow recoil	well-curv. pinna, soft but ready recoil	formed & firm with instant recoil	thick cartilage, ear stiff	
GENITALS Male	scrotum empty, no rugae		testes descend-ing, few rugae	testes down, good rugae	testes pendulous, deep rugae	
GENITALS Female	prominent clitoris & labia minora		majora & minora equally prominent	majora large, minora small	clitoris & minora completely covered	

Score is obtained by adding totals from Tables 37-1 and 37-2.

Gestation by Dates __________ wks

Birth Date ________ Hour ________ am pm

APGAR ________ 1 min ________ 5 min

MATURITY RATING

Score	Wks
5	26
10	28
15	30
20	32
25	34
30	36
35	38
40	40
45	42
50	44

SCORING SECTION

	1st Exam=X	2nd Exam=O
Estimating Gest Age by Maturity Rating	______ Weeks	______ Weeks
Time of Exam	Date ______ Hour ______ am pm	Date ______ Hour ______ am pm
Age at Exam	______ Hours	______ Hours
Signature of Examiner	______ M.D.	______ M.D.

Fig. 37-10 Newborn maturity rating and classification.

Mead Johnson & Co, Evansville, Indiana. Scoring section adapted from Ballard, JL, et al: Pediatr Res 11:374, 1977. Figures modified from Sweet, AY: Classification of the low-birth-weight infant. In Klaus, MH, and Fanaroff, AA: Care of the high-risk infant, Philadelphia, 1977, WB Saunders Co.

Table 37-3 *Preterm Infant's Potential Problems and Their Physiologic Bases*

Potential Problem	Physiologic Bases
Initiating and maintaining respirations	Paucity of functional alveoli; incomplete aeration of lungs caused by deficient surfactant Smaller lumen and greater collapsibility or obstruction of respiratory passages Weakness of respiratory musculature Insufficient calcification of bony thorax Absent or weak gag reflex Immature and friable capillaries in brain and lungs Few functional alveoli in infants less than 28 weeks' gestational age (usually nonviable); marginal function in infants at 29-30 weeks
Maintaining body temperature	Large surface area in relation to body weight (mass) Absent or poor reflex control of skin capillaries (no shiver response) Small, inadequate muscle mass activity; absent or minimum flexion of extremities on body Meager insulating subcutaneous fat Friable capillaries and immature temperature regulating center in brain The smaller the infant, the more difficult it is for her or him to maintain normal body temperature
Maintaining adequate nutrition	Mechanical feeding problems • Absent or weak sucking and swallowing reflexes; unsynchronized • Absent or weak gag and cough reflexes • Small stomach capacity • Immature cardiac sphincter (stomach) • Lax abdominal musculature Absorption and assimilation problems • Paucity of stored nutrients: vitamins A and C; calcium, phosphorus, iron; loss of fat and fat-soluble vitamins in stool • Immature absorption, decreased amount of hydrochloric acid • Impaired metabolism (enzyme systems) or enzyme pathology
Maintaining central nervous system (CNS) function	Birth trauma: damage to immature structures Fragile capillaries and impaired coagulation process; prolonged prothrombin time Recurrent anoxic episodes Tendency toward hypoglycemia
Maintaining renal function	Impaired renal clearance of metabolites and drugs Inability to maintain acid-base, fluid, and electrolyte homeostasis Impaired ability to concentrate urine Paucity of stored nutrients from mother
Resisting infection	Paucity of stored immunoglobulins from mother Impaired ability to synthesize antibodies Thin skin and fragile capillaries near surface Impaired ability to muster white blood cells
Resisting hematologic problems	Increased capillary friability and permeability Low plasma prothrombin levels (increased tendency to bleed) Relatively slowed erythropoietic activity in bone marrow Relatively increased rate of hemolysis Loss of blood for laboratory specimens
Maintaining musculoskeletal integrity	Weak, underdeveloped muscles Immature skeletal system (bones, joints) Meager subcutaneous fat with its cushioning effect
Maintaining retinal integrity	Immature vascular structures in retina Need for oxygen therapy

Table 37-4 *Differences in Experiences of Term and Preterm Delivery*

Term Delivery	Preterm Delivery
The parents have gone through the full developmental process of a 40-week pregnancy.	The parents have not completed the psychological and emotional growth of a 40-week-gestation pregnancy.
The infant is healthy and has the physiologic, motor, and state control and social capacities common to full-term infants.	The infant is small, immature, often physically unattractive, and sick.
The parents have an enormous surge of emotion postpartum, which is derived from a combination of feelings of achievement and pride in their own success and fulfilled expectations about the intactness and healthiness of their infant.	The parents are often overwhelmed by feelings of failure, loss, fear, and sadness.
Full-term infants in the first 1 to 2 hours after birth have a period of alert time during which they open their eyes, look around, breast-feed, and generally behave like or exceed most parent's fantasies of a little baby.	The infant has none of the cute, appealing behaviors of a full-term infant. The infant is not alert, does not suck, and may be too sick to be held at all.

From Sammons, W, and Lewis, J: Premature babies: a different beginning, St Louis, 1985, The CV Mosby Co.

viations are diagnosed also so that the parents can be assisted in their understanding and acceptance of the child. Deviations such as clumsiness, varying degrees of incoordination, slowness in reading and writing, and similar problems may be distressing to the child, parents, and other family members.

Parental Adaptation to Preterm Infant

Parents who experience the premature birth of their infant have a totally different experience from parents giving birth to a full-term infant (Sammons and Lewis, 1985). Because of this difference, parental attachment and adaptation to the parental role will be different also. Table 37-4 summarizes the key differences in the two experiences.

Parental Tasks. Parents face a number of psychologic tasks before effective relationships and parenting patterns can evolve. These tasks include the following:

1. *Anticipatory grief over the potential loss of an infant.* The parent grieves (see Chapter 28) in preparation for the infant's possible death, although the parent clings tenuously to the hope that the child will survive. This begins during labor and lasts until the infant dies or shows evidence of surviving.
2. *Acceptance by the mother of her failure to deliver a healthy, full-term infant.* Grief and depression typify this phase, which persists until the infant is out of danger and is expected to survive.
3. *Resumption of the process of relating to the infant.* As the baby begins to improve—gains weight, feeds by nipple, and is weaned from the incubator—the parent can begin the process of developing attachment to the infant that was interrupted by the infant's precarious condition at birth (Als and Brazelton, 1981; Goldberg, 1979).
4. *Learning how this baby differs in special needs and growth patterns.* Another parental task is to learn, understand, and accept this infant's caregiving needs and growth and development expectations (Sammons and Lewis, 1985).
5. *Adjusting the home environment to the needs of the new infant.* Grandparents and brothers and sisters also react to the birth of the preterm infant. Parents must reconcile the grief of grandparents and the bewilderment and anger of brothers and sisters at the disproportionate amount of parental time absorbed by the newborn.

Parental Responses. Two different approaches noted by Newman (1980) are *coping through commitment* and *coping through distance.* With the first approach parents take each day as it comes, recognizing and accepting the lessened responses of their infant and noting the gradual progress in their child's condition. With the second approach the parents pull away from emotional attachment to the infant; they postpone becoming attached until the infant is in better health.

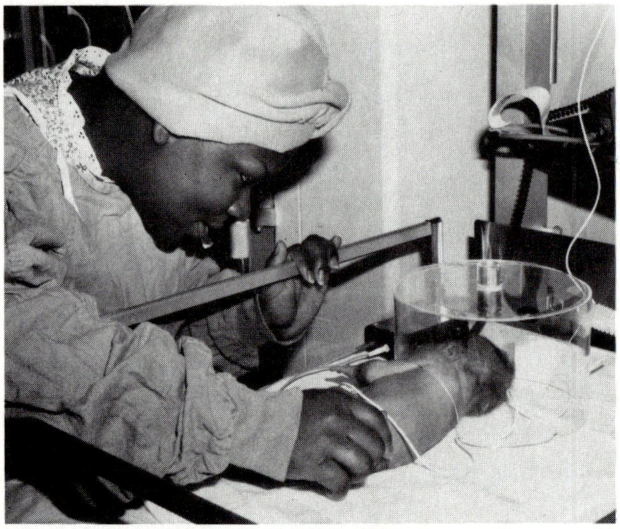

Fig. 37-11 Mother interacting with her baby using touch. Oxygen hood and overhead warmer are being used in place of incubator.

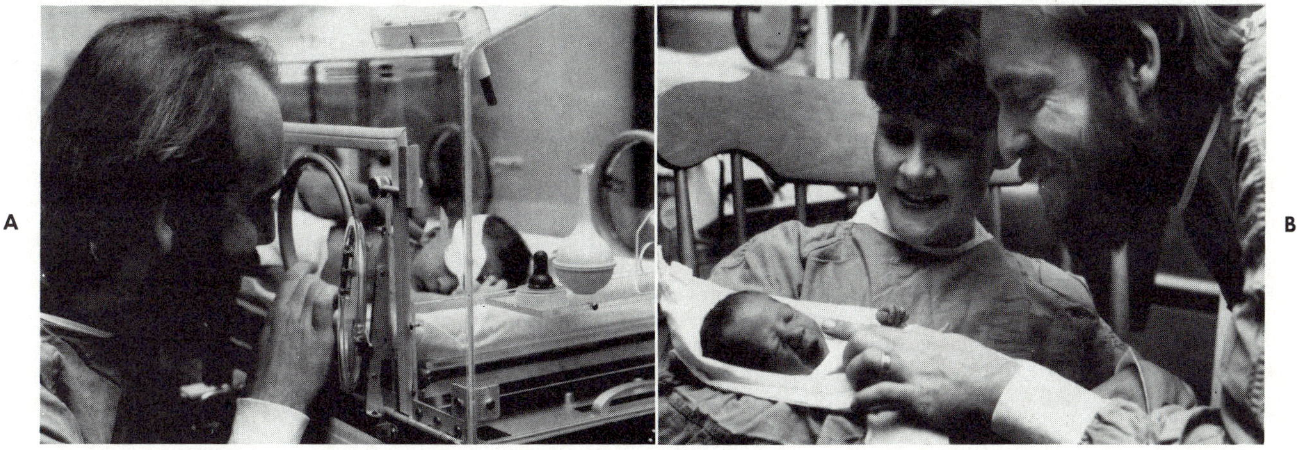

Fig. 37-12 Father interacts with his baby. **A**, Stroking baby's back. **B**, Touching baby with fingertip.

Parents have been observed to progress through stages as they spend more time with their infants. In the first stage they maintain an *en face* position, stroking and touching their infant (Figs. 37-11 and 37-12). In the second stage they assume some child care activities—feeding, bathing, changing the infant. In the third stage the infant becomes a person and is seen as a whole child (Schraeder, 1980). Sosa and Grua (1982) reported a personal communication with Brazelton in which he correlated parental behaviors with the previously noted three stages. In the first stage parents ask about *chemical data,* such as "What is his bilirubin today?" In the second stage they note their baby yawning, sneezing, hiccoughing, *reflexes* that mark their infant as human. At this time the infant is still not "claimed." In later stages they note their infant's *responses* to them and begin to feel that "this child is mine" and part of our family. Parents take on the role of advocate for their child.

Infant Responsiveness. The preterm infant's states of consciousness are more labile than the term infant's. The quiet alert state is less evident and unpredictable. Field (1979) noted that if a mother concentrated her interactions on imitation of the infant's behavior, the infant was increasingly attentive and interested. Too-active an involvement in child care tended to result in the infant's becoming disinterested and glancing away (gaze aversion). One young mother noted that "gentle stroking of her infant's head caused him to look at her." (She also reported that even at age 7 years, gentle head stroking calmed her child.)

Parenting Disorders. The incidence of physical and emotional abuse is three times greater toward the infant who, by virtue of prematurity or illness, was separated from the mother for a period of time after birth (Fomufod, 1976). Physical abuse includes varying degrees of poor nutrition and poor hygiene. Emotional abuse ranges from subtle to outright dislike of the child. There may be preferential treatment for brothers and sisters, nagging, extremely high expectations of the child, and various other types of overt or covert negative responses by one or both parents.

Factors surrounding the birth may predispose parents to subconsciously or overtly reject the child. These factors might include parental pain and anxiety, a heavy financial burden for the infant's care, unresolved anticipatory grief, threat to self-esteem, or unwanted pregnancy. The goal of the helping professionals is to reduce the incidence of child abuse and neglect.

Growth in the Parental Role. Sammons and Lewis (1985) describe the steps in adaptation of the mother or father to the parenting role with a preterm infant. They parallel the stages in parental change with the change in medical care of the infant (Table 37-5).

Nursing Diagnoses

To formulate nursing diagnoses, the nurse must analyze data obtained from continous monitoring of the infant and from observation of and discussions with the parents. The diagnoses may be physical, cognitive, or psychological. Examples of such diagnoses are as follows:

- Ineffective breathing pattern related to
  - Inadequate chest expansion, secondary to infant's position
- Parental knowledge deficit related to
  - Feeding the infant
- Situational low self-esteem related to
  - Mother's feelings of inadequacy in caring for the infant

Planning

The physiologic problems of immature body systems govern the plan of care of these infants. The infant is faced with many emergency treatments and procedures. Nursing care during this time of crisis is a critical factor in the infant's chances for survival and in the parents' eventual relationship with their child.

Table 37-5 *Parental and Medical Milestones*

	Parental Milestones	Medical Milestones
Preterm birth of baby Preterm termination of pregnancy	Deprived of last trimester of pregnancy, a time of major adjustment during which the following are accomplished: 1. Resolution of issues of competency of parenting 2. Formulation of future hopes for the child 3. Change in couple's relationship as they approach parenthood	Hospital admission
Parents apart—different areas of hospital or different hospital Isolation Issues of fault	Reverse of caregiving role: father there first Initial time is a period of extreme disorganization 1. Loss of family and community supports 2. Long period before social interaction with baby (parents may need this) 3. Sense of distance from baby Death issue Loss of fantasy child dream	Transport Ventilator Multiple procedures Intravenous or arterial catheters
Mother discharged from hospital	Adaptation to NICU* environment 1. Initial distance—uncertain where baby is 2. Numbers and machinery 3. Parents relate to different machine: breast pump	Baby physiologically unstable
Parents together	Observers of the nurse's role with the baby Begin to understand some of what the technicalities and the numbers mean Start to use the medical jargon on the telephone Start to see other people developing a relationship with the baby Dependent on relationships with nurse and physician	Getting better Nasogastric feedings Temperature instability Beginning of nursing and staff attachment to baby
Begin caregiving: adoption of the staff role	Competition with the staff Fathers start to perceive change in focus to mother-infant relationship Start to offer show of affection for the baby Signs Attachment to head "doughnut" support Toys Clothes	Baby off of major support systems Still on monitors Weight single focus of well-being
Attempts to read social cues of infant	Holding the baby; difficult to get to know the baby 1. Feeding problems 2. Caregiving but little attachment 3. Still feel like it is not "our baby" 4. Energy consumption: beginning to sense how to "help" the baby 5. Conflicting messages: "okay" but monitors just to make sure	Removal of last physical barriers Out of Isolette to bassinet
Changes in visiting patterns May visit separately	Need to form their own relationship—beginning of attachment 1. Subjective: not measureable by number of phone calls, duration of visits, etc. 2. What they want to do, not what they are told to do by staff Differentiation of mother and father roles 1. Different caregiving routines 2. Different visiting times 3. Competition over who had the "magic touch" at the last visit Reassessment of competency issues, parents' and infant's 1. Breast-feeding: continuation or failure 2. Less competition over caregiving 3. Joy at increased awake time 4. Joy at increased response to inanimate stimulation	Off monitors Feeling that the baby has made it Parallel questions of whether the parents are ready
Nesting behavior	Start forming identity of child 1. Push for discharge date, sometimes inappropriately soon before an emotional base established 2. Settle lingering medical and developmental concerns: apnea etc.; necessary for security to feel comfortable going home 3. Start to use name actively—not just she or he	Nursing detachment issues

From Sammons, W, and Lewis, J: Premature babies: a different beginning, St Louis, 1985, The CV Mosby Co.
*Neonatal intensive care unit.

Table 37-5 *Parental and Medical Milestones—cont'd*

	Parental Milestones	Medical Milestones
Start forming present role	Initial joy of predictable social response 1. Conflicting feelings of hope and risk 2. How do we form a relationship? Is it the same as for full-term infants? 3. Understanding child vs. understanding instructions, orders, and how to read behavior cues	
Grandparents and friends visit	Need to reestablish community and family supports	
Discharge	Final home preparations Often seem anxious—trying to adjust to facing new responsibilities Frequent questions	Medical discharge What to tell parents about high risk vs. recovery Is the premie normal?
Coming home: learning to live together	New sense of isolation—need to be self-sufficient Working out feeding and sleeping issues; new questions, uncertain answers Increased sense of competence of the parent-infant response system Predictability New feelings of crisis and doubt Medical visits or illnesses Grocery store at 6 months of age Overprotection, doubt about the premie Self-doubt	Visits to follow-up clinic
Answering questions about the future	Increasing sense of who the child is Independence vs. dependence issues New milestones: Smiles Laughter Talking Elicit attention Originate social games	
Feeling like the premie has made it	Personal time Another child Vacations	

Goals.

For the infant:

1. Maintain physiologic functioning
2. Maintain adequate nutrition
3. Minimize hematologic problems
4. Prevent infection
5. Prevent retinal problems
6. Prevent trauma to immature musculoskeletal system
7. Promote parent-infant attachment

For the parents:

1. Perceive the child as potentially normal (if this is medically substantiated)
2. Provide care comfortably
3. Experience pride and satisfaction in the care of the infant
4. Organize their time and energies to meet the love, attention, and care needs of the other members of the family and themselves as well

Implementation

The best environment for fetal growth and development is in the uterus of a healthy, well-nourished woman for 38 to 42 weeks. The extrauterine environment of the preterm newborn must approximate a healthy intrauterine environment for the normal sequence of growth and development to continue. The provision of such an environment is the basis for care of the preterm infant. Medical and nursing personnel and respiratory therapists work as a team to provide the intensive care needed. **The nurse acts as a constant in the infant's support system.**

Nursing actions are based on knowledge of the *physiologic problems* (Table 37-3) *imposed on the preterm infant and on the infant's need to conserve energy for repair, maintenance, and growth.* Assessment and reassessment of the infant's condition are requisites of nursing care. Nurses fulfill many roles in providing the intensive and extended care these infants require. They must interpret data, make decisions, and initiate therapy in short periods of time. Their actions as support persons and teachers are a part of the first phase of the parents' adjustment to the birth of the preterm baby.

Admission of a premature newborn to the intensive care nursery usually is an emergency situation. A rapid initial evaluation must be made to ascertain the need for lifesaving treatment. Resuscitative measures should be started in the delivery room. The newborn's need for warmth and oxygen must be ensured during transfer from the delivery room to the nursery.

Hospitals not equipped to care for high-risk infants arrange for their immediate transfer to specialized centers (see p. 909). During transport to a regional center the following are necessary to meet the infant's needs:

1. Prewarmed blankets, prewarmed incubator, or if incubator is not available, improvise: surround the infant with hot-water bottles at a distance of 5 to 10 cm from the infant's body.
2. Portable oxygen and suction apparatuses.
3. Bulb syringe or DeLee mucus-trap catheter.
4. Intravenous setup with a battery-powered infusion pump.
5. Medications as ordered by the physician.
6. Appropriate attendant or attendants.

The preterm infant is classified according to the degree of supportive care required, and the staff is assigned to the infant on that basis:

- Class A (severely compromised infant): 1 to 1 nurse to infant ratio.
- Class B (moderately compromised infant): 1 to 2 nurse to infant ratio.
- Class C (recovery and progress): 1 to 4 nurse to infant ratio.
- Class D (ready for normal newborn nursery): 1 to 8 nurse to infant ratio.

The nurse uses many modern technologic support systems to monitor body responses and maintain body function in the infant (Hansen, 1982). Gentle touch, concern for the traumatic effects of harsh lighting, and control of machinery noise are interwoven with the technical skill of the nurse in the intensive care nursery.

Physical Care

The premature infant's environmental support consists of the following:

1. Incubator control for body temperature.
2. Air or oxygen administration, depending on the infant's color and respirations.
3. Electronic monitors as needed for the observation of respiratory and cardiac functions and blood gases.

Metabolic support consists of measures such as the following:

1. Parenteral fluids to assist in supporting normal blood gas and acid-base homeostasis.
2. Parenteral fluids to facilitate antibiotic therapy if sepsis is a concern.
3. Blood specimen analyses to monitor blood gases, pH, hypoglycemia, and sepsis.

Infant Stimulation

Stimulation needs to be adjusted to the developmental level and tolerance of each infant (Gorski, Davison, and Brazelton, 1979). Infants in the early stages of development (less than 33 weeks) respond to stimulation with jerky limb extension, hyperflexion, and irregular vital signs. Stimulation for this group is kept to a minimum. They need to be handled with slow, sure motions. Their heads are supported and limbs held close to their body when changing position. This type of support reduces motor disorganization and stress. At age 34 to 36 weeks the infant will respond to visual and auditory stimuli in an alert state. At age 36 to 40 weeks infants are ready to respond to the caregiver's efforts to stimulate them.

Infant Feeding

The preterm infant may be fed by gavage or by bottle or breast, based on his developmental level (Chapter 23). Breast-feeding is recommended if the infant is able. The criteria for breast-feeding developed by Boggs and Rau (1983) are as follows:

- Weight at least 1500 g
- Awake for short periods
- Sucking, gagging, swallowing reflexes present
- Gavage feedings well tolerated
- Oxygen and ventilatory support not required

Nonnutritive Sucking

Nonnutritive sucking on a pacifier while gavage feeding has been demonstrated to have beneficial effects on preterm infants. As a result of this practice, the infants were ready for formula-feeding earlier, had better weight gain, were ready for discharge earlier, and suffered fewer complications (Field et al., 1982; Bernbaum et al., 1983). Makeshift pacifiers have been implicated in aspirations hazards (Milluncheck and McArtor, 1986). Ten deaths related to aspiration of baby bottle nipples were reported to the Consumer Product Safety Commission between 1975 and 1983. Nurseries and parents should buy only *one-piece pacifiers.*

Cardiopulmonary Resuscitation

Parents must be able to administer cardiopulmonary resuscitation (CPR) to their infant before taking the child home (Chapter 22). Preterm infants are 8 to 10 times more likely than term infants to develop sudden infant death syndrome (SIDS). Further, infants discharged from a neonatal intensive care unit are about twice as likely to die unexpectedly during the first year of life as are infants in the general population (Rehm, 1983). The phone number to be dialed in case of emergency should be posted near the phone.

Teacher/Counselor/Advocate

The nurse as support person and teacher shapes the environment and makes the caregiving more responsive to the needs of parents and child. Nurses are instrumental in helping parents learn who their infant is and to recognize behavioral cues in her or his development.

As soon as possible the parents should see and touch the infant so they can begin to acknowledge the reality of the event and reaffirm the infant's true appearance and condition. They will need encouragement to begin working through the psychologic tasks imposed by the preterm delivery.

A nurse or physician should be present when the parents visit the infant for the following reasons:

- To help them "see" the infant rather than focus on the equipment. The significance and function of the apparatus that surround the infant should be explained to them.
- To explain the characteristics normal for an infant of their baby's gestational age. In this way parents do not compare their child with a full-term healthy infant.
- To encourage the parents to express their feelings about the pregnancy, labor, and delivery.
- To assess the parents' perceptions of the infant to determine the appropriate time for them (especially the mother) to become actively involved in care.

Parents who have negative feelings about the pregnancy or the infant at risk need support. Their feelings can be acknowledged as valid, including the burden they are experiencing financially and emotionally and their understandable feelings toward the infant. (See Parenting Disorders discussion above.)

Soon after delivery, the parents are given the opportunity to meet the infant in the *en face* position, to touch the infant, and to see her or his favorable characteristics. As soon as possible, depending primarily on her physical condition, the mother is encouraged to visit the nursery at will and help with the infant's care. When she cannot be physically present, the staff devises appropriate methods to keep the family in almost constant touch with the newborn.

Some hospitals have instituted a parents' club for parents of infants in intensive care nurseries. These clubs encourage parents experiencing the same anxiety and grief to share their feelings. An "older" member often takes over a new member and provides additional support. Incorporating these actions into the infant's care plan acknowledges and supports nature's design by engaging and maintaining a bond between the mother and infant. This assures the infant the continued care she or he needs for physical and emotional survival at the optimum level.

Early discharge of some preterm infants is possible. The nurse's assessment, counseling, and teaching skills are invaluable for the success of home follow-up of infants after early hospital discharge (see research highlight).

Evaluation

Evaluation of the care given preterm infants and their families has to be multidimensional (Montgomery and Williams-Judge, 1986). In some families the infant dies despite all medical and nursing knowledge and skill (Kulkarni, 1978). In other families the sequelae of prematurity result in infants who will face lifetime disability. For these families evaluation criteria relate to the concepts of loss, grief, and self-concept (see Chapter 28).

For many other infants and families the immediate threat to well-being is overcome by intensive neonatal care.

RESEARCH HIGHLIGHT

A Randomized Clinical Trial of Early Hospital Discharge and Home Follow-up of Very-Low-Birth-Weight Infants

Purpose

To identify postdelivery concerns of parents of very low-birth-weight infants.

Sample

A sample of 72 mothers and 79 infants with birth weights of 1500 g (3 lb 5 oz) or less was randomly assigned to one of two groups. The control group (36 mothers and 40 infants) infants were discharged according to routine nursery policy. Infants in the experimental group (36 mothers and 39 infants) were discharged before they weighed 2200 g (4 lb $3\frac{1}{2}$ oz), as long as they met specific criteria.

Methodology

The early-discharge (experimental) group received home follow-up care provided by a perinatal nurse-specialist. The nurse-specialist met with the parents soon after the infant's birth; once a week during the infant's hospitalization; and during the first week after discharge and at 1, 9, 12, and 18 months. The nurse was in contact with the parents by telephone at least 3 times a week for the first 2 weeks and weekly thereafter for 8 weeks.

Findings

In addition to the nurse-initiated phone contacts, parents initiated more than 300 calls during the follow-up period. The five major areas of parental concern were (1) newborn health problems (30%), (2) concerns about routine care of the newborn (25%), (3) giving information (22%), (4) requesting information (13%), and (5) maternal concerns (10%).

Implications

The findings from this study demonstrated that programs of early-hospital discharge for low-birth-weight infants can potentially decrease iatrogenic illness and hospital-acquired infections, enhance parent-infant interaction, and decrease hospital costs for care. In fact, the average hospital charge for the early-discharge group was 27% less than that for the control group, and the average physician's charge was 22% less. The home follow-up care in the early-discharge group was $576, yielding a net savings of $18,560 for each infant.

From a nursing perspective the most important findings were reported as follows: there were no infants with failure to thrive because of parental neglect; there was no reported physical abuse of infants; and there were no foster placements among the infants in the early-discharge group who were observed by the nurse-specialist.

Brooten, D, et al: A randomized clinical trial of early hospital discharge and home follow-up of very-low-birth-weight infants, N Engl J Med 315:934, 1986.

The criteria for evaluation of the physical aspects of the care are the following:

1. Respirations are initiated and maintained
2. Body temperature is maintained
3. The infant is adequately nourished
4. CNS trauma is prevented or minimized
5. Infection is prevented
6. Renal function is supported
7. Hematologic problems are prevented or minimized
8. Musculoskeletal problems are prevented or minimized
9. Retinal damage is prevented or minimized

The criteria for evaluation of the psychosocial aspects of care include the following:

1. The mother retains a positive self-concept as a woman, mother, and sexual being
2. The mother, father, and family:
   a. Perceive the child as potentially normal (if this is medically substantiated)
   b. Provide the child with realistic care comfortably
   c. Experience pride and satisfaction in the care of the child
3. The parents are able to organize their time and energy to meet the needs for love, attention, and care of the other members of the family and themselves as well

RESPIRATORY DISTRESS SYNDROME

Respiratory distress syndrome (RDS) is a leading cause of morbidity and mortality among preterm infants. It affects about 20,000 infants each year in North America. Generally the smaller the preterm infant, the higher the mortality. RDS is seen almost exclusively in preterm infants, but occasionally a full-term newborn is affected.

The central problem in RDS is progressive atelectasis, which results from the development of a hyaline membrane within the newborn's terminal bronchial tree, that is, within the alveolar ducts and the alveoli. It occurs within a few hours after birth. The *membrane* is composed in part of fibrin derived from the pulmonary circulation and is not the result of aspirated fluid or an irritant. Accompanying problems such as hypoxia, metabolic and respiratory acidosis, and pulmonary hypoperfusion with right-to-left shunting (i.e., persistent fetal circulation) are secondary to atelectasis.

The cause of RDS is still unknown. The role of surfactant in preventing alveolar collapse at the end of expiration has been established. A deficiency in surfactant production may be the basis for RDS.

A deficiency in surfactant forces the infant to work to reexpand the lungs with each inspiration. The result is fatigue, depletion of energy reserves, hypoxia and hypercapnia, progressive atelectasis, and diminishing lung compliance (or increasing "stiffness"). Factors that impair the production of surfactant are hypoxia, acidosis, and reduced pulmonary blood circulation. Thus a vicious cycle is established. The normal newborn expends more calories and consumes more oxygen to breathe than does the adult. For the infant in respiratory distress this expenditure may be as much as six times that of the normal term newborn. The development of RDS may be expressed by the diagram shown in Fig. 37-13.

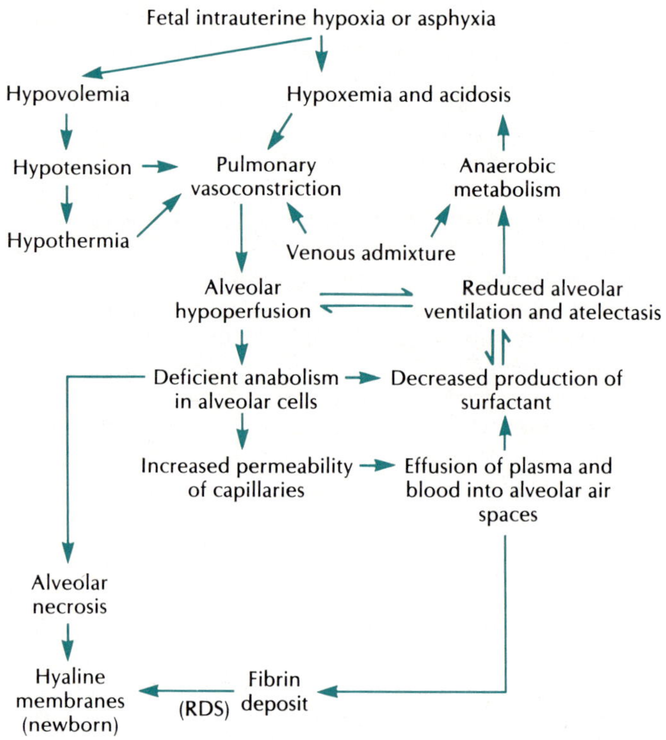

Fig. 37-13 Development of RDS.
Courtesy A. Hacket, Stanford University Medical Center, Stanford, Calif.

RDS may be apparent in the infant at birth. The newborn has a low Apgar score and commonly requires resuscitation and ventilatory assistance. Other symptoms generally appear within the first 6 hours. Initially expiratory grunting and nasal flaring are evident. As the disease progresses, tachypnea (60 breaths per min or more), retractions, and even cyanosis in room air may be noted. Hypotension and shock may be evident. Apneic pauses replace the expiratory grunting. An arterial PO_2 of 40 mm Hg or less in room air is a constant finding.

The diagnosis is confirmed by x-ray films, blood tests for pH, serum nonprotein nitrogen (NPN), potassium, and phosphorus. Tests for arterial blood gases are also used as diagnostic indicators for RDS.

Formerly, if the infant with RDS survived the first 48 to 72 hours, the clinical condition improved slowly until recovery at about 10 to 12 days. Newer methods and equipment have sustained the severely affected infant beyond 72 hours. Because of the more serious effects of the disease, death still may occur several weeks after birth. Therefore a guarded prognosis is given for several weeks.

Treatment. The following measures are important in the treatment of the infant with RDS:

1. A thermoneutral environment is provided so the infant's body temperature is maintained at 36.5° C (97.6° F).
2. Gentle handling of the newborn is necessary. This infant is disturbed as little as possible.

3. Caloric intake is sufficient to prevent catabolism (40 kcal/kg/24 hr or more).
4. Blood is replaced if an excessive amount is lost, usually as a result of samples taken for laboratory analysis.
5. Serum bilirubin levels are controlled by phototherapy, exchange transfusion, or both. Low serum albumin levels, hypoxia, and acidosis interfere with the albumin's binding to bilirubin and therefore subject these infants to kernicterus at low serum bilirubin levels (10 mg/dl or less; see Chapter 40).
6. Following are examples of specific respiratory therapies:
   a. Oxygen (60% or less) is administered by means of a hood (Fig. 37-11).
   b. Continuous positive airway pressure (CPAP) may be administered by means of an intratracheal tube, face mask, nasal prongs, or hood.
   c. Continuous negative airway pressure (CNAP) may be needed. CNAP is a respirator that works in the same manner as CPAP but exerts negative pressure on the newborn's body while the head is exposed. The newborn may breathe room air or an air-oxygen mix by means of a mask or prongs.
   d. Intermittent positive end expiratory pressure (PEEP) may be used.
7. Newer medical methods include the following:
   a. Administration of artificial surfactant or surfactant obtained from exogenous sources (Whaley and Wong, 1987). In recent years a number of controlled clinical trials of artificial surfactant in preterm infants have clearly shown its effectiveness, both as a preventative and as a therapy for RDS (Enhorning et al., 1985; Shapiro et al., 1985; Merritt et al., 1986; Gitlin et al., 1987). These studies used either human surfactant from amniotic fluid or a bovine-based preparation. Adverse side effects have been minimal to absent in the acute management of infants. Active research into a synthetic, protein-free material, which has been proved effective in animals, is under way (Durand et al., 1985). A bovine extract is expected to be commercially available soon. Surfactant replacement can then become routine care for the preterm infant in the delivery room (Lawson, 1987; Hodgman, 1987).
   b. Use of extracorporeal membrane oxygenation (ECMO) with a modified heart-lung machine (Bartlett et al., 1985) (Chapter 36).

COMPLICATIONS OF OXYGEN THERAPY

Bronchopulmonary dysplasia (BPD) and retinopathy of prematurity (ROP) are diseases of prematurity secondary to oxygen therapy (Bancalari and Gerhardt, 1986). Both conditions are relatively "new" disorders, recognized since the advent of methods of administering high concentrations of oxygen beginning in the 1940s. Although oxygen therapy may be lifesaving and occasionally must be given in high concentrations for extended periods of time, it is also potentially hazardous and must be administered judiciously. Other conditions besides BPD and ROP have become apparent. The mechanical creation of positive pressure in the lungs has increased the incidence of "air leaks." Use of oxygen apparatuses has also resulted in nasal, tracheal or pharyngeal perforation or inflammation (Whaley and Wong, 1987).

Bronchopulmonary Dysplasia

BPD is a common concomitant of lung disorders in infants, primarily preterm infants, in which focal areas of emphysema develop in the lungs. The cause is unknown, but the condition may develop as a sequela to alveolar damage caused by lung disease, use of high oxygen concentrations, and the prolonged use of CPAP or PEEP (Bancalari and Gerhardt, 1986).

Symptoms of respiratory distress, tachypnea, and increased effort appear. It is difficult to wean the infant from the positive pressure ventilator. This finding may be the first indication of the disease process.

The first sign that the infant is recovering from BPD is a decreasing dependence on oxygen therapy. Recovery may take several months. Mortality is between 30% and 50%; death may occur after the infant has been discharged from the hospital.

Retinopathy of Prematurity

The retinal changes in ROP were first described in 1942. The condition has been related to the use of high levels of oxygen and prolonged oxygen therapy. Judicious use of oxygen therapy and monitoring of Pao_2 levels have reduced the incidence of ROP, but the disease has not been eradicated.

Pao_2 between 50 and 70 mm Hg may be within safe limits. (The recently developed transcutaneous oxygen tension monitor [$tcPo_2$] is a noninvasive device that provides continuous oxygen tension values.) The most crucial period for toxic levels to occur is during the recovery phase from RDS and other respiratory distress. The exact level at which arterial oxygen tension becomes toxic and causes ROP is unknown.

Oxygen tensions that are too high for the level of retinal maturity initially result in vasoconstriction. After oxygen therapy is discontinued, neovascularization occurs in the retina and vitreous, with capillary hemorrhages, fibrotic resolution, and possible retinal detachment. Cicatricial (scar) tissue formation and consequent visual impairment may be mild or severe. The entire disease process in severe cases may take as long as 5 months to evolve. Examination by an ophthalmologist before discharge and a schedule for repeat examinations thereafter are recommended for the parents' guidance.

NECROTIZING ENTEROCOLITIS

NEC is an inflammatory disease of the gastrointestinal mucosa, commonly complicated by perforation. This often fatal disease appears in about 5% of newborns in intensive care nurseries. Although its cause is unknown, several possibilities are suspect:

1. Immaturity
2. Hypoxemia (postdelivery)

3. High-solute feedings
4. Excessive amounts of feedings
5. Perinatal asphyxia (commonly a historical antecedent)

Recent research suggests that reversal of asphyxia within 30 minutes may prevent gastrointestinal tract insult and so prevent the initiation of NEC pathophysiology. After 30 minutes, distribution of cardiac output tends to be directed more toward the heart and brain and away from the abdominal organs. Therefore prompt delivery of the intrauterine asphyxiated fetus of ventilation of the asphyxiated newborn may be beneficial to the gastrointestinal tract, as well as to other organs.

The onset is usually between 4 and 10 days. In the full-term infant the onset is almost always within the first 10 days. In the preterm infant the onset may be delayed up to 30 days. Signs of developing NEC are nonspecific, which is characteristic of many neonatal disease processes. Abdominal distension is probably the most common and regularly encountered sign. The infant's color is poor. Apneic periods increase in number. Commonly, there are gastric residuals of 2 ml or more before feedings. The stool may show occult blood (positive guaiac test). Diagnosis is confirmed by x-ray examination.

Treatment is supportive. Oral or tube feedings are discontinued to rest the gastrointestinal tract. Parenteral therapy (often by total parenteral nutrition [TPN]) is begun. NEC is an infectious disease, therefore control of infection is imperative. Antibiotic therapy may be instituted, and surgery is performed when necessary. Therapy may be prolonged, and recovery may be delayed by adhesions, complications of bowel resection (malabsorption), and intolerance of oral feedings.

SMALL-FOR-GESTATIONAL-AGE (DYSMATURE) INFANTS

Infants whose birth weight falls below the 10th percentile expected at term, for reasons other than heredity, are considered at high risk (mortality greater than 10%) (Korones 1986). Fetal growth retardation is attributable to the following possible causes:

- Deficient supply of nutrients (intrauterine malnutrition)
- Intrauterine infections
- Congenital malformations

Intrauterine growth retardation (IUGR) related to malnutrition will be discussed here. Two types of growth retardation are identified by the examination of cellular characteristics: IUGR may result from hypoplasia, a *deficient number of cells*, each containing the normal amount of cytoplasm. IUGR may also result from an adequate number of cells, each of which is diminished in size because of the *reduced amount of cytoplasm.*

Several physical findings are characteristic of the *growth-retarded neonate:*

- Generally has normal skull, but reduced dimensions of rest of body make skull look inordinately large
- Reduced subcutaneous fat
- Loose and dry skin
- Diminished muscle mass especially over buttocks and cheeks
- Sunken abdomen (scaphoid) as opposed to being normally well rounded
- Thin, yellowish, dry, and dull umbilical cord (normal cord is gray, glistening, round, and moist)
- Sparse scalp hair
- Wide skull sutures (inadequate bone growth)

The infant who is SGA as a result of intrauterine nutritional deficiency faces a number of physiologic problems.

Perinatal Asphyxia

Commonly, SGA infants have been exposed to chronic hypoxia for varying periods of time before labor and delivery. Labor is stressful to even a normal fetus and is more serious for one with growth retardation. The chronically hypoxic infant is severely compromised by even a normal labor and has difficulty compensating after birth. The alert, wide-eyed appearance of the newborn is attributed to prolonged prenatal hypoxia. Appropriate management and resuscitation are essential for the depressed infant.

The birth of SGA babies with perinatal asphyxia may be associated with a maternal history of heavy cigarette smoking; preeclampsia; low socioeconomic status; multiple gestation; gestational infections such as rubella, cytomegalovirus, and toxoplasmosis; advanced diabetes mellitus; and cardiac problems. When a woman with this background arrives in labor, the nursing staff must be alert to possible perinatal asphyxia.

Meconium Aspiration Syndrome

Two fetal responses to intrauterine hypoxia are the passage of meconium through a relaxed anal sphincter and reflex gasping. Gasping draws amniotic fluid and any particulate matter contained in the fluid deep into the bronchial tree. At birth, more aspiration may occur, and symptoms of respiratory distress often appear.

Hypoglycemia

Hypoglycemia is commonly encountered in SGA newborns, whether term or preterm. The incidence may be as high as 40%. Hypoglycemia in low-birth-weight infants is considered to be a glucose level of 20 mg/dl of blood or less. This disorder may occur anytime from birth until day 4 of life. If it is untreated, neurologic sequelae can be anticipated. Blood glucose levels are monitored by laboratory biochemical study and Dextrostix tests.

Heat Loss

Diminution of subcutaneous fat and a large body surface compared with body weight subject the SGA newborn to problems in thermoregulation. Cold stress jeopardizes recovery from asphyxia. The meagerness of fat and glycogen reserves increases such an infant's vulnerability to cold and other stress.

Nursing Care

Care of the SGA infant is based on the clinical problems present. The nursing care related to those problems is the same as for the preterm infant (see Implementation, p. 945).

POSTMATURE INFANT

Postterm, or *postdate,* refers to gestation prolonged beyond 42 *completed* weeks from the first day of the last menstrual cycle. *Postmaturity,* however, implies progressive placental insufficiency resulting in a dysmature newborn. *Not all postterm newborns are postmature.*

Weights of postmature infants usually fall within the normal range for gestational age. However, because of severe deteriorating metabolic exchange in the aging placenta the infant may be SGA. Fetal malnutrition and hypoxia result in the wasted appearance of this dysmature infant.

These newborns have a higher than normal incidence of fetal distress and perinatal death. The normal-appearing infants do well if fetopelvic disproportion (FPD) does not develop because of their increased size. A breakdown of infant deaths associated with prolonged pregnancy reveals that about one third occurred during pregnancy; approximately one half occurred during labor and delivery; and about one sixth during the puerperium.

Verification of Gestational Age

When a gravida is 2 weeks past her estimated date of delivery (EDD), one of the following possibilities and its implications apply:
- The pregnancy is not prolonged, and therefore there is no threat to the fetus.
- The pregnancy is prolonged, but the placenta continues to function efficiently and there is no threat to the fetus.
- The pregnancy is prolonged, and there is acute placental failure with threat to the fetus.
- The pregnancy is prolonged, there has been chronic placental insufficiency, and the threat to the fetus continues.

For safe delivery of the offspring, it becomes important to determine whether prolonged pregnancy actually has developed and whether there is any evidence of fetal jeopardy. Data for determining fetal gestational age is obtained from several sources and correlated (Chapters 21 and 22).

History and Interview. Verification of the time of the LMP or rejection of the LMP dates as inaccurate is important to the diagnosis of prolonged pregnancy. A correlation of the LMP with the estimated duration of pregnancy at two of the earliest obstetric examinations may lead to substantiation or recalculation of the EDD (see box, p. 268, and Chapters 21 and 22).

If the dates are accurate but the uterus is larger than expected for the duration of pregnancy, hydramnios or multiple pregnancy may be the cause. If the dates seem correct but the size of the fetus is disparate, fetal compromise, such as IUGR may be the problem, particularly when it occurs in association with preeclampsia.

The woman's medical status is reappraised. Diabetic women and women who have glucose intolerance of pregnancy have large babies, and this may confuse the estimate of gestational age. Amniocentesis to ascertain the true gestational age is also advised.

Certain groups of mothers are especially prone to carry beyond term. These groups include nulliparas, high parity mothers (gravida 4 or greater), and mothers whose preceding pregnancy was postterm.

Physical Examination. Physical examination may support the diagnosis of prolonged pregnancy; the following are examples of positive findings:
- Maternal weight loss in the last weeks of pregnancy (3 lb [1.3 kg] or more a week).
- Reduced rate of uterine and fetal growth.
- Palpation of a hard fetal head; lack of cephalic molding; high arrest of the fetal head.
- Meconium staining of the amniotic fluid.
- Oligohydramnios or decreased amniotic fluid (less than 300 ml).

Diagnostic Tests. Two serial *ultrasound examinations* and measurement of the *fetal biparietal diameter* should be accomplished 2 weeks apart from the twentieth week. This may confirm or reestablish the EDD. However, the EDD cannot be calculated when the initial biparietal diameter measures 9.5 cm or more (term size).

The fetal monitoring will include fetal activity determination (FAD), weekly estimate of fetal weight (EFW), nonstress test (NST) or oxytocin challenge test (OCT) and serial estriol determinations.

Medical Management

After confirmation of prolonged pregnancy the physician determines the protocol for delivery. A *trial of labor* by induction may be ordered (Chapter 33).

The postmature fetus (AGA or SGA) may tolerate the stress of labor poorly secondary to increasing placental insufficiency. Indices of fetal jeopardy are late fetal heart rate deceleration patterns with a slow return to the baseline rate, meconium-stained amniotic fluid, oligohydramnios, and a fetal scalp blood pH of 7.2 or less. Cephalopelvic or fetopelvic disproportion complicates some postterm labors. The oversized fetus may be exposed to excessive trauma during vaginal delivery, such as fractures and intracranial hemorrhage, and to asphyxia during labor (see Chapter 38 for birth trauma).

If induction is unsuccessful, if labor is unsatisfactory, or if fetal distress develops, cesarean delivery follows.

Nursing Care

During the antepartum period the nurse contributes to the assessment for identification of a prolonged pregnancy and often conducts nonstress tests to monitor fetal well-being. Identification and management of maternal reactions are important components of the nursing care plan. Emotional response of the woman can reflect feelings of fatigue, frustration, and anger as the pregnancy "never seems to end." She may experience negative feelings about her ability to cope and her "normalcy as a woman." Fears for the safety of her baby and the baby's future development can arise.

Intrapartum nursing care of the fetus is the same as for all other labors (Unit IV). It may be similar to that needed for fetopelvic disproportion and dystotic labor (Chapter 33). Parental fears are recognized, and support is offered. After birth, the neonate is assessed in the same manner as all newborns (Chapter 20).

Assessment

Most postterm and postmature infants are oversized but otherwise normal, with advanced development and bone age.

A postmature infant will have some but not necessarily all of the following physical characteristics:

- Generally has normal skull, but reduced dimensions of rest of body make skull look inordinately large
- Dry, cracked skin (desquamating), parchmentlike at birth
- Nails of hard consistency extending beyond fingertips
- Profuse scalp hair
- Subcutaneous fat layers depleted, leaving skin loose and giving an "old person" appearance
- Long and thin body contour
- Absent vernix
- Often meconium staining (golden yellow to green) of skin, nails, and cord
- May have an alert, wide-eyed appearance symptomatic of chronic intrauterine hypoxia

Nursing Diagnoses

The postmature infant's size and condition will determine whether the nursing diagnoses suitable for the "normal" newborn or those formulated for the preterm infant are appropriate. Examples include the following:

- Ineffective airway clearance related to
  - Meconium aspiration syndrome
- Potential hypothermia related to
  - Depleted stores of subcutaneous fat
- Potential for injury (permanent disability) related to
  - Birth trauma
- Potential for injury secondary to hypoglycemia related to
  - Depleted glycogen stores

Planning

Physiologic problems of postmaturity are reflected in the plan of care. *Immediate goals* are the initiation and maintenance of respiration, maintenance of body temperature and nutrition, prevention of CNS trauma and infection, and identification and treatment of birth trauma. The *long-term goal* is to prevent or minimize adverse sequelae to postmaturity.

Implementation

Immediate care is similar to that given to preterm infants (Affonso, 1980). Procedures to support physiologic function (e.g., respiration, body temperature, nutrition) are discussed in Chapters 22 and 36.

Evaluation

The nurse can be assured that care was effective when the goals for care have been met. Evaluation of the degree to which the long-term goal is achieved is delayed beyond the period of infancy.

SUMMARY

Infants whose gestational age and birth weight fall outside defined parameters of normal are considered to be at risk. The survival and well-being of the infant depend on the collaborative efforts of the medical and paramedical team. The nurse's skills in observing and recording often form the foundation for early diagnosis and appropriate treatment of medical and surgical conditions. Furthermore the nurse's role in facilitating the development of a positive parent-child relationship cannot be overemphasized.

KEY CONCEPTS

- Preterm infants are prone to develop problems related to the immaturity of organ systems.
- Nurses who work with preterm infants have an important role: to observe for respiratory distress and other early symptoms of physiologic functioning problems.
- Parental adaptation to preterm infants is different from that of parents who have given birth to full-term infants.
- Nurses have a vital role in facilitating the development of a positive parent-child relationship.
- Nurses' skills in interpreting data, making decisions, and initiating therapy in newborn intensive care units are crucial to the infant's survival.
- Parents need special instruction (CPR, oxygen therapy, suctioning, etc.) before they take a high-risk infant home.
- SGA infants are considered high risk secondary to fetal growth retardation.
- The high incidence of fetal distress among postmature infants is related to progressive placental insufficiency.

STUDY QUESTIONS AND ACTIVITIES

1. Discuss the reasons for problems with thermoregulation in preterm and postmature infants.
2. View and discuss one of the following (or similar film or tape): "Discussion with parents of a premature infant" (16 mm film, 32 min, Polymorph Films); "Vulnerabilities of the premature infant" (videotape, Health Sciences Consortium).

3. Discuss the complications that preterm infants can experience in response to therapy designed to support their physiologic functioning.
4. For several infants, perform and record assessment for gestational age.
5. Assist with the care of a compromised infant in the special care nursery. Identify the infant's physical characteristics. Observe the interactions of the parents and infant and describe the developmental task the parents are currently in. Develop a nursing care plan for the infant including supportive care for the parents.

References

Affonso, D, and Harris, T: Postterm pregnancy: implications for mother and infant, challenge for the nurse, JOGN Nurs 9:139, 1980

Als, H, and Brazelton, TB: A new model of assessing the behavioral organization in preterm and full term infants, J Am Acad Child Psychiatry 20;239, 1981

Bancalari, E, and Gerhardt, T: Bronchopulmonary dysplasia, Pediatr Clin North Am 33:1, 1986

Bartlett, RH, et al: Extracorporeal circulation in neonatal respiratory failure: a prospective randomized study, Pediatrics 76:479, 1985

Bennett, FC, Robinson, NM, and Sells, CJ: Growth and development of infants weighing less than 800 grams at birth, Pediatrics 71:319, 1983

Benzyl alcohol may be toxic to newborns: FDA Drug Bull 12:10, 1982

Bernbaum, JC, et al: Nonnutritive sucking during gavage feeding enhances growth and maturation in premature infants, Pediatrics 71:41, 1983

Boggs, KR, and Rau, PK: Breastfeeding the premature infant, Am J Nurs 83:1437, 1983

Dubowitz, LMS, et al: Gestational age of the newborn, J Pediatr 77:1, 1970

Durand, DJ, Clynam, RI, Heymann, MA, et al: Effects of a protein-free, synthetic surfactant on survival and pulmonary function in preterm lambs, J Pediatr 107:775, 1985

Enhorning, G, Shennan, A, Possmayer, F, et al: Prevention of neonatal respiratory distress syndrome by tracheal instillation of surfactant: a randomized clinical trial, Pediatrics 76:145, 1985

Field, TM: Interaction patterns of preterm and term infants. In Field, TM, editor: Infants born at risk, Jamaica, NY, 1979, Spectrum Publications

Field, T, et al: Nonnutritive sucking during tube feedings: effects on preterm neonates in an intensive care unit, Pediatrics 70:381, 1982

Fomufod, AK: Low birthweight and early neonatal separation as factors in child abuse, J Nat Med Assoc 68:106, 1976

Gitlin, JD, Soll, RF, Parad, RB, et al: Randomized controlled trial of exogenous surfactant for the treatment of hyaline membrane disease, Pediatrics 79:31, 1987

Goldberg, S: Premature birth: consequences of the parent-infant relationship, Am Sci 67:214, March/April 1979

Gorski, PA, Davison, MF, and Brazelton, TB: Stages of behavioral organization in the high-risk neonates: theoretical and clinical considerations, Semin Perinatol 3:61, 1979

Hansen, FH: Nursing care in the neonatal intensive care unit, JOGN Nurs 11:17, 1982

Hodgman, JE: Neonatology, JAMA 258(16):2254, 1987

Korones, S: High-risk newborn infants: the basis for intensive nursing care, ed 4, St Louis, 1986, The CV Mosby Co

Kulkarni, P, et al: Postneonatal infant mortality in infants admitted to a neonatal intensive care unit, Pediatrics 62:178, Aug 1978

Lawson, EE: Exogenous surfactant therapy to prevent respiratory distress syndrome, J Pediatr 110;492, 1987

Merritt, TA, Hallman, M, Bloom, B, et al: Prophylactic treatment of very premature infants with human surfactant, N Engl J Med 315:785, 1986

Milluncheck, E, and McArtor, R: Fatal aspiration of a make-shift pacifier Pediatrics 77:369, March 1986

Montgomery, LA, and Williams-Judge, S: An anticipatory support program for high-risk parents, Neonatal Network 5:33, Aug 1986

Philip, A: Neonatology: a practical guide, ed 3, Philadelphia, 1987, WB Saunders Co

Rehm, R: Teaching cardiopulmonary resuscitation to parents, MCN 8:411, Nov/Dec 1983

Sammons, W, and Lewis, J: Premature babies: a different beginning, St Louis, 1985, The CV Mosby Co

Schraeder, BD: Attachment and parenting despite lengthy intensive care, MCN 5:37, 1980

Shapiro, DL, Notter, RH, Morin, FC III, et al: Double-blind, randomized trial of a calf lung surfactant extract administered at birth to very premature infants for prevention of respiratory distress syndrome. Pediatrics 76:593, 1985

Sosa, R, and Grua, P: Perinatal responses to normal and premature birth experiences, J Calif Perinat Assoc 2:36, 1982

Whaley, LF, and Wong, DL: Nursing care of infants and children, ed 3, St Louis, 1987, The CV Mosby Co

Bibliography

Preterm Infant

Anderson, GC, et al: Effects of time-controlled non-nutritive sucking opportunities, Nurs Res 31:63, 1982

Barnard, KE, and Bee, HL: The impact of temporally patterned stimulation on the development of preterm infants, Child Dev 54:1156, 1983

Beaton, JL: A systems model of premature birth: implications for neonatal intensive care, JOGN Nurs 13:173, 1984

Clinical News: Breast is best—for preemies too, Am J Nurs 87(11):1403, 1987

Cole, CH: Prevention of prematurity: can we do it in America? Pediatrics 76:310, 1985

Cole, JG, and Frappier, PA: Infant stimulation reassessed. A new approach to providing care for the preterm infant, JOGN Nurs 14:471, 1985

Dubowitz, LMS, and Dubowitz, V: Gestational age of the newborn, Menlo Park, Calif, 1977, Addison-Wesley Publishing Co, Inc

Fanaroff, AA, and Martin, RJ: Neonatal-perinatal medicine: diseases of the fetus and infant, ed 4, St Louis, 1987, The CV Mosby Co

Ferrara, A, and Harin, A: Emergency transfer of the high-risk neonate: a working manual for medical, nursing, and administrative personnel, St Louis, 1980, The CV Mosby Co

Field, T, and Goldson, E: Pacifying effects of nonnutritive sucking on term and preterm neonates during heelstick procedures, Pediatrics 74:1012, 1984

Fria, JT: Assessment of hearing, Pediatr Clin North Am 28:757, 1981

Gerhardt, T, and Bancalari, E: Apnea of prematurity, I. Lung function and regulation of breathing, Pediatrics, 74:58, 1984

Gerhardt, T, and Bancalari, E: Apnea of prematurity. II. Respiratory reflexes, Pediatrics 74:63, 1984

Gross, SJ, and Eckerman, CO: Normative early head growth in very-low-birth-weight infants, J Pediatr 103:946, 1983

Harvey, D, et al: Abilities of children who were small-for-gestational-age babies, Pediatrics 69:296, 1982

Hawkins-Walsh, E: Diminishing anxiety in parents of sick newborns, MCN 5:30, 1980

Hirata, T, et al: Survival and outcome of infants 501 to 750 gm: a six-year experience, J Pediatr 102:741, 1983

Johnson, SH: Nursing assessment and strategies for the family at risk: high-risk parenting, ed 2, Philadelphia, 1986, JB Lippincott Co

Kuller, JM, Lund, C, and Tobin, C: Improved skin care for premature infants, MCN 8:200, 1983

Lieberman, E, Ryan, KJ, Monson, RR, and Schoenbaum SC: Risk factors accounting for racial differences in the rate of premature birth, N Engl J Med 317:743, Sept 1987

Magyary, D: Early social interactions: preterm infant-parent dyads, Issues Compr Pediatr Nurs 7:233, 1984

Mahan, CK: Care of the family of the critically ill neonate, Crit Care Q 4:89, 1981

Mahan, CK: The family of the critically ill neonate, Crit Care Update 10(6):24, 1983

Maloney, M, et al: A prospective controlled study of scheduled sibling visits to a newborn intensive care unit, J Am Acad Child Psychiatry 22:565, 1983

Manser, JI: Growth in the high-risk infant, Clin Perinatol 11:19, 1984

Marino, BL: When nurses compete with parents, JACCH 8:94, 1980

Miles, MS, and Carter, MC: Assessing parental stress in intensive care units, MCN 8:354, 1983

Moore, T, and Resnic, R: Special problems of VLBW infant, Contemp OB/GYN 23(6):174, 1984

Newman, L: Parents' perceptions of their low birth weight infants, Pediatrician 9:182, 1980

Perez, RH: Protocols for perinatal nursing practice, St Louis, 1981, The CV Mosby Co

Schraeder, BD: Attachment and parenting despite lengthy intensive care, MCN 5:37, 1980

Schwab, F, et al: Sibling visiting in a neonatal intensive care unit, Pediatrics, 71:835, 1983

Stengel, TJ: Infant behavior, maternal psychological reactions, and mother-infant interactional issues associated with the crises of prematurity: a selected review of the literature, Phys Occup Ther Pediatr 2(2/3):3, 1982

Infants with Problems Related to Gestational Age and Weight

Avery, ME: The argument for prenatal administration of dexamethasone to prevent respiratory distress syndrome, J Pediatr 104:240, 1984

Boros, SJ, et al: Using conventional infant ventilators at unconventional rates, Pediatrics 74:487, 1984

Boynton, BR, et al: Combined high-frequency oscillatory ventilation and intermittent mandatory ventilation in critically ill neonates, J Pediatr 105:297, 1984

Brown, EG, and Sweet, AY: Neonatal necrotizing entercolitis, Pediatr Clin North Am 29:1149, 1982

Cassady, G: Transcutaneous monitoring in the newborn infant, J Pediatr 103:837, 1983

Cohen, MA: Transcutaneous oxygen monitoring for sick neonates, MCN 9:324, 1984

Committee on Fetus and Newborn: Vitamin E and the prevention of retinopathy of prematurity, Pediatrics 76:315, 1985

Fuhrmann, K, et al: Prevention of congenital malformations in infants of insulin-dependent diabetic mothers, Diabetes Care 6:219, 1983

Gangitano, E: Protocol: hypoglycemia, J Perinatology 7(1):72, 1987

Garn, SM, et al: Effect of maternal cigarette smoking on Apgar scores, Am J Dis Child 135:503, 1981

Fox, WW, and Duara, S: Persistent pulmonary hypertension in the neonate: diagnosis and management, J Pediatr 103:505, 1983

Have ecmo, will travel: Am J Nurs 86:117, 1986

Heldt, GP, et al: Exercise performance of the survivors of hyaline membrane disease, J Pediatr 96:995, 1980

Hodgman, JE: Bronchopulmonary dysplasia. In Gellils, SS, and Kagan, BM: Current pediatric therapy, ed 12, Philadelphia 1986, WB Saunders Co

Huch, A, et al: Experience with transcutaneous O_2 ($tcpO_2$) monitoring of mother, fetus and newborn, J Perinat Med 2:51, 1980

Kaplow, R, and Fromme, LR: Nursing care plan for the patient receiving high-frequency jet ventilation, Crit Care Nurs 5:25, 1985

Kirkpatrick, BV, et al: Use of extracorporeal membrane oxygenation for respiratory failure in term infants, Pediatrics 72:872, 1983

Kleinman, JC, and Kessell, SS: Racial differences in low birth weight: trends and risk factors, N Engl J Med 317:749, Sept 1987

Levin, DL: Meconium inhalation syndrome. In Levin, DL, Morriss, FC, and Moore, GC: A practical guide to pediatric intensive care, ed 2, St Louis, 1984, The CV Mosby Co

Lucey, JF, and Dangman, B: A reexamination of the role of oxygen in retrolental fibroplasia, Pediatrics 73:82, 1984

Mammel, MD, et al: Comparison of high-frequency jet ventilation and conventional mechanical ventilation in a meconium aspiration model, J Pediatr 103:630, 1983

Meier, P, and Wilks, S: The bacteria in expressed mothers' milk, MCN 12(6):420, 1987

Meis, P, Ernest, JM, and Morre, M: Causes of low birth weight in public and private patients, Am J Obstet Gynecol 156(5):1165, 1987

Murphy, JD, Vawter, GF, and Reid, LM: Pulmonary vascular disease in fetal meconium aspiration, J Pediatr 104:785, 1984

Plapp, PR: Nursing implications in the early recognition of necrotizing enterocolitis, Issues Compr Pediatr Nurs 4(2):77, 1980

Purohit, DM, et al: Risk factors for retrolental fibroplasia experience with 3,025 premature infants, Pediatrics 76:339, 1985

Shohat, M, et al: Retinopathy of prematurity: incidence and risk factors, Pediatrics 72:159, 1983

Sims, ME, Jasani, N, and Hodgman, JE: Care of very low birth weight infants with neonatal nurse clinicians, J Perinatology 7(1):55, 1987

Walsh, M, and Kliegman, RM: Necrotizing enterocolitis: the spectrum of disease, Pediatr Basics, 40:4, March 1984

Weaver, KA, and Anderson, GC: Relationship between integrated sucking pressures and first bottle-feeding scores in premature infants, JOGN Nurs 17(2):113, 1988

Whiteman, L, Wuethrick, M, and Egan, E: Infants who survive necrotizing enterocolitis, Matern Child Nurs J 14(3):123, 1985

Wilson, R, et al: Age at onset of necrotizing enterocolitis: an epidemiologic analysis, Pediatr Res 16:82, Jan 1982

Wooten, B: Death of an infant, MCN 6:257, 1981

CHAPTER

38

Birth Trauma and Newborn of Diabetic Pregnancy

Learning Objectives

Correctly define the key terms listed.

Describe assessment of infants for birth trauma and for sequelae to a diabetic pregnancy.

Summarize the care of the newborn with soft tissue injuries.

Summarize the care of the newborn with skeletal injuries.

Summarize the care of the newborn with nervous system injuries.

Explain the mechanism of the process leading to problems from conception through birth for the infant of the diabetic mother.

Describe assessment of the infant of a diabetic mother.

Develop nursing care plans for each of the commonly associated conditions seen in infants of diabetic mothers.

Key Terms

birth trauma (injuries)
brachial paralysis
caput succedaneum
cardiomyopathy
cephalhematoma
discoloration of skin
facial paralysis
fetal hyperinsulinism
hypocalcemia
hypoglycemia
increased intracranial pressure
infant of diabetic mother (IDM)
infant of gestational diabetic mother (IGDM)
maternal ketoacidosis
macrosomia
phrenic nerve injury
respiratory difficulty in IDM
skeletal injuries

INFANT BIRTH TRAUMA

Birth injuries are those sustained during labor and delivery. The significance of birth injuries is most accurately assessed by review of mortality data from recent years. These data show a steady decline in birth injuries as a cause of neonatal mortality. In 1981 birth injuries ranked sixth among major causes of neonatal mortality, resulting in 23.8 deaths per 100,000 live births. In 1984 birth injuries caused 8.9 deaths per 100,000 live births, falling to eighth among leading causes. This apparent improvement has been attributed to refinements in obstetric techniques, the increased use of cesarean delivery over difficult vaginal deliveries, and elimination or decreased use of vacuum extractors and version and extraction. Despite this decrease, birth injuries still represent an important source of neonatal morbidity. Therefore the clinician should consider the broad spectrum of birth injuries in the differential diagnosis of neonatal clinical disorders (Fanaroff and Martin, 1987; Cyr, Usher, and McLean, 1984).

Most birth injuries may be preventable at least in theory. Careful attention to risk factors and the appropriate planning of delivery should reduce the incidence of birth injuries to a minimum. Ultrasonography allows for antepartum diagnosis of macrosomia, hydrocephalus, and unusual presentations. Particular pregnancies may then be delivered by controlled elective cesarean delivery to avoid significant birth injury (Merenstein and Gardner, 1985).

Often a small percentage of significant birth injuries may be unavoidable and occur despite skilled and competent obstetric care. Some injuries cannot be anticipated until the specific circumstances are encountered during delivery. Emergency cesarean delivery may provide a last-minute salvage, but in these circumstances the injury may truly be unavoidable. The same injury might be caused in several ways. Thus a cephalhematoma could be the result of an obstetric technique such as forceps delivery or vacuum extraction, or the same injury may occur secondary to the pressure of the fetal skull against the maternal pelvis. In the latter case, cephalhematoma may not be a birth injury (Eisenberg, Kirchner, and Perrin, 1984).

Many injuries are minor and readily resolve in the neonatal period without treatment. Other traumas require some degree of intervention. A few are serious enough to be fatal.

Classification of Birth Traumas

Birth traumas can be classified according to the following outline:

1. Soft tissue injuries
   a. Caput succedaneum
   b. Cephalhematoma
   c. Subcutaneous fat necrosis (pressure necrosis)
   d. Subconjunctival (scleral) hemorrhage
   e. Retinal hemorrhage
   f. Petechiae, erythema, abrasions, lacerations, ecchymoses, and edema
   g. Sternocleidomastoid muscle injury—congenital torticollis
   h. Hemorrhage into or rupture of abdominal organs
2. Skeletal injuries
   a. Molding of fetal skull bones
   b. Fractures
      (1) Skull (depressed or linear)
      (2) Clavicle, humerus, or femur
      (3) Dislocation, separation at joints
3. Peripheral nervous system injuries
   a. Brachial paralysis (Erb-Duchenne, Klumpke's)
   b. Facial paralysis
   c. Phrenic nerve injury (diaphragmatic paralysis)
   d. Vocal cord paralysis
4. Central nervous system injuries (intracranial hemorrhage or contusions, spinal cord injury)

The nurse's contributions to the welfare of the newborn begin with early observation and accurate recording. The prompt reporting of signs indicative of deviations from normal permits early initiation of appropriate therapy.

Assessment

Factors Predisposing to Injury

Several factors predispose an infant to birth injuries (Fanaroff and Martin, 1987; Merenstein and Gardner, 1985). *Maternal* factors include uterine dysfunction that leads to prolonged or precipitous labor, preterm or postterm labor, and cephalopelvic disproportion. Injury may result from dystocia caused by *fetal* macrosomia, multiple gestation, abnormal or difficult presentation (not caused by maternal uterine or pelvic conditions), and congenital anomalies. *Intrapartum events* that can result in scalp injury include the use of intrapartum monitoring of fetal heart rate (FHR) and collection of fetal scalp blood for acid-base assessment. *Obstetric delivery techniques* can cause injury. Forceps delivery, vacuum extraction, version and extraction, and cesarean delivery are all potential contributory factors.

Signs of Injury

The Apgar score may alert the caregiver to birth injuries. Flaccid muscle tone, regardless of cause, increases the risk of joint dislocations and separation during the birth process. Flaccid tone in extremities may be traced to nerve plexus injuries or long-bone fractures. A weak or hoarse cry is characteristic of laryngeal nerve palsy as a result of excessive traction on the neck during delivery. Marked bruising of the skin may preclude accurate assessment for color.

A complete physical assessment of the newborn is performed soon after birth (Chapter 21). Large-for-gestational-age (LGA) newborns may be preterm, term, postmature, or postterm; or children of diabetic (or prediabetic) mothers (see Figs. 37–1 and 37–2). Each of these categories has special concerns. Regardless of coexisting potential problems, the oversized infant or the infant too large for the maternal pelvis is at risk by virtue of size alone. Birth trauma, especially associated with breach or shoulder presentation, is a serious hazard for the oversized neonate. Asphyxia or central nervous system (CNS) injury or both may also occur.

An oversized infant traditionally has been one who weighs 4000 g (8 lb 13 oz) or more at birth. About 10% of newborns are of this weight, and about 2% weigh 4500 g (9 lb 15 oz) or more. Moreover, most of these newborns have other proportionately larger measurements. Many are delivered well after the estimated date of delivery (EDD). Since evidence of birth injury may not be apparent at the initial examination, assessment continues during each contact with the neonate.

Nursing Diagnoses

The nursing diagnoses will depend on the particular injury incurred. The following are therefore presented as examples only.

Parents

- Knowledge deficit related to
  - The injury
  - Cause of injury
  - Management and therapy
  - Prognosis
- Anticipatory grieving related to
  - Possible sequelae to the birth injury
- Spiritual distress related to
  - Occurrence of birth injury

Child

- Potential for impaired physical mobility related to
  - Brachial plexus injury
- Potential impaired gas exchange related to
  - Diaphragmatic paralysis (partial or complete)

Planning

Meeting the unique needs of the birth-injured newborn requires constant vigilance. Goals are established and prioritized. Nursing actions are selected in light of the particular disorder and individual needs of the infant and family.

Goals. The overall goals for care of infants with birth trauma are as follows:

1. Anticipate and diagnose premonitory or early sequelae of trauma
2. Minimize the effects of the disorder or avoid disability of the child
3. Treat injury or its sequelae promptly and appropriately when possible
4. Facilitate a positive parent-child relationship
5. Meet the parents' (family's) educational needs regarding the injury and its management

Implementation

Soft Tissue Injuries

Caput Succedaneum. Caput succedaneum is a localized edematous swelling of the scalp that persists for a few days after birth and then disappears. It has no pathologic significance (see Fig. 21-6, *A*).

Caphalhematoma. Cephalhematoma is a collection of blood from ruptured blood vessels between the periosteum and surface of the parietal bone (see Fig. 21-6, *B,* and discussion in Chapter 21). The swelling may appear unilaterally or bilaterally and disappears gradually in 2 to 3 weeks. Occasionally hyperbilirubinemia may result from breakdown of the accumulated blood.

Subcutaneous Fat Necrosis. Subcutaneous fat necrosis (pressure necrosis) results from pressure against the pelvis or from forceps (Chen et al., 1981). The lesion is clearly defined and is a firm mass (size varies) fixed to the overlying skin but movable over underlying tissue. Skin over the lesion may be reddish purple. These lesions usually resolve spontaneously in a few days.

Subconjunctival (Scleral) and Retinal Hemorrhages. Subconjunctival and retinal hemorrhages result from rupture of capillaries from increased intracranial pressure during birth. They clear within 5 days after birth and usually present no problems. However, parents need reassurance about their presence.

Discoloration and Injuries of the Skin. *Erythema, ecchymoses, petechiae, abrasions, lacerations,* and *edema* of buttocks and extremities may be present. Localized discoloration may appear over presenting or dependent parts. Ecchymoses and edema appear as bruises anywhere on the body. They can appear on the presenting part from the application of forceps. They can result from manipulation of the infant's body during delivery.

Bruises and ecchymoses over the face may be the result of face presentation (Fig. 38-1). The skin over the entire head may be ecchymotic and covered with petechiae secondary to a tight nuchal cord. Petechiae, or pinpoint hem-

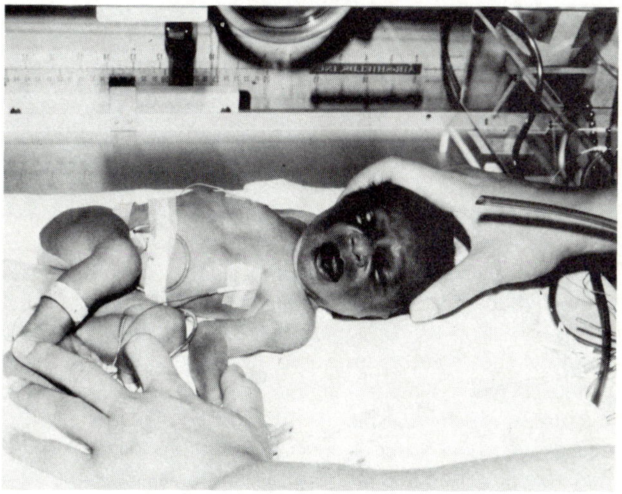

Fig. 38-1 Marked bruising of the entire face of 1490 g female born vaginally after face presentation. Less severe ecchymoses were present on the extremities. Despite use of phototherapy from the first day, icterus resulting from breakdown of the accumulated blood was noted on the third day, and exchange transfusions were required on the fifth and sixth days.

From Fanaroff, AA, and Martin, RJ, editors: Behrman's neonatal-perinatal medicine, ed 4, St Louis, 1987, The CV Mosby Co.

orrhagic areas, acquired during birth may extend over the upper trunk and face. These lesions are benign if they disappear within 2 days of birth and no new lesions appear. Ecchymoses and petechiae may be signs of a more serious disorder, such as thrombocytopenic purpura. If they do not disappear spontaneously in 2 days, the physician is notified. To differentiate hemorrhagic areas from skin rashes and discolorations, the nurse blanches the skin with two fingers. Because extravasated blood remains within the tissues, petechiae and ecchymoses do not blanch.

Trauma secondary to dystocia occurs over the presenting part; forceps injury occurs at the site of application of the instrument. Forceps injury commonly has a linear configuration across both sides of the face outlining the placement of the forceps. The affected areas are kept clean to minimize the risk of secondary infection. These injuries usually resolve spontaneously within several days with no specific therapy. The increased use of padded forceps blades may reduce the incidence of these lesions significantly (Fanaroff and Martin, 1987; Hebertson et al., 1985).

Accidental lacerations may be inflicted with a scalpel during cesarean delivery. These cuts may occur on any part of the body but are most often found on the scalp, buttocks, and thighs. Usually they are superficial, needing only to be kept clean. Butterfly adhesive strips will hold the edges of more serious lacerations together. Rarely, sutures are needed.

Hemorrhage into Abdominal Organs. Hemorrhage into abdominal organs or rupture of abdominal organs may occur after manipulation of the body during a difficult breech extraction. The liver is most susceptible to injury (French, 1982). The affected infant is pale, the liver enlarges progressively, and in some, a mass may be palpable. Rupture of the liver capsule occurs eventually, and the infant appears cyanotic and in shock. Surgical repair and blood transfusions are lifesaving.

Skeletal Injuries

Molding. The shaping of the head as it passes through the bony pelvis during labor is discussed in Chapter 16. This is a normal process that facilitates descent of the head.

Skull Fracture. The newborn's immature, flexible skull can withstand a great degree of deformation (molding) before fracture results. Considerable force is required to fracture the newborn's skull. Location of the fracture determines whether it is insignificant or fatal. If an artery lying in a groove on the undersurface of the skull is torn as a result of the fracture, increased intracranial pressure will ensue (p. 960). Unless a blood vessel is involved, linear fractures (which account for 70% of all fractures for this age group) heal without special treatment. The soft skull may become indented without laceration of either the skin or the dural membrane. These depressions, or "ping-pong ball" indentations, may occur during difficult deliveries from pressure of the head on the bony pelvis (Fig. 38-2). They can also occur as a result of injudicious application of forceps.

Fracture of the Clavicle. The clavicle is the bone most often fractured during delivery. Generally the break is in the middle third of the bone. Dystocia, particularly shoulder impaction, may be the predisposing problem. *Limitation of motion of the arm, crepitus of the bone, and no Moro's reflex on the affected side are diagnostic.* Except for use of gentle rather than vigorous handling, there is no accepted treatment for fractured clavicle. The figure-eight bandage appropriate for the older child should not be used for the newborn. The prognosis is good.

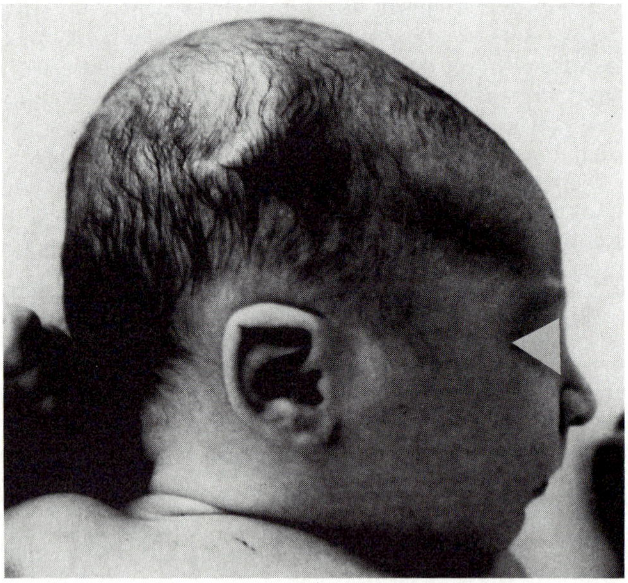

Fig. 38-2 Depressed skull fracture in a full-term male delivered after rapid (1 hour) labor. The infant was delivered by occiput-anterior presentation after rotation from occiput-posterior position.
From Fanaroff, AA, and Martin, RJ, editors: Behrman's neonatal-perinatal medicine, ed 4, St Louis, 1987, the CV Mosby Co.

Fracture of the Humerus or Femur. The humerus and femur are other bones that may be fractured during a difficult delivery. Fractures in newborns generally heal rapidly. Immobilization is accomplished with slings, splints, swaddling, and other devices.

The parents need support in handling these infants because they are often fearful of hurting them. Parents are encouraged to practice handling, changing, and feeding the affected newborn in the nursery under the guidance of personnel. This will increase their confidence and knowledge and facilitate attachment. A plan for follow-up therapy is developed with the parents so that the times and arrangements for therapy are workable and acceptable to them.

Peripheral Nervous System Injuries

Brachial Paralysis: Upper Arm. Erb-Duchenne paralysis (upper arm brachial paralysis) is the most common type of paralysis associated with a difficult delivery (Fig. 38-3). Typical symptoms are a flaccid arm with the elbow extended and the hand rotated inward, negative Moro's reflex on the affected side, sensory loss over the lateral aspect of the arm, and an intact grasp reflex.

A 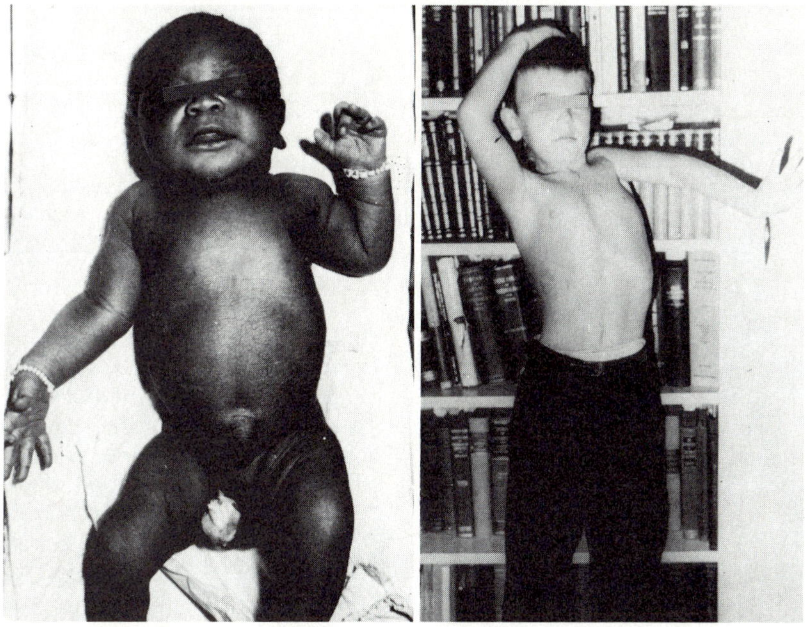 B

Fig. 38-3 A, Erb-Duchenne paralysis in newborn infant. Right upper extremity failed to participate in Moro's reflex. Recovery was complete. **B**, Residual of Erb-Duchenne paralysis. Left arm was short; it could not be raised above level shown.

From Shirkey, HC, editor: Pediatric therapy, ed 6, St Louis, 1975, The CV Mosby Co.

Treatment consists of intermittent immobilization, proper positioning, and exercise to maintain the range of motion of joints. Gentle manipulation and range-of-motion exercises are delayed until about the tenth day to prevent additional injury to the brachial plexus.

Immobilization may be accomplished with a brace or splint or by pinning the infant's sleeve to the mattress. The infant should be positioned for 2 or 3 hours at a time in the following manner: abduct the arm 90 degrees; externally rotate the shoulder; flex the elbow 90 degrees; and supinate the wrist with the palm directed slightly toward the face (Fig. 38-4). The arm should be freed periodically for good skin care. About the tenth day, gentle massage and range-of-motion exercises are begun to prevent contractures.

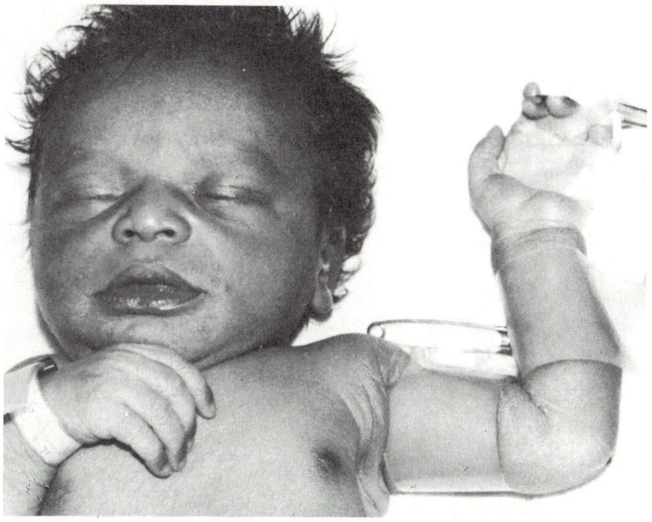

Fig. 38-4 Recommended corrective positioning for treatment of Erb-Duchenne paralysis. Note abduction and external rotation at shoulder, flexion at elbow, supination of forearm, and slight dorsiflexion at wrist.

From Behrmann, RE, editor: Neonatology: diseases of the fetus and infant, St Louis, 1973, The CV Mosby Co.

Brachial Paralysis: Lower Arm. Damage to the lower plexus, Klumpke's palsy, is less common. With lower arm paralysis, the wrist and hand are flaccid, the grasp reflex is absent, deep tendon reflexes are present, and dependent edema and cyanosis may be apparent (in the affected hand). Treatment consists of placing the hand in a neutral position, padding the fist, and gently exercising the wrist and fingers.

Parents are taught to position and immobilize the arm or wrist or both. They can gently massage and manipulate the muscles to prevent contractures while the arm is healing. If edema or hemorrhage is responsible for the paralysis, the prognosis is good and recovery may be expected in a few weeks. If laceration of the nerves has occurred and healing does not result in return of function within a few months (3 to 6 months or 2 years at the most), surgery may be indicated; however, little or no function will develop.

Facial Paralysis. Facial paralysis (Fig. 38-5) is generally caused by misapplication of forceps with pressure by one blade against the facial nerve during delivery. The face on the affected side is flattened and unresponsive to the grimace of crying or stimulation, and the eye will remain open. Moreover, the forehead will not wrinkle. Often the condition is transitory, resolving within hours or days of birth. Permanent paralysis is rare.

Treatment involves careful, patient feeding, prevention

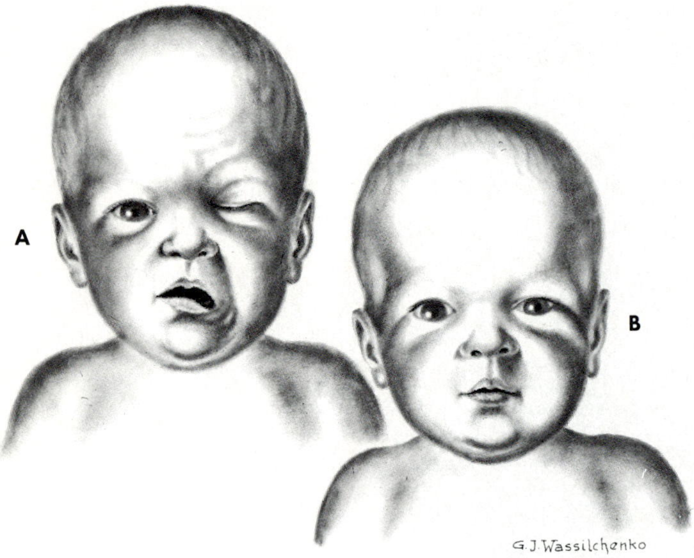

Fig. 38-5 **A**, Paralysis of right side of face 15 minutes after forceps delivery. Absence of movement on affected side is especially noticeable when infant cries. **B**, Same infant 24 hours later.

From Whaley, LF, and Wong, DL: Nursing of infants and children, ed 3, St Louis, 1987, The CV Mosby Co.

of damage to the cornea of the open eye, and supportive care of the parents. Commonly the infant looks grotesque, especially when crying. Feeding may be prolonged, with the milk flowing out of the newborn's mouth around the nipple on the affected side. The mother will need understanding and sympathetic encouragement while learning how to feed and care for the infant, as well as how to hold and cuddle the baby.

Phrenic Nerve Injury. Phrenic nerve injury almost always occurs as a component of brachial plexus injury. Injury to the phrenic nerve results in diaphragmatic paralysis. Cyanosis and irregular thoracic respirations with no abdominal movement on inspiration are characteristic of paralysis of the diaphragm. Babies with diaphragmatic paralysis usually require mechanical ventilatory support, at least for the first few days after birth. Occasionally this support is essential for several weeks until corrective surgery can be performed.

Central Nervous System Injuries

Intracranial Hemorrhage. Intracranial hemorrhage as a result of birth trauma is more likely to occur in the full-term, large infant. The hemorrhage occurs into the brain substance or as a subdural hematoma. The latter is the principal manifestation of intracranial hemorrhage. The signs and symptoms of intracranial hemorrhage are presented in the danger signs box at top, right. Subdural hematoma is seen with relative infrequency today because of the remarkable improvements in obstetric care in recent years.

Hypoxia and hypovolemia are the most common causes of intracranial hemorrhage. Hemorrhage from hypoxia occurs in the subarachnoid space or in the ventricles of the brain. *These intracranial hemorrhages, seen most commonly in premature infants, are not related to trauma.* The symptomatology varies. Abnormal respiration with cyanosis; hypotonia; reduced responsiveness (lethargy); irritability; a high-pitched, shrill cry; tense fontanel; twitching (Table 39-1); or convulsions may be noted.

General treatment consists of elevation of the head several inches higher than the hips, warmth, oxygen to relieve cyanosis, and administration of intravenous fluids or other suitable means of meeting the newborn's food and fluid needs. Minimum handling to promote rest should guide nursing care.

DANGER SIGNS

Intracranial Hemorrhage

1. Separation of the sutures
2. Bulging of the anterior fontanel

Table 38-1 *Possible Traumas Secondary to Vaginal Breech Delivery*

Trauma and Location	Resolution*
Petechiae	2-3 days
Head, neck, upper chest, lower back	
Ecchymoses, edema, hematomas	1 week
Presenting part	
Skull fracture	Variable; months
Occipital bone	
Fractures and dislocations	2-4 weeks
Facial bones, mandible bone/joint, nose, clavicle, humerus, epiphyseal separation	
Paralysis	
Vocal cords	Few months to years
Erb-Duchenne (C_{5-6})	3-6 months; or never
Diaphragm (phrenic nerve) (C_{3-5})	6 weeks to months
Spine, spinal cord	Death or permanent nerve sequelae
Torticollis	2-3 months
Sternocleidomastoid muscle	
Intraabdominal organs	
Liver rupture	Depends on recognition and therapy; death
Spleen rupture	Immediate if early recognition is followed by emergency surgery
Adrenal hemorrhage	Variable

*Resolution occurs only if damage is not permanent.

The treatment of subdural hemorrhage is aspiration or surgical removal of the blood collection. Repeated subdural taps for the evacuation of subdural blood is indicated whether or not the separation of sutures widens, the head size is increasing and the fontanel is bulging.

Spinal Cord Injuries. Spinal cord injuries may occur during manipulation of the newborn's body during breech extraction. Injury occurs when considerable traction force is required to deliver the shoulders or head or both. This injury is rarely seen today, since cesarean delivery is often used for delivery of a breech. Table 38-1 summarizes potential injuries secondary to difficult vaginal breech extraction.

Evaluation

The nurse can be assured that care has been effective if the goals for care have been met. Risk factors such as large fetal size and unusual presentations are identified before delivery. Mode of delivery is selected to prevent birth trauma. If injury is sustained, prompt identification permits early initiation of appropriate therapy. On a long-term basis, care has been effective if there are no residual adverse sequelae to birth injury as the child grows and develops.

INFANTS OF DIABETIC MOTHERS

Metabolic abnormalities of diabetes in pregnancy adversely affect embryonic and fetal development. Good diabetic control (Chapter 32) during critical embryonic development is possible for the woman whose glucose intolerance is known *and* well controlled before pregnancy. However, gestational diabetes is diagnosed after the crucial period of organogenesis is over. Consequently, the risk of hydramnios and congenital anomalies is greater for the woman with gestational diabetes. Correction of the metabolic abnormalities and individualizing the timing of delivery can minimize the incidence of stillbirths and neonatal deaths (Fanaroff and Martin, 1987). The mechanism of the process leading to problems from conception through birth is as follows.

In early pregnancy, fluctuations in blood glucose and episodes of ketoacidosis are thought to cause congenital anomalies. Later in pregnancy, when the mother's pancreas cannot release sufficient insulin to meet increased demands, maternal hyperglycemia results. The high levels of glucose cross the placenta and stimulate the fetal pancreas to release insulin. The combination of the increased supply of maternal glucose and other nutrients and increased fetal insulin results in excessive fetal growth called *macrosomia.* Hyperinsulinemia accounts for most of the problems seen. In addition, poor diabetic control or superimposed maternal infection adversely affects the fetus. *Normally, maternal blood has a more alkaline pH than does fetal blood* (with its excess of CO_2). This phenomenon encourages exchange of O_2 and CO_2 across the placental membrane. When the maternal blood is more acidotic than the fetal blood, no CO_2 or O_2 exchange occurs at the level of the placenta. The mortality for the unborn baby resulting from an episode of maternal ketoacidosis may be as high as 50% or greater (Fanaroff and Martin, 1987).

Prepregnancy and Prenatal Period. There is some indication that some neonatal conditions—macrosomia, hypoglycemia, hypocalcemia, hyperbilirubinemia, and perhaps fetal lung immaturity—may be eliminated or the incidence decreased by maintaining control over maternal glucose levels within narrow limits (Fuhrmann et al., 1983).

Infants with major congenital anomalies are born to diabetic women two to three times more often than they are to women in the general obstetric population. These anomalies most commonly arise during the first 7 weeks of embryonic life, before most women come under prenatal care and before metabolic control is normalized. Therefore

RESEARCH HIGHLIGHT

Maternal Prenatal Attachment in Normal and High-risk Pregnancies

Purpose

To compare maternal-fetal attachment in normal and high-risk pregnancies and to identify variables affecting the maternal attachment process during pregnancy.

Sample

The sample included 88 married participants in their third trimesters who were either attending a high-risk prenatal clinic or were participating in Lamaze classes.

Methodology

The women completed a demographic questionnaire providing descriptive data and information about the current pregnancy, and also completed Cranley's prenatal attachment tool.

Criteria identified for high-risk classification included: preterm labor, placenta previa, diabetes mellitus, gestational diabetes, fetal intrauterine growth retardation (IUGR), pregnancy-induced hypertension (PIH), and multiple criteria (two or more of above criteria).

Findings

No statistically significant differences in prenatal attachment were found between normal and high-risk groups. In addition there were no significant correlations between attachment scores and educational level, age, and race, as well as whether the pregnancy was planned or whether the women had a sonogram or ordinal position of the infant.

Implications

Data were collected during the third trimester. Other investigators found that prenatal affiliation increased after quickening. Therefore the findings from this study may be influenced by the timing of data collection. In conclusion, the investigators suggest that prenatal attachment seems to be a task that is accomplished during pregnancy regardless of whether the pregnancy is threatened.

Kemp, VH, and Page, CK, Maternal prenatal attachment in normal and high-risk pregnancies, JOGN Nurs 16(3):179, 1987.

there remains an irreducible minimum of perinatal mortality and morbidity that is secondary to fetal anomalies. Poor diabetic control in early pregnancy as evidenced by elevated maternal hemoglobin A_{Ic} ($\geq$8.5) is associated with an increased risk of major structural malformations. There is a growing body of evidence that the establishment of euglycemia before *conception* and *through the first trimester* will reduce the incidence of congenital anomalies to approximately that of the general obstetric population. Further reductions in perinatal mortality and morbidity beyond the "irreducible minimum" may in time be possible but only when care providers emphasize the need for prepregnancy planning and diabetes control (Fanaroff and Martin, 1987).

Maternal lack of food intake and dehydration act in concert to promote the production of ketone bodies and to decrease their rate of eventual excretion. Disturbances in oral intake coupled with nausea and vomiting set the stage for a ketoacidotic episode. This risk is heightened particularly during protracted nausea and vomiting in late gestation. Maternal acidosis is often reflected in uterine hyperactivity, together with a loss of FHR variability or the appearance of late decelerations. Hospitalization is required to prevent preterm birth or stillbirth. Metabolic stability is achieved with insulin, calories, fluids, and electrolytes.

This high-risk pregnancy places heavy demands on the gravida to ensure her well-being and that of her fetus. Maternal-fetal attachment in normal and high-risk pregnancies has been studied. The results of one such study are reported in the research highlight.

Table 38-2 lists a timetable for monitoring pregnancy complicated with diabetes mellitus.

Table 38-2 *Timetable: Monitoring Pregnancy Complicated with Diabetes Mellitus*

Assessment	Gestational Age
Out of hospital	
α-Fetoprotein	10 weeks
$Hb_{A_{Ic}}$ (glycosylated hemoglobin)	Weekly
Ultrasound	18 and 28 weeks for fetal growth
Serial urine or serum estriols	Weekly starting at 32 weeks
Nonstress test	Weekly starting at 34 weeks
Amniocentesis (lecithin/sphingomyelin ratio, phosphatidylglycerol)	36 weeks
Repeat amniocentesis for evaluation of lung maturity	If previous test showed immaturity
Hospitalization	
Protracted nausea and vomiting	Anytime for control of condition; at 36 weeks if good glucose/insulin control has not been achieved or if other risk develops
Infection (e.g., urinary tract infection)	
Inadequate diabetic control	

Perinatal Period. Perinatal management focuses on maternal hydration-calorie-insulin balance, adequate fetal perfusion and oxygenation, and prevention of maternal stress. Fetal hypoxia and acidosis can initiate or aggravate respiratory distress syndrome (RDS). Careful assessment of labor identifies a dystotic labor early so that appropriate interventions may be implemented for a safe vaginal or abdominal birth. Infusions given to the mother that contain dextrose require insulin to minimize the risk of fetal postnatal hypoglycemia and hyperbilirubinemia.

Postpartum Period. No single physiologic or biochemical event can explain the diverse clinical manifestions seen in the infants of diabetic mothers (IDMs) or infants of gestational diabetic mothers (IGDMs). For the conditions described previously, and those listed and discussed below the same principles of management pertain, whether they occur in the IDM or any other newborn. These conditions include macrosomia and birth trauma, congenital anomalies, hypoglycemia, hypocalcemia, lung immaturity—RDS, hyperbilirubinemia, hyperviscosity of blood, and cardiomyopathy.

Assessment

The mother's health and obstetric record is reviewed (Chapter 32). Observation and physical examination of the newborn reveals the conditions associated with pregnancies complicated by diabetes mellitus. Appropriate laboratory tests are performed.

Macrosomia

At birth the typical infant who is LGA has a round, cherubic ("tomato" or cushingoid) face, chubby body, and plethoric appearance (Fig. 38-6). This infant is **macrosomic**. The infant has enlarged viscera (hepatosplenomegaly, splanchnomegaly, cardiomegaly) and increased body fat (Fig. 38-7). The placenta and umbilical cord are larger than average. The brain is the only organ that is not enlarged. IDMs may be LGA but physiologically immature.

Insulin has been implicated as the primary growth hormone for intrauterine development. Maternal diabetes results in elevated maternal levels of amino acids and free fatty acids along with hyperglycemia. As the nutrients cross the placenta, the fetal pancreas responds by producing insulin to match the fuel supply. The resulting accelerated protein synthesis, together with a deposition of excessive glycogen and fat stores, is responsible for the typical macrosomic infant. This is the infant most at risk for the neonatal complications of hypoglycemia, hypocalcemia, hyperviscosity, and hyperbilirubinemia. *The excessive amounts of metabolic fuels presented to the fetus from the mother and the consequent fetal hyperinsulinism are now understood to represent the basic pathologic mechanism in the diabetic pregnancy* (Fanaroff and Martin, 1987).

Macrosomia (LGA infants) occurs in about 20% to 40% of class A, B and C diabetic pregnancies. Clinical efforts can only be focused on the control of maternal plasma glucose concentrations. With good prenatal care and control of di-

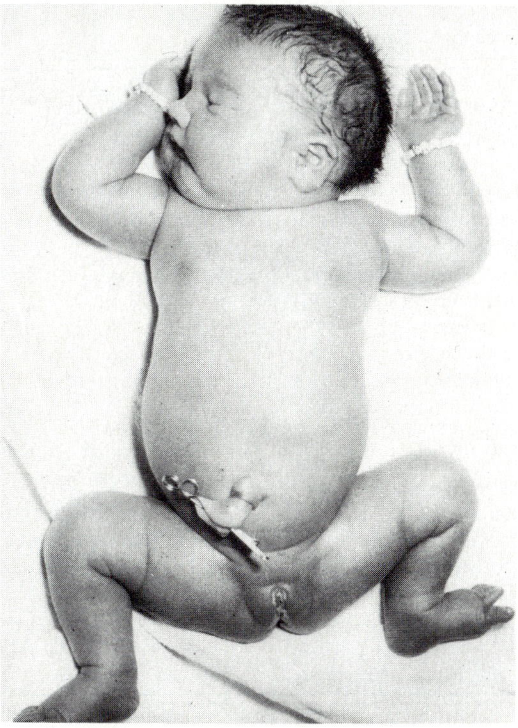

Fig. 38-6 "During their first 24 or more extrauterine hours they lie on their backs, bloated and flushed, their legs flexed and abducted, their tightly closed hands on each side of their head, the abdomen prominent and their respiration sighing. They convey a distinct impression of having had so much food and fluid pressed upon them by an insistent hostess that they desire only peace so that they may recover from their excesses."

From Shirkey, HC, editor: Pediatric therapy, ed 6, St Louis, 1980, The CV Mosby Co, Quotation from Whaley, LF, and Wong, DF: Nursing care of infants and children, ed 3, St Louis, 1987, The CV Mosby Co.

abetes mellitus, the incidence of macrosomia can be decreased.

The excessive size of these infants can and often does lead to dystocia because of fetopelvic disproportion. These infants, who may be born vaginally or by cesarean delivery after a trial of labor, may incur birth trauma.

Birth Trauma and Perinatal Asphyxia

Birth injury (secondary to macrosomia or to method of delivery) and perinatal asphyxia occur in 20% of IGDMs and 35% of IDMs. Examples of birth trauma include cephalhematoma; paralysis of the facial nerve (seventh cranial nerve) (Fig. 38-5); fracture of the clavicle or humerus (Fig. 38-7); brachial plexus paralysis, usually Erb-Duchenne (upper right arm) paralysis; and phrenic nerve paralysis, invariably associated with diaphragmatic paralysis. (See general nursing care plan, p. 966.)

Congenital Anomalies

Congenital anomalies occur in about 6% of IDMs.* Their incidence is two to four times that for normal controls. The incidence is greatest among the small for gestational age (SGA) newborns. IUGR leading to SGA infants is seen in infants of diabetic mothers with severe vascular disease. The most commonly occurring anomalies include CNS—anencephaly, encephalocele, meningomyelocele, hydrocephalus; caudal regression syndrome (CRS)—sacral agenesis with weakness or deformities of the lower extremities, malformation and fixation of the hip joints, and shortening or deformity of the femurs (Fig. 38-8); tracheoesophageal

*It has also been postulated that the mechanisms by which glucose causes teratogenic effects is mediated by a functional deficiency of arachidonic acid or *myo*-inositol at a critical period of organ differentiation (Fanaroff and Martin, 1987).

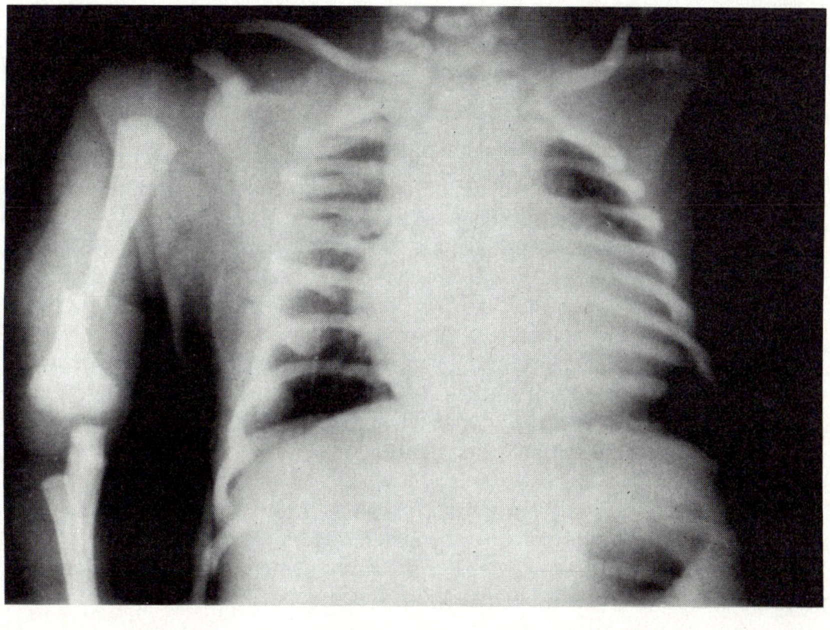

Fig. 38-7 Chest roentgenogram of a vaginally delivered full-term infant (4.7 kg) of a diabetic mother. Note cardiomegaly, hepatomegaly, congested lung fields, and fractures of the right humerus and left clavicle.

From Fanaroff, AA, and Martin, RJ, editors: Behrman's neonatal-perinatal medicine, ed 4, St Louis, 1987, The CV Mosby Co.

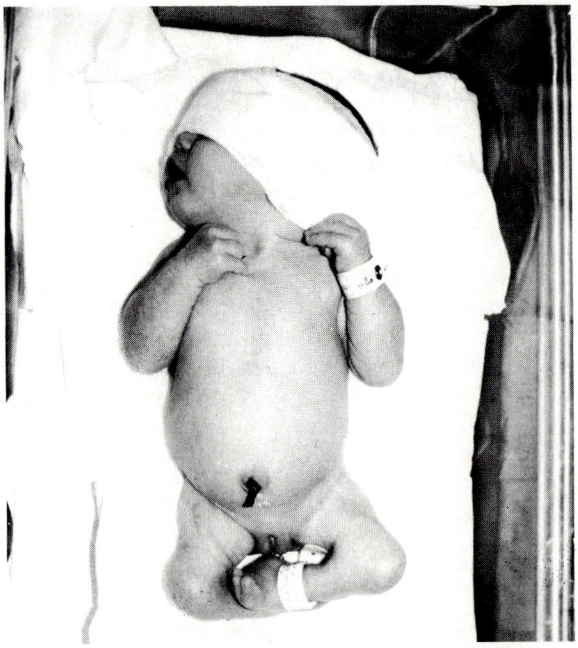

Fig. 38-8 Infant of diabetic mother with caudal regression syndrome (sacral agenesis).
From Fanaroff, AA, and Martin, RJ, editors: Neonatal-perinatal medicine: diseases of the fetus and infant, ed 4, St Louis, 1987, The CV Mosby Co.

Table 38-3 *Cardiomyopathy*

Hypertrophic Cardiomyopathy (HCM)	Nonhypertrophic Cardiomyopathy (NHCM)
Diagnostic echocardiogram:	**Diagnostic echocardiogram:**
Myocardium is hypercontractile	Myocardium is poorly contractile.
Myocardium (right ventricle and interventricular wall) is thickened	Myocardium is overstretched.
Decrease in size of ventricles	Increase in size of ventricles.
Outflow tract obstruction (poorly functioning mitral valve)	No outflow obstruction.
Treatment:	**Treatment:**
Medication: β-adrenergic blocker (e.g., propranolol to **decrease** contractility and heart rate)	Medication: cardiotonic (e.g., digoxin to **increase** contractility and **decrease** heart rate)
	Therapy for hypoglycemia/hypocalcemia and polycythemia

fistula; and congenital heart malformations or cardiomyopathy. Hypertrichosis on the pinnae has recently been added to the list of characteristic clinical features (Fanaroff and Martin, 1987).

Neonatal small left colon syndrome occurs in some IDMs and IGDMs. Neonatal small left colon syndrome is suspected when failure to pass meconium, abdominal distension, and bile-stained vomitus are noted. Contrast enemas show a markedly diminished caliber of the left colon from the splenic flexure. The syndrome is transient (Fanaroff and Martin, 1987).

Cardiomyopathy

The incidence of congenital heart lesions in these infants is five times higher than in the general population. Other lesions include transposition of the aorta and pulmonary artery, ventricular septal defects, and coarctation of the aorta. Maternal diabetic control is correlated with the incidence of lesions. Poor control is defined as maternal blood glucose greater than 300 mg/dl with glycosuria, ketonuria, or occasional ketoacidosis. Good control is defined as the maintenance of maternal blood glucose between 100 mg and 120 mg/dl. Careful diabetic management, especially in the second and third trimesters, decreases the severity of these lesions.

All IDMs need careful observation for cardiomyopathy; 50% of IDMs have cardiomegaly or congestive heart failure within 7 days of birth. Two types of cardiomyopathy are contrasted here. Clinicians must be alert to correctly identify the type of lesion so that appropriate therapy is instituted. Both types are associated with respiratory symptoms and congestive heart failure (Fanaroff and Martin, 1987). Hypertrophic cardiomyopathy (HCM) and nonhypertrophic cardiomyopathy (NHCM) are contrasted in Table 38-3 (Fanaroff and Martin, 1987; Gutgesell et al., 1980). The abnormality usually resolves in 3 to 12 months.

Hypoglycemia and Hypocalcemia

In hypoglycemia and hypocalcemia, separation of the placenta suddenly interrupts the constant infusion of glucose. The high level of circulating glucose at the time the umbilical cord is severed falls rapidly in the presence of fetal hyperinsulinism. *Asymptomatic* or symptomatic hypoglycemia occurs within the first 1 to 3 hours after birth. Hypocalcemia occurs in 30% of IDMs. In addition, hypocalcemia is associated with preterm delivery, birth trauma, and perinatal asphyxia. Symptoms of hypocalcemia, a prevalent finding in IDMs and IGDMs, are similar to those of hypoglycemia, but they occur between 24 and 36 hours of age. However, hypocalcemia must be considered if therapy for hypoglycemia is ineffective.

Jitteriness is one symptom of hypoglycemia and of hypocalcemia (Table 39-1). In many infants jitteriness remains despite therapy and cannot be explained by hypoglycemia or hypocalcemia (Fanaroff and Martin, 1987) (see box, p. 965, and general nursing care plan, p. 966).

Respiratory Difficulty

IDMs or IGDMs manifest a greater incidence of RDS than is found in normal infants of comparable gestational age. Synthesis of surfactant may be delayed because of the high fetal serum level of insulin (Philip, 1987). Fetal lung maturity as evidenced by a L/S ratio of 2 to 1 *is not reassuring* if the mother has diabetes mellitus or gestation-induced diabetes mellitus. For the infants of such mothers, an L/S ratio of 3 to 1 or more or the presence of **phosphatidylglycerol** in the amniotic fluid is more indicative of adequate lung maturity.

Respiratory distress without RDS also occurs. Transient tachypnea or "wet lung" syndrome is a cause of respiratory distress (Fanaroff and Martin, 1987; Pernoll, Benda, and Babson, 1986).

Hyperbilirubinemia

Hyperbilirubinemia develops in 50% of newborns of 32 to 34 weeks' gestation, and 15% of infants born at 37 weeks' gestation manifest this condition. Many newborns are plethoric because of polycythemia. *Polycythemia* increases blood viscosity, thereby impairing circulation. In addition, this increased number of red blood cells to be hemolyzed increases the potential bilirubin load that the newborn must clear. The excessive red blood cells are produced in extramedullary foci (liver and spleen) in addition to the usual sites in bone marrow. Therefore both liver function and bilirubin clearance may be adversely affected.

SUMMARY OF NURSING CARE OF INFANT WITH HYPOCALCEMIA, HYPOGLYCEMIA, OR SEPSIS

GOALS	RESPONSIBILITIES
Recognize early signs of pathophysiologic state	Assess each system for signs and symptoms suggestive of each condition; correlate findings with general impression of progress of infant (feeding, weight gain, response to stimuli, and sleeping patterns).
Prevent or decrease potential side effects of medical intervention	
Hypocalcemia	Administer calcium gluconate slowly; if heart rate falls below 100 beats per min, stop infusion. Prevent extravasation of calcium gluconate into tissues: Avoid scalp vein. Ensure placement of needle before administering drug. Tape needle securely at site of insertion. Apply pressure to puncture site after removal of needle. Counsel mother regarding infant feeding (breast-feeding or appropriate formulas).
Hypoglycemia	Begin oral feeding as soon as possible after birth. Administer glucose infusion carefully; avoid overloading the system by speeding up intravenous administration. Observe for signs of hyperglycemia (acidosis) and possible need for insulin. Decrease intravenous administration of glucose slowly to avoid hypoglycemia from physiologic hyperinsulinemia.
Sepsis	Observe for side effects of antibiotics. Regulate infusion carefully to allow for antibiotic to be administered within 1 hour. Use piggyback setup if main intravenous solution has added drugs.
Monitor environment to decrease factors that will complicate recovery from each condition	Maintain thermoregulation, hydration, and oxygenation of infant. Monitor vital signs and correlate with infant's progress.
Hypocalcemia	Reduce environmental stimuli. Organize care to ensure minimum handling of infant. Discuss with parents reasons for minimum holding. Institute seizure precautions.
Sepsis	Institute appropriate isolation techniques.
Observe for complications of disease	
Hypocalcemia	Observe for tetany and convulsions (Table 39-1).
Hypoglycemia	Check heel blood with Dextrostix. Check urine for glycosuria.
Sepsis	Observe for signs of meningitis, especially bulging anterior fontanel. Observe for pyarthrosis, usually evidenced by limited movement of affected joint. Observe for signs of shock, expecially fall in blood pressure.
Provide emotional support for parents	Allow parents the opportunity to express their feelings. Keep parents informed of infant's progress. Encourage frequent visiting and participation in care to foster parent-child attachment.

From Whaley, LF, and Wong, DL: Nursing care of infants and children, ed 3, St Louis, 1987, The CV Mosby Co.

Nursing Diagnoses

Following are examples of nursing diagnoses:

Newborn

- Potential for injury related to
  - Metabolic effects of maternal condition
  - Hypoglycemia, hypocalcemia, hyperbilirubinemia, hyperviscosity of blood
  - Birth trauma
- Potential for ineffective gas exchange related to
  - Lung immaturity
  - Cardiomyopathy
- Ineffective thermoregulation related to
  - Physiologic immaturity
- **Parents/Family**
- Anxiety, fear, or powerlessness related to
  - Uncertainty regarding neonate's prognosis
- Disturbance in self-concept related to
  - Experience of an "abnormal" pregnancy and compromised neonate
- Knowledge deficit related to
  - Neonate's condition, management, and prognosis

Planning

Ideally, planning for the infant of a diabetic mother begins during the antenatal period. Pediatric staff are present at the birth. For each child an individualized plan of care is developed.

Goals. Goals for the infant and family may include:

1. For the newborn: a birth without trauma or injury and a neonatal period without sequelae to trauma or pregnancy complicated by maternal diabetes mellitus.
2. For the family: an understanding of diabetes mellitus or the birth injury and willing compliance with management. If the newborn exhibits a disorder or dies, the grieving process is initiated.

Implementation

Implementation of care depends on the neonate's particular problems. General care of the compromised newborn is addressed in Chapter 36. A general nursing plan for newborns of diabetic mothers follows. Newborns exhibit general versus specific responses to some illnesses. Therefore a summary of nursing care of infants with hypocalcemia, hypoglycemia, or sepsis (Chapter 39) is presented in the box on p. 965.

Evaluation

The nurse can be assured that care has been effective if the goals of care are achieved. Prepregnancy counseling and excellent client collaboration in prenatal care and control of diabetes mellitus result in reduced congenital anomalies and macrosomia; the newborn is AGA, born at term, and suffers no sequelae seen in infants exposed to poorly controlled diabetes mellitus during pregnancy.

General Nursing Care Plan

COMPLICATIONS OF INFANTS OF DIABETIC MOTHERS

ASSESSMENT	NURSING DIAGNOSIS (ND)/ PLAN (P)/GOAL (G)	RATIONALE/ IMPLEMENTATION	EVALUATION
Review prenatal records, especially noting: maternal glucose control, ultrasound results for growth, nonstress test results, amniocentesis (L/S ratio, phosphatidyl-glycerol). Assess infant frequently within the first hours of life for (in order of incidence). Respiratory distress, and congenital anomalies or disorders. Birth trauma (cephalhematoma, paralysis of the facial nerve, fracture of the clavical).	ND: Altered breathing pattern related to lung immaturity as manifested by respiratory distress. ND: Altered breathing pattern related to secretions or meconium in airway after birth. P: Monitor continuously and modify plan of care as data emerge. G: Infant will maintain an open airway and show no signs of respiratory distress.	*To assure maintenance of an open airway, the nurse will:* Note maternal history, especially presence of phosphatidyl-glycerol (if obtained). Have oxygen and resuscitative equipment available. Note and report signs of respiratory distress. Monitor breath sounds every 15 minutes for 6 hours. Position newborn on side, with head slightly lower and neck slightly extended.	Infant maintains an open airway and respiratory distress is prevented or treated quickly. Infant suffers no birth trauma; or, trauma is promptly identified and treated with no adverse sequelae.

General Nursing Care Plan—cont'd

ASSESSMENT	NURSING DIAGNOSIS (ND)/ PLAN (P)/GOAL (G)	RATIONALE/ IMPLEMENTATION	EVALUATION
Meconium aspiration (amniotic fluid is stained, or if skin, nails, or cord is stained). Gestational age, weight (LGA, appropriate for gestational age [AGA], SGA), and degree of maturity (Tables 37-1, 37-2).		Suction neonate's mouth and nose as necessary and report meconium-stained secretions. Report and evaluate any birth trauma or congenital anomaly that might interfere with adequate ventilation. Treat infant as premature, regardless of weight, until gestational age and respiratory maturity are established.	Infant's gestational age is correctly determined and appropriate care is initiated.
Assess tests for **hypoglycemia**: Dextrostix, Clinistix. Procedure 22-1. 30 min of age. 1 ½ hr of age. 4 hr of age. 9 hr of age. 12 hr of age. 24 hr of age. Then once daily for 8 days. Evaluate serum blood glucose levels compared with Dextrostix value. Assess for signs of **hypoglycemia**: Feeding difficulty, hunger. Apnea. Irregular respiratory effort. Cyanosis. Weak, high-pitched cry. Jitteriness, twitching, eye rolling, seizures (Table 39-1). Lethargy	ND: Potential for injury related to hypoglycemia. ND: Altered nutrition: less than body requirements, related to hypoglycemia. P: Monitor closely and follow agency's protocols for care. G: Infant will maintain acceptable blood glucose levels and remain free from signs of hypoglycemia.	*To evaluate for hypoglycemia and prevent its occurrence, the nurse will:* Perform blood glucose test according to schedule. Obtain blood glucose test by laboratory once daily to compare with Dextrostix or if Dextrostix value <30 mg/dl during the first 72 hours of life or <45 mg/dl after first 3 days of life in the full term infant or <20 mg/dl in the preterm infant. Observe and report signs of hypoglycemia. If suck and swallow reflex is intact, feed the infant according to hospital protocol. Feedings should be in small frequent amounts beginning at 1 hour of age. Administer intravenous fluids as ordered if infant unable to feed. Report blood glucose <30 mg/dl; physician may administer 10% glucose in water intravenously.	Newborn suffers no hypoglycemic episodes. Newborn suffers no brain damage from hypoglycemia.
Assess blood levels for hypocalcemia (50% incidence with infants of insulin-dependent mothers). Assess signs of hypocalcemia within first 48 hours (edema, apnea, intermittent cyanosis, and abdominal distension). After 48 hours the classic symptoms of tetany may be noticed.	ND: Potential for injury related to hypocalcemia. P: Monitor closely and follow agency's protocols for care. G: Newborn will maintain acceptable blood calcium levels.	*To monitor calcium levels and treat hypocalcemia, the nurse will:* Obtain blood for serum calcium laboratory test once daily as ordered. Observe and report signs of hypocalcemia. Obtain intravenous access for calcium gluconate 10% solution as ordered (no scalp vein sites).	Newborn suffers no episodes of hypocalcemia. Newborn has no episodes of tetany.

Continued.

General Nursing Care Plan—cont'd

ASSESSMENT	NURSING DIAGNOSIS (ND)/ PLAN (P)/GOAL (G)	RATIONALE/ IMPLEMENTATION	EVALUATION
		Monitor calcium gluconate infusion. If heart rate < 100 beats/minute, discontinue infusion and notify physician. Apply firm pressure to intravenous site when catheter is removed from vein to avoid seepage of the calcium gluconate into surrounding tissues. Reduce environmental stimuli. Observe for (Table 39-1) and take precautions against seizures.	
Assess for polycythemia between 6 and 24 hr of life (if present).		*To assess for polycythemia the nurse will:* Obtain blood for complete blood cell count (CBC) and report results.	
If polycythemia is present, closely monitor for hyperbilirubinemia.		See hyperbilirubinemia care plan in Chapter 40.	
Assess for congenital anomalies or disorders (4% increased risk). Birth trauma (cephalhematoma, paralysis of the facial nerves, fracture of the clavical). Assess parent-newborn interactions. Assess educational needs for child care. See Perinatal Loss Care Plan p. 683.	ND: Knowledge deficit related to care of an IDM. ND: Anxiety, fear, grieving, powerlessness, situational low self-esteem, spiritual distress, ineffective individual or family coping, altered family processes—related to having, and caring for a child with a birth defect. P: Monitor closely and institute appropriate care (Chapter 40); be available to parents for discussion of questions; demonstrate care and observe return demonstration. G: Parents will verbalize understanding of the explained congenital anomalies or birth trauma and their effects or complications to the child's well being. G: Parents will verbalize feelings and concerns regarding their infant.	*To aid parents in adjusting to and caring for a child with an anomaly or transient birth injury, the nurse will:* Note and report congenital anomalies or birth trauma. Weigh newborn soon after delivery, then daily. Measure head and chest circumference. Explain all procedures to parents. Explain congenital anomalies or birth trauma and their effects on child. Answer questions and correct misconceptions. Encourage open communication. Demonstrate child care activities. Observe parent-infant interactions. Schedule appointments for lab studies and follow-up physical exam. Refer to outside resources (child care, homemaker, clergy, home health).	Parents verbalize understanding of instructions. Parents express feelings and concerns about their infant. If child has an anomaly or dies, parents experience appropriate grief response. Parents learn how to care for their child.

SUMMARY

Infants with birth injuries have a unique set of needs and problems. Primary nursing responsibility lies in assisting with the early identification of an injury. Implementation of care is based on the medical management and on the learning needs of parents and family members.

Perinatal mortality has improved presumably as a result of early identification and good control of diabetes, coupled with birth at or near term. Detection of excessive size and fetal monitoring during labor should lead to prevention of birth trauma and fetal asphyxia. Postneonatal mortality is higher than in normal controls, primarily because of an increased proportion of IDMs with congenital anomalies who survive the newborn period. Major determinants of poor outcome are poor diabetic control, early onset of diabetes and vascular complications, low birth weight and prematurity, and perinatal complications. Neurologic and developmental outcomes of IDMs are indefinite because of the lack of large prospective studies and because most studies do not encompass the period of improved antenatal, intrapartum, and neonatal management of the last decade. It is expected that future prospective studies will continue to demonstrate improved perinatal outcome, as well as improved quality of survival.

In addition to the areas discussed in this chapter, the care provider must also remember that the newborn belongs to a family that also has many needs.

KEY CONCEPTS

- A small percentage of significant birth injuries may be unavoidable and occur despite skilled and competent obstetric care.
- The same birth injury may be caused in several ways.
- Birth injuries range from those that are minor and resolve without treatment to those few that are serious enough to result in death.
- The nurse's primary contribution to the welfare of the newborn begins with early observation, accurate recording, and prompt reporting of signs indicative of deviations from normal.
- Metabolic abnormalities of diabetes mellitus in pregnancy adversely affect embryonic and fetal development.
- Prepregnancy planning and good diabetic control coupled with tight diabetic control during pregnancy may prevent the embryonic/fetal/neonatal conditions associated with pregnancies complicated by diabetes mellitus.
- Regardless of the infant's disorder or condition, the care provider must also remember that the newborn belongs to a family that also has many needs.

STUDY QUESTIONS AND ACTIVITIES

1. Assist with (or observe) the care of a compromised infant in the special care nursery. Identify the infant's physical characteristics. Observe the interactions of the parents and infant and describe the developmental task the parents are experiencing. In a group setting, develop a nursing care plan for the infant and her or his family.
2. Review and practice skills of assessment (e.g., physical examination, heel stick) that are necessary to identify the infant at risk.
3. Review and discuss the medical and nursing records of infants who experienced birth injury or whose mothers experienced a diabetic pregnancy. Identify the findings that identified the particular risk(s) to the infants. Discuss the nursing and medical management of the infants. Compare with text.

References

Birth Trauma

Chen, TH, et al: Subcutaneous fat necrosis of the newborn, Arch Dermatol 117:36, 1981

Cyr, RM, Usher, RH, and McLean, FH: Changing patterns of birth asphyxia and trauma over 20 years, Am J Obstet Gynecol 148:490, 1983

Eisenberg, D, Kirchner, SG, and Perrin, EC: Neonatal skull depression unassociated with birth trauma, AJR 143:1063, 1984

Fanaroff, AA, and Martin, RJ, editors: Neonatal-perinatal medicine: diseases of the fetus and infant, ed 4, St Louis, 1987, The CV Mosby Co

French, CE, and Waldstein, G: Subcapsular hemorrhage of the liver in the newborn, Pediatrics 69:204, 1982

Hebertson, RM, et al: Obstetric forceps pad designed to reduce infant trauma, Obstet Gynecol 65:275, 1985

Merenstein, GB, and Gardner, SL: Handbook of neonatal intensive care, St Louis, 1985, The CV Mosby Co

Infants of Diabetic Mothers

Fanaroff, AA, and Martin RJ, editors: Neonatal-perinatal medicine: diseases of the fetus and infant, ed 4, St Louis, 1987, The CV Mosby Co

Fuhrmann, D, et al: Prevention of congenital malformations in infants of insulin-dependent mothers, Diabetes Care 6:219, 1983

Gutgesell, HP, et al: Characterization of the cardiomyopathy in infants of diabetic mothers, Circulation 61:441, 1980

Pernoll, ML, Benda, GI, and Babson, SG: Diagnosis and management of the fetus and neonate at risk: a guide for team care, ed 5, St Louis, 1986, The CV Mosby Co

Bibliography

Birth Injuries

Bayne, O, and Rang, M: Medial dislocation of the radial head following breech delivery: a case report and review of the literature, J Pediatr Orthop 4:485, 1984

Bell, HJ, and Dykstra, DD: Somatosensory evoked potentials as an adjunct to diagnosis of neonatal spinal cord injury, J Pediatr 106:298, 1985

Cohen, AW, and Otto, SR: Obstetric clavicular fractures: a three-year analysis, J Reprod Med 25:119, Sept 1980
Cumming, WA: Neonatal skeletal fractures, birth trauma or child abuse? J Can Assoc Radiol 30:30, March 1979
Franck, LS: A national survey of the assessment and treatment of pain and agitation in the neonatal intensive care unit, JOGN Nurs 16(6):384, 1987
Garza-Mercado, R: Intrauterine depressed skull fractures of the newborn, Neurosurgery 10:694, 1982
Greenwald, AG, Schute, PC, and Shiveley, JL: Brachial plexus birth palsy: a 10-year report on the incidence and prognosis, J Pediatr Orthop 4:689, 1984
Gresham, EL: Birth trauma, Pediatr Clin North Am 22(2):317, 1975
Ingardia, CJ, and Cetrulo, CL: Forceps—use and abuse, Clin Perinatol 8:63, Feb 1981
Jain, IS, et al: Ocular hazards during birth, J Pediatr Ophthalmol Strabismus 17:14, Jan/Feb 1980
Korones, SB: High-risk newborn infants: the basis for intensive nursing care, ed 4, St Louis, 1986, The CV Mosby Co
Philip, AG, et al: Neonatal mortality risk for the eighties: the importance of birth weight/gestational age groups, Pediatrics 68:122, 1981
Wegman, ME: Annual summary of vital statistics—1984, Pediatrics 76:861, 1985
Whaley, LF, and Wong, DL: Nursing care of infants and children, ed 3, St Louis, 1987, The CV Mosby Co
Zelson, C, Lee, SJ, and Pearl, M: The incidence of skull fractures underlying cephalhematomas in newborn infants, J Pediatr 85:371, 1974.

Infants of Diabetic Mothers

Baker, L, et al: Diabetic embryopathy: mechanism involves myo-inositol and arachidonic acid (abstr) Pediatr Res 20:326A, 1986
Bohart, RD, et al: Continuous insulin infusion during the peripartum period; maternal and neonatal outcome, J Calif Perinat Assoc 2(1):26, 1982
Collins, JE, and Leonard, JV: Hyperinsulinism in asphyxiated and small-for-dates infants with hypoglycaemia, Lancet 2:311, 1984
Coustan, DR, and Carpenter, MW: Detection and treatment of gestational diabetes, Clin Obstet Gynecol 28:507, Sept 1985
Cowett, RM: Mechanism(s) of glucose disequilibrium in perinatal hypoxia, Pediatr Res 20:408A, 1986
Cowett, RM, and Schwartz, R: The infant of the diabetic mother, Pediatr Clin North Am 29:1213, 1982
Cowett, RM, Susa, JB, Giletti, B, et al: Glucose kinetics in infants of diabetic mothers, Am J Obstet Gynecol 146:781, 1983
Elseweidy, MM, Fadel, HE, and Abraham, EC: Glycosilated hemoglobin and plasma protein in newborns of normal and diabetic women, Pediatr Res 18:767, 1984
Feldman, F, et al: Glycosilated fetal hemoglobin: correlation with hyperglycemia and birth weight in infants of diabetic mothers, Diabetes 33:81, 1984
Golde, S, and Platt, L: Antepartum testing in diabetes, Clin Obstet Gynecol 28:516, Sept 1985
Grabauskas, P, et al: Helping the parents after a baby's death, RN, p 31, Aug 1987
Halliday, HL: Hypertrophic cardiomyopathy in infants of poorly-controlled diabetic mothers, Arch Dis Child 56:258, 1981
Hare, JW: Diabetes control to reduce congenital malformations, Contemp OB/GYN 20:(2):85, 1982
Hay, WW, and Sparks, JW: Placental, fetal and neonatal carbohydrate metabolism, Clin Obstet Gynecol 28:473, 1985
Kemp, VH, and Page, CK: The psychosocial impact of a high-risk pregnancy on the family, JOGN Nurs 15(3):232, 1986
Knight, G, Worth, RC, and Ward, JD: Macrosomy despite a well-controlled diabetic pregnancy (Letter), Lancet 2:1431, 1983
Korones, SB: High-risk newborn infants: the basis for intensive nursing care, ed 4, St Louis, 1986, The CV Mosby Co
Lagerlof, JM: Nurses and ethics, Calif Nurs Rev 9(5):12, 1987
McFadden, EA, Zaloga, GP, and Chernow, B: Hypocalcemia: a medical emergency, Am J Nurs 83:227, 1983
Merenstein, GB, and Gardner, SL: Handbook of neonatal intensive care, St Louis, 1985, The CV Mosby Co
Miller, E, Hare, JW, Cloherty, JP, et al: Elevated maternal hemoglobin A_{IC} in early pregnancy and major congenital anomalies in infants of diabetic mothers, N Engl J Med 304:1331, 1981
Mills, JL, et al: Lack of relation of increased malformation rates in infants of diabetic mothers to glycemic control during organogenesis, N Engl J Med 318(11):671, 1988
Morriss, FH, Jr: Infants of diabetic mothers: fetal and neonatal pathophysiology, Perspect Pediatr Pathol 8:223, 1984
Neave, C: Congenital malformation in offspring of diabetics, Perspect Pediatr Pathol 8:213, 1984
Nurses Association of the American College of Ostetricians and Gynecologists: Care of the infant of the diabetic mother, NAACOG Tech Bull, No 11, Sept 1981
Oh, W: Heading off problems in the diabetic's baby, Contemp OB/GYN, 19:91, 1982
Ouimette, J: Perinatal nursing: care of the high-risk mother and infant, Boston, 1986, Jones & Bartlett Publishers, Inc
Pedersen, JF, and Pedersen, LM: Early growth delay predisposes the fetus in diabetic pregnancy to congenital malformation, Lancet 1:737, 1982
Perlman, RH: The infant of the diabetic mother: pathophysiology and management, Prim Care 10:751, 1983
Perrine, SP, Greene, MF, and Faller, DV: Delay in the fetal globin switch in infants of diabetic mothers, N Engl J Med 312:334, 1985
Philip, AG: Neonatology: a practical guide, ed 3, Philadelphia, 1987, WB Saunders Co
Philip, AG, et al: Neonatal mortality risk for the eighties: the importance of birth weight/gestational age groups, Pediatrics 68:122, 1981
Plauche, WC, et al: Phosphatidylglycerol and lung maturity, Am J Obstet Gynecol 144:167, 1982
Queenan, JT: Managing polyhydramnios, Contemp OB/GYN 22:17, Aug 1983
Riblett, B: Insuring a safe pregnancy for your diabetic patient, RN 46(2):50, 1983
Sadler, ME: When your patient's baby dies before birth, RN, p 28, Aug 1987
Sexson, WR: Incidence of neonatal hypoglycemia: a matter of definition, J Pediatr 105(1):149, 1984
Srinivasan, G, et al: Plasma glucose values in normal neonates: a new look, J Pediatr 109:114, 1986
Teramo, K, and Hallman, M: Ways to head off RDS in diabetics/neonates, Contemp OB/GYN 21(6):127, 1983
Troy, P, et al: Sibling visiting in the NICU, Am J Nurs 88(1):68, 1988
Warram, JH, et al: Differences in risk of insulin-dependent diabetes in offspring of diabetic fathers, N Engl J Med 311:149, 1984
Whaley, LF, and Wong, DL: Nursing care of infants and children, ed 3, St Louis, 1987, The CV Mosby Co
Zeller, WP, Susa, JB, Widness, JA, et al: Glycosylation of hemoglobin in normal and diabetic mothers and their fetuses, Pediatr Res 17:200, 1983

CHAPTER

39

Infection and Drug Dependence

Learning Objectives

Correctly define the key terms listed.

List modes of transmission of pathogens.

Describe in detail the assessment of a newborn for infection.

Formulate nursing diagnoses for the infant and family for each type of infection.

Review implementation and evaluation of care of affected infants and their families.

Describe the care of the newborn with human immunodeficiency virus (HIV) infection.

Relate the assessment of a newborn for drug dependence.

Summarize general nursing care of the drug-dependent newborn.

Assess the effects of alcohol, heroin, methadone, marijuana, cocaine, phencyclidine, and smoking on the fetus and newborn.

Develop a care plan for the drug-dependent newborn and family.

Key Terms

AIDS dysmorphia syndrome
congenital rubella syndrome
fetal alcohol syndrome
fetal tobacco syndrome
focal infection
jitteriness
meningitis
mode of transmission
nosocomial infection
opportunistic infection
seizure
sepsis/septicemia
septic shock
thrush
TORCH infection
withdrawal syndrome

Sepsis continues to be one of the most significant causes of fetal wastage and neonatal morbidity and mortality. The newborn infant is uniquely susceptible to infection. Maternal immunoglobulin IgM does not cross the placenta. IgA and IgM require time to reach optimum levels after birth. Phagocytosis is less efficient. Serum complement levels are inadequate. Serum complement (C1 through C6) is involved in immunologic reactions (Table 6-10), some of which kill or lyse bacteria and enhance phagocytosis. Dysmaturity seen with intrauterine growth retardation (IUGR) and preterm and postterm birth further compromises the neonate's immune system. Special precautions for preventing infection, as well as prompt recognition when it occurs, are necessary for optimum management of the newborn.

Perinatal risk is also created by certain maternal behaviors. Maternal habits hazardous to the fetus and neonate are drug addiction, smoking, and alcohol abuse. Occasional withdrawal reactions have been reported in newborn infants of mothers who use to excess such drugs as barbiturates, alcohol, or amphetamines. Serious reactions are seen in newborns whose mothers abuse psychoactive drugs (Chapter 34) or are treated with methadone. Almost 50% of pregnancies of women addicted to opioids result in low-birth-weight (LBW) infants who are not necessarily preterm. Alcohol is a teratogen. Maternal ethanol abuse during gestation creates a readily identifiable fetal alcohol syndrome (FAS).

This chapter focuses on infection and substance abuse that place the fetus or neonate at risk.

INFECTION

Infections occur when a susceptible host comes in contact with a potentially pathogenic organism. When the organism proliferates and overcomes the host's defenses, infection results (Merenstein and Gardner, 1985).

Modes of Transmission

Newborn infections may be acquired in utero, during delivery, during resuscitation, and from within the nursery (Pernoll, Benda, and Babson, 1986; Fanaroff and Martin, 1987). Prenatal acquisition occurs by organisms placentally transferred directly into the fetal circulatory system and from infected amniotic fluid (e.g., herpes simplex virus [HSV], cytomegalovirus [CMV], rubella). Microorganisms ascend from the vagina and pass through the cervix. The membranes become infected and possibly rupture. Infection of the fetal skin and respiratory or gastrointestinal tract may result.

During delivery contact of the infant with an infected birth canal can result in generalized or local infection. The upper airway and gastrointestinal tract are again the principal pathways for generalized infections. The conjunctiva and oral cavity are the usual sites of local infection.

Postnatal infection may be acquired during resuscitation, usually from contamination of indwelling catheters or endotracheal tubes. Nursery-acquired infections may be transferred to the infant by hands of personnel or spread from contaminated equipment. The umbilicus is a receptive site for cutaneous infection leading to sepsis (Pernoll, Benda, and Babson, 1986; Fanaroff and Martin, 1987).

Certain pathogens have a predilection for the fetus. They may cause abortion, stillbirth, intrauterine infection, congenital malformations and acute disease. These pathogens may also cause chronic infection, with subtle manifestations that may be recognized only after a prolonged period. It is important to recognize the manifestations of infections in the neonatal period not only to treat the acute infection but also to anticipate the potential implication for the subsequent growth and development of the infant.

Scope of the Problem

Septicemia refers to a generalized infection in the blood stream. Septicemia, a common type of sepsis, affects between 1 in 500 to 1 in 1600 newborns. Pneumonia is the most common form of neonatal infection and one of the most important causes of perinatal death (Fanaroff and Martin, 1987). Bacterial meningitis affects one in 2500 live born infants. Gastroenteritis is sporadic, depending on epidemic outbreaks. Local infections such as conjunctivitis and omphalitis occur commonly but incidence rates are unavailable. Incidence rates of specific infections are given in the text when available. Infection continues to be a significant factor in fetal and neonatal morbidity and mortality.

Assessment

The *prenatal record* is reviewed for risk factors associated with and signs and symptoms suggestive of infection. Maternal vaginal or perineal infection may be transmitted directly to the infant during passage through the birth canal. Psychosocial history and history of sexually transmitted diseases (STDs) may strongly suggest possible acquired immune deficiency syndrome, (AIDS),* hepatitis B, or CMV infection.

The *perinatal events* are also reviewed. Premature rupture of membranes (PROM) may be secondary to maternal or intrauterine infection. Ascending infection may occur after prolonged rupture of membranes, prolonged labor, or intrauterine fetal monitoring. Resuscitation requiring intubation and deep suctioning may result in infection. The newborn's gestational age, maturity, birth weight, and gender all affect the incidence of infection. Sepsis occurs about twice as often in boys as in girls and results in a higher mortality in boys. The newborn is assessed for skin abscesses, rashes, cellulitis, and other indications of infection.

During the *postnatal period* the time of onset of suspicious signs is noted. Onset within the first 48 hours of life is more commonly associated with prenatal or perinatal predisposing factors. Onset after 2 or 3 days more commonly reflects disease acquired at or subsequent to delivery (Fanaroff and Martin, 1987).

The earliest clinical signs of neonatal sepsis are characterized by a lack of specificity. The nonspecific signs include lethargy, poor feeding, poor weight gain, or irritability. Or, the nurse or parent may also simply note that the

*The term "AIDS" is obsolete. "HIV infection" more correctly defines the problem.

infant is just not doing as well as before. Differential diagnosis may be confounded because of the similarity of signs of sepsis to noninfectious neonatal problems such as anemia or hypoglycemia (see box, p. 965). Additional clinical and laboratory information and appropriate cultures supplement the findings described.

Primary or secondary involvement of any organ system adds to the clinical signs. Hypothermia is as common as hyperthermia (fever) in response to infection. Tachypnea or apnea, cyanosis, tachycardia or bradycardia, and hypotension may be noted. Focal neurologic signs, tremors, seizures, or a full fontanel are seen in septic newborns even without meningitis. Other signs may be vomiting, abdominal distension, diarrhea, jaundice, pallor, or petechia. Jaundice occurs within the first 24 hours in the absence of hemolytic disease. Hemorrhage may be an associated sign in sepsis, which may be preceded or accompanied by focal infections such as omphalitis or conjunctivitis, or skin abscesses.

Laboratory studies are performed. Specimens for cultures include samples of blood, umbilical stump, naso-oropharynx, ear canals, skin, cerebrospinal fluid (CSF), stool, and urine. Increased direct (conjugated) bilirubin levels may be found, especially if the infecting microorganism is gram negative. Blood studies are performed to determine the presence of anemia, increased white blood cell count (WBC), or decreased red blood cell count (RBC) (an ominous sign). C-reactive protein may or may not be elevated (Table 6-10).

Vigilant assessment (e.g., parenteral fluid infusion) continues during and after treatment (Chapter 36). The newborn continues to be assessed for sequelae to septicemia.

Before the advent of antibiotics, 90% of newborns with sepsis died. Antibiotic therapy decreased mortality to between 13% and 45% depending on the causative organism.

Sequelae to septicemia include meningitis, pyarthrosis, and septic shock. **Meningitis**, a common sequela, may be evidenced by a bulging anterior fontanel (see discussion of signs of increased intracranial pressure, p. 960). Systemic antibiotics may not diffuse into CSF. Intrathecal infusion of a drug such as polymyxin may be initiated.

Pyarthrosis, which may affect any joint, usually localizes in the hips. Limitation in joint movement is one of the few signs of this condition.

Septic shock results from the toxins released into the bloodstream. The most common sign is a drop in blood pressure—a vital sign commonly overlooked in the care of the newborn. Other signs are rapid, irregular respirations and pulse (similar to septicemia in general).

Nursing Diagnoses

Any number of nursing diagnoses are possible depending on the infant's gestational age and birth weight, the organ systems involved, and the nature of the infection. Following are examples of nursing diagnoses:

Newborn

- Potential for infection related to
  - Need for resuscitation or inhalation therapy
  - Need for indwelling umbilical catheters, total parenteral nutrition (TPN), parenteral fluids
  - Intrauterine electronic fetal monitoring
  - Male gender
  - Dysmaturity, IUGR, gestational age
- Ineffective thermoregulation related to
  - Infection
- Impaired tissue integrity related to
  - Need for multiple supportive measures (e.g., biometric monitoring, TPN, inhalation therapy)
- Pain related to
  - Need for multiple supportive measures

Parents/Family

- Anxiety, fear, or anticipatory grieving related to
  - Uncertainty about child's prognosis
- Potential altered parenting related to
  - Feelings of inadequacy in caring for the child
- Powerlessness or spiritual distress related to
  - Perinatal events or newborn infant's condition
- Knowledge deficit related to
  - Newborn's condition, its course, and management

Planning

Planning begins with the development of standards for preventive measures in nurseries and protocols for diagnosis and treatment of infections. Individual assessment findings are utilized to plan care for each infant. Parents and family are encouraged to participate in planning.

Goals

1. Sepsis is prevented
2. Early signs of sepsis are recognized, and appropriate therapy is instituted
3. If therapy is necessary, no harmful sequelae result
4. Pathophysiologic sequelae to septicemia are avoided
5. Parents are able to form attachment to newborn
6. Parents' self-esteem is maintained
7. Staff establishes caring relationship with parents to foster their trust and to encourage continuing, active, positive interactions of family with members of health care system

Implementation

Preventive Measures

Virtually all controlled clinical trials have demonstrated that effective **handwashing** is responsible for the prevention of nosocomial infection in nursery units (Fanaroff and Martin, 1987). Nursing is directly or indirectly responsible for minimizing or eliminating environmental sources of infectious agents in the nursery. Measures to be taken include careful and thorough cleaning, frequent replacement of used equipment (e.g., changing intravenous tubing per hospital protocol, cleaning resuscitation and ventilation equipment), and disposal of excrement and linens in an appropriate manner. Overcrowding must be avoided in nurseries.

Skin Care. The skin, its secretions, and normal flora are natural defense mechanisms that protect against invading pathogens. The American Academy of Pediatrics (1983) supports a dry cleansing technique. The benefits of this approach are reduction of heat loss by exposure, decrease in skin trauma, limitation of exposure to agents with unknown toxicity, and reduction in nursing time. Initial cleansing is delayed until the newborn's temperature has stabilized. Sterile cotton sponges and sterile water or a mild nonmedicated soap are used to remove blood from the infant's face and head and meconium from the perineal area. The rest of the body is not cleansed unless a part is grossly soiled. The vernix caseosa is left in place. No single method of cord care has been shown to prevent colonization and subsequent disease. Alcohol, triple dye, or an antimicrobial agent is applied locally (Fanaroff and Martin, 1987; Merenstein and Gardner, 1985).

Curative Measures

Breast-feeding or feeding the newborn breast milk from the mother is encouraged. Protective mechanisms exist in breast milk. Colostrum contains agglutinins that are active against gram-negative bacteria. Human milk contains iron-binding protein that exerts a bacteriostatic effect on *Escherichia coli.* Human milk also contains macrophages and lymphocytes. The vulnerability of infants to common mucosal pathogens such as respiratory syncytial virus (RSV) may be reduced by passive transfer of maternal immunity in colostrum and breast milk. See Chapter 23 for assisting mothers with breast-feeding, maintenance of lactation until the newborn can breast-feed, and expression and storage of breast milk.

The mother's knowledge of the importance of her breast milk for the compromised newborn and her active involvement in this aspect of care benefits her in several ways as well. Bonding with the infant is facilitated. Self-concept and self-esteem are enhanced. Coping skills may be strengthened; if the infant succumbs, the mother's healthy grieving may be facilitated. If the mother cannot breast-feed or provide breast milk, the nurse provides support during the mother's bottle-feeding or other activity with the infant. The parents' activity with the infant is supported and appropriately guided and praised to achieve the benefits desired.

Emphasis is placed on following reliable surveillance to identify infection in newborns so that prompt isolation and appropriate therapy is instituted.

Eye and umbilical cord prophylaxis is discussed in Chapter 22. Monitoring intravenous infusion rate and administering antibiotics are the nurse's responsibility. It is important to administer the prescribed dose of antibiotic within 1 hour after it is prepared to avoid loss of drug stability. If the intravenous fluid the infant is receiving contains electrolytes, vitamins, or other medications, *do not* add antibiotics. The antibiotic (or other medication) may be deactivated or may form a precipitate. Instead, piggyback another bottle of the prescribed fluid to be infused and attach its tubing with a three-way stopcock to the needle at the infusion site. Remember to include the number of milliliters of fluid used from the piggyback bottle when calculating the newborn's intake.

Care must be taken when suctioning secretions from the newborn's oropharynx or trachea. These secretions may be infected. Clinicians who use mouth-suction-activated devices are potentially at risk for getting some of these secretions in their own mouths. Though no cases of virus transmission via this route have been documented, enough concern exists to make it seem prudent to use wall or bulb suction devices.

Isolation procedures are implemented according to hospital policy as indicated. See box for reminders about preventing the spread of infection. See Chapter 30 for universal precautions. The reader is reminded that changes in isolation protocols are occuring rapidly. Continuing education and inservices are suggested for the nurse to remain

REMINDERS: PREVENTION OF SPREAD OF INFECTION

CARE OF SPECIMENS AFTER COLLECTION

1. Place container on paper towel at bedside or sink area until after you have removed isolation gown and gloves.
2. Cleanse outside of container with alcohol swipe.
3. Place container on paper towel on isolation cart.
4. Affix addressographed sticker labeled "Isolation." **(Do not lick label!)**
5. Place specimen in a *single* plastic bag, marked "Isolation."
6. Attach requisition (also labeled "Isolation") with paper clip to outside of bag.
7. Send to appropriate laboratory.

LEAVING ISOLATION ROOM

1. Untie lower strings of gown.
2. Remove gloves and discard in trash container; if gloves have not been used, wash hands.
3. Untie upper strings of gown, remove, place in laundry or trash container.
4. Wash hands.
5. Use paper towel to turn off faucet and open door.
6. Remove mask and discard in trash container. **Mask shall not be worn around neck or reused.**
7. If there are hand-washing facilities immediately outside of the door, wash hands there rather than in isolation room—use paper towel to turn faucet.
8. Wash hands in utility room before continuing duties.

updated. See summary of nursing care of infant with hypocalcemia, hypoglycemia, or sepsis, p. 965.

For general care of the compromised infant see Chapter 36. For care related to a specific condition or therapy, see the Index.

Rehabilitative Measures

Rehabilitative measures will vary with the individual need of the neonate. Some newborns will need to be weaned from ventilatory support systems. Those who suffer sequelae such as mental retardation and epilepsy will require a knowledgeable family and supportive community resources. Other children will require corrective care for problems with dentition, vision, and hearing.

Evaluation

The nurse can be reasonably assured that care was effective if the goals for care are achieved. Sepsis is prevented. Or, if infection occurs, early signs are recognized and appropriate therapy is begun. No harmful sequelae develop to either the infection or its management. Parents are able to initiate a healthy attachment to their newborn and their self-esteem is maintained.

TORCH INFECTIONS

The occurrence of certain maternal infections during early pregnancy is well known to be associated with various congenital malformations and disorders (Chapter 30). The most common and best understood infections are represented by the acronym TORCH, for toxoplasmosis, other, rubella, cytomegalic virus, and herpes simplex (see box below). Herpes simplex may result in a severe systemic illness in newborns that is often fatal. Survivors of herpetic infection may have residual neurologic defects and chorioretinitis. The other congenital infections may also result in an encephalopathy with various anomalies, including microcephaly, chorioretinitis, intracranial calcifications, microphthalmia, and cataracts. To a certain extent the varied clinical manifestations of these infections overlap, but a specific diagnosis can be made by the constellation of clinical findings, as well as specific antibody studies (Fanaroff and Martin, 1987).

For maternal and fetal effects of TORCH and other infections, see chapter 30. For TORCH infections affecting newborns, see box below.

TORCH INFECTIONS AFFECTING NEWBORNS

T Toxoplasmosis
O Other: syphilis, varicella, group B β-hemolytic streptococcus, chlamydial infections, hepatitis B, AIDS
R Rubella
C CMV infections or cytomegalic inclusion disease (CMID)
H Herpes simplex

Toxoplasmosis

Toxoplasmosis is a multisystem disease caused by the protozoan *Toxoplasma gondii.* Cats who hunt infected birds and mice harbor the parasite and excrete the infective oocysts in their feces. Human infection follows hand-to-mouth contact, such as after disposal of cat litter or after handling or ingesting raw meat from cattle or sheep that grazed in contaminated fields.

About 30% of women who contract toxoplasmosis during gestation transmit the disease to their offspring. The diagnosis of toxoplasmosis in the newborn is supported by elevated cord blood serum IgM.

About 60% to 75% of affected newborns are asymptomatic. The clinical features of toxoplasmosis resemble cytomegalic inclusion disease in mother and infant. Both diseases are responsible for serious perinatal mortality and morbidity: 10% to 15% die; 85% have severe psychomotor problems or mental retardation by 2 to 4 years; and 50% have visual problems by 1 year.

Severe toxoplasmosis is associated with preterm birth, growth retardation, microcephalus or hydrocephalus, microphthalmia, chorioretinitis, central nervous system (CNS) calcification, thrombocytopenia, jaundice, and fever. Some clinical manifestations do not develop until later in life.

Treatment of toxoplasmosis during pregnancy is problematic. Pyrimethamine is the first-choice drug against *T. gondii.* However, it may be teratogenic, especially during the first trimester (Fanaroff and Martin, 1987). Sulfonamide therapy is effective, but the drug must be discontinued before delivery and even-exchange transfusion of the newborn may be necessary to avoid kernicterus. This may occur because sulfa drugs have a greater albumin-binding affinity than bilirubin, which may rise after delivery to critical levels. The newborn may be treated with pyrimethamine, but folinic acid supplement will be required to reduce the toxicity of the drug.

In congenital toxoplasmosis, maldevelopment or neurologic damage will not be affected by treatment. However, progression of the disease can be controlled by appropriate therapy. Regrettably, encysted (intramuscular) forms of *T. gondii* cannot be eradicated by any therapy and they may cause recurrence of the disease.

Hepatitis B Virus Infection

Hepatitis B virus (HBV), the most common etiologic agent of viral hepatitis, is implicated in 24% to 40% of cases. HBV infection during pregnancy is *not* associated with an increase in malformations, stillbirths, or IUGR; however, there is about a 32% increase in risk for preterm birth (Fanaroff and Martin, 1987). The transmission rate of HBV to the newborn may be as high as 90% (Beasley et al., 1983a). Transmission occurs transplacentally, serum to serum, and by contact with contaminated urine, feces, saliva, semen, or vaginal secretions during delivery. Infants are most commonly infected during birth or in the first few days of life. The rate of transmission is highest when the mother contracts the virus immediately before delivery. Transmission may possibly occur through breast milk, but bottle-fed infants also become antigen positive at the same or higher rate. Diagnosis is made by viral culture of amniotic fluid, presence of hepatitis B surface antigen, and by the presence of IgM in cord or baby's serum.

Neonatal and fetal effects are serious. Preterm birth exposes the neonate to the problems of prematurity. Infants may be asymptomatic at birth or show evidence of acute hepatitis with changes in liver function. Infants are at high risk of developing chronic hepatitis, cirrhosis of the liver, or liver cancer even years later (NAACOG, 1986).

The infant is initially treated with H-BIG 0.5 ml intramuscular (IM) injection within the first 12 hours of life, or with immune serum globulin. H-BIG vaccine, given in a course of three doses induces antibodies in 90% of recipients. The second dose is given at 1 month; and the third dose is given at 6 months. The vaccine should protect the child for up to 9 years. After the newborn has been cleansed thoroughly and has received the vaccine, breastfeeding may be allowed.

The Public Health Service defines women at high risk for hepatitis B as women who are Indochinese refugees, of Asian descent, or born in Haiti or South Africa; women with a history of liver disease; women who have occupational exposure to the HBV, such as laboratory technologists, nurses, and physicians; and women who work with mentally retarded individuals. Intravenous drug abusers, prostitutes, and household contacts of hepatitis B carriers are also at high risk (NAACOG, 1986).

There is now overwhelming evidence that screening pregnant women for hepatitis B surface antigen (HBsAg) will identify carriers of HBV (Marwick, 1987). Perinatal transmission of the virus can be reduced to 5% to 10% by using a series of immunizations (Beasley et al., 1983b; Wong et al., 1984; Stevens et al., 1985; Blocking, 1987). Screening all pregnant women for HBs-Ag would result in as many as 140 cases of acute neonatal hepatitis and as many as 1400 cases of chronic liver disease being prevented yearly per 100,000 pregnant women screened in the high risk groups, at a net annual savings of as much as $765 million (Arevalo, 1988).

Syphilis

Congenital and neonatal syphilis (Chapter 30) has reemerged in recent years as a significant health problem. Nationwide in 1987, 35,398 cases were reported. This represents an increase of 30% from the year before (Syphilis, 1988). The nationwide rate stands at 14.7 cases per 100,000. this is the highest figure since 1950. One significant cause for the increase may be the increase in prostitution by younger women who accept "crack"—a form of cocaine that can be smoked—as payment for sex, particularly in large urban regions (Morningstar and Chitwood, 1987) (Chapter 34).

Fetal infestation with the spirochete *Treponema pallidum* is blocked by Langhans' layer in the chorion until this layer begins to atrophy between 16 and 18 weeks' gestation. If spirochetemia is untreated, it will result in fetal death by midtrimester abortion or stillbirth in one out of four cases. All newborns in whom the infection occurs before 7 months' gestation are affected. Only 60% are affected if the infection occurs late in pregnancy. If maternal infection is adequately treated before the eighteenth week, newborns seldom demonstrate signs of the disease. Although treatment after the eighteenth week may cure fetal sphirochetemia, pathologic changes may not be prevented completely.

Because the fetus becomes infected after the period of organogenesis (first trimester), maldevelopment of organs does not result. Congenital syphilis may stimulate premature labor, but there is no evidence that it causes IUGR. Stigmas of congenital syphilis (Fig. 39-1) may include inflammatory and destructive changes in the placenta, in organs such as the liver, spleen, kidneys, adrenal glands, and in bone covering and marrow. Disorders of the CNS, teeth, and cornea may not become evident until several months after birth.

Assessment. The most severely affected newborns may be **hydropic** (edematous) and **anemic**, with enlarged liver and spleen. Hepatosplenomegaly is probably secondary to extramedullary hematopoietic activity stimulated by the severe anemia.

In some cases signs of congenital syphilis do not appear until late in the neonatal period. In these newborns early signs, such as poor feeding, slight hyperthermia, and snuffles, may be nonspecific. **Snuffles** refers to the copious clear serosanguineous mucous discharge from the obstructed nose. A mucopurulent discharge indicates secondary infection, usually by streptococci or staphylococci.

By the end of the first week of life, in untreated cases, a copper-colored maculopapular **dermal rash** appears. The rash is characteristically first noticeable on the palms of the hands, soles of the feet, and diaper area, and around the mouth and anus. The maculopapular lesions may become vesicular and confluent and extend over the trunk and extremities. **Condylomas** (elevated wartlike lesions) may be seen around the anus. Rough, cracked mucocutaneous lesions of the lips heal to form circumoral radiating scars known as **rhagades.**

Other involvement results in exfoliation (separation, flaking) of nails and loss of hair. Iritis and choroiditis are characteristic of infection of the eyes. Nephrotic syndrome secondary to renal infection, hepatitis with **jaundice**, lymphadenopathy, inflammation of the pancreas, testes, and colon, and a pseudoparalysis of the extremities may be noted. Laboratory tests may show a pleocytosis (usually lymphocytosis) and elevated CSF protein levels.

By 3 months of age, in 90% of infants (treated or untreated), periostitis and metaphyseal osteochondritis may be demonstrated by roentgenography. These bone lesions generally disappear by 10 months of age whether or not the infant receives antibiotic treatment.

After the physician determines that congenital syphilis is possible, the CSF (obtained by lumbar puncture) is examined with the FTA-ABS test (Table 6-10 and Chapter 30). If results are inconclusive, the physician will probably opt to treat the child as if the disease existed.

Medical Management. If the mother had been adequately treated before delivery and serologic testing of the newborn does not show syphilis, generally the newborn is not treated with antibiotics. In this case the newborn is

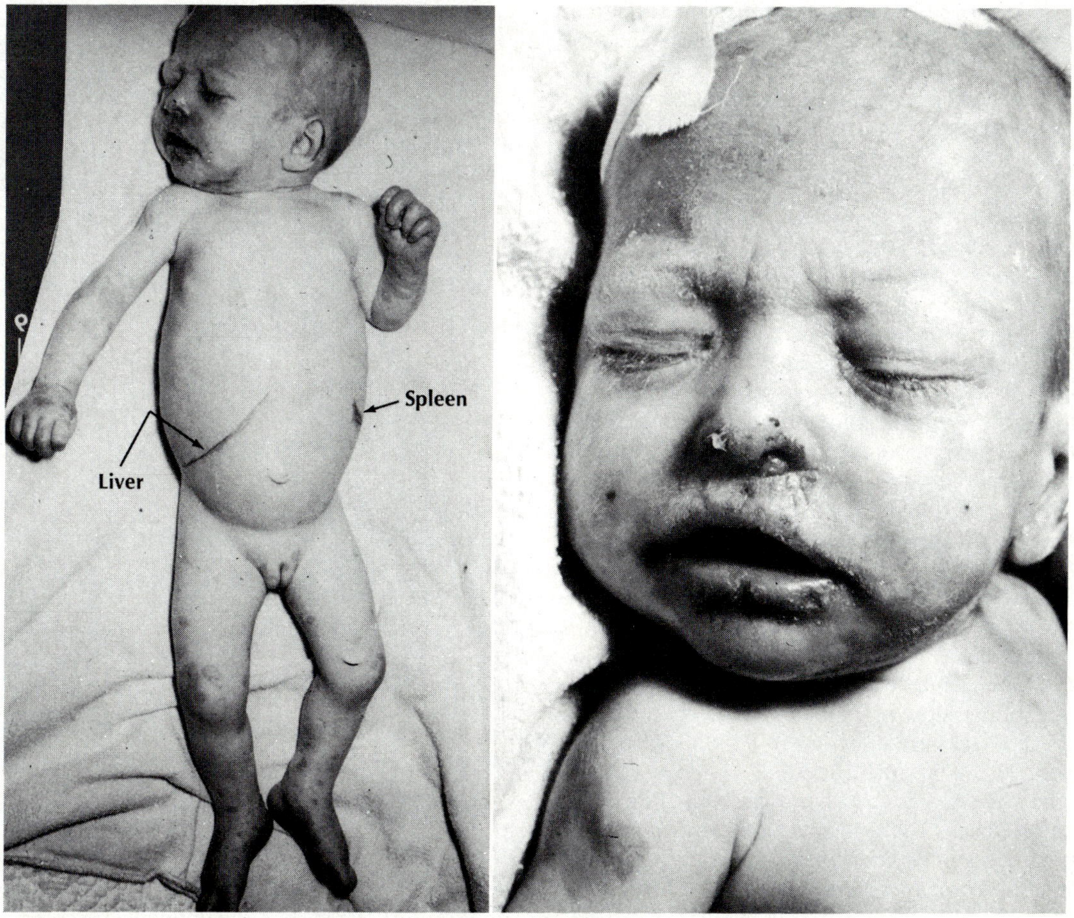

Fig. 39-1 Early congenital syphilis apparent at birth, which corresponds to secondary syphilis in the adult. (Late congenital syphilis, corresponding to tertiary syphilis, becomes apparent after 2 years of age.) **A,** Cutaneous lesions of congenital syphilis. Lines drawn on body indicate hepatosplenomegaly. No destruction of bridge of nose (common finding in congenital syphilis) is noted on this infant. **B,** Rhinitis (snuffles) resulting in rhagades and excoriation of upper lip. Red-colored rash is around mouth and on chin.

From Shirkey, HC, editor: Pediatric therapy, ed 6, St Louis, 1980, The CV Mosby Co.

checked for antibody titer (received from the mother via the placenta) every 2 weeks for 3 months, at which time the test result should be negative. Some physicians recommended antibiotic therapy for asymptomatic or inconclusive cases.

For antibiotic treatment to be effective, an "adequate" blood level must be maintained for an "adequate" period of time. Suggested medication protocol in the presence of symptomatic systemic disease differs from author to author and physician to physician. After 12 hours of antibiotic therapy, the child is not considered contagious. It is generally accepted that erythromycin is the substitute antibiotic of choice for newborns sensitive to penicillin.

Prognosis and Sequelae. In general, treatment of syphilis is more effective if it is begun early rather than late in the course of the disease. However, a recurrence rate of 5% can be expected. Even adequate treatment of congenital syphilis after birth does not always prevent late (5 to 15 years after initial infection) complications. Potential complications include neurosyphilis, deafness, Hutchinson's teeth (notched incisors), saber shins, joint involvement, saddle nose (depressed bridge), gummas (soft, gummy tumors) over the skin and other organs, and interstitial keratitis (inflammation of the cornea). The failure of therapy with the persistence of spirochetes in the eyes is not unusual. Antibiotics penetrate ocular tissue poorly. Mortality from congenital syphilis during early childhood is uncommon.

Rubella Infection

Congenital rubella infection is a major concern. The last epidemic in the United States occurred in 1964 and 1965. Of the 30,000 affected pregnancies, 20,000 resulted in infants with *congenital rubella syndrome,* and 10,000 fetal deaths or therapeutic abortions were recorded (Fanaroff and Martin, 1987). Since vaccination was begun in 1969, congenital rubella cases have been drastically reduced. Rubella immunity should be confirmed in all women before pregnancy (Table 6-10). Confirmation is determined either by verification of rubella immunization or by serologic determination of rubella-specific IgM in cord or baby's serum since history of rubella infection is unreliable (Chapter 12). Diagnosis is possible with viral cultures of amniotic fluid, placenta or baby's throat, urine, or spinal fluid.

Congenital rubella is not a static disease. More than two-thirds of infected infants show no apparent involvement at birth, but they develop consequences years later. Central and peripheral *hearing defects,* the most common result, appear to be progressive after birth. The major teratogenic effects of rubella involve the *cardiovascular* system (pulmonary artery hypoplasia, patent ductus arteriosus, and coarctation of the aortic isthmus) and *cataract* formation. Multiple other abnormalities commonly occur. These disorders include intrauterine and postnatal growth retardation, thrombocytopenic purpura (Fig. 39-2), dermal erythropoiesis, interstitial pneumonia, bony radiolucencies, retinopathy, and hepatosplenomegaly. Severe infections may result in fetal death. Delayed effects are manifested as thyroid dysfunction, diabetes mellitus, growth hormone deficiency, and progressive rubella panencephalopathy (Fanaroff and Martin, 1987).

The risk of a congenitally infected infant varies with the gestational age of the fetus when maternal infection occurs (Table 30-2). Anomalies are most severe if the mother contracts the virus during the first trimester.

The rubella virus has been cultured in babies for 1 to 1½ years after delivery. These infants are a serious source of infection to susceptible individuals, particularly potentially or actually pregnant women. Extended pediatric isolation is mandatory until the noncontagious stage of rubella has been reached. (Isolate newborn until pharyngeal mucus and urine are free of virus.)

For maternal vaccination in the puerperium, see Chapter 26. The use of Rh immune globulin does not interfere with effective rubella immunization.

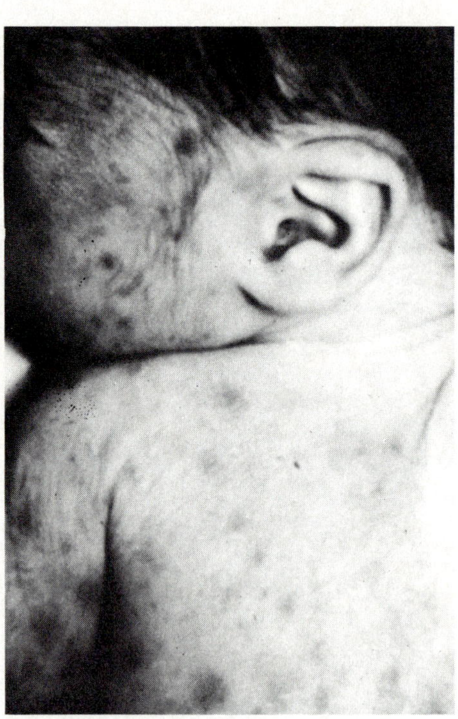

Fig. 39-2 Newborn with congenital rubella syndrome, showing multiple purpuric lesions over face, trunk, and upper arm.
From Fanaroff, AA, and Martin, RJ, editors: Behrman's neonatal-perinatal medicine: diseases of the fetus and infant, ed 4, St Louis, 1987, The CV Mosby Co.

Cytomegalovirus Infection

Cytomegalic inclusion disease (CMID) is a disorder caused by one or more of at least six strains of cytomegalovirus (CMV). CMV is deoxyribonucleic acid (DNA) virus of the herpes family. Maternal viremia during pregancy may result in abortion, stillbirth, or congenital or neonatal CMID in a live-born infant. It is the most common cause of congenital viral infections in humans, occurring in 1% of all newborns (Fanaroff and Martin, 1987). It is always a severely crippling disease of the infant.

Maternal infection with CMV may begin as a mononucleosis-like syndrome. However, in the majority of adults, the onset of the disease is uncertain. It may remain subclinical for years. Respiratory transmission is the major vector, but the virus has been recovered from semen, vaginal secretions, urine, or feces, and from bank blood. Maternal CMID may be diagnosed serologically. Many women, especially those in the lower socioeconomic classes, have antibody evidence of CMID. Women at risk for CMV infection include those who work in, or have children in, day care centers, institutions for the mentally retarded, or certain health fields (nursery, dialysis, laboratories, oncology).

The newborn with classic, full-blown CMID displays IUGR and has microcephaly. The newborn has a petechial rash, jaundice, and hepatosplenomegaly. Anemia, thrombocytopenia, and hyperbilirubinemia are to be expected. Intracranial, periventricular calcification often will be noted on x-ray films. Inclusion bodies ("owl's eye" figures) in cells sedimented from freshly voided urine or in liver biopsy specimens are typical. Elevated cord blood IgM, is suggestive evidence of disease. The virus may be isolated from urine or saliva of the newborn. Differential diagnosis includes other causes of jaundice, syphilis (positive VDRL), toxoplasmosis (positive Sabin-Feldman dye test), hemolytic disease of the newborn (positive Coombs' test), or coxsackie virus infection (culture).

Despite the extensive, endemic nature of the disease in women and men and its potential for havoc in perinatal life, critically affected newborns are only occasionally delivered. Milder forms of the disease may often result when the fetus is affected late in pregnancy. CMV can be transmitted through breast milk while the mother is experiencing acute CMV syndrome. Severe mental and physical handicaps mark virtually all infants who survive CMID.

Infants who are asymptomatic at birth are at risk for late sequelae. Hearing loss may not be apparent until after the first year of life. Chorioretinitis, microcephaly, mental retardation, and neuromuscular deficits may occur by 2 years of age. Some children are at risk for a defect in tooth enamel, resulting in severe caries.

No reasonable prevention or specific therapy exists for mother or infant (Fanaroff and Martin, 1987). Repeated pregnancies may be complicated by CMV infection.

Herpes Simplex Virus Infection

Herpes simplex virus (HSV) infections among newborns are being diagnosed more frequently. HSV infection is estimated to occur in as many as 1 in every 4000 to 5000 deliveries (Fanaroff and Martin, 1987).

The herpes viruses belong to a group of DNA viruses that cause latent infection, last for the lifetime of the individual, and result in periodic recurrences. Infected mothers are more likely to be white, non-Hispanic, unmarried, and less than 20 years old (NAACOG, 1986). Pregnancy increases both the frequency of infection and the persistence of the virus.

Modes of Transmission. The newborn may acquire the virus by any of four modes of transmission:

- Transplacental infection
- Ascending infection by way of the birth canal
- Direct contamination during passage through an infected birth canal
- Direct transmission, from infected personnel or family

Transplacental transmission of HSV infection to the newborn may occur during maternal viremia. However, an ascending transcervical infection first involves the intact fetal membranes causing chorioamnionitis. This infection then is likely to be the cause of premature rupture of membranes, rather than the sequel to PROM. Ascending transcervical infection of intact membranes may account for the triple rate of spontaneous abortions in the first 20 weeks of gestation with genital HSV infections, the development of neonatal infections despite cesarean birth with intact membranes, and the high rate of preterm birth (Brown et al., 1987). Transcervical infection can be accelerated by fetal monitoring electrodes. The electrodes break the fetal skin barrier and increase the risk of infection. Still the majority of infants show no evidence of infection in utero.

Congenital infection is rare. Congenital infection is marked by in utero destruction of normally formed organs. Affected infants are growth retarded. They have severe psychomotor retardation with intracranial calcifications, microcephaly, hypertonicity, and seizures. They suffer eye involvement, including microphthalmia, cataracts, chorioretinitis, blindness, and retinal dysplasia. Some infants have patent ductus arteriosus, limb anomalies, and recurrent skin vesicles, with a short life expectancy.

Most infants are infected directly during passage through the birth canal. The risk of infection during vaginal delivery in the presence of genital herpes has not been clearly delineated. It may be as high as 40% to 60% with active infection at term. Primary maternal infections after 32 weeks' gestation carry a higher risk (50%) for the fetus and newborn than recurrent infections (4%) (Fanaroff and Martin, 1987; Petit, 1987). The transmission rate of chronic vaginal herpes from the pregnant woman to her newborn is low, 8% or less (Bennett, 1987; Prober, 1987). Passive intrauterine immunity to herpes may be responsible. If the mother is asymptomatic at delivery, detectable infection may not be found in the infant.

Probably 10% of infants are infected postnatally. These infections occur most commonly via either airborne infection or direct contact with virus from labial lesions (cold sores) on the mother, father, or nursery personnel.

Disseminated and Local Infection. Clinically, neonatal infections have been classified as disseminated, with or without CNS involvement, or localized. Localized infections may involve the CNS, the eyes, the skin, or the oral cavity and occur in nearly one third of the infants.

Disseminated infections may involve virtually every organ system but predominantly the liver, adrenal glands, and lungs, the infants exhibit initial symptoms usually in the first week of life, but sometimes in the second week, with signs of bacterial sepsis or shock.

Clinical manifestations include skin vesicles in about 50% of infants (Fig. 39-3). Death results from progression of CNS involvement, respiratory distress and pneumonitis, shock, disseminated intravascular coagulation (DIC), and bleeding. Overall, the mortality without antiviral therapy is 82%.

Localized infections usually become apparent during the second to the fourth week of life. Lethargy, poor feeding, irritability, and focal or generalized seizures may be the initial manifestations. Half of the infants have skin vesicles, but some infants will never have mucocutaneous lesions. About 40% of infants die by 6 months of age from

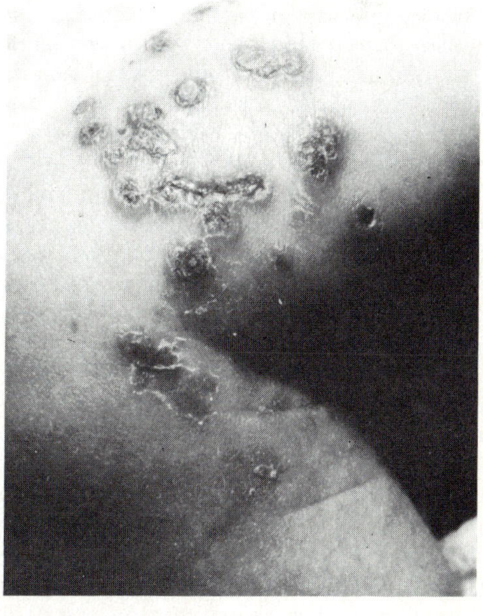

Fig. 39-3 Neonatal herpesvirus infection.

From Fanaroff, AA, and Martin, RJ, editors: Behrman's neonatal-perinatal medicine: diseases of the fetus and infant, ed 4, St Louis, 1987, The CV Mosby Co.

progressive neurologic deterioration. About the same percent survive with severe neurologic sequelae, including blindness.

Ocular involvement may occur alone and may be secondary to either HSV-1 or HSV-2. Ocular disease may not be discovered for months. Microphthalmia, cataracts, optic atrophy, and corneal scarring may result from chorioretinitis, keratitis, and retinal hemorrhage.

Management. Care of all newborn infants begins with parental prevention of genital infections. Spermicidal foams kill the virus, and condoms offer some protection against direct contact with lesions in the sexual partner. Maternal oral or intravenous acyclovir does shorten the viral shedding time but its effect on fetal safety is unknown. Therefore this agent is not recommended during pregnancy (Fanaroff and Martin, 1987).

Antepartum maternal cultures and antibody screening do not predict the infant's risk of exposure to HSV at delivery. The best time and route of delivery are still controversial. There is consensus that infants should be delivered by cesarean surgery when an active herpes infection is present at the onset of labor and the amniotic membranes have been ruptured less than 4 to 6 hours, regardless of whether the infection is primary or recurrent. Because of the possibility of transplacental and ascending transcervical infection, the mother must be informed that even cesarean delivery gives no guarantee that the baby will be free from infection (Fanaroff and Martin, 1987). Fetal scalp monitors are avoided.

During the postpartum period the nurse's main function is to teach the mother about the disease, recognition of lesions, and prevention of its transmission during care of the infant. Initially all infants should be isolated. Both gown and gloves should be worn by persons in contact with infants, until the results of the maternal cultures are determined negative. Nursery personnel with cold sores should practice strict handwashing and wear a mask. However there is no evidence to require their actual removal from the nursery (Fanaroff and Martin, 1987).

The newborn's eyes, oral cavity, and skin are inspected carefully for the presence of any lesions. Cultures are obtained from the mouth, the eyes, and any possible lesions. Circumcision is delayed until the infant is discharged. The infant may be discharged with the mother if the infant's cultures are negative. The mother is advised about the need for weekly pediatric appointments throughout the first month. As long as there are no suspicious lesions on the mother's breasts, breast-feeding is allowable. For the infant at risk, prophylactic topical eye ointment (vidarabine) is ordered to be administered for 5 days for prevention of keratoconjunctivitis.

Other than general supportive measures, the only therapy shown to have a significant effect on outcome is vidarabine, although a trial of acyclovir currently is being evaluated. There is no hyperimmune globulin available for use and there is little evidence to support the use of globulin (Fanaroff and Martin, 1987). Any infant who has lesions, is shedding virus, or has suspicious symptoms with a history of exposure to the virus should be treated immediately. Vidarabine is ordered in mg/kg/day. Therapy usually extends over 10 days. Vidarabine therapy has been credited with reduction in the mortality for disseminated herpes infection.

Chlamydial Infection

Chlamydia trachomatis is an **intracellular bacterium** that causes **neonatal conjunctivitis** and **pneumonia**. The conjunctivitis is first noted about 3 or 4 days after birth. If chlamydial disease is not treated, chronic follicular conjunctivitis with conjunctival scarring and corneal neovascularization may result.

If prenatal screening reveals infection with *C. trachomatis,* treatment of the mother is deferred until the early postpartum period to avoid exposing the fetus to the therapy. After delivery the mother is treated with tetracycline, 500 mg orally 4 times each day for 7 to 14 days. The newborn is also treated with tetracycline, 6 mg/kg/24 hr for 7 days, and ointment or solution of tetracycline is instilled into the conjunctival sac every 2 to 4 hours for 2 to 4 days. Sulfacetamide sodium (10%) drops or ointment may be used instead.

Prognosis is generally good. Ideally, the condition is diagnosed early, and both mother and newborn are treated in the immediate postpartum period.

Human Immunodeficiency Virus—Acquired Immune Deficiency Syndrome

Maternal infection with the retrovirus, human immunodeficiency virus (HIV), is presented in Chapter 30. The focus of this discussion is the newborn at risk for infection with HIV. The Public Health Service estimates that by 1991 about 3000 children will have the disease, and without new efficacious drug therapy, virtually all will die (Editorial, 1987). Pediatric acquired immune deficiency syndrome (AIDS) cases account for 1.4% of reported AIDS cases in the United States, but the numbers are expected to grow (Harris, 1986). The populations at risk for acquiring HIV have been identified (Chapter 30). Some women are unaware that they are in a high-risk group; these women are unaware that their sexual partners engage in high-risk behaviors (Landesman et al., 1987; Letters, 1987).

Transmission of HIV from the mother to the infant occurs transplacentally at various gestational ages, perinatally via maternal blood and secretions, and postnatally through breast milk or through other close contact (Pyun et al., 1987; Fanaroff and Martin, 1987).

Routine screening and counseling of all pregnant women is sparking considerable controversy (Landesman, 1987). Comparisons are being made between the frequency of perinatally transmitted AIDS with that of other perinatal diseases for which screening standards already exist. For example, the incidence of perinatally contracted herpes is between 1 in every 4000 to 5000 births to 1 in every 7500 to 10,000 births (Monif and Hardt, 1985), congenital rubella occurs once in 300,000 births (MMWR, 1986), and neural tube defects occur once in 1000 births

(Main and Mennuti, 1986). In one hospital in New York City, however, an HIV transmission rate of 33%, or 1 in every 150 births, was reported (Landesman et al., 1987).

The Centers for Disease Control has issued guidelines for counseling and antibody testing (MMWR, 1987). Several issues are being debated regarding routine screening. Many issues touch the core of the social fabric of the United States. These issues include the populations who have been identified to be at risk, including victims of child abuse; the adequacy and availability of social services, education and health care systems; the volatile issue of therapeutic abortion; the option of avoiding future pregnancies (Facing, 1987); and the reliability of current tests for HIV.

Diagnosis. *Diagnosis* of HIV infection in the newborn is the subject of intense research. Pyun et al. (1987) studied specific antibody responses by the neonate. Gravidas infected with HIV produce IgG antibodies. The IgG crosses the placenta to the fetus. Therefore cord blood is positive for antibody when tested by enzyme-linked immunosorbent assay (ELISA) or Western blot techniques. Because of their physiologically depressed immune response, newborns generally produce a less vigorous and more limited antibody response to HIV infection (Pahwa et al, 1986; Harnish et al., 1987; Johnson et al., 1987). The presence of HIV in the newborn currently must be verified either by culture or by demonstration of the presence of antigen (Harnish et al., 1987). Pyun et al. (1987) were able to demonstrate the early appearance of anti-HIV antibody of the IgM and later of the IgG3 class, suggesting perinatal infection.

Diagnosis is assisted by physical examination for stigmas of the *AIDS dysmorphia syndrome* (Marian et al., 1986; Klug, 1986). The neonate may be preterm or SGA. Some cranial and facial abnormalities have been identified (Fig. 39-4). These include microcephaly, a prominant box-like forehead, an increase in outer and inner canthal distance, mild slant to the eyes, a broad, flattened nasal bridge, a prominent triangular philtrum, and patulous lips.

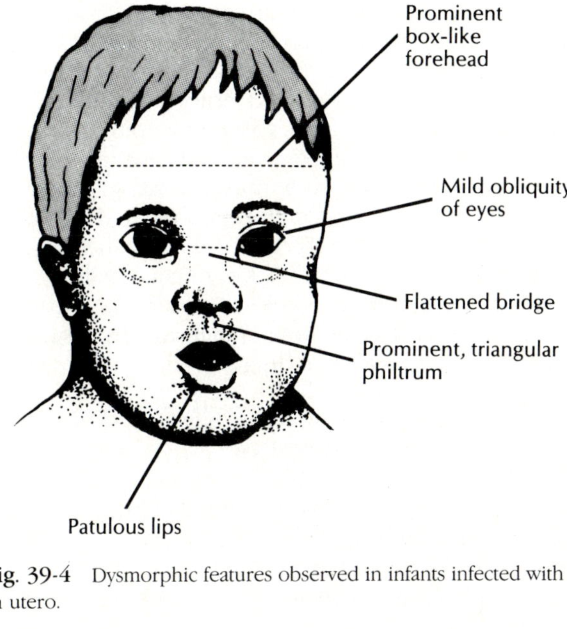

Fig. 39-4 Dysmorphic features observed in infants infected with HIV in utero.

The occurrence of an *opportunistic infection* in the newborn may alert the caregiver to the presence of HIV infection or assist in the confirmation of the diagnosis of HIV infection. In pediatrics, the presence of lymphoid interstitial pneumonitis is now considered a criterion for diagnosis (Fanaroff and Martin, 1987). The presence of oral candidiasis (thrush, p. 982) that is refractory to administration of topical antifungal agents carries a high index of suspicion for HIV infection (Prenatal, 1987).

Infected infants are usually symptomatic before 1 year of age with signs that are seen in adults. These signs include lymphadenopathy, hepatosplenomegaly, chronic diarrhea, interstitial pneumonitis, and persistent thrush. In addition, infants have failure to thrive, recurrent severe bacterial infections, and occasionally recurrent enlargement of the parotid glands. *Pneumocystis carinii* has occurred in 70% and Kaposi's sarcoma in 5% of affected children. Viral infection caused by cytomegalovirus and Epstein-Barr virus is commonly observed in children with AIDS. Bacterial sepsis also may be an initial manifestation (Fanaroff and Martin, 1987).

Infants who exhibit signs of HIV infection at birth tend to expire within a month. The disease progression has been slower and the mortality lower in infants with a later onset.

Differential diagnosis is crucial. Fanaroff and Martin (1987) suggest that in a symptomatic infant, ELISA testing of serum from the parents, siblings, and donors of any blood or blood products may be helpful. The immunodeficiency must be differentiated from congenital causes of immunodeficiencies, such as severe combined immunodeficiency, DiGeorge syndrome, Wiskott-Aldrich syndrome, neutrophil disorders, ataxia telangiectasia, and hypoagammaglobulinemia or agammaglobulinemia. Congenital rubella, CMV, toxoplasmosis, and herpes simplex infections in the first 6 months also must be eliminated.

Management. *Management* begins by implementing universal precautions and precautions for invasive procedures (Chapter 30) to prevent further transmission of HIV (MMWR, 1987; Jackson et al., 1987). Circumcision in males is avoided. Umbilical cord stumps are cleaned meticulously every day until healing is complete. Therapy includes prophylactic γglobulin, antimicrobial medications specific for the infections encountered, and corticosteroids in the presence of lymphoid interstitial pneumonitis. Azidothymidine (AZT) and ribavirin cross the brain barrier and may result in increase in weight and in the number of T-helper cells. For general care of the compromised newborn, see Chapter 36.

Counseling regarding the care of the women themselves, the family's care of the infant, and future pregnancies challenges the caregiver. Self-care involves avoiding at-risk behaviors during sexual encounters, avoiding substance abuse (Chapter 34), and avoiding future pregnancies. Regardless of proven risks and mass media education, "safe sex" practices have not been implemented by many people for a variety of reasons, including denial (Leishman, 1987).

The public health community has become aware that women who know that they carry HIV antibody still become pregnant for many reasons. These include denial of risk, desire to have a family depite the risk, and many more complex sociocultural considerations (Prenatal, 1987).

Some parents are opting to place the infected infants in foster homes despite the low risk for transmission among members of the same household. Social services are required in these cases. If the parent chooses to keep the infant, home health care is arranged. For more information and updated information parents are offerred the following resource: The National AIDS Hotline, 1-800-342-AIDS.

The family must be counseled about vaccinations. The child will not receive live vaccines against childhood diseases such as measles,* mumps, and rubella. The child will receive sabin polio vaccination, vaccination against pertussis and diphtheria, and tetanus toxoid.

Oral Thrush

Oral thrush, or mycotic stomatitis, is caused by *Candida albicans.* This infection results from direct contact with a contaminated birth canal, hands (mother's or others'), feeding equipment, breast, or bedding. The appearance of white plaques on the oral mucosa, gums, and tongue is characteristic. The white patches are easily differentiated from milk curds; the patches cannot be removed and tend to bleed when touched. In most cases the infant does not seem to be discomforted by the infection. A few newborns seem to have some difficulty swallowing.

Infants who are sick, debilitated, or receiving antibiotic therapy are more susceptible. Those with conditions such as cleft lip or palate, neoplasms, and hyperparathyroidism seem to be more vulnerable to mycotic infection.

The objectives of management are to eradicate the causative organism, control exposure to *C. albicans,* and improve the infant's resistance. Interventions include maintenance of scrupulous cleanliness to prevent reinfection (nursing personnel, parents, others.) Good hand-washing technique is always essential. Clean surfaces should be provided for newborns (newborn is never placed directly on sheets on which the mother has been sitting). Proper cleanliness of the equipment and environment is ensured. The compromised newborn's physiologic function (see Chapter 36) must be supported.

Medications are administered as ordered. Aqueous solution of gentian violet (1% to 2%) is applied with swab to oral mucosa, gums, and tongue. (Guard against permanent stain on skin, clothes, equipment. Warn parents about purple staining of baby's mouth.)

Nystatin (Mycostatin) is instilled into the newborn's mouth with a medicine dropper. Give infant sterile water to wash out milk before giving nystatin. Nystatin may also be swabbed over mucosa, gums, or tongue.

To give medication by medicine dropper, position the infant's head to the side or support the infant in a semi-Fowler's position. Insert the dropper into the oral cavity so that the tip rests against the cheek, alongside the tongue. Wait until the infant begins to suck on the dropper, then squeeze the rubber end slowly until the dropper is empty.

Gonorrhea

The incidence of gonococcal infection in gravidas has ranged from 2.5% to 7.3% in recent studies (Fanaroff and Martin, 1987). With this high incidence, it is not surprising that neonatal infection with *Neisseria gonorrhoeae* occurs frequently. After rupture of membranes, ascending infection can result in orogastric contamination of the fetus. The organism may also invade mucosal surfaces, such as the conjunctiva (ophthalmia neonatorum, Chapter 22), rectal mucosa, and pharynx. Contamination may occur as the infant passes through the birth canal or it may occur postnatally from an infected adult. Neonatal gonococcal arthritis, septicemia, meningitis, vaginitis, and scalp abscesses also occur.

Endocervical cultures for *N. gonorrhoeae* should be obtained routinely during pregnancy and appropriate treatment instituted when necessary to prevent fetal-neonatal infection. The newborn with a mild infection often recovers completely with appropriate treatment (see Chapter 30). Occasionally infants die in the early neonatal period from overwhelming infection.

DRUG DEPENDENCE

The adverse effects of exposure of the fetus to drugs are variable. They include transient behavioral changes such as fetal breathing movements or irreversible effects such as fetal death, IUGR, structural malformations, or mental retardation. Maternal use of drugs may be for the pharmacologic control of disease process (e.g., insulin) or for symptomatic relief of benign problems (e.g., aspirin). It has been shown that 92% to 100% of all obstetric clients take at least one physician-prescribed drug, and 65% to 80% also take self-prescribed drugs. In addition to the therapeutic use of drugs the nontherapeutic use of drugs, such as alcohol, nicotine, or narcotics, poses threats to fetal well-being. Critical determinants of the effect of the drug on the fetus include the specific drug, the dosage, the route of administration, the genotype of the mother or fetus, and the timing of the drug exposure (Chapter 34). Figs. 39-5 and 9-14 show critical periods in human embryogenesis and the teratogenic effects of drugs.

Assessment

Assessment of the newborn requires a review of the mother's prenatal record. A medical and social history of drug abuse and detoxication is noted. Some obstetric complications are seen in pregnancies complicated by substance abuse. The obstetric events include PROM, amnion-

*In the wake of six severe measles cases among children infected with the AIDS virus, federal health officials have reversed their earlier stand and recommend measles vaccinations for children with AIDS (Measles, 1988).

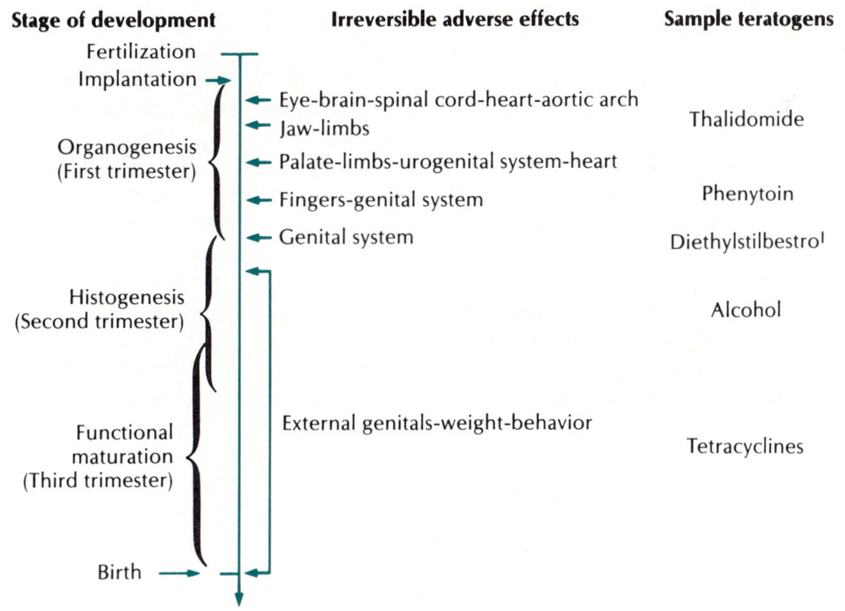

Fig. 39-5 Critical periods in human embryogenesis.
From Fanaroff, A, and Martin, R, editors: Behrman's neonatal-perinatal medicine: diseases of the fetus and infant, ed 4, St Louis, 1987, The CV Mosby Co.

itis, preterm labor, precipitous labor, abruptio placentae, placenta previa, and spontaneous abortion. Perinatal and neonatal mortality and morbidity are also seen. There is an increase in stillbirths and in the births of newborns diagnosed with IUGR, LBW, or preterm.

The woman who is addicted to narcotics may have infections that compound the risk to the infant. These infections include hepatitis, septicemia, and STDs, including AIDS (Niebyl, 1988).

The nurse is commonly the first to observe the signs of drug dependence in the newborn. The nurse's observations help the physician differentiate between drug dependence and other conditions: tracheoesophageal fistula, CNS disorder, sepsis, hypoglycemia, and electrolyte imbalance.

The neonate is assessed using the guidelines discussed in Chapter 21. The newborn's gestational age and maturity are noted (Chapter 37). In utero exposure to some drugs results in observable malformations or dysmorphia. Neonatal behavior may be suspect. Lethargy, decreased visual alertness and auditory response to the Brazelton Neonatal Behavioral Assessment Scale (BNBAS), or withdrawal symptoms are noted. Urine screening may be used to identify substances abused by the mother. Since many women are polydrug users, the newborn infant may initially exhibit a confusing complex of signs.

Nursing Diagnoses

Nursing diagnoses will depend on the assessment findings and are tailored to the individual needs of the newborn and the family. Following are examples of nursing diagnoses:

Newborn

- Potential for infection related to
  - Maternal risk behaviors
  - PROM
- Altered growth and development related to
  - Effects of maternal substance abuse
- Sleep pattern disturbance related to
  - Drug withdrawal

Parent(s)

- Actual or potential altered parenting related to
  - Continuation of substance abuse or detoxification program
  - Guilt for infant's condition
  - Inability to cope with care needs of a special infant
- Knowledge deficit related to
  - Care needs of an affected infant

Planning

Planning for care of the newborn presents a challenge to the health care team. Parents are included in the planning for the care of the newborn and are also encouraged to plan for their own care. A multidisciplinary approach is needed that includes home health or community resource people. Goals are stated in client-centered terms.

Goals

1. Newborn suffers no adverse sequelae to drug withdrawal
2. Malformations and dysfunction are identified and appropriate curative and rehabilitative measures are instituted

3. Parent(s) comes to terms with the newborn's condition and its management.

Implementation

Preventive Measures. Education and social support to prevent the abuse of drugs is the ideal approach. However, given the present scope of the drug abuse problem, total prevention is unrealistic.

Curative Measures. Nursing care of the drug-dependent newborn involves supportive therapy for fluid and electrolyte balance, nutrition, infection control, and respiratory care. Medications are given as ordered. The newborn's narcotic withdrawal signs may require a schedule of weaning from the drug. Phenobarbital, 6 mg/kg/24 hr IM may be ordered to be given or 2 mg orally 4 times a day for 3 or 4 days; the dose is reduced by one third every 2 days for about 2 weeks, at which time treatment is discontinued. Paregoric may be ordered to be given 2 to 4 drops/kg orally every 4 to 6 hours initially to as much as 20 to 30 drops/kg orally every 4 to 6 hours, depending on the symptomatology.

Swaddling, holding, reducing stimuli, and feeding as necessary may be helpful in easing withdrawal. See general nursing care plan, below.

Rehabilitative Measures. Drug dependence in the newborn is physiologic, not psychologic, so there is no predisposition to dependence later in life. However, the psychosocial environment in which the infant is raised may predispose to addiction.

The mother requires considerable support. Her need for and her abuse of drugs results in a decreased capacity to cope. The newborn's withdrawal signs and decreased consolability stress her coping abilities even further. Home health care, treatment for addiction, and education are important considerations. Sensitive exploration of the woman's options for the care of her infant and herself and for future fertility management may help her see that she has choices. Through this approach, respect is communicated to her as a person who can make responsible decisions.

General Nursing Care Plan

NEONATAL DRUG WITHDRAWAL

ASSESSMENT	NURSING DIAGNOSIS (ND)/ PLAN (P)/GOAL (G)	RATIONALE/ IMPLEMENTATION	EVALUATION
Note maternal drug history: length of drug habit; drug use during pregnancy; time and type of last drug taken. Assess patency of respiratory system: Note cough, swallow, and gag reflex. Note sneezing and nasal stuffiness. Note amount and color of mucus. Assess for congenital defects (esophageal atresia).	ND: Ineffective airway clearance related to mucous or anatomic obstruction. P: Monitor closely and intervene per doctor's orders or established protocols. G: Infant will maintain an open airway and possess no anatomic or mucous obstruction.	*To maintain an open airway, the nurse will:* Have resuscitative equipment available. Aspirate mouth and nose as indicated. Assess breath sounds frequently. Report tachypnea or signs of respiratory distress. Feed slowly in small amounts. Keep head elevated during feeding.	Infant maintains open airway and breathes easily.
Assess for respiratory distress. Note onset and duration of tachypnea respiratory rate > 60/minutes. Note heart rate frequently during tachypnea episodes. Note presence of respiratory distress (retractions, flaring of nostrils, apnea).	ND: Impaired gas exchange related to drug withdrawal effects. P: Monitor closely and intervene per doctor's orders or established protocols. G: Client will be able to maintain adequate ventilation by own respiratory effort.	*To support and monitor ventilation, the nurse will:* Place infant on cardiopulmonary monitor. Position for respiratory distress (head of bed elevated, prone, or side-lying). Report any increasing distress that alters heart rate or blood pressure.	Infant able to maintain oxygen intake and respirations by own effort.

General Nursing Care Plan—cont'd

ASSESSMENT	NURSING DIAGNOSIS (ND)/ PLAN (P)/GOAL (G)	RATIONALE/ IMPLEMENTATION	EVALUATION
Note color—pallor or cyanosis. Note mottling. Note symptoms indicating pathology (heart disease).		Provide oxygen therapy. Monitor blood gas values or transcutaneous oxygen and carbon dioxide values. Resuscitate and intubate as needed.	
Note hyperactive Moro's reflex. Symmetric or asymmetric. Moderately or markedly exaggerated. Has medication affected reflex? Does infant have high-pitched cry? Does crying stop or increase with soothing?	ND: Sensory perceptual alterations related to withdrawal as manifested by increased sensitivity to stimuli. ND: Pain related to withdrawal effects. P: Complete physical examination (Chapter 21 and Unit 8); intervene per physician's orders or hospital protocols. G: Infant will relax when stimuli is reduced or infant is medicated.	*To reduce CNS excitability, the nurse will:* Group care to allow for uninterrupted rest. Decrease environmental stimuli. Medicate or sedate as ordered. Swaddle infant with blankets, cuddle, and hold close.	Infant relaxes and sleeps. Crying diminishes.
Note tremors: Note occurrence with stimuli. Note location of tremors. Note degree of tremors. Observe for seizures: onset, origin, body involvement, clonic, tonic, (or both,) eye deviations, skin color. Note CNS signs: bulging fontanel at rest, increased head circumference, widely spaced sutures, fixation of gaze without blinking.	ND: Sensory/perceptual alterations related to withdrawal as manifested by seizures. ND: Potential for injury related to seizures. P: Monitor closely and intervene per physician's orders or hospital protocols. G: Infant will recover from seizures with minimal or no sequelae.	*To protect and monitor an infant with seizures, the nurse will:* Maintain a patent airway. Prevent trauma by confining child in a close, soft environment. Record and report frequency and duration of seizures. Medicate or sedate as ordered. Have resuscitative equipment available.	Infant recovers from seizures with minimal or no sequelae.
Note inability to sleep for long intervals. Assess sleep pattern. Assess effects of medication. Note yawning—onset and frequency.	ND: Sleep pattern disturbance related to withdrawal effect. P: Monitor closely and intervene per physician's orders or hospital protocols. G: Infant will be able to remain asleep for 3 to 4 hours.	*To promote rest, the nurse will:* Organize care to provide long rest periods. Reduce environmental stimuli. Swaddle infant with blankets, cuddle, or hold close.	Infant remains asleep for 3 to 4 hour periods.
Note suck, swallow, and gag reflex. Note "frantic" suck response. Assess sucking with different types of nipples. Assess for sucking blisters on lip or arms. Assess for causes of poor feeding (esophageal	ND: Altered nutrition: less than body requirements, related to inability to ingest or retain food. P: Monitor closely and intervene per physician's orders or hospital protocol. G: Client will ingest and	*To promote nutritional intake, the nurse will:* Feed small frequent amounts. Position nipple in mouth so sucking is effective. Keep head elevated during and after feeding. Avoid handling between feeding.	Infant ingests and retains sufficient nutrients for growth.

General Nursing Care Plan—cont'd

ASSESSMENT	NURSING DIAGNOSIS (ND)/ PLAN (P)/GOAL (G)	RATIONALE/ IMPLEMENTATION	EVALUATION
atresia, immaturity, hypoglycemia, sepsis). Note occurrence and frequency of regurgitation. Note intake and output (I&O).	retain sufficient nutrients to promote growth.	Medicate between feedings if possible. Monitor I&O. Correlate intake with condition, growth, and therapy. Protect arms with shirt to prevent sucking blisters. Offer safety pacifier.	
Note signs of dehydration: weight loss, sunken eyes and fontanel, poor skin tugor. Note characteristics of emesis or diarrhea (estimate fluid loss, color).	ND: Fluid volume deficit related to inability to retain fluids. P: Monitor closely and intervene per physician's orders or hospital protocol. G: Client will maintain adequate hydration and not demonstrate signs of dehydration.	*To maintain fluid and electrolyte balance, the nurse will:* Monitor I&O. Weigh every 8 hours or more often if vomiting and diarrhea continue. Give supplementary fluids if indicated for dehydration. Obtain blood for electrolyte levels as ordered.	Infant ingests and retains sufficient fluid or parenteral infusions provide sufficient fluids.
Note reddened areas over bony prominences. Note areas of skin breakdown. Note skin scratches.	ND: Impaired skin integrity related to withdrawal symptoms as manifested by excessive movement causing abrasions of the skin. ND: Potential for injury related to infection. P: Monitor closely and intervene per physician's orders or hospital protocol. G: Client will maintain intact skin free from infection.	*To maintain skin integrity, the nurse will:* Change position frequently. Provide skin care to reddened areas. Pad pressure areas with clothing. Keep finger nails trimmed. If skin is excoriated, treat for possible infection.	Infant's skin will remain intact and free from infection.

Evaluation

Final evaluation may not be possible. Goals may be met to some extent on a short-term basis. However, both the infant and the parent have long-term needs. The extent to which goals are met may not be known for years.

ABUSED SUBSTANCES

Alcohol

Reference to the association between fetal malformation and maternal alcoholism can be found in Greek and Roman mythology. Laws in Carthage and Sparta forbade consumption of alcohol by couples on their wedding night to prevent the conception of children with defects. Documentation of the fetal alcohol syndrome (FAS) can be found in the literature since the early part of the eighteenth century. The incidence of FAS in the United States is about 2.2 per 1000 live births and worldwide it is 1.9/1000 births (Niebyl, 1988; Abel and Sokol, 1988).

Predictable patterns of fetal and neonatal dysmorphogenesis are attributed to severe, chronic alcoholism in women who continue to drink heavily during pregnancy (Davis and Keith, 1983). The pattern of growth deficiency begun in prenatal life persists after delivery, especially in the linear growth rate, rate of weight gain, and growth of head circumferences (Zuspan, 1984). The box above, right summarizes the risks associated with maternal alcohol ingestion.

Ocular structural anomalies are common findings (Fig. 39-6). Limb anomalies, a variety of cardiocirculatory anomalies, especially ventricular septal defects, pose problems for the child. Mental retardation (IQ of 79 or below at 7 years of age), and fine motor dysfunction (poor hand-to-

RISKS ASSOCIATED WITH MATERNAL ALCOHOL INGESTION

Amount of Alcohol	Risks
Two or more drinks daily	IUGR
Includes:	
2 mixed drinks, 1 oz. liquor each	Immature motor activity
2 glasses of wine, 5 oz. each	Increased rate of anomalies
2 beers, 12 oz. each	Decreased muscle tone
	Poor sucking pressure
	Increased rate of stillbirths
	Decreased placental weight
Five or more drinks on occasion	Increased risk of structural brain abnormalities
Six or more drinks daily	FAS

From McCarthy, P: Am J Primary Health Care 8:34, 1983. Copyright the Nurse Practitioner: The American Journal of Primary Health Care.

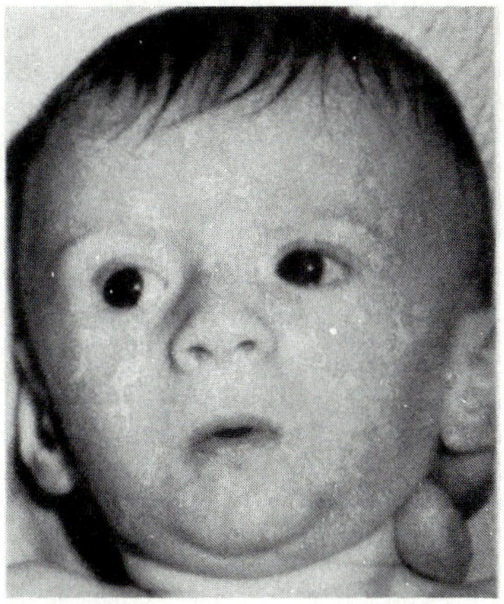

Fig. 39-6 Fetal alcohol anomaly.

Courtesy Dr. Charles Linder, Medical College of Georgia. From Goodman, RM, and Gorlin, RJ: Atlas of the face in genetic disorders, ed 2, St Louis, 1977, The CV Mosby Co.

mouth coordination, weak grasp) add to the handicapping problems that maternal alcoholism can impose. Genital abnormalities are seen in daughters of alcoholic mothers. Two thirds of newborns with FAS are girls; the cause of this altered sex birth ratio is unknown. Severe and chronic alcoholism (ethanol toxicity), not maternal malnutrition, is responsible for the severity and consistency of postdelivery performance problems (Fanaroff and Martin, 1987). High alcohol levels are lethal to the developing embryo. Lower levels cause brain and other malformations (McCarthy, 1983). Long-term prognosis (no studies are available as yet) is discouraging even in an optimum psychosocial environment, when one considers the combination of growth failure and mental retardation. The box at right summarizes the clinical findings.

Alcohol effects, however, depend not only on the amount of alcohol consumed but on the interaction of quantity, frequency, type of alcohol, and other drug abuse. Other drugs such as cigarettes, caffeine, and marijuana may potentiate the fetal effects of alcohol consumption during gestation (Fanaroff and Martin, 1987).

The infant of a mother who abuses alcohol is faced with a number of clinical problems. Identification of the problems leads to the medical diagnosis of FAS. The infant may suffer respiratory distress related to prematurity, neurologic damage, and a "floppy" epiglottis and small trachea. Tracheal-epiglottal anomalies may cause cardiopulmonary arrest. Feeding difficulties are related to prematurity, poor sucking ability, and possible cleft palate. The infant may exhibit brain dysfunction, microcephaly, and grand mal seizures.

Nursing care involves many of the same strategies used for the care of preterm infants (Chapter 37). Special efforts are made to involve the parents in their child's care and encourage opportunities for parent-child attachment. The application of the nursing process to the care of an infant with FAS is presented on p. 988.

MANIFESTATIONS OF THE PRINCIPAL FEATURES OF FETAL ALCOHOL SYNDROME

CNS Dysfunction	
Intellectual	Mild to moderate mental retardation
Neurologic	Microcephaly (small head size)
	Poor coordination
	Decreased muscle tone
Behavioral	Irritability in infancy
	Hyperactivity in childhood
Growth Deficiency	
Prenatal	Less than 3% for length and weight
Postnatal	Less than 3% for length and weight
	Failure to thrive
	Disproportionate-diminished adipose tissue
Facial Characteristics	
Eyes	Short palpebral fissures (small eye openings)
	Strabismus, ptosis, myopia
Nose	Short and upturned
	Hypoplastic philtrum (flat or absent groove above upper lip)
Mouth	Thinned upper vermilion (upper lip)
	Retrognathia in infancy (receding jaw)
Abnormalities in Other Systems	
Cardiac	Murmurs (atrial septal defects, ventricular septal defects, great-vessel anomalies, tetralogy of Fallot)
Skeletal	Limited joint movements (especially fingers and elbows and hip dislocations)
	Aberrant palmar creases
	Pectus excavatum
Renogenital	Kidney defects
	Labial hypoplasia
Cutaneous	Hemangiomas

From McCarthy, P: Am J Primary Health Care 8:34, 1983. Copyright The Nurse Practitioner: The American Journal of Primary Health Care.

Specific Nursing Care Plan

FETAL ALCOHOL SYNDROME (FAS)

Baby Albert was born 3 hours ago. His birth weight was 2464 grams (5½ lb). His mother, age 24, drank heavily during pregnancy. Bobby exhibits clinical problems of FAS (microcephaly, hypotonia, irritability, poor suck, and increased respiratory effort). Both his mother and father are anxious to care for their baby.

ASSESSMENT	NURSING DIAGNOSIS (ND)/ PLAN (P)/GOAL (G)	RATIONALE/ IMPLEMENTATION	EVALUATION
Increased respiratory effort. Note respiratory distress. Note apnea of prematurity with associated bradycardia. Monitor for seizure activity. Monitor cardiopulmonary response to distress: mottling, cool extremities, bradycardia, hypotension.	ND: Ineffective breathing pattern related to FAS. P: Complete physical examination (Chapter 21 and Unit 8); monitor closely and intervene per physician's orders or hospital protocols. G: Albert will maintain a patent airway. G: Albert will be able to maintain adequate ventilation by his own respiratory effort.	*To prevent or treat respiratory distress, the nurse will:* Place on cardiopulmonary monitor (set close alarm limits). Assess breath sounds frequently and report increasing distress. Place child in position where he exhibits least distress (prone or side). Suction mouth and nose as necessary. Have resuscitative equipment available. Observe for seizures and report. Implement seizure precautions.	Albert maintains a patent airway. Albert maintains adequate ventilation through his own respiratory effort.
Irritability. Poor suck. Assess suck, gag, and swallow reflex. Observe for potential aspiration (gagging, choking, cyanosis). Assess intake and output (I&O).	ND: Altered nutrition: less than body requirements, related to irritability and poor suck. P: Monitor closely and intervene per physician's orders or hospital protocol. G: Albert will ingest and retain nutrients sufficient for growth.	*To encourage successful feeding, the nurse will:* Elevate Albert's head during and following feeding. Feed in small frequent amounts. Evaluate different nipples for feeding. Burp well after feeds. Oral gavage feed as necessary. Obtain daily weight, maintain strict I&O. Keep suction ready to use; aspirate nares as circumstances require.	Albert takes and retains enough nutrients for growth.
Microcephaly, hypotonia, irritability, poor suck. Observe for other signs of brain dysfunction (tremulousness, hyperacusis).	ND: Altered family processes related to need to care for and love a child with a handicap. ND: Knowledge deficit related to infant's birth anomalies and their potential sequelae. P: Provide information; be available for discussion of concerns and questions; and refer to appropriate community	*To promote maternal-infant attachment to its optimum level, the nurse will:* Encourage frequent parental visits to the special care nursery and promote physical contact with the infant. Teach parents about Albert's anomalies and their possible sequelae. Help parents verbalize their concerns regarding anomalies.	Parents learn about Albert's anomalies and their possible effects on the child's future. Parents recognize and eventually accept Albert's handicaps.

Specific Nursing Care Plan—cont'd

ASSESSMENT	NURSING DIAGNOSIS (ND)/ PLAN (P)/GOAL (G)	RATIONALE/ IMPLEMENTATION	EVALUATION
	resources. (For care of mother's drug abuse problem, refer to Chapter 34.) G: Albert will be successfully cared for by his parents. G: Parents will learn about infant's special needs.	Be realistic when discussing Albert's potential for future physical, neurologic, and emotional development. Involve the parents in Albert's care (diapering, holding, bathing). Offer Albert appropriate auditory and sensory stimulation—do not overstimulate. Refer to outside resources (e.g., infant developmental/stimulation programs).	

Heroin

Heroin crosses the placenta. Of infants born to heroin-addicted mothers, 50% are of low birth weight (LBW), and 50% of these infants are small-for-gestational age (SGA). Heroin may have a direct growth-inhibiting effect on the fetus. There is an increased rate of stillbirths but not of congenital anomalies.

Detoxification is not advised before 14 weeks' gestation because of a potential risk of spontaneous abortion, and it is also not advised after the thirty-second week because of possible withdrawal-induced fetal distress (Niebyl, 1988).

Heroin withdrawal occurs in 50% to 75% of infants born to addicted mothers, usually within the first 24 to 48 hours of life. The signs depend on the length of maternal addiction, the amount of drug taken, and the time of injection before birth. The infant whose mother is on methadone may not demonstrate signs of withdrawal until a week or so after birth. The symptoms of infants whose mothers used heroin or methadone are similar in nature. Initially the infant may be depressed. The *withdrawal syndrome* may consist of a combination of any of the following signs. The newborn may be jittery and hyperactive. Table 39-1 gives a comparison between neonatal jitteriness and seizures. Commonly the infant's cry is shrill and persistent. The infant may yawn or sneeze frequently. The tendon reflexes are increased, but the Moro's reflex is decreased (Bartlett and Davis, 1980; Merker, Higgins, and Kinnard, 1985). The infant may exhibit poor feeding and sucking, tachypnea, vomiting, diarrhea, hypothermia or hyperthermia, and sweating. In addition, an abnormal sleep cycle with absence of quiet sleep and disturbance of active sleep has been described in these infants (Fanaroff and Martin, 1987).

Table 39-1 *Comparison of Newborn Jitteriness and Seizures*

Normal Newborn Jitteriness	Newborn Seizure
Dominant movement tremor	Clonic jerking that cannot be stopped by flexing the affected limbs
No ocular movement	Ocular movement
Highly sensitive to stimulation	Not sensitive to stimulation
Persists for about 4 days after birth	Persists beyond 4 days after birth

If withdrawal is not treated, the infant may develop fever, vomiting, diarrhea, dehydration, apnea, and convulsions. Death may follow. Therapy is individualized. Dehydration and electrolyte imbalance is prevented or treated. Usually one of the following drugs is ordered: phenobarbital; paregoric (compound tincture of opium); or diazepam, singly or in combination.

The long-term effect on these newborns is now being studied. Researchers have found that "many serious" mental and physical problems are evident in the child's first few months of life, as well as "numerous indications . . . [of] serious abnormalities in the brain structure that will not be revealed until later years" (Howard, 1986).

Methadone

Methadone, a synthetic opiate, has been the therapy of choice for heroin addiction since 1965. By blocking the euphoric effects, it reduces the craving for heroin. It does cross the placenta. An increasing number of infants have been born to methadone-maintained mothers, who seem to have better prenatal care and a somewhat better life-style than those taking heroin (Fanaroff and Martin, 1987). Multiple drug abuse, however, is a problem for many. The drugs include alcohol, barbiturates, tranquilizers, and other psychoactive drugs. Many are heavy smokers as well. Methadone withdrawal occurs in about 70% to 90% of infants born to these women. Methadone withdrawal resembles heroin withdrawal syndrome (p. 989), but tends to be more severe and prolonged. The incidence of seizures is higher, however. Seizures usually occur between days 7 and 10. The infants exhibit a disturbed sleep pattern similar to that seen in heroin withdrawal. The infants have higher birth weight and most are appropriate for gestational age (AGA). No increased incidence of congenital anomalies is seen.

Late-onset withdrawal occurs at 2 to 4 weeks and may continue for weeks or months. A higher incidence of sudden infant death syndrome (SIDS) has also been reported in these infants.

Therapy for methadone withdrawal is similar to that for heroin withdrawal. The few follow-up studies of these infants that are available reveal a higher incidence of hyperactivity, learning and behavior disorders, and poor social adjustment (Fanaroff and Martin, 1987). See the nursing care plan for neonatal drug withdrawal, p. 984.

Marijuana

Marijuana is thought to be the most abused drug in the United States with an estimated 20 million users. It crosses the placenta. Its use during pregnancy may result in a shortened gestation and a higher incidence of precipitate labor (<3 hours) (Niebyl, 1988). Some investigators have found a higher incidence of meconium staining (Greenland et al., 1984; Niebyl, 1988; Fanaroff and Martin, 1987). No increased incidence of congenital complications or effects on the infant's growth and physical parameters specific to marijuana use alone have been identified. However, when used with alcohol, decreased birth weight and a fivefold increase in risk for FAS is expected. Long-term follow-up studies on exposed infants are needed.

Cocaine

Cocaine is another commonly used drug in all social classes. It is the most powerfully addictive drug available (Chapter 34). Commonly it is used along with other drugs such as marijuana and alcohol. Its use is credited with a higher incidence of spontaneous abortion and abruptio placentae secondary to frequent episodes of vasospastic hypertension. It crosses the placenta and is found in breast milk. No congenital anomalies or effects on the infant's growth and physical parameters have been identified specific to cocaine.

Cocaine-dependent newborns often experience a significant and agonizing withdrawal syndrome that can last 2 to 3 weeks (Landry and Smith, 1987). The withdrawal signs have some of the same characteristics as heroin withdrawal. Irritability, marked jitteriness, rapid changes in mood, and hypersensitivity to noise and external stimuli characterize the infants. They exhibit poor feeding, irregular sleep patterns, tachypnea, tachycardia, and often diarrhea. Chasnoff et al. (1985) identified significant depression in interactive behavior and a poor organization response to environmental stimuli when assessing affected infants with the BNBAS.

The infants exposed to cocaine are typically lethargic, almost catatonic. They have visual attention problems in that they are unable to focus on their parent's face. These children often have been subjected to numerous small strokes because of abrupt changes in their mothers' blood pressure during pregnancy (Howard, 1986). Renal problems, lack of coordination, developmental retardation, and perhaps visual problems may be related. There may be an increased risk for SIDS. See the nursing care plan for neonatal drug withdrawal, p. 984.

Phencyclidine

Phencyclidine (PCP) (angel dust) is one of the most dangerous of the available abused drugs. It may have extremely unpredictable, bizarre, and violent effects, especially when combined with crack (cocaine free base) (a combination known as "space base") (Chapter 34). PCP increases the risk of injury to the user and therefore also to her passively dependent fetus. The user may be unaware that she is using PCP since it is commonly misrepresented as another drug of abuse or mixed with other drugs.

PCP crosses the placenta and is found in breast milk. Literature about newborns is limited. The infants exposed to PCP appear to be alert, active babies. "Their mothers often think they are smarter. They hold their heads up faster. . . . But, in fact, it is abnormal behavior. Although we aren't sure why, the tone of the muscles in the head is of the kind that we see in [children with] cerebral palsy," a disorder of the CNS characterized by spastic paralysis or other forms of defective motor ability (Bean, 1986).

Miscellaneous Substances

Amphetamine is one of the most potent stimulants available. It is used commonly by adolescents and young adults. The fetal and neonatal effects of maternal use of amphetamines in pregnancy are not well known. The effects appear to be dose related. Low birth weight, preterm birth, and perinatal mortality may be consequences of higher doses used throughout pregnancy. Newborns may be drowsy, jittery, and experience respiratory distress soon after birth. Lethargy may continue for several months, along with frequent infections, and poor weight gain. Emotional disturbances and delays in gross and fine motor coordination may be seen during early childhood.

Phenobarbital is another commonly abused drug in all social classes. It crosses the placenta readily and is subsequently found in high levels in the fetal liver and brain. Because of its slow metabolic rate, when withdrawal does occur, onset is generally at 2 to 14 days after birth and duration is about 2 to 4 months. Irritability, crying, hiccoughs, and sleepliness mark the initial response. During the second stage the infant is extremely hungry, regurgitates and gags frequently, and demonstrates episodic irritability, sweating, and a disturbed sleep pattern.

Treatment consists of swaddling, frequent feedings, and protection from noxious external stimuli. If there is no improvement with these methods, the infant should be given phenobarbital and then slowly withdrawn from this drug after control of symptoms (Fanaroff and Martin, 1987).

Caffeine has not been implicated as a teratogen in humans. After controlling for smoking and other habits (including alcohol consumption), demographic characteristics, and medical history, Linn et al. (1982) found no relationship between coffee consumption and any adverse outcomes of pregnancy. The Food and Drug Administration (FDA) (1980) suggests that "prudence dictates that pregnant women and those who may become pregnant avoid caffeine-containing products or use them sparingly."

Tobacco

Cigarette smoking in pregnancy has been found to be associated with birth weight deficits of up to 250 g for a full-term neonate (Stein and Sussler, 1984, Fanaroff and Martin, 1987). Maternal cigarette smoking is implicated in 21% to 39% of low-birth-weight infants. The rate of preterm birth is increased. Nicotine and cotinine, the two pharmacologically active substances in tobacco, are found in higher concentrations in infants whose mothers smoke (Luck et al., 1982). These substances can be secreted in breast milk for up to 2 hours after the mother has smoked. Cigarette smoke contains over 2000 compounds including carbon monoxide, dioxin, cyanide, and cadmium. Long-term studies show residual effects beyond the neonatal period (Niebyl, 1988). Deficits in growth, intellectual and emotional development, and behavior have been documented (DHHS 1983, Naeye and Peters, 1984).

The *fetal tobacco syndrome* is a diagnostic term applicable to infants who fit the following criteria (Nieberg et al., 1985):

1. The mother smoked five or more cigarettes a day throughout pregnancy.
2. The mother had no evidence of hypertension during pregnancy, specifically: (a) no preeclampsia and (b) documentation of normal blood pressure at least once after the first trimester.
3. The newborn has symmetric growth retardation at term (up to or greater than 37 weeks), defined as (a) a birth weight less than 2500 g and (b) a ponderal index ([weight in g]/[length in m]) greater than 2.32.
4. There is no other obvious cause of IUGR (e.g., congenital infection or anomaly).

Pregnant women need to be aware of the deleterious effects of smoking on their unborn baby's health. Mothers (and all others) need to refrain from smoking while near their newborn infant. Several studies have reported a positive association between maternal smoking and SIDS (Niebyl, 1988). It is not clear whether this association reflects in utero exposure or passive exposure postnatally, or both.

SUMMARY

The compromised newborn presents a challenge to the health care team. The nurse must have sound knowledge about conditions that place the newborn at risk, including problems related to infection and drug dependence. Constant vigilence, prompt reporting, and timely therapy are necessary to prevent serious sequelae to the disorder and its therapy.

The outcome for infants born to addicted mothers appears to depend on the interrelationships between many factors. These factors include not only intrauterine drug exposure but emotional, familial, and environmental instability that is so commonly associated with the drug culture.

The parents and other family members need a sensitive, thoughtful nurse to help them cope with the stress that arises from birth and care of a compromised newborn. The complex care of multiple problem clients requires an interdisciplinary approach that includes team members from home health care and community resources.

KEY CONCEPTS

- Some perinatal risk is directly related to maternal behaviors such as drug abuse and to maternal infection.
- Infection in the newborn may be acquired in utero, during delivery, during resuscitation, and from within the nursery.
- Sequelae to septicemia include meningitis, pyarthrosis, and septic shock.
- Rehabilitative measures are required for both the infant and the parent when the neonatal period is complicated by infection or drug dependence.
- The best known and most common maternal infections during early pregnancy that are associated with various congenital malformations are represented by the acronym TORCH.
- Transmission of HIV from the mother to the infant occurs transplacentally at various gestational ages, perinatally via maternal blood and secretions, and through breast milk or through other close contact.
- Critical determinants of the effect of maternal drug abuse on the fetus include the specific drug used, the dosage, the route of administration, the genotype of the mother or fetus, and the timing of the drug exposure.
- The nurse is commonly the first to observe the signs of drug dependence in the newborn.
- Rehabilitative measures must be included in the plan for care for the newborn and the parent to offer the infant an opportunity for optimum growth and development after discharge.
- Involvement of the family (including spouse or sexual partner, parents, children, or other close relatives living with or near the woman) and community resources must be considered in the implementation of care for the newborn suffering the effects of maternal infection or drug dependence.

STUDY QUESTIONS AND ACTIVITIES

1. Assign students to role-play the interations of a nurse with the parents of a child born with syphilis, AIDS, or other STD. Follow with group discussion.
2. Repeat the above assignment. The newborn is dependent on heroin, methadone, or cocaine.
3. Complete an assessment of community resources within the neighborhood that offer services to infants compromised by infection and drug dependence and their fam-

ilies. Identify services needed but not readily available or accessible.

4. Discuss social changes that may support the prevention of infection and drug addition. Consider the mass media, advertising, and other factors.

References

Neonatal Infections

American Academy of Pediatrics, American College of Obstetricians and Gynecologists; Guidelines of perinatal care, Evanston, Ill, 1983, American Academy of Pediatrics

Arevalo, JA, and Washington, AE: Cost-effectiveness of prenatal screening and immunization for hepatitis B virus, JAMA, 259(3):365, 1988

Beasley, RP, Hwang, LY, Stevens, CE, et al: Efficacy of hepatitis B immune globulin for prevention of perinatal transmission of the hepatitis B virus carrier state: final report of a randomized double-blind, placebo-controlled trial, Hepatology 3:135, 1983a

Beasley, RP, Hwang, LY, Lee, GC, et al: Prevention of perinatally transmitted hepatitis B virus infections with hepatitis B immune globulin and hepatitis B vaccine, Lancet 2:1099, 1983b

Bennett, EC: Sexually transmitted diseases: current approaches, NAACOG Newletter 14(8):1, 1987

Blocking hepatis B birth transmission, Med World News 28:17, 1987

Brown, AA, et al: Effects on infants of a first episode of genital herpes during pregnancy, N Engl J Med 317(2):1249, 1987

Facing the complex issues of pediatric AIDS: a public health perspective (editorial), JAMA 258(19):2736, 1987

Fanaroff, AA, and Martin, RJ, editors: Neonatal-perinatal medicine: diseases of the fetus and infant, ed 4, St Louis, 1987, The CV Mosby Co

Harnish, DG, Hammerberg, O, Walker, IR, and Rosenthal, KL: Early detection of HIV infection in a newborn, N Engl J Med, 316:272, 1987

Jackson, MM, et al: Clinical savvy: why not treat all body substances as infectious? Am J Nurs 87(9):1137, 1987

Johnson, JP, Nair, P, and Alexander, S: Early diagnosis of HIV infection in the neonate, N Engl J Med 316:273, 1987

Klug, RM: AIDS beyond the hospital: part two of a CE feature—children with AIDS, Am J Nurs 86(10):1126, 1986

Landesman, S, et al: Serosurvey of human immunodeficiency virus infection in parturients, JAMA 258(19):2701, 1987

Leishman, K: Heterosexuals and AIDS: the second stage of the epidemic, The Atlantic Monthly, p 39, Feb, 1987

MMWR: Public Health Service guidelines for counseling and antibody testing to prevent HIV infection and AIDS, MMWR 36:509, 1987

Main, D, and Mennuti, M: Neural tube defects: Issues in prenatal diagnosis and counseling, Obstet Gynecol 67:1, 1986

Marion, RW, et al: Human T cell lymphotrophic virus type III (HTLV-III) embryopathy: a new dysmorphia syndrome, Am J Dis Child 140:638, 1986

Marwick, C: Routine screening considered to end perinatal hepatitis transmission, JAMA, 257(15):1999, 1987

Measles shots advised for kids with AIDS, San Francisco Chronicle, April 4, 1988

Merenstein, GB, and Gardner, SL: Handbook of neonatal intensive care, St Louis, 1985, The CV Mosby Co

Monif, G, and Hardt, W: Management of herpetic vulvovaginitis in pregnancy, Semin Perinatol 7:16, 1985

NAACOG: Rubella/hepatitis B precautions advised, NAACOG Newsletter, 13(4):April, 1986

Pahwa, S, Kaplan, M, Fikrig, S, et al: Spectrum of human T-cell lymphotropic virus type III infection in children: recognition of symptomatic, asymptomatic, and seronegative patients, JAMA 255:2299, 1986

Pernoll, ML, Benda, GI, and Babson, SG: Diagnosis and management of the fetus and neonate at risk: a guide for team care, ed 5, St Louis, 1986, The CV Mosby Co

Petit, C: Stanford researchers find flaw in herpes text, San Francisco Chronicle, p 24, Jan 29, 1987

Prenatal care and HIV screening (letters to editor), JAMA 258(19):2693, 1987

Prober, CG: Low risk of herpes simplex virus infections in neonates exposed to the virus at the time of vaginal delivery to mothers with recurrent genital herpes simplex virus infections, N Engl J Med 316:240, 1987

Pyun, KH, et al: Perinatal infection with human immunodeficiency virus: specific antibody responses by the neonate, N Engl J Med 317(10):611, 1987

Stevens, CE, Toy, P, Tong, MJ, et al: Perinatal hepatitis B virus transmission in the United States: prevention by passive-active immunization, JAMA 253:1740, 1985

Syphilis cases up 35 percent in state, San Francisco Chronicle, p 4A, Jan 29, 1988

Wong, VCW, Ip, HMH, Reesink, HW, et al: Prevention of the HBsAg carrier status in newborn infants in mothers who are chronic carriers of HBsAg and HBeAg by administration of hepatitis B vaccine and hepatitis B immune globulin: double-blind randomized placebo-controlled study, Lancet 1:9821, 1984

Substance Abuse

Abel, EL, and Sokol, RJ: Incidence of fetal alcohol syndrome and economic impact of FAS-related anomalies, Drug Alcohol Depend, 1988 (In press)

Bartlett, D, and Davis, A: Recognizing fetal alcohol syndrome in the nursery, JOGN Nurs 9:23, 1980

Bean, Y: Report of ongoing research on the infants of mothers using cocaine and PCP, Los Angeles Times, January 1986

Chasnoff, IJ, et al: Cocaine use in pregnancy, N Engl J Med 313:666, 1985

Davis, RP, and Keith, L: Fetal alcohol syndrome: incurable but preventable, Contemp OB/GYN 21(3):57, 1983

DHHS: The health consequences of smoking for women: a report of the Surgeon General, Pub No 410-889/1284, Washington, DC, 1983, Department of Health and Human Services

Fanaroff, AA, and Martin, RJ: Neonatal-perinatal medicine: diseases of the fetus and infant ed 4, St Louis, 1987, The CV Mosby Co

Food and Drug Administration: Caffeine and pregnancy, FDA Drug Bulletin, 10:19, 1980

Greenland, S, et al: The effects of marijuana use during pregnancy. I. A preliminary epidemiology study, Am J Obstet Gynecol 150:23, 1984

Howard, J: Report of ongoing research on the infants of mothers using cocaine and PCP, Los Angeles Times, January 1986

Landry, M, and Smith, DE: CRACK: anatomy of an addiction, part 2, Calif Nurs Rev 9(3):28, 1987

Linn, S, et al: No association between coffee consumption and adverse outcomes of pregnancy, N Engl J Med 306:141, 1982

Luck, W, et al: Nicotine and cotinine: two pharmacologically active substances as parameters for the strain on fetuses and babies of mothers who smoke, J Perinatal Med 10:107, 1982

McCarthy, P: Fetal alcohol syndrome, Nurse Practitioner: Am J Primary Health Care 8:34, 1983

Merker, L, Higgins, P, and Kinnard, E: Assessing narcotic addiction in neonates, Pediatr Nurs 11:177, 1985

Morningstar, PJ, and Chitwood, DD: How women and men get cocaine: sex-role stereotypes and acquisition patterns, J Psychoactive Drugs 19(2):135, 1987

Naeye, RL, and Peters, EC: Mental development of children whose mothers smoked during pregnancy, Obstet Gynecol 64:60, 1984

Nieberg, L, et al: The fetal tobacco syndrome (commentary), JAMA 253:2998, 1985

Niebyl, JR: Drug use in pregnancy, ed 2, Philadelphia, 1988, Lea & Febiger

Stein, ZA, and Sussler, M: Intrauterine growth retardation: epidemiological issues and public health significance, Semin Perinatal 8:5, 1984

Zuspan, FP: When drugs and alcohol complicate pregnancy, Contemp OB/GYN 24(1):35, 1984

Bibliography

Neonatal Infections

Becker, L, and Lagomarsino, W: Isolation guidelines for perinatal patients: creating a new protocol, MCN 12(6):400, 1987

Bennett, J: AIDS: What precautions do you take in the hospital? Am J Nurs 86(8):952, 1986

Berman, SM, et al: Low birth weight, prematurity, and postpartum endometritis: association with prenatal cervical *Myoplasma hominis* and *Chlamydia trachomatis* infections, JAMA 257(9):1189, 1987

Bromberg, MH, and Hsia, LS: Rubella in the perinatal period, J Perinat Neonat Nurs 1(4):24, 1988

Buchs, S: Candida meningitis: a growing threat to premature and full-term infants, Pediatr Infect Dis 4:122, 1985

Bush, JJ: Protocol for tuberculosis screening in pregnancy, JOGN Nurs 15(3):225, 1986

California Nurses Association (CNA): Infection control precautions, (Correspondence) Sept, 1987, The Association

Carey, JC: Vaginal infections and prematurity, Birth, 14(2):91, 1987

Cohen, SP: Bacterial sepsis in the very low birth weight infant, J Perinat Neonat Nurs 1(4):66, 1988

Cushing, AH: Omphalitis in newborns, Contemp OB/GYN 30(5):53, 1987

Ferenczy, A, Silverstain, S, and Crum, CP: Papillomaviruses: importance of latency in HPV infections, Contemp OB/GYN 30(5):71, 1987

Foster, SD: Education, the best defense against AIDS, MCN 12(5):311, 1987

Freij, BJ, and Sever, JL: When is immunization in pregnancy really needed? Contemp OB/GYN 27:48, May 1986

Gaffney, SE, and Salinger, L: Group B streptococcus: the pregnant woman and her neonate, JOGN Nurs 16(2):91, 1987

Gennoro, S: Listerial infection: nursing care of mother and infant, MCN 5:390, 1980

Gerberding, JL, et al: Risk for transmitting the human imunodeficiency virus, cytomegalovirus, and hepatitis B virus to health care workers exposed to patients with AIDS and AIDS-related conditions, J Infect Dis 156:1, 1987

Gershon, A: Chickenpox: how dangerous is it? Contemp OB/GYN 31(3):41, 1988

Gordin, PC: Candida infection in the very low birth weight infant, J Perinat Neonat Nurs 1(4):47, 1988

Gravett, MG, et al: Independent associations of bacterial vaginosis and *Chlamydia trachomatis* with adverse pregnancy outcome, JAMA 256:1899, 1986

Guinan, ME, and Hardy, A: Epidemiology of AIDS in women in the United States: 1981 through 1986, JAMA 257(15):2038, 1986

Haggerty, L: TORCH: a literature review and implications for practice, JOGN Nurs 14:124, March/April, 1985

Hall, CB, et al: Ribavirin treatment of respiratory syncytial viral infection in infants with underlying cardiopulmonary disease, JAMA 254:3047, 1985

Hinman, AR: Prevention of congenital rubella infection: symposium summary, Pediatrics 75:1162, 1985

Ippolito, C, and Gives, RM: AIDS and the newborn, J Perinat Neonat Nurs 1(4):78, 1988

Kaunitz, AM, et al: Prenatal care and HIV screening, JAMA 258(19):2693, 1987

Klein, ME: Hepatitis B virus: perinatal management, J Perinat Neonat Nurs 1(4):12, 1988

Laga, M, et al: Prophylaxis of gonococcal and chlamydial ophthalmia neonatorum: a comparison of silver nitrate and tetracycline, N Engl J Med 318(11):653, 1988

Larson, E: Trends in neonatal infections, JOGN Nurs 16(6):404, 1987

Larson, E: Rituals in infection control: what works in the newborn nursery? JOGN Nurs 16(6):411, 1987

Letters: HIV infection and childhood sexual abuse, JAMA 259(15):2235, 1988

Lo, KJ, Tsai, YT, Lee, ST, et al: Immunoprophylaxis of infection with hepatitis B virus in infants born to hepatitis B surface antigen-positive carrier mothers, J Infect Dis 152:817, 1985

Loucks, A: Chlamydia: an unheralded epidemic, Am J Nurs 86(7):920, 1986

Loveman, A, Colburn, V, and Dobin, A: AIDS in pregnancy, JOGN Nurs 15(2):91, 1986

Marecki, MA: *Chlamydia trachomatis:* a developing perinatal problem, J Perinat Neonat Nurs 1(4):1, 1988

Marvin, C, and Slevin, A: Chlamydia—cause, prevention, and cure, MCN 12(5):318, 1987

Mendez, H, et al: Human immunodeficiency virus (HIV) infection in pregnant women and their offspring (abstract) Pediatr Res 21:1466A, 1987

Miles, PA: Sexually transmitted diseases, JOGN Nurs 13:102s, 1984

Miller, DS: Intravenous immune globulin for treating primary immunodeficiency disease, MCN 12(4):244, 1987

Minkoff, HL: Pregnant women with HIV, JAMA 258(19):2714, 1987

Minkoff, HL, et al: Pregnancies resulting in infants with acquired immunodeficiency syndrome: description of the antepartum, intrapartum, and postpartum course, Obstet Gynecol 69:285, 1987

Minkoff, HL, et al: Follow-up of mothers of children with AIDS, Obstet Gynecol 87:288, 1987

MMWR Supplement: Recommendations for prevention of HIV transmission in health-care settings, MMWR 36:2S, Aug, 1987

Olsen, TG: Your pregnant patient's rash: is it PUPP syndrome? Contemp OB/GYN 22:151, 1983

Paryani, SG, et al: Sequelae of acquired cytomegalovirus infection in premature and sick infants, J Pediatr 107:451, 1985

Pass, RF, et al: Young children as a probable source of maternal and congenital cytomegalovirus infection, N Engl J Med 316(22):1366, 1987

Questions and answers: Multiple genital papillomatosis: an indication for cesarean section? JAMA 258(22):3309, 1987

Report of the Surgeon General's workshop on children with HIV infection and their families, published DHHS-D-MC 87-1. US Dept of Health and Human Services, 1987

Ritter, SE, and Vermund, SH: Congenital toxoplasmosis, JOGN Nurs 14:435, Nov/Dec 1985
Samson, LF: Perinatal viral infection and neonates, J Perinat Neonat Nurs 1(4):56, 1988
Schachter, J, et al: Erythromycin in the routine treatment of chlamydial infections in pregnancy, N Engl J Med 314:276, Jan 30, 1986
Smith, H, and Congdon, P: Neonatal systemic candidiasis, Arch Dis Child 60:365, 1985
Sommers, GM, and Kao, MS: Pharmacology: chemotherapeutic agents used during pregnancy, Contemp OB/GYN 30(3):45, 1987
Stear, LA, and Elinger, SS: Understanding acquired immunodeficiency syndrome: implications for pregnancy, J Perinat Neonat Nurs 1(4):April 1988
Tafuro, P, and Gurevich, I: Prevention and management of varicella in high-risk individuals, MCN 9:314, Sept/Oct 1984
Troy, P, et al: Sibling visiting in the NICU, Am J Nurs 88(1):68, 1988
Washington, AE, Johnson, RE, and Sanders, LL: *Chlamydia trachomatis* infections in the United States: what are they costing us? JAMA 257(15):2070, 1987
Wetzel, AM, and Kirz, DS: Routine hepatitis screening in adolescent pregnancies: is it cost effective? Am J Obstet Gynecol 156(1):166, 1987
Winkler, B: Controlling chlamydial infections, Contemp OB/GYN 30(5):30, 1987
Witter, FR: Pharmacology: TB regimens during pregnancy, Contemp OB/GYN 23:101, 1984

Substance Abuse

Bingue, N, et al: Cocaine teratogenicity in humans, J Pediatr 110:93, 1987
Chasnoff, IJ, et al: Perinatal cerebral infarction and maternal cocaine use, J Pediatr 108:456, 1986
Dixon, SD, Coen, RW, and Crutchfield, S: Visual dysfunction in cocaine-exposed infants (abstract), Pediatr Res 21:359, 1987
Hingson, R, et al: Maternal marijuana use and neonatal outcome: uncertainty posed by self-reports, Am J Public Health 76(6):667, 1986
MacGregor, S, Keith, L, et al: Cocaine use during pregnancy: adverse perinatal outcome, Am J Obstet Gynecol 157(3), 686, 1987
Madden, JD, Payne, TF, and Miller, S: Maternal cocaine abuse and effect on the newborn, Pediatrics 77:209, 1986
Oro, AS, and Dixon, SD: Perinatal cocaine and methamphetamine exposure: maternal and neonatal correlates, J Pediatr 111(4):571, 1987
Ronkin, S, et al: Protecting mother and fetus from narcotic abuse, Contemp OB/GYN 31(3):178, 1988
Ryan, L, and Erlichs, FL: Outcome of infants born to cocaine-using drug-dependent women, Pediatr Res 20:338, 1986
Shanley, C: Management of narcotic dependent pregnancy, Aust Nurses J 16(2):50, 1986
Silver, H, et al: Addiction in pregnancy: high risk intrapartum management and outcome, J Perinatol 7(3):178, 1987
Sward, S: How babies suffer when mothers use cocaine, San Francisco Chronicle p B3, March 18, 1988
Woods, J, Plessinger, M, and Clark, K: Effect of cocaine on uterine blood flow and fetal oxygenation, JAMA 257:957, 1987

General Bibliography

Boynton, BR, and Boynton, CA: Discharge planning for high-risk infants, J Perinat 5:44, Fall 1985
Censullo, M: Home care of the high-risk newborn, JOGN Nurs 15:146, 1986
Consolvo, CA: Relieving parental anxiety in the care-by-parent unit, JOGN Nurs 15:154, March/April 1986
Gildea, J: A crisis plan for pediatric code, Am J Nurs 86:557, May 1986
Johnson, SH: Nursing assessment and strategies for the family at risk: high-risk parenting, ed 2, Philadelphia, 1986, JB Lippincott Co
Korones, SB: High-risk newborn infants: the basis for intensive nursing care, ed 4, St Louis, 1986, The CV Mosby Co
Ledger, KE, and Williams, DL: Parents at risk: an instructional program for perinatal assessment and preventive intervention, Victoria, B.C. Canada, 1981, Ministry of Health, Province of British Columbia, and Queen Alexandra Solarium for Crippled Children Society (Queen Alexandra Hospital, 2400 Arbutus Rd, Victoria, B.C., Canada V8N 1V7)
Merenstein, GB, and Gardner, SL: Handbook of neonatal intensive care, St Louis, 1985, The CV Mosby Co
Philip, AG: Neonatology: a practical guide, ed 3, Philadelphia, 1987, WB Saunders Co
Raff, BS: The use of homemaker-home health aides' perinatal care of high-risk infants, JOGN Nurs 15:142, March/April 1986
Raff, BS: Nursing care of high-risk infants and their families—introduction JOGN Nurs 15:141, March/April 1986
Segal, S, et al: The death of a child—parents' views of professional support, Can Med Assoc J 134:38, Jan 1, 1986
Whaley, L, and Wong, D: Nursing care of infants and children, ed 3, St Louis, 1987, the CV Mosby Co

CHAPTER

40

Hyperbilirubinemia and Congenital Anomalies

Learning Objectives

Correctly define the key terms listed.

Compare and contrast Rh and ABO incompatibility.

Explain management to prevent the pathologic consequences of hyperbilirubinemia.

Discuss assessment of the newborn for hyperbilirubinemia.

Develop a general plan of care for the prevention, identification, and management of hyperbilirubinemia in any newborn.

Review prenatal diagnosis of neonatal disorders.

Present assessment strategies during the postnatal period to aid in diagnosis of congenital disorders.

Describe general preoperative and postoperative care of the newborn.

Develop a general care plan for parents of a newborn with a defect or disorder.

Describe each congenital disorder presented in this chapter and identify the priority of care for each.

Key Terms

ABO
α-fetoprotein
choreoathetoid cerebral palsy
cleft lip or palate
congenital
Coombs' test
diaphragmatic hernia
epispadias
esophageal atresia
exchange transfusion
hemolytic disease of newborn
hip dysplasia
hydramnios
hydrocephalus
hypospadias
imperforate anus
inborn error of metabolism
intrauterine fetal transfusion
isoimmune hemolytic disease
kernicterus
microcephaly
neural tube defects
omphalocele
phocomelia
polydactyly
red blood cell antigenicity

HYPERBILIRUBINEMIA

The yellow discoloration of the skin and other organs caused by accumulation of bilirubin is termed *jaundice* or *icterus*. Jaundice in the newborn, a common sign of potential trouble, is primarily caused by unconjugated bilirubin, a breakdown product of hemoglobin (Hgb), after its release from hemolysed red blood cells (RBCs). The challenge of neonatal jaundice is to distinguish physiologic jaundice from a serious clinical pathologic condition.

Hyperbilirubinemia has a variety of etiologic factors. The main focus of this chapter is isoimmune hemolytic disease of the newborn secondary to Rh or ABO incompatibility (see Immunology, Table 6-8). Rh incompatibility is also known as erythroblastosis fetalis. Antibodies from the mother cross the placenta into fetal blood. Maternal antibodies attach to fetal RBCs and initiate a process that ends in hemolysis. Hemolysis of fetal RBCs leads to anemia and hyperbilirubinemia. Anemia decreases O_2 and CO_2 transport. It also favors movement of fluid out of the vascular bed to the extravascular compartment causing hypovolemia and edema. Elevated levels of serum unconjugated bilirubin result in the deposit of this pigment in body cells. Unconjugated bilirubin is cytotoxic to certain body cells; in the skin it is recognized as jaundice.

Rh Incompatibility

During antibody studies in the 1940s, it was observed that the injection of RBCs of rhesus monkeys into rabbits caused the production of an antiserum that agglutinated the RBCs of these monkeys and of most humans as well. Consequently RBCs that could be agglutinated by this specific antiserum possessed the rhesus (Rh) antigen and were called **Rh positive**. Those RBCs that did not possess the Rh factor (antigen) could not be agglutinated and were called **Rh negative**. Subsequently it was discovered that the Rh factor is not a single antigen but a complex blood system with a number of variants.

Six common Rh antigens are identified as follows: C, D, E, c, d, e. Antibody formation (sensitization) results from the presence of one or more of these (and other less common) antigens. Because two chromosomes are present in every cell, one derived from each parent, the genetic constitution of an individual with reference to these antigens might be, for example, DD, dd, or Dd.

Different combinations allow eight Rh genotypes, each with a single Rh chromosome (e.g., CDE, cde, cDE). Actually, 36 different combinations (genotypes) are possible. The order of antigenicity potency of these antigens is D, C, E, c, e, and d.

Soon after the Rh factor was reported, it was found that erythroblastosis fetalis, hydrops fetalis, and icterus gravis—variations of hemolytic disease of the newborn—were caused by the hemolysis of fetal Rh-positive RBCs by specific antibodies from an Rh-negative mother.

Between 10% and 15% of marriages of white persons will involve Rh-incompatible partners. About 5% of black couples will be Rh incompatible. It is rare than an Oriental couple will be similarly affected.

Not all Rh-positive men are homozygous for the Rh factor, nor will all children of Rh-positive men married to Rh-negative women be Rh positive. About 50% of the progeny of Rh-positive men who are heterozygous will be Rh positive; the remainder will be Rh negative. Rh negative offspring are in no danger because they are compatible with their mothers.

Some women have a greater antigenic (immune) response to the Rh factor. In the first pregnancy only 0.1% of mothers will be sensitized. In the second and third pregnancies 11% will be affected, and in the fourth or subsequent Rh-positive pregnancies, 15% of mothers will be affected. About 5% of Rh-incompatible matings produce affected infants.

Effects of sensitization are seen in subsequent pregnancies. The placenta of the seriously affected fetus is larger than normal. Increased villous size, persistence of Langerhans' cells, and foci of erythropoiesis are apparent. Commonly the amniotic fluid is yellowish, that is, pigment stained from the decomposition of bilirubin.

Severe Rh incompatibility results in marked fetal hemolytic anemia with erythroid hyperplasia of bone marrow and extramedullary (for example, spleen) hematopoiesis. The placenta clears the released blood pigments fairly well, however, so that only in extreme cases (such as icterus gravis) is the fetus icteric (yellow, or jaundiced). The marked anemia leads to cardiac decompensation, cardiomegaly, hepatomegaly, and splenomegaly. Edema, ascites, and hydrothorax develop. Severe anemia may lead to hypoxia. Intrauterine or early neonatal death may occur.

Once delivery has occurred, the erythroblastotic newborn becomes icteric (in severe cases, within 30 minutes after birth) because it cannot excrete the considerable residue of RBC hemolysis. Yellowish pigmentation of cerebral basal nuclei, hippocampal cortex, and subthalamic nuclei often develops (kernicterus). Kernicterus occurs when the serum bilirubin rises to levels toxic to the newborn, and serious central nervous system (CNS) abnormalities may develop and persist (such as, choreoathetoid cerebral palsy) if the infant survives. The most common sequela of kernicterus in the neonatal period is death.

ABO Incompatibility

ABO incompatibility is more common than Rh incompatibility, but the effects are generally less severe in the affected infant. ABO incompatibility occurs when type A, B, or AB fetal RBCs cause a type O mother to develop specific antibodies. These anti-A and anti-B antibodies are transferred across the placenta to the mother's fetus. In this situation even the firstborn infant may be affected. The newborn may show a weakly positive direct Coombs' test (p. 998, and Table 6-10). Cord bilirubin is usually less than 4 mg/100 ml and any hyperbilirubinemia can usually be treated with phototherapy as outlined in Procedure 22-10 and Fig. 22-10. Exchange transfusions are required in occasional cases only. Ongoing hemolysis may cause anemia, jaundice, and kernicterus and justifies serial hematocrit studies until stable.

Kernicterus

Kernicterus refers to bilirubin encephalopathy that results from the deposit of bilirubin, especially within the brain stem and basal ganglia. The yellow staining (jaundice of the brain tissue) and necrosis of neurons result from unconjugated bilirubin. Unconjugated bilirubin is readily capable of crossing the blood-brain barrier because of its high lipid solubility. Kernicterus may occur in certain newborns with no apparent clinical jaundice. Only one sequela in survivors is specific: **choreoathetoid cerebral palsy**. Other sequelae, such as mental retardation and serious sensory disabilities, may reflect hypoxic, vascular, or infectious injury that is often associated with kernicterus. About 70% of newborns who develop kernicterus die in the neonatal period.

The perinatal events that enhance the development of hyperbilirubinemia also increase the likelihood that kernicterus will develop, perhaps even in the presence of mild to moderate unconjugated hyperbilirubinemia. The perinatal events include hypoxia, asphyxia, acidosis, hypothermia, hypoglycemia, bacterial infection, certain medications, and hypoalbuminemia. These conditions interfere with conjugation or compete for albumin-binding sites.

Clinical manifestations of kernicterus commonly first appear between 2 and 6 days after birth. *Kernicterus is never present at birth.* Symptomatology changes as the disease process progresses. Four phases are recognized:

1. **Phase one:** the newborn is hypotonic and lethargic and exhibits a poor sucking reflex and depressed or absent Moro's reflex (some infants die during this phase).
2. **Phase two:** the newborn develops spasticity and hyperreflexia, often becomes opisthotonic, has a high-pitched cry, and may be hyperthermic. The newborn may convulse.
3. **Phase three:** at about 7 days of age, the newborn's spasticity lessens and may disappear.
4. **Phase four:** after the first month of life, the infant develops sequelae (e.g., spasticity, athetosis, partial or complete deafness, or mental retardation).

Rh_0(D) Human Immune Globulin

The more severe forms of isoimmune hemolytic disease result from Rh_0D^u group incompatibility. This form of hemolytic disease of the newborn occurred in 0.5% to 1% of all pregnancies in North America before prophylactic Rh_0(D) human immume globulin (RhoGAM) became available in the mid-1960s. Many children died or were seriously affected. Since immunization of Rh-negative women against this antigen began, the incidence of severe erythroblastosis has been drastically reduced.

Prophylaxis for Rh isoimmunization involves the use of Rh immune globulin as a preventive measure against Rh isoimmunization. It is not a treatment for Rh-negative women who are already sensitized, because it has no effect against antibodies already present in the maternal bloodstream. An injection of **Rh_O(D) immune globulin provides passive immunity,** which is transient and therefore will not affect a subsequent pregnancy. Rh_0(D) immune globulin (RhIG) prepares RBCs containing the Rh antigen for lysis by phagoctyes, before the recipient's immune system is activated to produce antibodies. **Production of one's own antibodies provides active immunity** (Table 6-8).

Antibodies formed by an active immune response remain within the individual's bloodstream, presumably for life. RhIG given to an Rh_0(D)-negative woman who is already sensitized would accomplish no purpose. Therefore it is recommended only for non-sensitized Rh-negative women at risk of developing Rh isoimmunization. Given to any Rh-positive person, an injection of RhIG would result in hemolysis of RBCs.

Assessment

Prenatal Events

Risk factors from the prenatal record are identified. The severity of physiologic jaundice differs greatly between *Oriental* and other ethnic populations. The mean serum levels of unconjugated bilirubin in Chinese, Japanese, Korean, and American Indian full-term newborns are between 10 and 14 mg/dl, or approximately double those for other non-Oriental populations. The incidence of bilirubin toxicity is also increased (Fanaroff and Martin, 1987).

Maternal infections often precede neonatal hyperbilirubinemia. Bacterial (e.g., syphilis), viral (e.g., rubella) and protozoal (e.g., toxoplasmosis) infections have a direct association. Maternal ingestion of sulfonamides or salicylates close to delivery affect the newborn's ability to remove bilirubin. Medical conditions such as *maternal diabetes mellitus* predispose the newborn to hyperbilirubinemia (Pernoll, Benda, and Babson, 1986).

Maternal blood type and Rh place the woman at risk for *isoimmunization,* (Chapter 6) which subsequently jeopardizes future pregnancies. *Women who are Rh negative are* at risk for developing antibodies to the Rh factor, a process called isoimmunization or sensitization. To develop antibodies, the mother will need to have been innoculated with Rh-positive RBCs. Therefore the woman's history is investigated for events that can lead to innoculation. These events include (1) transfusion with Rh-positive blood, (2) spontaneous or elective abortions ≥ 8 gestational weeks, (3) previous pregnancy(s) with an Rh-positive fetus, (4) amniocentesis for any reason, and (5) premature separation of the placenta (the latter is often difficult to identify).

Sensitization of the mother occurs promptly after an incompatible blood transfusion (improperly typed [Rh-positive] blood). Hematopoiesis (formation and development of blood cells) begins in the embryo during the sixth week after conception (i.e., during the eighth week after the last menstrual period [LMP]). Therefore a woman who has experienced one or more abortions 2 months or more since her LMP or has given birth has received innoculations of fetal blood generally at the time of placental separation.

During amniocentesis, the needle may cause localized damage to the single layer of cells that separates maternal and fetal circulation in the placenta, thus allowing some fetal RBCs into maternal circulation. If any of these events have occurred, the woman's record is checked for documentation of prophylaxis for isoimmunization (see p. 1000). The postnatal course(s) of a previous baby(s) is also assessed for evidence of maternal isoimmunization. Rh-negative women who receive prenatal care have blood drawn to screen for the presence of antibodies to antigens such as the Rh factor (i.e., the Hemantigen screen and Coombs' test). The *Hemantigen test* also screens for other less common RBC-antigens such as Kell, Duffy, and Kidd. Fortunately, serious fetal damage from these factors is unlikely.

Results of indirect *Coombs' tests* are reviewed. In this test the **maternal blood** serum is mixed with Rh-positive RBCs. The test is positive (maternal antibodies are present) if Rh-positive RBCs agglutinate (clump). The dilution of the specimen of blood at which clumping occurs (if it does occur) determines the titer (level of maternal antibodies). The titer determines the degree of maternal sensitization (isoimmunization). If the titer reaches 1:16, an amniocentesis for delta optical density (ΔOD) analysis is performed (Perry, Parer, and Inturrisi, 1986).

The first amniocentesis is usually performed between 18 weeks' (in the case of a high antibody titer and any previously affected fetuses) and 24 weeks' gestation (in the case of a low fixed antibody titer and any previously unaffected fetuses) (Perry, Parer, and Inturrisi, 1986). ΔOD is a spectrophotometric (color) analysis test (Chapter 27). This test determines the amount of bilirubin in the amniotic fluid.

Maternal blood type O may also place the newborn at risk (p. 996).

Perinatal Events

The perinatal record is reviewed for conditions that are associated with increased RBC destruction in the newborn and that may increase susceptibility (particularly from the immature infant) to the neurotoxic effect of bilirubin by (1) enhancing its passage across the blood-brain barrier and (2) reducing cellular integrity (Fanaroff and Martin, 1987). These factors include (1) perinatal asphyxia with a pH under 7.20, (2) an unstable physiologic condition of the newborn indicated by an Apgar score of 3 or less at 5 minutes, (3) hypothermia (temperature less than 35° C [95° F]), (4) deterioration of the infant's condition as indicated by clinical signs, and (5) hypoglycemia (also leads to acidosis).

All of these conditions adversely affect metabolism. Compromised metabolism in the neonate delays or interferes with bilirubin conjugation into a water-soluble form for excretion in urine and stool. Although the precise effects of these insults are undetermined, the increased risk to the newborn may be sufficient to justify treatment at lower levels of bilirubin.

Postnatal Events

The infant who has severe **erythroblastosis fetalis** may initially exhibit yellow-stained vernix or umbilical cord. The infant may have *hydrops fetalis.* Signs of this manifestation of severe hemolytic anemia include edema, pleural and pericardial effusions, and ascites; all of which indicate cardiac failure (many of these infants are stillborn). Placental enlargement is seen with severe disease.

There is an alteration of the average ratio of placental to fetal weight at term. The weight of the normal placenta is generally one sixth that of the fetus. With hemolytic disease of the newborn, the placenta may weigh as much as one half or three fourths the neonate's weight. Hepatosplenomegaly is commonly identified.

Preterm birth, low birth weight (LBW), and immaturity affect the newborn's ability to process bilirubin. *Immaturity* of, or defects in, the *glucuronyl transferase enzyme system* delays or interferes with the conjugation of bilirubin. Hepatic cell damage caused by infection or drugs also interferes with that enzyme system.

Other physiologic limitations of the newborn are diagnosed during investigation of hyperbilirubinemia. Congenital RBC abnormality (e.g., spherocytosis) or congenital enzyme deficiency (e.g., glucose-6-phosphate dehydrogenase [G6PD] deficiency) (Table 40-2) may be the basis for the newborn's hyperbilirubinemia. The incidence of G6PD deficiency is greater in Oriental populations and in people from the Greek islands of Lesbos and Rhodes.

Sequestered blood accounts for elevated bilirubin levels. Blood is sequestered (trapped or confined) in cephalhematomas, ecchymoses, and hemangiomas. As the blood is hemolyzed, levels of serum bilirubin rise.

Neonatal Jaundice

Jaundice is the visible demonstration of developmental limitations of bilirubin metabolism and transport in the neonatal period (Fanaroff and Martin, 1987). Approximately 50% of all full-term newborns are visibly jaundiced during the first 3 days of life. Serum bilirubin levels less than 5 mg/dl usually are not reflected in visible skin jaundice.

Physiologic hyperbilirubinemia characterized by a progressive increase in serum levels of unconjugated bilirubin from 2 mg/dl in cord blood to a mean peak of 6 mg/dl by 72 hours of age, followed by a decline to 5 mg/dl by day 5, and not exceeding 12 mg/dl. These serum values are within the normal physiologic limitations of the healthy term newborn who was not exposed to perinatal complications (such as hypoxia). No bilirubin toxicity develops.

Pathologic hyperbilirubinemia cannot be defined solely in terms of serum concentrations of unconjugated bilirubin. Pathologic hyperbilirubinemia refers to that level of serum bilirubin at which a particular newborn will sustain lesions in the brain tissue (kernicterus), renal tubular cells, intestinal mucosa, and pancreatic cells.

Every newborn is assessed for jaundice and hyperbilirubinemia. Findings are assessed from physical and behavioral examination and laboratory tests. The *blanch test* assists in the differentiation of cutaneous jaundice from skin color. To do the test, apply pressure with the thumb over a bony area (e.g., forehead) for several seconds to empty all the capillaries in that spot. If jaundice is present the blanched area will look yellow before the capillaries refill. The conjunctival sacs and buccal mucosa are assessed, especially in darker-skinned infants. It is preferable to assess for jaundice in daylight, because there is possible distortion of color from artificial lighting, reflection from nursery walls, and the like.

The nurse notes the infant's behavior. Changes in feeding and sleeping patterns, pallor, and dark color of stools and urine accompany hyperbilirubinemia. Neurologic signs of kernicterus are presented on p. 997.

Laboratory results add to the data base. Blood type, Rh factor, hemoglobin, hematocrit, and Coombs' test results identify maternal-fetal RBC incompatibility and erythroblastosis fetalis.

Laboratory reports that support the diagnosis of hyperbilirubinemia follow*:

1. Serum bilirubin levels increasing more than 5 mg/dl/24 hr
2. Full-term newborn: serum bilirubin level greater than 12 mg/dl, which represents the upper limit of peak concentration of physiologic jaundice (Chapter 21)
3. Low-birth-weight newborn: serum bilirubin levels of 10 to 12 mg/dl, even though the peak concentration of "physiologic jaundice" is 15 mg/dl
4. Premature newborn: all visible jaundice, even with serum bilirubin levels as low as 5 mg/dl

Blood from the umbilical cord is sent to the laboratory to establish the blood type and Rh status. Occasionally an Rh-positive infant is wrongly typed as Rh-negative because of so-called blocking antibodies covering the affected newborn's RBCs.

A **direct Coombs' test** is performed with **neonatal cord blood**. The neonate's RBCs are "washed" and mixed with Coombs' serum. The test is positive (maternal antibodies are present) if the infant's RBCs agglutinate. The dilution of the specimen of blood at which agglutination occurs (if it does occur) determines the titer of maternal antibodies in fetal serum. The titer determines the degree of maternal sensitization. If the titer is 1:64, an exchange transfusion is indicated.

Increased erythropoiesis with many nucleated RBCs are seen in hemolytic anemia of a progressive type. Hypoglycemia may be present and treated to avoid additional CNS insult (Chapter 38).

Transcutaneous bilirubinometry is a screening test for neonatal jaundice based on the relationship between the yellow color of the skin and total serum bilirubin level. This rapid, noninvasive transcutaneous procedure uses a spectrophotometric hand-held fiberoptic instrument that illuminates the skin and measures the intensity of its yellow color. The intensity of color is then displayed as a number that correlates with serum bilirubin concentration; it is *not* an absolute estimate of total bilirubin. This test screens for those jaundiced newborn infants with rising bilirubin levels whose condition may need further diagnostic investigation.

The small probe of the bilirubinometer is applied firmly against the newborn's skin over a bony surface of the forehead or the sternum. The photoprobe is held against the skin with enough pressure to blanch the skin. Then a pulse of light is transmitted through the skin to the subcutaneous tissues and the reflected color is recorded within a few seconds.

Skin pigmentation *does affect* the readings. Correlations between transcutaneous bilirubin index and serum bilirubin levels have been established for Japanese infants, American white infants, and American black infants at term. The different values for the preterm or LBW newborn of each racial group are not yet available. The instrument is not suitable for monitoring the newborn during or immediately after phototherapy or exchange transfusion.

No adverse effects on the newborn have been reported so far, and no short- or long-term effects are anticipated. The fiberoptic instrument releases a brief pulse of strong, cool, white light that does not harm underlying skin or tissues. The beam of light is absorbed mainly at the surface of the skin and underlying the subcutaneous tissue.

Nursing Diagnoses

Following are examples of nursing diagnoses for newborns at risk from hyperbilirubinemia:

- Potential for injury to neurons and cells in the kidney, pancreas, and intestine related to
  - Hyperbilirubinemia
- Impaired gas exchange related to
  - Hemolytic anemia
- Potential fluid volume deficit
  - Phototherapy
- Potential for parental anxiety related to
  - Hyperbilirubinemia, its management, and potential sequelae

Planning

Hospital protocols for care of hyperbilirubinemia are developed as a collaborative effort of the health care team. The health care team utilizes hospital protocols or standards when individualizing care for the infant and parents. Goals for care are stated in client-centered terms.

Goals

1. Prenatal and perinatal risk factors are identified and intervention implemented where appropriate
2. Hyperbilirubinemia and its sequela, kernicterus, are absent
3. There are minimal or no sequelae from hyperbilirubinemia and its treatment
4. Parents understand newborn's condition, therapies, and possible sequelae

*For the normal full-term newborn, serum bilirubin of 12 to 15 mg/dl is the cut-off point for phototherapy and 20 mg/dl for exchange transfusion. For sick or preterm newborns, it is best to prevent *any* rise in serum bilirubin altogether; no level can be regarded as "safe" in view of the possibility of opening the blood-brain barrier and the vulnerability of brain cells resulting from disease processes and inadequate energy reserves. For the sick or preterm newborn, phototherapy is advisable for visible jaundice, and exchange transfusion for serum bilirubin of 15 mg/dl (Wu, et al., 1985).

Implementation

Preventive Measures

Prevention is the primary focus of care. The nurse is not responsible for typing and cross-matching blood and blood products. However, the nurse is responsible for checking the product to be administered against the physician's order and the woman's blood type and Rh status.

Prenatal control of diabetes mellitus, prevention of infection, avoidance of sulfonamides and aspirin (when possible), and prevention of preterm birth reduce perinatal risks. Prevention of or prompt appropriate therapy for perinatal asphyxia, acidosis, cold stress, and hypoglycemia will decrease the newborn's risk of severe hemolytic disease and of susceptibility to neurotoxicity of bilirubin. Early feeding is initiated to stimulate the gastrocolic reflex to remove bilirubin through stooling (Chapter 22).

Prophylaxis for Rh isoimmunization is now available.

Antenatal Administration of Rh_0(D) Immune Globulin (Human). Rh sensitization is possible during pregnancy if the cellular layer separating fetal and maternal circulations is disrupted and fetal blood enters the maternal bloodstream. The cellular layer may be disrupted during amniocentesis or by placental abruption. For the woman who is Rh_0(D) negative D^u (allemorph variant) negative, and Coombs' negative, RhIG administered during the antenatal period after amniocentesis, at about 28 weeks' gestation and again within 72 hours after delivery can further reduce the incidence of maternal isoimmunization.

Postnatal Administration of Rh_0(D) Immune Globulin (Human). The United States Public Health Service recommendations are as follows:

1. RhIG is given only to a woman after delivery or abortion who is Rh_0(D) negative and D^u negative and whose fetus is Rh_0(D) positive or D^u positive. **It is *never* given to an infant or father.**
2. RhIG is not useful in a woman who has Rh antibodies.
3. RhIG should be given intramuscularly, not into fatty tissue or intravenously.

Prevention of isoimmunization of an Rh-negative woman to the Rh factor in her fetus is now possible in over 95% of cases. Prophylaxis is achieved by administering RhIG within 72 hours of evacuation of the uterus (by spontaneous or elective abortion or more advanced pregnancy).

Jaundice may not be apparent before the baby is discharged. Some baby's have sequestered blood (e.g., cephalhematoma). Therefore, especially if the mother is discharged with the infant soon after delivery, parents need to learn how to identify jaundice and know when to notify the physician (Locklin, 1987).

Curative Measures

Hyperbilirubinemia occurs in approximately 50% of normal newborns. *Phototheray* is conducted in the normal newborn nursery, usually for physiologic hyperbilirubinemia (see Procedure 22-10 and Fig. 22-10). A nursing care plan for an infant with hyperbilirubinemia is on p. 1001.

Some fetuses are candidates for *intrauterine transfusion* (Chapter 27). The transfusion is accomplished in the following manner.* Ultrasonography is used to locate the placenta. Then a needle is passed transabdominally into the amniotic sac, and radiopaque dye is injected. The fetus swallows the amniotic fluid. The radiopaque dye in the fetal gastrointestinal tract can be visualized by x-ray film. Then the physician injects packed RBCs directly into the fetal peritoneal cavity. The packed RBCs (drawn up into 10 ml units) are cross-matched with maternal serum. The **blood type used is Rh_0(D) negative and (usually) group 0.** Only blood that is negative for cytomegalovirus (CMV), hepatitis, and human immunodeficiency virus (HIV) is used (Perry, Parer, and Inturrisi, 1986). The fetus is able to absorb these RBCs into the fetal circulation via the lymphatic vessels and great veins and to utilize them to counteract the anemia; cardiac decompensation is thus forestalled. Results of this procedure are encouraging. The second transfusion is administered 10 days later, followed by transfusions every 3 weeks until delivery.

Exchange transfusion may be required in the immediate neonatal period. The nurse is alert to the fact that a significant risk for morbidity and a mortality risk of 0.1% to 1.0% exist with exchange transfusions. It is time consuming and expensive as well (see Procedure 40-1).

An exchange transfusion is accomplished by alternately removing a small amount of the infant's blood and replacing it with a like amount of donor blood. Depending on the infant's size, maturity, and condition, amounts of 5 to 20 ml at a time are slowly exchanged. The total amount of blood exchanged approximates 170 ml/kg of body weight (80 ml/lb) or 75% to 85% of the infant's total blood volume.

The staff observes infection control precautions for invasive procedures (Chapter 30).

Rehabilitative Measures

Planning for rehabilitative measures is necessary if kernicterus occurs. The family will need the services from many community resources to care for the affected child. An interdisciplinary approach that includes social services must be taken.

Evaluation

On a short-term basis care can be considered to be effective if unconjugated serum bilirubin levels do not reach or exceed toxic levels. These levels are arbitrarily set at $\geq$ 5mg/dl/24 hr, $\geq$ 12mg/dl in term neonates, and $\geq$ 15mg/dl in preterm neonates. Parents understand and are able to cope with hyperbilirubinemia and its management. Long-term evaluation of effective care rests in the absence of sequelae to hyperbilirubinemia (e.g., minimal brain dysfunction).

*Intrauterine exchange transfusion directly into umbilical cord vessels is being done in some hospitals.

Specific Nursing Care Plan

HYPERBILIRUBINEMIA

Bret Jackson is a 34-week-gestation premature infant born to a 26-year-old mother who came to the hospital 9 centimeters dilated in active labor. Bret was born via spontaneous vaginal delivery with apgar scores of 6 and 8. He has been cared for in the Special Care Nursery in a .40% oxyhood with mild retractions, occasional tachypnea and nasal flaring. Phototherapy was initiated 24 hours ago for a bilirubin level of 9.7 mg/dl, however, this morning's AM lab results are significantly higher at 14.0 mg/dl.

ASSESSMENT	NURSING DIAGNOSIS (ND)/ PLAN (P)/GOAL (G)	RATIONALE/ IMPLEMENTATION	EVALUATION
14.0 mg/dl serum bilirubin level. Assess color and consistency of stools; dark, concentrated urine. Assess for increasing pallor. Assess skin color in daylight and not artificial light, if possible. Assess signs of kernicterus: diminished Moro's reflex, poor suck, vomiting, hypotonia, high-pitched cry, lethargy, seizures.	ND: Potential for injury related to hyperbilirubinemia. P: Identify and treat hyperbilirubinemia promptly. G: Bret's hyperbilirubinemia is treated promptly and he will demonstrate no signs of kernicterus.	*To monitor and reduce serum bilirubin levels, the nurse will:* Record and report increasing bilirubin levels immediately for prompt treatment. Obtain blood for testing as ordered (bilirubin, Hgb & Hct, liver function tests, blood incompatibility studies, etc.). Obtain IV access and monitor IV infusion (adequate hydration is essential for bilirubin excretion). Maintain phototherapy as ordered (keep eyes patched and expose as much skin surface to light as possible, see p. 526). Child should only be removed from phototherapy for very brief periods. Test strength of bili lights while child is under phototherapy according to hospital and manufacturer policy. Note neurologic signs of kernicterus and report immediately. Set-up, assist, and monitor child during an exchange transfusion as indicated and ordered.	Bret's bilirubin levels decline with treatment and he demonstrates no signs of kernicterus or any iatrogenic complications of IV therapy, phototherapy, exchange transfusion, etc.
Assess parent's knowledge of hyperbilirubinemia, its treatment, and possible sequelae.	ND: Knowledge deficit related to hyperbilirubinemia, its treatment, and complications. P: Meet parents' knowledge needs. G: Parents learn about their newborn's condition, therapies, and possible sequelae. G: Parents participate in maintaining the treatment regime.	*To teach Bret's parents about hyperbilirubinemia, the nurse will:* Explain the different causes of hyperbilirubinemia and their potential sequelae. Explain the treatment modalities. Encourage parents to take an active role in the treatment plan (e.g., keeping eye patches in place and full skin exposed to light while under phototherapy, etc.). Encourage questions, feelings, or concerns.	Parents verbalize understanding of instruction. Parents participate in maintaining the treatment regime.

Procedure 40-1

EXCHANGE TRANSFUSION

DEFINITION

The introduction of whole blood in exchange for 75% to 85% of an infant's circulating blood that is repeatedly withdrawn in small amounts and replaced with equal amounts of donor blood

PURPOSE

1. Reduce serum bilirubin levels
2. Improve oxygen-carrying capacity of the blood:
   a. Remove red cells that are destined for hemolysis by circulating antibodies
   b. Correct the anemia
   c. Remove antibodies (or other causative agents) responsible for hemolysis
3. Correct acidosis

EQUIPMENT

1. Disposable exchange transfusion set
2. Fresh donor's blood (under 3 days old and heparinized), two units on hand in case of error or contamination
3. Monitoring equipment
4. Transfusion record
5. Water bath (38° C [100° F]) to warm the blood
6. Medications: **calcium gluconate** in 5 ml syringe with no. 24 needle; 50% glucose solution in 10 ml syringe with no. 24 needle; sodium bicarbonate in 10 ml syringe with no. 24 needle
7. Sterile gowns, drapes, gloves, caps, and masks
8. Cleansing solution with sterile cotton pledgets or gauze sponges
9. Adequate lighting
10. Heat source to keep the infant warm

NURSING ACTIONS	RATIONALE
Identify client and check physician's orders.	To provide the right therapy for the right person.
Wash hands before and after touching client or equipment. Glove, prn.	To prevent nosocomial infection and to implement universal precautions.
Prepare and adjust heat lamps or overhead radiant heat shield; have warmed blankets available for infant.	To prevent cold stress.
Give infant nothing orally for 3 or 4 hours, or stomach contents are aspirated by gastric tube.	To prevent aspiration.
Assemble resuscitative equipment: O_2 source, masks, breathing bag, airways, laryngoscope (extra batteries), endotracheal tube with obturator, suction, medication.	To have readily available if needed for immediate supportive therapy.
Position infant on back and restrain. Take and record vital signs.	To facilitate treatment. Prevents dislodging catheter and tissue trauma. Provides base line to evaluate change.
Assemble electronic monitoring equipment or stethoscope. Attach electrodes, or keep stethoscope over apex of heart. Monitor and record results continuously during procedure.	To identify hazards of procedure that include apnea, bradycardia (100 beats/min or less), cardiac arrhythmia or arrest.
Physician *and* nurse check donor blood: type, Rh, age, and free of sickle cell trait.	To minimize chance of error. Provides donor RBCs that are not affected by maternal antibodies present in the fetal system. Acts as precaution against fatal intravascular sickling.
Run tubing from bottle (bag) through warm water bath to infant.	To avoid cold stress, ventricular fibrillation, vasospasm, or decrease in blood viscosity.
Before starting transfusion, assist physician as necessary a. Cleanse site of cutdown (jugular or femoral artery) or umbilical stump (umbilical vein). b. Drape. c. Put on gown and gloves.	To prevent microbial contamination.
During transfusion:	*During transfusion:*
Physician measures central venous pressure (CVP) before initiating transfusion.	To act as precaution against heart failure from volume overload. Change from 10 to 12 cm pressure is indication to stop and reassess infant's status.
Nurse notes and records time exchange is begun.	To maintain accurate record.
For *each* successive withdrawal of infant's blood *and* injection of donor's blood, nurse records time, amounts in and out, cumulative amounts in and out.	To maintain accurate, continuous record to assist with ongoing procedure and provide index of infant's response.
After 100 ml has been exchanged, physician gives **calcium gluconate**: nurse monitors heart and respiratory rates and records them.	To minimize possibility of cardiac arrhythmias or arrest.

Procedure 40-1—cont'd

NURSING ACTIONS	RATIONALE
Nurse records pertinent comments.	To maintain accurate record.
Nurse records medications: time, type, amount, infant response.	To maintain accurate record.
After transfusion (catheter may be removed or left in place with dressing): Nurse finishes charting. Nurse continues to observe and record infant's behavior closely for 24 to 48 hours. (1) Vital signs: heart rate, respirations, temperatures, pedal pulses (2) Lethargy, jitteriness, convulsions (3) Dark urine (4) Edema	To identify complications. Infant is observed to prevent hemorrhage from site and to detect and treat promptly any complications of blood transfusion such as heart failure, hypocalcemia, acute hypercalcemia, hyperkalemia, hypernatremia, hypoglycemia and acidosis,* sepsis, shock, thrombus formation, transfusion mismatch reaction.

*Red blood cells continue anaerobic glycolysis with production of acid metabolites after removal from donor. Blood stored for longer than 2 days is likely to contain potentially dangerous levels of potassium and to be more readily subjected to hemolysis.

SUMMARY

In the United States Rh hemolytic disease of the newborn occurs once in approximately 150 to 200 full-term deliveries. At least 200,000 children are affected by Rh isoimmunization each year, of which 5000 are stillborn. If severe hemolytic disease of the newborn is untreated, about 10% of infants will develop kernicterus. With intrauterine (fetal) transfusions, about 40% of these children can be saved despite maternal and fetal hazards of the procedures. Amniocentesis studies, early delivery of affected fetuses, and exchange as well as replacement transfusions save many more. Complete recovery may be expected in most infants who do not develop kernicterus. If hyperbilirubinemia is treated promptly and effectively, most infants recover without residua or sequelae.

The parents require the nurse's support. Parents are involved in the plan of care and are kept informed of the child's condition throughout its management. Explanations of physiologic and pathologic hyperbilirubinemia are reinforced. The need for adequate fluid intake (such as water between feedings) and eye patches during phototherapy are clarified. The physician's explanations regarding the disease, its treatment, the infant's condition, and the possible prognosis are clarified and reinforced. See guidelines for client teaching: hyperbilirubinemia in Chapter 22.

CONGENITAL ANOMALIES

The desired and expected outcome of every wanted pregnancy is a normal, functioning infant with a good intellectual potential. Fulfillment of this hope depends on numerous factors, both hereditary and environmental. Probably all human characteristics have a genetic component, including those that produce unpleasant symptoms or unwelcome physical abnormalities that impair the fitness of the individual. Some diseases are produced through the action of a single gene or the combined action of many genes inherited from the parents; others are the result of the action of the environment on the genetic composition of the individual. In some instances the genetic component is obvious; in others it is subtle or scarcely discernible. Many disorders are apparent at birth; others do not become apparent for days, weeks, months, or even years. A disease or disorder that can be transmitted from generation to generation is termed *genetic* or *hereditary* (Chapter 9). A *congenital* disorder is one that is present at birth and can be caused by genetic or environmental factors or both.

Each year 250,000 infants are born with significant structural and functional disorders. Of all infants born, 0.5% to 1% have a congenital anomaly severe enough to end in death or require surgery to avoid death. Another 1% require definitve attention to avoid morbidity and handicapping (Pernoll, Benda, and Babson, 1986; Fanaroff and Martin, 1987). Major congenital defects are now the leading cause of death in term births where perinatal care is of good quality. With the fall in other causes of neonatal mortality, they now account for over 25% of all deaths.

The seriousness of this community health problem is reflected in the more than 6 million hospital days and $200 billion a year allocated to the care and treatment of these neonates. Prevention and detection procedures are being improved continuously. Methods of promoting the availability of these services to populations at risk challenge the community health care systems. An interdisciplinary team approach is imperative to provide holistic care: surgery, rehabilitation, and education of the child and social, psychologic, and financial assistance to the parents. Parental disappointment and disillusion and the nurse's own negative feelings toward (or stigmatization of) the infant's disorder add to the complexity of nursing care.

When studying and using this content, the reader is asked to keep an open mind. New data and technology are constantly being identified. Some of the appropriate procedures and treatments of the recent past are considered ineffective and even hazardous today. To support the goal of intact survival, therapy must be continuously reviewed and improved in light of progress.

Assessment

Prenatal Diagnosis

Recently refined testing procedures are available to monitor the development of the fetus. Prenatal diagnostic techniques such as amniocentesis, ultrasound, α-fetoprotein measurements (AFP), chorionic villi sampling (CVS), percutaneous umbilical cord blood sampling (PUBS), and gene probes contribute to the data base (Chapter 27). Although they comprise a valuable adjunct to prenatal care, these tests do not achieve 100% accuracy in detecting congenital defects (Table 27-9) (Cohen, 1987; Hershey, Craudall, and Perdue, 1986; Main and Mennuti, 1986; Kogan, Doherty, and Gitschier, 1987; Benacerraf, Gelman, and Frigoletto, 1987; Routine, 1987; Lewis and Mocarski, 1987). Some women choose to continue the pregnancy after positive identification of a congenital problem. The prenatal record is reviewed for documentation of parental wishes for the level of aggressiveness of management they would consider for the care of the infant. The record should also reveal the results of the parents' and hospital's advocate team's communication regarding assessment, education, and coordination of services for the infant (McLaughlin, et al., 1985).

Despite the status and availability of current technology, not all congenital disorders are or can be anticipated. The historical and medical information in the prenatal record is reviewed for factors that are associated with congenital disorders. These factors include various medical, surgical, and social conditions and their treatments (Chapter 34), maternal infection (Chapter 30), maternal endocrine and metabolic disorders (Chapters 32 and 38), and infection and drug dependence in the newborn (Chapter 39).

Perinatal Diagnosis

Many congenital anomalies require intervention soon after birth. Careful observations in the birth room or nursery will identify most of these conditions.

Volume of Amniotic Fluid. An excessive amount of amniotic fluid, **hydramnios**, is commonly associated with congenital anomalies in the newborn. The infant should be examined closely at the earliest possible time. In the presence of hydramnios, any of the following may be suspected:

1. Cephalocaudal malformations, such as hydrocephalus, microcephaly, anencephaly, and spina bifida
2. Orogastrointestinal malformations, such as cleft palate, esophageal atresia with or without a tracheal fistula, pyloric stenosis, volvulus, and imperforate anus
3. Miscellaneous conditions, such as Down's syndrome, congenital heart disease, deformed extremities, and infants of diabetic or prediabetic mothers
4. Preterm birth

Oligohydramnios (an insufficient amount of amniotic fluid) is primarily associated with those anomalies of the urinary tract that preclude normal micturition in utero. As a rule, renal agenesis or renal dysplasia is involved.

1. Urethral stenosis has also been reported to be associated with oligohydramnios.
2. Anomalies of the earlobes, rather than agenesis of the ear, are sometimes associated with renal abnormalities and are not direct results of oligohydramnios.
3. Potter's syndrome (renal agenesis) is the classic example of an association between oligohydramnios and renal anomalies. It includes a typical facies that involves abnormal earlobes.

Postnatal Diagnosis

An Apgar score and minimal assessment are completed as it is for each neonate after birth (p. 434). Any deviations from normal are reported to the physician immediately.

Respiratory System. Screening for congenital anomalies of the respiratory tract is necessary even for the infant who is apparently normal at birth. Respiratory distress at birth or shortly thereafter may be the result of lung immaturity or anomalous development. Congenital laryngeal web and bilateral choanal atresia (Fig. 40-1) are readily apparent at birth. Both require emergency surgery. Respiratory distress caused by diaphragmatic hernia and tracheoesophageal fistula appear immediately or may be delayed depending on the severity of the defect.

Neurologic System. Neurologic signs may reflect hid-

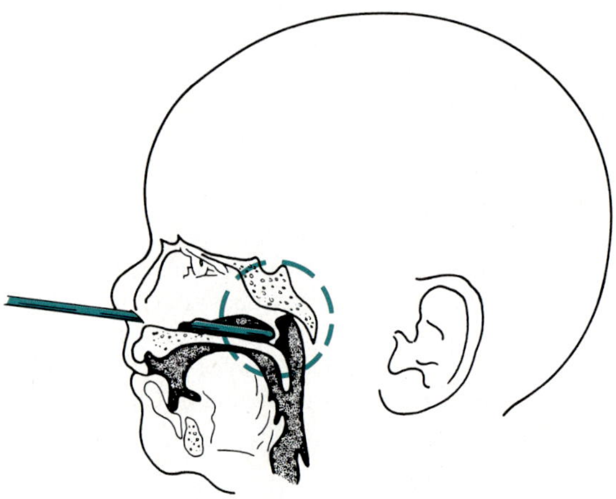

Fig. 40-1 Choanal atresia. Posterior nares are obstructed by membrane or bone either bilaterally or unilaterally. Infant becomes cyanotic at rest. With crying, newborn's color improves. Nasal discharge is present. Snorting respirations are often observed with increased respiratory effort. Newborn may be unable to breathe and eat at same time. Diagnosis is made by noting inability to pass small feeding tube through one or both nares.

Courtesy Ross Laboratories, Columbus, Ohio.

den congenital anomalies as well as numerous other conditions. Many neonatal responses are nonspecific. Each sign, such as high-pitched cry, hypotonia, jitteriness, low-set ears, and microcephaly or hydrocephaly, must be evaluated carefully before appropriate therapy can be instituted.

Some neural tube defects are obvious at first glance. The three main defects are anencephaly, spina bifida (which includes occult and visible meningocele and myelomeningocele), and encephalocele (p. 1014). These are defects in midline closures. If a neural tube defect is identified, the infant may have one or more of the other malformations in this group: cleft lip and palate, tracheoesophageal fistula, and diaphragmatic hernia.

Cardiovascular System. Severe congenital cardiovascular disorders often are evident immediately after birth, for example, severe cyanotic heart disease (Fig. 40-2). These infants usually are transferred directly to special nurseries or pediatric units. Some problems, such as a small patent ductus arteriosus or a minimal coarctation of the descending aorta, become apparent only as the infant is exposed to stresses such as growth demands of later infancy and early childhood, or infection. In about 75% of cases cardiovascular anomalies are unexpected.

Cardiovascular defects occur in 3 of every 1000 births. Congenital heart disease is implicated in approximately 50% of deaths from malformations during the first year of life. The etiologic factors are still unclear, although a famil-

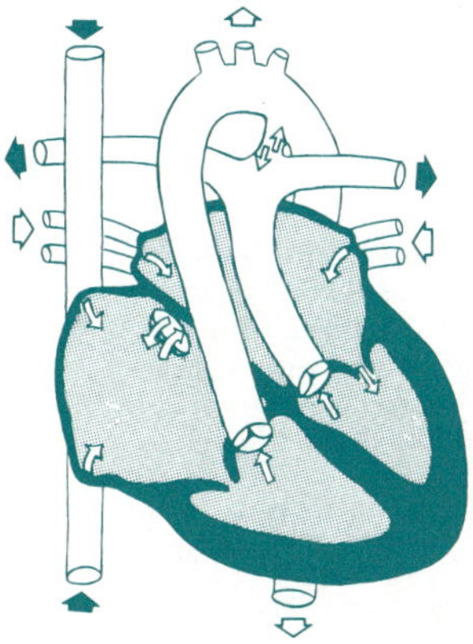

Complete transposition of great vessels

The anomaly is an embryologic defect caused by a straight division of the bulbar trunk without normal spiraling. As a result, the aorta originates from the right ventricle, and the pulmonary artery from the left ventricle. An abnormal communication between the two circulations must be present to sustain life.

Fig. 40-2 Congenital heart abnormalities.
Courtesy Ross Laboratories, Columbus, Ohio.

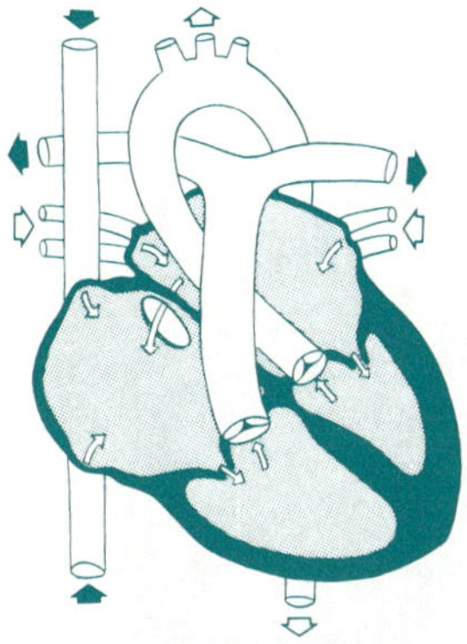

Atrial septal defects

An atrial septal defect is an abnormal opening between the right and left atria. Basically, three types of abnormalities result from incorrect development of the atrial septum. An incompetent foramen ovale is the most common defect. The high ostium secundum defect results from abnormal development of the septum secundum. Improper development of the septum primum produces a basal opening known as an ostium primum defect, frequently involving the atrioventricular valves. In general, left to right shunting of blood occurs in all atrial septal defects.

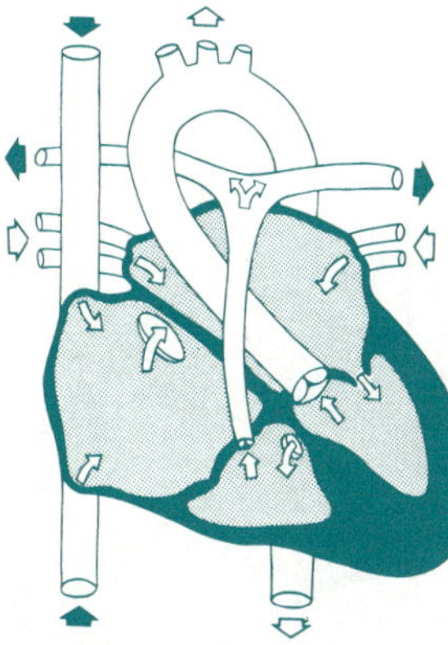

Tricuspid atresia

Tricuspid valvular atresia is characterized by a small right ventricle, large left ventricle, and usually a diminished pulmonary circulation. Blood from the right atrium passes through an atrial septal defect into the left atrium, mixes with oxygenated blood returning from the lungs, flows into the left ventricle, and is propelled into the systemic circulation. The lungs may receive blood through one of three routes: (1) a small ventricular septal defect, (2) patent ductus arteriosus, (3) bronchial vessels.

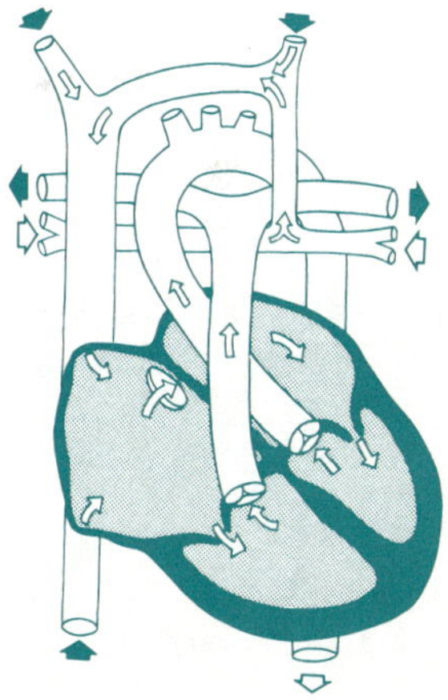

Anomalous venous return

Oxygenated blood returning from the lungs is carried abnormally to the right heart by one or more pulmonary veins emptying directly, or indirectly, through venous channels into the right atrium. Partial anomalous return of the pulmonary veins to the right atrium functions the same as an atrial septal defect. In complete anomalous return of the pulmonary veins, an interatrial communication is necessary for survival.

Continued.

Fig. 40-2—cont'd Congenital heart abnormalities.

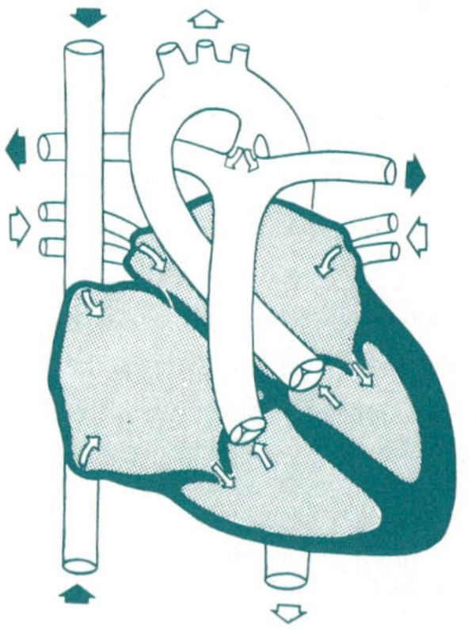

Patent ductus arteriosus

The patent ductus arteriosus is a vascular connection that, during fetal life, short circuits the pulmonary vascular bed and directs blood from the pulmonary artery to the aorta. Functional closure of the ductus normally occurs soon after birth. If the ductus remains patent after birth, the direction of blood flow in the ductus is reversed by the higher pressure in the aorta.

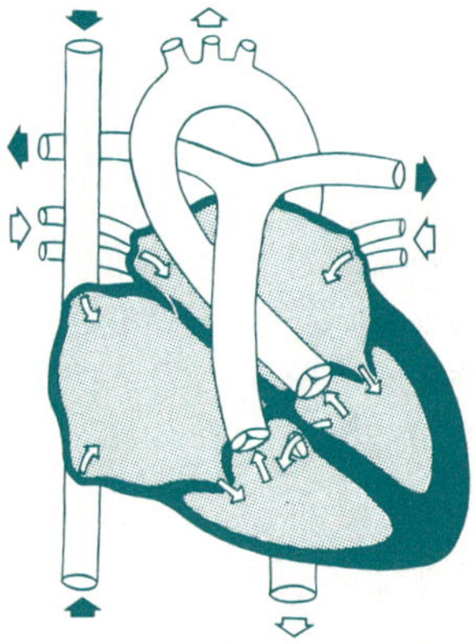

Ventricular septal defects

A ventricular septal defect is an abnormal opening between the right and left ventricle. Ventricular septal defects vary in size and may occur in either the membranous or muscular portion of the ventricular septum. Due to higher pressure in the left ventricle, a shunting of blood from the left to right ventricle occurs during systole. If pulmonary vascular resistance produces pulmonary hypertension, the shunt of blood is then reversed from the right to the left ventricle, with cyanosis resulting.

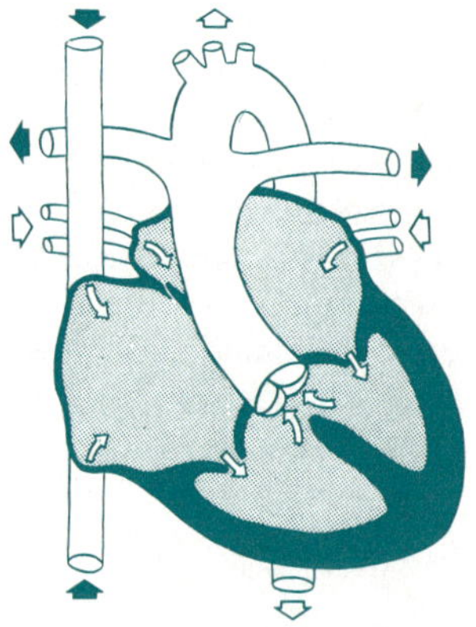

Truncus arteriosus

Truncus arteriosus is a retention of the embryologic bulbar trunk. It results from the failure of normal septation and division of this trunk into an aorta and pulmonary artery. This single arterial trunk overrides the ventricles and receives blood from them through a ventricular septal defect. The entire pulmonary and systemic circulation is supplied from this common arterial trunk.

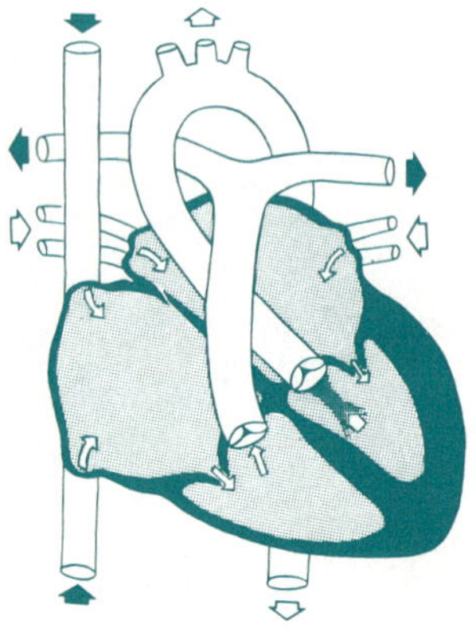

Subaortic stenosis

In many instances, the stenosis is valvular with thickening and fusion of the cusps. Subaortic stenosis is caused by a fibrous ring below the aortic valve in the outflow tract of the left ventricle. At times, both valvular and subaortic stenosis exist in combination. The obstruction presents an increased work load for the normal output of the left ventricular blood and results in left ventricular enlargement.

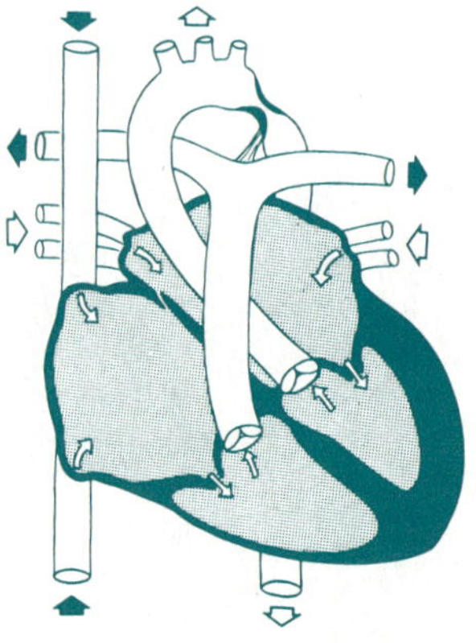

Coarctation of the aorta

Coarctation of the aorta is characterized by a narrowed aortic lumen. It exists as a preductal or postductal obstruction, depending on the position of the obstruction in relation to the ductus arteriosus. Coarctations exist with great variation in anatomic features. The lesion produces an obstruction to the flow of blood through the aorta causing an increased left ventricular pressure and work load.

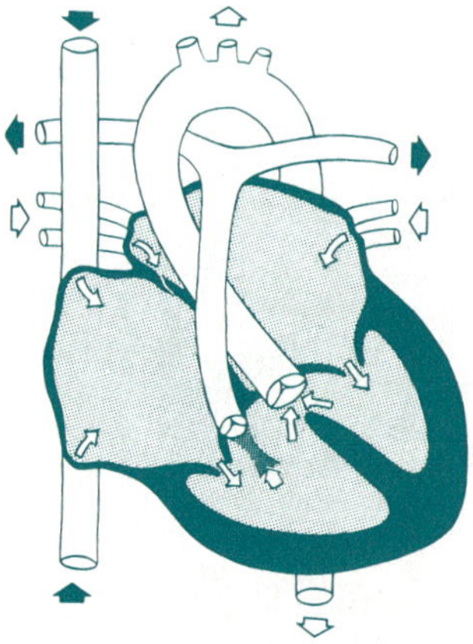

Tetralogy of Fallot

Tetralogy of Fallot is characterized by the combination of four defects: (1) pulmonary stenosis, (2) ventricular septal defect, (3) overriding aorta, (4) hypertrophy of right ventricle. It is the most common defect causing cyanosis in patients surviving beyond two years of age. The severity of symptoms depends on the degree of pulmonary stenosis, the size of the ventricular septal defect, and the degree to which the aorta overrides the septal defect.

ial tendency is evident in many cases. Coexisting congenital defects are common in newborns with cardiovascular anomalies. Maternal disease during pregnancy has been implicated. Symptoms characteristically are first evident after the umbilical cord is severed. The infant's *cry* is weak and muffled or loud and breathless. The newborn may be *cyanotic.* Cyanosis is usually generalized, it increases in the supine position, and is often unrelieved by oxygen. Cyanosis usually deepens with crying. The gray dusky color may be mild, moderate, or severe. Other infants may be *acyanotic,* pale, with or without mottling with exertion (such as crying).

The newborn's *activity level* varies from restless to lethargic. The infant may be unresponsive except to pain. The arms may be flaccid when eating. *Posturing* is significant. Hypotonia and flaccidity may be evident, even when sleeping. There may be hyperextension of the neck or opisthotonos. The newborn may be dyspneic when supine. Persistent *bradycardia* (120 beats per minute or less) or persistent *tachycardia* (160 beats per minute or more) may be noted.

Respirations are counted when the newborn is asleep. Findings may include tachypnea (60 respirations per minute or more), retractions with nasal flaring or tachypnea, and dyspnea with diaphoresis or grunting. Diaphoresis is an uncommon response in the normal newborn. Respirations may be gasping followed in 2 or 3 minutes by respiratory arrest if not treated promptly. Grunting may occur with exertion, such as crying or feeding by nipple.

These findings must be reported immediately. Children showing these types of signs are not cared for in the normal newborn nursery. They require prompt definite diagnosis and immediate appropriate therapy in a tertiary care pediatric unit.

Gastrointestinal System. Screening for gastrointestinal tract malformations is performed on a routine basis for all infants. Abdominal wall defects are apparent at birth. Omphalocele and gastroschisis are discussed on pp. 1013 and 1014. Intestinal obstruction, which occurs in about 1 in 3000 newborns, may occur in the presence of diaphragmatic hernia (p. 1012). A scaphoid (sunken) abdomen usually indicates a diaphragmatic hernia. A distended abdomen is particularly noteworthy in H-type tracheoesophageal fistula. These conditions require immediate surgery and are discussed later in this chapter.

Other malformations are apparent when further assessment is made. Malformation such as esophageal atresia and imperforate anus are discussed on pp. 1013 and 1014.

Urogenital System. Careful notation of perinatal events and observations such as oligohydramnios and absence of voiding aids in the identification and confirmation of existing congenital anomalies. In cases of ambiguous genitals (p. 1019), there is an urgent association between the parent-child relationship and the identification of the infant's sex. The identity of the newborn must be established as quickly as possible to facilitate initiation of a positive parent-child relationship.

Exstrophy of the bladder or the cloaca is rare (p. 1019).

Some infants have multiple congenital anomalies. A syndrome refers to a recognized pattern of malformations. The most familiar is Down's syndrome (Tables 27-9 and 40-1, and Fig. 40-3). Diagnosis is confirmed early in the neonatal period.

Five congenital anomalies require emergency surgery. These conditions and other malformations are presented under Implementation in this chapter. Although the surgery is the physician's responsibility, considerable nursing care is involved.

Table 40-1 *Common Autosomal Aberrations*

Syndrome	Chromosomal Abnormality and Nomenclature	Average Incidence	Major Clinical Manifestations
Cri-du-chat	Deletion of short arm of a B (no. 5) chromosome—46,XY,5p−		Distinctive weak, high-pitched mewlike cry resembling the cry of a cat; small head; hypertelorism; failure to thrive; severe mental retardation—profound with age
Trisomy 13 (Patau's)	Trisomy of a group D (no. 13) chromosome—47,XY,13+	1/15,000	Multiple anomalies, including cleft lip and palate (frequently bilateral); ear malformations; microphthalmia; polydactyly; eye defects; mental retardation; early death
Trisomy 18 (Edwards')	Trisomy of a group E (no. 18) chromosome—47,XY,18+	1/5000	Deformed and low-set ears; micrognathia; rocker-bottom feet; overlapping (index over third) fingers; prominent occiput; hypertelorism; failure to thrive and early death; mental retardation
Trisomy 21 (Down's)	Trisomy of a Group G (no. 21) chromosome—47,XY,21+ (trisomy); 46XY,D—G−, (Dq-Gq) + (translocation); 46,XY/47,XY,21 + (mosaic)	1/500	Brachycephaly with flat occiput; inner epicanthal folds; small ears, nose, and mouth with protruding tongue; muscular hypotonia; broad, short hands with stubby fingers and simian palmar crease; broad stubby feet with wide space between big and second toes; mental retardation; variable life expectancy

From Whaley, LF, and Wong, DL: Nursing care of infants and children, ed 3, St Louis, 1987, The CV Mosby Co.

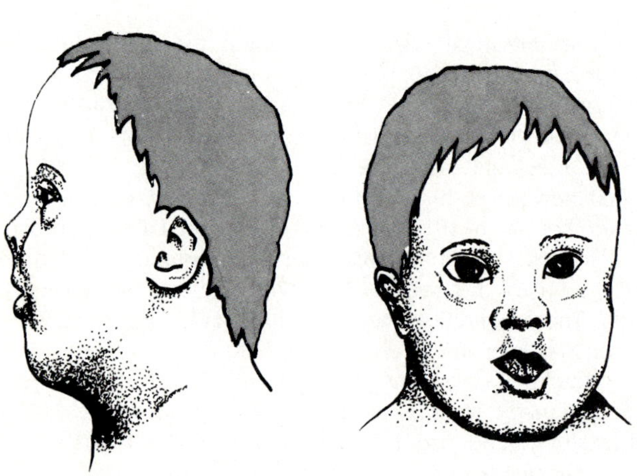

Fig. 40-3 Clinical features of Down's syndrome.

Genetic Diagnosis

Most diagnostic procedures for detection of genetic disorders are implemented after birth at any time from the postdelivery period through adulthood. The number and variety of these tests are too extensive to include here; therefore only those employed most frequently in the newborn period will be discussed.

Biochemical Tests. The most widespread use of postdelivery testing for genetic disease is the routine screening of newborn infants for phenylketonuria (PKU) (Appendix H), which is mandatory in most of the United States. The test is not valid until the infant has ingested an ample amount of the amino acid phenylalanine, a constituent of both human and cow's milk (Chapter 23). Similarly, galactosemia can be detected by measuring blood levels of galactose or the presence of reducing substances in the urine or affected infants who have ingested milk containing galactose.

In recent years many states in the United States have required routine screening for hypothyroidism. Thyroxine (T_4) is measured from a drop of blood obtained from a heel stick at 2 to 5 days of age. At this time the normally expected increase in T_4 is lacking in infants with hypothyroidism. The same blood sample can be used to test for all three of these metabolic disorders—**PKU**, **galactosemia** and **hypothyroidism** (Table 40-2 and Procedure 22-1).

Inborn errors of metabolism is a term applied to a large group of disorders caused by a metabolic defect that results from the absence of or change in a protein, usually an enzyme, because of gene action. These defects can involve any substrate produced from protein, carbohydrate, or fat metabolism.

Metabolic processes consist of a complex sequence of chemical reactions, each step of which is catalyzed by an enzyme. When an enzyme is absent or defective as a result of gene action, the normal process is interrupted and further reactions beyond that point are altered. All subsequent reactions are affected with variable consequences, depending on the enzyme involved. For example, (1) there may be a deficiency of the product, such as thyroxine in hereditary cretinism or melanin in albinism; (2) there may be an accumulation of the products preceding the blocks, such as galactose in galactosemia; or (3) alternate pathways may be used, with an increase in the products of these reactions, such as the increased production of phenyl ketones in PKU.

Inborn errors of metabolism are recessive disorders and, as such, require that the individual receive a defective gene from each parent. The parents are usually unaffected, because their normal, dominant gene directs the synthesis of sufficient protein to meet their metabolic needs under normal circumstances. With new biochemical techniques it is now possible to detect the presence of the abnormal gene in an increasing number of these disorders. A partial list of inborn errors of metabolism is outlined in Table 40-2.

Cytologic Studies. In most instances disorders resulting from chromosomal abnormalities can be diagnosed by clinical manifestations alone. Occasionally an infant is born whose clinical appearance is only suggestive. In these cases cytologic studies are more often carried out to confirm or rule out a tentative diagnosis. Sometimes all that is required are sex chromatin or fluorescent staining techniques. These stains can be prepared from any cells in the body. The most easily obtained and therefore the most commonly used are mucosal cells scraped from the inside of the cheek, placed on a glass slide, prepared, and stained (buccal smear).

Preparation of karyotype (Fig. 9-2) requires cells in the process of cell division. The most commonly used cells are those obtained from bone marrow, skin, or peripheral blood. The cells are grown in culture media. Division is arrested at the stage when cells are best visualized, then stained, photographed, and arranged in a karyotype for assessment. A karyotype is also requested in cases in which the sex of the infant is in doubt, since the assignment of a gender constitutes a social emergency (p. 1019). Some chromosomal abnormalities appear in Tables 40-1 and 40-3. Fig. 40-4 illustrates how the abnormalities arise and Fig. 40-5 illustrates one method of diagnosis.

Dermatoglyphics. The pattern formed by dermal ridges early in development is largely genetically determined by many genes on many chromosomes. Therefore addition or deletion of genetic material will produce alterations in the loops, swirls, and arches of the finger and toe prints, in the palm lines, and in the flexion creases on palms of the hands and soles of the feet (Fig. 40-6, *A*). Characteristic dermatoglyphic patterns have been noted in almost all the chromosomal abnormalities such as Down's syndrome (Fig. 40-6, *B*).

Characteristic palm creases have also been noted in a significant number of children with rubella syndrome and leukemia. The Sydney line (Fig. 40-6, *C*) has been observed more frequently in children with rubella syndrome than in children in a control group. Also this line is seen in approximately 15% of children with leukemia. Certain fingerprint patterns may be found in persons who suffer cardiac valvular problems later in life.

Table 40-2 *Some inborn errors of metabolism**

Disease	Basic Defect	Manifestations	Therapy
Adrenogenital syndrome†	21-hydroxylase deficiency; failure of hydrocortisone synthesis in adrenal cortex	Virilization	Hydrocortisone
Albinism	Deficiency of tyrosinase; failure to convert tyrosine to dopa and, hence, lack of melanin synthesis	Lack of pigment in skin, hair, and eyes; eye defects	None; avoid exposure to sunlight; ophthalmologic care
Crigler-Najjar syndrome	Glycyronyl transferase deficiency; inability to convert indirect bilirubin to direct bilirubin	Jaundice; spasticity; opisthotonos; early death	None
Cystic fibrosis	Unknown; defect in mucus-secreting glands; sweat glands secrete abnormal amounts of sodium chloride	Meconium ileus in newborn; celiac syndrome; pulmonary disease; failure to thrive	Inhalation therapy; antibiotics; pancreatic enzymes
Familial cretinism	Deficiency of iodotyrosine deiodinase	Lethargy; stunted growth; mental retardation	Early administration of thyroid hormone
Galactosemia†	Deficiency of galactose 1-phosphate uridyl transferase; inability to convert galactose to glucose	Failure to thrive; mental retardation; cataracts; jaundice; hepatomegaly; cirrhosis of liver	Eliminate galactose from diet
Glucose 6-phosphate dehydrogenase deficiency (G6PD)	Deficiency of G6PD	Asymptomatic under normal circumstances; hemolytic anemia and jaundice from ingestion of certain drugs (primaquine, acetanilid, sulfanilamide, and naphthalene) and fava beans	Avoid agents that precipitate clinical symptoms
Hypophosphatasia†	Deficiency of alkaline phosphatase	Skeletal abnormalities	None
Maple syrup urine disease†	Defective metabolism of branched chain amino acid	Onset in early infancy; neurologic disorders; odor of urine similar to that of maple syrup	Diet low in branched chain amino acids
McArdle syndrome	Deficiency of muscle phosphorylase	Muscle weakness	Glucagon injections
Phenylketonuria (PKU)	Deficiency of phenylalanine dehydrogenase	Blond hair, blue eyes, fair skin; mental retardation; bizarre behavior	Diet low in phenylalanine
Tay-Sachs disease†	Deficiency of hexosaminidase; defect in synthesis of gangliosides	Progressive neurologic deterioration; blindness: cherry-red spot in macula; early death	None
Tyrosinosis	Deficiency of *p*-hydroxy-phenylpyruvic acid oxidase	Hepatosplenomegaly	None
von Gierke's disease	Deficiency of G6PD; inability to reconvert glycogen to glucose.	Hematomegaly; vomiting; hypoglycemia, convulsions; coma; usually early death	High-protein diet; no definitive therapy
Werdnig-Hoffman syndrome	Unknown; atrophy of anterior horn cells in spinal cord and motor nuclei in brain stem	Usually apparent at birth; "floppy" infant; lies in frog position; fatal in early childhood	Symptomatic

*Autosomal-recessive inheritance pattern.
†Prenatal diagnosis is possible.

Many other diagnostic studies may be performed in the neonatal period to detect or rule out genetic defects, for example, x-ray studies for a variety of structural defects of bone and for gastrointestinal, renal, and neurologic disorders. Meconium ileus in the newborn is often the first manifestation of cystic fibrosis.

Parental Responses. Parental responses are carefully assessed. Signs and symptoms of initial grief responses are expected (Chapter 28). The family's understanding of the information that is being presented to them is assessed on an ongoing basis. The family's comprehension of the proposed management and risks, and of alternative courses of action are evaluated. The family's feelings about proposed management and their role in posttherapy care are explored. The family's emotional, social, and financial resources must be considered.

Table 40-3 *Common sex chromosome abnormalities*

Syndrome	Chromosomal Nomenclature	Phenotype	X Chromosome	Y Chromosome	Clinical Manifestations
Turner's	45,X	Female	0	0	Short stature; webbed neck; low posterior hairline; shield-shaped chest with widely spaced nipples; sterile, lymphedema of hands and feet in infant
Meta-female	47,XXX (can also be 48,XXXX or 49,XXXXX)	Female	+1 or more	0	Normal female characteristics; usually mentally retarded; mental deficiency in others; fertile
XYY male	47,XYY (can also be 48,XYYY or mosaic)	Male	0	+1 per Y	Usually normal sexual development; tendency to be tall with long head; poor coordination; may demonstrate aberrant behavior
Klinefelter's	47,XXY (48,XXYY, 48,XXXY, 49,XXXXY, etc. mosaics)	Male	+1 or more (1 per X)	+1 per Y	Tall with long legs; hypogenitalism; sterile; may have deficient male secondary sexual characteristics; may demonstrate aberrant behavior

From Whaley, LF, and Wong, DL: Nursing care of infants and children, ed 3, St Louis, 1987, The CV Mosby Co.

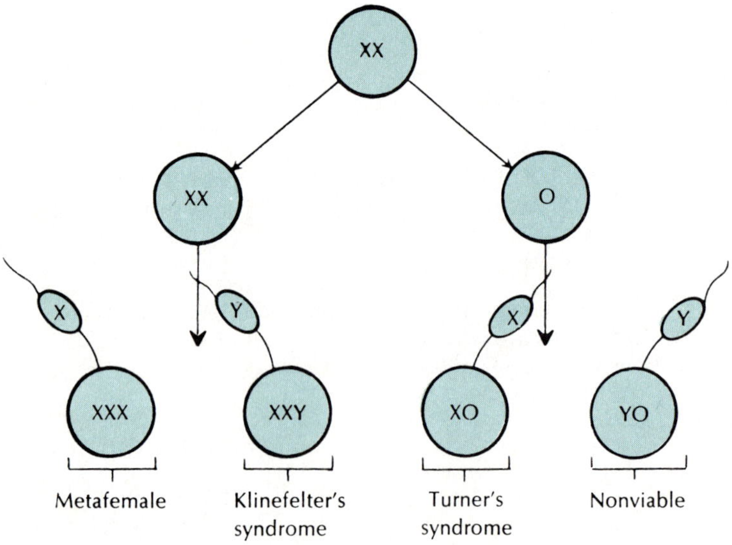

Fig. 40-4 Nondisjunction of X chromosomes in ovum fertilized by normal sperm to produce more common sex chromosomal aberrations.

From Whaley, LF, and Wong, DL: Nursing care of infants and children, ed 3, St Louis, 1987, The CV Mosby Co.

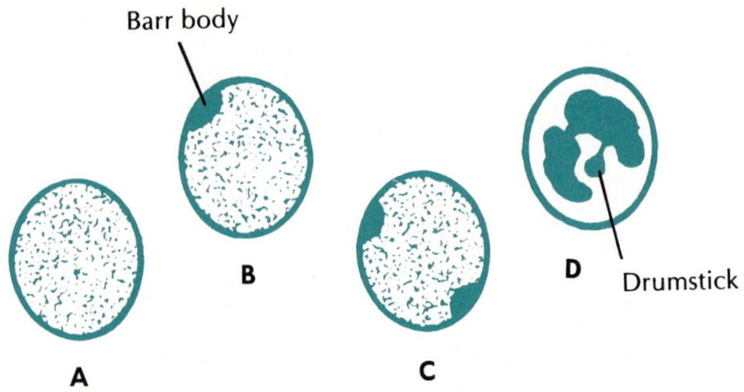

Fig. 40-5 Sex chromatin, or Barr body. **A,** No sex chromatin is found in normal male somatic cells. **B,** One Barr body is normal in female somatic cells. **C,** Two Barr bodies are found in cells with three X chromosomes (XXX or XXXY). **D,** "Drumstick" is found in many polymorphonuclear leukocytes of normal female.

From Whaley, LF, and Wong, DL: Nursing care of infants and children, ed 3, St Louis, 1987, The CV Mosby Co.

Nursing Diagnoses

Following are examples of nursing diagnoses to direct the care of newborns with congenital abnormalities.

Newborn

- Potential for injury or death related to
  - Presence of a congenital disorder
- Potential for infection related to
  - Anomaly or its treatment
- Potential for impaired gas exchange, nutrition, or mobility related to
  - Congenital anomaly
- Potential for altered growth and development related to
  - Inborn error of metabolism

Parents/Family

- Dysfunctional grieving or spiritual distress related to
  - Birth of a child with a defect
- Potential for ineffective individual/family coping related to
  - Birth of a child with a defect
- Anxiety related to
  - Uncertainty of prognosis or own ability to care for child
- Knowledge deficit related to
  - Cause
  - Management
  - Alternative courses of action
  - Community resources
  - Prognosis
  - Care needed by child after discharge

Planning

Planning for the care of a newborn with a congenital defect begins before the birth of the infant. Hospital protocols and standards of care are established so that definitive and prompt therapy is facilitated. Parents are involved

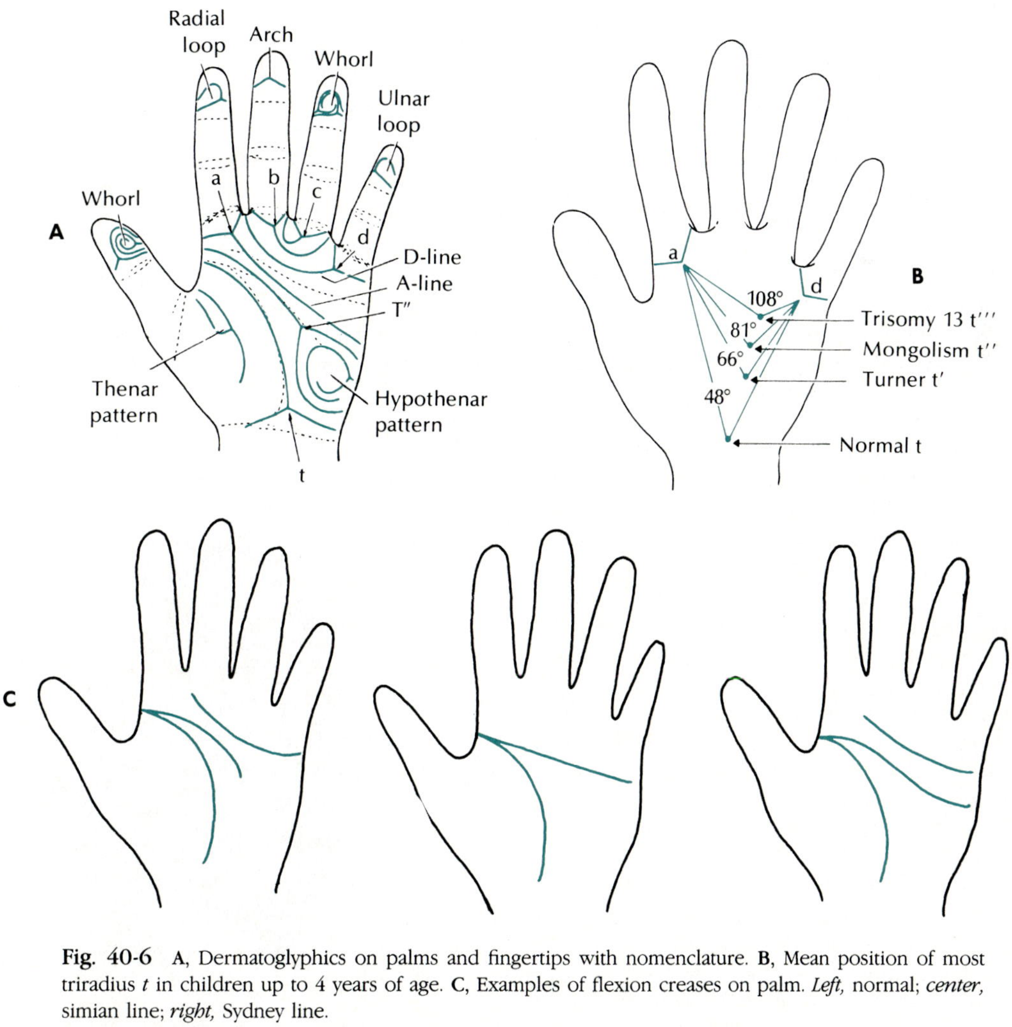

Fig. 40-6 **A**, Dermatoglyphics on palms and fingertips with nomenclature. **B**, Mean position of most triradius *t* in children up to 4 years of age. **C**, Examples of flexion creases on palm. *Left,* normal; *center,* simian line; *right,* Sydney line.

A and **B** from Penrose, LS: Nature 197:933, 1963; **C** from Whaley, LF: Understanding inherited disorders, St Louis, 1974, The CV Mosby Co.

in the plan for care to the extent possible. For some disorders, a collaborative health team approach that includes specialists (e.g., orthodontists, physical therapists, geneticists) and community services representatives is needed. Goals are stated in client-centered terms for the newborn and parents.

Goals

1. The newborn's disorder is recognized and appropriate therapy is initiated promptly.
2. The newborn suffers no adverse sequelae to the disorder or its management.
3. The parents understand the newborn's condition, its management and possible sequelae, as well as the anticipated prognosis.
4. The parents choose a course of action commensurate with their family's values and goals.

Implementation

General Preoperative and Postoperative Care

The newborn withstands the stress of surgery surprisingly well, provided it is done as soon after birth as feasible and the facilities available for care are adequately equipped and staffed. The medical-nursing team must be specially trained to anticipate and meet the newborn's physiologic needs (Chapter 36). The surgical team consists of the radiologist, surgeon, anesthesiologist, and nurse. Diagnostic studies are kept to a minimum, and consideration of the newborn's immaturity is kept in mind. Air may be used rather than standard radiopaque materials for diagnostic x-ray examinations to reduce the danger of regurgitation and aspiration. Microtechniques are utilized for the necessary blood chemistry studies (such as preoperative hemoglobin levels) to minimize blood loss.

The infant is transported to the operating room in an incubator with a self-contained power pack for the continuous provision of warmth. The infant is accompanied by an intensive care nursery nurse. Preanesthesia preparation includes hydration, administration of preoperative medications, usually minute amounts of atropine, insertion of an endotracheal tube, and gastric emptying.

During the operation, blood loss is constantly monitored. Blood is replaced milliliter for milliliter because the newborn's remarkable ability to maintain blood circulation through vasoconstriction means that vital signs remain unaltered until sudden and complete collapse occurs as the compensatory system is overtaxed. Temperature is maintained by positioning the infant on a thermal mattress and draping suitably.

Once the operation is completed, the infant is returned to the intensive care nursery. The first hour after the procedure is a crucial one; constant surveillance of recovery from the anesthesia is imperative. Body temperature is maintained between 36.1° and 36.7° C (97° and 98° F); optimum temperature is 36.5° C (97.6° F). An open airway is maintained by means of positioning of the head, suctioning, and use of high humidity. If the respiratory rate increases, suctioning is indicated. Oxygen dosage is prescribed on the basis of arterial blood gas values (such as Po_2). Fluid-electrolyte balance is monitored. Intravenous replacement is given as ordered. Postural drainage and percussion are ordered as necessary. The infant is turned from side to side to equalize pressure areas. An indwelling gastric catheter attached to intermittent suction removes gastric secretions. Removal of gastric contents prevents their possible aspiration because the infant's cough reflex is inadequate.

Most Common Surgical Emergencies

The following five congenital anomalies account for more than 90% of surgical emergencies of the newborn:

1. Diaphragmatic hernia
2. Tracheoesophageal anomalies
3. Omphalocele
4. Intestinal obstruction
5. Imperforate anus

Diaphragmatic Hernia. Diaphragmatic hernia is the most urgent of the neonatal emergencies. Incomplete embryonic development of the diaphragm allows herniation of abdominal viscera into the thoracic cavity (Fig. 40-7). The defect and herniation may be minimal and easily reparable or the defect may be so extensive that the viscera present in the thoracic cavity during embryonic life precluded the normal development of pulmonary tissue. Most cases involve a posterolateral defect, usually on the left. The extent of the defect and the severity and timing of the symptomatology determine the seriousness of the problem.

Signs that are suspicious of extensive diaphragmatic herniation can be assessed by the nurse. Signs include the following: constant respiratory distress from birth that becomes increasingly severe as bowels fill with air, large or

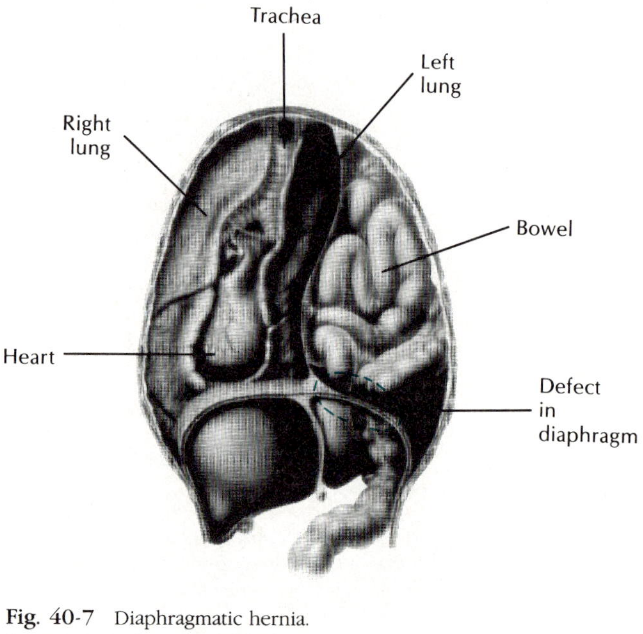

Fig. 40-7 Diaphragmatic hernia.
Courtesy Ross Laboratories, Columbus, Ohio.

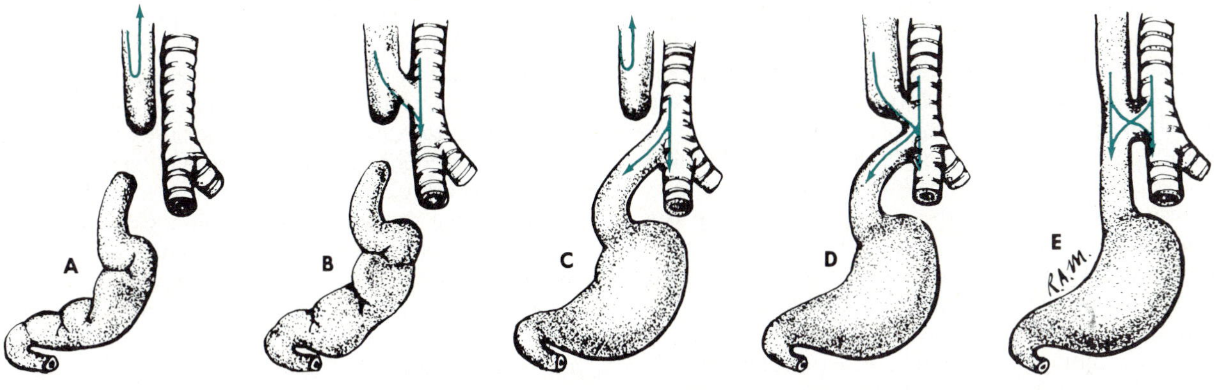

Fig. 40-8 Congenital atresia of esophagus and tracheoesophageal fistula. **A**, About 8%. Upper and lower segments of esophagus end in blind sac. **B**, Less than 1%. Upper segment of esophagus ends in atresia and connects to trachea by fistulous tract. Infant may drown with first feeding. **C**, About 87%. Upper segment of esophagus ends in blind pouch; lower segment connects with trachea by small fistulous tract. **D**, Less than 1%. Both segments of esophagus connect by fistulous tracts to trachea. Infant may drown with first feeding. **E**, About 4%. Esophagus is continuous but connects by fistulous tract to trachea; known as *H-type*.

From Whaley, LF, and Wong, DL: Nursing care of infants and children, ed 3, St Louis, 1987, The CV Mosby Co.

asymmetric chest contour, dullness to percussion on affected side, bowel sounds heard in thoracic cavity, and diminished breath sounds.

Prompt surgical repair is imperative after correction of acidosis, insertion of a nasogastric tube and aspiration, and oxygen therapy. The prognosis depends largely on the degree of pulmonary development and the success of diaphragmatic closure. Prognosis in severe cases is guarded.

Tracheoesophageal Anomalies. Esophageal atresia is an urgent congenital anomaly. Various types are recognized, depending on the presence or absence of an associated tracheoesophageal fistula, the site of the fistula, and the point and degree of esophageal obstruction (Fig. 40-8). The most common variety is associated with moderate hydramnios.

The following signs are suspicious for tracheoesophageal fistula: excessive oral secretions with drooling; progressive respiratory distress as unswallowed secretions spill over into trachea; and feeding intolerance. In feeding intolerance, choking, coughing, and cyanosis follow even a small amount of fluid taken by mouth. Soon after the first feeding is initiated, there is regurgitation of unaltered formula (unmixed with stomach secretions or bile).

Nursing actions are supportive. In the presence of excessive oral secretions and respiratory distress, **do not feed the infant orally** before consulting physician. In the presence of abdominal distension, place the newborn in semi-Fowler's position and raise the head 30 degrees or more (infant seat may be used). This position facilitates respiratory efforts and discourages reflux (spillage) of stomach secretions into the respiratory tree, with resultant chemical bronchitis and pneumonitis. On physician's order or per standing orders, insert a suction tube into the blind pouch. Connect the tube to low, intermittent suction.

Immediate surgical correction of the anomaly is mandatory. The prognosis depends on the degree of maturity of the newborn and the presence of a fistula or pneumonia.

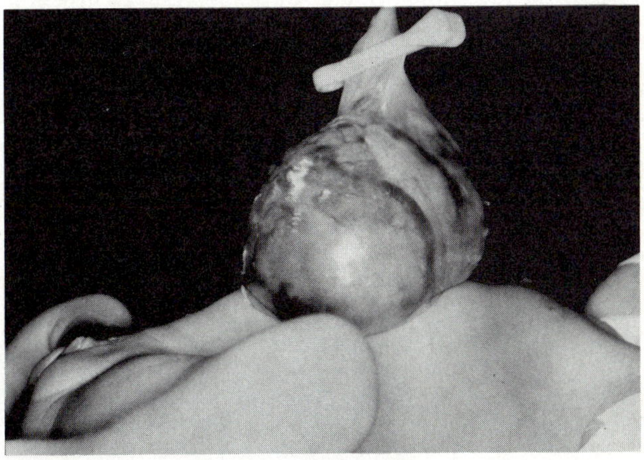

Fig. 40-9 Omphalocele containing liver.

Courtesy John R Campbell, MD, University of Oregon Health Sciences Center, Portland, Oregon.

Cardiac and other gastrointestinal anomalies commonly are associated with esophageal atresia.

Omphalocele. Omphalocele is a herniation noted at birth in which part of the intestine protrudes through a defect in the abdominal wall at the umbilicus (Fig. 40-9). Failure of migration of the midgut in embryonic development probably is responsible for omphalocele. The protruding bowel is covered only by a thin, transparent membrane composed of amnion.

Prompt closure of defects of less than 5 cm in diameter usually is successful. Larger defects may require closure in stages. The general prognosis is related to associated anomalies.

There is usually only a short span of time between the infant's birth and surgical intervention. Planning for the provision of support to the parents is an essential aspect of nursing care. In addition to the usual preoperative orders, preparation of the infant for surgery includes protecting the defect from infection, rupture, and drying. The physician prescribes that the omphalocele be protected by one of the following:

1. Sterile towels or sponges kept moist with sterile saline solution that has been warmed to body temperature.
2. Protective sterile petrolatum dressings and a firm plastic or metal dome covering.

Intestinal Obstruction. Congenital jejunal or ileal obstruction is suspected when distension and bile-stained or fecal vomiting occur in a newborn in the first 24 to 48 hours of life. Although this condition is uncommon, premature infants and those with other anomalies may be affected.

Nursing care is supportive: stop oral feedings and monitor intravenous therapy (see Procedure 36-4); prevent aspiration and suction gastric contents on physician's order (indwelling catheter to low, intermittent suction may be ordered); place infant in semi-Fowler's position to facilitate respiration.

X-ray films of the abdomen usually show a dilated small bowel without gas in the colon. A barium enema may be helpful in determining the cause of the obstruction. Hirschsprung's disease, ileus secondary to sepsis, meconium ileus, and volvulus must be considered in the differential diagnosis (Fig. 40-10). Prompt surgery usually provides good results.

Imperforate Anus. Imperforate anus is a congenital disorder that is more common in infant boys than infant girls (Fig. 40-11). About 85% of affected girls will have developed a small fistula (Fig. 40-12), but this is rare in boys. The obstruction may be of the low type (anal membrane) or the high type (anal or rectal atresia). Because some anomalies are not apparent by direct visualization, initial insertion of a probe (thermometer) into the anal canal is done with *extra* caution until patency is established.

Since continence for a lifetime may be dependent on the proper corrective surgery, a pediatric surgeon is consulted at once. Surgery may be as simple as an incision of an anal membrane. With anorectal agenesis, a prompt colostomy will be necessary.

Survival is expected. Continence, on the other hand, is dependent on several factors, including sacral anomalies and proper surgery.

Common Malformation

Meningomyelocele. **Meningomyelocele**, a neural tube defect, is a herniation of part of the meninges (containing cerebrospinal fluid [CSF] and CNS tissue) through a defect in the vertebral column or skull. The defect often occurs in the lower back (Fig. 40-13). In the accompanying spinal malformation, **spina bifida**, the meningomyelocele extrudes through the opening of the spinal column. The opening is the result of a congenital absence of one or more vertebral arches. Occasionally a familial history (5% recurrence rate) of this anomaly is identified. Most cases are of unknown (infectious?) origin. A **meningocele** is also a herniation of the meninges. A meningocele contains CSF but does not contain CNS tissue (cord or nerve roots). Prenatal diagnosis of neural tube defects (meningomyelocele, meningocele, anencephaly) is now possible (Chapter 27 and Table 27-9).

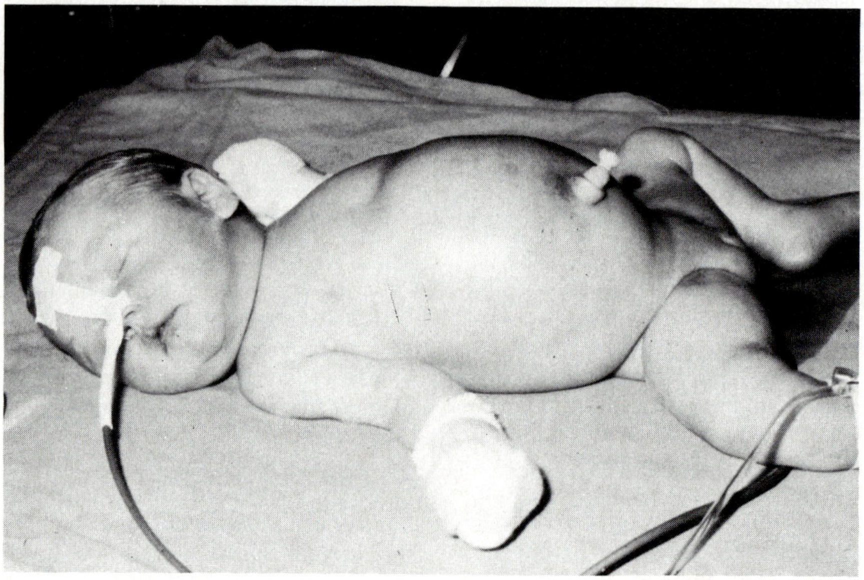

Fig. 40-10 Meconium ileus with midgut volvulus. Meconium ileus is frequently associated with cystic fibrosis. Normal meconium stool is not passed, and abdomen distends progressively. Treatment is directed at removal of mechanical obstruction and prevention of complications of cystic fibrosis.
Courtesy John R Campbell, MD, University of Oregon Health Sciences Center, Portland, Oregon.

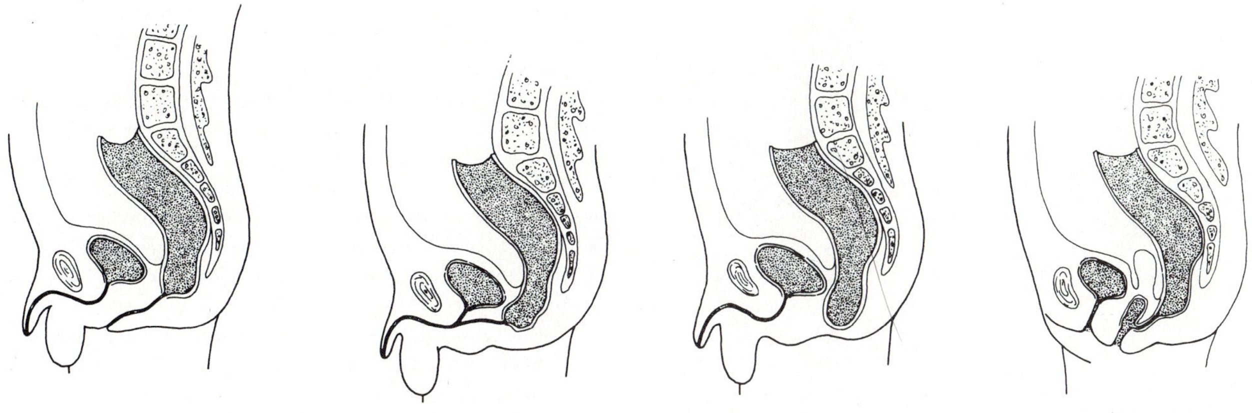

Fig. 40-11 Types of imperforate anus. Anal sphincter muscle may be present and intact. **A,** High lesion opening onto perineum through narrow fistulous tract. **B,** High lesion ending in fistulous tract to urinary tract. **C,** Low lesion in bowel passes through puborectal muscle. **D,** High lesion ending in fistulous tract to vagina.

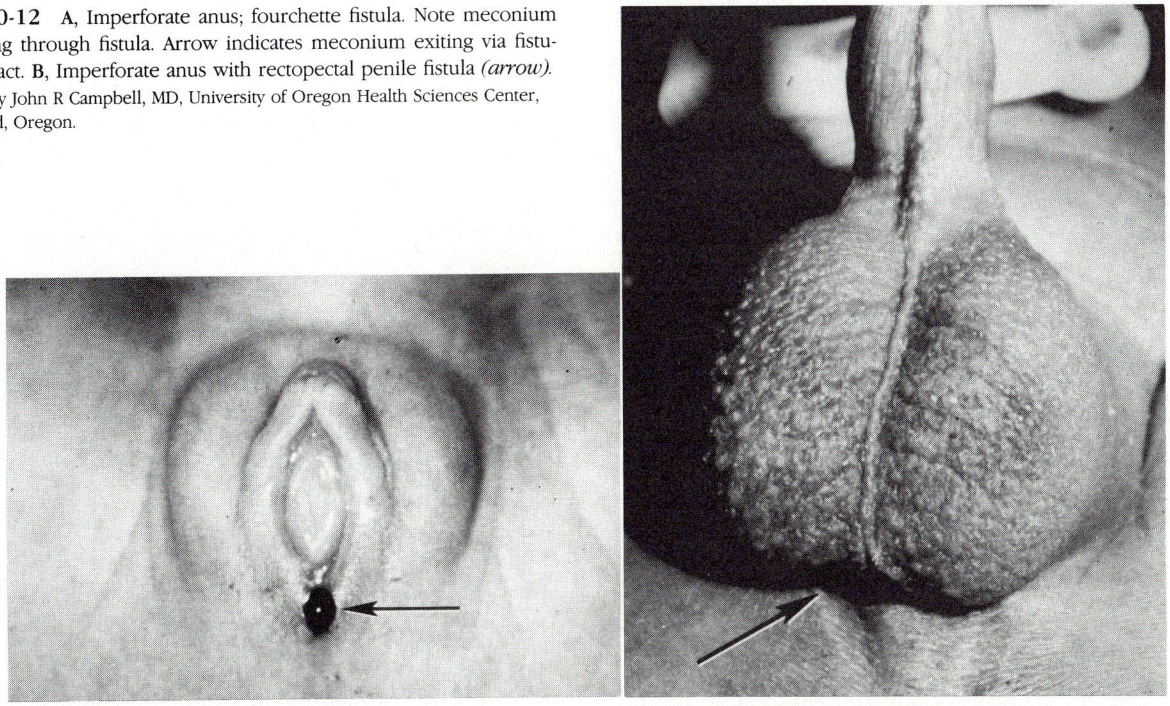

Fig. 40-12 **A,** Imperforate anus; fourchette fistula. Note meconium draining through fistula. Arrow indicates meconium exiting via fistulous tract. **B,** Imperforate anus with rectopectal penile fistula *(arrow).*
Courtesy John R Campbell, MD, University of Oregon Health Sciences Center, Portland, Oregon.

If the neonate is born with a large defect, the nurse aids in preventing its rupture and infection before surgery. Protection of the defect includes the following actions:

1. Position with care.
   a. Position prone or side-lying with rolled towels to prevent pressure or injury to defect, thereby providing portal of entry for infectious agents.
   b. Change position every hour to prevent pressure areas.
   c. If physician permits infant to be held, exercise caution to avoid injury to defect.
2. Provide skin care: skin around defect is cleansed and dried carefully to prevent breakdown, which would establish a portal of entry for infectious agents. Apply physician-ordered dressings, ointments, and so on.

The nurse assists in the diagnosis of a hidden defect. The nurse assesses neurologic function and notes the following: (1) paralysis of lower extremities, (2) flaccidity and spasticity of muscles below defect, and (3) sphincter control: character and number of voidings and stools; leakage of urine and stool.

Surgical repair often can be done in the neonatal pe-

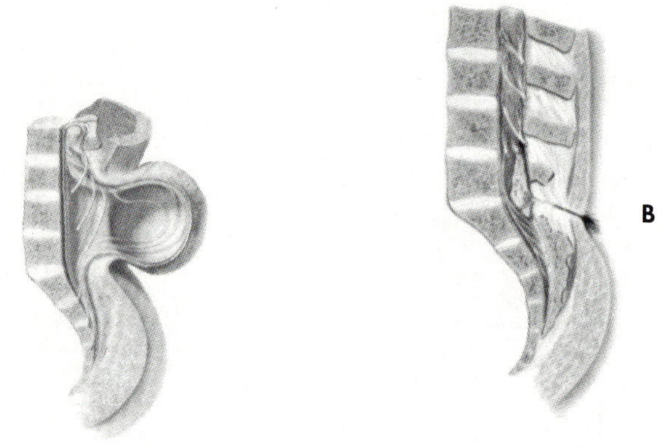

Fig. 40-13 A, Myelomeningocele. B, Dermal sinus tract with dermoid cyst, often associated with spina bifida occulta. Note also tuft of hair.
Courtesy Ross Laboratories, Columbus, Ohio.

riod. If other anomalies, such as hydrocephalus, are present, delayed correction may be elected. Permanent impairment of neuromuscular function below the level of the defect depends on the amount of CNS tissue involved. In severe cases, voluntary and involuntary functions are absent. The prognosis is guarded. Only about 60% of cases are operable. Many of these children die or achieve only partial function. Hydrocephalus ultimately develops in virtually all infants.

The parents will need considerable support and instruction regarding the infant's care. In some instances parents may require assistance in placing the child in a special care facility.

Congenital Hydrocephalus. Congenital hydrocephalus is macrocephaly caused by abnormal enlargement of the cerebral ventricles and skull. Head enlargement is the result of increased intraventricular CSF pressure. This condition is accompanied by enlargement of the head, prominence of the forehead, "setting sun" sign of the eyes, atrophy of the brain, weakness, and convulsions as the condition worsens.

Congenital hydrocephalus is encountered in approximately 1 in 2000 fetuses (about 12% of all malformations). Several types are known.

External hydrocephalus is caused by an abnormal accumulation of fluid between the brain and the dura mater. Obstruction of the CSF anywhere along its course may be responsible. Maldevelopment, infection, hemorrhage, neoplasia, or unknown causes must be considered. A history of maternal (and possibly fetal) bacterial or viral infection may be elicited. The most common lesion is atresia of the aqueduct between the third and fourth ventricles (Arnold-Chiari syndrome).

In *internal hydrocephalus* an excessive amount of CSF accumulates in the ventricular system of the brain. Rarely, oversecretion of CSF by a choroid plexus papilloma, rather than an obstruction, may result in internal hydrocephalus.

The fetus with hydrocephalus commonly assumes the breech presentation in utero. Severe dystocia caused by cephalopelvic disproportion (CPD) is encountered; cesarean delivery is warranted. When vaginal delivery is attempted, puncture of the fetal head and drainage of the excess fluid may be necessary before the head can be delivered. Fetal mortality after this procedure is approximately three deaths out of every four deliveries. Regardless of the route of delivery, the experience is emotionally traumatic for the parents and family.

X-ray films should confirm widening of the fontanels and sutures. Intracranial calcifications caused by cytomegalic viral (CMV) inclusion disease or toxoplasmosis (a protozoal infection) may be revealed (see TORCH, Table 30-2 and box on p. 975).

Subdural aspiration or transillumination of the head may disclose a subdural hematoma or tumor. The location and extent of obstruction usually can be identified by pneumoencephalography or ultrasonography.

Spina bifida occurs in approximately one-third of infants born with hydrocephalus.

Surgery is usually performed soon after birth. If surgical shunting is not accomplished, **increasing intracranial pressure**, evidenced by palpably widening fontanels and sutures, lethargy, irritability or vomiting, results in irreversible neurologic damage. A period of observation is necessary to determine the type of operation required. Meanwhile, nursing care is individualized.

Assessment for hydrocephalus includes notations describing the typical signs (see danger signs box, below).

DANGER SIGNS

Hydrocephalus

1. Changes in head size every day
   a. Width of sutures
   b. Size and tension of anterior fontanel
   c. Head circumference
2. Facial appearance
   a. Flat, broad bridge of nose
   b. Bulging forehead
   c. "Setting-sun" effect as eyes are displaced downward by pressure from accumulating fluid
3. Neurologic signs
   a. High-pitched, shrill cry
   b. Irritability or restlessness
   c. Poor feeding or changes in feeding pattern from good to poor
   d. Behavior changes
   e. Spina bifida

Nursing actions appropriate to the needs of a newborn with hydrocephalus include careful documentation of ongoing observations. Meticulous skin care is necessary to prevent pressure areas and infection of the skin of the head. Lamb's wool, sheepskin, or a flotation mattress is used under the infant. Frequent position changing and keeping the newborn clean and dry helps maintain skin integrity and health.

The newborn's heavy head is supported carefully when

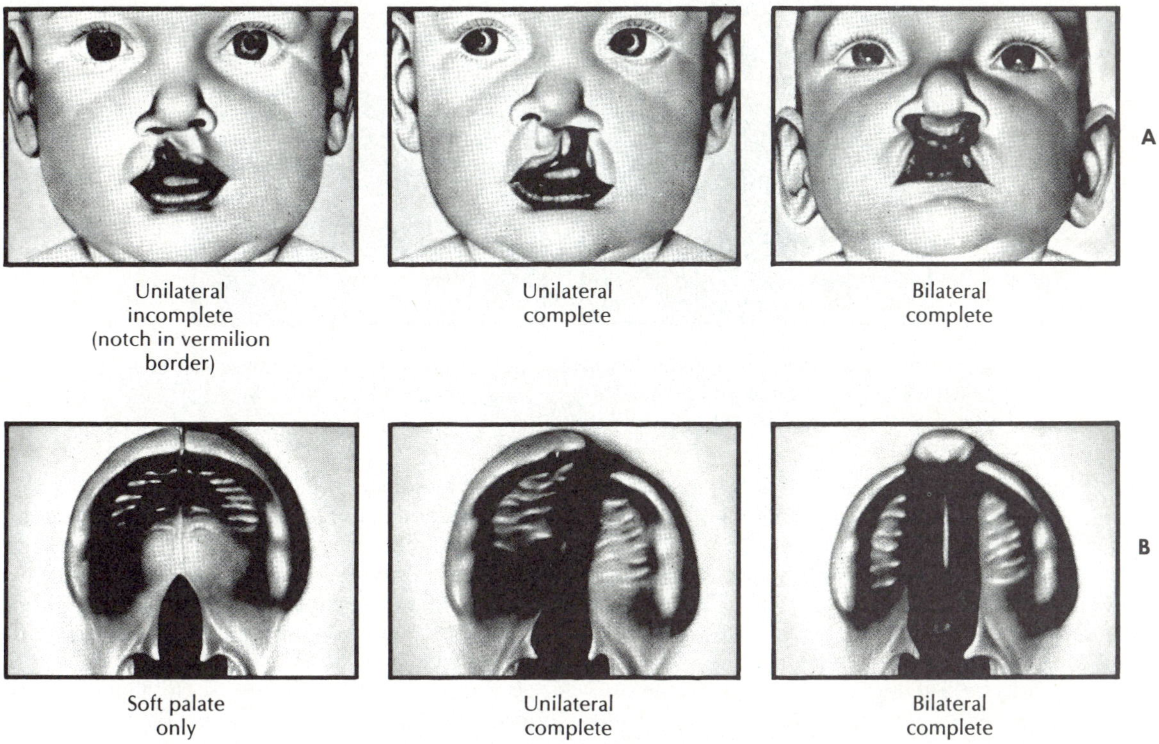

Fig. 40-14 **A**, Cleft lip. **B**, Cleft palate.
Courtesy Ross Laboratories, Columbus, Ohio.

being held or turned. The method, amount, and frequency of feeding are chosen to accomodate the infant's tolerance and energy level (Chapter 36). Care is taken to prevent vomiting and subsequent aspiration. Nonnutritive sucking, touching, and cuddling needs are met.

Damaged or destroyed brain tissue cannot be restored. Spontaneous arrest of hydrocephalus may occur, but often surgical shunting may be required to eliminate excess CSF. Despite arrest of the process, serious mental retardation and neurologic sequelae are common.

Anencephaly and Microcephaly. Anencephaly and microcephaly are congenital fetal deformities in which the head is considerably smaller than normal. In anencephaly there is complete or partial absence of the brain and of the overlying skull. Because the pituitary gland is absent or vestigial, the adrenal cortex is diminutive (for lack of adrenocorticotropic hormone [ACTH] stimulation). About 70% of anencephalic infants are girls. This condition is commonly accompanied by hydramnios. The cause of anencephaly is unknown, but multiple environmental factors have been postulated. A 3% recurrence rate in familial histories has been noted.

Anencephaly is incompatible with life; warmth and fluid are provided until the neonate's death, which is usually before the end of the first 24 hours after birth. Microcephalic infants require specific nursing care and medical observation to appraise the extent of psychomotor retardation that almost always accompanies this abnormality. The nurse's supportive role with parents is considerable.

In microcephaly the head generally is well formed but small. X-ray exposure of the woman may result in fetal microcephaly. Rubella, CMV, and perhaps other infectious processes are the causes in some cases.

Cleft-lip or Palate. Cleft lip or palate is a common congenital midline fissure, or opening, in the lip or palate; one or both deformities may occur (Fig. 40-14). The incidence is approximately 1 in 700 white neonates and 1 in 2000 black neonates. Polygenetic factors are causative in some cases, but fetal viral infection, maternal corticosteroid therapy, radiation, dietary influence, and hypoxia have been associated factors. The combination of cleft lip and palate affects more male than female infants.

Treatment requires special feeding techniques, for example, the use of uniquely designed nipples (Procedure 36-2). Cleft lip repair may be done soon after delivery if the newborn is free of infection, in good condition, and weighs 2500 g (5 lb, 9 oz). Cleft lip repair (Fig. 40-15, *A*) is best done when the infant weighs 4500 g (10 lb) or more since there is more tissue to work with. Advantages of earlier labial (lip) repair include facilitating a positive parent-child relationship and permitting the infant to learn to use and strengthen musculature around the mouth. Infants with palatolabial fissures often look grotesque and repulsive to the parents. After repair and with collaborative health team support, the mother commonly is able to assume responsibility for the newborn's care until palatal repair is feasible (Fig. 40-15, *B*). Repair is done usually between 16 and 24 months of age (9 kg [20 lb] body weight or more). The plastic surgeon, pediatrician, orthodontist, hospital and community nurses, speech therapist, and social worker

A 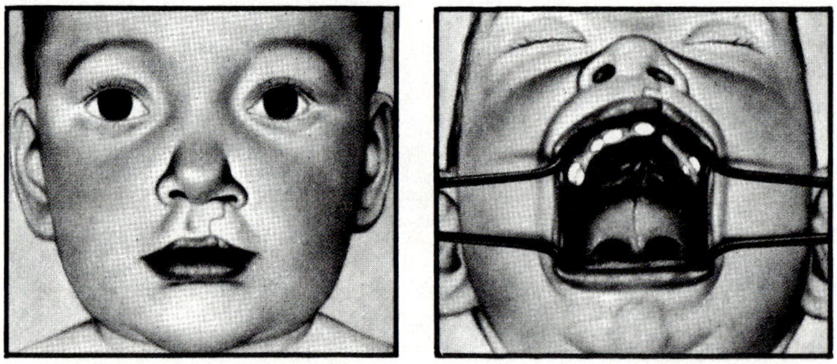 B

Fig. 40-15 Surgical repair of A, unilateral complete cleft lip and B, unilateral complete cleft palate.
Courtesy Ross Laboratories, Columbus, Ohio.

make up the collaborative health team that has made possible the effective treatment available today. Until repair of the palate is performed, a prosthesis is fitted to aid the infant's feeding and speech development and to reduce respiratory tract infections.

Musculoskeletal Disorders. The two most common musculoskeletal deviations seen in the neonatal period are congenital dysplasia of the hip and congenital clubfoot. Both conditions are easily recognized. Early detection and definitive treatment are mandatory for successful correction. Delay makes repair more difficult and prognosis less favorable.

Congenital Hip Dysplasia. Also known as *congenital dislocation of the hip,* this often hereditary disorder occurs more commonly in girls (Fig. 40-16) because of the structure of the pelvis. In this condition the acetabulum is abnormally shallow. The head of the femur becomes dislocated upward and backward to lie on the dorsal aspect of the ilium. The pressure of the displaced femoral head may form a false acetabulum on the ilium. A stretched joint capsule results, and ossification of the femoral head is delayed.

Before dislocation occurs, reduced movement, splinting of the affected hip, limited abduction, and asymmetry of the hip may be noted. After dislocation, all these signs will be present, together with the external rotation and shortening of the leg. A clicking sound may be noted on gentle forced abduction of the leg (Ortolani's sign, Fig. 21-21), and a bulge of the femoral head is felt or seen (Fig. 40-16, *B*). X-ray films will reveal a deformity in congenital dysplasia of the hip.

Treatment involves pressing the femoral head into the acetabulum to form an adequate socket before ossification is complete. The following methods are possible:

1. Thick diapers to abduct and externally rotate leg and flex hip (pin anterior flaps of diapers under posterior flaps).
2. Frejka pillow (apply diapers and plastic pants, and then apply pillow). Later this appliance will be followed by a spica cast in the most instances to maintain abduction, extension, and internal rotation, usually with the infant in a "frog-leg" position.

Talipes Equinovarus. Talipes equinovarus, or clubfoot, is a congenital fixed postural deformity in which the foot is twisted out of shape or position. The heel is turned inward from the midline of the leg, the sole of the foot is flexed at the ankle joint, and the Achilles tendon is shortened.

Before the infant is 2 months old, often during the first days of life, successive plaster casts are applied first to correct the heel inversion and adduction of the forefoot and later, the equinus deformity. Special shoes with lower legs braces will be necessary when the child learns to walk. Surgery may even be required in childhood if correction is incomplete. The prognosis depends on the extent of the deformity and the response to progressive orthopedic treatment.

Phocomelia. Phocomelia, or "seal-like limbs," is a developmental anomaly typified by absence of the arms or legs, or both, or stunting of the extremities. In the early 1960s the drug **thalidomide** was implicated as the causative agent for the limb deformities of many thousands of infants, especially in Germany. As a result the United States Food and Drug Administration tightened its regulations governing drug approval. Painfully apparent was evidence that drugs ingested during pregnancy may have tragic implications for fetal development. Thalidomide (and perhaps imipramine [Tofranil]) is a cause of this condition. Sporadic cases of congenital amputation or stunting are of unknown cause. The child born with these deformities requires special care.

Rehabilitative problems are often complex. The

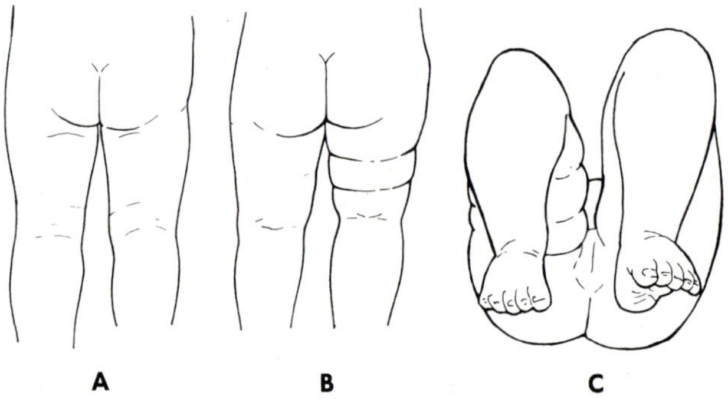

A B C

Fig. 40-16 Congenital dysplasia of hip. A, Normal gluteal and popliteal skin creases. B, Abnormal skin creases and asymmetry of skin folds. C, Apparent shortening of femur. Femur head is displaced.
Courtesy Ross Laboratories, Columbus, Ohio.

prostheses require frequent refitting as the child grows. The child requires careful guidance and training in achieving the optimum level of functioning possible. Approximately 15 child amputee centers are located throughout the United States.

Psychosocial developmental problems are significant. The kinesthetic satisfaction derived from kicking the legs and waving the arms is not possible. The hand-to-mouth movement behavior pattern, necessary for self-gratification and exploration of one's environment, is missing. The child learns about the environment by pushing the trunk up by the arms; a pillow prop under the infant's chest will compensate somewhat. The child's concerns about body image and obvious differences from others will require attention in later years. Any child reflects the attitudes and sentiments of those around her or him. Positive attitudes help the child incorporate these into a positive self-concept.

Supportive care of the parents must begin at the birth of the child and continue for years. After the initial grief reaction, the parents need information regarding the rehabilitative and psychosocial components of their child's care.

Polydactyly. Extra digits on the hands or feet occur occasionally (Fig. 40-17). In some instances polydactyly is hereditary. If there is little or no bone involvement, the extra digit is tied with silk suture soon after birth. The finger falls off within a few days, leaving a small scar. When there is bone involvement, surgical repair is indicated.

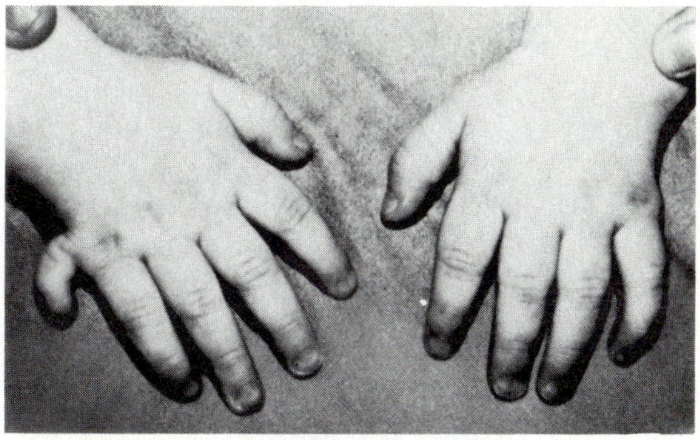

Fig. 40-17 Polydactyly: supernumerary digit of right hand. Most common congenital anomaly of upper extremity and is occasionally seen in conjunction with other congenital malformation.
Courtesy Mead Johnson & Co, Evansville, Indiana.

Genitourinary Tract Anomalies. Abnormally low-set or misshapen ears may indicate other, often genitourinary, anomalies (such as renal agenesis) (Fig. 21-18).

Exstrophy of the bladder. Exstrophy of the bladder (Fig. 40-18) is a congenital anomaly of unknown cause. With this anomaly a separation of the symphysis pubis and anterior abdominal wall structures results in exteriorization of the bladder trigone and surrounding mucosa. The exposed mucosa is deep red, has numerous folds, and is sensitive to touch. A direct passage of urine to the outside occurs. Associated anomalies, such as undescended testes, inguinal hernia, absence of the vagina, or bowel defects, should be sought. Surgical correction, often elimination of the bladder and construction of an ileal conduit, is rarely justified in the neonatal period. A prosthesis for collection of the urine and protection of the bladder may be employed.

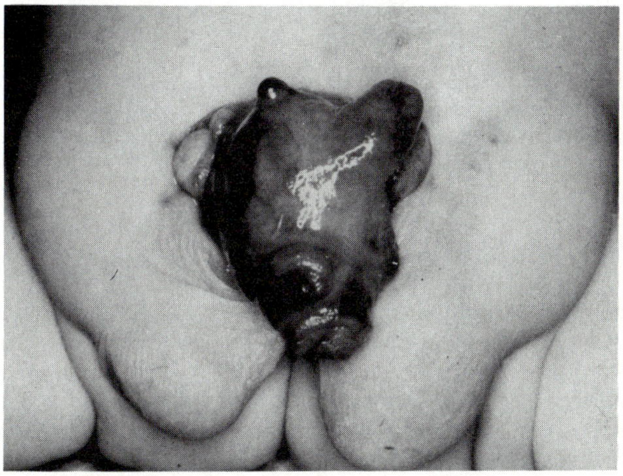

Fig. 40-18 Exstrophy of bladder.
Courtesy Edward S Tank, MD, Division of Urology, University of Oregon Health Sciences Center, Portland, Oregon.

Nursing management in the presence of exstrophy of the bladder focuses on the prevention of urinary tract infection and ulceration of adjacent skin from the constant seepage of urine. The child's touching and cuddling needs are met. Parents require considerable support and teaching to care for the defect if surgery is scheduled when the infant is several weeks or months of age.

Hypospadias and Epispadias. Hypospadias is a developmental anomaly in which the urethral meatus is placed lower than normal. In an infant boy the meatus opens in the midline of the undersurface of the penis or on the perineum. In an infant girl the meatus opens into the vagina. This condition tends to be hereditary.

Epispadias, also occurring in both sexes but predominating in boys, is a congenital absence of the upper urethral wall. In girls it is often associated with exstrophy of the bladder. In boys the meatal opening is located anywhere along the dorsum (upper side) of the penis.

Most instances of hypospadias are minor and require no corrective surgery. Pronounced defects require extensive urethroplasty. If needed, surgery is completed before the boy enters school so that he can urinate from a standing position like other boys. The more serious defects often coexist with other, multiple anomalies.

Nursing management of the physical care of the infant with hypospadias is the same as that for the normal infant. Should urethroplasty be required, no circumcision is done, since the foreskin is used in the surgical procedure. The parents are taught how to care for the urethral meatus and foreskin to prevent infection and promote cleanliness.

Sexual ambiguity. Sexual ambiguity in the newborn (Fig. 40-19) often is discovered by the nurse, who is usually the first one to perform a physical assessment. The obstetrician is still concentrating on the mother during the third stage of labor.

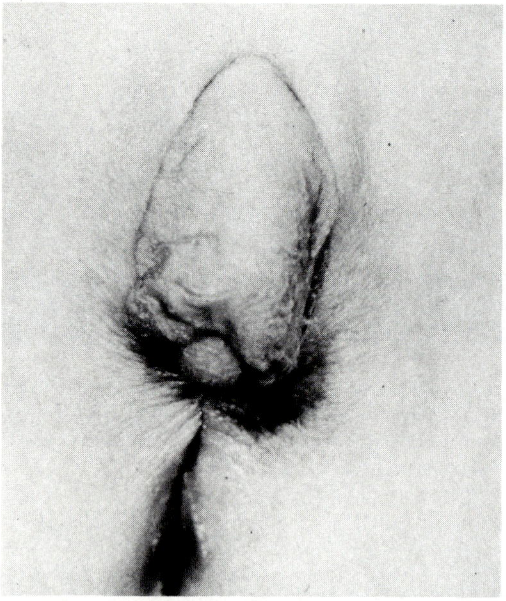

Fig. 40-19 Ambiguous external genitals (e.g., structure can be an enlarged clitoral hood and clitoris or a malformed penis).
Courtesy Edward S Tank, MD, Division of Urology, University of Oregon Health Sciences Center, Portland, Oregon.

Erroneous or abnormal sexual differentiation may be a genetic aberration (for example, congenital adrenal hypoplasia), or it may be caused by maternal problems (such as steroid sex hormone therapy for threatened abortion). It is imperative to establish the genetic sex and the sex of child rearing as soon as possible. Early identification is imperative to save embarrassment of reporting the birth of a (genetic) male who in fact is a female or the opposite. Early determination of genetic sex is important to permit the surgical correction of anomalies before an individual or social pattern is set. Prompt consultation with a surgeon who is experienced in the area of intersexuality should be arranged without delay. Meanwhile parents need supportive care as they await the decision.

Teratoma. Teratoma, a solid or semisolid neoplasm, is composed of the three embryonal tissue types (ectoderm, mesoderm, entoderm). A teratoma in the newborn may occur in the skull, mediastinum, or abdomen. A solid or semisolid tumor in the sacral area also may prove to be a teratoma. It is protected by sterile dressings before surgical removal. Many teratomas diagnosed in the newborn are malignant. If the lesion cannot be removed entirely by surgery, x-ray therapy and chemotherapy are used. Long-term survival rate for infants with sacrococcygeal teratoma is 85% after surgical removal in the neonatal period. The survival rate is only 50% if surgery is delayed until the infant is more than 1 month old. Rectal and anal function can always be preserved.

Disorders Not Apparent at Birth. Some disorders do not appear until some time after birth. The severity of the psychologic impact varies with the disorder and the time it appears. Together the parents and the affected child, if old enough, experience mourning, restructuring of self-image, and the reaction to stigmatization by society. Parents who had other children before the appearance of a disorder in an older child fear for the younger children. The middle-aged individual who develops Huntington's chorea, perhaps even after he has become a grandfather, fears for two generations of descendants. In many cases, affected individuals may experience anger and resentment toward the offending parents, just as parents of a child with a disorder feel resentment toward the child who "did this to us." If the mother unwittingly accepted therapy now shown to have adverse effects on her children (such as diethylstilbestrol [DES]), she may feel betrayed, angry, and afraid.

Genetic Disease

At the present time there is no cure for genetic disease, although remedies can be implemented to prevent or reduce the harmful effects of a few disorders. Structural defects can sometimes be modified to produce normal or near-normal function. Research is continually being carried out in the hope that methods can be devised to influence or change the genes directly, thereby preventing the disease process. However, at this time the major thrust in therapy is modification of the internal or external environment to minimize the effects of the disease. Rapid advances in the field of plastic and reconstructive surgery have reduced the impact of many functional and cosmetically displeasing physical defects. In some hereditary disorders, supplying the missing product that cannot be synthesized prevents the undesirable effects, for example, thyroid extract for hereditary cretinism, corticosteroids for adrenogenital syndrome, insulin for diabetes mellitus, and administration of missing blood factors for the hemophilias.

Diet modification may be required for infants with some inborn errors of metabolism. For example, a low phenylalanine diet reduces the harmful effects of that protein in phenylketonuria (PKU). Some female children successfully treated for PKU are now of reproductive age and present unique management challenges to caregivers (p. 801). Other examples are substitution of lactose-free products for milk fed to infants and children with galactosemia, and use of a diet low in branched chain amino acids for infants and children with maple syrup urine disease.

Support. Clarifying information and misunderstanding of information are important nursing functions. A newly diagnosed disorder often implies the implementation of a therapeutic regimen. For example, the disorder in question may be an inborn error of metabolism such as PKU or galactosemia that requires consistent and rigid adherence to a diet. The family may need help to secure the necessary formula and counseling from dietetic services. The importance of maintaining the diet, especially keeping an adequate supply of special preparations and avoiding unauthorized substitutions, must be impressed on the family.

Referrals to appropriate agencies are another essential part of the follow-up management. Many organizations and foundations help provide services and equipment for affected children, for example, the Cystic Fibrosis Foundation and the Muscular Dystrophy Association. Early Infant Stimulation Foundation programs are available for a child born with Down's syndrome. There are also numerous parent groups with whom the family can share experiences and derive mutual support from other families with a similar problem. Nurses need to become familiar with services available in their community that provide assistance and education to families with these special problems (Appendix K).

Probably the most important of all nursing functions is providing *emotional support* to the family during all aspects of the care of the child born with a defect or disorder. Feelings that are generated under the real or imagined threat posed by a genetic disorder are as varied as the persons being counseled. Responses may include all stress reactions, such as apathy, denial, anger, hostility, fear, embarrassment, grief, and loss of self-esteem (Chapter 28).

Parents benefit from seeing before and after pictures of other babies born with this defect. Coupled with other verbal and nonverbal supportive care, this visual reassurance is effective. Parents can be referred to other parents (or organizations of parents such as the Cleft Palate Club) for continuing mutual support.

Guilt and self-blame are universal reactions. Many look on the disorder as a stigma—especially if the disorder is visible to others. Persons involved with the family are often able to dispel fears and even absolve the family from guilt simply by explaining the random nature of cell division and segregation. Parents may derive comfort from knowing that everyone carries defective genes, which, when combined with the same genes in a partner, can produce undesirable consequences. Old wives' tales, superstitions, and long-held misconceptions are all factors that may influence a client's reaction to a disorder. Obstacles such as religious beliefs, intellectual level, and prior attitudes toward the disease affect the way in which families respond.

The attitude of other family members and relatives can have a significant impact on some persons—especially in situations where the blame can be pinpointed (such as a dominant or an X-linked disorder). Recessive disorders are less likely to cause blaming, since both partners carry the defective gene. Unfortunately most families tend to view a congenital disorder as a cause for shame. Its presence in a family may be cause to alter plans for marriage or childbearing even when the probability of recurrence is no more than a random risk. The way a family views the probability of recurrence varies tremendously. For example, one family will consider a 10% risk as reassuring, whereas another may consider it too great a risk to comtemplate marriage or childbearing.

The nature of a neonate's condition also influences the way families respond to a disorder. Factors such as the severity or chronicity of a disease, the age of onset, the threat of early death, a lengthy period of deterioration, presence or absence of pain, mental retardation, or cosmetic disfiguration all determine the impact that a condition will produce in a family. One family may risk a child with a disorder that produces a minor defect or even an early death but will not risk having a child with a lifelong physical or mental disability.

Sometimes counselors and other health personnel create barriers through their own attitudes toward a specific disease. It is often difficult to be nonjudgmental and objective in all instances. Nurses may intentionally or unintentionally influence families in making decisions. This is especially true when the client's intellectual level makes it difficult or impossible for that person to comprehend the ramifications of a situation. Even persons who can repeat information accurately often fail to grasp its significance in their case. Families may pressure the nurse to make decisions for them with questions such as, "What would you do if you were me?"

Families and individuals need ongoing education, guidance, and support (Johnson, 1986; Sammons and Lewis, 1985). They should be given the facts and possible consequences and all the assistance they need in problem solving, but the final decision regarding a course of action must be their own.

Evaluation

Care is evaluated by assessing the degree to which goals have been met. On the short-term basis, care has been effective if the neonate's disorder has been treated appropriately and the condition has stabilized within normal limits; when the parents have begun to cope with the situation, initiate attachment to the infant, and mobilize family support; and when appropriate community services have become involved therapeutically. Long-term evaluation is more difficult and is more relevant to pediatric and adult health care.

SUMMARY

Most infants make the transition from intrauterine to extrauterine life with little difficulty. For some, however, birth is complicated by many factors. Hyperbilirubinemia and congenital abnormalities place the newborn in jeopardy for intact survival.

The survival and well-being of these high-risk infants depends on advanced and often agressive nursing and medical management and a suitably controlled environment. The parents of the high-risk infant may experience feelings of lowered self-esteem and self-worth and alienation from the infant. Thus the nurse plays a vital role in the care of both the high-risk newborn and the parents.

KEY CONCEPTS

- Hyperbilirubinemia has a variety of etiologic factors including maternal-fetal Rh and ABO incompatibility.
- Erythroblastosis fetalis leads to anemia, edema, and cytotoxic effects of unconjugated bilirubin.
- Injection of Rho(D) immune globulin to Rh-negative and Coombs'-negative women bestows passive immunity and minimizes the possibility of isoimmunization.
- An Rh-negative woman receives Rh-positive RBCs from the fetus through disruption of the cellular layer separating fetal and maternal circulation and through an erroneous blood transfusion.

- Neonatal exchange transfusion with type O, Rh negative-RBCs serves to treat anemia and acidosis, and to remove bilirubin, maternal antibodies, and fetal RBCs that are beginning to hemolyze.
- Perinatal events such as hypoxia and cold stress increase the neonate's susceptibility to neurotoxic effects of bilirubin.
- Major congenital defects are now the leading cause of death in term neonates where perinatal care is of good quality.
- Hydramnios and oligohydramnios are associated with many congenital anomalies.
- Current technology permits prenatal diagnosis of many congenital anomalies and disorders.
- The curative and rehabilitative problems of a child with a congenital disorder are often complex, requiring a multidisciplinary approach to care.
- Supportive care to parents must begin at birth or at diagnosis and continue for years.

STUDY QUESTIONS AND ACTIVITIES

1. Visit a support group meeting for parents of infants with congenital defects; or, role-play interaction between a nurse and a family that has a newborn with a congenital defect; the parents reveal that this is the third child in the family to be born with the defect. Follow with group discussion.
2. Arrange a field trip to a community agency that offers rehabilitation to infants with congenital defects.
3. Observe or assist with an exchange transfusion.
4. Seek assignment to a neonate with a congenital anomaly, or a neonate receiving phototherapy for hyperbilirubinemia.
5. Practice assessment of neonates for congenital anomaly or jaundice.

References

Benacerraf, BR, Gelman, R, and Frigoletto, FD: Sonographic identification of second-trimester fetuses with Down's syndrome, N Engl J Med 317(22):1371, 1987
Cohen, FL: Neural tube defects: epidemiology, detection, and prevention, JOGN Nurs 16(2):105, 1987
Fanaroff, AA, and Martin, RJ, editors: Neonatal-perinatal medicine: diseases of the fetus and infant, ed 4, St Louis, 1987, The CV Mosby Co
Grannum, PA, et al: In utero exchange transfusion by direct intravascular injection in severe erythrobastosis fetalis, N Engl J Med 314(22): 1431, 1986
Hershey, DW, Crandall, BF, and Perdue, S: Combining maternal age and serum α-fetoprotein to predict the risk of Down syndrome, *Obstet Gynecol* 68:777, 1986
Johnson, SH: Nursing assessment and strategies for the family at risk: high-risk parenting, ed 2, Philadelphia, 1986, JB Lippincott Co
Kogan, SC, Doherty, M, and Gitschier, J: An improved method for prenatal diagnosis of genetic diseases by analysis of amplified DNA sequences, N Engl J Med 317:985, 1987
Lewis, C, and Mocarski, V: Obstetric ultrasound: application in a clinic setting, JOGN Nurs 16(1):56, 1987
Locklin, M: Assessing jaundice in full-term newborns, Pediatr Nurs 13(1):15, 1987
Main, DM, and Mennuti, MT: Neural tube defects: issues in prenatal diagnosis and counselling, *Obstet Gynecol* 67:1, 1986
McLaughlin, JF, Shurtleff, DB, Lamers, JY, et al: Influence of prognosis on decisions regarding the care of newborns with myelodysplasia, N Engl J Med 312:1589, 1985
Pernoll, ML, Benda, GI, and Babson, SG: Diagnosis and management of the fetus and neonate at risk: a guide for team care, ed 5, St Louis, 1986, The CV Mosby Co
Perry, SE, Parer, JT, and Inturrisi, M: Intrauterine transfusion for severe isoimmunization, MCN 11(3):182, 1986
Routine prenatal genetic screening (editorial), N Engl J Med 317(22):1407, 1987
Sammons, WA, and Lewis, JM: Premature babies: a different beginning, St Louis, 1985, The CV Mosby Co
Wu, PY, et al: Transcutaneous bilirubinometry: factors affecting the correlation of TcB index and serum bilirubin, J Perinatol 5:41, Summer 1985

Bibliography

Bone marrow transplantation for genetic diseases (editorial), N Engl J Med 316(17):1085, 1987
Bowman, JM: Controversies in Rh prophylaxis: who needs Rh immune globulin and when should it be given? Am J Obstet Gynecol 151(3):289, 1985
Boynton, BR, and Boynton, CA: Discharge planning for high-risk infants, J Perinat 5:44, Fall 1985
Brucker, M, and MacMullen, N: Chorionic villus sampling: counseling your patient, Nurse Pract 12(8):34, 1987
Cashore, WJ: Transcutaneous bilirubinometry, NAACOG Newsletter, 11:4, 1984
Censullo, M: Home care of the high-risk newborn, JOGN Nurs 15:146, March/April 1986
Chatterjee, MS: Parental age and Down's syndrome, Contemp OB/GYN 21(5):171, 1983
Consolvo, CA: Relieving parental anxiety in the care-by-parent unit, JOGN Nurs 15:154, March/April 1986
DiMaio, M, et al: Screening for fetal Down's syndrome in pregnancy by measuring maternal serum alpha-fetoprotein levels, N Engl J Med 317(6):342, 1987
Droegemueller, W, et al: Comprehensive gynecology, St Louis, 1987, The CV Mosby Co
Erlen, JA, and Holzman, IR: Anencephalic infants: should they be organ donors? Pediatr Nurs 14(1):60, 1988
Erythroblastosis fetalis: closing the circle (personal correspondence), N Engl J Med 314(22):1448, 1986
Field, T, and Goldson, E: Pacifying effects of nonnutritive sucking on term and preterm neonates during heelstick procedures, Pediatrics 74:1012, 1984
Gildea, J: A crisis plan for pediatric code, Am J Nurs 86:557, May 1986
Gross, SJ, et al: Sacrococcygeal teratoma: prenatal diagnosis and management, Am J Obstet Gynecol 156(2):393, 1987
Harris, SR: Early detection of cerebral palsy: sensitivity and specificity of two motor assessment tools, J Perinat 7(1):11, Winter 1987
Inturrisi, M, Perry, SE, and May, KA: Fetal surgery for congenital hydronephrosis, JOGN Nurs 14:271, July/Aug 1985
Kemp, V, and Page, C: Maternal prenatal attachment in normal and high-risk pregnancies, JOGN Nurs 16(3):179, 1987
Kricker, A, et al: Congenital limb reduction deformities and use of oral contraceptives, Am J Obstet Gynecol 155:1072, 1986
Korones, S: High-risk newborn infants: the basis for intensive nursing care, ed 4, St Louis, 1986, The CV Mosby Co

Larson, DR: Ethics: should anencephalic neonates be organ donors? AORN Journal, 47(3):778, 1988

Ledger, KE, and Williams, DL: Parents at risk: an instructional program for perinatal assessment and preventive intervention, Victoria, B.C. Canada, 1981, Ministry of Health, Province of British Columbia, and Queen Alexandra Solarium for Crippled Children Society (Queen Alexandra Hospital, 2400 Arbutus Rd., Victoria, B.C., Canada V8N 1V7)

Merenstein, GB, and Gardner, SL: Handbook of neonatal intensive care, St Louis, 1985, The CV Mosby Co

Niculescu, AM: Effects of *in utero* exposure to DES on male progency, JOGN Nurs 14:468, Nov/Dec 1985

Normal serum bilirubin levels in the newborn: effect of breast-feeding (abstract), Pediatr Currents 36(2):1, 1987

Palomaki, GE, and Haddow, JE: Maternal serum γ-fetoprotein, age, and Down syndrome risk, Am J Obstet Gynecol 156(2):460, 1987

Pernoll, ML, and Benson, RC: Current obstetric and gynecologic diagnosis and treatment, ed 6, Los Altos, Calif, 1987, Appleton & Lange

Porter, JB, et al: Drugs and stillbirth, Am J Public Health, 76:1428, 1986

Raff, BS: The use of homemaker-home health aides' perinatal care of high risk infants, JOGN Nurs 15:142, March/April 1986

Raff, BS: Nursing care of high-risk infants and their families—introduction, JOGN Nurs 15:141, March/April 1986

Seeds, JW, and Cefalo, RC: Anomalies with hydramnios: diagnostic role of ultrasound, Contemp OB/GYN 23:32, 1984

Segal, S, et al: The death of a child—parents' views of professional support, Can Med Assoc 134:38, Jan 1, 1986

Smith, K: Recognizing cardiac failure in neonates, MCN 4:98, 1979

Vintzileos, AM, et al: Congenital defects: let ultrasound guide your delivery plan, Contemp OB/GYN 24(2):46, 1984

Whaley, LF, and Wong, DL: Nursing care of infants and children, ed 3, St Louis, 1987, The CV Mosby Co

Resources for Down's Syndrome

The National Association for Down's Syndrome, Dept. N83, Box 63, Oak Park, Ill. 60303, and the Down's syndrome Congress, Dept. N83, 1640 W. Roosevelt Rd., Chicago, Ill. 60608. For additonal help, contact national and local associations for the mentally retarded

UNIT

IX

Women's Health and Gynecologic Care

Nursing care of the gynecologic client is preventive, curative, and rehabilitative in nature. It demands nursing skills that support women undergoing normal changes across the life span, as well as highly technical skills associated with care of the gynecologic-oncologic client.

In Chapter 41 abnormal conditions associated with menstruation, such as dysmenorrhea, premenstrual syndrome, and endometriosis are discussed. The climacterium, major disorders that arise with aging, and sequelae to childbirth are discussed.

Chapter 42 contains content basic to understanding fertility management. It includes care of clients relative to impaired fertility, control of fertility, surgical interruption of pregnancy, and termination of fertility.

Chapter 43 focuses on hazards to women's health in the environment and workplace. Violence, a major problem in the lives of many women, is discussed. This chapter discusses detection and diagnosis of the problems, care required, and community support available.

Chapter 44 discusses neoplasia, which, particularly in its malignant form, is part of the specialized oncologic care needed by gynecologic clients. The chapter reviews current concepts related to medical management, nursing care, the family, and community resources.

Nursing research highlights are included. Following are abstracts of examples of relevant nursing research.

Chapter 41: The effect of a support group on self-esteem of women with premenstrual syndrome; gastrointestinal symptoms and bowel patterns across the menstrual cycle in dysmenorrhea; and, age as a variable in an exercise program for the treatment of simple urinary stress incontinence.

Chapter 42: Relationship between weight change and diaphragm size change.

Chapter 43: The effectiveness of counseling services utilized by battered women.

Chapter 44: The effects of a patient education course in persons with a chronic illness, and social support in patients' and husbands' adjustment to breast cancer.

CHAPTER 41

Gynecologic and Urinary Concerns

Learning Objectives

Correctly define the key terms listed.

Develop a nursing care plan for a woman with primary dysmenorrhea.

Explain the pathophysiology of endometriosis that underlies the commonly associated symptoms.

Construct an assessment guide to use with women who are experiencing the climacterium.

Review factors to take into consideration when developing a plan of care for a woman exhibiting the symptomatology of the postclimacteric period.

Identify the types of problems a woman may have who has sustained levator ani injuries and anterior vaginal wall injuries during childbirth.

Describe nursing care of a woman with uterine displacement.

Describe nursing care of a woman who has genital fistulas.

Present an outline for client teaching about premenstrual syndrome.

Keeping the needs of the perimenopausal woman in mind, suggest types of community resources that would be helpful to people in this phase of growth and development.

Key Terms

atresia
climacterium
colpocele
cystocele
endometriosis
enterocele
fistula
hormone replacement therapy
hot flush (flash)
hypermenorrhea
hypogonadotropic amenorrhea
menopause
osteoporosis
pelvic relaxation
perineorrhaphy
pessary
premenstrual syndrome (PMS)
primary dysmenorrhea
procidentia
prostaglandin-synthesis inhibitor
secondary dysmenorrhea
stress urinary incontinence
urethrocele
uterine prolapse

Disorders associated with menstruation afflict a large percentage of women in the reproductive years. These conditions have a negative effect on the quality of the women's lives and on the lives of their families. The normal processes of the menstrual cycle are discussed elsewhere in this text. Special attention is directed to Chapter 6 for normal endocrine physiology not related to pregnancy and to Chapter 42 for conditions associated with infertility. This chapter deals with the most common gynecologic problems associated with the menstrual cycle—hypogonadotropic amenorrhea secondary to stress, dysmenorrhea, premenstrual syndrome, and endometriosis—long-term sequelae to childbirth trauma, and the difficulties encountered by women during the climacteric and postclimacteric periods that are the result of normal changes in the woman's reproductive and genitourinary systems. The gradual decline in ovarian function and cessation of menses characterize the normal climacterium. Events of the climacterium and the period that follows also significantly affect the quality of life of the woman and her family.

MENSTRUAL DISORDERS

Hypogonadotropic Amenorrhea

Hypogonadotropic amenorrhea reflects a problem in the central hypothalamic-pituitary axis. A diagnostic workup (Chapter 42) is necessary to identify the cause. Pituitary unresponsiveness caused by a rare pituitary lesion or an even more rare case of genetic inability to produce follicle-stimulating hormone (FSH) and luteinizing hormone (LH) is an infrequent occurrence. Levels of thyroid-stimulating hormone (TSH) and prolactin are measured, a radiographic view of the sella turcica is obtained, and a progestational challenge is done.

The most common category is hypogonadotropic amenorrhea resulting from hypothalamic suppression consequent to stress (e.g., pressures in the home, school, or workplace); underweight for height; rapid weight loss; eating disorders (anorexia nervosa, bulimia); strenuous exercise associated with competitive athletics or dancing (ballet). Two principal influences are recognized: (1) a critical body-fat-to-lean ratio and (2) the effect of stress itself. Menstrual regularity requires the maintenance of weight and body fat above a critical level.

The woman who is most likely to develop hypogonadotropic amenorrhea weighs less than 115 pounds and has lost 10 pounds or more through exercising. The serious female athlete may have an adequate weight but a reduced proportion of body fat. Peripheral levels of endorphins increase with physical stress (strenuous exercise) and perhaps with severe mental stress as well. Endorphins may exert a suppressive effect on the hypothalamus. The history, confirmed by physical examination, often reveals a weight-conscious woman engaging in significant physical exercise and concerned with control over her own body.

If counseling is ineffective in altering the client's life-style of exercise and weight control, regardless of her young age the woman may be a candidate for hormone replacement therapy (HRT). Women who fall into this category of hypogonadotropic amenorrhea tend to lose calcium from their bones; that is, their bone density is comparable to that of postmenopausal women. Prescribed therapy usually includes conjugated estrogen for days 1 through 24 of each month (starting with the first calendar day of the month) and medroxyprogesterone acetate (MPA)(Provera) for days 10 through 24; withdrawal bleeding usually occurs on day 27. Bone density is spared with this therapy. The woman receiving HRT needs to be reevaluated yearly for return of normal function. HRT does not protect against pregnancy if a return of normal menstrual function goes unsuspected.

If the woman's life-style of strenuous exercise and weight control does *not* result in menstrual changes and amenorrhea, no loss in bone density occurs and no intervention is indicated.

Dysmenorrhea

Dysmenorrhea is painful menstruation, one of the most common gynecologic problems in women of all ages. *Primary dysmenorrhea* occurs in the absence of organic disease; the initial episode occurs when ovulation begins, about 6 to 12 months after menarche. *Secondary dysmenorrhea* is associated with organic pelvic disease.

Primary dysmenorrhea begins when the ovary is fully developed, ova mature, and progestin is secreted; it often improves by age 25 or following pregnancy with vaginal delivery. Although psychogenic factors may be significant in the perception of and reaction to dysmenorrhea, a physiologic basis exists. Discomfort depends on ovulation; it does not occur when ovulation is suppressed.

If ovulation occurs, during the progesterone-induced luteal phase and subsequent menstrual flow, prostaglandin F_2 alpha ($PGF_{2\alpha}$) is found. Excessive secretion and subsequent excessive release of $PGF_{2\alpha}$ during menstrual shedding of the endometrium increase the amplitude and frequency of uterine contractions. Pain is described as a low abdominal aching. Cramplike cyclic pain of dysmenorrhea results from ischemia after strong muscle contractions. Increases production of $PGF_{2\alpha}$ may be responsible for systemic responses such as aching (back, lower abdomen, thighs), gastrointestinal symptoms (anorexia, nausea, vomiting, diarrhea), central nervous system (CNS) symptoms (dizziness, syncope, headache, poor concentration), weakness, and sweats. The initial event that causes prostaglandin release to precipitate symptoms remains unknown (Lublanezki and Fischer, 1987). See research highlight on gastrointestinal symptoms and dysmenorrhea, on p. 1028.

Secondary dysmenorrhea occurs in association with pathologic changes such as endometriosis, pelvic inflammatory disease, cervical stenosis, uterine or ovarian neoplasms or uterine polyps. The presence of an IUD is also a factor. Pregnancy must be ruled out to avoid confusion with complications of early pregnancy.

Primary Dysmenorrhea. For some women heat (heating pad, hot bath), massage, distraction, exercise, and sleep are sufficient to achieve relief for primary dysmenorrhea. Heat is especially effective because it reduces muscle tone and increases circulation; both effects relieve ischemia. For some women orgasm brings relief. Uterine contractions of orgasm facilitate menstrual flow and relieve pelvic vasocongestion. The pleasurable experience of orgasm can reduce tension and increase the woman's sense of well-being. The addition of natural diuretics to the diet helps some women reduce edema and related discomforts. Asparagus, parsley, and caffeine have a diuretic effect.

Several over-the-counter (OTC) menstrual pain preparations are available (Lublanezki and Fischer, 1987). Aspirin, a mild inhibitor of prostaglandin synthesis, may provide sufficient relief. Acetaminophen is useful for relief of noninflammatory pain associated with primary dysmenorrhea (Sohn, Korberly, and Tannenbaum, 1986). Relief is usually obtained with the recommended dosage, 650 mg every 4 hours not to exceed 4000 mg in a 24 hour period. Ibuprofen (Motrin, Advil, Nuprin) also inhibits prostaglandin synthesis. In doses of 200 to 400 mg every 4 to 6 hours, Ibuprofen is rated as superior to aspirin and acetaminophen as an analgesic by most women (Lublanezki and Fischer, 1987). These prostaglandin-synthesis* inhibitors are most effective if started several days before the onset of the menstrual flow. However, this could expose an early pregnancy to the drugs. Other commonly used prostaglandin-synthesis inhibitors include naproxen (Naprosyn and Anaprox) and mefenamic acid (Ponstel) (Droegemueller et al., 1987).

Some products, such as Cope and Midol, contain both aspirin and caffeine; Midol also contains cinnamedrine, a mild uterine relaxant. Many products contain pamabrom, which is similar to caffeine in its diuretic effect. Pyrilamine maleate, an antihistimine, is also in many OTC products. Its mechanism of action is unknown and has some sedative and analgesic effect. Pyrilamine is marketed only in combination with a diuretic or with a diuretic and analgesic.

Surgical intervention may be indicated as a last resort for women with intractable dysmenorrhea. Presacral neurectomy or sympathectomy brings relief to 70% of women who undergo the surgery.

RESEARCH HIGHLIGHT

Gastrointestinal Symptoms and Bowel Patterns Across the Menstrual Cycle in Dysmenorrhea

Purpose

Altered gastrointestinal function can produce distressful symptoms that may contribute to the loss of work and productivity and increased use of health care services. This study was designed to describe GI functional indicators across the menstrual cycle and to compare women with and without dysmenorrhea according to the GI functional indicators.

Sample

A convenient sample of 34 women between 19 and 37 years of age was studied for 2 menstrual cycles. Regular menstruation was defined as the woman's reported usual cycle length plus or minus 2 days. Women were divided into three groups: dysmenorrheic (14), non-pill-taking nondysmenorrheic (10), and nondysmenorrheic taking birth control pills (10).

Methodology

During the initial visit the Menstrual Distress Questionnaire was administered and subjects were instructed about the use of the GI Health Diary, which was developed for this study to measure GI function and symptoms.

Findings

Looser stools and stomach pains were more common during menses. There was a reported decreased food intake by dysmenorrheic women during menses. In fact more dysmenorrheic women had a history of menses-related GI symptoms.

Implications

These data suggest that GI function is related to menstrual cycle phase and there is an increased prevalence of GI symptoms close to and during menses. The investigators believe that this kind of information can assist in planning therapeutic interventions. For example, when women experience an illness, their history of GI symptoms and knowledge of their current menstrual cycle phase could influence interpretation of symptoms experienced during their current illness.

Heitkemper, MN, Shaver, JF, and Mitchell, ES: Gastrointestinal symptoms and bowel patterns across the menstrual cycle in dysmenorrhea, Nurs Res 37(2):109, 1988

Premenstrual Syndrome

Premenstrual syndrome (PMS) refers to a diffuse, loosely defined set of both physical and behavioral symptoms that begins approximately 7 to 10 days before menses and ends with the onset of menses (Table 41-1). Commonly there is a positive family history for PMS, although the relative influence of heredity versus environment is unclear.

PMS may be expressed positively in heightened creativity and ability to concentrate and in increased mental and physical activity. However, these reactions receive little notice in the media or literature.

To most people PMS refers to the variety of negative symptoms, among which are those related to edema or emotional instability: abdominal distension or bloating, pelvic fullness, swelling of extremities, breast tenderness, weight gain, irritability, depression, crying spells, insomnia, fatigue, feelings of unreality and panic, headache, and backache (O'Brien, 1982; Droegemueller et al., (1987). Some women feel more sexually arousable, whereas others react with indifference to even the thought of sex. For a small percentage of women PMS is so incapacitating that their normal activities are totally disrupted for 1 to 2 or more days during each cycle.

In part because of the elusiveness of the cause of PMS, there is little agreement and great variety in methods of management. Data from a careful, detailed history and a daily log of somatic symptoms and mood fluctuations spanning several cycles give direction to a plan for management. Cultural affective influences must be separated from physiologic influences (Fogel and Woods, 1981).

Psychosocial aspects may be the first priority for care. Support groups may affect the self-esteem of women with

*Prostaglandin-synthetase inhibitors block the effect of PGs on tissue.

Table 41-1 *Dysmenorrhea and Premenstrual Syndrome (PMS): Comparison of Onset and Duration, Range of Response, and Incidence*

	Dysmenorrhea	PMS
Onset and duration	Acute 24-48 hr before or coincident with onset of menses, with pelvic pain that decreases or ends with end of menses	Diffuse 7-10 days before menses; resolves with onset of menses
Range of response	From mild to severe and disabling for 24-48 hr	From awareness of physiologic changes to incapacitation or disruption of life-style
Incidence	Some discomfort: 80% of all women Severe enough to interfere with normal activities for 1-2 days: 35% of older adolescents; 25% of college women; 60%-70% of single women in their 30s and 40s Incapacitation: 10% of all women	5%-95% of all women

PMS (see research highlight). Lack of understanding of PMS may stress relationships to the breaking point. Couple counseling is scheduled before the anticipated onset of PMS.

Medications may be required for relief from some distress, for example, diuretics for edema. A well-balanced diet low in sodium or with addition of naturally diuretic foods may ease some symptoms.

Table 41-1 presents a comparison of onset and duration, range of response, and incidence of dysmenorrhea and PMS. A nursing care plan for women experiencing premenstrual syndrome is presented on p. 1033.

Endometriosis

Endometriosis is a disease characterized by the presence and growth of glands and stroma identical to the lining of the uterus, found outside the uterus (ectopic), attached to other organs or tissue in the woman's body (Fig. 41-1). The ectopic endometrial tissue includes both endometrial glands and stroma. The most common sites of implantation of ectopic endometrium are the ovaries, cul-de-sac, uterosacral ligaments, recto-vaginal septum, sigmoid colon, round ligaments, pelvic peritoneum, and urinary bladder. A chocolate cyst is a cystic area of endometriosis in the ovary. The dark coloring of the contents of the cyst is old blood.

The ectopic endometrial tissue responds to hormonal stimulation in the same way that uterine endometrium does. During the proliferative and secretory phases of the menstrual cycle, endometrium grows. During or immediately after menstruation, the tissue bleeds. To the surrounding tissue the bleeding is foreign, and this tissue responds by becoming inflamed. The inflammation develops into fibrosis. As the growth and shedding of the ectopic tissue is repeated each cycle, more bleeding causes more fibrosis. The fibrosis causes adhesions to adjacent organs. Scar tissue and distortion or blockage of surrounding organs may result.

Often this chronic, progressive disease remains asymptomatic and undiagnosed, eventually disappearing during the climacterium. However, for those women who have symptoms medical management and nursing intervention are required.

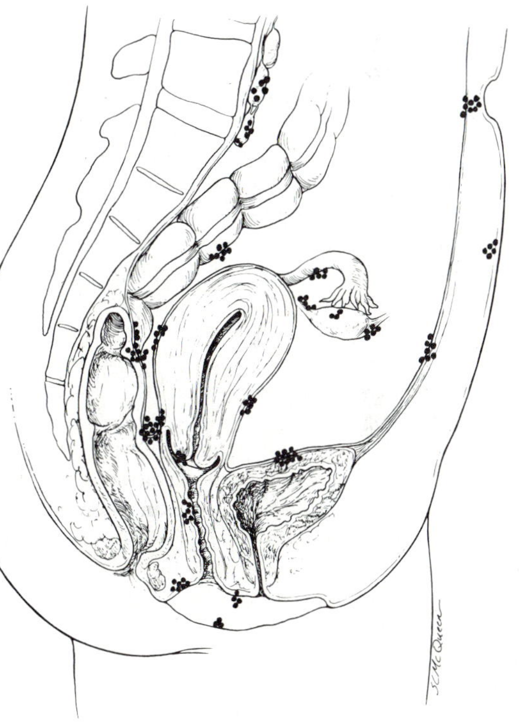

Fig. 41-1 Common sites of endometriosis.
From Droegemueller, W, et al: Comprehensive gynecology, St Louis, 1987, The CV Mosby Co.

Endometriosis is most common during the childbearing years. Although the exact number of women who have endometriosis is unknown, 5% to 15% of women who undergo pelvic surgery were observed to have endometriosis (Droegemueller et al; 1987). Bernhard (1982) states that this disease occurs most commonly in women between the ages of 25 and 40. It occurs regardless of parity, socioeconomic group, or cultural-ethnic background.

The cause of endometriosis is unknown. However, several theories have been suggested since 1860, when the disease was first described.

Transtubal migration or retrograde menstruation theory is the most popular explanation for endometriosis. It suggests that during menstruation endometrial tissue is regurgitated or mechanically transported from the uterus, up the uterine tubes, and into the peritoneal cavity. Implantation of endometrial tissue on the ovaries and other organs results from this backward propulsion of menstrual tissue.

Coelomic metaplasia doctrine is a theory that tries to account for the diversity of sites at which endometrial tissue may appear. It suggests that organs retain genetic material capable of developing endometrium. The coelom is the primitive base from which the ovary, peritoneum, and pleura derive. This might explain why endometriosis has been found in the lungs, lymphatics, and blood vessels.

Other theories include the following:

1. The lymphatic spread mechanism, in which endometriosis is carried by lymph to extrauterine sites.
2. The surgical implantation theory, in which endometrial tissue is implanted during pelvic surgery (e.g., cesarean delivery) in scar tissue.
3. The hematogenous route, in which endometriosis is transported by the circulatory system to extrauterine sites.

Symptoms of endometriosis vary among women and change over time. Often the severity of symptoms will be in inverse proportion to the extent and location of the endometriosis. Symptoms include secondary dysmenorrhea, dyspareunia, abnormal uterine bleeding, and impaired fertility (for a discussion of infertility, see Chapter 42).

The major symptom of endometriosis is **secondary dysmenorrhea**, or cramping associated with menstruation. Women describe it as dull pain or cramps in the lower abdomen or lower back or pain on defecation just before, during, or immediately after menstruation. Women may also have pain radiating into the thighs. Cramps may be progressive, becoming more painful each month. Eventually pain can become constant. Pelvic heaviness is described by some women.

A second, but less common, symptom is **dyspareunia**, or painful intercourse. The pain, experienced during deep penile penetration, may continue for several hours following intercourse. Endometriosis that includes adhesions around the vagina and ligaments decreases their flexibility during intercourse.

Another symptom although very rare, is **abnormal bleeding** in the form of hypermenorrhea, menorrhagia, or premenstrual staining. According to Ranney (1980), excessive menstrual flow might be the consequence of significant ovarian adhesions that have disrupted the normal ovarian hormone production.

Impaired fertility may result when endometrial tissue implants around the uterus. The ectopic tissues pull this organ into a fixed retroverted position. Adhesions result when bleeding from this tissue resolves. Adhesions around the uterine tubes decrease their motility and prevent the muscular tubes from moving spontaneously and carrying the ovum to the uterus. Tubes may also be blocked at the fimbriated ends by endometrial tissue, preventing the ovum from entering the tube. Approximately 30% to 45% of women with endometriosis are infertile, whereas this is the case for only 12% of women in the general population (Bernhard, 1982; Droegemueller et al., 1987).

The *diagnosis* of endometriosis is based on the findings of three procedures. Endometriosis is first suspected when a woman reports a history of menses-linked symptoms that have become worse over time. When a woman has been pregnant previously, the history may include an interval of 5 years since the last delivery.

A pelvic examination is the second diagnostic tool. Often nodular areas behind the cervix can be palpated. However, it is not appropriate to begin treatment for endometriosis until a third and definitive step has been taken.

The diagnosis of endometriosis can be made only after a laparoscopy has been performed. By inserting a laparoscope into the abdominal cavity, the surgeon can explore for growths and sometimes remove them. After a laparoscopy the woman and her physician can make informed decisions about treatment or pregnancy.

Classification of endometriosis according to severity has been proposed by several researchers in an effort to standardize the description of the disease and provide a tool for collecting meaningful data upon which treatments and prognosis may be based. However, none of the classification tools has been universally accepted. One example of classification for endometriosis is included here for information only (Table 41-2) (Acosta, 1973; Puleo and Hammond, 1983).

Treatment of endometriosis is based on the severity of the symptoms and the goals of the woman. For women without pain and without plans for pregnancy, no treatment, other than regular observation, is required. for those women with mild pain and with the capacity to become pregnant, analgesics are recommended.

For women who have severe pain and can postpone pregnancy, hormonal medications are used. High-dose contraceptive pills are prescribed at times, since they have been shown to shrink endometrial tissue. Progestogens, in the form of medroxyprogesterone acetate (MPA) in high doses, have also been used, but these are no longer approved by the Food and Drug Administration (FDA) for treatment of endometriosis. At the time of this writing the hormonal treatment of choice is danazol (Danocrine), a synthetic steroid derivative of ethisterone, studied since 1964. According to Michaels (1983), for the first month of treatment 600 mg/day is recommended. The first dose is started on the fifth day after the onset of menses. The dosage is reduced to 200 mg/day and remains at that level for as long as the woman is amenorrheic. The half-life of this oral drug is between 4 and 5 hours. Therefore it is best to take the prescribed daily amount in 4 equal doses. If menses resume, the dose is increased. According to Puleo and Hammond (1983), a majority of women note relief from pain within 6 weeks. Danazol is continued for 9 months. When it is discontinued, menstruation returns. Since ovulation may not be suppressed by danazol, a contraceptive should be used while this drug is being administered.

Danazol, a synthetic androgen, can produce masculiniz-

Table 41-2 *Classifications of Pelvic Endometriosis*

Classification	Characteristics
Mild	Scattered, fresh lesions (i.e., implants not associated with scarring or retraction of the peritoneum) in the anterior or posterior cul-de-sac or pelvic peritoneum Rare surface implant on ovary, with no endometrioma, without surface scarring and retraction, and without periovarian adhesions No peritubular adhesions
Moderate	Endometriosis involving one or both ovaries, with several surface lesions, with scarring and retraction, or small endometriomas Minimal peritubular adhesions associated with ovarian lesions described Superficial implants in anterior and/or posterior cul-de-sac with scarring and retraction; some adhesions, but no sigmoid invasion
Severe	Endometriosis involving one or both ovaries (usually both) with endometrioma $>2 \times 2$ cm One or both ovaries bound down by adhesions associated with endometriosis, with or without tubal adhesions to ovaries One or both tubes bound down or obstructed by endometriosis; associated adhesions or lesions Obliteration of the cul-de-sac from adhesions or lesions associated with endometriosis Thickening of the uterosacral ligaments and cul-de-sac lesions from invasive endometriosis with obliteration of the cul-de-sac Significant bowel or urinary tract involvement

From Acosta, IA, et al: Obstet Gynecol 42:19, 1973. Reprinted with permission from The American College of Obstetricians and Gynecologists.

ing traits, which often disappear when treatment is discontinued. Its side effects include weight gain, edema, decreased breast size, oily skin, hirsutism, deepening of the voice, decreased libido, vasomotor symptoms such as hot flushes, atrophic vaginitis, emotional lability, and seborrhea. Migraine headaches, dizziness, fatigue, and depression are also reported. Some women discontinue the drug because of these side effects.

Danazol is contraindicated in women with liver disease, and it should be used with care in women with cardiac and renal disease. Because it is an expensive drug, danazol may be out of the question for women without insurance or other financial resources. It should never be given when pregnancy is suspected, since the hormone may cause pseudohermaphroditism in female fetuses, giving rise to ambiguous genitals (Fig. 40-18).

It is important to note that endometriosis is not cured by hormonal treatments. When treatment is discontinued, pain returns within 3 to 9 months for 38% of women.

For women whose goal is to have children, another "treatment" for endometriosis is pregnancy. Both pregnancy and lactation are excellent prophylactic means in the presence of endometriosis because they suppress menstruation. During pregnancy and lactation the ectopic endometrium eventually shrinks. Many women find relief from pain for many years after pregnancy.

For those women who suffer from both severe pain and infertility as a result of endometriosis, surgery is another option. However, according to Wheeler and Malinak (1983), endometriosis recurred within 5 years in 40% of women who had undergone conservative surgery. Although endometriosis will recur in some women after surgery, conservative surgery does reduce the rate of spontaneous abortions in women who are attempting to bear children. Wheeler and associates (1983) found that the rate of miscarriage was higher in women with mild endometriosis and that surgical removal of the ectopic endometrial tissue produced a statistical decline in the spontaneous abortion rate.

None of the treatments described thus far can cure endometriosis. Neither conservative surgery nor hormonal medications can eliminate endometriosis and its symptoms, although they may relieve pain and infertility for a time. The only known cure for endometriosis is surgical removal of the uterus, uterine tubes, and ovaries.

If her symptoms are not too severe, a woman may want to wait until the climacterium for them to disappear. During the climacterium endometrial tissue atrophies and endometriosis ceases to be a problem. However, women who have had endometriosis and who chose to use HRT for complaints associated with menopause need to be aware that endometriosis can be reactivated for the length of time they undergo this therapy (p. 1039).

Assessment

A thorough history gives direction to the physical examination and to the specific diagnostic tests and procedures needed to establish a diagnosis (Chapter 8). For example, some women who take diazepam (Valium) develop menstrual irregularities or fail to ovulate. A menstrual history without consideration of life-style influences and patterns of coping can lead to a misdiagnosis. History based on recall alone may leave many questions unanswered. A useful diagnostic tool is a symptom diary. Emotional and behavioral descriptions are noted along with physical symptoms. Weight, diet, exercise, and rest patterns add valuable data. The woman's sexual, contraceptive, and obstetric history are important components of assessment. Previous pregnancy, method of delivery, elective abortions, use of an intrauterine device (IUD), and history of pelvic inflammatory disease (PID) must be considered. A history negative for each of these factors is meaningful.

Most people experiment with various home remedies and activities to relieve discomfort. The measures tried and the results achieved are noted. The woman's perceptions of her condition, cultural or ethnic influences, and experiences with other caregivers are elicited.

Nursing Diagnoses

Following are examples of nursing diagnoses that may emerge from assessment data from women experiencing disorders associated with menstruation:

- Potential for ineffective individual or family coping related to
  - Insufficient knowledge of the cause of the disorder
  - Emotional and physiologic effects of the disorder
  - Lack of knowledge regarding self-care and available therapy for the disorder
- Potential body image disturbance related to
  - Menstrual disorder
- Pain related to
  - Dysmenorrhea

Planning

After the data are collected and reviewed, the clinician meets with the women (or couple), mutual goals are established, and a plan of care is developed.

Goals

1. The woman (couple) understands and accepts her emotional and physical responses to her menstrual cycle or disorder.
2. The woman (couple) develops personal goals that benefit her (them) emotionally and physiologically.
3. The woman (couple) is able to choose appropriate therapeutic measures that meet her (their) goals.
4. Therapeutic or corrective measures are successful or woman (couple) effectively adapts to condition if cure is not possible.

Implementation

Actual therapy begins with the woman's first encounter with the clinician. The clinician's concern and recognition and acceptance of the woman's symptoms as valid are in themselves therapeutic. The woman (couple) is involved in the investigation of her problem during the history taking and examinations; she begins to see that she is not alone in this experience. Data developed through the use of a daily log of emotional status, subjective feelings, and physical state are correlated with objective evidence of physiologic changes (Table 6-1). The woman and her partner keep separate logs, which could also include how each perceives the other's responses day by day. The log serves as a tool through which feelings are ventilated, problems are identified and clarified, insights occur, and possible solutions begin to develop.

Often the man and the woman are surprised to note that *both* have cycles that must be considered in their relationship to themselves and to each other. When all data are collected, the clinician facilitates insights into causal relationships and suggests as many therapeutic alternatives as possible, and the woman (couple) makes choices that best achieve her (their) personal goals. See the research highlight below and nursing care plan for the woman with premenstrual syndrome, p. 1033.

Nurses are regarded by women as having information and support to share, and therefore nurses need to be prepared to discuss the options available for women with endometriosis. As teachers and counselors, nurses need to understand basic information about the sites, symptoms, and treatment of endometriosis. As caregivers in the operating room and recovery room, nurses need to be familiar with the procedures used for laparoscopy and laparotomy, as well as those for hysterectomy and salpingo-oophorectomy. A nursing care plan for endometriosis is on p. 1034.

RESEARCH HIGHLIGHT

The Effect of a Support Group on Self-esteem of Women with Premenstrual Syndrome

Purpose

To determine the effect of a support group on self-esteem of women with PMS.

Sample/Methodology

A small convenient sample of five women with diagnosed PMS who attended a support group was compared with a control group of six women with PMS who did not attend a group. The groups were compared for levels of self-esteem at 1 and 8 weeks using the Coopersmith self-esteem inventory.

Findings

There was no significant statistical difference in self-esteem from 1 to 8 weeks. However, the women who attended the support group had higher self-esteem mean (average) scores at 8 weeks after beginning the support group.

A total of 26 symptoms were reported by the sample. The women experienced an average of 10 symptoms each. The greatest number of symptoms (73%) were reported as emotional symptoms of anger or depression. Physical symptoms of headache and fatigue were reported by 27% of the sample.

Implications

In light of the small sample one cannot generalize the findings from this study. It was suggested that PMS support groups may affect women's level of self-esteem; therefore it would be advisable to replicate the study.

Walton J, and Youngkin, E: The effect of a support group on self-esteem of women with premenstrual syndrome, JOGN Nurs 16(3): 174, 1987

Specific Nursing Care Plan

PREMENSTRUAL SYNDROME (PMS)

Michele B, a 24-year-old nursing student identified herself as having premenstrual syndrome (PMS) by filling out a questionnaire given to her by the gynecology clinic director where she was doing her clinical experience. She recognized some of the symptoms as the ones she exhibits approximately 10 days before her menstruation begins. Some of those symptoms include: weight gain, bloating, depression, moodiness, breast tenderness, and a craving for sweets. The nurse in the clinic gave Michele the phone number of a PMS clinic where she could obtain help.

ASSESSMENT	NURSING DIAGNOSIS (ND)/ PLAN (P)/GOAL (G)	RATIONALE IMPLEMENTATION	EVALUATION
Single woman exhibiting physiologic and psychologic symptoms of PMS: Temporary water weight gain.	ND: Fluid volume excess related to hormonal influence and fluid retention 10 days before premenstruation. P: Minimize or prevent water weight gain. G: Michele relates a decrease in weight gain caused by water retention.	*To prevent or minimize premenstrual water weight gain Michele will:* Reduce or eliminate salty foods and added salt at the table. Consider pharmaceutical preparations (p. 1028) or natural diuretic foods.	Michele will show a reduction in water weight gain and edema premenstrually.
Breast tenderness.	ND: Pain, discomfort in breasts, related to influence of hormones and chemicals in diet. P: Minimize or prevent breast tenderness. G: Michele will relate increased breast comfort.	*To prevent or minimize breast tenderness Michele will:* Decrease caffeine intake in diet. Maintain a balanced diet rich in vitamins and minerals. Wear a comfortable supportive bra.	Michele verbalizes a decrease in breast tenderness.
Depression. Moodiness.	ND: Situational low self-esteem related to hormonal changes before menstrual period. P: Minimize or prevent depression and mood swings. G: Michele will relate less emotional distress.	*To decrease or prevent depression and mood swings Michele will:* Monitor vitamin intake. Avoid alcohol and cigarettes. Get plenty of exercise to decrease stress. Talk about feelings with someone close. Join a support group.	Michele verbalizes an understanding of information presented and experiences less depression. Michelle states she feels better about herself since she has become active in a support group.
Craving for sweets.	ND: Altered nutrition: potential for more than body requirements related to hormone-related change in carbohydrate metabolism. P: Use alternative activities and foods to reduce intake of foods high in simple sugars (glucose). G: Michele relates decreased need for and decreased intake of foods high in simple sugars (glucose).	*To minimize wide fluctuation in blood sugar levels, Michele will:* Reduce intake of simple sugars, candy, pastries, table sugar. Eat small, frequent meals and snacks of good nutritious value: i.e., fruit, cheese, etc; maintain a balanced diet. Monitor vitamin intake. Engage in enjoyable activities: social events, jogging or other sports.	Michele reduces intake of simple sugars, replacing sugar and salty snacks with more fruit and protein foods.

General Nursing Care Plan

ENDOMETRIOSIS

ASSESSMENT	NURSING DIAGNOSIS (ND)/ PLAN (P)/GOAL (G)	RATIONALE/ IMPLEMENTATION	EVALUATION
Dysmenorrhea with pelvic and abdominal pain which may radiate down thighs or be accompanied by sensation of pelvic fullness. Dysmenorrhea worsens with time.	ND: Pain related to endometriosis. ND: Knowledge deficit related to condition. ND: Body image disturbance, self-esteem disturbance related to symptomatology or diagnosis. P: Assist with diagnosis, meet knowledge needs, and provide opportunity to discuss feelings. G: Pain relieved or minimized; self-esteem is maintained; knowledge needs are met.	*To assist with knowledge needs, self-concept, and pain relief the nurse will:* Assess location, type, and duration of pain; history of discomfort. Provide pain medications as ordered: teach about use and side effects. Teach comfort measures: Heating pad to abdomen. Warm bath. Provide time to discuss feelings. Refer to support group.	Pain is localized and minimized. Woman uses medication correctly. Woman employs comfort measures at home.
Anxiety.	ND: Anxiety, mild to moderate, related to diagnosis. P: Decrease anxiety. G: Woman reports decreased anxiety.	*To decrease anxiety the nurse will:* Discuss feelings and concerns about diagnosis. Provide realistic hope. Be supportive. Provide complete, clear explanation of disease. Provide information about treatment plans. Assist as necessary with decisions about treatment.	Woman's anxiety is decreased through understanding. Woman verbalizes understanding of information presented.
Tiredness or weakness. Anemia.	ND: Activity intolerance related to anemia of hypermenorrhea. P: Relieve anemia and prevent recurrence. G: Blood studies show recovery from anemia; woman performs ADL without becoming overtired.	*To decrease tiredness and weakness secondary to anemia the nurse will:* Teach about and encourage diet high in iron and vitamin C. Provide information on iron supplements, if ordered (see guidelines for client teaching, Chapter 15). Discuss rest periods if possible. Encourage 8 hours of sleep per night.	Woman changes diet to include foods high in iron. Woman takes iron supplements as ordered.
Dyspareunia.	ND: Sexual dysfunction related to endometrial implants in cul-de-sac of Douglas. P: Meet knowledge needs, provide opportunity for discussion, and maintain or improve self-concept.	*To assist woman to cope with dyspareunia the nurse will:* Assess when pain occurs (during or after intercourse, with deep penetration). Discuss taking pain medication before sexual activity begins.	Woman has painless sexual intercourse.

General Nursing Care Plan—cont'd

ASSESSMENT	NURSING DIAGNOSIS (ND)/ PLAN (P)/GOAL (G)	RATIONALE/ IMPLEMENTATION	EVALUATION
	G: Painless sexual intercourse.	Suggest alternative positions where the woman has greater control over pressure exerted (woman superior, side lying). Counsel both partners together about need for clear communication before and during sexual intercourse to minimize discomfort and increase pleasure for both.	
Impaired fertility—unknown cause (see also Chapter 42).	ND: Knowledge deficit related to causes of impaired fertility. P: Meet knowledge needs. G: Pregnancy or unimpaired fertility.	*To help woman (couple) cope with impaired fertility the nurse will:* Discuss feelings about having children. Explain realistic potential of pregnancy with various treatments. Be supportive.	Woman (couple) verbalizes understanding of information.
Treatment therapies. Medications.	ND: Knowledge deficit related to treatment of endometriosis. P: Meet knowledge needs. G: Woman understands and takes medications appropriately.	*To explain treatment therapies; the nurse will:* Teach about medication used. Discuss reasons for using this drug. Explain which side effects to observe for and what to do if they occur. Make sure woman has accurate prescription and the right drug. Explain dosage schedule and importance of accuracy in taking.	Women understands about medication and takes the right dose on time.
Surgery (see also Chapter 34).	G: Accurate understanding of treatment regimens.	*To allay fears of surgery, the nurse will:* Teach about laparoscopy. Discuss minor vaginal bleeding afterward. Discuss belching or feeling bloated afterward because intraabdominal carbon monoxide. Teach preoperatively as with other surgery.	Woman comes through surgery with minimal or no problems.

An important resource for both nurses and women with endometriosis is the Endometriosis Association. First organized in Milwaukee in 1980, this association has developed a library of information on endometriosis, a data bank compiled from answers to a standardized questionnaire submitted by women with the disease, and a list of support groups around the United States.*

Another important resource for women with endometriosis is support groups organized by nurses. Nurses can use a local women's center or clinic to bring together women who want to learn more about endometriosis and give each other support as they try to cope with this enigmatic disease.

Evaluation

Menstruation-associated disorders can disrupt the quality of life for the affected woman and her family. Care of these disorders can be evaluated as having been successful when the woman reports an elimination of the problem or an acceptable improvement in the quality of her life. The nurse can be assured that care has been effective when the woman demonstrates skill in self-care and an improvement in self-concept and body image.

NORMAL CLIMACTERIUM AND POSTCLIMACTERIUM

As a result of medical breakthroughs in this century, most women can expect to live into their ninth decade. Consequently they will experience several stages of growth and development through which most women from previous centuries never had the opportunity to pass. These stages of growth and development are most likely uncharted territory for many women and can be a source of anxiety. Maturational changes often bring satisfaction, but the physical and social changes that accompany aging may encourage some women to seek support and information from nurses. One stage of development—the climacterium—can be a particular source of anxiety. Nurses can be effective in handling this anxiety if they are informed and supportive.

Climacterium derives from a Greek word meaning "rung of the ladder." It refers to the stage in women's lives when fertility is decreasing and the menstrual cycle becomes irregular and eventually stops. It also includes the period after ovulation ceases when symptoms associated with changing hormone levels appear. According to Van Keep (1983), the climacterium is that developmental phase during which a woman passes from the reproductive to the nonreproductive stage with regression of ovarian function.

Premenopause is the first phase of the climacterium. During this phase, women notice irregular menstruation or symptoms associated with menopause. Irregular cycles may last a few months or a few years. Complaints associated with menopause that may appear at this phase include vasomotor instability, fatigue, headaches, and emotional disturbances.

Menopause is the point at which menstruation ceases. Many people use the word to mean a stage, similar to the climacterium, but this usage is erroneous. The average age for menopause is 50. However, 10% of women stop menstruation by age of 40 and 5% do not stop until 60. Menopause is also a Greek word, meaning "month of cessation." Age at menopause is genetically predetermined and is not related to the number of ovulations, race, socioeconomic conditions, education, height, weight, age at menarche, or age at last pregnancy. The mean age of menopause is about 51 years (Droegemueller et al., 1987). Surgical menopause occurs with hysterectomy and bilateral oophorectomy.

Perimenopause includes the premenopause, the menopause, and at least a year after menopause. It is roughly the same time period as the climacterium.

Postmenopause is the phase that follows the menopause. During the postmenopause, women can develop symptoms associated with decreased gonadal hormones, such as vaginal atrophy and osteoporosis.

"Change of life" is a vernacular term referring to the climacterium.

Symptomatology: Climacterium

The following sections discuss symptoms associated with the climacterium. Not all women experience these symptoms, and some women (approximately 20% according to some researchers) never experience any symptoms. For the majority of women, symptoms are considered mild or moderate and rarely require medical attention. However, a small percentage of women have severe symptoms that require medical and nursing intervention. The next sections discuss the most commonly associated symptoms, the phases in which they appear, the frequency with which they appear, and their causes.

Vasomotor Instability. Vasomotor instability is the most common disturbance of the climacterium. The term means changeable vasodilation and vasoconstriction. During the perimenopause women experience vasomotor instability as *hot flushes* (flashes) and night sweats. A hot flush is a sudden explosive systemic physiologic phenomenon that takes place over a period of 30 seconds to 5 minutes. The flush is preceded by an increase in digital perfusion, which is followed by increases in peripheral skin temperature, circulating norepinephrine and LH levels, and heart rate. With each flush there are increases in LH, adrenocorticotropic hormone (ACTH), and cortisol but not FSH or estradiol. The LH increase is an effect of the change in the hypothalamic-pituitary axis and not a cause of the hot flush, because women without a pituitary gland also have hot flushes (Droegemueller et al., 1987).

Women with vasomotor instability experience the hot flush differently. The starting location of the flush varies. Most commonly it starts in the neck, head, scalp, or ears. Women report that it also starts below the breasts or "all over." A feeling of heat spreads up or down or all over the body. The intensity of the heat varies also. Women describe the hot flushes as either mild, moderate, or severe. *Mild* hot flushes do not interfere with daily activities. Women report that the sensation of heat is brief and bearable and that they barely notice elevated temperature. *Moderate* hot

*For more information, write to the Endometriosis Association, PO Box 92817, Milwaukee, Wis 53202.

flushes are less bearable, and women report being uncomfortable with noticeable elevated temperature. Perspiration may also be produced in a few areas of the body. Women feel as if they have a fever. *Severe* hot flushes produce an intense feeling of heat and make women feel extremely uncomfortable. These women at times feel as if they are suffocating and seek relief by opening windows, removing outer layers of clothing, and fanning themselves. Severe hot flushes make it difficult for women to continue activities of daily living without interruption. Vasoconstriction may immediately follow, so that some women experience cold chills after the hot flush. Usually the blood pressure remains the same throughout the episode.

Hot flushes can occur often throughout the day, and may continue for several months or years. Women report that several factors can stimulate an episode. These factors include eating spicy foods, entering a crowded or stuffy room, drinking hot tea, coffee, or soup, and being in close proximity to a source of heat. Being under stress may also initiate hot flushes.

Night sweats are another form of vasomotor instability associated with menopause. These are experienced by many women during the perimenopause as profuse perspiration as well as heat radiating from the body during the night. Sleep is interrupted, as night clothes and bed linens may be soaked and in need of changing. These episodes may occur nightly and many women complain of not being able to go back to sleep. One member of a menopause study described her experience (Miller, 1984):

> I had hot flushing several times a day with profuse sweating. I also had disturbance of sleep . . . waking several times a night with a chemical "rush" of some kind followed by an intense sensation of hot flushing all over. I needed to throw off the covers. Then I would get chilled by perspiration.

Women's complaints of interrupted sleep have led some to link vasomotor instability to insomnia, another frequent complaint women report during perimenopause. Some studies have found that many of women's waking episodes during sleep may be associated with nocturnal hyperthermia, or night sweats.

Other vasomotor symptoms associated by women with the perimenopause include dizziness, numbness and tingling in fingers and toes, and possibly headaches. All of these symptoms may be caused by fluctuations of vasoconstriction or vascular spasms. Headaches will be discussed further in a separate section. There is little research to substantiate that headaches are a result of vasomotor instability; much more research needs to be done.

Several other disturbances are associated with perimenopause. Their cause and relationship to changing levels of gonadal and pituitary hormones is unclear. However, because these disturbances generate much concern, annoyance, and at times, disability for women during the climacterium they will be discussed in the hope that nurses and other health professionals will not ignore them.

Emotional Disturbances. Mood swings, irritability, anxiety, and depression are among the emotional disturbances women associate with perimenopause. Women state that they feel more emotionally labile, more nervous, or more agitated. They complain that they feel out of control of their emotions. A few women become severely depressed. (Miller, 1984):

> I became very moody. I was very loving one minute, then the next minute, I would turn into a bitch. I got really mad for small reasons, up to the point where I might throw things or not talk to anyone for a whole day. For instance, seeing one dirty dish on the kitchen sink would cause me to yell at my two teenage children and my husband. Fortunately, he understood what I was going through; my moodiness was definitely caused by menopause.

Three factors may influence this change in women's affect during the climacterium: physiologic and biochemical changes, midlife stress, and cultural messages.

Physiologic and Biochemical Changes. It is known that rapidly changing hormones may effect postpartum mood swings and precipitate postpartum depression. Researchers have tried to find a similar link between mood swings during the climacterium and shifting hormones. Women often associate the mood swings and irritability of the climacterium with the feelings they experienced during and immediately after pregnancy. According to Miller (1984), Mrs. S mentioned that she had been depressed and irritable around menopause but that she had been at other times in her life also. "I was usually sensitive with all my pregnancies—12 of them!" Other women stated that the lability they felt was similar to postpartum depression, which they had also experienced. Mrs. T said she felt out of control and for no reason that she could understand, other than "unbalanced hormones." Mrs L who underwent menopause at age 54, said:

> The most obvious symptoms to me was the change in my emotions. I became very moody. One minute I would feel great, and the next I was depressed and crying. My moodiness reminded me of when I was pregnant. I remember my emotions were quite unstable then. Either feeling great or awful—no in-between. I believe my emotions were caused by menopause. I wasn't going through any traumatic times, that I can think of, that would have caused the changes. I was pretty happy with my life. I know there's a lot of hormonal changes that go on during menopause, just as there are in pregnancy, so I think that was the cause.

What women believe has been substantiated by only a handful of researchers. Greenblatt and colleagues (1979) agree that disturbances of mood are a consequence of decreasing hormones and recommend estrogen replacement therapy (ERT) to prevent or relieve depression. Schneider (1977) related decreasing endogenous estrogen to depression and found that giving ERT relieved mild to moderate depression. However, ERT did not reverse severe depression, which suggests that there are other causes for emotional disturbances during the climacterium. Like other researchers, Anderson (1987) reported that the large number of emotional symptoms experienced strongly suggest a significant impact of physical complaints on the psyche. As yet, no one has determined what the biochemical process is that underlies the variation in emotional responses.

Midlife Stress. Stress is a factor in all stages of growth and development, but the stresses that occur during middle adulthood may aggravate or overwhelm a woman trying to cope with menopause. Women in their 40s and 50s have many changes with which to cope. These changes include dealing with teenage children, having teenagers leave home, helping aging parents, become widowed or divorced, and grieving for friends and family who are ill or dying. Also, the spouse may be having difficulty with his own midlife crisis. All of these stresses may increase the woman's risk of having somatic as well as affective disorders (Miller, 1984):

> I was newly divorced and under a great deal of pressure to find a job and make a home for myself and my child. I was terribly depressed and angry and got headaches, nausea, hot flashes, and leg pains.

The ability to cope with the stress that accompanies change involves three factors: understanding of the events that are taking place (perceptions), support systems, and coping mechanisms. The presence or absence of any of these factors affects the success with which a woman copes with stress. For a woman who seeks help for climacterium complaints that seem to be the result of stress, the nurse first assesses how much more information about the climacterium should be provided. Second, the nurse encourages the woman to discuss the stressful experiences she is having so that her perception of the situation becomes more realistic and her coping skills are reintroduced.

Cultural Messages. For many women menopause is a symbol of loss, for example, the loss of the ability to bear children. For women who have accepted childbearing and childrearing as their major role or profession, menopause symbolizes an ending, a termination. Other women see menopause as the first step to old age and associate with it the loss of attractiveness, of physical ability, and of energy. Unlike some other cultures, Western culture values youth and relegates the elderly to positions without status. For women whose identity is based on nurturing children and caring for a family or on sexual attractiveness, menopause is not a welcome sign. In cultures were postmenopausal women gain status, such as India, the Far East, and the South Pacific Islands, depression among menopausal women is not observed. However, in Western culture, no rituals give older women a special place and function. The wisdom gained from life experience is not valued as much as are youth and physical attractiveness. Women do not become a part of men's rituals after menopause, as they do in Bali or Rajput, India. Many women have little to compensate for the losses they accumulate: loss of youth, loss of attractiveness, loss of strength and vigor, and loss of function and role.

For women who perceive menopause as a time of loss, depression is inevitable and a natural phase of the grieving process. In fact, depression may be the normal reaction, given the youth-oriented culture, and a necessary stage in the process of readjustment. Because this depression is simply a phase in the period of readjustment rather than a disease, no cure is possible.

For many women menopause is not a loss or a symbol of losses, but a relief instead. Anderson et al., (1987) reported that it was rare for a woman, employed or unemployed, to express sadness or regret that her children had left home. Menopause is a relief from fear of pregnancy, the hassle of menstruation, and the inconveniences of contraception. Women who see the positive side of menopause realize that as they grow older, they gain more than they lose (Miller, 1984):

> I didn't experience any of the symptoms of the menopause. Maybe I didn't notice it. I only felt a sense of relief.

Fatigue. Fatigue is another disturbance mentioned commonly by women during the perimenopause, and many indicate that it can be a problem. Fatigue is described as "feeling tired" or "feeling weak" most of the time for 1 to 2 years, until a few months after menopause. After menstruation ceases, the fatigue disappears and energy to cope with daily stresses returns. Mrs. L (Miller, 1984) stated:

> I was in very good health before menopause. I got up around 5 AM and went to bed around 11 PM. I worked very hard and was busy all the time, but that never tired me. During the period of menopause, between 1975 and 1976, I got tired easily. I knew that this was caused by menopause.

The cause of fatigue is unknown. Whether it is related to hormonal changes is speculative, but a significant number of women relate fatigue to the perimenopause.

Headaches. Headaches are a problem for a small number of women during the perimenopause. Many women suffer from headaches, especially during the premenstrual phase, but often they state that these become worse during the climacterium. Headaches associated with menopause do not return during the postmenopause. Mrs. T's statement is typical of this group of women (Miller, 1984):

> I also had headaches that lasted an entire day at the beginning and an hour or two about a month later. These headaches came a short time after my menopause started. I was really stumped because I had never had a headache in my life.

Symptomatology: Postclimacteric Period

Several symptoms associated with menopause manifest themselves in the postmenopausal phase (the postclimacterium), when women are in their late 50s, 60s and 70s. These symptoms are related to genital atrophy and osteoporosis.

Genital Atrophy. *Genital atrophy* (atrophic vaginitis) means shrinking of the reproductive organs. After menopause, when the reproductive organs are no longer being stimulated by large quantities of estrogen, they grow smaller. At times, the shrinking of the uterus, vagina, vulva, and distal portion of the urethra leads to several disturbances. The symptoms include itching, dyspareunia, urinary frequency, dysuria, uterine prolapse, stress incontinence, and constipation. Not all women experience these symptoms, but they are irritating to those who do.

Itching around the vulva may be a postmenopausal complaint. As estrogen decreases, vulvar tissue becomes thinner, less elastic and more prone to irritation and inflammation. Women complain of an intense, constant itch that they can make worse by scratching.

Dyspareunia, or painful intercourse, can occur as the vagina becomes smaller, the vaginal walls become thinner and dryer, and lubrication during sexual stimulation takes longer. Intercourse may become irritating or painful. Postcoital bleeding also may indicate vaginal atrophy. Often women at this time decide to forego intercourse altogether: however, this is not necessary, as will be discussed later.

Urinary frequency occurs sometimes after menopause because the distal portion of the urethra, which has the same embryologic origin as the reproductive organs, shortens and shrinks. Irritants have easier access to the urinary tract with its shorter urethra; the irritants may cause urinary frequency. At times, irritation will lead to cystitis and necessitate medical treatment. Although urinary frequency and dysuria (painful or difficult urination) are often symptoms of bladder infection, urine cultures for postmenopausal women often reveal the absence of any pathogens. In the event that urinary frequency and dysuria persist, urine cultures are a sensible means of determining whether nonhormonal treatment is indicated.

Urinary incontinence and *uterine displacement* are other common findings during this period. Urinary incontinence is discussed on page 1051, and uterine displacement on page 1052. *Constipation* or pain during bowel movements may indicate that a rectocele has occurred (p. 1048).

Not all women experience symptoms of genital atrophy. Endogenous estrogen has been found to provide stimulation a decade after menopause. Women often do not associate urinary tract infections during the postmenopause with changes during the climacterium. However, hormone replacement therapy (below, and p. 1046) often brings relief.

Osteoporosis. Osteoporosis means increased porosity of the bone. The major cause of this pathologic condition is withdrawal of estrogen as a result of regression of the ovaries. Approximately 25% of women, most of whom are fair, small boned, and thin, will be plagued by this condition after menopause. Women at risk also include those with another family member who had the disease. Black women are not at risk for osteoporosis; the reason for this is not known.

Usually the first sign of osteoporosis is loss of height (Fig. 41-2). Women who notice that they have lost an inch or more may be having vertebral column collapse. Another early symptom is back pain, especially in the lower back. Later signs of osteoporosis include dowager's hump, in which the vertebrae can no longer support the upper body in an upright position, and fractured hip, in which the fracture often precedes the fall. Loss of bone mass progresses at a rate of 1% to 1.5% per year after menopause in nonobese white and Oriental women (Droegemueller, et al., 1987). This rate of loss per year diminishes after approximately 10 years.

Unfortunately, osteoporosis cannot be detected by x-ray studies until 50% of the bone mass has already been lost. However, blood tests for serum levels of calcium, phosphate, alkaline phosphatase, and protein can provide conclusive answers regarding the presence of the osteoporotic process. Women who have access to hospitals with computerized axial tomography (CAT scan) have an advantage in that the CAT scan can more accurately identify osteoporosis at an earlier phase than x-rays.

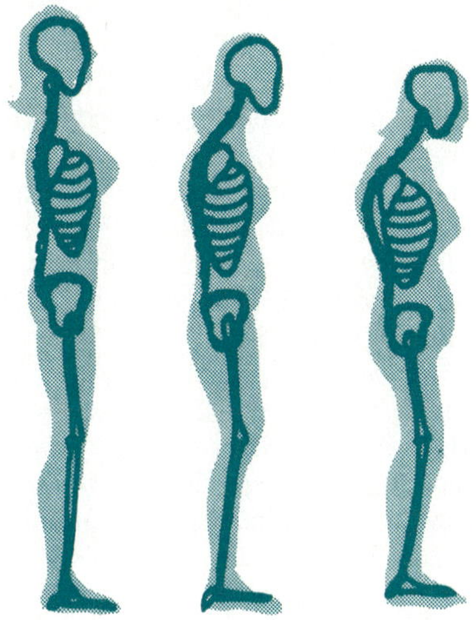

Fig. 41-2 Skeletal changes secondary to osteoporosis assessed by height and body shape at **A**, age 55; **B**, age 65; and **C**, age 75.

Because the cause of osteoporosis is complex, only a simplified description will be presented here. Estrogen performs two functions that ensure healthy bone. First, estrogen is vital in the changing of vitamin D into a powerful and necessary chemical (calcitonin) that enables absorption of calcium by the intestine. After menopause, vitamin D is at low levels in the intestine, leading to less absorption of dietary calcium from the gut. Most of the serum calcium is then derived from bone.

A second function of estrogen is that it stimulates the osteoblasts, the cells that form bone. Bone formation decreases as a consequence of decreasing levels of estrogen. Old bone deteriorates faster than new bone is formed, which leads to gradually decreasing thickness of the cortex of bones and increase of marrow. During the decades after menopause, in addition to the interruption of calcium absorption from nutritional sources, the slow thinning of the bones places many women at risk for problems associated with osteoporosis.

Therapy

Hormonal Treatment. Estrogen increases calcitonin levels and calcitonin prevents bone resorption and maintains bone density. To prevent osteoporosis, estrogen replacement must be maintained as long as the woman is ambulatory (Droegemueller et al., 1987). Several retrospective epidemiologic studies have shown that estrogens reduce the incidence of fractures (Kiel et al., 1987). Weiss et al. (1980) and Paganini-Hill et al. (1981) reported that a reduction in fractures occurred mainly in women who had taken estrogen for more than 5 years. The minimum dose of estrogen needed to prevent osteoporosis is 0.625 mg of conjugated equine estrogens. Bone density studies with other estrogen formulations have not been published. In addition to estrogen replacement, calcium supplementation and weight-bearing exercise are of ancillary benefit in preventing postmenopausal osteoporosis. Women with osteoporosis treated with various regimens with and without vitamin D had no difference in incidence of osteoporotic fractures.

In summary, estrogen increases calcium absorption and reduces the rate of bone resorption. It will not stimulate new bone growth but will stabilize osteoporosis if it is present. It will prevent osteoporosis if therapy is started at the time of menopause. It cannot reverse bone thinning that has already occurred. For women at risk to develop osteoporosis, specifically nonobese white or Oriental women, estrogen replacement therapy is the keystone to the three-pronged approach of *estrogen, calcium supplementation,* and possibly *weight-bearing exercise* as a method to prevent the debilitating and painful disease.

On the basis of initial studies, it seems unwise to make confident recommendations for the prophylactic use of exercise for the express purpose of preventing osteoporosis. The types of exercise programs that will have the greatest benefit to the skeleton have not been established. More vigorously designed prospective studies to determine the specific role of exercise in building and maintaining bone mass must be undertaken. However, exercise may have an impact on reducing the incidence of fractures aside from its effect, if any, on bone mass. Exercise reduces the likelihood of falls from the elderly and improves one's ability to cope with injuries consequent to falls. Research in this area is needed. Until results of studies are available, it is prudent to refrain from indiscriminately counseling individuals to undertake programs of exercise with the hope of preventing osteoporosis (Block et al., 1987).

Effects of Hormone Replacement

Metabolism. With any drug there is a benefit-risk ratio, but the risks of estrogen replacement therapy are minimal (Droegemueller et al., 1987). Metabolic changes are related to the dosage and type of estrogen ingested. The type of estrogen used for postmenopausal hormone replacement therapy is much less potent than ethinyl estradiol used in oral hormone contraceptives. For prevention of osteoporosis, bone density studies have shown that at least the equivalent of 0.625 mg of conjugated equine estrogen needs to be taken. Women with hot flushes sometimes need to receive a higher dose, the equivalent of 1.25 mg of conjugated equine estrogen, or greater, for relief of these symptoms (Droegemueller et al., 1987).

Estrogen appears to have little effect on glucose metabolism. Recent studies have not shown a decrease in glucose tolerance in women treated with doses of estrogen as high as 1.25 mg of conjugated equine estrogen. Some studies have shown a statistically increased risk of gallbladder disease in postmenopausal estrogen users; other studies have not substantiated those findings (Droegemueller et al., 1987). Estrogens may, however, accelerate the formation of cholelithiasis in susceptible individuals.

Cardiovascular System. Although oral contraceptive use increases the blood pressure of some women, there is no evidence that the doses of natural oral estrogens used to treat postmenopausal women cause an increase in blood pressure (Barrett-Connor et al., 1979; Wren and Routledge, 1983). Findings from these two studies indicate that postmenopausal women with hypertension are candidates for estrogen replacement therapy. If their blood pressure increases while they are receiving this treatment, it is unlikely that the conjugated equine estrogen is the cause of the blood pressure elevation.

Ethinyl estradiol in oral contraceptives does produce a hypercoagulable state. However, natural estrogens in the doses used for hormone replacement do not increase clotting factors (Aylwood et al., 1971). There is no evidence of an increased incidence of thrombophlebitis or thromboembolism in postmenopausal women who use estrogen as compared with control subjects. Also there is no evidence that postmenopausal women with a history of thrombophlebitis have an increased incidence of thrombophlebitis when taking estrogen.

When compared with the increased risk of myocardial infarction found in women over 35 years of age who smoke and ingest high doses of oral contraceptives, the use of estrogen replacement has been demonstrated to reduce the risk of myocardial infarction. Diabetes mellitus, hypertension, and smoking increase the chance of death from ischemic heart disease (Ross et al., 1987). Estrogens decrease the chance of death from that disorder. These findings demonstrate a protective effect of estrogens against myocardial infarction, even in women who smoke. Several other studies have also demonstrated a reduction in risk of coronary heart disease in estrogen users (Ross et al., 1987). In addition, many studies have demonstrated that there is about a 50% reduction in myocardial infarction in estrogen users (Droegemueller et al., 1987).

The mechanism whereby estrogen prevents myocardial infarction has not been determined. However, the demonstrated reduction in this major cause of mortality in women is a major beneficial effect of estrogen (Ottoson, Johansson, and Von Schoultz, 1985). Bilateral oophorectomy increases the risk of coronary heart disease, but this increase appears to be prevented by estrogen replacement therapy (Colditz et al., 1987).

Neoplastic Effects. Neoplastic risks of postmenopausal estrogen replacement therapy has raised much concern. Neoplasia of the *breast* and *endometrium* are of particular concern since these are the target tissues of estrogen. The possibility exists that estrogen can stimulate a nonpalpable breast neoplasm. Carcinoma of the breast may exist in the preclinical state for as long as 8 years before it is palpable. Based on this knowledge it is advisable to obtain a mammogram to rule out subclinical breast neoplasia for all women before initiating estrogen therapy. If no tumor is found however, current evidence indicates that oral estrogen will not increase the risk of developing breast cancer (Droegemueller et al., 1987).

Endometrial cancer that develops in women who use estrogens is nearly always well differentiated and is usually cured by a simple hysterectomy (Collins et al., 1980). The risk of developing endometrial carcinoma for women taking estrogen replacement can be markedly reduced by concurrent use of progestogens. The duration of progestin therapy is more important than the dosage. Small amounts of progestin taken for more than 10 days each month have also been shown to reduce the incidence of endometrial carcinoma (Gambrell et al., 1979; and Hammond et al., 1979). There is evidence that ingestion of progestins lowers the chances of postmenopausal estrogen users' developing cancer of the endometrium. Therefore if the women has a uterus, she can reduce her risk of endometrial carcinoma by concurrent use of progestins.

Treatment Regimens. The treatment regimen commonly used in the United States is 0.625 mg of conjugated equine estrogen or estrone sulfate for the first 25 days of each month. Beginning on days 12 to 15 of estrogen use, 5 to 10 mg of medroxyprogesterone acetate (MPA) is added daily for 10 to 13 days. With this pattern, about one-half of women will experience regular *withdrawal bleeding.* Many postmenopausal women find this withdrawal bleeding an annoying problem. Other therapeutic regimens are also used. One protocol prescribes 0.625 mg of conjugated equine estrone or estrone sulfate together with 2.5 to 5 mg of MPA administered daily or every day Monday through Friday. This regimen reduces the chance of developing breakthrough bleeding. It also avoids a week-off treatment during which symptoms may appear. Preliminary data indicate that most women do not bleed with the latter protocol and their endometrium remains atrophic. Several authorities recommend that progestins not be given to women without a uterus because of the adverse effects on lipids (i.e., progestin counters the beneficial effect of lipid reduction found when estrogen alone is taken).

Intramuscular and once-a-week oral estrogen regimens are available. These methods result in higher initial blood levels of estrogen than oral estrogen methods do. To keep estrogen levels low, oral daily medication appears safer. Transdermal and subdermal estradiol administration provides a relatively constant level of estrogen. Some women prefer this method; however, some women develop skin irritation in the area of the patch or injection. Conjugated estrogens are also available in cream and suppository form. Estrogen in vaginal suppository form can relieve urinary tract problems (such as urinary frequency) when they are caused by atrophy of reproductive tissue around the bladder and urethra. This form of therapy can be used to alleviate vaginal pruritis and dyspareunia that is secondary to withdrawal of ovarian production of estrogen. If the woman has a uterus, oral progestins are usually ordered. A routine pretreatment endometrial biopsy is usually unnecessary (Droegemueller et al., 1987). Routine annual endometrial biopsies are not considered to be necessary unless breakthrough bleeding occurs.

In summary, the indications for estrogen replacement therapy in the postmenopausal woman include the presence of vasomotor symptoms, as well as prevention or reversal of atrophic vaginitis, atrophic urethritis, and osteoporosis. Estrogen appears to retard the onset of myocardial infarction. Should these data be confirmed further, estrogen replacement therapy may be considered for nearly all postmenopausal women. Contraindications to estrogen replacement are uncommon. Physical findings that would contraindicate replacement therapy include a history of breast cancer, recent history of endometrial cancer, active liver disease, or thrombophlebitis.

Sexuality

There is no truth to the rumor that sex ends at menopause. Enjoyment of sexual expression can continue through the final stage of human growth. However, several factors may influence whether women and their partners change their expression of sexuality during and after menopause. These factors are physical changes, physiologic changes, changes in the partner, and cultural messages.

Physical appearance changes as the body ages. There is no way to prevent the inevitable aging process that hair, skin, eyes, and other parts of the body undergo. For some people, these changes represent losses that may influence whether they continue to take pleasure in expression of their sexuality. For those who see aging as a loss, sexuality may become difficult to incorporate into what they perceive to be a less attractive identity.

Physiologic changes that are influenced by ovarian atrophy and reduced endogenous gonadal hormone production occur after menopause. These changes are apparent in the reduced size of the vagina and clitoris. According to Masters and Johnson (1966), after menopause, the vagina is less expansive, the vaginal walls are thinner, and the length and width are decreased. During intercourse, vaginal lubrication is decreased in quantity and takes longer to develop. As a result, women may complain that it takes much longer to reach orgasm, or that intercourse is painful. Intercourse may become too bothersome, and as a result women may give it up entirely.

However, it has also been found that the capacity for orgasm is not decreased and the libido is not changed by shifts in hormones. Women who have intercourse at least twice a week do not seem to lose vaginal lubrication as they grow older.

A significant factor in the expression of sexuality for many women is the *partner.* Several events can interfere with this expression. First, physiologic changes occurring in the man may influence whether he continues to want sex (Anderson et al., 1987). As men age, they too take longer to reach orgasm. Erections take longer to occur and are less firm, sperm production decreases, and ejaculations become sporadic. Men may believe thay are becoming impotent or ill and give up sexual activity as too frustrating. Women may believe that their partners are losing interest in them, although this is not the case at all. Changes in the man may simply be a result of the influence of decreasing testosterone production. Couples need counseling to understand the physiologic bases for these changes.

Another event that influences sexual expression after menopause is the availability of a partner. Unfortunately the climacterium may be complicated by the loss of the partner through divorce or death. Widowed and divorced women find renewing sexual activity with another partner more difficult than men who are widowed or divorced. Primarily, sexual partners are not available for older women as they are for older men. Socially, older women have fewer opportunities to develop relationships because they are less sought as sexual partners. Of all the factors discussed, the loss of one's partner has the most devastating effect on sexual expression and the most difficult for nurses to influence and correct.

Cultural messages affect sexuality. Some women interpret the loss of reproductive ability as a sign to discontinue sexual intercourse because it has become a duty rather than a source of satisfaction. As long as some women are able to bear children, they accept intercourse as part of their responsibility as wives. Menopause frees some women from this duty and they choose to forego intercourse. For other women the freedom from pregnancy is a relief. Libido may increase without the fuss of contraceptives, fear of pregnancy, or interruption from the menstrual cycle. Libido increases because the only possible consequence of intercourse is pleasure. Sexual satisfaction increases as the pressures and inconveniences of fertility disappear. According to Seidlitz (1978):

> Menopause is not the end of female sexuality, as the myth would have it, but only the end of childbearing. Properly treated, it can be the beginning of a life of freedom to shift our concern from the needs of others to ourselves, the freedom to explore new directions, to pursue old or new interests, and to become involved in whatever relationships and activities we desire.

Assessment

A thorough health history, physical examination, and laboratory tests are essential to establish a complete data base (Chapter 8). The focus of assessment is to separate pathologic states from the normal climacterium. Personal or familial history of breast or uterine cancer, hypertension, thrombophlebitis, liver or gallbladder disease, undiagnosed uterine bleeding, or other acute or chronic disease must be considered in the plan of care. Hysterectomy and bilateral oophorectomy are noted. Recent changes in menstrual history are elicited to identify the phase of the climacterium the woman is experiencing. Signs and symptoms of the climacterium are described.

A careful history and physical examination will determine whether risk factors for development of osteoporosis are present. Factors known to increase the risk of osteoporosis are as follows (Droegemueller et al., 1987; Anderson et al., 1987):

- Race: white or Oriental
- Reduced weight for height
- Early spontaneous menopause
- Early surgical menopause
- Family history of osteoporosis
- Diet: low calcium intake, low vitamin D intake, high caffeine intake, high alcohol intake, and high protein intake
- Cigarette smoking
- Sedentary life-style

The woman's perception of this stage of life, ethnic and cultural factors, and knowledge and concerns about sexuality and available care are all documented.

Nursing Diagnoses

Following are examples of nursing diagnoses that may emerge from data submitted by a woman experiencing a normal climacterium.

- Potential for ineffective individual and family coping related to
    - Changes of the climacterium
- Potential for altered growth and development related to
    - Insufficient knowledge of climacterium
- Potential for pain related to
    - Regression of ovarian function
- Potential for injury related to
    - Osteoporosis
- Potential for sexual dysfunction related to
    - Events associated with the climacterium
- Potential for situational low self-esteem related to
    - Physical and emotional responses during the climacterium

Planning

Planning requires sensitivity to as well as knowledge of events characteristic of the climacterium. Planning should occur collaboratively with the woman and her spouse/partner and family members as necessary. Knowledge of community resources is helpful. Goals are stated in client-centered terms.

Goals

1. Symptoms of climacterium are managed to the woman's satisfaction.
2. Osteoporosis is prevented or minimized.
3. Woman and family cope effectively with events of the climacterium.
4. Woman's and family's knowledge needs are met.
5. Woman and family view the complaints of the climacterium as part of a normal phase of growth and development instead of treating it as a deficiency disease.

Implementation

Most women know little about the menopause. Some women find relief in the knowledge that many women experience similar complaints and that these symptoms have a normal physiologic basis. With this knowledge, women become informed partners in making decisions regarding therapy. Women do not adhere to medical and nursing advice that has not been adequately explained and with which they do not agree or understand. This is especially true of the climacterium, which is not life-threatening but which involves the quality of life. Women who are prescribed hormone therapy but are not given sufficient explanation and information do not follow the regimen for long (Anderson et al., 1987). Treatment of women experiencing the climacterium must be individualized for the specific woman. Menopause clinics are needed where research on the effects of various treatments can be planned, developed, and evaluated. In such a clinic, group support is possible. In addition, the involved specialties of endocrinology, radiology, psychosocial resources, exercise physiology, and nutrition can be more effectively coordinated. This type of clinic is a logical progression from family planning or fertility management clinics.

Nursing Roles

The nurse who has an understanding of the climacterium and postclimacterium can be effective in helping women and their spouses through a phase of their lives that may be confusing and depressing for them. The nurse has three major roles in working with women who are between the ages of 40 and 60. The nurse is an information-giver, a supportive listener, and an encourager of realistic coping methods.

Information-giver. Enough basic information about the perimenopause is available that no woman has to suffer from lack of information or misinformation. Old wives' tales can cause anxiety in women who are approaching premenopause, and experiencing climacteric complaints arouses fear about the normalcy of the changes occurring in their bodies. Nurses can help women in any health care setting or in the community by giving them the correct information. Nurses can help find the appropriate contraceptive, explain that sexual intercourse need not be forsaken, demonstrate why hot flushes occur, and provide details on many other aspects of menopause that will help women decide what action is needed (see nursing care plan for women experiencing the postmenopausal period, on p. 1044).

Contraception is still an issue for women through menopause. Ovulation may not cease until 12 months after the last menstrual cycle. Menopausal women can become pregnant. One of the barrier methods is recommended for women whose partners have not had a vasectomy. Neither birth control pills nor IUDs are recommended for women after the age of 40.

The nurse is responsible for imparting factual information and offering supportive and nonjudgmental guidance for women who indicate that factors associated with the menopause have changed the *methods and patterns of expressing their sexuality*. The nurse's attitude toward sex and the older adult is important. A negative attitude toward sex and the older client can reinforce the client's misgivings about maintaining an active sex life.

Many people do not realize that maintaining an active and satisfying sex life may require only small adjustments. For the couple who is grieving over lost youth and attractiveness, nurses can help them recognize the grieving process, support the couple through acceptance of these changes, and reassure them of the body's unchanging capacity for sexual satisfaction. For women with dyspareunia, vaginal preparations that relieve painful intercourse are available. Couples can also be reassured of the naturalness of having desire for sex into old age. Couples are referred to counselors for specific suggestions to remedy functional sexual problems.

Supportive Listener. Women often need validation that their complaints are not unusual and that they are not alone in what they are experiencing. Nurses can encourage women to discuss their fears and anxiety and to find other women with whom they can share their concerns. Developing a supportive network can ease the stress of change.

Encourager of Realistic Coping Methods. Nurses can do many things that help women cope with the climacterium. They not only can start women's groups that focus on menopause, they can also identify women who need to talk to a physician when medical intervention seems indicated and can help family members become more supportive of the woman who is having climacteric complaints. Nurses need to be familiar with local resources and direct women to classes that supply the appropriate information and support. Nurses' provision of more classes and groups for women who want to discuss menopause would also be helpful.

Midlife Support Groups

"Women feel so isolated," reported Theresa, 48 years old. "I have no older female relatives and no one to turn to. I can't go up to someone on the street who looks the right age and ask her about menopause. It really helps to have a group to share experiences with." (Rutzick, 1980)

Recently women's centers and clinics have been offering support groups and classes for women who want to discuss menopause and other midlife events. Their objectives are to provide knowledge that allays fears and anxiety related to menopause and to provide support for women who are having similar experiences and who eventually can support each other. These groups have become a popular means for helping women understand and cope with midlife changes.

Topics presented include factual information about anatomy and physiology of the climacterium, research on HRT, sexuality, and alternatives for coping with climacteric complaints. Women are eager to learn about themselves and what they consider a natural process. They bring to the group not only their unique experiences but also a highly sophisticated understanding of what they see happening to women in general. They are encouraged to recognize how much they have learned about menopause through experiencing the phenomenon themselves and noting it in other women.

Although groups and classes often start by presenting information, women soon start to provide emotional support for each other as they talk about personal concerns. Members of a group are comforted to learn that others are feeling some of the same complaints and having the same fears. Often discussing hot flushes can lessen the anxiety associated with their occurrence.

Several cities in the United States provide groups and classes for women. If no group or class is available in the community, nurses need to consider starting one. It is an effective way to relieve anxiety about menopause and provide support for those who have little or no support system.

Text continued on p. 1046.

General Nursing Care Plan

NORMAL CLIMACTERIUM

ASSESSMENT	NURSING DIAGNOSIS (ND)/ PLAN (P)/GOAL (G)	RATIONALE/ IMPLEMENTATION	EVALUATION
Vasomotor Instability Hot flashes	ND: Pain related to vasomotor disturbances. P: Minimize discomfort, and discuss self-care techniques. G: Woman reports increased comfort. ND: Knowledge deficit related to common symptomatology. P: Discuss symptomatology. G: Woman learns signs and symptoms.	*To help woman understand the climacterium and management of symptoms, the nurse will:* Assess what symptoms woman is experiencing. Discuss physiology of these symptoms. Explain any medications physician orders. Be a good listener. Discuss self-care techniques.	Woman understands these symptoms are normal. Woman uses comfort measures at home.
Night sweats Insomnia	ND: Sleep pattern disturbance related to night sweats and insomnia. P: Minimize or prevent sleep difficulties. G: Woman relates decrease in distress related to sleep pattern disturbance.		
Dizziness Tingling in extremities	ND: Sensory-perceptual alteration related to paresthesia of fingers and toes and dizziness. P: Minimize or prevent problems resulting from paresthesia and dizziness. G: Woman does not experience effects of sensory-perceptual alterations.		
Emotional disturbances Mood swings, irritability Depression Anxiety, nervousness, and agitation	ND: Ineffective individual coping related to the changes of climacterium. P: Assist woman to improve coping mechanisms. G: Woman relates increased ability to accept or cope with changes. ND: Body image disturbance related to changes in body functions. P: Provide opportunity to discuss feelings. G: Woman focuses on positive aspects of this time of her life.	*To facilitate client acceptance of her changing psyche the nurse will:* Discuss stress in the woman's life at the present. Teach relaxation techniques. Teach stress reduction. Validate woman's feelings, reassure her she is not going crazy or losing her mind. Discuss methods to help woman to cope effectively with her changing body and roles in life. Refer woman to support group.	Woman verbalizes problems and discusses possible solutions. Woman uses stress reduction and relaxation techniques.

General Nursing Care Plan—cont'd

ASSESSMENT	NURSING DIAGNOSIS (ND)/ PLAN (P)/GOAL (G)	RATIONALE/ IMPLEMENTATION	EVALUATION
	ND: Anxiety, mild, related to the stresses of midlife and changing body patterns. P: Relieve anxiety by facilitating verbalization of problems and concerns. G: Woman relates decrease in anxiety.		
Fatigue Tiredness Weakness	ND: Increased activity intolerance related to change in body functions and interrupted sleep. P: Teach relaxation techniques and stress reduction (Chapter 13). G: Woman learns and implements self-care techniques.	*To help woman relieve fatigue the nurse will:* Discuss daily activities. Assess use of time. Suggest nap in afternoon, if possible. Suggest clustering chores, and resting in between. Discuss diet. Discuss mild exercise.	Woman understands information presented and uses suggestions at home.
Genital atrophy Dyspareunia Vaginal discharge	ND: Sexual dysfunction related to physical and physiologic changes. P: Correct or compensate for physical impairments. G: Woman expresses satisfaction with sexual activity.	*To help woman in understanding and dealing with these changes the nurse will:* Discuss sexual patterns. Offer suggestions on new positions. Discuss use of a lubricating jelly (not Vaseline—water soluble).	Woman speaks openly with nurse and employs suggestions.
Urinary frequency Stress incontinence	ND: Altered patterns of urinary elimination, related to normal changes or to cystocele. P: Prevent or minimize problems. G: Woman retains normal pattern of urinary elimination.	Teach/encourage Kegel's exercises. Review physiologic and anatomic changes. Review treatment modalities.	Woman retains or regains an acceptable pattern of urinary elimination.
Urinary tract infection	ND: Potential for infection, related to changes in urinary patterns. P: Teach how to prevent infection (Chapter 8). G: Woman does not develop infection.	Review prevention of urinary tract infection (Chapter 8).	Woman does not develop infection.
Constipation or painful bowel movements	ND: Constipation, related to possible rectocele. P: Teach woman how to minimize or correct problem. G: Woman's bowel elimination pattern resumes within normal limits.	Review self-care techniques of exercise, fluids, diet, routine habits. Discuss physiologic and anatomic basis. Review physician's suggested treatment modalities.	Woman retains or regains her normal pattern of bowel elimination through self-care or surgery.

Continued.

General Nursing Care Plan—cont'd

ASSESSMENT	NURSING DIAGNOSIS (ND)/ PLAN (P)/GOAL (G)	RATIONALE/ IMPLEMENTATION	EVALUATION
Headaches	ND: Pain, related to headache. P: Identify cause, minimize or prevent pain. G: Woman experiences fewer headaches. Woman uses self-care techniques to cope with headaches.	*To help woman avoid or minimize headaches the nurse will:* Assess type and position of headache. Ascertain when headaches are the worst. Discuss use of medication as ordered by physician.	Headaches are relieved.
Osteoporosis	ND: Knowledge deficit related to causes and prevention of osteoporosis. P: Identify those at risk, teach prevention. G: Woman uses self-care techniques and takes medications as ordered.	*To inform woman about causes and prevention, the nurse will:* Explain about estrogen withdrawal. Discuss woman's risk for osteoporosis. Discuss the part calcium intake plays in preventing significant bone loss.	Woman understands information presented.
Menopause	ND: Knowledge deficit related to cessation of menstruation. P: Teach woman about the menopause. G: Woman verbalizes understanding about menopause.	*To teach woman about cessation of menstruation, the nurse will:* Discuss importance of birth control at this time. Discuss ovarian function. Discuss cessation of hormones and the effects on the body. Point out positive aspects of this time of the woman's life. Dispell old wives tales.	Woman takes on a more positive outlook. Woman does not become pregnant at this time.

Hospitalization of the Elderly

Nurses need to be aware of the impact of separation of an elderly couple on their expression of sexuality. Interrupted regular sexual activity because of prolonged hospitalization means that the couple will have difficulty renewing sexual activity when hospitalization is over. It is important that the couple is aware of this consequence of separation. Another area in which nurses can help couples maintain their usual sexual activity after they are admitted to a nursing home is encouraging placement of the couple together. There is no reason why the elderly who have enjoyed a healthy sex life should be forced to give it up when they become too old to care for other aspects of their lives.

Alternative Methods of Management

Hormone replacement therapy (HRT) may be prescribed for some women. As indicated earlier, HRT is indicated for severe vasomotor instability, genital atrophy when symptoms impede activities of daily living, and osteoporosis prevention. However there are many women who cannot or will not take HRT. Other products are available. Nurses need to be aware of them as alternatives for coping with premenopausal and postmenopausal complaints. These women may obtain relief from one of the alternatives available.

Drugs. *Bellergal* tablets have been prescribed for the last decade for hot flushes. The tablet is composed of phenobarbital, ergotamine tartrate, and belladonna. According to Sandoz, the pharmaceutical producer, symptoms are eliminated or significantly reduced because autonomic nervous system activity is reduced. However, women taking Bellergal may have side effects, especially drowsiness. Barbiturates not only produce a sedative effect, they also can be addictive, and this must be considered if women plan to take the tablet for a long time. Also, this form of therapy is contraindicated for women with peripheral vascular disease, coronary heart disease, hypertension, impaired hepatic or renal function, sepsis, glaucoma, or hypersensitivity to any of the components.

Clonidine is generally used for hypertensive clients, but at smaller doses than those used for lowering blood pressure, it has been found effective in reducing the number of hot flushes experienced.

Vitamin E. Vitamin E has been a popular alternative among women who do not take HRT but who do want relief from hot flushes and fatigue. Seaman and Seaman (1977) note that women who take vitamin E regularly reported relief from hot flushes, leg cramps and loss of energy. However, Blatt et al. (1953) found that vitamin E works for as many women as does a placebo in relieving perimenopausal complaints.

Vitamin E is found in a variety of foods, including spinach, peanuts, wheat germ, vegetable oils, and soybeans. For women who chose to supplement their diet and reduce hot flushes, 100 IU daily has been recommended by Seaman and Seaman (1977). Dosage however varies widely depending on the source of the recommendation. Nachtigall (1977) recommends that 1 to 2 teaspoons of wheat germ oil every day provides an adequate amount of vitamin E without danger of overdosage. Between 50 and 400 IU can be taken daily, during meals, when fat is also ingested, without any ill effects.

Herbs. For centuries, women have been seeking relief from hot flushes and other menstrual complaints by using the leaves and roots of local plants. From Chinese herbal medicine, European folk medicine, and American Indian medicine have come indications that certain plants may contain properties that relieve hot flushes. No scientific research substantiates any claims for any of the herbs mentioned, however, it presents fascinating possibilities for future research. Some of the herbs and roots that have been used traditionally were included by Lydia Pinkham (1819-1883) in her Vegetable Compound (Burton, 1949). Its popularity among Victorian women may be accounted for in part by the alcohol (18%) used to preserve the herbs in solution. Whether it actually helped relieve complaints associated with the climacterium is debatable. The Pinkham family maintained that when administered during the change of life, it greatly decreased the number of hot flushes experienced each day, but the Federal Trade Commission reported in 1938 that it could not substantiate most of the family's claims for the herbal concoction. Shortly thereafter, estrogen became available and Lydia Pinkham's Vegetable Compound lost popularity. Currently the herbal mixture is produced by Cooper Laboratories and is available with the following ingredients: jamaica dogwood, pleurisy root, black cohosh, life root, licorice, dandelion, and gentian. Licorice has been found to contain vegetable estrogens. Other plants (e.g., pussy willow, sarsaparilla, wild cherry, and yucca) contain estrogenic material or can be converted to estrogen by chemical means within the body.

Genseng and Dong Quai are Oriental herbs that some women use to prevent hot flushes. Scientific research to substantiate popular wisdom would be helpful; until that time dosages and side effects are unknown.

Coping with Genital Atrophy. Preventive measures are available for several problems that result from genital atrophy. These measures will not cure problems that already exist, but they may be effective in preventing problems such as prolapsed uterus and dyspareunia. Generally these measures neither are harmful nor have side effects.

Kegel's Exercises. After menopause occurs, muscle tone around the reproductive organs may decrease. Kegel's exercises can strengthen these muscles and improve muscle tone. If practiced on a regular basis, the exercises help prevent prolapsed uterus and stress incontinence. Women can be taught to do Kegel's exercises easily and in any position (see also client teaching: Kegel's exercises, Chapter 8).

Water-soluble Lubricants. For women who experience loss of lubrication because of vaginal atrophy and who chose not to use estrogen cream, water-soluble lubricants are helpful. They are applied directly to the vulva and the penis. K-Y Lubricating Jelly and coconut oil are two examples of water-soluble lubricants. Women who use them often get relief from pain and discomfort during intercourse. Oil-based lubricants such as petroleum jelly (Vaseline) should not be used because they clog vaginal glands, which then can be sites for bacterial infection.

Fluid Intake Measures and Other Dietary Suggestions. Another consequence of genital atrophy is urinary frequency and dysuria. For women for whom HRT is contraindicated, increasing daily fluid intake may prevent infections. At least eight glasses of water are recommended daily. This decreases urine concentration and bacterial multiplication.

Prevention of Infection. Another consequence of genital atrophy is bladder or urinary tract infections resulting in urinary urgency, frequency, and dysuria. Many older women develop a type of asymptomatic bacteriuria; they do not have cramping, pain, or burning on voiding. However, the other symptoms may be present. Most urinary tract infections are limited to the urethra and the bladder. Occasionally a urinary tract infection involves the kidney, a serious complication. Signs of serious infection include fever, chills, vomiting, and pain in the back over the kidneys (costovertebral angle tenderness) (see client teaching: urinary tract infections, Chapter 8).

Prevention of Complaints Associated with Osteoporosis. Another problem that develops after menopause is osteoporosis. No preventive measure other than HRT is known yet. However, the following suggestions may retard the disease.

Calcium. Adding calcium supplements to the diet retards the development of osteoporosis in women after menopause. Although calcium cannot reverse losses of bone mass or prevent fractures from eventually occurring, it can slow down the osteoporotic process. It is recommended that calcium be taken daily by mouth as early as the premenopause by women who are at risk. The dose recommended is 1.5 g daily usually taken before sleep (at bed time). Calcium is available as calcium carbonate, calcium lactate, and calcium gluconate. At times vitamin D is recommended as a supplement because it aids in the metabolism of calcium in the intestine. Fluoride is not recommended: it has produced gastrointestinal irritation in women who have used it. Women taking calcium supplements should increase water intake. Calcium is not recommended for women with kidney disease because it may lead to hypercalcemia.

Nutrition. To promote bone strength, it is recommended that women after menopause eat food high in calcium and low in phosphorus and avoid excessive intake of protein. Phosphorus tends to promote bone breakdown. Dairy products are high in phosphorus and are not ordinarily recommended for postmenopausal women. However, dairy products should not totally be eliminated. Fat free milk and yogurt are good sources of calcium and vitamin D. It is recommended that women drink 3 glasses (750 ml) each day. Other foods that contain calcium but are low in phosphorus include sesame seeds, spinach, turnip greens, and seaweed. Excessive amounts of protein should be avoided because the body's calcium balance can be adversely effected. No more than 1 g/kg body weight is needed per day. Another suggestion related to nutrition is avoidance of excessive amounts of alcohol. Excessive use of alcohol interferes with preservation of bone tissue.

Exercise. Although regular exercise is important in the maintenance of a healthy cardiovascular system and strong bones and muscles, it cannot prevent osteoporosis. Osteoporosis is caused principally by biochemical changes and may be influenced by a sedentary life-style, but it cannot be prevented or reversed by daily periods of exercise.

Evaluation

Evaluative criteria of care reflect physiologic, anatomic, psychologic, and emotional progress toward the goals of care. Effective individual and family coping, alleviation of signs and symptoms, and prevention of osteoporosis are all indicators that management has been successful.

SEQUELAE OF CHILDBIRTH TRAUMA

Alterations in Pelvic Support

The term *pelvic relaxation* refers to the weakening and lengthening of fascial supports of the bladder and urethra, the uterus and vaginal wall, and the rectum. Although relaxation may occur in any woman, young or old, parous or nulliparous, or sexually active or virginal, in most cases it is the delayed but direct result of parturition. Pelvic trauma, stress and strain, and the aging process are also implicated (Droegmueller et al., 1987). Evidence of extensive damage is noted, and repairs are made shortly after delivery. More often, symptoms of pelvic relaxation appear during the perimenopausal period, when the tonic effects of ovarian hormones on pelvic tissues are lost and atrophic changes in the fascial supports begin. Pelvic relaxation is regarded in the same way that a hernia is regarded elsewhere: (1) both are sequelae to weakness in supporting tissues and both are progressive, and (2) neither exercise nor rest will correct the problem or restore normal anatomic relations and physiologic function.

Generally, symptoms of pelvic relaxation relate to the structure involved: urethra, bladder, uterus, vagina, cul-de-sac, or rectum. The most common complaints women offer are pulling and dragging sensations, pressure, protrusions, and fatigue. Low backache, commonly associated with pelvic relaxation, is probably secondary to postural adjustments made in the attempt to relieve symptoms.

Several symptoms characterize structural support problems or uterine displacement or both: stress urinary incontinence, pelvic discomfort or pressure, and a sensation of fullness in the pelvis, especially after prolonged periods of standing or deep penile penetration during coitus. Symptoms are progressive over time.

There are several types of pelvic relaxation: rectocele, enterocele, cystocele, urethrocele, and uterine prolapse.

Levator Ani Injuries. During distension of the birth canal and lower vagina, levator ani bundles separate and levator fascia is stretched. In spite of the natural resiliency of this layer, often it does not stretch enough to permit vaginal delivery without some injury and therefore does not return completely to its predelivery state of intactness. The clinician needs to remember that although external damage may be minimal or not visible, extensive damage may have occurred in the deep supporting structures. When lacerations occur in the levator muscles (Figs. 6-15 and 6-16), the muscle fibers contract, causing the muscle to separate and retract laterally and destroy the perineal body, thereby eliminating the normal support of the rectum.

The perineal and vaginal lacerations that usually occur along with lacerations in the levator ani damage the fascial layer in the rectovaginal septum, destroying the anterior support of the rectum. Levator ani fibers may also detach from the lateral walls of the rectum, destroying the rectum's lateral support. The episiotomy that is delayed until the perineum is overstretched and blanched offers no protection, because the underlying structures have already been stretched to their maximum.

Permanent defects in support may be a sequel to childbirth regardless of obstetric management and may occur also in women who have never been pregnant. Rectocele and enterocele are two such defects.

Rectocele. With this defect, especially when the woman is on her feet, the weight of abdominal contents causes the posterior wall to sag anteriorly. Each time she strains during bowel evacuation, the feces are forced against the thinned rectovaginal wall, stretching it more. Gradually, rectal herniation of the anterior wall through the relaxed or ruptured vaginal fascia and rectovaginal septum increases (Fig. 41-3) until, eventually, a large bulge may be seen through the relaxed introitus. Most rectoceles are small and produce few symptoms; some are so huge that they protrude outside the vagina when the woman stands up. The woman may experience symptoms for the first time after menopause, when tissue atrophy in response to withdrawal of estrogen permits a rapid increase in the size of the rectocele.

Disturbances in bowel function, the sensation of "bearing down" or that the pelvic organs are falling out, and awareness of a protrusion in the vagina are characteristic of this structural defect. With a very large rectocele, women find it difficult to evacuate the rectum. Some women facilitate bowel evacuation by applying digital pressure vaginally to hold up the rectal pouch. Symptoms are usually absent when the woman is lying down.

Rectoceles that produce symptoms are repaired surgically. The operative procedure to approximate the separated levator muscles and their fascia with the perineal body in the midline is performed through the vagina. This

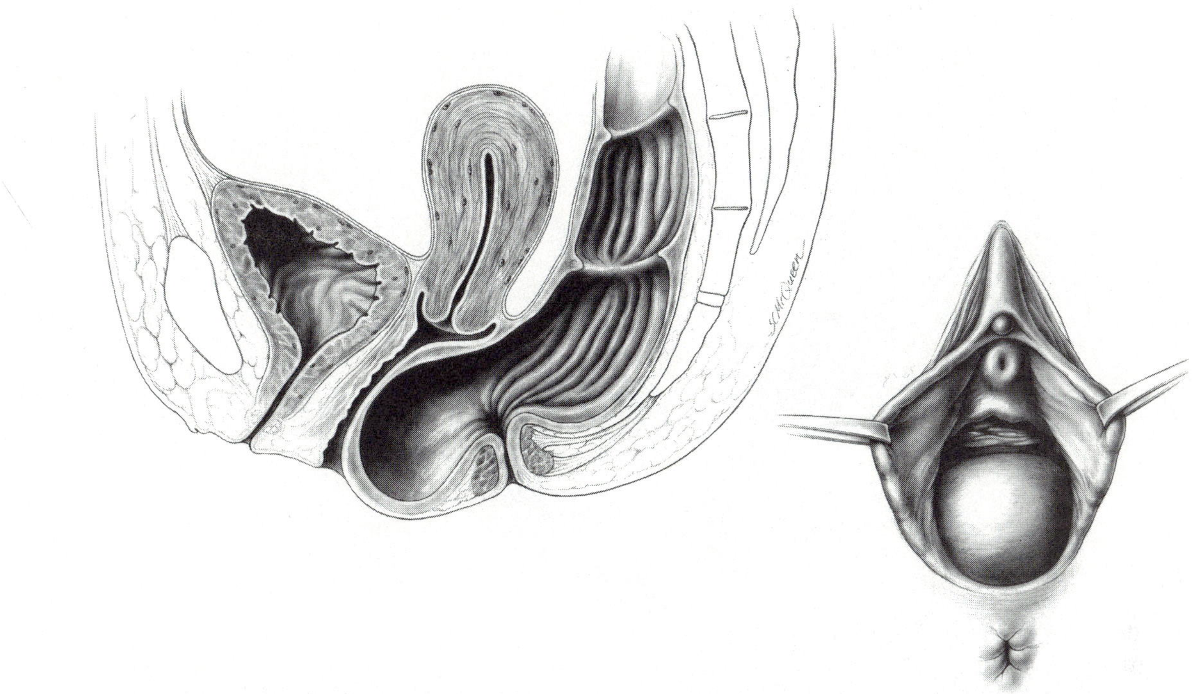

Fig. 41-3 Side and direct views of rectocele.
Redrawn from Symmonds, RE: Relaxations of pelvic supports. In Benson, RC, editor: Current obstetric and gynecologic diagnosis and treatment, ed 5, Los Altos, Calif, 1984, Lange Medical Publications.

surgery is called *perineorrhaphy, posterior colpoplasty,* or more simply, *posterior vaginal repair.*

Enterocele. Enterocele (Fig. 41-4), or posterior vaginal hernia, is the herniation of the peritoneum of the posterior cul-de-sac between the uterosacral ligaments into the rectovaginal septum. The sacculation contains loops of small bowel but no rectum. This condition is seen commonly with uterine prolapse and after vaginal hysterectomy for relaxation. Depending on its size and extent, the woman may be unaware of the problem or may complain of pressure or a bearing-down or dragging sensation and low backache.

The enterocele may be diagnosed during a rectovaginal examination. Characteristically, the deficit is first noticed as an increased thickness of the rectovaginal septum and a perception of pressure on the examiner's fingertip when the woman is asked to increase intraabdominal pressure by coughing. A vaginal approach is used to close the defect surgically by approximating the uterosacral ligaments and the levator muscles in the midline.

Anterior Vaginal Wall Injury. As the lower uterine segment elongates during labor (Fig. 16-14), the bladder, attached to the anterior surface of the uterus (Fig. 6-9), is pulled up out of the pelvis. As a consequence, only the urethra, the vesical neck, and a portion of the bladder wall are vulnerable to injury. During descent of the fetal presenting part and vaginal dilation, the structures of the vesicovaginal septum are stretched and may be torn in numerous areas beneath the vaginal epithelium. With fetopelvic disproportion or a precipitous delivery, structures of the vesical and vaginal walls are stretched and may be injured. The bladder neck and urethra may be compressed between the presenting part and the pubic bones or forced downward, ahead of the presenting part. A prolonged expulsive stage also increases the chance of injury to the bladder neck and urethral wall.

Since soft tissue damage usually occurs behind an intact vaginal epithelium, there is nothing visible to repair. The emphasis of care is on prevention, for example, avoiding bladder distension during labor, performing an adequate episiotomy at the appropriate time, and judiciously using low forceps for delivery of the fetal head. Cystocele, urethrocele, and vaginal prolapse are possible sequelae.

Cystocele. Cystocele (Fig. 41-5), the protrusion of the bladder downward into the vagina, develops when supporting structures in the vesicovaginal septum are injured. Anterior wall relaxation, not apparent immediately after delivery, gradually develops over a period of time—often after the woman has given birth to several babies.

When the woman stands up, the weakened anterior vaginal wall cannot support the weight of the urine in the bladder; the vesicovaginal septum is forced downward, the bladder is stretched, and its capacity is increased. With time the cystocele enlarges until it protrudes into the vagina. Complete emptying is difficult if not impossible because the cystocele sags below the bladder neck. Cystocele is often accompanied by rectocele, and the bladder descends when the uterus prolapses. Some women are unaware of the condition or may complain of a bearing-down sensation or a protrusion of a mass from the vagina.

The condition is recognized as a bulging of the anterior wall of the vagina; the size of the cystocele is best appreciated when the woman is standing. Unless the bladder neck and urethra are damaged, urinary continence is unaffected. Women with large cystoceles complain of having to push upward on the sagging anterior vaginal wall to be able to

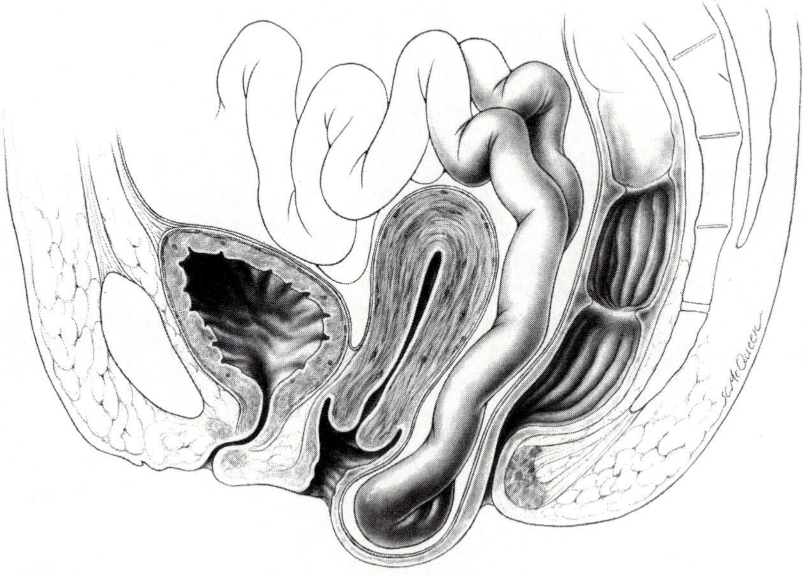

Fig. 41-4 Lateral view of enterocele and prolapsed uterus.
Redrawn from Symmonds, RE: Relaxations of pelvic supports. In Benson, RC, editor: Current obstetric and gynecologic diagnosis and treatment, ed 5, Los Altos, Calif, 1984, Lange Medical Publications.

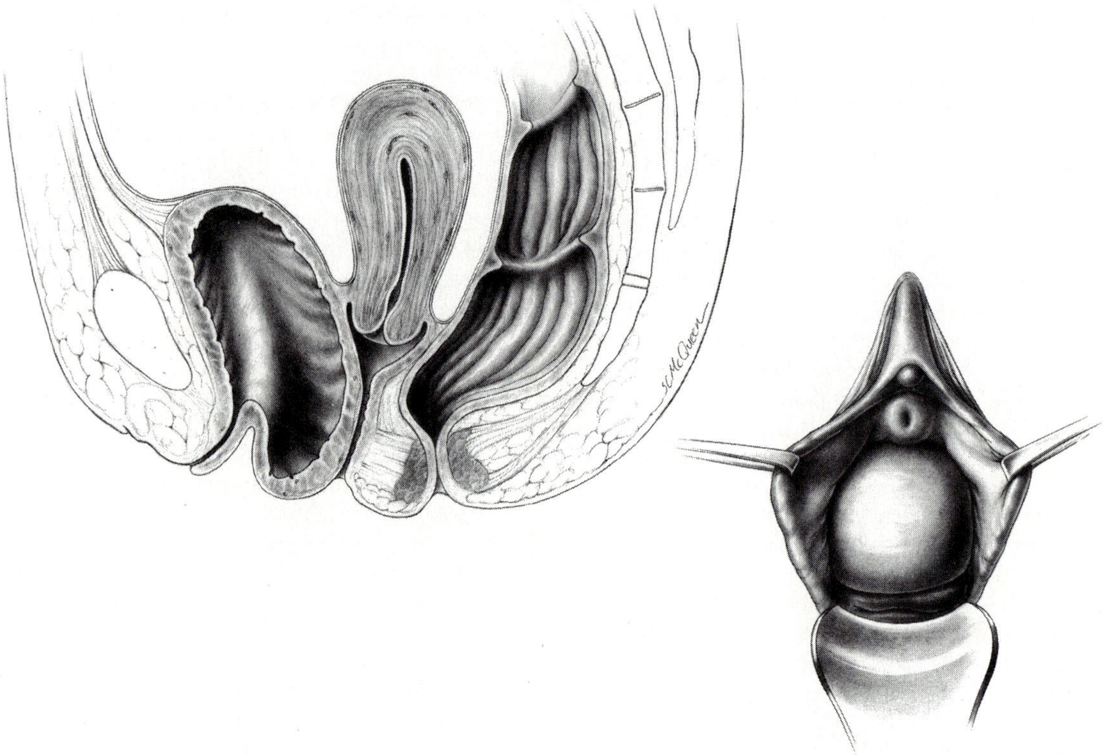

Fig. 41-5 Side and direct views of cystocele.
Redrawn from Symmonds, RE: Anatomy of the female reproductive system. In Benson, RC, editor: Current obstetric and gynecologic diagnosis and treatment, ed 5, Los Altos, Calif, 1984, Lange Medical Publications.

void at all. Recurrent cystitis is a common complication when urine is retained for long periods in a cystocele; ascending urinary tract infection may also develop.

Surgical support can be accomplished only through the vagina, which permits the only access to the area to be repaired. Plication (taking a fold, or tuck, or a running stitch to gather material together) of the bladder wall reduces the cystocele. Surgical intervention is necessary only when symptoms exist.

Urethrocele. Herniation of the paravaginal fascia under the urethra allows the urethra to protrude into the vagina. As with cystocele, the condition may be asymptomatic or the woman may be aware of a vaginal mass or protrusion or may complain of stress urinary incontinence if there is relaxation of fascial supports in the area of the posterior urethrovesical angle.

Vaginal Prolapse. Prolapse of the vagina (hernia in vagina), *colpocele,* an uncommon but greatly distressing condition, may occur after vaginal or abdominal hysterectomy. In almost all cases it coexists with enterocele and often with cystocele.

Vaginal Atresia. Childbirth injury may result in vaginal atresia at any level in the vagina but usually occurs along a lateral wall in the upper third. Palpation reveals a sharp, annular, constricting band of tissue. Causes include faulty repair of a laceration, failure to perform a needed repair, and anterior and posterior colporraphy. Removal of too much redundant vaginal wall tissue, excessive tightening of the levator ani muscles during the posterior wall repair, or perineorrhaphy may contribute to the distressing problem.

Surgical correction may be as simple as incising some annular bands of tissue or employing graduated obturators to dilate a constricting band in the lower one third of the vagina. More extensive vaginal plastic surgery may be needed in more severe vaginal atresia.

Urinary Incontinence

Uncontrollable leakage of urine is experienced by many women. Although this condition may be the result of injury sustained during childbirth, other factors may be considered. Five categories of conditions can disturb urinary control (Willson et al., 1988):

1. *Stress urinary incontinence.* The loss of urine occurs with sudden increases in intraabdominal pressure, such as that generated by sneezing, or from sudden jarring movement. The loss is caused by structural injuries to the urethra and bladder neck.
2. *Detrusor dyssynergia.* The incontinence results from involuntary detrusor activity, which is triggered by a variety of stimuli.
3. *Urge incontinence.* Urge incontinence is characterized by the inability to keep from urinating when the urge to void occurs suddenly. Urge incontinence usually is caused by intrinsic disorders of the bladder and urethra, the most common being urethritis and urethral stricture, trigonitis, and cystitis.
4. *Neuropathies.* Neurologic disorders, such as multiple sclerosis, diabetic neuritis, and diseases of or injuries to the spinal cord, disturb the nerve control of bladder function. Such disorders usually cause overflow or uninhibited detrusor incontinence.
5. *Congenital and acquired urinary tract abnormalities.* Urinary tract abnormalities include congenital defects, such as ectopic ureter, abnormal muscular development of the vesical neck, and neurologic disorders, and acquired lesions, such as urinary fistulas and destruction of all or part of the urethra. The incontinence is usually constant and unrelated to voiding, to activity, or to position.

Stress urinary incontinence and acquired urinary tract abnormalities are discussed in this section. Cystocele and urethrocele have already been discussed.

Stress Urinary Incontinence. This is a disturbance in urinary control wherein the woman loses urine in response to increased intraabdominal pressure that occurs when she coughs, laughs, or sneezes. It is common for many multiparas to experience stress incontinence, especially in conjunction with menstruation. Some women may experience stress incontinence after the first vaginal delivery, whereas others have no symptoms until after several vaginal deliveries. The symptoms become more annoying after menopause, when tissues atrophy.

Stress urinary incontinence may follow injury to bladder neck structures. A sphincter mechanism at the bladder neck compresses the upper urethra, pulls it upward behind the symphysis, and forms an acute angle at the junction of the posterior urethral wall and the base of the bladder (Fig. 41-6, *A*). This angle aids urine retention even if the intravesical pressure is increased over normal. When a person wishes to empty the bladder, the sphincter complex relaxes and the internal urethral orifice is opened by the muscles of the trigone. The trigone contracts to expand the opening and to pull the contracting bladder wall upward; urine is forced out.

The sphincter mechanism must be intact to maintain continence; that is, muscles must be intact and must function in unison. The angle between the urethra and the base of the bladder is lost (Fig. 41-6, *B*) or increased if the supporting pubococcygeus muscle is injured; this change, coupled with failure of urethral compression (urethrocele), results in severe incontinence. Diagnosis is confirmed if urine spurts out when the woman is in the lithotomy position and is requested to bear down, cough, or hold her breath; the test can be repeated with the woman standing. Other causes must be ruled out, for example, neurogenic bladder dysfunction, detrusor dyssynergia, urinary tract fistulas, urinary tract infection, and urethral strictures.

If there is minimal descent of the bladder and urethra, stress urinary incontinence can be relieved by systematic muscle exercise (Kegel's exercises, p. 1047, and Chapter 8) 80 to 100 times per day (see research highlight). Hormone replacement therapy (estrogen and progesterone) may improve urinary control for affected women after menopause if local atrophic change is the primary factor. Surgical correction is reserved for those for whom other therapy has been unsuccessful: defects such as cystocele, urethrocele, and uterine prolapse are corrected and structural supports are shortened and strengthened. The anticipated result is restoration of the urethrovesical angle and narrowing of the internal urethral orifice.

RESEARCH HIGHLIGHT

Age as a Variable in an Exercise Program for the Treatment of Simple Urinary Stress Incontinence

Purpose

To compare the effectiveness of biofeedback on pubococcygeal muscle strengthening and simple urinary stress incontinence in older and younger women.

Sample/Methodology

A convenient sample of 9 women 55 years or older (mean, 64 years) and 5 women aged 54 years or younger (mean, 38 years) participated in a study in which Kegel's exercises, using biofeedback, were taught for the treatment of simple urinary stress incontinence. The instrument used for biofeedback and measurement in this study was the Personal Perineometer. The Personal Perineometer measures the pressure exerted by the pubococcygeal muscle in increments of 0 to 60 μV during contractions of the muscle.

Subjects had weekly clinic visits for 8 weeks. They completed the self-assessment of continence questionnaires and were measured for pubococcygeal strength with the Personal Perineometer.

Findings

Data were analyzed descriptively because of the small sample size. All women in both the younger and older groups reported improvements in the frequency or amount of stress incontinence during the study. On the last clinic visit, six of nine subjects in the older group and four of five subjects of the younger group reported no incidence of stress incontinence during the preceeding week. In addition, the younger group eliminated incontinence at a lower μV reading than did the older group, indicating that less muscle strength was required to effect a cure in younger women than was needed in the older women.

Implications

The responsibility for teaching Kegel's exercises for the treatment of simple urinary stress incontinence, with or without sophisticated biofeedback equipment, falls within the scope of nursing practice.

Henderson, JS, and Taylor, KH: Age as a variable in an exercise program for the treatment of simple urinary stress incontinence, JOGN Nurs 16(4):266, 1987.

Injuries to Pelvic Joints

Separation of the *symphysis pubis* occurs to some degree during delivery. If forcible extraction or delivery of a large baby occurs, serious injury is likely. After delivery, when the woman attempts to move or stand on her feet, she suffers severe pain in the area of the symphysis pubis and *sacroiliac joints.* Palpation reveals tenderness over the symphysis, wide separation of the ends of the pubic bones, and unusual mobility (several centimeters) of the bone ends when she shifts her weight from one foot to the other.

Uterine Displacement

Prolapse. The cardinal (Mackenrodt's) ligaments (Fig. 6-10) provide the major support for the uterus and vagina. These ligaments may be unduly stretched if the fetus is large or if forceps delivery is attempted before full cervical dilation.

If the cardinal ligaments do not return to normal after delivery, the uterus will sag backward and downward into the vagina. The uterus usually forms an acute angle with the axis of the vagina, which in itself tends to prevent prolapse. Prolapse of the uterus occurs when the cardinal ligaments and other supporting structures (e.g., uterosacral ligaments) relax and the relationship of the axis of the uterus to that of the vagina is altered (Fig. 41-7).

Congenital defects account for descensus (prolapse) of the uterus in infants and nulliparas, but childbirth injury is responsible for its gradual development in multiparas. Cystocele and rectocele, which almost always accompany uterine prolapse, enlarge and pull down on the uterus and cervix, adding to the stress on the weakened cardinal ligaments. The more severe prolapses are seen in postmenopausal women when tissue atrophy eliminates whatever residual support existed. Degrees of prolapse are classified as follows:

1. *First-degree prolapse.* Cervix is situated between the level of the ischial spines and the vaginal introitus.
2. *Second-degree prolapse.* Cervix protrudes through introitus, but corpus remains within the vagina.
3. *Third-degree prolapse.* Complete prolapse; cervix and body of uterus protrude through vagina, and vagina is inverted. The extent of the defect is best evaluated by asking the woman to strain while lying down, by exerting traction on the cervix with a tenaculum, or by examining her while she is in an upright position.
4. *Procidentia.* Uterus, vaginal vault, rectum, and bladder, and perhaps the posterior cul-de-sac as well, protrude.

Symptoms of uterine prolapse reflect sensations produced by the weight of the descending structures and their protrusion through the vaginal introitus. Third-degree prolapse may eventuate in cervical ulceration and bleeding.

Transvaginal surgical correction of the defect is preferable, but in selected individuals (e.g., those who are aged and debilitated) a pessary may be inserted to stabilize the uterus (Fig. 41-8). The goals of operative procedures are to correct the cystocele and rectocele, return the uterus to a forward position, shorten the elongated cervix, and shorten the cardinal ligaments. Several procedures accomplish these goals: (1) Manchester-Fothergill: amputation of the cervix, shortening of the cardinal ligaments, and plastic repair of the vagina; (2) vaginal hysterectomy; and (3) colpocleisis (Le Fort's procedure): obliteration of the vagina by approximation of the anterior and posterior walls.

Retroversion and Lateral Displacement. Displacement indicates a movement from front to back (Fig. 6-8) or from side to side, rather than a descent, as in prolapse. The two types of displacement are (1) a change in the long axis of the uterus, for example, anteflexion, malposition, and retroflexion; and (2) a change in the direction of the long

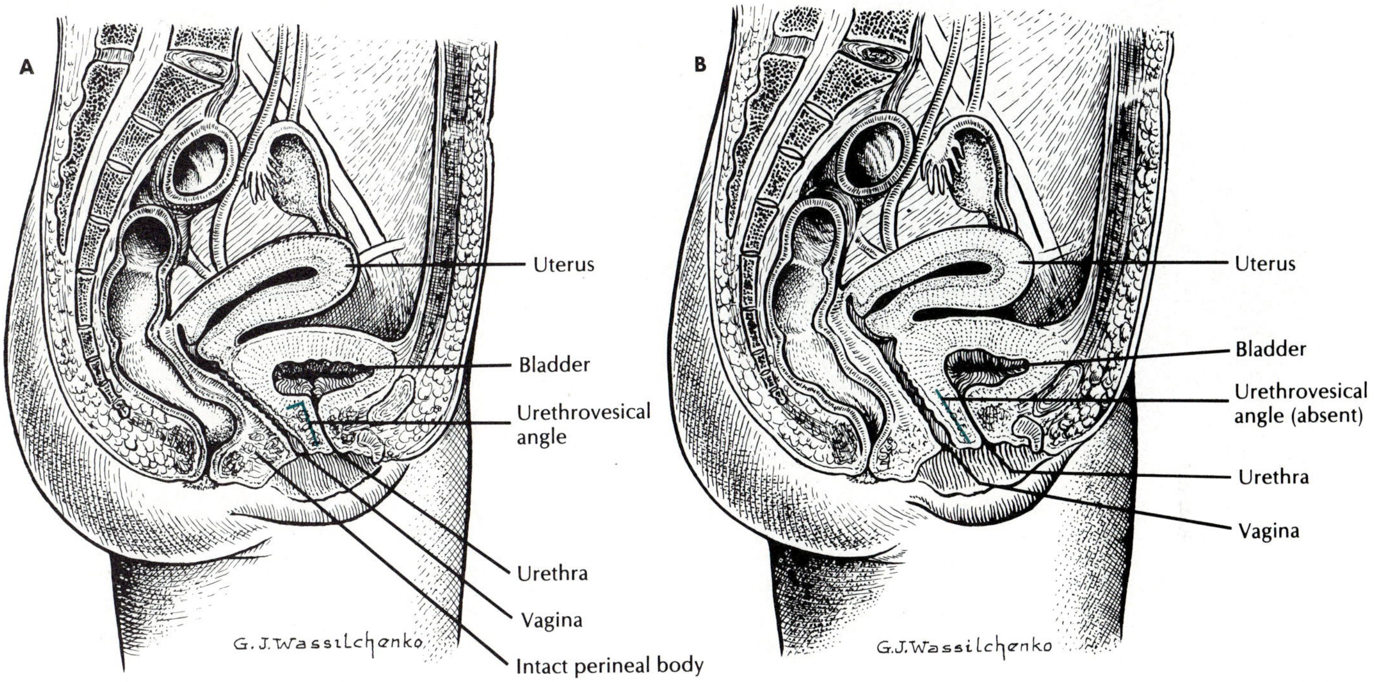

Fig. 41-6 Urethrovesical angle. **A**, Normal angle. **B**, Widening (absence) of angle.

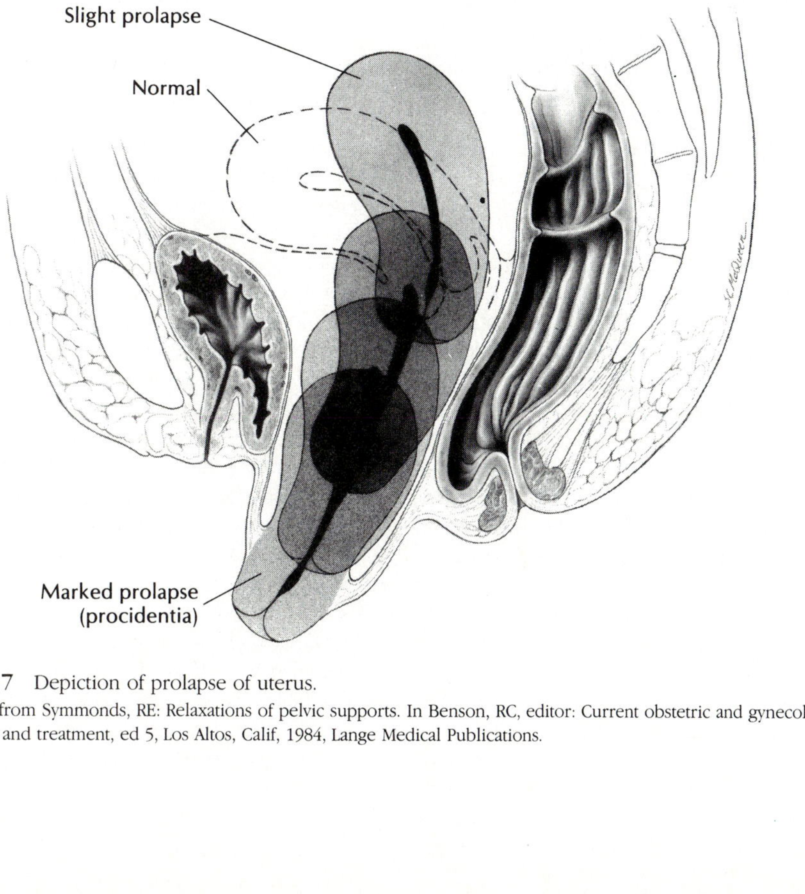

Fig. 41-7 Depiction of prolapse of uterus.

Redrawn from Symmonds, RE: Relaxations of pelvic supports. In Benson, RC, editor: Current obstetric and gynecologic diagnosis and treatment, ed 5, Los Altos, Calif, 1984, Lange Medical Publications.

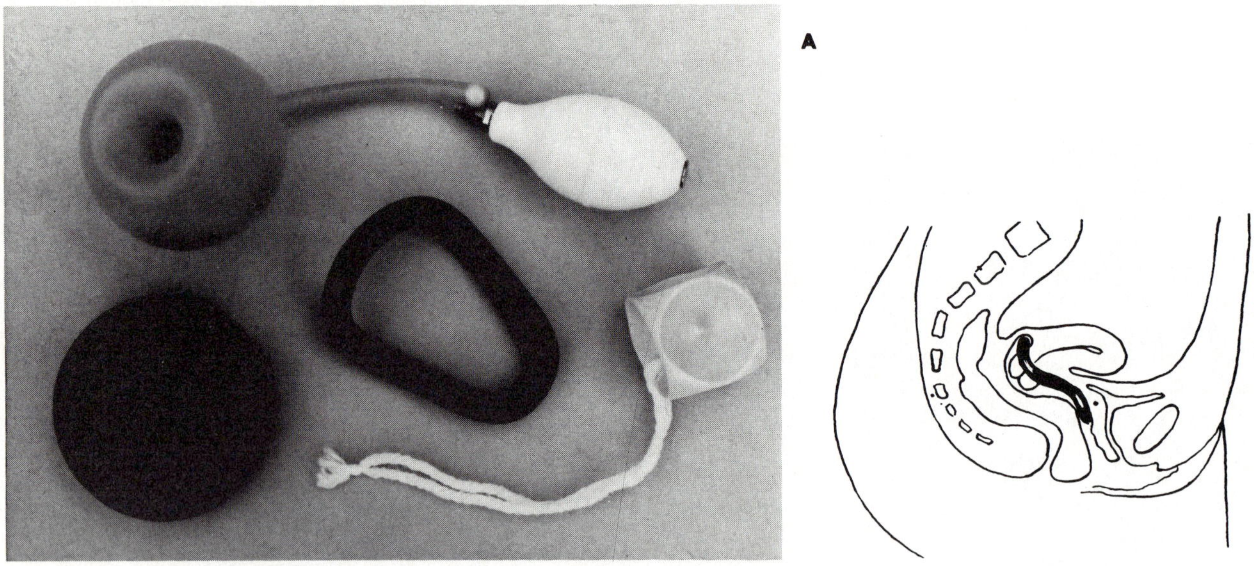

A

B

Fig. 41-8 A, Examples of pessaries (Smith-Hodge, donut, inflatable types). B, Pessary in place to hold posterior vaginal fornix and, with it, attached cervix well backward and upward in pelvis.
A from Droegemueller, W, et al: Comprehensive gynecology, St Louis, 1987, The CV Mosby Co. B from Beacham, DW, and Beacham, WD: Synopsis of gynecology, ed 10, St Louis, 1982, The CV Mosby Co.

axis of the uterus in relation to the vaginal canal, for example, lateral displacement, anteversion (the most common position), retroversion, and retrocession.

Most positional differences are simple anatomic variations. They are asymptomatic and have no clinical significance. *Retroversion* is the most common simple displacement caused by factors that are congenital or acquired after childbirth. Cul-de-sac disease may be responsible and is of clinical significance. *Lateral displacement* may signal adnexal disease such as large ovarian tumor on the opposite side or pulled over to the side of the inflammatory process or scar tissue.

The supporting ligaments that hold the uterus in anteversion are the round and uterosacral ligaments. The uterosacral ligaments pull the cervix backward and upward; the round ligaments hold the fundus in the anterior position (Fig. 6-9). These ligaments gradually regain their length and return the uterus to anteversion in two thirds of women within approximately 2 months after delivery; in one third of women the uterus remains retroverted.

Uncomplicated retroversion as a sequel to childbirth is rarely symptomatic; low backache is not a symptom. Occasionally it may be difficult to conceive because the cervix points toward the anterior vaginal wall and away from the posterior fornix containing seminal fluid after coitus in the supine position. Retrodisplacement is also clinically significant because it must occur first before the uterus can prolapse.

Infrequently, chronic pelvic congestion may accompany a chronically retroverted uterus and is credited as the cause of deep pelvic and low back pain, difficulty with evacuation of the rectum, menstrual abnormalities associated with an exaggeration of premenstrual tension, and dyspareunia. The uterus may become boggy and congested, and the tubes and ovaries (often containing multiple follicular cysts) often prolapse posteriorly into the cul-de-sac.

Surgical correction is necessary only if the woman has symptoms that may be related to uterine position. A properly placed *pessary* (Fig. 41-8) replaces the uterus in the anterior position. If symptoms are relieved, it can be assumed that uterine displacement had contributed to the symptoms. Even though pessaries are retained for short periods of time, the woman needs to follow principles of good hygiene to avoid vaginal infection. Some women can be taught to remove the pessary at night, cleanse it, and replace it when they get up in the morning. This practice helps reduce the likelihood of pressure necrosis from irritation against the vaginal wall. If the pessary is always to be left in place, regular douching (Chapter 44) may be recommended to remove the increased secretions its presence may cause and to help prevent infection. The woman is encouraged to visit her health care provider frequently while the pessary is in place. Fortunately, for most women the pessary may not be required after a period of treatment, after which the woman is symptom free. After childbirth, surgery for displacement of a previously normal uterus is rarely necessary.

Genital Fistulas

A fistula is an abnormal or unnatural communication between one hollow viscus and another or from one hollow viscus to the outside. Genital fistulas are located between the bladder and the genital tract (vesicovaginal, vesicocervical, vesicouterine), between the ureter and the vagina (ureterovaginal), and between the rectum or sigmoid colon and other structures (enterovesical, enterouterine, enterovaginal). Congenital anomaly, gynecologic surgery, obstetric trauma, cancer, radiation therapy, gynecologic trauma, and infection are etiologic factors. Discussion of obstetric-related urinary tract and rectovaginal fistulas follows.

Urinary Tract Fistulas. The most common urinary tract fistula (vesicovaginal) forms in the anterior vaginal wall (Fig. 41-9). Historically, necrosis of the vesicovaginal septum from pressure during delayed labor was responsible for the fistula formation; this is seldom the case today because such labors would dictate cesarean delivery. Today, operative injury near the uterovesical junction during radical hysterectomy for cancer is the primary cause of a fistula between the uterus and the bladder. The woman with this abnormal opening is partially or completely incontinent, and urine passes through the vagina. A transvaginal surgical repair is possible in most cases.

Rectovaginal Fistulas. The most common causes of this abnormal communication between the rectum and vagina are infection in the episiotomy, a suture placed through the rectal wall during repair, or an unrecognized rectal injury during parturition or vaginal repair. Fistulas may form subsequent to extension of cervical cancer or radiation therapy. Trauma-induced fistulas are usually located near the introitus; those induced by cancer tend to be located higher in the reproductive structures.

Surgical repair is possible but complicated by infection, which delays healing or causes the repair to break down. Preoperative preparation is necessarily prolonged to allow for 2 days of liquid diets, enemas, and antibiotic therapy. A temporary colostomy may be indicated before surgical correction of a complicated rectovaginal fistula.

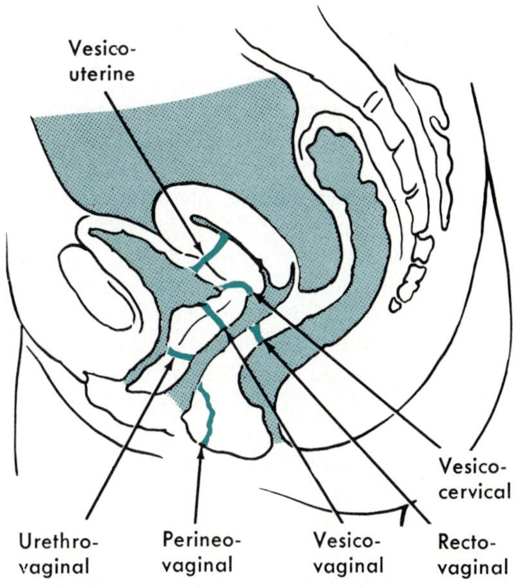

Fig. 41-9 Types of fistulas that may develop in vagina, uterus, and rectum.

From Phipps, WJ, et al: Medical-surgical nursing: concepts and clinical practice, ed 3, St Louis, 1987, The CV Mosby Co.

Assessment

A complete health history, physical examination, and laboratory tests are performed to obtain a data base (Chapter 8). Assessment for sequelae to childbirth trauma and uterine displacement focuses primarily on the reproductive tract, the genitourinary tract, bowel elimination, and psychosocial and sexual factors. Data is accumulated to substantiate a diagnosis of the specific anatomic and functional disorder involved. The woman's knowledge of her disorder, its management, and its possible prognosis is assessed.

Nursing Diagnoses

Following are examples of nursing diagnoses for the woman experiencing late sequelae of childbirth trauma and uterine displacement.

- Constipation, diarrhea related to
  - Anatomic changes
- Pain related to
  - Changes in anatomy and elimination patterns
- Ineffective individual coping related to
  - Changes in body image
- Altered family processes or interpersonal relationships related to
  - Woman's anatomic and functional changes
- Stress incontinence related to
  - Anatomic and physiologic changes
- Potential injury related to
  - Lack of skill in self-care procedures
  - Lack of understanding of rationale behind need to comply with therapy
- Social isolation, spiritual distress, body image disturbance, or situational low self-esteem related to
  - Anatomic and physiologic changes.

Planning

Planning requires sensitive consideration in collaborating with the woman for her care. The nurse bases plans on a broad base of knowledge of psychosocial, medical, and surgical nursing and skill in the application of that knowledge. Goals for care are established and stated in client-centered terms.

Goals

1. Women are knowledgeable about possible childbirth sequelae and symptoms and participate in yearly physical examinations that facilitate early diagnosis and implementation of corrective intervention.
2. Women implement appropriate hygienic actions.
3. Women accept change in body functions without loss of positive body image, self-concept, and self-esteem.
4. Medical and surgical interventions are successful in the repair of anatomic defects and the control of reproductive and genitourinary tract dysfunction.

Implementation

Nursing care of women with pelvic relaxation problems and fistulas requires sympathetic understanding and encouragement because the women's emotional reactions are often intense. Women with vesicovaginal or rectovaginal fistulas may become withdrawn or, conversely, hostile because of embarrassment about odors and soiling of their clothing beyond their control. Occasionally the woman becomes so accustomed to the odors that she is no longer aware of them; the nurse needs to use a sensitive approach in suggesting hygienic practices that reduce these odors. Several deodorizing douches are available: commercial ones may be prescribed by the physician, or noncommercial solutions, such as chlorine solution (5 ml or 1 teaspoon of chlorine household bleach to 1 L or 1 quart of water), may be used. The chlorine solution is also appropriate for external perineal irrigation. Sitz baths and thorough washing of the surrounding skin with unscented, uncolored, mild soap and warm water are helpful. Sparse dusting with deodorizing powders such as sodium borate can be used. Hygienic care is time consuming and must be repeated frequently throughout the day; protective pads or pants must be worn. All of these activities may be demoralizing to the woman and frustrating to herself and to her family.

If the woman has a rectovaginal fistula, there is a constant oozing of fecal material into the vagina, which may be temporarily lessened by giving a high enema; preoperatively, the woman is encouraged to do this before going out of the house. A soft rubber catheter is used if enemas are given in the preoperative period and should be directed carefully on the side of the rectum opposite the fistula. The tubing must extend beyond the fistula, or the enema fluid will return through the vagina with no benefit to the woman. Although a constipating diet will give temporary relief by discouraging fecal material from entering the vagina through the fistula, constipation will eventually cause pressure and may possibly aggravate the condition; it may even cause the fistula to enlarge. Therefore the woman is advised against restricting diet and fluids in an effort to control bowel action. After surgery, enemas are contraindicated until healing is complete.

Perioperative Care

It is fruitless to perform surgery until inflammation and induration have subsided. This preoperative period may extend to 3 to 4 months. Surgical repair is made through a suprapubic incision into the bladder. The fistulous tract is then dissected out and closed.

In the first postoperative week the woman can expect drainage from the bladder through a suprapubic and a urethral catheter, usually connected to a suction apparatus set at gentle negative pressure. In the rare instance when catheter irrigation is indicated, very gentle pressure is mandatory. Urinary and vaginal drainage are noted. Vaginal douches may be ordered; douching is accomplished gently and with gentle fluid pressure. Bed rest or restriction to the hospital room may be needed for several days because the drainage tubes need to be suctioned. The nurse is challenged to institute measures to prevent physical complications of immobility (especially pneumonia, thrombus formation, constipation, and loss of calcium from bones) and emotional discomfort from sensory deprivation.

Repair of fistulas is not always successful, and repeat surgeries may be needed. The nurse needs to employ a variety of techniques and understanding patience when a woman's anxiety and irritation are expressed. The woman needs encouragement from the nursing and medical staff, and she needs assurance that they understand her problem. When fistulas persist, couples have special problems that require patience and understanding. The couple is encouraged to communicate with one another regarding interference with their sexual relationship; joint counseling may be necessary.

When the surgery involves the vagina, postoperative care is directed to prevent pressure on the vaginal suture line and to prevent wound infection. Perineal dressings are rarely needed.

Perineal cleansing is done at least twice daily and after each voiding and defecation. Several methods are acceptable: sterile cotton balls moistened with benzalkonium chloride, bichloride of mercury, and normal saline solution may be used, or the woman may sit on a douche pan and have the solution poured over the perineum.

A heat lamp, used 15 to 20 minutes 3 times per day, encourages healing of the perineum. The heat lamp is used after perineal care to aid in drying the area to prevent sloughing of tissue. Local application of an ice pack helps reduce swelling and promotes comfort. Ice packs are always covered before application to the skin. A disposable glove filled with ice serves as an adequate ice pack and is easily made and inexpensive to use. The use of moist heat (e.g., Sitz baths, varies among physicians), Sitz baths may not be ordered until after sutures have been removed.

An indwelling catheter attached to continuous drainage may be in place for 24 to 48 hours. Urinary output and character of urine are monitored. After removal of the catheter, the woman is encouraged to void in the usual way.

Within 7 to 10 days after surgery, daily vaginal douching with normal saline solution may be prescribed. Whether douches are ordered immediately after surgery or at a later date, sterile equipment and sterile solution is used. The douch nozzle is inserted very gently and rotated slowly and gently during administration of the fluid (see procedure, Chapter 44).

Discharge planning includes instruction for continued douching at least once per day, followed by a tub bath. Laxatives are to be taken to keep stools soft and prevent constipation to minimize stress on the surgical site. The woman is encouraged to follow up her medical care by keeping scheduled appointments. The physician will counsel her regarding the appropriate time to discontinue vaginal douching and to determine when it is safe for her to resume sexual relations. As with counsel given to women after other types of gynecologic surgery, women are reminded to avoid jarring activities and lifting heavy objects for at least 6 weeks postoperatively.

Evaluation

Care can be evaluated as effective if the anatomic defect is repaired and function is restored. If function cannot be fully restored through surgery, medication, or other therapy, care is deemed effective if the woman retains self-esteem and her family processes are perceived as satisfactory.

SUMMARY

Common menstrual disorders are discussed, especially hypogonadotropic amenorrhea, dysmenorrhea, premenstrual syndrome, and endometriosis. The normal climacterium and postclimacterium are described. Conditions involving pelvic support, urinary continence, and genital fistulas occur in women as late sequelae to childbirth trauma or accompany changes resulting from withdrawal of ovarian hormones. Emphasis is on etiologic factors, symptomatology, and the nursing process with women experiencing gynecologic and urinary concerns.

KEY CONCEPTS

- Disorders associated with menstruation have a negative effect on the quality of life for affected women and their families.
- Premenstrual syndrome (PMS) refers to a diffuse, loosely defined set of symptoms that begins approximately 7 to 10 days before menses and ends with the onset of menses.
- Symptoms of endometriosis include secondary amenorrhea, dyspareunia, abnormal uterine bleeding, and infertility.
- The climacterium is a normal developmental phase during which a woman passes from the reproductive to the nonreproductive stage with the regression of ovarian function.
- During the climacterium, women seek care for symptoms that arise from vasomotor instability, emotional disturbances, fatigue, genital atrophy, and changes related to sexuality.
- Osteoporosis is a progressive loss of bone mass, especially in nonobese white and Oriental women, that is a direct result of the decreasing levels of estrogen after menopause and that can be prevented or minimized with hormone replacement therapy.
- Estrogen increases calcitonin levels and calcitonin prevents bone resorption and maintains bone density; dietary calcium supplementation and exercise may have a role in maintaining bone density, but conclusions await further study.
- There is no truth to the rumor that sexuality and ability for sexual expression comes to an end at menopause.
- Pelvic relaxation and lengthening of fascial supports may occur in any woman, young or old, parous or nulliparous, or sexually active or virginal; or they may be the delayed sequelae of childbirth trauma.
- Nursing care of women with pelvic relaxation problems and fistulas requires sympathetic understanding and encouragement because the women's emotional reactions are often intense.

STUDY QUESTIONS AND ACTIVITIES

1. Care for a woman with endometriosis. What treatments has she undergone? Assess her psychological well-being as related to the acceptance of her condition.
2. Determine if there is a PMS support group in your community. If so, attend a meeting. If no group is available, interview at least three women to determine their responses to PMS. How do their responses differ? Did any of the three describe the positive aspects of PMS?
3. Seek assignment to a client undergoing gynecologic surgery and follow her through the perioperative phase. Describe her fears, acceptance of body image changes, possible sterilization, and discharge planning. Describe your feelings regarding reproductive tract surgery. What attitudinal changes may make you more comfortable?
4. Develop a plan of care for the above client based on nursing diagnoses. Be sure to include emotional aspects of care in your plan. Share and discuss your interventions with students who have cared for similar clients.
5. In a group, discuss your feelings about or experiences with any of the conditions presented in this chapter. Discuss how the nurse's feelings, values, and beliefs can affect nursing care.

References

Acosta, AA, et al: A proposed classification of pelvic endometriosis, Obstet Gynecol 42:19, 1973

Anderson, E, et al: Characteristics of menopausal women seeking assistance, Am J Obstet Gynecol 156(2):428, 1987

Aylwood, M, Maddock, J, Lewis, PA, et al: Oestrogen replacement therapy and blood clotting, Curr Med Res Opin 4(suppl 3):83, 1971

Barrett-Connor, E, Brown, WV, Turner, J, et al: Heart disease risk factors and hormone use in postmenopausal women, JAMA 241:2167, 1979

Bernhard, LA: Endometriosis, JOGN Nurs 11:300, 1982

Blatt, M, et al: Vitamin E and climacteric syndrome, AMA Arch Intern Med 91:799, 1953

Burton, J: Lydia Pinkham is her name, New York, 1949, Farrar, Strauss & Co

Colditz, GA, et al: Menopause and the risk of coronary heart disease in women, N Engl J Med 316:1105, April 30, 1987

Collins, J, Donner, A, Allen, LH, and Adams, O: Oestrogen use and survival in endometrial cancer, Lancet 2:961, 1980

Block, JE, et al: Does exercise prevent osteoporosis? (Commentary), JAMA 257(22):3115, 1987

Droegemueller, W, et al: Comprehensive gynecology, St Louis, 1987, The CV Mosby Co

Fogel, DI, and Woods, NF: Health care of women: a nursing perspective, St Louis, 1981, The CV Mosby Co

Gambrell, RD, Jr, Massey, FM, Castaneda, TA, et al: Reduced incidence of endometrial cancer among postmenopausal women treated with progestogens, J Am Geriatr Soc 27(9):389, 1979

Greenblatt, R, et al: Update on the male and female climacteric, J Am Geriatr Soc 27:481, 1979
Hammond, CB, Jelovsek, FR, Lee, KL, et al: Effects of long-term estrogen replacement therapy. II. Neoplasia Am J Obstet Gynecol 133:537, 1979
Kiel, DP, et al: Hip fracture and the use of estrogens in postmenopausal women, N Engl J Med 317(19):1169, 1987
Lublanezki, N, and Fischer, RG: Pediatric drug information, Pediatr Nurs 13(6):435, 1987
Masters, W, and Johnson, V: Human sexual response, Boston, 1966, Little, Brown & Co, Inc
Michaels, R, editor: Rule out pregnancy before using danazol, Nurse's Drug Alert 7(2):10, 1983
Miller, LL: Interviews with women about menopause, unpublished paper, San Jose State Univ 1984
Nachtigall, L: The Lila Nachtigall report, New York, 1977, GP Putnam's Sons, Inc
O'Brien, PM: The premenstrual syndrome: a review of the present status of therapy, Drugs 24:140, 1982
Ottosson, UB, Johansson, BG, and Von Schoultz, B: Subfractions of high-density lipoprotein cholesterol during estrogen replacement therapy: a comparison between progestogens and natural progesterone, Am J Obstet Gynecol 151:746, 1985
Paganini-Hill, A, Ross, RK, Gerkins, VR, et al: A case control study of menopausal estrogen therapy and hip fractures, Ann Intern Med 95:28, 1981
Puleo, J, and Hammond, C: Conservative treatment of endometriosis externa: the effects of danazol therapy, Fertil Steril 40:164, 1983
Ranney, B, editor: Symposium on endometriosis, Clin Obstet Gynecol 23(3):863, 1980
Ross, RK, Paganini-Hill, A, Mack, TM, and Henderson, BE: Estrogen use and cardiovascular disease. In Mishell, DR, Jr, editor: Menopause: physiology and pharmacology, Chicago, 1987, Year Book Medical Publishers, Inc
Rutzick, B: Menopause support groups, Broomstick 2(9):5, 1980
Schneider, M, et al: The effect of exogenous estrogens on depression in menopausal women, Med J Aust 2:162, 1977
Seaman, B, and Seaman, G: Women and the crisis in sex hormones, New York, 1977, Rawson Associates, Publishers
Seidlitz, S: An interview, Midlifery 2:4, April 1978
Sohn, C, Korberly, B, and Tannenbaum, R: Menstrual products, Handbook of Nonprescription Drugs 17:371, 1986
Van Keep, PA: Maturitas 5(1):64, 1983
Weiss, NS, Ure, CL, Ballard, JH, et al: Decreased risk of fractures of the hip and lower forearm with postmenopausal use of estrogen, N Engl J Med 303:1195, 1980
Wheeler, J, and Malinak, LR: Recurrent endometriosis: incidence, management and prognosis, Am J Obstet Gynecol 146:247, 1983
Wheeler, J, et al: The relationship of endometriosis to spontaneous abortion, Fertil Steril 39:656, 1983
Willson, JR, et al: Obstetrics and gynecology, ed 7, St Louis, 1983, The CV Mosby Co
Wren, BG, and Routledge, AD: The effect of type and dose of oestrogen on the blood pressure of post-menopausal women, Maturitas 5:135, 1983

Bibliography

Albanese, JA, and Nutz, PA: Mosby's nursing drug cards, St Louis, 1988, The CV Mosby Co
Barbieri, RL (editorial): New therapy for endometriosis, Engl J Med 318(8):512, 1988
Brown, MA, and Woods, NF: Correlates of dysmenorrhea: a challenge to past stereotypes, JOGN Nurs 13(4):259, 1984
Budoff, PW: No more hot flashes and other good news, New York, 1983, GP Putnam's Sons
Byyny, RL: The women over 50: guidelines for preventive medicine, Contemp OB/GYN 31(Special issue):43, April, 1988
Creasman, WT, and Soper, JT: The undiagnosed adnexal mass after the menopause, Clin Obstet Gynecol 29(2):446, 1986
Chesnut, CH: Noninvasive techniques for measuring bone mass: a comparative review, Clin Obstet Gynecol 30(4):812, 1987
Dalsky, GP: Exercise: its effect on bone mineral content, Clin Obstet Gynecol 30(4):820, 1987
Davis, MR: Screening for postmenopausal osteoporosis, Fertil Steril 156:1, 1987
Delaney, J, et al: The curse: a cultural history of menstruation, New York, 1976, New American Library
Dwyer, JM: Manual of gynecologic nursing, Boston, 1986, Little, Brown & Co, Inc
Eagan, A: The selling of pre-menstrual syndrome, Ms Oct 1983
Eastell, R, and Riggs, BL: New approaches to the treatment of osteoporosis, Clin Obstet Gynecol 30(4):860, 1987
Ebersole, P, and Hess, P: Toward healthy aging: human needs and nursing response, ed 2, St Louis, 1985, The CV Mosby Co
Engel, NS: Menopausal stage, current life change, attitude toward women's roles, and perceived health status, Nurs Res 36(6):353, 1987
Fortier, KJ: Postmenopausal bleeding and the endometrium, Clin Obstet Gynecol 29(2):440, 1986
Gass, KA: Coping strategies of widows, J Gerontol Nurs 13(8):29, 1987
Graham, H, Hammond, J, and Ballard, J: The effects of physical activity and estrogen therapy upon bone loss in postmenopausal females, aged 50 to 68 years, JOGN Nurs 16(5):365, 1987
Griffith-Kenney, J: Contemporary women's health: a nursing advocacy approach, Menlo Park, Calif, 1986, Addison-Wesley Publishing Co, Inc
Halbreich, U, Alt, IH, and Paul, L: Premenstrual changes: impaired hormonal homeostasis. From Brown, WA, editor: Neurologic clinics, 6(1):173, 1988
Hammond, CB, and Maxson, WS: Estrogen replacement therapy, Clin Obstet Gynecol 29(2):407, 1986
Haney, AF: The "physiology" of the climacterium, Clin Obstet Gynecol 29(2):397, 1986
Havens, B, and Swenson, I: Menstrual perceptions and preparation among adolescent females, JOGN Nurs 15(5):406, 1986
Heaney, RP: The role of nutrition in prevention and management of osteoporosis, Clin Obstet Gynecol 30(4):833, 1987
Henderson, BE, Ross, RK, Paganini-Hill, A, and Mack, TM: Estrogen use and cardiovascular disease, Am J Obstet Gynecol 154:1181, 1986
Hodgkinson, CP: Rectovaginal fistual repair: succeeding on the second try, Contemp OB/GYN 23:93, March 1984 (Special issue)

Hoeffer, B: Predictors of life outlook of older single women, Res Nurs Health 10(2):111, 1987
Jaffe, MS, and Melson, KA: Laboratory and diagnostic cards: clinical implications and teaching, St Louis, 1988, The CV Mosby Co
Kaye, W, and Neff, S: Could her irregular menses be caused by bulimia? Contemp OB/GYN 21:97, May 1983 (Special issue)
Keating, SB, and Kelman, GB: Home health care nursing, Philadelphia, 1988, JB Lippincott Co
Lindsay, R: The menopause: sex steroids and osteoporosis, Clin Obstet Gynecol 30(4):847, 1987
Lublanezki, N, and Fischer, RG: OTC-menstrual pain preparations, Pediatr Nurs 13(6):435, 1987
Masterson, BJ: The women over 50: surgical evaluation of the gyn patient, Contemp OB/GYN 31(Special Issue):99, April 1988
Mezrow, G, and Rebar, RW: The women over 50: tailoring ERT to fit the patient, Contemp OB/GYN 31:51, April 1988 (Special issue)
Muggah, HF, and Staseson, S: The gynecological teaching associates program, Canadian Nurse, p 28, Feb, 1988
Nichols, DH: Preventing and treating enterocele, Contemp OB/GYN 23:16, March 1984 (Special issue)
Nichols, DH: Sacrospinous support after total vaginal prolapse, Contemp OB/GYN 23:42, March 1984 (Special issue)
Nichols, DH: The women over 50: managing prolapse with or without surgery, Contemp OB/GYN 31(Special Issue):159, April 1988
Notelovitz, M: The climacteric and osteoporosis, Clin Obstet Gynecol 30(4):787, 1987
Notelovitz, M, Kitchens, C, Ware, M, et al: Combination estrogen and progestogen replacement therapy does not adversely affect coagulation, Obstet Gynecol 62:596, 1983
Options in estrogen replacement therapy (Symposium), Contemp OB/GYN 31(3):190, 1988
Orque, MS, et al: Ethnic nursing care: a multicultural approach, St Louis, 1983, The CV Mosby Co
Parfitt, AM: Bone remodeling and bone loss: understanding the pathophysiology of osteoporosis, Clin Obstet Gynecol 30(4):789, 1987
Parker, RT, and Piscitelli, J: Gynecological surgery in the elderly patient, Clin Obstet Gynecol 29(2):453, 1986
Parker, RT: Woman: the climacterium and the years that follow, Clin Obstet Gynecol 29(2):341, 1986
Peterson, HB, Lee, NC, and Rubin, GL: Genital neoplasia. In Mishell, DR, Jr, editor: Menopause: physiology and pharmacology, Chicago, 1987, Year Book Medical Publishers, Inc
Prevention and treatment of postmenopausal osteoporosis, Med Lett 29(746):Aug 1987
Raisz, LG: Local and systemic factors in the parthogenesis of osteoporosis, N Engl J Med 318(13):818, 1988
Raymond, C: Hormone replacement: gynecologists consider the heart, JAMA 258(12):1573, 1987
Remondet, JH, and Hansson, RO: Assessing a widow's grief—a short index, J Gerontol Nurs 13(4):31, 1987
Richardson, DA, and Ramahl, A: The women over 50: typical urinary tract disorders, 31:145, April 1988 (Special issue)
Riis, B, Thomsen, K, and Christiansen, C: Does calcium supplementation prevent postmenopausal bone loss? N Engl J Med 316:173, 1987
Scully, D, and Bart, P: A funny thing happened on the way to the orifice: women in gynecology textbooks, Am J Soc 78:1045, 1973
Shelley, S, and Anderson, C: The influence of selected variables on the experience of menstrual distress in alcoholic and nonalcoholic women, JOGN Nurs 15(6):484, 1986
Smith, DH, and Rosenthal, MB: Sexuality and changes with aging, Contemp OB/GYN 31(6):88, 1988
Soper, JT, and Creasman, WT: Vulvar dystrophies, Clin Obstet Gynecol 29(2):431, 1986
Speroff, L: The women over 50: a new challenge for the gynecologist, Contemp. OB/GYN 31:22, April 1988 (Special issue)
Steege, JF: Sexual function in the aging woman, Clin Obstet Gynecol 29(2):462, 1986
Swenson, I, and Havens, B: Menarche and menstruation: a review of the literature, J Community Health Nurs 4(4):199, 1987
Vanzyl York, P: Nutritional needs of women. The Melpomene Report. A Journal for Women's Health Research, 6(2):10-14, 1987
Walton, J, and Youngkin, E: The effect of a support group on self-esteem of women with premenstrual syndrome, JOGN Nursing (16(3):174, May/June 1987
Wilhelm-Haas, E: Premenstrual syndrome: its nature, evaluation, and management, JOGN Nurs 13:223, 1984
Wilson, MA: Menstrual disorders: premenstrual syndrome, dysmenorrhea, amenorrhea, JOGN Nurs 13(2):11s, 1984

CHAPTER 42

Fertility Management

Barbara Derwinski-robinson

Learning Objectives

Correctly define the key terms listed.

List common causes of impaired fertility.

Discuss the psychologic impact of impaired fertility.

List common diagnoses and treatments for impaired fertility.

Describe the different methods of contraception.

State the advantages and disadvantages of commonly used methods of contraception.

Explain the common nursing actions that facilitate contraceptive use.

Evaluate the alternatives available to a woman experiencing an unplanned pregnancy.

Describe the techniques used for surgical interruption of pregnancy.

Recognize the various ethical and legal considerations of impaired infertility, control of fertility, and termination of fertility.

Key Terms

basal body temperature (BBT)
calendar method
cervical cap
cervical mucus method
condom
contraception
dilation and curettage (D&C)
diaphragm
elective abortion
fertile period
GIFT
impaired fertility
intrauterine device (IUD)
in vitro fertilization-embryo transplant
male contraception
oral contraceptives
periodic abstinence
predictor tests
referred shoulder pain
safe period
semen analysis
spinnbarkheit
therapeutic intrauterine insemination
thermal shift
vacuum (suction) curettage
vaginal sponge
withdrawal bleeding

This chapter addresses several fertility-related issues, associated tests, and common therapies. The reproductive spectrum is addressed covering everything from impaired fertility, to voluntary control of fertility, to surgical interruption of pregnancy.

IMPAIRED FERTILITY

The inability to conceive and bear a child comes as a surprise to 10% to 15% of otherwise healthy adults. It is difficult to be denied the experiences of pregnancy and birth, parenthood, and the expression of love through the care and nurturing of another human being. Disturbance in one's sexual self-concept is often experienced. Couples requesting assistance with impaired fertility problems have already decided that they want a child. They seek acceptance and assistance from the nurse and physician in coping with and possibly resolving these problems.

The traditional definition of impaired fertility is the inability to conceive after at least 1 year of adequate exposure when no contraceptive measures were used. It is also the inability to deliver a live infant after three consecutive conceptions. A contemporary definition does not consider a time limit. It is the inability to conceive or carry to live birth at a time the couple has chosen to do so.

Impaired fertility is *primary* if the woman has never been pregnant or the man has never impregnated a woman. It is *secondary* if the woman has been pregnant at least once but has not been able to conceive again or sustain a pregnancy. The incidence of impaired fertility seems to be increasing, probably because of (1) the trend to delay pregnancy until later in life when fertility decreases naturally, (2) the increase in pelvic inflammatory disease, and (3) the increase in substance abuse.

The following time frame during which 100 couples having unprotected intercourse might expect to become pregnant has been described by Hatcher et al. (1986). Approximately 25 of 100 couples will conceive in the first month; 35 additional couples will conceive in the second through the sixth month; 20 couples will conceive during the seventh through the seventeenth month; and an additional 10 couples will conceive during the eighteenth through the twenty-fourth month. When or if conception will occur for the remaining ten couples remains unknown. Impaired fertility testing is usually not begun until couples have experienced at least 1 year of unprotected intercourse. However, for the anxious couple or the older couple (woman over 30 years and man over 40 years), a 6-month effort is sufficient before fertility studies are begun.

Investigation of fertility and identification of the conditions that may be responsible for the infertile state constitute a long and tedious process. Impaired fertility may occur when a single fertility factor is absent. At other times a combination of factors, female and male, is necessary to impair fertility. Female and male factors each separately account for about 40% of impaired fertility. Factors from both partners are responsible for the remaining 20%. (Hatcher et al., 1986):

Male factor	40% to 50%
Tubal factor	20% to 25%
Ovulatory factor	20% to 25%
Cervical factor	1% to 2%
Uterine factor	1%
Unexplained	10%
Multifactorial	20% to 30%

The percentages equal more than 100% because the cause of impaired fertility for approximately one-third of couples involves multiple causality.

Of those couples seeking assistance for impaired fertility from any health care provider (i.e., nurse clinician, general medical practitioner, a "generalist" practitioner of obstetrics and gynecology, or an andrologist [a urologist who specializes in impaired fertility]), Kilmann (1984) reports that 40% will discover the cause, correct the cause, and conceive. An uncorrectable cause will be discovered by 40%, and for 20% of couples neither a cause can be determined nor will they conceive. Of infertile women seeking care from specialist, 50% will become pregnant. Of the remaining 50%, the cause will be found for approximately 90%. However, not all of these causes are correctable. Despite knowing the cause, approximately 40% of these women will be unable to conceive. For 10% of women seeking assistance from specialists, no known cause for their impaired fertility will be found. Couples with 4 or more years of impaired fertility have a poor conception prognosis, even if no demonstrable pathology is ever found. Diagnosis and treatment of impaired fertility require considerable physical, emotional, and financial investment over an extended period of time.

Some of the data needed to investigate impaired fertility are of a sensitive, personal nature. Obtaining these data may be viewed as an invasion of privacy. The tests and examinations are occasionally painful and intrusive and can take the romance out of lovemaking. A high level of motivation is needed to endure the investigation. The attitude, sensitivity, and caring nature of those who are involved in the assessment of impaired fertility lay the foundation for the client's ability to cope with the subsequent therapy and management. All members of the health team must respect the clients' rights to privacy and the confidentiality of client records.

Religious Considerations

Civil laws and religious proscriptions about sex must always be kept in mind by the clinician. For example, the Orthodox Jewish husband and wife may face infertility investigation and management problems because of religious laws that govern marital relations. According to Jewish law the couple may not engage in marital relations during menstruation and through the following 7 "preparatory days." The wife then is immersed in a ritual bath (Mikvah) before relations can resume. The 5 menstrual days and 7 preparatory days collectively are called the "nida state." Any vaginal bleeding of physiologic origin marks the beginning of the nida state. Fertility problems can arise when the woman has a short cycle (i.e., a cycle of 24 days or less, when ovulation would occur on day 10 or earlier). Small doses of estrogen may delay ovulation to allow for the time needed to complete the nida state. Other procedures that induce bleeding may delay intercourse for another 12 days to allow for the nida state. Thus Orthodox Jewish clients, as well as observant Catholics, may at times question proposed diagnostic and therapeutic procedures because of religious proscriptions. These clients are encouraged to consult their rabbi or priest for a ruling.

In the book of Genesis, God commanded Adam and Eve to be fruitful and multiply. Ever since, humankind has tried to heed that command. Some religions view procreation as the sole purpose of sexual intercourse. Furthermore, parenthood is seen as a way to purge sexual intercourse of its sinfulness. According to some religious teachings, a woman must bear children to reach heaven, or to free souls from bondage, or to purge herself from sin. Other religions teach that a marriage can be annulled if a woman is found to be infertile, though the reverse is not true if a man is found to be infertile. Religious influences over fertility and hence impaired fertility account for many of the sociocultural attitudes displayed toward childless couples (Menning, 1977).

Cultural Considerations

Worldwide cultures continue to employ symbols and rites that celebrate fertility. One fertility rite that persists today is the custom of throwing rice at the bride and groom. Other fertility symbols and rites include the passing out of congratulatory cigars by a new father, and baby showers held in anticipation of a child's birth. Last but not least is the American image of motherhood. Though Americans do not worship motherhood as an icon as in ancient cultures, mothers and motherhood are paid homage, especially in the communications media of the United States. It is no wonder that Mother's Day is the busiest day for telephone companies and one of the busiest for florists. (Fogel and Woods, 1981).

The person without children in Samoa is pitied. According to Borwnlee (1978), in many cultures a woman's inability to conceive may be due to her sins, to evil spirits, or to the fact that she is an inadequate person. The virility of a man in some cultures remains in question until he demonstrates his ability to reproduce by having at least one child.

Determination of a culturally defined cause for sterility is usually accompanied by a culturally proposed solution for the problem. These proposed solutions may or may not be effective. For example, Vietnamese men thought sterility was caused by loss of sperm, or spermatorrhea, during nocturnal emissions (wet dreams) or through daytime discharge (Coughlin, 1965). Tonics consisting of licorice, aconite, and ginseng might be used to counteract the effect. Certain foods such as cereal were to be eaten, and substances such as alcohol were to be avoided.

In most cultures, responsibility for impaired fertility is usually attributed to the woman. If infertility is believed to be caused by a misplaced uterus, methods are used to replace it. A Samoan woman may go to a bush doctor who will massage the abdomen over the uterus with oil and attempt to put it back in place (Clark and Howland, 1978).

For Mexican-American women and others who subscribe to heat/cold balance and imbalance theories, barrenness is considered to result from having a "cold womb" (Clark, 1970). The cold womb may be heated through external and internal means. Clark (1970) describes two methods used by Mexican-American women. One method requires a barren woman to sit over a washtub of hot water, to which rosemary is added, so that the vapors warm the womb. The other method attempts to build up body heat over a period of 3 days. This is done by avoiding cold foods and water, using a belladonna plaster over the sacral area, and ingesting cathartic pills and hot chocolate.

Assessment

The nurse assists in obtaining data relevant to fertility through interview and physical examination (see Chapter 8, Table 42-1, and boxes, pp. 1064 and 1065). The data base needs to include information to identify whether infertility is primary or secondary. Religious, cultural, and ethnic data are noted.

Many couples have already visited various physicians and have read extensively on the subject. Their previous experiences are recorded. The depth and breadth of their knowledge base is explored.

Factors Associated with Impaired Fertility

Investigation of fertility and identification of the conditions that may be responsible for the infertile state constitute a long and tedious process (usually 3 months or more). Impaired fertility may occur when a single fertility factor is absent. At other times a combination of factors, female and male, is necessary to impair fertility. In Table 42-1 each factor essential to fertility is presented along with a listing of conditions associated with impaired fertility. Assessment for fertility factors in the woman and in the man are outlined in the boxes on pp. 1064 and 1065.

Nursing Diagnoses

Following are examples of nursing diagnoses that may become apparent from the data base.

- Knowledge deficit related to
  - Anatomy and physiology of reproduction
  - Investigtion of impaired fertility
  - Cause, course, management, and expected prognosis of condition
- Potential for altered individual/family coping related to
  - Need for and methods used in the investigation of impaired fertility
- Potential self-esteem disturbance related to
  - Impaired fertility
- Potential for social isolation or spiritual distress or dysfunctional grieving related to
  - Impaired fertility, its investigation, and management

Planning

Planning requires sensitivity to the client's needs. Based on knowledge of impaired fertility, the nurse is equipped to assist with the development of a plan of care for the couple with impaired fertility. The plan is developed in collaboration with the physician in light of the nurse's level of expertise and with other members of the health team and the couple to achieve certain mutually determined goals. The goals are phrased in client-centered terms.

Goals

1. Couple is educated in the anatomy and physiology of the reproductive system.
2. Any abnormalities identified through various tests and examinations are treated (e.g., infections, blocked uterine tubes, sperm allergy, varicocele).
3. Couple receives an estimate of their chances to conceive.
4. Couple resolves guilt feelings and does not need to focus blame.

Table 42-1 *Factors Associated with Fertility and Impaired Fertility*

Factor Required for Fertility	Conditions Associated with Impaired Fertility
Development of reproductive tract is normal.	Congenital or developmental factors Abnormal external genitals (e.g., enlarged clitoris or fused labia) which may suggest masculinization Gynetresia (e.g., absence of vagina or shallow vagina) Vaginal anomalies (e.g., double vagina with single or double cervix and single or double uterus or with one vaginal canal ending blindly, the other vaginal canal ending at entrance to a uterus) Unusual uterus (e.g., congenitally small, or "infantile," uterus) Uterine and tubal defects from exposure to DES as embryo/fetus Abnormalities of ovaries (see ovulation)
Ovulation: hypothalamus-pituitary-gonadal axis is normal. An ovum is released from a mature ovarian follicle.	Absence of ovulation Malfunctioning of axis with menstrual irregularities Abnormal ovaries are seen in Turner's syndrome or Stein-Leventhal syndrome Hormonal suppression of hypothalamus-pituitary-gonadal axis with birth control medication Emotional problems (e.g., severe psychoneurosis or psychosis or anorexia nervosa, which may be responsible for anovulatory cycles, commonly associated with amenorrhea or oligomenorrhea) Menstrual irregularities from vigorous exercise (jogging, sports), especially in thin women
Tubal: ovum enters uterine tube promptly after ovulation. Sperm migrate into uterine tube, where fertilization takes place. Fertilized ovum finds its way down tube into endometrial cavity to implant into hormone-prepared endometrium 7 to 10 days after ovulation.	Uterine tube is blocked or its function is altered Blockage of tube by scar tissue formation after infection (pelvic inflammatory disease, ruptured appendix followed by peritonitis) or pelvic surgery Blockage of tube by compression or kinking by abnormal growth such as endometriosis and neoplasms Alteration in tubal motility by birth control medication or from emotional stress
Uterine: endometrium is adequately prepared to receive fertilized ovum.	Uterus is malformed or endometrium is unreceptive to fertilized ovum (malfunction of hypothalamus-pituitary-gonadal axis; presence of endometrial infection; presence of intrauterine device [IUD])
Vaginal-cervical mucus is receptive and supportive to sperm. Cervix is competent.	Absence of mucous characteristics receptive and supportive to sperm Altered vaginal pH from feminine hygiene preparations or douches, infections, antibiotic chemotherapy, disease states (e.g., diabetes mellitus), poor hygiene, or emotional stress Presence of spermicidal foams or other preparations used for contraception Development of antibodies (an immunologic response) against a specific male's sperm (see discussion of sperm, in assessments of the woman and the man)
Sperm are normal, adequate in number, and ejaculated into female reproductive tract.	Sperm factors discussed later in this chapter
Conceptus develops normally, reaches viability, and is delivered in good condition.	

5. Couple conceives or, failing to conceive, decides on an alternative acceptable to both of them (e.g., childlessness, adoption, or therapeutic intrauterine insemination).
6. Couple finds acceptable methods for handling pressures they may feel from peers and relatives regarding their childless state.

Implementation

Nursing actions vary with the nurse's level of education, position held, and policies of the agency. Basic to all nursing actions is knowledge of those factors that are essential to or contribute to fertility, of assessment strategies (history, examinations, and tests), and of management and therapy for infertility. The nurse acts on the client's readiness to learn and her or his level of understanding of impaired fertility. Although primary responsibility for teaching the client or clients rests with the physician, the nurse assists in the identification of the client's gaps in knowledge, clarifies information, and reinforces the physician's explanations and instructions. Occasionally the nurse acts as the client's advocate by helping the client state a concern or question or request further explanation from the physician or technician.

The nurse's nonverbal behavior before and during the procedure can reassure and support the client. Often the client feels inadequate because of the necessity for testing and the intimidating nature of the tests.

Written and verbal instructions for specific preparation

ASSESSMENT OF THE WOMAN

History

1. Duration of impaired fertility: length of contraceptive and noncontraceptive exposure
2. Fertility in other marriages of self or spouse
3. Obstetric
   a. Number of pregnancies and abortions
   b. Length of time required to initiate each pregnancy
   c. Complications of any pregnancy
   d. Duration of lactation
4. Gynecologic: detailed menstrual history and leukorrheal history
5. Previous tests and therapy done for infertility
6. Medical: general medical history including chronic and hereditary disease; drug use
7. Surgical: especially abdominal or pelvic surgery
8. Sexual history in detail: libido, orgasm capacity, techniques, frequency of intercourse, and postcoital practices
9. Psychosomatic evaluation
   a. General
   b. As regards impaired fertility, particularly her reason for seeking advice at this time

Physical Examination

1. General: careful examination of other organs and parts of body; special attention given to habitus, fat and hair distribution, acne
2. Genital tract: state of hymen (full penetration); clitoris; vaginal infection, including trichomoniasis and candidiasis; cervical tears, polyps, infection, patency of os, accessibility to insemination; uterus, including size and position, mobility; adnexae, tumors, evidence of endometriosis

Laboratory Data

1. Routine urine, complete blood count, and serologic test for syphilis; additional laboratory studies as indicated
2. Basic endocrine studies in women with irregular menstrual cycles or in amenorrhea, hirsutism, acne, or excessive weight gain

Irregular Menstrual Cycles	*Amenorrhea*
Protein-bound iodine (PBI) or other thyroid tests	Tomographic x-ray films of skull
17-Ketosteroids	T_4 or other thyroid tests
17-Hydroxycorticoids	17-Ketosteroids
4-Hour glucose tolerance test	17-Hydroxycorticoids
Endometrial biopsy	4-Hour glucose tolerance test
	Endometrial biopsy
	Gonadotropin determination
	Buccal smear and chromosomal studies

   Other laboratory tests added as desired for a more complete diagnosis of endocrine problems
3. RH factor and antibody titer tests—important in abortion and premature delivery problems
4. Sperm antibody agglutination studies. Special laboratory procedure involves obtaining a fresh semen specimen from man and a blood sample from the woman. Sperm are incubated in the blood serum of the woman and checked at intervals for agglutination; the test is negative if no agglutinated sperm are found.

for tests will increase the client's feeling of adequacy. Supportive nursing actions include providing privacy while giving instructions for obtaining specimens and changing clothes, draping, creating a comfortable physical environment, padding the stirrups of the examination table, efficiency in use of equipment, warming the speculum, and coaching for relaxation.

In addition to discussing the specifics of common tests for impaired fertility, nurses can provide sensory information about these future tests. McHugh, et al. (1982) define sensory information as "information about our environment that is acquired by way of our sensory modalities-sight, hearing, touch, taste, and smell". To acquire descriptions of commonly used tests, nurses can interview current clients and ask them to describe their tests in sensory terms. Then nurses can share the most frequently occurring descriptions with future clients. Providing preparatory information can help clients form a mental image of what an experience will include and thus help make the testing experience more tolerable and less distressing.

Women often experience anxiety when undergoing a pelvic examination (Chapter 8). After any procedure, often the client is fully dressed and comfortably seated (at the same level as the nurse and physician), she or he benefits

ASSESSMENT OF THE MAN

History

1. Fertility in other marriages of self or spouse
2. Medical: general medical history, including venereal infections, mumps orchitis, chronic diseases, recent fever, drug use
3. Surgical: herniorraphy, injuries to genitals, or other surgery in genital area
4. Occupational: exposure to chemicals, x-ray equipment, or extreme therapy changes; physical nature of occupation; vacations and work habits
5. Previous tests and therapy done for study of impaired fertility
6. Duration of impaired fertility
7. Sex history in detail, with discussion of actual coital techniques; such as frequency and ability to ejaculate
8. Adequacy of erection

Physical Examination

1. General examination: careful examination of other organs and parts of body, with special attention given to habitus, fat and hair distribution
2. Genital tract: penis and urethra; scrotal size; position, size, and consistency of testes; epididymides and vasa deferentia; prostate size and consistency
3. Careful search for varicocele, with man in both supine and upright positions

Laboratory Data

1. Routine urine, complete blood count, and serologic test for syphilis
2. Complete semen analysis—essential
   a. Liquefaction: usually complete within 10 to 30 minutes
   b. Semen volume — 2-5 ml (range: 1 to 7 ml)
   c. Semen pH — 7.2 to 7.8
   d. Sperm density — 20 to 200 million/ml
   e. Normal morphology (%) — ≥60%
   f. Motility (important consideration in sperm evaluation); percentage of forward-moving sperm estimated in relationship to abnormally motile and nonmotile sperm. This requires evaluation by a technician with some degree of experience but as the test provides a more accurate diagnosis; it is well worth the time involved; ≥50% is normal
   g. Cell count: average normal, 60 million or more per milliliter or a total of 150 to 200 or more million per ejaculate; minimum normal standards: 40 million/ml, with a total count of at least 125 million per ejaculate (average of counts on two or preferably three separate specimens)

   NOTE: These values are not absolute, but only relative to the final evaluation of the couple as a single reproductive unit.
3. Additional laboratory studies as indicated
   a. Basic endocrine studies indicated in men with oligospermia or aspermia:
      (1) Tomographic x-ray films of skull
      (2) T_4 or other thyroid tests
      (3) 17-Ketosteroids
      (4) Gonadotropin determination
      (5) 17-Hydroxycorticoids and pregnanediol
      (6) Buccal smear and chromosome studies, for example, Klinefelter's syndrome, XXY sex chromosomes
      (7) Test for sperm antibodies; autoimmunization. Autoimmune antibodies (produced by the man against his own sperm) agglutinate or immobilize sperm is less than 5% of men with impaired fertility
   b. Testicular biopsy, where correct interpretation is available (may give a more accurate diagnosis and prognosis in cases of azoospermia and severe oligospermia), vasography if indicated and available

from an opportunity to talk about the experience in an unhurried manner. Not only do these behaviors help the client relax, but also they indicate that the recipient of such care is worthy and thus helps build self-esteem. The goal of nursing-medical *care* is to encourage the client to become an active partner in care as well as to establish rapport to ensure that therapy and eventual counseling is facilitated.

The nurse needs to know the correct method for obtaining, labeling, and transporting specimens to the laboratory. A mishandled specimen may lead to misdiagnosis or the need to obtain another specimen. These errors create added expense to the client as well as significant time delays before therapy can be instituted.

Feelings connected to impaired fertility are many and complex.* The origin of some of these feelings are myths, superstitions, misinformation, or "magical" thinking about the cause of infertility. Other feelings arise from the need to undergo many tests and examinations and from being "different" from others.

Menning (1977) and Speroff et al. (1983) have tried to debunk some common myths. These myths include:

1. *Infertility has a psychologic origin.* For 80% to 90% of all cases of impaired fertility, there is a discernible physiologic explanation.
2. *Adopting improves a couple's chance of conceiving.* A classic, often quoted, study by Rock et al. (1965) found no significant increase in conception among 113 couples with impaired fertility who had adopted and 249 couples who had not adopted.
3. *Being infertile is a sexual disorder.* For most couples, impaired fertility is not related to their ability to perform sexual intercourse.
4. *It is immoral to wish to bear children and to actively pursue that goal.* For those who wish to have children, their impaired fertility is an involuntary barrier to their choice of parenthood.

Veevers' (1973) report on the social meaning of parenthood and nonparenthood provides further insight into the psychosocial impact of impaired fertility. To the extent to which a society perceives nonparenthood as unnatural, as an avoidance of responsibility, a rejection of gender role, a sign of immaturity, or a hindrance to positive marital adjustment is the extent to which couples with impaired fertility may perceive their society as being nonsupportive. Under such circumstances, an infertile couple might have problems not only accepting their impaired fertility but also in discussing their feelings with health care providers.

Nurses can help clients express and talk about their feelings as honestly as possible. Ventilation may help couples unburden themselves of negative feelings. Professional referral may be necessary.

The myriad of psychologic responses to a diagnosis of impaired fertility may tax a couple's giving and receiving of physical and sexual closeness. The prescriptions and proscriptions for achieving conception may add tension to a couple's sexual functioning. Couples are instructed about frequency and timing of intercourse as well as use of certain coital positions. It is no wonder that couples complain of decreased desire for intercourse, orgasmic dysfunction, or midcycle erectile disorders. A once spontaneous act of expressing love has become a mechanical act for creating a baby.

During evaluation of impaired fertility, the previously private act of intercourse becomes a topic of discussion. Even in the sexually liberated culture of the 1980s, few people eagerly share the frequency of coitus and positions used during intercourse.

To be able to deal comfortably with a couple's sexuality, nurses must be comfortable with their own sexuality. Nurses need to resolve their sexual identity, have up-to-date factual knowledge about human sexual practices, be able to accept the preferences and activities of others without being judgmental, acquire skill in interviewing and in therapeutic use of self, develop sensitivity to the nonverbal cues of others, and be knowledgeable of the couple's sociocultural and religious tenets. Once nurses are comfortable with their own sexuality, they can better help couples understand why the private act of lovemaking needs to be shared with health care professionals.

Because of the interference with the spontaneity of coitus, many infertility specialists limit the period of investigation. These specialists have found that the shorter the diagnostic period, the less the disruption of a couple's sexual lifestyle.

The woman or couple facing impaired fertility exhibits behaviors that resemble the *grieving process* that is associated with loss (Chapter 28). The loss of one's genetic continuity with the generations to come leads to loss of self-esteem, of a sense of adequacy as a woman (or man), of control over one's destiny, and of a sense of self. The investigative process leads to a loss of spontaneity and control over the couple's marital relationship and sometimes over one's progress toward career and life goals. All people do not experience every one of the reactions described below nor can the length of time be predicted that any one reaction will last for an individual.

The nurse may feel at a loss in knowing how to assist. Table 42-2 presents characteristic behaviors of people experiencing the psychologic impact of impaired fertility along with some suggestions for nursing (or other health professionals') actions.

The support systems of the couple with impaired fertility need to be explored. This exploration should include persons available to assist, their relationship to the couple, their ages, their availability, and the cultural or religious support that is available. This type of assessment is suitable for a health team conference where representatives of several disciplines can share ideas and work cooperatively in developing a plan for management.

If the couple conceives, nurses need to be aware that the concerns and problems of the previously infertile couple may not be over. Many couples are overjoyed with the pregnancy. However, some are not. Some couples rearrange their lives, sense of self, and personal goals within their acceptance of their infertile state. The couple may feel that those who worked with them to identify and treat impaired fertility expect them to be happy with the pregnancy. The couple may be shocked to find that they them-

*See Chapter 7 for psychosocial aspects and Chapter 28, Loss and Grief.

Table 42-2 *Nursing Actions: Behavior Associated with Impaired Fertility*

Behavioral Characteristic	Nursing Actions
Surprise: each person assumes she or he is fertile and that pregnancy is an option.	Point out resemblance to grieving process—a normal, expected reaction to loss. Refer to support group.* Prepare them for length of time it may take to grieve, types of feelings (psychologic, somatic) to expect. Encourage and allow time to talk of past and present feelings of sexuality, self-image, and self-esteem.
Denial: "It can't happen to me!"	Allow time for denial because it gives the body and mind time to adjust a little at a time. Do not feed into the client's denial; instead say, "It must be hard to believe such a devastating report."
Anger: toward others (perhaps even at the nurse) or themselves.	Explain that the reaction to loss of control and to a feeling of helplessness is often anger, which can easily be projected onto another person. Without release, anger can lead to chronic depression. Anger is a natural feeling. Allow time to express anger at losing their sense of control over their bodies and destinies; identify and direct energy directly at the problem. Airing one's own anger often eases the intensity of the emotion. A helpful approach may be, "It's OK to be angry . . . at those who are pregnant, at people who want abortions, at self, at mate, at caregivers, and so forth."
Bargaining: "If I get pregnant, I'll dedicate the child to God.	Accept bargaining statements without comment.
Depression:	
Isolation: personal.	Allow time for both woman and man to talk about how it feels whenever a sight, event, or word serves as a reminder of own state of impaired fertility. Develop role playing situations to practice interactions with others under various circumstances to increase the couple's ability to cope and to problem solve (increases their self-confidence). The nurse may say, "You must feel so terribly alone sometimes."
Guilt/unworthiness.	Allow time to identify feelings that may be based on earlier behaviors (e.g., abortion, premarital sex, contact with sexually transmitted disease [STD]). Goal: couple or person comes to the realization that "unworthiness" and impaired fertility are unrelated.
Acceptance (resolution).	Clients need to know that grief feelings are never laid away forever; they may be activated by special reminders (e.g., anniversaries).

*RESOLVE, Inc, PO Box 474, Boston, Mass 02178.

selves feel resentment because the pregnancy, once a cherished dream, now necessitates another change in goals, aspirations, and identities. The normal ambivalence toward pregnancy (Chapter 12) may be perceived as reneging on the original choice to become parents. The couple may choose to abort the pregnancy at this time (see p. 1103). If the couple wishes to continue with the pregnancy, they will need the care pregnant couples need (see Unit III). The couple may need extra preparation for the realities of pregnancy, labor, and parenthood, because they have developed fantasies about childbearing when they thought it was beyond their reach. *A history of impaired fertility is considered to be a risk factor for pregnancy.* The couple who has a history of impaired fertility before this pregnancy faces another label, that of being at high risk for this pregnancy (see Chapter 27).

The couple too may desire information about contraception after the birth of this baby. If the previously infertile couple desires additional children, the couple is advised about those contraceptive methods that are least likely to cause damage and impair fertility.

If the couple does not conceive, they are assessed regarding their desire to be referred for help with adoption, therapeutic intrauterine insemination, or with choosing childlessness. The couple would find a list of such agencies within their particular community helpful. Examples of community agencies, besides RESOLVE, are OURS* and ARENA* (organizations for those who wish to adopt), and National Organization for Nonparents* (for those who choose to remain childless).

Evaluation

The nurse can be reasonably assured that care was effective when the client-centered goals have been achieved:

1. Couple increases their knowledge of anatomy and physiology of reproduction.
2. Couple collaborates with the investigation of impaired fertility.
3. Any abnormalities identified through various tests and examinations are treated successfully.

*Lists of such groups throughout the United States can be obtained from OURS, Inc, 20140 Pine Ridge Dr, Anoaka, MN 55303.

4. Couple resolves guilt feelings and does not need to focus blame.
5. If the couple conceives, the couple accepts their responses to pregnancy, realigns their goals, aspirations, and identities, and is comfortable with their decisions regarding the pregnancy.
6. If the couple does not conceive, they decide on an acceptable alternative and seek support as necessary. They find acceptable methods for handling pressures they may feel from peers and relatives regarding their childless state, and they receive a list of community agencies that assist with adoptions or provide appropriate support.

Investigation of Female Infertility

There are several examinations and tests for impaired fertility. Each method of assessment is discussed under the following headings: which partner is involved in testing or in collection of the specimen, why the test is done, when the test is scheduled, how and where the test is accomplished, the risks involved, the information that is sought, and specific medical and nursing actions pertinent to the situation. Nurses can alleviate some of the mystery associated with impaired fertility by telling the clients of the timing and rationale for each test (Table 42-3).

Self-assessment of basal body temperature (BBT) and cervical mucus (pp. 1087 and 1089) involves touching oneself and one's discharges. Therefore self-assessment can be emotionally uncomfortable for some women. The nurse may also be uneasy teaching self-assessment techniques to others. Fertility test findings favorable to fertility are summarized on p. 1078.

Congenital or Developmental Factors. If the woman has abnormal external genitals, surgical reconstruction of abnormal tissue and construction of a functional vagina may permit normal intercourse. If internal reproductive tract structures are absent, there is no hope for fertility. Surgical intervention depends entirely on the anatomic development, the surgical feasibility, and the individual's actual gender role. Laparoscopy is one surgical technique that is used for both diagnosis and treatment of intraabdominal disorders (see box, p. 1069).

Vaginal and uterine anomalies and their surgical repair vary from individual to individual. If a functional uterus can be reconstructed, pregnancy may be possible. After surgical repair of the uterus, cesarean delivery is necessary to prevent uterine rupture during labor. Women with ovarian agenesis or dysgenesis are sterile, and no treatment will improve their fertility.

Ovarian Factors

Review of Ovarian Function. Within healthy ovaries, graafian follicles respond to follicle-stimulating hormone (FSH) and luteinizing hormone (LH) by the maturation of an ovum and ovulation. The graafian follicle produces estrogen; the empty graafian follicle becomes the corpus luteum and produces estrogen and progesterone.

Impairment of Ovarian Function. Anovulation may be primary. *Primary anovulation* may be caused by a pituitary ot hypothalamic hormone disorder or an adrenal gland disorder such as congenital adrenal hyperplasia. *Secondary anovulation* may be caused by ovarian disease. In amenorrheic states and instances of anovulatory cycles, hormone studies usually reveal the problem (see boxes, p. 1071).

Table 42-3 *Tests for Impaired Fertility: Timing and Rationale*

Menstrual Cycle Days	Test/Examination	Rationale
1-4	Hysterosalpingogram Tubal insufflation (Rubin test)	Late follicular, early proliferative phase will not disrupt a fertilized ovum. May open uterine tubes before time of ovulation.
Peak cervical mucus flow*	Postcoital (Sims-Huhner test)	Ovulatory late proliferative phase—look for normal motile sperm in cervical mucus.
	Sperm immobilization antigen-antibody reaction	Immunologic test to determine sperm and cervical mucus interaction.
	Assessment of cervical mucus	Cervical mucus should have low viscosity, high spinnbarkheit.
Ovulation	Ultrasound observation of follicular collapse	Collapsed follicle is seen after ovulation.
20-25	Serum assay of plasma progesterone	Midluteal midsecretory phase—check adequacy of corpus luteal production of progesterone.
	Basal body temperature (BBT)	Elevation occurs in response to progesterone.
26–27	Endometrial biopsy	Late luteal, late secretory phase—check endometrial response to progesterone and adequacy of luteal phase.

*Exogenous estrogen may be given to induce mucus flow if spontaneous and reasonably regular ovulation does not occur.

LAPAROSCOPY

Who: Woman and a driver to take her home

Why: To assess visually the organs in the interior of the abdomen; and to perform minor surgical procedures

How: A small telescope is inserted through a small incision in the anterior abdominal wall using cold fiberoptic light sources that allow for superior visualization of the internal pelvis (Fig. 42-1)

When: Laparoscopy is timed depending on the purpose: if tubal patency is to be assessed, it is done 2 to 6 days following cessation of menses; if sites of endometriosis are to be treated, any day of the cycle is appropriate

Where: In a surgical suite with an anesthesiologist present (may be done on an outpatient basis)

Risk:
1. Usually general anesthesia is used
2. A pneumoperitoneum is established by insufflation of carbon dioxide gas via a needle inserted through the abdominal wall
3. Complications are rare (about 1 in 500): infection; electric burns of intraabdominal tissue
4. Postoperative shoulder (referred) pain or subcostal discomfort may occur for a short time

Procedure

- Woman signs informed consent and is prepared verbally for the examination.
- Woman is usually admitted a few hours before surgery having taken nothing by mouth (NPO) for 8 hours.
- Woman voids just before surgery.
- Woman's pubic area is shaved only if examination is likely to be followed by laparotomy.
- Anesthesia is given: general anesthesia with intubation; occasionally, local.
- Woman is placed in a modified lithotomy position, with the legs at 45 degrees.
- The vagina, perineum, and abdomen are prepared and draped, and the area from the umbilicus to the vagina is exposed.
- An intrauterine probe is inserted except in cases where intrauterine pregnancy may be present.
- A needle is inserted and a pneumoperitoneum with carbon dioxide gas is established to elevate the abdominal wall from the organs creating an empty space that permits visualization and exploration with laparoscope. Rubin's cannula is used for injections of methylene blue dye to assess for tubal patency. The needle may be inserted at lower border of umbilicus.
- Examination or procedure is performed.
- After surgery, deflation of most of gas is done by direct expression. Trocar (and needle) sites are closed with a single subcuticular absorbable suture or a skin clip, and an adhesive bandage is applied.
- Postoperative recovery requires taking of vital signs, assessing level of consciousness, preventing aspiration, monitoring intravenous fluids, and reassuring client regarding shoulder discomfort. Discharge from hospital usually occurs in 4 to 6 hours.
- Shoulder or subcostal discomfort (from pneumoperitoneum) usually lasts only 24 hours and is relieved with a mild analgesic.
- Caution the woman against heavy lifting or strenuous activity for 4 to 7 days, at which time she is usually asymptomatic.

Information Sought

Findings favorable to fertility:
1. No developmental abnormalities of pelvic structures.
2. No lesions, infections, or adhesions.
3. No complications occur as a result of the examination or procedure.
4. If tubal insufflation is done, the tubes are found to be patent.
5. If there is a reparable problem (e.g., adhesions that are kinking the uterine tubes), the problem is repaired through the laparoscope.

Fig. 42-1 Laparoscopy.

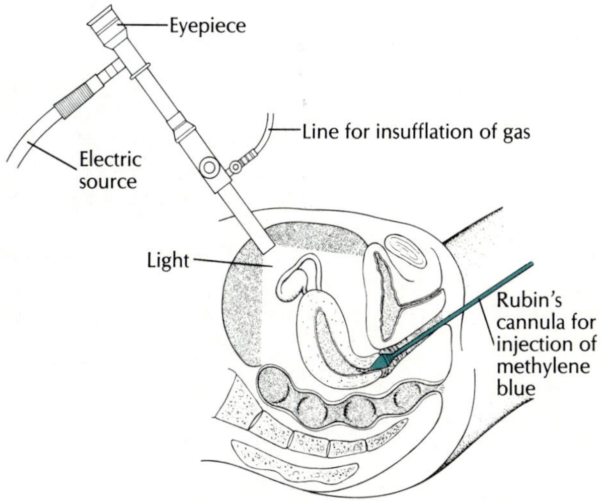

ULTRASOUND PELVIC EXAMINATION

Who: Woman

Why: To visualize pelvic tissues for a variety of reasons (e.g., to identify abnormalities, to verify follicular development and maturity to determine timing for retrieval of ova for preparation of in vitro fertilization or for planning of therapeutic intrauterine insemination, to confirm intrauterine [vs. ectopic] pregnancy)

When: Timing depends on the purpose

How: Use of static scanner or a real-time scanner (Chapter 27); if indicated, a bimanual examination may be performed under ultrasound observation

Where: Clinic or office

Risk: Low, diagnostic ultrasound is physically safe; no anesthesia is needed

Procedure	Information Sought
• Woman's bladder is full to permit visualization of uterus and adnexa if abdominal ultrasound is used. • Bladder need not be full if vaginal ultrasound is used (FIg. 42-2). • Woman is positioned comfortably and the examination is performed. • Findings are discussed with woman.	Findings favorable to fertility: 1. Size, shape, position of reproductive structures are within normal limits. 2. Ovarian changes of follicle development, ovulation, and formation of corpus luteum can be documented and occur within normal limits. 3. No abnormalities such as ovarian cysts, tubal pathology, masses, or foreign bodies (broken intrauterine devices [IUDs]) are seen.

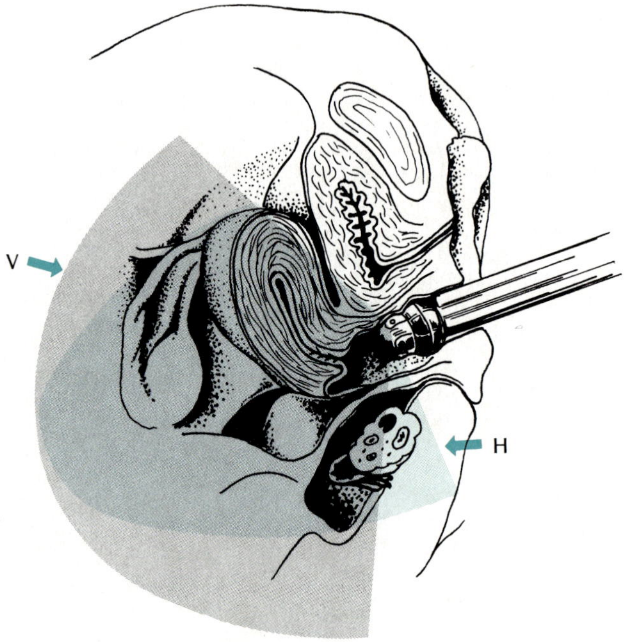

Fig. 42-2 Vaginal ultrasonography. Major scanning planes of transducer: H = horizontal, V = vertical.

HORMONE ANALYSIS

Who: Woman
Why: To assess endocrine function
How: Blood and urine specimens are obtained
When: At varying times during menstrual cycle
Where: Clinic, physician's office, or hospital laboratory
Risk: 1. Low
2. Discomfort from venipuncture
3. Inconvenience of collecting urine and taking to laboratory (when urine specimens are used)

Procedure	Information Sought
• Blood sample is drawn.	Findings favorable to fertility: 1. Levels of progesterone, estrogen, FSH and LH are all appropriate.
• Urine specimen is obtained.	2. Levels of 17-ketosteroids and 17-hydroxycorticosteroids are within normal limits.

TIMED ENDOMETRIAL BIOPSY

Who: Woman and a driver to take her home
Why: To assess function of corpus luteum and receptivity of endometrium for implantation; and to check for tuberculosis*
How: Sample of endometrium is removed for histologic study
When: Late in menstrual cycle; 3 to 4 days before expected menses
Where: Clinic or hospital surgical suite
Risk: 1. Analgesia and anesthesia (paracervical block, Chapter 17 and p. 1108) may be needed
2. Discomfort from uterine cramping

Procedure	Information Sought
• Couple is cautioned to abstain from intercourse during preceding "fertile" period to avoid dislodging a possible pregnancy during procedure. • Cervix is dilated with laminaria† 4 to 24 hours before procedure (requires no analgesia). • Woman assumes lithotomy position, is draped, and has a speculum inserted. • Laminaria are removed. • If not previously dilated with laminaria, cervix is dilated now with metal rod dilators. Analgesia/anesthesia is often necessary. • Small specimen of endometrium is removed from side wall in fundus to avoid an embryo should conception have occurred.‡	Findings favorable to fertility: 1. Endometrium is negative for tuberculosis, polyps, or inflammatory conditions. 2. Endometrium reflects secretory changes normally seen in presence of adequate luteal (progesterone) phase.

*The incidence of tuberculosis is high today because large numbers of recent refugees have come to the United States with the disease.
†Laminaria are small, thin inserts of packed seaweed, which, when inserted into the cervix, absorb moisture and thus dilate the cervix (Fig. 42-11).
‡When implantation occurs, it is usually high in the fundus, either in the anterior or in the posterior portion.

Treatment and Prognosis. In some instances endocrine therapy with so-called fertility drugs such as oral clomiphene citrate (Clomid) or with intramuscular human menopausal gonadotropin (hMG) (Pergonal) may induce ovulation in anovulatory women (Table 42-4).

Ovarian tumors must be excised; whenever possible, functional ovarian tissue is left intact. Chronic infection, which may cover much or all of the ovary, usually necessitates surgery to free and expose the ovary so that ovulation can occur.

An increasing number of young women are experiencing *secondary amenorrhea.* Their history reveals a serious interest in jogging and other sports or a considerable weight loss that has been followed by menstrual irregularities (see also Chapter 41). Their dietary history may reveal meals that consist of lean red meat and calorie-free soda drinks. Examination results commonly reveal amenorrhea or menstrual irregularities and osteoporosis (from loss of calcium). The woman who engages in vigorous exercise with normal menstrual cycle does not need to be concerned about osteoporosis (see also Chapter 41). She may have actually increased her calcium levels in bones and thereby increased their healthy density. Any woman who has missed two or three periods, however, is urged to consult a reproductive endocrinologist or an obstetrician-gynecologist.

Thyroid gland dysfunction may be associated with menstrual abnormalities, impaired fertility, or recurrent fetal waste. Therapy consists of management of the thyroid condition coupled with careful scrutiny of BBT charts (p. 1087) for synchrony of sperm deposition with ovulation before fertilization. Continuous monitoring and management of thyroid function during pregnancy is also carried out. The same thyroid aberrations have occasionally been associated with unaltered reproductive ability.

In the presence of severe emotional problems the woman is referred to a mental health therapist. Her condition may require the teamwork of the mental health therapist, the endocrinologist, and an obstetrician-gynecologist.

Diazepam (Valium) ingestion may be responsible for menstrual irregularities or failure to ovulate, changes in libido, and gynecomastia, possibly by raising estrogen levels. These effects can be reversed simply by withdrawing from the drug.

Tubal (Peritoneal) Factors

Review of Tubal Function. The fingerlike processes of the fimbriated end of the uterine tube and the tube itself need to be freely movable to approach the ovary to "catch" the ovum. The tube must be open, sufficiently long, and capable of ciliary action and peristalsis to carry the ovum into and down the tube. In most cases fertilization occurs in the ampulla of the tube. Some unknown factor, possibly an enzyme, supplied by the ampulla of the tube seems to be required for the physiologic change or "conditioning" of the sperm called capacitation (see Chapter 9).

Impairment of Tubal Function. The motility of the tube and its fimbriated end may be reduced or absent as a result of infections, adhesions, or tumors (Chapter 30). In rare instances there may be congenital absence of one tube. It is also possible to find one tube relatively shorter than the other. This condition is often associated with an abnormally developed uterus.

Inflammation within the tube or involving the exterior of the tube or the fimbriated ends represents a major cause of impaired fertility. Tubal adhesions resulting from pelvic infections (e.g., ruptured appendix) may impair fertility. Infection with purulent discharge eventually heals by scar formation. In the process the tube may be blocked anywhere along its length. Tubal patency is assessed by methods such as the Rubin test (box below, p. 1074; Fig. 42-3). It can be closed off at the fimbriated end, or it can be distorted and kinked by adhesions. Adhesions may permit the tiny sperm to pass through the tube but may prevent a fertilized egg from completing the journey into the intrauterine cavity. This results in an ectopic pregnancy that may completely destroy the tube (see discussion of ectopic pregnancy).

In other cases, adhesions of the tubes to the ovary or bowel may follow *endometriosis.* Endometriosis is a disease in which endometrial tissue, ordinarily found only within the uterus, is present outside the uterus attached to other organs or tissue in the woman's body (Chapter 41). The ectopic endometrial tissue responds to hormonal stimulation in the way that uterine endometrium does. In endometriosis, periodic monthly bleeding from endometrial implants causes dense adhesions, making pregnancy difficult or impossible.

Treatment and Prognosis. Treatment must include prevention and early adequate management of infection with appropriate antibiotics. Surgery may be necessary when drainage of a serious focus of infection is required. Hysterosalpingography is useful for identification of tubal obstruction and also for the release of blockage. During laparoscopy, delicate adhesions may be divided and removed and endometrial implants may be destroyed by electrocoagulation. Laparotomy and even microsurgery may be required to do extensive repair of the damaged tube. Prognosis is dependent on the degree to which tube patency and function can be restored.

Uterine Factors

Review of Uterine Functions. The uterus must be of sufficient size and shape to permit maintenance of a pregnancy to term. The endometrium must be prepared by estrogen and progesterone and must be healthy for implantation to occur.

Impairment of Uterine Function. *Congenital abnormalities* of the uterus are far more common than might be expected. Minor developmental anomalies of the uterus are fairly common; major anomalies occur rarely (Fig. 42-4). Hysterosalpingography may reveal a double uterus or other anomalous congenital variations that include a T-shaped uterus and a boxlike uterus (see box, p. 1075). These types of uteruses have been described in daughters of women who took diethylstilbestrol (DES) during the early months

Table 42-4 *Drug Therapy for Female Infertility*

Drug	Indications	Nursing Actions
Ovulatory Stimulants		
Clomiphene citrate (Clomid; Serophene) (O)—follicular maturing agents	Anovulation caused by hypothalamic suppression (but with an intact hypothalamic-pituitary-ovarian axis)	Counsel regarding oral ingestion of Clomid or Serophene, maintenance of BBT chart for evidence of ovulation, and potential side effects: ovarian cyst formation, vasomotor effects; visual disturbances, partial alopecia, abdominal disturbances, and multiple pregnancies.
Bromocriptine (Parlodel), a synthetic ergot alkaloid	Anovulation caused by elevated levels of prolactin (inhibits release of prolactin)	Counsel regarding oral ingestion of drug with food to reduce its side effects: nausea, vomiting, lightheadedness, dizziness (tolerance develops within a few weeks; menstruation resumes in 75% of women in 6 to 8 weeks). Should not be taken with drugs that elevate prolactin levels, for example, psychotropic agents. Monitor BBT so that drug is discontinued if pregnancy occurs.
Thyroid stimulating hormone (TSH)	Anovulation caused by hypothyroidism	Counsel regarding medical regimen: medication and assessment of blood levels of TSH.
Human menopausal gonadotropin (hMG) (Pergonal; Profasi HP)	Anovulation caused by hypogonadotropic amenorrhea	Administer or test self-injection of hMG.
Gonadotropin-releasing hormone (GnRH), alone or preceded by clomiphene citrate or hMG	Anovulation caused by hypothalamic-pituitary dysfunction, hypothalamic failure, or failure to ovulate with use of Clomid or Serophene	Assist with daily injection or teach woman self-injection. Overall success rate is 15% to 20%.
Hormone Replacement Therapy		
Conjugated estrogens and medroxyprogesterone	Hypoestrogenic condition: high stress level, decreased level of body fat caused by eating disorder (e.g., anorexia nervosa) or excessive exercise	Counsel regarding oral ingestion—estrogens on days 1 to 24 and progesterone on days 15 to 24; possible side effects (e.g., fluid retention); stress reduction and so on.
Hydroxyprogesterone supplementation (vaginal suppositories or IM)	Luteal phase defects	Counsel regarding administration: start 3 to 4 days after estimated ovulation and continue to menses (if no menses, a serum pregnancy test is done).
	Endometriosis	Assist with protocol of care (Chapter 41).
Other		
Prednisone (O) (a glucocorticoid)	Congenital adrenal hyperplasia	Counsel regarding oral ingestion regimen and associated side effects.
Danazol	Endometriosis	Assist with counseling woman regarding daily dosages and possible side effects: weight gain, hot flushes, night sweats, decrease in breast size, bloody vaginal discharge, atrophic vaginitis.
Mefenamic acid; Naproxen	Dysmenorrhea with pain, nausea, vomiting, headaches, fainting, diarrhea that are induced by danazol therapy for endometriosis	Counsel regarding need to start therapy 48 hours before onset of dysmenorrhea.
Antimicrobial Therapy	Infection	Implement usual actions when administering antimicrobial medications.

RUBIN TEST

Who: Woman and a driver to take her home
Why: To assess patency of uterine tube or tubes
How: Tubal insufflation with carbon dioxide gas (Fig. 42-3)
When: 2 to 6 days after menses to avoid forcing possible fertilized ovum through tube into peritoneal cavity; in the absence of infection to avoid forcing infectious material through tube into abdomen
Where: Clinic or physician's office
Risk: 1. Low; no exposure to radiation
2. Discomfort: uterine cramping during procedure; referred shoulder pain after procedure
3. False-positive readings

Procedure	Information Sought
• Woman assumes lithotomy position and is draped. • Analgesia may be required. • Vaginal speculum is inserted; cannula is inserted into cervical os; carbon dioxide gas is passed through cervix to uterus and tubes with the rate and pressure under careful control.	Findings favorable to fertility: 1. Woman experiences referred shoulder pain. 2. Auscultation of abdomen reveals passage of air through tubes. 3. Carbon dioxide pressure is below 150 mm Hg. *False results* (tube is patent, but gas flow is obstructed) may result from poor technique or spasms of the tubes. *Possible therapeutic effects* of test: passage of carbon dioxide may clear out tubes or straighten out kinked tubes.

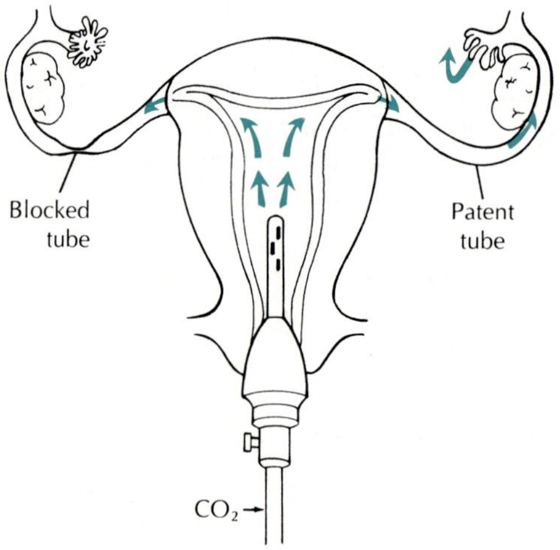

Fig. 42-3 Rubin test. Carbon dioxide escapes into abdominal cavity through patent left uterine tube.

of pregnancy. Endometrial and myometrial *tumors* (e.g., polyps or myomas) may also be revealed by x-ray studies of infertile women.

Asherman's syndrome, uterine adhesion or scar tissue, is characterized by hypomenorrhea or amenorrhea. The adhesions, which may partially or totally obliterate the uterine cavity, are sequelae to surgical interventions such as too vigorous curettage (scraping) after an abortion (elective or spontaneous). The hysteroscope is useful in the verification of intrauterine scars as well as for the localization and removal of displaced or broken intrauterine devices (IUDs).

Endometritis (inflammation of the endometrium) may result from any of the causes of infection of the uterine tubes. Women who use an IUD are more susceptible to endometrial infection than are nonusers.

Treatment and Prognosis. A woman with a relatively small uterus may become pregnant, but the uterus may be

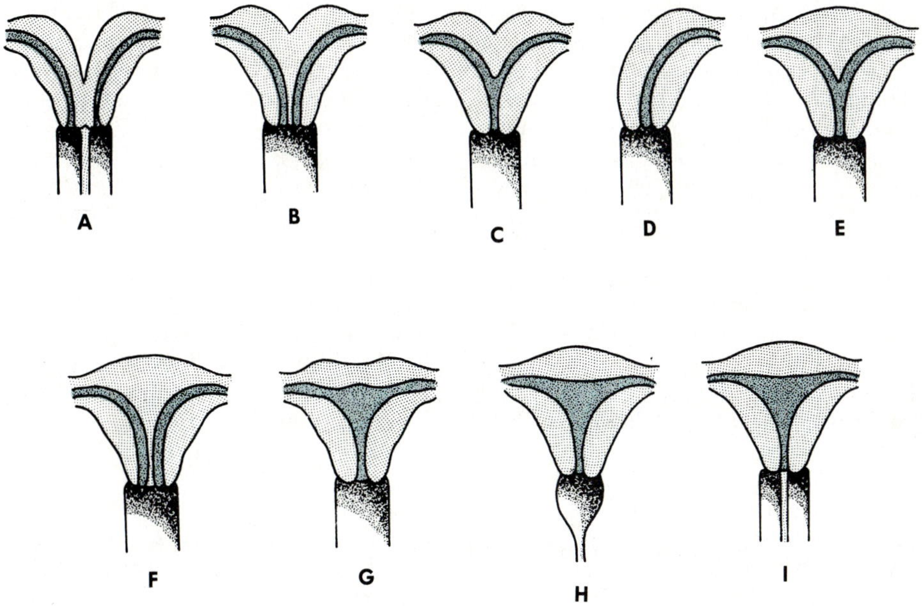

Fig. 42-4 Abnormal uteruses. **A**, Uterus didelphys bicollis (septate vagina). **B**, Uterus bicornis bicollis (vagina simplex). **C**, Uterus bicornis unicollis (vagina simplex). **D**, Uterus unicornis. **E**, Uterus subseptus. **F**, Uterus septus. **G**, Uterus arcuatus. **H**, Congenital stricture of vagina. **I**, Septate vagina.
Modified from Willson, JR, and Carrington, ER: Obstetrics and gynecology, ed 6, St Louis, 1979, The CV Mosby Co.

HYSTEROSALPINGOGRAPHY

Who: Woman and a driver to take her home
Why: To assess tubal patency and endometrial cavity to a lesser degree; to assess uterine mobility
How: Fluoroscopic visualization (image intensification fluoroscopy) or spread of radiopaque dye
When: 2 to 6 days after menstruation to avoid flushing a fertilized ovum out through a tube into the perionteal cavity; if the woman has pelvic inflammatory disease (PID), she is treated with antibiotics first, and the test is rescheduled in 2 to 3 months
Where: Radiology department
Risk: 1. Allergy to radiopaque dye
2. Possible need for premedication
3. Exposure to radiation
4. Discomfort: uterine cramping during procedure; referred shoulder pain after procedure
5. Need for someone to drive her home if medicated or in pain

Procedure	Information Sought
• Woman may be premedicated. • Woman assumes lithotomy position and is draped. • Vaginal speculum is inserted. • Dye is instilled into uterus with a special cannula inserted into the cervical canal. Dye (Ethiodol*) is injected under controlled pressure. • Usually three films are taken: 1. Before dye instillation 2. As dye spills out from one or both tubes. 3. After dye has spread throughout cavity. • The shoulder pain: 1. Subsides with position change. 2. Disappears usually within 12 to 24 hours. 3. Is controlled by mild analgesics. • Perineal pad is applied to protect clothing from dye.	Findings favorable to fertility: 1. Spilling of dye into peritoneum within 10 to 15 minutes. 2. Spread of dye throughout peritoneal cavity. 3. Referred shoulder pain. Shoulder pain is indicative of subphrenic irritation from the chemical if the chemical spilled into peritoneal cavity. Possible therapeutic effects of test: 1. Passage of dye may clear tubes of mucous plugs, straighten kinked tubes, or break up adhesions. 2. Cilia may be stimulated in the lining of the tubes. 3. It may aid healing as a result of the bacteriostatic effect of dye (iodine).

*Ethiodol, a liquid, oil-based dye, produces a better picture, has a lower incidence of injection pain, and results in better post-hysterosalpingography pregnancy rates than does water-soluble sodium acetrizoate (Salpix). Embolization and possible death are extremely rare but have occurred after hysterosalpingography with either Ethiodol or Salpix. Therefore informed consent should state this fact.

incapable of accommodating the enlarging fetus, and a spontaneous abortion may result. In such cases recurrent or habitual (three or more) spontaneous abortions often occur. No medical therapy has been effective for the enlargement of an abnormally small uterus. Observation suggests that women who do become pregnant but who miscarry often abort at a later time with each successive pregnancy. Finally, after two or three pregnancy losses, they may deliver a viable infant. Apparently actual "growth" of the uterus occurs with each pregnancy. Plastic surgery—for example, the unification operation for bicornuate uterus—often improves a woman's ability to conceive and carry the fetus to term.

Impaired fertility may result from infections such as endometrial tuberculosis (from an acid-fast bacillus) or schistosomiasis (from a fluke parasite), which are significant health problems in many parts of the world including the Near East, Puerto Rico, and South America. These disorders often involve the tubes and ovaries. Medical cure of the infection may permit pregnancy despite some scarring of the endometrium.

Surgical removal of tumors involving the endometrium or uterus often improves the woman's chance of conceiving and maintaining the pregnancy to viability. Surgical treatment of uterine tumors or maldevelopment that results in successful pregnancy requires delivery by cesarean surgery near term. The uterus may rupture as a result of weakness of the area of surgical healing.

Vaginal-Cervical Factors

Review of Vaginal-Cervical Function. Vaginal fluid is acid (pH of 4 or less), whereas cervical mucus is normally alkaline (pH of 7 or more). Ejaculation should place the sperm at or near the cervical os. The alkalinity of cervical mucus helps support sperm and permits the ascending transportation of sperm at the time of ovulation.

In addition, endocervical mucus normally obstructs or plugs the cervix, acting as a barrier against infection. The latter is important because, in the woman, ascending infection to the peritoneum is virtually unimpeded with a normally patent genital tract. Alkaline mucus in the cervix not only controls procreation but also is a specific protection to life and health. The amount of cervical mucus and its characteristics are influenced by the hormones estrogen and progesterone (see Table 10-3 and Figs. 6-26 and 6-27).

Impairment of Vaginal-cervical Function. Vaginal-cervical infections (e.g., *Trichomonas* vaginitis chlamydial infection) increase the acidity of the vaginal fluid and reduce the alkalinity of the cervical mucus. Thus vaginal infection often destroys or drastically reduces the number of viable, motile sperm before they enter the cervical canal. The amount of mucus and its physical changes are influenced by the presence of blood, pathogenic bacteria, and such irritants as an IUD or a tumor. Severe emotional stress, antibiotic therapy, and diseases such as diabetes mellitus alter the acidity of mucus.

About 20% of infertile women have sperm antibodies.* Sperm may be immobilized within the cervical mucus, or they become incapable of migration into the uterus (see postcoital test, box, p. 1077). A greater incidence of sperm agglutination occurs in women with otherwise unexplained impaired fertility. However, the true significance and reliability of tests for sperm immobilization or agglutination are uncertain.

Treatment and Prognosis. Therapy for lower genital infection requires the elimination of vaginitis or cervicitis (Chapter 30). Appropriate antibiotic or chemotherapeutic drugs generally resolve this problem. In addition to antibiotics, radial chemocautery (destruction of tissue with chemicals) or thermocautery (destruction of tissue with heat, usually electrical) of the cervix, cryosurgery (destruction of tissue by application of extreme cold, usually liquid nitrogen), or conization (excision of a cone-shaped piece of tissue from the endocervix) is effective in eliminating chronic infection. When the cervix has been deeply cauterized or frozen or when extensive conization has been performed, extreme limitation of mucus production by the cervix may result. Therefore sperm migration may be difficult or impossible because of the absence of a mucous "bridge" from the vagina to the uterus. Therapeutic intrauterine insemination may be necessary to carry the sperm directly through the *internal os* of the cervix.

If the cervical os is unusually small, it is often called a pinhole os. In such cases, gentle dilation of the cervix or several shallow radial incisions followed by dilation are often sufficient to open the lower cervix. In contrast, if the cervix is grossly lacerated after delivery and widely gapping, suturing the cervix (trachelorrhaphy) or cryosurgery may be required to reduce the size of the external os. Prevention of recurrent infection helps maintain a column of mucus.

Good general hygiene must be practiced to minimize vaginal infections. The woman benefits from good hand washing before and after elimination of urine and stool. To avoid self-contamination, she must wipe from front to back once with each tissue and never wipe back and forth over the perineal area. Feminine deodorants, soaps that are heavily colored and perfumed, bubble-bath salts that cause chemical irritation, and tight clothing that provide a dark damp milieu favorable to microbial growth are avoided. Good nutrition is practiced with the avoidance of large amounts of unrefined sugars which raise the pH of vaginal fluids. To maintain a healthy vaginal-cervical pH during antibiotic therapy, the woman may insert one or two applicators full of cultured yogurt (not pasteurized) once or twice daily. As a general rule, douching is avoided unless by prescription from a physician (Chapter 44).

Good mental health helps prevent some forms of vaginitis that could become secondarily infected. Stress from anxiety, worry, and emotional discomfort increases the vaginal pH so that vaginal infections are more likely to take hold. Concurrent medical conditions such as diabetes mellitus must be controlled to maintain vaginal-cervical pH within normal range.

Treatment is available for women who have *immunologic reactions to sperm.* Exposure to semen via the orogenital and anal modes is avoided. The use of condoms during genital intercourse for 6 to 12 months will reduce

*The production of antibodies by one member of a species against something that is commonly found within that species is termed *isoimmunization.*

POSTCOITAL TEST

Who: Both the woman and the man

Why: To test for adequacy of coital technique, cervical mucus, sperm, and degree of sperm penetration

How: Assessment of specimen of cervical mucus following ejaculation of semen into vagina

When: 8 to 24 hours after sexual intercourse that is synchronized with expected time of ovulation (as determined from evaluation of BBT, cervical mucus changes, and usual length of menstrual cycle); performed only in the absence of vaginal infection

Where: Clinic or office

Risk:
1. Low; physically safe; no anesthesia is needed because having this test feels about the same as having a Papanicolaou smear
2. May be difficult to have intercourse with ejaculation "on schedule"; sex "on demand" may strain the couple's interpersonal relationship
3. Expected day of ovulation may occur when facilities or physician is unavailable

Procedure	Information Sought
• Couple is asked to abstain from intercourse for 48 hours before test commences. • Then intercourse with ejaculation into vaginal vault should occur within the 8 hours before the test. • Woman may shower but not bathe between time of intercourse and test. • Within 24 hours after intercourse, but preferably 8 hours, in the office or clinic: 1. Woman is positioned in lithotomy position and draped; speculum is inserted without lubrication (no lubrication is needed at this time because mucus is abundant and the lubricant may alter the viscosity of the cervical mucus and invalidate the results); cervix is cleansed. 2. Mucus is removed with a syringe, cannula, or cotton-tipped swab from the internal and the external cervical os and examined for macroscopic and microscopic characteristics.	Findings favorable to fertility: 1. Coital technique is adequate if sperm is found. 2. Mucus is supportive if many sperm are motile. 3. If more than 20 motile sperm are found, male most likely produces at least 20 million/ml.* 4. Mucus is clear and abundant, with good spinnbarkheit. 5. A drop of each specimen is used for the fern test; with high estrogen at ovulation, fern pattern (arborization) is seen (Fig. 6-27, *A*).

*Postcoital test is *not* a substitute for semen analysis.

female antibody production in the majority of women who have elevated antisperm antibody titers. After the serum reaction subsides, condoms are used at all times except at the expected time of ovulation. Approximately one third of couples with this problem conceive by following this course of action. A summary of fertility test findings favorable to fertility is outlined in the box on p. 1078.

The prognosis for the infertile woman is generally good provided a serious genital or inflammatory disorder is not identified. Most women present numerous so-called minor problems that, although compounded, may be relatively easy to correct (e.g., chronic cervicitis, hypothyroidism). If successful treatment has not been achieved after a year, for example, other alternatives may be considered (e.g., adoption, childlessness, therapeutic insemination, or in vitro fertilization).

In Vitro Fertilization and Embryo Transfer (IVF-ET)

The first successful term delivery of an infant conceived by in vitro fertilization (test-tube pregnancy) in 1978 was the culmination of years of study and experimentation by Robert Edwards and Patrick Steptoe in England. Since then several other "laboratory conceived" and normal-appearing newborns have been delivered.

Many women whose uterine tubes either are obstructed or have been removed are not potential candidates for similar treatment. However, because of the complexity and cost of the procedure, the likelihood is that this approach to impaired fertility must remain limited for the near future. The following steps, ultrasimplified, are necessary for in vitro fertilization.

1. Ovulation is induced by gonadotropin therapy (clomiphene citrate).
2. Mature follicles are identified by laparoscopy, and needle aspiration of ova is carried out.
3. Ova are transferred to tissue culture media.
4. Before laparoscopy semen is collected. Freshly ejaculated sperm cannot fertilize an ovum; they must be capacitated. A simple process in humans, capacitation involves only a short incubation period in a culture medium. After capacitation, sperm are added to the ova (Pernoll and Benson, 1987).
5. After fertilization a second tissue culture transfer allows division to approximately a 12-cell blastocyst (3 to 6 days).

SUMMARY OF FERTILITY TEST FINDINGS FAVORABLE TO FERTILITY

1. Follicular development, ovulation, and luteal development are supportive to pregnancy:
   a. BBT (presumptive evidence of ovulatory cycles)
      (1) Is biphasic
      (2) Reveals temperature elevation that persists for 12 to 14 days just before menstruation
   b. Cervical mucus characteristics change appropriately during phases of the menstrual cycle
   c. Findings from endometrial biopsies taken at different times during menstrual cycle are consistent with day of cycle
   d. Laparoscopic visualization of pelvic organs verifies follicular and luteal development
2. The luteal phase is supportive to pregnancy:
   a. Levels of plasma progesterone are adequate
   b. Endometrial biopsy findings indicate a secretory endometrium
3. Cervical factors are receptive to sperm during expected time of ovulation:
   a. Cervical os is open
   b. Cervical mucus is clear, watery, abundant, and slippery and demonstrates good spinnbarkheit and arborization (fern pattern)
   c. Cervical examination is negative for lesions and infections
   d. Postcoital test findings are satisfactory (adequate number of live, motile, normal sperm present in cervical mucus)
   e. No immunity to sperm can be demonstrated
4. The uterus and uterine tubes are supportive to pregnancy:
   a. Uterine and tubal patency is documented by
      (1) Passage of carbon dioxide into peritoneal cavity
      (2) Spillage of dye into peritoneal cavity
      (3) Outlines of uterine and tubal cavities of adequate size and shape with no abnormalities
   b. Laparoscopic examination verifies normal development of internal genitals and absence of adhesions, infections, endometriosis, and other lesions
5. Semen is supportive to pregnancy:
   a. Sperm are adequate in number per milliliter of ejaculate
   b. Majority of sperm show normal morphology
   c. Sperm are motile
   d. No autoimmunity exists
   e. Seminal fluid is normal

6. Progesterone therapy in the interval induces a late secretory type of endometrium, whereupon the blastocyst is transferred to the uterus, where the implantation (nidation) of the zygote occurs and embryonic development proceeds.

Within an 18-month period, overall success rates for in vitro fertilization worldwide have risen from 1% to 8% to almost 20%. This vast improvement is attributable to increased precision in predicting ovulation and in retrieving the ovum. The conventional methods of predicting ovulation—calendar, BBT, cervical mucus, fertility awareness, and laboratory tests such as vaginal cytology and serum hormone determination—can only approximate the moment of ovulation. The more precise methods are beyond the scope of this text but are mentioned here for interest. These methods are (1) stimulating ovulation with clomiphene citrate (Clomid) or human menopausal gonadotropin (hMG) (Pergonal) given at a precise time during the cycle, (2) monitoring ovulatory function with realtime ultrasound, and (3) performing rapid radioimmunoassay for estrogen level. Through a laparoscope the ovum is retrieved by inserting an aspiration needle into the ripened follicle and removing the ovum. The husband's semen is collected and treated before its use for fertilization of the ovum. The complete procedure is described by Marrs (1982). Pace-Owens (1985) found that in vitro fertilization costs from $3000 to $6000 per treatment.

Human experimentation and manipulation of this type have been sanctioned by the United States Department of Health and Human Services. The Roman Catholic Church is strongly opposed to in vitro fertilization. Legal aspects of in vitro fertilization are discussed in Chapter 4.

Gamete Intrafallopian Tube Transfer

Gamete intrafallopian (uterine) tube transfer (GIFT) is similar to IVF-ET. Ovulation is induced as in IVF-ET; an hCG injection is given; and the oocytes are aspirated from follicles via laparoscopy or minilaparotomy (Pernol and Benson, 1987; Asch, et al., 1984). Before laparoscopy, semen is collected. Sperm are capacitated using the same technique as for IVF-ET. The eggs are identified in the laboratory. Capacitated sperm are then mixed with the ova and drawn up into a catheter. The ova and sperm are then transferred to the uterine tubes, permitting natural fertilization and cleavage, with subsequent successful pregnancies. A 20% to 30% pregnancy rate per cycle has been reported for this technique.

GIFT is only useful for women who have normal tubal function. The success of this technique has not been compared with the less complicated technique of simple induced ovulation combined with therapeutic intrauterine insemination. GIFT is more expensive to perform than IVF-ET using ultrasound egg aspiration.

Other Techniques. *Ovum or embryo transfer* involves inseminating a donor female with semen from the husband of an infertile woman (Bustillo et al., 1984). After 4 days, when the fertilized (or unfertilized) egg reaches the uterus, it is lavaged out of the donor female and placed into the uterus of the infertile wife. The infertile woman carries the pregnancy. Term pregnancy rate is only 3%.

Embryos have been *donated* from one woman to another with resultant live births. These women are not candidates for IVF-ET because of severe pelvic adhesions or absence of functional ovaries. In the latter case, the endometrium must be primed with estrogen and progesterone before transfer to the donated embryo. Progesterone supplementation must be maintained for 10 weeks.

Freezing and preservation of the embryo for thawing and transfer in a later cycle have been successful in cattle but have had limited success in humans. Oocyte cryopreservation has not been successful in any species. No one advocates the discarding of embryos (see ethical issues, Chapter 4).

These, as well as the other procedures, have enormous future potential but create many ethical and legal concerns.

Complications. Other than the established risks associated with laparoscopy and general anesthesia, few risks are associated with IVF-ET, GIFT, or other techniques. Congenital anomalies occur no more frequently than in normally conceived embryos. Ectopic pregnancies, however, do occur, and these carry a significant maternal risk.

Investigation of Male Infertility

Factors Implicated in Male Infertility. Male reproductive failure may be caused by many of the difficulties that also affect women, such as nutritional, endocrine, and psychologic disorders. In Table 42-1 each factor essential to fertility is presented, along with a listing of conditions associated with impaired fertility. Assessment for male fertility factors is outlined on p. 1065. Substance abuse may have adverse effects on male infertility (Table 42-5).

Semen is analyzed early in the diagnostic process: A sperm analysis is done at least twice to determine whether oligospermia or other abnormalities are likely. Before collecting a specimen the man avoids ejaculation for 2 to 3 days. Then he collects a specimen from masturbation in a clean glass jar and takes the sealed jar to the laboratory within 2 hours after emission. Warming or chilling the specimen is not required. The Roman Catholic man may prefer to remove ejaculated sperm from the woman's vagina with a Doyle (vaginal) spoon. A condom should not be used for collection of the semen (unless a special sheath manufactured by the Milex Corporation is used), since any residual rubber solvents and sulfur present would alter the specimen. The semen is examined for gross appearance and other characteristics (pp. 1065 and 1078).

A summary of infertility factors, tests, and nursing actions are presented in Table 42-6. Fertility test findings favorable to fertility are summarized on p. 1078.

General Therapies. *Medical therapy* for male infertility has been disappointing, especially when pituitary or testicular diseases are discovered. Occasionally it is possible to suppress the production of sperm with injections of testosterone and in that way cause a reduction in the number of autoimmune antibodies present in the man. Following the reduction in sperm autoantibodies, sperm quality improves, and a pregnancy sometimes occurs. Drug therapy for male infertility is discussed in Table 42-7.

The difficulty may be caused by timing and frequency of intercourse. The couple is taught about the menstrual cycle, the peak cervical mucus symptom, and appropriate timing of intercourse.

Penile intromission is often difficult because of chordee and obesity. In these situations the couple is advised to alter positions used for intercourse. Heavy use of alcohol makes penile erection difficult to achieve and maintain until ejaculation. The man is advised to avoid imbibing alcohol during the time of the woman's ovulation.

Infections (e.g., T mycoplasma) are identified and treated promptly. Poor nutritional state is corrected if it exists. Problems with the thyroid or adrenal glands are corrected.

Table 42-5 ***Substance Abuse and Male Infertility***

Substance	Possible Effects
Alcohol	Causes erectile problems ("impotence").
Marijuana *(Cannabis sativa)*	Adversely affects spermatogenesis: decreases number and motility, decreases percentages of sperm with the normal oval configuration. Potential permanent damage to germ cells (does not seem to affect testosterone production, however). Causes gynecomastia, especially if taken in combination with psychoactive and antidepressant drugs.
Monoamine oxidase (MAO) (antidepressant)	Adversely affects spermatogenesis.
Amyl nitrate, butyl nitrate, ethyl chloride, methaqualone (used to prolong orgasm)	Results in changes in spermatogenesis.
Heroin, methadone, barbiturates	Decreases libido.

Table 42-6 *Male Infertility Factors, Tests, and Nursing Actions*

Infertility Factor	Tests	Nursing Actions
Physical		
Semen composition	Microscopic analysis: sperm density, motility, structure	Counsel regarding collection of specimen
Absence or decreased number of sperm: ambiguous genitals; disparity of testicular size	Testicular biopsy	Preoperative preparation for general anesthesia Postoperative: ice bag to scrotum, suspensory, mild analgesics
Small gonads, inadequate virilization	Karyotyping for chromosomal abnormality Determination of gonadotropin levels	Assist with protocol of care
Obstructive lesions of vas and epididymis	Vasography often done with testicular biopsy or x-ray examination using contrast medium	Preoperative and postoperative care as above.
Integrity of hypothalamic-pituitary-testicular axis	Clomiphene citrate (Clomid or Serophene) stimulation of pituitary to release LH and FSH	Counsel regarding oral ingestion for the 5-7 days preceding the test
	Gonadotropin-releasing hormone (GnRH) stimulation* of pituitary to release LH and FSH	Assist in office or clinic
	Human chorionic gonadotropin (hCG) stimulation of Leydig cell function and increased testosterone production	Assist with protocols for test in office or clinic
Infections—viral (mumps) or bacterial (tuberculosis or gonorrhea)	Assessment for current infection	Counsel regarding need to follow directions for antibiotic therapy; use of oral lactinex or lacto-bacillus or cultured yogurt to prevent intestinal upset from antibiotic therapy
Semen volume	Measurement of volume after 2-3 days of abstinence from ejaculation	Counsel regarding protocols for abstention, collection, and transportation to laboratory
Sperm agglutination and *sperm immobilization antigen-antibody reaction*	Assessment for infection *(Escherichia coli);* Kibrick (agglutination) and Isojima (immobilization) test for circulating and seminal sperm agglutinating autoantibodies	Assist with protocols for tests.
Sperm antibodies	Serum tests (e.g., Kibrick, Isojima)	Assist with protocols for tests
Retrograde ejaculation†	Measurement of ejaculate volume and assessment for sperm in urine after ejaculation	Assist with protocols for tests
Varicocele	Physical examination	Assist as indicated
Trauma—long-term catheterization, foreign objects in urethra (e.g., hair-pin)	Physical examination	Assist as indicated
Testis torsion	Physical examination; history of sudden onset with intense pain or recurrent, less severe orchidynia (pain)	Assist as indicated; prepare for surgery as above
Psychosocial		
Male sexual dysfunction	Psychiatric and physical work-up	Provide caring, nonjudgmental attitude and an unrushed and confidential milieu; assist the physician to dispel misinformation and reassure client regarding her/his behavior‡
Religious proscriptions	History	Assist as indicated; counsel regarding approaching clergy/rabbi with problems/concerns

*Experimental.
†Passage of semen deposited into prostatic urethra during emission back up into the bladder through an incompetent bladder neck.
‡Requires special education and skills.

Table 42-7 *Drug Therapy for Male Infertility*

Drug	Indications	Nursing Actions
Testosterone enanthate (Delatestryl) and testosterone cypionate (Depo-Testerone) by injection	Stimulate virilization, especially the adolescent	Teach self-administration, or administer every 2 weeks
hCG (Pregnyl), IM (LH activity)	Virilize a hypogonadotropic male to restore Leydig cell function and spermatogenesis	Administer three times a week, perhaps for 18 months
FSH (human menopausal gonadotropin [hMG], Pergonal or Profasi HP)	Aid hCG for completion of spermatogenesis	Administer three times a week
Bromocriptine (ergot derivative and dopamine agonist, Parlodel)	Treat hypogonadotropic hypogonadism-associated prolactin-producing hypothalamic or pituitary tumors; may reduce the tumor	Counsel regarding oral ingestion with food to decrease side effects: dizziness, fainting, hypotension, headache, nausea, vomiting
Adrenal corticoids specific for the condition	Addison's disease Cushing's disease Congenital adrenal hypoplasia	Practice general medical nursing
Clomiphene citrate (Clomid or Serophene)	Idiopathic subfertility	Counsel regarding oral ingestion every day or every other day in cyclic fashion (25 days followed by 5-day rest period; repeat)
Vitamin C (ascorbic acid, a reducing agent)	Sperm agglutination where there are no autoantibodies	Counsel regarding oral ingestion of 500 mg three times a day indefinitely
Methylprednisolone (Medrol)	Steroid immunosuppression of sperm autoantibodies	Counsel regarding oral ingestion: 96 mg/day for 7 days starting the first regimen on day 21 of the woman's cycle, then every 4 weeks for 3 months
Sputolysin (mucolytic agent)	Increased seminal viscosity; used to wash semen before artificial seminal liquefaction	Counsel regarding use as precoital douching agent by female sexual partner
α-Amylase	Delayed seminal liquefaction	Counsel regarding use as precoital douching agent or cocoa-butter vaginal suppository by femal sexual partner

Surgical repair of varicocele* has been relatively successful. A varicocele on the left side is found in a substantial number of subfertile men. Ligation of the varicocele does lead to improvement of the sperm quality and commonly to pregnancy.

Simple changes in life-style may be effective in the treatment of subfertile men. High temperatures in the groin area reduce the number of sperm produced. High temperatures may be caused by the wearing of brief shorts and tight jeans that keep the scrotal sac pressed against the body regardless of environmental temperature changes. The testes are kept at temperatures too high for efficient spermatogenesis. Frequent and prolonged hot tubbing has also been implicated in relative infertility. It must be remembered that these conditions only led to relative infertility and should not be employed as a means of contraception.

Therapeutic Insemination

The term *homologous insemination* (insemination by husband) denotes the use of the husband's semen. The term *heterologous insemination* (insemination by donor) denotes the use of the semen of a donor other than the husband.

When the husband's sperm has poor quality or motility, several semen samples are collected from him. The samples consist of split ejaculates, that is, the sperm-rich *first portion* only is collected for freezing and later pooling for therapeutic insemination (husband). Rapid freezing with liquid nitrogen and subsequent thawing do not cause genetic damage even after 10 years' storage using glycerol. Pooling should increase the sperm count and improve the placement of a portion of the total semen specimen at the cervical os.

Assuming normal female fertility, therapeutic insemination (husband) at or about the time of ovulation has resulted in pregnancy in as many as 70% of cases. Numerous inseminations may be necessary to ensure proper timing at ovulation. The BBT and cervical mucus record help determine when to attempt insemination. Approximately 50% of pregnancies with therapeutic insemination (donor) will occur within 2 months; almost 90% occur within 6 months.

Insemination directly into the uterine cavity should be avoided because of severe cramping (prostaglandin effect) and possible infection. The recommended procedure is the instillation of about 0.5 ml of the specimen into the cervical canal with the remainder deposited in a cleanly washed

*Varicocele refers to varicose veins on the spermatic vein in the groin. The swollen, distended veins press on the testes and impair their function.

contraceptive diaphragm to be worn by the woman for about an hour.

Insemination with the husband's semen presents no legal problems, but insemination with donor sperm may involve many legal, ethical, and emotional aspects. The couple must know there is no guarantee of pregnancy and that in either case the spontaneous abortion rate is approximately the same as in a control population. There is no increase in maternal or perinatal complications; the same frequency of anomalies (about 5%) and obstetric complications (between 5% and 10%) that accompanies normal insemination applies also to therapeutic insemination.

The decision for therapeutic insemination with donor sperm should be made only after thorough consideration and discussion. The implications for the long-term welfare of the child as well as the parents must be considered.

Surrogate Motherhood

Surrogate motherhood can be achieved by two methods. One way is to have the surrogate mother inseminated with semen from the infertile woman's husband and carry the baby to delivery. Then the baby is formally adopted by the infertile couple. A less common method is to retrieve an ovum from the infertile woman, fertilize it with her husband's sperm, and place it into the uterus of the surrogate mother-to-be.

These newer interventions cause some legal and ethical problems (Chapter 4). For therapeutic insemination, the two major problems are donor selection and record keeping. Donor selection could result in eugenic decisions being made for a couple. Inadequate record keeping may prevent tracing of potential birth defects. Because of inadequate record keeping, it would be possible for one donor to father several children. In time two of them, who would be half siblings, might meet and marry. Their offspring would be at increased risk for genetic problems.

There are also two major issues surrounding human in vitro fertilization with resultant embryo transfer. The first issue is "Do human beings have the right to interfere so drastically in natural reproduction?"; and the second issue is "Is it permissible to deliberately destroy blastocysts before transfer to the woman's uterus if they are found to be defective?" (Fromer, 1983). The two ethical issues associated with surrogate motherhood are (1) should the surrogate mother be paid, and (2) to whom does the resulting child belong? The lengthy 1987 court trial involving Baby M. was probably only the beginning of the ethical problems that will eventually find their way to court.

For couples who can give up the quest for biologic parenthood, adoption is also an option. However, with increasing numbers of single mothers keeping their babies, this option may take 3 or more years.

Summary. For nurses to help a couple adapt to and live with their impaired fertility, nurses must be knowledgeable about the causes of impaired fertility and the common psychosociocultural and sexual responses. By being knowledgeable and sensitive, nurses can intervene more effectively. Though all couples cannot have a biologic child, all couples can work toward achieving and maintaining a satisfactory interpersonal and psychosexual relationship.

CONTROL OF FERTILITY: FAMILY PLANNING AND CONTRACEPTION

Contraception is the voluntary prevention of pregnancy having both individual and social implications. It has been established that more than 90% of couples in the United States have used or intend to use some method of contraception (birth control). Family planning is accepted in principle by all religions.

The availability of reliable and safe techniques for fertility management has meant that parenthood, with its tasks and responsibilities as well as its pleasures, can be willingly assumed by adults who wish to do so. Recent advances in the physiologic safety of prenatal, perinatal, and postnatal existence can now be combined with the psychologic safety of being a wanted child.

Spacing of children is important for promotion of health not only of the mother but also of her children. Quality of the offspring rather than quantity is now emphasized. Moreover, to control excessive world population, voluntary limitation of family size has become important.

Religious Considerations

Some strict protestant denominations, Hasidic Jews, and Roman Catholics believe that family planning can be achieved by periodic abstinence alone. Religion, however, may not be as great a barrier as once believed. Ostling (1984) reported that according to the National Center for Health Statistics a majority of Catholic women under age 45 have used contraceptive methods not approved by the Catholic Church. Samoans represent a variety of religions, but for them contraceptive practices are not highly valued (Clark and Howland, 1978). Rather, priority is placed on demonstration of male and female fertility through childbirth.

Cultural Considerations

Cross-cultural information about contraceptive practices is limited. Before modern times, probably the most effective contraception resulted from sexual taboos. Postpartum taboos were generally effective. Kay (1982) points out that the Mexican-Americans she studied continued to place a 40-day restriction on sexual intercourse after childbirth.

In the past, American Indians used herbs as oral contraceptives (Vogel, 1973). Information about these herbs was useful in the development of today's oral contraceptives. Some American Indian groups today favor the use of contraceptives, but others believe that they are against God's will. Although the Japanese were one of the earliest cultural groups to accept the use of birth control and abortion (Okamoto, 1978), Japanese couples are reluctant to use contraception until they have borne one child (Bernstein and Kidd, 1982).

Some subcultural groups in the United States and in third-world countries believe that the great emphasis placed on family planning is based on the desire of the white middle class to limit minority groups. Darity and Turner (1972) report that a significant group of black Americans is wary of methods used for fertility management.

The ability to control fertility is based on an understanding of the menstrual cycle. According to Scott (1978) a majority of Bahamians, Cubans, Haitians, and Puerto Ricans believe the function of menstruation to be that of ridding the person of unclean waste or unnecessary blood. A large number of Bahamians believe that menstruating means a person is healthy. Less bleeding means that something is wrong. Snow's research (1974) among blacks in parts of the western and northern United States also indicates the prevalent belief in impure blood.

If the belief that menstrual flow indicates health or lack of it, anything that would interfere with menstruation would be considered undesirable. Hormonal contraception, which often reduces the amount of and duration of menstrual-like flow, is considered dangerous to one's health. The IUD often affects the cycle and is also considered dangerous.

Family planning and contraception have posed numerous problems for nurses working with persons whose belief systems place a high value on having children. Nevertheless, many persons with these belief systems are interested in learning about contraception and will listen to explanations if they include respect for another's values. According to Dougherty (1972), health care innovations are accepted or rejected depending on how they fit into the client's cultural pattern.

Assessment

A history, physical examination, and laboratory tests precede the initiation of some forms of contraception. A complete gynecologic examination is performed (Chapter 8). Menstrual, contraceptive, and obstetric histories are taken. The woman's knowledge about contraception and her sexual partner's commitment to any particular method are determined. Data are required about the frequency of coitus (once every so often or several times per week), whether the woman has one sexual partner or several, the level of involvement the woman wishes to assume, and her (their) objections to any methods. The woman's level of comfort and willingness to touch her genitals and cervical mucus are assessed. Myths are identified. Religious and cultural factors are determined. The woman's verbal and nonverbal responses to hearing about the various available methods are carefully noted. An individual's reproductive-life plan needs to be considered. Individuals need to consider the following questions. How sad would they be if they could never become biologic parents? How concerned would they be if they were to become pregnant before they were ready to biologically childbear? If they became pregnant before they wanted to be, would abortion be an alternative?

Nursing Diagnoses

Nursing diagnoses reflect the assessment findings. Following are examples of nursing diagnoses that may emerge.

- Knowledge deficit related to
  - The number and nature of options available
  - The advantages, disadvantages, modes of action, and effectiveness of methods
  - Responsibility of woman and partner for a chosen method
  - Side effects to report to health care provider
- Potential for decisional conflict related to
  - Unplanned pregnancy
- Potential for infection or injury related to
  - Inappropriate use of contraceptive method
- Potential for altered sexuality patterns related to
  - Inappropriate method of contraception
  - Inappropriate use of chosen method of contraception

Planning

Planning is a collaborative effort among the woman, her sexual partner (when appropriate), the physician, and the nurse. The goals are determined and stated in client-centered terms.

Goals

1. The woman learns accurate information about contraceptive methods.
2. The woman is comfortable and satisfied with the chosen method.
3. If further childbearing is desired, pregnancy occurs at the time planned.
4. No adverse sequelae occur as a result of the chosen method of contraception.

Implementation

Client teaching (Chapter 2) is fundamental to initiating and maintaining any form of contraception. A care-provider relationship based on trust is an important facet in client compliance. The nurse counters myths with facts, clarifies misinformation, and fills in gaps of knowledge. There are various contraceptive techniques used in North America. The ideal contraceptive should be safe, easily available, economical, acceptable, simple to use, and promptly reversible. Although no means or method may ever achieve all these objectives, impressive progress has been made recently. The woman or couple must be fully informed of the risks (Tables 42-8 and 42-9), effectiveness, reversibility, and the alternatives (Table 42-10) (see discussion of informed consent, Chapter 4). An outdated way of calculating effectiveness is the Pearl index (failures per 100 women per years of exposure). The major problem with the Pearl index is that the longer a researcher runs a study the lower the failure rates will be. This means that the low failure rates may be misleading. Failure rates decrease over time either because a user will gain experience with and use a method more appropriately or the less effective users will drop out of the study. Table 42-10 lists the failure rates observed in the first year of use of a given contraceptive. The table data provide answers to two questions: (1) Of 100 users who start out the year using a given method and who use it correctly, how many will become pregnant in the first year? and (2) Of 100 typical users who start the

Table 42-8 *Estimated Annual Deaths Associated with Fertility Control and No Control per 100,000 Fertile Women*

Method	Age (years)					
	15-19	20-24	25-29	30-34	35-39	40-44
No method	5.5	5.2	7.1	14.0	19.3	22
Abortion only (legal)	2.3	2.5	2.5	5.2	9.8	6.6
Oral contraceptive only (nonsmoker)	1.3	1.4	1.4	2.2	4.5	3.1
Oral contraceptive only (smoker)	1.5	1.6	1.6	10.8	13.4	59
IUD only	1.1	1.2	1.2	1.4	1.6	1.4
Traditional contraception* only	1.1	1.4	1.9	3.7	4.7	4.0
Traditional contraception with abortion	0.3	0.4	0.4	0.8	1.4	0.8

*Family planning methods, spermicides, and condoms.

Table 42-9 *Risk Factors and Degree of Associated Risk by Age for Users of Oral Contraceptives*

Risk	Age (years)		
	≤29	30-39	≥40
Heavy smokers (≥15 cigarettes)	2	3	4
Light smokers (≤14 cigarettes)	1	2	3
Nonsmokers with no added risk conditions	1	1,2	2
Nonsmokers with added risk conditions	2	2,3	3,4

1 = Use associated with low risk; 2 = use associated with moderate risk; 3 = use associated with high risk; 4 = use associated with very high risk.

year using a given method, how many will become pregnant by the end of the year?

Contraception employs one or more of the following methods:

1. Methods available to people without prescription
   a. Biologic periodic abstinence: natural family planning
   b. Chemical barriers: spermicidal creams, gels, or vaginal suppositories and sponges
   c. Mechanical barrier: condoms or sheaths
2. Methods that require periodic medical examination and prescription*
   a. Hormonal therapy: estrogen or progestogen preparations or a combination of these compounds
   b. Mechanical barrier: cervical uterine occlusion by diaphragms or caps
   c. Intrauterine contraceptive devices
3. Methods that require surgical intervention
   a. Female sterilization
   b. Male sterilization

Elective interruption of pregnancy is a surgical procedure that requires sensitivity as well as expert technical skill from health care providers. Methods of elective abortion appropriate for each trimester will be discussed.

The nurse supervises return demonstrations and practice to assess client understanding. The client is given written instructions and phone numbers for questions. If the client has difficulty with written instructions, the woman (couple) is offered graphic material and a phone number to call as necessary, or an offer to return for further instruction (see guidelines for client teaching: general contraception).

*Certified nurse-midwives and some certified nurse-practitioners may be educated to provide this service.

Evaluation

The nurse can be reasonably assured that care was effective if the goals of care have been achieved: the woman (couple) learns about the various methods of contraception; pregnancy occurs only when it has been planned; and no adverse sequelae occur as a result of the chosen method of contraception.

Table 42-10 *Contraceptive Methods and Pregnancies per 100 Women*

Method of Contraception	Contraceptive Failures (number of pregnancies)*
No method	60-80
Calendar only	14-47
Periodic abstinence	1-47
Jellies/creams	4-36
Condom	3-36
Aerosol foams	2-29
Mucous method	1-25
Diaphragm with spermicide	2-20
BBT only	1-20
BBT with intercourse during post-ovulatory time	1-7
IUD	1-6
Combination oral contraceptives	1-3

*The fewer the number of pregnancies, the greater the effectiveness.

Guidelines for Client Teaching

GENERAL CONTRACEPTIVE METHODS

ASSESSMENT

1. Complete physical assessment and history appropriate for each method.
2. Assessment of woman's (couple's) knowledge of method selected.
3. Assessment of body image.
4. Assessment of motivation needed for method selected.
5. Assessment of life-style and discussion whether method selected fits into daily life.

NURSING DIAGNOSES

Knowledge deficit related to method selected.
Potential for pregnancy or injury related to knowledge deficit or ignorance of method selected.
Potential for infection related to not adhering to proper guidelines of method selected.
Altered nutrition: less than body requirements related to side effects of oral contraceptives.

GOALS

Short-term

Woman (couple) develops a trusting relationship with care provider.
Nurse identifies myths, clarifies information, and dispells misinformation.
Woman (couple) becomes comfortable in the use of the method.
Woman learns relevant information regarding the method being used (i.e., use, action, advantages, disadvantages, side effects, and effectiveness).

Intermediate

Woman (couple) confers with care provider when questions arise regarding use or desire to change to another method.
Women reports side effects or complications or suspected pregnancy immediately.
Woman returns to care provider for periodic checkups or when a change in the method is warranted (e.g., pregnancy is desired, diaphragm needs to be refitted after birth of baby or gain or loss of more than 4.5 kg (10 lb).

Long-term

Woman remains in good health while using chosen method.
Woman achieves desired objective for contraception, that is no children, or desired number of children.
Woman indicates satisfaction with chosen method and care received.

REFERENCES AND TEACHING AIDS

Inserts from packages of chosen method.
Hospital or clinic teaching pamphlets or booklets.
Flip chart showing anatomy of pelvic structures or total body plastic medical model.
Audiovisuals or films for teaching.
Samples of contraceptive device (i.e., BBT charts and thermometer)
Fresh egg white for teaching about cervical mucus.
Mirror.
Handouts of printed material.

CONTENT/RATIONALE	TEACHING ACTION
To meet information needs: Provide general discussion about selected method, its mode of action, and reasons for choosing it. Establish basis and direction for cognitive, psychomotor, and affective learning needs. Teach at the client's level without being condescending.	*Encourage general discussion through use of the following:* Provide time, privacy, and assurance regarding confidentiality. Create a receptive, nonjudgmental atmosphere. Consider appropriate cultural/ethnic, intellectual/educational, and developmental factors pertinent to the woman (couple).
Supply information about action, advantages, disadvantages, side effects, and effectiveness.	*Using references and equipment listed above, implement the following:* Discuss information about method selected.
Discuss method, its placement, locus of action.	Indicate on illustration or medical model the placement of the device (IUD, diaphragm, cervical cap or sponge, condom), loci of action (hormonal contraceptive versus diaphragm).
To assist client in developing competence and confidence with chosen method: Learning is reinforced if content is taught in a variety of ways. Time and hands-on experience with chosen method reinforces learning. Confidence and mastery of content and experience before woman leaves the care provider are more likely to result in use of method.	Demonstrate appliance (diaphragm with spermicide), characteristics of "fertile" cervical mucus (egg white), entering temperature on BBT graph, calculating fertile times. Supervise client's return demonstration and practice. Assess client's recall of content taught or its availability on printed material provided.
To reaffirm health care provider's caring and woman's motivation: Review the material presented.	Ascertain that client has appropriate phone numbers for questions and suggest client call back, prn, after implementing method at home.

EVALUATION Woman (couple) demonstrate competence and ask appropriate questions regarding method of choice; goals are met within an appropriate time frame.

Methods Available Without Prescription

Several nonprescription methods for control of fertility are practiced. Prescription and supervision are unnecessary for barrier methods, that is, condom, foam, spermicide, vaginal sponges, and for periodic abstinence. In 1982, among women aged 15 to 44 years practicing contraception, the condom was used by 12.2%, foam by 2.4%, and periodic abstinence by 4% (Bachrach, 1984). Two methods were practiced that are *not* recommended: withdrawal (coitus interruptus), 2%, and douching, 0.2% (Bachrach, 1984).

Periodic Abstinence or "Natural" Family Planning. Periodic abstinence was practiced by 4% of women aged 15 to 44 years practicing contraception in 1982 (Bachrach, 1984). The term *periodic abstinence* is preferred over "natural family planning" for contraceptive methods that rely on avoidance of intercourse during presumed fertile days on the menstrual cycle. Many couples find abstinence for 7 to 18 or more consecutive days of each menstrual cycle to be unnatural (Klaus, 1982).

Periodic abstinence methods employ a combination of the following:

1. Rhythm or calendar method
2. BBT method
3. Cervical mucus (Billings, ovulation) method
4. Sympto-thermal method
5. Fertility awareness method
6. Predictor test for ovulation

These methods depend on the continuous observation and recording of events of the menstrual cycle. The woman or couple must be able to assess hormone-induced signs and symptoms that indicate whether she is in the fertile or infertile part of the menstrual cycle. While teaching a woman about fertility awareness, the nurse uses this opportunity for helping the woman or couple learn a great deal about their bodies.

The *mode of action* for these methods of contraception is abstention from intercourse during the fertile period.*

The human ovum can be fertilized no later than 24 to 48 hours after ovulation. Motile sperm have been recovered from the uterus and the oviducts as long as 60 hours after coitus. However, their ability to fertilize the ovum probably lasts no longer than 24 to 48 hours. Pregnancy is unlikely to occur if a couple abstains from intercourse for 4 days before and for 3 or 4 days after ovulation *(fertile period).* Unprotected intercourse on the other days of the cycle *(safe period)* should not result in pregnancy. The principal problems with this method are that the exact time of ovulation cannot be predicted accurately. Couples may also find it difficult to exercise restraint for several days before and after ovulation.

*The World Health Organization (Liskin, 1981) concluded in 1979 that the cervical mucus and sympto-thermal methods "had very limited application, particularly in developing countries, and recommended that the World Health Organization Programme devote no further research to measuring their effectiveness." Similarly, the International Planned Parenthood Federation concluded in 1982 that "couples electing to use periodic abstinence should, however be clearly informed that the method is not considered an effective method of family planning."

Ovulation usually occurs about 14 days before the onset of menstruation. Therefore variations in the length of menstrual cycles are usually a result of differences in the length of the preovulatory phases. The fertile period can be anticipated by the following:

1. Calculating the time at which ovulation is likely to occur based on the lengths of previous menstrual cycles *(calendar method)*
2. Recording the rise in basal body temperature (BBT), a result of the thermogenic effect of progesterone *(temperature method)*
3. Recognizing the changes in cervical mucus at different phases of the menstrual cycle *(ovulation or Billings method)*
4. Using a predictor test for ovulation
5. Utilizing a combination of several methods

Unique developments of monoclonal antibody technology have added the *predictor test* for ovulation. This type of test is a major addition to the periodic abstinence methods to help women who want to plan the time of their pregnancies and those who are trying to conceive.

Rhythm or Calendar Method. With the *calendar method* the fertile period is determined after accurately recording the lengths of menstrual cycles for 1 year. According to the Ogino formula the first unsafe day (beginning of the fertile period) can be determined by subtracting 18 days from the length of the shortest cycle. The last unsafe day (beginning of postovulatory safe period) can be calculated by subtracting 11 days from the length of the longest cycle. If the shortest cycle is 24 days and the longest is 30 days, application of the formula is as follows:

Shortest Cycle	*Longest Cycle*
24	30
−18	−11
6th day	19th day

To avoid conception the couple would abstain during the "fertile" period, days 6 through 19.

If the woman has very regular cycles of 28 days each, the formula indicates the fertile days to be:

Shortest Cycle	*Longest Cycle*
28	28
−18	−11
10th day	17th day

To avoid pregnancy, the couple abstains from day 10 through 17 because ovulation occurs on day 14. A major drawback of the calendar method is that one is trying to predict future events with past data. The predictability of the menstrual cycle to be unpredictable is also not taken into consideration.

Basal Body Temperature. The BBT during the menses and for approximately 5 to 7 days thereafter usually varies from 36.2° to 36.3° C (97.2° to 97.4° F). If ovulation fails to occur, this pattern of lower body temperature continues throughout the cycle. Infection, fatigue, less than 3 hours of sleep per night, awakening late, and anxiety may cause temperature fluctuations, altering the expected pattern. If a new BBT thermometer is purchased, this fact is noted on the chart because the readings may vary slightly. Jet lag, alcohol taken the evening before, or sleeping in a heated water bed must also be noted on the chart because each will affect the BBT (see guidelines for client teaching).

About 24 to 36 hours *before* ovulation the temperature may drop 0.2° to 0.3° F and then rise 0.7° to 0.8° F within 24 to 48 hours *after* ovulation. The temperature remains on an elevated plateau until 2 to 4 days before menstruation. Then it drops to the low levels recorded during the previous cycle.

The drop and subsequent rise in temperature are referred to as the *thermal shift.* When the entire month's tem-

Guidelines for Client Teaching

BASAL ("RESTING") BODY TEMPERATURE

ASSESSMENT

1. Woman having trouble conceiving for pregnancy.
2. Need for presumptive evidence of ovulation and an adequate luteal (progesterone) phase.
3. Woman interested in learning how to determine her ovulation time.

NURSING DIAGNOSES

Knowledge deficit related to BBT, the procedure to take it and keep a graph.

Potential self-esteem disturbance related to the inability to conceive a child.

Sexual dysfunction related to possible infertility and anovulation.

GOALS

Short-term

Woman learns what BBT is and how to take and record it.

Intermediate

Woman maintains a record of BBT, fever, stress, cervical mucus characteristics.

Long-term

Woman is motivated enough to obtain and maintain BBT graph for several months.

REFERENCES AND TEACHING AIDS

Pamphlets, booklets, diagrams, any printed material depicting the taking and recording of the BBT.

BBT thermometer.

CONTENT/RATIONALE	TEACHING ACTION
To provide content related to BBT: In an ovulating woman, there is a variation in the BBT during the course of her menstrual cycle because of hormones working in her body. The BBT is lower during the first part of the menstrual cycle, the proliferative phase. As ovulation approaches, and the effects of LH and progesterone take over, the BBT rises. If fertilization of the ovum takes place, the BBT remains elevated. However, if fertilization does not take place, the corpus luteum deteriorates and the BBT falls to the lower level again, until the next ovulation occurs.	Discuss BBT with the woman. Show woman a diagram depicting the phases of the menstrual cycle. Discuss the different hormones in the woman's body that are responsible for her menstrual cycle and ovulation. Leave time for questions. Show woman a sample BBT graph and the biphasic line seen in ovulatory cycles.
The BBT thermometer is calibrated in tenths rather than fifths. If woman doesn't want to buy a BBT thermometer, a regular oral thermometer may be used, but it must be left in the mouth under the tongue for 5 minutes.	Show the client the BBT thermometer, and how it is calibrated.
Discuss the procedure woman will follow every day. Before going to bed, shake the thermometer down and leave it on the bedside table. On awakening the following morning, the woman will put the thermometer under her tongue and not move any more. After 3 minutes she will take the thermometer out of her mouth and replace it on the night stand. On arising, the woman will read the thermometer and record the temperature on the graph. Using a snooze alarm on the woman's clock is a convenient way to time the temperature taking.	Provide a demonstration. Encourage woman to demonstrate taking and reading the thermometer and how she will graph the temperature while nurse watches. Encourage woman to start a log at the same time that keeps track of any other activity that might interfere with her true BBT.

EVALUATION Woman verbalizes understanding of the instructions given, provides a return demonstration, asks appropriate questions, and meets all goals mutually set. When woman returns after 2 or 3 cycles, she brings a completed log and graph and can identify phases of her menstrual cycle by using these data.

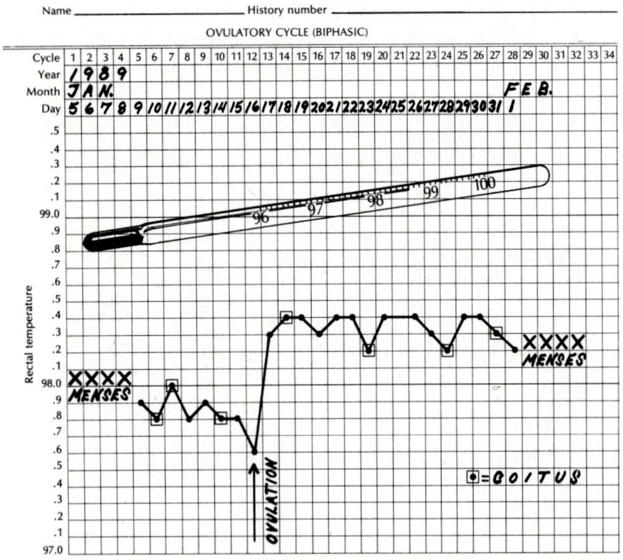

Fig. 42-5 A, Special thermometer for recording BBT, marked in tenths to enable person to read more easily. B, Basal temperature record shows drop and sharp rise at time of ovulation. Biphasic curve indicates ovulatory cycle.

peratures are recorded on a graph, the pattern described above is more apparent. It is more difficult to perceive day-to-day variations without the entire picture (Fig. 42-5). To determine if a rise in temperature is indeed the thermal shift, the woman must be aware of other signs approaching ovulation while she continues to assess the BBT. See discussion of sympto-thermal method below for other indicators of ovulation.

Cervical Mucus Method. The cervical mucus method, also called the *Billings method* or the *ovulation method,* depends on the characteristic changes in the amount and consistency of cervical mucus at the time of ovulation (see Table 6-1 and Figs. 6-26 and 6-27).

Drs. John and Evelyn Billings (1975) of Australia recognize two absolutes about conception. These are that cervical mucus always accompanies ovulation and that cervical mucus is necessary for viability and motility of sperm. They believe that without adequate cervical mucus coitus will not result in conception. These changes are easily learned by most couples (see guidelines for client teaching). The first task is to learn to distinguish changes in the cervical mucus. To ensure accurate assessment of changes, the cervical mucus should be free of semen, contraceptive gels or foams, and blood or discharge from vaginal infections for at least one full cycle. Other factors that create difficulty in identifying mucous changes include douches and vaginal deodorants, being in the sexually aroused state (which thins the mucus), and medications such as antihistamines, which dry up the mucus.

It is difficult to evaluate the mucus in the presence of semen or discharge from vaginal infection. Therefore the woman double checks for fertility by assessing her BBT record and other symptoms of fertility. (NOTE: Each woman has her own unique pattern of mucous changes.)

Whether or not the individual wants to use this method for contraception, it is to the woman's benefit to learn to recognize mucus characteristics at ovulation. Assessing changes in cervical mucus can be useful diagnostically for any of the following purposes:

1. To alert the couple to the reestablishment of ovulation while breast-feeding and after discontinuation of oral contraception
2. To note anovulatory cycles at any time and at the commencement of menopause
3. To assist couples in planning a pregnancy

Sympto-thermal Method. The sympto-thermal method combines the BBT and cervical mucus methods with awareness of secondary, cycle phase–related symptoms. Both partners take responsibility for assessments, recordings, and evaluation of their findings. Together they determine the days for abstinence. Couples who use the sympto-thermal method commonly report an improvement in their sexual relationship.

The couple gains fertility awareness as they learn the woman's individual psychologic and physiologic symptoms. These symptoms mark the relatively infertile period (menstrual), fertile period (secretory phase), and infertile period (proliferative phase). Secondary symptoms (see Table 6-1) include increased libido, midcycle spotting, mittelschmerz, pelvic fullness, or tenderness, and vulvar fullness. The couple, perhaps using a speculum, looks at the cervix to assess for changes indicating ovulation: that is, the os dilates slightly, the cervix softens and rises in the vagina, and cervical mucus is copious and slippery. To complete their records, the couple notes days on which coitus, changes in routine, illness, and so on have occurred (Fig. 42-6).

Effectiveness of the sympto-thermal method with abstinence during the fertile period ranges between 73% and 97%.

Fertility Awareness Method. The fertility awareness method is a combination of the sympto-thermal method and barrier contraception. During the fertile period the couple has the choice of abstinence from genital-genital contact or the use of barrier contraception. After ovulation the couple may enjoy freedom from contraception for the remaining nonfertile days of the menstrual cycle.

Predictor Test for Ovulation. This test detects the sudden surge of LH that occurs approximately 12 to 24 hours before ovulation. Unlike BBT, the test is not affected by illness, emotional upset, or physical activity. Available for home use, a test kit contains sufficient material for several days' testing during each cycle. A positive response indicative of an LH surge is noted by color change that is easy to read. Directions for use of this home test kit vary with the manufacturer.

Chemical Barriers. A vaginal spermicide is a physical barrier to sperm penetration that also has a chemical action on sperm. *Nonoxynol 9* and octoxynol 9 are the most commonly used spermicidal chemicals. Intravaginal spermicides are marketed as aerosol foams, foaming tablets, suppositories, creams and gels (Fig. 42-7). Preloaded, single-dose applicators small enough to be carried in a small purse are available (Grimes, 1986). This form of contraceptive must be placed deeply in the vagina in contact with the

Guidelines for Client Teaching

CERVICAL MUCUS CHARACTERISTICS

ASSESSMENT

1. Woman (couple) wants to know how cervical mucus changes with the menstrual cycle.
2. Woman (couple) wants to know how to tell period of maximum fertility by using the changes in cervical mucus.

NURSING DIAGNOSIS

Knowledge deficit related to the changes in cervical mucus during the menstrual cycle and how changes affect fertility.

GOALS

Short-term

Woman learns how to assess for peak mucus sign.

Intermediate

Woman learns to check for mucus several times per day.
Woman learns to record observations daily as to quantity, consistency, color, and sensation from last day of menstrual flow.

Long-term

Woman records findings along with BBT for several menstrual cycles.
Woman (couple) knows when peak mucus sign occurs for maximum fertility.

REFERENCES AND TEACHING AIDS

Pamphlets and booklets distributed by hospitals, clinics, or physicians.
Raw egg white.

CONTENT/RATIONALE	TEACHING ACTION
To provide content related to cervical mucus: Explain to woman (couple) how cervical mucus changes throughout the menstrual cycle. Right before ovulation, the watery, thin, clear mucus becomes more abundant and thick. Feels like a lubricant and can be stretched 5+ cm; this is called spinnbarkheit. This indicates the period of maximum fertility. Sperm deposited in this type of mucus can survive until ovulation occurs.	Show charts of menstrual cycle along with changes in the cervical mucus. Have woman practice with raw egg white. Show findings favorable to fertility (Figs. 6-26 and 6-27).
To teach assessment technique: Explain to woman (couple) that assessment of cervical mucus characteristics is best learned when mucus not mixed with semen, contraceptive jellies or foams, or discharge from infections.	Couple asked to refrain from ejaculation of semen into or near vaginal opening for at least one infection-free cycle.
Woman is to assess cervical mucus several times a day for several cycles. Mucus can be obtained from vaginal introitus, no need to reach into vagina to cervix.	**Good hand washing is imperative** to begin and end all self-assessment. From last day of menstrual flow the woman starts her observations.
Woman records her findings on the same record on which her BBT is entered. Woman records any other events also.	Supply her with a BBT log and graph, if she doesn't already have one.

EVALUATION Woman (couple) follows your directions, asks appropriate questions, and all goals are met. When woman returns after two or three cycles, she can describe the changes in her cervical mucus during each phase.

cervix before each coitus. Special precautions must be taken. The can of foam must be shaken to distribute the spermicide before use. Tablets and suppositories take from 10 to 30 minutes to dissolve. Maximum spermicidal effectiveness lasts usually no longer than 1 hour. If intercourse is to be repeated, reapplication of additional spermicide must precede it. Douching must be avoided for at least 6 hours after coitus (Grimes, 1986).

Mode of Action. Spermicides provide a physical and chemical barrier that prevents viable sperm from entering the cervix. The effect is local, within the vagina.

Advantages. Ease of application, safety, low cost, and ready availability without prescription or previous medical examination characterize this method. The delicate vaginal mucosa is not harmed unless the woman is allergic to a particular preparation. Spermicides aid in lubrication of the

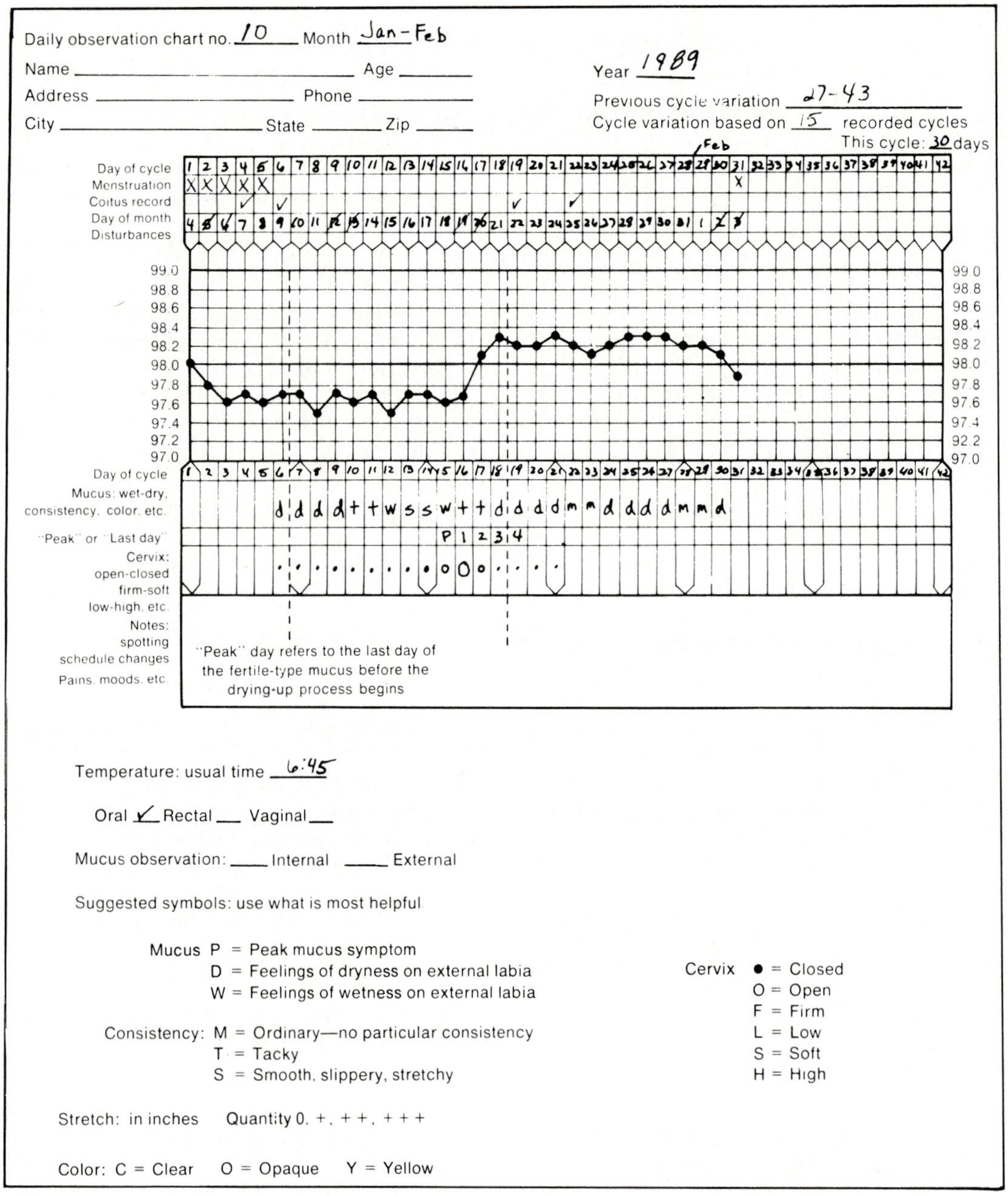

Fig. 42-6 Example of completed sympto-thermal method chart.
From Fogel, C, and Woods, NF: Health care of women, St Louis, 1981, The CV Mosby Co.

vagina. Because their effect is local, spermicides offer an alternative to hormonal contraception (e.g., for the nursing mother [to avoid interfering with lactation], for the premenopausal woman [to prevent masking symptoms of onset of the climacterium], and as a backup for the woman who forgets to take her oral contraceptive). There is evidence that spermicides provide some protection against sexually transmitted disease through bacteriostatic action. The addition of spermicides increases the effectiveness of the other forms of contraception (e.g., condoms, diaphragms).

Disadvantages and Side Effects. Users of this method may complain of its "messiness," unpleasant "fizz," stickiness, or unpleasant taste. Allergic response or irritation of vaginal or penile tissue may occur. Some users experience decreased tactile sensation. The need to wait 10 minutes to 30 minutes before coitus initially and to reapply additional spermicide before repeated intercourse is not acceptable to all people.

Effectiveness. According to Pritchard, MacDonald, and Gant (1985) the high pregnancy rate seen with this method is probably the result of inconsistent use of the spermicide. Of 100 users who start out the year using vaginal spermicides and who use them correctly, the lowest observed failure rate has been 3 to 5. Of 100 typical users the number of pregnancies by the end of the first year will be 18 (Table 42-10).

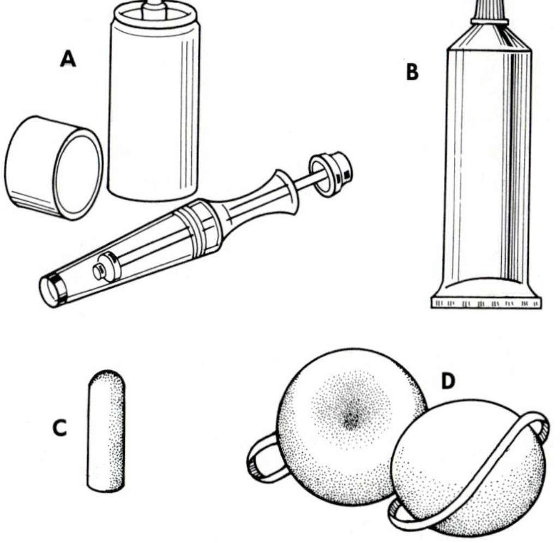

Fig. 42-7 Vaginal spermicides. **A**, Foam with applicator. **B**, Gel or cream. **C**, Suppository, **D**, Sponge.

Nursing Actions. The nurse encourages open communication between the sexual partners to discuss intravaginal contraception. Clients are offered the opportunity to see and handle a variety of samples. To maximize learning, the woman is given the opportunity to insert one application into a medical model or her vagina. The male partner sometimes indicates an interest in learning how to insert the spermicide into his female partner. The nurse needs to feel comfortable teaching him as well.

Vaginal Sponge. The polyurethane sponge was approved by the Food and Drug Administration in 1983 (Fig. 42-6, *D*). Water is added to activate the spermicide and facilitate insertion. Spermicide is released continuously for 24 hours. A woven loop is used for retrieval from the vagina. It is recommended that at least 6 hours lapse between last intercourse and removal (Grimes, 1986).

Mode of Action. The mode of action is the same as that for the spermicides.

Advantages. Like the other spermicides, the sponge is an over-the-counter (OTC) product. It offers spontaneity and is less "messy" than other spermicide delivery systems. Reapplication of spermicide during the 24 hours the sponge is in place is unnecessary.

Disadvantages and Side Effects. The only reported effects were allergic reactions (2% to 3%) or irritation (2% to 3%) that typically occur with all nonoxynol 9 products. Six percent of users reported difficulty in removing the sponge (Grimes, 1986).

Effectiveness. A relatively high failure rate has been reported during the first year of use, especially in parous women (Grimes, 1986). Of 100 users who start out the year using a contraceptive sponge and who use it correctly and consistently, the lowest observed failure rate has been 9 to 11 pregnancies. The failure rate is higher than with the contraceptive diaphragm, which when used correctly and consistently has a failure rate of 2 (Table 42-10).

Nursing Actions. Nursing actions are similar to those for other spermicides. Clients are reminded that each sponge is to be used once, for 24 hours only. It is left in place for 6 hours after coitus, and discarded. The woman is coached to "bear down" to facilitate removal of the sponge.

Condom. The condom is a thin, stretchable sheath to cover the penis (Fig. 42-8, *A*). Four basic features differ among condoms marketed in the United States. These features are material, shape, lubricants, and spermicides. Ninety-nine percent are made of rubber. A functional difference in condom shape is the presence or absence of a sperm reservoir tip. To enhance vaginal stimulation, some condoms have lateral ribs. A wet jelly or dry powder lubricates some condoms. Since 1982, spermicide (0.5 g of nonoxynol 9) has been added to the interior or exterior surfaces of some condoms.

The sheath is applied over the erect penis before insertion or loss of preejaculatory drops of semen. Conception is made possible even if preejaculatory drops fall around the external vaginal opening because sperm are contained in these drops.

Mode of Action. Used correctly, condoms prevent sperm from entering the cervix. Spermicide-coated condoms cause ejaculated sperm to be immobilized rapidly.

Advantages. Condoms are safe, without side effects, and are readily available. Premalignant changes in the cervix can be prevented or ameliorated in women whose partners use condoms (Pritchard, MacDonald, and Gant, 1985). If the condom is used throughout the act of intercourse and there is no unprotected contact with female genitals, condoms can act as a protective measure against spread of sexually transmitted diseases (STDs). The STDs include gonorrhea, syphilis, herpes, chlamydia, acquired immune deficiency syndrome (AIDS),* and trichomoniasis (Grimes, 1986; Pritchard, MacDonald, and Gant, 1985; Willson, Car-

*The combination of spermicide and the condom seems to create a synergistic action against a number of sexually transmitted diseases (Grimes, 1986).

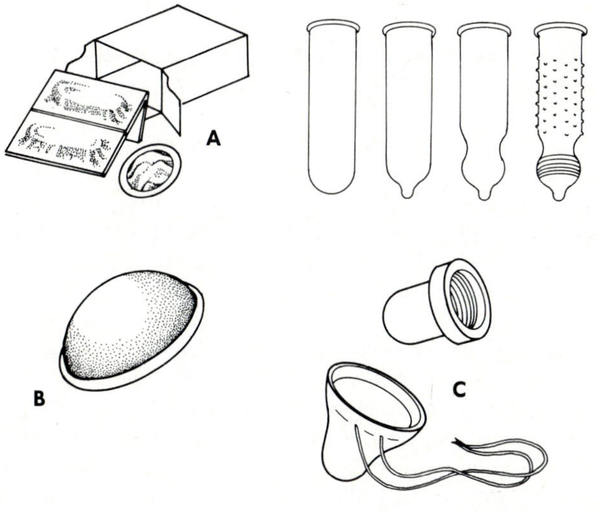

Fig. 42-8 Mechanical barriers. **A**, Condoms (no prescription required); types of condoms. **B**, Diaphragm. **C**, Cervical caps.

rington, and Ledger, 1987; and *San Francisco Chronicle,* 1/14/86). The unique feature of this method is that the male assumes a major role in contraception (Grimes, 1986).

Disadvantages and Side Effects. If condoms are used improperly, spillage of sperm can result in pregnancy. Some couples object to interrupting lovemaking to apply the sheath or complain that sensation is blunted. On occasion, condoms have torn during intercourse.

Effectiveness. Of 100 users who start out the year using a condom and who use one correctly and consistently, the lowest observed failure rate is 2 pregnancies. For 100 typical users, the number of pregnancies by the end of the year will be 10 (Table 42-10). Condoms with spermicide are highly effective at killing sperm within the condom. The effectiveness of the spermicides on the outside of the condom in case a condom breaks has not been evaluated (Hatcher et al., 1986).

Nursing Actions. Both the female and male partner benefit from a discussion of their feelings about this method of contraception. Samples of condoms with different features, a price list, and demonstration of the application and removal of a condom using a medical model offer the clients a focus for discussion and a basis for choice. Clients need to be alerted to the mode of action, advantages, disadvantages, and effectiveness of this method.

NOTE: Coitus interruptus, a method practiced for centuries, is mentioned here only to caution couples against this type of unreliable method. This method requires the man to withdraw before ejaculation. Extreme self-discipline is needed, and the sexual relationship may be strained. The danger of pregnancy from sperm in the pre-ejaculatory drops is ever present. No advantages are given for this method, which has the lowest rate of effectiveness, comparable to the use of no contraceptive method.

Methods Requiring Periodic Medical Examination and Prescription

Several methods for the control of fertility require prescription and supervision. Interview, physical examination, and occasionally laboratory tests are prerequisites for some forms of contraception. These methods of contraception include hormonal therapy, use of diaphragms or caps, and IUDs.

Hormonal Contraception. Steroidal contraceptives are available in several preparations. Some are described in Table 42-11.

Oral hormonal contraceptives were used by 28.6% of women aged 15 to 44 years practicing contraception during 1982 (Bachrach, 1984). The minipill accounts for only 1% of oral contraceptives sold. Because of the wide variety of preparations available the woman and nurse need to read the package insert for information about specific products prescribed.

Mode of Action. Activation of the hypothalamus and pituitary to release FSH and LH depends on fluctuation in the blood concentration of ovarian estrogen and progesterone. The contraceptive action is a combined effect of ovulation inhibition, endometrial changes, and alteration in cervical mucus, and perhaps altered tubal function (Willson, Carrington, Ledger, 1987). The medication suppresses anterior pituitary secretion of the gonadotropins FSH and LH, thereby inhibiting ovulation. It also has a direct effect on the endometrium, so that from 1 to 4 days after the last steroid tablet is taken the endometrium sloughs and bleeds as a result of hormone withdrawal. The *withdrawal bleeding* usually is less profuse than that of normal menstruation and may last only 2 to 3 days. Some women have no bleeding at all.

The cervical mucus remains thick as a result of the effect of the progestin. Cervical mucus under the effect of progesterone does not provide as suitable an environment for sperm penetration as does the thin, viscid mucus at ovulation (Willson, Carrington, and Ledger, 1987).

Advantages. For motivated women it is easy to take an oral contraceptive (OC) at about the same time each day. Taking the pill does not relate directly to the sexual act; this fact increases its acceptability to some women. Commonly, there is an improvement in sexual response once the possibility of pregnancy is not an issue. For some, it is convenient to know when to expect the next "menstrual" flow. The regular cyclic stimulation of the endometrium may help regulate menstrual cycles and make it possible for conception to occur at a later time. Occasionally, using oral hormone therapy for a period of time may decrease or eliminate premenstrual tension and dysmenorrhea (menstrual cramps).

There has been little publicity about the advantages of hormonal contraceptives. Mishell (1982) and Ory (1982) list the noncontraceptive health benefits of oral contraceptives. The benefits include decreased menstrual blood loss and resultant iron-deficiency anemia, regulation of irregular cycles, protection against endometrial adenocarcinoma, reduced incidence of benign breast disease, protection against the development of functional ovarian cysts, protection against acute salpingitis* and pelvic inflammatory disease (PID) caused by gonorrhea, and possible protection against ovarian cancer and rheumatoid arthritis. However, there is biologic and epidemiologic evidence that PID caused by *Chlamydia* is enhanced by oral contraceptives (Washington, et al., 1985). Combination oral contraceptives have been used to treat such medical conditions as idiopathic thrombocytopenia purpura and endometriosis.

Since ovulation is suppressed, the risk for ectopic pregnancy is about one-tenth that of women not using contraceptives. This form of contraception is associated with minimum risk for women aged 15 to 29 years. The mortality is 1.2 and 1.4/100,000 for nonsmoking and smoking women, respectively.

Women taking steroidal contraceptives are examined before the medication is prescribed and yearly thereafter. The examination includes medical and family history, weight, blood pressure, general physical and pelvic examination, screening cervical cytologic analysis, and hemoglobin determination. Consistent medical surveillance is valuable in the detection of noncontraception-related disorders as well, so that timely treatment can be initiated.

*Wolner-Hanssen et al. (1985) suggest that this protection may apply to both gonococcal and chlamydial salpingitis.

Table 42-11 *Hormonal Contraception*

Composition	Route of Administration	Duration of Effect
Combination of an estrogen and a progestin:	Oral	Not more than 24 hours
Biphasic: constant dose of estrogen and an increase in progestin on day 11		
Triphasic: 3 different products on market—in 2, estrogen is constant and progestin varies; in 1, amounts of both vary. Total hormone dose per cycle is lower than in biphasic combinations		
Sequential: estrogen during first half of cycle, progestin during second half; not sold in United States		
Minipill: progestin (norethindrone, 0.35 mg) only	Oral	24 hours
Morning-after pill: estrogen (diethylstilbestrol [DES]) in very high levels—25 mg	Oral	Taken within 72 hours of unprotected coitus during fertile period; because of DES effect on fetus, abortion advised if method fails
Depo-Provera: progestin only (medroxyprogesterone acetate), 150 mg	Intramuscular injection	From 3 to 6 months
Norplant system: progestin (Levonorgestrel) in silastic containers	Implant, subdermal	Up to 5 years

Disadvantages and Side Effects. Women must be screened for conditions that present absolute or relative contraindications to oral contraceptive use. *Absolute contraindications* include a history of thromboembolic disorders, cerebrovascular or coronary artery disease, breast cancer, estrogenic-dependent tumors, undiagnosed abnormal genital bleeding, known or suspected pregnancy, liver tumor, sickle cell disease, or migraine headaches (Grimes, 1986; Hatcher et al., 1984; Kols et al., 1982). *Relative contraindications* include age of 40 years or older, diabetes mellitus, hypertension, heavy smoking (more than 15 cigarettes per day), gallbladder disease, gestational cholestasis, history of renal disease, impaired liver function, and hyperlipidemia (Grimes, 1986). The main causes of hospitalization and death are cardiovascular problems (e.g., myocardial infarction [heart attack], cerebrovascular accident [stroke], and thromboembolism) (Grimes, 1986).

Certain side effects of anovulatory drugs are attributable to estrogen and progestin or both. Side effects of *estrogen excess* include nausea and vomiting, dizziness, edema, leg cramps, increase in breast size, chloasma (mask of pregnancy), visual changes, hypertension, and vascular headache. Side effects of *estrogen deficiency* include early spotting (days 1 to 14), hypomenorrhea, nervousness, and atrophic vaginitis leading to painful intercourse (dyspareunia). Side effects of *progestin excess* include increased appetite, tiredness, depression, breast tenderness, vaginal yeast infection, oily skin and scalp, hirsutism, and postpill amenorrhea. Side effects of *progestin deficiency* include late spotting and breakthrough bleeding (days 15 to 21), heavy flow with clots, and decreased breast size.

In the presence of side effects, especially those that are bothersome to the woman, a different product, a different drug content, or another method of contraception may be required. The "right" product for a woman contains the lowest dose of sex steroid hormones that prevents ovulation and that has the fewest and least harmful side effects. There is no way to predict the "right" dose* for any particular woman; trial and error is the main method for prescribing OCs, starting with the lowest possible estrogen dose.

The *changes in glucose tolerance* that occur in some women taking OCs are similar to those changes that occur during pregnancy. OCs challenge the islets of Langerhans to produce more insulin. If the individual is prediabetic, the use of oral contraception can induce the frank expression of diabetes mellitus.

The OC also affects the woman's *general nutritional needs,* especially for B vitamins. There is considerable evidence that OCs are implicated in deficiencies of vitamin B_6 (pyridoxine) and folic acid in about 20% to 30% of users. Among some OC users, symptoms such as headaches, nausea and vomiting, and emotional disturbances and depression have been alleviated by dietary supplementation of vitamin B_6.

Symptoms of folic acid deficiency are rare, since folate is plentiful in the North American diet. However, if a pregnancy occurs soon after the pill is discontinued, folic acid deficiency is to be expected. Clinical symptoms of folic acid deficiency are those of megaloblastic anemia: increasing fatigue, pallor, moderate depapillation of the tongue, and changes in peripheral blood and bone marrow. Symptoms are rapidly reversed with supplementation of folic acid or if the OC is discontinued.

Although not yet proven, there may be some deficiency of vitamin C and vitamin B_{12} (cobalamin). Vitamins whose metabolism is suspected of being altered by OCs are vitamin A, vitamin B_2, and niacin.

*Warn women, young and old, that using another woman's OCs may not prevent ovulation, if the dose is not correct for them.

Some women complain of *edema,* which is associated with administration of estrogens; however, if the dose of estrogen is sufficiently low, fluid retention is not likely to occur or can be compensated for by decreasing the oral intake of sodium compounds.

Women who discontinue oral contraception for a planned pregnancy commonly ask whether they should wait before attempting to conceive.* Although data are controversial, there does seem to be some evidence of increased incidence of chromosomal changes in abortuses when pregnancy occurs during the first few (usually one or two) cycles after discontinuation of oral contraception.

After discontinuing oral contraception there is usually a delay before ovulation and menstrual cycles recur. However, *postpill amenorrhea* exceeding 6 months should be investigated.

Some neoplasms of the breast, benign or malignant, may be stimulated by estrogen. If another hormone-dependent tumor is suspected (e.g., of the endometrium), oral contraception is contraindicated.

There is an association between long-term use of contraceptive pills by women over 30 years of age and the occurrence of a liver tumor known as hepatocellular adenoma (HCA). The risk of developing HCA is higher with increasing use of OCs. The annual incidence of HCA is approximately 3 or 4 per 100,000 long-term users of OCs. In comparison the annual occurrence rate is approximately 1 to 1.3 per 1 million in women aged 16 to 30 years and in women aged 31 to 34 who have never used OCs or have used them for 24 months or less. Of the women who develop HCA, 88% are long-term users of OCs. The development of HCA can be minimized when the lowest possible dose that provides protection against pregnancy is used. Hepatic adenomas are also associated with the use of OCs. Because hepatic adenomas may rupture and cause death through hemorrhage, they should be considered in women with abdominal pain and tenderness, an abdominal mass, or shock.

Infrequently *hypertension* is first noted after the woman begins oral contraception, especially if she is 30 years of age or older. In some women, higher blood levels of angiotensinogen and plasma renin have been found. It is thought that these factors play a part in the hypertension experienced by some women. After discontinuing oral contraception, hypertension subsides.

Some *laboratory values* may be altered in women taking OCs. These changes are listed, not for memorization, but only for interest and to alert the nurse to the need to ask about contraceptive use when taking a health history. The following laboratory values may be increased: bromsulphalein (BSP), serum glutamic oxaloacetic transaminase (SGOT), serum glutamic pyruvic transaminase (SGPT), alkaline phosphatase, and thyronine-binding protein (a thyroid hormone).

Some conditions are aggravated by fluid retention. Women susceptible to *migraine headaches* may notice an increase in headaches when taking the pill. Since headaches are also symptomatic of cerebral thrombosis, there may be confusion with correct diagnosis. Therefore women who experience migraine headaches are counseled to use other forms of contraception. Although many women with *epilepsy* tolerate OCs well, others tend to have an increase in the incidence of seizures.

Some women who wear *contact lenses* experience a change in the curvature of the cornea. Although the reason for this change is unknown, the woman is advised to discontinue use of the contact lenses while taking OCs.

More serious *neuroocular lesions* are associated with use of OCs. Optic neuritis, or retinal thrombosis, although rare, has been reported. Symptoms such as sudden or gradual and partial or complete loss of vision and double vision require immediate diagnosis and treatment. **Women must stop taking OCs at the first sign of visual disorders.**

There is an increased risk of *gallbladder disease* after 2 years of use of OCs. The risk doubles after 4 to 5 years of pill use.

The effectiveness of OCs is decreased along with an increased possibility of break-through bleeding if the woman is receiving any of the following drugs:

- Barbiturates (for sedation)
- Phenylbutazone (for arthritis or bursitis; treatment for superficial thrombophlebitis)
- Phenytoin sodium (for seizure disorders)
- Ampicillin (for infections)

Long-term use of OCs slows diazepam (Valium) clearance by the liver; therefore higher blood levels of the drug increase the risk of an overdose of diazepam. Planned Parenthood facilities keep current information about newly identified drug interactions as it becomes available.

Effectiveness. Taken exactly as directed, OCs prevent ovulation, and pregnancy cannot occur; the overall effectiveness rate is almost 100%. Of 100 users who start the year using combination OCs and who use them correctly and consistently, the lowest observed failure rate is 0.5 pregnancies. For 100 typical users the failure rate is 2 pregnancies in 1 year (Table 42-11). Almost all failures (i.e., pregnancy occurs) are caused by omission of one or more pills during the regimen. The minipill is slightly less effective than the combination pill but can reach 98% reliability if taken exactly as prescribed.

The woman being considered for therapy with the morning-after pill is advised that should pregnancy occur anyway, elective abortion by cervical dilation and curettage (D and C) may be considered. This is because of the adverse effects of DES on the fetus. The effectiveness of the morning-after pill reaches 100% if hormone therapy is followed by D and C.

Nursing Actions. There are many different preparations of oral hormone contraceptives. The nurse needs to review the prescribing information in the package insert with the client. Some dosage regimens stipulate that the first pill be taken on day 5 of the menstrual cycle; others start on day 1 or on Sunday. Because of the wide variations, each woman must be clear about the unique dosage regimen for the preparation prescribed for her. Directions for care after missing one or two tablets also vary. In general, recent findings indicate that if one or two tablets are

*For discussion of effect of the pill on the fetus when the woman continues with oral contraception after conception, see Appendix G.

missed, another form of contraception needs to be used until the required regimen is reestablished. Typical counseling regarding missed doses follows:

The woman needs to take the pill at the same time each day to maintain constant blood levels of estrogen and progesterone for 21 days. If one pill is missed, the woman takes that pill as soon as she remembers it. She takes the next pill at the regularly scheduled time. If the woman misses two pills, she takes both as soon as she remembers to do so. A second form of contraceptive (e.g., diaphragm with spermicide) for the rest of that cycle is advised. If three pills are missed, the remainder of the pills in that packet are discarded and use of a back-up type of contraceptive is advised. A new packet of pills is begun on the fifth day of the next cycle (bleeding should begin within 2 to 3 days after she misses the pills; day 1 of the new cycle is the first day of bleeding.)

Withdrawal bleeding (periods) tends to be short and scanty when some combination OCs are taken. A woman may see no fresh blood at all. Some women may have only a drop of blood or a brown smudge on their tampon or underwear. This counts as a period. This fact may explain why some women have difficulty remembering the first day of their last period.

No more than 50% to 70% of women who start taking OCs are still taking them after 1 year. It is therefore important that nurses recommend that all women choosing to use the OC also be provided with a second method of birth control and that women be instructed and comfortable with this backup method. Most women stop taking OC's for nonmedical reasons; that is, they *choose* to stop; not because they develop a complication or a serious side effect.

Before OCs are prescribed and periodically throughout hormone therapy, the woman is alerted to stop taking the pill and to report any of the following symptoms to the physician immediately. The word *aches* helps in retention of this list:

A—Abdominal pain: may indicate a problem with the liver or gallbladder
C—Chest pain or shortness of breath: may indicate possible clot problem within lungs or heart
H—Headaches (sudden or persistent): may be caused by cardiovascular accident or hypertension
E—Eye problems: may indicate vascular accident or hypertension
S—Severe leg pain: may indicate a thromboembolic process

A general teaching tool for contraceptive methods is presented in guidelines for client teaching on p. 1085.

Diaphragm with Spermicide. The vaginal diaphragm is a shallow, dome-shaped rubber device with a flexible wire rim that covers the cervix. There are four main styles of diaphragms available in a wide range of diameters (50 to 95 mm). Diaphragms differ in the inner construction of the circular rim. The four types of rims are flat spring, coil spring, arcing spring, and wide seal. The wide seal rim is relatively new. It has a flexible flange approximately 1.5 cm wide attached to the inner edge. The purpose of the flange is to hold the spermicide in place and to create a better seal between the diaphragm and vaginal wall. The diaphragm should feel comfortable. The use of a contraceptive gel or cream with the diaphragm offers both mechanical and chemical barriers to pregnancy.

Mode of Action. The diaphragm is a mechanical barrier preventing the meeting of the sperm with the ovum. The diaphragm holds the spermicide in place against the cervix for the 6 hours it takes to destroy the sperm.

Advantages. Except for occasional allergic responses to the diaphragm or spermicide, there are no side effects from a well-fitted device. The diaphragm can be inserted several hours before intercourse. The woman who engages in intercourse infrequently may choose this barrier method. The spermicide does offer additional lubrication if it is needed. A decreased incidence of vaginitis, cervicitis (including cervicitis caused by *Chlamydia* and *Gonorrhea*), PID and cervical intraepithelial neoplasia is noted among women who use contraceptive creams, foams, and gels with the diaphragm.

Disadvantages and Side Effects. This method is contraindicated for the woman with relaxation of her pelvic support (uterine prolapse) or a large cystocele. It is also not advised for the woman who is "uninformed."

Disadvantages include the reluctance of some women to insert and remove the diaphragm. A cold diaphragm and a cold gel temporarily reduce vaginal response to sexual stimulation if insertion of the diaphragm occurs immediately before intercourse. Some women or couples object to the "messiness" of the spermicide. These annoyances of diaphragm usage, along with failure to insert the device once foreplay has begun, are the most common reasons for failures of this method. Side effects may include irritation of tissues related to contact with spermicides. Urethritis and recurrent cystitis caused by upward pressure of the diaphragm rim against the urethra may be increased by the use of the contraceptive diaphragm.

Effectiveness. Of 100 users who start out the year using a contraceptive diaphragm with spermicide and who use it correctly and consistently, the lowest observed failure rate is 2 pregnancies. For 100 typical users, the number of pregnancies by the end of the first year of use will be 19 (Table 42-11). Highly motivated women may achieve contraception rates of 99% after the first year.

Nursing Actions. The woman is informed that she needs an annual gynecologic examination and that the device may need to be refitted after the loss or gain of 4.5 kg (10 lb) or more or if she gives birth (see research highlight, p. 1099). Since there are various types of diaphragms on the market, the nurse uses the package insert for teaching the woman how to use and care for the diaphragm. The directions for one product are given on p. 1096.

Toxic shock syndrome (TSS) (Chapter 30) can occur in association with the use of the contraceptive diaphragm. The nurse should instruct the woman about ways to reduce her risk for TSS. These measures include not leaving the diaphragm in place for more than 24 hours; not using the diaphragm during menses; and learning and watching for danger signs of TSS. These danger signs include temperature of 38.4°C (101°F), diarrhea, vomiting, muscle aches, and sunburn-like rash.

Text continued on p. 1098.

USE AND CARE OF THE DIAPHRAGM

Positions for Insertion of Diaphragm

Squatting

This is the most frequently used position and most women find this position satisfactory.

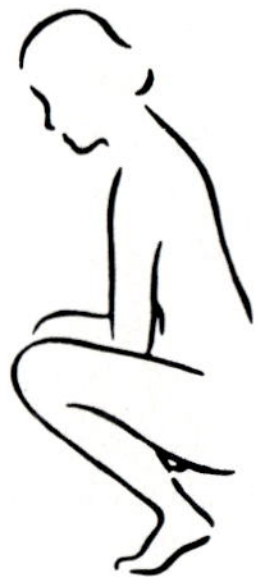

Leg Up Method

A position to suit the convenience of particular women is to raise the left foot (if right hand is used for insertion) on a low stool, and in a bending position the diaphragm is inserted.

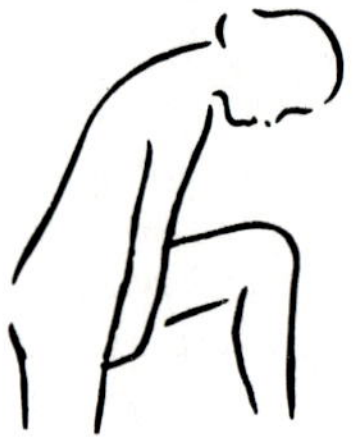

Chair method

A practical method for diaphragm insertion is for the woman to sit far forward on the edge of a chair.

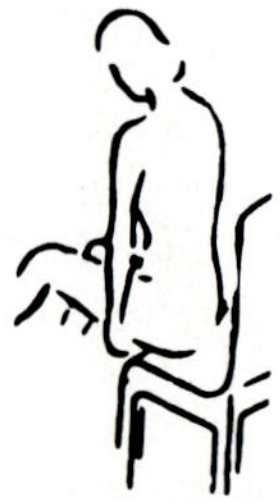

Reclining

In some instances, certain women prefer to insert the diaphragm while in a semi-reclining position in bed.

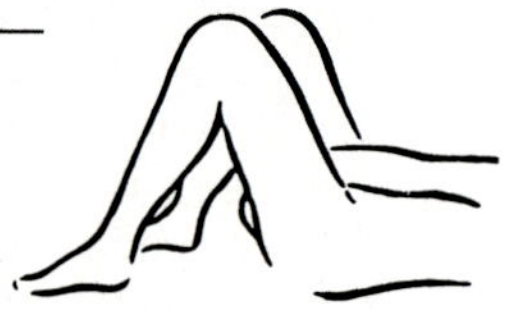

Inspection of Diaphragm

Your diaphragm must be inspected carefully before each use. The best way to do this is:

Hold the diaphragm up to a light source. Carefully stretch the diaphragm at the area of the rim, on all sides, to make sure there are no holes. Remember, it is possible to puncture the diaphragm with sharp fingernails.

Another way to check for pinholes is to carefully fill the diaphragm with water. If there is any problem, it will be seen immediately.

If your diaphragm is "puckered," especially near the rim, this could mean thin spots.

The diaphragm should not be used if you see any of the above . . . consult your physician.

Preparation of Diaphragm

Your diaphragm must always be used with a spermicidal lubricant in order to be effective. Pregnancy cannot be prevented effectively by the diaphragm alone.

Always empty your bladder before inserting the diaphragm. Place about 2 teaspoonsful of contraceptive gel, contraceptive jelly, or contraceptive cream on the side of the diaphragm that will rest against the cervix (or whichever way you have been instructed). Spread it around to coat the surface and the rim. This aids in insertion and offers a more complete seal. Many women also spread some gel (jelly) or cream on the other side of the diaphragm. See Fig. A.

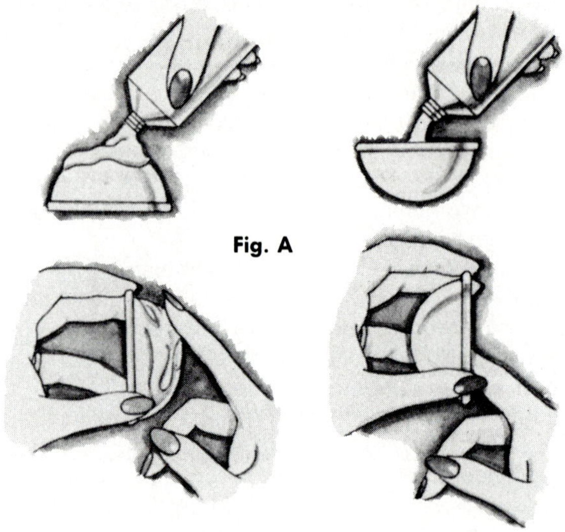

Fig. A

Insertion of Diaphragm

The diaphragm can be inserted as much as 6 hours before intercourse. Hold the diaphragm between your thumb and fingers. The dome can either be up or down, as directed by your physician. Place your index finger on the outer rim of the compressed diaphragm. See Fig. B. Use the fingers of the other hand to spread the labia (lips of the vagina). This will assist in guiding the diaphragm into place.

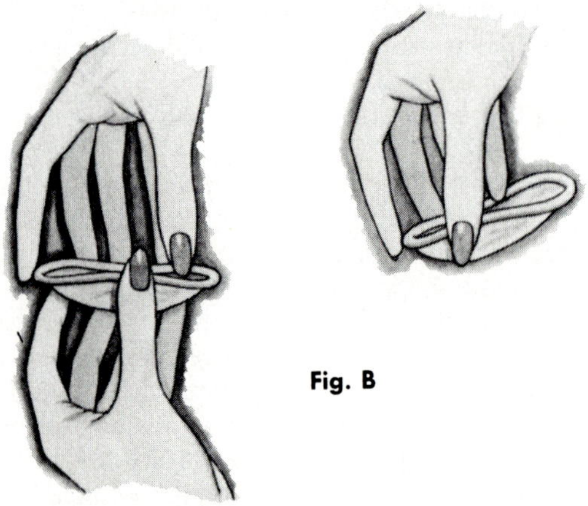

Fig. B

USE AND CARE OF THE DIAPHRAGM—cont'd

Insert the diaphragm into the vagina. Direct it inward and downward as far as it will go to the space behind and below the cervix. See Fig. C.

Fig. C

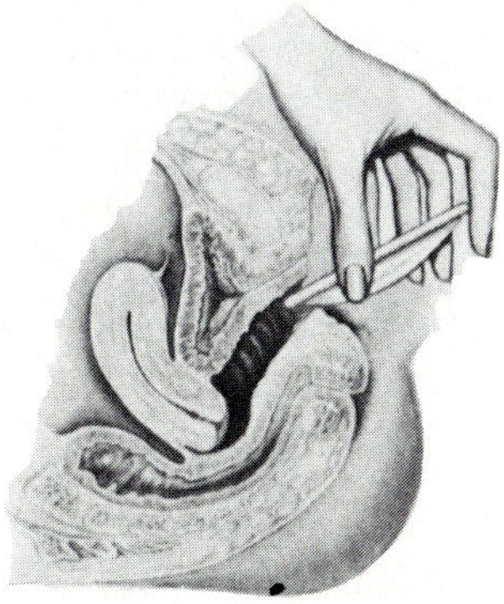

Tuck the front of the rim of the diaphragm behind the pelvic bone so that the rubber hugs the front wall of the vagina. See Fig. D.

Fig. D

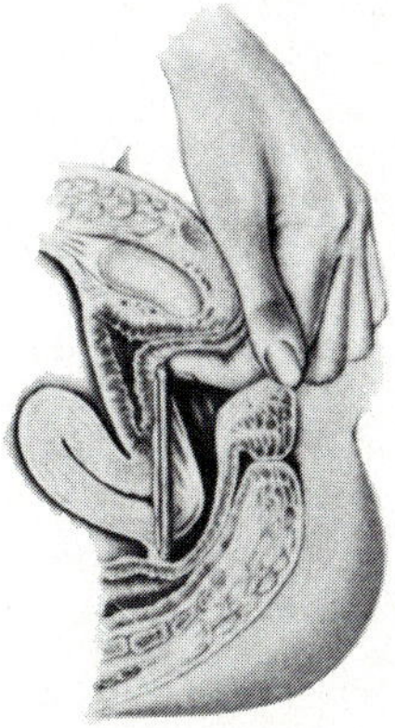

Directions for Insertion With Diaphragm Introducer

Hold the introducer in either hand. Compress the diaphragm, dome up, with the fingers of your other hand. Place one end of the rim in the grooved end of the introducer. See Fig. E.

Fig. E

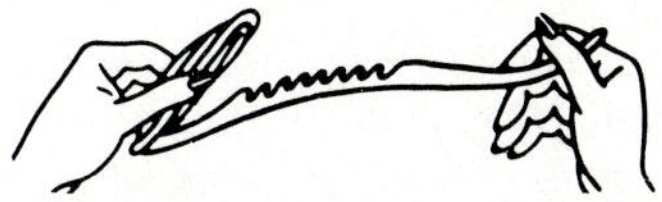

Fit the other end of the diaphragm over the notch corresponding to the diaphragm size. See Fig. F. Squeeze approximately 1 tablespoonful of gel, jelly, or cream into the folds of the diaphragm. Spread a small amount around the rim.

Fig. F

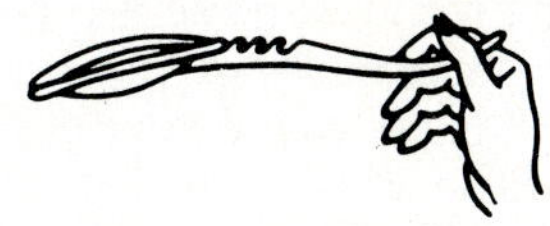

The diaphragm may be inserted while you are lying flat with your legs drawn up. However, any position may be used if more convenient. See positions for insertion of diaphragm.

Insert the diaphragm in a downward direction as far back as it will comfortably go . . . past the cervix. See Fig. G.

Fig. G

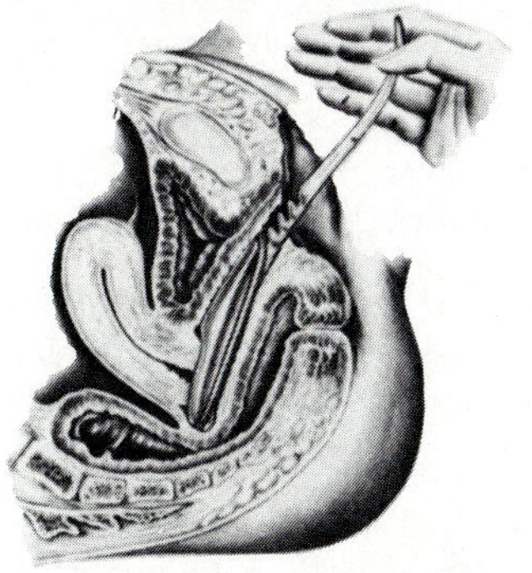

To release the diaphragm, rotate the introducer to the right or left and gently withdraw it. See Fig. H. After the introducer is removed, tuck the front rim of the diaphragm behind the pelvic bone. See Fig. D.

Fig. H

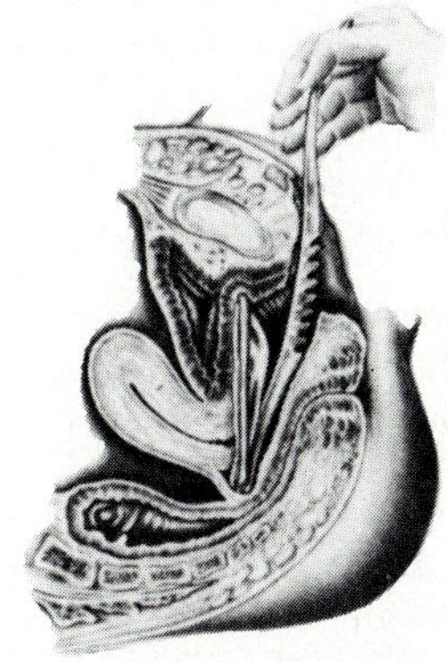

Feel for your cervix through the diaphragm to be certain it is properly placed and securely covered by the rubber dome. See Fig. 1.

Fig. I

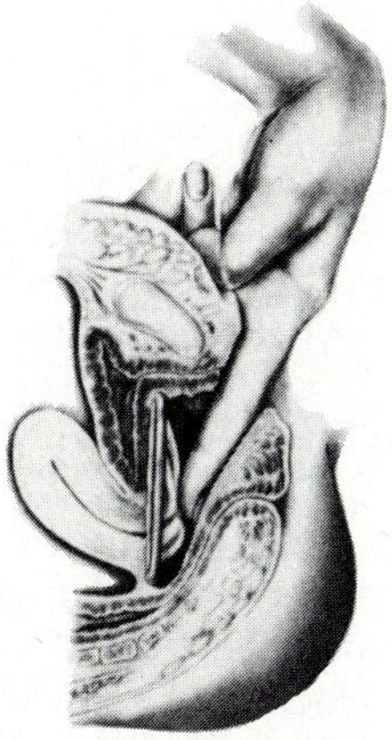

To clean the introducer, wash with mild soap and warm water, rinse and dry thoroughly.

Continued.

USE AND CARE OF THE DIAPHRAGM—*cont'd*

Final Checking

Whether the diaphragm is inserted manually or with the introducer, the finger test must always be made to see that the outer rim of the diaphragm is tucked firmly behind the pelvic bone (see Fig. D). At the same time, you must check to see that the small round knob of the cervix (mouth of the womb) is securely covered by the rubber dome of the diaphragm. See Fig. I.

Repeated Intercourse

Without removing the diaphragm, an additional applicatorful of gel (jelly) or cream must be used if intercourse takes place more than 6 hours after the diaphragm has been inserted or for each repeated intercourse. The diaphragm must remain in place for at least 6 hours after the last intercourse.

General Information

Regardless of the time of the month, this method of contraception must be used each and every time intercourse takes place. Your diaphragm must be left in place for at least 6 hours after the last intercourse. If you remove your diaphragm before the 6-hour time period, your chance of becoming pregnant could be greatly increased. You should not leave your diaphragm in place for more than 24 hours, to do so may encourage growth of bacteria that could result in infection or toxic shock syndrome.

Douching is not necessary after the use of the diaphragm. However, if desired or recommended by your physician, you must wait the full 6 hours after the last intercourse.

Removal of Diaphragm

The only proper way to remove the diaphragm is to insert your forefinger up and over the top side of the diaphragm, and slightly to the side.

Next, turn the palm of your hand downward and backward hooking the forefinger firmly on top of the inside of the upper rim of the diaphragm, *breaking the suction.*

Pull the diaphragm down and out. This avoids the possibility of tearing the diaphragm with the fingernails. The diaphragm *should not* be removed by trying to catch the rim from *below* the dome. See Fig. J.

Fig. J

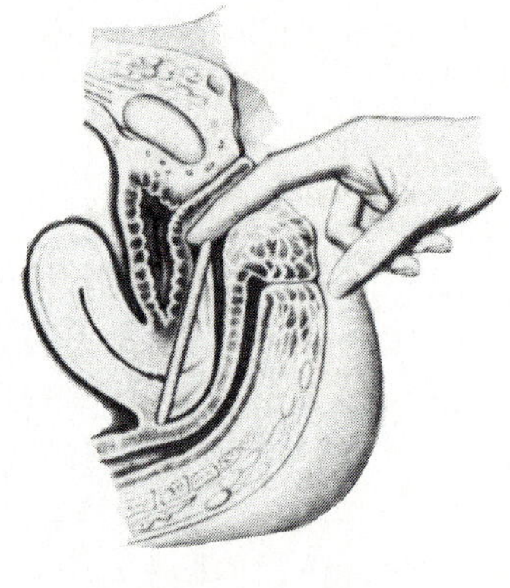

Care of Diaphragm

When using a vaginal diaphragm, avoid using products that may contain petroleum such as certain body lubricants, vaginal lubricants, or vaginitis preparations. These products can weaken rubber.

A little care means longer wear for your diaphragm. After each use the diaphragm should be washed in warm water and Ivory soap. Do not use detergent soaps, cold cream soaps, deodorant soaps, and soaps containing petroleum as they can weaken the rubber. *Ivory soap should be the only soap used.*

After washing, the diaphragm should be dried thoroughly. All water and moisture should be removed with your towel. The diaphragm should then be dusted with *cornstarch.* Scented talc, body powder, baby powder, and the like, should not be used because they can weaken the rubber. Remember, only *cornstarch* for dusting.

The diaphragm should then be placed back in the plastic case for storage. It should not be stored near a radiator or heat source, or exposed to light for an extended period of time.

Cervical Cap. Cervical caps come in two types: one is presized in small, medium, and large, and one is custom fitted. The custom cervical cap is a plasticlike cap about 2.5 cm (1 in) in diameter and is fitted to conform to the individual woman's cervix. This cap has several advantages: (1) It can be made in the physician's office in approximately 20 minutes. A mold of the cervix is made with a nontoxic substance used to make contact lenses. A plaster cast is made of the mold, and then the cap is fitted onto the cast. (2) Its design allows menstrual flow out through the cervix and self-cleaning with natural mucous flow, while preventing sperm from entering the cervix. (3) No foreign-matter reaction has been noted in users of this device. (4) It can be left in place indefinitely.

The presized cervical cap, however, cannot be left in place indefinitely (Fig. 42-8, *C*). In 1988, the U.S. Food and Drug Administration (FDA) approved the cervical cap for general use. The FDA has recommended that users remove the cap after 48 hours, though some studies indicate that the cap can safely be left in place for up to 7 days (Kleinmann, 1988).

Effectiveness. Of 100 users of the cervical cap who start out the year using it and who use it correctly and consistently, the lowest observed failure rate has been 2. For 100 typical users, the number of pregnancies by the end of the year will be 13 (Table 42-11).

Intrauterine Devices. An intrauterine device (IUD) is a small device inserted into the uterine cavity. Medicated

RESEARCH HIGHLIGHT

Relationship Between Weight Change and Diaphragm Size Change

Purpose

To determine the necessity and scientific validity of the practice of having women who use a vaginal diaphragm have the fit of the diaphragm checked by a clinician after a weight gain of 10 or more pounds.

Sample/Methodology

A sample of 125 charts were selected from active files in 2 family planning agencies. The subjects selected included: diaphragm users who had 2 or more fittings of at least 6 weeks apart, had not given birth or had not had a second trimester abortion during the intervening time, had not undergone pelvic surgery, and had no physical anomalies such as cystocele or rectocele.

The mean time between visits was 16.56 months. The sample had a weight variance range of 53 pounds, with a maximum gain of 28 pounds and a maximum loss of 25 pounds. There was no change in diaphragm size in 70% of the sample.

Findings

A Pearson r value ($r = 0.058$) indicated that there was no relationship between weight change and diaphragm size change for this sample.

The extreme variances in size change (plus or minus 10 mm or 15 mm) occurred almost exclusively for those with weight losses. No size change greater than 5 mm occurred in this group, and the subject with the maximum gain of 28 pounds did not require any size change.

The group of subjects exhibiting minimum weight change was as likely to have a different size diaphragm fitted as were subjects exhibiting substantial weight change.

Implications

Because of the small sample of women who gained or lost more than 10 pounds, these results should not be generalized to diaphragm users experiencing a weight change of more than 20 pounds.

Kugel, C, and Verson, H: Relationship between weight change and diaphragm size change, JOGN Nurs 15:123, March/April 1986.

IUDs have taken the place of nonmedicated IUDs (Grimes, 1986).* Medicated IUDs are loaded with either copper† (Fig. 42-9) or a progestational agent. These chemically active substances are released continuously to the endometrium, for example, copper-bearing devices for 3 to 4 years (at present) and progesterone devices for 1 year. IUDs are impregnated with barium sulfate for radiopacity.

Mode of Action. IUDs alter the endometrium locally and thereby discourage implantation should fertilization

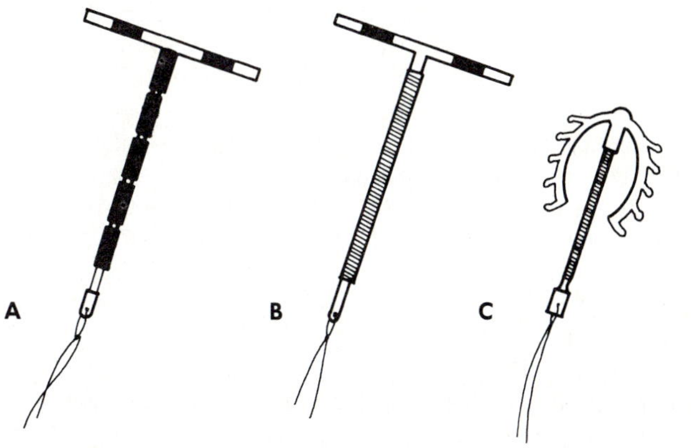

Fig. 42-9 Intrauterine devices. **A**, Copper-T 220. **B**, Copper-T 380A contains 380 square millimeters of copper mounted on a polyethylene base (approved by FDA), now being marketed by GynoMed Pharmaceutical, Inc. **C**, Multiload devices come in different sizes and are prepared with different loads of copper. Not yet available in the United States, they are widely available outside of the United States.

occur. Because the effect is local, there is no disruption of the woman's ovulatory pattern.

Advantages. The IUD offers constant contraception without the need to remember to take pills each day or engage in other manipulation before or between coital acts. If pregnancy can be excluded, an IUD may be placed at any time during the menstrual cycle. An IUD may be inserted immediately after abortion (Liskin and Fox, 1982).

The absence of interference with hormonal regulation of menstrual cycles makes the IUD more appropriate than hormonal contraception for heavy smokers, women over 35, or those with a history of vascular disease or familial diabetes. Contraceptive effects are reversible. When pregnancy is desired, the IUD may be removed by the physician.

Disadvantages and Side Effects. The use of an IUD is contraindicated for women with a history of PID, known or suspected pregnancy, undiagnosed genital bleeding, suspected genital malignancy, or a distorted intrauterine cavity. IUDs are associated with perforation of the uterus, embedment in endometrium or myometrium, uterine cramping and bleeding, iron-deficiency anemia secondary to blood loss, pelvic infections, pregnancy with IUD in place, and pregnancy following undetected expulsion. Some women allergic to copper develop a rash, necessitating the removal of the copper-bearing IUD.

The incidence of perforation is minimized by delaying insertion until a woman finishes lactation (Liskin and Fox, 1982). Except for the Dalkon Shield, the risk of IUD-associated PID is largely limited to the first few months after insertion (Lee et al., 1983). PID occurs in approximately 1% to 3% of women wearing IUDs of all types (Zatuchni, 1985). PID is linked with involuntary infertility (Daling et al., 1985). The risk of PID and primary tubal infection is minimized if a medicated device is used by a woman who has only one sexual partner (Cramer et al., 1985).

The presence of the IUD threads must be checked after menstruation and at the time of ovulation as well as before

*The last nonmedicated plastic IUD (the Lippes loop) was discontinued by its manufacturer in 1985.

†Searle and Company removed CU-7 and TATUM-7 from the United States market on February 1, 1986.

coitus to rule out expulsion of the device. If pregnancy occurs with IUD in place, it should be removed immediately, if possible (Grimes, 1986). Retention of the IUD increases the risk of septic spontaneous abortion and other obstetric problems (Liskin and Fox, 1982). Because the IUD reduces the absolute number of pregnancies overall, current IUD wearers have only 40% the risk for ectopic pregnancy experienced by women not using contraception (Ory, 1981).

The mean blood loss is increased for the copper IUD but not for the Progestesert. This blood loss may be clinically significant in undernourished populations.

The use of medical diathermy (shortwave and microwave) in a woman with a metal-containing IUD may cause heat injury to surrounding tissue. Therefore medical diathermy to the abdominal and sacral areas should not be used on women using copper-bearing IUDs. Additional amounts of copper available to the body from copper containing IUDs may precipitate symptoms in women with undiagnosed Wilson's disease. The incidence of Wilson's disease (an inborn error of metabolism) is 1 in 200,000.

Because of the litigious nature of American contemporary society, most health care providers are requiring lengthy detailed consent forms to be signed by any woman requesting an IUD. In 1988 a new copper IUD (Tatum-T) was released on the U.S. market (Fig. 42-8, *B*). Family planning experts recommend that only women who are involved in stable, monogamous relationships and who have at least one child are appropriate candidates for IUDs. The manufacturer does not recommend women using the Copper-T 380A if they are either under 25, have never had children, or are involved in anything but an exclusive, monogamous relationship (Copper-bearing, 1988).

Effectiveness. Effectiveness and length of effectiveness vary with the type of copper-containing device. The Copper-T 220 and 380 and the multiload Copper 250 (not available in the United States, but probably the world's largest selling IUD) have lower pregnancy rates than the currently available Copper-T 200 (Zatuchni, 1985). Both the Copper-T 220 and 380 have copper sleeves on the transverse arms of the T as well as copper around the vertical arm (Fig. 42-9, A, B,).The local effect of copper is extended to the fundal endometrium, where implantation is most likely to occur.

According to Hatcher (1986), of 100 users who start out the year using an IUD and who use it correctly and consistently, the lowest observed failure rate will be 1.5 pregnancies. For 100 typical users, the number of pregnancies by the end of the first year will be 5 (Table 42-10).

Nursing Actions. The nursing actions related to the IUD are presented in the form of teaching tools. A general teaching tool for contraceptive methods is given (p. 1085).

Methods Requiring Surgical Intervention: Sterilization

Sterilization refers to surgical procedures intended to render the person infertile. Most procedures involve the occlusion of the passageways for the ova and sperm (Fig. 42-10). For the female the oviducts (uterine tubes) are occluded; for the male the sperm ducts (vas deferens) are occluded. Only surgical removal of the ovaries (oophorectomy) or uterus (hysterectomy) or both will result in ab-

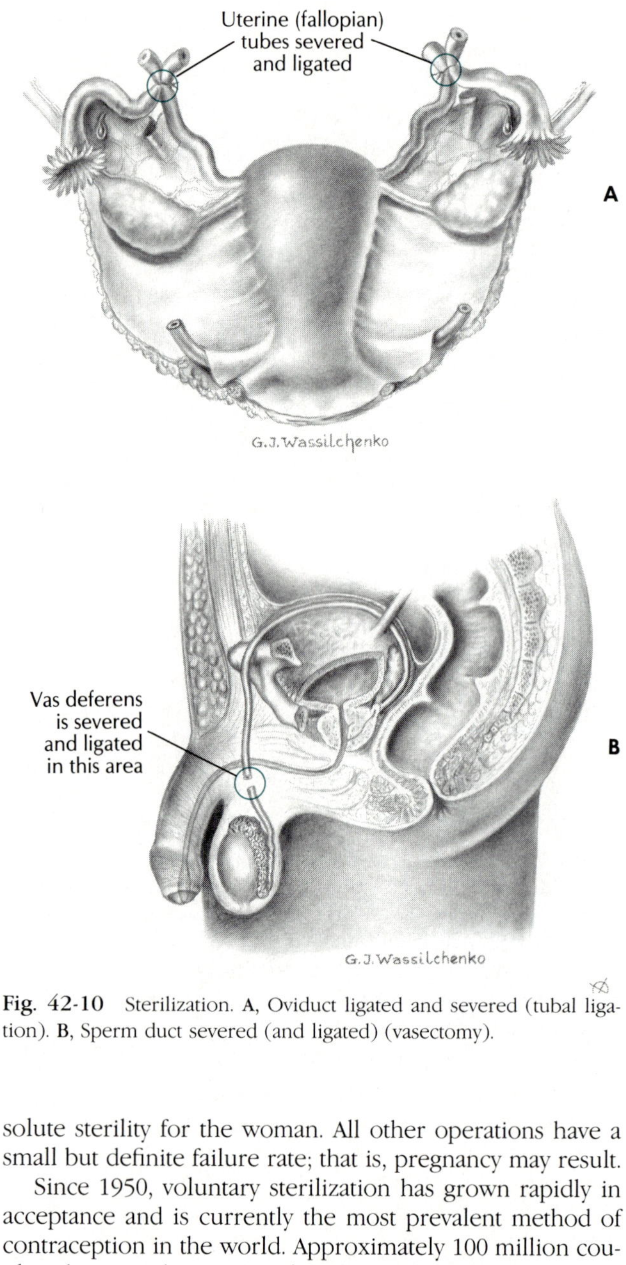

Fig. 42-10 Sterilization. **A**, Oviduct ligated and severed (tubal ligation). **B**, Sperm duct severed (and ligated) (vasectomy).

solute sterility for the woman. All other operations have a small but definite failure rate; that is, pregnancy may result.

Since 1950, voluntary sterilization has grown rapidly in acceptance and is currently the most prevalent method of contraception in the world. Approximately 100 million couples choose voluntary sterilization, and the demand is expected to grow during this century. In the United States, voluntary sterilization is the most common choice of contraception for couples who are 30 years of age or older.

Motivation for Sterilization. Motivation for elective sterilization includes (1) personal preference, (2) obstetric reasons, such as multiparity, (3) medical reasons such as hypertensive, cardiovascular, or renal disease in the woman or recurrent acute epididymitis in the man, and (4) diagnosis of inheritable disease.

Sterilization as a means of contraception may be requested by couples who have almost come to the end of their childbearing years and have the desired number of children. It is also chosen by young adults who have decided not to bear children. Persons in the first group are generally acceptive of the procedure even though there may be some feelings of regret because one of life's phases is over. Persons in the second group need the opportunity to explore the consequences of their choice.

Laws and Regulations. All states have strict regulations for informed consent (see Chapter 4). Now many states in the United States permit voluntary sterilization of any mature, rational woman without reference to her marital or pregnancy status. Although the partner's consent is not required, the client is encouraged to discuss the situation with her or his partner.

Sterilization of minors or mentally incompetent females is restricted by most states. The operation often requires the approval of a board of eugenicists or other court-appointed individuals.

If federal funds are used, the person must be at least 21 years of age and mentally competent. Some state and federal regulations govern Medicaid funds for elective sterilization; for example, counseling and a waiting period after the decision is made are mandatory.

Assessment

Motivation for sterilization and the result of exploration of alternatives are explored. The client's knowledge of the sterilization methods and of the chosen method is assessed. Gaps in knowledge and misinformation are noted.

History, physical examination, and laboratory data are collected (Chapter 8). The record is reviewed for the signed informed consent, and the client's understanding is verified (Chapter 4). General preoperative, operative, and postoperative assessments are performed (Chapter 34).

Nursing Diagnoses

Following are examples of nursing diagnoses for the woman undergoing surgical sterilization.

- Knowledge deficit related to
  - Alternatives
  - Method chosen
  - Preoperative and postoperative events
- Pain related to
  - Postoperative period
- Potential spiritual distress related to
  - Reason for choosing sterilization

Planning

Planning is a collaborative effort among the woman, her sexual partner (where appropriate), the physician, and the nurse. Depending on the motivation for sterilization, other physicians may need to be part of the health care team. Goals are determined and stated in client-centered terms.

Goals

1. Client has received and understood all information necessary to give informed consent
2. Procedure is successful and recovery is uneventful
3. Client continues to be satisfied with the decision for sterilization, the procedure, and the experience with the health care team

Implementation

The nurse plays an important role in assisting people with decision making so that all requirements for informed consent are met. People seek information about the various methods of sterilization. Table 42-12 summarizes expected actions, advantages and side effects, and effectiveness for each method. The table is used as a basis for teaching and counseling. The nurse also provides information about alternatives to sterilization, for example, contraception.

The nurse acts as a sounding board for people who are exploring the possibility of choosing sterilization and their feelings about and motivation for this choice. The nurse records this information, which may be the basis for referral to a family planning clinic, a psychiatric social worker, or another professional health care provider.

Information about what is entailed in various procedures, how much discomfort or pain can be expected, and what type of care is needed must be given. Many individuals fear sterilization procedures because of the imagined effect on their sexual life. They need reassurance concerning the hormonal and psychologic basis for sexual function and the fact that uterine tube occlusion or vasectomy has no biologic sequelae in terms of sexual adequacy.

Preoperative Preparation. Printed instructions are usually available for clients from the physician. The physician performs the preoperative health assessment, which includes a psychologic assessment, physical examination, and laboratory test. The nurse assists with the health assessment, answers questions, and confirms the client's understanding of printed instructions (e.g., NPO [nothing by mouth] after midnight). Ambivalence and extreme fear of the procedure are reported to the physician.

Postoperative Care. Postoperative care depends on the procedure performed, for example, laparoscopy,* laparotomy, hysterectomy, or vasectomy. General care includes postanesthesia recovery, vital signs, fluid-electrolyte balance (intake and output, laboratory values), prevention of or early identification and treatment for infection or hemorrhage, control of discomfort, and assessment of emotional response to the procedure and recovery.

Discharge Planning. Discharge planning depends on the type of procedure performed. In general, the client is given written instructions about observing for and reporting symptoms and signs of complications, the type of recovery to be expected, and the date and time for a follow-up appointment.

Evaluation

The nurse can be reasonably assured that care was effective when the goals of care are achieved: the client has received and understood all information necessary to give in-

*See p. 1068 for discussion of laparoscopy.

Table 42-12 *Summary of Sterilization Methods: Basis for Counseling*

Method and Action	Advantages	Disadvantages and Side Effects	Effectiveness
Woman			
Tubal occlusion: uterine tubes ligated and severed, banded or clipped, or fulgurated, to prevent passage of egg	Abdominal surgery using 2.5 cm (1 in) incision and laparoscopy. Ovaries and endometrium remain intact; menstruation continues	Major surgery with possible complications of anesthesia, infection, hemorrhage, and trauma to other organs Psychologic trauma in some women Sperm may enter peritoneal cavity if tubal ligature slips, and ectopic (abdominal) pregnancy may ensue	100% effective if ligatures, bands, or clips do not slip or cut through
Hysterectomy with salpingo-oophorectomy; no egg produced	No further menstruation	Abrupt loss of ovarian hormones, simulating menopause Possibility of major surgical complications Pyschologic trauma if there is a perceived loss of femininity and sexuality	100% effective
Man			
Vasectomy: vas deferens ligated and severed or banded to interrupt passage of sperm	Relatively simple surgical procedure Does not affect endocrine production or function of testosterone Does not alter volume of ejaculate	Possibility of impotence in some men because of psychologic response to procedure Reversible in many cases Even if procedure is reversed, man may remain infertile if he has developed an autoimmune response (antibodies) to his sperm	100% effective after ejaculate is free of sperm that was in vas deferens (about 6 weeks or 10 ejaculations)

formed consent; the procedure was successful and recovery was uneventful; and the client continues to be satisfied with the decision for sterilization, the procedure, and the experience with the health care team.

Female Sterilization

Timing of Female Sterilization. Female sterilization may be done immediately after delivery (within 24 to 48 hours), concomitantly with abortion, or as an interval procedure (during any phase of the menstrual cycle). Most sterilization procedures are performed immediately after a pregnancy, probably because of heightened motivation or increased practicality. Usually the woman is already in the hospital and all preoperative preparations (blood work, physical examination, etc.) have been completed.

However, all sterilization procedures have the lowest morbidity and failure rates when accomplished at a time other than immediately after a pregnancy. Tissue edema continues during the early postpartum period, which may permit the sutures to cut through the tubal wall and leave an opening into the tube.

Tubal Occlusion. The operation used commonly is the laparoscopic tubal fulguration (destruction of tissue by means of an electric current). See box (p. 1068) for laparoscopy examination, a procedure of entering the abdomen for access to the uterine tubes. A minilaparotomy may be used for tubal ligation (Fig. 42-11) or for the application of bands or clips. Bands (e.g., Falope ring) and clips (e.g., Hulka-Clemens) are placed around the tubes to block them. Fulguration and ligation are considered to be permanent methods. Use of the bands or clips have the theoretic advantage of possible removal and return of tubal patency.

For the minilaparotomy approach the woman is admitted the morning of surgery, having received nothing by mouth (NPO) since midnight. Preoperative sedation is given. The procedure may be carried out with local anes-

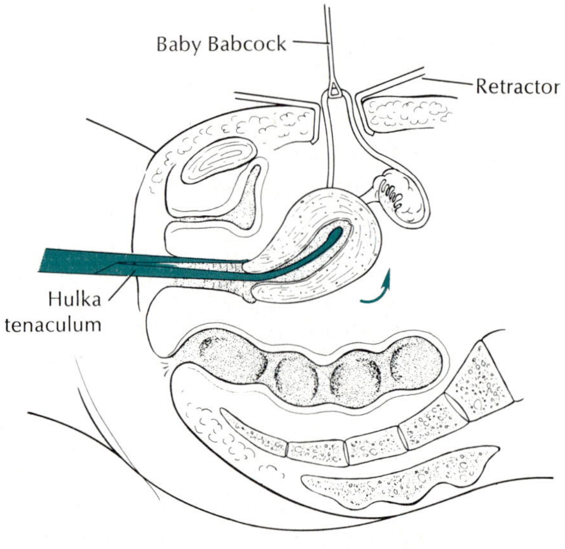

Fig. 42-11 Use of minilaparotomy to gain access to oviducts for tubal occlusion procedures. Tenaculum is used to lift uterus upward *(arrow)* toward incision.

thesia. A small vertical incision is made in the abdominal wall below the umbilicus. The woman may experience sensations of tugging but no pain, and the operation is completed within 20 minutes. She may be discharged 4 hours later if she has recovered from anesthesia. Any abdominal discomfort usually can be controlled with a mild analgesic (e.g., aspirin). Within 10 days the scar is almost invisible.

Major medical complications after elective sterilization are rare. Dysfunctional uterine bleeding or ovarian cyst formation may occur after tubal surgery, presumably because of disturbance of the utero-ovarian circulation.

Tubal Reanastomosis. Tubal continuity is not difficult to reestablish except after laparoscopic tubal fulguration. The incidence of successful pregnancy after reanastomosis is only about 15%. The loss of a segment of tube necessary for sperm capacitation and fertilization is the probable cause.

Male Sterilization. Vasectomy is the easiest and most commonly employed operation for male sterilization. In the United States since 1975, 1 million men undergo vasectomy each year. Vasectomy can be carried out with local anesthesia and on an out-of-hospital basis.

In vasectomy, short right and left incisions are made into the anterior aspect of the scrotum above and lateral to each testis over the spermatic cord (Fig. 42-10, *B*). Each vas deferens is identified and doubly ligated with fine nonabsorbable sutures. Then each vas deferens is incised between the ligatures. Occasionally the surgeon fulgurates the cut stumps of the sperm ducts. Many surgeons bury the cut ends into scrotal fascia to lessen the chance of reunion. Then the skin incisions are closed. Usually one nonabsorbable suture is used for closure of each skin incision. A dressing is applied.

The man is instructed in self-care to promote a safe return to routine activities. To reduce swelling and relieve discomfort, ice packs are applied to the scrotum intermittently for a few hours postoperatively. A suspensory, or bandage, is applied to decrease discomfort by supporting the scrotum. Moderate inactivity for about 2 days is advisable because of local scrotal tenderness. The skin suture can be removed 5 to 7 days postoperatively. Sexual intercourse may be resumed as desired.

Some sperm will remain in the proximal portions of the sperm ducts after vasectomy. At least 10 ejaculations and about 6 weeks are required to clear the ducts of sperm. Therefore contraception is needed until the sperm count in the ejaculate is down to zero.

Vasectomy has no effect on potency (ability to achieve and maintain an erection) or volume of ejaculate. Endocrine production of testosterone continues so that secondary sex characteristics are not affected. Sperm production continues. Men occasionally may develop a hematoma, discharge, or infection. Less common are painful granulomas from accumulation of sperm. Sperm unable to leave the epididymis are lyzed by the immune system.

Complications after bilateral vasectomy are uncommon and usually not serious. They include bleeding (usually external), suture reaction, and reaction to anesthetic agent. Sterilization failures, usually caused by a recanalization, are rare, occurring in about 2 per 1000 men.

Tubal Reanastomosis. Microsurgery to reanastomose the sperm ducts can be accomplished successfully in 90% of cases (i.e., sperm in the ejaculate) (Jarow, 1987). However, the fertility (pregnancies) rate is much lower, 40% to 60% in most series. The length of obstructive interval is the determining factor. The rate of success decreases as the time since the procedure increases. The vasectomy may result in permanent changes in the testes that leave men unable to father children. The changes are those ordinarily seen only in the elderly (e.g., interstitial fibrosis [scar tissue between the seminiferous tubules]) (Jarow et al., 1985). Some men develop antibodies against their own sperm (autoimmunization). The role of antisperm antibodies in fertility after vasectomy reversal has not been completely determined. Women with antibodies have been fertile; however, women with higher antisperm antibody titers take longer to conceive (Jarow, 1987).

Summary. Personnel who function in infertility and birth control clinics or in hospitals must be carefully selected. Studies indicate that attitudes of personnel significantly affect the client's perception of the quality of care received (World Health Organization, 1971). This consideration is important in planning for the overall delivery of health services. Seeking help for infertility and fertility control is often the only contact some people have with the health care system. Positive perceptions of the interest, concern, and technical skill of health workers in this instance may induce wider use of health facilities and care in the future.

SURGICAL INTERRUPTION OF PREGNANCY

Elective abortion is the purposeful interruption of a previable pregnancy. Indications for elective abortion are as follows:

1. Preservation of the life or health of the mother (e.g., class III or IV heart disease)
2. Avoidance of the birth of an offspring with a serious developmental or hereditary disorder (e.g., Tay-Sachs disease)
3. Elective abortion (e.g., because of inability of the parents to support or care for the child, rape, mental incompetence, or because of severe emotional problems)

The control of birth, dealing as it does with human sexuality and the question of life and death is one of the most highly emotionalized components of health care. Abortion as one of the surgical alternatives to contraception is regulated in most countries. Regulations exist presumably to protect the mother from the complications of abortion or because of religious constraints. The U.S. Supreme Court set aside previous antiabortion laws in January 1973, holding that first-trimester abortion is permissible in this country inasmuch as the mortality from interruption of early gestation is now less than the mortality after normal term delivery. Second-trimester abortion was left to the discretion of the individual states. Roman Catholic hospitals and some of those maintained by strict fundamentalists forbid abortion (and often sterilization) despite legal challenge.

Before the legalization of abortion, many illegal abortions took place, with little-documented sequelae other than death from infection or hemorrhage or both. Although studies indicate that biologic sequelae do occur after abortion, rates of biologic complications tend to be low, especially if the woman aborts during the first trimester. Studies related to psychologic sequelae reveal that they are short lived. Sequelae are related to circumstances surrounding the abortion, such as rape or the attitudes reflected by friends, family, and health workers. It must be remembered that the woman facing an abortion is pregnant and will exhibit the emotional responses shared by all pregnant women, including postdelivery depression.

In an attempt to regulate the conflict between professional responsibilities and personal ethics the Nurses' Association of the American College of Obstetricians and Gynecologists (NAACOG) published a position paper on the nurse's role with the abortion client in May 1972, in which the simultaneous rights of each were described (Tyrer, 1973). Women have the right to expect and receive supportive, nonjudgmental care. Nurses have the right to refuse to assist with abortions or sterilizations in keeping with their own moral or religious beliefs, unless the woman's life is in danger.

The values, beliefs, and moral convictions of the nurse are involved to the same extent as those of the pregnant woman. The conflicts and doubts of the nurse can be readily communicated to women who are already anxious and overly sensitive. Health professionals need assistance to identify and come to terms with their own feelings. It is not uncommon for confusion to arise as beliefs are challenged by the reality of care. A nursing student reacted to learning experiences associated with in-hospital abortions in the following manner:

> I really feel I believe in the rightness of therapeutic abortion, but when I watched the physician insert the needle and then inject the dose of prostaglandin, I felt an unreasoning rage sweep over me. I could have attacked him. Funny, I felt no anger toward the girl at all. I really need to rethink my beliefs.

Responses can also change with life experiences. A nurse who before her marriage had worked as counselor in a municipal clinic established a reputation as a supportive and concerned counselor of young persons with regard to birth control. Four years later she remarked:

> I've been trying to get pregnant for the past 3 years. I didn't realize how important it would be to me. You know I can't counsel about abortion any more. I can't be objective. I keep feeling, "Have your baby and please give it to me." I am more concerned about myself now, not them [the pregnant women], and counseling won't work that way.

Assessment

A thorough assessment is conducted through history, physical examination, and laboratory tests (Chapter 8). Compelling medical, surgical, or psychiatric indications for elective abortion, though not numerous, are possible factors. The following conditions probably would qualify: class III coronary heart disease; fulminating (pelvic) Hodgkin's disease; stage 1B carcinoma of the cervix; and Marfan's syndrome with early aortic aneurysm. The length of pregnancy and the condition of the woman need to be determined to select the appropriate type of abortion procedure (Table 42-13).

The woman's understanding of alternatives, the types of abortions, and expected recovery is assessed. Misinformation and gaps in knowledge are identified. The record is reviewed for the signed informed consent and the client's understanding is verified (Chapter 4). General preoperative, operative, and postoperative assessments are performed (Chapter 34).

Nursing Diagnoses

Following are examples of nursing diagnoses for the woman undergoing interruption of pregnancy.

- Knowledge deficit related to
  - Alternatives to abortion
  - Types of abortion
  - Preoperative and postoperative events
- Potential for infection related to
  - The procedure itself
  - Lack of understanding of preoperative and postoperative self-care
- Potential pain related to
  - The procedure
- Potential self-esteem disturbance related to
  - The procedure

Planning

Planning is a collaborative effort among the woman, her sexual partner (as appropriate), the physician, and the nurse. Depending on the motivation for elective abortion, other physicians may need to be part of the health care team. Goals are established collaboratively and should be stated in client-centered terms.

Goals

1. Client has received and understood all information necessary to give informed consent
2. Procedure is successful and recovery is uneventful
3. Client continues to be satisfied with the decision for elective abortion, the procedure, and the experience with the health care team

Implementation

Counseling about abortion includes help for the woman in identifying how she perceives the pregnancy; information about the choices available, that is, having an abortion or carrying the pregnancy to term and then either keeping the child or giving it up for adoption; and information about types of abortion procedures (Table 42-13). *The goal is to assist the woman in coming to a decision that is her own.* She will need help to explore the meaning of the

Table 42-13 *Interruption of Pregnancy: Basis for Counseling*

Methods*	Advantages	Disadvantages and Side Effects	Effectiveness
First-trimester Procedures			
Menstrual extraction: forced endometrial extraction through undilated cervix	Performed up to 14 days after missed period No legal proscriptions	Cervical trauma may occur, may lead to incompetence Hemorrhage	100% if implantation site is not missed
Prostaglandin: Intravenous (IV) administration or injection into cul-de-sac of Douglas or by vaginal suppository or pessary	Stimulates smooth muscle Causes degeneration of corpus luteum	Requires about 24 hours to take effect May cause vomiting, diarrhea, chills, local tissue reaction Retained placenta necessitates D and C	100%
Vacuum (suction) curettage: cannula suction after cervical dilation, under local anesthesia	Effective with relatively few complications: minimum bleeding, minimum discomfort 5-15 minutes duration Done on out-of-hospital or same-day surgery basis	Pregancy 12 weeks or less Possibility of cervical trauma (decreased if dilation accomplished by insertion of laminaria tent 4-24 hours before procedure); endometrial trauma possible Hazards: possible uterine perforation, hemorrhage, or infection	100% if implantation site is not missed and if other reproductive tract anomaly (double uterus) does not exist
Dilation and curettage (D and C): cervix dilated, endometrium scraped with spoonlike instrument	Duration of 15 minutes Usually few complications	Pregnancy 12 weeks or less Hazards: uterine perforation, infection (25%), effects of general anesthesia, cervical trauma	100% if implantation site is not missed
Second-trimester Procedures			
Intraamniotic infusion: between week 14 and 23 or 24 (uterus in abdominal cavity and sufficient amniotic fluid present)	Does not require laparotomy	Increase in complications proportionately with weeks of gestation	Fetal death within 1 hour of injection; abortion completed within 36-40 hours
Transabdominal extraction: amniotic fluid extracted; replaced with equal amount of saline solution (20%) (or 30% urea in 5% dextrose in water)	Ambulation until labor starts (within 24 hours) and during early labor	Reaction to saline solution (hypernatremia): tinnitus, tachycardia, and headache Water intoxication: edema, oliguria ($\leq$200 mg/8 hours), dyspnea, thirst, and restlessness Induced labor, occasionally explosive with an unripe cervix; fetus passes out of posterior vault of vagina and forms fistula Hazards requiring hospitalization (6% readmitted for complications): Hemorrhage and possible D and C May require postabortal D and C or vacuum extraction as well Fever with sepsis	Two thirds of fetuses aborted within 24 hours
Instillation of 40-45 mg prostaglandins $PGF_2\alpha$, E_2	Labor usually shorter than with saline solution Avoid complications of water intoxication and hypernatremia	May cause vomiting, diarrhea, nausea Fetus may be born alive D and C may be required to remove placental fragments	100%
Dilation and evacuation (D and E)	Hospitalization shortened With skilled operator, complication rate lower than with intraamniotic infusion methods	24 hours before procedure, 2 or 3 laminaria tents used to dilate cervix to required 2 cm Fetus possibly born alive	100%

*Prophylaxis against Rh isoimmunization, $Rh_0(D)$ immune globulin, is given within 72 hours to every Rh-negative, Du-negative, unsensitized (Coombs' negative) woman.

Continued.

Table 42-13 *Interruption of Pregnancy: Basis for Counseling—cont'd*

Methods*	Advantages	Disadvantages and Side Effects	Effectiveness
Second- and Third-trimester Procedures			
Hysterotomy: cesarean incision	Preferred method if woman wishes tubal ligation or hysterectomy to follow	Complications after major surgery—hemorrhage and infection Fetus possibly born alive, opening ethical, moral, religious, and legal problems Mortality risk—combination hysterotomy-hysterectomy 10% greater than with D and C	100%
Hysterectomy: at or before 24 weeks without first emptying uterus	As above	As above	100%

various alternatives and consequences to herself and her significant others. It is often difficult for a woman to express her true feelings (e.g., what abortion means to her now and in the future, and what support or regret her friends and peers may demonstrate). A calm, matter-of-fact approach on the part of the nurse can be helpful (e.g.: "Yes, I know you are pregnant, I am here to help. Let's talk about alternatives.") Listening to what the woman has to say and encouraging her to speak are essential. Neutral responses such as "Oh," "Uh-huh," and "Umm" and nonverbal encouragement such as nodding, maintaining eye contact, and use of touch are helpful in setting an open, accepting environment. Clarifying, restating, and reflecting statements, use of open-ended questions, and giving feedback are communication techniques that can be used to maintain a reality focus on the situation and bring the woman's problems into the open. Once a decision has been made, the woman must be assured of continued support. Information about what is entailed in various procedures (Table 42-13), how much discomfort or pain can be expected, and what type of care is needed must be given. If family or friends cannot be involved, scheduling time for the nursing personnel to give the necessary support is an essential component of the care plan.

Preoperative preparation, postoperative care, and discharge planning parallel the methods used for sterilization (see p. 1101).

Evaluation

The nurse can be reasonably assured that care was effective when the goals of care have been met: the client has received and understood all information necessary to give informed consent; the procedure is successful, recovery is uneventful, and the client continues to be satisfied with the decision for elective abortion, the procedure, and the experience with the health care team.

Early Abortion

Methods for performing early therapeutic abortion include the following:

1. Menstrual extraction—early aspiration of the endometrium in women who have not yet missed a period
2. Surgical D and C when newer aspiration equipment is unavailable
3. Uterine aspiration after one or two missed periods

The insertion of a small laminaria tent retained by a vaginal tampon for 4 to 24 hours usually will facilitate the purposeful interruption of a first-trimester pregnancy by dilating the cervix atraumatically (Fig. 42-12). On removal of the moist, expanded laminaria, the cervix will have dilated two or three times its original (dry) diameter. Rarely will further mechanical dilation of the cervix be required. The insertion of an adequate-sized aspiration cannula (8.5 to 10.5 mm) is almost always possible. Cervical laceration and bleeding are reduced by the use of laminaria. A disadvantage is the delay necessary and the need for an additional visit to the physician's office or clinic.

The woman comes to the clinic or physician's office the day before the abortion procedure. An antiseptic solution is used to prepare the pelvic area. A vaginal speculum is inserted, and the vaginal canal and cervix are cleansed. Injection of a local anesthetic agent into the cervix may follow (see paracervical block, Chapter 17, and p. 1108). Again the area is cleansed, and the laminaria tent is inserted into the endocervical canal. Prophylactic use of an antibiotic is usually begun. Some women experience a mild cramping or have light spotting from the anesthetic injection. Discomfort can usually be controlled with analgesics.

Aspiration abortion may be performed in the physician's office or in the hospital setting. If the woman chooses a hospital setting, she is admitted the day after insertion of the laminaria tent and is given preoperative sedation. The vaginal area is cleansed (shaving is not necessary). The suction procedure for accomplishing an early elective abortion

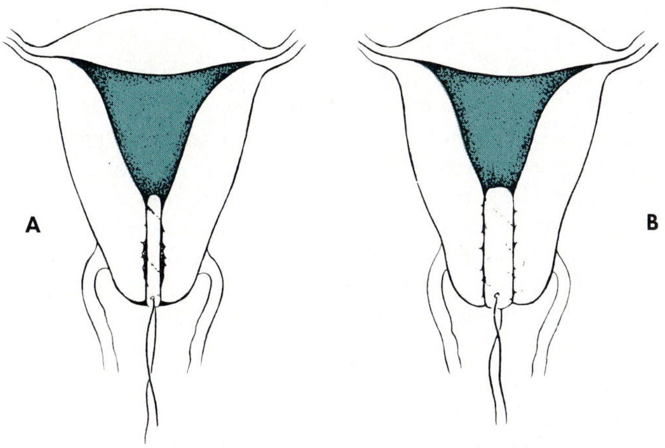

Fig. 42-12 Laminaria tents. **A**, Inserted through narrow cervical canal beyond the internal os. **B**, Cervix dilated 4 to 12 hours later.
From Sanberg, EC: Synopsis of obstetrics, ed 10, St Louis, 1978, The CV Mosby Co.

(ideal time is 8 to 10 weeks since last menstrual period) usually requires less than 5 minutes and can easily be effected under paracervical block anesthesia and single sedation. During the procedure the nurse or physician keeps the woman informed as to what to expect next, for example, menstrual-like cramping, sounds of suction machine. The nurse assesses the woman's vital signs and observes her for vagal response (p. 145). The aspirated uterine contents must be carefully inspected to ascertain whether all fetal parts and adequate placental tissue have been evacuated. A single dose of oxytocin is usually sufficient to control bleeding. The woman may remain in the hospital 3 or 4 hours for detection of excessive cramping or excessive bleeding and then is discharged. If the procedure is done in the physician's office, preoperative sedation is usually not given, and the anesthetic of choice is usually paracervical block. After the abortion the woman rests on the table until she is ready to get up. Then she remains in the waiting room until she feels she can travel. She may be discharged in the company of a relative or friend.

Bleeding after the operation normally is about the equivalent of a heavy menstrual period, and cramps are rarely severe. Infection such as endometritis or salpingitis occurs in about 8% of women. Subsequently a D and C procedure for bleeding or sepsis caused by retained placental tissue is necessary in about 2% of women. Serious depression or other psychiatric problems are rare.

Postabortal instructions differ with the institution (e.g., use of tampons may be denied for only 3 days or for up to 6 weeks, and resumption of sexual intercourse may be permitted within 1 week or discouraged for 6 weeks). The woman may bathe or shower daily. Instruction is given to watch for excessive bleeding, cramps, or fever and to avoid douches of any type. The woman may expect her menstrual period to resume 4 to 6 weeks from the day of the procedure. The nurse offers information about the birth control method the woman prefers if this has not been done previously during the counseling interview that usually precedes the decision to have an abortion. The woman must be strongly encouraged to return for her follow-up visit so that complications can be avoided and an acceptable contraceptive method prescribed.

Second- and Third-trimester Abortions

There are four types of techniques used for second- and third-trimester abortions:

1. *Transabdominal intrauterine injection of hypertonic sodium chloride.* The woman is admitted to the hospital for this procedure. Amniocentesis is performed. The physician determines where the needle (an 18-gauge, 7.5 cm [3 in] spinal needle) will be inserted. The area is cleansed, and if desired, a local anesthetic agent is given. Approximately 200 ml of amniotic fluid is withdrawn, and a similar amount of sterile 20% sodium chloride is injected. The woman is instructed to report when uterine contractions begin—generally, within 8 to 48 hours. In most cases augmentation with oxytocin is necessary to effect uterine evacuation in a reasonable time. Occasionally reinjection is required. Labor begins, in theory at least, because the hypertonic saline solution releases the placental uterine progesterone blockade that normally prevents the onset of labor. The same careful monitoring of uterine contractions is as necessary as for a term delivery. Instruction in relaxation and breathing techniques is indicated, and analgesia can be administered for discomfort. The assistance of a supportive person at the time of birth of the dead fetus is essential. If the woman wishes to see the fetus, emotional support should be provided before and after the procedure. Many woman are relieved to find the fetus normal and commonly inquire as to its sex. After the delivery the standard observations and postpartum care are carried out (see Chapter 26). Contraceptive counseling is given before discharge. The woman is advised to return should excessive bleeding occur.

Complications of hypertonic saline injection for second-trimester abortion may occur. Complications with the approximate frequency of their occurrence include infection (10%), need for D and C to remove retained tissue (15%), failure to abort (10%), and excessive bleeding, necessitating transfusion (2%). Rarely, disseminated intravascular coagulation (DIC) or expulsion of the fetus through the uterine isthmus occurs.

2. *Injection of urea solution after amniocentesis.* After the removal of about 200 ml of amniotic fluid, 200 ml of 30% solution of urea in 5% dextrose in water is introduced into the uterus by gravity drip. After 1 hour a solution of 5 units of oxytocin in 500 ml of 5% dextrose in water is started intravenously. Fetal death occurs, and delivery ensues in most cases within 12 hours. Complications are less common and are less serious than with hypertonic saline solution.

3. *Transabdominal intrauterine injection of* $PGF_{2\alpha}$ The undesirable side effects of hypertonic saline solution, such as hypernatremia or DIC, do not occur with prostaglandins; therefore it has become the treatment of choice. However, nausea and vomiting are common problems. Abortion usu-

ally takes place within 18 to 24 hours after injection. If it does not occur, the procedure is repeated, but only half the dosage is used.

4. *Abdominal or vaginal hysterotomy.* Hysterotomy may be chosen after more than 14 to 16 weeks of pregnancy, after failure of intrauterine injection of saline solution or $PGF_{2\alpha}$, and when sterilization is desired. The vaginal approach is employed when transabdominal surgery should be avoided. The management is comparable to that of cesarean delivery.

RU 486 (Mifepristone)

Progesterone is essential for the maintenance of pregnancy. RU 486 is a progesterone antagonist that prevents implantation of a fertilized egg. It is most effective in early gestation, during the luteal phase, within 10 days of the expected onset of what would be the first missed period after conception. It can be taken up to 5 weeks after conception. However, it is considered to be an effective and safe method for termination of early pregnancy. The medication should be used only under close medical supervision (Couzinet et al., 1986).

Uterine bleeding begins within 4 days of administration of the first dose. Usually a period of painless heavy bleeding is reported. Termination of pregnancy occurs for most women. For the woman in whom abortion does not occur, evacuation of the uterus by aspiration is facilitated by the softening of the uterine cervix. RU 486 is responsible for cervical softening. Some women experience slight nausea and fatigue during the period of bleeding.

The present results are similar to those reported in investigations in which prostaglandin analogues were used to terminate early pregnancy. Although the success rate with prostaglandins also approaches 85%, this method is associated with painful uterine contractions and gastrointestinal side effects in approximately 50% of subjects. In contrast, RU 486 is well tolerated. Supporters of this method feel that even with known disadvantages, RU 486 offers a reasonable alternative to surgical abortion, which carries the risks of anesthesia, surgical complications, infertility, and psychological sequelae (Couzinet et al., 1986; Debate 1987a). Others have taken a strong stand against the use of RU 486 (mifepristone) (Debate, 1987b).

Anesthesia for Gynecologic Procedures: Paracervical (Uterosacral) Block. Paracervical block anesthesia is used for a variety of obstetric (Chapter 17) and gynecologic procedures (Fig. 17-1, *B*). Tests for infertility such as endometrial biopsy and aspiration abortion are two such procedures. Complications may include vasovagal syncope and intravascular injection.

The procedure is explained to the woman. She is asked to void if her bladder is full. Her vital signs are checked and recorded. The sight of the long needle used to inject the anesthesia may be frightening (Fig. 17-18). The woman can be reassured that only the tip of the needle will be inserted. For this sterile procedure the physician or anesthesiologist will need the nurse's assistance in positioning the woman (dorsal recumbent position with knees flexed), handling supplies, and helping the woman to remain immobile while the injection is made.

SUMMARY

The roles of the nurse vary in the care of clients requiring treatment for infertility, control of fertility, termination of fertility, and interruption of pregnancy. A solid knowledge base of anatomy and physiology, mastery of nursing skills, and the nurse's self-awareness are all essential factors in meeting client needs. Professional satisfaction is the reward for the nurse who is able to assist clients coping with reproductive issues. Seeking help for infertility and fertility control is commonly the only contact some people have with the health care system. Positive perceptions of the interest, concern, and technical skill of health care providers in this instance may induce wider use of health facilities and care in the future.

KEY CONCEPTS

- Impaired fertility is the inability to conceive and carry a child to term after 1 year of unprotected sexual intercourse. Impaired fertility affects between 10% to 15% of otherwise healthy adults.
- Male and female factors each separately account for 40% of impaired fertility. Factors from both partners are responsible for the remaining 20%.
- Common etiologic factors of impaired fertility include decreased sperm production, interference with hypothalamic-pituitary-ovarian axis, tubal occlusion, and varicocele.
- It is estimated that 40% to 50% of couples with impaired fertility who seek assistance will be able to become pregnant and carry the child to viability.
- Less conventional ways of achieving parenthood include therapeutic intrauterine insemination, in vitro fertilization-embryo transplant, GIFT, and surrogate motherhood.
- There are a variety of contraceptive methods and various effectiveness ratings, advantages, and disadvantages.
- Nurses need to help couples choose the contraceptive method or methods best suited to them.
- Proper concurrent use of spermicides and latex condoms provides protection against AIDS.
- Tubal ligations and vasectomies are permanent sterilization methods used by increasing numbers of women and men.
- Abortion accomplished in the first trimester is 10 times safer than carrying a pregnancy to term.

STUDY QUESTIONS AND ACTIVITIES

1. Compare the various fertility control methods with regard to effectiveness, advantages, and disadvantages.
2. Write a teaching plan to specifically instruct a couple about the use of one nonpermanent method of contraception.
3. Discuss three ways a nurse can help a couple cope with a diagnosis of infertility.
4. Discuss the ethical issues resulting from therapeutic intrauterine insemination, in vitro fertilization-embryo transplant, GIFT, or surrogate motherhood.

References

Asch, RH, et al: Pregnancy after translaparoscopic gamete intrafallopian transfer [GIFT] (Letter) Lancet 2:1034, 1984

Bachrach, CA: Contraceptive practice among American women: 1973-1982, Fam Plann Perspect 16:253, 1984

Bernstein, JL, and Kidd, YA: Childbearing in Japan. In Kay, MA, editor: Anthropology of human birth, Philadelphia, 1982, FA Davis Co

Billings, J: Natural family planning: the ovulation method, ed 3, Collegeville, Minn, 1975, The Liturgical Press

Brownlee, AT: Community, culture, and care: a cross-cultural guide for health workers, St Louis, 1978, The CV Mosby Co

Bustillo, M, et al: Nonsurgical ovum (embryo) transfer as a treatment in infertile women: preliminary experience, *JAMA* **251**:1171, 1984

Clark, M: Health in the Mexican-American culture: a community study, Berkeley, 1970, University of California Press

Clark, AL, and Howland, IH: The American Samoan. In Clark, AL, editor: Culture/childbearing/health professionals, Philadelphia, 1978, FA Davis Co

Copper-bearing IUD introduced in United States, NAACOG Newsletter 15(1):9, 1988

Coughlin, R: Pregnancy and birth in Vietnam. In Hart, D, et al, editors: Southeast Asian birth customs: three studies in human reproduction, New Haven, Conn, 1965, Human Relations Area Files

Couzinet, B, et al: Termination of early pregnancy by the progesterone antagonist RU 486 (Mifepristone), N Engl J Med 315(25):1565, 1986

Cramer, DW, et al: Tubal infertility and the intrauterine device, N Engl J Med 312:941, 1985

Daling, JR, et al: Primary tubal infertility in relation to the use of an intrauterine device, N Engl J Med 312:937, 1985

Darity, WA, and Turner, CB: Family planning, race consciousness and the fear of genocide, Am J Pub Health 62:1454, 1972

The debate: abortion pill (RU 486). We should test this drug in the USA, USA Today p 10A, Jan 15, 1987

The debate: abortion pill. Keep this chemical killer out of the USA (an opposing view, JC Willke), USA Today, p 10A, Jan 15, 1987b

Dougherty, MC: A cultural approach to the nurse's role in health-care planning, Nurs Forum 11:310, 1972

Fogel, CI, and Woods, NF: Health care of women: a nursing perspective, St Louis, 1981, The CV Mosby Co

Grimes, DA: Reversible contraception for the 1980s, JAMA 255(1):69, 1986

Hatcher, RA, et al: Contraceptive technology, ed 13, New York, 1986, Irvington Publishers, Inc

Hatcher, RA, Contraceptive technology 1984-1985, New York, 1984, Irvington Publishers, Inc

IPPF International Medical Advisory Panel: Statement on intrauterine devices, IPPF Med Bull no 6, vol 15, 1981

Jarow, JP: Vasectomy: autoimmunity and reversal, JAMA 257(15):2087, 1987

Jarow, JP, et al: Quantitative pathologic changes in the human testis after vasectomy, N Engl J Med 313(20):1252, 1985

Kay, MA, editor: Anthropology of human birth, Philadelphia, 1982, FA Davis Co

Kilmann, PR: Human sexuality in contemporary life, Boston, 1984, Allyn & Bacon, Inc

Klaus, H: Natural family planning: a review, Obstet Gynecol Surv 37:128, 1982

Kleinmann, L: Cervical cap approved at last, Health 20(7):8, 1988

Kols, A, et al: Oral contraceptives in the 1980s, Popul Rep [A], no 6, 1982

Lee, NC, et al: Type of intrauterine device and the risk of pelvic inflammatory disease, Obstet Gynecol 62:1, 1983

Liskin, LS, and Fox, G: Periodic abstinence: how well do new approaches work: Popul Rep [I], no 3, 1981

Liskin, LS, and Fox, G: IUDs: an appropriate contraceptive for many women, Popul Rep [B], no 4, 1982

Marrs, RP: In vitro fertilization's future looks bright, Contemp OB/GYN 20:135, 1982

Marrs, RP, editor: Human in-vitro fertilization, Clin Obstet Gynecol 29:117, 1986

McHugh, NC, et al: Preparatory information: what helps and why, Am J Nurs 82:780, 1982

Menning, B: Infertility: a guide for the childless couple, Englewood Cliffs, NJ, 1977, Prentice-Hall, Inc

Mishell, DR: Noncontraceptive health benefits of oral steroidal contraceptives, Am J Obstet Gynecol 248:184, 1982

Modica, MM, and Timor-Tritsch, IE: Transvaginal sonography provides a sharper view into the pelvis, JOGNN Nurs 17(2):89, 1988

Okamoto, NJ: The Japanese American, In Clark, A, editor: Culture-childbearing/health professionals, Philadelphia, 1978, FA Davis Co

Ory, HW: The Women's Study: ectopic pregnancy and intrauterine contraceptive devices: new perspectives, Obstet Gynecol 57:137, 1981

Ory, HW: The noncontraceptive health benefits from oral contraceptive use, Fam Plann Perspect 14:182, 1982

Pace-Owens, S: In vitro fertilization and embryo transfer, JOGN Nurs 14:44s, 1985

Pernoll, ML, and Benson, RC, editors: Current obstetric and gynecologic diagnosis and treatment, ed 6, Los Altos, Calif, 1987, Appleton & Lange

Population Reports: IUDs: an appropriate contraception for many women, series B, no 4, July 1982

Pritchard, JA, MacDonald, PC, and Gant, NF: Williams obstetrics, ed 17, Norwalk, Conn, 1985, Appleton-Century-Crofts

Rock, J, et al: Effects of adoption on infertility, Fertil Steril 16:305, 1965

San Francisco Chronicle, Jan 14, 1986, and Feb 1, 1986

Scott, CS: The theoretical significance of a sense of well-being for the delivery for gynecological health care. In Bauwens, EE, editor: The anthropology of health, St Louis, 1978, The CV Mosby Co

Snow, L: Folk medical beliefs and their implications for care of patients, Ann Intern Med 81:82, 1974

Speroff, L, et al: Clinical gynecologic endocrinology and infertility, Baltimore, 1983, Williams & Wilkins

Tyrer, L: The new morality, ethics, and nursing, JOGN Nurs 2:54, 1973

Veevers, JE: The social meaning of parenthood, Psychiatry, 36:291, 1973

Vogel, G: American Indian medicine, New York, 1973, Ballantine Books, Inc

Washington, AE, et al: Oral contraceptives, *Chlamydia trachomatis* infection, and pelvic inflammatory disease, JAMA 253:2246, 1985

Willson, JR, Carrington, ER, and Ledger, WJ: Obstetrics and gynecology, ed 8, St Louis, 1987, The CV Mosby Co

Wolner-Hanssen, P, et al: Laparoscopic findings and contraceptive use in women with signs and symptoms suggestive of acute salpingitis, Obstet Gynecol 66:233, 1985

World Health Organization: Induced abortion as public health program: report on working group, Copenhagen, 1971, Regional Office for Europe

Zatuchni, G: New devices for intrauterine contraception, Contemp OB/GYN 24 (special issue: technology 1985): 77, Oct 1985

Bibliography

A fresh look at barrier contraceptives, Contemp OB/GYN 31(3):132, 1988

Alexander, NJ, and Schlaff, W: Insemination: some cautions, Contemp OB/GYN (Special Issue):99, 1987

Annas, GJ: Baby M: babies (and justice) for sale, Hastings Cent Rep 17(3):13, 1987

Ausbacher, R: Immunologically triggered ovarian failure, Contemp OB/GYN (Special Issue):25, 1987

Berkowitz, R, et al: Selective reduction of multifetal pregnancies in the first trimester, N Engl J Med 318(16):1043, 1988

Berry, WR, et al: Transmission of hepatatis B virus by artificial insemination, JAMA 257(8):1079, 1987

Cabrol, D, Bouvier, D'Yvoire, M, et al: Induction of labour with mifepristone after intrauterine fetal death, Lancet 2:1019, 1985

Caillouette, J, and Koehler, A: Phasic contraceptive pills and functional ovarian cysts, Am J Obstet Gynecol 156:1538, June 1987

Carey, M, and Brown, S: Infertility surgery for pelvic inflammatory disease: success rates after salpingolysis and salpingostomy, Am J Obstet Gynecol 156(2):296, 1987

Christianson, C: Support groups for infertile patients, JOGN Nurs 15:293, 1985

Clark, JB, et al: Pharmacological basis of nursing practice, St Louis, 1986, The CV Mosby Co

Clinical News: DES daughters: fighting fear with facts, Am J Nurs 85:639, June 1985

Clinical News: The latest in the search for a perfect contraceptive, Am J Nurs 85:126, Feb 1985

Creighton, H: In vitro fertilization, Nurs Manage 16:12, April 1985

Cupit, LG: Contraception: helping patients choose, JOGN Nurs 13:23s, 1984

Daniell, JF: Tailoring the laser for infertility surgery, Contemp OB/GYN (Special Issue):133, 1987

Darland, NW: Infertility associated with luteal phase defect, JOGN Nurs 14:212, May/June 1985

Davis, DC: A conceptual framework for infertility, JOGN Nurs 16(1):30, 1987

DeMoya, D, and DeMoya, A: Best contraceptive for paraplegic women, RN 48:56, Dec 1985

Dirubbo, NE: The condom barrier, Am J Nurs 87(10):1306, 1987

Dodson, MG: A detailed program review of in vitro fertilization with a discussion and comparison of alternative approaches, Surg Gynecol Obstet 162:89, Jan 1986

Do oral contraceptives prevent rheumatoid arthritis? JAMA 256(2):215, 1986

Droegemueller, W, et al: Comprehensive gynecology, St Louis 1987, The CV Mosby Co

Drug Dispatches: A modified pill, Nurs '86, 16:76, Jan 1986

Dugan, KA: Diagnostic laparoscopy under local anesthesia for evaluation of infertility, JOGN Nurs 14:363, Sept/Oct 1985

Elias, S, and Annas, GJ: Social policy considerations in noncoital reproduction, JAMA 255:62, 1986

Eschenbach, DA: Infertility caused by infection, Contemp OB/GYN (Special Issue):29, 1987

Estok, PJ, and Rudy, EB: Intensity of jogging: relationship with menstrual/reproductive variables, JOGN Nurs 13:390, Nov/Dec 1984

Hammond, MG: Monitoring ovulation, Contemp OB/GYN (Special Issue):59, 1987

Goldbaum, G, et al: The relative impact of smoking and oral contraceptive use on women in the United States, JAMA 258(10):1339, 1987

Hearn, MT, et al: Psychological characteristics of in vitro fertilization participants, Am J Obstet Gynecol 156(2):269, 1987

Horsley, JE: Can you refuse to assist in abortions? RN, p 65, May 1987

Infertility: female factors. Harvard Medical School Health Letter 12(8):5, 1987

Infertility: Harvard Medical School Health Letter 12(7):6, 1987

Intravaginal transducer developed for infertility studies. NAACOG Newsletter 13(6):9, 1986

Jones, HW, Jr, Jones, GS, Hodgen, GD, and Rosenwaks, Z, editors: In vitro fertilization, Norfolk, Baltimore, 1986, Williams & Wilkins

Kaunitz, AM, Grimes, DA: The woman over 50: endometrial sampling in older women, Contemp OB/GYN 31(Special Issue):85, April 1988

Keye, WR: Guiding infertile patients, Contemp OB/GYN (Special Issue):151, 1987

Kraus, S: Making babies (IVF). Stanford Medicine, P 26, Winter 1987

Kugel, C, and Verson, H: Relationship between weight change and diaphragm size change, JOGN Nurs 16:123, 1986

LeMaire, GS: The luteinized unruptured follicle syndrome: anovulation in disguise, JOGN Nurs 16(2):116, 1987

Magil, B: Monoclonals: new frontiers in reproductive medicine, Contemp OB/GYN 26(special issue: technology 1986):75, Oct 1985

Malpractice Update: Fathers' rights cloud abortion issue, Contemp OB/GYN 31(6):136, 1988

Mascola, L, and Guinan, ME: Screening to reduce transmission of sexually transmitted disease in semen used for artificial insemination, N Engl J Med 314:1354, 1986

Mattson, RH, et al: Use of oral contraceptives by women with epilepsy, JAMA 256(2):238, 1986

Minnesota firm introduces new contraceptive condom, NAACOG Newsletter 13(9):11, 1986

Mishell, DR, Jr: Current status of intrauterine devices, N Engl J Med 312:984, 1985

The missed-period pill (RU 486), Harvard Medical School Health Letter 12(5):1, 1987

Modica, MM, and Timor-Tritsch, IE: Transvaginal sonography provides a sharper view into the pelvis, JOGN Nurs 17(2):89, 1988

New copper IUD. Med Lett 30(760):1, 1988

New guidelines for the use of semen donor insemination: 1986, Fertil Steril 46:95S, 1986

North, BB, and Vorhauer, BW: Use of the Today contraceptive sponge in the United States, Int J Fertil 30:81, 1985

Northwestern University Program for Applied Research on Fertility Regulation: Immunologic methods of fertility regulation—report of a workshop, Res Frontiers Fertil Reg 3:1, 1985

Nurses' Drug Alert: Adverse effects of contraceptive sponges, Am J Nurs 85:171, Feb 1985

Nurses' Drug Alert: Vaginal sponge and toxic shock; oral contraceptive failure; spermicides and congenital malformations: no relation, Am J Nurs 85:693, June 1985

Olshansky, EF: Identity of self as infertile: an example of theory-generating research, ANS 9:54, 1987

Orne, B, and Hawkins, JA: Reexamining the oral contraceptive issues, JOGN Nurs 14:30, Jan/Feb 1985

Orque, MD, Bloch, B, and Monrroy, LS: Ethnic nursing care: a multicultural approach, St Louis, 1983, The CV Mosby Co

Ostling, RN: A bold stand on birth control, Time. In Hass, K, and Haas, A: Understanding sexuality, St Louis, 1987, Times Mirror/Mosby College Publishing

Problem-patient conference: Habitual aborters, Contemp OB/GYN 27:147, Feb 1986
Timing of postpartum tubal ligation, JAMA 259(2):275, 1988
Quin, PA, et al: Prevalence of antibody to *Chlamydia trachomatis* in spontaneous abortion and infertility, Am J Obstet Gynecol 156(2):291, 1987
Realini, JP, and Goldzieher, JW: Oral contraceptives and cardiovascular disease: a critique of the epidemiologic studies, Am J Obstetrics Gynecol 152(6): whole issue (part 2), 1985
Roland, R: Technology and motherhood: reproductive choice reconsidered, SIGNS 12(3):512, 1987
Rosenberg, MJ, et al: Effect of the contraceptive sponge on chlamydial infection, gonorrhea, and candidiasis, JAMA 257(17):2308, 1987
Rosenthal, MB: Grappling with the emotional aspects of infertility, Contemp OB/GYN 26:7, July 1985
Sandelowski, M: The color gray: ambiguity and infertility, Image 19:70, 1987
Sandelowski, M, and Pollock, C: Women's experiences of infertility, Image 18:140, 1986
Sauer, MV: Measuring sperm motility, Contemp OB/GYN 30 (special issue):83, Oct 1988
Seibel, MM: A new era in reproductive technology: in vitro fertilization, gamete intrafallopian transfer, and donated gametes and embryos, N Engl J Med 318(13):828, 1988
Shapiro, S: Oral contraceptives—time to take stock, N Engl J Med 315(7):450, 1986
Sherrod, RA: Coping with infertility: a personal perspective turned professional, MCN 13(3):191, 1988
Smith, PM: Ovulation induction, JOGN Nurs 14:37s, 1985
Speroff, L: The woman over 50: a new challenge for the gynecologist, Contemp OB/GYN, 31(Special Issue):22, April 1988
Speroff, L, and Wallach, EE: The changing face of infertility, Contemp OB/GYN (Special Issue):8, 1987
Tatum, HJ: Contraception and family planning. In Pernoll, ML, and Benson, RC, editors: Current obstetric and gynecologic diagnosis and treatment, ed 6, Los Altos, Calif, 1987, Appleton & Lange
Ullman, K: A GIFT for infertile couples, Am J Nurs 87(9):1130, 1987
Utian, WH: OCs for women over 40, Contemp OB/GYN 30(6):67, 1987
Wallach, EE: Fertility drugs—what effects on the fetus? Contemp OB/GYN 26:171, Aug 1985
Wedell, MA, Billings, T, and Fayez, JA: Endometriosis and the infertile patient, JOGN Nurs 14:280, July/Aug 1985
Weisman, CS, et al: Delivery of fertility control services by male and female obstetrician-gynecologists, Am J Obstet Gynecol 156(2):464, 1987
Contraceptives: a buying guide, University of California, Berkeley, Wellness Letter 3(5):3, 1987
White, JE: Influence of parents, peers, and problem-solving on contraceptive use, Pediatr Nurs 13(5):317, 1987
Zimmet, JA, et al: An historical look at a contemporary question: the cervical cap, Health Educ 17(5):53, 1986

CHAPTER

43

Hazards to Women's Health

Learning Objectives

Correctly define the key terms listed.

Review how personality characteristics of victim and abuser complement each other.

List three kinds of family interaction patterns that make a woman vulnerable to wife battering.

Identify the myths about abuse and battering and how they might influence nursing care.

Explain the cycle of violence and the nursing process for each phase.

Describe the five categories of rape and the rape trauma syndrome.

Develop a nursing care plan for the immediate and follow-up care for rape victims.

Compile a list of substances that are hazardous to reproductive health.

Develop a nursing care plan for women who may be or have been exposed to reproductive health hazards.

Key Terms

absence of consent
abuse
alleged rape
anger rape
battered woman
blitz rape
confidence rape
cost-benefit analysis
cycle of violence
domestic violence
incest
learned helplessness
mutagenic effect
power rape
rape kit
rape trauma syndrome
reproductive health hazards
sadistic rape
sexual assault
sick-building syndrome
Stockholm syndrome
toxicology screen

Hazards to women's health cover a wide spectrum. Battering, sexual assault, incest, rape, and hazards in the environment and workplace are significant problems with each carrying the potential for serious physical, psychologic, and emotional injury or impairment.

Battering of women refers to assault, a violent physical attack. Clinical findings include bruises, lacerations, burns, hematomas, and fractures. A sexual assault is any aggressive or violent act involving sexual intimacy performed by one person on another without that person's consent. Abuse of women is defined as physical, emotional, or sexual mistreatment: aggressive behavior, including acts of a sexual or physical nature, verbal belittling, or intimidation. Battery, abuse, and assault are often used interchangeably.

Accurate statistics are not available as the following estimates demonstrate. An estimated 1 million to 6 million women per year will suffer abuse (Chez, 1987). According to Federal Bureau of Investigation (FBI) estimates, 25 million wives are abused by their husbands each year (Whitkin-Lanoil, 1987). Data from a National Crime Survey reveal an average yearly rate of assault by spouses or former spouses of 2.7 per 1000 women during the period from 1973 to 1981. These numbers are impressive despite the fact that assault within families is the most underreported of all crimes (Hillard, 1986; Klaus, 1984). Delgaty (1985) reports that 1 in 10 married Canadian women is physically abused each year. This conservative statistic does not include the number who are psychologically or emotionally abused. Pregnancy is a time of increased battering episodes (Hillard, 1985). It has been estimated that in the United States, 1 women is beaten every 18 seconds (Battered, 1987). Every 3½ minutes (Battered 1987) to every 6 minutes (Riesenberg, 1987) a woman is a victim of rape or attempted rape. About 50% of all rapes of women over 30 years are part of the battering syndrome. Rape constitutes an estimated 10% to 20% of all reported crime (Hicks, 1981); about 80% of rapes go unreported, and many of the victims do not seek health care. An estimated 100,000 cases or more of incest occur per year; 12% to 24% of the female victims become pregnant (Zdanuk, Harris, and Wisian, 1987). The overwhelming physical evidence of the prevalence of these serious crimes precludes the need to identify them as major issues in current society.

Although both women and men may take on either role or both roles—abuser and/or victim—this chapter focuses only on women (from adolescence through old age) as victims of violence. The vast areas of child abuse and molestation and of men as victims of spouse battering and rape are beyond the scope of this text.

Hazards to reproductive health in the environment and workplace affect everyone. The hazards exist whether the woman works in or outside the home. Pollution with chemicals, fumes, and noise and direct and indirect effects from equipment, furniture, buildings, and grounds have become major health concerns.

Nurses will see victims in all age groups and in every area of their practice. Because of the magnitude of the problems of violence against women and environmental hazards to reproductive health, maternity and gynecologic nurses cannot ignore this reality of client care. There is a need to focus on prevention, effective nursing actions, and long-term counseling of victims.

See other areas of this text for specifics regarding anatomy and physiology, genetics and fetal development, the gynecologic examination, care during the prenatal and perioperative periods, fertility management, and infection.

BATTERED WOMEN

Women should have the right to move about within the confines of their homes among those persons with whom they share the most intimate, interpersonal relationships without fearing for their safety and well-being, or for life itself. In general, women accept and expect that right as a given (Drake, 1982). Battering is a criminal act; in a marriage, it is a fundamental betrayal of trust (Delgaty, 1985).

The abuse of spouses occurs at all socioeconomic levels, as well as all educational levels. The myth that only persons in the low socioeconomic classes or that those with little education are the primary perpetrators of wife abuse has been refuted. Wives are most likely to be abused than are husbands, although it is not entirely unknown for a man to report physical or emotional abuse by his spouse.

The problem of wife abuse is particularly significant because 90% of homicides in families are preceded by family violence. Battering precipitates one in every four suicides by all women and half of all suicides by black women in the United States.

It is estimated that 50% of all women will be battered at some time. Since nurses come from the general population, how many have themselves been abused (or have been abusers)? What effect has the experience had on their ability to cope with the crisis state presented by victims who have come for medical care?

Wife battering, spouse abuse, and domestic (family) violence are all terms applied to physical trauma inflicted by the male partner on the female partner in a marriage or marital-like relationship. An extraordinary variety of other definitions have been formulated for this behavior. Some common elements in these definitions are (1) repetition of episodes, (2) some demonstrable injury or injuries resulting from the violence, and (3) violence that is deliberate and severe.

These elements preclude the occasional physical acts of shoving, shaking, or restraining that occur in some marriages. At present, family violence generally is considered a part of family life by both the law and large numbers of women. Some people are socialized to believe that domestic violence is an acceptable way of dealing with the stresses of family life (Martin, 1976; Mandel, 1986; Stuart and Sundeen, 1987; Battered, 1987); for example, women have reported that they believe it is acceptable for a husband to beat his wife "every once in a while."

Initial studies of wife abuse began in the early 1970s. Several disciplines approached the problem from different viewpoints. For example, researchers in *psychiatry* were concerned with the causative factors that drive a man to beat his wife and the reasons that women who are repeatedly beaten will stay with the spouse. Researchers in *sociology* looked at the factors in society and the institution of marriage that would keep a woman captive in a violent marriage. The *health care providers* were concerned with case finding, documentation, and physical care.

Characteristics of Victims and Abusers

Every socioeconomic group is represented among abused wives. As noted earlier in this chapter, race, religion, social background, age, and educational level are not significant factors in differentiating women at risk.

Battered wives may feel they are to blame for their situation because they are "not good-enough wives." They fear societal rejection if they discuss their problem openly. This fear is justified in many cases because society has stereotyped these women as masochistic. It is impossible for many people to comprehend why a woman would remain in a situation where she is repeatedly beaten and injured.

One explanation may be the tendency for some victims to form a symbiotic relationship, sometimes called the victim-victimizer bond or the *Stockholm syndrome*. This type of relationship is named after a female bank teller in Stockholm who was abducted and became romantically involved with her captor. After being released, a hostage suffering from this bond exhibits the negative effects of the syndrome: nightmares, tremors, sweating, substance (drug, food) abuse, various phobias, and stress reactions such as ulcers, hypertension, allergies, and depression. These psychosomatic responses are attributed to a growing realization of the humiliation and demoralization suffered during the experience.

Elbow (1977) has identified four types of men who become abusive husbands and has categorized them as the Controller, the Defender, the Approval Seeker, and the Incorporator.

Controller. The Controller strives for autonomy through the control of others. He is not emotionally reciprocal in his relationships; he usually gets his way and is never to blame when things go wrong. He sees other people in terms of what they can do for him. When the Controller feels he can no longer dominate, he will use violence as an attempt to regain control. It is possible that his wife represents his extremely domineering parent(s), who did not permit him to be autonomous as a child.

Defender (Protector). Having a spouse to harm, love, and forgive is a fundamental need of the Defender. His fear is that he will be harmed, and he strikes out before he is struck. He needs a wife who is totally dependent on him, clings to him, and is defenseless so that he can protect her. He believes, however, that his wife will try to punish him for being assertive or sexual. He tries, through violence, to keep his wife powerless, thereby reducing his own vulnerability.

Approval Seeker. Continued reaffirmation of self-esteem is required by the Approval Seeker. He has a low self-image and expects rejection. He may even precipitate rejection by his mate through his behavior. Violence occurs when he feels the most criticized.

Incorporator. The need of the Incorporator is to draw another individual's strengths into his own psyche to fill his emotional gaps. His desperation can be observed in several ways. He may cling to his mate, have public displays of anger, and have suicidal ideation. Any attempt by the wife to withdraw from the situation increases his desperation and may lead to violence.

Complementary personality characteristics and childhood influences are found in couples who are susceptible to development of abuser/victim relationships (Table 43-1).

Significance of Family of Origin

Women who were victims of incest or whose mothers were victims of domestic violence are at significant risk for battering. Similarly, men who, as children, observed their fathers abuse their mothers or sisters are more likely to abuse their wives.

It appears that some women are not "innocent victims," nor do they consciously precipitate violence, but, rather, they unconsciously or subconsciously collaborate with their mates to initiate violent episodes. Such a woman may seek a particular type of mate with whom she will reenact her own childhood family experience. In one study Parker and Schumacher (1977) found that battered wives come from families that exhibited one of three types of interaction patterns: families in which mothers used subtle methods of control and fathers were merely figureheads; families in which mothers were submissive and fathers were dominant; and families consisting of disturbed mothers and multiple "fathers."

Subtly Controlling Mothers and Figurehead Fathers. In this type of family the daughter observes how her mother manipulates her father into following her wishes and assuming them to be his own. The mother gives subtle approval or disapproval to her husband while using him as an authority figure and principal disciplinarian over the children.

Daughters from this type of family verbalize that they want a husband who is decisive, is respected, and has direction in life. If the man fails to live up to the wife's expected image of him, she may attempt to manipulate him through means she sees as encouragement but he perceives as criticism. When violence occurs, she accepts it much as she accepted punishment from her father.

Ironically, these marriages appear to be relatively stable. The couples with these characteristics who have acknowledged domestic violence as a problem in their lives appear to be primarily concerned with avoiding legal problems resulting from the violence—not with tactics to avoid the violence itself.

Submissive Mothers and Dictatorial Fathers. These battered wives come from families in which the fathers were physically and verbally abusive to the mothers. The mothers, who were usually unassertive and dependent, were unable to protect themselves or their children from attack. The fathers were generally irritable and harsh, with no pattern to their episodes of punishment and abuse. These daughters tended to identify with their fathers in an attempt to avoid their anger and were often classified as "tomboys."

As women, they seem to choose their husbands impersonally and usually marry men they know have violent tendencies. They seem to view their husbands' rages as a nor-

Table 43-1 *Characteristics of Victim and Abuser*

Victim	Abuser
Childhood Influences	**Childhood Influences**
Many raised to be submissive, passive, and dependent	Raised in family where males rein supreme
Likely to accept traditional female role in marriage	As children may have used violence to problem-solve
Accepts female sex-role stereotypes	Accepts "macho" values
Personality Characteristics	**Personality Characteristics**
Attributes beating to some personal inadequacy	Feelings of inadequacy, inferiority, and insecurity
Low self-esteem and feelings of worthlessness	Emotionally immature and/or aggressive (Zdanuk, 1987)
Learned helplessness reduces problem-solving ability	Extremes in behavior and overreacting are typical
Low tolerance for frustration	Low self-esteem with high degree of self-loathing
Easily upset, critical, aloof, and reserved	Intolerant of having masculinity threatened (White, 1985)
Severe stress reactions and psychophysiologic symptoms	Lacks respect for women
Can't trust anyone	Poor impulse control
Some attempt suicide	Excessive possessiveness and jealousy (Hillard, 1986)
Punishment justified if marriage fails	Some use aggressive sexual attacks to punish and enhance own self-esteem
Lifestyle Factors	**Lifestyle Factors**
Isolated from family and friends	No particular profession, occupation, or socioeconomic group
Totally dependent on husband for financial and emotional support	Often has difficulties at work
	Severely restricts freedom and mobility of wife

mal consequence of life and seldom involve the authorities in episodes of violence.

Disturbed Mothers and Multiple "Fathers." Daughters of women who are chronically emotionally disturbed and who have had many mates are at risk of becoming battered wives. Their mothers often choose mates who drink heavily and who abuse both themselves and their daughters. The daughters are commonly neglected and shuffled around from one caregiver to another. They may even witness sexual promiscuity and actual sexual acts by their mothers or be victims of incest by their assorted father figures.

In their quest to fill the need for the ideal fantasized father, they form quick, intense, dependent relationships with men. Often they find men who are ineffectual and unable to support them financially. As the relationship becomes more intolerable, violence erupts.

Myths About Battered Women

Health professionals often become frustrated by women who remain in battering relationships. As with other human dynamics that are not easily explained, a number of myths have emerged to account for this perceived self-destructive behavior (Collier, 1987; Griffith-Kenney, 1986). Table 43-2 lists a series of myths and facts about abuse and battering.

Cycle of Violence

When the woman is asked why she remains with a battering mate, she may say that there are times when their relationship is fine. A cyclic pattern to the battering behavior has been described as a period of increasing tension leading to the battery, followed by an aftermath characterized by kind, loving behavior and a plea for forgiveness by the husband (Hillard, 1986).

Phase I: The Tension Building State. This phase is characterized by minor incidents that result in shaking, shoving, throwing objects, berating, and other aggressive behaviors. A chance comment, a frown in response to a statement, buying the wrong kind of cookies, a speck of dust found on a table are all examples of the kinds of minor behaviors that precipitate aggression.

To avoid brutality the woman becomes more compliant and withdrawn. She often feels partially responsible for the man's anger and becomes his accomplice in her efforts to prevent him from hurting her more.

Phase II: The Acute Battering Incident. The batterer loses control and unleashes his rage on the victim to "teach her a lesson." The beatings usually last between 2 and 24 hours. However, some victims have reported abuse for a week or more. The man stops when the women "has learned her lesson."

Table 43-2 *Myths and Facts About Abuse and Battering*

Myth	Fact
Battering occurs in a small percentage of the population.	Physical assault reportedly occurred in 28% of all American homes in 1976 (Strauss et al., 1980).
Battering occurs only in lower-class families.	Although lower class families have a higher incidence of battering (Gelles, 1979), it also occurs in middle and upper income families. Incidence not really known because of tendency of middle and upper income families to hide their battering.
Battered women like to be beaten and deliberately provoke the attack. They are masochistic.	Women are terrified of their assailants and go to great lengths to avoid a confrontation. In some cases the woman may provoke her husband to release tension that, if left unchecked, might lead to a more severe beating and possible death.
Batterers are uneducated men who are unable to cope with the world.	Many batterers are successful professionals, including politicians, ministers, physicians, and lawyers.
Men who batter their wives also beat their children.	Two thirds of wife-batterers do not beat their children.
Battered women were battered children.	This myth holds true in only a few cases. Most battered women report that their husbands were the first person to beat them.
Alcohol and drug abuse causes battering.	Gelles (1976) and Delgaty (1985) proposed that batterers use alcohol as an excuse to batter and shift the blame from themselves to the alcohol.
Once a battered wife, always a battered wife.	Many women who have battering relationships do not marry again. Those who stay in the relationships do so out of fear and financial dependence. Shelters have long waiting lists.
Batterers and battered women cannot change.	Counseling can effectively help resocialize both batterers and battered women.

Most women do not seek medical treatment unless the situation is an emergency. Instead they minimize or deny the severity of their injuries. This is often done to protect the batterer and themselves from retaliation.

The victim is usually in a state of shock and experiences both physical and psychologic stress. She feels trapped with no place to go and no help from authorities. For example, in an article titled "Woman victimized twice—by her ex-lover and the system" (Mandel, 1986), a woman who was being beaten by her husband telephoned 911 and said there was a battering in progress. The dispatcher told her there were real crimes going on and that "we don't have time to come out for that."

Phase III: Kindness and Contrite, Loving Behavior. The reconciliation is characterized by loving behavior and promises never to do it again. The batterer believes that he has taught the woman a lesson and will not have to repeat the experience. The victim wants to believe that the man loves her and is serious about not hurting her again.

Women in chronic battering situations may also stay with the batterer because they have no job skills, are economically dependent, are afraid of being alone, or are even fearful of retaliation if they leave. Gelles (1976) reported that the less power and resources the woman has the more likely she is to stay in the situation.

Pfouts (1978) described a "cost-benefit analysis" employed by abused women as they choose a method for coping with the abuse. This analysis involves a decision-making process wherein the woman weighs the benefits of remaining in the relationship against the costs. She then compares these findings with the benefits she expects to obtain if she chooses an alternative. Four principal alternatives emerge for abused wives:

1. The self-punishing response: the wife assumes the blame and stays in the relationship.
2. The aggressive response: the wife becomes violent.
3. The early disengagement response: the wife leaves the situation shortly after the violence begins or enacts control mechanisms over the husband's behavior.
4. The reluctant midlife disengagement response: the wife leaves the relationship after a lengthy time.

The cylce of violence often begins in the first year of marriage (Lichtenstein, 1981). Many victims remain in the abusive situation for an average of 6 to 7 years, especially when there are small children involved.

Many women report that they were first beaten when their husbands learned of their pregnancy. The blows are often directed toward the breasts, abdomen, and genitals. It has been hypothesized that jealousy of the baby's intrusion on the couple's relationship and the increased strain

RESEARCH HIGHLIGHT

The Effectiveness of Counseling Services Utilized by Battered Women

Purpose

To determine the effectiveness of counseling services utilized by battered women.

Sample/Methodology

Recruited to participate in this study were 1000 predominantly white, married, middle class battered women. The response rate was high with 85% usable questionnaires. Additional data were obtained from 146 interviews.

Findings

Severity of beating did not appear to predict counseling utilization. Most of the women received help from social service/counseling agencies as opposed to clergy or women's groups. Women reported, however, that women's groups are more effective than traditional forms of counseling utilized by battered wives.

Implications

A control group study with extended follow-up periods is recommended. If objective measures of effectiveness prove to be consistent with the subjective measures reported in this study, it would be appropriate to recommend shifting resources from traditional agencies to women's groups. Agencies would be encouraged to restaff and retool to place increased emphasis on modeling, direct material aid, and the use of indigenous paraprofessionals.

Bowker, L, and Maurer, L: The effectiveness of counseling services utilized by battered women, Women and Therapy 5(4):65, 1986.

on the marriage either triggers or exacerbates abuse.

The battered pregnant woman should be treated as a high-risk obstetric client because she often has more medical, social, or psychologic needs (Mercer, 1977) that require special attention. She is at additional risk for repeated physical trauma and for psychologic trauma because of a deficient support system.

Pregnancy is a time of increased battering episodes for a variety of reasons: (1) The biopsychosocial stresses of pregnancy may strain the relationship beyond the couple's ability to cope; frustration is followed by violence. (2) The man may be jealous of the fetus, resenting its intrusion into the couple's relationship. As one expectant father succinctly stated, "I don't get the TLC I got before that thing came along." (3) The beating may be the man's conscious or subconscious attempt to end the pregnancy. After delivery the mother may be so physically and emotionally drained that she may have difficulty bonding with her infant. She is considered at risk of becoming an abusive mother whether she chooses to stay in the abusive relationship or not. If she remains with her husband, the chances are 1 in 3 or 4 that he will batter the child as well.

Reaching Out for Help

Battered women are reluctant to seek help for various reasons: the need to avoid the stigma associated with the nature of the family violence, the fear that they will not be believed, the fear of reprisal from their husbands, and in some states in which battering is a reportable crime, the wish to avoid involvement with police. A study by Bowker and Maurer (1986) reports on the kind of counseling services that battered women deem most effective (research highlight).

Exactly what drives a woman to seek assistance is not clear, but apparently it may be the result of a behavioral change in the woman. The women who display any of the following three characteristics are more likely to seek assistance:

1. Women who are beaten frequently and severely
2. Women who have not experienced or witnessed family violence in their family of origin
3. Women who see an alternative to life in their marriages—specifically, women with jobs

Assessment

Careful assessment of all clients, pregnant or not, may reveal findings that alert the nurse or physician to the possibility of battering. The diagnosis is missed in a significant number of cases. The *history* may contain data with a high index of suspicion for battering: drug or child abuse; repeated injury to the head, face, neck, chest, abdomen, and upper extremities; a time delay between the injury and seeking treatment; previous abuse; and chronic depression. Women who wear sunglasses should be asked to remove them for an assessment for bruises around the eyes. The presenting problem may be broken bones, serious bleeding injuries (nosebleed, lacerations), and/or burns from a variety of sources. Women may be vague or evasive in their account of the cause of the injuries.

If the woman is seen during the tension-building period of the battering cycle, her symptoms usually contain an emotional element (e.g., chest pain, hyperventilation, gastrointestinal disorders, and headache).

Interviewing skills are essential. The validating interview should take place in a quiet, private area. In a nonjudgmental, caring manner, the interviewer may comment that the woman's signs and symptoms do not fit with the description of the accident but that they are consistent with injury inflicted by another person. The nurse may then comment that it is not uncommon to find such injuries when wives are hurt by their husbands. Finally, the nurse can ask the woman if, indeed, she was hurt by her husband (Finley, 1981). Types of questions that could be asked include: Do you and your partner fight? Does the fighting ever become physical? Is there a history of abuse in your partner's family? How did this happen? Did someone do this to you?

As stated earlier, pregnancy increases the likelihood of domestic abuse. Therefore a clustering of the following situations may indicate a battering situation: incidence of abortion, miscarriage, or preterm delivery; injuries or bruises acquired during pregnancy; sexual dysfunction during pregnancy; divorce or separation during pregnancy; persistent gynecologic complaints (especially abdominal pain or dyspareunia); attempted suicide; and repeated missed office visits and/or alcohol or other substance abuse (Chez, 1987).

Nursing Diagnoses

Nursing diagnoses are individualized for each woman. Following are examples of potential nursing diagnoses for battered women.

- Knowledge deficit related to
  - The phenomenon of battering
  - Cycle of violence
  - Community resources for protection and support
- Ineffective individual and family coping related to
  - Persistence of victim-abuser relationship
- Actual injury related to
  - Battering episode
- Self-esteem disturbance related to
  - Continuing victim-abuser relationship
- Spiritual distress related to
  - Continuing victim-abuser relationship.

Planning

To develop an effective plan, the caregiver must be comfortable working with the victim and her family. In addition, the caregiver must have a broad knowledge base of this phenomenon, excellent communication skills, and access to appropriate community resources. If possible, continuity of care is planned with the health care provider(s) with whom the woman develops a relationship of trust.

Goals. Goals are formulated in client-centered terms. Following are examples of goals for care.

1. The battered woman is identified
2. The woman is protected from further abuse
3. The woman perceives herself as deserving of respect and not as "deserving" to be victimized
4. The woman reestablishes a feeling of control
5. The woman identifies her areas of strength and develops goals for herself
6. The woman increases her knowledge of the following:
   a. Alternatives, options, and choices
   b. Community resources (shelters, financial aid, child care, education, etc.)
   c. Roles of members of the health care team
7. Physical injuries are treated promptly
8. If the woman is pregnant or has children, the fetus and children are protected from abuse.

Implementation

If the woman is pregnant, a support network is developed with the other maternity nurses who will be involved in her care during the peripartum period. Each nurse can plan care that will point out the woman's strengths and raise her self-esteem. The husband is welcomed to attend prenatal visits and classes and is included in other ways if the woman choses to stay with him. Counseling services are offered to both spouses. The first days after delivery are particularly crucial—the mother is physically and emotionally vulnerable and usually tired, and the baby's crying may be intolerable to both the father and the mother. The danger of abuse to mother and child is acute during this time. A support network of maternity and pediatric staff, community health nurses, and parental crisis center personnel is needed to coordinate efforts to provide support during this crucial period.

The nurse *does* do the following:

1. Treat the woman with dignity and concern, to help her reduce her feelings of isolation, embarrassment, shame, and guilt.
2. Encourage the woman to refer to herself specifically, using statements such as "I am" rather than referring to herself in general terms (Finley, 1981).
3. Indicate sensitivity to and acceptance of the woman's state of confusion.
4. Indicate that hope exists. As the woman develops a sense of hope, her ability to formulate realistic goals increases.
5. Help the woman identify and explore her options; for example, remaining in the relationship is one option among several. The woman's feeling of being controlled by the situation may be reduced as she considers her choices.
6. Offer family planning counseling, since unplanned or unwanted pregnancy is a precipitating factor in wife abuse.
7. Offer referrals for treating substance abuse and for learning problem-solving behaviors and techniques for "fighting fair" to replace violence.

The nurse *does not* do the following:

1. Berate the woman's husband. The woman may be very protective of him, and negative input from the nurse may force her to sever therapeutic ties.
2. Urge or encourage the woman to leave home. She alone must make this decision. Leaving before a commitment to a different way of life is firm can bring the woman back into the situation. Studies indicate that this is a high-risk time for homicide (Elbow, 1977).

A woman indicates her readiness to leave the relationship when she indicates she is capable of planning for herself, investing in herself as a person, recognizing that the abuse is part of a continuing pattern, and is able to express the desire to leave when no abuse is occurring at the moment.

Many nurses become frustrated when women return time after time with injuries. As client advocates, nurses must be sensitive to the battered woman's problems and be able to tolerate their own empathic feelings of fear and terror (Griffith-Kenney, 1986). This is particularly true for the nurse who is herself a battered woman (Collier, 1987). A nursing care plan for the postpartum mother who was battered follows.

Specific Nursing Care Plan

BATTERED POSTPARTUM WOMAN

Rosemary P. has just been admitted to the postpartum floor. As the nurse is helping her into the bed she notices bruises, scars, and scratches covering parts of Rosemary's body. When the nurse questions Rosemary she replies, "I fell down the steps." Rosemary appears withdrawn and does not make eye contact with the nurse when speaking to her.

Twelve hours postdelivery Rosemary is still requesting that her baby stay in the nursery. Her husband has not visited, but a dozen roses were delivered to her from him. The floor and nursery staff recognize some difficulty with bonding and suspect problems with her relationship. The nurse manager calls the physician, who asks the social service department to visit Rosemary. When Marge, the social worker, comes to see Rosemary, the husband is in the room. When he finds out who she is he becomes angry, ejecting Marge from the room and throwing the water pitcher at the door after her. As Marge is leaving the room she notices Rosemary cowering and sobbing in bed.

ASSESSMENT	NURSING DIAGNOSIS (ND)/ PLAN (P)/GOAL (G)	RATIONALE/ IMPLEMENTATION	EVALUATION
Physical and emotional fatigue. Rosemary not bonding with infant.	ND: Activity intolerance: decreased, related to potential physical abuse, labor, and delivery of infant. P: Provide safe and restful environment. G: Woman is able to rest to regain physical strength.	*To assist Rosemary with rest and to increase energy reserves the nurse will:* Provide a quiet nonthreatening environment.	Rosemary sleeps.
		Cluster and assist with procedures and activities of daily living (ADL).	Rosemary begins to ambulate and take responsibility for own ADL.
		Display a nonjudgmental attitude.	
		Limit visitors with Rosemary's permission.	
		Reassure Rosemary she can call the nurse at any time for any thing she may want or need.	Rosemary calls on nurses for assistance, to converse, and to share information.
	ND: Altered parenting related to lack of attachment behaviors. P: Provide safe, caring environment to facilitate beginning attachment to newborn. G: Woman begins to show attachment behaviors.	*To assist with bonding the nurse will:* Bring infant to mother after she has awakened from sleep so she is well rested.	Mother begins to touch, stroke, and kiss infant.
		Sit and feed infant while mother observes or strokes or touches infant.	Mother asks questions about infant care.
		Allow infant to sleep in room beside mother's bed.	
		Allow time for questions.	
		Have mother observe baby care if she is too tired to do it herself.	Mother begins to feed and care for infant without prompting from nurses.
Avoiding making eye contact with person speaking to her.	ND: Self-esteem disturbance related to feelings of worthlessness. P: Provide care and environment to bolster her self-esteem. G: Rosemary starts to feel good about herself.	*To promote good self-esteem the nurse will:* Praise Rosemary's accomplishments.	Rosemary starts making eye contact.
		Ask Rosemary's opinion about care of herself and her infant.	Rosemary smiles.

Continued.

Specific Nursing Care Plan—cont'd

ASSESSMENT	NURSING DIAGNOSIS (ND)/ PLAN (P)/GOAL (G)	RATIONALE/ IMPLEMENTATION	EVALUATION
		Promote trust by respecting Rosemary's beliefs and providing helpful assistance. Be sincere in behavior. Provide choices.	Rosemary starts conversation with nurse.
Anxious and fearful.	ND: Anxiety, moderate, related to potential or real family relationship problems. P: Decrease anxiety. G: Rosemary appears to be and verbalizes that she feels "better"	*To decrease anxiety:* Provide support. Provide reassurance. Inquire about support systems in the family. Assist Rosemary with obtaining community support. Provide compassionate treatment.	Rosemary's verbal and nonverbal cues are less anxious.
Husband-wife relationship strained.	ND: Ineffective individual and family coping related to problems with husband-wife relationship. P: Assist woman with coping strategies. G: Rosemary accepts assistance.	*To assist Rosemary with individual coping the nurse can:* **Not take sides.** Provide support. Counsel Rosemary about seeking outside help. Be nonjudgmental when Rosemary resists assistance. Keep a sense of humor. Keep a sense of reality.	Rosemary accepts assistance and speaks to social worker about networking for support and assistance.
Stays to self, doesn't socialize with roommate.	ND: Social isolation related to fear and low self-esteem. P: Provide care and environment to bolster self-esteem. G: Rosemary begins to converse with roommate and staff.	*To encourage Rosemary to socialize or converse the nurse will:* Respect Rosemary's right to privacy. Not force the issue. Speak to roommate—tell her it is nothing personal with her. Let Rosemary make the first move, but set limits.	This may not resolve itself in the 2 to 3 days woman is in the hospital. However, even a good morning to the roommate is a step forward.
Bruises and cuts on body. Episiotomy.	ND: Pain, related to bruises, wounds, and episiotomy. P: Prevent or minimize pain. G: Rosemary states she is more comfortable.	*To increase comfort the nurse can:* Provide comfort measures. Provide medication as ordered.	Rosemary verbalizes increased comfort.
	ND: Impaired skin integrity related to cuts on body and episiotomy. P: Prevent infection, promote healing. G: Infection does not occur.	*To prevent infection and promote healing of open skin areas the nurse will:* Teach Rosemary how to keep areas clean. Teach good pericare. Give antibiotics as ordered. Promote good nutrition to assist healing process.	Rosemary does not develop infection.

Specific Nursing Care Plan—cont'd

ASSESSMENT	NURSING DIAGNOSIS (ND)/ PLAN (P)/GOAL (G)	RATIONALE/ IMPLEMENTATION	EVALUATION
Suspected victim of wife abuse. Possible perpetuation of violence.	ND: Potential for violence: directed at others, related to being abused. P: Prevent violence in the home; promote a healthier personal and family environment. G: Violence in the family is prevented.	*To help Rosemary recognize the possibility of her infant being a victim of abuse also, the nurse can:* Discuss this openly with Rosemary in a nonaccusatory manner. Contact social service department with physician's order. Consult a psychiatrist or psychologist to speak to Rosemary. Refer to appropraite community agencies (Appendix K).	Rosemary speaks freely with nurse. Rosemary agrees to seek help. Representative of community agency visits with Rosemary (and her husband if he wishes to be present).

Evaluation

Evaluation may be somewhat difficult because some changes are hard to evaluate objectively or because the woman (family) may not return for care. Intervention can be considered effective if the woman (couple) has developed self-esteem and a sense of self-worth, no longer views herself as a deserving victim, affirms her own individuality, has developed problem-solving behaviors, and is comfortable with her choices, and when no further battering or abusive episodes occur.

RAPE, SEXUAL ASSAULT, AND INCEST

Forcible rape is a crime that women may fear more than any other. **Rape**, a legal, not a medical entity, is defined differently from state to state. In many jurisdictions, rape, in its strictest sense, is the penile penetration of the female sex organ, or labia in some states, without her consent. Penetration by any other male appendage or other object or penile penetration of any other orifice constitutes **sexual assault**, another legal term. Hymenal penetration or ejaculation does not have to occur. The key feature to establish rape is the *absence of consent;* threat or coercion implies the lack of consent. The victim who is mentally retarded, is unconscious or otherwise physically unable to move, has been drugged without her knowledge, or is a minor (statutory rape) is not capable of giving consent. It is up to the court to prove absence of consent; hence the term *alleged rape* or *alleged sexual assault* is used in medical records.

Incest has been defined by Warner (1980) as "inappropriate sexual behavior among surrogate family members." This includes sexual contact from an adult to a child (such as rape), genital fondling, or oral-genital contact. In addition, sexual contact between nuclear or extended family members (either biologic or step relations) is included in the definition of incest.

Although incest is a universal taboo, an estimated 100,000 cases or more of incest occur each year in the United States. Pregnancy occurs in 12% to 24% of the female victims. Simens (1982) reports that 20% to 35% of all adult women surveyed were sexually molested as children. Nurses who work in schools, public health, pediatrics, obstetrics, and emergency rooms are in an excellent position to identify victims and strategically intervene (Zdanuk, 1987).

Several states have laws defining rape in terms of a *perceived threat* to the victim's well-being. Sometimes the threat is simple to describe. If the rapist uses a weapon such as a gun or knife, the threat is obvious; if he first engages the intended victim in conversation or is admitted by her into her home and then rapes her without a weapon, the threat she perceives may be more difficult to prove. Cases are brought to court only to be dismissed because the victims cannot prove the presence of a threat. Defense attorneys have used the argument that the woman gave implicit consent for intercourse by the fact that she let the rapist into her apartment, engaged in conversation with him in a bar, or made no attempt to get help during the attack.

Some couples willingly engage in violent sexual acts, considered perverse by many; legal defense could focus on showing that the victim gave consent to enter into sexual behaviors in spite of the potential for injury.

Rape is a violent crime on the increase. Since there are many reasons that deter a woman from reporting the crime, accurate statistics concerning psychosocial and demographic variables relating to rape are not available.

Women do not report rape because of the associated stigma or out of embarrassment, guilt that in some way they provoked the assault, fear of retribution from the rapist or his friends, dread of being humiliated and figuratively "raped" again by the police or the court, and discouragement generated by the dismally small number of convictions, to name a few reasons. Victims often fear the reactions of husbands, lovers, friends, family, and children and prefer to suffer alone.

The true incidence will not be known until women feel free to report the crime.

Violent Nature of Rape

Myths about rape continue to exist; for example, "there is no such thing as a *real* rape," "women *want* to be taken by force," women "ask for it" by dressing and acting in sexually provocative ways, and, the most dangerous of the myths, "it can't happen to me."

Rape is not an act of lust, nor is it an overzealous release of passion. Rape is a violent, aggressive assault on the body and integrity of the victim. As one victim said: "No matter how terrible people think rape is, it's worse than they know. It's like a bomb going off at the center of your soul."

The rapist has no regard for his victim's age, race, sexual attraction, or physical condition—10-day-old infants, as well as handicapped elderly women confined to wheelchairs, have been raped. Most rapes occur *intra*racially rather than *inter*racially. The victim often knows her attacker as a casual acquaintance or as a friend of long standing, or he may be a complete stranger to her.

Socialization into violence may be a key. In 1935 Margaret Mead (a sociologist) noted that in cultures where males are socialized to be nurturant, not aggressive, rape is unknown.

Nichaus (1986) describes 5 categories of rape:

Blitz rape: victim and assailant are strangers. A woman pulled into an alley is blitz raped.

Confidence rape: deceit is the major characteristic of confidence rape; for example, the date who uses coersion to obtain sex when the partner is a reluctant, unconsenting acquaintance. This kind of rape is common and seldom reported because the woman is afraid of being considered an accomplice to the rape.

Power rape: the man's victims are usually strangers attacked in a blitz rape. By dominating his victim, the man places the woman in the powerless position he experiences and despises. He fantasizes sexual conquest as a demonstration of his strength and potency. He believes that the woman enjoys the experience.

Anger rape: this is a revenge rape. The assailant uses rape to symbolically punish a significant woman in his life. These are impulse rapes characterized by considerable brutality and trauma.

Sadistic rape: sadism usually characterizes all of the sadistic rapist's relationships. They eroticize their aggression. They abuse and torture the woman until they are completely out of control. In a frenzy, he may commit a "lust murder."

Rape Trauma Syndrome

Regardless of the absence of severity of physiologic trauma present, rape is a serious psychologic emergency; priority consideration in the emergency department is imperative. The degree of support the woman receives in the immediate posttrauma period may have long-range consequences.

Burgess and Holmstrom (1975) described the progressive manifestations of rape trauma syndrome, presented in the following outline:

1. Acute phase: disorganization
   a. Impact reactions, with two styles of response; *expressed,* evidenced in behaviors such as crying or restlessness; and *controlled,* reflected in a calm, composed, or subdued affect
   b. Somatic reactions: physical discomfort, skeletal muscle tension, gastrointestinal irritability, and genitourinary disturbance (itching or burning on urination)
   c. Emotional reactions: fear, humiliation, degradation, and embarrassment; anger, need for revenge, and self-blame; not uncommonly, mood swings
2. Long-term process: reorganization
   a. Increased motor activity: changing residence and/or phone number
   b. Nightmares
   c. Trauma phobia: fear of indoors or outdoors (depending on site of rape), of being alone, of crowds, or of people walking or standing behind the woman; sexual fears

Burgess and Holmstrom (1974a,b) have been instrumental in educating professional and lay people about the victim, the physical and psychologic effects of rape, and therapeutic management of rape victims. The victim's crisis response after a rape develops in four stages (Foley and Davies, 1983):

1. Tension rises as the victim tries her habitual problem-solving techniques
2. The woman's stress and discomfort increase because she cannot cope and cannot restore homeostasis
3. The additional stress acts as an internal stimuli to mobilize the woman's internal and external resources to solve her problem, and
4. If disequilibrium continues and cannot be resolved or avoided, tension increases and major disorganization and/or disintegration of personality occurs

In the therapeutic management, Foley and Davies (1983) emphasize crisis intervention to protect the victim from further psychologic trauma.

Welch (1977) describes rape as a psychologic emergency, after which recovery follows a devious course. Each of three identified phases can last days, months, or years. In the first phase the victim's *acute reaction* is manifested by shock, dismay, generalized anxiety, fear, and immobilization. To the casual observer the victim in the second phase appears outwardly to have *adjusted;* for example, she indicates that she has no further need of help. Now she just wants to forget the incident and return to her previous activities at work and in the home. During the third phase, *ultimate integration and resolution,* the woman who is unfamiliar with symptoms of this phase of recovery may be surprised by the onset of depression and disrupted eating and sleep patterns and by a renewed need to talk about the experience. Surprises can be ego weakening, whereas prior preparation for this eventuality can be ego strengthening.

Hilberman (1976) discusses the often-overwhelming feelings of powerlessness and helplessness described by rape victims.

Responses of Those Close To Rape Victim

Rape affects everyone who comes in contact with the victim. The family also experiences the two phases of response: an acute reaction and a long-term reorganization process (Burgess and Holmstrom, 1974a).

Assessment

Sexual assault treatment centers usually have a standard form for obtaining and recording pertinent data (Shepard, 1983).

Consent forms must be signed before evidence can be collected and released to the police and before photographs can be taken. If the victim is under 16 years of age, a pediatrician is notified. A parent or guardian is required to sign the consent forms. The children's protective service may need to be called to facilitate consent.

History. The history include the client's age, allergies, and *menstrual* history, including the age of menarche, date of last menstrual period (LMP), and menstrual pattern. If LMP was not normal, the woman is asked to describe it. Her *obstetric* history is determined: gravidity, parity, date of termination of last pregnancy, and, if she thinks she may be pregnant now, symptoms she is experiencing. She is asked to describe her *sexual* history: the date and time of the most recent coitus before the alleged assault and whether a condom was used, her current mode of contraception, whether she was a virgin before the assault, whether she uses tampons, whether she uses douches, and the date of the last douche.

The woman is asked to describe the *assault* (she may need support and assistance in verbalizing the offender's acts): Did the penis enter the vagina? Did he have an orgasm? Was there oral or anal penetration? Did he wear a condom? She is asked to recount her *activity since the assault;* Did she douche, bathe or shower, or defecate or urinate? How, when, and from whom did she seek assistance afterward?

Physical Examination and Laboratory Tests. The physical examination is conducted after the procedure is explained to the woman. She remains clothed* while her vital signs and blood pressure are determined, and her clothing is inspected for stains, tears, and foreign material. She is assisted to undress and is draped; a female attendant, rape counselor, or other person of her choice may remain with her during the examination. The physician informs her of every step of the procedure. Her body is inspected for bruises, swelling, scratches, lacerations, stab wounds, and body lice. A head-to-toe examination is performed. Special attention is given to the area assaulted (e.g., pelvic structures and genitals).

External genitals, thighs, buttocks, and lower abdomen are assessed, and if there are injuries, photographs may be taken or drawings made. A new test, not yet acceptable to the courts, is toluidine blue staining; a positive toluidine blue staining of the vulva occurs in a significant percentage of rape victims but rarely in women who have coitus with consent (Lauber and Souma, 1982; Shepard, 1983).

A speculum examination (no lubricant is used) is performed gently to detect tears or bruises and to collect appropriate specimens. The cervix is scraped for *Neisseria gonorrhoeae* culturing, and vaginal fluid is obtained for analysis. One slide is fixed and dried to be stained and examined for sperm, a swab of fluid is placed in saline solution for potential sperm serovaring and a sample is assayed for acid phosphatase.*

A bimanual pelvic examination is performed carefully to determine the size and position of the uterus and adnexa. If a pelvic mass is palpated, it may be caused by bleeding into the broad ligament. If pregnancy is a possibility, a pregnancy test is done. Internal pelvic assessment is ended with a rectovaginal examination.

Blood is drawn for a Venereal Disease Research Laboratory (VDRL) test. Any x-ray films or photographs that were taken are noted at this time.

Additional specimens are obtained for evidence to document the identity of the offender.

1. Swabs are taken from all orifices if she is unconscious, or as deemed appropriate from the woman's history. Slides are prepared from the material on the swabs and allowed to air-dry. The slides are placed into mailers; the swabs are put into one test tube.
2. Contents of the vaginal vault are aspirated and put into another test tube.
3. The woman's pubic hair is combed; the comb and adhering hair are placed into an envelope, sealed, and labeled "combings." At least 12 of her pubic hairs are pulled out by the roots (or hair is clipped very close to the skin), placed into an envelope, and labeled "pubic hair samples."
4. Fingernail scrapings are placed into a separate envelope and labeled.

All slides, envelopes, test tubes, and slide mailers must be labeled personally by the examining physician with a Carborundum pencil, with the woman's name, the date and time, and the site from which the specimen was taken. Her clothes are put into a paper bag, sealed, and labeled. All

*An ultraviolet light (Wood's lamp) will cause semen to fluoresce even if the man has had a vasectomy. The fluorescent areas of the body and clothing can then be identified for further examination and for sources of specimens for acid phosphatase determination. Specimens can be aspirated or scraped off, appropriately packaged, and labeled.

*Acid phosphatase is an enzyme found in high concentrations in seminal fluid.

transactions—obtaining her specimens, packaging them, labeling them, and giving them over to either the police or a laboratory technician—are witnessed and signed by both the giver and the receiver; the time and date are also noted.

During the examination the woman's *emotional status* is assessed and findings are recorded; which impact reactions she is exhibiting, her orientation to time and place, and her attention span, affect, and verbal description and feelings about the assault. The availability of family or peer support systems is assessed. She is asked about her plans to report or not report the crime to the police.

Nursing Diagnoses

Following are nursing diagnoses for the immediate and later posttrauma periods.

Immediate posttrauma period:

- Anxiety/fear related to
  - The experience itself
  - The interactions with police, caregivers
  - The physical examination to assess injury and collect evidence
- Pain related to
  - The experience itself
  - The examination
- Rape trauma syndrome, silent or compound reaction, related to
  - The experience
- Potential for injury related to
  - The experience
- Self-esteem disturbance related to
  - Posttrauma syndrome
- Potential for decisional conflict related to
  - Possible pregnancy

Later posttrauma period:

- Posttrauma response (phobias) related to
  - Posttrauma syndrome
- Potential for infection with sexually transmitted diseases (STDs) related to
  - The experience
- Potential for impaired social interaction related to
  - Rape trauma syndrome

Planning

Planning for care for victims of rape, sexual assault, or incest requires the same sensitivity, understanding, and knowledge as that needed for the care of the battered woman.

Priorities of personnel who provide care to victims of rape or sexual assault in hospital-based sexual assault centers or in community-based rape crisis centers should include the following (Klingbeil et al., 1976):

1. An emotional support system for the family, friends, and parents, as well as for the victim
2. A sensitive health care system to provide optimum care and to document objective data
3. Presentation of information and education sessions to health care providers, educators, students, members of criminal justice systems, and community groups
4. Interaction and effective communication with the criminal justice system at all levels
5. Involvement with community interest groups concerned with the problems of sexual assault

Goals

1. The woman's care is provided in a nonjudgmental, caring, and unhurried manner
2. All evidence is collected during the examination, and all laboratory specimens are individually packaged and carefully labeled, dated, and sealed; receipts are obtained from the laboratory technicians and police
3. The woman does not perceive herself to be victimized by the health care providers
4. The woman understands the phases of the rape trauma syndrome
5. Antimicrobial prophylaxis for infection (e.g., for STD following rape; for tetanus or other infection following trauma from assault) is successful in preventing infection
6. Pregnancy is prevented, or if pregnancy occurs, the woman is able to make an informed decision about its management
7. Physical injuries heal without disfigurement or loss of function
8. The woman participates in scheduled follow-up care
9. The woman successfully passes through all the stages in the rape trauma syndrome
10. Family bonds are strengthened; family members are supportive of each other

Implementation

Medical management includes (1) treating the physical injuries, (2) providing prophylaxis for infection (e.g., gonorrhea, tetanus) and (3) providing prophylaxis for pregnancy if the woman is not pregnant already. If physical trauma is life-threatening, appropriate intervention takes precedence over collecting evidence.

Immediate Care. If the victim is menarchal, is using no contraception, and is at a time of high risk for pregnancy in her cycle, hormonal therapy may be prescribed for her. Hormonal therapy such as ethinyl estradiol (Estinyl) is prescribed for 5 days to prevent pregnancy if the assault occurred within the previous 48 hours. She is told that the drug can cause nausea and that she should expect withdrawal bleeding shortly after finishing the therapy. Antinauseant therapy in the form of a prochlorperazine preparation (Compazine) is also prescribed to counter the side effects of high doses of estrogens. She is apprised of the availability of abortion or menstrual extraction as a backup measure. If she misses a menstrual period in spite of therapy or if she fails to have withdrawal bleeding from the estrogens, she is assessed for the β-subunit of human chorionic gonadotropin in 2 to 3 weeks (a highly accurate test for pregnancy). She has the option of continuing a pregnancy if pregnancy does occur but is warned about the teratogenic effects of estrogen in these doses.

If the woman is pregnant at the time of the assault, she should be observed for several hours for uterine contractility.

Psychologic support is provided by the manner in which the woman is signed into the emergency room, the respect she is shown, the privacy that is provided for the examination and consultation, and the manner in which the examination is carried out. Access to supplies (including mouth wash) and facilities in which to clean up, clothes to wear home, money as needed, and transportation to wherever she is staying (an alternate place may need to be found for her) add to the woman's comfort and perception of being in control.

In some facilities the social worker is notified the moment a victim is admitted; other facilities contact local rape crisis centers, usually staffed by specially trained volunteers on 24-hour call for just these types of emergencies. The victim needs to be informed of all the steps involved in the rape examination and follow-up. Rape counselors provide ongoing support in a variety of ways. In addition to providing emotional support, transportation, etc., the counselor helps her interact with her family, friends, and various authorities, informs her of the rape trauma syndrome, and finds other resources for her as needed. Male volunteers help to counsel male members of the victim's family and peers.

One rape crisis center developed "A Note to Those Closest to Rape Victims: Families, Lovers, and Friends" (see box, p. 1126).

Discharge. The woman is discharged with medications and printed instructions about their use, printed instructions for self-care, and names and phone numbers of resource people should she require assistance. Medical follow-up in the gynecology or pediatric clinic is scheduled for 1 week for a repeat culture for gonorrhea, at 6 weeks for assessment of healing of injuries, and at 8 weeks for a repeat VDRL test and test for acquired immune deficiency syndrome (AIDS) antibodies. Repeat tests are rescheduled as necessary (Chapter 30). The woman and her counselor determine whether there is a need for additional medical or psychologic follow-up between the scheduled visits. The woman has a choice of site for follow-up—some women choose to continue with the physician who first performed the examination, others prefer their private physician, and still others need referral to a clinic in the area (city, state) to which they have moved.

After Discharge. Because of the phases of recovery, follow-up telephone contact is continued until the woman has no further need of such help.

A bill for laboratory work and treatment, if sent to the victim, adds insult to injury. Not only can the bill impose a financial burden, but it is a tangible reminder of the assault and adds the indignity of having to pay a financial penalty for being a victim. Today, many municipalities are assuming the cost of examination and treatment for rape.

Evaluation

The nurse can be reasonably assured that care was effective when priorities of care (p. 1124) have been met. The woman receives care that is nonjudgmental and caring. The examination is accomplished in a nonhurried manner and meets all legal specifications. The woman does not perceive herself as a victim; she receives anticipatory guidance regarding delayed reactions; STDs and pregnancy are prevented; and family bonds are supported and strengthened. Later the woman has no adverse physical, psychologic, or emotional sequelae.

REPRODUCTIVE HEALTH HAZARDS IN THE WORKPLACE AND ENVIRONMENT

The purpose of this chapter is not to generate global anxiety but to alert the nurse to a line of investigation, to keep the nurse informed, and to help the nurse communicate information. Information is the foundation for decision-making in personal health goals.

Potentially harmful materials in the workplace and environment have become an increasing concern. Some substances adversely affect factors required for fertility. These substances have a selective effect on chromosomes, gamete formation, ovulation, fertilization, implantation, embryogenesis, fetal development, and parturition (Chapter 9). Other materials affect reproduction by reducing libido (marijuana) or sexual performance (alcohol) (Chapters 34 and 42). Substances may have a *mutagenic effect* on chromosomes at any time during the male's or female's life span. Mutagens such as plastic-vinyl chloride cause permanent genetic changes in gametes of females and males. Other agents have a *teratogenic effect*. Teratogenes affect embryogenesis in the current pregnancy only. Well known teratogens are alcohol and thalidomide (Chapter 40, and Appendix G), rubella (Chapters 30 and 39), and poorly controlled diabetes mellitus (Chapter 38).

Substances that can be inhaled from the air are the most common concern. Also worrisome are materials that can be absorbed through the skin and those that can enter the body by mouth, such as lead dust that has settled on the fingers. Other potential threats arise from *physical forces:* eye stress from working at a video display terminal (VDT) all day, temperature, atmospheric pressure, oxygen content of the air, noise, vibration, acceleration, and ionizing radiation. *Social forces* that emphasize slimness and set styles of dress pose potential threats. Slimness and excessive exercise alter the woman's ovulation, high heels affect balance, tight pants create the warm, moist environment needed for genital infections in the woman and reduced spermatogenesis in the male. Jobs that entail lifting heavy weights or working on slick floors, and working at high elevations or in unusual body positions may also pose hazards to the gravida or new mother (Chapter 13) (Bond, 1986). *Emotional forces* such as severe stress affect the hypothalamic-pituitary-gonadal axis. Anovulation and irregular menstrual cycles may result.

Whether or not a substance or condition produces de-

A NOTE TO THOSE CLOSEST TO RAPE VICTIMS: FAMILIES, LOVERS, AND FRIENDS

How does rape affect a woman? How does rape affect those closest to a victim? How can those closest to a rape victim do "the right thing"? We have some ideas which we wish to share with you, and we hope they will offer a beginning for giving effective support to rape victims. More than anyone else, it is those closest to a victim who influence how she will deal with the attack.

Most women who have been raped do not react to the sexual aspects of the crime, but instead they react to the terror and fear that is involved. Often an immediate reaction of the woman is "I could have been killed." Many of those around her, particularly men, may find themselves concerned with the sexual aspects of the crime. The more this preoccupation is communicated to the woman, the more likely she is to have difficulties in dealing with her own feelings. Probably the best way to understand her feelings is to try to remember or imagine a situation where you felt powerless and afraid. You may remember feeling very alone, fearful and needing comfort.

Often the raped woman needs much love and support the first few days. Affection seems to be important. Stroking or caressing can be comforting. They help break down the loneliness and alienation. This, of course, leads to the question of sex. It is impossible to generalize about how the woman will feel about sex, nor should you guess. If you have been involved sexually with the woman, try to discuss, at an appropriate time, how she feels in general about the attack, about you, and about sex. (An appropriate time is not right after the rape. Let her comments to the first two questions guide you in deciding whether you have chosen a good time to discuss it or whether you would be pushing the point too soon.) Some women will be anxious to resume normal sexual relations as a way of forgetting the rape; others will be more hesitant.

In the case of virgin rapes, female support seems most important. It is a good time to discuss the pleasure involved in sex—as well as to reassert the woman's right to decide when and with whom she wishes to have sex. Hopefully, a woman's mother will feel comfortable about this; if not, a friend or sister—especially if she has been raped—might help.

It seems advisable for the woman to talk about the rape; however, it is not possible to generalize about how much she should be encorged to talk about it. Women do not seem to appreciate specific questions; they tend to be too probing and callous. To probe in these areas may only worsen any problems the woman may have in dealing with the rape.

Instead, questions about how she feels now and what bothers her the most are more useful. They are not threatening and should allow her to talk about her most immediate concerns. Remember, too, the woman wants to talk about other things. Often the rape may leave a woman concentrating on other problems and it is important that she talk about these. Probably the most practical suggestion is that you communicate your own willingness to let her talk. Because of your closeness to her, the woman may be more sensitive to your feelings. If the rape distresses her, it may be impossible for her to talk to you. She may also try to protect you. In these and other cases, where she really will not be able to talk with you, encourage her to speak with someone she trusts. Remember that the rape has brought up feelings of powerlessness, and encouraging her to talk to whom she wants, when she wants, is more helpful than feeling that it is necessary to talk to you.

If the rape is treated as a serious crime and not a heinous experience, women would probably have less difficulty in dealing with it. The woman survived the attack and one would suppose that she would want to resume living a "normal" life as quickly as possible. In a healthy, supportive environment, most women will find the rape meshes with other unhappy experiences in their lives. Because of others' reactions, or their own life situations at the time of the rape, other women will find the rape was indeed a traumatic milestone. If, after a reasonable amount of time, a woman seems unable to cope with the day-to-day problems of life, professional help may be sought.

Whether or not professional counseling is sought, it is not a replacement for warm, concerned, loving communications. A professional counselor may help, but he or she cannot replace your role in the relationship. Rape not only affects the woman, but also you, as it plays upon your own fears and fantasies. Try to recognize the fears for what they are; otherwise you may end up projecting them on the woman and cause some serious problems for her and your relationship.

Finally, it should be noted that, if the woman has pressed charges, the whole process involves numerous hassles and stresses. Your awareness of the legal processes and problems involved and your support will be helpful.

Reprinted with permission and courtesy of the Washington, DC, Rape Crisis Center, PO Box 21005, Kalorama St. Station, Washington, DC 20009.

tectable effects depends in part on exposure level, dose, or length of exposure. Some individuals are more susceptible than others. Genetic factors, general health, and life-style (including smoking and diet) can also affect susceptibility to chemicals and conditions in the environment.

Nonionizing radiation in microwave ovens and ultrasound have different characteristics and biologic effects than ionizing radiation (e.g., x-rays). Nonionizing radiation in microwaves and ultrasound diagnostic equipment does *not* have sufficient energy to ionize molecules and disrupt cellular deoxyribonucleic acid (DNA) (Jankowski, 1986). There is no evidence of mutagenic or carcinogenic effects from properly constructed microwave ovens or from diagnostic ultrasound (Brent, 1980; Bond, 1986; ACOG, 1984; NIOSH, 1981). Magnetic resonance imagery (MRI) VDTs also do *not* represent reproductive health hazards (Budinger, 1981; Thomas and Morris, 1981; Bond, 1986; Hirning and Aitken, 1982; Droegemueller et al., 1987).

The chemicals to worry about are those that come from industrial waste, landfill seepage, agricultural herbicides and pesticides, gasoline and oil, and common household solvents and cleaners (Shavelson, 1987; Ferguson, 1986). Methylene chloride is the best liquid paint and grease remover on the market. It is a common component of aerosol propellents in such products as hair spray, pesticides, paints, and lubricants. It is used in the electronic industry to clean printed circuit boards and is the solvent of choice for decaffeinating coffee. Absorbed in the body, it generates carbon monoxide, which interferes with the body's ability to pick up and deliver oxygen. Inhalation of low levels for short periods (minutes to hours) may cause dizziness, nausea, headache, and confusion. At high levels, methylene chloride may cause unconsciousness and death (Hazards, 1986).

Drinking water may contain arsenic, benzene, cadmium, carbon tetrachloride, dioxin, lead, and vinyl chloride among others. Certain geographic areas contain greater concentrations of these pollutants than others. Under-the-sink filtering systems filter out some of the substances (How, 1987).

Women are exposed to potentially hazardous substances in their homes and workplaces. Homemakers and domestic workers are exposed to alkalis, bleaches, detergents, and solvents that emit fumes. Fresh paint increases levels of hydrocarbons in the environment especially if ventilation is poor. Sealers used to prevent plumbing leaks at joints often contain arsenic to retard growth of mold. This arsenic and other chemicals may be leached from plumbing systems.

People working in office buildings have displayed symptoms that have been termed the *sick-building syndrome.* Newer designs and construction to conserve energy have compromised ventilation. The result is an increase in concentrations of dust, ozone from copying machines, tobacco smoke, and hydrocarbons. Carbonless paper irritates the skin. Fumes accumulate from cleaning fluids. In some buildings the air contains levels of pollutants 50 times higher than that accepted by the Environmental Protection Agency (EPA) for air-quality for out-of-doors.

Noise is everywhere. Sound is a form of energy with the potential to damage tissues (Noise, 1986). Women report fetal startle responses to loud noises such as telephone rings and some forms of music. Some women experience excessive and extremely uncomfortable fetal movements in response to hard rock music. Newborns in intensive care nurseries show better weight gain when the noise level is controlled. Long term damage has not been identified.

Hospital staff are exposed to gases, x-rays, antineoplastic medications, needle accidents, and weight-related and other accidents (Moses, 1987; Munley et al., 1986). Vehicle drivers breathe carbon monoxide and other combustion products of gasoline, as well as polynuclear aromatics. They are also subjected to physical stress, vibration, and accidents. Electronics assemblers are exposed to trichloroethylene, lead, tin, methylene chloride, antimony, epoxy resins, and methyl ethyl ketones. Hairdressers work with acetone, aerosol propellents (e.g., freon), benzyl alcohol, ethyl alcohol, and hair dyes. Cigarette smoke is encountered commonly. Animal handlers, including meat cutters, inspectors, and teachers, are exposed to infections and flea and tick preparations.

Lead is a potential hazard to potters, artists, ceramists, and glass workers. Lead poisoning is still a threat (Lead, 1988). Lead poisoning is responsible for menstrual abnormalities, spontaneous abortion, decreased fertility in females and males, stillbirths, infants to low birth weight (LBW), and poor neurobehavioral development in children (Bellinger et al., 1987).

Assessment

A complete assessment always provides a basis for research, especially when related to reproductive hazards in the home and workplace. Such careful assessment recently uncovered a peculiar finding in a population of wives of Navy airforce navigators—all reported births of females only. Study into the possible cause of this phenomenon continues.

Findings from the woman's present health status, including an extensive reproductive health history, are accumulated. Nonoccupational exposure to drugs (smoking, alcohol, "recreational" chemicals) and infection, geographic location and proximity to toxic disposal sites and industries, and spouse's occupation are noted. The woman's and her partner's current and past occupational histories are vital to detection of hazards to the reproductive system. The time, length of exposure, work conditions, and symptomatology related to work are identified. Wives of asbestos and agricultural workers inhale fibers and pesticides from work clothes; wives of those who work with anesthetic and other gases inhale metabolites in the spouse's breath; farm workers absorb and inhale pesticides used on plants; people eat foods (fish, vegetables) from water and soil with high levels of toxic substances (Shavelson, 1987).

A toxicology screen is ordered if it is indicated. The presence and level of toxins, and the number and condition of blood components may need to be assessed. If exposure of either parent to a mutagen is suspected, a karyotype may be ordered. Investigation of the cause of a defect includes a search for possible environmental agents. A retrospective approach often yields data that are difficult to validate so that an association may be suspected but not conclusive.

Nursing Diagnoses

Following are examples of nursing diagnoses of the woman that may emerge from assessment data.

- Potential for impaired gas exchange related to
  - Inhalation of toxic substances aided by injudicious use of chemicals, inadequate ventilation, and inappropriate disposal of chemical wastes, including equipment such as rags, brushes
- Potential for injury related to
  - Toxic substances ingested, inhaled, or absorbed through the skin
- Knowledge deficit related to
  - Toxicity of substances in the environment
  - Use of chemicals
  - Avoidance of exposure
  - Alternatives to some commonly used chemicals
  - Safe use and disposal of chemicals
- Anxiety or grief related to
  - Evidence of toxic exposure (e.g., impaired fertility, birth of a child with a defect)

Planning

Effective planning requires a world-wide effort to prevent pollution and the spread of infection. Personal and professional involvement is needed on local, state, and national levels to control hazards to reproductive health. A care plan is developed to meet the individual's needs and the goals for care are stated in client-centered terms.

Goals

1. Females and males suffer no mutagenic insults
2. Impaired fertility associated with environmental hazards to reproductive health is prevented
3. Gravidas are not exposed to insults teratogenic to their unborn babies
4. People implement health practices that prevent or minimize effects of environmental hazards to reproductive health

Implementation

Prevention should be the focus of self-care in any care plan. Several preventive measures are discussed in Chapter 13 (e.g. exercise tips for pregnant women, client teaching for good posture and body mechanics, and standards for maternity care and employment).

Preventive measures are suggested for infection, nutrition, substance abuse, and other health-related concerns throughout this text. Cleanliness, ventilation, adherence to manufacturer's directions for use and disposal of materials, use of protective gear to shield against known and unknown hazards, and avoidance of exposure are examples of strategies to reduce risk.

In some instances safer materials can be substituted for potentially hazardous ones. Most household cleaning needs can be met with baking soda, table salt, distilled white vinegar, lemon juice, trisodium phosphate (TSP) (which does not emit fumes), a plunger, and some common sense. These substances clean drains, wash windows, degrease, prevent mold and mildew, disinfect, and scour (Dadd, 1987).

Impaired fertility and the birth of a child with a defect present special challenges to the nurse and health care team (Green and Malin, 1988). Curative and rehabilitative measures appropriate to these situations are presented in several parts of this text, especially in Chapters 28, 40, and 42.

Industrial nurses must be alert to conditions in the workplace that may affect reproductive health of workers and their spouses. Stress reduction through relaxation and guided imagery, and moderate exercise and rest are useful (see index for these content areas).

As private citizens nurses must become involved in their professional and political organizations to promote and support legislation to control pollution of the environment. Nurses can teach about alternative ways to clean the home and care for yards and gardens to reduce exposure to potentially harmful substances.

Evaluation

Evaluation of short-term results is possible to some extent. The birth of a healthy baby with no apparent disorder or disease, the uncomplicated recovery of the new mother, continued fertility, and demonstration of a life-style that supports good reproductive health are some indicators that care was effective. However, the long-term effects may not be known for many years or generations.

SUMMARY

Violence against women is a major social problem. Society and health professionals must move beyond mere recognition of the problem to understand the dynamics of violence against women. Nurses as client advocates can intervene in the cycle of violence by helping victimized women recognize their options and take appropriate action.

Reproductive health hazards exist in the environment and workplace. The content in this chapter alerts the nurse to current information and presents a line of investigation. The information is intended to assist the nurse with decisions about personal health goals and with nursing care plans for clients and their families.

KEY CONCEPTS

- It has been estimated that one out of every six U.S. couples engage in family violence at least once a year.
- Pregnancy is a time of increased battering episodes.
- The abuse of spouses occurs at all socioeconomic levels, as well as at all educational levels.
- Battered women may feel that they are to blame for their situation.
- Complementary personality characteristics and childhood influences are found in couples who are susceptible to development of abuser/victim relationships.
- To develop an effective plan, the caregiver must be comfortable working with the victim (of rape, incest, or battering) and her family.
- Although incest is a universal taboo, an estimated 100,000 cases or more of incest occur each year in the United States.
- The true incidence of rape will not be known until women feel free to report the crime.
- The rapist has no regard for his victim's age, race, sexual attraction, or physical condition.
- Rape is not just a woman's problem; it is a community problem.
- Pollution of the environment is a serious and growing hazard to reproductive health.

STUDY QUESTIONS AND ACTIVITIES

1. Visit a rape crisis center and observe the care given a victim. Describe the supportive role of the nurse. What procedures are carried out in collection of evidence? Obtain the "rape kit" used and review the use and purpose of the contents. Describe your feelings regarding the victim.
2. If possible, attend a rape trial. What mechanisms are in place that offer support to the victim? Describe your feelings regarding treatment of the victim by the legal system.
3. Visit or volunteer time at a battered women's shelter or a victims' hotline.
4. Set up and conduct the following role-playing situations in class:
   a. An adolescent pregnant as a result of incest
   b. A nursing student raped in the dorm
   c. A woman brought to the emergency room with black eyes, a broken leg, and multiple cuts and bruises
5. Make a list of the household chemicals used in your home. In a group seminar compile a master list. Select some examples from the list, identify their purpose, describe why they are hazardous, and list what alternatives can be substituted to accomplish the same purpose.

References

Violence to Women

Battered wives testify—'no legal recourse,' San Francisco Chronicle, p A18, Sept 17, 1987

Bowker, L, and Maurer, L: The effectiveness of counseling services utilized by battered women, Women and Therapy 5(4):65, 1986

Burgess, AW, and Holmstrom, LL: Crisis and counseling requests of rape victims, Nurs Res 23:196, 1974

Burgess, AW, and Holmstrom, LL: Rape: victims of crisis, Bowie, Md, 1974b, Robert J Brady Co

Burgess, AW, and Holmstrom, LL: Rape trauma syndrome: coping behavior of the rape victim, Nurs Dig 3:17, May/June 1975

Chez, RA, moderator: If you suspect a patient is a victim of abuse, Contemp OB/GYN 29(6):132, 1987

Collier, JA: When you suspect your patient is a battered wife, RN, p 33, May 1987

Delgaty, K: Battered women: the issues for nursing, NAACOG Newsletter, 12(10):9, 1985

Drake, VK: Battered women: a health care problem in disguise, Image 14:40, June 1982

Elbow, M: Theoretical considerations of violent marriages, Social Casework, p 515, Nov 1977

Finley, B: Nursing process with the battered woman, Nurse Pract 6(4):11, 1981

Foley, TS, and Davies, MA: Rape: nursing care of victims, St Louis, 1983, The CV Mosby Co

Gelles, RJ: Abused wives: why do they stay, J Marriage Fam, Nov 1976

Gelles, RJ: The myths of battered husbands, Ms 8(4):65, 1979

Griffith-Kinney, J: Contemporary women's health: a nursing advocacy approach, Menlo Park, Calif, 1986, Addison-Wesley Publishing Co, Inc

Hicks, DJ: Sexual battery: management of the rape victim. In Sciarra, JJ, editor: Obstetrics and gynecology, New York, 1981, Harper & Row, Publishers, Inc

Hilberman, E: The rape victim, New York, 1976, Basic Books

Hillard, PJ: Physical abuse in pregnancy, Obstet Gynecol 66:185, 1985

Hillard, PJ: Physical abuse and pregnancy, Fam Prac Recertification 8(9):89, 1986

Klaus, PA, and Rand, MR: Family violence, Bureau of Justice Statistics (special report), Washington, DC, 1984

Klingbeil, KS, et al: Multidisciplinary care for sexual assault victims, Nurs Pract 1(6):21, 1976

Lauber, AA, and Souma, ML: Use of toluidine blue for documentation of traumatic intercourse, Obstet Gynecol 60:644, 1982

Lichtenstein, VR: The battered women: guideline for effective nursing intervention, Issues Ment Health Nurs 3:237, 1981

Mandel, B: Woman victimized twice—by her ex-lover and the system, San Francisco Examiner, Nov 2, 1986

Martin, D: Battered wives, New York, 1976, Pocket Books (Also published by New Glide Publications)

Mercer, RT: Nursing care for parents at risk, Thorofare, NJ, 1977, Charles B Slack, Inc

Nichaus, MA: Rape. In Griffith-Kenney, J: Contemporary women's health, Menlo Park, Calif, 1986, Addison-Wesley Publishing Co, Inc

Parker, B, and Schumacher, DN: The battered wife syndrome and violence in the nuclear family of origin: a controlled pilot study, Am J Public Health 67:760, 1977

Pfouts, JH: Violent families: coping responses of abused wives, Child Welfare 57:101, 1978

Riesenberg, D: Treating a societal malignancy—rape, JAMA 257(6):726, 1987

Shepard, M: Guide to managing the victim of rape, Contemp OB/GYN 22(3):253, 1983

Simens, S, and Brandzel, RC: Sexuality: nursing assessment and intervention, Philadelphia, 1982, JB Lippincott Co

Straus, MA, et al: Behind closed doors: violence in the American family, Garden City, NY, 1980, Anchor Books

Stuart, GW, and Sundeen, SJ: Principles and practice of psychiatric nursing, ed 3, St Louis, 1987, The CV Mosby Co

Warner, CG: Rape and sexual assault, Germantown, Penn, 1980, Aspen Publishers, Inc

Welch, MS: Rape and the trauma of inadequate care, Nurs Dig 5:50, Spring 1977

White, EC: Chain, chain, change: for black women dealing with physical and emotional abuse, Seattle, 1985, The Seal Press, New Leaf Series

Witkin-Lanoil, G: Too close to home, Health, p 6, Jan 1987

Zdanuk, JM, Harris, CC, and Wisian, NL: Adolescent pregnancy and incest: the nurse's role as counselor, JOGN Nurs 16(2):99, 1987

Environmental Hazards

ACOG American College of Obstetricians and Gynecologists: Video display terminals and reproductive health—a statement to the US House of Representatives' Subcommittee on Health and Safety, Washington, DC, 1984

Bellinger, D, et al: Longitudinal analyses of prenatal and postnatal lead exposure and early cognitive development, N Engl J Med 316(7):1037, 1987

Bond, MB: Reproductive hazards in the workplace, Contemp OB/GYN 28(3):57, 1986

Brent, RL: X-ray, microwave and ultrasound: the real and unreal hazards, Pediatr Ann 9:469, Dec 1980
Budinger, TF: Nuclear magnetic resonance (NMR) in vivo studies: known thresholds for health effects, J Comput Assist Tomogr 5:800, Dec 1981
Dadd, DL: Nontoxic cleaners for your home, San Francisco Chronicle, p C8, April 1, 1987
Droegemueller, W, et al: Comprehensive gynecology, St Louis, 1987, The CV Mosby Co
Ferguson, S: Birth defects and the environment—finding the connection, CBE Environmental Rev, P8, Fall 1986
Green, D, and Malin, J: Prenatal diagnosis: when reality shatters parents' dreams, Nurs '88 18(2):61, 1988
Hazards of methylene chloride, Harvard Medical School Health Letter 11(10):5, 1986
Hirning, CR, and Aitken, JH: Cathode-ray tube x-ray emission standard for video display terminals, Health Phys 43:727, Nov 1982
How to tell if your water is pure, San Francisco Chronicle, p C1, Feb 4, 1987
Lead poisoning still a threat, state says, San Francisco Chronicle, p A2, Feb 6, 1988
Moses, M: Reproductive health in the workplace: health workers and reproductive hazards, BIRTH 14(3):153, 1987
Munley, AJ, Railton, R, Gary, WM, et al: Exposure of midwives to nitrous oxide in four hospitals, Br Med J 293:1063, 1986
National Institute for Occupational Safety and Health: Potential health hazards of video display terminals, US Department of Health and Human Services, 1981, NIOSH Pub #81-129
Noise pollution: irritant or hazard? Harvard Medical School Health Newsletter 11(8):1, 1986
Thomas, A, and Morris, PG: The effects of NMR exposure in living organisms. Part I. A microbial assay, Br J Radiol 54:615, July 1981
Shavelson, L: Poisoned lives: six stories from toxic California, Image, p 22, July 26, 1987

Bibliography

Violence to Women

Binder, RL: Why women don't report sexual assault, J Clin Psychiatry 42:437, 1981
Bowker, L, and Maurer, L: The effectiveness of counseling services utilized by battered women, Women and Therapy, 5(4):65, 1986
Aguilera, DC, and Messick, JM: Crisis intervention: theory and methodology, ed 5, St Louis, 1985, The CV Mosby Co
Alexander, P: A systems theory conceptualization of incest, Fam Process 24:79, 1985
Bowker, L, and Maurer, L: The effectiveness of counseling services utlized by battered women, Women and Therapy 5(4):65, 1986
Cohen, T: The incestuous family revisited, Soc Casework 64:154, March, 1983
Correspondence: Sexually transmitted diseases in victims of sexual assault, N Engl J Med 316(16):1023, 1987
de Chesnay, M: Father-daughter incest, J Psychosoc Nurs Ment Health Serv 22:9, 1984
Ewing, WA: Domestic violence and community health care ethics: reflections on systemic intervention, Fam Commun Health 10(1):54, 1987
Fenton, MV: Development of the scale of humanistic nursing behaviors, Nurs Res 36(2):82, 1987
Ferris, E: Long term consequences of adult rape responses to violence in the family and sexual assault, Rockville, Md, National Center for the Prevention and Control of Rape, 6(1):Jan/Feb 1983
Finkelhor, D, Gelles, RJ, Hotaling, GT, et al: The dark side of families, Beverly Hills, Calif, 1983, Sage Publications, Inc
Fiora-Gormally, N: Battered wives who kill: double standard out of court, single standard in? Law Hum Behav 2(2):133, 1978
Goodstein, R, and Page, A: Battered wife syndrome: overview of dynamics and treatment, J Psychiatry 138:8, Aug 1981
Greany, GD: Is she a battered woman? A guide for ER response, Am J Nurs 84:724, 1984
Gross, TP, and Rosenberg, ML: Shelters for battered women and their children: an underrecognized source of communicable disease transmission, Am J Public Health 77(9):1198, 1987
Heinrich, KT: Effective responses to sexual harassment, Nurs Outlook 35(2):70, 1987
Helton, A: Battering during pregnancy, Am J Nurs 86(8):910, 1986
Helton, AS, and Snodgrass, FG: Battering during pregnancy: intervention strategies, BIRTH 14(3):142, 1987
Higgins, SD: Caring for the injured pregnant patient, Contemp OB/GYN 21(3):32, 1983 (Special issue)
Hogan, N, and Juhasz, A: The detection of incest, Home Health Care Nurse 2:20, 1984
Houghton, BD: Domestic violence training: treatment of adult victims of family violence, J NY State Nurses Assoc 12(4):25, 1981
Jennings, BH: Social support: a way to a climate of caring, Nurs Adm Q 11(4):63, 1987
Johnson, SH: High-risk parenting: nursing assessment and strategies for the family at risk, ed 2, Philadelphia, 1986, JB Lippincott Co
Martin, PY, et al: Services to rape victims in Forida 1984: a needs assessment study, Tallahassee, 1984, State of Florida, Department of Health and Rehabilitative Services
Matteson, PS: Pregnant and battered, Childbirth Educator 5(2):46, 1985-86
Moleti, CA: Caring for socially high-risk pregnant women, MCN 13(1):24, 1988
Okun, L: Woman abuse: facts replacing myths, Albany, New York, 1986, State University of New York Press
Parker, S, and Parker, H: Early years bonding can help avert later abuse, University of Utah Review, 1985
Payne, JS, Downs, S, and Newman, K: Helping the abused woman, Nurs '86, 16(9):52, 1986
Reedy, NJ: Trauma in pregnancy, NAACOG update series, lesson 23, Vol 1, 1984
Sammons, LN: Battered and pregnant, MCN 6:246, July/Aug 1981
Sanday, PR: The sociocultural context of rape: a cross-cultural study, J Soc Issues 37(4):5, 1981
Sexually transmitted diseases in victims of sexual assault (correspondence), N Engl J Med 316(16):1023, 1987
Snodgrass, F: Where do women turn? Am J Nurs 86(8):912
Sredl, DR, et al: Offering the rape victim real help, Nurs '79, p 38, July 1979
Stanko, E: Intimate intrusions—women's experience of male violence, Boston, 1985, Routledge & Kegan Paul, Inc
Stark, E, et al: Wife abuse in the medical setting, Rockville, Md, 1981, National Clearinghouse on Domestic Violence
Swearingen, P, editor: The Addison-Wesley photo-atlas of nursing procedures, Menlo Park, Calif, 1984, Addison-Wesley Publishing Co, Inc

Tilden, V, and Shepherd, P: Increasing the rate of identification of battered women in an emergency department: use of a nursing protocol, Res Nurs Health 10(4):209, 1987

Urbaneic, J: Incest trauma, J Psychosoc Nurs Ment Health Serv 25(7):33, 1987

Walker, LE: The battered woman syndrome, New York, 1984, Springer Publishing Co, Inc

Zdanuk, J, Harris, C, and Wisian, N: Adolescent pregnancy and incest: the nurse's role as counselor, JOGN Nurs 16(2):99, 1987

Environmental Hazards

Anonymous. OSHA work-practice guidelines for personnel dealing with cytotoxic (antineoplastic) drugs, Am J Hosp Pharm 43:1193, 1986

Bingol, N, et al: Terotogenicity of cocaine in humans, J Pediatr 110:93, 1987

Council on Scientific Affairs, AMA: Effects of pregnancy on work performance, JAMA 251:1995, 1984

Council on Scientific Affairs, AMA: Effects of toxic chemicals on the reproductive system, JAMA 253, 1985

Council on Scientific Affairs, AMA: Effects of physical forces on the reproductive cycle, AMA, 1985

Council on Scientific Affairs, Advisory Panel on Reproductive Hazards in the Workplace, AMA: Effects of toxic chemicals on the reproductive system, AMA, 1985

Driscoll, ME: AIDS: legal aspects of occupational exposure, Calif Nurs Review 10(3):10, 1988

Dupre, L: Safety in the workplace. Part I. Handling chemotherapy drugs, Calif Nurs Rev 10(2):12, 1988

Estok, P, and Rudy, E: Marothon running: comparison of physical and psychosocial risks for men and women, Res Nurs Health 10(2):79, 1987

Foster, SD: MCN patient teaching, MCN 12(2):131, 1987

Freivogel, W: High court upholds special pregnancy benefits, St Louis Post Dispatch, Jan 14, 1987

Griffith-Kenney, J: Contemporary women's health: a nursing advocacy approach, Menlo Park, Calif, 1986, Addison-Wesley Publishing Co, Inc

Health status of Vietnam veterans, III: reproductive outcomes and child health, JAMA 259(18):2715, 1988

Howard, J: Report of ongoing research on the infants of mothers using cocaine and PCP, Los Angeles Times, January 1986

Krakoff, IH: Cancer chemotherapeutic agents, Cancer 37:93, 1987

Luck, W, et al: Nicotine and cotinine: two pharmacologically active substances as parameters for the strain on fetuses and babies of mothers who smoke, J Perinatal Med 10:107, 1982

McDonald, AD, et al: Visual display units and pregnancy: evidence from the Montreal survey, J Occup Med 28(12):1226, 1986

McDonald, AD, et al: Spontaneous abortion and occupation, J Occup Med 28(12):1232, 1986

McKee, D: New Milner-Fenwick Program addresses pregnant working woman, Patientvision Update, p 8, Summer 1987

Meurer, J, Sr: The impact of environmental hazards on reproduction, NAACOG Update Series 1(25):issue, 1984

Miller, SA: Chemotherapy drug handling safety, Calif Nurs Review 10(2):12, 1988

MMWR: Outbreak of occupational hepatitis—Connecticut, JAMA 257(11):1453, 1987

NAACOG: Reproductive health hazards: women in the workplace, 11:issue, Feb 1985

Pregnant women banned from AT&T chip lines, St. Louis Post Dispatch, Jan 14, 1987

Riordan, J, and Riorday, M: Drugs in breast milk, Am J Nurs 84(3):328, 1984

Schuyt, HC, Brakel, K, Oostendorp, SGLM, et al: Abortions among dental personnel exposed to nitrous oxide, Anaesthesiology 41:82, 1986

Selevan, SG, Lindbohm, ML, CandPolSci, et al: A study of occupational exposure to antineoplastic drugs and fetal loss in nurses, N Engl J Med 313:1173, 1985

Safety of antimicrobial drugs in pregnancy, Med Lett Drugs Ther 29(743):issue, 1987

Stockwell, H, and Lyman, G: Cigarette smoking and the risk of female reproductive cancer, Am J Obstet Gynecol 157(1):35, 1987

FOR MORE INFORMATION

National Coalition Against Domestic Violence
Suite 305
2401 Virginia Avenue, NW
Washington, DC 20037

National Center on Women and Family Law
799 Broadway, Room 402
New York, NY 10003

National Coalition Against Sexual Assault
c/o Fern Ferguson, President
Volunteers of America of Illinois
8787 State St., Suite 202
East St. Louis, IL 62203

Project SHARE
US Department of Health and Human Services
P.O. Box 2309
Rockville, MD 20852

National Crime Prevention Council
The Woodward Building
733 15th St., NW, Room 540
Washington, DC 20005

CHAPTER

44

Neoplasia

Learning Objectives

Correctly define the key terms listed.

Discuss the emotional impact of cancer.

Develop a nursing care plan for a woman who has a lump in her breast.

Prepare a nursing care plan for a woman with cancer of the uterus and vagina.

Explain procedures, in client-centered terms, to detect and diagnose cancer.

Explain treatments for preinvasive and invasive conditions.

Review preventive measures that reduce risk for developing cancer.

Assess cancer and pregnancy.

Develop a nursing care plan for a woman with gestational trophoblastic disease.

Key Terms

benign
biopsy
cancer
carcinoma
chemotherapy
conization
cryosurgery
diethylstilbestrol (DES)
gestational trophoblastic disease (GTD)
hysterectomy
in situ
laser surgery
malignant
mammary dysplasia
mammography
mastectomy
melanoma
metastasis
neoplasia
Papanicolaou smear
radiotherapy
sarcoma

Neoplasia refers to an abnormal body state characterized by the growth of tumors, benign or malignant. Malignant growth, or cancer, is a prevalent disease in all living organisms. The health or life of plants and animals, as well as humans, is endangered by this disorder. All nurses will encounter people with cancer regardless of their area of nursing practice. Most people fear the diagnosis of cancer. When cancer is diagnosed, the nurse is in a unique position to play a therapeutic role. As knowledge of the prevention, diagnosis, and therapy of cancer increases and discussion of feelings becomes more open, everyone including the nurse is more likely to develop a positive, hopeful attitude toward the disorder and its treatment.

The knowledge and expertise that nurses gain about cancer can be used in creating public awareness and acceptance of its primary and secondary prevention. In addition, nurses provide nursing care to people during the acute and chronic phases of cancer and can play a signficant role in providing physical and emotional comfort and guidance to these people and their families.

Cancers may be classified according to their cell type origin. Two main types are those of epithelial and of mesenchymal (connective tissue) origin. The term *carcinoma* denotes a malignant tumor of epithelial cells, and the term *sarcoma* denotes a malignant tumor of connective tissue cells. When a malignant tumor contains all three types of embryonal tissue, it is called a *teratoma.* Some tumors are known by the names of the scientists who first described them, for example, Hodgkin's disease (Phipps, Long, Woods, 1987).

This chapter presents a discussion of neoplasia of the woman's reproductive tract and breasts in the nongravid and gravid states. Many other chapters contain information that complements the discussion in this chapter, especially Chapter 6 (section on immunology), Chapter 34 (section on surgical complications and pregnancy), and Chapter 28 (loss and grief).

THE EMOTIONAL IMPACT OF CANCER*

The wearing effects of a long illness combined with the wrenching experience of acute episodes produce an emotional impact that few other illnesses have. Cancer once carried a great stigma, and many people still associate it with suffering, disfigurement, hopelessness, and certain death. Not only is the person affected; family, friends, and medical professionals are all touched by various aspects of the disease and its treatment.

The woman and her loved ones face the threat to life, the large expense, the loss of usual work and play patterns, changes in body functions or appearance, prolonged disability and/or discomfort, and shifts in social and family roles. Intense feelings are engendered by cancer; and the manifold disruptions caused by the disease alter each person's ability to cope with these feelings. Despair, fear, and shame may be magnified because many women have never experienced these strong emotions and find them difficult to discuss and manage. Yet failure to examine these deep feelings or share them with others can only increase the sense of isolation, loneliness, and bewilderment. When the emotional turmoil is not recognized by the woman and those around her, associated "negative" behaviors may be misinterpreted and condemned, and the woman may alienate her loved ones and lose the support she so desperately needs.

Cancer can also have positive effects. Today, more and more people are accepting and adjusting to cancer. They are finding that many kinds of cancer are compatible with career, marriage, parenthood, and that a full, productive, and happy life is possible with a diagnosis of cancer. For some, having cancer enhances the experiences of daily life, by enabling them to focus on what is most important and meaningful.

The Woman's Responses

How the woman learns her diagnosis and prognosis, as well as the time of this disclosure, are of utmost importance. Many women have tremendous internal resources, and these can be summoned when the diagnosis is revealed with compassion and hope. Although it is the physician's responsibility to inform the woman and her family of the diagnosis, treatment plan, and prognosis, it is the nurse's responsibility to clarify this information in response to questions the woman will ask when she is ready to learn more about her condition. Knowing the woman and how she has handled crises in the past, and understanding what cancer means to her will give the health team clues to the emotional support she needs. Nurses can be of great help as they let the woman talk, listening and evaluating what she is really saying and helping her express fears and other feelings.

When confronted with the diagnosis of cancer; most people react with anguish and shock. One described it thus: "I felt as though the sky had fallen on me." Another said, "It was like being hit with a locomotive, only somehow I was alive and hurting." This stage of reaction is followed by disbelief and denial. The woman rationalizes that laboratory reports were in error or actually were those of another person. As she slowly relinquishes this crutch, the woman may be angry, grief-stricken, or depressed. Positive attitudes, if they develop at all, come later, depending on the woman's personality, her past experiences, the extent of her illness and its prognosis, and the support she receives.

At the time of the diagnosis the woman is distracted by worry, and yet this is the time when hospital personnel want her to plan for her future. Obviously, treatment decisions must be made immediately, but many other decisions can wait and, in fact, will be sounder if the woman is rested and relatively unshaken as she considers them. The nurse can help by providing time for the newly diagnosed woman to adjust to a changed future, to mourn, and to assess her profound feelings of fear and loss. This is, above all, a time to be with the woman, offering the special sense of closeness of an authentic, empathic relationship.

*From: A cancer source book for nurses, rev ed, New York, 1981, American Cancer Society, Inc.

Family Reactions

Families often suffer as much or more than the woman herself. Those who never enjoyed warm relationships may be consumed with remorse over past injustices or missed opportunities; or their rancor may be so deep that the thought of investing time, money, and emotion in the care of the woman is intolerable. Some relatives are jealous of the attention the sick person receives, and many, exhausted by the responsibilities the illness places on them, are angry and resentful. Other families, bound by affection, may deplore the present, dread the future, and set impossible standards of care based on self-abnegation.

Some families facing cancer, while crushed by the initial blow, are united and strengthened by all the resources they bring to the situation. Together they find support and meaning in adversity, emerging from the crisis with added stature. Positive family attitudes can be cultivated by the nurse's strong assurance that family members are very important to the woman, and by acceptance of their feelings as natural rather than either admirable or repugnant.

Nurses often hear the wistful remark, "If only there were something I could do . . . ." Although there are many helpful activities to become involved in, families may need help in recognizing them. Relatives who want to share in the physical care of the woman should be taught to do so; others may find this distasteful, and their caring can be expressed in such ways as driving the woman to appointments, returning books to the library, arranging a birthday party, assisting with child care, selecting gifts, or helping the woman with a project. Family members also need time away from the woman, to attend to responsibilities and personal interests, and to regain emotional strength.

Most important is the contribution family members and friends make to the woman's sense that she is still loved and needed. Frequent short visits, during which community and family news is discussed, can help the woman feel valued and worthwhile. Opportunities to recall their youth are welcomed by older people, who enjoy reminiscing with an attentive relative.

As with most human interactions, what is done is less important than how it is done.

The Dying Woman

At one time death and dying was a taboo subject, and the principal interests and efforts of health care providers were directed toward those for whom there was some hope of recovery. The early work of Elizabeth Kübler-Ross helped expand awareness of the many needs of the terminally ill and of the interventions that can be used in their care. Today, persons in the final stage of life are included as fully in the scope of nursing concerns as are any other clients.

Early treatment of cancer is aggressive, hopeful, and seeks a cure; when a cure or remission cannot be achieved, the focus of care shifts to supportive, palliative measures that alleviate symptoms of the progressing disease and provide comfort and maximum function during the woman's remaining time. Because the period between a focus on cure and a focus on palliation is often prolonged, the woman with cancer is apt to experience most of the stages described by Kübler-Ross and to require support through each.

After diagnosis, the woman experiences denial, then anger. As treatment begins, she may "bargain" for a cure. If treatment is successful and death is forestalled by remission or cure, the process of adjustment to terminality ceases and the woman again focuses on life and its challenges. When treatment fails to secure a cure or remission ends, the woman must turn again to the task of adjustment.

Grieving for relatives, friends, possessions, and all of the familiar and pleasant aspects of living that are to be lost, the woman is profoundly depressed. She may regret unaccomplished tasks, unfulfilled dreams, mistakes, and marred relationships, and be deeply frustrated. Time has run out for her, and it is likely that there will be no second chances. Starting alone on a long journey to the unknown, she is afraid. Seeing healthy people all about her apparently destined for a long life, she may be angry and jealous. Sometimes, in approaching death, she finds greater meaning in life and gains much strength, communicating this to others. Many finally accept dying as an inevitable, sad, but meaningful final phase of living.

Family and friends also experience diverse feelings. When grieving is prolonged, as it often is when the woman has cancer, the stress can be enormous and can interfere with other interpersonal relationships. The hospital environment may further intrude on relationships, limiting privacy and access to the woman and hindering opportunities for caring gestures.

Because these factors may diminish the woman's chances for a dignified and peaceful death, alternative modes of health care delivery for the terminally ill are being explored. These approaches include home care, with provisions for supportive medical and nursing services as needed, and hospice care, where the woman is not abandoned once cure is no longer the focus of medical intervention. Hospice care may take place in a specific institutional setting, bringing together dying people in a single building or building complex, or it may exist within an acute care facility. Regardless of setting, the principles of care include support of normalcy for as long as possible, adequate relief of pain and other discomforts, removal of barriers to interaction with family and loved ones, and sustained emotional and spiritual support.

Reactions of Health Professionals

Many health professionals find cancer depressing, viewing it as a hopeless disease. These professionals are trained to promote healthfulness and cure disease, but the nature of cancer thwarts their self-image as helping healing persons. Unfortunately, in dismissing the disease as hopeless, they are dismissing the woman too.

Others view cancer as a challenge to be combated with all the treatment possibilities medical technology can provide. The danger here is that the woman becomes a casualty in the battle, an interesting specimen upon which to test new or radical treatments long after hope of cure has been abandoned.

Still others see cancer care as an opportunity to fully use their knowledge and skills in the care of a complex disease. For these professionals, hope is always present, advanced therapies are administered within a framework of total nursing care, and palliative measures are offered when oppressive therapy is no longer appropriate.

Caring for women with cancer on an ongoing basis can be emotionally draining. It is to nurses that desperate family members and women with cancer turn with their pleas and complaints. Sometimes, nurses identify closely with the woman with cancer; having cared for her through many devastating episodes, the final loss is severe and personal. Nurses are particularly taxed when groups of people on the hospital unit or in the nurse's case load compete for attention and energies. Nurses must seek emotional support from peers, superiors, and others within and outside the hospital or clinic to regain emotional strength.

BENIGN BREAST DISEASE

The most common of the benign breast lesions, **mammary dysplasia** (fibrocystic breast disease or chronic cystic mastitis) occurs in approximately 1 in 3 premenopausal women. Ovarian hormones may be an etiologic factor because new cysts are rare after menopause. Some women experience premenstrual pain or tenderness. However, most women are asymptomatic and seek medical advice after they palpate a lump.

A simple cyst may occur, although multiple cysts of varying sizes occur bilaterally. Cysts near the skin surface may be mobile. Deeper cysts, especially aggregations of many cysts, are indistinguishable by palpation from carcinoma. *Surgical biopsy* is required to differentiate malignant disease from benign breast disease.

Therapy for mammary dysplasia ranges from simple measures, to medical management and surgery (Droegemueller et al., 1987). For some women, the pain and tenderness may be relieved with padded brassieres, analgesics, and certain dietary measures—caffeine restriction and vitamin E supplementation. Reduction in caffeine (methylxanthine) is recommended for the woman with mammary dysplasia although Lubin et al. (1985) found *no* association between caffeine ingestion and benign breast disease. Many foods and drugs contain caffeine. Many products are also now being produced that have had caffeine and other ingredients removed. People withdrawing from caffeine need to be reassured that the headache that occurs during the withdrawal phase lasts only a few days.

Occasionally, simple measures do not suffice. The most significant medical management of fibrocystic disease is the use of *danazol* (Danocrine) (see discussion of endometriosis, Chapter 41).

The total daily dosage of danazol capsules (Danocrine) for mammary dysplasia of the breast ranges from 100 mg to 400 mg given in four divided doses depending on tissue response. *Therapy should begin during menstruation,* or *appropriate tests should be performed to rule out pregnancy.* A nonhormonal method of contraception is recommended when this drug is taken at this dose, otherwise, ovulation may not be suppressed. For most women, pain and tenderness decrease significantly by the first month and are eliminated in 2 to 3 months. Usually elimination of nodularity requires 4 to 6 months of uninterrupted therapy. Regular menstrual patterns, irregular menstrual patterns, and amenorrhea each occur in approximately one third of women treated with 100 mg of danazol (Danocrine) per day. Irregular menstrual patterns and amenorrhea are seen more frequently when the dosage is higher. When the drug is discontinued, about 50% of women may show evidence of recurrence of symptoms within 1 year; in this event, treatment may be reinstated.

Surgical removal of nodules is attempted only in selected cases. In the presence of multiple nodules, the surgical approach would involve multiple incisions and tissue manipulation and not prevent the development of more nodules.

Intraductal papilloma is a rare, benign condition that develops within the terminal nipple ducts. Usually too small to be palpated, the characteristic sign is nipple discharge that is serous, serosanguinous, or bloody. After malignancy is ruled out, the affected segments of the ducts and breasts are surgically excised.

Lipoma is a common benign tumor that may resemble a malignant lesion because of its firm consistency and poor encapsulation. After biopsy confirmation of lipoma, surgical excision is the only therapy needed.

Occasionally, a blow to the breast causes a contusion that leads to fat necrosis. **Fat necrosis** is a firm, irregularly shaped mass that can cause skin retraction and thus mimic a malignancy. Usually the woman recalls no antecedent trauma.

Hypertrophy may occur. It is most often caused by hormone level fluctuations during the menstrual cycle. NOTE: This normal occurrence is often mistakenly diagnosed as mammary dysplasia.

MALIGNANT BREAST DISEASE

The United States has one of the highest rates of breast carcinoma in the world. Presently in the United States approximately 130,000 new cases are diagnosed, and approximately 41,000 deaths occur yearly from breast carcinoma. The specific risk to an American woman of developing a breast carcinoma is 1 in 10 (10%) during her lifetime. The risk for an American woman without a single risk factor is 1 in 17 (6%) (Droegemueller et al., 1987). In women ages 35 to 39 the rate of breast carcinoma is 55/100,000 women per year (Berg, 1984). The cause of breast carcinoma is poorly understood despite extensive investigation. Some risk factors that predispose the woman to or promote the induction of breast cancer have been identified. The risk factors fall into several categories: age, hormones, nutrition, demography, radiation, and previous breast disease. Genetic predisposition (family history in mother or sister), environmental carcinogens, viral agents, and radiation exposure are also considered.

The age at which a woman delivers her first child is more important as a risk factor than parity. If a woman's first term birth occurs before age 20, she has 50% less risk than a nulliparous woman. If the first term pregnancy occurs after 35, the risk is 1.5 times greater than that for women who give birth to their first baby before age 26. For many years it was believed that breast-feeding decreased a woman's risk for the future development of breast neoplasia. Subsequent studies have found that breast-feeding is neither a positive nor a negative risk factor. Findings from recent studies do *not* indicate a relationship between the use of medications such as reserpine (elevates prolactin levels), cigarette smoking, and exogenous estrogen either in oral contraceptives or given to postmenopausal women (Rosenberg and Schwingl et al., 1984; Rosenberg and Miller et al., 1984) (Chapter 41). Risk factors identify *only* 25% of women who will eventually develop breast carcinoma.

Two problems obscure a clear understanding of the risk factors of breast cancer. One is the long latent period, 15 to 25 years, before the development of clinically recognizable carcinoma. The other is the consideration both of the duration and the intensity of factors that may induce or promote cancer. Many risk factors are additive. Although there are limits in the clinical applicability of risk factors, women at increased risk should be screened at more frequent intervals.

Detection and Diagnosis. Asymptomatic women are assessed at periodic intervals to detect breast neoplasms. Early detection and diagnosis reduce mortality because the cancers are smaller in size, lesions are more localized, and there tends to be a lower percentage of positive nodes. Established methods of detection include breast self-examination (BSE), periodic physician examination, and mammography (Rudolph and McDermott, 1987).

The characteristics of growth in breast carcinoma are important for understanding screening and detection. The average breast mass doubles in volume every 100 days and doubles in diameter every 300 days. A breast carcinoma grows for 6 to 8 years before reaching a diameter of 1 cm. In slightly less than another year the carcinoma will reach 2 cm in diameter. The mean diameter of a breast mass discovered by women who perform BSE at monthly intervals is 2 cm (Droegemueller et al., 1987).

Palpation of the breast has an estimated accuracy of 65% to 75% and is considered to be the first step in the diagnostic process. BSE has the major advantages of no cost to the woman and convenience (see guidelines for client teaching, Chapter 8). Physical examination and mammography are complementary procedures to detect neoplasia.

Mammography is the single most accurate diagnostic test currently available: it is 85% accurate. However, a negative mammogram does not rule out breast carcinoma. *Open breast biopsy,* at 100% accuracy, is the definitive diagnostic test. *Needle aspiration* diagnoses a cyst with 99% accuracy. Occasionally, external bruising or ecchymosis occurs as a result of the procedure, for which the woman may need reassurance.

Transillumination, thermography, and ultrasound breast imaging are unproven as methods to detect early breast carcinoma and should be considered experimental. Research with magnetic resonance imaging is just beginning.

Diagnostic techniques and equipment used in mammography have eliminated the controversy of this test. In 1983 the American Cancer Society expanded its recommendations for mammography (Kopans, Meyer, and Sadowsky, 1984; Kopans, 1987). A baseline mammogram is recommended for all women between 35 and 40 years. From 40 to 49 years, women should have mammography at 1- to 2-year intervals. For the woman 50 years or older, an annual mammogram is recommended. Physical examination by a practitioner is recommended at 3-year intervals for women 20 to 40 years, then annually. Physical examination and mammograms are scheduled depending on individual risk factors and the finding of precursors of breast carcinoma.

New investigative serum assay, breast cancer radioimmunoassay (RIA), is being used in research for detecting and monitoring breast cancer. This development is part of the emerging technology involving monoclonal antibodies.

Treatment. The prognosis and treatment of breast malignancies are related primarily to the stage of the disease and the extent of spread to regional nodes (Fig. 44-1). The three major objectives of treating breast carcinoma are control of local disease, treatment of distant metastasis, and improved quality of life for the woman treated for the disease (Veronesi et al., 1981).

Local disease is treated by several methods. However, no difference in long-term survival rates has been documented, regardless of the extent of surgical therapy or aggressiveness of local radiotherapy (Droegemueller et al., 1987; Recht and Harris, 1987). Chemotherapy is appropriate for women with proven metastatic disease and for those at high risk for recurrent disease. Recent emphasis on conservative surgery with radiation therapy to control multiple

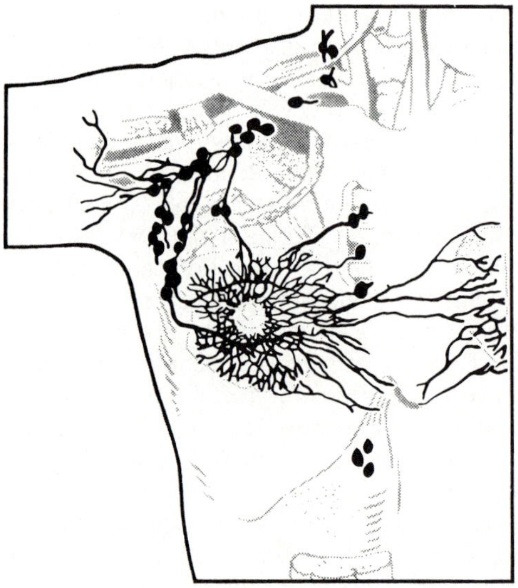

Fig. 44-1 Lymphatic spread of breast cancer.
From: A cancer source book for nurses, rev ed, New York, 1981, American Cancer Society, Inc.

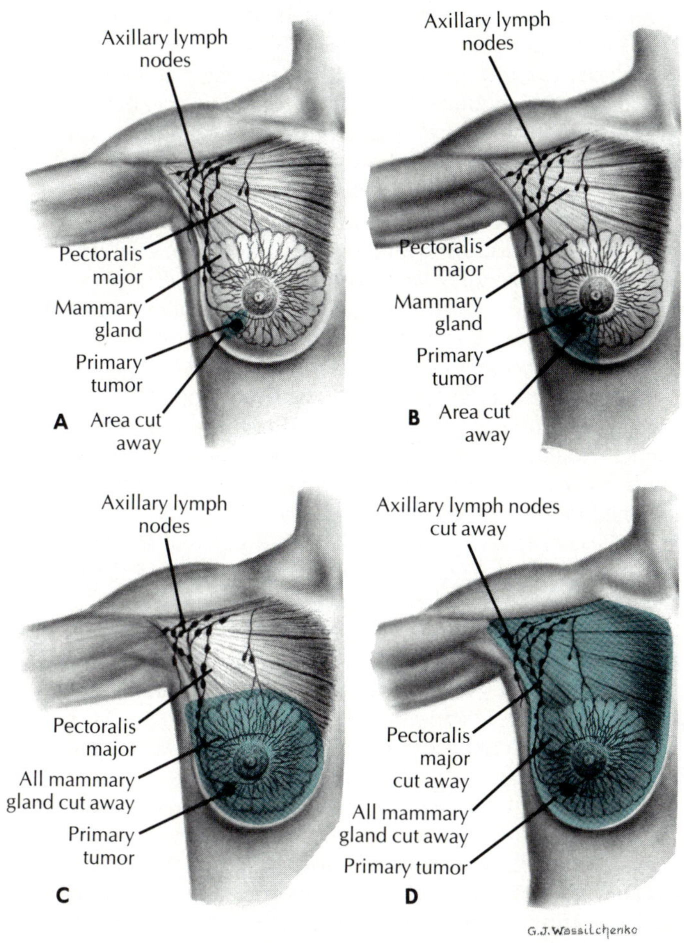

Fig. 44-2 Four ways to deal surgically with cancer of breast: **A**, lumpectomy (tylectomy), **B**, quadrectomy (segmental resection), **C**, total (simple) mastectomy, and **D**, radical mastectomy.

foci of cancer within the same breast or after simple mastectomy has improved the quality of life.

Surgical Therapy. The most conservative surgery is illustrated in Fig. 44-2, *A* and *B*. Total (simple) mastectomy (Fig. 44-2, *C*) and axillary dissection is an equivalent alternative to radical mastectomy (Fig. 44-2, *D*) for primary operable breast carcinoma. Only the mammary tissue and most of the axillary lymph nodes are removed. Preservation of the pectoral muscles leaves their function intact. Not only is the cosmetic effect better, but breast reconstruction using a plastic implant within 6 to 12 months is facilitated. The cure rate for both the radical and modified radical procedures seems to be the same.

It is important to offer every woman alternatives in treatment with complete disclosure of the advantages and risks.

Medical Therapy. Hormone therapy is used when the cancer is sensitive to estrogen or progesterone (i.e., estrogen or progesterone receptor-positive). Bilateral oophorectomy is common in a premenopausal woman; tamoxifen, an oral antiestrogen, is an alternative to oophorectomy (castration). Oral estrogens, depo-medroxyprogesterone, androgens, and danazol have also been used to treat breast carcinoma.

Combined hormonal therapy and chemotherapy may improve the cytotoxicity of chemotherapy (Levine and Lippman, 1984; Levin et al., 1988). Combinations of cytotoxic drugs are superior to a single agent. The chemotherapeutic agents chosen most often for breast cancer are cyclophosphamide, methotrexate, Adriamycin, 5-fluorouracil, and vinblastine. In addition to their antineoplastic qualities, these cytotoxins have some immunosuppressive side effects. Episodes of thrombosis can be expected to occur in women undergoing chemotherapy for breast cancer (Levine et al., 1988).

The 5-year survival of a woman whose breast carcinoma is believed to be localized to the breast with negative axillary nodes is 85%; when axillary nodes are positive, 5-year survival is 53%. Chemotherapy substantially prolongs survival (Henderson, 1988).

CANCER OF THE CORPUS UTERI

After breast and colorectal malignancy, *endometrial carcinoma* is third in frequency. Uterine adenocarcinoma originates from epithelial tissues of the endometrium. This condition usually affects mature women with a peak incidence between 50 and 64 years of age. Overall, about 1 woman in 100 will develop this disease during her lifetime. Carcinoma originating from other histologic components of the uterus is rare (5%), and prognosis is poor.

Factors that increase the risk for developing endometrial carcinoma are numerous. Three of the most important factors are obesity, nulliparity, and menopause over the age of 52 years. Unapposed estrogen stimulation from medications or from polycystic ovary syndrome (Stein-Leventhal syndrome) and feminizing ovarian tumors are also associated with increased risk. The incidence of endometrial cancer among white women is approximately twice the rate in black women (Drogemueller et al., 1987). However, white women have a higher survival rate (Christopherson, Connelly, and Alberhasky, 1983). Diabetes increases the risk by 2.8%.

Detection and Diagnosis. The cardinal sign of endometrial cancer is abnormal uterine bleeding (e.g., postmenopausal bleeding, premenopausal recurrent metrorrhagia). Thirty percent of postmenopausal bleeding is caused by carcinoma. After metastases to the vagina, a mucosanguineous discharge may be seen. Cervical polyps, usually a benign condition, may be the cause of bleeding (see p. 1139).

Histologic examination is used for diagnosis. *Papanicolaou test* of cellular material obtained by aspiration of the endocervix will identify two thirds of cases. The woman is instructed not to douche during the 24 hours preceding the tests. The *Gravlee Jet Washer* is an instrument used for diagnostic screening for uterine cancer. Uterine cells are collected by washing the uterine cavity with normal saline and collecting the washed material in a reservoir attached to the jet. This method is reserved primarily for women over 35. Some uterine cramping may occur during the procedure. *Fractional curettage* yields the most accurate results. Fractional curettage involves scraping of the endocervix and endometrium for histologic evaluation to determine the grade of neoplasm and its stage (extent). Perforation of the uterus is a possible complication. *Endometrial biopsy* will identify about 90% to 92% of cases.

Acceptable miscellaneous methods include palpation, inspection of uterus (laparoscopy) and vagina, colposcopy, hysteroscopy, cystoscopy, intravenous pyelogram (IVP [intravenous urography]), proctosigmoidoscopy, barium enema, bone and liver scans, arteriography, venography, lymphangiography, and biopsy of areas suspected to have been invaded.

Adenocarcinoma spreads by several routes. It may spread by direct extension along endometrium into cervical canal or through myometrium to the serosa and into the peritoneal cavity. It may pass through uterine tubes to the ovaries, broad ligaments, and peritoneum. Spread may also occur via the blood stream and/or lymphatics.

Treatment. For adenocarcinoma of the endometrium, in its early stages, total abdominal hysterectomy (TAH) and bilateral salpingo-oophorectomy (BSO) is the usual treatment of choice. The woman who is given the diagnosis and a thorough explanation of the proposed surgery in a caring and personalized manner is more likely to experience an uncomplicated recovery physically and emotionally.

For more extensive disease, radiotherapy, steroid hormones, and chemotherapy are used singly or in combination or as adjunctive therapy to surgery. These therapies are discussed in greater detail later in this chapter.

CANCER OF THE CERVIX UTERI

The accessible location of the cervix and upper vagina make it possible to investigate premalignant lesions of these structures. This process has resulted in improved detection and treatment. Cytology to identify neoplasia and use of the colposcope as an instrument to localize the site of change and allow directed biopsy have contributed to improvement of the management of these disorders. The squamocolumnar junction is an important landmark where neoplastic change occurs in the cervix (Fig. 6-13).

There are several commonalities among women who develop cervical carcinoma, the second most common malignancy of the reproductive tract (Cashavelly, 1987; Lovejoy, 1987). Women are generally between 40 and 45 years of age. They are more likely to be from lower socioeconomic groups. The risk for cervical cancer is increased in women who experience first intercourse at an early age (18 years or less), experience frequent coitus, and have multiple sex partners. Males with multiple sex partners also increase the risk of neoplasia for a female sex partner. Cigarette smoking appears to increase the risk of cervical neoplasia (Droegemueller et al., 1987). Typically women report a history of cervical infections. Infections most commonly linked to subsequent cervical carcinoma are caused by herpes simplex virus II, human papilloma virus types 16, 18, and 31, and perhaps cytomegalovirus. These viruses alter the deoxyribonucleic acid (DNA) of nuclei of immature cervical cells. The addition of semen (sperm) from many different partners promotes the initiation of a process that ends in dysplasia; years later, carcinoma results.

Some women have been exposed to *diethylstilbestrol* (DES) in utero. Administration of DES or another nonsteroidal estrogen to a pregnant woman may be followed by developmental or functional genital problems in both female and male progeny (Fig. 6-2). The abnormalities are rare, when one considers the estimate that about 500,000 pregnant women received DES between 1940 and 1970. Single or multiple abnormalities may be noted. Some abnormalities develop or are recognized after puberty. Curiously, most individuals who were exposed prenatally appear to have been unaffected. Hence, an association rather than an actual cause-and-effect relationship is likely and a trigger factor or factors are being sought.

In DES-exposed girls the following developmental or functional disorders have been described: circumferential vaginal ridges; cervical deformity, for example, "cock's comb" cervix, hooding, clefts, pseudopolyps; hypoplastic or T-shaped uterus; constricting bands within the uterus; tubal anomalies; vaginal or cervical adenosis, dysplasia, or cervical incompetence. There appears to be an increased frequency of oligomenorrhea and a lower incidence of pregnancy in these women also. Most critical is the assessment that about 1 out of 1000 women exposed to DES prenatally develop vaginal or cervical **clear-cell adenocarcinoma**, usually during adolescence.

Approximately 90% of cervical malignancies are squamous cell carcinomas; 10% are adenocarcinomas.

In DES-exposed males the most common gross lesions reported are epididymal cysts, hypotrophic testes, or testicular capsular thickening. In addition, sperm analyses have revealed low volume of ejaculate, oligospermia, diminished sperm density, and the lower motile sperm count per milliliter. No equivalent of female clear-cell carcinoma or increase in male genitourinary cancer has been noted, however.

Detection and Diagnosis. A thorough health history identifies the woman at increased risk for cervical cancer. Physical examination, enhanced by colposcopic techniques, reveals dysplasia.

Papanicolaou Test. Papanicolaou tests detect about 90% of early cervical neoplasia. Early detection and treatment of preinvasive neoplasia is responsible for reducing deaths from this cause by 50% (Droegemueller et al., 1987). However, 2 out of 5 women do not have routine Papanicolaou tests. *For the woman at average risk, a Papanicolaou test is recommended once every 3 years after two initial negative tests 1 year apart* (American Cancer Society, 1984).

Papanicolaou test results in the past have been recorded in one of five categories. Since some laboratories still use these categories they are presented here.

Class I	No abnormal cells present
Class II	Atypical cells are identified; inflammation must be ruled out
Class III	Suspicious abnormal cells present
Class IV	Malignant cells present—carcinoma in situ
Class V	Malignant cells present—invasive cancer

Current practice utilizes a descriptive classification. The descriptive terminology is as follows:

Normal
Metaplasia

Inflammation
Minimal atypia—koilocytosis
Mild dysplasia
Moderate dysplasia
Severe dysplasia—carcinoma in situ
Invasive carcinoma

Reexamination is warranted following treatment for infection. Additional diagnostic procedures (e.g., biopsy) are advised as necessary.

Biopsy. The value of the cervical Papanicolaou cytologic smear is not in diagnosis, but in screening; diagnosis rests with a *tissue biopsy.* Pathologic areas are identified for biopsy by colposcopic inspection in 85% of cases. If colposcopy is unavailable, abnormal areas may be identified by staining the cervix with an iodine solution, for example, Lugol's (strong iodine) or Schiller's (potassium iodide 2 g, iodine 1 g, and water 3000 ml).

Cervical intraepithelial abnormalities range from simple dysplasia to carcinoma in situ. Three categories of cervical intraepithelial neoplasia (CIN) are recognized:

CIN I Mild dysplasia
CIN II Moderate dysplasia
CIN III Severe dysplasia, and carcinoma in situ

Cervical polyps are pedunculated (footed) tumors that usually originate from the lining of the cervical canal, but may arise from the external cervical mucosa as well. Usually these reddish or purplish growths occur singly and remain relatively small. Occasionally, they may grow so long that they will protrude from the vagina. Polyps are often asymptomatic and are found on routine examination. Sometimes they are the cause of intermenstrual bleeding, bleeding after coitus, or bleeding while straining at stool. Biopsy confirms their benign nature. These growths can be removed by tying them off and allowing them to necrose and slough away. Rarely they are malignant.

Cervical Conization. Histologic study of tissue obtained by cervical conization (Fig 44-3) or amputation assists in the staging of cervical carcinoma. *Minimal* cervical dysplasia refers to abnormal cellular proliferation in the lower one third of the epithelium; this dysplasia tends to be self-limiting and generally regresses to normal. *Severe* cervical dysplasia involves the lower two thirds of the epithelium and often progresses to carcinoma in situ. *Carcinoma in situ* (CIS) is diagnosed when the full thickness of epithelium shows abnormal cells. *Invasive carcinoma* is the diagnosis when abnormal cells penetrate the basement membrane and invade the stroma. Invasive carcinoma spreads via the lymphatics to distant tissues and by direct extension to surrounding structures.

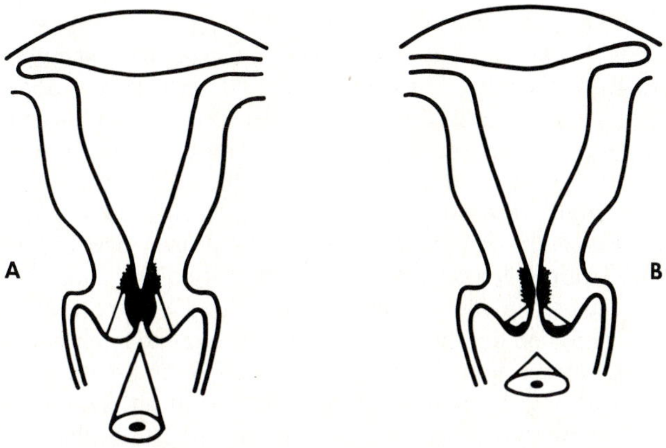

Fig. 44-3 **A**, Cone biopsy for endocervical disease. Limits of lesion were not seen colposcopically. **B**, Cone biopsy for CIN of the exocervix. Limits of lesion were identified colposcopically.
From DiSaia, PJ, and Creasman, WT: Clinical gynecologic oncology, ed 3, St Louis, 1989, The CV Mosby Co.

Fractional Curettage. Out-of-hospital *cervical punch biopsy* and *endocervical curettage* accurately identify about 90% of cases. In-hospital *cold knife cone biopsy* and *fractional curettage* with anesthesia may be necessary if results from other methods are inconclusive.

There are two advantages to a cone biopsy. It can be used (1) to establish the diagnosis and (2) to effect a cure. If carcinoma in situ is diagnosed, and if the woman wishes to retain her childbearing capacity, conization removes the abnormal tissue; further treatment is unnecessary. The woman is monitored with Papanicolaou tests every 3 months to ensure that all abnormal tissue has been removed and that there is no recurrence.

Ultrasound. *Ultrasonography* contributes to the recognition, staging, and assessment of recurrence in carcinoma of the uterus, ovary, and cervix (Droegemueller et al., 1987). Ascites is easily recognized with ultrasound. For a discussion of ultrasound, see Chapter 27.

Treatment For Preinvasive Conditions

Cryosurgery. Cryosurgery (*cryo-*, a combining form meaning cold, freezing) is an out-of-hospital procedure that requires no analgesia or anesthesia. Cryosurgery is scheduled within 1 week after cessation of last menstrual period to avoid treating a woman with an early pregnancy. The preferred refrigerant is nitrous oxide. The largest speculum tolerable to the woman is used to permit the best visualization and to keep the vaginal walls out of the way. All mucus and cellular debris is removed from the vagina and cervix with cotton balls soaked in 3% acetic acid solution. The probe tip freezes the abnormal tissue and a small amount of surrounding normal tissue. The frozen tissue becomes necrotic and sloughes off in a few days.

Posttreatment side effects are usually few and not of a serious nature. The profuse watery discharge that persists for 2 to 4 weeks is usually viewed only as a nuisance. Follow-up examination and Papanicolaou test is scheduled in 4 months. Because repair may still be in progress the finding of "abnormal" cells should be reassessed at 6 months. Persistent abnormal cells require reevaluation and plans are made for repeat cryosurgery or other therapy. Rarely, spotting or cervical stenosis are complications.

Endocervical cells seem to regenerate, leaving a normal cervical canal in most instances. Surveillance with frequent Papanicolaou tests and colposcopic examination must continue indefinitely after this type of conservative therapy.

Laser* Surgery. The carbon dioxide (CO_2) laser is currently in clinical use. Its electrical discharge, produced

**Laser*, *l*ight *a*mplification by *s*timulated *e*mission of *r*adiation.

from a mixture of carbon dioxide, nitrogen, and helium, gives rise to a continuous invisible infrared beam. The CO_2 laser has been used in neurosurgery, for debridement of third-degree burns, and to control bleeding ulcers. It may replace cryosurgery and cauterization for many gynecologic conditions. Unlike healing after cryosurgery, cervixes treated with CO_2 laser show epithelial regrowth beginning by 2 days. Cervixes are reepithelialized within 3 weeks, with healing complete by 6 weeks. The original architecture of the cervix is preserved and the squamocolumnar junction remains visible. For treatment of the cervix (relatively insensitive tissue), the woman may need no anesthesia. Some women complain of a burning or cramping sensation that is tolerable for most women.

The treated vulva and vagina also heal rapidly. Vulvar healing is painful however, especially during urination. Pain intensifies for about 3 to 4 days postoperatively and usually disappears by 2 weeks. Sitz baths, whirlpool baths, soaking, and local anesthetic/antibiotic creams bring relief from discomfort and aid healing. A squeeze bottle can be used to spray water over the perineum *during* urination to decrease discomfort. Also, the woman can urinate through the cardboard tube from toilet tissue held up around the meatus and in this way keep the urine off the perineum. Hair dryers are used to dry the area.

Recurrence rates after laser surgery are lower than with cryosurgery. The procedure has two disadvantages: (1) for tissue other than the cervix, it is too painful to be done without analgesia or anesthesia; and, (2) the procedure takes longer.

The CO_2 laser may be used for several lesions on the cervix: CIN, chronic cervicitis, condylomata, cysts, hemangiomas, polyps; and to relieve stenosis. The following lesions in the vagina may be treated with the laser: adenosis, condylomata, DES lesions, endometriosis, granuloma, herpesvirus infection, and vaginal intraepithelial neoplasia (VAIN). A vaginal speculum designed for laser therapy is seen in Fig. 44-4. The vulva may be treated for the following: benign nevi, carbuncles, condylomata, dystrophy, hemangioma, herpesvirus infection, molluscum contagiosum, and vulvar intraepithelial neoplasia (VIN).

The CO_2 laser may also be used for internal lesions during hysteroscopy and laparoscopy and for infertility surgery (lysis of adhesions and endometriosis), among others.

Cervical Conization. The extent of epithelial involvement is determined on the ectocervix and clearly delimited by colposcopy or Schiller's staining. The incision is made to include all the abnormal and some normal surrounding tissue (Fig. 44-3). Bleeding can be lessened by a prior injection of a dilute solution of phenylephrine (Neo-Synephrine) along the proposed incision line. Hemorrhage, uterine perforations, and anesthesia present immediate risks; rare complications include delayed bleeding, cervical stenosis, cervical incompetence, or impaired fertility.

To retain optimum fertility, cryosurgery, laser surgery, or local excision is indicated. If multiple lesions are present, therapeutic conization is preferred. Once a woman has had carcinoma in situ, she will always be at greater risk and needs to be monitored carefully. Removal of the cervix or uterus continues to be the definitive therapy in women who do not wish to retain their reproductive capacity.

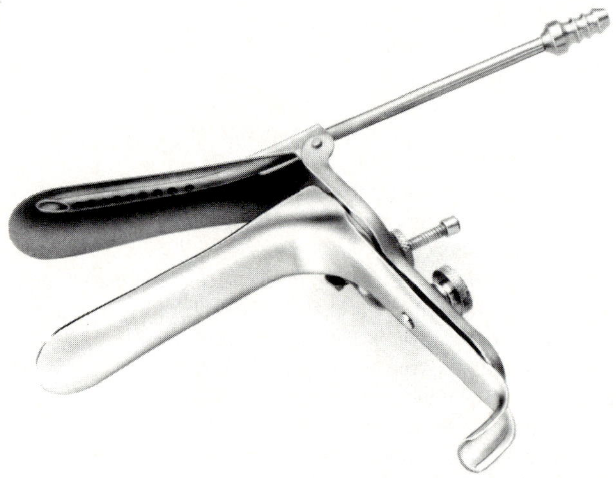

Fig. 44-4 Smoke caused by laser-induced tissue vaporization can be drawn out of the vagina with an instrument such as the Smoke Removal Tube (SRT), a malleable stainless steel tube permanently fixed to the speculum blade. The SRT is open at the distal end and has a number of holes along the length of the tube for gathering the smoke. Its proximal end has a standard hose fitting for connection to a suction machine.
Courtesy Amko Manufacturing Co, Bellmawr, NJ.

Treatment For Invasive Conditions

Radiotherapy. Radiation may be delivered by radium applications to the cervix followed by external radiation therapy that includes lymphatics of the pelvic side wall. Major complications include radiation cystitis and proctitis and rectovaginal and vesicovaginal fistula formation (Fig 41-9).

The use of hydroxyurea as a radiosensitizer may improve survival for those treated for cervical carcinoma with radiation (Piver, 1984). In preparation for radiotherapy, the woman needs to be in good nutritional status and maintained with a high protein-vitamin and high caloric diet. Anemia, if present, should be corrected before the initiation of radiotherapy.

External irradiation and intracavity radium therapy is used in various combinations for the best results, and tailored to each woman and her particular lesion. Megavoltage machines such as cobalt, linear accelerators, and the betatron have the distinct advantage of providing a more homogeneous dose to the pelvis. The hard, short rays of megavoltage pass through the skin without much absorption by the skin and therefore cause little dermal injury.

Radium is the isotope that has traditionally been used in the treatment of cancer of the cervix; cesium and cobalt have been added to therapy regimens. There are three intracavity techniques using specially designed applicators (Fig 44-5) and the fourth technique involves the application of radium in the form of needles directly into the tumor.

In advanced carcinoma of the cervix, conventional intracavitary applicators are not applicable. Interstitial therapy employs a template to guide the insertion of a group of 18-gauge hollow steel needles into the lesion transperineally (Fig 44-6). After the needles are placed, the iridium wires are inserted when the woman is returned to her hospital room.

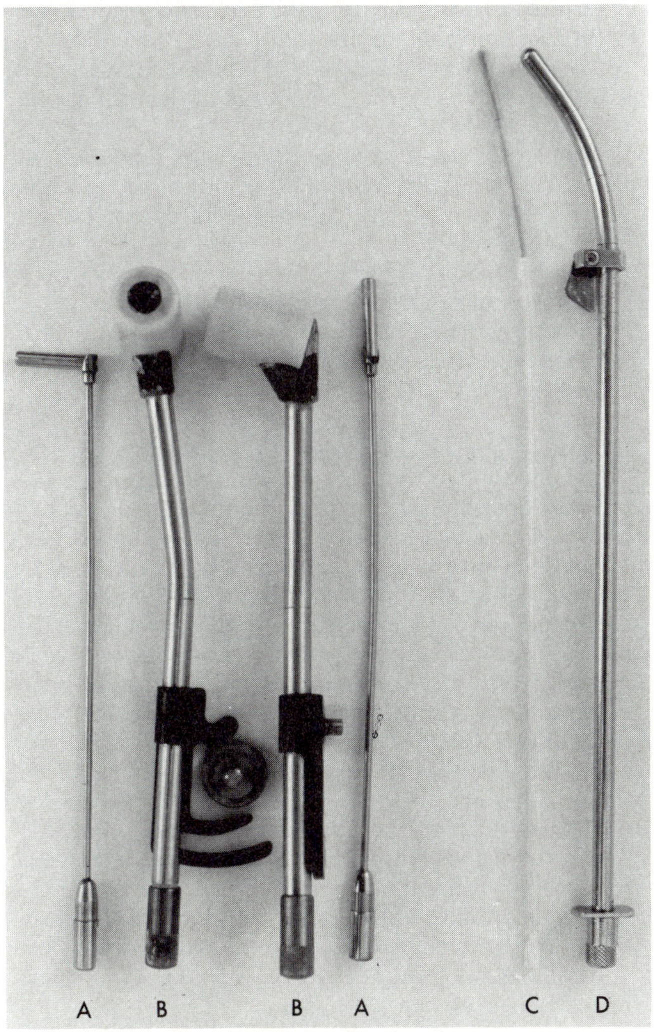

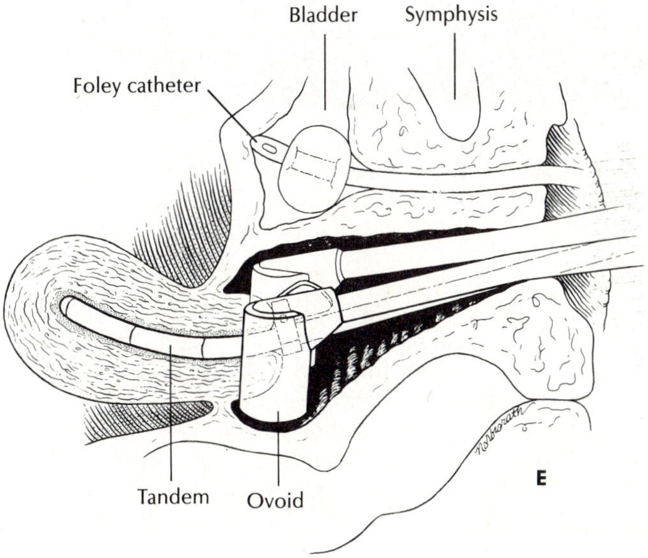

Fig. 44-5 Intracavitary implant. **A**, Inserts for colpostats to insert radium or cesium. **B**, Colpostats. **C**, Teflon tubing to insert radium or cesium into tandem. **D**, Tandem. **E**, Placement of tandem and colpostats before vaginal packing.

From Phipps, WJ, et al, editors: Medical-surgical nursing: concepts and clinical practice, ed 3, St Louis, 1987, The CV Mosby Co.

A

B

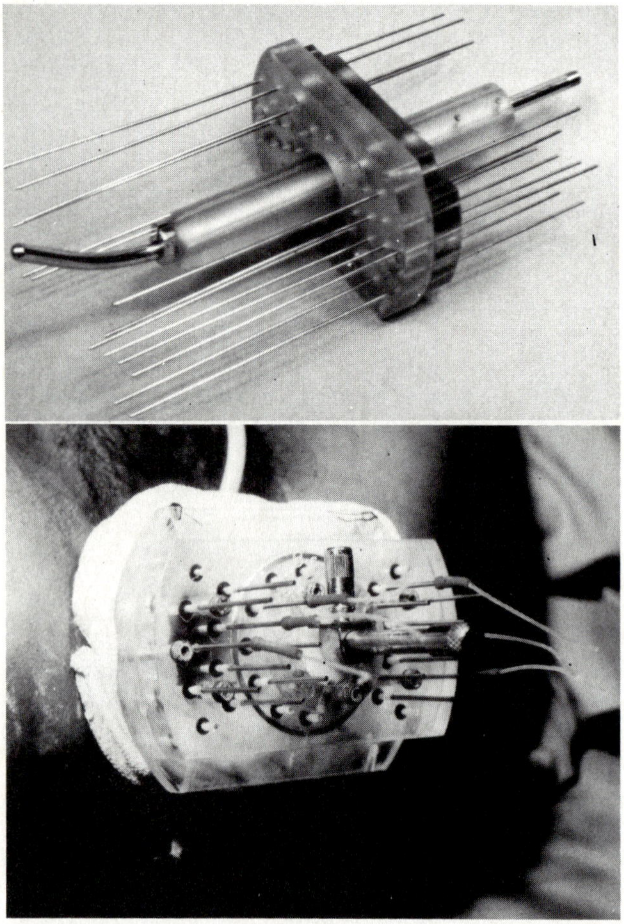

Fig. 44-6 **A**, Interstitial-intracavitary implant (Syed/Neblett applicator). **B**, Implant procedure completed.
From DiSaia, PJ, and Creasman, WT: Clinical gynecologic oncology, ed 3, St Louis, 1987, The CV Mosby Co.

Complications of Radiation Therapy. Morbidity as a direct result from properly conducted therapy is usually minimal. Some of the morbidity seen may be caused by the uncontrolled tumor and not to the therapy. Acute treatment complications occurring during or shortly following therapy, include irritation of the rectum, small bowel, and bladder, reactions in the skin folds, and mild bone marrow suppression. Dysuria and frequency may occur. Late irradiation sequelae including damage to the rectum and bladder are less common. Symptoms of radiation proctitis may follow as asymptomatic interval of many months to years after treatment. The symptoms of small bowel injury (postprandial crampy abdominal pain and anorexia) should not be confused with recurrence of the tumor; diversion surgery yields good results.

Radical Hysterectomy. In early stages, comparable survival rates are obtained by both radiotherapy and surgery. Radiotherapy is applicable to virtually all clients; radical surgery excludes certain medically inoperable clients. Surgery may be the method of choice for those women with stage I and stage IIA disease for whom preservation of ovarian function is desired. Complications of less than 1% can be expected postoperatively. Surgery is necessary when radiation is contraindicated, for example, in the presence of pelvic inflammatory disease (PID) or inflammatory disease of the bowel, concurrent pregnancy, and client preference. Some lesions are not radiosensitive.

With modern techniques of surgery, anesthesia, antibiotics, and electrolyte balance, morbidity after radical hysterectomy is between 1% and 5%. Radical hysterectomy involves removal of the uterus, tubes, ovaries, upper third of the vagina, entire uterosacral and uterovesicle ligaments, and all of the parametrium on each side, along with pelvic node dissection encompassing the four major pelvic lymph node chains: ureteral, obturator, hypogastric, and iliac. Dissection serves to preserve the bladder, rectum, and ureters while removing as much of the remaining tissue of the pelvis as is feasible.

Women with positive pelvic nodes usually receive postoperative whole-pelvis irradiation, although there is no evidence that it alters the incidence of recurrence in the pelvic area. However, there does seem to be a lesser incidence of distant metastases in the irradiated group.

Major complications following radical hysterectomy are formation of ureteral fistulas and lymphocysts, pelvic infection, and hemorrhage; the incidence of complications is decreasing steadily.

Recurrent and Advanced Carcinoma of the Cervix

Approximately 1 of 3 women with invasive cervical cancer will have recurrent or persistent disease after therapy; prognosis is discouraging with a survival rate of between 10% and 15% for 1 year. Irradiation of mestastatic areas is commonly successful in providing local control and symptomatic relief; irradiation for recurrent disease is usually not considered. Chemotherapy has not proved to be beneficial in most cases for a variety of reasons (e.g., the previously irradiated area is fibrotic and avascular, thus precluding a high blood level and tissue concentrations of the drug, and many drugs are nephrotoxic and require an unobstructed ureter, not often seen in these clients). If drugs are tried, mitomycin, vincristine, and bleomycin may be used; or adriamycin used in conjunction with cyclophosphamide and 5-fluorouracil. Squamous cell carcinoma (constituting most of cervical cancers) has generally been one of the histologic varieties least responsive to most chemotherapeutic agents.

CANCER OF THE UTERINE TUBES

Primary carcinoma of the uterine tube (usually the distal one third) is rare with a peak incidence between the ages of 50 and 60. The cause is unknown. Vague abdominal discomfort (from pressure on the bladder or rectum) and an enlarging unilateral pelvic mass or ascites are often misdiagnosed as ovarian carcinoma. Diagnosis of cancer of the uterine tubes follows surgery. Early in the disease, radiation is used. Later, total abdominal hysterectomy, bilateral salpingo-oophorectomy, and omentectomy is followed by chemotherapy.

CANCER OF THE VAGINA

Vaginal carcinomas account for only 1% of gynecologic malignancy, with a peak incidence between the ages of 45 to 65. Almost all (95%) are squamous cell carcinomas; 5% are primary and secondary adenocarcinomas, secondary squamous cell carcinomas (older women), clear cell adenocarcinomas (young women, especially following intrauterine exposure to DES [p. 1138]), and sarcoma botryoides (embryonal rhabdomyosarcoma) in infants and children. The lesion, usually seen in the upper one third of the vagina, often extends into the bladder and rectum.

Bleeding after coitus or examination, dyspareunia, and watery discharge are characteristic of vaginal cancer. Bladder involvement results in urinary frequency or urgency; rectal extension causes painful defecation.

Papanicolaou test and biopsy of Schiller stained areas disclose the diagnosis.

Therapy for vaginal cancer is directed by the extent of the lesion and the age and condition of the female; radical hysterectomy and removal of the upper vagina with dissection of the pelvic nodes, or radium and external radiation. The 5-year survival rate is less than one in three women who develop this disease.

CANCER OF THE OVARY

Ovarian carcinomas comprise 18% of gynecologic malignancies. The peak incidence is found in women in their 30s. The cause is unknown.

Ovarian cancer has been called a silent disease because early warning symptoms that would send a woman to her physician are absent (e.g., no bleeding or other discharge and no pain). Vague lower abdominal discomfort and mild digestive complaints are the early symptoms for some. An ovary enlarged to 5 cm or more found during routine examination requires careful diagnostic work-up. The accompanying increase in abdominal girth (caused by ovarian enlargement or ascites) is usually attributed to an increase in weight, or a 'shift in weight' that is seen commonly in women entering their middle years. Pelvic pain, anemia, and cachexia are late findings. (Ovarian cancer is often found in an advanced stage so that prognosis is poor.)

The physical signs and symptoms described above, a positive Papanicolaou test of vaginal, pleural, or peritoneal fluids, and lung and bone scans establish the diagnosis. Clinical staging gives direction to treatment and prognosis (Droegemueller et al., 1987; Phipps; Long, Woods, 1987).

Therapeutic management of ovarian carcinoma is influenced adversely by the many histologic types of malignancy, late identification, commonly seen widespread metastases, involvement of both ovaries, and direct extension to the uterus and adjacent structures. Surgical removal of as much of the tumor as possible is the first step in therapy. This may involve just the removal of one ovary and tube or radical excision of uterus, ovaries, tubes, and omentum. Chemotherapy follows surgery. Alkylating agents of choice are cyclophosphamide, melphalan, thiotepa, and chlorambucil. Ovarian malignancy is highly sensitive to several chemotherapeutic agents.

When metastasis is localized, an experimental chemotherapeutic approach has been initiated. Antineoplastic drugs (e.g., *cis*-platinum and adriamycin) or nonspecific immunostimulant agents (e.g., interferon) are administered into the peritoneal cavity. Abdominal pain or discomfort, the major problem during the period of treatment, may arise from catheter-caused peritoneal irritation, drug-induced chemical peritonitis, or peritonitis from infection. Immunostimulants often provoke a painful inflammatory response.

CANCER OF THE VULVA

Vulvar carcinoma accounts for 3% to 4% of all gynecologic malignancies and occurs most often in women after menopause. Although easily visible, many women wait up to 3 years before seeking medical attention. About 90% of lesions are squamous cell carcinoma; 4%, basal cell carcinoma; 6%, Paget's disease, adenocarcinoma of Bartholin's glands, fibrosarcoma, and melanoma. Squamous cell carcinoma in situ (CIS) today is diagnosed in women between 20 and 40 years of age. Age at diagnosis of CIS 15 to 20 years ago was between 50 and 60. This shift may presage a downward shift in the mean age of occurrence (Richart, 1988).

Each woman is screened for a history of sexually transmitted diseases (STDs). There may be a relationship between infections with herpes simplex virus and human papilloma viruses types 16, 18, and 31 and perhaps 6 and 11.

The vulvar lesion is usually asymptomatic until it is 1 to 2 cm in diameter. CIS is usually pruritic (itchy). Necrosis and infection of the lesion result in ulceration with bleeding or watery discharge.

Vulvar intraepithelial neoplasms are usually multifocal. Initially, growth is superficial but later extends into the urethra, vagina, and anus. In approximately 50% of late cases, superficial inguinal and femoral lymph nodes become involved.

Simple biopsy with histologic evaluation reveals the diagnosis. The areas of pathology are identified by staining the vulva with toluidine blue (1%), allowing an absorption time of 3 to 5 minutes, then washing with acetic acid (2% to 3%); abnormal tissue retains the dye. Biopsy is necessary to rule out such conditions as STD (e.g., chancroid, granuloma inguinale, syphilis), basal cell carcinoma, and CIS. In situ malignancies are initially small, red, white, or pigmented friable papules. In Paget's disease, the lesions are red, moist, and elevated. Melanomas appear as bluish-black, pigmented, or papillary lesions. Melanomas metastasize through the blood stream and lymphatics.

Therapy of squamous cell carcinoma depends on the size of the vulvar lesion. The more extensive the lesion, the greater the involvement of the lymph nodes. Radical vulvectomy with dissection of the superficial and femoral nodes is often required for this malignancy. If deep pelvic nodes are involved, prognosis for 5-year survival is dismal. Lymphedema is a postoperative problem for about a year. If the lesion is inoperable, radium needle implants may be the treatment of choice. *Basal cell carcinoma* of the vulva is treated with local excision. *Paget's disease* requires total vulvectomy. Surgical incision for CIS varies with the extent of the lesion and the woman's age, (e.g., local excision to total vulvectomy). Split-thickness skin grafts and rotational and myocutaneous flaps help maintain anatomy and functional integrity of the perianal area after radical surgery for vulvar cancer (Lacey and Stern, 1988).

Assessment

Baseline data is obtained through a health history, physical examination, and laboratory tests (Chapter 8). Many complex changes are involved related to the disease process and its management. These changes affect the woman's ability to meet her physiologic, psychologic, and social health needs.

The woman may initially exhibit one of the seven warning signs of cancer. Recall of the signs is aided by the use of the acronym, CAUTION:

Change in bowel and bladder habits
A sore that does not heal
Unusual bleeding or discharge
Thickening or a lump in the breast or elsewhere
Indigestion or difficulty in swallowing
Obvious change in a wart or mole
Nagging cough or hoarseness

The findings of the physical examination assist in differentiating between a benign and a malignant neoplasm. In general, the difference can be discerned by comparison of characteristics (Phipps, Long, and Woods, 1987):

Benign	*Malignant*
Limited growth potential	May proliferate rapidly or grow slowly
Localized	Spreads (metastasizes) throughout the body
Fibrous capsule	No enclosing capsule
Rarely recurs after removal	May recur even after treatment
Usually regular in shape	Irregular shape with poorly defined border
Cells similar to cell of parent tissue (well differentiated)	Cells much different from parent cells (poorly differentiated)
Expansive growth	Infiltrative growth

The woman is assessed for her mode of coping (e.g., does she function best by seeking information, knowing the prognosis) (Miller and Powers, 1988). What are her internal and external resources. What are her responses and the family's reactions (pp. 1133 to 1135).

Nursing Diagnoses

Following are examples of nursing diagnoses relevant to women experiencing dysplasia and neoplasia.

- Knowledge deficit related to
  - Disease process, management, prognosis, and self-care activities
- Ineffective individual and family coping related to
  - The condition
- Pain related to
  - The disease or its therapy
- Impaired physical mobility, altered sexuality patterns, body image disturbance, altered role performance, altered nutrition: less than body requirements related to
  - The disease process, its management, and prognosis
- Potential for spiritual distress related to
  - The threat of bodily mutilation, pain, and death

Planning

Women and their families have the right to participate in planning for care. Depending on their coping styles when facing difficult situations, women and their families vary in their desired degree of privacy, participation, and communication. Their coping styles must be respected and considered in their care plan. Where possible, goals are mutually derived. Goals are stated in clientcentered terms.

Goals*

1. Primary prevention of cancer is accomplished through healthful practices that avoid exposure to known carcinogenic agents
2. Secondary prevention of cancer is achieved through participation in programs for early detection and prompt initiation of therapy when cancer is in its earliest stages and a cure is more likely
3. Case finding occurs through astute assessment by health care providers
4. Anxieties, fears, and discomfort are minimized during the diagnostic period
5. After the diagnosis of cancer is confirmed, the woman receives appropriate assistance with reactions of loss and grief and with preparation for therapy and posttherapy recovery
6. The woman is maintained in optimum psychologic and physical condition before, during, and after therapy
7. Therapy results in cure, and permanent disability is avoided or minimal
8. Rehabilitation is optimized (e.g., activities of daily living, intrapersonal and interpersonal relationship, career goals, sexuality and sexual expression) within the context of the surgical alteration
9. Should recurrence occur, it is detected and treated expeditiously.
10. If the disease advances, the woman and her family are assisted toward optimum health during the dying process

Implementation

Preventive Measures. Teaching for health is an important role of the nurse. Good *nutrition* is imperative to support the function of the immune system. The obese woman

*Based on recommendations of the American Cancer Society: A cancer sourcebook for nurses, rev ed, New York, 1981, The Society.

can be counseled for weight reduction or referred to a weight-reduction program. The woman who abuses alcohol requires nutritional support to counter the associated deficiencies (Chapter 34), and the woman who smokes requires referral to a quit-smoking program such as Fresh Start sponsored by the American Cancer Society. All females are advised to delay sexual activity until after cervical and vaginal anatomic and physiologic maturity is achieved (about 18 years). The risk of adverse sequelae to premature sexual activity is somewhat reduced if the female has only one male partner who himself has no other sexual partner. Sexual partners need to be able and willing to identify STDs promptly and receive treatment immediately. Exposure to environmental hazards should be avoided (Chapter 43). Through these activities, risk factors for breast and gynecologic neoplasia are reduced.

Teaching and encouraging self-care is part of every care plan. BSE and physical examination by a practitioner that includes a Papanicolaou smear are discussed in Chapter 4. For various reasons, some women do not participate in screening programs (Leathar and Roberts, 1985; Williams, Edwards, and Hane, 1987). Nurses must have the ability to suspend their own beliefs and refrain from even hinting that these women are remiss. Condemnation from the nurse may compound her guilt or other negative feelings. These negative responses are stressors that weaken the immune system. The woman's collaboration in her own care could be compromised. Women and their families can be best served through sensitivity and respect.

Each woman needs to tune into her own natural body rhythms and body characteristics so that changes can be noted and reported promptly. Each woman should know her complete family history. Women who are placing their children for adoption should compile a pertinent health history to accompany the records of these children.

Preventive measures are also appropriate with women undergoing therapy or during the process of dying. Teaching self-care and relaxation and being a caring, supportive listener may help a woman and her family cope in a manner that helps them come to terms with their situation (Mast, Meyers, and Urbanski, 1987a, b, c; Hickey, 1986; Larson, 1986; Hauck, 1986; Bluhm, 1987; Stetz, 1987; Miller and Powers, 1988).

Curative Measures. Curative measures can be physiologic, anatomic, psychologic, or social. People need to have their existing coping skills supported or receive support if their coping ability is inadequate to meet their needs. Since each woman's and her family's reactions to cancer and its diagnosis and management are unique, there is no simple formula for care. One mode of coping is information seeking. Acquiring information is used to master new situations by problem-solving and by controlling or reducing emotional stress (Hopkins, 1986). Information is beneficial for those who cope this way typically, but will increase the anxiety for those who avoid information (Derdiarian, 1987). The diagnosis of cancer generally has adverse effects on spousal relationships. The nurse can facilitate open communication about their fears, doubts, and feelings. Grief responses, guilt, sense of isolation, sexual dysfunction, and fantasies of death and dying all require attention from caregivers (Chapter 28).

Curative measures accompany the discussion of each condition. The skills of many members of the health team are required. Clear, concise communication of ideas about care and planned interventions is essential for coordination, continuity, and integration of care (Phipps, Long, and Woods, 1987). The social worker, physical and occupational therapists, clergy, and psychologist may all be needed to contribute to the well-being of the woman and her family.

The diagnostic and therapeutic procedures must be described in simple terms to women and their families. Complex equipment and injections or ingestion of various substances are involved in diagnosis and care. The nurse's ability to give factual information clearly and concisely often help the woman cope with anxiety. Several conditions and their management are discussed in the following section.

External Radiotherapy

Pretreatment Care. The radiologist will meet with the woman to discuss the treatment with her and to answer her questions, and the area to be treated will be indicated with indelible ink.

The woman's anxiety may be such that she may not be able to understand all that she hears or sees so that the nurse may need to assess for and fill in (or alert the physician or radiologist to fill in) gaps, especially related to the following: the equipment, which is like that used for x-ray examination except larger, the hyperbaric oxygen chamber, which may be used to increase cellular oxygen and thus make tumor cells more radiosensitive; the radiotherapist, who will be behind a shield, but still close by and in communication with her; the position she will be put in and asked to maintain for some minutes; and the therapy, which is painless.

During Therapy. The woman is counseled regarding maintaining general good health. She is more vulnerable to infection; therefore she is reminded of general measures to avoid infection (e.g., practice good hygiene, avoid people with infection, avoid large crowds, keep environment clean). To maintain good skin care the woman is taught to assess her skin often; avoid soaps, ointments, cosmetics, deodorants if axilla is being irradiated, etc., because these may contain metals that would alter the dose she receives and could lead to skin breakdown; wear loose clothing over the area; use air mattress or cover mattress with foam pads or sheep skin; and of course, avoid removing the markings made by the radiologist. If her skin becomes red or itchy, it is treated with remedies prescribed by radiologist (e.g., sprays, A & D ointment, or lanolin). To treat skin that is broken or desquamating the woman is shown how to use remedies prescribed by radiologist (e.g., irrigation with equal parts peroxide and saline; application of antibiotic or lanolin ointment; exposure to air; and application of loose dressing but avoiding use of adhesive [or any] tape directly on the target area of skin).

To maintain good nutrition the woman is reminded to maintain a daily record of weight; use high-protein supplements; eat small, attractive, appetizing meals, probably bland in nature; take vitamins; and keep environment light, airy, clean, and quiet (especially before and after meals). If the woman is ill enough to be hospitalized, she may need total parenteral nutrition or tube feedings. Nausea interferes with adequate intake; therefore the woman may take antiemetics, as necessary. Maintain high daily fluid intake (2000 to 3000 ml) as suggested if not contraindicated. To increase her comfort, minimize infection, and promote adequate food intake, the woman is encouraged to perform frequent oral hygiene.

The nurse explains, as necessary, the need for blood studies to monitor white blood cell count (to determine degree of immunosuppression).

Posttreatment Care. Before discharge (if the woman is in the hospital during treatment) or the posttherapy care, the woman's need for information is met. The woman has a continued need to avoid infection and to report symptoms of infection to her physician immediately. She will need to maintain good nutrition and fluid intake. She and her family are forewarned of the persistence of radiation effects for 10 to 14 days after last treatment and to expect signs of healing in about 3 weeks. Good skin and mouth care are needed to support a sense of well-being and prevent infection. The woman and her family are informed of symptoms to report to the physician: continued gastrointestinal symptoms (nausea, vomiting, anorexia, diarrhea) and increasing skin irritation at the site of therapy (redness, swelling, pain, pruritis). She will need clear, explicit instructions about the medications she is to take (name, dose, times, purpose, side effects) and instructions to avoid any medications not prescribed by her physician. The woman and her family are reassured that she is not "radioactive"!

Internal Radiotherapy

Internal radiotherapy requires hospitalization. The radiation safety officer determines the precautions to be observed in each situation. Printed instruction sheets are usually available stating precautions to be followed for each type of radiation substance used. A precaution sign is placed on the door to the person's room. Personnel who come in direct contact with anyone receiving radiotherapy may be required to wear isolation gowns, rubber gloves, and a film badge (worn under the gown) to monitor the amount of exposure received.

If no contact is permitted, the room must be equipped with an intercom, a telephone, and a radio and television set. Food and other articles are given to the woman through a special porthole.

Nurses and those receiving radiotherapy need to know how unsealed radioactive substances (not discussed in this chapter) are eliminated so that the woman does not get the impression that she will be a danger to others idefinitely. This misconception could increase her feelings of isolation and cause her to be fearful of returning to her family. Before therapy is begun, the woman's room is prepared, that is, it is stocked with linens, extra pillows and blankets, and

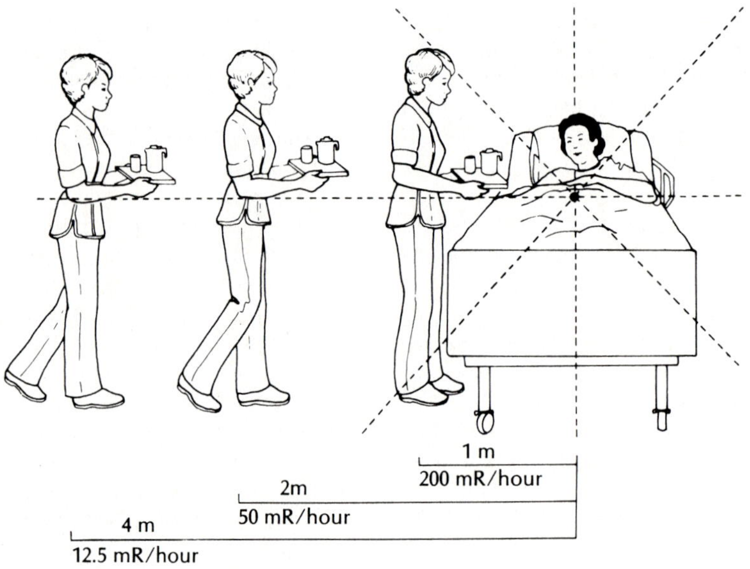

Fig. 44-7 Nurse nearest source of radioactivity (woman) is exposed to more radioactivity. Some hospitals have movable shield that can be placed between care provider and source of radioactivity.
Modified from Bouchard-Kurtz, R, and Speese-Owens, N: Nursing care of the cancer patient, ed 4, St Louis, 1981, The CV Mosby Co.

equipment, and everything (including the window blinds) is checked for workability.

Nurses must protect themselves from overexposure to radiation. Precautions include the following behaviors:

1. Careful isolation techniques: avoiding putting one's possibly contaminated hands into the mouth, carefully handling the woman's secretions and excrement (if she is receiving unsealed radioactive chemotherapy), and observing good handwashing technique. These behaviors reflect knowledge that alpha and beta rays cannot pass through skin but may be in body fluids and excrement.
2. Careful planning of nursing activity to limit time (to 30 minutes or less per shift) spent in close proximity to the woman (Fig. 44-7) to avoid exposure to gamma rays, which can penetrate several inches of lead.

Exposure to radiation is controlled in three ways—distance, time and shielding (with lead). Increasing the distance from the source decreases exposure. Brief communication from an open doorway is permissible and reassures the woman (Phipps, Long, and Woods, 1987).

Familiarity with applicators is a *must* for all nurses working with people receiving radiotherapy so that if a "strange object" is found in the linen or on the floor, it is not touched.

EXAMPLE: One of the authors was a nursing supervisor at night several years ago. The unit nurse on an oncology floor held the charts on her lap as she gave report on each person in turn—total report time, 20 minutes. When she replaced the last chart, she lifted a folded paper towel from her lap, extended the towel to show what it held and asked, "What is this?" She had found the "strange object" (about 1 hour and 20 minutes before report) on the bathroom floor of a woman receiving intrauterine radiotherapy. At the time, the nurse was 23 years old, engaged to be married, and looking forward to having a family. The nurse was told to drop the object immediately and leave the nurses' station. The radiologist arrived wearing a lead apron and gloves, pushing a lead-lined container, and carrying long forceps with which he lifted and replaced the "strange object" into the lead container.

Orientation to this type of unit mandates thorough orientation to safety precautions to be implemented at all times by all personnel.

Today most hospital protocols include having a lead container and forceps in the room for use should a radioactive implant become dislodged. For the person with sealed radiotherapy, a movable lead screen is available that can be placed between the area in which the therapeutic applicator is located and the personnel. The lead screen is also used to protect visitors from radiation. Refer to medical-surgical nursing texts for more extensive discussion.

Sealed Internal Radiotherapy

Irradiation with radium (cesium) is delivered to the cervix sealed in a mold, an afterloader, colpostat, Ernst applicator, or other applicators that can be placed and left in position for a specified length of time. Since radium is so costly, it is being replaced with other radioactive materials such as cobalt.

Unsealed radioactive chemotherapy (with radioactive iodine or phosphorus for example) is not discussed here. The reader is directed to medical-surgical texts.

Preinsertion Care. The woman is prepared for insertion with the following care, which is accompanied by an explanation for each activity. To reduce the need for an enema or attention to bowel elimination for a few days, the gastrointestinal tract is prepared using low-residue diet, enemas, and sometimes bowel sedation. The vaginal vault is prepared with an antiseptic douche such as povidone-iodine. The woman may be asked to prepare the vaginal vault by douching before admission. See guidelines for client teaching: vaginal douching. A vaginal douche is usually ordered after hospital admission.

An indwelling urinary bladder catheter is inserted, as ordered. The woman is assured that pain will be managed.

During Radiation Therapy. The applicator is inserted in surgery with the woman under general anesthesia if necessary. The usual postanesthesia recovery care follows and she is returned to her room. The woman is positioned on her back. There the applicators are loaded with the radioactive substance.

A lead shield is placed next to the woman's pelvic area. Vital signs are monitored every 4 hours. Active range of motion exercises and deep breathing are encouraged every 2 hours; she is not permitted to turn from side to side. The head of the bed is elevated about 35 degrees.

Her diet is progressed from clear liquid to low residue, as ordered. Parenteral or oral fluids are given up to 3000 ml daily. Intake and output are measured. The woman is given a partial bath, washing only above her waist—no perineal or catheter care is given. Massage is restricted to her shoulders and neck. Linen is changed only as absolutely necessary. Any linen or equipment used is retained in the room until therapy is complete to prevent loss of an applicator or seed.

If vaginal or rectal bleeding or hematuria occurs, the physician is notified immediately.

Emotional support is provided by planning to be with her for short periods, encouraging her to verbalize concerns and needs, encouraging family members, clergy, or others to visit for short periods daily or to communicate by phone. Pregnant women and children are not permitted to visit.

After the radium is removed, bladder function is monitored, oral fluid intake is encouraged at least to 3000 ml daily, douches and enemas are given as needed, and the woman is allowed to shower. The woman and her family are assured that she is not radioactive.

Discharge Planning. Before discharge, the woman (and her family) need counseling and receive printed instructions for the following:

1. Maintenance of good nutrition and fluid intake to 3000 ml daily (unless contraindicated) to promote healing and to avoid urinary tract infection and constipation
2. Maintenance of a balance between rest and exercise
3. Maintenance of good hygiene, (e.g., daily showers, daily douches until discharge stops)
4. Sexuality and sexual expression:

Guidelines For Client Teaching

VAGINAL DOUCHING

ASSESSMENT

1. Vaginal douching has been prescribed by the physician.
2. Vaginal douche must be used to deliver medication to the vagina or cervix.
3. Preoperative vaginal douche ordered.

NURSING DIAGNOSIS

Knowledge deficit related to vaginal douching.

GOALS

Short-term

Woman verbalizes understanding of vaginal douching procedure.

Intermediate

Woman implements vaginal douching per physician's order.

Infection is cured or prevented.

Long-term

Woman does not have a recurrence of condition that required vaginal douching.

REFERENCES AND TEACHING AIDS

Printed instructions

Douche equipment

CONTENT/RATIONALE	TEACHING ACTION
To confirm reasons for douching, the nurse reviews: Woman's condition. Physician's order.	Provide information and allow time for discussion.
To teach safe and effective method of douching the nurse presents the following:	
Void and wash hands before douching.	Emphasize good hygiene.
Use the following position to place fluid properly: a. The optimum position is semirecumbent in a clean tub (after a bath) or in bed (Fig. 44-8). A douche pan may be used in a tub as well. b. The woman can douche while seated on the toilet; however, the labia should be held together to permit solution to fill the entire vaginal vault.	Use illustration to clarify proper placement of fluids.
Prepare solution for optimum comfort and effectiveness. The temperature should be 40° to 43°C (105° to 110°F), comfortably warm to the inner aspect of wrist.	Read over the instructions on package of douche medication, answer questions, clarify information.
Allow some solution to flow out of nozzle to lubricate tip, or lubricate with K-Y jelly or other water-soluble lubricant.	Demonstrate technique to woman and allow her to ask questions. Watch woman give a return demonstration.
Hold or place solution container 60 cm (2 ft) above the hips to avoid greater heights, which increase the pressure of the flow. *Do not* use a bulb syringe (or exert excessive force if using a disposable douche with an attached nozzle), fluid or air embolus may result and death may ensue.	Discuss how woman will implement method at home; for example, does she have a bathtub, storage space for the equipment? Observe return demonstration of force of fluid flow.
To bathe the vaginal vault with fluid, insert nozzle upward and backward for 7.6 cm (3 in). a. Rotate nozzle so that fluid flushes entire mucosa, including that of the posterior fornix. Rotation of the nozzle also reduces the chance of forcing fluid into the cervix.	Use illustration to reinforce verbal description of anatomic position of vagina and of filling vaginal vault with fluid.
b. When douching seated on the toilet, hold labia together to fill the vaginal vault, then allow fluid to exit rapidly to flush out debris. Repeat until fluid is used up.	Encourage woman to ask questions. Promote discussion pertaining to the two methods of administration.
c. Hold labia together for specified period of time if the objective of the douche is to expose the mucosa to medication or moist heat.	Make sure woman understands this point. Repeat this instruction if necessary.
Sitting up and leaning forward aid in emptying the vagina.	Use illustration to aid understanding.
For proper care of equipment and to prevent possible spread of infection, wash douche equipment with warm soap and water, and store in a well-ventilated place away from extremes of temperature.	Stress the importance of keeping the equipment clean and dry.
Wash hands to maintain good hygiene.	Discuss simple asepsis with the client (e.g., how bacteria may be transferred from dirty hands to other areas on the body without realizing).

EVALUATION The nurse knows that teaching was effective when woman's return demonstration is accurate, no fluid or air embolus occurs, and there is no spread of infection. Prevention of or resolution of infection may reflect teaching effectiveness.

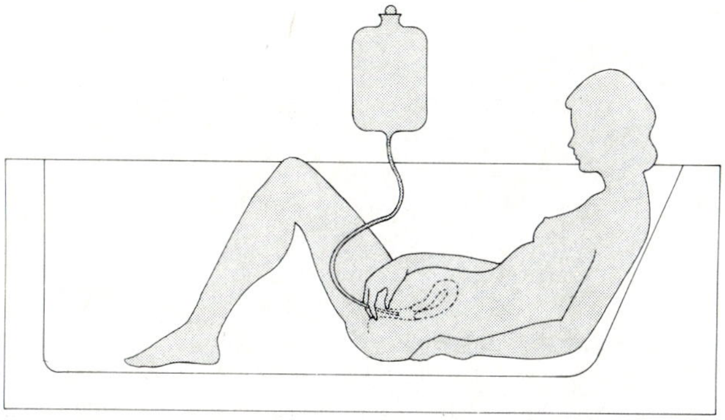

Fig. 44-8 Woman can lie in bathtub while douching. Vaginal douching is contraindicated during pregnancy.

a. Resumption of sexual intercourse in 6 weeks or at time designated by the physician
b. Use of vaginal dilator if needed and ordered
c. Expectation that sterilization and cessation of menstruation usually occur

5. Symptoms to report immediately: bleeding (vaginal, rectal, or in urine), foul-smelling vaginal discharge, fever, abdominal distension or pain, signs and symptoms of menopause.

Chemotherapy

Most chemotherapeutic agents disrupt cell development and reproduction. The accelerated rate of growth and reproduction of malignant cells renders them more susceptible than the slower growing, normal cells. Some normal cells reproduce constantly (e.g., cells of the bone marrow, gastrointestinal tract, and hair follicles). These cells are affected by the drugs giving rise to the familiar side effects—immunosuppression, nausea, vomiting, and anorexia, and alopecia (hair loss).

Knowledge of the replication pattern (phases of maturation) of cell "generations" has made it possible to schedule drug infusions (or ingestion) at appropriate times to achieve progressive eradication of malignant cells.

Among drugs that may hold promise as chemotherapeutic agents include L-asparaginase (an enzyme), streptozotocin (a nitrosourea), and interferon (a naturally occurring human glycoprotein).

The nurse who handles and administers antineoplastic drugs requires additional preparation for this function (Miller, 1988). The following nursing actions are general in scope and represent basic concepts of care. Many of the interventions are similar to those given to people receiving radiotherapy because there are some similarities in client response, for example, immunosuppression, gastrointestinal disturbances, and fatigue. Women need the same type of honesty about the effects of therapy and encouragement to maintain good hygiene, nutrition, and fluid intake. Fears and concerns that accompany chemotherapy are also similar except that chemotherapy involves physical discomfort during the administration of the drugs. Antiemetics, antacids, and good mouth care add to the woman's comfort. The nurse can suggest the use of scarves and wigs to cover hair loss. Laboratory evaluations may reveal the need for platelets and red blood cells; urine and stool must be assessed for bleeding; and ingestion of aspirin is avoided. During chemotherapy, nursing care for the primary condition continues and the woman's needs—physical, anatomic, safety, spiritual, and others—must be met.

NOTE: The nurse is cautioned to follow hospital protocols to prevent inadvertant exposure to this potent environmental hazard (Chapter 43).

Radical Mastectomy

The discussion that follows is pertinent specifically to the care required by a woman after surgical excision of the mammary tissue, pectoral muscles, lymph nodes, and all fat, fascia, and adjacent tissue. Less radical surgery does not require some of the care discussed; the care of a woman with less radical surgery is scaled down accordingly.

Preoperative Care. General preoperative teaching and care is given (see Chapter 34 for general care) including emotional support. Some emotional support may be obtained by arranging for a visit from a member of Reach for Recovery, Inc. The woman is reminded that when she awakens after surgery, her arm on the affected side will feel tight. A nursing care plan for a single, young woman with breast cancer is on p. 1150.

Immediate Postoperative Care. After recovery from anesthesia, the woman is returned to her room. Special precautions must be observed to prevent or to minimize lymphedema of the affected arm. When vital signs are taken, the blood pressure cuff is never applied on the affected arm. The affected arm is elevated with pillows above the level of her right atrium. Blood is not drawn from nor are parenteral fluids given in this arm. Early arm movement is encouraged. Pressure dressings may be needed. If a pressure dressing is used, circulation in the hand is monitored by assessing for color, sensation, and motion in fingers and hand; the dressing is released only on direct order from physician. Any increase in the circumference of that arm is reported immediately.

Nursing care of the wound involves immediate therapy for signs of hemorrhage (dressing, drainage tubes, and Hemovac), shock, and infection. Dressings are reinforced as necessary. Since the nipple may be "stored" on another body site (abdomen) pending future reimplantation over reconstructed breast, this site is observed for hemorrhage and infection every hour and care is given exactly as ordered.

The woman is asked to turn (alternating between unaffected side and back), cough (while nurse or woman applies support to chest), and deep breathe every 2 hours. Breath sounds are auscultated every 4 hours. Active range of motion exercise of legs is encouraged. Parenteral fluids are given until adequate oral intake is possible. Emotional support is continued.

Convalescent Care. Care given during the immediate postoperative period is continued as necessary. Early ambulation is encouraged not only to improve circulation and ventilation and prevent loss of calcium from bone but also

Specific Nursing Care Plan

SINGLE, YOUNG WOMAN WITH BREAST CANCER

Mary L. is a 32-year-old single woman who has been working in a dry cleaning plant for 10 years. While showering 5 months ago she noticed a hard lump in her breast. She now has a pinkish-watery discharge from her right nipple. She has not come to the clinic until now because she was afraid. An aspiration biopsy was done and the report revealed advanced malignancy. The physician has spoken to her about coming into the hospital for a mastectomy and possible chemotherapy. She has a casual relationship with a male friend in the neighborhood but her only support is her 68-year-old mother who is chronically ill with hypertension and arthritis.

ASSESSMENT	NURSING DIAGNOSIS (ND)/ PLAN(P)/GOAL(G)	RATIONALE IMPLEMENTATION	EVALUATION
Young woman with advanced breast cancer. Mary states she does not remember hitting her breast so she doesn't know how she got cancer; she is afraid of surgery, mutilation, and having cancer; and she is afraid of dying.	ND: Knowledge deficit related to diagnosis of breast malignancy. P: Provide time to discuss diagnosis; questions, and concerns. G: Mary speaks of disease in more realistic terms.	*To meet Mary's information needs, the nurse will:* Assess readiness to learn. Assess information given to her by the physician. Review information from physician. Provide written materials from American Cancer Society pertaining to her diagnosis.	Mary verbalizes understanding of information presented by both nurse and physician.
Mary is afraid to tell mother about diagnosis.	ND: Potential ineffective coping (family and individual) related to condition and its management. P: Facilitate problem-solving and communication between daughter and mother. G: Mary accepts diagnosis, shares it with mother, gains support during illness. ND: Anxiety related to insufficient information of available therapies. P: Provide information. G: Mary makes an informed decision.	*To assist Mary with coping mechanisms, the nurse will:* Bring mother into clinic to speak to physician. Arrange a meeting among a social worker, Mary, and her mother. *To assist Mary in anxiety reduction, the nurse will:* Provide time to discuss feelings and to supply information. Review therapies being considered by physician.	Mary begins to accept her diagnosis. Mary and mother support each other and draw strength from one another Mary confirms reduced anxiety and satisfaction with role in decision-making.
Mary is unaware of available therapies for breast cancer. Mastectomy is therapy of choice. Requests information about postoperative care.	ND: Knowledge deficit related to postoperative care. P: Provide needed teaching and time to discuss feelings, concerns. G: Mary relates accurate understanding of information from preoperative teaching.	*To assist Mary to meet learning needs, the nurse will:* Discuss upcoming surgery with physician and Mary. Arrange for Mary to meet with a woman from Reach to Recovery close to her age. Speak with clergyman. Implement guidelines for client teaching, p. 1152	Mary gains some insight into what the surgery is like, and verbalizes feelings.

for the psychologic benefits of the upright position (e.g., mood elevation, decrease of perception of self as continuing in the sick role). Arm exercises are encouraged at least 4 times daily (see box, below). Exercise is increased as tolerated and is stopped at the point of pain. Initially, the woman alternately clenches and extends her fingers, then progresses to wrist and elbow exercises, gradually abducting her arm and raising it up to and over her head. She is encouraged to exercise by assisting with her care—washing her face, brushing teeth, eating with her affected hand and arm. Physical therapy is usually prescribed. A representative of Reach for Recovery, Inc. often visits, reinforces the woman's exercise efforts, assists with providing emotional support relating to her change in body image (anatomic, physiologic, sexual) and may assist with teaching wound care.

Discharge Planning. Before discharge considerable time should be spent counseling the woman (and her family) about the following aspects of self-care (printed instructions should be available) (see client teaching: discharge after mastectomy, p. 1152).

POSTMASTECTOMY ARM EXERCISES*

Exercise: Climbing the Wall

1. Stand facing wall with toes close to wall
2. Bend elbows and place palms of hands against wall at shoulder level
3. Move both hands parallel to each other up the wall as far as possible until incisional pull or pain occur
4. Move both hands down to starting position
5. Goal is complete extension with elbow straight
6. Activities that use the same action: reaching top shelves, hanging out clothes, washing windows, hanging curtains, setting hair

Exercise: Arm Swinging

1. Bend forward from waist, permitting both arms to relax and hang naturally
2. Swing arms together left to right (motion comes from shoulder)
3. Swing arms in circles parallel to floor, clockwise and counterclockwise
4. Stand up slowly

Exercise: Rope Pull

1. Attach a rope over a shower rod or hook
2. Grasp each end of rope, alternately pulling on each end, raising affected arm to a point of incisional pull or pain
3. Shorten rope over time until affected arm is raised almost directly overhead

Exercise: Elbow Spread

1. Clasp hands behind neck
2. Raise elbows to chin level, holding head erect; move slowly and rest when incisional pull or pain occur
3. Gradually spread elbows apart; rest when pull or pain occur

*From American Cancer Society: Reach to Recovery, New York, The Society.

1. Care of the arm on the affected side: increase exercise but always stop at the point pain; elevate arm on pillows several times per day and at night, if possible; report swelling immediately; resume housekeeping gradually; recognize that arm may feel numb so that unrecognized injury may occur while handling tools, hot or cold things, carrying purse; inform others not to use that arm for injections or for drawing blood, etc.

   NOTE: Swelling of the arm emerged as an unanticipated problem 12 months after surgery for a significant number of women (Life, 1987).
2. Good hygiene (daily showers) is encouraged but underarm deodorant on affected side should be avoided until physician approves of its use.
3. Necessity of follow-up care and monthly BSE.
4. Resumption of sexuality depends on woman and her partners but pressure on her chest wall is to be avoided.
5. Symptoms that should be reported to the physician: evidence of infection (fever, redness, pain), swelling, drainage.
6. Prostheses available: early use of temporary breast forms and a well-fitted brassiere improve her appearance and her mental outlook; prostheses are fitted later after healing is complete.
7. Community services available (some, such as Visiting Nurse or even Reach for Recovery, need a physician's referral).

Radical Hysterectomy

Radical hysterectomy involves surgical excision of ovaries, tubes, uterus (complete with cervix), parametrial tissue, and lymph node dissection. In the premenopausal woman, some ovarian tissue may be preserved.

Preoperative Care. General preoperative teaching and care and emotional support is given (Chapter 34).

For this extensive surgery, the woman may enter the hospital 2 days before the scheduled surgery. The surgical area is prepared by cleansing enema and a vaginal douche each evening before surgery, daily showers or baths with antibacterial soap, and a clear liquid diet. During this time, emotional (including spiritual) support is continued.

During this preoperative period, teaching continues regarding postsurgical events, for example, intravenous fluids, pain management, drainage tubes, dressings, indwelling urinary bladder catheter, breathing exercises, coughing, turning, and early ambulation. The woman needs to be prepared to see a suprapubic catheter, which may remain in place for 1 to 8 weeks. The woman needs reassurance that bladder function will return.

Immediate Postoperative Care. After recovery from anesthesia, the woman is returned to her room. Vital signs and blood pressure are assessed every 4 hours for 48 hours and then 4 times daily during her hospitalization. She receives nothing by mouth, except for some ice chips unless they are contraindicated, until she passes flatus and bowel sounds are heard. Mouth care is provided frequently to add to her comfort. Her diet is then increased to clear liquids and her tolerance is assessed. She usually has a nasogastric tube to intermittent suction to prevent distension of the

Guidelines For Client Teaching

DISCHARGE AFTER MASTECTOMY

ASSESSMENT

1. Woman has had a mastectomy.
2. Woman needs instruction on activities postdischarge.

NURSING DIAGNOSES

Knowledge deficit related to discharge activities after mastectomy.

Potential activity intolerance related to postoperative recovery.

Potential for impaired physical mobility related to mastectomy.

Potential self-care deficit; bathing hygiene, dressing/grooming, related to mastectomy.

Pain, related to postoperative healing.

Body image disturbance related to mastectomy.

Situational low self-esteem related to amputation of breast, change in body image, and diagnosis of cancer.

Potential for ineffective individual/family coping related to diagnosis of surgery and amputation of breast.

Potential altered sexuality patterns related to impaired self-image and mastectomy.

Potential sensory-perceptual alterations (tactile) of affected arm; hot-cold, numbness, pressure, pain, related to mastectomy.

GOALS

Short-term

Woman takes part in self-care activities.

Woman can verbalize feelings about her surgery and her diagnosis.

Woman begins to use prosthesis in brassiere.

Woman continues exercises at home to strengthen and stretch muscles on affected side.

Intermediate

Woman recognizes symptoms that should be reported to the physician that signal problems.

Woman/couple can verbalize feelings together.

Woman begins to accept altered body image.

Woman assumes complete self-care.

Long-term

Woman has positive body image.

Couple resumes sexual contact.

Woman continues monthly BSE.

Woman keeps follow-up appointments with physician.

REFERENCES AND TEACHING AIDS

Books and pamphlets from the American Cancer Society and Reach to Recovery, Inc. that give instructions on exercises, activities of daily living, tips on dressing, etc.

CONTENT/RATIONALE	TEACHING ACTION
To counsel woman/couple on care at home: Discuss activities of daily living, hygiene. Daily baths or showers are encouraged. Use of talcum powders and deodorant should be avoided until recovery from surgery and radiation is complete and the physician approves.	Use pamphlets and printed instructions, encourage discussion.
To develop strength and maintain joint mobility: Teach postmastectomy exercises, p. 1151.	Demonstrate to the woman/couple the exercises that are most beneficial for her recovery. Usually it will be the ones she has already started while in the hospital. Ask for a return demonstration, guiding her through them and telling her to stop when she experiences pain.

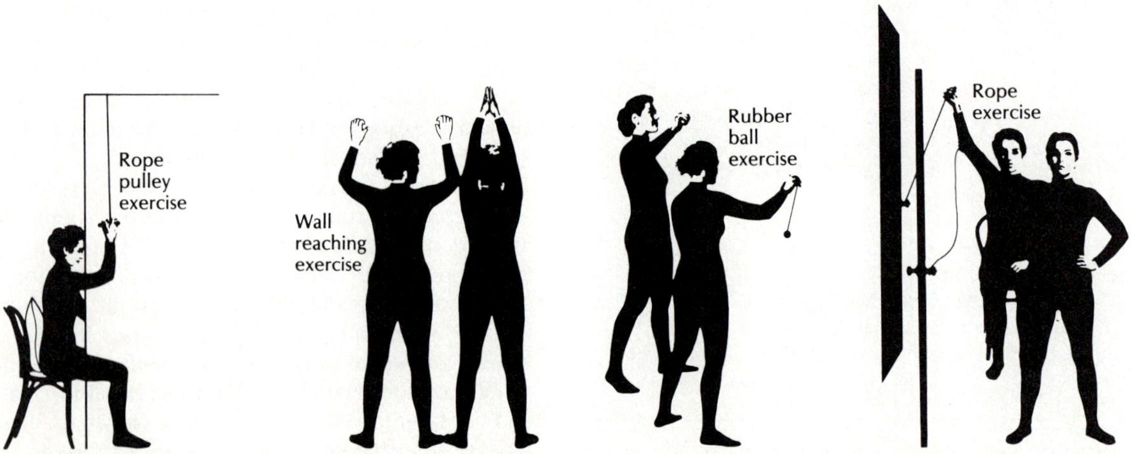

Continued.

Guidelines For Client Teaching—Cont'd.

CONTENT/RATIONALE	TEACHING ACTION
To instruct woman on wound care:	
Provide information on signs and symptoms that should be reported to the physician immediately.	Following physician's discharge orders, demonstrate wound care; write down the instructions for woman to take home. Provide a list of signs and symptoms that she should report to the physician (i.e., fever, redness, pain, swelling, drainage from wound). Tell woman these are signs of infection.
To assist woman with her bra and the prosthesis:	
Contact physician or Reach to Recovery representative.	Reinforce teaching done by physician and representative from Reach to Recovery.
To prevent injury:	
Discuss elevation of the arm on the affected side. Instruct woman to tell others not to use the arm for blood work, injections, etc. Caution woman about possible injury to arm as a result of numbness or decrease in sensation.	Show woman with a picture or diagram how her arm should be elevated on pillows for sleep and periodically during the day. Instruct woman to report swelling of the arm immediately.
To facilitate couple's relationship and maintain self-esteem:	
Discuss resumption of sexual activity according to physician's orders and how woman is feeling.	Encourage couple to verbalize feelings. Do not push this subject if woman/couple appears uncomfortable with it. Review process of and time frame for grieving.
Discuss follow-up care.	Reaffirm woman's return appointment with physician and emphasize importance of follow-up care.
Provide information on community support systems, nurses, housekeepers, Reach to Recovery, Inc.	Discuss this with the couple.

EVALUATION Woman/couple verbalizes understanding of information presented, asks appropriate questions, and keeps follow-up appointments. All goals are reached within time.

gastrointestinal tract, to prevent stretching of the incision line, and to promote comfort. Parenteral fluids are given until fluids are tolerated by mouth; intake and output is carefully monitored to prevent over and underhydration.

The woman will need to be reminded to turn and deep breathe; assistance is given as needed. Breath sounds are assessed and any deviations from normal reported immediately. The most significant single cause of morbidity and prolonged hospitalization after major procedures are respiratory complications. Anesthesia and surgery alter breathing patterns and ability to cough. Atelectasis, pneumonia, and pulmonary embolus may occur.

Hemorrhage is always a possible complication after surgery. The Hemovac is emptied every 1 to 2 hours and the amount and character is recorded. Drainage from any tubes is also assessed for bleeding. Vaginal drainage, if any, should be serosanguineous. Hematuria is noted and recorded. The physician is kept apprised of any deviations from normal expectations.

Drainage of urine is monitored closely. The nurse reports any seepage of urine around the suprapubic catheter; the vaginal discharge is assessed for urine drainage.

Care of infusion sites for parenteral fluids and exercise of the lower extremities and early ambulation help prevent thrombus formation, thrombophlebitis, and thromboembolism.

Paralytic ileus is expected after surgery in which the intestinal tract has been manipulated. The nasogastric tube, early ambulation, and withholding oral fluids until bowel sounds are heard support the return of gastrointestinal function. An enema or a Harris flush may bring relief from flatus and stimulate return of function. Oral laxatives should not be given until the lower bowel is functioning.

Sitting may result in pelvic congestion so that the high Fowler's position is avoided. Pelvic congestion is discouraged by putting the bed flat for 10 minutes every 2 hours for the first 24 hours and avoiding the use of the knee gatch (or pillow). Antiembolic stockings may be applied as ordered. Passive leg exercises should also be part of routine care and can be done during the complete bed bath as well as at other times during the day.

Comfort measures, such as massage, repositioning, use of pillows for positioning, and attention to the woman's emotional needs are helpful adjuncts to pharmacologic control of discomfort during this time. The nurse needs to keep in mind that some analgesics have a constipating effect. Cleanliness, fresh linen, perineal care, and offering wet washcloths after the woman has used a bedpan all contribute to the woman's comfort.

Convalescent Care. The same care that was given during the immediate postoperative period is continued as necessary. The woman's diet is progressed to high protein or high residue, as ordered. High fluid intake to 3000 ml is urged, if not contraindicated. If the urinary catheter is removed, the woman is assessed for urinary retention. Progressive ambulation is encouraged, whereas sitting for long periods of time is discouraged. Rectal tube, Harris flush, and enemas are used to bring relief from distension from gas accumulation resulting from paralytic ileus; stool softeners, mild laxatives, or suppositories are ordered as necessary.

Some women benefit from an abdominal binder especially when walking, but this is no longer a routine measure; the woman is encouraged to use her own abdominal muscles to support her abdomen.

Estrogen therapy is usually started as soon as the woman can take oral fluids. The nurse can take this opportunity to remind the woman she will no longer have menstrual periods and to encourage her to verbalize questions or concerns she may have about hormone replacement therapy (see discussion of hormone replacement therapy, p. 1039).

The woman needs continuous emotional support. She may have fears of death; permanent disfigurement and change in functioning; altered feelings of self as a woman; concerns regarding her femininity, sexuality, and loss of reproductive capacity; and questions arising from things she has heard about posthysterectomy changes (e.g., facial hair, going mad, or becoming depressed).

Discharge Planning. If the woman is to have a suprapubic catheter for a period of time, she and her family need to learn how to care for it. Feelings about needing and having the catheter must be addressed before the woman can mobilize herself to learn about its care.

She and her family will need counseling regarding the following aspects of her care:

1. Good nutrition and fluid intake are maintained.
2. A balance between rest and exercise is maintained with limitation of sitting for long periods of time; driving or heavy lifting is avoided for about 6 weeks; dancing or other activities that may increase pelvic congestion is avoided. (Desired activities need to be approved by the physician.)
3. Rationale for estrogen therapy is discussed as well as the fact that the surgery has resulted in the ending of ovarian and menstrual function. (She should have understood this well before signing the informed consent, but she may need this information reinforced.)
4. Resumption of intercourse, douching, and tub baths are deferred until after the follow-up examination at about 6 weeks. Counseling of the couple may be indicated, especially regarding the use of alternative means of achieving sexual satisfaction until healing takes place.
5. The following symptoms should be reported to the physician: wound infection, vaginal bleeding, gastrointestinal changes, or persistence of postoperative symptoms (cramping, distension, change in bowel habits).
6. If the woman is to take medication, she should know its name, dose, time of administration, purpose, and side effects.

Radical Vulvectomy and Lymphadenectomy

Radical vulvectomy is the surgical excision of the vulva and dissection of lymph nodes in the presence of invasive cancer.

Skinning vulvectomy with skin graft or *laser surgery* may be performed for cancer in situ when only the upper layers of the vulva need to be excised. The preoperative and postoperative care is similar to that for radical vulvectomy. Even though the surgery is not as extensive, the woman needs the same type of emotional support as any woman undergoing surgery.

Preoperative Care. The woman enters the hospital 2 to 3 days before surgery so that the bowel can be cleansed with enemas each evening and the vagina cleansed with antiseptic douches. Baths, sitz baths, and showers with antibacterial soap are taken daily. A clear liquid, low residue diet is maintained until surgery. Some physicians advocate beginning antibiotic therapy during the 24 to 48 hours before surgery. General preoperative teaching and care and emotional support are given (Chapter 34).

With this surgery the woman needs to expect to remain flat in bed for 24 to 48 hours. She may be on an alternating pressure air mattress or other type of mattress to prevent pressure sores (decubiti) and she may need to wear antiembolic stockings. A pressure dressing with drainage tubes or Hemovac are common with this type of wound; an indwelling urinary catheter is needed. To prevent respiratory complications she will need to learn how to cough and deep breathe, to do leg exercises, and to use the overhead trapeze bar to help her move in bed.

Immediate Postoperative Care. After recovery from anesthesia, the woman is returned to her room. Vital signs and blood pressure are assessed every 2 hours for 6 hours, then every 4 hours for 4 days, then every 8 hours. Closer monitoring of vital signs is necessary because of the prolonged bed rest with the bed flat. She will need to be assisted to turn every 2 hours; a pillow is kept between her legs during turning. Deep breathing and coughing are encouraged at frequent intervals. Breath sounds are auscultated every 2 to 4 hours. Pain is managed as necessary.

Parenteral fluids (and good mouth care) are given for as long as the woman cannot have fluids by mouth. Some women may receive heparin therapy (low doses) temporarily to forestall thrombus formation caused by immobility. The woman's popliteal and pedal pulses are assessed. Passive exercises of the lower extremities help maintain good circulation. Antiembolic stockings may be ordered; they are reapplied at least once per shift.

Drainage from tubes or in Hemovac and on dressings are monitored. Dressings may need to be reinforced but are never removed without a physician's order.

The skin is assessed and skin care is given every 2 to 4 hours and as necessary for comfort and to prevent breakdown of tissues. Bowel sounds are assessed at least once per shift. Catheter drainage is assessed. A careful record of her intake and output is maintained.

Immobility and the nature of the surgery mandate that the environment around the woman be kept therapeutic (e.g., ventilated, privacy [as desired], deodorized as necessary, and nurses available to listen to her and to encourage her to discuss her questions and concerns).

Convalescent Care. Defecation should be avoided while dressings are in place; paregoric may be ordered to delay need for bowel evacuation. When dressings are removed, the woman is given stool softeners, suppositories, or enemas as needed; her perineal area is irrigated with antiseptic solution after each elimination. Routine irrigation of the surgical site may be ordered often with a solution of one part saline to one part peroxide or plain normal saline solution; the area is then dried with a hand-held hair dryer or a heat lamp. Care must be taken to avoid burning the area! Sitz baths or whirlpool baths are soothing and aid healing.

The full Fowler's position is avoided, as well as pressure under the knees from pillows or raising the knee gatch on the bed. Active range of motion exercises of the lower extremities are encouraged frequently. The woman is allowed to walk as ordered and cautioned against sitting for prolonged periods or crossing her legs while sitting.

Between the fifth and tenth day, the urinary catheter is removed; she is assessed for urinary retention. She is encouraged to maintain a daily fluid intake of approximately 3000 ml. A high-protein diet is encouraged.

Discharge Planning. The woman and her family are counseled about the following postoperative activities: balance of rest and exercise, feelings of loss and grief that are common following this type of surgery, good hygiene, antiembolic stockings, high-protein, high-carbohydrate diet, medications she is to take, and activities to avoid. She should not cross her legs when sitting, lift heavy objects, or sit or stand for prolonged periods. Periodically during the day and at night, she needs to elevate her legs to prevent pelvic congestion. She and her sexual partner may need counseling regarding the need to abstain from intercourse until the physician gives approval and provides instruction for alternative methods of achieving sexual satisfaction.

She may go home with a urinary catheter in place and therefore would need to learn catheter care. She is also instructed to report symptoms of infection: Unusual odors, pain, or vaginal bleeding; fever (above 100° F [37.8° C]); swelling in the groin; frequency or urgency of urination, or cramping.

This surgery does not affect the woman's fertility.

Pelvic Exenteration

Pelvic exenteration refers to the surgical excision of all reproductive organs and adjacent tissues and includes radical hysterectomy, pelvic node dissection, cystectomy with formation of ileal conduit (Fig. 44-9), vaginectomy, and rectal resection with colostomy. This procedure is reserved for those women with recurrent or persistent carcinoma within the pelvis after irradiation. Women are carefully selected for this procedure; 5-year survival rates average around 20% to 35%. Many of the complications that follow this surgery are those that follow any form of major surgery, for example, pulmonary embolism, pulmonary edema, myocardial infarction, and cerebrovascular accidents. These complications are seen immediately after surgery. Infection originating in the pelvic cavity usually occurs later, if it occurs.

One of the most serious postoperative complications is small bowel obstruction related to the denuded pelvic floor; about 50% of these women need repeat surgery for this complication and about half of them die as a result.

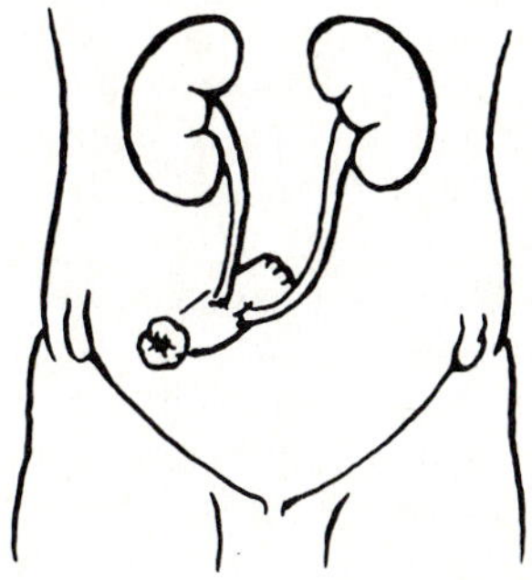

Fig. 44-9 Ileal conduit or ileal bladder construction: transplantation of ureters into isolated section of ileum that then serves as bladder. Another ostomy is formed for fecal drainage (not shown).
From: A cancer source book for nurses, rev ed, New York, 1981, American Cancer Society, Inc.

It is encouraging that technical advances continue to reduce the operative morbidity and mortality associated with pelvic exenteration. Many women who undergo this prodcedure not only can be cured but also rehabilitated to functional and comfortable lives.

Preoperative Care. Preoperative care is extensive because of the nature of this radical procedure. The woman enters the hospital up to 5 days before the scheduled surgery. During that time, she will bathe daily with antibacterial soap, douche with antiseptic solution, and maintain a low-residue diet until about 48 hours before surgery when she will begin a clear liquid diet. Cathartics are started about 48 hours before surgery; cleansing enemas are given for 1 or 2 evenings. Usually she begins antibiotic and vitamin K therapy for 2 or 3 days before surgery. To further decompress the gastrointestinal tract, a nasogastric tube may be placed and connected to low intermittent suction as early as 72 hours before surgery.

Continuous emotional support is an absolute must. If the hospital is so staffed, a "stoma" nurse is notified of the woman's admission so that a preoperative visit can be made. The spouse and other family members are encouraged to participate as well. Many concerns and questions arise that deal with bowel and bladder emptying and with sexuality and sexual expression after surgery—a vagina may be constructed during the original surgery or at a later date.

Preoperative teaching is also more extensive: the woman needs to be prepared to remain in bed for up to 1 week, to cough and deep breathe frequently, to have bulky dressings in place, to have many tubes in place, to have a colostomy or ileostomy and a urinary conduit opening out onto the abdomen, and to wear antiembolic stockings. She needs reassurance that pain will be managed.

Immediate Postoperative Care. After recovery from anesthesia, the woman is returned to her room. The vital signs and blood pressure are assessed every hour for approximately 48 hours; then every 4 hours for 7 days or as necessary. Temperature is assessed by mouth or axillae; rectal temperature taking is contraindicated. Parenteral therapy is maintained up to 4000 ml daily; total parenteral nutrition may be required for a period of time. Mouth care is given every 2 hours. All intake and output is measured. Pain is managed. Blood or blood component transfusions may be required 2 to 3 times during the first postoperative week.

The prolonged bed rest requires careful attention to the prevention of problems of immobility. The woman is assisted to cough, deep breathe, and turn every 2 hours. Breath sounds are auscultated at least every 4 hours. An intestinal decompression tube is connected to intermittent low suction. Popliteal and pedal pulses are assessed every 2 to 4 hours. Antiembolic stockings are reapplied at least every shift. Passive range of motion is performed with all extremities every 4 hours and as necessary. Skin care to all body surfaces, but especially to pressure areas, is undertaken every 2 to 4 hours. The bowel is auscultated at least once per 8-hour shift.

The operative site, the dressings, and drainage apparatuses are checked and findings recorded every hour for the first 48 hours. Dressings are reinforced and changed as necessary.

For the care of ostomies and urinary diversion conduits the nurse should see texts on medical-surgical nursing or hospital protocols for care.

The immediate environment is kept as therapeutic as possible: clean, fresh, deodorized, and private. Emotional support is continuous: the woman is encouraged to verbalize her fears and concerns, communication with loved ones is facilitated, and discussions about body image changes and loss and grief evoked by the experience are discussed openly with the woman and with interested family members.

Convalescent Care. Care given during the immediate postoperative period is continued as necessary. Vital signs and blood pressure assessments are done every 4 hours. Before the physician removes the intestinal decompression tube, the woman's tolerance for a clear liquid diet is assessed for 24 hours. The woman's fluid and nutritional status is constantly assessed and parenteral fluids, electrolytes, and total parenteral nutrition interventions are implemented as necessary. After the decompression tube is removed, the woman can take her vitamin and mineral tablets, urinary antiseptics, and antibiotics by mouth. She is encouraged to maintain a fluid intake of up to 4000 ml daily. A high-protein diet consisting of several meals and snacks per day is encouraged.

After dressings and packings have been removed, the woman's perineal area is irrigated (as ordered, usually with solution of one part saline to one part peroxide), patted dry or dried with a hand-held hair dryer on low or a heat lamp (25 watt bulb no closer than 18 inches to prevent burning). She is assisted with active range of motion exercises to all extremities at least 4 times daily. Sitz baths may be taken when she is able to walk and can tolerate them. She is assisted to walk as tolerated but chair sitting is avoided.

The woman continues to receive ostomy care. She and other family members are involved in the care of the ostomies in preparation for discharge.

Emotional (including spiritual) care is continuous.

Discharge Planning. The woman and her family are counseled about the following activities (written instructions are available):

1. Ostomy and urinary diversion care; wound irrigations
2. Sitz baths that are to be taken at least twice per day
3. Symptoms to report to the physician: unusual odor or drainage, fresh bleeding, unusual pain, fever (temperature above 100° F [37.8° C]), upper respiratory symptoms of infection, and increased swelling in groin or elsewhere in body
4. Antiembolic stockings or supportive hosiery
5. Balancing exercise with rest; knowledge that fatigue for a considerable period of time following surgery is common
6. High-protein, high-carbohydrate diet
7. Estrogen replacement therapy
8. Sexuality and sexual expression: alternative ways to achieve sexual satisfaction until new vagina is constructed and healing has occurred
9. Other medications she may be receiving: time, dosage, means of administration, and side effects
10. Community agencies available: American Cancer Society, other (some need physician referral)

Prostaglandins and Cancer

Prostaglandins (PGs), their metabolites, and related compounds have a vital function in almost every aspect of human physiology. The biosynthesis, mode of action, and pharmacologic configuration of these compounds have important implications in cell biology and clinical medicine. Their possible role in cancer may be related to biologically important interactions in carcinogenesis, the rate of proliferation and differentiation of tumor cells, tumor cell metastasis, the host-tumor relationship, and cancer therapy (Karmali, 1983).

Two processes are identified in chemical carcinogenesis: initiation by chemical reactive carcinogens, and promotion by a promoting agent. PGs may be implicated in both processes. Excessive PGs have been found in several types of malignant neoplasias. PGE_2 has been associated with symptoms commonly seen with breast cancer, for example, metastatic spread to bone and hypercalcemia. Carcinomas of the breast and lung produce more PG-like material than do normal tissues. In some people with cancer, PG production by tumor cells causes immunosuppression.

Research continues on the role of PGs in neoplasia and drugs that may influence the synthesis and action of PGs in such a way as to suppress carcinogenesis and metastasis.

Rehabilitative Measures

Rehabilitative and curative measures overlap in some instances. Discharge planning encompasses rehabilitative actions. Rehabilitation of the woman with cancer to an optimum level of functioning through the efforts of many health team members results in a more satisfying life for the woman and her family (Phipps, Long, and Woods, 1987). Reconstructive and plastic surgery or physical therapy may be required. Home health care and community

RESEARCH HIGHLIGHT

The Effects of a Patient Education Course in Persons With a Chronic Illness

Purpose

This study was conducted to measure the effects of a structured patient-centered education program in a chronically ill person's knowledge of specific aspects of her or his cancer and its ramifications. The study was designed to answer questions about the subjects: self-reported state of anxiety, knowledge of the disease, and perceived purpose and "meaningfulness" of life.

Sample

A sample of 52 persons were randomly selected from a group of persons aged 18 and older who had been newly diagnosed or rediagnosed within the year as having cancer. Individuals were paired (experimental and control) using pretest scores on the three dependent variables.

Methodology

The experimental (treatment) group attended 8 90-minute structured education sessions over a period of 4 weeks. Topics covered in the "I Can Cope" course were (1) learning about the disease, (2) coping with daily health problems, (3) communicating with others, (4) liking yourself, (5) living with limits, and (6) finding resources that can help.

Findings/Implications

When compared, every measure of preprogram and postprogram differences favored the treatment group. This study suggests that patient education is an important factor in helping people with cancer develop realistic expectations and attitudes. The study demonstrates that the "I Can Cope" program can help adults live with their chronic disease.

Johnson, J: The effects of a patient education course in persons with a chronic illness, Cancer Nurs 5:117, 1982.

health nurses may need to be involved to give care, teach, counsel, and support the woman and her family.

Ambulatory health care services are used for follow-up. Nurse-led programs such as "I Can Cope" have proven effective for teaching about the disease and in helping the women cope (see research highlight). Other therapeutic support groups vary with community resources and can be found by calling the local chapter of the American Cancer Society.

Evaluation

Evaluation of effectiveness of care is an ongoing process. Goals of care serve as evaluative criteria against which to measure the extent to which care has been effective. That is, the woman demonstrates appropriate decision-making and self-care during various therapies. Pain is alleviated or is tolerable with the measures available to her. Nutrition and hydration are maintained. Physical injury, bleeding, trauma, infection, and edema are treated, minimized, or eliminated. An optimum level of mobility for the woman's physical condition is maintained. The woman suffers no problems with bowel and bladder elimination, ventilation, sexuality, self-perception, self-concept, and role-relationships (Cooley, Yeomans, and Cobb, 1986; Cooley and Cobb, 1986; Stetz, 1987). The woman and her family come to terms with their values and beliefs and do not suffer spiritual distress.

CANCER AND PREGNANCY

Fortunately the peak incidence for most malignant diseases does not occur during the reproductive years (DiSaia, 1983). The most common cancers reported during pregnancy in order of frequency are breast cancer, leukemia and lymphoma, melanoma, various gynecologic cancers, and bone tumor. A brief discussion follows.

Cancer of the Breast

Approximately 1% to 2% of women are pregnant or lactating at the time of diagnosis of cancer of the breast (Pernoll and Benson, 1987). Breast cancer complicates about 1 in 3000 pregnancies. Diagnosis is often delayed because the normal changes in the breast obscure the disease. Pregnancy or lactation is not a contraindication to surgery. Treatment is the same as for the nonpregnant woman. For advanced disease in the second or third trimester, alkylating agents, 5-fluorouracil, and vincristine are relatively safe for the fetus (DiSaia, 1983). Chemotherapy may significantly improve the survival of these women.

After diagnosis, breast-feeding is contraindicated on two counts: (1) if one of the oncogens for breast cancer is a virus, as many have postulated, then the remaining breast may be contaminated and the virus may be passed to the newborn and may act as a latent inducer of breast carcinoma, and (2) lactation increases vascularity in the remaining breast, which may contain a neoplasm.

The question of subsequent pregnancies depends on the disease-free interval and the status of the lymph nodes (Morrow and Townsend, 1987). A disease-free interval of 2 years, no evidence of metastatic disease, and negative nodes are good prognostic signs. That is, prognosis is not adversely affected by a subsequent pregnancy (Harvey et al., 1981; Morrow and Townsend, 1987).

A 70% 5-year survival rate is anticipated after therapy when the neoplasm is confined to the breast. If axillary metastases are present, the 5-year survival rate after therapy is 30% to 40%. Earlier diagnosis in pregnant women and improved therapy underlie the improvement in the overall survival rate.

Leukemia

The average age for gravidas with acute leukemia is 28; incidence during pregnancy is not specified, but the incidence in the general population in the United States is 10 in 100,000.

Pregnancy seems to have no specific effect on the course of the disease, except that vigorous therapy is detrimental to early gestation. Preterm labor and postpartum hemorrhage are associated with acute leukemia. Acute myelocytic leukemia (90% of cases) has a more fulminant course and requires immediate therapy; in the presence of chronic myelocytic leukemia, therapy can be delayed somewhat. Some gravidas with the chronic form of the disease who had chemotherapy and radiotherapy directed at the spleen have delivered apparently healthy infants. The decision to terminate the pregnancy rests with the woman and her family; however, prompt, aggressive therapy is always advisable if remission is to be achieved.

Hodgkin's Disease (Lymphoreticuloma)

Hodgkin's disease is a malignant lymphoma that affects many younger people and complicates about one in 6000 pregnancies. Younger women (under 40) have a better prognosis.

Although pregnancy in the early stages does not appear to affect the course of the disease adversely, aggressive therapy has improved overall survival considerably. Radiotherapy and chemotherapy now are responsible for the care or control of Hodgkin's disease for long periods of time. Unless gestation is well into the third trimester, delay in initiating therapy should be minimal. Radiotherapy to diseased areas above the diaphragm can be initiated during the third trimester with proper shielding of the fetus. Chemotherapy is strongly contraindicated during the first trimester and is relatively contraindicated in the second and third trimesters.

If the gravida and her family refuse any therapy until pregnancy terminates naturally, the physician has no choice. However, termination of the pregnancy before initiating radiotherapy or chemotherapy is most desirable (DiSaia, 1983).

Melanoma

Malignant melanoma may be one of the rare cancers that can be affected adversely by pregnancy. Maternal adaptations to pregnancy (Chapter 10) are implicated:

1. Melanocyte-stimulating hormone (MSH) increases after 8 weeks gestation.
2. Adrenocorticotropic production increases also and ACTH heightens MSH activity.

Although pregnancy has been implicated in the more rapid metastases to regional lymph nodes, stage for stage, there does not seem to be a significant difference in the survival of gravid and nongravid women.

Diagnosis is established by biopsy. Therapy consists of radical local excision.

For most other malignancies, the placenta is unexplainably resistant to invasion by maternal cancer. Though melanoma accounts for few cases of malignant disease during pregnancy, almost 50% of the *placental metastases* and almost 90% of *fetal metastases* occur from maternal melanoma.

Bone Tumors

Ewing's sarcoma and osteogenic sarcoma are the most common primary malignant bone tumors seen in pregnancy. Usually the areas involved are the clavicle, sternum, spine, humerus, and femur. A lump or mass, local pain, and disability are characteristic manifestations.

Osteogenic sarcoma affects areas of high bone turnover (during growth spurts especially); Ewing's sarcoma is a rare condition that develops within bone marrow. Pregnancy does not affect nor is affected by the disease.

Surgical excision is usually well tolerated during pregnancy; adjuvant chemotherapy is delayed until after delivery if the cancer is diagnosed near term. With prompt chemotherapy (within a few weeks of diagnosis), 50% to 70% (compared with 5% before the advent of chemotherapy) of affected women are disease-free at 5 years. If the disease recurs, it usually does so within 3 years. Therefore women are counseled to defer pregnancy during this time.

Pelvic Malignancies

Cancer of the Vulva. The diagnosis of preinvasive (vulvular intraepithelial neoplasia) disease during pregnancy is not uncommon. Therapy is postponed until the postpartum period.

If invasive disease is diagnosed during the first trimester, vulvectomy with bilateral groin dissection may be done after the fourteenth week. When it is diagnosed in the third trimester, local wide excision is done deferring definitive surgery until after delivery. Pregnancy does not alter the course of the disease.

After radical vulvectomy and bilateral inguinal lymphectomy, several women who have become pregnant again carried the pregnancies to term and delivered vaginally. If local fibrosis is present and could impede delivery, abdominal delivery is advisable.

Cancer of the Vagina. Except for clear-cell adenocarcinoma of DES-exposed women, cancer of the vagina is not common. If clear-cell adenocarcinoma of the cervix and vagina or sarcoma are found in the upper vagina, the preferred surgery is radical hysterectomy, upper vaginectomy, and bilateral pelvic lymphadenectomy, followed by chemotherapy. If disease is advanced, the preferred treatment is to empty the uterus and begin radiotherapy.

Cancer of the Cervix. Rarely an invasive carcinoma of the cervix is discovered during pregnancy. It has been thought that pregnancy may have an adverse effect on cervical carcinoma, but this has not proven to be the case. An additional concern has been that giving birth through a cervix invaded by carcinoma might worsen the prognosis. Although there has been concern about the spread of tumor cells in such cases, there is no clear evidence to indicate that tumor dissemination is caused by the birth process. The major risk to the woman of delivery through a cervix containing invasive carcinoma is the risk of hemorrhage as a result of tearing of the tumor during cervical dilation and delivery. Therefore abdominal surgical delivery is preferred (Droegemueller et al., 1987).

The cancer itself does not harm the pregnancy: stage for stage, the outcome for the gravida with cervical cancer is roughly the same as for the nonpregnant woman (DiSaia and Creasman, 1989; Droegemueller et al., 1987). Carcinoma of the cervix is curable if diagnosed and treated in its early stages. Diagnosis and therapy is the same whether or not the woman is pregnant. Further diagnosis and treatment for CIS and dysplasia are deferred until the puerperium.

The therapy of invasive carcinoma of the cervix during pregnancy is affected by many factors. The stage of the disease and the trimester in which the cancer is diagnosed are important. Equally important are the beliefs and desires of the woman and her family in terms of initiating therapy that can interrupt the pregnancy as opposed to postponing the therapy until fetal viability is achieved. If the carcinoma is diagnosed in the first trimester or early in the second trimester (before 20 weeks), treatment is preferably undertaken immediately. The main concern is that a delay of over 4 months would lead to tumor progression or spread.

For pregnancies beyond the twentieth week of gestation a decision regarding initiating therapy immediately or delaying until fetal viability must be made. If it is desired to continue the therapy, the health of the fetus and its maturity is assessed. Appropriate ultrasound studies and amniotic fluid analysis are used to ensure fetal lung maturity. After cesarean delivery, therapy is completed by surgery, radiation, or chemotherapy with the same considerations of tumor size, stage, and invasiveness for any woman who is treated before the twentieth week of pregnancy. If immediate treatment is to be undertaken, hysterotomy is first performed and then surgery or radiation therapy completed. The gravida who is diagnosed during the first trimester has a better prognosis than those diagnosed during the third trimester.

Cancer of the Uterus. Endometrial carcinoma during pregnancy is rare; only a few cases have been documented since 1900. Diagnosis was usually an incidental finding after therapeutic abortion or surgery and the lesions were minimally or not invasive. Recommended therapy is total abdominal hysterectomy and bilateral salpingo-oophorectomy and adjuvant radiotherapy.

Cancer of the Uterine Tube. With a peak incidence between 50 and 55 years, concurrent pregnancy is only a remote possibility. Should it occur, the recommended therapy (total abdominal hysterectomy and bilateral salpingo-oophorectomy with postoperative radio- or chemotherapy) is the same as for the nongravid woman. A few cases have been first diagnosed following tubal ligation during routine histologic evaluation of the small resected segment.

Cancer of the Ovary. Ovarian tumors are infrequent complications during pregnancy. Serious complications may develop: pelvic impaction, obstructed labor, torsion of the ovarian pedicle, hemorrhage into the tumor, rupture of a cyst, and infection; or they may be malignant (only 2% to 5% of all ovarian neoplasms are found during pregnancy). The peak incidence of cancer of the ovary is over 50, therefore it is less likely to be seen during a pregnancy.

Differential diagnosis, especially during the second half of pregnancy, is difficult. Abdominal palpation and ultrasonography are the tools. The most common complication is torsion, which occurs most often when the uterus is rising rapidly (8 to 16 weeks) or involuting during the puerperium. Indicators of torsion are lower abdominal pain, tense and tender abdomen with guarding, nausea, vomiting, and shock-like symptoms.

An ovarian tumor may be first diagnosed at delivery because the enlarged uterus obscured its presence. If it falls back into the cul-de-sac, it may obstruct the birth canal and during labor may be traumatized. Hemorrhage into the tumor is followed by necrosis and suppuration (pus formation).

Malignancy of the ovary occurs approximately once in 8000 to 20,000 deliveries. The pregnancy does not alter the woman's prognosis if an aggressive therapeutic approach is taken. Fortunately, ovarian germ cell neoplasms occurring in pregnancy are usually benign (DiSaia and Creasman, 1989).

Chemotherapy During Pregnancy

Many cytotoxic agents are teratogenic early in pregnancy and would result in either spontaneous abortion or fetal abnormality. In addition, these drugs theoretically are mutogenic, abortifactants, and lethal to the fetus at any time. Nothing is known about the long-term effects of in utero exposure should the child survive. Chemotherapy with some drugs (aminopterin and methotrexate) in the second and third trimesters may not cause observable harm to the fetus.

Radiotherapy During Pregnancy. During embryonic development, tissues are extremely radiosensitive. If cells are genetically altered or killed during this time, the child either will fail to survive or will be deformed. From a radiologic stance there are three significant periods in embryonic development:

1. *Preimplantation:* If irradiation does not destroy the fertilized egg, it probably does not affect it significantly.
2. *Critical period of organogenesis:* During this period, especially between days 18 and 38, the organism is most vulnerable; microcephaly, anencephaly, eye damage, growth retardation, spina bifida and foot damage may occur.
3. *After day 40:* Large doses may still cause observable malformation and damage to the central nervous system.

Irradiation of gonads involves genetic damage—gene mutation and chromosome breakage—even at relatively low doses. Most mutations are recessive so that mutant effects may not surface for many generations.

GESTATIONAL TROPHOBLASTIC DISEASE

Gestational trophoblastic disease (GTD) is a morphologic continuum with the first deviation from normal implantation at one end, followed by hydatidiform mole (a benign condition) (see Chapter 31), evolving into invasive mole, and finally, ending with choriocarcinoma, the most proliferative and aggressive stage. Trophoblastic disease follows pregnancy (ectopic or intrauterine). In choriocarcinoma, the villi are absent and the neoplasm is composed of sheets of malignant trophoblast. Hemorrhage and necrosis, common in choriocarcinoma, result from the lack of vascular supply.

Before 1956, metastatic GTD had a short clinical course and was fatal. In 1956, complete remission with methotrexate in some women was reported (Li, Hertz, and Spencer). In 1960, actinomycin D (dactinomycin), when given sequentially with methotrexate, increased the remission rate from 50% to approximately 75%. These drugs remain the drugs of choice.

Hertz is credited with conceptualizing GTD as a disease continuum. Recognition that the benign hydatidiform mole has the potential to persist or recur as a proliferative and highly metastatic malignancy has improved cure rates by improving diagnosis.

Radioimmunoassay based on the β-subunit of human chorionic gonadotropin (hCG) permits detection of a very low level, and identifies those who need chemotherapy or those in whom persistent neoplasia mandates further therapy.

Evacuation of the intact mole is the initial therapy. The uterus is evacuated with a cervical dilation and curettage (D and C) accompanied by oxytocin infusion to stimulate uterine contractions that facilitate emptying of the uterus. Hysterectomy is an option if retention of reproductive capacity is not an issue. This procedure results in a cure rate of 90%.

Chemotherapy is begun if the hCG level rises, plateaus, or persists. After evacuation of a mole, the woman is monitored with radioimmunoassay for hCG at weekly intervals.

Some women are at greater risk for malignancy: the woman with complete versus partial mole, the woman whose molar disease is complicated by excessive bleeding after evacuation or by pulmonary symptoms, the older woman, and the woman with high parity. Women are categorized to be at low, moderate, or high risk based on limitation of metastasis to lungs and pelvis, metastasis to brain or liver, and level of hCG.

The woman receiving combination drug therapy must be monitored for white blood cell and platelet counts. The regimen is withheld if absolute polymorphonuclear leukocyte counts drop below $1500/mm^3$, the platelet count goes below $100,000/mm^3$, or if there is evidence of hepatic or renal impairment. The intravenous infusion must be inspected frequently for extravascular infiltration; infiltration results in tissue necrosis and sloughing.

Each woman is followed until three consecutive hCG β-subunit of hCG radioimmunoassay tests are negative. Women are counseled to avoid pregnancy for 1 year so the hCG levels, if found, are not confused with pregnancy. Long-term follow-up is warranted.

SUMMARY

Cancer and tumor are two words that evoke a multitude of images, mostly negative, in all who hear them. It is devastating to hear the terms in relation to oneself. The content of this chapter is intended to give the nurse an overview of cancer of the breast, cancer of the structures of the reproductive tract and perineum, and gestational trophoblastic disease. Nursing care of the woman with cancer and her family presents the nurse with energy-draining challenges. This challenge also offers the potential of fulfillment on both a professional and personal level.

KEY CONCEPTS

- One out of ten American females (10%) develop breast carcinoma during their lifetime.
- Risk factors identify only 25% of women who will eventually develop breast carcinoma.
- Mammography is the only nonexperimental screening method of detecting breast cancer at an early and highly curable stage; biopsy is the only definitive method for diagnosis.
- Women between 34 and 40 years of age should have one baseline mammogram plus annual physical examinations that should continue for life; women between 40 and 49 years of age should have a mammogram at 1 to 2 year intervals; after 50 years of age, annual mammograms are recommended.
- Important risk factors for endometrial carcinoma include obesity, nulliparity, menopause after the age of 52 years, and diabetes mellitus.
- The primary symptom of endometrial carcinoma is abnormal uterine bleeding, especially postmenopausal bleeding.
- Papanicolaou smear screening is thought to be the primary reason for the decreased frequency of invasive carcinoma of the cervix by 50% in the past 20 years.
- Risk factors for cervical neoplasia include multiple sex partners, sexually transmitted diseases, (herpes simplex virus, type II, cytomegalovirus, human papillomavirus-16, 18, 31) and cigarette smoking.
- At the present time there are four major forms of curative or palliative therapy: surgery, radiotherapy, chemotherapy, and immunotherapy.
- Cancer and its therapy are emotionally and physically draining on the woman, her family, and the caregiver.

STUDY QUESTIONS AND ACTIVITIES

1. Seek assignment to a woman preparing for surgery for a malignant condition. Follow her through the perioperative phase. What types of support systems are available to her? What coping mechanisms does she use? Identify the special needs of her family.
2. Develop a plan of care for the above woman and her family. Identify your feelings regarding malignancy in the female, and incorporate your responses into the plan of care.
3. Visit the American Cancer Society in your community. Interview a staff member to determine the types of services available to clients. Report your findings back to your group.
4. Attend a support group for people with cancer. Describe support given and received within the group. Identify your feelings during the meeting.
5. Informally interview other students on your campus regarding knowledge and use of screening methods for detection of neoplasia. Write an article based on your findings and submit it for publication in your school's newspaper. Your goal: increased awareness in your community.

References

American Cancer Society: Cancer facts and figures, New York, 1984

Berg, JW: Clinical implications of risk factors for breast cancer, Cancer 53:589, 1984

Bluhm, J: Helping families in crisis hold on, Nurs 87 17(10):44, 1987

Cashavelly, BJ: Cervical dysplasia: an overview of current concepts in epidemiology, diagnosis, and treatments, Cancer Nurs 10(4):199, 1987

Christopherson, WM, Connelly, PJ, and Alberhasky, RC: Carcinoma of the endometrium. V. An analysis of prognosticators in patients with favorable subtypes and stage I disease, Cancer 51:1705, 1983

Cooley, ME, Yeomans, AC, and Cobb, SC: Sexual and reproductive issues for women with Hodgkin's disease. II. Application of PLISSIT model, Cancer Nurs 9(5):248, 1986

Cooley, ME, and Cobb, SC: Sexual and reproductive issues for women with Hodgkin's disease. I. Overview of issues, Cancer Nurs 9(4):188, 1986

Derdiarian, A: Informational needs of recently diagnosed cancer patients: a theoretical framework. Part 1. Cancer Nurs 10(2):107, 1987

DiSaia, PJ, and Creasman, WT: Clinical gynecologic oncology, ed 4, St Louis, 1989, The CV Mosby Co

DiSaia, PJ: Vulvular diseases: a better way to manage CIS, Contemp Obstet Gynecol 21:127, 1983

Droegemueller, W, et al: Comprehensive gynecology, St Louis, 1987, The CV Mosby Co

Harvey, JC, et al: The effect of pregnancy on the prognosis of carcinoma of the breast following radical mastectomy, Surg Gynecol Obstet 153:723, 1981

Hauck, SL: Pain: problem for the person with cancer, Cancer Nurs 9(2):66, 1986

Henderson: Adjuvant therapy for breast cancer, N Engl J Med 318(7):443, 1988

Hickey, SS: Enabling hope, Cancer Nurs 9(3):133, 1986

Hopkins, MB: Information-seeking and adaptational outcomes in women receiving chemotherapy for breast cancer, Cancer Nurs 9(5):256, 1986

Karmali, RA: Prostaglandins and cancer: CA 33:322, 1983

Kopans, DB, Meyer, JE, and Sadowsky, N: Breast imaging, N Engl J Med 310:960, 1984

Kopans, DB: The role of mammography in the diagnosis of breast cancer, Updates 1(11):1, 1987

Lacey, CG, and Stern, JL: Tailor radical surgery to meet patient needs: vulvar cancer, Contemp OB/GYN 31(2):97, 1988

Larson, PJ: Cancer nurses' perceptions of caring, Cancer Nurs 9(2):86, 1986

Leathar, DS, and Roberts, MM: Older women's attitudes towards breast disease, self examination, and screening facilities: implications for communication, Br Med J 290:668, 1985

Levine, MN, et al: The thrombogenic effect of anticancer drug therapy in women with stage II breast cancer, N Engl J Med 318(7):404, 1988

Levine, RM, and Lippman, ME: Breast cancer management: Recent advances and recommendations, Adv Intern Med 29:215, 1984

Li, M, Hertz, R, and Spencer, DB: Effects of methotrexate therapy upon choriocarcinoma and chorioadenoma, Proc Soc Exp Biol Med 93:361, 1956

Life after cancer. This World, San Francisco Chronicle, p 15, June 21, 1987

Lovejoy, NC: Precancerous lesions of the cervix: personal risk factors, Cancer Nurs 10(1):2, 1987

Lubin, F, Ron, E, Wax, Y, et al: A case-control study of caffeine and methylxanthines in benign breast disease, JAMA 253:2388, 1985

Mast, D, Meyers, J, and Urbanski, A: Relaxation techniques: a self-learning module for nurses: Unit 1, Cancer Nurs 10(3):141, 1987a

Mast, D, Meyers, J, and Urbanski, A: Relaxation techniques: a self-learning module for nurses: Unit II, Cancer Nurs 10(4):217, 1987b

Mast, DE, Meyers, J, and Urbanski, A: Relaxation techniques: A self-learning module for nurses: Unit III, Cancer Nurs 10(5):Oct 1987c

Morrow, CP, and Townsend, DE: Synopsis of gynecologic oncology, ed 3, New York, 1987, John Wiley & Sons

Miller, JF, and Powers, MJ: Development of an instrument to measure hope, Nurs Res 37(1):6, 1988

Miller, SA: Chemotherapy drug handling safety, Calif Nurs Review 10(2):12, 1988

Pernoll, ML, and Benson, RC, editors: Current obstetric and gynecologic diagnosis and treatment, Los Altos, Calif, 1987, Lange Medical Books

Phipps, WJ, Long, BC, and Woods, NF: Medical-surgical nursing: concepts and clinical practice, ed 3, St Louis, 1987, The CV Mosby Co

Piver, MS: Promise of hydroxyurea for cervical Ca, Contemp Obstet Gynecol 23:45, 1984

Recht, A, and Harris, JR: Conservative surgery and radiation therapy for early breast cancer, Updates 1(9):1, 1987

Richart, RM, moderator: Treatment priorities for vulvar neoplasia, Contemp OB/GYN 31(2):79, Feb 1988

Rosenberg, L, Schwingl, PJ, Kaufman, DW, et al: Breast cancer and cigarette smoking, N Engl J Med 310:92, 1984

Rosenberg, L, Miller, DB, Kaufman, DW, et al: Breast cancer and oral contraceptive use, Am J Epidemiol 119:167, 1984

Rudolph, AL, and McDermott, RJ: The breast physical examination: its value in early cancer detection, Cancer Nurs 10(2):100, 1987

Stetz, KM: Caregiving demands during advanced cancer: the spouse's needs, Cancer Nurs 10(5):260, 1987

Veronesi, V, Sacozzi, R, Del Vecchio, M, et al: Comparing radical mastectomy with quadrantectomy, axillary dissection, and radiotherapy in patients with small cancers of the breast, N Engl J Med 305:6, 1981

Williams, ED, Edwards, K, and Hane, N: Barriers to breast cancer screening in older women, Community Health 10(3):51, 1987

Bibliography

Albanese, JA, and Nutz, PA: Mosby's nursing drug cards, St Louis, 1988, The CV Mosby Co

Anderson, J: Facing up to mastectomy, Nurs Times, 84(3):36, 1988

Bergeron, C: Bowenoid papulosis is intraepithelial neoplasia, Contemp OB/GYN 29(6):27, 1987

Boothby, RA, and Lovecchio, JL: Chemotherapy for endometrial Ca, Contemp OB/GYN 30(5):145, 1987

Breast cancer treatment: promising new agents, Contemp OB/GYN 30(1):61, 1987

Breast Ca treatment: reasons for optimism, Contemp OB/GYN 29(6):55, 1987

Carenza, L, Villani, C, and Porpora, MG: Surgical techniques: hysterectomy's role in endometrial Ca, Contemp OB/GYN 30(2):153, 1987

Chao, Y: Folk curing and caring activities practiced concomitantly by hospitalized gynaecological patients receiving radiotherapy. In Cancer Nursing in the 80's, Proceedings of the Third International Conference on Cancer Nursing, Melbourne, March 1984

Coates, A, et al: Improving the quality of life during chemotherapy for advanced breast cancer, N Engl J Med 317(24):1490, 1987

DePetrillo, AD: Gestational trophoblastic disease: an update, Contemp OB/GYN 29(1):199, 1987

Dische, S: When tumors resist radiotherapy, Contemp OB/GYN 29(1)183, 1987

Eddy, DM, et al: The value of mammography screening in women under 50 years, JAMA, 259(10):1512, 1988

Eggland, ET: Nurse's guide to home health care, Nurs '87 17(10):75, 1987

Eich, SJ: Promising early breast cancer treatment—without mastectomy, Cancer Nurs, p 51, Feb 1985

Endometrial cancer: state of the art, Contemp OB/GYN 31(6):107, 1988

Feller, WF, et al: Modified radical mastectomy with immediate breast reconstruciton, Am Surg 52:129, March 1986

Fernsler, J: A comparison of patient and nurse perceptions of patients' self-care deficits associated with cancer chemotherapy, Cancer Nurs 9(2):50, 1986

Finkler, NJ, Bast, RC, and Knapp, RC: Tumor markers in gynecologic cancer, Contemp OB/GYN 30(3):29, 1987

Fisher, B, et al: Five-year results of a random clinical trial comparing total mastectomy and segmental mastectomy with or without radiation in the treatment of breast cancer, N Engl J Med 312(11):665, 1985

Foley, SF: Preventive gynecologic nursing in an inpatient setting, J Obstet Gynecol Neonat Nurs 16:160, May/June 1987

Fox, SA, et al: Breast cancer screening recommendations: Current status of women's knowledge, Community Health 10(3):39, 1987

Friedlander, M, and Richart, RM: Objectively assessing neoplastic cells, Contemp OB/GYN 31(3):59, 1988

Funch, DP: Socioeconomic status and survival for breast and cervical cancer, Women Health 11:37, Fall/Winter 1986

Greifzu, S: Breast cancer: the risks and the options, RN, p 26, Oct 1986

Harris, RE, and Wynder, EL: Breast cancer and alcohol consumption: a study of weak associations, JAMA 259(19):2867, 1988

Heintz, AP: What causes ovarian cancer? Contemp OB/GYN 29(3):25, 1987

Hilgers, RD: Improving the outcome of high-risk gestational trophoblastic neoplasia, Contemp OB/GYN 29(5):73, 1987

Hulka, BS: Breast disease: what influences breast cancer risk? Contemp OB/GYN 29(4):91, 1987

Indman, PD: Office laser surgery for cervical disease, Contemp OB/GYN 29(3):45, 1987

Jankowski, CF: The risks of radiation during pregnancy, Am J Nurs 86(3):260, 1986

Johnson, SR: The woman over 50: how to evaluate perimenopausal bleeding, Contemp OB/GYN 31(Special Issue):67, April 1988

Keating, SB, and Kelman, GB: Home health care nursing, Philadelphia, 1988, JB Lippincott Co

Lee, GF: Fine-needle aspiration of the breast: the outpatient management of breast lesions, Am J Obstet Gynecol 156:1532, June 1987

Lindsey, AM, et al: Endocrine mechanisms and obesity; influences in breast cancer, Oncol Nurs Forum 14:47, March/April 1987

Lovecchio, JL: A new way to detect malignant cells, Contemp OB/GYN p 91, Oct 1987 (Special issue)

Macfee, MS: The woman over 50: two nonmalignant vulvar entities, Contemp OB/GYN 31(Special Issue):113, April 1988

Marchant, DJ: The woman over 50: breast cancer after menopause, Contemp OB/GYN 31(Special Issue):126, April 1988

Martin, BA, and Belcher, JV: Influence of cultural background on nurses' attitudes and care of the oncology patient, Cancer Nurs 9(5):230, 1986

Mattison, DR, Angtuaco, T, and Long, C: Magnetic resonance imaging in ob-gyn, Contemp OB/GYN 29(1):48, 1987

McGee, IE: Management of cervical dysplasia in pregnancy, Nurse Pract 12:34, March 1987

Mechcatie, E: Fibrocystic breasts: long-term care. Patient Care 21:41, March 1987

Modica, MM, and Timor-Tritsch, IE: Transvaginal sonography provides a sharper view into the pelvis, JOGN Nurs 17(2):89, 1988

Muggah, HF, and Staseson, S: The gynecological teaching associates program, Can Nurse, p 28, Feb 1988

Nichols, DH: Steps to assure safe vaginal hysterectomy, Contemp OB/GYN, p 91, June 1987 (Special issue)

Ozols, RE: Chemotherapy of ovarian cancer, Updates 2(1):1, 1988

Perreault, RM, and Starkey, EA: Intraperitoneal chemotherapy, Nurs '87, 17(9):112, 1987

Richart, RM, moderator: Vulvectomy techniques and challenges, Contemp OB/GYN 31(1):128, 1988

Rubin, D: Gynecologic cancer: uterine and ovarian malignancies, RN, p 52, June 1987

Rutledge, DN: Factors related to women's practice of the breast self-examination, Nurs Res 36:117, March/April 1987

Schlesselman, JJ, et al: Breast cancer in relation to early use of oral contraceptives: no evidence of a latent effect, JAMA 259(12):1828, 1988

Schnitt, SJ, et al: Ductal carcinoma in situ (intraductal carcinoma) of the breast, N Engl J Med, 318(14):898, 1988

Senekjian, EK, and Herbst, AL: Update on DES exposure, Contemp OB/GYN 29(2):29, 1987

Shingleton, WW, and McCarty, K: Breast disease: what you should know about breast pathology, Contemp OB/GYN 29(2):89, 1987

Spitzer, M, and Krumholz, BA: Pap screening for teenagers, Contemp OB/GYN 31(1):33, 1988

Stockwell, H, and Lyman, G: Cigarette smoking and the risk of female reproductive cancer, Am J Obstet Gynecol 157(1):35, 1987

Twiggs, LB, and Savage, JE: Nonmetastatic GTD: a curable disease, Contemp OB/GYN 29(5):61, 1987

Weeks, DD, et al: When leukemia complicates pregnancy, MCN 13(1):28, 1988

White, E: Projected changes in breast cancer incidence due to the trend toward delayed childbearing, Am J Pub Health 77(4):495, 1987

FOR MORE INFORMATION

American Cancer Society, Inc.
National Headquarters
777 Third Ave.
New York, New York 10017

Ca—A Cancer Journal for Clinicians
777 Third Avenue
New York, New York 10017

Cancer Nursing by Raven Press
1185 Avenue of the Americas
New York, New York 10036.

For additional information and answers to questions you have about breast lumps, call the following toll-free telephone number and you will be automatically connected to the Cancer Information Service office serving your area: 1-800-4-Cancer. In Alaska, call 1-800-638-6070; in Washington, D.C. (and suburbs in Maryland and Virginia) call 636-5700; on Oahu call 524-1234 (Neighbor Islands call collect). Spanish-speaking staff members are available to callers from the following areas (daytime hours only): California (area codes 213, 714, 619, and 805), Florida, Georgia, Illinois, Northern New Jersey, New York City, and Texas.

The American Society of Plastic and Reconstructive Surgeons, Inc.
Patient Referral Service
233 North Michigan Avenue, Suite 1900
Chicago, Illinois 60601

Appendices

APPENDIX

A

The Pregnant Patient: Bill of Rights

The Pregnant Patient has the right to participate in decisions involving her well-being and that of her unborn child, unless there is a clear-cut medical emergency that prevents her participation. In addition to the rights set forth in the American Hospital Association's "Patient's Bill of Rights" (which has also been adopted by the New York City Department of Health), the Pregnant Patient, because she represents *two* patients rather than one, should be recognized as having the additional rights listed below.

1. *The Pregnant Patient has the right,* prior to the administration of any drug or procedure, to be informed by the health professional caring for her of any potential direct or indirect effects, risks, or hazards to herself or her unborn or newborn infant which may result from the use of a drug or procedure prescribed for or administered to her during pregnancy, labor, birth or lactation.

2. *The Pregnant Patient has the right,* prior to the proposed therapy, to be informed, not only of the benefits, risks and hazards of the proposed therapy, but also of known alternative therapy, such as available childbirth education classes which could help to prepare the Pregnant Patient physically and mentally to cope with the discomfort or stress of pregnancy and the experience of childbirth, thereby reducing or eliminating her need for drugs and obstetric intervention. She should be offered such information early in her pregnancy in order that she may make a reasoned decision.

3. *The Pregnant Patient has the right,* prior to the administration of any drug, to be informed by the health professional who is prescribing or administering the drug to her that any drug she receives during pregnancy, labor and birth, no matter how or when the drug is taken or administered, may adversely affect her unborn baby, directly or indirectly, and that there is no drug or chemical which has been proven safe for the unborn child.

4. *The Pregnant Patient has the right,* if cesarean section is anticipated, to be informed prior to administration of any drug, and preferably prior to her hospitalization, that minimizing her and, in turn, her baby's intake of nonessential preoperative medicine, will benefit her baby.

5. *The Pregnant Patient has the right,* prior to the administration of a drug or procedure, to be informed if there is *no* properly controlled follow-up research which has established the safety of the drug or procedure with regard to its direct and/or indirect effects on the physiological, mental and neurological development of the child exposed, via the mother, to the drug or procedure during pregnancy, labor, birth or lactation (this would apply to virtually all drugs and the vast majority of obstetric procedures).

6. *The Pregnant Patient has the right,* prior to the administration of any drug, to be informed of the brand name and generic name of the drug in order that she may advise the health professional of any past adverse reaction to the drug.

7. *The Pregnant Patient has the right* to determine for herself, without pressure from her attendant, whether she will accept the risks inherent in the proposed therapy or refuse a drug or procedure.

8. *The Pregnant Patient has the right* to know the name and qualifications of the individual administering a medication or procedure to her during labor or birth.

9. *The Pregnant Patient has the right* to be informed, prior to the administration of any procedure, whether that procedure is being administered to her for her or her baby's benefit (medically indicated) or as an elective procedure (for convenience or teaching purposes).

10. *The Pregmant Patient has the right* to be accompanied during the stress of labor and birth by someone she cares for, and to whom she looks for emotional comfort and encouragement.

From Haire, D.B.: The Pregnant Patient's Bill of Rights, J. Nurs. Midwife, 20:29, Winter, 1975. This article is not reproduced here in its entirety.

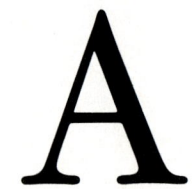

11. *The Pregnant Patient has the right* after appropriate medical consultation to choose a position for labor and for birth which is least stressful to her baby and to herself.

12. *The Obstetric Patient has the right* to have her baby cared for at her bedside if her baby is normal, and to feed her baby according to her baby's needs rather than according to the hospital regimen.

13. *The Obstetric Patient has the right* to be informed in writing of the name of the person who actually delivered her baby and the professional qualifications of that person. This information should also be on the birth certificate.

14. *The Obstetric Patient has the right* to be informed if there is any known or indicated aspect of her or her baby's care or condition which may cause her or her baby later difficulty or problems.

15. *The Obstetric Patient has the right* to have her and her baby's hospital medical records complete, accurate and legible and to have their records, including Nurse's Notes, retained by the hospital until the child reaches at least the age of majority, or, alternatively, to have the records offered to her before they are destroyed.

16. *The Obstetric Patient,* both during and after her hospital stay, has the right to have access to her complete hospital medical records, including Nurses' Notes, and to receive a copy upon payment of a reasonable fee and without incurring the expense of retaining an attorney.

It is the obstetric patient and her baby, not the health professional, who must sustain any trauma or injury resulting from the use of a drug or obstetric procedure. The observation of the rights listed above will not only permit the obstetric patient to participate in the decisions involving her and her baby's health care, but will help to protect the health professional and the hospital against litigation arising from resentment or misunderstanding on the part of the mother.

RESPONSIBILITIES

In addition to understanding her rights the Pregnant Patient should also understand that she too has certain responsibilities. The Pregnant Patient's responsibilities include the following:

1. *The Pregnant Patient is responsible* for learning about the physical and psychologic process of labor, birth, and postpartum recovery. The better informed expectant parents are the better they will be able to participate in decisions concerning the planning of their care.

2. *The Pregnant Patient is responsible* for learning what comprises good prenatal and intranatal care and for making an effort to obtain the best care possible.

3. *Expectant parents are responsible* for knowing about those hospital policies and regulations that will affect their birth and postpartum experience.

4. *The Pregnant Patient is responsible* for arranging for a companion or support person (husband, mother, sister, friend, etc.) who will share in her plans for birth and who will accompany her during her labor and birth experience.

5. *The Pregnant Patient is responsible* for making her preferences known clearly to the health professional involved in her care in a courteous and cooperative manner and for making mutually agreed-upon arrangements regarding maternity care alternatives with her physician and hospital in advance of labor.

6. *Expectant parents are responsible* for listening to their chosen physician or midwife with an open mind, just as they expect him or her to listen openly to them.

7. Once they have agreed to a course of health care, *expectant parents are responsible,* to the best of their ability, for seeing that the program is carried out in consultation with others with whom they have made the agreement.

8. *The Pregnant Patient is responsible* for obtaining information in advance regarding the approximate cost of her obstetric and hospital care.

9. *The Pregnant Patient* who intends to change her physician or hospital is responsible for notifying all concerned, well in advance of the birth if possible, and for informing both of her reasons for changing.

10. In all their interactions with medical and nursing personnel, *the expectant parents should* behave toward those caring for them with the same respect and consideration they themselves would like.

11. During the mother's hospital stay *the mother is responsible for* learning about her and her baby's continuing care after discharge from the hospital.

12. After birth, *the parents should* put into writing constructive comments and feelings of satisfaction and/or dissatisfaction with the care (nursing, medical and personal) they received. Good service to families in the future will be facilitated by those parents who take the time and responsibility to write letters expressing their feelings about the maternity care they received.

APPENDIX B

NAACOG's Standards for Obstetric, Gynecologic, and Neonatal Nursing

I: NURSING PRACTICE

STANDARD: Comprehensive obstetric, gynecologic, and neonatal (OGN) nursing care is provided to the individual, family, and community within the framework of the nursing process.

INTERPRETATION: The nurse is responsible for decisions and actions within the domain of nursing practice. Comprehensive nursing care includes helping the person meet physical, psychosocial, spiritual, and developmental needs. Systematic use of the nursing process, which encompasses assessment, nursing diagnosis, planning, implementation, and evaluation will meet the patient's needs. Individualized nursing care is best achieved by collaboration with patient, family, and other members of the health-care team. Complete and accurate documentation of all nursing care and patient response is essential for continuity of care and for meeting legal requirements. The nurse must promote a safe and therapeutic environment for the individual, family, and community.

II: HEALTH EDUCATION

STANDARD: Health education for the individual, family, and community is an integral part of obstetric, gynecologic, and neonatal nursing practice.

INTERPRETATION: The nurse is responsible for providing pertinent information to the individual, family, and community so they may participate in and share responsibility for their own health promotion, maintenance, and restorative care. The nurse plans, implements, and evaluates health education based on principles of teaching and learning. To enhance health care and promote continuity of health education, the nurse uses the educational resources within the community and collaborates with other health-care providers.

Health education should be documented and evaluated. Evaluation is based on individualized goals and set criteria.

III: POLICIES AND PROCEDURES

STANDARD: The delivery of obstetric, gynecologic, and neonatal nursing care is based on written policies and procedures.

INTERPRETATION: Policies and procedures define the boundaries of nursing practice within the health-care setting and indicate the qualifications of personnel authorized to perform OGN nursing procedures. The qualifications may include educational preparation and/or certification. The policies and procedures should be in accordance with the philosophy of the agency, state nurse practice act, governmental regulations, and other applicable standards or regulations.

A multidisciplinary framework should be used in writing policies and procedures. Policies and procedures should be evaluated on an ongoing basis and revised as necessary. The policies and procedures should be readily accessible to the health-care providers within the health-care setting.

IV: PROFESSIONAL RESPONSIBILITY AND ACCOUNTABILITY

STANDARD: The obstetric, gynecologic, and neonatal nurse is responsible and accountable for maintaining knowledge and competency in individual nursing practice and for being aware of professional issues.

INTERPRETATION: Maintaining both the knowledge and skills required to achieve excellence in OGN nursing is incumbent upon the nurse. The nurse should be cognizant of changing concepts, trends, and scientific advances in OGN care. Updating knowledge and skills is achievable through formal education, professional continuing education, and the use of or participation in nursing research. Knowledge of specialty nursing can be recognized through certification.

The nurse should be aware of governmental policies and legislation affecting health care and nursing practice. Participating in legislative and regulatory processes is appropriate for the nurse.

Responsibilities defined in written position descriptions and performance demonstrated by the OGN nurse should be regularly evaluated and documented. In addition, criteria for the evaluation of OGN nursing practice should be drawn from applicable statutes, the ethics of the profession, and current standards of practice.

V: PERSONNEL

STANDARD: Obstetric, gynecologic, and neonatal nursing staff are provided to meet patient care needs.

INTERPRETATION: The obstetric, gynecologic, and neonatal nursing management determines the staff required for the provision of individualized nursing care commensurate with demonstrated patient needs, appropriate nursing interventions, qualifications of available nursing personnel, and other factors that must be considered. These factors may include nursing care needs; number of deliveries; number and types of surgical procedures; average inpatient census; volume of ambulatory patients; percentage of high-risk patients; educational, emotional, and economic needs of the patients; provision for staff continuing education; medical staff coverage, ancillary services available; size and design of facilities; responsibilities of nursing staff; and ongoing research.

Personnel in each OGN unit should be directed by a registered nurse with educational preparation and clinical experience in the specific OGN area of practice. This nurse is responsible for management of nursing care and supervision of nursing personnel.

When nursing, medical, or other specialty students are assigned to the unit for clinical experience, their roles and responsibilities should be clearly defined in writing. Nursing students should not be included in the unit's staffing plan.

Written position descriptions that identify standards of performance for OGN nurses should be developed and used in periodic personnel evaluations. Documentation should reflect each nurse's participation in orientation and verify knowledge and expertise in those skills required for OGN nursing practice. Orientation and evaluation of personnel for whom the registered nurse is held accountable should be documented as well.

Written policies for the reassignment of OGN nursing personnel should exist to accommodate both increases and decreases of inpatient days and ambulatory visits. The policies should include a contingency plan for staffing during peak activity periods.

APPENDIX C

NANDA-Approved Nursing Diagnoses (Through the 8th Conference, 1988)

Activity intolerance
Activity intolerance, potential
Adjustment, impaired
Airway clearance, ineffective
Anxiety
Aspiration, potential for
Body image disturbance
Body temperature, altered, potential
Breast-feeding, ineffective
Breathing pattern, ineffective
Cardiac output, decreased
Communication, impaired verbal
Constipation
Constipation, colonic
Constipation, perceived
Coping, defensive
Coping, family: potential for growth
Coping, ineffective family: compromised
Coping, ineffective family: disabling
Coping, ineffective individual
Decisional conflict (specify)
Denial, ineffective
Diarrhea
Disuse syndrome, potential for
Diversional activity deficit
Dysreflexia
Family processes, altered
Fatigue
Fear
Fluid volume deficit (1)
Fluid volume deficit (2)
Fluid volume deficit, potential
Fluid volume excess
Gas exchange, impaired
Grieving, anticipatory
Grieving, dysfunctional
Growth and development, altered
Health maintenance, altered
Health seeking behaviors (specify)
Home maintenance management, impaired
Hopelessness
Hyperthermia
Hypothermia
Incontinence, bowel
Incontinence, functional
Incontinence, reflex
Incontinence, stress
Incontinence, total
Incontinence, urge
Infection, potential for
Injury, potential for
Knowledge deficit (specify)
Mobility, impaired physical
Noncompliance (specify)
Nutrition, altered: less than body requirements
Nutrition, altered: more than body requirements
Nutrition, altered: potential for more than body requirements
Oral mucous membrane, altered
Pain
Pain, chronic
Parental role conflict
Parenting, altered
Parenting, altered, potential

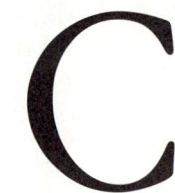

Personal identity disturbance
Poisoning, potential for
Post-trauma response
Powerlessness
Rape-trauma syndrome
Rape-trauma syndrome: compound reaction
Rape-trauma syndrome: silent reaction
Role performance, altered
Self care deficit, bathing/hygiene
Self care deficit, dressing/grooming
Self care deficit, feeding
Self care deficit, toileting
Self-esteem disturbance
Self-esteem, chronic low
Self-esteem, situational low
Sensory/perceptual alterations (specify) (visual, auditory, kinesthetic, gustatory, tactile, olfactory)
Sexual dysfunction
Sexuality patterns, altered
Skin integrity, impaired
Skin integrity, impaired, potential
Sleep pattern disturbance
Social interaction, impaired
Social isolation
Spiritual distress (distress of the human spirit)
Suffocation, potential for
Swallowing, impaired
Thermoregulation, ineffective
Thought processes, altered
Tissue integrity, impaired
Tissue perfusion, altered (specify type) (renal, cerebral, cardiopulmonary, gastrointestinal, peripheral)
Trauma, potential for
Unilateral neglect
Urinary elimination, altered patterns
Urinary retention
Violence, potential for: self-directed or directed at others

APPENDIX

D

Expected Date of Delivery (EDD)

Find the date of the last menstrual period in the top line (light-face type) of the pair of lines. The dark number (bold-face type) in the line below will be the expected day of delivery.

Jan.	1	2	3	4	5	6	7	8	9	10	11	12	13	14	15	16	17	18	19	20	21	22	23	24	25	26	27	28	29	30	31	
Oct.	8	9	10	11	12	13	14	15	16	17	18	19	20	21	22	23	24	25	26	27	28	29	30	31	(1	2	3	4	5	6	7	Nov.
Feb.	1	2	3	4	5	6	7	8	9	10	11	12	13	14	15	16	17	18	19	20	21	22	23	24	25	26	27	28				
Nov.	8	9	10	11	12	13	14	15	16	17	18	19	20	21	22	23	24	25	26	27	28	29	30	(1	2	3	4	5				Dec.
Mar.	1	2	3	4	5	6	7	8	9	10	11	12	13	14	15	16	17	18	19	20	21	22	23	24	25	26	27	28	29	30	31	
Dec.	6	7	8	9	10	11	12	13	14	15	16	17	18	19	20	21	22	23	24	25	26	27	28	29	30	31	(1	2	3	4	5	Jan.
April	1	2	3	4	5	6	7	8	9	10	11	12	13	14	15	16	17	18	19	20	21	22	23	24	25	26	27	28	29	30		
Jan.	6	7	8	9	10	11	12	13	14	15	16	17	18	19	20	21	22	23	24	25	26	27	28	29	30	31	(1	2	3	4		Feb.
May	1	2	3	4	5	6	7	8	9	10	11	12	13	14	15	16	17	18	19	20	21	22	23	24	25	26	27	28	29	30	31	
Feb.	5	6	7	8	9	10	11	12	13	14	15	16	17	18	19	20	21	22	23	24	25	26	27	28	(1	2	3	4	5	6	7	Mar.
June	1	2	3	4	5	6	7	8	9	10	11	12	13	14	15	16	17	18	19	20	21	22	23	24	25	26	27	28	29	30		
Mar.	8	9	10	11	12	13	14	15	16	17	18	19	20	21	22	23	24	25	26	27	28	29	30	31	(1	2	3	4	5	6		April
July	1	2	3	4	5	6	7	8	9	10	11	12	13	14	15	16	17	18	19	20	21	22	23	24	25	26	27	28	29	30	31	
April	7	8	9	10	11	12	13	14	15	16	17	18	19	20	21	22	23	24	25	26	27	28	29	30	(1	2	3	4	5	6	7	May
Aug.	1	2	3	4	5	6	7	8	9	10	11	12	13	14	15	16	17	18	19	20	21	22	23	24	25	26	27	28	29	30	31	
May	8	9	10	11	12	13	14	15	16	17	18	19	20	21	22	23	24	25	26	27	28	29	30	31	(1	2	3	4	5	6	7	June
Sept.	1	2	3	4	5	6	7	8	9	10	11	12	13	14	15	16	17	18	19	20	21	22	23	24	25	26	27	28	29	30		
June	8	9	10	11	12	13	14	15	16	17	18	19	20	21	22	23	24	25	26	27	28	29	30	(1	2	3	4	5	6	7		July
Oct.	1	2	3	4	5	6	7	8	9	10	11	12	13	14	15	16	17	18	19	20	21	22	23	24	25	26	27	28	29	30	31	
July	8	9	10	11	12	13	14	15	16	17	18	19	20	21	22	23	24	25	26	27	28	29	30	31	(1	2	3	4	5	6	7	Aug.
Nov.	1	2	3	4	5	6	7	8	9	10	11	12	13	14	15	16	17	18	19	20	21	22	23	24	25	26	27	28	29	30		
Aug.	8	9	10	11	12	13	14	15	16	17	18	19	20	21	22	23	24	25	26	27	28	29	30	31	(1	2	3	4	5	6		Sept.
Dec.	1	2	3	4	5	6	7	8	9	10	11	12	13	14	15	16	17	18	19	20	21	22	23	24	25	26	27	28	29	30	31	
Sept.	7	8	9	10	11	12	13	14	15	16	17	18	19	20	21	23	24	25	26	27	28	29	30	31	(1	2	3	4	5	6	7	Oct.

APPENDIX

E

Standard Laboratory Values: Pregnant and Nonpregnant Women

	Nonpregnant	Pregnant
Hematologic values		
Complete blood count (CBC)		
Hemoglobin, g/dl	12-16*	10-14*
Hematocrit, PCV, %	37-47	32-42
Red cell volume, ml	1600	1900
Plasma volume, ml	2400	3700
Red blood cell count, million/mm^3	4-5.5	4-5.5
White blood cells, total per mm^3	4500-10,000	5000-15,000
Polymorphonuclear cells, %	54-62	60-85
Lymphocytes, %	38-46	15-40
Erythrocyte sedimentation rate, mm/h	≤	30-90
MCHC, g/dl packed RBCs (mean corpuscular hemoglobin concentration)	30-36	No change
MCH/(mean corpuscular hemoglobin per picogram [less than a nanogram])	29-32	No change
MCV/μm^3 (mean corpuscular volume per cubic micrometer)	82-96	No change
Blood coagulation and fibrinolytic activity†		
Factors VII, VIII, IX, X		Increase in pregnancy, return to normal in early puerperium; factor VIII increases during and immediately after delivery
Factors XI, XIII		Decrease in pregnancy
Prothrombin time (protime)	60-70 sec	Slight decrease in pregnancy
Partial thromboplastin time (PTT)	12-14 sec	Slight decrease in pregnancy and again decrease during second and third stage of labor (indicates clotting at placental site)
Bleeding time	1-3 min (Duke) 2-4 min (Ivy)	No appreciable change
Coagulation time	6-10 min (Lee/White)	No appreciable change
Platelets	150,000 to 350,000/mm^3	No significant change until 3-5 days after delivery, then marked increase (may predispose woman to thrombosis) and gradual return to normal
Fibrinolytic activity		Decreases in pregnancy, then abrupt return to normal (protection against thromboembolism)
Fibrinogen	250 mg/dl	400 mg/dl

*At sea level. Permanent residents of higher levels (e.g., Denver) require higher levels of hemoglobin.

†Pregnancy represents a hypercoagulable state.

	Nonpregnant	Pregnant
Mineral/vitamin concentrations		
Serum iron, µg	75-150	65-120
Total iron-binding capacity, µg	250-450	300-500
Iron saturation, %	30-40	15-30
Vitamin B_{12}, folic acid, ascorbic acid	Normal	Moderate decrease
Serum proteins		
Total, g/dl	6.7-8.3	5.5-7.5
Albumin, g/dl	3.5-5.5	3.0-5.0
Globulin, total, g/dl	2.3-3.5	3.0-4.0
Blood sugar		
Fasting, mg/dl	70-80	65
2-hour postprandial, mg/dl	60-110	Under 140 after a 100 g carbohydrate meal is considered normal
Cardiovascular determinations		
Blood pressure, mm Hg	120/80*	114/65
Peripheral resistance, dyne/s-cm^{-5}	120	100
Venous pressure, cm H_2O		
Femoral	9	24
Antecubital	8	8
Pulse, rate/min	70	80
Stroke volume, ml	65	75
Cardiac output, L/min	4.5	6
Circulation time (arm-tongue), sec	15-16	12-14
Blood volume, ml		
Whole blood	4000	5600
Plasma	2400	3700
Red blood cells	1600	1900
Plasma renin, units/L	3-10	10-80
Chest x-ray studies		
Transverse diameter of heart	—	1-2 cm increase
Left border of heart	—	Straightened
Cardiac volume	—	70 ml increase
Electrocardiogram	—	15° left axis deviation
V_1 and V_2	—	Inverted T-wave
V_4	—	Low T
III	—	Q + inverted T
aVr	—	Small Q
Hepatic values		
Bilirubin total	Not more than 1 mg/dl	Unchanged
Cephalin flocculation	Up to 2+ in 48 h	Positive in 10%
Serum cholesterol	110-300 mg/dl	↑ 60% from 16-32 weeks of pregnancy; remains at this level until after delivery
Thymol turbidity	0-4 units	Positive in 15%
Serum alkaline phosphatase	2-4.5 units (Bodansky)	↑ from week 12 of pregnancy to 6 weeks after delivery
Serum lactate dehydrogenase		Unchanged
Serum glutamic-oxaloacetic transaminase		Unchanged
Serum globulin albumin	1.5-3.0 g/dl	↑ slight
	4.5-5.3 g/dl	↓ 3.0 g by late pregancy
A/G ratio		Decreased
α_2-globulin		Increased
β-globulin		Increased
Serum cholinesterase		Decreased
Leucine aminopeptdidase		Increased
Sulfobromophthalein (5 mg'kg)	5% dye or less in 45 min	Somewhat decreased

*For the woman about 20 years of age
10 years of age: 103/70.
30 years of age: 123/82.
40 years of age: 126/84.

Continued.

	Nonpregnant	Pregnant
Renal values		
Bladder capacity	1300 ml	1500 ml
Renal plasma flow (RPF), ml/min	490-700	Increase by 25%, to 612-875
Glomerular filtration rate (GFR), ml/min	105-132	Increase by 50%, to 160-198
Nonprotein nitrogen (NPN), mg/dl	25-40	Decreases
Blood urea nitrogen (BUN), mg/dl	20-25	Decreases
Serum creatinine, mg/kg/24 hr	20-22	Decreases
Serum uric acid, mg/kg/24 hr	257-750	Decreases
Urine glucose	Negative	Present in 20% of gravidas
Intravenous pyelogram (IVP)	Normal	Slight to moderate hydroureter and hydronephrosis; right kidney larger than left kidney
Miscellaneous laboratory values		
Total thyroxine concentration	5-12 μg/dl thyroxine	↑ 9-16 μg/dl thyroxine (however, unbound thyroxine not greatly increased)
Ionized calcium		Relatively unchanged
Aldosterone		↑ 1 mg/24 hr by third trimester
Dehydroisoandrosterone	Plasma clearance 6-8 L/24 hr	↑ plasma clearance tenfold to twentyfold

APPENDIX

F

Standard and Deviations from Standard Weight for 17- to 24-Year-Old Nonpregnant Women

Height		Underweight (<85%)		Standard Weight		Overweight (>120%)	
cm	in	kg	lb	kg	lb	kg	lb
140	52.2	38.0	84	45	99	53.8	118
142	56.0	39.0	86	46	101	55.0	121
144	56.7	40.0	88	47	103	56.4	124
146	57.5	40.7	90	48	105	57.6	127
148	58.3	41.8	92	49	108	59.0	130
150	59.1	42.8	94	50	110	60.4	133
152	60.0	43.8	96	51	112	61.8	136
154	60.7	44.6	98	52	115	63.0	139
156	61.5	45.6	100	53	117	64.4	142
158	62.2	46.6	103	55	121	65.8	145
160	63.0	47.7	105	56	123	67.4	148
162	63.8	49.0	108	57	126	69.1	152
164	64.6	50.0	110	58	129	70.6	155
166	65.4	51.0	112	59	131	72.1	159
168	66.2	52.0	114	61	134	73.6	162
170	66.9	53.4	118	63	138	75.4	166
172	67.7	54.6	120	64	141	77.2	170
174	68.5	56.0	124	66	145	79.1	174
176	69.3	57.5	127	68	149	81.2	179
178	70.1	59.1	130	69	152	83.4	184
180	70.9	60.6	134	71	157	85.6	189
182	71.7	61.9	137	73	161	87.4	193
184	72.4	63.2	139	74	163	89.3	197
186	73.2	64.5	142	76	167	91.1	201
188	74.0	65.7	145	78	171	92.8	205
190	74.8	66.7	147	79	173	94.2	208
192	75.6	67.7	149	80	175	95.6	211
194	76.4	68.7	152	81	179	97.0	214
196	77.2	69.5	153	82	180	98.2	217
198	78.0	70.4	155	83	182	99.4	219
200	78.7	71.2	157	84	185	100.6	222
202	79.5	72.0	159	85	187	101.6	224

Adapted from Task Force on Nutrition: Assessment of maternal nutrition, Chicago, 1978, The American College of Obstetricians and Gynecologists and the American Dietetic Association.

APPENDIX G

Human Fetotoxic Chemical Agents

Maternal Medication	Reported Effects on Fetus or Neonate
Analgesics	
Indomethacin (Indocin)	Prolongs gestation (monkey); in neonates, used to close patent ductus arteriosus
Narcotics	70% of maternal level; death, apnea, depression, bradycardia, hypothermia
Salicylates	Death in utero; hemorrhage, methemoglobinemia, ↓ albumin-binding capacity, salicylate intoxication, difficult delivery, ? prolonged gestation
Anesthesia	
Conduction	Indirect effect of maternal hypotension; direct effect—convulsions, death, acidosis, bradycardia, myocardial depression, fetal hypotension, methemoglobinemia
General Ether Halothane (Fluothane) Trichloroethylene (Trilene)	Apnea, depression (prolonged inhalation by gravid female), ? congenital malformations, chromosomal abnormality*; ether has direct narcotic effect on infant
Hypnosis	Indirect effect of maternal hyperventilation and excessive bearing down
Local	
Paracervical	Methemoglobinemia, fetal acidosis, bradycardia, neurologic depression, myocardial depression
Anticoagulants	
Coumarins	Fetal death, hemorrhage, calcifications
Anticonvulsant agents	
Barbiturates	Irritability and tremulousness 4-5 months after delivery; hemorrhage, enzyme inducer
Paramethadione (Paradione)	CHD, microphthalmia, mental retardation, abortion
Phenytoin and barbiturate	Congenital malformations, cleft lip and palate, congenital heart disease (CHD), CNS and skeletal anomalies, failure to thrive, enzyme inducer, hemorrhage
Trimethadione (Tridione)	
Antidiabetics	*See* hypoglycemic agents
Antimalarial	
Quinine	? Congenital anomalies of CNS and extremities, thrombocytopenia, hypoplastic optic nerve, congenital deafness
Antimicrobials	All antimicrobials cross placenta
Ampicillin	↓ Maternal urinary and plasma estriol levels
Cephaloridine	Blood levels maintained for hours after delivery; ? false positive direct Coombs' test
Chloramphenicol	Crosses placenta with no reported effect; interferes with biotransformation of tolbutamide, phenytoin, biohydroxycoumarin (i.e., hypoglycemia may occur if used in combination)
Chloroquine	Death, deafness, retinal hemorrhage
Erythromycin	Possible hepatic injury

Modified from Babson, S.G., et al.: Diagnosis and management of the fetus and neonate at risk: a guide for team care, ed. 4, St. Louis, 1980, The C.V. Mosby Co., p. 26; and Perinatal pharmacology, Mead Johnson Symposium and Perinatal and Developmental Medicine (no. 5), Vail, Colo., 1974.

*Pregnant nurses working in operating rooms have shown a higher incidence of abortion, stillbirths, and congenital anomalies for unknown reasons.

Maternal Medication	Reported Effects on Fetus or Neonate
Nitrofurantoin	Megaloblastic anemia, G6PD deficiency
Novobiocin	Hyperbilirubinemia
Quinine, quinidine	Possible ototoxicity, thrombocytopenia
Streptomycin	Therapeutic levels reached, nerve deafness
Sulfonamides	
Long and short acting	Icterus, hemolytic anemia, kernicterus, ? growth retardation, thrombocytopenia
Tetracycline	Placental transfer after 4 months' gestation; enamel hypoplasia, delay in bone growth, ? congenital cataract
Antituberculosis	
Isoniazid	Toxic blood level in fetus; no reported effect; mother should be on pyridoxine supplement
Pyridoxine	*See* vitamins
Belladonna derivatives	
Atropine	Intrauterine tachycardia; dilated, nonreacting pupils
Scopolamine	? Delays labor, ? delays respiration, deleterious to premature infant
Cancer chemotherapeutic agents	
Aminopterin Busulfan Cyclophosphamide 6-Mercaptopurine Methotrexate	Abortion, congenital anomalies (first trimester); combination of drugs detrimental to fetus; skeletal and cranial malformations, hydrocephalus; questionable long-term effects = slow somatic growth; ovarian agenesis; ↓ immune mechanisms
Cardiovascular agents	
Digitoxin	Placental transfer, no reported effect
Propranolol	Indirect effect of delay in cervical dilation
Cholinesterase inhibitors	Myasthenia-like symptoms for 1 week; muscle weakness in 10% to 20% of infants
Cigarette smoking	Effect equal to number of cigarettes smoked; ↑ incidence of stillbirth; low birth weight; ? effect on later somatic growth and mental development; reduction in O_2 transport to fetus
Diuretics	
Ammonium chloride Benzothiazides Chlorothiazide Thiazide	Maternal and fetal acidosis; thrombocytopenia, hemorrhage, hypoelectrolytemia, convulsions, respiratory distress, death, hemolysis
Diazoxide	Hypertrichosis lanuginosa, alopecia, ? hypoglycemia
Drugs of abuse (usually multiple drugs consumed)	
Alcohol	Blood level equal to mother's; convulsions, withdrawal syndrome, hyperactivity, crying, irritability, poor sucking reflex, low birth weight; cleft palate, ophthalmic malformation, malformation of extremities and heart; poor mental performance; microencephaly, small-for-dates, growth deficiency
Barbiturates	Withdrawal symptoms, convulsions, onset immediately after birth or at 2 weeks of age
Glutethimide	Small-for-dates, irritability
LSD (lysergic acid)	Chromosome breakage, limb and skeletal anomalies
Narcotics Heroin Methadone	Small-for-dates, 4% to 10% mortality, habituation, withdrawal symptoms, convulsions, sudden death, indirect effect of maternal complications (i.e., infection, hepatitis, venereal disease), ? permanent effect on somatic growth
Fluorine	Placental transfer—utilized for growth and development of bones and teeth of fetus
Hormones	
Androgens Estrogens Progestins	Labioscrotal fusion before week 12; after 12 weeks, phallic enlargement; ? other anomalies; ? ↑ bilirubin, vaginal cancer; cleft lip and palate; CHD; tracheoesophageal fistula; and atresia; cancer and prostate, testes, and bladder
Corticosteroids	Adrenal insufficiency, cleft palate, small-for-dates infant
Ovulatory agents	? Anencephaly, ? chromosomal abnormalities in abortus, multiple pregnancy
Hypoglycemic agents	
Chlorpropamide	Higher fetal mortality, prolonged hypoglycemia, competes for albumin-binding sites
Insulin	Insulin coma, ? increased fetal damage
Tolbutamide	? Potentiates hypoglycemia in newborn, thrombocytopenia
Hypotensive agents	
Hexamethonium	Paralytic ileus, perforation; death
Reserpine	1% to 15% of infants have symptoms; nasal stuffiness, bradycardia, respirtory distress, hypothermia, abnormal muscle tone (in mice, hyperactivity and increased emotionalism)

Continued.

Maternal Medication	Reported Effects on Fetus or Neonate
Insecticide and pesticides	
Organochlorine	Present in fetus, ? enzyme induction, ? premature labor
Intravenous alcohol	Hypoglycemia; abnormal bone marrow morphology in premature infant
Intravenous fluids	Excessive fluids—hyponatremia, seizures
Muscle relaxants	
Curare	Paralysis in utero (prolonged use), position deformities
Narcotic antagonist	
Nalorphine (Nalline) Levallorphan (Lorfan)	Not effective unless large doses of narcotics administered to mother; act as respiratory depressant if cause of depression is other than narcotic
Oxytocin	Thrombocytopenia, fetal bradycardia, water intoxication, ? ↑ bilirubin level; abortions (ergot)
Psychotropic drugs	
Antidepressants	
Aventyl Chloropyramine Imipramine Nortriptyline	Withdrawal, coliclike syndrome, cyanosis, irritability, weight loss, hyperhydrosis, respiratory distress, craniofacial anomalies, CNS and skeletal anomalies, urinary retention
Diazepam (Valium)	High fetal levels; hypotonia, poor sucking reflex, hypothermia; ↑ low Apgar score; ↑ resuscitation, ↑ assisted deliveries; dose related
Lithium carbonate	Neonatal serum levels reach adult toxic range; lethargy, cyanosis for 10 days; teratogenic—dose related
Phenothiazine	? Effect on eyes; withdrawal; extrapyramidal dysfunction; delay in onset of respiration; maternal hypotension, ? prolongs labor, ↓ effective uterine contraction; ? chromosomal breakage; hypotonia, hyperactivity
Radiation	Microencephaly, mental retardation, many unknown effects; nondisjunction of chromosomes
Radiopaque media	Elevated parathyroid hormone inhibition (PHI), depressed ^{131}I uptake
Sedatives	
Barbiturate	Apnea, depression, depressed EEG, poor sucking reflex, slow weight gain; concentration of drug in brain; enzyme inducer = lower bilirubin level
Bromides	Growth failure, lethargy, dilated pupils, dermatitis, hypotonia, ? effect on mental development
Magnesium sulfate	Neonatal blood level does not correlate with clinical condition; respiratory depression, hypotonia, convulsions, death; exchange transfusion may be required
Paraldehyde	Apnea, depression
Thalidomide	Administered between days 34-50 of gestation causes phocomelia, malformation of cord, angiomas of face, CHD, intestinal stenosis, eye defects, absence of appendix
Thyroid medications	
Iodine Thioureas	Normal or goitrous; euthyroid, hyperthyroid, or hypothyroid; respiratory distress due to tracheal compression; thrombocytopenia
^{131}I	Uptake of fetal thyroid after 12 weeks' gestation; exophthalmos, arrest of brain development
Toxins	
Carbon monoxide	Stillbirth, brain damage equal to anoxia
Heavy metals	
Arsenic	Concentrated in brain
Lead	Abortion, growth retardation, congenital anomalies, sterility
Mercury	Cerebral palsy, mental retardation, convulsions, involuntary movements, defective vision; mother asymptomatic
Naphthalene	Hemolysis
Vitamins	
A and D	Congenital anomalies
K (water-soluble analogs)	Icterus, anemia, kernicterus
Pyridoxine	Withdrawal seizures

APPENDIX H

Standard Laboratory Values in the Neonatal Period

1. Hematologic values

	Neonatal
Clotting factors	2 min
Activated clotting time (ACT)	2 min
Bleeding time (Ivy)	1-8 min
Clot retraction	Complete 1-4 hr
Clotting time	
2 tubes	5-8 min
3 tubes	5-15 min
Fibrinogen	150-300 mg/dl*
Fibrinolysin (plasminogen)	Lysis of clot
Partial thromboplastin (PTT)	<90-120 sec
Prothrombin time, one-stage (PT)	12-21 sec
Thromboplastin generation test (TGT)	8-24 sec in 6 min tube

	Term	*Preterm*
Hemoglobin (g/dl)	17-19	15-17
Hematocrit (%)	57-58	45-55
Sedimentation rate, erythrocytes (ESR) min/hr	0-2	1-5
Reticulocytes (%)	3-7	Up to 10
Fetal hemoglobin (% of total)	40-70	80-90
Nucleated RBC/mm^3 (per 100 RBC)	200(0.05)	(0.2)
Platelet count/mm^3	100,000-300,000	120,000-180,000
WBC/mm^3	15,000	10,000-20,000
Neutrophils (%)	45	47
Eosinophils and basophils (%)	3	
Lymphocytes (%)	30	33
Monocytes (%)	5	4
Immature WBC (%)	10	16

2. Biochemical values

		Neonatal
Ammonia		100-150 μg/dl
Amylase		0-1000 IU/hr
Antistreptolysin O titer, group B		
Normal		12-100 Todd units
Recent streptococcal infection		200-2500 Todd units
Bilirubin, direct		0-1 mg/dl
Bilirubin, total	Cord:	<2 mg/dl
	Peripheral blood: 0-1 day	6 mg/dl
	1-2 day	8 mg/dl
	3-5 day	12 mg/dl

1 to *6* from Pierog, S.H., and Ferrara, A.: Medical care of the sick newborn, ed. 2, St. Louis, 1976, The C.V. Mosby Co.
*dl refers to deciliter (1 dl = 100 ml); this conforms to the SI system: international measurements that have been standardized.

Continued.

Blood gases	Arterial:	pH 7.31-7.45
		P_{CO_2} 33-48 mm Hg
		P_{O_2} 50-70 mm Hg
	Venous:	pH 7.28-7.42
		P_{CO_2} 38-52 mm Hg
		P_{O_2} 20-49 mm Hg
Calcium, ionized		
Calcium, total		
Catecholamines (μg/24 hr)		
Neonatal: norepinephrine, 2-12; epinephrine, 1-2		
Newborn: Norepinephrine, 2-4; epinephrine, 0-1		2.1-2.6 mEq/L
		4-7.0 mEq/L
Ceruplasmin (*p*-phenylenediamine dihydrochloride, 37 C)		
Chloride		
Cholesterol, esters		
Cholesterol, total		1-30 mg/dl
Copper		95-110 mEq/L
Cortisol		42% to 71% of total
		45-170 mg/dl
		20-70 μg/dl
AM specimen		15-25 μg/dl
PM specimen		5-10 μg/dl
C-reactive protein (CRP)		0
Creatine		
Creatine phosphokinase (CPK) (creatine phosphate, 30 C)		0.2-1 mg/dl (higher in females)
Creatinine		10-300 IU/L
Electrophoresis, total protein		0.3-1 mg/dl
		Preterm: 4.3-7.6 g/dl
		Newborn: 4.6-7.4 g/dl
Preterm: albumin, 3.1-4.2; α_1-globulin, 0.1-0.5; α_2-globulin, 0.3-0.7; β-globulin, 0.3-1.2; γ-globulin, 0.3-1.4		
Newborn: albumin, 3.6-5.4; α_1-globulin, 0.1-0.3; α_2-globulin, 0.2-0.5; β-globulin, 0.2-0.6; γ-globulin, 0.2-1.2		
Fatty acids, free		0.4-1 mg/L
α_1-fetoprotein		0
Fibrinogen		150-300 mg/dl
Glucose, fasting (FBS)		
Hepatitis-associated (Australia) antigen		
Immunoglobulin levels, serum, newborn		
IgG 645-1.244		
Igm 5-30		
IgA 0-11		0
		660-1.439 mg/dl
Iodine, butanol extractable (BEI)		
Iodine, T_4-by-column (thyroxine)		
Iodine, T_4 (competitive protein-binding thyroxine)		
Iodine, total serum organic (PBI)		
Iron		
Iron-binding capacity (IBC)		
17-Ketogenic steroids (17-KGS)		
17-Ketosteroids (17-KS)		
Lactic dehydrogenase (LDH) (pyruvate, 30 C)		

Lipids, total
Lipoproteins, newborn (mg/dl)
Alpha 70-180
Beta 50-160
Chylo 50-110

3-13 μg/dl
3-12 μg/dl
3-12 μg/dl
4-14 μg/dl
100-200 μg/dl
60-175 μg/dl
2.4 mg/24 hr
0.5-2.5 mg/24 hr
300-1500 IU/L
170-450 mg/dl

Magnesium
Malate dehydrogenase (MDH) (oxaloacetic acid, 37 C)
Phosphatase, acid
Phosphatase, alkaline
Phospholipids
Phosphorus
Potassium
Pregnanediol
Protein, total
Sodium
Transaminases, serum

1.4-2.9 mEq/L
41-68 IU/L
10.4-16.4 IU/L
50-275 IU/L
75-170 mg/dl
3.5-8.6 mg/dl
4-7 mg/L
0 mg/24 hr
4.3-7.6 g/dl
140-160 mEq/L

Glutamic-oxaloacetic (SGOT) (aspartate, 30 C)
Glutamic-pyruvic (SGPT)
Triglycerides
Urea nitrogen (BUN)
Vanillylmandelic acid (VMA)

5-70 IU/L
5-50 IU/L
5-40 mg/dl
5-15 mg/dl
0-1 mg/24 hr

3. Urinalysis

Volume: 20-40 ml excreted daily in the first few days; by 1 week, 24 hr urine volume close to 200 ml
Protein: may be present in first 2-4 days
Casts and WBCs: may be present in first 2-4 days
Osmolarity (mOsm/L): 100-600
pH: 5-7
Specific gravity: 1.001-1.020

4. Cerebrospinal fluid

Calcium
Cell count

2-3 mg/L
WBCs/mm^{3}0-15
RBCs/mm^{3}0-500

Chloride
Color
Glucose

Continued.

	110-120 mg/L
	May be xanthochromic
	24-40 mg/dl
Lactate dehydrogenase (LDH)	5-80 IU/L
Magnesium	3-3.3 mg/dl
Pándy's test (for excess globulins)	Negative
pH (at 37° C)	7.33-7.42
Pressure	50-80 mm Hg
Protein, total	20-120 mg/dl
Sodium	130-165 mg/L
Specific gravity	1.007-1.009
Transaminase, glutamic-oxaloacetic (GOT)	2-10 IU/L
Volume	5 ml

5. Cardiorespiratory determinations

Blood pressure at birth
  Term: systolic, 78 mm Hg; diastolic, 42 mm Hg
  Preterm: systolic, 50-60 mm Hg; diastolic 30 mm Hg
Respiratory rate: 30-60 min
Heart rate, fetus
  Baseline: 120-160/min
    Tachycardia: >160 beats/min (with maternal complications)
    Bradycardia: <120 beats/min (with maternal hypotension and hypoxia)
    Acceleration: tachycardia > 160 beats/min with uterine contraction—normal (usually)
  Beat-to-beat variability: disappears with fetal distress
  With uterine contraction
    Early deceleration: bradycardia with onset of contraction—benign
    Variable deceleration: bradycardia due to cord compression—usually benign
    Late deceleration: bradycardia after lag period due to fetal hypoxia—ominous sign
Heart rate, term infant: 140 ± 20 beats/min

6. Urine screening tests for inborn errors of metabolism

Benedict's test: for reducing substances in the urine—glucose, galactose, fructose, lactose; phenylketonuria, alkaptonuria, tyrosyluria, and tryosinosis may give positive Benedict's test.

Ferric chloride test: an immediate, green color for phenylketonuria, histidinemia, and tyrosinuria, a gray to green color for presence of phenothiazines, isoniazid, red to purple color for presence of salicylates or ketone bodies.

Dinitrophenylhydrazine test: for phenylketonuria, maple syrup urine disease, Lowe's syndrome.

Cetyltrimethyl ammonium bromide test: for mucopolysaccharides: immediate positive reaction in gargoylism (Hurler's syndrome); delayed, moderately positive reaction for Marfan's, Morquio-Ullrich, and Murdoch syndromes.

Metachromatic stain (or *urine sediment*): Granules: (free or as inclusion bodies in cells) are seen in metachromatic leukodystrophy; may also be seen rarely in Tay-Sachs and other lipid diseases of the central nervous system.

Amino acid chromatography: Aminoaciduria may be normal in newborns; chromatography may be helpful to detect hypophosphatasia and argininosuccinicaciduria.

Diaper test, Phenistix test, and *Dinitrophenyl-hydrazine (DNPH) test:* simple, inexpensive tests for PKU (phenylketonuria); used for screening; most useful when infant is at least 6 weeks of age.

7. Blood serum phenylalanine tests

Guthrie inhibition assay methods: drops of blood placed on filter paper; laboratory uses bacterial growth inhibition test; phenylalanine level above 8 mg/dl blood: diagnostic of PKU. Effective in newborn period; used also to monitor PKU diet; blood easily obtained by heel or finger puncture; inexpensive; used for wide-scale screening

APPENDIX I

Relationship of Drugs to Breast Milk and Effect on Infant

Drug	Excreted in Milk	Amount in Milk After Therapeutic Dose	Effect on Infant
Analgesics and antiinflammatory drugs (nonnarcotic)			
Acetaminophen (Datril, Tylenol)	Yes		Detoxified in liver. Avoid in immediate postdelivery period, otherwise no problems with therapeutic dose.
Aspirin	Yes	1-3 mg/dl*	Long history of experience shows complications rare. Can cause interference with platelet aggregation and diminished factor XII (Hageman factor) at birth. When mother requires high, continuing level of medication for arthritis, aspirin is drug of choice. Observe infant for bruisability. Platelet aggregation can be evaluated. Salicylism only seen in maternal overdosing. Mother should increase vitamin C and vitamin K intake.
Donnatal (phenobarbital, hyoscyamine sulfate, atropine sulfate, hyoscine hydrobromide)	Yes		Consider for its component parts. Can be given to children but can accumulate in neonate.
Flufenamic acid (Arlef)	Yes	0.50 μg/ml (mean)†	No apparent effect on infant when maternal dosage was 200 mg, three times a day. Infant able to excrete via urine.
Indomethacin (Indocin)	Yes		Convulsions in breast-fed neonate (case report). Used to close patent ductus arteriosus. Insufficient data as to effect on other vessels. May be nephrotoxic.
Mefenamic acid (Ponstel)	Yes	Trace amounts‡	No apparent effect on infant at therapeutic doses; infant able to excrete via urine.
Naproxen (Naproxyn, synaxyns, naprosine, naxen, proxen)	Yes	1% of maternal plasma; binds to plasma protein	Less toxic in adults than some other organic derivatives.

Modified from Lawrence, RA: Breastfeeding: a guide for the medical profession, ed 2, St Louis, 1985, The CV Mosby Co pp. 509-529.

*Plasma level was 1-5 mg/dl.

†Shown when mean maternal plasma level was 6.41 μg/ml. Mean level in infant's plasma was 0.12 μg/ml; In infant's urine, 0.08 μg/ml. (Maternal plasma level was 50 times that of infant).

‡0.91 μg/ml mean maternal plasma level showed 0.21 μg/ml mean milk level. Mean infant plasma level was 0.08 μg/ml and mean urine level, 9.8 μg/ml.

Continued.

Drug	Excreted in Milk	Amount in Milk After Therapeutic Dose	Effect on Infant
Oxyphenbutazone (Tandearil)	Yes	In milk of 2 of 55 mothers, 10% to 80% of maternal plasma level	No known effect.
Pentazocine (Talwin)	No		Withdrawal in neonatal period from ingestion during pregnancy.
Phenylbutazone (Butazolidin)	Yes	0.63 mg ml 90 min after 750 mg given IM	Very potent drug; risk to infant not well defined but considerable. Not given directly to children; may accumulate in infant.
Propoxyphene (Darvon)	Yes	0.4% of maternal* dose	Only symptoms detectable would be failure to feed and drowsiness. On daily, around-the-clock dosage, infant could consume 1 mg/day.
Antibiotics			
Amantadine (Symmetrel)	Yes	Not defined	Vomiting, urinary retention, rash. Contraindicated.
Ampicillin (Polycillin, Amcill, Omnipen, Penbritin)	Yes	0.07 μg/ml	Sensitivity due to repeated exposure; diarrhea or secondary candidiasis.
Carbenicillin (Pyopen, Geopen)	Yes	0.265 μg/ml 1 hr after 1 g given	Levels not significant. Drug is given to neonate.
Cefazolin (Ancef, Kefzol)	Yes	1.5 μg/ml (0.075% of dose)	Probably not significant.
Cephalexin (Keflex)	No		
Cephalothin (Keflin)	No		
Chloramphenicol (Chloromycetin)	Yes	Half blood level; 2.5 mg/dl	Gray syndrome. Infant does not excrete drug well, and small amounts may accumulate. Contraindicated. May be tolerated in older infant with mature glycuronide system.
Chloroquine (Aralen)	Yes	2.7 mg in 2 days†	Can be used to *treat* child under 6 months of age who is wholly breast fed.
Colistin (Colymycin)	Yes	0.05-0.09 mg/dl	Not absorbed orally.
Demeclocycline (Declomycin)	Yes	0.2-0.3 mg/dl	Not significant in therapeutic doses. Can be given to infants.
Erythromycin (Ilosone, E-Mycin, Erythrocin)	Yes	0.05-0.1 mg/dl; 3.6-6.2 μg/ml	Higher concentrations have been reported in milk than in plasma. Should not be given under 1 month of age because of risk of jaundice. Dose in milk higher when given IV to mother.
Gentamicin	Unknown		Not absorbed from gastrointestinal tract, may change gut flora. Drug is given to newborns directly.
Isoniazid (Nydrazid)	Yes	0.6-1.2 mg/dl‡	Infant as risk for toxicity, but need for breast milk may outweigh risk.
Kanamycin (Kantrex)	Yes	18.4 μg/ml after 1 g given IM	Infant absorbs little from gastrointestinal tract. Infants can be given drug.
Lincomycin (Lincocin)	Yes	0.5-2.4 mg/dl	Not significant in therapeutic doses to affect child.
Mandelic acid	Yes	0.3 g/24 hr after dose of 12 g/day	Not significant in therapeutic doses to affect child.
Methacycline (Rondomycin)	Yes	½ plasma level; 50-260 μg/dl	Same precautions as with tetracycline.
Methenamine (Hexamine)	Yes		Not significant in therapeutic doses to affect child.
Metronidazole (Flagyl)	Yes	Level comparable to serums§	Caution should be exercised because of its high milk concentrations. Contraindicated when infant under 6 months may cause neurologic disorders and blood dyscrasia.
Nalidixic acid (Neggram)	Yes	0.4 mg/dl	Not significant in therapeutic doses beyond neonatal period. Hemolytic anemia in an infant attributed to nalidixic acid in G6PD deficiency or when mother has renal failure.

*Shown by animal experiments. Milk plasma ratio (M/P) = ½.
†Peaks in 6 hr.
‡Same concentration in milk as in maternal serum.
§Gives serum levels in infants of 0.05 to 0.4 μg/ml.

Drug	Excreted in Milk	Amount in Milk After Therapeutic Dose	Effect on Infant
Nitrofurantoin (Furadantin)	Yes	Trace to 0.5 μg/ml	Not significant in therapeutic doses to affect child except in G6PD deficiency.
Novobiocin (Albamycin, cathomycin)	Yes	0.36-0.54 mg/dl	Infant can be given drug directly.
Nystatin (Mycostatin)	No	Not absorbed orally	Can be given to infant directly
Oxacillin (Prostaphlin)	No		
Para-aminosalicylic acid	No		
Penethamate (Leocillin)	No	27-74 μg/dl	Animal study suggests it be avoided
Penicillin G, benzathine (Bicillin)	Yes	10-12 units/dl	Clinical need should supersede possible allergic responses.
Penicillin G, potassium	Yes	Up to 6 units/dl; 1.2-3.6 μg/dl	Infant can be given penicillin directly. Parents should be told to inform physician that infant has been exposed to penicillin because of potential sensitivity.
Pyrimethamine (Daraprim)	Yes	0.3 mg/dl (3% of dose)	Significant in therapeutic doses when infant under 6 months and entirely breast-fed.
Quinine sulfate	Yes	0-0.1 mg/dl after maternal dose of 300-600 mg	In therapeutic doses, no effect on child except rare thrombocytopenia.
Sodium fusidate	Yes	0.2 μg/ml	Not significant in therapeutic doses to affect child.
Streptomycin	Yes	Present for long periods in slight amounts when given as dihydrostreptomycin	Not to be given more than 2 weeks. Ototoxic and nephrotoxic with long use. Is given to infants directly.
Sulfanilamide	Yes	9 mg/dl after dose of 2-4 g/24 hr	Not significant in therapeutic doses; may cause a rash or hemolytic anemia. Should be avoided for first month after delivery.
Sulfapyridine	Yes	3-13 mg/dl after dose of 3 g/24 hr	To be avoided; has caused skin rash.
Sulfathiazole	Yes	0.5 mg/dl after dose of 3 g/24 hr	Not significant in therapeutic doses to affect child after 1 month of age.
Sulfisoxazole (Gantrisin)	Yes	Concentration similar to plasma level	To be avoided during first month after delivery; may cause kernicterus.
Tetracycline HC1 (Achromycin, Panmycin, Sumycin)	Yes	0.5-2.6 μg/ml after dose of 500 mg four times a day	Not enough to treat an infection in an infant. May cause discoloration of the teeth in the infant; the antibiotic, however, may be largely bound to the milk calcium. Do not give longer than 10 days or repeatedly.
Anticoagulants			
Coumarin derivatives Dicumarol (bishydroxycoumarin) Warfarin (Panwarfin)	Yes	Probably little but may be cumulative*	Monitor prothrombin time. Give vitamin K to infant. Discontinue if surgery or trauma occurs. Drug of choice if mother to continue nursing.
Ethyl biscoumacetate (Tromexan)	Yes	0-0.17 mg/dl†	Hemorrhage around umbilical stump and cephalhematoma reported Prothrombin normal in infants with hemorrhage. Vitamin K has no effect. Contraindicated while nursing.
Heparin	No		Heparin ineffective orally.
Phenindione (Hedulin)(Dindevan)	Yes		Breast milk a major route of excretion. Reports of serious hemorrhage in infant. Prothrombin times prolonged in infant. Contraindicated while nursing.
Anticonvulsants and sedatives‡			
Barbital (Veronal)	Yes	8-10 mg/L after 500 mg dose	May produce sedation in infant, in general, barbiturates pass into milk but do not sedate infant. Watch for symptoms.

*Reports conflict.
†No correlation with dosage, continues in milk after plasma clear.
‡All barbitals appear in breast milk.

Continued.

Drug	Excreted in Milk	Amount in Milk After Therapeutic Dose	Effect on Infant
Carbamazepine (Tegretol)	Yes	60% of plasma levels*	Animal studies show lack of weight gain, unkempt appearance.
Chloral hydrate (Noctec, Somnos)	Yes	Up to 1.5 mg/dl	No significant symptoms, can be given to infants directly.
Phenytoin (Dilantin)	Yes	1.5 to 2.6 μg/ml after 300 mg/24 hr dose	One case of hemolytic reaction reported. Other infants appear to tolerate the small doses. Therapeutic plasma level 10-20 μg/ml.
Mephenytoin (Mesantoin)(hydantoin homologue of mephobarbital)	Unknown		Detoxified in liver. No information.
Pentobarbital (Nembutal)	Yes		Depends on liver for detoxification so may accumulate in first week of life until infant is able to detoxify. No problem for older infant in usual doses.
Phenobarbital (Luminal)	Yes	0.1-0.5 mg when plasma level 0.6-1.8 mg	Sleepiness and decreased sucking possible. On usual analeptic doses infants alert and feed well. On hypnotic doses infants depressed and difficult to rouse.
Phensuximide (Milontin)			No specific data.
Primidone (Mysoline)	Yes		Causes drowsiness and decreased feeds. May cause bleeding due to hypoprothrombinemia. Infant needs vitamin K. Avoid drug during lactation.
Sodium bromide (Bromo-Seltzer and across-the-counter sleeping aids)	Yes	Up to 6.6 mg/dl	Drowsy, decreased crying, rash, decreased feeding.
Trimethadione (Tridione)			No specific data.
Antihistaminics Brompheniramine (Dimetane) Diphenhydramine (Benadryl) Methdialzine (Tacaryl) Tripelennamine (Pyribenzamine)	Yes	No specific data available; all pass into milk	Drug is used in neonates. May cause sedation, decreased feeding, or may produce stimulation and tachycardia. Should avoid long-acting preparations, which may accumulate in infant. When combined with decongestants, may cause decrease in milk.
Autonomic drugs			
Atropine sulfate†	Yes	0.1 mg/dl	Hyperthermia, atropine toxicity, infants especially sensitive; also inhibits lactation. Infant dose 0.01 mg/kg.
Carisoprodol (Soma, Rela)	Yes	2-4 times maternal plasma level	Blocks interneuronal activity in descending reticular formation and spinal cord; drowsiness, hypotonia, poor feed.
Ergot (Cafergot)	Yes	Unknown	90% of infants had symptoms of ergotism: vomiting and diarrhea to weak pulse and unstable blood pressure. Short-term therapy for migraine should not exceed 6 mg. Cafergot also contains 100 mg caffeine.
Mepenzolate bromide (Cantil)	No		Postganglionic parasympathetic inhibitor used to diminish gastric acidity and decrease spasm of colon. Oral absorption low.
Methocarbamol (Robaxin)	Yes	Minimum	Too little in milk to produce effect.
Neostigmine	No		No known harm to infant.
Proprantheline bromide (Pro-Banthine)	No	Uncontrolled data indicate no measurable levels	Drug rapidly metabolized in maternal system to inactive metabolite. Mother should avoid long-acting preparations, however.
Scopolamine (Hyoscine)	Yes		Usually given as single dose and of no problem to neonate. No data on repeated doses.
Cardiovascular drugs			
Diazoxide (Hyperstat)			Arteriolar dilators and antihypertensive, only given IV, not active orally.
Dibenzyline‡			No data available

*When plasma 13.0 μmole/L, 7.5 μmole/L in milk.
†Ingredient in many prescription and nonprescription drugs.
‡α-blocking agent.

Drug	Excreted in Milk	Amount in Milk After Therapeutic Dose	Effect on Infant
Digoxin	Yes	0.96-0.61 ng/m*	Dixogin 20% bound to protein; infant receives <1/100 of dose. If mother at toxic level of 5 ng/ml, milk would have a 4.4 ng/ml and infant would receive only 1/20 daily dose.
Guanethidine (Ismelin)†	Yes		Not significant in therapeutic doses to affect child.
Hydralazine (Apresoline)	Yes		Jaundice, thrombocytopenia, electrolyte disturbances possible.
Methyldopa (Aldomet)†	Yes		Galactorrhea. No specific data except as affects mother's milk production.
Propranolol (Inderal)‡	Yes	40 ng/ml of maternal plasma§	Insignificant amount. Infants reported had no symptoms noted. Should watch for hypoglycemia and/or "β-blocking" effects.
Quinidine	Yes		Arrhythmia may occur.
Reserpine (Serpasil)‖	Yes		May produce galactorrhea, lethargy, diarrhea, or nasal stuffiness.
Cathartics			
Aloin	Yes	Low	Occasionally caused colic and diarrhea in infant.
Anthraquinone laxatives such as dihydroxyanthraquinone (Dorbane and Dorbantyl)	Yes	High	Caused colic and diarrhea in infant.
Calomel	No	None	None.
Cascara	Yes	Low	Caused colic and diarrhea in infant.
Milk of magnesia	No	None	No effect.
Mineral oil	No	None	No effect
Phenolphthalein	Unknown	Unknown¶	Reported to cause symptoms in some.
Rhubarb	Unknown	None	None in syrup form. Fresh rhubarb may give symptoms of colic and diarrhea.
Saline cathartics	No	None	No effect.
Senna	No	None	None.
Stool softeners and bulk-forming laxatives	No	None	No effect.
Suppositories (for constipation)	No	None	Not absorbed
Diagnostic materials and procedures			
Barium		No	Not absorbed
Iopanoic acid (Telepaque)	Yes		Not sufficient to produce problem in infant on single dose. Does contain iodine radical.
Radioactive compounds			
Radioactive sodium	Yes	0.5% to 1.3% of dose/L**	Diminished after 24 hr; discontinue nursing 24 hr.
[^{67}Ga] citrate	Yes		Discontinue nursing until ^{67}Ga has cleared, usually 24 hr.
^{125}I, ^{131}I	Yes	M/P = 0.13 μCi/0.002 μCi††	^{131}I content in milk proportional to amount of milk. Most excreted in 24 hr. Discontinue nursing for 48 hr or check milk before resuming feeding if under 48 hr.
^{90}Sr	Yes	M/P = 1/10	Less than in cow's milk. Bottle infant doubles stores in 1 month.
^{99m}Tc	Yes		Reported to clear in 6-22 hr. Discontinue breast-feeding 24 hr. ^{99m}Tc preferentially picked up by breast tissue.

*Peak level occurs 4-6 h after dose given. Maternal plasma level was higher, M/P = 0.9 and 0.8; infant's plasma level was 0.
†Adrenergic blocking agent.
‡β-blocking agent.
§Total daily dose to infant via milk is 15-20 μg.
‖Adrenergic blocking agent.
¶Reports differ.
**Peak in 2 hr; detectable for 96 hr.
††27% of dose in 48 hr.

Continued.

Drug	Excreted in Milk	Amount in Milk After Therapeutic Dose	Effect on Infant
Tuberculin test	No		Tuberculin-sensitive mothers can adoptively immunize their infants through breast milk, and that immunity may last several years.
X-ray films	No		No effect.
Diuretics			
Acetazolamide (Diamox)	Probable	No specific data available but probably similar to sulfonamide	Acts as enzyme inhibitor on carbonic anhydrase nonbacteriostatic sulfonamide. Observe only for dehydration and electrolyte loss by monitoring urine and turgor.
Furosemide (sulfamoylanthranilic acid) (Lasix)	No		Drug is given to children under medical management.
Mercurial diuretics (Dicurin, Thiomerin)	Yes		In addition to diuretic effect, there is risk of mercury deposition. However, drug not absorbed orally.
Spironolactone (Aldactone)	Yes	Canrenone, a metabolite, appears	Acts as antagonist of aldosterone; causes sodium excretion and potassium retention. The metabolite apparently has some activity.
Thiazides (Diuril, Enduron, Esidrix, Hydrodiuril, Oretic, Thiuretic tables)	Yes	>0.1 mg/dl*	Risk of dehydration and electrolyte imbalance, especially sodium loss, which would require monitoring. Watching weight and wet diapers and taking an occasional specific gravity reading of the urine and serum sodium would indicate status of infant. Risk, however, is extremely low, May suppress lactation due to dehydration in mother.
Environmental agents			
Aldrin	Yes	Varies by location	Not a reason to wean from breast. No need to test milk unless inordinate exposure.
Benzene hexachloride (BHC)	Yes	Varies by location	Not a reason to wean from breast. No need to test milk unless inordinate exposure.
Dichlorodiphenyltrichloroethane (DDT or DDE)	Yes	Varies by location	Not a reason to wean from breast. No need to test milk unless inordinate exposure.
Dieldrin	Yes	Varies by location	Also found in permanently mothproofed garments. Avoid these. Not a reason to wean.
Hexachlorobenzene (HCB)	Yes	Varies by location	Not a reason to wean from breast. No need to test milk unless inordinate exposure.
Heptachlorepoxide	Yes	Varies by location	Not a reason to wean from breast. No need to test milk unless inordinate exposure.
Methyl mercury	Yes	500-1,000 ng/ml†	Infant blood level 600 ng/ml in heavy exposure. Only in excessive exposure is testing and/or weaning necessary.
Polybrominated biphenyl (PBB)	Yes	Varies by location	If mother at high risk from the environment or the diet, milk sample should be measured. If level in milk is high, then breast-feeding should be discontinued. Those at risk are (1) workers who handle PBB/PCB and (2) individuals who eat game fish from contaminated waters. Crash diets mobilize fats and should be avoided especially if PBB or PCB present.
Polychlorinated biphenyl (PCB)	Yes	Varies by location	
^{90}Sr, ^{89}Sr (strontium)	Yes	1/10 of that in maternal diet	Cow's milk has six times as much as human milk. Cow's milk-fed infant doubles amount in body in 1 month.
Heavy metals			
Arsenic	Yes	Can be measured for given woman	Can accumulate. Check infant's blood level if there is reason to suspect exposure.
Copper	Yes		
Fluorine	Yes		Monitor for excessive dose.
Gold thiomalate (Myocrisin)	Yes	0.022 μg/ml when mother given 50 mg/week	No proteinuria or aminoaciduria observed

*Linear relationship between plasma and milk. In 1 L of milk at 0.1 mg/dl there would be 1 mg/24 hr. Infant dose is 20 mg/kg/24 hr.
†M/P = 8.6% in heavy exposure.

Continued.

Drug	Excreted in Milk	Amount in Milk After Therapeutic Dose	Effect on Infant
Halothane	Yes	2 ppm	Nursing mothers who work in environment with halothane should be checked.
Iron	Yes		
Lead	Unknown		Nursing contraindicated if maternal serum 40 μg; conflicting reports, breast milk not always cause of lead poisoning in breast-fed infant.
Magnesium	Yes		Not sufficient to be toxic.
Mercury	Yes		Hazardous to infant.
Hormones and contraceptives			
Carbimazole (Neo-Mercazole)	Yes		Antithyroid effect may cause goiter.
Chlorotrianisene (Tace)	Yes		Has estrogenic effect although does not change consistency of milk. May have feminizing effect on infant.
Contraceptives (oral) Ethinyl estradiol Mestranol 19-Nortestosterone Norethindrone (Norlutin) Norethynodrel (Enovid)	Yes		May diminish milk supply. May decrease vitamins, protein, and fat in milk. One author showed no difference when mothers took norethindrone. Most significant concern is long-range impact of hormone on young infant, which is not certain. Reports of feminization of infant.
Corticotropin	Yes		Destroyed in gastrointestinal tract of infant. No effect.
Cortisone	Yes		Animal studies show 50% lower weight than controls and retarded sexual development and exophthalmos.
Dihydrotachysterol (Hytakerol)			May cause hypercalcemia; need monitoring of infant serum and urine calcium.
Epinephrine (Adrenalin)	Yes		Destroyed in GI tract of infant.
Estrogen	Yes	0.17 μg/dl after 1 g	Risks as with oral contraceptives.
Fluoxymesterone (Halotestine, Ora-Testryl, Ultrandren)	Yes		Suppress lactation; masculinizing
Insulin	Unknown		Destroyed in gastrointestinal tract.
Liothyronine (Cytomel)	No		Synthetic form of natural thyroid.
Medroxyprogesterone acetate (Provera)	No		
Phenformin HC1	Yes	Minimum	Not sufficient to cause symptoms in infant. Does not cause hypoglycemia in normal infants. No case reports available.
Prednisone	Yes	0.07-0.23% dose/L after 5 mg dose*	Minimum amount not likely to cause effect on infant in short course.
Pregnanediol	Yes		Unknown risk as with other female hormones over a long period of time.
Tolbutamide (Orinase)	Yes		Not recommended in the childbearing years.
Narcotics			
Codeine		0 to trace after 32 mg every 4 hr (6 doses)	No effect in therapeutic level and transient usage. Can accumulate. Individual variation. Watch for neonatal depression.
Heroin	Yes		13 of 22 infants had withdrawal. Historically breast-feeding had been used to wean addict's infant. This is no longer recommended.
Marijuana *(Cannabis)*	Yes		Shown in laboratory animals to produce structural changes in nursling's brain cells; impairs DNA and RNA formation. Infant at risk of inhaling smoke during feeding or when held by person who is smoking.
Meperidine (Demerol)	Yes	>0.1 mg/dl†	Trace amounts may accumulate if drug taken around the clock when infant is neonate. Watch for drowsiness and poor feeding

*0.16 μg/ml after 10 mg dose; 2.67 μg/ml after 2 hr.
†Plasma 0.07-0.1 mg/dl.

Continued.

Drug	Excreted in Milk	Amount in Milk After Therapeutic Dose	Effect on Infant
Methadone	Yes	0.03 μg/ml or 0.023-0.028 mg/24 hr*	When dosage not excessive, infant can be breast-fed if monitored for evidence of depression and failure to thrive.
Morphine	Yes	Trace	Single doses have minimum effect. Potential for accumulation. May be addicting to neonate. Breast feeding no longer considered appropriate means of weaning infant of an addict.
Percodan (oxycodone [derived from opiate thebaine] aspirin, phenacetin, caffeine)	Yes		Consider for its component parts. In neonatal period sleepiness and failure to feed, which increase maternal engorgement and neonatal weight loss, have been observed, probably caused by oxycodone.
Psychotropic and mood-changing drugs			
Alcohol	Yes	Similar to plasma level	Ordinarily no problem and can be therapeutic in moderation, infants are more susceptible to effects. Chronic drinking reported to cause obesity in infant. Ethanol in doses of 1-2 g/kg to mother causes depression of milk-ejection reflex (dose dependent). No acetaldehyde found in infants.
Amphetamine	Yes		Has caused stimulation in infants with jitteriness, irritability, sleeplessness. Long-acting preparations cumulative.
Benzodiazepines† Chlordiazepoxide HC1 (Librium)	Yes		Not sufficient to affect infant first week when glucuronyl system needed for detoxification. May accumulate. Older infant, no apparent problem.
Diazepam (Valium)	Yes	90 μg/L‡	Detoxified in glucuronyl system. In first weeks of life may contribute to jaundice. Metabolite active. Effect on infant: hypoventilation, drowsiness, lethargy, and weight loss. Single doses over 10 mg contraindicated during nursing. Accumulation in infant possible.
Pineazepam	Yes	Metabolite, 5-11.2 ng/ml; pineazepam, >1.0 ng/ml§	No data, probably similar to diazepam.
Haloperidol (Haldol)	Yes	Unknown	A butyrophenone antidepressant; animal studies in nurslings show behavior abnormalities.
Lithium carbonate (Eskalith, Lithane, Lithonate)	Yes	⅓-½ maternal plasma level‖	Measurable lithium in infant's serum. Infant kidney can clear lithium; however, lithium inhibits adenosine 3′:5:-cyclic monophosphate, significant for brain growth. Also affects amine metabolism. Real effects not measurable immediately. Report of cyanosis and poor muscle tone and ECG changes in nursing infant.
Monomine oxidate (MAO) inhibitors (Eutonyl, Nardil)			Inhibits lactation.
Meprobamate (Miltown, Equanil)	Yes	2-4 times maternal plasma level	If therapy continued, infant should be followed closely.
Penfluridol¶	Yes	Unknown	Animal studies show learning abnormalities in sucklings. This is a potent long-acting oral neuroleptic drug.
Phenothiazines Chlorpromazine (Thorazine)	Yes	⅓ plasma level**	Can be safely nursed; minimum in milk. Increase maternal prolactin. No symptoms in infants reported; 5-year follow-up showed infants normal.
Mesoridazine (Serentil)	Yes	Minimum	
Piperacetazine (Quide)	Yes	Minimum	Probably no effect

*Mother received 50 mg/24 hr; M/P = 0.83. Peak level 4 hr after oral dose. Results obscured if addict also taking the herbal root golden seal.
†Alcohol enhances effect of this group.
‡10 mg or less yields 45 mg of diazepam/ml and 85 ng of metabolite/ml. P/M ratio is variable. Mean P/M ratio of diazepam is 6.14; of metabolite is 3.64. Effect lasts about 4 days.
§Both drug and active metabolite appear for about 4 days after dose.
‖0.030 mmol/L in infant's serum, 0.57 mmole/L in infant's urine. Milk level was half of maternal serum level in one case report.
¶Neuroleptic drug.
**If dose <200 mg, milk contains bare trace. Dose of 1200 mg showed trace.

Drug	Excreted in Milk	Amount in Milk After Therapeutic Dose	Effect on Infant
Thioridazine (Mellaril)	Yes	No information	Thioridazine is less potent in general than other phenothiazines. Probably quite safe.
Trifluoperazine (Stelazine)	Yes	Minimum	
Tricyclic antidepressants	Yes		Apparently no accumulation. No infants that have been observed showed symptoms. Watch for depression or failure to feed. Increase maternal prolactin secretion.
Amitriptyline HC1 (Elavil)	Yes	Minimum amounts	
Desipramine HC1 (Norpramin, Pertofrane)		Minimum amounts	
Imipramine HC1 (Tofranil)	Yes	0.1 mg/dl*	
Stimulants			
Caffeine	Yes	1% of dose	Accumulates when intake moderate and continual . Causes jitteriness, wakefulness, and irritability. Caffeine present in may hot and cold drinks. Consider if infant very wakeful.
Theobromine	Yes	3.7-8.2 mg/L after 240 mg dose†	No adverse symptoms observed in the infants. Chocolate most common cause of exposure.
Theophylline	Yes	10% of maternal dose‡	Irritability, fretfulness.
Thyroid and antithyroid medications			
Carbimazole (Neo-Mercazole)	Yes		May cause goiter.
Methimazole (Tapazole)	Yes	M/P >1	Inhibits synthesis of thyroid hormone but does not inactivate existing thyroid. Can inhibit infant thyroid. ⅛ grain/day of thyroid can be given to infant simultaneously.
Potassium iodide	Yes	3 mg/dl§	May alter thyroid function of infant; may cause goiter in infant.
Propylthiouracil	Yes	0.077% of dose	Risk of goiter and agranulocytosis. With present microtechniques for T_3, T_4 and TSH, close monitoring of infant is possible, as with methimazole.
Radioactive iodine ^{125}I, ^{131}I (as a treatment)	Yes	M/P >1	*Treatment* doses are excreted via the breast for 1-3 weeks. Milk can be checked by Geiger counter if there is a question. Breast feeding should be discontinued until milk is clear.
Thiouracil	Yes	9-12 mg/d‖	Same as for propylthiouracil
Thyroid and thyroxine	Yes		Does not produce adverse symptoms on long-range follow-up. Noted to improve milk supply of hypothyroid mothers. No contraindication.
Miscellaneous			
Cyclophosphamide	Yes	Present¶	Antineoplastic agent. Any amounts contraindicated.
DPT	Yes	Minimum	Does not interfere with immunization schedule.
Methotrexate	Yes	Minor route of excretion: M/P = 0.08/1.0	Antimetabolite. Infant would receive 0.26 μg/dl, which researchers consider nontoxic for infant.
Nicotine	Yes	Mean 91 ppb (20-512 ppb)**	Decreases milk production. No apparent effect on infant—perhaps a tolerance is developed in utero. Smoking may interfere with let-down reflex if smoking started before onset of a feeding.
Poliovirus vaccine	No		Live vaccine taken orally. Not necessary to withhold nursing 30 min before and after dose. Provide booster after infant no longer nursing.
Rh antibodies	Yes		Destroyed in gastrointestinal tract; not effective orally.
Rubella virus vaccine	Yes	Minimum	Will not confer passive immunity. Mother should not be given vaccine when at risk for pregnancy.
Smallpox vaccine	No		Exposure is by direct contact. Live virus. No longer given.

*Plasma level 0.2-1.3 mg/dl.
†113 g chocolate bar.
‡M/P = 0.7.
§Dose was 325-650 mg three times a day.
‖Maternal plasma level was 3.4 mg/dl after a 1 g dose; M/P = 3.
¶Single 500 mg IV dose in milk at 1,3,5, and 6 h after injection.
**At ½-1½ packs/day. Large variation from single donor.

APPENDIX J

Recommended Schedule for Active Immunization of Normal Infants and Children

Recommended Age	Immunization(s)	Comments
2 months	DTP,[1] OPV[2]	Can be initiated as early as 2 weeks of age in areas of high endemicity or during epidemics
4 months	DTP,OPV	2-month interval desired for OPV to avoid interference from previous dose
6 months	DTP (OPV)	OPV is optional (may be given in areas with increased risk of polio exposure)
15 months	Measles, mumps, rubella, (MMR)[3]	MMR preferred to individual vaccines; tuberculin testing may be done
18 months	DTP,[4,5] OPV[5]	
24 months	HBPV[6]	
4-6 years[7]	DTP,OPV	At or before school entry
14-16 years	Td[8]	Repeat every 10 years throughout life

From American Academy of Pediatrics: Report of the Committee on Infectious Diseases, III., ed. 20, 1986. Copyright American Academy of Pediatrics, 1986.

[1]DTP—Diptheria and tetanus toxoids with pertussis vaccine.

[2]OPV—Oral, poliovirus vaccine contains attenuated poliovirus types 1,2, and 3.

[3]MMR—Live measles, mumps, and rubella viruses in a combined vaccine.

[4]Should be given 6 to 12 months after the third dose.

[5]May be given simultaneously with MMR at 15 months of age.

[6]Haemophilus b polysaccharide vaccine.

[7]Up to the seventh birthday.

[8]Td—Adult tetanus toxoid (full dose) and diptheria toxoid (reduced dose) in combination.

APPENDIX K

Resources

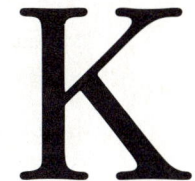

This appendix contains the following resources:
Audiovisual materials/computer assisted instruction (CAI)
Community and national resources
Nursing organizations
National clearinghouses
Nursing journals

AUDIOVISUAL MATERIALS/COMPUTER ASSISTED INSTRUCTED (CAI)

Nursing Perspectives

Patient Advocacy in Nursing Practice
Career Aids, Inc.

Problem-Oriented Medical Record
American Journal of Nursing Co.

Nursing Care Plans
American Journal of Nursing Co.

Nurse, Ethics and the Law
Trainex

Medical-Ethical Legal Issues (includes issues on amniocentesis and surrogate mothering)
American Journal of Nursing Co.

Cultural Psychosocial, and Biologic Aspects of Human Sexuality

Human Reproduction: Male and Female Anatomy and Conception
Career Aids, Inc.

Reproduction
Career Aids, Inc.

Memories of Family (family relationships)
Polymorph Films

Heredity, Health and Genetic Disorders
Ibis Media

Genetics: Fundamental Principles
Career Aids, Inc.

Heredity, Health and Genetic Disorders
Career Aids, Inc.

Hormones and Chromosomes in Man
Prentice-Hall Media

Infertility
Trainex

The Gynecologic Exam
American Journal of Nursing Co.

Birth Control—Update
Trainex

The Pill and IUD
Cinema Medica

The Normal Prenatal Period

Fetal and Maternal Development: From Conception to Birth
Career Aids, Inc.

Fetal Development
Trainex

The First Days of Life (development inside the woman; by fiberoptic photography)
Cinema Medica

Pregnancy
Career Aids, Inc.

First Trimester—9 Months to Motherhood
Second Trimester—6 Months to Motherhood
Third Trimester—3 Months to Motherhood
Trainex

Pregnancy: Maternal Body Changes and Stresses
Career Aids, Inc.

Emotional Changes and Sexuality in Pregnancy and Postpartum
Career Aids, Inc.

Pregnant Fathers
Joseph T. Anzalone Foundation

Fathers
American Society for Psychoprophylaxis in Obstetrics

Nicholas and the Baby
Centre Productions, Inc.

A Shared Beginning (Lamaze)
Judy Christiansen

The Ties That Bind (portrays how relationships between parent and infant are experienced in pregnancy and during and immediately after birth; discusses bonding to a premature infant; discusses needs of the newborn's older siblings)
Polymorph Films

Drugs During Pregnancy: Are Any Really Safe?
University of Michigan

Building a Healthy Baby: The First Trimester
Robert J. Brady Co.

Prenatal Care: Months Four through Nine
Robert J. Brady Co.

Prenatal Care
Pyramid Films

Prenatal Exam: General, Obstetrical and Fetal Assessment
Career Aids, Inc.

Minor Discomforts of Pregnancy: Prevention and Relief
Career Aids, Inc.

Assessment of the Pregnant Abdomen
American Journal of Nursing Co.

Nutrition in Pregnancy
Cinema Medica

Nutrition During Pregnancy for Mother and Child
Career Aids, Inc.

Great Expectations (nutrition during pregnancy and lactation)
Society for Nutrition Education

Preparing for Easier Childbirth
Career Aids, Inc.

Prenatal Exercises and Body Conditioning
Career Aids, Inc.

Introduction to Prepared Childbirth
Trainex

Essential Exercises for the Childbearing Year
Polymorph Films

Normal Childbirth

Process of Labor and Delivery: Anatomy and Physiology
Career Aids, Inc.

Labor
Trainex

Decisions—The Patient in Labor
Trainex

Labor and Delivery
Trainex

Not Me Alone
Polymorph Films

Childbirth
Career Aids, Inc.

The Labor-Delivery Series
Career Aids, Inc.

A Shared Beginning (Lamaze)
Judy Christiansen

The Story of Eric (Lamaze)
Centre Films

Gentle Birth (Leboyer)
Polymorph Films

Birth in the Squatting Position
Polymorph Films

Modern Obstetrics: Normal Delivery
Wexler Film Productions

Delivery
Trainex

Childbirth for the Joy of It: Part II
Cinema Medica

Human Birth Film (seven birth presentations)
J.B. Lippincott Co.

Second State: Giving Birth
BABES

Decisions—The Patient After Delivery
Trainex

Care of the Newborn: Forces of Labor and Fetal Heart Rate Monitoring
Trainex

Recognition of Fetal Distress
Career Aids, Inc.

Fetal Monitoring
BABES

Anesthesia for Delivery
J.B. Lippincott Co.

Alternative settings for childbirth

Happy Birthday (birth in homelike hospital setting)
Cinema Medica

Birth Centers
Cinema Medica

Children at Birth (birth in hospital and home settings)
Cinema Medica

Primum Non Nocere (natural childbirth at home)
Cinema Medica

Alternative Childbirth (all the choices in childbirth available today: hospital, birth center, and attended and unattended home births)
Cinema Medica

Not by Chance (realistic home birth)
Cinema Medica

Five Women Five Births (choices in childbirth)
Davidson Films, Inc.

Nicholas and the Baby (family-centered childbirth)
American Journal of Nursing Co.

And Then There Were Four (homelike birth in a hospital setting)
Barias/Walker Associates

Together, with Love (birthing room)
Centre Films, Inc.

Welcome, Emily! (birthroom, midwife)
Diane Gant

The Normal Newborn

Nursing Care of the Newborn: Circulation of the Fetus and Transitional Circulation of the Newborn
Trainex

Amazing Newborn (behavioral development already present at birth)
Polymorph Films

Nursing Care of the Newborn: Assessing Cardiac Status
Trainex

Nursing Care of the Newborn: Physical Exam of the Newborn
Trainex

From Birth to One Month: Physical Assessment
Health Media Corp.

From Birth to One Month: Nursing Assessment
Health Media Corp.

Appraisal of the Newborn
American Journal of Nursing Co.

Dubowitz Assessment of Newborn Gestational Age
Polymorph Films

Assessment of Neonatal Transition
Career Aids, Inc.

Introduction to Newborn Nursing
Health Media Corp.

First 12 Hours
Health Media Corp.

Thermal Environment of the Neonate
University of Michigan

Prevention of Neonatal Cold Injury
Career Aids, Inc.

Newborn nutrition and feeding

Breastfeeding: A Special Closeness (includes specific problems such as sexuality, working mothers, male attitudes, breastfeeding in public)
American Journal of Nursing Co.

Breastfeeding: A Practical Guide
American Journal of Nursing Co.

Aspects in Maternal Care: Development and Function of the Breast and Highlights in the Care of the Nursing Mother
Trainex

Breastfeeding Your Baby
Trainex

Breastfeeding: Prenatal and Postpartal Preparation
Polymorph Films

Learning to Breastfeed
Polymorph Films

Breastfeeding for the Joy of It
Cinema Medica

Talking About Breastfeeding (breast-feeding in spite of obstacles)
Polymorph Films

Breastfeeding, A Special Love
"Questions, Father's Role," 22 min
"Breastmilk," 16 min
"Art of Breastfeeding," 23 min
Medirec

Bottlefeeding Your Baby
Trainex

First Foods
"Essential Nutrients for Babies and How to Supply Them"
"When and How to Introduce Semi-solid Foods"
"How to Safely and Economically Prepare Baby Foods at Home"
"How to Select and Use Commercial Baby Foods"
Society for Nutrition Education

The Normal Postdelivery Period

Postpartum Care 207
Trainex

Postpartum Period
Career Aids, Inc.

Emotional Changes and Sexuality in Pregnancy and Postpartum
Career Aids, Inc.

Now That You're Postpartum (physical changes, importance of outside help and support, emotional closeness)
Polymorph Films

Family Bonding: Pregnancy, Birth and the First Hours
Career Aids, Inc.

Birth and Bonding
Career Aids, Inc.

The Nurturing Father
Career Aids, Inc.

Family Following Childbirth
Trainex

Make Room for Dad
Trainex

Adapting to Parenthood
Polymorph Films

The Ties That Bind (relationships between parent and infant during pregnancy, during and after birth)
Polymorph Films

Nicholas and the Baby
Centre Productions, Inc.

Help, I'm a New Parent
Fathers
Making Decisions About Sex
Churchill Films

2 A.M. Feeding (transition into parenting) film
New Day

High-Risk Pregnancy

High-risk mothers and newborns

Babies and Special Considerations (basic care of high-risk infant)
Career Aids, Inc.

Pregnancy After 35
Polymorph Films

Patients at Risk of Delivering Low Birth Weight Infants
University of Michigan

Prematurity

Immediate Care of the Preterm Infant
University of Michigan

Care of the Preterm Infant
University of Michigan

Nutrition for the Low Birth Weight Infant
University of Michigan

Respiratory Problems of the Newborn
Health Media Corp.

Respiratory Distress Syndrome
University of Michigan

Age Minus 60 Days
Bandera Enterprises

Loss and Grief

Death and Dying
Trainex

When a Baby Dies
Career Aids, Inc.

Death of a Newborn (grieving process, support of medical staff)
Polymorph Films

Discussion with Parents of a Malformed Baby
Polymorph Films

Discussions with Parents of Premature Infants
Polymorph Films

Prematurity: Emotional Aspects

Mothers and the Premature Baby
Trainex

Premature Infants—The 7% Dilemma
Trainex

Prematurely Yours (premature infant behavior and personality)
Polymorph Films

To Have and Not to Hold (helping parents of prematures cope)
Polymorph Films

The Role of Parents (emotional needs of parents of preterm infants)
University of Michigan

Complications

Deviations from the Normal Progress of Pregnancy
University of Michigan

Complications of Pregnancy
Trainex

Modern Obstetrics: Pre-eclampsia, Eclampsia
Wexler Film Productions

Modern Obstetrics: Postpartum Hemorrhage
Wexler Film Productions

Shock: The Final Pathology
American Journal of Nursing Co.

Introduction to Shock
Trainex

Hypovolemic Shock
Trainex

Hypertension During Pregnancy (pregnancy-induced hypertension and chronic hypertension)
University of Michigan

Management of the Postdate Pregnancy
University of Michigan

Diabetes in Pregnancy
University of Michigan

Prevention and Identification of Premature Labor
University of Michigan

Management of Premature Labor
University of Michigan

Nutritional Management of the High Risk Pregnancy
Society for Nutrition Education

Complications of Labor—Diagnostic Testing
Trainex

Diagnostic Amniocentesis
University of Michigan

Disorders of the Female Reproductive System—Complications of Labor. On Rounds in Obstetrics—Dystocia: An Overview
Trainex

Disorders of the Female Reproductive System and Complications of Labor: A Trial of Labor
Trainex

Newborn Complications

Jaundice in the Newborn
The Neurogically Suspect Infant
Anemia in the Newborn
Respiratory Distress Syndrome
Hypoglycemia in the Newborn
Health Media Corp.

Neurological Insults in the Neonate
Career Aids, Inc.

Adolescent Parenthood

Teenage Pregnancy and Prevention
"Part I: The Problem"
"Part II: the Choices"
"Part III: The Solutions"
Ibis Media

When Teens Get Pregnant (emotional aspects)
Polymorph Films

Teens Having Babies (care of the pregnant teenager)
Polymorph Films

Sociocultural Risk Factors

Drugs, Smoking, and Alcohol During Pregnancy
Polymorph Films

Should RN's Initiate Change in Nursing Practice in Poverty Areas?
American Journal of Nursing Co.

Cesarean Birth

Complications of Labor—Cesarean Section: A Surgical Alternative
Trainex

Cesarean Childbirth (family centered)
Cinema Medica

Birth by Cesarean (includes diagnostic testing)
Career Aids, Inc.

Deliverance: A Family's Cesarean Experience
Polymorph Films

Having A Section Is Having a Baby (all aspects of a cesarean delivery)
Polymorph Films

A Shared Cesarean Beginning (emphasizes father's involvement)
Judy Christiansen

Cesarean Bonding Experience
Tri-County Cesarean Parents Association

ADDRESSES FOR ORDERING

American Academy of Husband-Coached Childbirth (AAHCC)
P.O. Box 5224
Sherman Oaks, CA 91413
(213) 788-6662, (800) 423-2397 (outside California)

American Journal of Nursing Company
AJN Company Rental Library
% USCAN International
110 West Hubbard St.
Chicago, IL 60610
(312) 828-1146

The American Society for Psychoprophylaxis in Obstetrics (ASPO)
33429 Farragut Station
Washington, DC 20033
(202) 783-7050

Joseph T. Anzalone Foundation
P.O. Box 5206
Santa Cruz, CA 95063

BABES (Bay Area Birth Education Series)
% Deanna Sollid
59 Berens Dr.
Kentfield, CA 94907

Bandera Enterprises
P.O. Box 1107
Studio City, CA

Burias/Walker Associates
15 Lacosta Dr.
Natick, MA 01760
(617) 893-3553

Robert J. Brady Co. (A Prentice-Hall Co.)
Bowie, MD 20715
(301) 262-6300 or (800) 638-0220

Career Aids, Inc.
8950 Lureine Ave. Dept. P8
Chatsworth, CA 91131

Centre Films, Inc.
1103 N. El Centro Ave.
Hollywood, CA 90038
(213) 466-5123

Centre Productions, Inc.
1312 Pine St.
Suite 4
Boulder, CO 80302

Childbirth Graphics, Ltd.
1210 Culver Rd.
Rochester, NY 14609
(716) 482-7940

Judy Christiansen
2068 Cynthia Way
Los Altos, CA 94022
(415) 961-6692

Churchill Films
662 N. Robertson Blvd.
Los Angeles, CA 90069
(213) 657-5110

Cinema Medica
2335 West Foster Ave.
Chicago, IL 60625
(800) 621-5147
In Illinois, call collect (312) 784-7686

Davidson Films, Inc.
850 O'Neill Ave.
Belmont, CA 94002
(415) 591-8319

Diane Gent
445 South Green Rd.
South Euclid, OH 44121
(216) 561-6281

Health Media Corp.
P.O. Box 167
Tulsa, OK 74101
(918) 743-9777

Ibis Media
Box 308
Pleasantville, NY 10570

J.B. Lippincott Co.
East Washington Square
Philadelphia, PA 19105

Mead Johnson
Nutritional Division
2404 W. Pennsylvania St.
Evansville, IN 46285

Medirec
4731 S. State St.
Murray, UT 84107
(801) 266-1114

The C.V. Mosby Co.
11830 Westline Industrial Dr.
St. Louis, MO. 63146

New Day Films
P.O. Box 315
Franklin Lakes, NJ 07417
(201) 891-8240

Merrell-National Laboratories
Division of Richardson-Merrell
Cincinnati, OH 45215
Offers informational publications regarding vaginal conditions and therapy and free loan of films such as "Vaginitis" and "Laparoscopy: The View Within."

Polymorph Films
118 South St.
Boston, MA 02111
(617) 542-2004

Prentice-Hall Media
Serv Code BT ABC
150 White Plains Rd.
Tarrytown, NY 10591

Pyramid Films
Box 1048
Santa Monica, CA 90406
(213) 828-7577

Marjorie Pyle, RNC
Lifecircle
2378 Cornell Dr.
Costa Mesa, CA 92626

Ross Laboratories
Division Abbott Laboratories
Creative Services and Information
625 N. Cleveland Ave.
Columbus, OH 43216
Offers informational publications in several languages regarding nutrition for pregnant women and newborns and free loan of films such as "Amazing Newborn" and "Death of a Newborn."

Society for Nutrition Education
1736 Franklin St.
Oakland, CA 94612

Trainex
P.O. Box 116
Garden Grove, CA 92642
(800) 854-2485, (800) 472-2479 in California
(714) 898-2561 in Canada (collect)
telex: 68:5595
slides/cassettes, filmstrips/cassettes
price: 1 ato 4, $110 each
5 or more, $100 each
rental $20

Tri-County Cesarean Parents Association
℅ Joan M. Possiel
1 St. James Rd.
Budd Lake, NJ 07828

Media Library,
University of Michigan Medical Center
R4440 Kresge I, Box 56
Ann Arbor, MI 48109
(313) 763-2074

Wexler Film Production
801 N. Seward St.
Los Angeles, CA 90038

Wyeth Laboratories
P.O. Box 8299
Philadelphia, PA 19101

COMMUNITY AND NATIONAL RESOURCES

Online Computer Services

BRS Information Technologies
1200 Route 7
Latham, NY 12110
(800) 833-4707; (518) 583-1161

DIALOG Information Services, Inc.
3460 Hillview Avenue
Palo Alto, CA 94304
(800) 982-5838; (800) 227-1927; (415) 858-2700

National Library of Medicine
MEDLARS Management Section
Bldg 38A, Room 4N-421
8600 Rockville Pike
Bethesda, MD 20894
(800) 638-8480; (301) 496-6193

Agencies

AASK (Aid to the Adoption of Special Kids)
3530 Grand Avenue
Oakland, CA 94610
(415) 451-1748

AIDS Medical Foundation
10 East 13th Street, Suite LD
New York, NY 10003
(212) 206-0670

Al-Anon/Alateen
P.O. 862
Midtown Station
New York, NY 10018
(212) 254-7230

Alcoholics Anonymous
P.O. Box 459
Grand Central Station
New York, NY 10017
(212) 686-1100

American Academy of Husband-Coached Childbirth
P.O. Box 5224
Sherman Oaks, CA 91413
(818) 788-6662
Teaches Robert A. Bradley's method of "Husband-Coached Childbirth," an offshoot of Grantly Dick-Read's method.

American Academy of Pediatrics
Publications Dept.
P.O. Box 927
Elk Grove, IL 60009-0927
(312) 869-9327
Provides literature for families, parents, and health profession groups related to child health, illness, and welfare.

American Cancer Society
90 Park Avenue
New York, NY 10016
(212) 736-3030
Provided brochures on Papanicolaou (Pap) smears, smoking during pregnancy, and breast self-examination.

American Cleft Palate Association
331 Salk Hall
Pittsburgh, PA 15261
(412) 681-9620

American College of Obstetricians and Gynecologists
600 Maryland Avenue, SW
Suite 300 East
Washington, DC 20024
(202) 638-5577
Provides extensive lists of publications and resources.

American Dietetic Association
430 N. Michigan Ave.
Chicago, IL 60611

American Fertility Foundation
2131 Magnolia Avenue
Suite 201
Birmingham, Al 35256
(205) 251-9764

American Foundation for Maternal and Child Health, Inc.
(research on the perinatal period)
30 Beekman Place
New York, NY 10022
(212) 759-5510

American Heart Association
7320 Greenville Avenue
Dallas, TX 75231
(214) 750-5300

American Hospital Association
Dept. of Order Processing
840 N. Lakeshore Dr.
Chicago, IL 60611

American Institute of Family Relations
4942 Vineland Ave.
North Hollywood, CA 91601

American Medical Association
535 North Dearborn Street
Chicago, IL 60610
(312) 645-5000

American Red Cross
17th and E Streets
Washington, DC 20006
(202) 737-8300

American Society for Deaf People
814 Thayer Avenue
Silver Springs, MD 20910
(301) 585-5400

American Society for Psychoprophylaxis in Obstetrics (ASPO)
1840 Wilson Blvd.
Suite 204
Arlington, VA 22201
(703) 524-7802
Teaches Lamaze technique of prepared childbirth to interested couples; prepares qualified people for teaching this method. Offers brochures, publications, teaching materials, and audiovisual aids.

Association for the Aid of Crippled Children
345 East 46th St.
New York, NY 10017
Devoted to the prevention of crippling diseases and conditions and to improvement in the care of disabled children and youth and their adjustment in society.

Association of Birth Defects in Children
3201 E. Crystal Lake Ave.
Orlando, FL 32806

Association for Childbirth at Home, International
P.O. Box 39498
Los Angeles, CA 90039
(213) 667-0839
See also Childbirth

Association of Voluntary Sterilization, Inc. (AVS)
(provides information on sterilization and referral service)
122 E. 42nd
New York, NY 10168
(212) 351-2500

Boston Women's Health Book Collective
47 Nichols Avenue
Watertown, MA 02172
(617) 921-0271

Canadian Institute of Child Health
410 Laurier Avenue
Suite 803
West Ottawa, Ont. KIR 7T6

Centers for Disease Control
1600 Clifton Road, N.E.
Atlanta, GA 30333
(404) 329-1819 (404) 329-3286

Center for the Study of Multiple Birth
333 East Superior Street
Suite 463-5
Chicago, IL 60611
(312) 266-9093

Channing L. Bete Co., Inc.
Greenfield, MA 01301
Publishes material regarding childbearing in cartoon form.

Child Study Association of America
9 East 89th St.
New York, NY 10028
Provides parent education materials.

Compassionate Friends
(Following death of an infant)
P.O. Box 1347
Oak Brook, IL 60521
(312) 990-0010

COPE (Coping with the Overall Pregnancy/Parenting Experience)
37 Clarendon Street
Boston, MA 02116
(617) 357-5588

C/SEC, Inc. (Cesarean/Support Education and Concern)
22 Forest Road
Framingham, MA 01701
(617) 877-8266

Department DES
National Cancer Institute
Office of Cancer Communications
Bldg. 31, Room 10A19
Bethesda, MD 20892
(800) 4-CANCER

Ed-U-Press
760 Ostrum Ave.
Syracuse, NY 13210
Offers series of excellent cartoon books for adolescents and parenting classes.

Educational and Scientific Plastics, Ltd.
76 Holmethorpe Ave.
Holmethorpe, Red Hill Surrey, RH1, 2PF, England
Offers numerous plastic models.

Endometriosis Association
238 West Wisconsin Avenue
P.O. Box 92187
Milwaukee, WI 53202
(414) 962-8972

Environmental Protection Agency (EPA)
Public Information Center
Room PM 211-B
401 M Street, SW
Washington, DC 20460
(202) 382-7550

Equal Rights for Fathers
P.O. Box 90042
San Jose, CA 95109-3042
(415) 848-2323

Family Research in Health Care
National Council on Family Relations
1910 W. County Road B.
Suite 147
St. Paul, MN 55113
(612) 633-6933

Family Service Association of America
11700 Westlake Park Drive
Milwaukee, WI 53223
(414) 359-2111

Fertility Research Foundation (FRF)
1430 Second Avenue
Suite 103
New York, NY 10021
(212) 744-5500

Florence Crittenton Association of America
608 South Dearborn St.
Chicago, IL 60605
Unites in forming an effective and continuing organization; develops and maintains standards of service; in general, assists in bringing about a greater understanding of factors relating to unmarried mothers and adolescent girls with other problems in adjustment.

Hazardous Waste Hotline
(800) 424-9346

Heart Information Center
National Heart Institute
U.S. Public Health Service
9000 Rockville Pike
Bldg 31, Room 4A21
Bethesda, MD 20892

Home Oriented Maternity Experience (HOME)
511 New York Ave.
Takoma Park, MD 20012

International Childbirth Education Association (ICEA)
P.O. Box 20048
Milwaukee, WI 55420
Assists individuals and childbirth groups who are interested in family-centered maternity: film and record directory, books and pamphlets and an annotated catalogue of resources.

La Leche League International, Inc.
9615 Minneapolis Ave.
Franklin Park, IL 60131
(312) 455-7730
Provides support and brochures for nursing mothers and pattern for making a baby carrier.

Maternal Health Society
Box 46563, Station G
Vancouver, B.C. V6R 4G8

Maternity Center Association, Inc.
48 East 92nd St.
New York, NY 10028
(212) 269-7300
Publishes free brochure describing their many publications and pattern for knitted uterus.

Medic-Alert Foundation International
2323 Colorado Ave.
Turlock, CA 95380

National Abortion Rights Action League
1101 14th Street, NW
Washington, DC 20005
(202) 371-9779
Pro-choice political action group

National American Diabetes Association
1660 Duke Street
Alexandria, VA 22314
(703) 549-1500

Nurses Association of the American College of Obstetricians and Gynecologists
409 12th Street, SW
Washington, DC 20024-2191
(202) 638-0026

National Association of Childbirth Education, Inc. (NACE)
3940 Eleventh St.
Riverside, CA 92501

National Association for Down's Syndrome (NADS)
1800 Dempster
Park Ridge, IL 60068-1146
(312) 823-7550

National Association of Parents and Professionals for Safe Alternatives in Childbirth (NAPSAC)
P.O. Box 267
Marble Hill, MO 63764
(314) 238-2010

National Center on Child Abuse
Office of Child Development
P.O. Box 1182
Washington, DC 20013
(703) 821-2086

National Center for Education in Maternal and Child Health
38th and R Streets, NW
Washington, DC 20057
(202) 625-8400

National Center for Health Statistics (NCHS)
Scientific and Technical Information Branch
Department of Health and Human Services
3700 East-West Highway
Room 1-57
Hyattsville, MD 20782
(301) 436-8500
Source of vital and health statistics for the United States

National Childbirth Trust
9 Queensborough Terrace
London, W2, England
Offers books, films, and other aids for use in classes or in labor.

National Conference of Catholic Charities
1346 Connecticut
Washington, DC 20036
Gives particular emphasis to service for children and youth; i.e., foster care, counseling (unmarried parents), adoption services (statewide), short-term counseling to families and youth, emergency material assistance.

National Foundation/March of Dimes
1275 Mamaroneck Ave.
White Plains, NY 10605
(914) 428-7100
Publishes a directory of genetic services. It is involved in professional education, as well as research on genetic defects. The Foundation also sponsors programs for purchase of teaching and disseminating information to the general public.

National Foundation for Jewish Genetic Diseases, Inc.
250 Park Ave., Suite 1000
New York, NY 10177

National Genetics Foundation
555 W. 57th St.
New York, NY 10019

National Institute of Child Health and Human Development (NICHD)
National Institutes of Health
9000 Rockville Pike
Bldg 31, Room 2A32
Bethesda, MD 20892
(301) 496-4000

National Institute of Environmental Health Sciences
P.O. Box 12233
Research Triangle Park, NC 27709
(919) 541-3345
See also Occupational Health

National Institutes of Marriage & Family Relations
6116 Rolling Rd., Suite 316
Springfield, VA 22152

National Library of Medicine (NLM)
Public Information Office
8600 Rockville Pike
Bethesda, MD 20894
(301) 496-6308
Source for biomedical information and indexes of Journal and research literature related to biomedical fields.

National Mental Health Association
1021 Prince St.
Alexandria, VA 22341-2971

National Organization of Mothers of Twins Clubs, Inc.
12404 Princess Jeanne, NE
Albuquerque, NM 87112
(505) 275-0955

National Rehabilitation Association
633 S. Washington St.
Alexandria, VA 22314

National Right to Life Committee
419 7th Street, NW
Suite 402
Washington, DC 20004
(202) 626-8800
Pro-life political action group.

National Safety Council
444 N. Michigan Ave.
Chicago, IL 60611

National Sudden Infant Death Syndrome Foundation
2320 Glenview Road
Glenview, IL 60025
(312) 657-8080

National Women's Health Network
224 Seventh Street, SE
Washington, DC 20003
(202) 543-9222

Parenthood After Thirty
451 Vermont
Berkeley, CA 94707
(415) 524-6635

Parents of Prematures
℅ Houston Organization for Parent Education, Inc.
2990 Richmond
Suite 204
Houston, TX 77098
(713) 524-3089

Parents Without Partners
8807 Colesville Road
Silver Spring, MD 20910
(301) 588-9354

Patient Counseling Library
Budlong Press Co.
5428 N. Virginia Ave.
Chicago, IL, 60625
(212) 541-7800
Provides videotapes (e.g., "A doctor discusses. . . ") suitable for clinics or waiting rooms covering topics such as pregnancy, infant care, sexuality, breast-feeding, and weight control.

Planned Parenthood Federation of America, Inc.
810 Seventh Ave.
New York, NY 10019
Provides leadership for universal acceptance of family planning as an essential element of responsible family life through education, service, and research.

Premenstrual Syndrome Action
P.O. 16292
Irving, CA 92713
(714) 854-4407

Reach to Recovery (breast cancer)
American Cancer Society

Resolve, Inc. (impaired fertility)
5 Water Street
Arlington, MA 02174
(617) 643-2424

Runaway Hotline
(800) 231-6946; in Texas (800) 392-3352

Save the Children Federation, Inc.
345 East 46th St.
New York, NY 10017
Helps eliminate the causes of poverty among children in the United States and overseas while maintaining efforts to ameliorate the effects of poverty in those areas where the needs are greatest.

SHARE (Source of help in Airing and Resolving Experiences) for parents who have suffered loss of newborn baby
℅ St. John's Hospital
800 E. Carpenter Street
Springfield, IL 62760
(217) 544-6464

SIECUS
Human Science Press
72 Fifth Ave.
New York, NY 10011
Provides publications (e.g., "Sexual relations in pregnancy and postpartum") and teaching aids.

Society of Obstetricians and Gynaecologists of Canada
14 Prince Arthur Avenue
Suite 109
Toronto, Ont. M5R 1A9

United States Government
Children's Bureau
U.S. Department of Health and Human Services
Washington, DC 20402
Consumer Product Safety Commission
Washington, DC 20207
Printing Office
Washington, DC 20402
Public Documents Distribution Center
Consumer Information
Pueblo, CO 81009

Public Health Service
200 Independence Avenue, SW
Washington, DC 20201
(202) 245-6867
Provides information and publications on many aspects related to pregnancy.

Spina Bifida Association of America
1700 Rockville Pike
Suite 540
Rockville, MD 20852
(800) 621-3141

Stepfamily Association of America
602 E. Joppa Road
Baltimore, MD 21204
(301) 823-7570

Victims Anonymous
9514-9 Reseda Blvd. #607
Northridge, CA 91324
(818) 993-1139

VBAC (Vaginal Birth After Cesarean)
10 Great Plain Terrace
Needham, MA 01292

Women Against Rape
P.O. Box 02084
Columbus, OH 43202
(614) 291-9751

Women Against Violence Against Women (WAVAW)
543 North Fairfax Avenue
Los Angeles, CA 90036

Women in Transition (WIT)
112 South 16th Street
Philadelphia, PA 19102
(215) 922-7500

The Women's Health Forum (Healthright)
175 Fifth Ave.
New York, NY 10010

Women's Occupational Health Resource Center
School of Public Health
Columbia University
701 West 168th Street
New York, NY 10032
(212) 305-2500

Women's Sports Foundation
(800) 227-3988

NATIONAL CLEARINGHOUSES

American Foundation for Maternal and Child Health
(research on the perinatal period)
300 Beekman Place
New York, NY 10022
(212) 759-5510

Arthritis Information Clearinghouse
P.O. Box 9782
Arlington, VA 22209

Cancer Information Clearinghouse
National Cancer Institute
Office of Cancer Communications
Building 31, Room 10A-18
9000 Rockville Pike
Bethesda, MD 20892
(800) 4-CANCER

Clearinghouse on the Handicapped
Switzer Building, Room 3132
330 C. St., S.W.
Washington, DC 20202

Clearinghouse for Occupational Safety and Health Information
National Institute for Occupational Safety and Health
4676 Columbia Parkway
Cincinnati, OH 45226
(513) 533-8236

Consumer Information Center
18th and E Streets, NW
Washington, DC 20405
(202) 566-1794

Food and Drug Administration (FDA)
Office of Consumer Affairs
Public Inquiries
5600 Fishers Lane(HFE-88)
Rockville, MD 20857
(301) 443-3170

Family Resource Clearinghouse
Child Development Center
Box 85
Metropolitan State College
1006 11th Street
Denver, CO 80204
(303) 556-8362

Food and Nutrition Information Center
National Agricultural Library Building, Room 304
Beltsville, MD 20705

Health Information Resources
National Health Information Clearinghouse
P.O. Box 1133
Washington, DC 20013

High Blood Pressure Information Center
120/80 National Institutes of Health
Bethesda, MD 20892

National Center on Women and Family Law
799 Broadway
Room 402
New York, NY 10003
(212) 674-8200

National Clearinghouse for Alcohol Information
P.O. Box 2345
Rockville, MD 20857
(301) 468-2600

National Clearinghouse for Drug Abuse Information
P.O. Box 416
Dept. DQ
Kensington, MD 20795
(800) 638-2045; in Maryland (800) 492-6605

National Clearinghouse for Family Planning Information
P.O. Box 12921
Arlington, VA 22209
or
P.O. Box 10716
Rockville, MD 20850
(703) 558-4990

National Clearinghouse for Mental Health Information
Public Inquiries Section
5600 Fishers Lane, Room 15C-17
Rockville, MD 20857

National Diabetes Information Clearinghouse
Box NDIC
Bethesda, MD 20892
(301) 468-2162

National Health Information Clearinghouse "Healthfinder"
P.O. Box 1133
Washington, DC 20013-1133
(800) 336-4797; in Virginia, call collect (703) 522-2590

National Institute of Mental Health
Public Inquiries Branch
Parklawn Building, Room 15C-05
5600 Fishers Lane
Rockville, MD 20857

National Library Service for the Blind and Physically Handicapped
Library of Congress
Washington, DC 20542

National Maternal and Child Health Clearinghouse
3520 Prospect St., N.W., Ground Floor
Washington, DC 20057

National Rehabilitation Information Center
4407 8th St., N.E.
Washington, DC 20017

National Self-Help Clearinghouse
33 W 42nd St., Room 1210
New York, NY 10036
(212) 840-1259

Office on Smoking and Health
Technical Information Center
Park Building, Room 1-10
5600 Fishers Lane
Rockville, MD 20857

President's Council on Physical Fitness and Sports
450 5th St., N.W., Suite 7103
Washington, DC 20001

Self-Help Center
1600 Dodge Ave., Suite S-122
Evanston, IL 60201

Sudden Infant Death Syndrome Clearinghouse
8201 Greensboro Dr., Suite 600
McLean, VA 22102

NURSING JOURNALS

Birth: Issues in Prenatal Care and Education (formerly **Birth and Family Journal**)
110 El Camino Real
Berkeley, CA 94705
Quarterly publication, sponsored by International Childbirth Education Association (ICEA) and American Society of Psychoprophylaxis in Obstetrics (ASPO)
(415) 658-5099

Bookmarks
ICEA Supplies Center
P.O. Box 20048
Minneapolis, MN 55420
Complimentary annotated catalogue of book reviews published several times per year

Canadian Nurse
The Canadian Nurses' Association
50 The Driveway
Ottawa, Canada K2PIE2

Journal of the California Perinatal Association
16952 Ventura Blvd.
Encino, CA 91316

Journal of Obstetric, Gynecologic and Neonatal Nursing
Harper & Row, Publishers
Medical Department
2350 Virginia Ave.
Hagerstown, MD 21740
Journal of the Nurses' Association of the American College of Obstetricians and Gynecologists

Journal of Nurse-Midwifery
Editor
82 Willow Ln.
Tenafly, NJ 07670
or
American Elsevier Publishing Co.
52 Vanderbilt Ave.
New York, NY 10017
Official publication of the American College of Nurse-Midwives

Maternal/Newborn Advocate
The National Foundation/March of Dimes
P.O. Box 2000
White Plains, NY 10602
Complimentary quarterly publication of the National Foundation/March of Dimes

MCN The American Journal of Maternal Child Nursing
555 W. 57th St.
New York, NY 10019

Nurse Practitioner: A Journal of Primary Nursing Care
3845 42nd Ave., N.E.
Seattle, WA 98105

Nursing Research
555 W. 57th St.
New York, NY 10019

Perinatal Press
Perinatal Press Subscriptions
The Perinatal Center
Sutter Memorial Hospital
52nd and F Sts.
Sacramento, CA 95819

Women's Health Nursing Scan
J.B. Lippincott Co.
Downsville Pike, Rte 3, Box 20-B
Hagerstown, MD. 21740

Sources for pamphlet and articles printed in various languages and for various ethnic groups may be obtained by checking with the local representatives of the following:

American Red Cross
17th and D. St., N.W.
Washington, DC 20006

NURSING ORGANIZATIONS

American College of Nurse Midwives
1522 K Street, NW
Suite 1120
Washington, DC 20005
(202) 347-5445

American Nurses Association
1101 14th Street, NW
Suite 200
Washington, DC 20005
(202) 789-1800

Canadian Nurses Association
50 The Driveway
Ottawa, Ont. K2P 1E2

Midwives Alliance of North America
United States and Canada
% Concord Midwifery Service
30 South Main Street
Concord, NH 03301
(603) 225-9586

National League for Nursing (NLN)
Ten Columbus Circle
New York, NY 10019
(212) 582-1022
See also Nurse-Widwifery

Nurses Association of the American College of Obstetricians and Gynecologists (NAACOG)
409 12th Street, S.W.
Washington, DC 20024-2191
(202)638-0026
Toll free 1-800-533-8822

Glossary

abdominal Belonging or relating to the abdomen and its functions and disorders.
- **a. delivery** Birth of a child through a surgical incision made into the abdominal wall and uterus; cesarean delivery.
- **a. gestation** Implantation of a fertilized ovum outside the uterus but inside the peritoneal cavity.
- **a. hysterectomy** Surgical removal of the uterus through an abdominal wall incision.
- **a. pregnancy** See *abdominal gestation.*

ablatio placentae See *abruptio placentae.*

abortion Termination of pregnancy before the fetus is viable and capable of extrauterine existence, usually less than 21 to 22 weeks' gestation (or when the fetus weighs less than 600 g).
- **complete a.** Abortion in which fetus and all related tissue have been expelled from the uterus.
- **criminal a.** Termination of pregnancy performed by unqualified people usually under septic conditions. Women may resort to this if therapeutic abortions are unavailable.
- **elective a.** Termination of pregnancy chosen by the woman that is not required for her physical safety.
- **habitual (recurrent) a.** Loss of three or more successive pregnancies for no known cause.
- **incomplete a.** Loss of pregnancy in which some but not all the products of conception have been expelled from the uterus.
- **induced a.** Intentionally produced loss of pregnancy by woman or others.
- **inevitable a.** Threatened loss of pregnancy that cannot be prevented or stopped and is imminent.
- **missed a.** Loss of pregnancy in which the products of conception remain in the uterus after the fetus dies.
- **septic a.** Loss of pregnancy in which there is an infection of the products of conception and the uterine endometrial lining, usually resulting from attempted termination of early pregnancy.
- **spontaneous a.** Loss of pregnancy that occurs naturally without interference or known cause.
- **therapeutic a.** Pregnancy that has been intentionally terminated for medical reasons.
- **threatened a.** Possible loss of a pregnancy; early symptoms are present (e.g., the cervix begins to dilate).
- **voluntary a.** See *abortion, elective.*

abortus Fetus usually less than 21 weeks' gestational age and under 600 g.

abruptio placentae Partial or complete premature separation of a normally implanted placenta.

abstinence Refraining from sexual intercourse periodically or permanently.

accreta, placenta See *placenta accreta.*

acculturation Process of adopting the cultural traits or social patterns of another group.

acetonuria Presence of acetone and diacetic bodies in the urine.

acidosis Increase in hydrogen ion concentration resulting in a lowering of blood pH below 7.35.
- **metabolic a.** Increase in hydrogen ion concentration caused by increased acids from (1) abnormal metabolism (too many acids produced), (2) renal malfunction (acids not being excreted), or (3) excessive loss of base (diarrhea).

acini cells Milk-producing cells in the breast.

acme Highest point (e.g., of a contraction).

acrocyanosis Peripheral cyanosis; blue color of hands and feet in most infants at birth that may persist for 7 to 10 days.

acromion Projection of the spine of the scapula (forming the point of the shoulder); used to explain the presentation of the fetus.

adenomyoma Type of tumor affecting glandular and smooth muscle tissue, such as uterine musculature.

adnexa Adjacent or accessory parts of a structure.
- **uterine a.** Ovaries and fallopian tubes.

adult respiratory distress syndrome (ARDS) Set of symptoms including decreased compliance of lung tissue, pulmonary edema, and acute hypoxemia. The condition is similar to respiratory distress syndrome of the newborn.

afibrinogenemia Absence or decrease of fibrinogen in the blood such that the blood will not coagulate. In obstetrics, this condition occurs from complications of abruptio placentae or retention of a dead fetus.

afterbirth Lay term for the placenta and membranes expelled after the birth or delivery of the child.

afterpains Painful uterine cramps that occur intermittently for approximately 2 or 3 days after delivery and that result from contractile efforts of the uterus to return to its normal involuted condition.

AGA Appropriate (weight) for gestational age.

agalactia Absence or failure of milk secretion after childbirth.

agenesis Failure of an organ to develop.

alae nasi Nostrils.

albuminuria Presence of readily detectable amounts of albumin in the urine.

alkalosis Abnormal condition of body fluids characterized by a tendency toward an increased pH, as from an excess of alkaline bicarbonate or a deficiency of acid.

allantois Tubular diverticulum of the posterior part of the embryo's yolk sac that passes into the body stalk, accompanied by the allantoic blood vessels that develop and become the umbilical vein and paired umbilical arteries; later, after fusing with the chorion, it helps to form the placenta.

allele One of two or more alternative forms of a gene at the same site on a chromosome; alleles determine alternative characters in inheritance. Alleles that occur at the same position, or locus, on a chromosome pair may produce different effects during development.

alveoli, fetal Terminal pulmonary sacs that in fetal life are filled with fluid. This fluid is a transudate of fetal plasma.

ambient Surrounding; around.

amenorrhea Absence or suppression of menstruation.

amnesia Loss of memory.

amnii, liquor See *liquor amnii.*

amniocentesis Procedure in which a needle is inserted through the abdominal and uterine walls into the amniotic fluid; used for assessment of fetal health and maturity and for therapeutic abortion.

amniography Procedure used primarily to detect placenta previa by x-ray examination, entailing injection of radiopaque dye into amniotic fluid.

amnion Inner membrane of two fetal membranes that form the sac and contain the fetus and the fluid that surrounds it in utero.

amnionitis Inflammation of the amnion, occurring most frequently after early rupture of membranes.

amniotic Pertaining or relating to the amnion.

a. fluid Fluid surrounding fetus derived primarily from maternal serum and fetal urine.

a. sac Membrane "bag" that contains the fetus before delivery.

amniotomy Artificial rupture of the fetal membranes (AROM).

anaerobic catabolism In the absence of free oxygen, the breakdown of organized substances into simpler compounds, with the resultant release of energy.

analgesia Lack of pain without loss of consciousness.

analgesic Any drug or agent that will relieve pain.

androgen Substance that produces masculinizing effects (e.g., testosterone).

androgynous personality Having some characteristics of both sexes.

android pelvis Male type of pelvis.

anencephaly Congenital deformity characterized by the absence of cerebrum, cerebellum, and flat bones of skull.

anesthesia Partial or complete absence of sensation with or without loss of consciousness.

anomaly Organ or structure that is malformed or in some way abnormal with reference to form, structure, or position.

anorexia nervosa Psychoneurotic disorder characterized by a prolonged refusal to eat, resulting in emaciation, amenorrhea, emotional disturbance concerning body image, and an abnormal fear of becoming obese.

anovular menstrual period Cyclic uterine bleeding not accompanied by the production and discharge of an ovum.

anovulatory Failure of the ovaries to produce, mature, or release eggs.

anoxia Absence of oxygen.

antenatal Occurring before or formed before birth.

antepartal Before labor.

anterior Pertaining to the front.

a. fontanel See *fontanel, anterior.*

anteroposterior repair Operation in which the upper and lower walls of the vagina are reconstructed to correct relaxed tissue.

anthropoid pelvis Pelvis in which the anteroposterior diameter is equal to or greater than the transverse diameter.

antibody Specific protein substance developed by the body that exerts restrictive or destructive action on specific antigens, such as bacteria, toxins, or Rh factor.

anticipatory grief Grief that predates the loss of a beloved object.

antigen Protein foreign to the body that causes the body to develop antibodies. Examples: bacteria, dust, Rh factor.

Apgar score Numeric expression of the condition of a newborn obtained by rapid assessment at 1, 5, and 15 minutes of age; developed by Dr. Virginia Apgar.

apnea Cessation of respirations for more than 10 seconds associated with generalized cyanosis.

Apt test Differentiation of maternal and fetal blood when there is vaginal bleeding. It is performed as follows: Add 0.5 ml blood to 4.5 ml distilled water. Shake. Add 1 ml 0.25N sodium hydroxide. Fetal and cord blood remains pink for 1 or 2 minutes. Maternal blood becomes brown in 30 seconds.

areola Pigmented ring of tissue surrounding the nipple.

secondary a. During the fifth month of pregnancy, a second faint ring of pigmentation seen around the original areola.

arthralgia Any pain that affects a joint.

articulation Fastening together or connection of the various bones of the skeleton; a joint. The articulations of the bones are classified as (1) immovable (synarthrosis), (2) slightly immovable (amphiarthrosis), and (3) freely movable (diarthrosis).

artificial insemination Introduction of semen by instrument injection into the vagina or uterus for impregnation.

Aschheim-Zondek test Pregnancy determination in which a woman's urine is injected into a mouse. After 5 days the animal is killed and its ovaries are examined. Enlarged ovaries and maturing follicles indicate pregnancy.

asphyxia Decreased oxygen and/or excess of carbon dioxide in the body.

fetal a. Condition occurring in utero, with the following biochemical changes: hypoxemia (lowering of Po_2), hypercapnia (increase in Pco_2), and respiratory and metabolic acidosis (reduction of blood pH).

a. livida Condition in which the infant's skin is characteristically pale, pulse is weak and slow, and reflexes are depressed or absent; also known as *blue asphyxia.*

a. pallida Condition in which the infant appears pale and limp and suffers from bradycardia (80 beats/min or less) and apnea.

aspiration pneumonia Inflammatory condition of the lungs and bronchi caused by the inhalation of vomitus containing acid gastric contents.

aspiration syndrome See *meconium aspiration syndrome.*

asynclitism Oblique presentation of the fetal head at the superior strait of the pelvis; the pelvic planes and those of the fetal head are not parallel.

ataractic Drug capable of promoting tranquility; a tranquilizer.

atelectasis Pulmonary pathosis involving alveolar collapse.

atherosclerosis Common arterial disorder characterized by yellowish plaques of cholesterol, lipids, and cellular debris in the inner layers of the walls of large and medium-sized arteries, resulting in reduced circulation in organs and areas normally supplied by the artery.

athetosis Neuromuscular condition characterized by slow, writhing, continuous, and involuntary movement of the extremities, as seen in some forms of cerebral palsy and in motor disorders resulting from lesions in the basal ganglia.

atony Absence of muscle tone.

atresia Absence of a normally present passageway.

biliary a. Absence of the bile duct.

choanal a. Complete obstruction of the posterior nares, which open into the nasopharynx, with membranous or bony tissue.
esophageal a. Congenital anomaly in which the esophagus ends in a blind pouch or narrows into a thin cord, thus failing to form a continuous passageway to the stomach.
attachment Relationship between two persons (e.g., a parent and a child).
attitude Body posture or position.
fetal a. Relation of fetal parts to each other in the uterus (e.g., all parts flexed, all parts flexed except neck is extended, etc.).
auscultation Process of listening for sounds produced within the body.
autoimmunization Development of antibodies against constituents of one's own tissues (e.g., a man may develop antibodies against his own sperm).
autosomes Any of the paired chromosomes other than the sex (X and Y) chromosomes.
axis Line, real or imaginary, about which a part revolves or that runs through the center of a body.
pelvic a. Imaginary curved line that passes through the centers of all the anteroposterior diameters of the pelvis.
azoospermia Absence of sperm in the semen.

bacteremic shock Shock that occurs in septicemia when endotoxins are released from certain bacteria in the bloodstream.
bag of waters Lay term for the sac containing amniotic fluid and fetus.
ballottement (1) Movability of a floating object (e.g., fetus). (2) Diagnostic technique using palpation: a floating object, when tapped or pushed, moves away and then returns to touch the examiner's hand.
Bandl's ring Abnormally thickened ridge of uterine musculature between the upper and lower segments that follows a mechanically obstructed labor, with the lower segment thinning abnormally.
Barr body (sex chromatin) Chromatin mass located against the inner surface of the nucleus in females, possibly representing the inactive X chromosome.
Bartholin's glands Two small glands situated on either side of the vaginal orifice that secrete small amounts of mucus during coitus and that are homologous to the bulbourethral glands in the male.
basalis, decidua See *decidua basalis.*
Bell's palsy See *palsy, Bell's.*
bicornuate uterus Anomalous uterus that may be either a double or single organ with two horns.
biliary atresia See *atresia, biliary.*
bilirubin Yellow or orange pigment that is a breakdown product of hemoglobin. It is carried by the blood to the liver, where it is chemically changed and excreted in the bile or is conjugated and excreted by the kidneys.
Billings method See *ovulation method.*
bimanual Performed with both hands.
b. palpation Examination of a woman's pelvic organs done by placing one hand on the abdomen and one or two fingers of the other hand in the vagina.
biopsy Removal of a small piece of tissue for microscopic examination and diagnosis.
birthing chair Chair used in labor and delivery to promote the comfort of the mother and the efficiency of parturition. The chair may be specially designed, having many technical features, or it may be a simple three-legged stool with a high, slanted back and a circular seat with a large central hole in it.
blastoderm Germinal membrane of the ovum.
b. vesicle Stage in the development of a mammalian embryo that consists of an outer layer, or trophoblast, and a hollow sphere of cells enclosing a cavity.
bleeding diathesis See *diathesis, bleeding.*
blood-brain barrier Obstruction that prevents passage of certain substances from blood into brain tissue.
bloody show Vaginal discharge that originates in the cervix and consists of blood and mucus; increases as cervix dilates during labor.
body image Person's subjective concept of his or her physical appearance.
bonding See *attachment.*
born out of asepsis (BOA) Pertaining to birth without the use of sterile technique.
Bradley method Preparation for parenthood with active participation of father and mother.
Braxton Hicks sign Mild, intermittent, painless uterine contractions that occur during pregnancy. These contractions occur more frequently as pregnancy advances but do not represent true labor.
Braxton Hicks version One of several types of maneuvers designed to turn the fetus from an undesirable position to a more acceptable one to facilitate delivery.
Brazelton assessment Criteria for assessing the interactional behavior of a newborn.
breakthrough bleeding Escape of blood occurring between menstrual periods; may be noted by women using chemical contraception (birth control pill).
breast milk jaundice See *jaundice, breast milk.*
breech presentation Presentation in which buttocks and/or feet are nearest the cervical opening and are born first; occurs in approximately 3% of all deliveries.
complete b.p. Simultaneous presentation of buttocks, legs, and feet.
footling (incomplete) b.p. Presentation of one or both feet.
frank b.p. Presentation of buttocks, with hips flexed so that thighs are against abdomen.
bregma Point of junction of the coronal and sagittal sutures of the skull; the area of the anterior fontanel of the fetus.
brim Edge of the superior strait of the true pelvis; the inlet.
bronchopulmonary dysplasia Emphysematous changes caused by oxygen toxicity.
brown fat Source of heat unique to neonates that is capable of greater thermogenic activity than ordinary fat. Deposits are found around the adrenals, kidneys, and neck, between the scapulas, and behind the sternum for several weeks after birth.
bruit, uterine Sound of passage of blood through uterine blood vessels, synchronous with fetal heart rate.
cachexia Severe generalized weakness, malnutrition, and emaciation.
caked breast See *engorgement.*
calcemia See *hypercalcemia.*
Candida vaginitis Vaginal, fungal infection; moniliasis.
capsularis, decidua See *decidua capsularis.*
caput Occiput of fetal head appearing at the vaginal introitus preceding delivery of the head.
c. succedaneum Swelling of the tissue over the presenting part of the fetal head caused by pressure during labor.
carrier Individual who carries a gene that does not exhibit itself in physical or chemical characteristics but that can be transmitted to children (e.g., a female carrying the trait for hemophilia, which is expressed in male offspring).
catamenia Menses.
caudal anesthesia Type of regional anesthesia used in childbirth in which the anesthetic agent is injected into the caudal area of the spinal canal through the sacral hiatus, affecting the caudal nerve roots and thereby anesthetizing the cervix, vagina, and perineum. Medication does not mix wtih cerebrospinal fluid (CSF).

caul Hood of fetal membranes covering fetal head during delivery.
cautery Method of destroying tissue by the use of heat, electricity, or chemicals.
centesis suffix pertaining to a surgical puncture or perforation.
cephalhematoma Extravasation of blood from ruptured vessels between a skull bone and its external covering, the periosteum. Swelling is limited by the margins of the cranial bone affected (usually parietals).
cephalic Pertaining to the head.
  c. presentation Presentation of any part of the fetal head.
cephalopelvic disproportion (CPD) Condition in which the infant's head is of such a shape, size, or position that it cannot pass through the mother's pelvis.
cervical amputation Removal of the neck of the uterus.
cervical cap (custom) Individually fitted contraceptive covering for the cervix.
cervical cauterization Destruction (usually by heat or electric current) of the superficial tissue of the cervix.
cervical conization Excision of a cone-shaped section of tissue from the endocervix.
cervical erosion Alteration of the epithelium of the cervix caused by chronic irritation or infection.
cervical mucus method See *ovulation method*.
cervical os "Mouth" or opening to the cervix.
cervical polyp Small tumor on a stem (pedicle) attached inside the cervix.
cervical stenosis Narrowing of the canal between the body of the uterus and the cervical os.
cervicitis Cervical infection.
cervix Lowest and narrow end of the uterus; the "neck." The cervix is situated between the external os and the body or corpus of the uterus, and its lower end extends into the vagina.
cesarean delivery Birth of a fetus by an incision through the abdominal wall and uterus.
cesarean hysterectomy Removal of the uterus immediately after the cesarean delivery of an infant.
Chadwick's sign Violet color of mucous membrane that is visible from about the fourth week of pregnancy; caused by increased vascularity of the vagina.
change of life See *climacterium*.
chemotaxis Response involving movement that is positive (toward) or negative (away from) to a chemical stimulus.
chloasma Increased pigmentation over bridge of nose and cheeks of pregnant women and some women taking oral contraceptives; also known as *mask of pregnancy*.
choanal atresia See *atresia, choanal*.
cholecystitis Acute or chronic inflammation of the gallbladder.
cholelithiasis Presence of gallstones in the gallbladder.
choreoathetoid cerebral palsy Condition characterized by both choreiform (jerky, ticlike twitching) and athetoid (slow, writhing) movements.
chorioamnionitis Stimulated by organisms in the amniotic fluid, which then become infiltrated with polymorphonuclear leukocytes.
chorioepithelioma Carcinoma of the chorion; rapid malignant proliferation of the epithelium of the chorionic villi.
chorion Fetal membrane closest to the intrauterine wall that gives rise to the placenta and continues as the outer membrane surrounding the amnion.
chorionic villi See *villi, chorionic*.
chromosome Element within the cell nucleus carrying genes and composed of DNA and proteins.
circumcision Excision of the male's prepuce (foreskin).
cleft lip Incomplete closure of the lip; harelip.
cleft palate Incomplete closure of the palate or roof of mouth; a congenital fissure.
climacterium (change of life) Period when the human body undergoes significant psychologic and physiologic changes, such as the termination of reproductive function in the woman.
clitoris Female organ analogous to male penis; a small, ovoid body of erectile tissue situated at the anterior junction of the vulva.
  prepuce of the c. see *prepuce of the clitoris*.
coccyx Small bone at the base of the spinal column.
coitus Penile-vaginal intercourse.
  c. interruptus Intercourse during which penis is withdrawn from vagina before ejaculation.
colostrum Yellow secretion from the breast containing mainly serum and white blood corpuscles preceding the onset of true lactation 2 or 3 days after delivery.
colpectomy Surgical excision of the vagina.
colporrhaphy (1) Procedure of suturing the vagina. (2) Procedure whereby the vagina is denuded and sutured for the purpose of narrowing the vagina.
colpotomy Any surgical incision into the wall of the vagina.
communicating hydrocephalus See *hydrocephalus, communicating*.
complement Naturally occurring blood component that is a factor in the destruction of bacteria.
complementary feeding Supplemental feeding given to the infant if he is still hungry after breast feeding.
complete abortion See *abortion, complete*.
complete breech presentation See *breech presentation, complete*.
compliance, lung Degree of distensibility of the lung's elastic tissue.
conception Union of the sperm and ovum resulting in fertilization; formation of the one-celled zygote.
conceptional age In fetal development, the number of completed weeks since the moment of conception. Because the moment of conception is almost impossible to determine, conceptional age is estimated at 2 weeks less than gestational age.
conceptus Embryo or fetus, fetal membranes, amniotic fluid, and the fetal portion of the placenta.
concurrent sterilization Method of preparing formula in which all the ingredients and equipment are sterilized prior to mixing.
condom Mechanical barrier worn on the penis for contraception; "rubber."
condyloma Wartlike growth on the skin usually seen near the anus or external genitals. There is a pointed type, and there is the flat, broad, moist papule of secondary syphilis.
confinement Period of childbirth and early puerperium.
congenital Present or existing before birth as a result of either hereditary or prenatal environmental factors.
conjoined twins See *twins, conjoined*.
conjugate
  diagonal c. Radiographic measurement of distance from *inferior border* of SP to sacral promontory; may be obtained by vaginal examination; 12.5 to 13 cm.
  true c. (c. vera) Radiographic measurement of distance from *upper margin* of symphysis pubis (SP) to sacral promontory; 1.5 to 2 cm less than diagonal conjugate.
conjunctivitis Inflammation of the mucous membrane that lines the eyelids and that is reflected onto the eyeball.
consanguinity Existing blood relationship between persons.
contraception Prevention of impregnation or conception.
contraction ring See *Bandl's ring*.
Coombs' test Indirect: determination of Rh-positive antibodies in maternal blood; direct: determination of maternal Rh-positive antibodies in fetal cord blood. A positive test result indicates the presence of antibodies or titer.

coping mechanism Any effort directed at stress management. It can be task oriented and involve direct problem-solving efforts to cope with the threat itself or be intrapsychic or ego defense oriented with the goal of regulating one's emotional distress.

copulation Coitus; sexual intercourse.

corpus Discrete mass of material; body

c. cavernosum Term referring to one of two cylinders of spongy tissue within the penis or tissue within the clitoris that engorges with blood during sexual excitement resulting in erection.

c. luteum Yellow body. After rupture of the graafian follicle at ovulation, the follicle develops into a yellow structure that secretes progesterone in the second half of the menstrual cycle, atrophying about 3 days before sloughing of the endometrium in menstrual flow. If impregnation occurs, this structure continues to produce progesterone until the placenta can take over this function.

c. spongiosum One of the spongy cylinders of tissue within the penis; has a protective function.

cotyledon One of the 15 to 28 visible segments of the placenta on the maternal surface, each made up of fetal vessels, chorionic villi, and an intervillous space.

couvade Custom whereby the husband goes through mock labor while his wife is giving birth.

Couvelaire uterus See *uterus, Couvelaire*.

CPAP Continuous positive airway pressure.

cradle cap Common seborrheic dermatitis of infants consisting of thick, yellow, greasy scales on the scalp.

craniotabes Localized softening of cranial bones.

creatinine Substance found in blood and muscle; measurement of levels in maternal urine correlates with amount of fetal muscle mass and therefore fetal size.

Crede's method Obsolete method by which the placenta is expelled by downward manual pressure on the uterus through the abdominal wall. The thumb is placed on the posterior surface of the fundus of the uterus and the flat of the hand on the anterior surface. Pressure is applied in the direction of the birth canal.

Crede's prophylaxis Instillation of 1% silver nitrate solution into the conjunctivas of newborn infants immediately after birth to prevent ophthalmia neonatorum, particularly that caused by gonorrheal organisms.

crepitus (1) Noise produced when pressure is applied to tissues containing abnormal amounts of air. (2) Grating sound heard when broken bone ends are moved. (3) Noise of gas being expelled from the intestines.

crib death Unexpected and sudden death of an apparently normal and healthy infant that occurs during sleep and with no physical or autopsic evidence of disease. Also referred to as sudden infant death syndrome (SIDS).

cri-du-chat syndrome Rare congenital disorder recognized at birth by a kittenlike cry, which may prevail for weeks, then disappear. Other characteristics include low birth weight, microcephaly, "moon face," wide-set eyes, strabismus, and low-set misshaped ears. Infants are hypotonic; heart defects and mental and physical retardation are common. Also called cat-cry syndrome.

crowning Stage of delivery when the top of the fetal head can be seen at the vaginal orifice.

cryo- Prefix meaning cold, freezing.

cryosurgery Local freezing and removal of tissue without injury to adacent tissue and with minimum blood loss, done with special equipment.

cryptochidism Failure of one or both of the testicles to descend into the scrotum. Also called undescended testis.

cul-de-sac of Douglas Pouch formed by a fold of the peritoneum dipping down between the anterior wall of the rectum and the posterior wall of the uterus; also called *Douglas' cul-de-sac, pouch of Douglas,* and *rectouterine pouch*.

culdocentesis Use of needle puncture or incision to remove intraperitoneal fluid (blood, purulent material) by way of the vagina.

culdotomy Incision or needle puncture of the cul-de-sac of Douglas by way of the vagina.

Cullen's sign Faint, irregularly formed, hemorrhagic patches on the skin around the umbilicus. The discolored skin is blue-black and becomes greenish brown or yellow. Cullen's sign may appear 1 to 2 days after the onset of anorexia and the severe, poorly localized abdominal pains characteristic of acute pancreatitis. Cullen's sign is also present in massive upper gastrointestinal hemorrhage, ruptured ectopic pregnancy.

culture The total learned way of life of a society.

curettage Scraping of the endometrium lining of the uterus with a curet to remove the contents of the uterus (as is done after an inevitable or incomplete abortion) or to obtain specimens for diagnostic purposes.

cutis marmorata Transient vasomotor phenomenon occurring primarily over extremities when the infant is exposed to chilling. It appears as a pink or faint purple capillary outline on the skin. Occasionally it is seen if the infant is in respiratory distress.

cyesis Pregnancy.

cystocele Bladder hernia; injury to the vesicovaginal fascia during labor and delivery may allow herniation of the bladder into the vagina.

cytogenics Branch of genetics concerned primarily with the study of chromosomes and correlations with associated gene behavior.

cytology The study of cells, including their formation, origin, structure, function, biochemical activities, and pathology.

death Cessation of life.

fetal d. Intrauterine death. Death of a fetus weighing 500 g or more of 20 weeks' gestation or more.

infant d. Death during the first year of life.

maternal d. Death of a woman during the childbearing cycle.

neonatal d. Death of a newborn within the first 28 days after birth.

perinatal d. Death of a fetus of 20 weeks' gestation or older or death of a neonate 28 days old or younger.

decidua Mucous membrane, lining of uterus, or endometrium of pregnancy that is shed after giving birth.

d. basalis Maternal aspect of the placenta made up of uterine blood vessels, endometrial stroma, and glands. It is shed in lochial discharge after delivery.

d. capsularis That part of the decidual membranes surrounding the chorionic sac.

d. vera Nonplacental decidual lining of the uterus.

decrement Decrease or stage of decline, as of a contraction.

deletion Loss of a piece of a chromosome that has broken off.

delivery Expulsion of the child with placenta and membranes by the mother or their extraction by the obstetric practitioner.

abdominal d. See *abdominal delivery*.

ΔOD_{450} (read delta OD_{450}) Delta optical density (or absorbance) at 450 nm, obtained by spectral analysis of amniotic fluid. This prenatal test is used to measure the degree of hemolytic activity in the fetus and to evaluate fetal status in women sensitized to Rh(D).

deoxyribonucleic acid (DNA) Intracellular complex protein that carries genetic information, consisting of two purines (adenine and guanine) and two pyrimidines (thymine and cytosine).

dermatoglyphics Study of skin ridge patterns on fingers, toes, palms of hands, and soles of feet.

DES Diethylstilbestrol, used in treating menopausal symptoms. Exposure of female fetus predisposes her to reproductive tract malformations and (later) dysplasia.

desquamation Shedding of epithelial cells of the skin and mucous membranes.

developmental crisis Severe, usually transient, stress that occurs when a person is unable to complete the tasks of a psychosocial stage of development and is therefore unable to move on to the next stage.

developmental task Physical or cognitive skill that a child must accomplish during a particular age period in order to continue developing, as walking, which precedes the development of sense of autonomy in the toddler period.

diaphragmatic hernia Congenital malformation of diaphragm that allows displacement of the abdominal organs into the thoracic cavity.

diastasis recti abdominis Separation of the two rectus muscles along the median line of the abdominal wall. This is often seen in women with repeated childbirths or with a multiple gestation (triplets, etc.). In the newborn it is usually due to incomplete development.

diathesis Hereditary condition, tendency, or susceptibility of an individual to some abnormality or disease.

bleeding d. Predisposition to abnormal blood clotting.

DIC Disseminated intravascular coagulation.

Dick-Read method An approach to childbirth based on the premise that fear of pain produces muscular tension, producing pain and greater fear. The method includes teaching physiological processes of labor, exercise to improve muscle tone, and techniques to assist in relaxation and prevent the fear-tension-pain mechanism.

dilatation of cervix Stretching of the external os from an opening a few millimeters in size to an opening large enough to allow the passage of the infant.

dilatation and curettage (D and C) Vaginal operation in which the cervical canal is stretched enough to admit passage of an instrument called a *curet*. The endometrium of the uterus is scraped with the curet to empty the uterine contents or to obtain tissue for examination.

discordance Discrepancy in size (or other indicator) between twins.

disparate twins See *twins, disparate*.

disseminated lupus erythematosus Chronic inflammatory disease affecting many systems of the body. The pathophysiology of the disease includes severe vasculitis, renal involvement, and lesions of the skin and nervous system. The primary cause of the disease has not been determined; viral infection or dysfunction of the immune system has been suggested. Also called systemic lupus erythematosus (SLE).

diverticulum Pouch-like herniation through muscular wall of a tubular organ. A diverticulum may be present in the stomach, small intestine, or, most commonly, in the colon.

dizygotic Related to or proceeding from two zygotes (fertilized ova).

dizygous twins See *twins, dizygous*.

Döderlein's bacillus Gram-positive bacterium occurring in normal vaginal secretions.

dominant trait Gene that is expressed whenever it is present in the heterozygous gene state (e.g., brown eyes are dominant over blue).

Douglas' cul-de-sac See *cul-de-sac of Douglas*.

Down's syndrome Abnormality involving the occurrence of a third chromosome, rather than the normal pair (trisomy 21), that characteristically results in a typical picture of mental retardation and altered physical appearance. This condition was formerly called *mongolism* or *mongoloid idiocy*.

dry labor Lay term referring to labor in which amniotic fluid has already escaped. A "dry birth" does not exist.

Dubowitz assessment Estimation of gestational age of a newborn, based on criteria developed for that purpose.

ductus arteriosus In fetal circulation, an anatomic shunt between the pulmonary artery and arch of the aorta. It is obliterated after birth by a rising Po_2 and change in intravascular pressures in the presence of normal pulmonary function. It normally becomes a ligament after birth but in some instances remains patent.

ductus venosus In fetal circulation, a blood vessel carrying oxygenated blood between the umbilical vein and the inferior vena cava, bypassing the liver. It is obliterated and becomes a ligament after birth.

Duncan's mechanism Delivery of placenta with the maternal surface presenting, rather than the shiny fetal surface.

dura (dura mater) Outermost, toughest of the three meninges covering the brain and spinal cord.

dynamic ileus Spastic ileus; intestinal obstruction characterized by recurrent and continuous spasms (sudden muscular contractions).

dys- Prefix meaning abnormal, difficult, painful, faulty.

dyscrasia Incompatible mixture (e.g., fetal and maternal blood incompatibility).

dysfunction, placental See *placental dysfunction*.

dysfunctional uterine bleeding Abnormal bleeding from the uterus for reasons that are not readily established.

dysmaturity See *intrauterine growth retardation (IUGR)*.

dysmenorrhea Difficult or painful menstruation.

dysmorphogenesis Development of ill-shaped or malformed structures.

dyspareunia Painful sexual intercourse.

dystocia Prolonged, painful, or otherwise difficult delivery or birth because of mechanical factors produced by either the passenger (the fetus) or the passage (the pelvis of the mother) or because of inadequate powers (uterine and other muscular activity).

placental d. Difficulty in the delivery of the placenta.

ecchymosis Bruise; bleeding into tissue caused by direct trauma, serious infection, or bleeding diathesis.

eclampsia Severe complication of pregnancy of unknown cause and occurring more often in the primigravida; characterized by tonic and clonic convulsions, coma, high blood pressure, albuminuria, and oliguria occurring during pregnancy or shortly after delivery.

ectoderm Outer layer of embryonic tissue giving rise to skin, nails, and hair.

ectopic Out of normal place.

e. pregnancy Implications of the fertilized ovum outside of its normal place in the uterine cavity. Locations include the abdomen, fallopian tubes, and ovaries.

EDC Expected date of confinement; "due date."

effacement Thinning and shortening or obliteration of the cervix that occurs during late pregnancy or labor or both.

effleurage Gentle stroking used in massage.

ejaculation Sudden expulsion of semen from the male urethra.

elective abortion See *abortion, elective*.

electroshock (therapy) Induction of a brief convulsion by passing an electric current through the brain for the treatment of affective disorders, especially in clients resistant to psychoactive drug therapy. Also called electroconvulsive therapy (ECT).

embolus Any undissolved matter (solid, liquid, or gaseous) that is carried by the blood to another part of the body and obstructs a blood vessel.

embryo Conceptus from the second or third week of development until about the eighth week after conception, when mineralization (ossification) of the skeleton begins. This period is characterized by cellular differentiation and predominantly hyperplastic growth.

empathy Projection of one's own consciousness and awareness onto that of another so as to obtain an objective awareness of and insight into the emotions, feelings, and behavior of another person and their meaning and significance. Empathy may be distinguished from sympathy in that sympathy is usually nonobjective and noncritical, whereas the state of empathy includes relative freedom from emotional involvement.

endocervical Pertaining to the interior of the canal of the cervix of the uterus.

endocrine glands Ductless glands that secrete hormones into the blood or lymph.

endometriosis Tissue closely resembling endometrial tissue but aberrantly located outside the uterus in the pelvic cavity. Symptomatology may include pelvic pain or pressure, dysmenorrhea, dyspareunia, abnormal bleeding from the uterus or rectum, and sterility.

endometrium Inner lining of the uterus that undergoes changes caused by hormones during the menstrual cycle and pregnancy; decidua.

engagement In obstetrics, the entrance of the fetal presenting part into the superior pelvic strait and the beginning of the descent through the pelvic canal.

engorgement Distention or vascular congestion. In obstetrics, the process of swelling of the breast tissue brought about by an increase in blood and lymph supply to the breast, which precedes true lactation. It lasts about 48 hours and usually reaches a peak between the third and fifth postdelivery days.

engrossment Sustained involvement of a parent with an infant.

entoderm Inner layer of embryonic tissue giving rise to internal organs such as the intestine.

entrainment Phenomenon observed in the microanalysis of sound films in which the speaker moves several parts of the body and the listener responds to the sounds by moving in ways that are coordinated with the rhythm of the sounds. Infants have been observed to move in time to the rhythms of adult speech but not to random noises or disconnected words or vowels. Entrainment is thought to be an essential factor in the process of maternal-infant bonding.

epicanthus Fold of skin covering the inner canthus and caruncle that extends from the root of the nose to the median end of the eyebrow; characteristically found in certain races but may occur as a congenital anomaly.

episiotomy Surgical incision of the perineum at the end of the second stage of labor to facilitate delivery and to avoid laceration of the perineum. (See also *perineotomy*.)

epispadias Defect in which the urethral canal terminates on dorsum of penis or above the clitoris (rare).

Epstein's pearls Small, white blebs found along the gum margins and at the junction of the soft and hard palates. They are a normal manifestation and are commonly seen in the newborn. Similar to Bohn's nodules.

epulis Tumorlike benign lesion of the gingiva seen in pregnant women.

equilibrium A state of balance or rest owing to the equal action of opposing forces, as calcium and phosphorus in the body. In psychiatry, a state of mental or emotional balance.

Erb-Duchenne paralysis Paralysis caused by traumatic injury to the upper brachial plexus, occurring most commonly in childbirth from forcible traction during delivery. The signs of Erb's paralysis include loss of sensation in the arm and paralysis and atrophy of the deltoid, the biceps, and the branchialis muscles. Also called Erb's palsy.

ergot Drug obtained from *Claviceps purpurea,* a fungus, which stimulates the smooth muscles of blood vessels and the uterus, causing vasoconstriction and uterine contractions.

erythema toxicum Innocuous pink papular neonatal rash of unknown cause, with superimposed vesicles appearing within 24 to 48 hours after birth and resolving spontaneously within a few days.

erythroblastosis fetalis Hemolytic disease of the newborn usually caused by isoimmunization resulting from Rh incompatibility or ABO incompatibility.

erythropoiesis Erythrocyte (RBC) production, which involves the maturation of a nucleated precursor into a hemoglobin-filled, nucleus-free erythrocyte regulated by erythropoietin, a hormone produced by the kidney.

escutcheon Pattern of distribution of pubic hair.

esophageal atresia See *atresia, esophageal.*

estradiol An estrogen.

estrangement, psychologic Reaction to the birth of and subsequent separation from a sick and/or premature infant, whereby the mother is diverted from establishing a normal relationship with her baby.

estriol Major metabolite of estrogen that increases during the second half of pregnancy with an intact fetoplacental unit (normal placenta, normal fetal liver and adrenals) and normal maternal renal function.

estrogen Female sex hormone produced by the ovaries and placenta.

estrus Cyclic period of sexual activity in mammals other than primates; state of being in heat.

ethnocentrism Belief in the inherent superiority of the race or group to which one belongs. Also a proclivity to consider other ethnic groups in terms of one's own racial origins.

eu- Prefix meaning normal, good, well, easy.

eugenics Science that deals with the improvement of the human race through control of hereditary (genetic) factors by voluntary social action.

euthenics Science that deals with the improvement of the human race through the control of environmental factors (pollution, drug abuse, malnutrition, and disease).

eutocia Normal or natural labor or birth.

exchange transfusion Replacement of 75% to 85% of circulating blood by withdrawing the recipient's blood and injecting a donor's blood in equal amounts, the purposes of which are to prevent an accumulation of bilirubin in the blood above a dangerous level, to prevent the accumulation of other by-products of hemolysis in hemolytic disease, and to correct anemia.

exocervix Outer layer of the portion of the cervix that protrudes into the vagina; ectocervix.

exostosis Benign cartilage-covered hump on the surface of a bone, often resulting from chronic irritation.

expulsive Having the tendency to drive out or expel.

- **e. contractions** Labor contractions that are characteristic of the second stage of labor.

exstrophy Eversion; the turning inside out of a part.

extension Straightening of a body part; opposite of flexion.

extraperitoneal Occurring or located outside the peritoneal cavity.

extrauterine Occurring outside the uterus.

- **e. pregnancy** Ectopic pregnancy in which the fertilized ovum implants itself outside the uterus.

facies Pertaining to the appearance or expression of the face; certain congenital syndromes typically present with a specific facial appearance.

FAD Fetal activity determination.

failure to thrive Condition in which neonate's or infant's growth and development patterns are below the norms for age.

fallopian tubes Two canals or oviducts extending laterally from each side of the uterus through which the ovum travels, after ovulation, to the uterus.

false labor Uterine contractions that do not result in cervical dilatation, are irregular, are felt more in front, often do not last more than 20 seconds, and do not become longer or stronger.

false pelvis The part of the pelvis superior to a plane passing through the linea terminalis.

familial Pertaining to a condition present in more members of a family than would be expected by chance.

fecundation Act of fertilization or impregnation.

fecundity Ability to bear children frequently and in large numbers.

Ferguson's reflex Reflex contractions of the uterus after stimulation of the cervix.

ferning (arborization) test The appearance of a fernlike pattern in dried smears of uterine cervical mucus, indicating the presence of estrogen.

- **ovulation f. t.** Test in which cervical mucus, placed on a slide, dries in a branching pattern in the presence of high estrogen levels at the time of ovulation.
- **pregnancy f. t.** Test in which cervical mucus, placed on a slide, does not dry in a branching pattern because of high levels of progesterone along with estrogen.

fertility Quality of being able to reproduce.

fertility rate Number of births per 1000 women aged 15 through 44 years.

fertilization Union of an ovum and a sperm.

fetal Pertaining or relating to the fetus

- **f. alcohol syndrome** Congenital abnormality or anomaly resulting from maternal alcohol intake above 3 oz. of absolute alcohol per day. It is characterized by typical craniofacial and limb defects, cardiovascular defects, intrauterine growth retardation, and developmental delay.
- **f. alveoli** See *alveoli, fetal.*
- **f. attitude** See *attitude, fetal.*
- **f. asphyxia** See *asphyxia, fetal.*
- **f. death** See *death, fetal.*
- **f. distress** Evidence such as a change in the fetal heartbeat pattern or activity indicating that the fetus is in jeopardy.
- **f. lie** Relation of the fetal spine to the maternal spine; i.e., in vertical lie, maternal and fetal spines are parallel and the fetal head or breech presents; in transverse lie, fetal spine is perpendicular to the maternal spine and the fetal shoulder presents.
- **f. presentation** The part of the fetus that presents at the cervical os.

fetofetal transfusion See *parabiotic syndrome.*

α-fetoprotein (AFP) Fetal antigen; elevated levels in amniotic fluid associated with neural tube defects.

fetotoxic Poisonous or destructive to the fetus.

fetus Child in utero from about the eighth week after conception, until birth.

fibroid Fibrous, encapsulated connective tissue tumor, especially of the uterus.

fimbria Structure resembling a fringe, particularly the fringe-like end of the fallopian tube.

FiO_2 (fraction of inspired oxygen) Percentage of oxygen a person is receiving.

fissure Groove or open crack in tissue.

fistula Abnormal tubelike passage that forms between two normal cavities, possibly congenital or caused by trauma, abscesses, or inflammatory processes.

flaccid Having relaxed, flabby, or absent muscle tone.

flaring of nostrils Widening of nostrils (alae nasi) during inspiration in the presence of air hunger; sign of respiratory distress.

flexion In obstetrics, resistance to the descent of the baby down the birth canal causes the head to flex, or bend, so that the chin approaches the chest. Thus the smallest diameter (suboccipitobregmatic) of the vertex presents.

fluid, amniotic See *amniotic fluid.*

folic acid deficiency anemia Anemia caused by lack of folic acid in the diet.

follicle Small secretory cavity or sac.

- **graafian f.** Mature, fully developed ovarian cyst containing the ripe ovum. The follicle secretes estrogens, and after ovulation, the corpus luteum develops within the ruptured graafian follicle and secretes estrogen and progesterone.

follicle-stimulating hormone (FSH) Hormone produced by the anterior pituitary during the first half of the menstrual cycle. Stimulates development of the graafian follicle.

fomites Nonliving material on which disease-producing organisms may be conveyed (e.g., bed linen).

fontanel Broad area, or soft spot, consisting of a strong band of connective tissue contiguous with cranial bones and located at the junctions of the bones.

- **anterior f.** Diamond-shaped area between the frontal and two parietal bones just above the baby's forehead at the junction of the coronal and sagittal sutures.
- **mastoid f.** Posterolateral fontanel usually not palpable.
- **posterior f.** Small, triangular area between the occipital and parietal bones at the junction of the lambdoidal and sagittal sutures.
- **sagittal f.** Soft area located in the sagittal suture, halfway between the anterior and posterior fontanels; may be found in normal newborns and in some neonates with Down's syndrome.
- **sphenoid f.** Anterolateral fontanel usually not palpable.

footling (incomplete) breech presentation See *breech presentation, footling.*

foramen ovale Septal opening between the atria of the fetal heart. The opening normally closes shortly after birth, but if it remains patent, surgical repair usually is necessary.

foreskin Prepuce, or loose fold of skin covering the glans penis.

fornix Any structure with an arched or vaultlike shape.

- **f. of the vagina** Anterior and posterior spaces, formed by the protrusion of the cervix into the vagina, into which the upper vagina is divided.

fossa Shallow depression.

fourchette Tense band of mucous membranes at the posterior angle of the vagina connecting the posterior ends of the labia minora.

Fowler's position Posture assumed by client when head of bed is raised 18 or 20 inches and individual's knees are elevated.

frank breech presentation See *breech presentation, frank.*

fraternal twins Nonidentical twins that come from two separate fertilized ova.

frenulum Thin ridge of tissue in midline of undersurface of tongue extending from its base to varying distances from the tip of the tongue.

Friedman's curve Labor curve; pattern of descent of presenting part and of dilatation of cervix; partogram.

Friedman's test Modification of the Aschheim-Zondek pregnancy test: the urine of a woman suspected of pregnancy is injected into a mature, unmated female rabbit. If at the end of 2 days of these injections, the ovaries of the rabbit contain fresh corpora lutea or hemorrhagic corpora, the test is positive, signifying that the woman is pregnant.

frigidity Archaic term designating a woman's inability to achieve orgasm; orgasmic dysfunction.

FSH See *follicle-stimulating hormone.*

fulguration Destruction of tissue by means of electricity.

fundus Dome-shaped upper portion of the uterus between the points of insertion of the fallopian tubes.

funic souffle See *souffle, funic.*

funis Cordlike structure, especially the umbilical cord.

galacto-, galact- Combining form denoting milk.

galactorrhea Excessive flow or secretion of milk.

galactosemia Inherited, autosomal recessive disorder of galactose metabolism, characterized by a deficiency of the enzyme galactose-1-phosphate uridyl transferase.

gamete Mature male or female germ cell; the mature sperm or ovum.

gastroschisis Abdominal wall defect at base of umbilical stalk.

gastrostomy Surgical creation of an artificial opening into the stomach through the abdominal wall, performed to feed a client when oral feeding is not possible.

gastrula Early embryonic stage of development that follows the blastula.

gate control theory Proposed in 1965 by Melzack and Wall, this theory explains the neurophysical mechanism underlying the perception of pain.

gavage Feeding by means of a tube passed to the stomach.

gender identity The sense or awareness of knowing to which sex one belongs. The process begins in infancy, continues throughout childhood, and is reinforced during adolescence.

gene Factor on a chromosome responsible for hereditary characteristics of offspring.

generative Capable of reproduction.

genetic Dependent of the genes. A genetic disorder may or may not be apparent at birth.

genetic counseling Process of determining the occurrence or risk of occurrence of a genetic disorder within a family and of providing appropriate information and advice about the courses of action that are available, whether care of a child already affected, prenatal diagnosis, termination of a pregnancy, sterilization, or artificial insemination is involved.

genetics Biologic science that deals with the genetic transmission of physical and chemical characteristics from parents to offspring, as well as the influence of environmental agents on genes and genetic expression.

genitalia Organs of reproduction.

genotype Hereditary combinations in an individual determining his physical and chemical characteristics. Some genotypes are not expressed until later in life (e.g., Huntington's chorea); some hide recessive genes, which can be expressed in offspring; and others are expressed only under the proper environmental conditions (e.g., diabetes mellitus appearing under the stress of obesity or pregnancy).

gestation Period of intrauterine fetal development from conception through birth; the period of pregnancy.

  abdominal g. See *abdominal gestation.*

gestational age In fetal development, the number of completed weeks counting from the first day of the last normal menstrual cycle.

glabella Bony prominence above the nose and between the eyebrows.

glans penis Smooth, round head of the penis, analogous to the female glans clitoris.

glomerulonephritis Noninfectious disease of the glomerulus of the kidney, characterized by proteinuria, hematuria, decreased urine production, and edema.

glycosuria Presence of glucose (a sugar) in the urine.

gonad Gamete-producing, or sex, gland; the ovary or testis.

gonadotropic hormone Hormone that stimulates the gonads.

Goodell's sign Softening of the cervix, a probable sign of pregnancy, occurring during the second month.

gossypol Oral contraceptive produced from cotton plants; currently in experimental stage of use by males in the United States.

graafian follicle (vesicle) See *follicle, graafian.*

gravid Pregnant.

grieving process A complex of somatic and psychological symptoms associated with some extreme sorrow or loss, specifically the death of a loved one.

grunt, expiratory Sign of respiratory distress (hyaline membrane disease [respiratory distress syndrome, or RDS] or advanced pneumonia) indicative of the body's attempt to hold air in the alveoli for better gaseous exchange.

gynecoid pelvis Pelvis in which the inlet is round instead of oval or blunt; heart shaped. Typical female pelvis.

gynecology Study of the diseases of the female, especially of the genital, urinary, and rectal organs.

habitual (recurrent) abortion See *abortion, habitual.*

habituation An acquired tolerance from repeated exposure to a particular stimulus. Also called negative adaptation; a decline and eventual elimination of a conditioned response by repetition of the conditioned stimulus.

habitus Indications in appearance of tendency or disposition to disease or abnormal conditions.

harlequin sign Rare color change of no pathologic significance occurring between the longitudinal halves of the neonate's body. When infant is placed on one side, the dependent half is noticeably pinker than the superior half.

Hawthorne effect A general beneficial effect on a person or group of people as a result of a therapeutic encounter with a health care provider or as a result of a change in the environment (lighting, temperature, type of room [family-centered versus four-bed unit]).

Hegar's sign Softening of the lower uterine segment that is classified as a probable sign of pregnancy and that may be present during the second and third months of pregnancy and is palpated during bimanual examination.

hematocrit Volume of red blood cells per deciliter (dl) of circulating blood; packed cell volume (PCV).

hematoma Collection of blood in a tissue; a bruise or blood tumor.

hemoconcentration Increase in the number of red blood cells resulting from either a decrease in plasma volume or increased erythropoiesis.

hemoglobin Component of red blood cells consisting of globin, a protein, and hematin, an organic iron compound.

  h. electrophoresis Test to diagnose sickle cell disease in newborns. Cord blood is used.

hemorrhagic disease of newborn Bleeding disorder during first few days of life based on a deficiency of vitamin K.

hereditary Pertaining to a trait or characteristic transmitted from parent to offspring by way of the genes; used synonymously with *genetic.*

hermaphrodite Person having genital and sexual characteristics of both sexes.

heterologous insemination Insemination in which the semen specimen is provided by an anonymous donor. The procedure is used primarily in cases where the husband is sterile.

heterozygous Having two dissimilar genes at the same site, or locus, on paired chromosomes (e.g., at the sites for eye color, one chromosome carrying the gene for brown, the other for blue).

high risk An increased possibility of suffering harm, damage, loss, or death.

hirsutism Condition characterized by the excessive growth of hair or the growth of hair in unusual places.

Homans' sign Early sign of phlebothrombosis of the deep veins of the calf in which there are complaints of pain when the leg is in extension and the foot is dorsiflexed.

homoiothermic Referring to the ability of warm-blooded animals to maintain internal temperature at a specified level regardless of the environmental temperature. This ability is not fully developed in the human neonate.

homologous Similar in structure or origin but not necessarily in function.

homologous insemination Insemination in which the semen specimen is provided by the husband. The procedure is used primarily in cases of impotence or when the husband is incapable of sexual intercourse because of some physical disability.

homozygous Having two similar genes at the same locus, or site, on paired chromosomes.

hormone Chemical substance produced in an organ or gland that is conveyed through the blood to another organ or part of the body, stimulating it to increased functional activity or secretion. See specific hormones.

hour-glass uterus Uterus in which a segment of circular muscle fibers contracts during labor. The resultant "constriction ring" dystocia is characterized by lack of progress in spite of adequate contractions; by pain experienced prior to palpation of a uterine contraction and persisting after the observer feels the contraction end; and by recession of the presenting part during a contraction, instead of descent of the presenting part.

human chorionic gonadotropin (HCG) See *prolan*.

human chorionic somatomammotropin (HCS) Another term for human placental lactogen (HPL) and placental growth hormone.

hyaline membrane disease (HMD) Disease characterized by interference with ventilation at the alveolar level, theoretically caused by the presence of fibrinoid deposits lining alveolar ducts. Membrane formation is related to prematurity (especially with fetal asphyxia) and insufficient surfactant production (L/S ratio less than 2:1). Otherwise known as *respiratory distress syndrome (RDS)*.

hydatidiform mole Abnormal pregnancy characterized by a degenerative process in the chorionic villi that produces high levels of human chorionic gonadotropin (HCG), multiple cysts, and rapid growth of the uterus with hemorrhage. Signs and symptoms include vaginal bleeding, the discharge containing grapelike vesicles. Sequela may be chorioadenoma, a highly malignant neoplasm.

hydramnios (polyhydramnios) Amniotic fluid in excess of 1.5L; often indicative of fetal anomaly and frequently seen in poorly controlled, insulin-dependent, diabetic pregnant women even if there is not coexisting fetal anomaly.

hydremia Excess of watery fluid in the blood.

hydrocele Collection of fluid in a saclike cavity, especially in the sac that surrounds the testis, causing the scrotum to swell.

hydrocephalus Excessive accumulation of cerebrospinal fluid within the ventricles of the brain resulting from interference with normal circulation and absorption of the cerebrospinal fluid and especially from the destruction of the foramens of Magendie and Luschka because of congenital anomaly, infection, injury, or brain tumor. In infants, the increased head diameter is possible because the sutures of the skull have not closed.

communicating h. Hydrocephalus in which normal communication between the fourth ventricle and the subarachnoid space is maintained, allowing cerebral fluid to circulate into the lumbar thecal space.

noncommunicating h. Failure of the ventricular fluid to empty into the lumbar thecal space because of an obstruction.

hydropic Dropsical or pertaining to dropsy; abnormal accumulation of serous fluid in the body tissues and cavities.

hydrops fetalis Most severe expression of fetal hemolytic disorder, a possible sequela to maternal Rh isoimmunization; infants exhibit gross edema (anasarca), cardiac decompensation, and profound pallor from anemia and seldom survive.

hymen Membranous fold that normally partially covers the entrance to the vagina in the virgin.

hymenal caruncles Small, irregular bits of tissue that are remnants of the hymen.

hymenal tag Normally occurring redundant hymenal tissue protruding from the floor of the vagina that disappears spontaneously in a few weeks after birth.

hymenotomy Surgical incision of the hymen.

hyperbilirubinemia Elevation of unconjugated serum bilirubin concentrations.

hypercalcemia Excess of calcium in the blood.

hypercapnia Excessive arterial P_{CO_2} caused by inadequate ventilation. In greater degrees it acts as a respiratory depressant.

hypercarbia Greater than normal amounts of carbon dioxide in the blood. Also called hypercapnia.

hyperemesis gravidarum Abnormal condition of pregnancy characterized by protracted vomiting, weight loss, and fluid and electrolyte imbalance.

hyperesthesia Unusual sensibility to sensory stimuli, such as pain or touch.

hyperlipidemia Excessive amount of fats in the blood.

hypermagnesemia Excessive amount of serum magnesium; in obstetrics, it occurs in the mother or fetus or both after the mother is treated with magnesium sulfate for preeclampsia-eclampsia.

hyperplasia Increase in number of cells; formation of new tissue.

hyperreflexia Increased action of the reflexes.

hypertrophy Enlargement, or increase in size, of existing cells.

hyperventilation Rapid, shallow (or prolonged, deep) respirations resulting in respiratory alkalosis: a decrease in H^+ concentration and P_{CO_2} and an increase in the blood pH and the ratio of $NaHCO_3$ to H_2CO_3. Symptoms may include faintness, palpitations, and carpopedal (hands and feet) muscular spasms. Relief may result from rebreathing in a paper bag or into one's cupped hands to replace the CO_2 "blown off" during hyperventilation.

hypocalcemia Deficiency of calcium in the serum that may be caused by hypoparathyroidism, vitamin D deficiency, kidney failure, acute pancreatitis, or inadequate plasma magnesium and protein.

hypochlorhydria Diminished secretion of hydrochloric acid.

hypofibrinogenemia Deficient level of a blood clotting factor, fibrinogen, in the blood; in obstetrics, it occurs following complications of abruptio placentae or retention of a dead fetus.

hypogastric Pertaining to the lower middle of the abdomen or hypogastrium.

hypogastric arteries Branches of the right and left iliac arteries carrying deoxygenated blood from the fetus through the umbilical cord, where they are known as *umbilical arteries,* to the placenta.

hypoglycemia Less-than-normal amount of glucose in the blood, usually caused by administration of too much insulin, excessive secretion of insulin by the islet cells of the pancreas, or by dietary deficiency.

hypospadias Anomalous positioning of urinary meatus on undersurface of penis or close to or just inside the vagina.

hypotensive drugs Drugs that lower the blood pressure.

hypothalamus Portion of the diencephalon of the brain forming the floor and part of the lateral wall of the third ventricle. It activates, controls, and integrates the peripheral autonomic nervous system, endocrine processes, and many somatic functions, as body temperature, sleep, and appetite.

hypothenar Fleshy elevation on the ulnar (little finger) side of the palm of the hand. Also called *hypothenar eminence.*

hypotonia Reduced tension; relaxation of arteries. Also, loss of tonicity of the muscles or intraocular pressure.

hypoxemia Reduction in arterial Po_2 resulting in metabolic acidosis by forcing anaerobic glycolysis, pulmonary vasoconstriction, and direct cellular damage.

hypoxia Insufficient availability of oxygen to meet the metabolic needs of body tissue.

hysterectomy Surgical removal of the uterus.

- **abdominal h.** See *abdominal hysterectomy.*
- **panhysterectomy** Removal of entire uterus, but ovaries and tubes remain.
- **subtotal h.** Removal of fundus and body of the uterus, but the cervical stump remains.
- **total h.** Removal of entire uterus, including the cervix, but the ovaries and tubes remain.

hysterosalpingography Recording by x-ray of the uterus and uterine tubes after injecting them with radiopaque material.

hysterotomy Surgical incision into the uterus.

iatrogenic Caused by a physician's words, actions, or treatment.

icterus gravis Acute yellow atrophy of the liver with cerebral disorders.

icterus neonatorum Jaundice in the newborn.

idiopathic respiratory distress syndrome (hyaline membrane disease) Severe respiratory condition found almost exclusively in premature infants and in some infants of diabetic mothers regardless of gestational age. See also *hyaline membrane disease (HMD).*

IDM Infant of a diabetic mother.

IgA Primary immunoglobulin in colostrum.

IgG Transplacentally acquired immunoglobulin that confers passive immunity against the infections to which the mother is immune.

IgM Immunoglobulin neonate can manufacture soon after birth. Fetus produces it in the presence of amnionitis.

iliopectineal line Bony ridge on the inner surface of the ilium and pubic bones that divides the true and false pelvises; the brim of the true pelvic cavity; the inlet.

immature baby Infant usually weighing less than 1134 g (2½ lb) and who is considerably underdeveloped at birth.

implantation Embedding of the fertilized ovum in the uterine mucosa; nidation.

impotence Archaic term designating a man's inability, partial or complete, to perform sexual intercourse or to achieve orgasm; erectile dysfunction.

impregnate To fertilize, or make pregnant.

inanition Pathophysiologic condition of the body resulting from lack of food and water; starvation.

inborn error of metabolism Hereditary deficiency of a specific enzyme needed for normal metabolism of specific chemicals (e.g., deficiency of phenylalanine hydroxylase results in phenylketonuria [PKU]; a deficiency of hexosaminidase results in Tay-Sachs disease).

incompetent cervix Cervix that is unable to remain closed until a pregnancy reaches term, because of a mechanical defect in the cervix resulting in dilatation and effacement usually during the second or early third trimester of pregnancy.

incomplete abortion See *abortion, incomplete.*

increment An increase, or buildup, as of a contraction.

incubator Apparatus used for an infant in which the temperature may be regulated.

induced abortion See *abortion, induced.*

induction Artificial stimulation or augmentation of labor.

inertia Sluggishness or inactivity; in obstetrics, refers to the absence or weakness of uterine contractions during labor.

inevitable abortion See *abortion, inevitable.*

infant A child who is under 1 year of age.

infantile uterus Uterus that has failed to attain adult characteristics.

infertility Decreased capacity to conceive.

infiltration Process by which a substance such as a local anesthetic drug is deposited within the tissue.

inhalation analgesia Reduction of pain by administration of anesthetic gas. Occasionally given during the second stage of labor. Consciousness is retained to allow the woman to follow instructions and to avoid the adverse effects of general anesthesia.

inlet Passage leading into a cavity.

- **pelvic i.** Upper brim of the pelvic cavity.

innominate Without a name.

- **i. bone** The hip bone.

internal os Inside mouth or opening.

interstitial cell-stimulating hormone (ICSH) Hormone that stimulates production of testosterone; analogous to LH in the female.

intertuberous diameter Distance between ischial tuberosities. Measured to determine dimension of pelvic outlet.

intervillous space Irregular space in the maternal portion of the placenta, filled with maternal blood and serving as the site of maternal-fetal gas, nutrient, and waste exchange.

intrapartum During labor and delivery.

intrathecal Within the subarachnoid space.

intrauterine device (IUD) Small plastic or metal form placed in the uterus to prevent implantation of a fertilized ovum.

intrauterine growth retardation (IUGR) Fetal undergrowth of any etiology, such as deficient nutrient supply or intrauterine infection, or associated with congenital malformation.

introitus Entrance into a canal or cavity such as the vagina.

intrômission Insertion of one part or object into another (e.g., introduction of penis into vagina).

intussusception Prolapse of one segment of bowel into the lumen of the adjacent segment.

in utero Within or inside the uterus.

in vitro fertilization Fertilization in a culture dish or test tube.

inversion Turning end for end, upside down, or inside out.

- **i. of the uterus** Condition in which the uterus is turned inside out so that the fundus intrudes into the cervix or vagina, caused by a too vigorous removal of the placenta before it is detached by the natural process of labor.

involution (1) Rolling or turning inward. (2) Reduction in size of the uterus after delivery and its return to its normal size and condition.

iontophoretic pilocarpine test Sweat test, usually a diagnostic test for cystic fibrosis (mucoviscidosis).

ischium Lower lateral two fifths of the acetabulum and the short, stout column of bone that supports it.

isoimmune hemolytic disease Breakdown (hemolysis) of fetal/neonatal Rh-positive RBCs because of Rh antigens formed by an Rh-negative mother who had been previously exposed to Rh-positive RBCs.

isoimmunization Development of antibodies in a species of animal with antigens from the same species (e.g., development of anti-Rh antibodies in an Rh-negative person).

ITP Abbreviation for idiopathic thrombocytopenic purpura.

jaundice Yellow discoloration of the body tissues caused by the deposit of bile pigments (unconjugated bilirubin); icterus.

- **breast milk j.** Yellowing of infant's skin from pregnanediol (in mother's milk) inhibition of enzyme (glucuronyl transferase) necessary for conjugation of bilirubin.

pathologic j. Jaundice noticeable within 24 hours after birth; caused by some abnormal condition such as an Rh or ABO incompatibility and resulting in bilirubin toxicity (e.g., kernicterus)

physiologic j. Jaundice usually occurring 48 hours or later after birth, reaching a peak at 5 to 7 days, gradually disappearing by the seventh to tenth day, and caused by the normal reduction in the number of red blood cells. The infant is otherwise well.

Kahn test Precipitation or flocculation test for the diagnosis of syphilis.

kalemia Presence of potassium in the serum.

karyotype Schematic arrangement of the chromosomes within a cell to demonstrate their numbers and morphology.

Kegel exercises Exercises to strengthen the pubococcygeal muscles.

kernicterus Bilirubin encephalopathy involving the deposit of unconjugated bilirubin in brain cells, resulting in death or impaired intellectual, perceptive, or motor function, and adaptive behavior.

Kernig's sign Stiffness of the back; nuchal rigidity.

ketoacidosis Acidosis accompanied by an accumulation of ketones in the body, resulting from faulty carbohydrate metabolism.

ketonemia Acetone bodies in the blood, causing the characteristic fruity breath odor of ketoacidosis.

ketosis Increase in ketone bodies (acetone) from incomplete metabolism of fatty acids.

kin group People related by blood or marriage.

Klumpke's palsy Atrophic paralysis of forearm.

labia Lips or liplike structures.

l. majora Two folds of skin containing fat and covered with hair that lie on either side of the vaginal opening and from each side of the vulva.

l. minora Two thin folds of delicate, hairless skin inside the labia majora.

labor Series of processes by which the fetus is expelled from the uterus; parturition; childbirth.

laceration Irregular tear of wound tissue; in obstetrics, it usually refers to a tear in the perineum, vagina, or cervix caused by childbirth.

lactase Enzyme necessary for the digestion of lactose.

lactation Function of secreting milk or period during which milk is secreted.

lactogen Drug or other substance that enhances the production and secretion of milk.

lactogenic Stimulating the production of milk.

l. hormone Gonadotropin produced by anterior pituitary and responsible for promoting growth of breast tissue and lactation; prolaction; luteotropin.

lactose intolerance Inherited absence of the enzyme lactose.

lactosuria Presence of lactose in the urine during late pregnancy and during lactation. Must be differentiated from glycosuria.

Lamaze method Method of psychophysical preparation for childbirth developed in the 1950s by a French obstetrician, Fernand Lamaze. It requires classes, practice at home, and coaching during labor and delivery.

lambdoid Having the shape of the Greek letter lambda.

l. suture Suture line extending across the posterior third of the skull, separating the occipital bone from the two parietal bones, and forming the base of the triangular posterior fontanel.

laminaria tent Cone of dried seaweed that swells as it absorbs moisture. Used to dilate the cervix nontraumatically in preparation for an induced abortion or in preparation for induction of labor.

lanugo Downy, fine hair characteristic of the fetus between 20 weeks' gestation and birth that is most noticeable over the shoulder, forehead, and cheeks but is found on nearly all parts of the body except the palms of the hands, soles of the feet, and the scalp.

laparoscopy Examination of the interior of the abdomen by inserting a small telescope through the anterior abdominal wall.

laparotomy Incision into the abdominal cavity.

large for dates (large for gestational age [LGA]) Exhibiting excessive growth for gestational age.

lavage Washing out of a cavity such as the stomach.

lecithin A phospholipid that decreases surface tension; surfactant.

lecithin/sphingomyelin ratio Ratio of lecithin to sphingomyelin in the amniotic fluid. This is used to assess maturity of the fetal lung.

Leopold's maneuver Four maneuvers for diagnosing the fetal position by external palpation of the mother's abdomen.

let-down reflex Oxytocin-induced flow of milk from the alveoli of the breasts into the milk ducts.

leukorrhea White or yellowish mucous discharge from the cervical canal or the vagina that may be normal physiologically or caused by pathologic states of the vagina and endocervix (e.g., *Trichomonas vaginalis* infections).

LH See *luteinizing hormone (LH)*.

libido Sexual drive.

lie Relationship existing between the long axis of the fetus and the long axis of the mother. In a longitudinal lie, the fetus is lying lengthwise or vertically, whereas in a transverse lie the fetus is lying crosswise or horizontally in the mother's uterus.

ligation Act of suturing, sewing, or otherwise tying shut.

tubal l. Abdominal operation in which the fallopian tubes are tied off and a section is removed to interrupt tubal continuity and thus sterilize the woman.

lightening Sensation of decreased abdominal distention produced by uterine descent into the pelvic cavity as the fetal presenting part settles into the pelvis. It usually occurs 2 weeks before the onset of labor in nulliparas.

linea nigra Line of darker pigmentation seen in some women during the latter part of pregnancy that appears on the middle of the abdomen and extends from the symphysis pubis toward the umbilicus.

linea terminalis Line dividing the upper (false) pelvis from the lower (true) pelvis.

lingua Tongue or tonguelike structure.

l. frenata Tongue with a very short frenulum, resulting in tongue-tie, an extremely rare condition.

liquor Any fluid liquid.

l. amnii Amniotic fluid that surrounds the fetus within the amniotic sac.

lithotomy position Position in which the woman lies on her back with her knees flexed and abducted thighs drawn up toward her chest.

live birth Birth in which the neonate, regardless of gestational age, manifests any heartbeat, breathes, or displays voluntary movement.

livida, asphyxia See *asphyxia livida*.

lochia Vaginal discharge during the puerperium consisting of blood, tissue, and mucus.

l. alba Thin, yellowish to white, vaginal discharge that follows lochia serosa on about the tenth postdelivery day and that may last from the end of the third to the sixth postdelivery week.

l. rubra Red, distinctly blood-tinged vaginal flow that follows delivery and lasts 2 to 4 days after delivery.

l. serosa Serous, pinkish brown, watery vaginal discharge that follows lochia rubra until about the tenth postdelivery day.

L/S ratio (lecithin/sphingomyelin ratio) Test for fetal lung maturity.

lunar month Four weeks (28 days).

lutein Yellow pigment derived from the corpus luteum, egg yolk, and fat cells.

l. cells Ovarian cells involved in the formation of the corpus luteum and that contain a yellow pigment.

luteinizing hormone (LH) Hormone produced by the anterior pituitary that stimulates ovulation and the development of the corpus luteum.

luteotropin (LTH) Lactogenic hormone; prolactin; an adenohypophyseal hormone.

lysis of adhesions Operation to free adhesions (bands of scar tissue) that have caused organs to be abnormally drawn or tied to each other.

lysozyme Enzyme with antiseptic qualities that destroys foreign organisms and that is found in blood cells of the granulocytic and monocytic series and is also normally present in saliva, sweat, tears, and breast milk.

maceration (1) Process of softening a solid by soaking it in a fluid. (2) Softening and breaking down of fetal skin from prolonged exposure to amniotic fluid as seen in a postterm infant. Also seen in a dead fetus.

macroglossia Hypertrophy of tongue or tongue large for oral cavity; seen in some preterm neonates and in neonates with Down's syndrome.

macrophage Any phagocytic cell of the reticuloendothelial system including Kupffer cell in the liver, splenocyte in the spleen, and histocyte in the loose connective tissue.

macrosomia Large body size as seen in neonates of diabetic or prediabetic mothers; macrosomatia.

magnesemia Presence of serum magnesium.

malpractice Professional negligence that is the proximate cause of injury or harm to a client, resulting from a lack of professional knowledge, experience, or skill that can be expected in others in the profession or from a failure to exercise reasonable care or judgment in the application of professional knowledge, experience, or skill.

mammary gland Compound gland of the female breast that is made up of lobes and lobules that secrete milk for nourishment of the young. Rudimentary mammary glands exist in the male.

manic depressive psychosis Major affective disorder characterized by episodes of mania and depression. One or the other phase may be predominant at any given time; one phase may appear alternately with the other; or elements of both phases may be present simultaneously. Also called bipolar disorder.

mask of pregnancy See *chloasma*.

mastalgia Breast soreness or tenderness.

mastectomy Excision, or removal, of the breast.

mastitis Inflammation of mammary tissue of the breasts.

maternal mortality Death of a woman related to childbearing.

maturation (1) Process of attaining maximum development. (2) In biology, a process of cell division during which the number of chromosomes in the germ cells (sperm or ova) is reduced to one half the number (haploid) characteristic of the species.

maturational crisis Crisis that arises during normal growth and development, e.g., puberty.

meatus Opening from an internal structure to the outside (e.g., urethral meatus).

mechanism Instrument or process by which something is done, results, or comes into being; in obstetrics, labor and delivery.

meconium First stools of infant: viscid, sticky; dark greenish brown, almost black; sterile; odorless.

m. aspiration syndrome Function of fetal hypoxia: with hypoxia, the anal sphincter relaxes and meconium is released; reflex gasping movements draw meconium and other particulate matter in the amniotic fluid into the infant's bronchial tree, obstructing the air flow after birth.

m. ileus Lower intestinal obstruction by thick, puttylike, inspissated meconium that may be the result of deficiency of trypsin production in the newborn with cystic fibrosis.

m.-stained fluid In response to hypoxia, fetal intestinal activity increases and anal sphincter relaxes, resulting in the passage of meconium, which imparts a greenish coloration.

megaloblastic anemia Hematologic disorder characterized by the production and peripheral proliferation of immature, large, and dysfunctional erythrocytes.

meiosis Process by which germ cells divide and decrease their chromosomal number by one half.

-melia Pertaining to a limb or part of a limb or extremity, as in amelia (absence of a limb) or phocomelia (absence of part of arms or legs).

membrane Thin, pliable layer of tissue that lines a cavity or tube, separates structures, or covers an organ or structure; in obstetrics, the amnion and chorion surrounding the fetus.

membrane rupture Tearing of the fetal membranes (amnion and chorion) with the release of amniotic fluid.

menarche Onset, or beginning, of menstrual function.

meningomyelocele Saclike protrusion of the spinal cord through a congenital defect in the vertebral column.

menopause From the Greek word *men* (month) and *pausis* (to stop), the actual permanent cessation of menstrual cycles.

menorrhagia Abnormality profuse or excessive menstrual flow.

menses (menstruation) Periodic vaginal discharge of bloody fluid from the nonpregnant uterus that occurs from the age of puberty to menopause.

mentum Chin, a fetal reference point in designating position (e.g., "Left mentum anterior" [LMA], meaning that the fetal chin is presenting in the left anterior quadrant of the maternal pelvis).

mesoderm Embryonic middle layer of germ cells giving rise to all types of muscles, connective tissue, bone marrow, blood, lymphoid tissue, and all epithelial tissue.

metabolic acidosis See *acidosis, metabolic*.

metritis Inflammation of the endometrium and myometrium.

metrorrhagia Abnormal bleeding from the uterus, particularly when it occurs at any time other than the menstrual period.

microcephaly Congenital anomaly characterized by abnormal smallness of the head in relation to the rest of the body and by underdevelopment of the brain, resulting in some degree of mental retardation.

micrognathia Abnormal smallness of mandible or chin.

midwife One who practices the art of helping and aiding a woman to give birth.

migration In obstetrics, the passage of the ovum from the ovary into the fallopian tubes and thence into the uterus.

milia Unopened sebaceous glands appearing as tiny, white, pinpoint papules on forehead, nose, cheeks, and chin of a neonate that disappear spontaneously in a few days or weeks.

milk-leg See *phlegmasia alba dolens*.

miscarriage Spontaneous abortion; lay term usually referring specifically to the loss of the fetus between the fourth month and viability.

missed abortion See *abortion, missed*.

mitleiden Suffering along with.

mitochondria Slender microscopic filaments or rods found in the cell cytoplasm; the principal sites of oxidative reactions by which the cell is provided with energy.

mitosis Process of somatic cell division in which a single cell divides, but both of the new cells have the same number of chromosomes as the first.
mittelschmerz Abdominal pain in the region of an ovary during ovulation, which usually occurs midway through the menstrual cycle. Present in many women, mittelschmerz is useful for identifying ovulation, thus pinpointing the fertile period of the cycle.
molding Overlapping of cranial bones or shaping of the fetal head to accommodate and conform to the bony and soft parts of the mother's birth canal during labor.
mongolian spot Bluish gray or dark nonelevated pigmented area usually found over the lower back and buttocks present at birth in some infants, primarily nonwhite. The spot fades by school age in black or Oriental infants and within the first year or two of life in other infants.
mongolism, See *Down's syndrome*.
moniliasis Infection of the skin or mucous membrane by a yeastlike fungus, *Candida albicans*. see *thrush*.
monitrice One trained in psychoprophylactic methods and who supports women during labor.
monosomy Chromosomal aberration characterized by the absence of one chromosome from the normal diploid complement.
monozygotic Originating or coming from a single fertilized ovum, such as identical twins.
monozygous twins See *twins, monozygous*.
mons veneris Pad of fatty tissue and coarse skin that overlies the symphysis pubis in the woman and that, after puberty, is covered with short curly hair.
Montgomery's glands tubercles Small, nodular prominences (sebaceous glands) on the areolas around the nipples of the breasts that enlarge during pregnancy and lactation.
morbidity (1) Condition of being diseased. (2) Number of cases of disease or sick persons in relationship to a specific population; incidence.
morning sickness Nausea and vomiting that affect some women during the first few months of their pregnancy; may occur at any time of day.
Moro's reflex Normal, generalized reflex in a young infant elicited by a sudden loud noise or by striking the table next to the child, resulting in flexion of the legs, an embracing posture of the arms, and usually a brief cry. Also called startle reflex.
mortality (1) Quality or state of being subject to death. (2) Number of deaths in relation to a specific population; incidence.
 fetal m. Number of fetal deaths per 1000 births (or per live births). See also *death, fetal*.
 infant m. Number of deaths per 1000 children 1 year of age or younger.
 maternal m. Number of maternal deaths per 100,000 births.
 neonatal m. Number of neonatal deaths per 1000 births (or per live births). See also *death, neonatal*.
 perinatal m. Combined fetal and neonatal mortality. See also *death, perinatal*.
morula Developmental stage of the fertilized ovum in which there is a solid mass of cells resembling a mulberry.
mosaicism Condition in which some somatic cells are normal, whereas others show chromosomal aberrations.
mucous membrane Specialized thin layer of tissue lining certain cavities and passages that is kept moist by the secretion of mucus.
mucous-trap suction apparatus Device consisting of a catheter with a mucous trap that prevents mucus aspirated from the newborn infant's nasopharynx and trachea from being sucked or drawn into the operator's mouth.
mucus Viscid fluid secreted by the mucous membranes.
multigravida Woman who has been pregnant two or more times.
multipara Woman who has carried two or more pregnancies to viability, whether they ended in live infants or stillbirths.
multiple pregnancy Pregnancy in which there is more than one fetus in the uterus at the same time.
multiple sclerosis (MS) Progressive disease characterized by disseminated demyelination of nerve fibers of the brain and spinal cord.
mutation Change in a gene or chromosome in gametes that may be transmitted to offspring.
myasthenia gravis Abnormal condition characterized by the chronic fatigability and weakness of muscles, especially in the face and throat, as a result of a defect in the conduction of nerve impulses at the myoneural junction.

Naegele's rule Method for calculating the estimated date of confinement (EDC), or "due date."
natal Relating or pertaining to birth.
navel Depression in the center of the abdomen, where the umbilical cord was attached to the fetus; umbilicus.
necrotizing bronchitis Pathologic death of cells within the bronchi.
necrotizing enterocolitis (NEC) Acute inflammatory bowel disorder that occurs primarily in preterm or low-birth-weight neonates. It is characterized by ischemic necrosis (death) of the gastrointestinal mucosa that may lead to perforation and peritonitis.
negligence Commission of an act that a prudent person would not have done or the omission of a duty that prudent person would have fulfilled, resulting in injury or harm to another person. In particular, in a malpractice suit a professional person is negligent if harm to a client results from such an act or such a failure to act, but it must be proved that other prudent persons of the same profession would ordinarily have acted differently under the same circumstances.
neonatal hypovolemic shock Cardiovascular collapse due to a diminished volume of circulating fluid in the cardiovascular system.
neonatal mortality Statistical rate of infant death during the first 28 days after live birth, expressed as the number of such deaths per 1,000 live births in a specific geographic area or institution in a given period of time.
neonatology Study of the neonate.
nephroureterolithiasis Stones in the kidneys and ureters.
neurofibromatosis Congenital condition transmitted as an autosomal dominant trait, characterized by numerous neurofibromas of the nerves and skin, by cafe-au-lait spots on the skin, and, in some cases, by developmental anomalies of the muscles, bones, and viscera.
neutral temperature range That grouping of environmental conditions in which the neonate's oxygen consumption is at a minimum and his temperature is within normal limits.
nevus Natural blemish or mark; a congenital circumscribed deposit of pigmentation in the skin; mole.
 n. flammeus Port-wine stain; reddish, usually flat, discoloration of the face or neck. Because of its large size and color, it is considered a serious deformity.
 n. vasculosus (strawberry hemangioma) Elevated lesion of immature capillaries and endothelial cells that regresses over a period of years.
nidation Implantation of the fertilized ovum in the endometrium, or lining, of the uterus.
nondisjunction Failure of homologous pairs of chromosomes to separate during the first meiotic division or of the two chromatids of a chromosome to split during anaphase of mitosis or the second meiotic division. The result is an abnormal number of chromosomes in the daughter cells.

nonshivering thermogenesis Infant's method of producing heat by increasing his metabolic rate.
nonstress test (NST) Evaluation of fetal response (fetal heart rate) to natural contractile uterine activity or to an increase in fetal activity.
nosocomial Pertaining to a hospital.
nucleotide Single segment of helical strand of DNA.
nulligravida Woman who has never been pregnant.
nullipara Woman who has not yet carried a pregnancy to viability.
nursing practitioner Registered nurse who has additional education to practice nursing in an expanded role.
nystagmus Constant, involuntary, rhythmic oscillation of the eyeball. The movements may be in any direction.

obstetrix Midwife; from *obstare,* to stand before.
occipitobregmatic Pertaining to the occiput (the back part of the skull) and the bregma (junction of the coronal and sagittal sutures) or anterior fontanel; the smallest diameter of the fetal head.
occiput Back part of the head or skull.
oligohydramnios Abnormally small amount or absence of amniotic fluid; often indicative of fetal urinary tract defect.
oliguria Diminished secretion of urine by the kidneys.
omphalic Concerning or pertaining to the umbilicus.
omphalitis Inflammation of the umbilical stump characterized by redness, edema, and purulent exudate in severe infections.
omphalocele Congenital defect resulting from failure of closure of the abdominal wall or muscles and leading to hernia of abdominal contents through the navel.
oocyesis Ectopic ovarian pregnancy.
oocyte Primordial or incompletely developed ovum.
oophorectomy Excision or removal of an ovary.
operculum Plug of mucus that fills the cervical canal during pregnancy.
ophthalmia neonatorum Infection in the neonate's eyes usually resulting from gonorrheal or other infection contracted when the fetus passes through the birth canal (vagina).
opisthotonos Tetanic spasm resulting in an arched, hyperextended position of the body.
oral GTT Test for blood sugar following oral ingestion of a concentrated sugar solution.
orchitis Inflammation of one or both of the testes, characterized by swelling and pain, often caused by mumps, syphilis, or tuberculosis.
orgasmic platform Congestion of the lower vagina during sexual intercourse.
orifice Normal mouth, entrance, or opening, to any aperture.
os Mouth, or opening.
  external o. (o. externum) External opening of the cervical canal.
  internal o. (o. internum) Internal opening of the cervical canal.
  o. uteri Mouth, or opening, of the uterus.
ossification Mineralization of fetal bones.
-otomy Combining form meaning cutting, incision, section.
outlet Opening by which something can exit.
  pelvic o. Inferior aperture, or opening, of the true pelvis.
ovary One of two glands in the female situated on either side of the pelvic cavity that produces the female reproductive cell, the ovum, and two known hormones, estrogen and progesterone.
ovulation Periodic ripening and discharge of the unimpregnated ovum from the ovary, usually 14 days prior to the onset of menstrual flow.
  o. method Evaluation of cervical mucus throughout the menstrual cycle; ovulation occurs just after the appearance of the peak mucus sign; Billings method.
ovum Female germ, or reproductive cell, produced by the ovary; egg.
oxygen toxicity Oxygen overdosage that results in pathologic tissue changes (e.g., retrolental fibroplasia, bronchopulmonary dysplasia).
oxytocics Drugs that stimulate uterine contractions, thus accelerating childbirth and preventing postdelivery hemorrhage. They may be used to increase the let-down reflex during lactation.
oxytocin Hormone produced by the posterior pituitary that stimulates uterine contractions and the release of milk in the mammary gland (let-down reflex).
  o. challenge test (OCT) Evaluation of fetal response (fetal heart rate) to contractile activity of the uterus stimulated by exogenous oxytocin (Pitocin).

$Paco_2$ Partial pressure of carbon dioxide in arterial blood.
pallida, asphyxia See *asphyxia pallida.*
palpation Examination performed by touching the external surface of the body with the fingers or palmar surface of the hand.
  bimanual p. See *bimanual palpation.*
palsy Permanent or temporary loss of sensation or ability to move and control movement; paralysis.
  Bell's p. Peripheral facial paralysis of the facial nerve (cranial nerve VII), causing the muscles of the unaffected side of the face to pull the face into a distorted position.
  Erb's p. See *Erb-Duchenne paralysis.*
panhysterectomy See *hysterectomy.*
Pao_2 Partial pressure of oxygen in arterial blood.
Papanicolaou (Pap) smear Microscopic examination using scrapings from the cervix, endocervix, or other mucous membranes that will reveal, with a high degree of accuracy, the presence of premalignant or malignant cells.
para Term used to refer to past pregnancies that reached viability regardless of whether the infant was dead or alive at birth.
parabiotic syndrome Fetofetal blood transfer caused by placental vascular anastomoses occurring in a small plethoric twin (polycythemia) and one pale twin (anemia).
parametritis Inflamed condition of the cellular tissue or parmetrium of the uterus; pelvic cellulitis.
parametrium Flat, smooth muscle, and loose connective tissue lying around the uterus and extending laterally between the layers of the broad ligaments.
parenteral Administration or injection of nutrients, fluids, or drugs into the body by any way other than the digestive tract.
parity Number of pregnancies that reached viability.
parovarian Pertaining to the residual structure in the broad ligament between the fallopian tubes and the ovary.
parturient Woman giving birth.
parturition Process or act of giving birth.
patent Open.
pathogen Substance or organism capable of producing disease.
pathognomonic Characteristic or distinctive symptom or sign of a disease that facilitates recognition or differentiation from other conditions.
pathologic hyperbilirubinemia High (toxic) levels of serum bilirubin due to a disease process causing hemolysis (e.g., Rh incompatibility); jaundice apparent within first 24 hours.
pathologic jaundice See *jaundice, pathologic.*
pathosis A disease condition.
patulous Open or spread apart.
peak mucus sign Lubricative, cloudy-to-clear-egg white cervical mucus occurring under high estrogen levels close to time of ovulation; ferns; good spinnbarkheit.
pedigree Shorthand method of depicting family lines of individuals who manifest a physical or chemical disorder.

pelvic Pertaining or relating to the pelvis.
p. axis See *axis, pelvic.*
p. inlet See *inlet, pelvic.*
p. outlet See *outlet, pelvic.*

pelvimeter Device for measuring the diameters and capacity of the pelvis.

pelvimetry Measurement of dimensions and proportions of the pelvis to determine its capacity and ability to allow the passage of the fetus through the birth canal.

pelvis Bony structure formed by the sacrum, coccyx, innominate bones, and symphysis pubis, and the ligaments that unite them.
android p. See *android pelvis.*
anthropoid p. See *anthropoid pelvis.*
false p. Pelvis above the linea terminalis and symphysis pubis.
gynecoid p. See *gynecoid pelvis.*
platypelloid p. See *platypelloid pelvis.*
true p. Pelvis below the linea terminalis.

pemphigus An uncommon, serious disease of the skin and mucous membranes, characterized by thin-walled bullae arising from apparently normal skin or mucous membrane. The bullae rupture easily, leaving raw patches. The person loses weight, becomes weak, and is subject to major infections.

pemphigus neonatorum Neonatal impetigo.

penis Male organ used for urination and copulation.

perforation of the uterus Accidental puncture of the uterus, usually with a curet and occasionally by an intrauterine device (IUD).

peridural anesthesia Injection of anesthetic outside the dura mater (anesthetic does not mix with spinal fluid); epidural anesthesia.

perinatal Of or pertaining to the time and process of giving birth or being born.

perinatal period Period extending from the twentieth or twenty-eighth week of gestation through the end of the twenty-eighth day after birth.

perinatologist Physician who specializes in fetal and neonatal care.

perineorrhaphy Suture or operation used in repairing a laceration of the perineum, usually following labor.

perineotomy Surgical incision into the perineum. In obstetrics the perineotomy is usually called an *episiotomy* and is done at the end of the second stage of labor to avoid laceration of the perineum and to facilitate delivery. (See also *episiotomy.*)

perineum Area between the vagina and rectum in the female and between the scrotum and rectum in the male.

periodic breathing Sporadic episodes of cessation of respirations for periods of 10 seconds or less not associated with cyanosis commonly noted in premature infants.

peritoneum Strong serous membrane reflected over the viscera and lining the abdominal cavity.

pessary Device placed inside the vagina to function as a supportive structure for the uterus or a contraceptive device.

petechiae Pinpoint hemorrhagic areas caused by numerous disease states involving infection and thrombocytopenia and occasionally found over the face and trunk of the newborn because of increased intravascular pressure in the capillaries during delivery.

pH Hydrogen ion concentration.

phenotype Expression of certain physical or chemical characteristics in an individual resulting from interaction between genotype and environmental factors.

phenylketonuria (PKU) Recessive hereditary disease that results in a defect in the metabolism of the amino acid phenylalanine caused by the lack of an enzyme, phenylalanine hydroxylase, that is necessary for the conversion of the amino acid phenylalanine into tyrosine. If PKU is not treated, brain damage may occur, causing severe mental retardation.

phimosis Tightness of the prepuce, or foreskin, of the penis.

phlebitis Inflammation of a vein with symptoms of pain and tenderness along the course of the vein, inflammatory swelling and acute edema below the obstruction, and discoloration of the skin because of injury or bruise to the vein, possibly occurring in acute or chronic infections or after operations or childbirth.

phlebothrombosis Formation of a clot or thrombus in the vein; inflammation of the vein with secondary clotting.

phlebotomy Incision of a vein for the letting of blood, as in collecting blood from a donor.

phlegmasia alba dolens Phlebitis of the femoral vein with thrombosis leading to a venous obstruction, causing acute edema of the leg, and occurring occasionally after delivery; also called *milk-leg.*

phocomelia Developmental anomaly characterized by the absence of the upper portion of one or more limbs so that the feet or hands or both are attached to the trunk of the body by short, irregularly shaped stumps, resembling the fins of a seal.

phototherapy Utilization of lights to reduce serum bilirubin levels by oxidation of bilirubin into water-soluble compounds that are then processed in the liver and excreted in bile and urine.

physiologic hyperbilirubinemia Hemolysis of excessive fetal RBCs in the early neonatal period; jaundice not apparent during first 24 hours. Levels are nontoxic to the individual.

physiologic jaundice See *jaundice, physiologic.*

pica Unusual craving during pregnancy (e.g., of laundry starch, dirt, red clay).

pinna Ear cartilage.

placenta Latin, flat cake; afterbirth; specialized vascular disc-shaped organ for maternal-fetal gas and nutrient exchange. Normally it implants in the thick muscular wall of the upper uterine segment.
abruptio p. See *abruptio placentae.*
battledore p. Umbilical cord insertion into the margin of the placenta.
circumvallate p. Placenta having a raised white ring at its edge.
p. accreta Invasion of the uterine muscle by the placenta, thus making separation from the muscle difficult if not impossible.
p. previa Placenta that is abnormally implanted in the thin, lower uterine segment and that is typed according to proximity to cervical os: total—completely occludes os; partial—does not occlude os completely; and marginal—placenta encroaches on margin of internal cervical os.
p. succenturiata Accessory placenta.

placental Pertaining or relating to the placenta.
p. dysfunction Failure of placenta to meet fetal needs and requirements; placental insufficiency.
p. dystocia See *dystocia, placental.*
p. infarct Localized, ischemic, hard area on the fetal or maternal side of the placenta.
p. souffle See *souffle, placental.*

platypelloid pelvis Broad pelvis with a shortened anteroposterior diameter and a flattened, oval, transverse shape.

plethora Deep beefy red coloration ("boiled lobster" hue) of a newborn caused by an increased number of blood cells (polycythemia) per volume of blood.

pneumomediastinum Accumulation of air around the heart and vena cava.

pneumothorax Escaped air from affected lung into the pleural space, displacing the heart and mediastinum toward the unaffected side of the chest.

podalic Concerning or pertaining to the feet.
p. version Shifting of the position of the fetus so as to bring the feet to the outlet during labor.

polycythemia Increased number of erythrocytes per volume of blood, which may be caused by large placental transfusion, fetofetal transfusion, or maternal-fetal transfusion, or it may be due to hypovolemia resulting from movement of fluid out of vascular into interstitial compartment.
polydactyly Excessive number of digits (fingers or toes).
polygenic Pertaining to the combined action of several different genes.
polyhydramnios See *hydramnios*.
polyuria Excessive secretion and discharge of urine by the kidneys.
position Relationship of an arbitrarily chosen fetal reference point, such as the occiput, sacrum, chin, or scapula on the presenting part of the fetus to its location in the front, back, or sides of the maternal pelvis.
positive sign of pregnancy Definite indication of pregnancy (e.g., hearing the fetal heartbeat, visualization and palpation of fetal movement by the examiner, sonographic examination).
posterior Pertaining to the back.
p. fontanel See *fontanel, posterior*.
postmature infant Infant born at or after the beginning of week 43 of gestation or later and exhibiting signs of dysmaturity.
postnatal Happening or occurring after birth.
postpartum Happening or occurring after birth.
Potter's syndrome Silicosis.
precipitate delivery Rapid or sudden labor of less than 3 hours' duration beginning from onset of cervical changes to completed birth of neonate.
preeclampsia Disease encountered during pregnancy or early in the puerperium characterized by increasing hypertension, albuminuria, and generalized edema; pregnancy-induced hypertension (PIH): toxemia.
pregnancy Period between conception through complete delivery of the products of conception. The usual duration of pregnancy in the human is 280 days, 9 calendar months, or 10 lunar months.
abdominal p. See *abdominal gestation*.
ectopic p. See *ectopic pregnancy*.
extrauterine p. See *extrauterine pregnancy*.
premature infant Infant born before completing week 37 of gestation, irrespective of birth weight; preterm infant.
premenstrual syndrome Syndrome of nervous tension, irritability, weight gain, edema, headache, mastalgia, dysphoria, and lack of coordination occurring during the last few days of the menstrual cycle preceding the onset of menstruation.
premonitory Serving as an early symptom or warning.
prenatal Occurring or happening before birth.
prepartum Before delivery; prior to giving birth.
prepuce Fold of skin, or foreskin, covering the glans penis of the male.
p. of the clitoris Fold of the labia minora that the glans clitoris.
presentation That part of the fetus which first enters the pelvis and lies over the inlet: may be head, face, breech, or shoulder.
breech p. See *breech presentation*.
cephalic p. See *cephalic presentation*.
presenting part That part of the fetus which lies closest to the internal os of the cervix.
pressure edema Edema of the lower extremities caused by pressure of the heavy pregnant uterus against the large veins; edema of fetal scalp after cephalic presentation (caput succedaneum).
presumptive signs Manifestations that suggest pregnancy but that are not absolutely positive. These include the cessation of menses. Chadwick's sign, morning sickness, and quickening.
preterm infant See *premature infant*.
previa, placenta See *placenta previa*.
priapism Continuous erection of the penis, not usually accompanied by sexual feeling, which may appear in conjunction with leukemia, renal calculi, and spinal cord lesions.
primigravida Woman who is pregnant for the first time.
primipara Woman who has carried a pregnancy to viability without regard to the child's being dead or alive at the time of birth.
primordial Existing first or existing in the simplest or most primitive form.
probable signs Manifestations or evidence which indicates that there is a definite likelihood of pregnancy. Among the probable signs are enlargement of abdomen. Goodell's sign, Hegar's sign, Braxton Hicks' sign, and positive hormonal tests for pregnancy.
proband Individual in a family who comes to the attention of a genetic investigator because of the occurrence of a trait; the index case, or propositus.
prodromal Serving as an early symptom or warning of the approach of a disease or condition (e.g., prodromal labor).
progesterone Hormone produced by the corpus luteum and placenta whose function is to prepare the endometrium of the uterus for implantation of the fertilized ovum, develop the mammary glands, and maintain the pregnancy.
projectile vomiting Extremely forceful, expulsive vomiting.
prolactin See *lactogenic hormone*.
prolan Hormone produced by chorionic villi, now called *human chorionic gonadotropin (HCG),* that is found in the serum and urine of pregnant women and forms the basis of the biologic and immunologic pregnancy tests.
prolapsed cord Protrusion of the umbilical cord in advance of the presenting part.
proliferative phase of menstrual cycle Preovulatory, follicular, or estrogen phase of the menstrual cycle.
promontory of the sacrum Superior projecting portion of the sacrum at the junction of the sacrum and the L-5.
prophylactic Pertaining to prevention or warding off of disease or certain conditions; condom, or "rubber."
propositus See *proband*.
prostaglandin (PG) Substance present in many body tissues; has a role in many reproductive tract functions.
proteinuria Excretion of protein into urine.
pruritis Itching.
pruritis gravidarum Itching of the skin caused by pregnancy.
pseudocyesis Condition in which the woman has all the usual signs of pregnancy, such as enlargement of the abdomen, cessation of menses, weight gain, and morning sickness, but is not pregnant; phantom or false pregnancy.
pseudopregnancy See *pseudocyesis*.
pseudoprematurity See *intrauterine growth retardation (IUGR)*.
psychologic miscarriage Absence or lack of love for one's infant.
psychoprophylaxis Mental and physical education of the parents in preparation for childbirth, with the goal of minimizing the fear and pain and promoting positive family relationships.
ptyalism Excessive salivation.
puberty Period in life in which the reproductive organs mature and one becomes functionally capable of reproduction.
pubic Pertaining to the pubis.
pubis Pubic bone forming the front of the pelvis.
pudendal block Injection of a local anesthetizing drug at the pudendal nerve root in order to produce numbness of the genital and perianal region.
pudendum External genitalia of either sex; Latin, "that of which one should be ashamed."
puerperal sepsis Infection of the pelvic organs during the postdelivery period; childbed fever.
puerperium Period of time following the third stage of labor and lasting until involution of the uterus takes place, usually about 3 to 6 weeks.

pulse pressure Difference between systolic and diastolic blood pressure.

pyloric stenosis Narrowing of the pyloric sphincter at the outlet of the stomach, causing an obstruction that blocks the flow of food into the small intestine.

quickening Maternal perception of fetal movement; usually occurs between weeks 16 and 20 of gestation.

rabbit test See *Friedman's test.*

radium insertion Introduction of metallic element radium (Ra) into the uterus or cervix to treat cancer.

rales Crackling sounds heard as air passes through the fluid present within the terminal bronchioles and alveoli.

raphe A line of union of the halves of various symmetrical parts, as the abdominal raphe of the linea alba or the raphe penis, which appears as a narrow, dark streak on the inferior surface of the penis.

RDS See *respiratory distress syndrome (RDS).*

recessive trait Genetically determined characteristic that is expressed only when present in the homozygotic state.

rectocele Herniation or protrusion of the rectum into the posterior vaginal wall.

rectovaginal ligament A posterior ligament.

reflex Automatic response built into the nervous system that does not need the intervention of conscious thought (e.g., in the newborn, rooting, gagging, grasp).

regional block anesthesia Anesthesia of an area of the body by injecting a local anesthetic to block a group of sensory nerve fibers.

regurgitate Vomiting or spitting up of solids or fluids.

residual urine Urine that remains in the bladder after urination.

respiratory distress syndrome (RDS) Condition resulting from decreased pulmonary gas exchange, leading to retention of carbon dioxide (increase in arterial P_{CO_2}). Most common neonatal causes are prematurity, perinatal asphyxia, and maternal diabetes mellitus; hyaline membrane disease (HMD).

restitution In obstetrics, the turning of the fetal head to the left or right after it has completely emerged from the introitus as it assumes a normal alignment with the infant's shoulders.

resuscitation Restoration of consciousness or life in one who is apparently dead or whose respirations or cardiac function or both have ceased.

retained placenta Retention of all or part of the placenta in the uterus after delivery.

reticulocytosis Increase in number of reticulocytes in circulating blood.

retraction (1) Drawing in or sucking in of soft tissues of chest, indicative of an obstruction at any level of the respiratory tract from the oropharynx to the alveoli. (2) Retraction of uterine muscle fiber. After contracting, the muscle fiber does not return to its original length but remains slightly shortened, a unique attribute of uterine muscle that aids in preventing postdelivery hemorrhage and results in involution.

retroflexion Bending backward

- **r. of the uterus** Condition in which the body of the womb is bent backward at an angle with the cervix, whose position usually remains unchanged.

retrolental fibroplasia (RLF) Retinopathy of prematurity associated with hyperoxemia, resulting in eye injury and blindness.

retroversion Turning or a state of being turned back.

- **r. of the uterus** Displacement of the uterus; the body of the uterus is tipped backward with the cervix pointing forward toward the symphysis pubis.

Retrovirus A single piece of RNA surrounded by a protein coat, or envelope. A unique enzyme, reverse transcriptase, allows this RNA retrovirus to go backward, *against the 'flow of life.'* The RNA becomes a piece of DNA, which infects the cell's DNA nucleus and remains in the cell until its death. (The normal flow of genetic information in life is from DNA to RNA to protein.)

Rh factor Inherited antigen present on erythrocytes. The individual with the factor is known as *positive* for the factor.

rhonchi Coarse, snorelike sounds produced as air passes through the fluid in the large bronchi, frequently heard after aspiration of oral secretions or feedings.

rhythm method Contraceptive method in which a woman abstains from sexual intercourse during the ovulatory phase of her menstrual cycle and at least 3 days before and 1 day after the ovulation date.

ribonucleic acid (RNA) Element responsible for transferring genetic information within a cell; a template, or pattern.

risk factors Factors that cause a person or a group of people to be particularly vulnerable to an unwanted, unpleasant, or unhealthful event.

Ritgen maneuver Procedure used to control the delivery of the head.

role playing Psychotherapeutic technique in which a person acts out a real or simulated situation as a means of understanding intrapsychic conflicts.

rooming-in unit Maternity unit designed so that the newborn's crib is at the mother's bedside or in a nursery adjacent to the mother's room.

rooting reflex Normal response in newborns when the cheek is touched or stroked along the side of the mouth to turn the head toward the stimulated side, to open the mouth, and to begin to suck. The reflex disappears by 3 to 4 months of age but in some infants may persist until 12 months.

rotation In obstetrics, the turning of the fetal head as it follows the curves of the birth canal downward.

Rubin's test Transuterine insufflation of the fallopian tubes with carbon dioxide to test their patency.

rugae Folds of vaginal mucosa.

Rupture of membranes (ROM)

- **Artificial (AROM)** Deliberate rupture of membranes by physician, usually to induce or augment labor.
- **Premature (PROM)** Most commonly refers to rupture of membranes anytime before onset of labor irrespective of whether the duration of pregnancy at time of rupture is 24 weeks or 44 weeks.
- **Preterm** Rupture of membranes remote from term gestation (e.g., ≤ 37 weeks).
- **Prolonged** Rupture of membranes ≥ 24 hours before delivery.
- **Spontaneous (SROM)** Rupture of membranes without artificial means

sac, amniotic See *amniotic sac.*

sacroiliac Of or pertaining to the sacrum and ilium.

sacrum Triangular bone composed of five united vertebras and situated between L-5 and the coccyx; forms the posterior boundary of the true pelvis.

saddle block anesthesia Type of regional anesthesia produced by injection of a local anesthetic solution into the cerebrospinal fluid intrathecal (subarachnoid) space in the spinal canal.

sagittal suture Band of connective tissue separating the parietal bones, extending from the anterior to the posterior fontanel.

salpingo-oophorectomy Removal of a fallopian tube and an ovary.

scaphoid abdomen Abdomen with a sunken interior wall.

schizophrenia Any one of a large group of psychotic disorders characterized by gross distortion of reality, disturbances of language and communication, withdrawal from social interaction, and the disorganization and fragmentation of thought, perception, and emotional reaction.

Schultze's mechanism Delivery of the placenta with the fetal surfaces (shiny in appearance) presenting (archaic).

sclerema Hardening of skin and subcutaneous tissue that develops in association with such life-threatening disorders as severe cold stress, septicemia, and shock.

scrotum Pouch of skin containing the testes and parts of the spermatic cords.

sebaceous glands Oil-secreting glands found in the skin.

secondary areola See *areola, secondary*.

secretory phase of menstrual cycle Postovulatory, luteal, progestational, premenstrual phase of menstrual cycle; 14 days in length.

secundines Fetal membranes and placenta expelled after childbirth; afterbirth.

segmentation Process of cleavage or division by which the fertilized ovum multiplies before differentiating into layers.

semen Thick, white, viscid secretion discharged from the urethra of the male at orgasm; the transporting medium of the sperm.

sensitization Development of antibodies to a specific antigen.

septic abortion See *abortion, septic*.

shake test "Foam" test for lung maturity of fetus; more rapid than determination of L/S ratio.

Sims' position Position in which the client lies on the left side with the right knee and thigh drawn upward toward the chest.

singleton Pregnancy with a single fetus.

situational crisis Crisis that arises suddenly in response to an external event or a conflict concerning a specific circumstance. The symptoms are transient, and the episode is usually brief.

Skene's glands Paraurethral glands situated on each side of urethral meatus.

small for dates (small for gestational age [SGA]) Refers to inadequate growth for gestational age.

smegma Whitish secretion around labia minora.

socioeconomic status Combined social and economic level of individuals or groups.

souffle Soft, blowing sound or murmur heard by auscultation.

- **funic s.** Soft, muffled, blowing sound produced by blood rushing through the umbilical vessels and synchronous with the fetal heart sounds.
- **placental s.** Soft, blowing murmur caused by the blood current in the placenta and synchronous with the maternal pulse.
- **uterine s.** Soft, blowing sound made by the blood in the arteries of the pregnant uterus and synchronous with the maternal pulse.

sperm Male sex cell. Also called spermatozoon.

spermatic cord Structure supporting the testis and containing blood vessels, nerves, muscle fibers, and the vas deferens.

spermatogenesis Process by which mature spermatozoa are formed, during which the diploid chromosome number (46) is reduced by half (haploid, 23).

spermicide Chemical substance that kills sperm by reducing their surface tension, causing the cell wall to break down by a bactericidal effect or by creating a highly acidic environment. Also called spermatocide.

spina bifida occulta Congenital malformation of the spine in which the posterior portion of laminas of the vertebras fails to close but there is no herniation or protrusion of the spinal cord or meninges through the defect. The newborn may have a dimple in the skin or growth of hair over the malformed vertebras.

spinnbarkheit Formation of a stretchable thread of cervical mucus under estrogen influence at time of ovulation.

splanchnic engorgement Excessive filling or pooling of blood within the visceral vasculature that occurs following the removal of pressure from the abdomen, e.g., birth of a child, removal of an excess of urine from bladder (1000 ml), removal of large tumor.

spontaneous abortion See *abortion, spontaneous*.

square window Angle of wrist between hypothenar prominence and forearm; one criterion for estimating gestational age of neonate.

station Relationship of the presenting fetal part to an imaginary line drawn between the ischial spines of the pelvis.

sterility (1) State of being free from living microorganisms. (2) Complete inability to reproduce offspring.

sterilization Process or act that renders a person unable to produce children.

stillborn Born dead.

striae gravidarum ("stretch marks") Shining reddish lines caused by stretching of the skin, often found on the abdomen, thighs, and breasts during pregnancy. These streaks turn to a fine pinkish white or silver tone in time in fair-skinned women and brownish in darker-skinned women.

stroma Supporting tissue.

subculture Group having social, economic, ethnic, or other traits distinctive enough to distinguish it from others within the same culture or society.

subinvolution Failure of a part (e.g., the uterus) to reduce to its normal size and condition after enlargement from functional activity (e.g., pregnancy).

subluxation Incomplete dislocation.

subtotal hysterectomy See *hysterectomy, subtotal*.

succedaneum See *caput succedaneum*.

superfecundation Successive fertilization of two or more ova formed during the same menstrual cycle by the sperm of the same father or different fathers.

superfetation Fertilization of an ovum when the woman is already pregnant.

supernumerary nipples Excessive number of nipples varying in size from small pink spots to the size of normal nipples and usually not associated with underlying glandular tissue.

supine hypotension Shock; fall in blood pressure caused by impaired venous return when gravid uterus presses on ascending vena cava, when woman is lying flat on her back; vena caval syndrome.

suppuration Process by which pus is formed.

surfactant Phosphoprotein necessary for normal respiratory function that prevents the alveolar collapse (atelectasis). See also *lecithin* and *L/S ratio*.

suture (1) Junction of the adjoining bones of the skull. (2) Operation uniting parts by sewing them together.

symphysis pubis Fibrocartilaginous union of the bodies of the pubic bones in the midline.

syndactyly Malformation of digits, commonly seen as a fusion of two or more toes to form one structure.

synostosis Articulation by osseous tissue of adjacent bones; union of separate bones by osseous tissue.

taboo Proscribed (forbidden) by society as improper and unacceptable.

tachypnea Excessively rapid respiratory rate (e.g., in neonates, respiratory rate of 60 breaths/min or more).

talipes equinovarus Deformity in which the foot is extended and the person walks on the toes.

telangiectasia Permanent dilatation of groups of superficial capillaries and venules.

telangiectatic nevi ("stork bites") Clusters of small, red, localized areas of capillary dilatation commonly seen in neonates at the nape of the neck or lower occiput, upper eyelids, and nasal bridge that can be blanched with pressure of a finger.

teratogenic agent Any drug, virus, or irradiation, the exposure to which can cause malformation of the fetus.

teratogens Nongenetic factors that cause malformations and disease syndromes in utero.

teratoma Tumor composed of different kinds of tissue, none of which normally occur together or at the site of the tumor.

term infant Live infant born between weeks 38 and 42 of completed gestation.

testis One of the glands contained in the male scrotum that produces the male reproductive cell, or sperm, and the male hormone testosterone; testicle.

tetany, uterine Extremely prolonged uterine contractions.

tetralogy of Fallot Congenital cardiac malformation consisting of pulmonary stenosis, intraventricular septal defect, dextroposed aorta that receives blood from both ventricles, and hypertrophy of the right ventricle.

thalassemia Hemolytic anemia characterized by microcytic, hypochromic, and short-lived red blood cells (RBCs) caused by deficient hemoglobin synthesis. It is an autosomal recessive, genetically transmitted disease occurring in two forms.

t. major (homozygous form) evident in infancy, it is recognized by anemia, fever, failure to thrive, and splenomegaly and confirmed by characteristic changes in the RBCs on microscopic examination.

t. minor (heterozygous form) it is characterized only by a mild anemia and minimal RBC changes.

therapeutic abortion See *abortion, therapeutic.*

thermogenesis Creation or production of heat, especially in the body.

thermoneutral environment Environment that enables the neonate to maintain a body temperature of 36.5° C (97.7° F) with minimum use of oxygen and energy.

threatened abortion See *abortion, threatened.*

thrombocytopenia Abnormal hematologic condition in which the number of platelets is reduced, usually by destruction of erythroid tissue in bone marrow owing to certain neoplastic diseases or to an immune response to a drug.

thrombocytopenic purpura Hematologic disorder characterized by prolonged bleeding time, decreased number of platelets, increased cell fragility, and purpura, which result in hemorrhages into the skin, mucous membranes, organs, and other tissue.

thromboembolism Obstruction of a blood vessel by a clot that has become detached from its site of formation.

thrombophlebitis Inflammation of a vein with secondary clot formation.

thrombus Blood clot obstructing a blood vessel that remains at the place it was formed.

thrush Fungal infection of the mouth or throat characterized by the formation of white patches on a red, moist, inflamed mucous membrane and is caused by *Candida albicans.*

toco- (toko-) Combining form that means childbirth or labor.

tocolytic drug Drug used to suppress premature labor.

tocotransducer Electronic device for measuring uterine contractions.

tongue-tie Congenital shortening of the frenulum, which, if severe, may interfere with sucking and articulation; a rare condition.

TORCH organisms Organisms that damage the embryo or fetus; acronym for *t*oxoplasmosis, *o*ther (e.g., syphilis), *r*ubella, *c*ytomegalovirus, and *h*erpes simplex.

torticollis Congenital or acquired stiff neck caused by shortening or spasmodic contraction of the neck (sternocleidomastoid) muscles that draws the head to one side with the chin pointing in the other direction; wryneck.

total hysterectomy See *hysterectomy, total.*

toxemia Term previously used for disorders occurring during pregnancy or early puerperium, known as *preeclampsia-eclampsia,* that are characterized by one or all of the following: edema, hypertension, proteinuria, and, in severe cases, convulsion and coma; pregnancy-induced hypertension (PIH).

tracheoesophageal fistula Congenital malformation in which there is an abnormal tubelike passage between the trachea and esophagus.

transition Last phase of first stage of labor; 8 to 10 cm dilatation.

translocation Condition in which a chromosome breaks and all or part of that chromosome is transferred to a different part of the same chromosome or to another chromosome.

trauma Physical or psychic injury.

Trichomonas vaginitis Inflammation of the vagina caused by *Trichomonas vaginalis,* a parasitic protozoon and characterized by persistent burning and itching of the vulvar tissue and a profuse, frothy, white discharge.

trimester Time period of 3 months.

trisomy Condition whereby any given chromosome exists in triplicate instead of the normal duplicate pattern.

trophectoderm See *trophoblast.*

trophoblast Outer layer of cells of the developing blastodermic vesicle that develops the trophoderm or feeding layer which will establish the nutrient relationships with the uterine endometrium.

tubal ligation See *ligation, tubal.*

tubercles of Montgomery Small papillae on surface of nipples and areolae that secrete a fatty substance that lubricates the nipples.

twins Two neonates from the same impregnation developed within the same uterus at the same time.

conjoined t. Twins who are physically united; Siamese twins.

disparate t. Twins who are different (e.g., in weight) and distinct from one another.

dizygous t. Twins developed from two separate ova fertilized by two separate sperm at the same time; fraternal twins.

monozygous twins Twins developed from a single fertilized ovum; identical twins.

ultrasonography High frequency sound waves to discern fetal heart rate or placental location or body parts.

umbilical cord (funis) Structure connecting the placenta and fetus and containing two arteries and one vein encased in a tissue called *Wharton's jelly.* The cord is ligated at birth and severed; the stump falls off in 4 to 10 days.

umbilical vasculitis Inflammation of the umbilical cord and its blood vessels.

umbilicus Navel, or depressed point in the middle of the abdomen that marks the attachment of the umbilical cord during fetal life.

urachus Epithelial tube connecting the apex of the urinary bladder with the allantois. Its connective tissue forms the median umbilical ligament.

urethra Small tubular structure that drains urine from the bladder.

urinary frequency Need to void often or at close intervals.

urinary meatus Opening, or mouth, of the urethra.

uterine Referring or pertaining to the uterus.

u. adnexa See *adnexa, uterine.*

u. bruit Abnormal sound or murmur heard while auscultating the uterus.

u. ischemia Decreased blood supply to the uterus.

u. prolapse Falling, sinking, or sliding of the uterus from its normal location in the body.

u. souffle See *souffle, uterine.*

uterus Hollow muscular organ in the female designed for the implantation, containment, and nourishment of the fetus during its development until birth.

Couvelaire u. Interstitial myometrial hemorrhage following premature separation (abruptio) of placenta. A purplish-bluish discoloration of the uterus and boardlike rigidity of the uterus are noted.

inversion of the u. See *inversion of the uterus.*

retroflexion of the u. See *retroflexion of the uterus.*

retroversion of the u. See *retroversion of the uterus.*

vagina Normally collapsed musculomembranous tube that forms the passageway between the uterus and the entrance to the vagina.

vaginismus Intense, painful spasm of the muscles surrounding the vagina.

varices (varicose veins) Swollen, distended, and twisted veins that may develop in almost any part of the body but are most commonly seen in the legs, caused by pregnancy, obesity, congenital defective venous valves, and occupations requiring much standing.

vasectomy Ligation or removal of a segment of the vas deferens, usually done bilaterally to produce sterility in the male.

VDRL test Abbreviation for Venereal Disease Research Laboratory test, a serological flocculation test for syphilis.

venous Pertaining or relating to the veins.

vera, decidua See *decidua vera.*

vernix caseosa Protective gray-white fatty substance of cheesy consistency covering the fetal skin.

version Act of turning the fetus in the uterus to change the presenting part and facilitate delivery.

podalic v. See *podalic version.*

vertex Crown or top of the head.

v. presentation Presentation in which the fetal skull is nearest the cervical opening and born first.

vesicle Tiny blister; a small, thin-walled raised skin lesion containing clear fluid.

vesicle, blastoderm See *blastoderm vesicle.*

vestibule Area at the entrance to another structure.

v. of vagina Space between the labia minora where the urinary meatus and vaginal introitus are located.

viable Capable of living, such as a fetus that has reached a stage of development, usually 24 to 28 weeks, which will permit it to live outside the uterus.

villi Short, vascular processes or protrusions growing on certain membranous surfaces.

chorionic v. Tiny vascular protrusions on the chorionic surface that project into the maternal blood sinuses of the uterus and that help to form the placenta and secrete hCG.

voluntary abortion See *abortion, elective.*

volvulus Twisting of the bowel on itself, causing intestinal obstruction.

vulva External genitalia of the female that consist of the labia majora, labia minora, clitoris, urinary meatus, and vaginal introitus.

vulvectomy Removal of the external genitalia of the female.

well-baby clinics Clinics that offer medical supervision and services to healthy infants.

Wharton's jelly White, gelatinous material surrounding the umbilical vessels within the cord.

witch's milk Secretion of a whitish fluid for about a week after birth from enlarged mammary tissue in the neonate, presumably resulting from maternal hormonal influences.

womb See *uterus.*

X chromosome Sex chromosome in humans existing in duplicate in the normal female and singly in the normal male.

X linkage Genes located on the X-chromosome.

Y chromosome Sex chromosome in the human male necessary for the development of the male gonads.

zero fluid balance Equality of amount of intake and amount of output.

zero population growth In a given year, live births equal to total number of deaths (i.e., no population increase for that year).

zona pellucida Inner, thick, membranous envelope of the ovum.

zygote Cell formed by the union of two reproductive cells or gametes; the fertilized ovum resulting from the union of a sperm and an ovum.

Index

*Page numbers followed by *b* indicate boxed material; page numbers followed by *f* indicate illustrations; page numbers followed by *t* indicate tables.

D

M

P

S

V

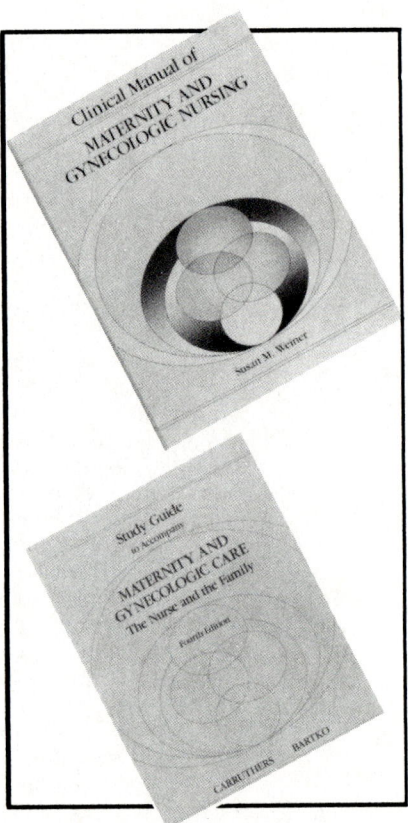

ACYCLOVIR/ACYCLOVIR SODIUM▲

(ay-sye-kloe-veer)

CATEGORY: *Antiviral* — Rx; Preg Cat C

BRAND NAMES
Zovirax (Burroughs-Wellcome)

DOSAGE FORMS
Capsule: 200mg
Powder for injection (IV)▲: 500mg/vial
Ointment: 5%

ACTION: Antiviral activity due to interference c̄ virus DNA polymerase, and DNA replication in virus-infected host cells; selective for herpesvirus (HSV-1, HSV-2). **USE:** Management of herpes genitalis (HSV-2), mucocutaneous herpes simplex (HSV-1) in immunocompromised pts.

PHARMACOKINETICS

Half-life	Protein binding	Excretion
2-3.5h	9%-33%	Urine via tubular secretion, glomerular filtration primarily as unchanged drug

CONTRAINDICATIONS: *Hypersensitivity.*

DOSAGE

Topical	Apply ointment 6 times/d for 7d
Pediatric *IV*	250mg/m² administered at constant rate for 1h q8h for 7d
Adult *IV*	5mg/kg administered at constant rate for 1h q8h for 7d
PO	Initial genital herpes: 200mg q4h 5 times/d for 10d while awake (total 50 capsules) Long-term suppression/recurrent disease: 200mg tid for 6mo; some pts may require 5 doses daily for 6mo. Intermittent treatment: 200mg q4h while awake 6 times/d for 5d (total 25 capsules)

SIDE/ADVERSE EFFECTS: CNS: agitation, confusion, hallucinations, lethargy, tremors, ***seizures/coma*** (all systemic) ▪ CV: *inflammation or phlebitis* at infusion site, hypotension ▪ INT: *burning/stinging* at application site (topical), rash hives, pruritus.

DRUG INTERACTIONS: Probenecid will ↓ urinary excretion of acyclovir, causing accumulation c̄ potential

*Available in Canada only.
Note: Side/adverse effects: common in *italic;* serious in ***boldface italic.***

ERGONOVINE MALEATE

(er-goe-noe-veen)

CATEGORY: *Oxytoxic* — Rx; Preg Cat NA

BRAND NAME
Ergotrate Maleate (Lilly)

DOSAGE FORMS
Injection (IM/IV): 0.2mg/ml
Tablet: 0.2mg

ACTION: Oxytoxic effect due to direct stimulation of uterine smooth muscle, resulting in intense contractions followed by periods of relaxation; accordingly, ↑ uterine tone ↓ postpartum uterine bleeding; drug can occasionally produce severe hypertensive episodes, esp in toxemic pts. **USE:** Treatment/prevention of postpartum/postabortal hemorrhage due to uterine atony.

PHARMACOKINETICS

Onset PO	Onset IM	Onset IV	Duration	Elimination
10m	2-5m	Immediate	Up to ≥3h	Primarily via feces

CONTRAINDICATIONS: Hypersensitivity, threatened spontaneous abortion.

DOSAGE

Adult *PO*	Initial dose 0.2mg, usually IM, followed by 0.2-0.4mg PO q6-12h until danger of atony is over (approximately 48h)
IM	0.2mg; may be repeated for severe hemorrhage
IV	Route should be restricted to excessive hemorrhage because of higher rate of side effects, esp nausea, vomiting

SIDE/ADVERSE EFFECTS: CNS: headache ▪ CV: hypertension, particularly when administered IV ▪ GI: nausea, vomiting ▪ Other: possible symptoms of ergot poisoning.

DRUG INTERACTIONS: Concurrent/sequential use c̄ vasoconstrictors/regional anesthesia may affect BP.

NURSING MANAGEMENT
ADMINISTRATION: *Not* routinely used before delivery ▪ Assess BP ▪ Assess serum calcium; IV calcium gluconate if hypocalcemic ▪ PO: avoid excessive moisture in storage ▪ Injection: store in cold place (<46° F); do

*Available in Canada only.
Note: Side/adverse effects: common in *italic;* serious in ***boldface italic.***

BROMOCRIPTINE MESYLATE

(broe-moe-krip-teen)

CATEGORY: *Dopaminergic:* dopamimetic, prolactin inhibitor — Rx; Preg Cat NA

BRAND NAME
Parlodel (Sandoz)

DOSAGE FORMS
Capsule 5mg, tablet 2.5mg

ACTION: Dopaminergic receptor activity, esp c̄ D-2 dopamine receptors in CNS, produces significant amelioration of hyperprolactinemia, Parkinson disease; bromocriptine may cause symptoms of acromegaly to subside. **USE:** Treatment of idiopathic Parkinson disease ▪ Short-term treatment of amenorrhea/galactorrhea associated c̄ hyperprolactinemia ▪ Treatment of female infertility associated c̄ hyperprogalactinemia ▪ Prevention of lactation; some pts may experience mild/moderate rebound lactation ▪ Treatment of acromegaly.

PHARMACOKINETICS

PO absorption	Peak	Protein binding	Excretion
28%	1-1.5h	90%-96%	Via bile (feces) as metabolites

CONTRAINDICATIONS: Hypersensitivity to drug/ergot alkaloids.

DOSAGE
Adult *PO*

Parkinson disease	Initial dose 1.25mg bid. Dosage may ↑ every 14-28d by 2.5mg/d. Do *not* exceed 100mg/d
Amenorrhea/galactorrhea	2.5mg 2-3 times/d. Therapy usually started c̄ 2.5mg/d. Should *not* exceed 6mo
Infertility	2.5mg 2-3 times/d. Therapy usually started c̄ 2.5mg, ↑ during first wk of treatment
Lactation prevention	Therapy should start no sooner than 4h after delivery in pts c̄ stable VS. Usual dose 2.5mg bid for 14-21d
Acromegaly	Initial dose 1.25-2.5mg hs c̄ food for 3d; c̄ 1.25-2.5mg increments q3-7d until satisfactory response obtained. Usual range 20-30mg/d. Do *not* exceed 100mg/d

SIDE/ADVERSE EFFECTS: CNS: *dizziness, headache,* fatigue, lethargy, ***epileptiform seizures,*** nightmares, con-

*Available in Canada only.
Note: Side/adverse effects: common in *italic;* serious in ***boldface italic.***

ERYTHROMYCIN OPHTHALMIC OINTMENT

(eh-rith-roe-mye-sin)

CATEGORY: *Antibiotic:* macrolide antibiotic — Rx

BRAND NAMES	DOSAGE FORMS
Ak-Mycin (Akorn)	Ophthalmic ointment: 0.5% (5mg/g)
Ilotycin (Dista), (Lilly in Canada)	Ophthalmic ointment: 0.5% (5mg/g)

ACTION: Bacteriostatic activity due to inhibition of ribosomal protein synthesis in susceptible microorganisms; topical ophthalmic application has limited tissue penetration, may fail to protect against gonococcal penicillinase-producing strains of *Neisseria gonorrhoeae.* **USE:** Treatment of ophthalmic infections due to susceptible organisms ▪ Prophylaxis of gonococcal/chlamydial ophthalmia neonatorum.

CONTRAINDICATIONS: Hypersensitivity.

DOSAGE

Ophthalmic infection	Apply ribbon (approximately 1cm) of ointment to infected eye(s), usually in conjunctival sac, ≥1 times/d
Ophthalmia neonatorum	Use new tube for each infant. Apply ribbon (0.5-1cm) of ointment in each conjunctival sac *not* later than 1h after delivery

SIDE/ADVERSE EFFECTS: EENT: local ophthalmic irritation ▪ Other: possible overgrowth of nonsusceptible organisms.

NURSING MANAGEMENT
ADMINISTRATION: Assess for hx of hypersensitivity ▪ Avoid contamination of ointment tube tip ▪ Use new tube of ointment for each neonate ▪ Apply thin strip into lower conjunctival sac after delivery ▪ Do *not* flush from eye after administration ▪ Avoid excessive heat, light in storage; do *not* freeze.

EVALUATION: Observe for signs of local hypersensitivity; notify physician.

*Available in Canada only.
Note: Side/adverse effects: common in *italic;* serious in ***boldface italic.***

not exceed 60d at room temperature ▪ Do *not* administer discolored/precipitated solutions ▪ IV: use infusion control device; administer *slowly* ▪ Have emergency support equipment available ▪ Provide emotional support.

EVALUATION: Monitor BP, pulse ▪ Monitor serum calcium ▪ Observe for signs of ergotism (nausea, vomiting, dizziness, cramps, headache, confusion) ▪ Postpartum: monitor fundal height/tone; assess amount/character of lochia.

EDUCATION: Explain procedure, rationale to pt, family ▪ Occurrence of contractions ▪ Relaxation techniques ▪ Comfort measures ▪ Store in tightly closed container ▪ Avoid smoking ▪ Notify physician of infection, signs of ergotism (cramps, vomiting, thirst, weakness, tingling in extremities).

NOTES:

toxicity ▪ Use c̄ caution c̄ interferon/methotrexate; neurologic rxs may occur.

NURSING MANAGEMENT
ADMINISTRATION: Parenteral: administer only by IV infusion over 1h; use infusion control device; avoid rapid/bolus dose; dilute 500mg vial c̄ 10ml sterile H_2O for injection (50mg/ml); shake vial well until solution is clear, stable for 12h (room temperature); further dilute c̄ dextrose/electrolyte solutions to ≥70mg (7mg/ml), use w/in 24h (room temperature); precipitate occurs c̄ refrigeration, will redissolve at room temperature ▪ Topical: use glove to prevent herpes transmission ▪ Maintain hydration ▪ Avoid exposure to heat/moisture in storage ▪ Administer at *end* of hemodialysis.

EVALUATION: Monitor F/E, hepatic, renal status ▪ Assess for ↑ BUN, serum creatinine (IV).

EDUCATION: Take exactly as directed by physician ▪ Take PO form c̄ food ▪ Dizziness may occur; use caution when engaging in potentially hazardous activities ▪ ↑ Fluid intake (8-10 glasses/d) ▪ Use condoms if sexually active ▪ Information on herpes (symptoms, hygiene, transmission) ▪ Women: avoid breastfeeding ▪ Store in tightly closed container ▪ Procedure for topical application.

NOTES:

EDUCATION: Explain procedure, rationale to family ▪ Report signs of local hypersensitivity (redness, tearing, irritation) immediately ▪ Avoid using common towels/wash cloths among family members ▪ Procedure for ophthalmic administration.

NOTES:

fusion ▪ CV: hypotension, edema, palpitations ▪ EENT: nasal congestion, visual disturbances ▪ GI: *N/V/D*, cramps, anorexia, constipation, dyspepsia, dry mouth, metallic taste ▪ GU: urinary frequency ▪ Other: symptoms of ergotism.

DRUG INTERACTIONS: Use c̄ hypotensive agents can produce significant hypotension ▪ Use c̄ levodopa can ↑ frequency of visual/auditory hallucinations ▪ Phenothiazines can ↑ prolactin levels, are best avoided.

NURSING MANAGEMENT
ADMINISTRATION: Assess for hx of ergot alkaloid hypersensitivity ▪ Avoid exposure to heat, moisture, light in storage ▪ Administer c̄ meals/milk ▪ Assess BP for stability before administration.

EVALUATION: Monitor hepatic/neuropsychiatric status ▪ Monitor VS, esp BP ▪ Pregnancy test at periodic intervals ▪ Assess serum FSH, LH, prolactin, urinary retention, pregnanediol prn ▪ Assess visual fields.

EDUCATION: Take c̄ meals ▪ Avoid alcohol ▪ May cause dizziness; use caution in potentially hazardous activities ▪ Avoid changing positions (lying/sitting/standing) rapidly ▪ Women: use birth control during therapy (unless for fertility), do *not* use oral contraceptives; avoid use if breastfeeding ▪ Keep scheduled appointments c̄ physician ▪ May take >6wks for menses to recur ▪ Missed dose: if remembered >4h, do *not* take; do *not* double dose; resume regular dose schedule ▪ Store in tightly closed container.

NOTES:

ESTROGENS, CONJUGATED

(ess-troe-jenz)

CATEGORY: *Estrogenic agent* — Rx; Preg Cat X

BRAND NAMES / **DOSAGE FORMS**

**C.E.S. (ICN)*
Premarin (Ayerst) — Powder for injection (IM/IV): 25mg/vial; Tablet: 0.3, 0.625, 0.9, 1.25, 2.5mg; Vaginal cream: 0.625mg/g

ACTION: Estrogens required for development, maintenance of female reproductive system, secondary sex characteristics. **USE:** Treatment of moderate/severe symptoms associated c̄ menopause ▪ Treatment of atrophic vaginitis, kraurosis vulvae, female hypogonadism, female castration, breast/prostatic cancer palliation, primary ovarian failure ▪ Prevention of postpartum breast enlargement ▪ Probably effective for estrogen deficiency-induced osteoporosis in conjunction c̄ diet.

PHARMACOKINETICS: Rapid PO absorption, wide tissue distribution, high protein binding, urinary excretion.

CONTRAINDICATIONS: Known/suspected pregnancy, estrogen-dependent neoplasms, breast cancer except in appropriately selected pts; abnormal genital bleeding, active past hx estrogen associated thrombophlebitis/thromboembolic disorders, (except for breast/prostatic cancer treatment).

DOSAGE

Adult *PO*	
Menopause	1.25mg/d. If pt is menstruating, start on day 5 of bleeding for cyclic administration
Atrophic vaginitis, kraurosis vulvae	≥0.3mg/d, depending on response. Administer cyclically
Hypogonadism	2.5-7.5mg/d divided, for 20d, followed by rest period of 10d
Castration, ovarian failure	1.25mg/d, cyclically
Postpartum breast enlargement	3.75mg q4h for 5 doses. 1.25mg q4h for 5d
Prostatic cancer	1.25-2.5mg tid
Breast cancer	10mg tid for at least 3mo
IM/IV	
Abnormal uterine bleeding	25mg, repeat in 6-12h prn. Start PO doses as soon as possible

*Available in Canada only.
Note: Side/adverse effects: common in *italic;* serious in ***boldface italic.***

MAGNESIUM SULFATE (INJECTION)

(mag-nee-zhum sul-fate)

CATEGORY: *Anticonvulsant* — Rx; Preg Cat A

AVAILABLE PREPARATIONS / **DOSAGE FORMS**

Magnesium Sulfate (various) — Injection (IM/IV): 10%, 12.5%, 50%

ACTION: Anticonvulsant activity due to inhibition of peripheral neuromuscular transmission. **USE:** Anticonvulsant for seizures associated c̄ epilepsy, pregnancy-induced hypertension ▪ Treatment of Mg deficiency.

PHARMACOKINETICS

	Onset	Duration	Excretion
IV	Immediate	30m	Via urine
IM	1h	3-4h	Via urine

CONTRAINDICATIONS: Heart block/myocardial damage (parenteral), severe renal impairment.

DOSAGE

Anticonvulsant	
Pediatric *IM*	20-40mg/kg
Adult *IM*	1-5g prn
IV	1-4g
Infusion	4g in 250ml 5% dextrose at ≤3ml/m
Cerebral edema	To 2.5g IV
Mg deficiency	
Pediatric	2-10m/Eq/d
Adult	4-24m/Eq/d

SIDE/ADVERSE EFFECTS: CNS: depression of deep tendon reflexes ▪ CV: hypotension, depressed cardiac function, circulatory collapse ▪ GI: diarrhea ▪ INT: sweating, flushing ▪ RESP: respiratory depression.

DRUG INTERACTIONS: Use c̄ CNS depressants may ↑ effects ▪ Use c̄ great caution in dig pts.

NURSING MANAGEMENT

ADMINISTRATION: IM: do *not* exceed 50% solution in adults; 1% procaine may be added to ↓ injection

*Available in Canada only.
Note: Side/adverse effects: common in *italic;* serious in ***boldface italic.***

HYDRALAZINE HYDROCHLORIDE

(hye-dral-a-zeen)

CATEGORY: *Antihypertensive* — Rx; Preg Cat C

BRAND NAMES / **DOSAGE FORMS**

Alazine (Major) — Tablet: 10, 25, 50mg
Apresoline HCl (Ciba) — Injection (IM/IV): 20mg/ml; Tablet: 10, 25, 50, 100mg

COMBINATION PRODUCTS

Apresazide 25/25 (Ciba), Aprozide 25/25 (Major)	Hydralazine HCl/hydrochlorothiazide per capsule: 25mg/25mg
Apresazide 50/50 (Ciba), Aprozide 50/50 (Major),	Hydralazine HCl/hydrochlorothiazide per capsule: 50mg/50mg
Apresazide 100/50 (Ciba), Aprozide 100/50 (Major)	Hydralazine HCl/hydrochlorothiazide per capsule: 100mg/50mg
Ser-Ap-Es (Ciba)	Reserpine/hydralazine HCl/hydrochlorothiazide per tablet: 0.1mg/25mg/15mg

ACTION: Antihypertensive effect due to direct relaxing, vasodilation of arteriolar smooth muscle. **USE:** Treatment of hypertension as sole agent/in combination c̄ other antihypertensives.

PHARMACOKINETICS

PO absorption	Peak	Half-life	Protein binding	Excretion
Rapid	1-2h	3-7h	87%	Via urine primarily as metabolites

CONTRAINDICATIONS: Hypersensitivity, coronary artery disease, mitral valvular/rheumatic heart disease.

DOSAGE

Pediatric *PO*	0.75mg/kg divided, increase slowly for 2-3wks to daily maximum 7.5mg/kg prn
Adult *PO*	Initial dose 10mg qid for 2-4d, increase to 25mg qid for balance of wk, 50mg qid wk2. Adjust to lowest effective dose for maintenance
IM/IV	20-40mg, repeat prn. Switch to PO as soon as possible

*Available in Canada only.
Note: Side/adverse effects: common in *italic;* serious in ***boldface italic.***

MEDROXYPROGESTERONE ACETATE

(me-drox-ee-proe-jess-te-rone)

CATEGORY: *Progestational hormone* — Rx; Preg Cat X

BRAND NAMES / **DOSAGE FORMS**

Amen (Carmick) — Tablet: 10mg
Provera (Upjohn) — Tablet: 2.5, 5, 10mg

ACTION: Progestational agents effect pituitary gland, uterus, vaginal mucosa, mammary glands; inhibit pituitary gonadotropin, resulting in ovarian suppression; uterine effects incl relaxation of uterine smooth muscle, secretory phase of endometrial development; vaginal mucosa exhibits increased mucification; other effects incl stimulation of mammary tissue growth, progesterone withdrawal resulting in menstruation. **USE:** Amenorrhea ▪ Abnormal uterine bleeding due to hormonal imbalance in absence of organic disease.

PHARMACOKINETICS: Good PO absorption excreted as conjugated metabolites via urine.

CONTRAINDICATIONS: Hypersensitivity, past hx of thrombophlebitis, thromboembolic disorders, cerebral apoplexy, suspected breast/genital malignancy, liver disease.

DOSAGE

Adult *PO*	
Amenorrhea	5-10mg/d for 5-10d. Withdrawal bleeding usually w/in 3-7d after ending therapy
Uterine bleeding	5-10mg/d for 5-10d beginning on calculated d 16 or 21 of menstrual cycle. Withdrawal bleeding usually w/in 3-7d after ending therapy

SIDE/ADVERSE EFFECTS: CV: edema, thrombophlebitis, pulmonary embolism ▪ END: galactorrhea ▪ GU: breakthrough bleeding, spotting, menstrual flow change, amenorrhea, cervical erosion/secretions ▪ HEP: cholestatic jaundice ▪ INT: acne, alopecia, hirsutism, urticaria, pruritus, rash ▪ PSYCH: depression.

DRUG INTERACTIONS: Possible ↓ in glucose tolerance, antidiabetic agents; may require dose adjustments in diabetics.

*Available in Canada only.
Note: Side/adverse effects: common in *italic;* serious in ***boldface italic.***

pain; *deep* gluteal injection ▪ IV: do *not* exceed 20% solution, 150mg/m ▪ Assess patellar reflex (knee jerk); hold dose until (+) response obtained ▪ Assess respirations; do *not* administer if <16/m ▪ Institute seizure precautions ▪ Do *not* administer discolored/precipitated solutions ▪ Do *not* leave pt unattended ▪ Place pt in left lateral position if pregnant ▪ Assess urinary output (>25ml/h) ▪ Have emergency support equipment available ▪ Avoid abrupt withdrawal ▪ Provide emotional support.

EVALUATION: Monitor CV, renal status ▪ Monitor BP continuously ▪ Monitor serum Mg^{++} levels ▪ Observe for seizure activity; record details (duration, characteristics, pt response) ▪ Monitor respirations (toxicity; <16/m) ▪ Assess patellar reflex; notify physician if hyporeflexic ▪ Monitor urinary output ▪ Assess neonate for Mg^{++} toxicity ▪ Therapeutic serum Mg^{++} concentration: 4-6mEq/L.

EDUCATION: Explain procedure, rationale to pt, family ▪ Safety precautions ▪ Comfort measures.

OVERDOSE MANAGEMENT: Symptoms: hypotension, ↓ respirations/respiratory paralysis, absence of deep tendon reflexes, ↓ fetal heart rate ▪ Treatment: administer IV 10ml 10% aqueous solution calcium gluconate over 3m; *Warning*—do *not* give to dig pts (arrhythmias may occur) ▪ Emergency artificial ventilation may be necessary.

NOTES:

Cream	
Atrophic vaginitis, kraurosis vulvae	1/2-1 applicator (2-4g) intravaginally/topical

SIDE/ADVERSE EFFECTS: CNS: headache, migraine, dizziness, mental depression ▪ EENT: intolerance to contact lenses ▪ GI: nausea, vomiting, abdominal cramps, bloating ▪ GU: amenorrhea, breakthrough bleeding, dysmenorrhea, candidiasis, ↑ size of uterine fibromyomas ▪ INT: melasma, ***erythema multiforme***/nodosum, alopecia, hirsutism, urticaria ▪ MET: ↓ carbohydrate tolerance ▪ Other: weight changes, porphyria exacerbation.

DRUG INTERACTIONS: Use c̄ tricyclic antidepressants may produce toxic rxs.

NURSING MANAGEMENT
ADMINISTRATION: Administer cyclically (3wks on, 1wk off) c̄ meals ▪ Avoid abrupt withdrawal ▪ Parenteral: reconstitute by withdrawing 5ml air from container, inject 5ml sterile diluent against container side, gently agitate, do *not* shake; compatible c̄ normal saline, dextrose, invert sugar solutions; *not* compatible c̄ acidic solutions; stable for 60d refrigerated, protect from light ▪ IM: administer *deep, slowly* into gluteal UOQ; use dry syringe, 21-gauge needle for oil preparations ▪ IV: preferred route; administer *slowly;* do *not* administer oil preparations IV ▪ Vaginal: Apply c̄ plastic dose applicator.

EVALUATION: Monitor BP, PT ▪ Assess for endometrial cancer (Pap test, physical exam) ▪ Diabetics: careful urine testing ▪ Assess for behavior changes, depression ▪ Monitor pt weight; observe for edema.

EDUCATION: Nausea may occur during first 2wks of therapy ▪ Women: avoid pregnancy, breastfeeding ▪ Breast self-exam (incl men) ▪ Avoid smoking ▪ Take c̄ food ▪ Notify physician/dentist of use before treatment ▪ Keep appointments c̄ physician ▪ Avoid direct sunlight, UV light ▪ Stop taking drug, notify physician if pregnancy suspected ▪ Vaginal: apply hs; use sanitary napkin ▪ Notify physician *immediately* of chest/leg pain, unusual vaginal bleeding, difficult breathing, slurred speech ▪ Men: enlarged breasts, impotence (reversible).

NOTES:

NURSING MANAGEMENT
ADMINISTRATION: Assess for hx of progestin hypersensitivity ▪ PO: administer c̄ meals ▪ Avoid exposure to light in storage.

EVALUATION: Monitor VS, esp BP, pulse ▪ Monitor hydration status (I&O, daily weight) ▪ Assess emotional status (mental depression) ▪ Monitor hepatic status.

EDUCATION: Review package insert c̄ pt ▪ Take as directed by physician ▪ Avoid exposure to direct sunlight, UV light (sun lamps); use sunscreen ▪ Keep scheduled appointments c̄ physician/for Pap/pelvic exams ▪ Notify physician/dentist of use before therapy ▪ Women: avoid breastfeeding, pregnancy; menstrual changes may occur ▪ Procedure for breast self-exam ▪ Symptoms of thrombotic episodes (sudden shortness of breath, migraine headache, chest pain, diplopia).

NOTES:

Combination Products	Dosage must be adjusted for each pt, in general 1-2 U (caps/tabs) 1-3 times/d

SIDE/ADVERSE EFFECTS: CNS: *headache,* peripheral neuritis, dizziness, tremors, anxiety, psychotic rxs ▪ CV: *palpitations, tachycardia, angina pectoris,* edema, paradoxical hypertension ▪ EENT: nasal congestion, conjunctivitis ▪ GI: *anorexia, N/V/D,* constipation, paralytic ileus ▪ GU: difficult urination ▪ HEM: anemia, leukopenia, ***agranulocytosis,*** lymphadenopathy ▪ HEP: hepatitis ▪ INT: rash, urticaria, pruritus ▪ RESP: dyspnea.

DRUG INTERACTIONS: Use c̄ adrenergic drugs may antagonize hypotensive effect ▪ Use c̄ other antihypertensives, MAO-I produces additive hypotensive effects.

NURSING MANAGEMENT
ADMINISTRATION: Assess for hx of hypersensitivity ▪ Assess renal function; ↓ dosage if impaired ▪ PO: administer c̄ meals; switch from parenteral form w/in 48h ▪ IV: administer *slowly* (10mg/m); monitor BP, heart rate ▪ Elderly may require ↓ dosage ▪ Avoid abrupt withdrawal ▪ Have pyridoxine (vitamin B_6) available for neurotoxicity.

EVALUATION: Monitor VS, esp BP, electrolyte status, I&O, daily weight ▪ Assess for edema in extremities; mental status (depression, disorientation, anxiety).

EDUCATION: Dizziness/drowsiness may occur; use caution in potentially hazardous activities ▪ Avoid changing positions rapidly ▪ Take as ordered by physician even if symptom free; do *not* skip doses ▪ Take c̄ meals ▪ Do *not* stop taking w/out notifying physician ▪ Check c̄ physician/pharmacist before taking OTC/Rx preparations ▪ Notify physician *immediately* of tingling/numbness of hands/feet; stop taking drug ▪ Physician may order vitamin B_6 supplements to alleviate neurotoxic effects ▪ Avoid high-Na^+ foods ▪ Avoid ↑ exercise, temperature extremes, smoking ▪ Used to control, *not* cure, hypertension ▪ Maintain optimum weight ▪ Do *not* use c̄ alcohol, other CNS depressants ▪ Keep scheduled appointments c̄ physician; have BP checked regularly ▪ Check for swelling in feet/legs daily ▪ Men: impotence may occur.

NOTES:

MEPERIDINE HYDROCHLORIDE

(me-per-i-deen)

CATEGORY: *Narcotic:* synthetic opiate — Rx C-II; Preg Cat NA

BRAND NAMES
Demerol HCl (Winthrop-Breon), (Winthrop in Canada)

DOSAGE FORMS
Injection (IM/IV/SC), syrup, tablet

ACTION: Narcotics produce analgesia, euphoria, sedation; equianalgesic doses of meperidine, morphine produce same amount of euphoria, respiratory depression, sedation, addiction liability; PO administration significantly less effective; 70mg equivalent to 10mg morphine. **USE:** Relief of moderate/severe pain ▪ Pre-op sedation, post-op analgesic, obs analgesia, support of anesthesia.

DOSAGE

Analgesic	
Pediatric *PO/IM/SC*	0.5-0.8mg/lb q3-4h prn
Adult *PO/IM/SC*	50-150mg q3-4h prn
OB *IM/SC*	50-100mg when pain is regular. May be repeated every 1-3h
Anesthesia	Titrated against pt needs by IV injection/continuous infusion
Pre-op	
Pediatric *IM/SC*	0.5-1mg/kg 30-90m before anesthesia
Adult *IM/SC*	50-100mg 30-90m before anesthesia

PHARMACOKINETICS

	Onset	Peak	Duration	Protein binding	Half-life	Excretion
PO	15-20m	60m	2-4h	60%-70%	4-8h	Renal as metabolites, 5% unchanged
IM	10m	40-60m	2-4h	60%-70%	4-8h	
SC	10m	30-50m	2-4h	60%-70%	4-8h	

CONTRAINDICATIONS: Hypersensitivity, c̄ MAO-I therapy, nursing mothers.

*Available in Canada only.
Note: Side/adverse effects: common in *italic;* serious in ***boldface italic.***

METHOTREXATE/METHOTREXATE SODIUM▲ (AMETHOPTERIN, MTX)

(meth-oh-trex-ate)

CATEGORY: *Antineoplastic:* antimetabolic, folic acid antagonist — Rx; Preg Cat D

BRAND NAMES
Folex (Adria), Mexate (Bristol-Myers), Methotrexate (Lederle)

DOSAGE FORMS
Injection (IM/IV), powder for injection▲ (IM/IV), tablet

ACTION: Antimetabolic activity due to competitive inhibition of dehydrofolate reductase, which inhibits folic acid synthesis. **USE:** Treatment of gestational choriocarcinoma, chorioadenoma destruens, hydatiform mole, lymphoblastic/meningeal leukemias ▪ Treatment of breast cancer, epidermoid cancer of head/neck, lung cancer ▪ Treatment of Burkitt lymphoma, advanced states (III, IV) of lymphosarcoma, advanced mycosis fungoides, disabling psoriasis.

PHARMACOKINETICS: PO peak 1-2h excreted unchanged.

CONTRAINDICATIONS: Psoriasis in pregnant pts or pts c̄ preexisting blood dyscrasias, liver, kidney impairment.

DOSAGE: Must be individualized.

Trophoblastic tumor	15-30mg/d *PO/IM* for 5d, repeated 3-5 times c̄ ≥1 rest wks between courses
Lymphoblastic leukemia	3.3mg/M² c̄ prednisone 60mg/M²/d. After remission, 30mg/M² *PO/IM* twice/wk or 2.5mg/kg *IV* every 14d
Meningeal leukemia	12mg/M² *intrathecal* q2-5d
Lymphoma	10-25mg/d *PO* for 4-8d for several courses c̄ 7-10d rest periods
Mycosis fungoides	2.5-10mg/d *PO* for wks/mo
Psoriasis	10-25mg/wk as single *PO/IM/IV* dose. Do not exceed dose of 50mg/wk

SIDE/ADVERSE EFFECTS: CNS: headache, drowsiness, aphasia, paresis, ***convulsions,*** blurred vision ▪ GI: *N/V/D, abdominal distress,* ***ulcerative stomatitis,*** anorexia, gingivitis, ***bleeding, hematemesis*** ▪ GU: ***renal failure,*** azotemia, cystitis, ***hematuria,*** menstrual dysfunction, abortion, fetal teratogenesis, severe nephropathy

*Available in Canada only.
Note: Side/adverse effects: common in *italic;* serious in ***boldface italic.***

NALOXONE HYDROCHLORIDE

(nal-ox-one)

CATEGORY: *Narcotic antagonist* — Rx; Preg Cat B

BRAND NAME
Narcan (DuPont)

DOSAGE FORMS
Injection (IM/IV/SC): 0.4mg/ml
Neonatal injection (IM/IV/SC): 0.02mg/ml

ACTION: Narcotic antagonism primarily due to competition c̄ narcotics for CNS receptor sites. **USE:** Induce complete/partial reversal of narcotic depression (incl respiratory) induced by natural/synthetic narcotics, propoxyphene, narcotic agonist/antagonists nalbuphine, pentazocine, butorphanol ▪ Diagnosis of suspected acute opioid overdosage.

PHARMACOKINETICS: IM/SC onset 2-5m, IV 1-2m; half-life 60-90m in adults, longer in infants; excreted via urine primarily as metabolites.

CONTRAINDICATIONS: Hypersensitivity.

DOSAGE

Pediatric *IM/IV/SC*	
Overdose	0.01mg/kg IV. Subsequent dose 0.1mg/kg may be given IV prn
Post-op	0.005-0.01mg/kg IV. Repeat at 2-3m intervals to desired degree of reversal Neonate: 0.01mg/kg. Repeat at 2-3m intervals to desired degree of reversal
Adult *IM/IV/SC*	
Overdose	0.4-2mg IV. Repeat at 2-3m intervals to desired degree of reversal
Post-op	0.1-0.2mg/kg IV. Repeat at 2-3m intervals to desired degree of reversal

SIDE/ADVERSE EFFECTS: GI: nausea, vomiting (rare) c̄ high doses post-op ▪ Other: withdrawal symptoms in narcotic-dependent pt.

*Available in Canada only.
Note: Side/adverse effects: common in *italic;* serious in ***boldface italic.***

OXYCODONE HYDROCHLORIDE

(ox-i-koe-done)

CATEGORY: *Narcotic:* semisynthetic opiate — Rx C-II; Preg Cat NA

BRAND NAMES
Oxycodone HCl (various)

DOSAGE FORMS
PO solution: 5mg/5ml
Tablet: 5mg

COMBINATION PRODUCTS — Rx C-II

Percocet (DuPont)	Oxycodone HCl 5mg/acetaminophen 325mg per tablet
Percodan (DuPont)	Oxycodone 4.88mg/aspirin 325mg per tablet
Percodan-Demi (DuPont)	Oxycodone 2.44mg/aspirin 325mg per tablet
Tylox (McNeil)	Oxycodone HCl 5mg/acetaminophen 500mg per capsule

ACTION: Narcotics produce analgesia, euphoria, sedation. **USE:** Relief of moderate/severe pain.

PHARMACOKINETICS: Good PO absorption c̄ onset at 10-15m, peak about 1h, duration 4-6h; excretion via urine.

CONTRAINDICATIONS: Hypersensitivity; use c̄ extreme caution in head injuries.

DOSAGE
Adult *PO* — 5mg q6h. All fixed combination products, usual dose 1 tablet/capsule q6-8h

SIDE/ADVERSE EFFECTS: CNS: *sedation, lightheadedness,* euphoria, dysphoria, tremors, disorientation, ↓ convulsive threshold ▪ CV: hypotension, palpitations, flushing of face ▪ EENT: miosis ▪ GI: *nausea, vomiting,* dry mouth, constipation, biliary tract spasm ▪ GU: urine retention ▪ INT: pruritus, urticaria ▪ RESP: ***respiratory depression.***

DRUG INTERACTIONS: Use c̄ alcohol, antihistamines, barbiturates, benzodiazepines, methotrimeprazine, phenothiazines, other CNS depressants produces additive CNS depression; ↓ dosage may be required ▪ Use c̄ tricyclic antidepressants may produce additive respiratory depression.

NURSING MANAGEMENT
ADMINISTRATION: Assess for hx of opioid hypersensitivity ▪ Assess quality, intensity, location of pain ▪ Store under double lock/key; document use accurately ▪

*Available in Canada only.
Note: Side/adverse effects: common in *italic;* serious in ***boldface italic.***

NURSING MANAGEMENT

ADMINISTRATION: Mix c̄ sterile H_2O for injection prn ▪ Do *not* leave pt unattended ▪ Have emergency support equipment available ▪ Store in original container; avoid exposure to light.

EVALUATION: Monitor VS, esp respirations ▪ Observe for ↓ respirations after treatment, because duration of action of narcotic may be longer than that of naloxone ▪ Observe for signs of narcotic withdrawal (restlessness, muscle spasms, ↑ VS, lacrimation) ▪ Assess for ↑ PTT ▪ Assess ABGs.

EDUCATION: Explain procedure, rationale to pt, family ▪ Safety precautions ▪ Comfort measures.

NOTES:

SIDE/ADVERSE EFFECTS: CNS: *sedation, lightheadedness,* euphoria, dysphoria, weakness, tremor, disorientation, transient hallucinations ▪ CV: hypotension, palpitation, flushing of face, phlebitis after IV administration ▪ GI: *nausea, vomiting,* dry mouth, biliary tract spasm, constipation ▪ GU: urinary retention ▪ INT: *sweating,* pruritus, urticaria ▪ RESP: respiratory depression ▪ Other: addiction.

DRUG INTERACTIONS: Use c̄ alcohol, antihistamines, barbiturates, benzodiazepines, methotrimeprazine, phenothiazines, depressants can produce additive CNS depression; dosage reductions may be required.

NURSING MANAGEMENT

ADMINISTRATION: Assess for hx of hypersensitivity ▪ Store under double lock/key; document use accurately ▪ Check compatibility chart for mixing pre-op IM preparations ▪ Do *not* administer if respirations <12/m ▪ IM: inject *deep* into muscle; rotate sites ▪ IV: dilute; administer *slowly* ▪ Have narcotic antagonist, support measures available ▪ Avoid administration in pts c̄ suspected head injury ▪ Administer *before* pt has intense pain ▪ Utilize + power of suggestion ▪ Avoid abrupt withdrawal c̄ long-term use ▪ Elderly may require ↓ dosage.

EVALUATION: Monitor respirations, circulatory function ▪ Assess bowel function, abdominal distention ▪ Assess renal function, urinary retention ▪ Check for signs of dependence (↑ drug request) ▪ Assess for potentiation of CNS depressant effect ▪ Assess for nausea/vomiting; administer antiemetic ▪ Assess for signs of overdose (coma, pinpoint pupils, respiratory depression.

EDUCATION: Avoid changing positions (lying/sitting/standing) rapidly ▪ Avoid excessive sensory stimulation ▪ Keep bedrails up when nonambulatory ▪ Obtain assistance as needed when ambulatory ▪ Turn, cough, deep-breath after surgery ▪ Constipation may occur; ↑ fluids, bulk-containing foods ▪ Avoid potentially hazardous activities ▪ Avoid smoking ▪ Indiscriminate use may lead to severe dependence ▪ Avoid use c̄ alcohol, other CNS depressants.

OVERDOSE MANAGEMENT: *See* Narcotics category card.

NOTES:

Assess hepatic function; may require ↓ dosage if impaired ▪ Do *not* administer if respirations are <12/m ▪ Have narcotic antagonist (naloxone), support measures available ▪ Avoid administration in pts c̄ suspected head injury ▪ Administer *before* pt has intense pain ▪ Administer around clock to pts c̄ severe, chronic pain ▪ Administer c̄ food/milk ▪ PO liquid: may mix c̄ juices; avoid freezing ▪ Utilize + power of suggestion ▪ Avoid abrupt withdrawal c̄ long-term use; D/C gradually ▪ Elderly may require ↓ dosage.

EVALUATION: Monitor respirations, circulatory function, esp BP ▪ Assess bowel function, abdominal distention ▪ Assess renal function, urinary retention ▪ Check for signs of dependence (↑ drug request) ▪ Assess for potentiation of CNS depressant effect ▪ Assess for nausea, vomiting; administer antiemetic ▪ Assess for signs of overdose (coma, pinpoint pupils, respiratory depression) ▪ May produce ↑ CSF pressure.

EDUCATION: Avoid changing positions (lying/sitting/standing) rapidly ▪ Avoid excessive sensory stimulation ▪ Keep bedrails up when nonambulatory ▪ Turn, cough, deep breathe after surgery ▪ Constipation may occur; ↑ fluids, bulk-containing foods ▪ Avoid potentially hazardous activities ▪ Avoid smoking ▪ Indiscriminate use may lead to severe dependence ▪ Avoid use c̄ alcohol, other CNS depressants ▪ Take as ordered by physician; do *not* ↑ dose ▪ PO liquid: may mix c̄ juice; do *not* freeze ▪ Notify physician/dentist of use before treatment.

OVERDOSE MANAGEMENT: Principal symptoms are respiratory depression, stupor/coma ▪ Acute overdose results in apnea, circulatory collapse, cardiac arrest, possible death ▪ Emergency treatment: maintain respiration; remove drug by gastric lavage; administer naloxone HCl 0.01mg/kg IV; administer IV fluids to maintain adequate BP; because narcotics ↓ convulsive threshold, use of stimulants should be avoided.

NOTES:

▪ HEM: ***bone marrow depression,*** *leukopenia,* ***thrombocytopenia,*** anemia, hypogammaglobulinemia, hemorrhage, septicemia ▪ HEP: hepatic toxicity ▪ INT: erythematous rash, pruritus, urticaria, photosensitivity, depigmentation, alopecia ▪ RESP: ***interstitial pneumonitis, chronic interstitial obstructive pulmonary disease.***

DRUG INTERACTIONS: Use c̄ PO hypoglycemics, phenylbutazone, salicylates, sulfonamides, thiazides can ↑ MTX toxicity due to protein storage site displacement ▪ Use c̄ alcohol, other hepatotoxic drugs ↑ toxic effect ▪ Salicylates, probenecid ↓ MTX renal excretion ▪ Folic acid preparations (vitamins) can antagonize antineoplastic effect ▪ Use c̄ PO anticoagulants may enhance their effects.

NURSING MANAGEMENT

ADMINISTRATION: Check pt hx for recent course of radiation/antineoplastic agents ▪ Assess oral cavity for ulceration ▪ Assess renal function; may require ↓ dosage if impaired ▪ Administer antiemetic before therapy ▪ PO: administer 1h ac/2h pc ▪ Parenteral: dilute according to manufacturer's directions; administer by *slow* IV push ▪ Avoid exposure to moisture, light in storage.

EVALUATION: Monitor CBC; neurologic, hepatic function ▪ Assess for infection, bleeding, anemia ▪ May produce hyperglycemia; monitor diabetics closely ▪ Assess hydration status.

EDUCATION: Store in dry, tightly closed, light-resistant container ▪ ↑ Fluid intake (8-10 glasses/d) ▪ Avoid exposure to infection ▪ Check c̄ physician before immunization ▪ Diet as tolerated; avoid spicy foods ▪ Maintain good oral hygiene; use soft-bristled toothbrush ▪ Notify physician of symptoms of bone marrow depression (fever, sore throat, bruising, bleeding, lethargy) ▪ Avoid exposure to direct sunlight, UV light ▪ Loss of hair may occur (reversible) ▪ Compliance c̄ prescribed dosage regimen ▪ Women: avoid breastfeeding ▪ Check c̄ physician/pharmacist before taking OTC preparations ▪ Avoid alcohol ▪ Use contraception (during & for up to 8 wks after therapy).

NOTES:

OXYTOCIN
(ox-i-toe-sin)

CATEGORY: *Oxytoxic* — Rx

BRAND NAMES / **DOSAGE FORMS**

Pitocin (Parke-Davis) — Injection (IM/IV): 5U/0.5ml, 10U/ml

Syntocinon (Sandoz), (Sandoz Pharma in Canada) — Injection (IM/IV): 10U/ml; Nasal spray: 40U/ml (2, 5ml bottle)

ACTION: Oxytoxic effect due to ↑ sodium ion permeability in uterine smooth muscle cells, which ↑ number of contracting myofibrils, enables uterus to contract; uterine sensitivity to oxytocin gradually ↑ during pregnancy, reaching peak before parturition. **USE:** Antepartum: initiation/augmentation of uterine contractions ▪ Stimulate uterine contractions during stage 3 of labor, control postpartum hemorrhage ▪ Initiate milk let-down reflex (spray).

PHARMACOKINETICS

IM absorption	Onset	Duration	Excretion
Excellent	3-5m	2-3h	Via urine primarily as metabolites

CONTRAINDICATIONS: Hypersensitivity, cephalopelvic disproportion, unfavorable fetal position, obstetrical emergencies that favor surgical intervention, fetal distress when delivery not imminent, prolonged use in uterine inertia/severe toxemia, hypertonic uterine patterns, when vaginal delivery is contraindicated; nasal spray during pregnancy.

DOSAGE

Adult *IM/IV*

Antepartum	Start c̄ infusion rate 1-2mU/m. Slowly ↑ until contractions reach desired rate, intensity
Postpartum	10-40U in 100ml, infused at sufficient rate to control uterine atony. 3-10U after delivery of placenta
Nasal spray	1 spray in one/both nostrils 2-3m before nursing/pumping breasts

SIDE/ADVERSE EFFECTS: CV; ***cardiac arrhythmia,*** postpartum hemorrhage, fetal bradycardia ▪ GI: nausea, vomiting ▪ GU: pelvic hematoma; uterine hypertonicity, spasms, tetanic contractions, rupture.

*Available in Canada only.
Note: Side/adverse effects: common in *italic;* serious in ***boldface italic.***

RITODRINE HYDROCHLORIDE
(ri-toe-dreen)

CATEGORY: *Sympathomimetic:* $beta_2$ adrenergic, uterine relaxant — Rx; Preg Cat B

BRAND NAMES / **DOSAGE FORMS**

Yutopar (Astra), (Bristol in Canada) — Injection (IV): 10mg/ml; Tablet: 10mg

ACTION: Sympathomimetic activity selective for beta receptors, esp $beta_2$ adrenoreceptors of bronchial tree, peripheral vascular beds, uterus; predominant betamimetic effect on uterine smooth muscle, which ↓ intensity, frequency of contractions; placental drug transfer occurs, limited $beta_1$ activity results in transitory ↑ in maternal, fetal heart rates. **USE:** Management of preterm labor in suitable labor.

PHARMACOKINETICS

PO availability	Peak	Half-life	Protein binding	Excretion
30%	30-60m	1.3-20h	32%	Via urine as unchanged drug, metabolites

CONTRAINDICATIONS: Before wk 20 of pregnancy, conditions in which continuation of pregnancy is hazardous, incl antepartum hemorrhage requiring immediate delivery; chorioamnionitis; eclampsia, severe preeclampsia; intrauterine fetal death; maternal cardiac disease, hyperthyroidism, controlled diabetes; pulmonary hypertension ▪ Preexisting maternal medical conditions seriously affected by ritodrine betamimetic activity, incl asthma already treated c̄ beta adrenergics/steroids; cardiac arrhythmias associated c̄ tachycardia/drug toxicity; hypovolemia; pheochromocytoma; ritodrine hypersensitivity; uncontrolled hypertension.

DOSAGE

IV infusion — Usual starting dose 50-100μg/m, ↑ q10m by 50μg/m until desired effect obtained. Usual effective range 150-350μg/m. Treatment should continue for at least 12h after uterine contractions cease

*Available in Canada only.
Note: Side/adverse effects: common in *italic;* serious in ***boldface italic.***

Rh_o (D) IMMUNE GLOBULIN

CATEGORY: *Immunosuppressant:* biological — Rx; Preg Cat C

BRAND NAMES

Standard dose	Microdose
Gamulin Rh (Armour)	*Mini-Gamulin Rh*
HypRho-D (Cutter)	*HypRho-D Minidose*
**Rho (D) Immune Globulin (Connaught)*	*RhoGam (Ortho)*
**WinRho (Winn Rh Institute)*	

ACTION: Sterile solution of immunoglobulin [IgG anti-Rh_o (D)] obtained from fractionated human plasma, used to suppress immune response in nonsensitized pts c̄ Rh– blood who receive Rh+ blood cells because of fetomaternal hemorrhage, transfusion accident. **USE:** Microdose preparation: Used to suppress antibody formation in women c̄ Rh⁻ blood after abortion/pregnancy termination up to and incl week 12 of gestation unless father has Rh⁻ blood. Standard preparation: Used to suppress antibody formation in women c̄ Rh⁻ blood after delivery, abortion/pregnancy termination, abdominal trauma during pregnancy ▫ Used to suppress antibody formation after transfusion accident.

PHARMACOKINETICS: Not applicable.

CONTRAINDICATIONS: Hypersensitivity, previously sensitized individuals; micropreparation for genetic amniocentesis at wk 15-18, antepartum prophylaxis at wk 28.

DOSAGE

OB	IM injection of total contents of single vial w/in ≤72h. Multiple dose required when fetomaternal hemorrhaging >30ml
Transfusion	IM injection of total contents of single vial(s) w/in ≤3 days. Specific dose dependent on volume of blood Rhpositive transfused

SIDE/ADVERSE EFFECTS: CNS: lethargy ▪ MS: myalgia, localized stiffness/tenderness at injection site ▪ Other: limited allergic reactions including anaphylaxis.

NURSING MANAGEMENT

ADMINISTRATION: Assess for hx of hypersensitivity ▪ Preadministration criteria (type, cross-match neonatal cord blood): mother must be Rh_o (D) –, D^u –; Mother should *not* have been previously sensitized to Rh_o factor: Infant must be Rh_o (D) +, D^u +, direct

*Available in Canada only.
Note: Side/adverse effects: common in *italic;* serious in ***boldface italic.***

ZIDOVUDINE
(zy-doe-view-deen)

CATEGORY: *Antiviral* — Rx; Preg Cat C

BRAND NAME / **DOSAGE FORMS**

Retrovir (Burroughs Wellcome) — Capsule: 100mg

ACTION: Antiviral activity due to inhibition of viral replication in selected retroviruses incl human immunodeficiency virus (HIV/HTLV III), etiological agent of AIDS, ARC; drug is thymidine analogue that inhibits HIV reverse transcriptase enzymes, required for DNA synthesis. **USE:** Management of AIDS and advanced ARC in pts c̄ confirmed *Pneumocystis carinii* pneumonia, (PCP), or lymphocyte (T_4 cells) count <200/mm³.

PHARMACOKINETICS

PO absorption	Peak	Half-life	Excretion
52%-75%	0.5-1.5h	0.78-1.93h	Via urine as metabolites (GAZT)

CONTRAINDICATIONS: Hypersensitivity.

DOSAGE

Adult *PO* — Starting dose 200mg q4h around clock. Treatment ranged from 12-26wks during initial clinical studies

SIDE/ADVERSE EFFECTS: CNS: anxiety, loss of mental acuity, vertigo, nervousness ▪ CV: vasodilation ▪ EENT: pharyngitis, sinusitis, hoarseness, rhinitis, amblyopia, hearing loss, photophobia ▪ GI: constipation, oral ulcers, flatulence, dysphagia, bleeding from gums/rectum ▪ GU: dysuria, polyuria, urinary frequency/hesitancy ▪ HEM: *anemia, granulocytosis* ▪ INT: acne, pruritus, urticaria ▪ MS: arthralgia, muscle spasm/tremor.

DRUG INTERACTIONS: Use c̄ acetaminophen can ↑ incidence of granulocytopenia ▪ Use c̄ nephrotoxic, cytotoxic, bone marrow depressants can result in additive toxicity ▪ Use c̄ probenecid may reduce zidovudine renal excretion.

*Available in Canada only.
Note: Side/adverse effects: common in *italic;* serious in ***boldface italic.***

PO maintenance	10mg 30m before termination of IV therapy. Usual dosage for first 24h 10mg q2h. Usual maintenance dose 10-20mg q4-6h. Do *not* exceed 120mg/d

SIDE/ADVERSE EFFECTS: CNS: nervousness, anxiety, emotional upset, tremor, headache ■ CV: dose-related changes in maternal BP; maternal, fetal heart rates; pulmonary edema ■ GI: N/V/D, epigastric distress, constipation ■ Other: rash, dyspnea, hyperventilation, lactic acidosis ■ Fetal: hypoglycemia, ileus.

DRUG INTERACTIONS: Use c̄ corticosteroids can produce pulmonary edema ■ Use c̄ beta blockers antagonizes therapeutic effects ■ Use c̄ anesthetics can ↑ hypotensive effects ■ Use c̄ sympathomimetics produces additive effects.

NURSING MANAGEMENT
ADMINISTRATION: Assess VS ■ Do *not* use saline diluents unless dextrose undesirable (diabetics) ■ Use solution w/in 48h of preparation ■ Do *not* administer discolored/precipitated solution ■ Place pt in left lateral position ■ IV: use infusion control device ■ Restrict fluids per physician's order ■ Store parenteral form at room temperature; do *not* freeze ■ Provide emotional support.

EVALUATION: Monitor I&O ■ Monitor VS, esp BP, respiratory rate (labored breathing) ■ Monitor uterine contractions, fetal heart rate ■ Observe for pulmonary edema; D/C drug if present ■ Assess for ↑ serum glucose, esp diabetics.

EDUCATION: Explain procedure, rationale to pt, family ■ Relaxation techniques ■ Comfort measures ■ Check c̄ physician before using OTC preparations ■ Notify physician of contractions, rupture of membranes.

NOTES:

DRUG INTERACTIONS: Use c̄ vasopressors can produce severe hypertension.

NURSING MANAGEMENT
ADMINISTRATION: Fetal monitoring: assess fetal maturity, position ■ Administer by only *one* route, *not* simultaneous routes ■ IV: use infusion pump; do *not* give IV push ■ Place pt in left lateral position ■ Do *not* leave pt unattended ■ Have emergency support equipment available ■ Avoid overstimulation of uterus ■ Do *not* administer discolored/precipitated solutions ■ Parenteral: store in original container, avoid freezing.

EVALUATION: Monitor BP, pulse q15m ■ Monitor fetal heart rate, intrauterine pressure ■ Assess uterine rupture, fetal distress ■ Monitor uterine contractions; stop if very frequent (<q2m)/prolonged ■ Monitor I&O; assess hydration status (continuous infusion, PO fluids can lead to H_2O intoxication) ■ Postpartum: monitor fundal height/tone.

EDUCATION: Explain procedure, rationale to pt, family ■ Occurrence of contractions ■ Relaxation techniques ■ Comfort measures ■ Procedure for use of nasal spray.

NOTES:

NURSING MANAGEMENT
ADMINISTRATION: Assess for hx of hypersensitivity ■ Avoid administration of acetaminophen during therapy ■ Avoid exposure to light.

EVALUATION: Monitor VS, esp temperature ■ Monitor hepatic, renal status ■ Monitor WBC counts (anemia, granulocytopenia); repeated blood transfusions may be necessary.

EDUCATION: Take as ordered by physician at intervals around clock to maintain blood levels; do *not* ↑ dose ■ Do *not* share drug ■ Women: avoid breastfeeding ■ Used to control, *not* cure, HIV infections ■ Check c̄ physician of any change in health status ■ Avoid concurrent use of acetaminophen (↑ toxicity) ■ Check c̄ physician/pharmacist before taking OTC preparations ■ Avoid sexual contact/blood donation (risk of HIV transmission) ■ Keep scheduled appointments c̄ physician for blood work.

NOTES:

Coombs –; Verify that lot numbers are same for cross-match solution, preparation to be administered ■ Cross-match 5% suspension of mother's RBCs c̄ 2gtt cross-match solution ■ Administer w/in 72h after Rh-incompatible delivery, terminated incomplete pregnancy, blood transfusions ■ Administer IM (deltoid); do *not* administer IV ■ Check preparation c̄ another nurse ■ Do *not* administer to infant ■ Do *not* administer discolored/precipitated solutions ■ Store in refrigerator ■ Provide emotional support.

EVALUATION: Assess for tenderness at injection site ■ Assess for ↑ body temperature ■ Assess for lethargy, myalgia if >1 dose administered.

EDUCATION: Explain procedure, rationale to pt, family ■ Importance of screening both parents for Rh incompatibility.

NOTES:

Temperature Equivalents

Celsius	Fahrenheit	Celsius	Fahrenheit
34.0	93.2	38.6	101.4
34.2	93.6	38.8	101.8
34.4	93.9	39.0	102.2
34.6	94.3	39.2	102.5
34.8	94.6	39.4	102.9
35.0	95.0	39.6	103.2
35.2	95.4	30.8	103.6
35.4	95.7	40.0	104.0
35.6	96.1	40.2	104.3
35.8	96.4	40.4	104.7
36.0	96.8	40.6	105.1
36.2	97.1	40.8	105.4
36.4	97.5	41.0	105.8
36.6	97.8	41.2	106.1
36.8	98.2	41.4	106.5
37.0	98.6	41.6	106.8
37.2	98.9	41.8	107.2
37.4	99.3	42.0	107.6
37.6	99.6	42.2	108.0
37.8	100.0	42.4	108.3
38.0	100.4	42.6	108.7
38.2	100.7	42.8	109.0
38.4	101.1	43.0	109.4

To convert Fahrenheit to Celcius:
(Temperature minus 32) $\times \frac{5}{9}$
Example: To convert 98.6 degrees Fahrenheit to Celsius:
$98.6 - 32 = 66.6 \times \frac{5}{9} = 37$ degrees

To convert Celcius to Fahrenheit
$\frac{9}{5} \times$ temperature $+ 32$
Example: To convert 40 degrees Celsius to Fahrenheit: $\frac{9}{5} \times 40 = 72 + 32 = 104$ degrees

Conversion of Pounds and Ounces To Grams for Newborn Weights*

Pounds	Ounces 0	1	2	3	4	5	6	7	8	9	10	11	12	13	14	15	Pounds
0	—	28	57	85	113	142	170	198	227	255	283	312	430	369	397	425	0
1	454	482	510	539	567	595	624	652	680	709	737	765	794	822	850	879	1
2	907	936	964	992	1021	1049	1077	1106	1134	1162	1191	1219	1247	1276	1304	1332	2
3	1361	1389	1417	1446	1474	1503	1531	1559	1588	1616	1644	1673	1701	1729	1758	1786	3
4	1814	1843	1871	1899	1928	1956	1984	2013	2041	2070	2098	2126	2155	2183	2211	2240	4
5	2268	2296	2325	2353	2381	2410	2438	2466	2495	2523	2551	2580	2608	2637	2665	2693	5
6	2722	2750	2778	2807	2835	2863	2892	2920	2948	2977	3005	3033	3062	3090	3118	3147	6
7	3175	3203	3232	3260	3289	3317	3345	3374	3402	3430	3459	3487	3515	3544	3572	3600	7
8	3629	3657	3685	3714	3742	3770	3799	3827	3856	3884	3912	3941	3969	3997	4026	4054	8
9	4082	4111	4139	4167	4196	4224	4252	4281	4309	4337	4366	4394	4423	4451	4479	4508	9
10	4536	4564	4593	4621	4649	4678	4706	4734	4763	4791	4819	4848	4876	4904	4933	4961	10
11	4990	5018	5046	5075	5103	5131	5160	5188	5216	5245	5273	5301	5330	5358	5386	5415	11
12	5443	5471	5500	5528	5557	5585	5613	5642	5670	5698	5727	5755	5783	5812	5840	5868	12
13	5897	5925	5953	5982	6010	6038	6067	6095	6123	6152	6180	6209	6237	6265	6294	6322	13
14	6350	6379	6407	6435	6464	6492	6520	6549	6577	6605	6634	6662	6690	6719	6747	6776	14
15	6804	6832	6860	6889	6917	6945	6973	7002	7030	7059	7087	7115	7144	7172	7201	7228	15
	0	1	2	3	4	5	6	7	8	9	10	11	12	13	14	15	
								Ounces									

*To convert pounds and ounces to grams, multiply the pounds by 453.6 and the ounces by 28.35; add the totals.
To convert grams into pounds and decimals of a pound, multiply the grams by 0.0022.
To convert grams into ounces, divide the grams by 28.35 (16 oz = 1 lb).